Comprehensive Neonatal Nursing Care

Carole Kenner, PhD, RNC-NIC, NNP, FAAN, is nationally and internationally known for her policy-setting work to establish rights of the neonate, standards for the care of the neonate, and the reduction of infant mortality worldwide. Dr. Kenner holds many titles, including Dean/Professor, School of Nursing, and Associate Dean, Bouvé College of Health Sciences, at Northeastern University, Boston. She also serves as President, Consultants with Confidence, Inc., West Roxbury, MA; Executive Director and Founder of the Council of International Neonatal Nurses, Inc.; and Trainer, End-of-Life Nursing Education Consortium in Pediatric Palliative Care (ELNEC), Washington, DC. She has published more than 100 peer-reviewed journal articles, 30 books, and at least 80 book chapters. Dr. Kenner has participated as PI, Co-PI, or Consultant on nearly 60 research grants. She is a member of four honorary organizations, including the American Academy of Nursing (AAN) (elected 1994) and is a member of numerous review panels, editorial boards, and consultant groups. In 2010 Dr. Kenner received the prestigious Audrey Hepburn Award for Contributions to the Health and Welfare for Children, from Sigma Theta Tau International.

Judy Wright Lott, DSN, NNP-BC, FAAN, is the Founding Dean of the nursing program at Wesleyan College in Macon, GA. She served as Dean, Baylor University Louise Herrington School of Nursing (TX) from 2002 to 2012. Dr. Lott has served as a Neonatal NP (NNP) (2004–2005); Associate Professor of Nursing and Director of NNP Specialty, at the University of Cincinnati College of Nursing (1996–2002); and Assistant Professor, Neonatal Graduate specialty, University of Florida College of Nursing (1986–1990). She has worked in the clinical setting in various capacities since 1976. From 1992 to 1996, she was the NNP Service Director/Associate Professor of Nursing (joint appointment) at the Children's Hospital Medical Center, University of Cincinnati College of Nursing, where she also was responsible for the administration of the NNP Service of the Level III NICU (1992–1996); and NNP Coordinator, Carolinas Medical Center, Charlotte, NC, where she was responsible for 12 NNPs. Dr. Lott was inducted into the AAN (2003), the AACN Fuld Leadership for Academic Nursing Program (2003–2004), and Visiting Professor for the Perinatal Society of Australia and NZ (2001). Dr. Lott has coauthored three editions of *Comprehensive Neonatal Nursing Care* with Dr. Kenner. Dr. Lott has been invited to deliver over 40 presentations, over 60 presentations at national professional meetings, and 17 research presentations. She has published over 20 peer-reviewed journal articles, 30 book chapters, and has been awarded 6 funded research grants, including a $260,000 grant from NINR.

Comprehensive Neonatal Nursing Care

Fifth Edition

Editors
Carole Kenner, PhD, RNC-NIC, NNP, FAAN
Judy Wright Lott, DSN, NNP-BC, FAAN

SPRINGER PUBLISHING COMPANY
NEW YORK

Springer Publishing Company, LLC
11 West 42nd Street
New York, NY 10036
www.springerpub.com

Acquisitions Editor: Margaret Zuccarini
Composition: diacriTech

ISBN: 978-0-8261-0975-0
e-book ISBN: 978-0-8261-0976-7

13 14 15 16 / 5 4 3 2 1

The author and the publisher of this Work have made every effort to use sources believed to be reliable to provide information that is accurate and compatible with the standards generally accepted at the time of publication. Because medical science is continually advancing, our knowledge base continues to expand. Therefore, as new information becomes available, changes in procedures become necessary. We recommend that the reader always consult current research and specific institutional policies before performing any clinical procedure. The author and publisher shall not be liable for any special, consequential, or exemplary damages resulting, in whole or in part, from the readers' use of, or reliance on, the information contained in this book. The publisher has no responsibility for the persistence or accuracy of URLs for external or third-party Internet websites referred to in this publication and does not guarantee that any content on such websites is, or will remain, accurate or appropriate.

Library of Congress Cataloging-in-Publication Data
Comprehensive neonatal nursing care / editors, Carole Kenner, Judy Wright Lott.—Fifth edition.
p. ; cm.
Preceded by: Comprehensive neonatal care / [edited by] Carole Kenner, Judy Wright Lott. 4th edition. c2007.
Includes bibliographical references and index.
ISBN 978-0-8261-0975-0—ISBN 978-0-8261-0976-7 (e-book)
I. Kenner, Carole, editor of compilation. II. Lott, Judy Wright, 1953- editor of compilation.
[DNLM: 1. Neonatal Nursing. 2. Infant, Newborn, Diseases—nursing. WY 157.3]
RJ253
618.92'01—dc23
2013020803

Printed in the United States of America by Bang Printing.

I wish to first express my appreciation, love, and support for my Dad who turned 101 in 2012. He still gets excited when a new edition is published. Thank you, Dad, from both of us as Judy also has grown close to you over the years.

Carole

I would like to thank my daughter, husband, and sisters for their love, support, and patience through not only this edition, but the previous editions as well.

Judy

Together we would like to express our appreciation for the assistance of Margaret Zuccarini, from Springer Publishing Company, who is a longtime trusted colleague who guided this project to a successful birth. Thank you for believing in this project. A special thank you goes to Chris Teja from Springer for all your assistance and guidance through the development and publication. We really enjoyed working with both of you. Also, we would like to thank Jan Zasada for her tireless efforts to try to keep us organized and on track. And of course, thanks to all the authors who provided their expertise. Finally, we want to thank the professionals across the globe who take care of the babies and their families.

Judy Wright Lott and Carole Kenner

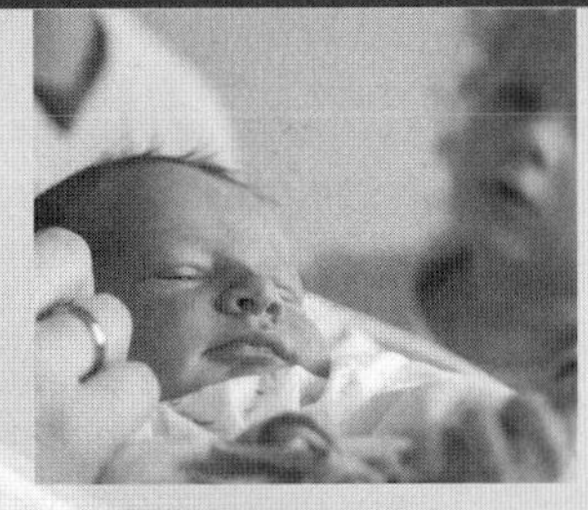

Contents

UNIT VI: ENVIRONMENTAL HEALTH AND FAMILY-CENTERED CARE IN THE NICU AND BEYOND

UNIT VII: NEONATAL CARE IN THE NEW MILLENNIUM: CHALLENGES AND OPPORTUNITIES

UNIT VIII: NEONATAL DIAGNOSTIC AND CARE PROTOCOLS

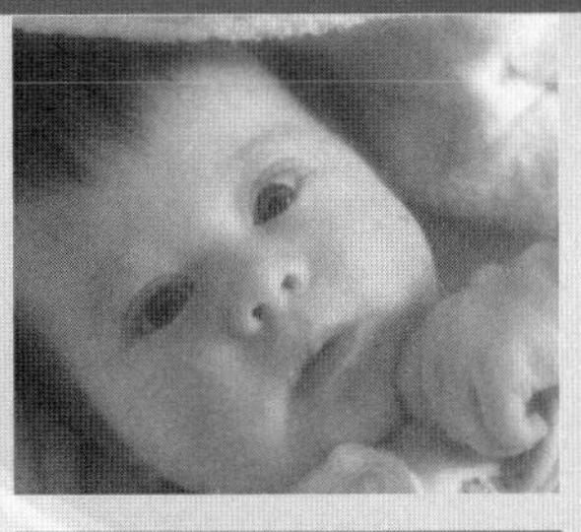

Contributors

Leslie Altimier, MSN, RN
Director of Clinical Marketing, Mother and Child Care; Patient Care and Clinical Informatics
Phillips Healthcare
Andover, MA

Diane M. Anderson, PhD, RD
Associate Professor
Baylor College of Medicine
Houston, TX

Jennifer Arnold, MD, MSc, FAAP
Assistant Professor
Division of Neonatology
Baylor College of Medicine
Houston, TX

Gail A. Bagwell, RN, MSN, CNS
Clinical Nurse Specialist
Nationwide Children's Hospital
Columbus, OH

Susan Tucker Blackburn, PhD, RN FAAN
Professor Emeritus
University of Washington
Seattle, WA

Mary Beth Bodin, DNP, CRNP, NNP-BC
Assistant Professor and NNP Track Coordinator
University of Alabama at Birmingham
Birmingham, AL

Beverly Bowers, PhD, APRN-CNS, ANEF
Assistant Dean for the Center for Educational Excellence and Associate Professor
University of Oklahoma College of Nursing
Oklahoma City, OK

Marina Boykova, MSc, RN
Doctoral Student
University of Oklahoma
College of Nursing
Oklahoma City, OK

Caitlin Bradley, MS, NNP-BC, RN
Staff Development Specialist
Children's Hospital Boston
Boston, MA

Joyce M. Butler, MSN, NNP-BC
Instructor, Department of Pediatrics
University of Mississippi Medical Center
Jackson, MS

Waldemar A. Carlo, MD
Professor, Director, Division of Neonatology; Director, Newborn Nurseries
University of Alabama at Birmingham
Birmingham, AL

Tony C. Carnes, PhD
Senior Technical Fellow, Integrated Patient Intelligence Group, Respiratory and Monitoring Solutions
Covidien
Mansfield, MA

Terri A. Cavaliere, DNP, NNP-BC, RN
Neonatal Nurse Practitioner at Schneider Children's Hospital, North Shore University Hospital and Assistant Professor Stony Brook University
Stony Brook, NY

Mary E. Coughlin, MS, BSN, APN, CCRN
Director of Professional Practice, Education, Research
Steward Health Care
Carney Hospital
Dorchester, MA

Sergio DeMarini, MD
Neonatologist
IRCCS Burlo Garofolo
Trieste, Italy

Georgia R. Ditzenberger, PhD, NNP-BC, APNP
Assistant Professor, CHS
Department of Pediatrics
Neonatology Division
University of Wisconsin
School of Medicine and Public Health
Madison, WI

Willa H. Drummond, MD, MS (Medical Informatics)
Professor of Pediatrics, Physiology and Large Animal Clinical Sciences
University of Florida
Gainesville, FL

Wakako Eklund, MS, NNP, RN
Neonatal Nurse Practitioner
Pediatrix Medical Group, Inc.
Nashville, TN

Susan Ellerbee, PhD, RNC-OB
Associate Professor
University of Oklahoma, College of Nursing
Oklahoma City, OK

Jody A. Farrell, RN, MSN
Director, Fetal Treatment Center
University of California, San Francisco Benioff Children's Hospital
San Francisco, CA

Kathleen Haubrich, PhD, RN
Associate Professor
Miami University
Hamilton, OH

Diane Holditch-Davis, PhD, RN, FAAN
Associate Dean for Research Affairs
Duke University School of Nursing
Durham, NC

Linda MacKenna Ikuta, MN, RN, CCNS, PHN
Neonatal Clinical Nurse Specialist
Packard Children's Hospital
Palo Alto, CA

Jamieson E. Jones, MD
Staff Neonatologist
Desert Regional Medical Center Hospital
San Diego, CA

Kathleen P. Juco, BSN, CCTN **(Certified Clinical Transplant Nurse)**
Staff Nurse, Perioperative Services
Lucile Packard Children's Hospital at Stanford
San Jose, CA

Nadine A. Kassity-Krich, MBA, BSN, RN
Adjunct Professor
University of San Diego
San Diego, CA

Carole Kenner
Dean/Professor
Northeastern University
School of Nursing
Associate Dean Bouve College of Health Sciences
Boston, MA

Joanne McManus Kuller, RN, MS
Neonatal Clinical Nurse Specialist
Children's Hospital & Research Center Oakland
Oakland, CA

Judith A. Lewis, PhD, RN, WHNP-BC, FAAN
Professor Emerita
Virginia Commonwealth University, School of Nursing
Richmond, VA

Cindy M. Little, PhD, WHNP-BC, CNS
Assistant Clinical Professor
Drexel University
Philadelphia, PA

Judy Wright Lott, DSN, NNP-BC, FAAN
Dean of Nursing
Wesleyan College
Macon, GA

Carolyn Houska Lund, RN, MS, FAAN
Neonatal Clinical Nurse Specialist
Children's Hospital & Research Center Oakland
Oakland, CA

Maureen F. McCourt, MS, RN, NNP, PNP
Instructor NNP Program
Northeastern University
Boston, MA
Neonatal Nurse Practitioner Supervisor
Women & Infants Hospital
Providence, RI

Jacqueline M. McGrath, PhD, RN, FNAP, FAAN
Associate Dean for Research and Scholarship Professor
School of Nursing
University of Connecticut
Storrs, CT

Kathryn R. McLean, MSN, RNC, NNP
Neonatal Nurse Practitioner
Women & Infants Hospital
Providence, RI

Sheryl J. Montrowl, MSN, NNP-BC
Clinical Coordinator Pediatrics,
Neonatal Nurse Practitioner
Division of Neonatology
Department of Pediatrics
University of Florida
Gainsville, FL

Samual Mooneyham, BSN, RN
Neonatal Nurse Practitioner Student
Northeastern University
School of Nursing
Boston, MA

Merry K. Moos, BSN, FNP, FAAN
Professor, Department of OB/GYN
University of North Carolina Chapel Hill
School of Medicine
Chapel, Hill NC

Dorothy M. Mullaney, DNP, MHSc, ANPRN, NNP-BC, RN
Neonatal Nurse Practitioner
Dartmouth Hitchcock Medical Center
Hanover, NH

Beth Mullins, MSN, NNP-BC
Neonatal Nurse Practitioner
Instructor, Department of Pediatrics
University of Mississippi Medical Center
Jackson, MS

Susan K. Newbold, PhD, RN-BC, FAAN, FHIMSS
Healthcare Informatics Consultant
Franklin, TN

Debra M. Parker, MSN, APRN-NP
Lead Neonatal Nurse Practitioner
Methodist Women's Hospital
Omaha, NE

Leslie A. Parker, PhD, NNP-BC
Clinical Assistant Professor
University of Florida
Gainesville, FL

Lyn S. Prater, PhD, RN
Senior Lecturer and Undergraduate Clinical Coordinator
Baylor University
School of Nursing
Dallas, TX

Shahirose S. Premji, RN, BSc, BScN, MScN, PhD
Associate Professor
University of Calgary
Faculty of Nursing
Public Health Nurse, Alberta Health Services
Adjunct Associate Professor
University of Calgary, Faculty of Medicine, Department of Community Health Sciences
Alberta Children's Hospital Research Institute for Child and Maternal Health, Member
Calgary, Alberta, Canada

Jana L. Pressler, PhD, RN
Professor and Associate Dean of Graduate Programs
East Carolina University, College of Nursing
Greenville, NC

Linda L. Rath, PhD, RN, NNP-BC
Associate Professor
University of Texas at Tyler
Tyler, TX

Cheryl Riley, MSN, RN, NNP-BC
Coordinator of the Neonatal Nurse Practitioner Program
Baylor University
School of Nursing
Dallas, TX

Rachel Ritter, BSN, RN
Staff Nurse
Neonatal Intensive Care Unit
Children's Hospital Boston
Boston, MA

Lori Baas Rubarth, PhD, APRN, NNP-BC
Associate Professor and NNP Program Coordinator
Creighton University School of Nursing
Omaha, NE

Debra A. Sansoucie, Ed.D, ARNP, NNP-BC
Vice President, Advanced Practitioner Program
Pediatrix Medical Group
Sunrise, FL

Elizabeth L. Sharpe, DNP, ARNP, NNP-BC
Neonatal Nurse Practitioner
Pediatrix Medical Group, Inc.
West Palm Beach, FL

Beth Shields, PharmD
Pediatric Clinical Pharmacist
Rush University Medical Center
Chicago, IL

Thomas D. Soltau, MD
Assistant Professor
University of Alabama at Birmingham
Birmingham, AL

Kaye Spence, AM, RN, MN, FCN
Clinical Nurse Consultant
The Children's Hospital at Westmead
Westmead, Australia

Becky Spencer, MSN, RN, IBCLC
Lecturer
Baylor University
School of Nursing
Dallas, TX

Kathleen R. Stevens, RN, EdD, ANEF, FAAN
Professor and Director
Academic Center for Evidence-Based Practice www.ACESTAR.uthscsa.edu and Improvement Science Research Network www.ISRN.net
University of Texas Health Science Center San Antonio
San Antonio, TX

Laura A. Stokowski, RNC, MS
Staff Nurse
Inova Fairfax Hospital for Children
Falls Church, VA

Tanya Sudia-Robinson, RN, PhD
Professor
Georgia Baptist College of Nursing of Mercer University
Atlanta, GA

Marlene Walden, PhD, RN, NNP-BC, CCNS
Nurse Scientist and Neonatal Nurse Practitioner
Texas Children's Hospital
Assistant Professor, Pediatrics-Newborn
Baylor College of Medicine
Houston, TX

Robert D. White, MD
Director, Regional Newborn Program
Newborn ICU, Memorial Hospital
South Bend, IN

Lynda Law Wilson, RN, PhD, FAAN
Professor and Assistant Dean for International Affairs
The University of Alabama at Birmingham
School of Nursing
Birmingham, AL

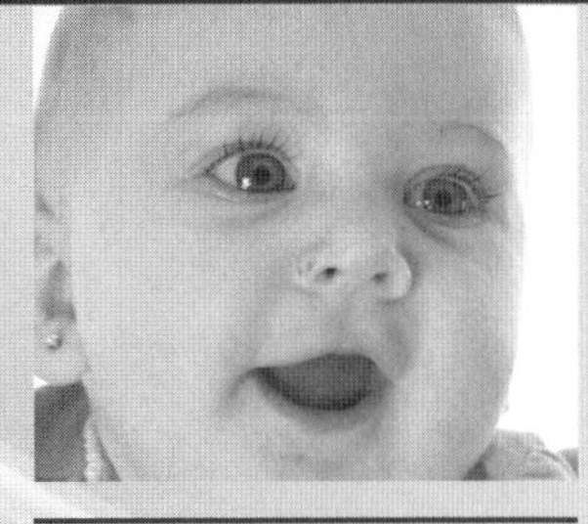

Past Contributors to the Fourth Edition

Kathy Bergman, MSN, RNC, CNS
Nursing Faculty, Department of Nursing
Coordinator, Learning Resource Center
Xavier University
Cincinnati, OH

Dorothy Brooten, PhD, RN, FAAN
Professor
School of Nursing
Florida International University
Principal
The Research A-Team, LLC
Miami, FL

Javier Cifuentes, MD
Neored-Clinica Indisa
Providencia, Santiago
Associate Professor
Department of Pediatrics
Catholic University of Chile
Santiago, Chile

Deborah L. Fike, MSN, RNC, NNP
Neonatal Nurse Practitioner
Pediatrix Medical Group of Ohio
Miami Valley Hospital
Dayton, OH

Rebecca Lynn Roys Gelrud, MS, RN, BC
Clinical Informatics Consultant
ICU Data Systems, Inc.
Richmond, VA

Karen Kavanaugh, PhD, RN, FAAN
Professor
Department of Maternal Child Nursing
University of Illinois at Chicago
Chicago, IL

Kristie Nix, EdD, RN
Associate Professor
University of Tulsa
Tulsa, OK

Frances Strodtbeck, DNS, RNC, NNP, FAAN
Director, Graduate Program in Nursing
Professor and Coordinator
Advanced Neonatal Nursing Program
Louise Herrington School of Nursing
Baylor University
Dallas, TX

Janet Thigpen, MN, RNC, CNNP
Neonatal Nurse Practitioner
Division of Neonatology
Department of Pediatrics
Emory University School of Medicine
Atlanta, GA

Sara Rich Wheeler, DNS, BC, RN, LCPC
Dean of Nursing
Lakeview College of Nursing
Danville, IL
Principal
Grief, Ltd.
Covington, IN

Pamela Holtzclaw Williams, RN, JD
Research Staff Member
University of Oklahoma
College of Nursing
Department of Case Management
Norman, OK

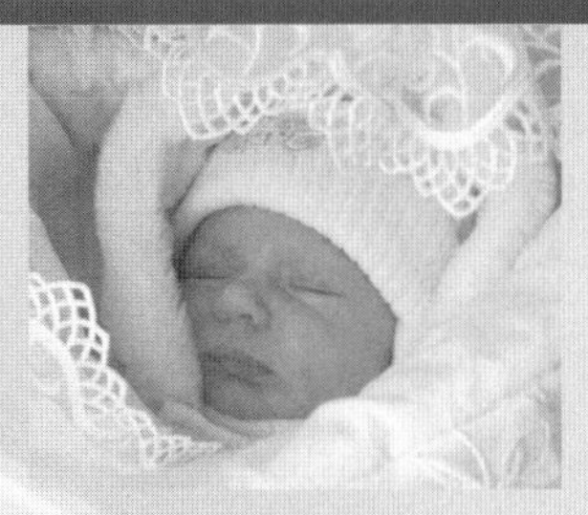

Foreword

When the first edition of *Comprehensive Neonatal Nursing Care* was published in 1993, it was a time of rapid expansion in neonatal care. The knowledge needed for the practice of neonatal nursing had grown tremendously, not only in depth but in breadth, and there was no one "go to" textbook that really captured the science and art of neonatal nursing in a way that could serve the learner in the classroom and the practitioner in clinical care. *Comprehensive Neonatal Nursing Care* filled that gap then, and 20 years and four editions later; it is still the go-to reference for both novice and expert neonatal nurses.

The new fifth edition includes the latest information on hot topics, such as emerging infections, neuroprotection and care of the late preterm infant, as well as updates in all other aspects of neonatal embryology, physiology, medical, surgical, and psychosocial care. The textbook is organized with a focus on integrative management of the newborn and family. There is extensive use of research findings in each of the chapters to provide evidence to support practice strategies and clinical decision making. Complete references are found at the end of each chapter.

The fifth edition of *Comprehensive Neonatal Nursing Care* is the first major textbook to fully embrace the globalization of neonatal nursing care, and it addresses the varying approaches but similar goals and knowledge needs of low- and high-resource countries in which neonatal care is delivered. Although remaining responsive to the individual circumstances of the infant, family, and setting of care, we are now more than ever being called upon to demonstrate that competent neonatal nursing improves patient outcomes and is cost effective. There will be many opportunities and challenges in the coming years to meet the nursing care needs of infants and families within health care systems that worldwide are undergoing rapid and sometimes dramatic transformation. As it has for the past 20 years, *Comprehensive Neonatal Nursing Care* continues to provide the specialty with an accurate compass for staying on a true course toward better outcomes for neonates and families. The editors and authors have done a fantastic job of putting together a truly *comprehensive* textbook to guide us all, novice and expert alike, in our global quest to deliver high-quality neonatal nursing care.

Linda S. Franck, PhD, RN, FRCPCH, FAAN
Professor and Chair, Department of Family Health Care Nursing
University of California, San Francisco

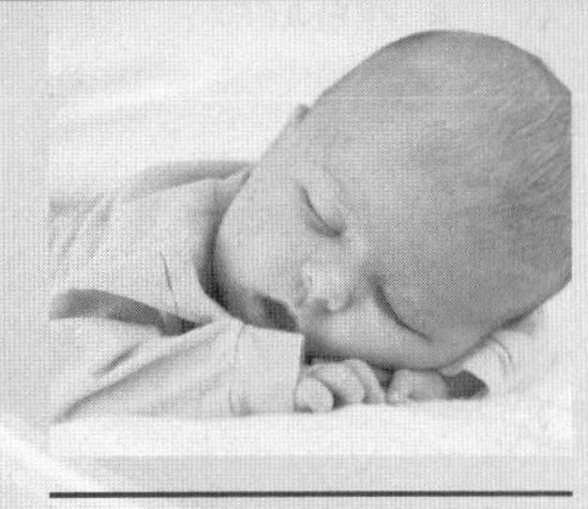

Preface

One of the most complex issues in health care is the care of sick or premature infants and infants with multiple, severe congenital anomalies. Despite advanced technology and knowledge, preterm delivery continues to be a significant problem in the United States. Maternal risk factors have changed over the past decade. For example, more women with chronic illnesses such as diabetes or sickle cell anemia are giving birth to infants with consequent health problems. The rise of in vitro fertilization has resulted in increased multiple births and prematurity. Many infants in neonatal intensive care units (NICUs) have been exposed to substances or are born to mothers with other risk factors such as delayed childbearing or childhood cancers. The care of these at-risk infants requires the use of more and more complex technology. Surfactant administration, nitric oxide administration, high-frequency jet ventilators, dialysis, organ transplantation, and other extraordinary measures are becoming commonplace. However, in the midst of these high-tech interventions, developmentally supportive care interventions such as dimming lights, using visible rather than audible alarms, using more physiologically and developmentally appropriate positioning and skin-to-skin care, and cobedding multiples are emerging as important interventions, due to increasing evidence regarding the importance of maintaining a developmentally supportive NICU environment for improved long-term infant/child outcomes. The family is considered a partner in care, and family-centered care, which has been a buzz word for two decades, is really being operationalized as part of developmentally supportive care.

Providers of neonatal care need accurate, comprehensive information as a basis for providing care to newborns. A thorough understanding of normal physiology as well as the pathophysiology of disease processes is necessary for well-designed care practices. Knowledge about associated risk factors, genetics, critical periods of development, principles of nutrition and pharmacology, and current neonatal research findings are all essential for providing optimal care for neonates. The concept of a family-centered approach to care is important too; parents are an integral part of the care team. Care practices need to be based on the best evidence available, rather than on tradition. A multidisciplinary approach has been replaced by an integrated interprofessional approach to care. All these elements form the foundation for assessment, planning, implementation, and evaluation of the effectiveness of neonatal care.

The nurse plays a vital role in the provision of integrated health care to newborns. During the past decade, the nurse's role has included added responsibilities, which are recognized at both the staff and advanced practice levels. For the purposes of this book, two definitions of advanced practice are being used. They are the National Association of Neonatal Nurses' (NANN) definitions of clinical nurse specialist (CNS) and neonatal nurse practitioner (NNP) (NANN, Position Statement, 1990). The association reaffirmed these in 2000, and in 2009 another position statement was issued that defines the NNP competencies (NANN, 2009).

CLINICAL NURSE SPECIALIST

The CNS is a registered nurse with a master's degree who, through study and supervised practice at the graduate level, has become an expert in the defined clinical area of nursing. The CNS provides for the diagnosis and treatment of human responses to actual or potential health problems of patients and their families within the specialized area through direct patient care and clinical consultation. In addition, the CNS may act in an educational, research, liaison, or leadership role to promote optimal nursing care for the patients served.

NEONATAL NURSE PRACTITIONER

The NNP is a registered nurse with clinical expertise in neonatal nursing who has received formal education with supervised clinical experience in the management of sick newborns and their families. The NNP manages a caseload of neonatal patients with consultation, collaboration, and general supervision from a physician. Using extensive knowledge of pathophysiology, pharmacology, and physiology, the NNP exercises independent or intradependent (in collaboration with other health professionals) judgment in the assessment, diagnosis, and initiation of certain delegated medical processes and procedures. As an advanced practice neonatal nurse, the NNP is additionally involved in education, consultation, and research at various levels.

The American Association of Colleges of Nurses (AACN) has proposed a change in the educational preparation for advanced practice nurses. The proposal recommends that the nurse practitioner be prepared at a "doctor of nursing practice" (DNP) level. This will likely affect the NNP role, as well as other advanced practice nurses, over the next few years.

The neonatal staff nurse role requires accurate and thorough assessment skills, excellent ability to communicate with other health professionals and patients' families, and a broad understanding of physiology and pathophysiology on which to base management decisions. It requires highly developed technical skills as well as critical decision-making skills. With health care delivery changes, the role also requires supervision of ancillary personnel and an informed delegation of certain patient-oriented tasks. These changes require the staff nurse to possess even better assessment skills and sound knowledge of physiology and pathophysiology than in the past because some decision making will be done in concert with other, less highly trained personnel.

PURPOSE AND CONTENT

The fifth edition of this book provides a comprehensive examination of the care of neonates from a physiologic and pathophysiologic approach appropriate for any health professional concerned with neonatal care.

This text provides a complete physiologic and embryologic foundation for each neonatal body system. Additionally, it includes medical, surgical, and psychosocial care because the integrative management approach is absolutely imperative to the well-being of the newborn and family. Appropriate diagnostic tests and their interpretation are included in each organ-system chapter. There is extensive use of research findings in the chapters to provide evidence to support practice strategies and demonstrate the rationale for clinical decision making. Complete references for more in-depth reading are found at the end of each chapter so that the reader may pursue more specific information on a topical area. Use of tables and illustrations to support material that is presented in the narrative portions is sure to be another help to the practicing neonatal nurse.

The thread of integrative management is interwoven throughout the text. Foundational topics such as genetics, physiologically critical periods of development, nutrition, and parenting are included, as are topics of recent interest such as iatrogenic complications, neonatal pain, use of computers or other technology in neonatal care, and neonatal AIDS. Now more than ever, neonatal care providers must examine patient outcomes and nurse outcomes to meet the demands for providing cost-effective and high-quality care. Research is critical to support both the art and science of neonatal care. Whenever possible, the contributors remind the reader of areas in need of further study. Chapters address evidence-based practice and new trends in neonatal care, such as hospice and palliative care, management of the NICU environment, evidence-based nursing, care of the extremely-low-birth-weight infant, complementary therapies, and competency-based neonatal nursing education. Another feature is the Preemie Bill of Rights, which we felt was important as we put more emphasis on the consumer and his or her needs. Of course, for neonatal care, the consumer is the newborn/infant and family. This book is not a quick reference; it provides comprehensive in-depth discussions along with detailed physiologic principles and collaborative management strategies. It provides a sound basis for safe and effective neonatal care; however, the new format should make the information easier to find.

Each organ system is discussed in depth, including the respiratory system, its complications and new technologies, followed by assessment of and management strategies for the cardiovascular system; nutrition and the gastrointestinal system; and metabolic, endocrine, immunologic, hematopoietic, neurologic, musculoskeletal, genitourinary, integumentary, auditory, and ophthalmic systems. General areas of neonatal care—the new health care delivery environment, regionalization today, evidence-based nursing, legal/ethical issues, collaborative research, competency-based neonatal nursing education, family-centered care, bereavement, and hospice and palliative care—are included as appropriate. Bereavement and chronic sorrow are discussed along with the newer field of neonatal hospice and palliative care because a happy ending is not always possible in perinatal and neonatal nursing. Human genetics is introduced, and the impact of environmental influences on the developing fetus, as well as the nursing implications of the Human Genome Project, is discussed. This provides the transition into the aspects of perinatal care, the high-risk pregnancy, and the effects of labor on the fetus. The text then deals with more specific neonatal topics, starting with stabilization, managing the NICU environment, newborn and infant neurobehavioral development, monitoring neonatal biophysical parameters, computer technology, and assessment. This edition includes the most up-to-date information from the American Heart Association's Neonatal Resuscitation Program as well as elements of the S.T.A.B.L.E.® program used for infants undergoing transport. Diagnostic imaging and diagnostic test and laboratory values represent the section of the text that highlights the evaluative measures used by practitioners to identify the neonatal problem and its progress. This edition continues with the surgical neonate, neonatal pain, neonatal AIDS, the drug-exposed neonate, and care of the extremely-low-birth-weight infant. Because neonatal nurses are seeing more and more extremely-low-birth-weight infants, we wanted to address this population's unique care needs. The final group of chapters covers the discharge phase. Topics include principles of newborn and infant drug therapy, systematic assessment and home follow-up, neonatal behavior, assessment and management of neonatal behavior, the transition to home and, finally, home care. One topic that has been added to this edition is complementary therapies. Never before has there been so much interest in or controversy over such interventions. We address what is known and where the gaps are in this area of neonatal care. This section recognizes that many neonatal nurses now care for infants through the first year of life. It also acknowledges the need for technology in the home and some guidelines for families who feel as if they have set up mini-NICUs in their homes.

In this edition, each of the chapters and sections has been updated to include the newest techniques, such as the latest trends in fetal therapy; progress with the mapping of human genes; use of computers, including Internet connections that open up global neonatal care issues for examination and discussion; the latest issues in health care reform and the impact on nursing care; and the latest research findings appropriate to each of the sections.

To provide depth to these topical areas, physicians, nurses, infant developmental specialists, and other health professionals concerned with neonatal care from across the country and around the world are contributors in all editions. The attempt was made not only to tap the experts in the neonatal field but also to have them represent as wide a geographic area as possible. We hope that the broad geographic distribution of contributors and reviewers will help minimize the effect of regional differences in clinical practice as reflected in the text. The fifth edition recognizes that neonatal nursing and care are global issues. The book's format changed to reflect moving from prenatal considerations, then into intrapartal and postal periods; the latter section includes new information on the Helping Babies Breathe program from the American Academy of Pediatrics for low-resourced countries and the S.T.A.B.L.E. program. This edition includes information on emerging infections, the newest information on the late preterm infant—a hot topic. The last section is new and includes the new millennium challenges and opportunities. Selected neonatal evidence-based protocols are found in a separate section, so they are easy to find and use.

We hope that you will find the information contained in this text very useful and helpful to you in providing care to newborns and their families.

Carole Kenner, PhD, RNC-NIC, NNP, FAAN
Judy Wright Lott, DSN, NNP-BC, FAAN

REFERENCE

National Association of Neonatal Nurses (NANN). (2009). Requirements for advanced neonatal nursing practice in neonatal intensive care units. Position Statement #3042. Glenview, IL: NANN.

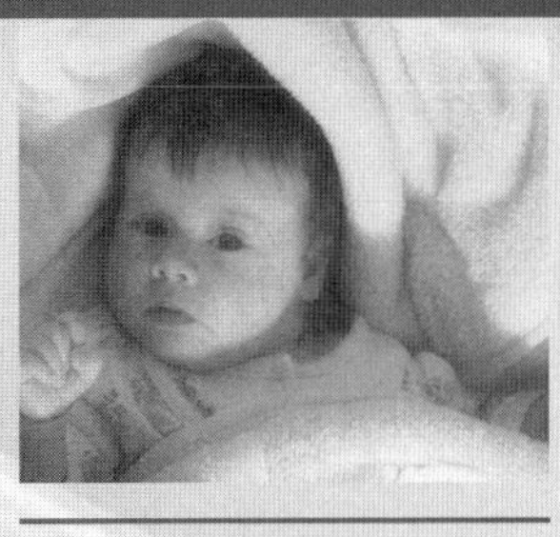

Acknowledgments

The idea for this book was born in the basement office of one of the editors (Kenner) in Cincinnati, Ohio. The other editor (Lott) had flown up from her home in Georgia for a long weekend to work on just an article and presentation. As we were researching that topic, we had a difficult time finding the references we needed. We could find many medical references for the condition, but we found few references written about the nursing care needed. Over the course of those few days we recognized there was no comprehensive book about the nursing care for neonates. As those of you who know Dr. Kenner are aware, once a need is identified, she will set about meeting that need. Further, she will provide opportunities for colleagues to assist in the process. I was so lucky to be in that basement office when we decided to write the first comprehensive neonatal nursing care reference. My collaboration with Dr. Kenner has led to so many opportunities throughout my career. So, I want to express my great admiration, appreciation, and gratitude for Dr. Kenner's influence upon my professional and personal life. Thanks, Carole. You are awesome.

Judy Wright Lott

Dr. Lott, I appreciate your kind words and your sense of humor as we pulled this book together. We are laying new ground for neonatal nurses, and I am so pleased you took the chance with me. Thank you for a great 20-year journey with this book! You too are awesome.

Carole Kenner

UNIT I: PRENATAL CONSIDERATIONS AND CARE

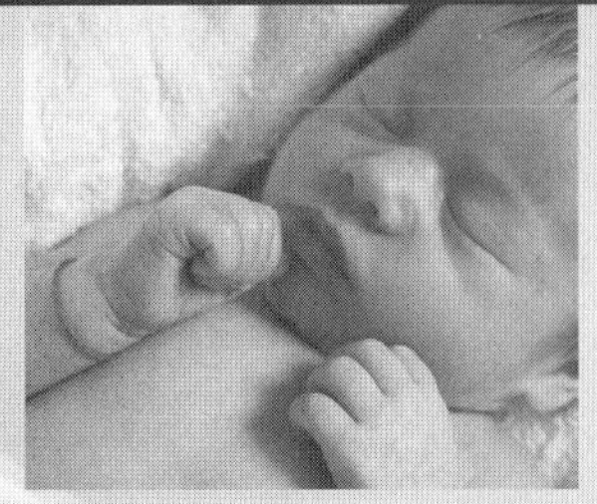

CHAPTER 1

Fetal Development: Environmental Influences and Critical Periods

■ Cindy M. Little

In this chapter, the major events of prenatal development are described, and critical development periods for the major organ systems are identified. A brief review of the events beginning with fertilization is included, but the reader is referred to an embryology text for a more thorough account. Human genetics is discussed in Chapter 38.

EARLY FETAL DEVELOPMENT

The process of human development begins with the fertilization of an ovum (female gamete) by a spermatocyte (male gamete). The fusion of the ovum and sperm initiates a sequence of events that causes the single-celled zygote to develop into a new human being. During the 38 to 42 weeks of gestation, dramatic growth and development occurs that is unequaled during any other period of life.

Fertilization

Large numbers of spermatozoa are necessary to increase the chances for conception because the spermatozoa must traverse the cervical canal, the uterus, and the uterine (fallopian) tubes to reach the ovum; approximately 200 to 600 million sperm are deposited in the posterior fornix of the vagina during ejaculation. The usual site of fertilization is in the ampulla, the widest portion of the uterine tubes, located near the ovaries. Sperm are propelled by the movement of the tails, aided by muscular contractions of the uterus and fallopian tubes. The spermatozoa undergo two physiologic changes in order to penetrate the corona radiata and zona pellucida, the barriers around the secondary oocyte. The first change is capacitation, an enzymatic reaction that removes the glycoprotein coating from the spermatozoa and plasma proteins from the seminal fluid. Capacitation generally occurs in the uterus or uterine tubes and takes about 7 hours. The second change, the acrosome reaction, occurs when a capacitated sperm passes through the corona radiata, causing structural changes that result in the fusion of the plasma membranes of the sperm and the oocyte. Progesterone released from the follicle at ovulation stimulates the acrosome reaction. Three enzymes are released from the acrosome to facilitate entry of the sperm into the ovum. Hyaluronidase allows the sperm to penetrate the corona radiata, whereas trypsin-like enzymes and zona lysin digest a pathway across the zona pellucida (Moore & Persaud, 2008; Sadler, 2010).

Only about 300 to 500 spermatozoa actually reach the ovum. When a spermatozoon comes into contact with the ovum, the zona pellucida and the plasma membrane fuse, preventing entry by other sperm. After penetration by a single sperm, the oocyte completes the second meiotic cell division, resulting in the haploid number of chromosomes (22,X) and the second polar body. The chromosomes are arranged to form the female pronucleus (Moore & Persaud, 2008; Sadler, 2010).

As the spermatozoon moves close to the female pronucleus, the tail detaches and the nucleus enlarges to form the male pronucleus. The male and female pronuclei fuse forming a diploid cell called the zygote. The zygote contains 23 autosomes and one sex chromosome from each parent (46,XX or 46,XY). The genetic sex of the new individual is determined at fertilization by the contribution of the father. The male parent (XY) may contribute either an X or a Y chromosome. If the spermatozoon contains an X chromosome, the offspring is female (46,XX). If the spermatozoon receives one Y chromosome, the offspring is male (46,XY). Individual variation is the result of random or independent assortment of the autosomal chromosomes (Moore & Persaud, 2008; Sadler, 2010).

Cleavage

Mitotic cell division occurs after fertilization as the zygote passes down the uterine tube, resulting in the formation of two blastomeres (Figure 1.1). The cells continue to divide,

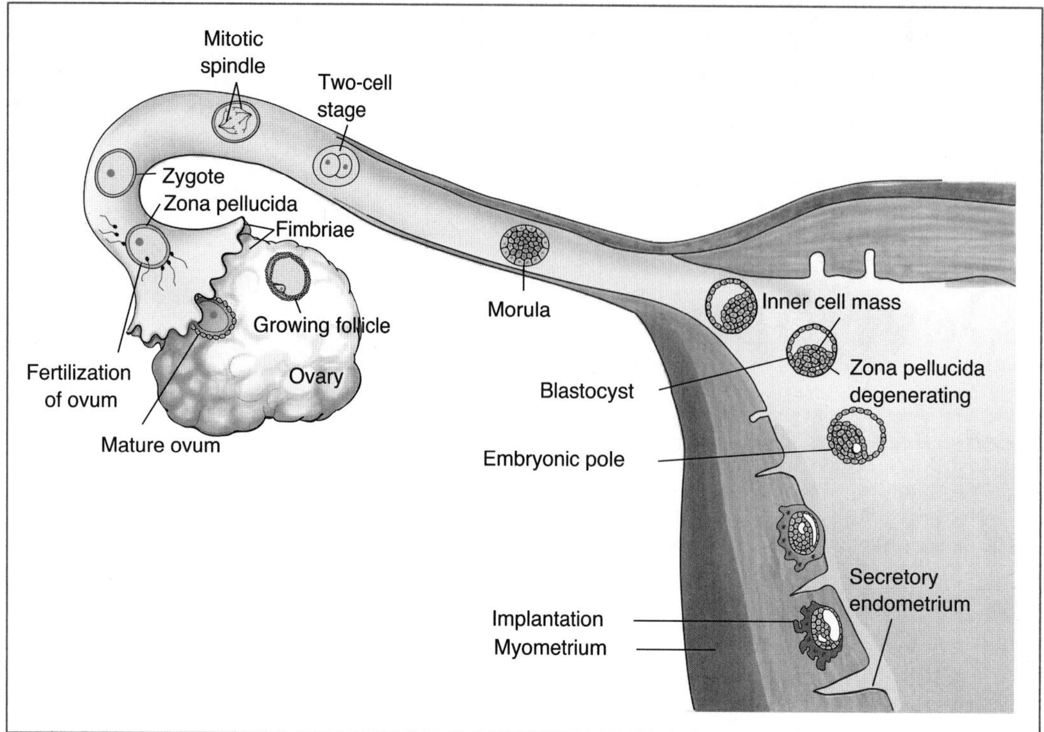

FIGURE 1.1 Fantastic voyage: From fertilization to implantation. The journey through the fallopian tubes takes approximately 4 days. During this time, mitotic cell division occurs. Implantation occurs on about day 9 through day 12.

increasing in number, although decreasing in size. The term *cleavage* is used to describe the mitotic cell division of the zygote (Figure 1.2). When the number of cells reaches approximately 16 (usually on the third day), the zygote is called a morula, because of its resemblance to a mulberry. The zygote reaches the morula stage about the time it enters the uterus. The morula consists of groups of centrally located cells called the inner cell mass and an outer cell layer. At this stage, the individual cells are called blastomeres. The outer cell layer forms the trophoblast, from which the placenta develops. The inner cell mass, called the embryoblast, gives rise to the embryo (Moore & Persaud, 2008; Sadler, 2010).

After the morula penetrates the uterine cavity, fluid enters through the zona pellucida into the intercellular spaces of the inner cell mass. The fluid-filled spaces fuse, forming a large cavity known as the blastocyst cavity about the fourth day after fertilization. The morula is now called the blastocyst. This outer cell layer known as the trophoblast forms the wall of the blastocyst, which later becomes the placenta, and the embryoblast projects from the wall of the blastocyst into the blastocyst cavity. The uterine secretions nourish the blastocyst until implantation occurs (Moore & Persaud, 2008; Sadler, 2010).

Implantation

Degeneration of the zona pellucida occurs on about the fifth day after fertilization, allowing the blastocyst to attach to the endothelium of the endometrium on about the sixth day. The trophoblasts then secrete proteolytic enzymes that destroy the endometrial endothelium and invade the endometrium. Two layers of trophoblasts develop; the inner layer is made up of cytotrophoblasts, and the outer layer is composed of syncytiotrophoblasts. The syncytiotrophoblast has finger-like projections that produce enzymes capable of further eroding the endometrial tissues. By the end of the seventh day, the blastocyst is superficially implanted (Figure 1.3).

Formation of the Bilaminar Disk

Implantation is completed during the second week. The syncytiotrophoblast continues to invade the endometrium and becomes embedded. Spaces in the syncytiotrophoblast, called lacunae, fill with blood from ruptured maternal capillaries and secretions from eroded endometrial glands. This fluid nourishes the embryoblast by diffusion. The lacunae give rise to the uteroplacental circulation. The lacunae fuse to form a network that then becomes the intervillous spaces of the placenta. The endometrial capillaries near the implanted embryoblast become dilated and eroded by the syncytiotrophoblast. Maternal blood enters the lacunar network and provides circulation and nutrients to the embryo. Maternal-embryonic blood circulation provides the developing embryo with nutrition and oxygenation and removes waste products before the development of the placenta. Finger-like projections, primary chorionic villi, of the chorion develop into the chorionic villi of the placenta at about the same time (Moore & Persaud, 2008; Sadler, 2010).

The inner cell mass differentiates into two layers: the hypoblast (endoderm), a layer of small cuboidal cells, and the epiblast (ectoderm), a layer of high columnar cells. The two layers form a flattened, circular bilaminar embryonic disk. The amniotic cavity is derived from spaces within the epiblast. As the amniotic cavity enlarges, a thin layer of epithelial cells covers the amniotic cavity. During the development of the amniotic cavity, other trophoblastic cells form a thin extracoelomic membrane, which encloses

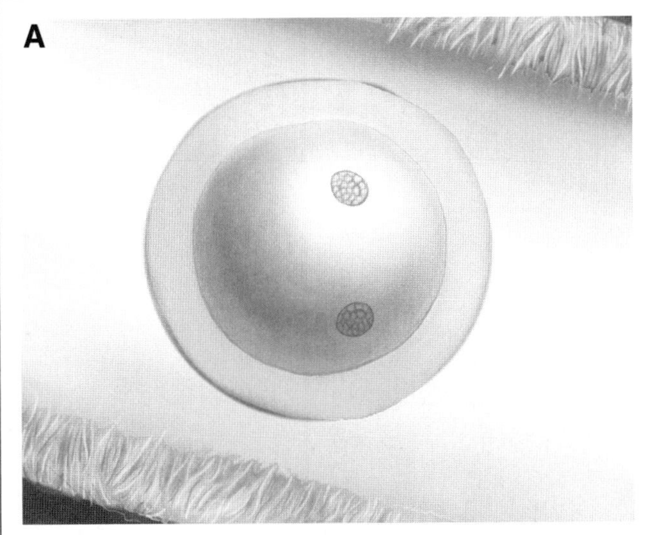

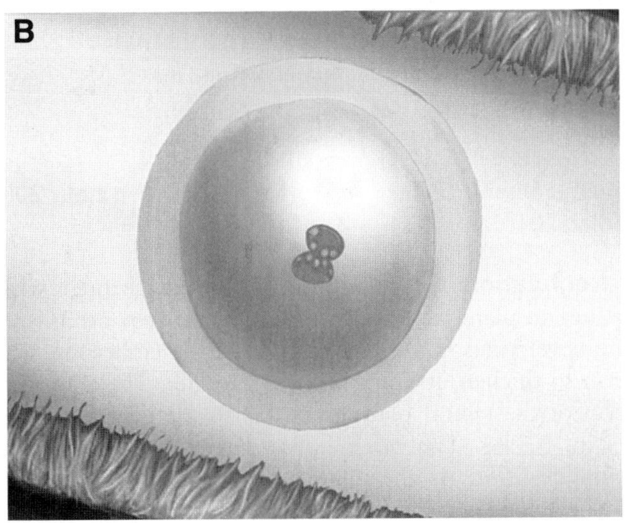

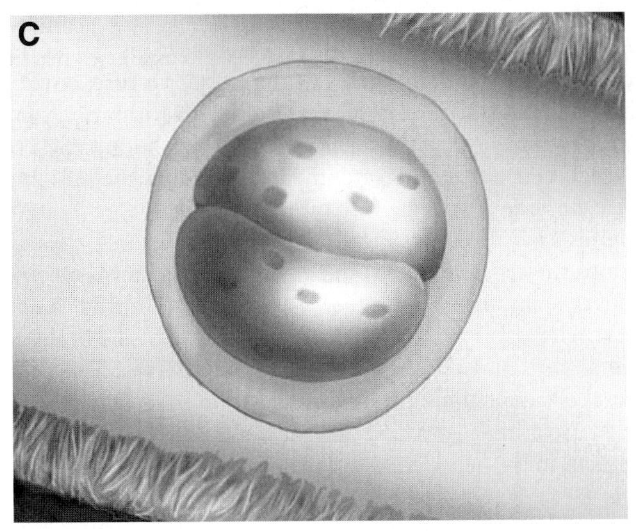

FIGURE 1.2 Stages of cell division: cleavage. (A) Zygote. (B) Zygote undergoing first cleavage. (C) Two-cell blastomere state.

the primitive yolk sac. The yolk sac produces fetal red blood cells. Other trophoblastic cells form a layer of mesenchymal tissue, called the extraembryonic mesoderm, around the amnion and primitive yolk sac. Isolated coelomic spaces in the extraembryonic mesoderm fuse to form a single, large, fluid-filled cavity surrounding the amnion and yolk sac, with the exception of the area where the amnion is attached to the chorion by the connecting stalk. The primitive yolk sac decreases in size, creating a smaller secondary yolk sac (Moore & Persaud, 2008; Sadler, 2010).

Two layers of extraembryonic mesoderm result from the formation of the extraembryonic cavity. The extraembryonic somatic mesoderm lines the trophoblast and covers the amnion, and the extraembryonic splanchnic mesoderm covers the yolk sac. The chorion is made up of the extraembryonic somatic mesoderm, the cytotrophoblast, and the syncytiotrophoblast. The chorion forms the chorionic sac, in which the embryo and the amniotic and yolk sacs are located. By the end of the second week, there is a slightly thickened area near the cephalic region of the hypoblastic disk, known as the prochordal plate, which marks the location of the mouth (Moore & Persaud, 2008; Sadler, 2010).

Formation of the Trilaminar Embryonic Disk: The Third Week of Development

The third week of development is marked by rapid growth, the formation of the primitive streak, and the differentiation of the three germ layers, from which all fetal tissue and organs are derived (Moore & Persaud, 2008; Sadler, 2010) (Figure 1.4).

■ **Gastrulation.** Gastrulation is the process through which the bilaminar disk develops into a trilaminar embryonic disk. Gastrulation is the most important event of early fetal formation; it affects all of the rest of embryologic development. During the third week, epiblast cells separate from their original location and migrate inward, forming the mesoblast, which spreads cranially and laterally to form a layer between the ectoderm and the endoderm called the intraembryonic mesoderm. Other mesoblastic cells invade the endoderm, displacing the endodermal cells laterally, forming a new layer, the embryonic ectoderm. Thus, the hypoblastic ectoderm produces the embryonic ectoderm, embryonic mesoderm, and the majority of the embryonic endoderm. These three germ layers are the source of the tissue and organs of the embryo (Moore & Persaud, 2008; Sadler, 2010).

■ **Primitive Streak.** Over days 14 to 15, a groove and thickening of the ectoderm (epiblast), called the primitive streak, appears caudally in the center of the dorsum of the embryonic disk. The primitive streak results from the migration of ectodermal cells toward the midline in the posterior portion of the embryonic disk. The primitive groove develops in the primitive streak. When the primitive streak begins to produce mesoblastic cells that become intraembryonic mesoderm, the epiblast is referred to as the embryonic ectoderm and the hypoblast is referred to as the embryonic mesoderm (Moore & Persaud, 2008; Sadler, 2010).

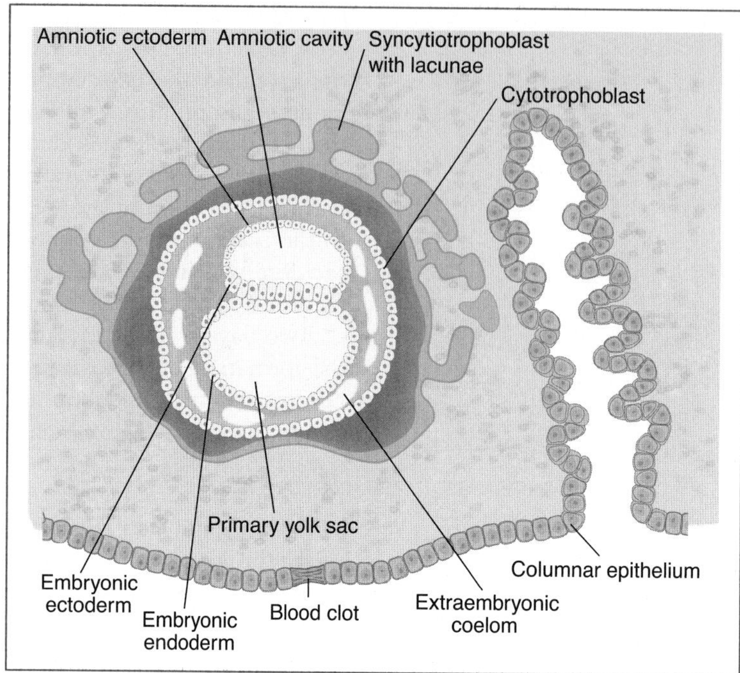

FIGURE 1.3 Cross section of a blastocyst at 11 days. Two germ layers are present. The trophoblast has differentiated into the syncytiotrophoblast and the cytotrophoblast.

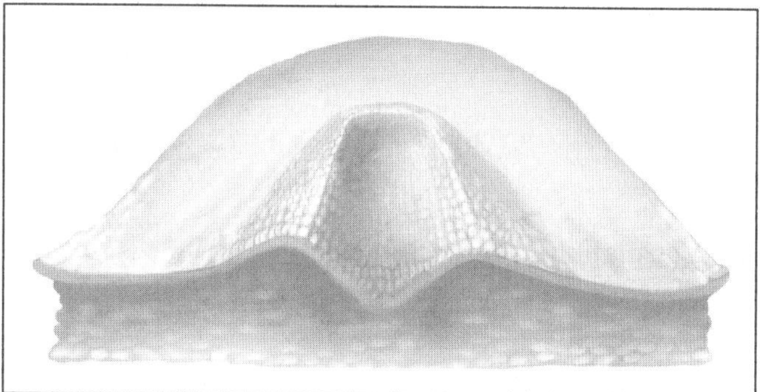

FIGURE 1.4 Formation of the trilaminar embryonic disk: gastrulation. During gastrulation, the bilaminar embryonic disk is changed to a trilaminar embryonic disk, consisting of the epiblast (ectoderm), hypoblast (endoderm), and mesoblast (mesoderm).

■ Notochordal Process. Cells from the primitive knot migrate cranially and form the midline cellular notochordal process. This process grows cranially between the ectoderm and the endoderm until it reaches the prochordal plate, which is attached to the overlying ectoderm, thus forming the oropharyngeal membrane. The cloacal membrane, caudal to the primitive streak, develops into the anus (Moore & Persaud, 2008; Sadler, 2010).

The primitive streak produces mesenchyme (mesoblasts) until the end of the fourth week. The primitive streak does not grow as rapidly as the other cells, making it relatively insignificant in size when compared with the other structures that continue to grow. Persistence of the primitive streak or remnants is the cause of sacrococcygeal teratomas (Moore & Persaud, 2008; Sadler, 2010).

The notochord is a cellular rod that develops from the notochordal process. The notochord is the structure around which the vertebral column is formed. It forms the nucleus pulposus of the intervertebral bodies of the spinal column (Figure 1.5) (Moore & Persaud, 2008; Sadler, 2010).

■ Neurulation. Neurulation is the process through which the neural plate, neural folds, and neural tube are formed. The developing notochord stimulates the embryonic ectoderm to thicken, forming the neural plate. The neuroectoderm of the neural plate gives rise to the central nervous system (CNS). The neural plate develops cranial to the primitive knot. As the neural plate elongates, the neural plate gets wider and extends cranially to the oropharyngeal membrane. The neural plate invaginates along the central axis to form a neural groove with neural folds on each side. The neural folds move together and fuse, forming the neural tube showing the first indication of brain development (Figure 1.6). The neural tube detaches from the surface ectoderm, and the free edges of the ectoderm fuse, covering the posterior portion of the embryo. With formation of the neural tube, nearby ectodermal cells lying along the crest of each neural fold migrate inward, invading the mesoblast on each side of the neural tube. These irregular, flattened masses are called the neural crest. This structure's cells give rise to the spinal ganglia, the ganglia of the autonomic nervous system, and cranial nerves V, VII, IX, and X. Neural crest cells also form the meningeal covering of the brain and spinal cord and the sheaves that protect nerves. The neural crest cells contribute to the formation of pigment-producing cells, the adrenal medulla, and skeletal and muscular development in the head (Moore & Persaud, 2008; Sadler, 2010).

■ Development of Somites. Another important event of the third week is the development of somites, which give rise to most of the skeleton and associated musculature and much of the dermis of the skin. During formation of the neural tube, the intraembryonic mesoderm on each side thickens, forming

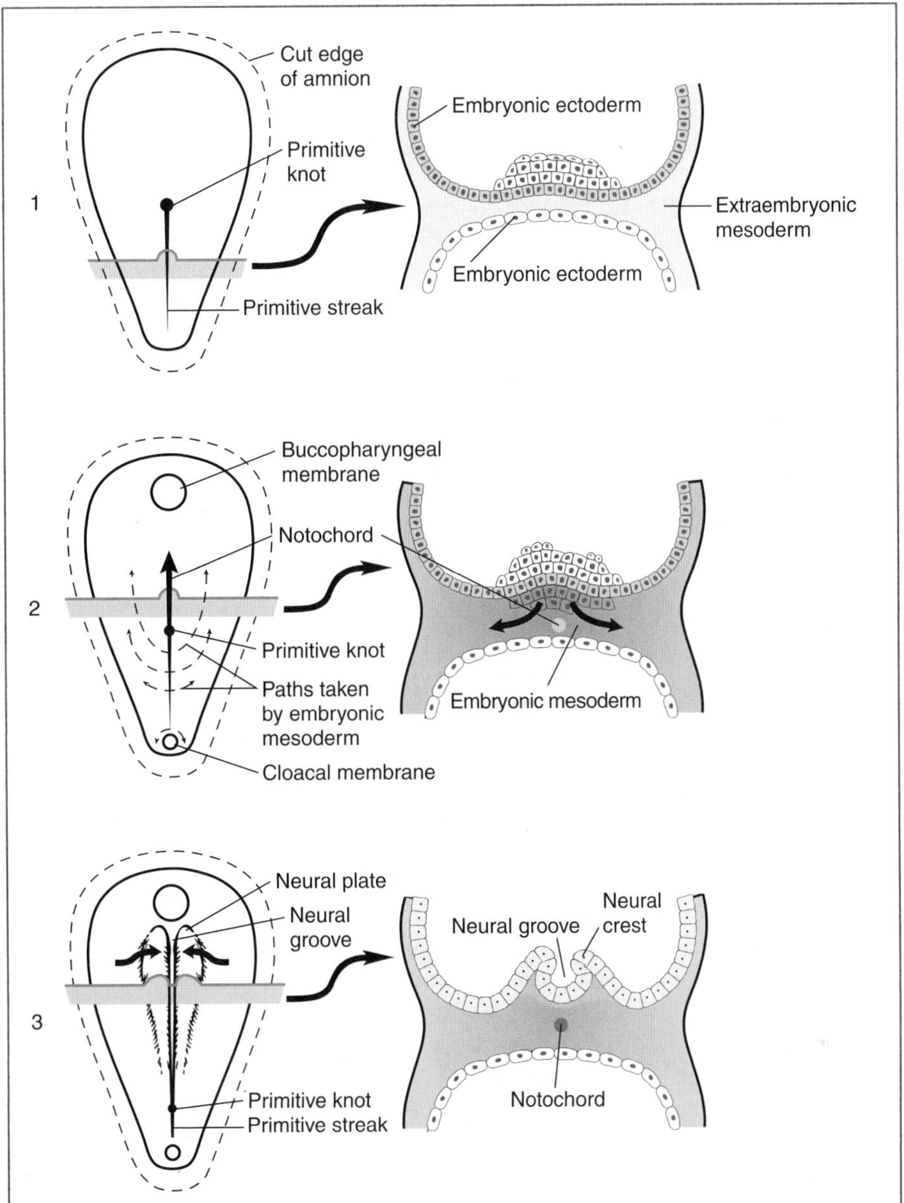

FIGURE 1.5 Formation of primitive streak, primitive knot, notochord, and neural groove.

longitudinal columns of paraxial mesoderm. At about 20 days, the paraxial mesoderm begins to divide into paired cuboidal bodies known as somites. In all, 42 to 44 somites develop, in a craniocaudal sequence, although only 38 develop during the "somite" period. These somite pairs can be counted and give an estimate of fetal age before a crown-rump measurement is possible (Moore & Persaud, 2008; Sadler, 2010).

■ **Intraembryonic Cavity.** Another significant process is the formation of the intraembryonic cavity. This structure first appears as a number of small spaces within the lateral mesoderm and the cardiogenic mesoderm. These spaces combine to form the intraembryonic cavity; it is horseshoe-shaped and lined with flattened epithelial cells that eventually line the peritoneal cavity. The intraembryonic cavity divides the lateral mesoderm into the parietal (somatic) and visceral (splanchnic) layers. It gives rise to the pericardial cavity, the pleural cavity, and the peritoneal cavity (Moore & Persaud, 2008; Sadler, 2010).

PLACENTAL DEVELOPMENT AND FUNCTION

The rudimentary maternal-fetal circulation is intact by the fourth week of gestation. Growth of the trophoblast results in numerous primary and secondary chorionic villi, covering the surface of the chorionic sac until about the eighth week of gestation. At about the eighth week, the villi overlying the conceptus (decidua capsularis) degenerate, leaving a smooth area (smooth chorion). The villi underlying the conceptus (decidua basalis) remain and increase in size, producing the chorion frondosum, or fetal side of the placenta. The maternal side of the placenta is made up of the chorion and the chorionic villi. On implantation of the conceptus, maternal capillaries of the decidua basalis rupture, causing maternal blood to circulate through the developing fetal placenta (chorion frondosum). As growth and differentiation progress, extensions from the cytotrophoblast invade the syncytial layer and form a cytotrophoblastic shell, surrounding the conceptus and chorionic villi.

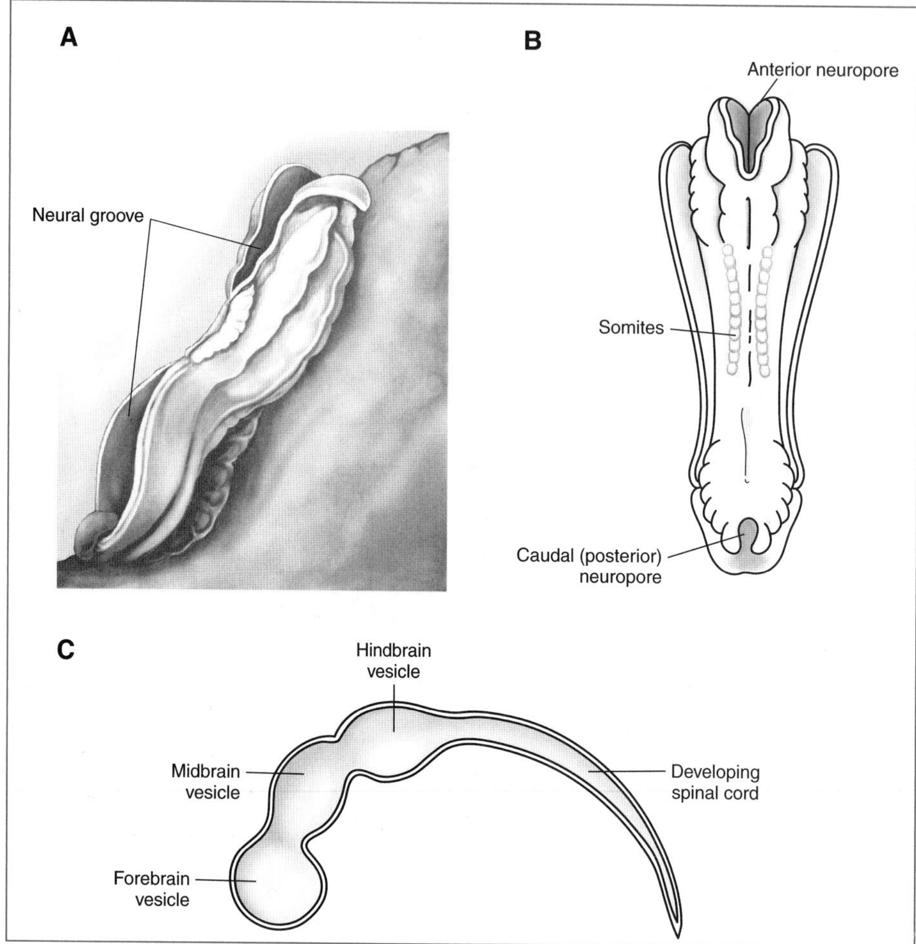

FIGURE 1.6 Formation of the neural tube. (A) Neural groove. (B) Closure of the neural tube almost completed. (C) Dilation of the neural tube forms the forebrain, midbrain, and hindbrain.

This shell is continuous but has communications between maternal blood vessels in the decidua basalis and the intervillous spaces of the chorion frondosum. The latter is attached to the maternal side of the placenta (decidua basalis) by the cytotrophoblastic shell and anchoring villi. The placenta is mature and completely functional by 16 weeks of development (Figure 1.7). If the corpus luteum begins to regress prior to the 16th week and fails to produce enough progesterone (the hormone responsible for readying the uterine cavity for the pregnancy), the pregnancy is aborted because the placenta is not capable of supporting the pregnancy on its own until about this time (Moore & Persaud, 2008; Sadler, 2010).

Placental-Fetal Circulation

A simple ebb-and-flow circulation is present in the embryo, yolk sac, connecting stalk, and chorion by 21 days of gestation. By 28 days, unidirectional circulation is established. Deoxygenated fetal blood leaves the fetus via the umbilical arteries and enters the capillaries in the chorionic villi where gaseous and nutrient exchange takes place. Oxygenated blood returns to the fetus through the umbilical veins. At first there are two arteries and two veins, but one vein gradually degenerates, leaving two arteries and one vein. If only one artery is present, a congenital anomaly, especially a renal one, should be suspected (Moore & Persaud, 2008; Sadler, 2010).

Placental Function

Normal growth and development of the embryo depend on adequate placental function. The placenta is responsible for oxygenation, nutrition, elimination of wastes, production of hormones essential for maintenance of the pregnancy, and transport of substances. In addition, the placenta synthesizes glycogen, cholesterol, and fatty acids, which provide nutrients and energy for early fetal development. Transport across the placental membrane occurs primarily through simple and facilitated diffusion, active transport, and pinocytosis. Oxygen, carbon dioxide, and carbon monoxide cross the placenta through simple diffusion. The fetus is dependent on a continuous supply of oxygenated blood flowing from the placenta (Moore & Persaud, 2008; Sadler, 2010).

Water and electrolytes cross the placenta freely in both directions. Glucose is converted to glycogen in the placenta as a carbohydrate source for the fetus. Amino acids move readily across the placental membranes for protein synthesis in the fetus. Free fatty acids are transferred across the placenta by pinocytosis. There is limited or no transfer of maternal cholesterol, triglycerides, and phospholipids. Water- and fat-soluble vitamins cross the placenta and are essential for normal development (Moore & Persaud, 2008).

The placenta produces and transports hormones that maintain the pregnancy and promote growth and development of the fetus. Chorionic gonadotropin, a protein

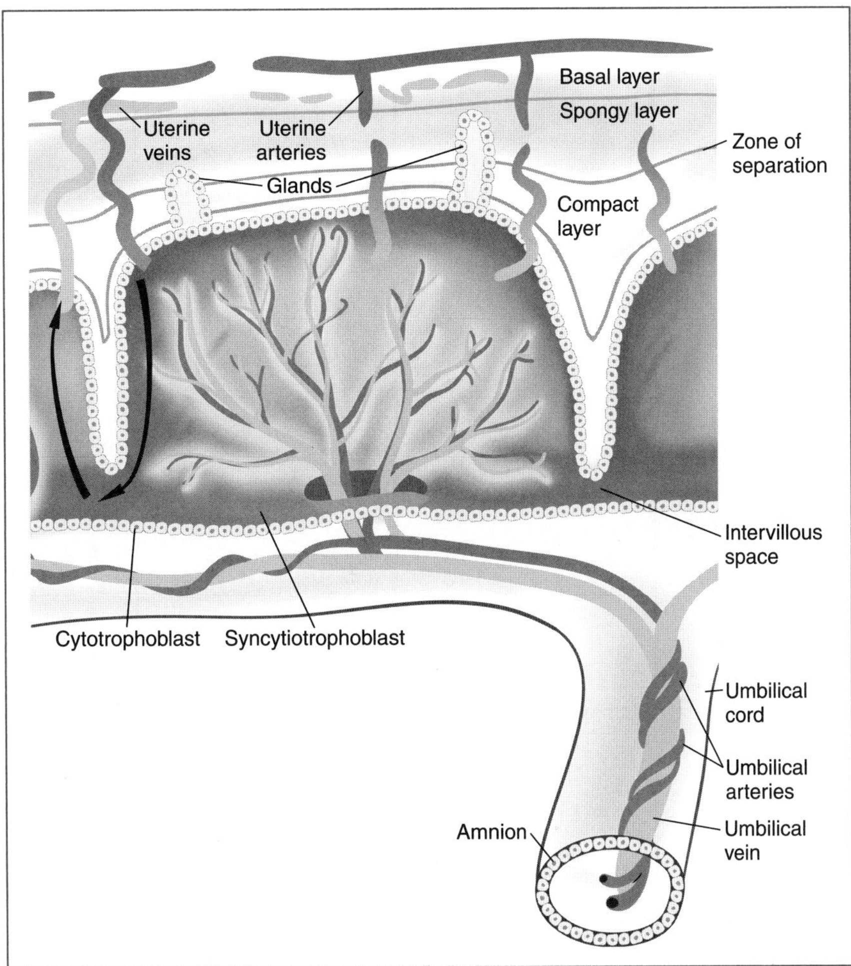

FIGURE 1.7 Formation of the placenta. The fetal and maternal sides of the placenta. Separation of the placenta from the uterus occurs at the site indicated by the black line labeled zone of separation.

hormone produced by the syncytiotrophoblast, is excreted in maternal serum and urine. The presence of human chorionic gonadotropin is used as a test for pregnancy. Human placental lactogen, also a protein hormone produced by the placenta, acts as a fetal growth-promoting hormone by giving the fetus priority for receiving maternal glucose (Moore & Persaud, 2008; Sadler, 2010).

The placenta also produces steroid hormones. Progesterone, produced by the placenta throughout gestation, is responsible for maintaining the pregnancy. Estrogen production by the placenta is dependent on stimulation by the fetal adrenal cortex and liver. Placental transport of maternal antibodies provides the fetus with passive immunity to certain viruses. IgG antibodies are actively transported across the placental barrier, providing humoral immunity for the fetus. IgA and IgM antibodies do not cross the placental barrier, placing the neonate at risk for neonatal sepsis. However, failure of IgM antibodies to cross the placental membrane explains the lower incidence of a severe hemolytic process in ABO blood type incompatibilities when compared with Rh incompatibilities. The latter result when an Rh-negative mother has an Rh-positive fetus. If the mother is sensitized to the Rh-positive fetal blood cells, the mother produces IgG antibodies. IgG is transferred from the maternal to fetal circulation, and hemolysis of fetal red blood cells occurs (Moore & Persaud, 2008; Sadler, 2010).

The placenta is selective in the transfer of substances across the placenta; however, this selectivity does not screen out all potentially harmful substances. Viral, bacterial, and protozoal organisms can be transferred to the fetus through the placenta. Toxic substances such as drugs and alcohol can also be transferred to the fetus. The effects of these substances depend on the stage of gestation and type and duration of exposure, as well as the interaction of these and other factors, such as nutrition.

EMBRYONIC PERIOD: WEEKS 4 THROUGH 8

The embryonic period lasts from the beginning of gestational week 4 through the end of week 8. Organogenesis, which is the formation of all major organs, occurs during this period. The shape of the embryo changes as the organs develop, taking a more human shape by the end of the eighth week. The major events of the embryonic period are the folding of the embryo and organogenesis (Figure 1.8).

Folding of the Embryo

In the trilaminar embryonic disk, the growth rate of the central region exceeds that of the periphery so that the slower growing areas fold under the faster growing areas, forming body folds. The head fold appears first, as a result of craniocaudal elongation of the notochord and growth of the

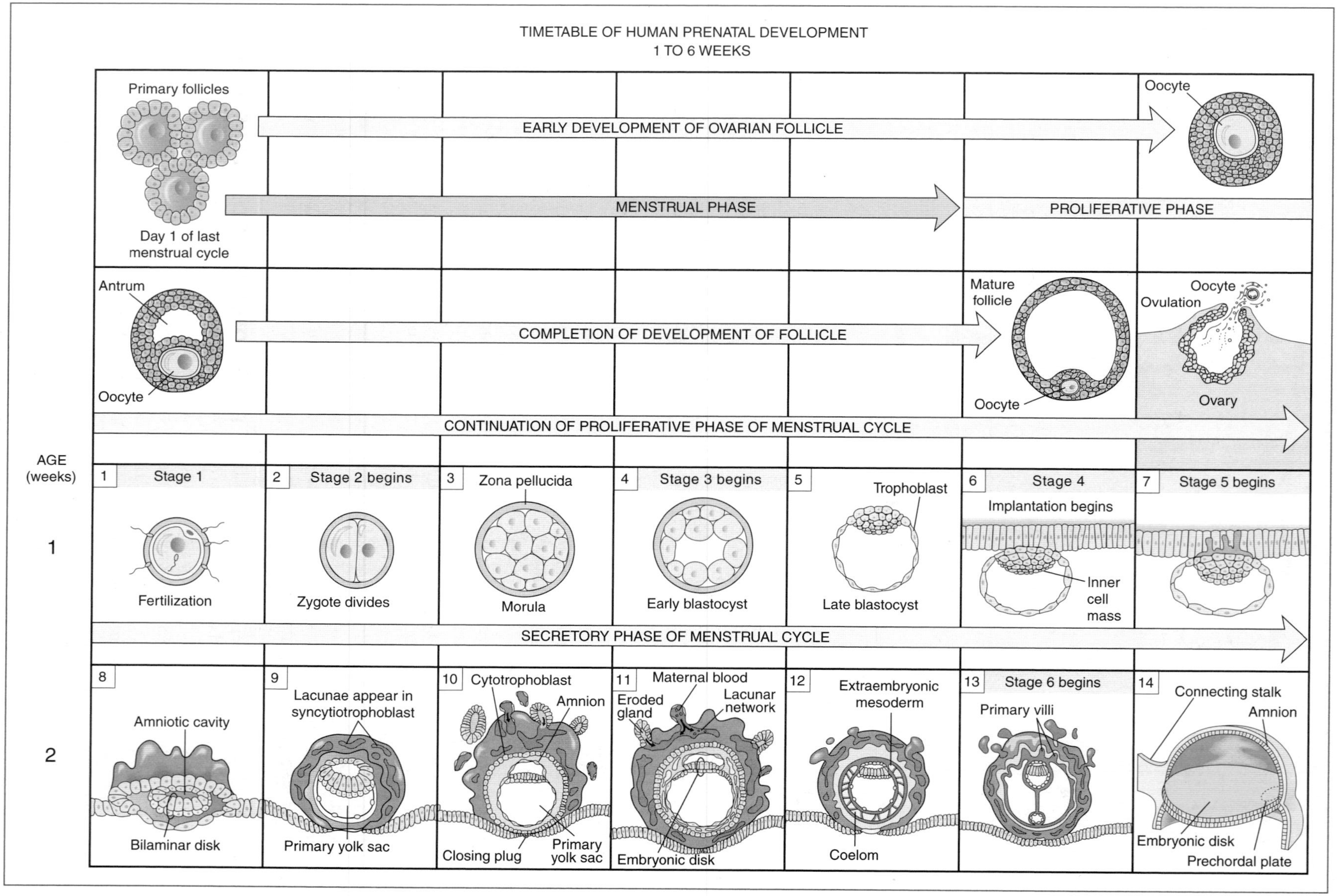

FIGURE 1.8 Critical periods of development.

From Moore and Persaud (2008). Reprinted with permission.

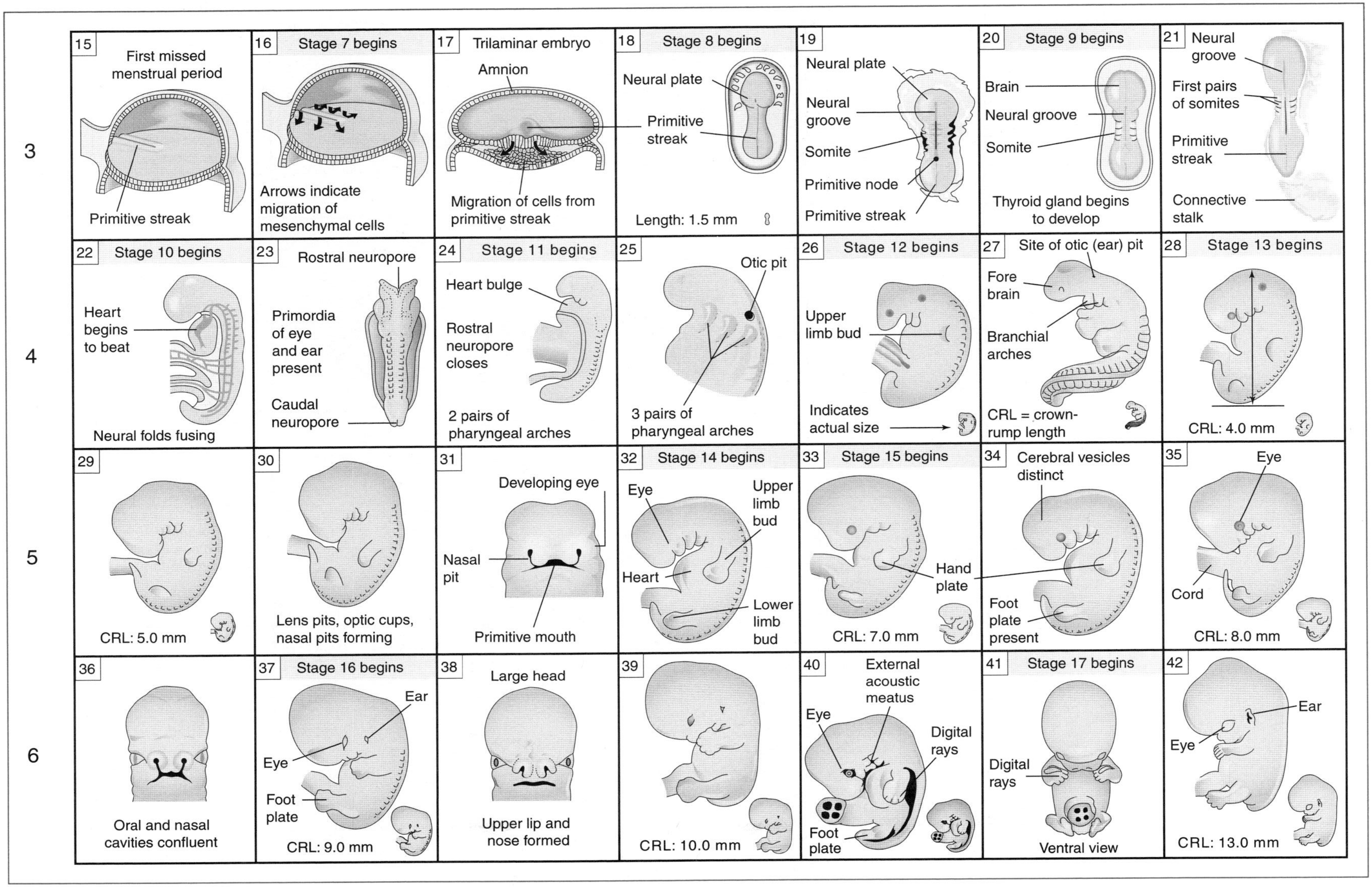

Week							
3	15 First missed menstrual period; Primitive streak	16 Stage 7 begins; Arrows indicate migration of mesenchymal cells	17 Trilaminar embryo; Amnion; Migration of cells from primitive streak	18 Stage 8 begins; Neural plate; Primitive streak; Length: 1.5 mm	19 Neural plate; Neural groove; Somite; Primitive node; Primitive streak	20 Stage 9 begins; Brain; Neural groove; Somite; Thyroid gland begins to develop	21 Neural groove; First pairs of somites; Primitive streak; Connective stalk
4	22 Stage 10 begins; Heart begins to beat; Neural folds fusing	23 Rostral neuropore; Primordia of eye and ear present; Caudal neuropore	24 Stage 11 begins; Heart bulge; Rostral neuropore closes; 2 pairs of pharyngeal arches	25 Otic pit; 3 pairs of pharyngeal arches	26 Stage 12 begins; Upper limb bud; Indicates actual size →	27 Site of otic (ear) pit; Fore brain; Branchial arches; CRL = crown-rump length	28 Stage 13 begins; CRL: 4.0 mm
5	29 CRL: 5.0 mm	30 Lens pits, optic cups, nasal pits forming	31 Developing eye; Nasal pit; Primitive mouth	32 Stage 14 begins; Eye; Upper limb bud; Heart; Lower limb bud	33 Stage 15 begins; Hand plate; CRL: 7.0 mm	34 Cerebral vesicles distinct; Foot plate present	35 Eye; Cord; CRL: 8.0 mm
6	36 Oral and nasal cavities confluent	37 Stage 16 begins; Ear; Eye; Foot plate; CRL: 9.0 mm	38 Large head; Upper lip and nose formed	39 CRL: 10.0 mm	40 External acoustic meatus; Eye; Digital rays; Foot plate	41 Stage 17 begins; Digital rays; Ventral view	42 Ear; Eye; CRL: 13.0 mm

FIGURE 1.8 Critical periods of development. *(continued)*

From Moore and Persaud (2008). Reprinted with permission.

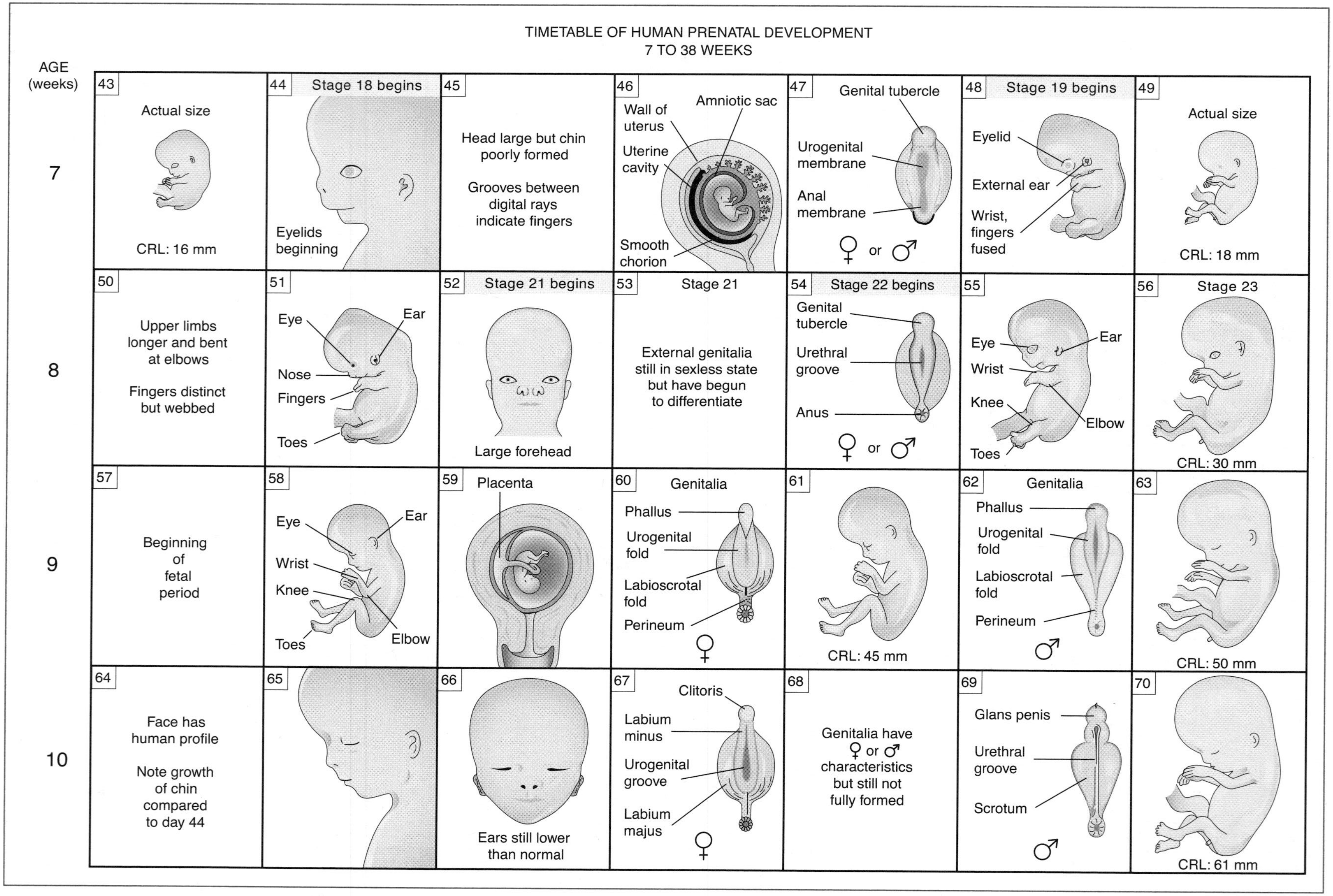

TIMETABLE OF HUMAN PRENATAL DEVELOPMENT
7 TO 38 WEEKS

AGE (weeks)							
7	43 Actual size; CRL: 16 mm	44 Stage 18 begins; Eyelids beginning	45 Head large but chin poorly formed; Grooves between digital rays indicate fingers	46 Wall of uterus; Amniotic sac; Uterine cavity; Smooth chorion	47 Genital tubercle; Urogenital membrane; Anal membrane; ♀ or ♂	48 Stage 19 begins; Eyelid; External ear; Wrist, fingers fused	49 Actual size; CRL: 18 mm
8	50 Upper limbs longer and bent at elbows; Fingers distinct but webbed	51 Eye; Ear; Nose; Fingers; Toes	52 Stage 21 begins; Large forehead	53 Stage 21; External genitalia still in sexless state but have begun to differentiate	54 Stage 22 begins; Genital tubercle; Urethral groove; Anus; ♀ or ♂	55 Eye; Ear; Wrist; Knee; Elbow; Toes	56 Stage 23; CRL: 30 mm
9	57 Beginning of fetal period	58 Eye; Ear; Wrist; Knee; Toes; Elbow	59 Placenta	60 Genitalia; Phallus; Urogenital fold; Labioscrotal fold; Perineum; ♀	61 CRL: 45 mm	62 Genitalia; Phallus; Urogenital fold; Labioscrotal fold; Perineum; ♂	63 CRL: 50 mm
10	64 Face has human profile; Note growth of chin compared to day 44	65	66 Ears still lower than normal	67 Clitoris; Labium minus; Urogenital groove; Labium majus; ♀	68 Genitalia have ♀ or ♂ characteristics but still not fully formed	69 Glans penis; Urethral groove; Scrotum; ♂	70 CRL: 61 mm

FIGURE 1.8 Critical periods of development. *(continued)*
From Moore and Persaud (2008). Reprinted with permission.

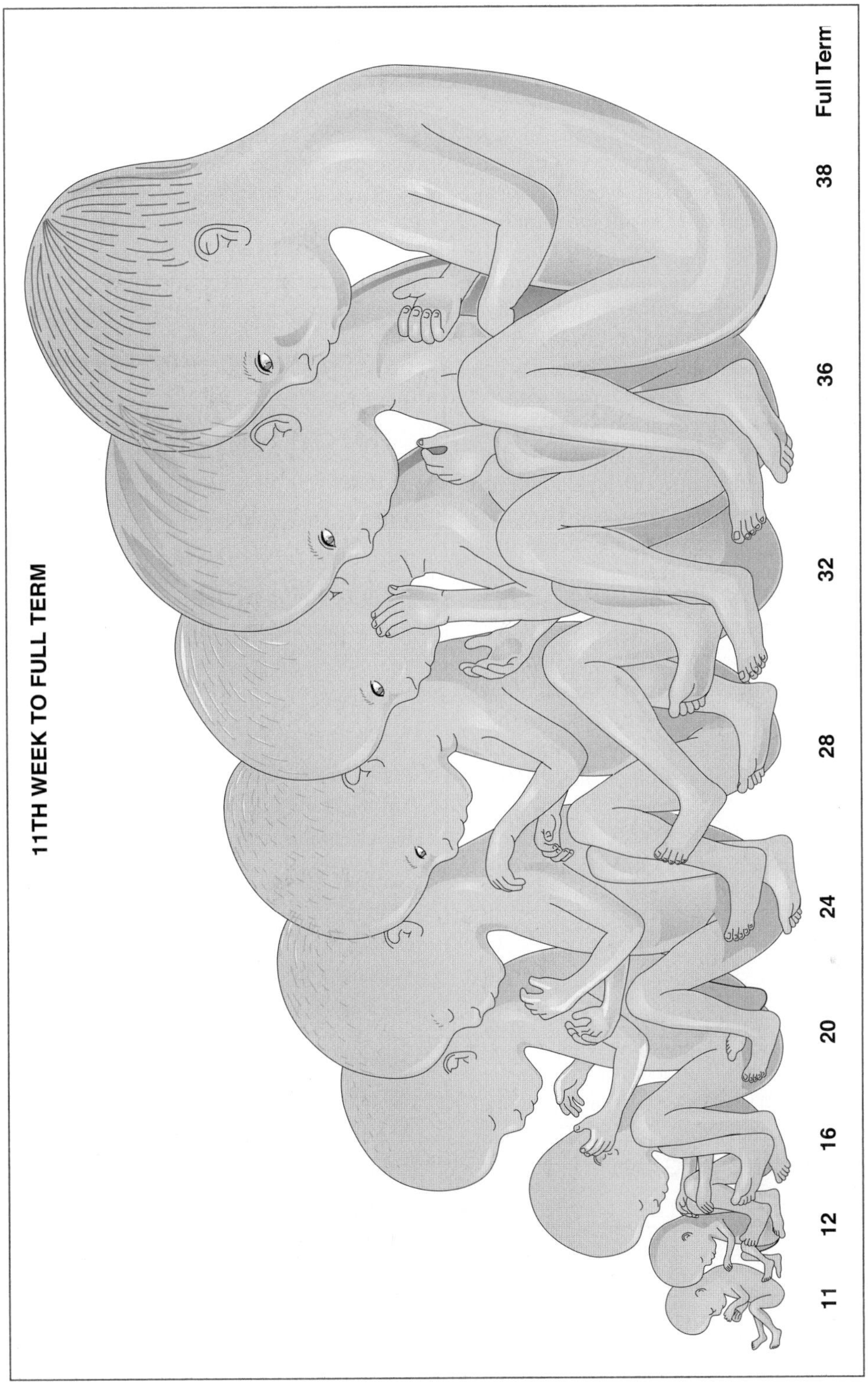

FIGURE 1.8 Critical periods of development. *(continued)*
From Moore and Persaud (2008). Reprinted with permission.

brain, which projects into the amniotic cavity. The folding downward of the cranial end of the embryo forces the septum transversum (primitive heart), the pericardial cavity, and the oropharyngeal membrane to turn under onto the ventral surface. After the embryo has folded, the mass of mesoderm cranial to the pericardial cavity, the septum transversum, lies caudal to the heart. The septum transversum later develops into a portion of the diaphragm. Part of the yolk sac is incorporated as the foregut, lying between the heart and the brain. The foregut ends blindly at the oropharyngeal membrane, which separates the foregut from the primitive mouth cavity (stomodeum) (Moore & Persaud, 2008; Sadler, 2010).

The tail fold occurs after the head fold as a result of craniocaudal growth progression. Growth of the embryo causes the caudal area to project over the cloacal membrane. During the tail folding, part of the yolk sac is incorporated into the embryo as the hindgut. After completion of the head and tail folding, the connecting stalk is attached to the ventral surface of the embryo, forming the umbilical cord. Folding also occurs laterally, producing right and left lateral folds. The lateral body wall on each side folds toward the median plane, causing the embryo to assume a cylindrical shape. During the lateral body folding, a portion of the yolk sac is incorporated as the midgut. The attachment of the midgut to the yolk sac is minimal after this fold develops. After folding, the amnion is attached to the embryo in a narrow area in which the umbilical cord attaches to the ventral surface (Moore & Persaud, 2008; Sadler, 2010).

Organogenesis: Germ Cell Derivatives

The three germ cell layers (ectoderm, mesoderm, and endoderm) give rise to all tissues and organs of the embryo. The germ cells follow specific patterns during the process of organogenesis. The main germ cell derivatives are listed in Box 1.1. The development of each major organ system is discussed separately. The embryonic period is the most critical period of development because of the formation of internal and external structures. The critical periods of development for the organs are also discussed in the section on specific organ development.

DEVELOPMENT OF SPECIFIC ORGANS AND STRUCTURES

Nervous System

The origin of the nervous system is the neural plate, which arises as a thickening of the ectodermal tissue about the middle of the third week of gestation. The neural plate further differentiates into the neural tube and the neural crest. The neural tube gives rise to the CNS. The neural crest cells give rise to the peripheral nervous system (Figure 1.9) (Moore & Persaud, 2008; Sadler, 2010).

The cranial end of the neural tube forms the three divisions of the brain: the forebrain, the midbrain, and the hindbrain. The cerebral hemispheres and diencephalon arise from the forebrain; the pons, cerebellum, and medulla oblongata arise from the hindbrain. The midbrain makes up the adult midbrain (Moore & Persaud, 2008; Sadler, 2010).

The cavity of the neural tube develops into the ventricles of the brain and the central canal of the spinal column. The neuroepithelial cells lining the neural tube give rise to nerves and glial cells of the CNS. The peripheral nervous system consists of the cranial, spinal, and visceral nerves and the ganglia. The somatic and visceral sensory cells of the peripheral nervous system arise from neural crest cells. Cells that form the myelin sheaths of the axons, called Schwann cells, also arise from the neural crest cells (Moore & Persaud, 2008; Sadler, 2010).

Cardiovascular System

The fetal cardiac system appears at about 18 to 19 days of gestation, and circulation is present by about 21 days.

BOX 1.1

GERM CELL DERIVATIVES

Ectoderm

CNS (brain, spinal cord)
Peripheral nervous system
Sensory epithelia of eye, ear, and nose
Epidermis and its appendages (hair and nails)
Mammary glands
Subcutaneous glands
Teeth enamel
Neural crest cells
Spinal, cranial, and autonomic ganglia cells
Nerve sheaths of peripheral nervous system
Pigment cells
Muscle, connective tissue, and bone of branchial arch origin
Adrenal medulla
Meninges

Mesoderm

Cartilage
Bone
Connective tissue
Striated and smooth muscle
Heart, blood, and lymph vessels and cells
Gonads
Genital ducts
Pericardial, pleural, and peritoneal lining
Spleen
Cortex of adrenal gland

Endoderm

Epithelial lining of respiratory and gastrointestinal tracts
Parenchyma of tonsils, thyroid, parathyroid, liver, thymus, and pancreas
Epithelial lining of bladder and urethra
Epithelial lining of tympanic cavity, tympanic antrum, and auditory tube

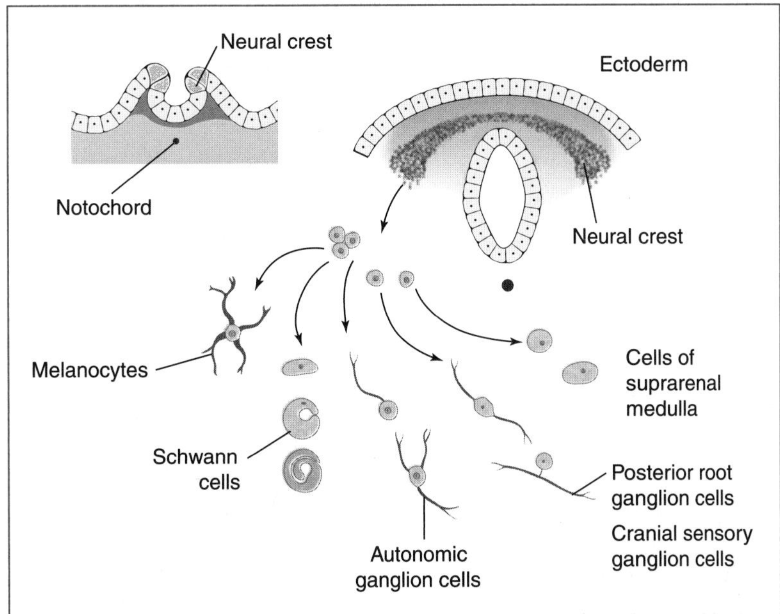

FIGURE 1.9 Differentiation of the nervous system. The cells of the neural crest differentiate into the cells of the ganglia, Schwann cells, and the cells of the suprarenal medulla and melanocytes.

The cardiovascular system is the first organ system to function in utero. The heart starts to beat at the beginning of the fourth week. The heart and blood develop from the middle layer (mesoderm) of the trilaminar embryonic disk. Tissue from the lateral mesoderm migrates up the sides of the embryonic disk, forming a horseshoe-shaped structure that arches and meets above the oropharyngeal membrane. With further development, paired heart tubes form, which then fuse into a single heart tube (Figure 1.10). The vessels that make up the vascular system throughout the body develop from mesodermal cells that connect to each other, with the developing heart tube and the placenta. Thus, by the end of the third week of gestation, there is a functional cardiovascular system (Moore & Persaud, 2008; Sadler, 2010).

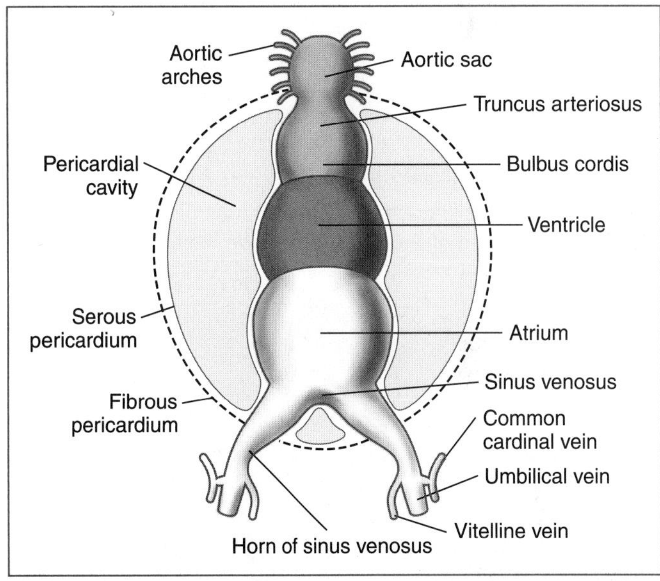

FIGURE 1.10 Formation of the single heart tube. The appearance of the single heart tube inside the pericardial cavity. Note that the atrium and sinus venosus are outside the pericardial cavity.

As the heart tube grows, the folding of the embryonic disk results in the movement of the heart tube into the chest cavity. The heart tube differentiates into three layers: the endocardial layer, which becomes the endothelium; the cardiac jelly, which is a loose tissue layer; and the myoepicardial mantle, which becomes the myocardium and pericardium. The single heart tube is attached at its cephalic end by the aortic arches and at the caudal end by the septum transversum. The attachments limit the length of the heart tube. Continued growth results in dilated areas and bulges, which become specific components of the heart. The atrium, ventricle, and bulbus cordis can be identified first, followed by the sinus venosus and truncus arteriosus. To accommodate continued growth, two separate bends in the heart occur. It first bends to the right to form a U shape, and the next bend results in an S-shaped heart. The bending of the heart is responsible for the typical location of cardiac structures (Figure 1.11) (Moore & Persaud, 2008; Sadler, 2010).

Initially, the heart is a single chamber; partitioning of the heart into four chambers occurs from the fourth to sixth weeks of gestation. The changes that cause the partitioning of the heart occur simultaneously. The atrium is separated from the ventricle by endocardial cushions, which are thickened areas of endothelium that develop on the dorsal and ventral walls of the open area between the atrium and ventricle. The endocardial cushions fuse with each other to divide the atrioventricular canals into right and left atrioventricular canals. Partitioning of the atrium occurs through invagination of tissue toward the endocardial cushions, forming the septum primum. As the septum primum grows toward the endocardial cushions, it becomes very thin and perforates, becoming the foramen ovale. The septum primum does not fuse completely with the endocardial cushions; it has a lower portion that lies beside the endocardial cushions. Overlapping of the septum primum and the septum secundum forms a wall if

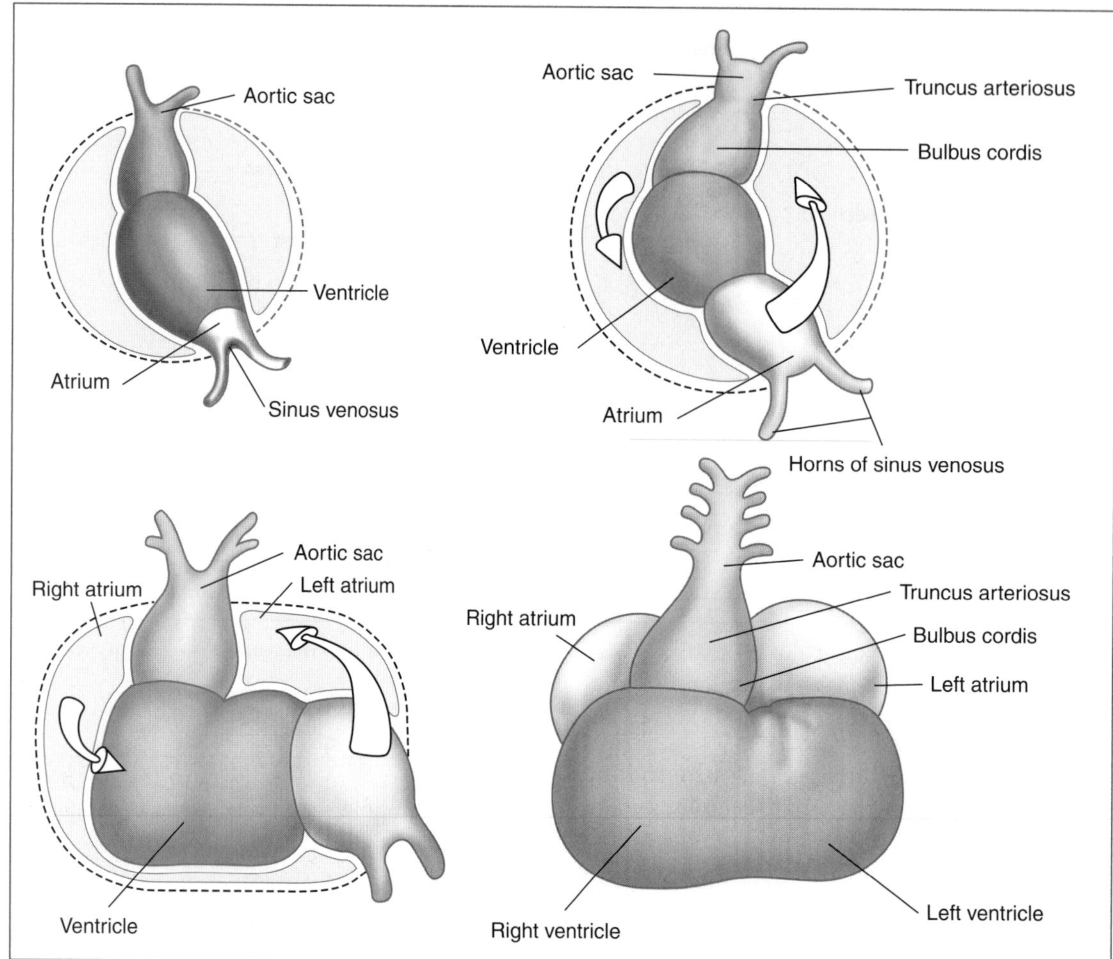

FIGURE 1.11 Bending of the heart tube inside the pericardial cavity. The bending of the heart tube brings the atrium into the pericardial cavity. The sinus venosus is taken into the right atrium and the coronary sinus.

the pressure in both atria is equal. In utero, the pressure on the right side is increased, allowing blood to flow across the foramen ovale from the right side of the heart to the left side (Figure 1.12) (Moore & Persaud, 2008; Sadler, 2010).

The ventricle is also partitioned by a membranous and muscular septum. The muscular portion of the septum develops from the fold of the floor of the ventricle. With blood flowing through the atrioventricular canal, ventricular dilation occurs on either side of the fold or ridge, causing it to become a septum. The membranous septum arises from ridges inside the bulbus cordis. These ridges, continuous into the bulbus cordis, form the wall that divides the bulbus cordis into the pulmonary artery and the aorta. The bulbar ridges fuse with the endocardial cushions to form the membranous septum. The membranous and muscular septa fuse to close the intraventricular foramen, resulting in two parallel circuits of blood flow. The pulmonary artery is continuous with the right ventricle, and the aorta is continuous with the left ventricle (Figure 1.13) (Moore & Persaud, 2008; Sadler, 2010).

The blood flowing through the bulbus cordis and truncus arteriosus in a spiral causes the formation of ridges. The ridges fuse to form two separate vessels that twist around each other once. Thus, the pulmonary artery exits the right side of the heart and is in the left upper chest; the aorta exits the left side of the heart and is located close to the sternum (Moore & Persaud, 2008; Sadler, 2010).

The pulmonary veins grow from the lungs to a cardinal vein plexus. Concurrently, a vessel develops from the smooth wall of the left atrium. As the atrium grows, the pulmonary vein is incorporated into the atrial wall. The atrium and its branches give rise to four pulmonary veins that enter the left atrium. These pulmonary vessels, connected to the plexus of the cardinal vein, provide a continuous circulation from lung to heart. The pulmonary and aortic valves (semilunar valves) develop from dilations within the pulmonary artery and aorta. The ebb-and-flow circulation through these structures causes them to hollow out to form the cusps of the valves. The tricuspid and mitral valves develop from tissue around the atrioventricular canals that thicken and then thin out on the ventricular sides, forming the valves (Figure 1.14) (Moore & Persaud, 2008; Sadler, 2010).

Respiratory System

The development of the respiratory system is linked to the development of the face and the digestive system. The respiratory system is composed of the nasal cavities, nasopharynx, oropharynx, larynx, trachea, bronchi, and lungs (Figure 1.15). Development of the lungs occurs in four

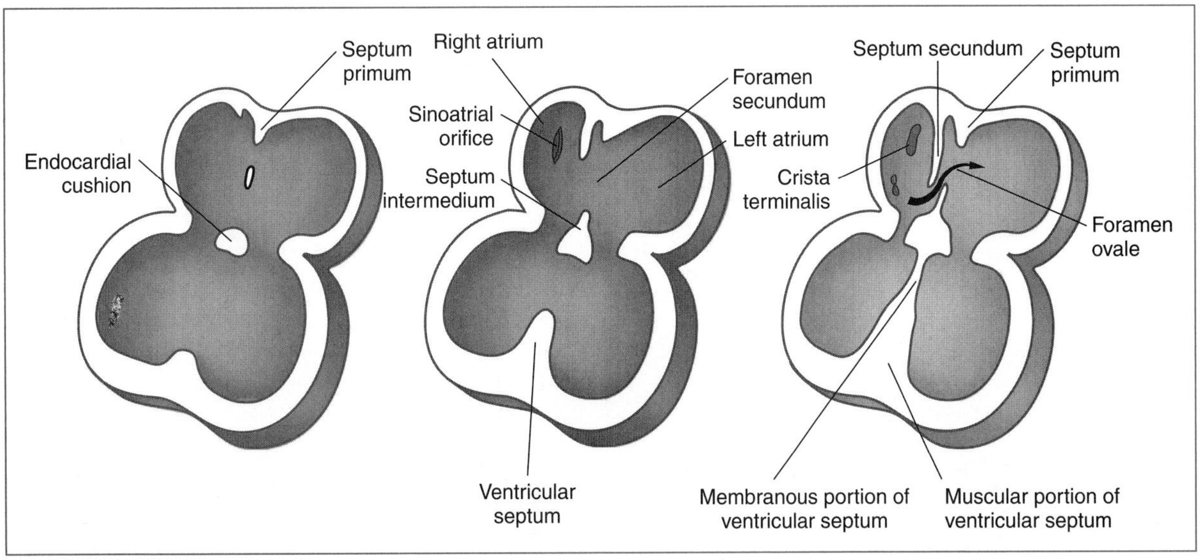

FIGURE 1.12 Partitioning of the atrium. The partitioning of the atrium into the right and left atria through septation.

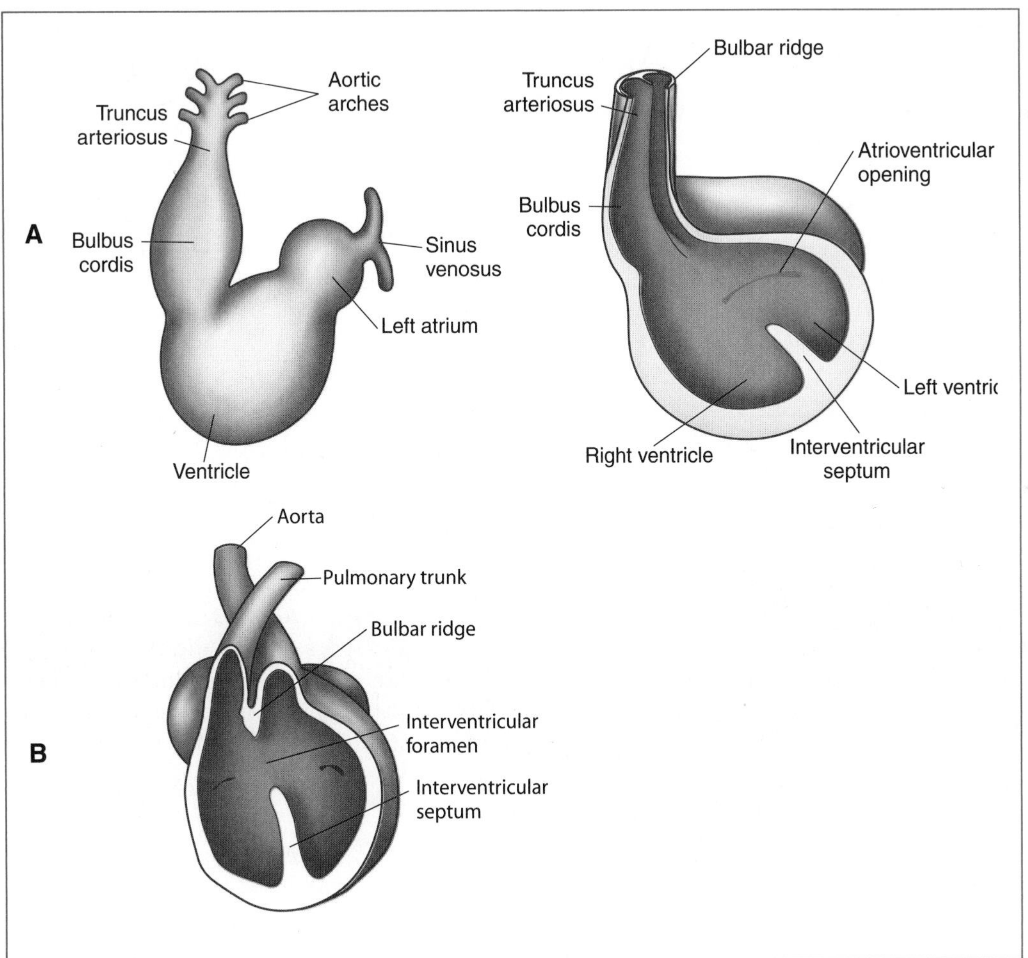

FIGURE 1.13 Partitioning of the ventricles. (A) Five chambers are present in the heart at 5 weeks gestation. (B) At 6 weeks the bulbus cordis has been taken into the ventricles and the interventricular septum has partitioned the ventricles into right and left sides.

overlapping stages, which extend from the fifth week of gestation until about 8 years of life. The stages are listed in Table 1.1. At term birth, the normal respiratory system functions immediately. For adequate functioning of the respiratory system, there must be a sufficient number of alveoli, adequate capillary blood flow, and an adequate amount of surfactant produced by the secretory epithelial cells or the type II pneumatocytes. It is the surfactant that prevents alveolar collapse and aids in respiratory gas exchange. Production of surfactant begins around 20 weeks but does

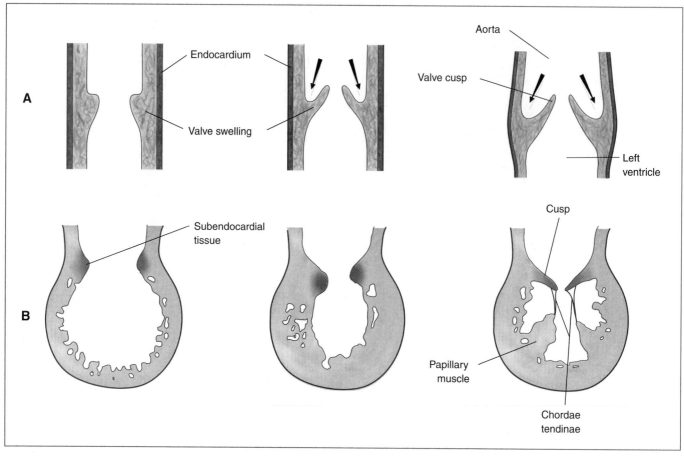

FIGURE 1.14 Formation of the heart valve. (A) Formation of the semilunar valves of the aorta and the pulmonary artery. (B) Formation of the cusps of the atrioventricular valves.

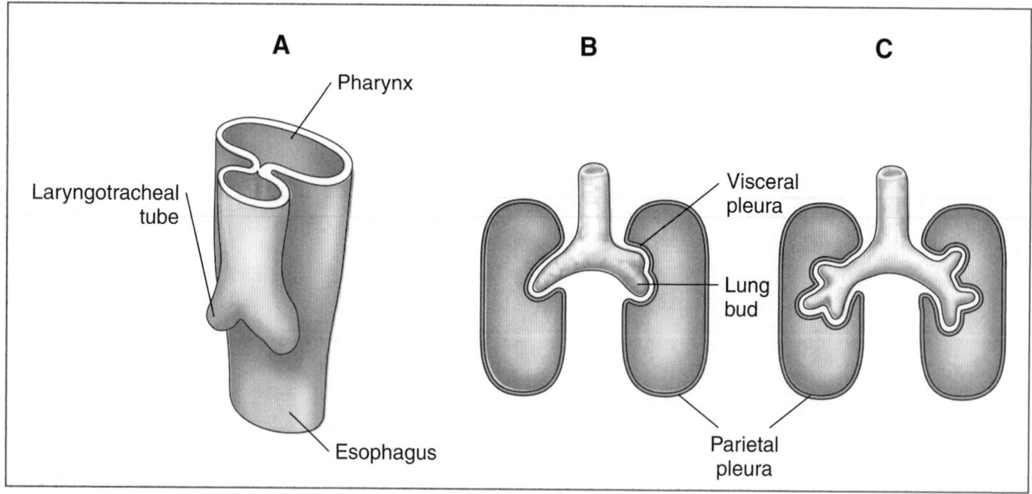

FIGURE 1.15 Development of the pulmonary system. (A) The laryngotracheal groove and tube have formed; the margins of the laryngotracheal groove fuse, forming the laryngotracheal tube. (B) Invagination of the lung buds into the intraembryonic cavity. (C) Division of the lung buds into the right and left mainstem bronchi.

not reach adequate levels until late in gestation. In addition, work to identify the role of epidermal growth factor (EGF) in the development of the fetal respiratory system has determined that EGF indirectly promotes branching morphogenesis of the lung epithelium through a direct effect on the mesenchyme (Moore & Persaud, 2008; Sadler, 2010).

Muscular System

The muscular system develops from mesodermal cells called myoblasts. Striated skeletal muscles are derived from myotomal mesoderm (myotomes) of the somites. The majority of striated skeletal muscle fibers develop in utero. Almost all striated skeletal muscles are formed by 1 year of age.

TABLE 1.1

STAGES OF LUNG DEVELOPMENT

Stage	Critical Events
Stage 1: Pseudoglandular period weeks 5–7	Development of the conducting airway
Stage 2: Canalicular period weeks 13–25	Enlargement of the bronchial lumina and terminal bronchioles Vascularization of lung tissue Development of respiratory bronchioles and alveolar ducts Development of a limited number of primitive alveoli
Stage 3: Terminal sac period week 24 to birth	Development of primitive pulmonary alveoli from alveolar ducts Increased vascularity Type II pneumatocytes begin to produce surfactant by about 24 weeks
Stage 4: Alveolar period late fetal period until about 8 years of age	Pulmonary alveoli formed by thinning of terminal air sac lining One eighth to one sixth of adult number of alveoli present at term birth Number of alveoli increase until age 8 years

Growth is achieved by an increase in the diameter of the muscle fibers, rather than the growth of new muscle tissue. Smooth muscle fibers arise from the splanchnic mesenchyme surrounding the endoderm of the primitive gut. Smooth muscles lining vessel walls of blood and lymphatic systems arise from somatic mesoderm. As smooth muscle cells differentiate, contractile filaments develop in the cytoplasm, and the external surface is covered by an external lamina. As the smooth muscle fibers develop into sheets or bundles, the muscle cells synthesize and release collagenous, elastic, or reticular fibers (Figure 1.16) (Moore & Persaud, 2008; Sadler, 2010).

Cardiac muscle develops from splanchnic mesenchyme from the outside of the endocardial heart tube. Cells from the myoepicardial mantle differentiate into the myocardium. Cardiac muscle fibers develop from differentiation and growth of single cells rather than fusion of cells. Cardiac muscle growth occurs through the formation of new filaments. The Purkinje fibers develop late in the embryonic period. These fibers are larger and have fewer myofibrils than do other cardiac muscle cells. The Purkinje fibers function in the electrical conduction system of the heart (Moore & Persaud, 2008; Sadler, 2010).

Skeletal System

The skeletal system develops from mesenchymal cells. In the long bones, condensed mesenchyme forms hyaline cartilage models of bones. By the end of the embryonic period, ossification centers appear, and these bones ossify by endochondral ossification. Other bones, such as the skull bones, are ossified by membranous ossification in which the mesenchyme cells become osteoblasts (Figure 1.17).

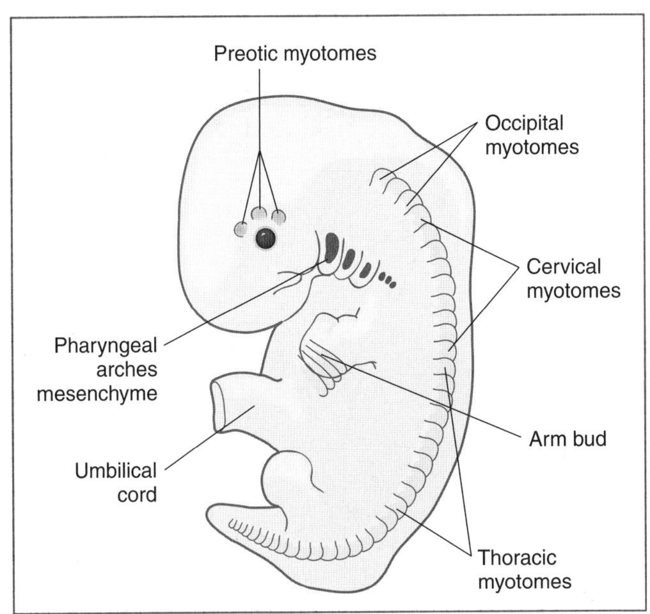

FIGURE 1.16 Origin of the muscles of the head and neck.

The vertebral column and the ribs arise from the sclerotome compartments of the somites. The spinal column is formed by the fusion of a condensation of the cranial half of one pair of sclerotomes with the caudal half of the next pair of sclerotomes. The skull can be divided into the neurocranium and the viscerocranium. The neurocranium forms the protective covering around the brain. The viscerocranium forms the skeleton of the face. The neurocranium is made up of the flat bones that surround the brain and the cartilaginous structure, or chondrocranium, that forms the bones of the base of the skull. The neurocranium (chondrocranium) is made up of a number of separate cartilages, which fuse and ossify by endochondral ossification to form the base of the skull (Moore & Persaud, 2008; Sadler, 2010).

Gastrointestinal System

The gastrointestinal system is primarily derived from the lining of the roof of the yolk sac. The primitive gut, consisting of the foregut, midgut, and hindgut, is formed during the fourth gestational week (Figure 1.18). The structures that arise from the foregut include the pharynx, esophagus, stomach, liver, pancreas, gallbladder, and part of the duodenum. The esophagus and trachea have a common origin, the laryngotracheal diverticulum. A septum, formed by the growing tracheoesophageal folds, divides the cranial part of the foregut into the laryngotracheal tube and the esophagus. Smooth muscle develops from the splanchnic mesenchyme that surrounds the esophagus. The epithelial lining of the esophagus, derived from the endoderm, proliferates, partially obliterating the esophageal lumen. The esophagus undergoes recanalization by the end of the embryonic period (Moore & Persaud, 2008; Sadler, 2010).

The stomach originates as a dilation of the caudal portion of the foregut. The characteristic greater curvature of the stomach develops because the dorsal border grows faster

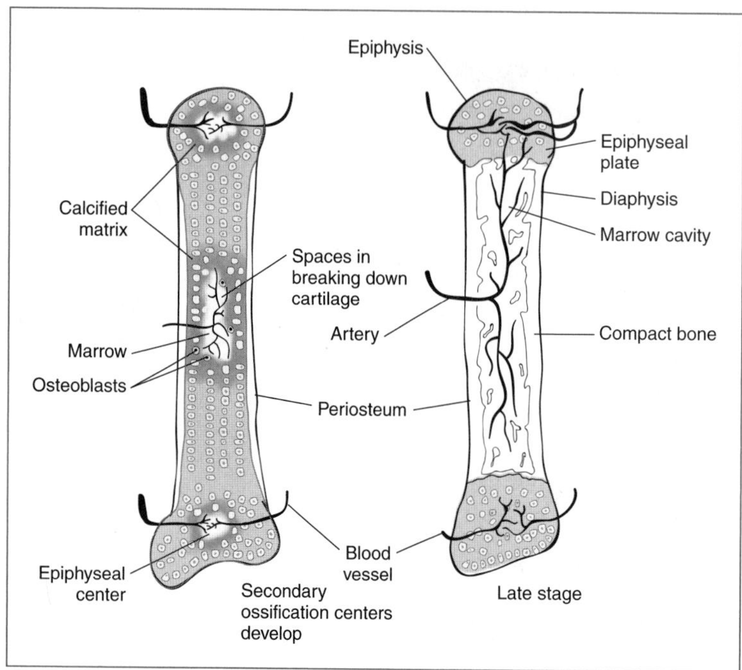

FIGURE 1.17 Endochondral ossification of bones.

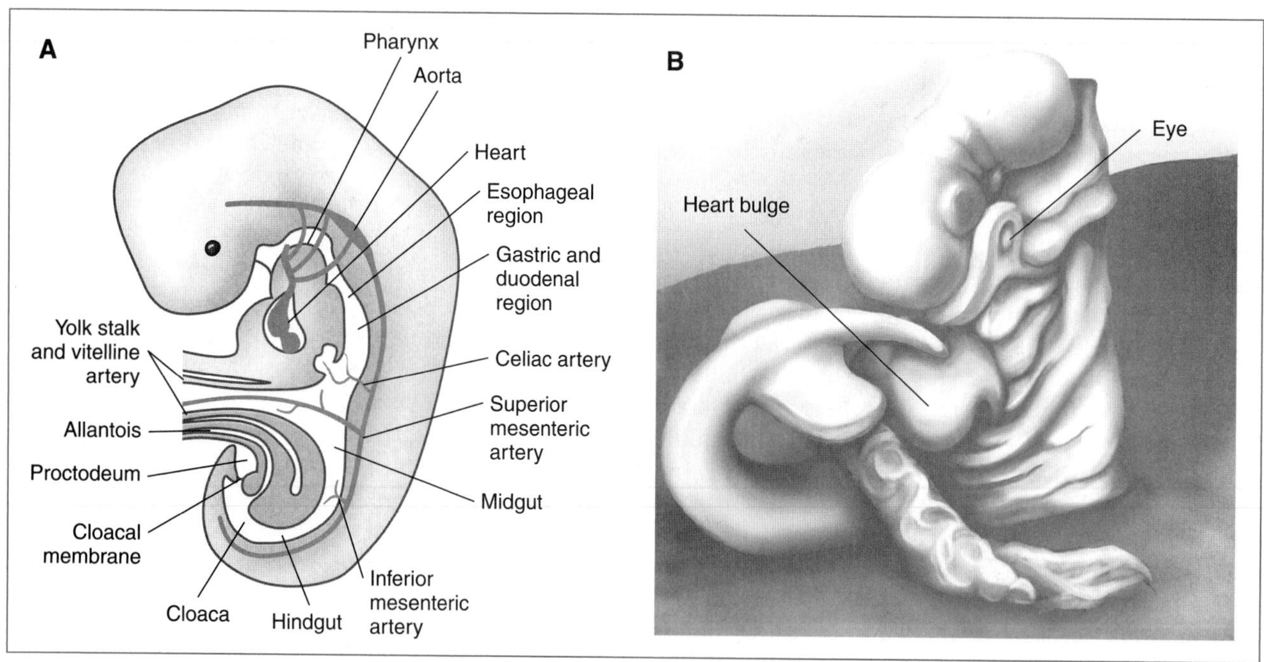

FIGURE 1.18 (A, B) The primitive gut. The early gastrointestinal system present in an embryo at about 4 weeks gestation.

than the ventral border. As the stomach develops further, it rotates in a clockwise direction around the longitudinal axis. The duodenum is derived from the caudal and cranial portions of the foregut and the cranial portion of the midgut. The junction of the foregut and midgut portions of the duodenum is normally distal to the common bile duct (Moore & Persaud, 2008; Sadler, 2010).

The liver, gallbladder, and biliary ducts originate as a bud from the caudal end of the foregut. The liver is formed by growth of the hepatic diverticulum, which grows between the layers of the ventral mesentery, forming two parts. The liver forms from the largest, cranial portion. Hepatic cells originate from the hepatic diverticulum. Hematopoietic tissue and Kupffer cells are derived from the splanchnic mesenchyme of the septum transversum. The liver develops rapidly and fills the abdominal cavity. The liver begins its hematopoietic function by the sixth gestational week (Moore & Persaud, 2008; Sadler, 2010).

The smaller portion of the hepatic diverticulum forms the gallbladder. The common bile duct is formed from the stalk connecting the hepatic and cystic ducts to the duodenum. By the 12th week, bile formation begins by the hepatic cells. The pancreas is derived from the pancreatic buds that arise from the caudal part of the foregut. Insulin secretion begins at week 10 (Moore & Persaud, 2008; Sadler, 2010).

The structures that are derived from the midgut include the remainder of the duodenum, the cecum, the appendix, the ascending colon, and the majority of the transverse colon. The intestines undergo extensive growth during the first weeks of development. The liver and kidneys occupy the abdominal cavity, restricting the space available for intestinal growth. The growth of the intestines is accommodated through a migration out of the abdominal cavity via the umbilical cord. A series of rotations occurs before the intestines return to the abdomen. The first rotation is counterclockwise, around the axis of the superior mesenteric artery. At about the 10th week, the intestines return to the abdomen, undergoing further rotation. When the colon returns to the abdomen, the cecal end rotates to the right side, entering the lower right quadrant of the abdomen. The cecum and appendix arise from the cecal diverticulum, a pouch that appears in the fifth week of gestation on the caudal limb of the midgut loop (Figure 1.19) (Moore & Persaud, 2008; Sadler, 2010).

The hindgut is that portion of the intestines from the midgut to the cloacal membrane. The latter structure consists of the endoderm of the cloaca and the ectoderm of the anal pit. The cloaca is divided by the urorectal septum. As the septum grows toward the cloacal membrane, folds from the lateral walls of the cloaca grow together, dividing the cloaca into the rectum and upper anal canal dorsally and the urogenital sinus ventrally. By the end of the sixth week the urorectal septum fuses with the cloacal membrane, forming a dorsal anal membrane and a larger ventral urogenital membrane. At about the end of the seventh gestational week, these two membranes rupture, forming the anal canal (Moore & Persaud, 2008; Sadler, 2010).

Urogenital System

The development of the urinary and genital systems is closely related. The urogenital system develops from the intermediate mesenchyme, which extends along the dorsal body wall of the embryo. During embryonic folding in the horizontal plane, the intermediate mesoderm is moved forward and is no longer connected to the somites. This mesoderm forms the urogenital ridge on each side of the primitive aorta. Both the urinary and genital systems arise from this urogenital ridge. The area from which the urinary system is derived is called the nephrogenic cord. The genital ridge is the area from which the reproductive system is derived (Moore & Persaud, 2008; Sadler, 2010).

There are three stages of development of the kidney: the pronephros, the mesonephros, and the metanephros. The pronephros, a nonfunctional organ, appears in the first month of gestation and then degenerates, contributing only a duct system for the next developmental stage. The mesonephros uses the duct of the pronephros and develops caudally to the pronephros (Figure 1.20). The mesonephros begins to produce urine during development of the meta-

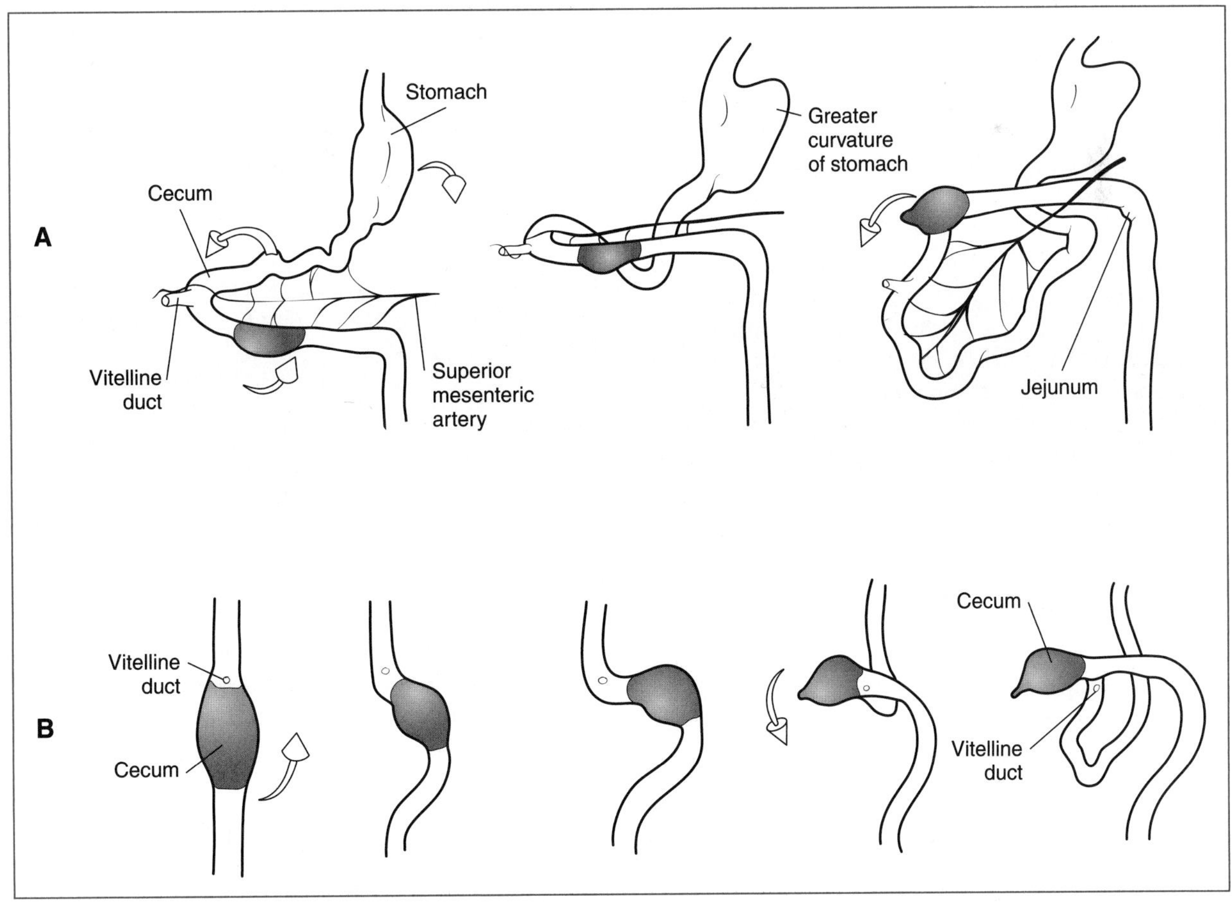

FIGURE 1.19 Migration and rotation of the midgut. (A) Counterclockwise 90-degree rotation of midgut loop and "herniation" into extraembryonic cavity. (B) Counterclockwise 180-degree rotation of midgut loop on return to the abdominal cavity.

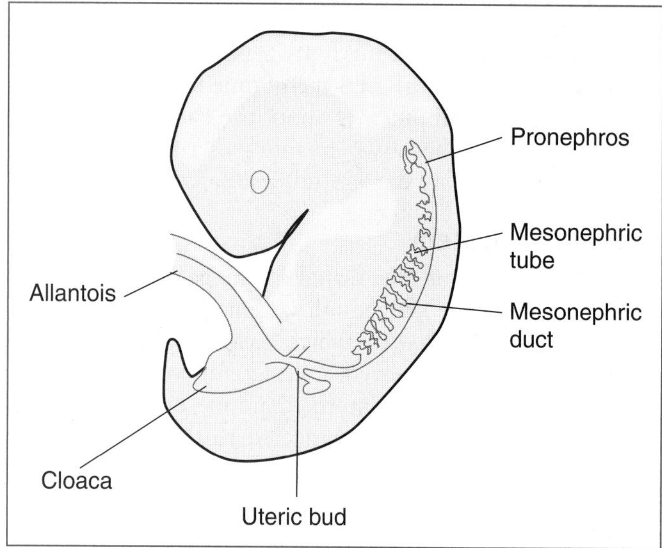

FIGURE 1.20 Development of the kidney. The locations of the pronephros and mesonephros.

nephros. The mesonephros degenerates by the end of the embryonic period. Remnants of the mesonephros persist as genital ducts in males or vestigial structures in females. The metanephros appears in the fifth week of gestation and becomes the permanent kidney. The metanephros begins to produce urine by about the 11th week of gestation. The number of glomeruli increases until week 32 when the fetal kidney becomes subdivided into lobes. The urinary bladder and the urethra arise from the urogenital sinus and the splanchnic mesenchyme. The caudal portion of the mesonephric ducts is incorporated into the bladder, giving rise to the ureters (Moore & Persaud, 2008; Sadler, 2010).

Although the genetic sex of the embryo is determined at conception, the early development of the genital system is indistinguishable until the seventh week of gestation. Beginning in the seventh week, the gonads begin to differentiate. The ovaries and the testes are derived from the coelomic epithelium, the mesenchyme, and the primordial germ cells. Development of female sexual organs occurs in the absence of hormonal stimulation precipitated by the H-Y antigen gene carried on the Y chromosome. If the Y chromosome is present, testes develop; otherwise, ovaries develop (Moore & Persaud, 2008; Sadler, 2010).

FETAL PERIOD: WEEK 9 THROUGH BIRTH

The fetal period begins at the start of week 9 following conception and continues through the duration of pregnancy. It is characterized by further growth and development of the fetus and the organs formed during the embryonic period.

Week 9 to 12

At the beginning of this period, the head is large and the body begins growing faster than the head. The face is broad and characterized by a wide nose and widely spaced eyes. The mouth is formed and palate formation is complete. Tooth buds appear for the baby teeth. Fingernails are present and the fetus can curl his fingers to make a fist. The intestines enter the abdomen from the umbilical cord. By the end of the 12th week, blood formation shifts from the liver to the spleen. The fetus can produce urine and excretes it into the amniotic fluid. By the end of the 12th week, the sex of the fetus can be identified by appearance of the external genitalia. By week 12 the fetus weighs 45 g (1.6 oz) and has a crown-rump (C-R) length of 8 cm (3.2 in) (Moore & Persaud, 2008).

Week 13 to 16

During this time of rapid growth, the fetal head becomes smaller in proportion to the body. The appearance of hair patterning is forming on the head, and *lanugo*, a fine downy hair, is found on the body. Fingerprints are now developed. The fetus can now open his mouth, make a sucking motion, and swallow amniotic fluid. Ossification of the fetal skeleton is active during this time. Reflex response and muscular activity begin. The lower limbs lengthen during this time, and limb movement is more coordinated. In females, the ovaries differentiate and contain primordial follicles. At 16 weeks the fetal weight is about 200 g (7 oz) and the C-R length is 13.5 cm (5.4 in) (Moore & Persaud, 2008; Sadler, 2010).

Week 17 to 20

This marks a period of slower growth. The skin is covered in fatty, cheese-like substance called *vernix caseosa* that protects it from exposure to amniotic fluid. The limbs are in proportion to the rest of the body and muscles are well developed. Myelination of the spinal cord begins at 20 weeks. Lanugo now covers the body, and brown fat begins to form in the base of the neck, behind the sternum, and around the kidneys. Fetal movement is usually felt by the mother around 18 weeks. The uterus is formed in the female fetus by 18 weeks and at 20 weeks the testes begin to descend in the male fetus. At 20 weeks the fetus has a crown to heel (C-H) length of 25 cm (10 in) and a weight of 435 g (15 oz) (Moore & Persaud, 2008; Sadler, 2010).

Week 21 to 25

During this period there is substantial weight gain but the fetus is thin and has little subcutaneous fat. The skin is wrinkled and translucent red because the capillaries are close to the surface of the skin. The fetus has a grasp and startle reflex and rapid eye movements begin. Eyebrow and eyelashes are fully formed. Teeth that will become second molars are forming. At 24 weeks the lungs begin to produce surfactant. IgG levels reach maternal levels. At 24 weeks the fetus has a C-H length of 28 cm (11.2 in) and a weight of 780 g (1 lb 11 ½ oz) (Moore & Persaud, 2008; Sadler, 2010).

Week 26 to 29

The fetal lungs, pulmonary capillaries, and CNS are more mature, and the fetus is likely to survive if born after 24 to 25 weeks. Blood formation (erythrocyte production) shifts from the spleen to the bone marrow. The CNS is now mature enough that it can direct breathing movements and control body temperature. There is now enough subcutaneous fat to help maintain body temperature. The eyelids that have been closed since 9 weeks gestation start to open. In males, the testes descend into the inguinal canal and upper scrotum. At 28 weeks, the fetus has a C-H length of 35 cm (14 in) and a weight of 1,200 to 1,250 g (2 lb 12 oz) (Moore & Persaud, 2008; Sadler, 2010).

Week 30 to 34

This period marks a rapid increase in body fat and muscle. Bones are fully developed but are soft and pliable. The lungs are not yet mature but developed enough to provide gas exchange if the fetus were to be born during this period. Surfactant production is not quite at mature levels. The fetus exhibits rhythmic breathing movements as a result of a more mature CNS. The pupillary light reflex is present at 30 weeks. The fetal skin is smooth and pigmented, and the fingernails reach the fingertips. At 32 weeks, the fetus has a C-H length of 38 to 43 cm (15.2–17.2 in) and weighs 2,000 g (4 lb 7 oz) (Moore & Persaud, 2008; Sadler, 2010).

Week 35 to 36

Growth of all body systems continues until birth but at a slower rate. The circumference of the head and abdomen is approximately equal by 36 weeks. The fetus starts to look "plump" and the skin is less wrinkled. Lanugo is disappearing. In males the testes are in the scrotum. In both males and females, breasts are enlarged. At 36 weeks, the fetus has a C-H length of 42 to 48 cm (16.8–17.2 in) and a weight of 2,500 to 2,750 g (5 lb 8 oz–6 lb 1 oz) (Moore & Persaud, 2008; Sadler, 2010).

Week 37 to 40

The fetus is considered *full term* between 38 and 40 weeks. During the last few weeks of gestation, the fat increases in the fetus at a rate of 14 g/d; however, white fat makes up 16% of her total weight. Amniotic fluid decreases to 500 mL or less as the fetal mass fills the uterus. The measurement of the fetal foot is slightly larger than the femur and this is used as an alternate measurement to confirm fetal age. The chest is more prominent but slightly smaller than the diameter of the head. The earlobes are firm, and the skin has a smooth polished appearance. Vernix caseosa is present in the deep folds and creases of the skin. The lungs are well developed and have the ability to exchange gases. The lecithin-sphingomyelin (L/S) ratio is approaching 2:1, indicating lung maturity. At term, the fetus weighs 3,200 g or more and is 48 to 52 cm (19–21 in) long (Moore & Persaud, 2008; Sadler, 2010).

DEVELOPMENTAL RISKS

The fetus is at less risk for structural defects caused by teratogenic factors than is the embryo; however, there is still a risk for functional impairment of existing structures. This risk is addressed in the section on environmental factors. Changes in specific organs or organ systems during the fetal period are discussed in the section on the development of specific organs (Moore & Persaud, 2008; Sadler, 2010). For a summary of prenatal development, see Box 1.2.

BOX 1.2

THREE PERIODS OF FETAL DEVELOPMENT

Embryonic Period

Extends from the fertilization of the ovum

Period 1: Preembryonic Period

Extends from the fertilization of the ovum to the formation of the embryonic disk with three germ layers—week 1 to week 3.

Period 2: Embryonic Period

Period of rapid growth and differentiation; formation of major organ systems occurs—week 4 to week 8.

Period 3: Fetal Period

Further growth and development of organ systems—extends from week 9 to week 40 (term).

Data from Moore and Persaud (2008).

Congenital Defects

Congenital defects or anomalies are structural or anatomic abnormalities present at birth. Congenital defects vary in severity and location, ranging from minor insignificant defects to major organ system defects and are attributed to genetic or chromosomal abnormalities or to maternal or environmental factors. Most congenital defects result from an interaction between genetic and environmental factors, or multifactorial inheritance. Congenital defects caused by single-gene disorders and chromosomal abnormalities are discussed in Chapter 38. The influence of the environment on embryonic development is discussed in this section.

Moore and Persaud (2008) listed six mechanisms that can cause congenital defects: (1) too little growth, (2) too little resorption, (3) too much resorption, (4) resorption in the wrong location, (5) normal growth in an abnormal position, and (6) overgrowth of a tissue or structure. Embryonic organs are most sensitive to noxious agents during a period of rapid cell growth and differentiation. Damage to the primitive streak at about 15 days of gestation could cause severe congenital malformations of the embryo because of its role in the production of intraembryonic mesoderm, from which all connective tissue is formed. Biochemical differentiation occurs before morphologic differentiation, so organs or structures are sensitive to the action of teratogens before they can be identified.

Critical Periods of Human Development

Environmental influences during the first 2 weeks after conception may prevent successful implantation of the blastocyst and cause spontaneous abortion of the embryo. The most sensitive period for the embryo, known as the *critical period*, is the period of organogenesis, during the first 8 weeks of development. Each organ has a critical period during which its development is most likely to be adversely affected by the presence of teratogenic agents; however, some organs such as the brain are sensitive throughout fetal development (see Figure 1.8 for critical periods for each major organ system) (Moore & Persaud, 2008).

The terms *congenital anomaly, congenital malformation*, and *birth defect* are used synonymously to describe structural abnormalities in an infant; however, according to Moore and Persaud (2008), there are four classifications of congenital anomalies: malformation, disruption, deformation, and dysplasia. A malformation is a structural defect of an organ or larger body region. Usually a malformation is a defect of a morphogenic or developmental field and may result in complex or multiple malformations. A disruption is an interruption of a normal developmental process. This may be caused by a teratogen such as a drug or virus; however, it is not inherited. A deformation is an alteration in form or shape that results from mechanical forces in otherwise healthy tissue. Dysplasia is abnormal development of tissue and may affect several organs.

Birth defects are a leading cause of infant death, accounting for more than 20% of all infant deaths. The generally reported incidence of congenital defects is about 2% to 3%. The actual incidence is higher because some defects are not apparent at birth. Close to 12% of birth defects are not discovered until after the newborn period. The incidence of all defects (including both minor and major defects) is approximately 14% (Lewis, 2008; Moore & Persaud, 2008).

Environmental Factors

Environmental factors cause 7% to 10% of congenital anomalies. During the critical period, or the first 8 weeks, when cell division, cell differentiation, and morphogenesis take place, the fetal structures are most sensitive to environmental agents known as *teratogens*. Each organ or structure has its own critical period in which exposure to teratogens can cause malformations of functional disturbances in varying severity depending on the timing and the teratogen. Teratogens are agents such as chemicals, viruses, radiation, drugs, maternal disease, and other environmental factors that cause birth defects (Lewis, 2008; Moore & Persaud, 2008).

Infectious Agents

Several viral agents including rubella, cytomegalovirus (CMV), herpes simplex (HSV), and human immunodeficiency virus (HIV) have been positively identified as teratogenic to the developing fetus. Rubella (German measles) is a viral infection spread through the air or by close contact. The virus can cross the placenta and during the first trimester can cause cataracts, permanent hearing loss, cardiac malformations (especially patent ductus arteriosis and pulmonary stenosis), and congenital rubella syndrome in the fetus. If exposed in the second or third trimester, the fetus can develop learning disabilities or speech and hearing problems. Prevention is the goal; however, women should be tested to determine if the rubella antibody is present, and if not, she should be vaccinated as long as she is not pregnant and will avoid pregnancy for at least six months.

CMV is a virus belonging to the herpes family. It is transmitted by direct contact of body fluids including urine, saliva, blood, semen, and breast milk. Approximately 30% to 50% of women have never been infected with CMV, and infected women have no symptoms (Sadler, 2010). One third of women who have a primary infection during pregnancy will pass it to the fetus as it crosses the placenta (Centers for Disease Control and Prevention [CDC], 2010). If exposed in early gestation, the embryo will likely spontaneously abort. At least 20% of infants who are infected will have microcephaly, meningoencephalitis, which causes hearing and vision loss, mental retardation, and seizures (CDC, 2010).

HSV is one of the most common sexually transmitted infections among adult women and is transmitted across broken skin and mucus membrane by direct exposure to the virus. If a woman has a primary outbreak during late pregnancy, there is a 30% to 50% risk of transmission to the fetus. Infection to the fetus is transmitted during birth 85% of the time. An infected fetus has a mortality rate of 50%. Infants who survive may have significant neurological defects, blindness, and seizures (Moore & Persaud, 2008; Sadler, 2010).

HIV is the virus that causes acquired immunodeficiency syndrome (AIDS). HIV is transmitted through body fluids: blood, semen, genital fluids, and human milk and can cross the placenta in pregnancy. Almost all pediatric cases of HIV are acquired in utero or through breastfeeding. Women who are treated in pregnancy with an antiretroviral medication reduce the risk of transmission to 2% (CDC, 2010; Cooper et al., 2002). Anomalies associated with HIV are microcephaly, growth factor, and craniofacial features.

Toxoplasmosis is caused by a protozoan, *Toxoplasma gondii*, and when exposed in utero can cause hydrocephalus, cerebral calcification, microphthalmia, and ocular defects in the fetus. *T. gondii* can be contracted from raw or undercooked meat, by handling feces of infected cats, or from the soil. The risk and severity depend on the timing of the exposure in pregnancy (Moore & Persaud, 2008; Sadler, 2010).

Untreated primary maternal infections of *Treponema pallidum*, the spirochete that causes syphilis, can result in serious congenital anomalies or stillborn. Congenital syphilis is classified as early or late. Early is defined as in the first three months of life and may cause vesiculobullous lesions, rash, lymphadenopathy, hepatosplenomegaly, and a mucopurulent nasal discharge known as "snuffles." Late congenital syphilis occurs around or after age 2 and includes symptoms such as gummatous ulcers on the nose, septum, and palate, bossing of frontal and parietal bones, optic atrophy leading to blindness, interstitial keratitis, and sensorineural deafness. Treatment must be as early as possible to prevent complications and transmission of the infection to the fetus (Moore & Persaud, 2008).

Other viral agents have been implicated as causes of congenital malformations. Such malformations have been reported following maternal infection with mumps, varicella, echovirus, coxsackie virus, and influenza virus. The incidence of congenital malformations following these infections is unknown, but is suspected to be low (Sadler, 2010). (For further information on viral agents, see Chapter 11.)

Drugs/Medications

Drug safety is a primary concern during pregnancy, especially in women with pregestational disease. Safety of a medication cannot be tested on pregnant women for obvious ethical reasons as it could expose a fetus to possible teratogens.

Few drugs are known to be teratogenic; however, no drug can be considered completely safe. The Food and Drug Administration (FDA) has established five categories of medications in pregnancy: (1) Category A means that studies have failed to demonstrate a risk to the fetus; (2) Category B indicates that animal studies have not demonstrated a risk to the fetus; however, there are no well-controlled studies in pregnant women; (3) Category C indicates that animal studies have shown an adverse effect on the fetus; however, there are no studies on humans and benefits to mother may outweigh risks to fetus; (4) Category D shows there is positive evidence of human fetal risk and risk may outweigh benefits; and (5) Category X indicates that there is positive evidence of fetal anomalies or risks that clearly outweigh any possible benefit in pregnant women (Fredericksen, 2011).

Drugs that are known teratogens that can cause birth defects include antibiotics streptomycin and tetracycline; antineoplastic agents; anticoagulants, anticonvulsants; hormones such as adrenocorticoids and diethylstilbestrol (DES); antithyroid drugs; psychotropics; antianxiety agents such as diazepam; and retinoic acid (vitamin A).

Hormonal agents are also implicated in the incidence of congenital defects. Androgenic agents (progestins) may cause masculinization of female fetuses. DES, a synthetic estrogen used to prevent abortion in the 1940s and 1950s, has been found to cause an increased incidence of vaginal and cervical cancer in female children exposed to the drug in utero. There are associated abnormalities of the reproductive system, often causing reproductive dysfunction (Moore & Persaud, 2008; Sadler, 2010).

Amphetamines are associated with oral clefts and heart defects. Salicylates (aspirin), a commonly used medication during pregnancy, may be harmful to the fetus if taken in large amounts or may lead to bleeding problems. Isotretinoin, a drug used to treat acne, causes craniofacial abnormalities, cleft palate, thymic aplasia defects, and neural tube defects (Sadler, 2010).

Illicit Drugs

Social or recreational drugs are highly suspected of contributing to congenital defects and the risk of spontaneous abortion. Drugs such as lysergic acid diethylamide (LSD) have been associated with limb abnormalities and CNS abnormalities. Other drugs that may be teratogenic include phencyclidine and marijuana. "Crack" cocaine has been associated with preterm birth (PTB), low birth weight (LBW), premature rupture of membranes (PROMs) placental abruption, and sudden infant death syndrome (SIDS) (Gouin, Murphy, & Shah 2011). The tendency of drug abusers to use multiple drugs, combined with poor nutritional habits and lack of prenatal care, makes it difficult to establish the effects of the drugs individually.

As yet, no teratogenic effects of marijuana have been reported. Research on the teratogenicity of marijuana is difficult since it is an illegal substance. There is strong evidence that marijuana crosses the placenta and can result in intrauterine growth restriction (IUGR). Infants who have been exposed have exhibited a transient neonatal syndrome that includes lethargy, hypotonia, tremors, and blunted response to visual stimuli (Hansen et al., 2008). Researchers continue to follow marijuana use in pregnancy to determine its teratogenicity.

■ **Alcohol.** The term *fetal alcohol syndrome* (FAS) is used to describe the cluster of defects characteristic of maternal ingestion of alcohol. A major factor in the development of FAS is timing, amount, and frequency of alcohol consumption during pregnancy. The characteristic pattern of development in FAS includes craniofacial abnormalities; microcephaly; limb deformities; smooth philtrum; thin upper lip; small palpebral fissures; and short nose. CNS abnormalities include cognitive impairment; impaired fine motor skills; developmental disabilities; attention deficit disorder; and seizure disorder (Day, 2012).

Fetal alcohol spectrum disorder (FASD) is a modern term that describes the range of permanent effects of alcohol use in pregnancy. The FDA lists alcohol as a Category D drug; therefore, it is contraindicated in pregnancy. There is no level of alcohol consumption that can be considered safe; therefore, it is recommended that alcohol be avoided throughout the perinatal period (Warren, Hewitt, & Thomas, 2011).

■ **Tobacco.** The dangers of smoking cigarettes in pregnancy have been well documented. The use of tobacco during pregnancy can lead to PTB, LBW, PROMs, placenta previa, placental abruption, or stillbirth. The fetus can suffer from growth restriction because of the vasoconstrictive properties of nicotine, which decreases the oxygenated blood to the fetus. Smoking can cause adverse effects on development in children and may include mood or conduct disorders, an increase in behavioral problems, anxiety, depression, and obesity (Murin, Rafii, & Bilello, 2011).

■ **Ionizing Radiation.** There is no established "safe" level for radiation. Large amounts of exposure during pregnancy can be detrimental to the fetus; however, this is a rare occurrence.

The severity of radiation-induced defects depends on the duration and timing of exposure. Radiation exposure during the first trimester of pregnancy most like will result in loss of the embryo. High levels of radiation can cause microcephaly, microphthalmia, growth restriction, skeletal and visceral abnormalities, retinal changes, cataracts, and cleft palate. There is no evidence that the small amount of radiation required for modern radiographic studies is harmful; however, caution is used to minimize the exposure to the fetus because of the potential for cumulative effects of radiation exposure throughout the life span (Groen, Bae, & Lim, 2012).

■ Heavy Metals. Prenatal exposure to lead can lead to neurological deficits in children. Other reported effects of exposure to lead during pregnancy include spontaneous abortion, LBW, PTB, and developmental delays. Lead can be found in lead crystal glassware, arts and crafts supplies, paint (banned as a paint additive in the United States in 1978), lining of cans used for canned foods, cigarette smoke, and cosmetics. Other contaminants such as herbicides, pesticides, and fungicides have been shown to cause PTB, reduced fetal growth, and congenital CNS, circulatory, respiratory, urogenital, and musculoskeletal anomalies when women are exposed during pregnancy (Stillerman, Mattison, Giudice, & Woodruff, 2008).

Evidence has shown that mercury may be harmful to a fetus depending on timing of exposure. Mercury can cause severe neurological symptoms including behavioral disturbances. High levels of mercury exposure may cause fetal abnormalities and neurotoxicity including microcephaly, severe mental and physical developmental retardation, and blindness. Pregnant women should avoid eating fish with high levels of mercury such as swordfish, shark, and king mackerel (Karagas et al., 2012).

■ Bisphenol-A. Bisphenol-A (BPA) is an organic compound used to make polycarbonate plastic, epoxy resins, and dental sealants. BPA can be found in plastic baby bottles, plastic lining in canned foods, and polycarbonate plastic containers. The chemical structure of BPA is similar to estrogen and may have the same effect on the body. High levels of BPA found in blood have been associated with recurrent miscarriages, preeclampsia, IUGR, and PTB. Plastics with a recycle code of 1, 2, 4, 5, and 6 are not likely to contain BPA; however, more plastic packaging is stating whether the item contains BPA. Women who are trying to conceive should avoid using plastic items that contain BPA (Stillerman, Mattison, Giudice, & Woodruff, 2008).

Maternal Disease

Pregestational maternal disease can be teratogenic to a fetus. Women with poorly controlled pregestational diabetes have a three to four times higher risk of having a fetus with a birth defect than women in the general population. Anomalies typically occur between weeks 5 and 8 and can include brain anomalies, skeletal defects, developmental abnormalities, and congenital heart defects.

Thyroid deficiency during the last two trimesters of pregnancy and first months after birth can result in mental retardation or other neurologic deficits in the neonate. Untreated maternal hypothyroidism can adversely affect the developing fetus. Maternal hypothyroidism is associated with spontaneous abortion, preterm labor (PTL) and PTB, gestational hypertension, anemia, placental abruption, postpartum hemorrhage, and fetal death. Uncontrolled hyperthyroidism during pregnancy is associated with some of the same complications, as well as LBW, stillbirth, fetal growth restriction (FGR), maternal heart failure, congenital hypothyroidism, fetal thyrotoxicosis, and neonatal hyperthyroidism (Yazbeck & Sullivan, 2012).

Women with phenylalanine hydroxylase deficiency (phenylketonuria [PKU]) and hyperphenylalaninemia are at risk of having a fetus with congenital anomalies if the phenylalanine levels are elevated in pregnancy. High maternal levels of phenylalanine during pregnancy can result in microcephaly, delayed speech, mental retardation, and neurologic damage. More than 40% of pregnant women are obese. Pregnant obese women have a high risk of having poor maternal, fetal, or neonatal outcomes. Nutritional deficiencies, poor metabolic control, and coexisting medical conditions may interfere with organogenesis and complicate the pregnancy. Congenital anomalies include microcephaly, cleft lip and palate, neural tube defects, cardiac anomalies, anorectal atresia, diaphragmatic hernia, hydrocephalus, and hypospadias (Gunatilake & Perlow, 2011).

Other

Another teratogenic factor is hyperthermia caused by maternal use of hot tubs or saunas or by maternal febrile illness during pregnancy. Hyperthermia can increase the incidence of embryonic resorption and malformations. The type and severity of congenital defect depends on the amount of temperature elevation, duration of the exposure, and stage of embryonic development. If the mother is exposed during the critical period (the first 8 weeks) when the CNS is particularly vulnerable to hyperthermia, congenital defects of the CNS may occur. Other defects that may occur involve cardiac, renal, limbs, and teeth. It is recommended that women avoid hot tubs and saunas during pregnancy and monitor and treat febrile illness (Crinnon, 2011).

Good nutrition has long been considered essential for proper growth and development of the fetus. Dietary habits have a profound effect on pregnancy outcomes. However, with the exception of folic acid, in which there is evidence that deficiencies are causally related to defects of the neural tube, there is little known about the role of micronutrients on fetal development. Supplementation of vitamins and minerals must occur within the appropriate critical period of development to be effective. Little is known about nutritional imbalances in pregnant women. Fowles, Timmerman, Bryant, and Kim (2011) found that women whose diets consisted mainly of fast food were more likely to be obese, depressed, and stressed. Fast-food consumption is associated with excessive caloric intake and excessive weight gain in pregnancy. Suliga (2011) found that pregnant women consumed inadequate amounts of fruits, vegetables, whole grain cereals, milk, dairy, and fish. Evidence of dietary quality in pregnancy suggests that poor dietary quality during the critical period of pregnancy may predispose the infant to heart disease, altered insulin metabolism and type 2 diabetes, obesity, and hypertension as an adult. This is caused by a phenomenon called reprogramming of the fetal phenotype that results in permanent changes in the child's physiology (Fowles et al., 2011).

Finally, advanced paternal age has recently been associated with an increased risk of complex disorders such as autism, schizophrenia, autism spectrum disorder, and cancer (Hultman, Sandin, Levine, Lichtenstein, & Reichenberg, 2011; Toriello & Meck, 2008). Other anomalies associated with advanced paternal age include neural tube defects, congenital heart defects, malformation of extremities, hydrocephalus, and orofacial clefts (Green et al., 2010).

Environmental factors that have yet to be identified may exert influence on the development of the fetus. It is essential to consider the environment of the fetus in terms of the uterine environment and the environment of the mother in assessment of the influences on fetal development.

SUMMARY

This chapter has provided an overview of embryologic and fetal development, outlined the critical periods of development, and described the more common congenital defects. Knowledge of embryologic and fetal development is essential as a foundation for understanding the role of environment, genetics, physical, or other factors that may have an impact upon anatomy, physiology, or pathophysiology of the organism. The future health of the individual is in large part dependent upon numerous events that take place during gestation. As knowledge of genetics, development, and human pathophysiology improves, better health care technologies may emerge that can significantly reduce morbidity and mortality and improve quality of life.

CASE STUDY

A 19-year-old female at approximately 19 weeks of gestation presents to the high-risk clinic by referral from her primary obstetrician. She had a morphology scan at her doctor's office at 18 weeks with intracranial calcifications noted as well as probably hyperechogenic bowel. She and her husband had moved to North Carolina from a small town in Mississippi. They had married immediately after graduation from high school and he had joined the Army. They had neither family in the area nor any other social support systems. Her primary obstetrician had forwarded prenatal records that described a 24- to 48-hour viral illness between 16 and 17 weeks with a fever of 102°F and flu-like symptoms including myalgia and malaise. Detailed ultrasounds demonstrated numerous intracranial calcifications, microcephaly, pleural effusions, and decreased amniotic fluid. The perinatologist discussed with the couple the probability that she had been exposed to and developed CMV, which was passed on to the fetus. The couple refused amniocentesis following a prolonged discussion with family members in Mississippi because they had decided to continue with the pregnancy regardless of the outcome. The infant was born at 37 weeks and was diagnosed with blindness, deafness, and is likely to have severe mental disabilities.

- How would you explain the CMV infection?
- How would you explain the potential outcomes for the baby as well as the extent of care that would be required for optimal developmental outcome?
- How would you prepare the parents for the care of an infant with multiple serious disabilities?

■ **CMV.** When a woman is infected with CMV for the first time during pregnancy (primary infection), the risk that her baby will get infected is as high as 50%. Primary maternal CMV infections occur in 0.15% to 2.0% of all pregnancies. Infants born with CMV are at risk for long-term disabilities such as mental retardation, learning disabilities, epilepsy, cerebral palsy, hearing impairment or deafness, and visual impairment or blindness. Congenital CMV infection is transmitted to the fetus by maternal viremia and placental infection. Maternal immunoglobulin G (IgG) transports the virus across the placental syncytiotrophoblast. In a primary infection in which the placenta becomes infected with CMV, the ability to provide nutrients and oxygen to the fetus is impaired. The placenta becomes enlarged, and tissue damage occurs due to viral placentitis and revascularization. Many symptoms in the newborn are due to the infection of the placenta rather than the direct effect of the virus on the fetus. A primary CMV infection in the first trimester is associated with the worst outcomes. A maternal infection that occurs prior to conception is unlikely to pass to the fetus.

Although the majority (85%–90%) of congenital infections are asymptomatic, 5% to 20% of infants born to mothers with primary CMV infection are overtly symptomatic. Only 10% to 15% of these babies will show symptoms of infection at birth. Symptoms may include petechia, jaundice, hepatosplenomegaly, microcephaly, IUGR, chorioretinitis, thrombocytopenia, and anemia. Babies born with CMV are also at risk for long-term effects such as sensorineural hearing loss, vision problems, and psychomotor development delay. CMV-infected children have a mortality rate of about 5%, and severe neurologic morbidity occurs in 50% to 60% of survivors. Asymptomatic infants are also at risk of developing long-term neurodevelopment morbidity, but the risk is much lower than in symptomatic neonates.

Diagnosis is made by viral culture of amniotic fluid and by ultrasound examination. Amniocentesis is essential for prenatal diagnosis and CMV isolation from amniotic fluid is the gold standard for prenatal diagnosis. A high viral load in the amniotic fluid may indicate a poor outcome; however, it may also be related to gestational age at the time of sampling. Once a fetal infection has been diagnosed, the fetus should be closely monitored by ultrasound. Abnormal ultrasound findings include: abnormalities in amniotic fluid such as polyhydramnios or oligohydramnios, IUGR, hydrocephaly or microcephaly, intracranial calcifications, ventricle cerebral ventriculomegaly or atrophy, hyperechogenic bowel, pseudomeconium ileus, hepatosplenomegaly, ascites or hydrops, and/or necrotic, cystic, or calcified lesions in the brain or liver. Some babies that have been infected with CMV during pregnancy will show signs of problems on ultrasound; however, the absence of sonographic findings does not guarantee a normal outcome. Some fetuses with CMV will not show any signs of infection on ultrasound. Once a fetus is diagnosed with a CMV infection, ultrasounds should be done every 2 to 4 weeks to watch for signs that may predict the outcome. Routine serologic testing is not recommended and should be used only when a pregnant woman develops a flu-like illness or if a CMV infection is suspected following an ultrasound.

Currently, there is no effective therapy for CMV infection, and women can be offered the option of pregnancy termination once a fetal infection is detected by ultrasound or amniocentesis and once a fetus is determined or suspected to be affected. Research on the use of CMV-specific hyperimmune globulin in pregnant women with a primary infection has been reported to improve outcomes; however, further studies are needed. There is also some evidence that ganciclovir treatment of babies with symptoms of congenital CMV may be beneficial for prevention or amelioration of hearing loss.

There are currently no vaccines for CMV and no clinical trials of new vaccines. Prevention of congenital CMV infection by practicing good personal hygiene is crucial. Pregnant women should avoid intimate contact with saliva and urine from young children and use good hand washing after changing diapers and wiping secretions. At least one third of women in the United States have direct contact with children less than 3 years old. Children and staff who care for children in day care centers are especially likely to be infected; therefore, pregnant women who have children in day care settings are especially vulnerable. One should assume that all children under age 3 have CMV in their urine and saliva. Other recommendations include not sharing cups, plates, or toothbrushes, not kissing children on or near the mouth, and not sharing towels or washcloths with a young child.

References

Nigro, G., & Adler, S. P. (2011). Cytomegalovirus infections during pregnancy. *Current Opinion in Obstetrics and Gynecology, 23*, 123–128.

Yinon, Y., Farine, D., & Yudin, M. H. (2010). SOGC practice guideline: Cytomegalovirus infection in pregnancy. *Journal of Obstetrics and Gynecology Canada, 240*, 348–354.

EVIDENCE-BASED PRACTICE BOX

BPA is a synthetic estrogenic chemical that is used in the production of several consumer products including polycarbonate plastic and resins, flame retardants, and dental sealants. It is found in plastic food and drink containers and in the lining of some canned goods. Plastics marked with recycling codes 1, 2, 4, 5, and 6 are unlikely to contain BPA; however, plastics with codes 3 and 7 may contain the chemical. There are no government labeling requirements for products containing BPA. BPA is a weak endocrine disruptor with properties similar to estrogen. In 2010, the FDA warned about possible hazards to fetuses, infants, and young children. Ehrlich et al. (2012) found a positive association between urinary concentrations of BPA and implantation failure in women undergoing in vitro fertilization. Perera et al. (2012) found evidence that BPA is a neurodevelopmental toxicant. Their study of 198 children (87 boys and 111 girls) included measuring urine concentrations of BPA during pregnancy and up to 5 years of age. Elevated exposure in boys was associated with emotionally reactive and aggressive behavior consistent with similar studies in laboratory animals. Girls demonstrated an inverse association for anxiety and depression. These findings suggest that child behavior may be affected by prenatal BPA exposure. Because little is known about the overall effects of BPA, pregnant women should be advised to avoid products with BPA and to use products labeled "Contains no BPA" for their infants and children.

References

Ehrlich, S., Williams, P. L., Missmer, S. A., Flaws, J. A., Berry, K. F., Calafat, A. M., . . . Hauser, R. (2012). Urinary bisphenol A concentrations and implantation failure among women undergoing in vitro fertilization. *Environmental Health Perspectives, 120*(7), 978–983.

Perera, F., Vishnevetsky, J., Herbstman, J. B., Calafat, A. M., Xiong, W., Rauh, V., & Wang, S. (2012). Prenatal bisphenol A exposure and child behavior in an inner-city cohort. *Environmental Health Perspectives, 120*(8), 1190–1194.

ONLINE RESOURCES

Basic Embryology Review Program/University of Pennsylvania: This web page follows development from fertilization through birth. This site has been selected in two well-known "Best of the Web" reviews.
http://www.med.upenn.edu/meded/public/berp

Centers for Disease Control and Prevention: Information on birth defects and literature and statistics for health care professionals.
http://www.cdc.gov/ncbddd/birthdefects/index.html

Clinical Teratology Website: A project of the TERIS (Teratogen Information System) at University of Washington. Designed to serve as a resource guide for health care professionals.
http://www.depts.washington.edu/~terisweb

College of Medicine; University of Cincinnati
http://www.med.uc.edu/embryology/contents.htm#Chapter1

The Teratology Society: This multidisciplinary scientific society was founded in 1960. Members study the causes and biologic processes leading to abnormal development and birth defects at the fundamental and clinical levels, as well as appropriate measures for prevention.
http://www.teratology.org

REFERENCES

Centers for Disease Control and Prevention. (2010). Cytomegalovirus (CMV) and congenital CMV infection. Retrieved from http://www.cdc/cmv/congenital-infection.html

Cooper, E. R., Charurat, M., Mofenson, L., Hanson, I. C., Pitt, J., Diaz, C., . . . Blattner, W. (2002). Combination antiretroviral strategies for the treatment of pregnant HIV-1-infected women and prevention of perinatal HIV-1 transmission. *Journal of Acquired Immune Deficiency Syndrome*, *29*(5), 484–494.

Crinnon, W. J. (2011). Sauna as a valuable clinical tool for cardiovascular, autoimmune, toxicant-induced, and other chronic health problems. *Alternative Medicine Review, 16*(3), 215–225.

Day, S. (2012). Alcohol consumption during pregnancy: The growing evidence. *Developmental Medicine & Child Neurology, 54*(3), 200.

Fowles, E. R., Timmerman, G. M., Bryant, M., & Kim, S. H. (2011). Eating at fast food restaurants and dietary quality in low-income pregnant women. *Western Journal of Nursing Research, 33*(5), 630–651.

Fredericksen, C. T. (2011). The new FDA pregnancy labeling requirements for drugs. *Journal of Midwifery and Women's Health, 56*(3), 303–307.

Gouin, K., Murphy, K., & Shah, P. S. (2011). Effects of cocaine use during pregnancy on low birth weight and preterm birth: Systemic review and metaanalyses. *American Journal of Obstetrics and Gynecology, 204*, e1–e12.

Green, R. F., Devine, O., Crider, K. S., Olney, R. S., Archer, N., Olshan, A. F., & Shapira, S. K. (2010). Association of advanced paternal age and risk for major congenital anomalies. *Annals of Epidemiology, 20*(3), 241–249.

Groen, R. S., Bae, J. Y., & Lim, K. J. (2012). Fear of the unknown: Ionizing radiation exposure during pregnancy. *American Journal of Obstetrics & Gynecology, 206*(6), 456–462.

Gunatilake, R. P., & Perlow, J. H. (2011). Obesity and pregnancy: Clinical management of the obese gravida. *American Journal of Obstetrics and Gynecology, 204*(2), 106–119.

Hansen, H. H., Krutz, B., Sifringer, M., Stefovska, V., Bittigau, P., Pragst, F., . . . Ikonomidou, C. (2008). Cannabinoids enhance susceptibility of immature brain to ethanol neurotoxicity. *Annals of Neurology, 64*(1), 42–52.

Hultman, C. M., Sandin, S., Levine, S. Z., Lichtenstein, P., & Reichenberg, A. (2011). Advanced paternal age and risk of autism: New evidence from a population based study and a meta-analysis of epidemiological studies. *Molecular Psychiatry, 16*, 1203–1212.

Karagas, M. R., Choi, A. L., Oken, E., Horvat, M., Schoeny, R., Kamai, E., . . . Korrick, S. (2012). Evidence on the human health effects of low-level methylmercury exposure. *Environmental Health Perspectives, 120*(6), 700–806.

Lewis, R. (2008). *Human genetics: Concepts and applications.* New York, NY: McGraw Hill.

Moore, K. L., & Persaud, T. V. N. (2008). *The developing human: Clinaically oriented embryology.* Philadelphia, PA: Saunders.

Murin, S., Raffi, R., & Bilello, K. (2011). Smoking and smoking cessation in pregnancy. *Clinics in Chest Medicine, 32*(1), 75–91.

Sadler, T. W. (2010). *Langman's medical embryology* (11th ed.). Philadelphia, PA: Lippincott William & Wilkins.

Stillerman, K. P., Mattison, D. R., Giudice, L. C., & Woodruff, T. J. (2008). Environmental exposures and adverse outcomes: A review of the science. *Reproductive Sciences, 15*(7), 631–650.

Suliga, E. (2011). Nutritional behaviors of pregnant women. *Pediatric Endocrinology, Diabetes, and Metabolism, 17*(2), 76–81.

Toriello, H. V., & Meck, J. M. (2008). Statement on guidance for genetic counseling in advanced paternal age. *Genetics in Medicine, 10*(6), 457–460.

Warren, K. R., Hewitt, B. G., & Thomas, J. D. (2011). Fetal alcohol spectrum disorder: Research challenges and opportunities. *Alcohol Research & Health, 34*(1), 4–14.

Yazbeck, C. F., & Sulllivan, S. D. (2012). Thyroid disorders during pregnancy. *Medical Clinics of North America, 96*(2), 235–256.

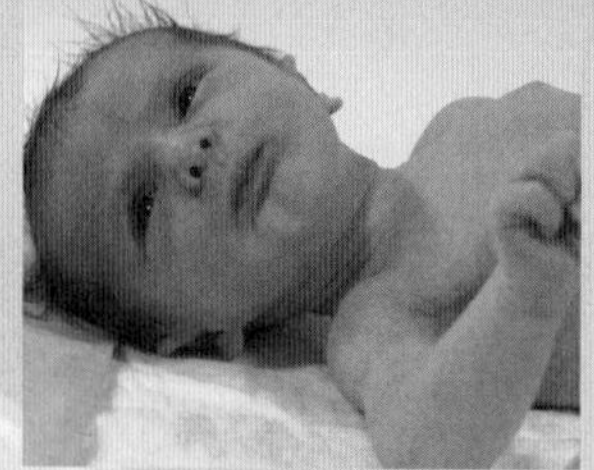

CHAPTER

2

Prenatal, Intrapartal, and Postpartal Risk Factors

■ Beverly Bowers

Most pregnancies are normal and result in a healthy newborn. However, it is not always the case. Pregnant women can be unknowingly exposed to potentially harmful physical, psychosocial, behavioral, or environmental conditions that can increase pregnancy risk. As our understanding of genomics and epigenetics advances, there is growing evidence of the genetic influence upon some perinatal risk factors and of a link between exposure to environmental triggers and perinatal outcomes. Even with optimal prenatal care, the fetus can experience adverse perinatal outcomes like preterm birth (PTB), low birth weight (LBW), congenital anomalies, neonatal morbidity, or neonatal mortality. After birth, maternal-related risk factors may continue to put neonates at risk for illness or injury. There is growing evidence that the consequences of being born premature or LBW can impact the individual's health over their lifetime.

Perinatal care providers must engage in continuous systematic assessment of potential maternal risk factors from prepregnancy through the postpartum period in order to optimize perinatal outcomes. Patient education, emotional support, and assistance with lifestyle alterations necessary for healthy pregnancy are key components of prenatal care. This chapter presents an overview of risk factors that contribute to adverse perinatal and neonatal outcomes in the prenatal, intrapartum, and postpartum periods. Global perspectives as well as the perspectives of the United States are reviewed.

MILLENNIUM DEVELOPMENT GOALS

Global efforts to improve health indicators for the poorest countries were determined to be a priority by members of the United Nations. The eight Millennium Development Goals (MDGs) were developed to unite efforts by countries and development agencies to achieve progress toward dramatically improving international health by 2015. The MDGs serve as benchmarks to measure progress toward health initiatives. All MDGs have a relationship to improving maternal–infant health (World Health Organization [WHO], Howson, Kinney, & Lawn, 2012).

MDG 1—Eradicate extreme poverty and hunger
MDG 2—Achieve universal primary education
MDG 3—Promote gender equality and empower women
MDG 4—Reduce child mortality
MDG 5—Improve maternal health
MDG 6—Combat HIV/AIDS, malaria, and other diseases
MDG 7—Ensure environmental sustainability
MDG 8—Form a global partnership for development

PERINATAL OUTCOMES INDICATORS

When examining risk factors, certain indicators are used for comparison of perinatal outcomes between populations. PTB, infant weight including intrauterine growth restriction (IUGR), and infant mortality rate (IMR) will be discussed as some of the more commonly cited indicators.

Preterm Birth

According to the WHO et al. (2012), PTB is defined as birth before 37 weeks of completed gestation. It is further subdivided into moderately PTB defined as 32 to less than 37 weeks completed gestation, which includes late preterm defined as 34 to less than 27 weeks completed gestation. Very PTB is defined as 28 to less than 32 weeks of completed gestation, and extremely preterm is considered as less than 28 weeks of completed gestation. Rarely, preterm infants as young as 21 weeks and 6 days gestational age have survived after months of aggressive neonatal intensive care. PTB can also be classified as spontaneous or provider-initiated, such as due to maternal conditions which necessitate early delivery for health of the mother and the fetus.

Fetal gestational age prior to delivery can be estimated based on maternal menstrual history or early prenatal ultrasound. Neonatal gestational age after birth can be estimated through assessment of physical and neuromuscular maturational characteristics using a scale such as the Dubowitz or New Ballard score. The New Ballard has been demonstrated to provide a reliable estimate of gestational age which correlates closely to gestational age based on last menstrual period (LMP) for extremely premature infants as young as 26 weeks gestation (Ballard et al., 1991). One concern is there may be ethnic variation in maturity ratings which can affect Ballard scores leading to overestimation of gestational age in non-White newborns with possible failure to identify at-risk newborns (Ahn, 2008; Taylor, Denison, Beyai, & Owens, 2010).

It is estimated that 10% of births worldwide are preterm. Each year 15 million babies are *Born Too Soon*, and more than a million infants die due to complications of prematurity (WHO et al., 2012). The preterm rate ranges from 8% to 18% globally. More than 60% of PTBs occur in 10 countries from sub-Saharan Africa, South Asia, and the United States. European countries have the lowest rates of PTB. The outcomes for premature infants born in low-income countries are not as favorable as for those born in high-income countries. Many preterm infant survivors are left with hearing, vision, or intellectual problems that last a lifetime (WHO et al., 2012).

About a half million infants were born prematurely in the United States in 2010, representing a 12% prematurity rate. The U.S. prematurity rate ranked 131 out of 184 nations globally, and was the highest prematurity rate for a high-income nation, comparable to rates of some low income nations (WHO et al., 2012). In the United States 45% of all PTBs occur spontaneously, 25% to 30% occur due to spontaneous premature rupture of membranes (PROM), and 30% to 35% result from inductions or cesarean sections (MacDorman & Mathews, 2011). Provider-initiated PTBs, including late PTBs, represent from 28% to 40% of all PTBs in the United States, with rates having increased in recent years (Wong & Grobman, 2011).

The percentage of PTBs in the United States is higher than other developed nations. Ethnic disparities exist in PTB rates. In 2008, non-Hispanic Black (NHB) women were more likely to deliver a preterm infant (18.3%) than non-Hispanic White (NHW) women (11.5%). NHB women were more than twice as likely to deliver a very preterm infant (<32 weeks gestation) than a NHW woman: 4.1% as compared with 1.6%. Because very preterm infants are at increased risk for neonatal death, more NHB infants are at increased risk for neonatal death. Preterm related infant deaths were three times higher for NHB infants than for NHW infants. Asian/Pacific Islander women have the lowest incidence of PTB; almost 5% lower than NHW women (MacDorman & Mathews, 2011).

The causes of PTB are complex, multifactorial, and not certain. Causes of prematurity may vary between high-income and lower income nations. Multiple variables have been associated with increased risks for preterm delivery including social stress and ethnicity, infection and inflammation, and genetic factors (Muglia & Katz, 2010). The most predictive risk factor is a history of a previous preterm delivery. Use of a prematurity screening tool for risk factors, fetal fibronectin testing, or identification of shortened cervical length by ultrasound may all be helpful in identification of women at risk for premature labor; however, a perfect screening tool does not exist (Norwitz & Caughey, 2011). Even women with several risk factors may not deliver prematurely. Currently, exciting research is ongoing to attempt to unlock the secrets of premature labor. Large-scale studies aim to identify potential biological pathways of spontaneous preterm labor (PTL) through exploration of contributions of maternal and fetal gene–gene or gene–environment interactions to PTL. Other studies seek to identify and track biomarkers of stress or infection, or to identify polymorphisms of candidate genes that may help provide early identification of women at risk for PTL (Muglia & Katz, 2010; Williamson et al., 2008).

In order to have the best chances for survival, many preterm infants require intensive medical treatment and nursing care. There are differences in how preterm infants are medically treated in high-income and low-income nations. The high cost of providing neonatal intensive care for vulnerable preterm infants adds a huge financial burden to the health care system. As gestational age decreases, the overall costs of care increases. Care costs more for extremely preterm infants who require more diagnostic or medical procedures, medications, and longer hospital stays (Blosky et al., 2010). The Institute of Medicine (IOM, 2007) estimates that the care of infants born at less than 28 weeks gestation costs as much as 20 times that of infants born at 32 to 37 weeks gestation. Preterm infants are also more at risk for hospital readmission within 6 weeks of birth, adding more to the financial burden (Martens, Derksen, & Gupta, 2004). There are additional societal costs of prematurity which are seldom entered into the equation, such as early intervention services, special education, and disability services for infants who survive with residual problems and loss of productivity by parents and caregivers (IOM, 2007). The reality is that not all countries have the infrastructure or finances to aggressively treat all preterm infants. Some cultures are more accepting of infant death than others and do not expect all infants to survive no matter what the cost. However, there are some initial interventions that can be performed in any setting which can increase chances of survival for many premature infants, even in lower income nations.

Birth Weight and IUGR

Birth weight is one of the most important determinants of the infant's future health (WHO et al., 2012). LBW is defined as an initial birth weight of less than 2,500 g and is further categorized as either very low birth weight (VLBW) or extremely low birth weight (ELBW). VLBW is defined as an initial birth weight of less than 1,500 g, and ELBW is defined as birth weight of less than 1,000 g. Ideally birth weight should be measured within the first hour of birth before significant postnatal losses occur. In some cases, when the infant is in distress, the birth weight might be estimated until an accurate weight can be determined. The incidence of LBW in the United States is about 8.7% (Mathews, Miniño, Osterman, Strobino, & Guyer, 2011). LBW infants are at higher risk for neonatal and postnatal morbidity and mortality. Being born LBW has implications for health as an adult and has been linked to obesity, hypertension, diabetes mellitus, and decreased fertility later in adult life (Okah, Cai, & Hoff, 2005). While survival for ELBW infants has improved with advances in neonatal care, the risk for neurodevelopmental impairment has increased (Wilson-Costello, Friedman, Minich, Fanaroff, & Hack, 2005). As many as 50% of children born extremely preterm or at ELBW have residual effects of prematurity with cognitive, academic, or psychological problems when they are of school age (Anderson & Doyle, 2003).

The macrosomic or large for gestational age (LGA) fetus also has risks. Pregnancy risk factors for being LGA include maternal obesity, maternal age older than 35, maternal diabetes, prolonged pregnancy longer than 41 weeks, abnormally tall or short maternal stature, and male fetus. Potential complications for the mother include prolonged labor with increased risk for cephalopelvic disproportion and need for cesarean section. During vaginal delivery, the LGA infant is at a five times risk for injury as the result of shoulder dystocia due to fracture of the clavicle or brachial plexus injury (Nahum, Talavera, Legro, Gaupp, & Smith, 2011). After delivery, the macrosomic infant is at risk for hypoglycemia, polycythemia, and hyperbilirubinemia.

After birth, the neonate's weight, frontal occipital head circumference, and length at birth are plotted on a graph to evaluate appropriateness of growth based on gestational age. Gestational age can be based upon maternal history, ultrasound, or physical assessment. The infant is categorized as appropriate for gestational age (AGA) if birth weight falls between the 10th and 90th percentile for their gestational age; small for gestational age (SGA) if birth weight falls into the lower 10th percentile for weight based upon gestational age; or LGA if birth weight is greater than 90th percentile for weight based upon gestational age, or more than 4,000 g. Identification of infants who are SGA or LGA helps assure they receive proper monitoring of blood glucose and early feedings if indicated.

Before birth, an estimated fetal weight (EFW) can be determined via ultrasound. As many as 40% of fetuses who are classified as SGA (i.e., EFW below 10% for growth) might actually be healthy and genetically small. Another 20% may be intrinsically small secondary to a chromosomal or environmental condition such as trisomy 18, fetal alcohol syndrome (FAS), or infection, such as cytomegalovirus. The remaining 40% have increased perinatal risk and have IUGR (Ross, Mansano, Talavera, & Smith, 2011).

IUGR can be caused by maternal, fetal, or placental problems. Maternal causes include conditions such as preeclampsia; smoking or taking certain drugs can result in progressive uteroplacental insufficiency and limit the normal delivery of oxygen and nutrients to the fetus. Inadequate maternal nutrition, low prepregnancy weight, low weight gain in pregnancy, or inadequate prenatal care are other maternal causes of IUGR. Fetal conditions that can contribute to IUGR include fetal genetic factors, congenital infection, intrauterine crowding from multiple pregnancy, Rh isoimmunization, or twin-to-twin transfusion. Placental causes of IUGR include cord pathology, placental infarcts, or implantation issues such as placenta previa or abruption placenta (Faraci et al., 2011; Ross et al., 2011). Severe uteroplacental insufficiency restricts blood flow to the fetus and affects fetal growth and oxygenation. To spare function of vital organs, the fetus enters a brain-sparing mode which accounts for changes in fetal growth. Oxygen and nutrients are prioritized to the brain, heart, adrenals, and placenta, away from the kidneys, lungs, muscles, bone marrow, and gastrointestinal tract (Ross et al., 2011).

Fetuses with IUGR must be identified and closely monitored with nonstress testing, biophysical profiles, amniotic fluid volume estimates, contraction stress tests, and Doppler studies of maternal and umbilical vessels. Preterm IUGR with the presence of oligohydramnios (amniotic fluid volume index <5) or abnormal umbilical Doppler results (absent or reverse end-diastolic flow) were modestly predictive of poor perinatal outcomes (Scifres, Stamilo, Macones, & Obido, 2009). Early delivery is indicated if signs of fetal stress or distress are present. After birth, infants with IUGR often have problems with low blood glucose or thermoregulation due to a lack of subcutaneous fat. They also are at increased risk for necrotizing enterocolitis, thrombocytopenia, and renal failure because during fetal development, blood was shunted away from the gastrointestinal and renal system to the brain, heart, and other vital organs as a protective mechanism. IUGR infants whose birth weights fall within the third to fifth percentile for gestational age are more at risk for adverse outcomes (Zhang, Merialdi, Platt, & Kramer, 2010). IUGR infants who are exposed to suboptimal conditions in utero are more at risk as adults to develop a metabolic syndrome with adult type 2 diabetes, obesity, hypertension, hypercholesterolemia, and heart disease (Barker, 2006; Joss-Moore & Lane, 2009; Ross et al., 2011).

IMR

It is estimated that 86% of all newborn deaths worldwide are due to one of three causes: infection, asphyxia, and PTB (United Nations Children's Fund [UNICEF], 2009). Neonatal deaths during the first 28 days of life account for 40% of deaths of children under age 5 (WHO et al., 2012). Worldwide, one million infants die in the first month of life because of prematurity (Muglia & Katz, 2010). The world IMR is estimated at 42.09 deaths per 1,000 live births (Central Intelligence Agency [CIA], 2012). Infants from low- or middle-income countries represent 98% of all neonatal deaths within the first 28 days of life (UNICEF, 2009). Reducing neonatal deaths will have a major impact on progress toward achieving the United Nations MDG 4, which aims to reduce child mortality worldwide. Because of a high percentage of PTBs, the United States ranked 30th internationally in infant mortality in 2005, lagging behind many European countries (MacDorman & Mathews, 2011). Differences in interpretation of what constitutes fetal viability can account for some differences in how neonatal deaths are reported.

The U.S. IMR in 2008 was 5.98 infant deaths per 1,000 live births (CIA, 2012). The leading causes of infant mortality in the United States differ from worldwide causes of infant mortality and include: (1) congenital malformations, deformations, and chromosomal abnormalities; (2) disorders related to short gestation and LBW, not elsewhere classified; and (3) sudden infant death syndrome (SIDS) (Murphy, Xu, & Kochanek, 2012). The highest IMR rate was reported in infants born to NHB mothers (13.35 deaths per 1,000 live births) as compared with infants born to NHW mothers (5.58 per 1,000 live births) (Mathews et al., 2011). Based on 2007 birth data in the United States, infants of NHB mothers have a 2.4 higher rate of infant mortality for all causes and a 3.9 higher rate of infant mortality due to consequences of LBW as compared with infants of NHW mothers (MacDorman, Mathews, National Center for Health Statistics & Centers for Disease Control, 2011). Disparities also exist within the Hispanic population based upon country of origin. Infant mortality for infants of Hispanic mothers ranged from 4.8 deaths/1,000 live births for infants of mothers from Central and South American to 7.7 deaths/1,000 live births for infants of Puerto Rican mothers, which was a 1.4 higher risk of infant mortality for infants of Puerto Rican mothers (MacDorman et al., 2011). In 2008, the IMR for multiple births was 28.73, five times that of singleton births (5.83) (Mathews & MacDorman, 2012).

Ethnic disparities are also evident related to neonatal mortality during the first 28 days of life. Comparison rates for NHB and NHW infants for the three leading causes of neonatal death show infants will demonstrate the disparities that exist. Infants of NHB mothers had the highest rate of neonatal deaths related to prematurity or LBW (2.99 deaths/1,000 live births) as compared with infants of NHW mothers (0.76 deaths/1,000 live births), while infants of Asian or Pacific Islander mothers had the lowest rate (0.59 deaths/1,000 live births). Infants of NHB mothers had the highest rate (1.20 deaths/1,000 live births) of neonatal deaths due to congenital malformations as compared with infants of NHW mothers (0.95 deaths/1,000 live births), and infants of Asian or Pacific Islander mothers had the lowest rate (0.57 deaths/1,000 live births). Infants of NHB mothers had the highest neonatal death rate (0.90 deaths/1,000 live births) due to being affected by maternal complications of pregnancy as compared with infants of NHW mothers (0.32 deaths/1,000 live births); infants of Asian or Pacific Islander mothers had the lowest rate (0.19 deaths/1,000 live births) (Hauck, Tanabe, & Moon, 2011).

Preterm infants account for most neonatal deaths, and if they do survive have increased risks for morbidity. Prematurity and LBW place infants at an increased risk for disability, neonatal death, or the development of lifetime chronic health problems. Prevention of PTB and LBW has the potential to save lives, prevent long-term health problems associated with prematurity, and provide significant savings of health care dollars.

Epidemiologic Paradox

Birth outcomes can't always be predicted by the presence of maternal risk or sociodemographic factors (MacDorman & Mathews, 2011). For example, Mexican women who immigrate to the United States have demographic and socioeconomic factors such as high rates of teen pregnancy, less educated mothers, and higher rates of no prenatal care or late prenatal care in the third trimester that put them at high risk for poor perinatal outcomes. On the other hand, Asian Indian women who immigrate to the United States have demographic and socioeconomic risk factors similar to White women that put them at low risk. Asian Indian women have higher education levels with more college graduates, less teenaged pregnancy, and are more likely to get adequate prenatal care. However an "epidemiologic paradox" occurs, and outcomes do not occur as predicted. African American women have the highest incidence of LBW, SGA, and fetal and neonatal deaths in the United States at rates almost twice that of White women. Foreign-born Mexican women with demographic and socioeconomic risk factors comparable to African American women have better than expected perinatal outcomes, including less LBW and less neonatal deaths than White women. In comparison, Asian Indian women have higher incidences of prematurity, LBW, SGA, and fetal death than White women. This "epidemiologic paradox" suggests that there might be other factors that give foreign-born women either a perinatal advantage or disadvantage such as environmental factors, diet or lifestyle factors, or genetic factors (Gould, Madan, Qin, & Chavez, 2003).

MATERNAL RISK FACTORS

Evaluation of maternal risk factors can help anticipate many of the neonates who will be at increased risk for problems at birth. There is no way to accurately predict every neonate who will be at risk since a cause-and-effect relationship between high-risk maternal characteristics or behaviors and poor outcomes is not always clearly defined. For example, there have been cases of identical twins where one twin was born healthy and the other one required admission to the neonatal intensive care unit (NICU). Although both babies had similar genetic makeup, gestational age, and exposure to the same in utero environment, only one of them had problems.

One of the most essential ways to decrease problems of prematurity, LBW, and perinatal death is to promote optimal pregnancy health. The ideal state is for all women considering pregnancy to seek preconceptual counseling. During the preconceptual visit, the woman can learn about risk factors that could potentially cause birth defects or problems with pregnancy. Risk factors may be either modifiable or nonmodifiable. Examples of modifiable risk factors that can be changed include diet, smoking, alcohol use, or substance abuse. Nonmodifiable risk factors are intrinsic factors that can't be changed such as maternal age, ethnicity, genetic inheritance, or preexisting health problems. Risk factors usually do not occur in isolation. The presence of one risk factor may lead to other risk factors causing an additive effect. For example, a pregnant woman who lacks financial resources might also have a poor obstetric history, an inadequate nutritional intake, increased stress, and nicotine addiction. Some maternal risk factors can be modified through patient education, counseling, lifestyle changes, and support. The purpose of preconceptual care is to help the woman who is contemplating pregnancy get into optimal physical condition for childbearing prior to conception. Unfortunately, preconceptual counseling is not the norm. Therefore, all women of childbearing age must be encouraged to live healthy lifestyles and to seek early prenatal care in the first trimester of pregnancy. Even the first trimester of pregnancy is not too late to implement interventions or modify lifestyle risk factors that will maximize positive pregnancy outcomes.

Maternal risk factors consist of demographic, behavioral, and psychosocial factors, as well as maternal medical conditions and pregnancy related conditions. Demographic risk factors include ethnicity, age, socioeconomic status, occupation, and environmental or work-related exposures. Psychosocial risk factors include social, behavioral, stress-related, or maternal psychological conditions. The IOM categorizes medical risk factors for prematurity into immutable factors which can't be changed and mutable factors which can possibly be altered (Alexander, 2007). Examples of immutable factors include factors which predate the pregnancy such as obstetric history (i.e., previous history of infertility, PTB, or pregnancy loss), maternal characteristics such as short stature, low prepregnancy weight, low body mass index (BMI), or pregnancy-related conditions that only happen during pregnancy such as multiple gestation, pregnancy-induced hypertension (PIH), or gestational diabetes. Mutable risk factors include behavioral risk factors the mother has either prior to or during pregnancy that can possibly be harmful to the fetus, such as inadequate dietary intake, smoking, or substance abuse (drugs or alcohol).

A complete maternal history done at the first prenatal visit will help identify important demographic and medical risk factors that might influence the outcomes of the pregnancy. A variety of demographic factors are related to neonatal outcomes. The presence of risk factors should serve as a warning. Many women with identifiable high-risk factors will give birth to healthy infants without problems. The potential influence of demographic risk factors of age, ethnicity, obstetric history, and the health-compromising behaviors (HCBs) of nutrition, smoking, alcohol, and drug use upon pregnancy will be further discussed.

Maternal Age

Maternal age is considered to be a risk factor for poor perinatal outcomes at either end of the childbearing age spectrum. The maternal childbearing age range has widened over the past decade partially due to advances in assisted reproductive technology (ART) that have made it possible for women to achieve pregnancy, even into the fifth or sixth decade of life, if desired. Worldwide, the maternal age at the time of the birth of the first child ranges from an average of 15.5 to 20.5 years in traditional forager, agricultural, and horticultural societies and from 25.1 to 29.9 years in more developed nations (Kramer & Lancaster, 2010).

There is conflicting evidence that teen pregnancy increases the risk of adverse outcomes. Some adverse outcomes could be due to societal socioeconomic conditions. Teen mothers may have up to a twofold risk of adverse outcomes from pregnancy such as preterm delivery, LBW, low 5-minute Apgar score, or early neonatal death (Kongnyuy et al., 2008). Adverse perinatal outcomes are more likely in very young teen mothers (Kramer & Lancaster, 2010). Adolescent mothers younger than age 15 are considered to be especially high risk because they are biologically immature, and their growing body is competing with the fetus for nutrient resources. They have not had the chance to complete their own physical growth and reproductive development. If teens become pregnant within 2 years of menarche, they are reproductively immature which can increase risks of a fetal loss, PTB, or infant death (Fraser, Brockert, & Ward, 1995).

In 2010, the U.S. teen birth rates for ages 15 to 19 years declined dramatically to its lowest point since 1946 to a rate of 34.4 births per 1,000 births (Hamilton, Martin, & Ventura, 2011). Even so, the United States has one of the highest teen birth rates worldwide compared with other developed nations. Numbers of teen and adolescent births globally are difficult to estimate, but rates are higher in countries where child marriage is allowed. However, there are many countries where unmarried teen pregnancy rates are high. Teen mothers and their infants have increased perinatal risks including higher risk of dying during childbirth as compared with 20-year-old women. Infants of teen mothers have a 60% increased risk of dying within the first year of life (Rowbottom, 2007). There are also lifelong disadvantages for younger teen mothers who have less years of formal education. Education is known to be a factor related to promotion of positive pregnancy behaviors. Pregnant adolescents who are uneducated most likely will not use contraception, may not recognize danger signs in pregnancy that something is wrong, or may not even seek prenatal care. In the United States, teen mothers are more likely to be unmarried and therefore require financial support for the pregnancy from parents or social agencies. In 2010, 88% of teen mothers were not married at the time of the birth (Hamilton et al., 2011). Many teen mothers find it difficult to return to school full time once they assume the parenting role without support or help with day care from their parents. Dropping out of school can destine them to a lifetime of working in low-paying jobs unless they complete their education. Some teen girls drop out of school or leave home due to poor family relationships even before getting pregnant. Preexisting maternal disadvantages, not young maternal age, are more likely to account for negative outcomes of teen parenting for mothers and infants (Smith-Battle, 2006). After birth, infants of younger mothers (< 19 years of age) had an increased risk for readmission to the hospital within the first 6 weeks after newborn discharge (Martens et al., 2004). Teen mothers are also more likely to have a repeat teen pregnancy. In 2010, about 19% of teen births in the United States were the mother's second, third, or fourth child (Hamilton et al., 2011).

Advanced maternal age refers to women who are older than 35 at the estimated date of delivery. Women may have problems conceiving secondary to infertility, or some women may choose to delay childbearing voluntarily while pursuing educational or professional goals. A recent trend has been an increase in the number of women in the advanced maternal age group who are having babies. Advances in reproductive science, such as oocyte donation, have made it possible for women who are postmenopausal in their 50s or 60s to conceive. The birth rate for women ages 40 to 44 was 9.9 births per 1,000 women and the birth rate for women ages 45 to 49 increased in 2008 to 0.7 births per 1,000 women (Mathews et al., 2011). Advanced maternal age poses increased risks for decreased fertility, chromosomal abnormalities in the infant, spontaneous abortion, ectopic pregnancy, preterm delivery, or stillbirth (Andersen, Wohlfahrt, Christens, Olsen, & Melbye, 2000; Cleary-Goldman et al., 2005; Heffner, 2004; Salihu, Wilson, Alio, & Kirby, 2008; Yaniv et al., 2011). Late fetal and early perinatal death rates are higher for pregnant women between ages 45 and 54 than for any other age groups. Pregnant women older than 45 have a rate of spontaneous abortion that is nine times higher than pregnant women between the ages of 20 to 24 (Andersen et al., 2000). Women older than 40 are at increased risk for placental abruption and perinatal mortality (Cleary-Goldman et al., 2005). Although fertility tends to decline with advanced maternal age, women between the ages of 35 and 39 actually have an increased risk of conceiving twins without the assistance of fertility treatments, another factor that increases their risk status (Andersen et al., 2000). Women over age 45 are at more risk to have a preterm infant than younger age groups at each gestational age (i.e., <32 weeks, <34 weeks, and <37 weeks). Older women also are more likely to have multifetal pregnancies due to use of assistive reproductive technologies which could account for the increased prematurity rates (Yogev et al., 2010).

Older pregnant women are at an increased risk for medical problems associated with aging such as diabetes or PIH (Yaniv et al., 2011). The rates of medical complications including gestational diabetes and preeclampsia toxemia were reported to be significantly higher in pregnant woman over age 45, and risk increases as maternal age advances (Yaniv et al., 2011; Yogev et al., 2010). Diabetes increases their risk for delivery of a macrosomic infant. They also have increased risks for placenta previa, preterm delivery, or delivery of a LBW infant (Aliyu et al., 2005; Ananth, Wilcox, Savitz, Bowes, & Luther, 1996). Women older than 40 tended to gain less weight during pregnancy, a factor that could contribute to the increased risk of LBW.

Some studies have not found any worse outcomes due to increased maternal age. Some women as old as 60 years of age have had healthy pregnancies and healthy infants. Kanungo et al. (2011) reported that neonates born to older mothers had improved odds of survival without major morbidity or mortality due to conditions such as bronchopulmonary dysplasia, necrotizing enterocolitis, or sepsis. Possibly older women who choose to get pregnant make a conscious decision to get pregnant, start pregnancy in optimal health, are well educated, have better social and economic support, and have increased surveillance and medical care during pregnancy.

Advanced maternal age creates genetic risks because as the woman gets older the genetic material contained within her ova ages. The prevailing theory is that all females are born with all of the oocytes they will ever have which contain the genetic material that she will pass on to her progeny. According to maternal aging theory, as the woman ages, her oocytes and the genetic material contained within also age. Aging genetic material is more likely to have errors occur during cell division and migration during meiosis that can result in aneuploidy (an abnormal number of chromosomes), lower implantation rates, decreased fertility, or increased risk of spontaneous abortion (Gleicher, Weghofer, & Barad, 2011). Trisomy 21 (Down syndrome), trisomy 18, and trisomy 13 are examples of genetic problems resulting from errors in cell division. The risk for having an infant with Down syndrome increases with advanced maternal age. For example, a 30-year-old woman's risk to have an infant with Down syndrome is 1 in 885, at age 35 the risk is 1 in 365, and at age 40 the risk is 1 in 109 (Hook & Lindsjo, 1978).

PATERNAL FACTORS

Certain paternal factors have been associated with adverse perinatal outcomes. Extremes of paternal age—younger than 20 years or older than 40 years—may be associated with LBW (Shah et al., 2010). Advanced paternal age greater than 45 has been associated with increased risk of stillbirth (Amina et al., 2012). Advanced paternal age should also be considered when evaluating prenatal risks, as it has been associated with rare congenital anomalies in offspring due to dominant mutations such as neural tube defects, congenital cataracts, upper limb reduction defects, and Down syndrome (MacIntosh, Olshan, & Baird, 1995). Older fathers are more likely to have offspring with autosomal dominant genetic conditions such as Marfan syndrome, achondroplasia, Huntington's chorea, and von Willebrand disease (Heffner, 2004). A careful assessment of family history of both parents will help alert the health care provider to these potential risks.

Paternal environmental or occupational exposure to certain chemicals can lead to developmental outcomes including PTB, altered growth, structural or functional abnormalities, or death. Some effects may be expressed across the lifetime of the child (Mattison, 2010). High levels of paternal occupational exposure to lead have been linked to LBW and PTB (Shah et al., 2010). Paternal exposure to environmental toxins may not only affect fetal development but may have consequences for the child throughout his or her lifetime (Mattison, 2010).

LIFE COURSE DETERMINANTS OF BIRTH OUTCOMES AND WEATHERING

The life course theory (LCT) is an approach being used to explain health, disease, and health disparities across populations and over time. Rather than focusing on ethnic or genetic differences or an individual's choices to explain health disparities, the LCT focuses on social, economic, and environmental factors as key determinants that help shape health or disease in communities and populations. The LCT acknowledges the importance of intergenerational preprogramming (i.e., maternal preconceptual health) and prenatal preprogramming (i.e., the in utero environment) in influencing fetal and child health. While health can be impacted at any time, there are critical and sensitive periods when events can have a maximal impact on lifetime health such as during fetal development, early childhood, or adolescence. The goal would be to promote interventions during these sensitive times to maximize health (U.S. Department of Health and Human Services [USDHHS], 2010).

Applying the LCT perspective to preterm delivery would propose that reproductive and birth outcomes are the product of circumstances and events that occur not only during pregnancy but throughout the life of the mother, beginning either before or at the time when she was conceived. The LCT perspective acknowledges the possibility that early-life experiences can shape health across an entire lifetime and could potentially influence the health of future generations (Braveman & Barclay, 2009). According to the LCT perspective, it is not enough to assess the woman's experiences during the immediate preconceptual and prenatal period to determine risks for poor outcomes. Assessment of major events during her entire life course and the effects of material deprivation, social disadvantage, discrimination, and marginalization must be explored. The health consequences of poverty and race-based discrimination and the health effects of chronic stress from having inadequate resources to meet demands must also be considered. For example, exposure to poor nutrition as a child, or even as a developing fetus could impact a woman's pregnancy outcomes. The life course perspective aligns with the developmental origins of health and disease approach which posits the important role of the fetal in utero environment in development of structure and functions of organs of the body. For example, a lack of folic acid during development can lead to neural tube defects; exposure to tobacco can lead to LBW or short gestation; and exposure to maternal antidepressants may cause cardiac malformations, alter neonatal blood pressure, or change infant behavior (Swanson, Entringer, Buss, & Wadhwa, 2009). Components of a perinatal life course risk assessment tool are not yet developed; however, this area of study offers intriguing promise to unravel some possible explanations for health care disparities.

PSYCHOLOGICAL STRESS IN PREGNANCY

Maternal mental health and psychological stress are increasingly being studied as possible sources of adverse perinatal outcomes. Stress is an interaction between the person and environment in which there is a perceived discrepancy between the demands of the environment and the individual's resources (i.e., psychological, social, or biological) for dealing with it. During pregnancy women may experience many types of stressors. Life stressors include stress about finances, work situations, difficult relationships, health concerns of self or other family members, or other factors. Emotional stress may include feelings of anxiety, fear, tension, depressions, or sadness (Tegethoff, Greene, Olsen, Schaffner, & Meinlschmidt, 2011). Acute stressors during pregnancy include situational crisis or natural disasters. There is a growing body of evidence related to the effects of acute and chronic maternal stress during pregnancy on gestational length and birth weight. Other evidence points to associations between preconceptual stress and accumulated life stress on birth outcomes.

Acute stressors can occur due to life events such as the death or serious illness of a loved one. Death of the father of the developing fetus or of a first-degree relative of the mother during mid-pregnancy was found to be related to shortened gestation, LBW, and SGA (Class, Lichtenstein, Langstrom, & D'Onofrio, 2011). Timing of the stressor during the pregnancy seemed to predict the outcome. There was increased risk for shortened gestation if the stressor occurred in the fourth or fifth month of pregnancy, while vulnerability to LBW or SGA increased if the stressor happened in the fifth or sixth month of pregnancy (Class et al., 2011). Another study reported maternal exposure to severe life events, such as death or serious illness in close relatives as early as 6 months before conception increased the risk of PTB or very PTB (Khashan et al., 2009). Studies of pregnant women who experience economic shocks, such as job loss or downturns in the economy and natural disasters such as earthquakes during the first trimester, have demonstrated a relationship between these acute stressors and LBW (Margerison-Zilko, Catalano, Hubbard, & Ahern, 2011; Torche, 2011).

Pregnancy-related anxiety is a form of anxiety specific to pregnant women and includes worries about the health and well-being of the baby, impending labor and birth, hospital and health care experiences and one's own health and survival, and about parenting and the maternal role. Based on several large-scale studies, pregnancy-related anxiety is emerging as a risk factor for PTB in African American, Hispanic, and White populations (Dunkel Schetter, 2011). Pregnancy-specific stress includes: (1) positive or negative feelings about the pregnancy, (2) pregnancy-related concerns about the health of the baby, labor, and delivery or body size and body image, (3) pregnancy-specific support, and (4) pregnancy-related symptoms and attitudes toward whether the current pregnancy was intended or wanted (Wadhwa, Entringer, Buss, & Lu, 2011). There may be critical periods during fetal development where there is increased vulnerability to the effects of maternal stress (Wadhwa et al., 2011).

Major stressors such as life events, major catastrophes, chronic strain, neighborhood stress, and multiple stressors contribute to PTB, gestational age, or gestational length. The exact mechanism by which maternal stress causes PTL is not fully understood, but it is thought to occur by one of two mechanisms. Corticotrophin-releasing hormone released as a by-product of maternal stress could stimulate neuroendocrine pathways within the maternal-fetal-placental unit that trigger labor; or maternal stress could cause increased maternal and fetal susceptibility to inflammation and infection, triggering labor through an immune-inflammatory pathway (Hogue & Bremner, 2005; Rich-Edwards & Grizzard, 2005). These interactions between neuroendocrine, immune, and behavioral processes may be tempered by maternal resilience resources (ego strength, personality, social, coping, cultural values, and world view) and endowed factors (health, height, weight, and childhood socioeconomic status [SES]), (Dunkel Schetter, 2011). Hardiness, resilience, and social support might act as stress buffers in some women, lessening the impact of stress (Patrick & Bryan, 2005).

Not all women are affected in the same way by stress, which could account for difficulty with prediction of outcomes. Critical periods may occur during pregnancy where there is altered vulnerability to the effects of prenatal stress. Women reporting high levels of psychosocial stress in pregnancy as compared to those reporting low levels of stress have a 25% to 60% increased risk for PTB (Wadhwa et al., 2011).

The cumulative effects of lifetime exposure to acute stress and experiences of chronic day-to-day stress increase the risk of stress-related disease during pregnancy and may help explain some ethnic disparities in birth outcomes (Hogue & Bremner, 2005). Noting that infants of teenaged African American women had a survival advantage over infants of older African American women Geronimus (1992) proposed maternal "weathering" or premature aging caused by stress (stress age), as a possible explanation for this disparity. The weathering hypothesis proposes that socioeconomic disadvantage contributes to an earlier decline in the health of African American women, including the reproductive system. Therefore, if women delay childbearing past this optimal time, then their aging reproductive systems do not function as efficiently (Geronimus, 1996). Furthermore, prepregnancy chronic stress might lead to accelerated physiological aging of the female reproductive system thus leading to poor pregnancy outcomes. Women who experience added stress during pregnancy have increased risks for delivery of preterm or LBW infants due to the decreased efficiency of their reproductive systems (Rich-Edwards, Buka, Brennan, & Earls, 2003). While more research is needed to test the weathering hypothesis, it aligns well with the life course perspective and offers a promising direction to explain ethnic disparities related to PTB and LBW.

The added stress of being Black and subject to racial discrimination has been proposed as another possible cause of ethnic disparities in perinatal outcomes. Experiences with racial and gender discrimination and violence are encountered by many Black American women throughout their life course. Racial discrimination may be a chronic stressor which contributes to racial disparities in birth outcomes and has been linked to PTB, LBW, and VLBW (Giurgescu, McFarlin, Lomax, Craddock, & Albrecht, 2011). Childhood experiences with discrimination seem to stand out and have enduring effects on these women. They anticipate future racial encounters will occur or that they will be treated unfairly; therefore they are in a chronic hypervigilant state which could have effects on multiple organs or immune defenses which could affect birth outcomes (Nuru-Jeter et al., 2009). Black American women also experience added stress during pregnancy due to having multiple identities as women, Black, and pregnant, which subjects them to stereotype threats. They experience added distress, and worry that they are being perceived in a negative, stereotypical manner, such as being thought of as a "welfare mom" when they are pregnant (Rosenthal & Lobel, 2011). Due to increased lifetime stress, Black American women may experience increased "stress age" that could influence pregnancy outcomes, which are stress sensitive. Researchers have established links between some pregnancy-related diseases and later chronic illness, such as women with gestational diabetes have an increased risk for type 2 diabetes later in life, lending support to weathering. A possible explanation is that poor pregnancy outcomes represent initial signs of aging of the endocrine, immune, and reproductive systems (Rich-Edwards & Grizzard, 2005). The "weathering hypothesis" offers an interesting explanation for the increased incidence of preterm delivery and LBW infants for older childbearing women or women who are under stress. As we learn more about the impact of psychological stressors on pregnancy outcomes, this life course perspective makes sense. These theories may be worth exploring in other countries where disparities in birth outcomes exist, including poverty, racial or gender discrimination, or violence against women.

OBSTETRIC FACTORS

Obstetric history is a good indicator of the presence of maternal risk factors. Women with previous obstetric complications are more at risk for problems with the current pregnancy. Previous obstetric history of infertility, stillbirth, preterm infant, infant with growth restriction or congenital anomalies/genetic problems, complications during pregnancy or birth, or other poor outcomes are clues that indicate that the pregnancy must be closely monitored. Prepregnancy health status is another factor associated with the risk of preterm delivery. Women who are in poor physical condition prior to conception (i.e., underweight, having poor prepregnancy physical function, chronic hypertension, or smoking before pregnancy) have an increased risk for preterm delivery (Haas et al., 2005). Important obstetric factors that can compound pregnancy risk are the adequacy of prenatal care, the number of previous pregnancies, interpregnancy level, the use of assistive reproductive technology (ART), and postterm pregnancy.

PRENATAL CARE

Prenatal care that begins in the first trimester of pregnancy and continues until birth helps promote good birth outcomes. Most women seek prenatal care during the first trimester of pregnancy. Only about 8% of U.S. women start prenatal care during the last trimester or have no prenatal care, with higher rates of late or no prenatal care seen in NHB and Hispanic women as compared with NHW women (Mathews et al., 2011). UNICEF and WHO have set a worldwide goal for a minimum of four prenatal visits during pregnancy. Worldwide, approximately 72% of women have at least one prenatal visit, and 42% of women (excluding China) have four or more prenatal visits (UNICEF, 2009).

Inadequate prenatal care increases the risk for LBW, PTB, and perinatal death (Fraser et al., 1995; Vintzileos, Ananth, Smulian, Scorza, & Knuppel, 2002). High postneonatal death rates seen in infants of women who did not have prenatal care might be associated with lack of access to care providers or lack of use of pediatric medical care (Vintzileos et al., 2002).

The decision to seek prenatal care is influenced by the woman's attitudes toward pregnancy, cultural preference, or lifestyle factors. For some women, access to prenatal care is limited due to financial constraints or geographic availability of a trained practitioner. Having six prenatal visits prior to delivery was a protective factor against LBW and prematurity. A systematic review and meta-analysis of women who received group prenatal care demonstrated lower rates of PTB than for women who had traditional prenatal care, although there were no differences in incidence of LBW or IUGR between the groups (Ruiz-Mirazo, Lopez-Yarto, & McDonald, 2012).

Providing care of the mother at delivery by a skilled birth attendant could also improve outcomes through early recognition of problems during labor and intervention. Worldwide there are many countries where a majority of women deliver at home with or without assistance of a trained practitioner. Countries with the highest rates of unattended births also have the highest rates of infant mortality (UNICEF, 2009). The United Nations MDG 5 seeks to provide universal access for all women to reproductive care including access to prenatal care and family planning information.

PARITY

Parity or number of previous deliveries is another risk factor to consider. Parity is difficult to disassociate from age as women with higher parity are usually older. The risk for having a LBW infant, a preterm delivery, an abruptio placenta, or placenta previa increases as parity increases (Aliyu et al., 2005). In general primiparous women older than 35 years of age and multiparous teens younger than 18 years of age have an increased risk for PTB at any gestational length; however, there are some racial differences. Both primiparous and multiparous Black and Hispanic women have an increased risk for very PTB starting at a younger age (25 years). Primiparous teenagers tend to have the highest risk of having an extremely PTB (EPTB). The incidence of EPTB is higher in older primiparous Black and Hispanic women as compared with teenagers. On the other hand, in White women EPTB risk is highest at either end of the age spectrum for both teenagers and older primiparas. However, for all races, the risks for any type of PTB increase as women are older than 40 years of age (Schempf, Branum, Lukacs, & Schoendorf, 2007).

INTERPREGNANCY LEVEL

Interpregnancy level is defined as the amount of time between delivery of a baby and the subsequent conception of another child. Short interpregnancy level of less than 6 months increases the risk for maternal complications, including third-trimester bleeding, PROM, puerperal endometritis, anemia, and maternal death. Women with longer interpregnancy levels have the highest risk for preeclampsia, eclampsia, and gestational diabetes, again probably related to older maternal age. The risk for prematurity is increased when the interpregnancy level is less than 18 months or greater than 59 months (Fuentes-Afflick & Hessol, 2000). Worldwide, increasing the interpregnancy level to 24 months or more would help decrease numbers of prematurity, LBW, and neonatal deaths (UNICEF, 2009).

ASSISTIVE REPRODUCTIVE TECHNOLOGY

ART is any procedure or medical treatment used to assist a woman to achieve pregnancy. ART is an option for many couples who have a history of infertility. ART methods include the use of medications to stimulate ovulation and release of eggs, or procedures where eggs and sperm are removed and mixed outside of the body to achieve fertilization. Some techniques require that the fertilized egg remain outside the body for a few days before being implanted back into the woman's body. In some cases, the eggs, sperm, or embryos might be frozen for later use or manipulated with instrumentation during the earliest stages of cell formation.

According to the Centers for Disease Control (CDC), about 1% of U.S. pregnancies are conceived using ART (CDC, 2011). ART increases the risk for multiple pregnancy, prematurity, and LBW. Most types of ART procedures result in high rates of multiple pregnancies since couples may choose to have multiple embryos implanted to maximize their chances for success. In 2006, 49% of ART pregnancies were multiples as compared with 3% in the general U.S. population. As numbers of fetuses increased, the risk of prematurity increased. For example, 14% of singleton births after ART were delivered prematurely as compared with 65% of ART twins and 95% of ART triplets (Sunderam et al., 2009). Multiple gestation pregnancy naturally increases risks for PTL, cesarean delivery, and LBW and provides one explanation for the increase in number of LBW and preterm infants over the past few years. However, the risk for prematurity and LBW exists for even singleton pregnancies conceived with ART (Lung, Shu, Chiang, & Lin, 2009). In 2006, about 13% of ART infants were born prematurely as compared with 11% in the general U.S. population. Additionally 9% of ART infants were LBW at birth as compared with 6% in the general population (Martin et al., 2009). A large Danish study compared infants of infertile couples who conceived either naturally or with ART and reported they had increased incidence of malformations of the nervous system, digestive system, and musculoskeletal system in both groups, pointing to a possible association between subinfertility and infertility and increased prevalence of congenital malformations in children. Congenital malformations in infants of untreated infertile couples who conceived naturally increased as the time to attain pregnancy increased. Infants who were conceived by ART had a higher incidence of genital organ malformations. Intracytoplasmic sperm injection, a procedure used with men who have suboptimal sperm counts or motility, was associated with a higher incidence of congenital malformations (Zhu, Basso, Obel, Bille, & Olsen, 2006). There have been case reports associating ART with rare imprinting disorders such as Beckwith–Wiedemann syndrome, Angelman syndrome, and retinoblastoma which require further studies (Manipalviratn, DeCherney, & Segars, 2009).

Couples who electively conceive through ART with a large number of embryos may have to make tough ethical decisions, including options for selective reduction later in the pregnancy, in order to protect the health of compromised fetuses. The risk for prematurity and LBW increases as numbers of fetuses increase, increasing risks of poor outcomes for the infants. The decision to maintain a pregnancy with a large number of fetuses can be economically and emotionally catastrophic for the family. Outcomes for the babies who survive depend in part upon the number of fetuses and gestational age at delivery. Some countries have set mandatory limits on the numbers of embryos that can be implanted during ART procedures to help address some of these issues (Green, 2004). Continued research to improve ART techniques to assure success of singleton pregnancies will do much to impact outcomes of ART pregnancies.

POSTTERM PREGNANCY

Postterm pregnancy is defined as a pregnancy that continues past 42 weeks (294 days) or 14 days past the estimated due date (American College of Obstetricians and Gynecologists [ACOG], 2004). Incidence is in about 7% of all pregnancies. The cause of postterm pregnancy is not known, but it occurs more often with male fetuses and may have a genetic basis. Some cases of postterm pregnancy can be attributed to inaccurate dates used to calculate the estimated date of confinement. Ultrasound dating of pregnancy is considered to be accurate if done during the first trimester; however, ultrasound dating of pregnancy has a margin of error.

Postterm infants are more likely to have macrosomia, with increased risks for prolonged labor or cephalopelvic disproportion (CPD) with increased risk for cesarean section, or shoulder dystocia with increased risks of possible musculoskeletal injury (i.e., fractured clavicle or brachial plexus injury). Postmaturity also predisposes to uteroplacental insufficiency in about 20% of cases. These infants present with chronic IUGR and are more at risk for cord compression due to oligohydramnios and presence of thick meconium (Morantz & Torrey, 2004). Adverse outcomes are more likely in the presence of oligohydramnios (ACOG, 2004). Postterm pregnancy has also been related to lower umbilical artery pH levels and lower Apgar scores (Caughey, Washington, & Laros, 2005). The risk for cesarean section due to nonreassuring heart rate or CPD increases weekly as gestational age goes beyond 39 weeks (Caughey, Stotland, Washington, & Escobar, 2007). ACOG recommends close surveillance of postterm pregnancies between 41 and 42 weeks due to increased risks of complications as gestational age advances. Postterm fetuses should be evaluated by nonstress testing or biophysical profiles. Delivery is not indicated as long as test results are reassuring (ACOG, 2004). Cervical ripening and induction of labor at 41 weeks is an alternative approach for management of postterm pregnancies (Norwitz, Snegovskikh, & Caughey, 2007).

HCBs

HCBs such as smoking, illicit drug use, or alcohol use can compromise overall maternal health during pregnancy and can negatively influence fetal well-being. Prepregnancy maternal health status and health behaviors may play a role in PTL risk. Babies born to mothers who smoke, drink alcohol, or take drugs weigh less than babies of mothers who do not smoke, drink, or take drugs (Okah et al., 2005). Inadequate nutrition, over-the-counter or prescribed drug consumption, and environmental factors may create other HCBs and increase risks during pregnancy.

Smoking

Smoking is a major predictor of LBW possibly due to impaired oxygen delivery (hypoxia) and nutrient delivery from the mother to fetus (Chiriboga, 2003). Infants of mothers who smoke have an increased risk of spontaneous abortion, late fetal death, preterm delivery, and neonatal mortality. Women who smoke are more likely to use alcohol or illicit drugs during pregnancy than those who do not smoke. Smoking rate during pregnancy has been estimated at 10.4% with ethnic variations. More NHW women (16.3%) smoke during pregnancy as compared with NHB women (10.1%) and Hispanic women (2.1%) (Mathews et al., 2011).

Substance Abuse

Substance abuse is a concern for childbearing women of all ages. More teenagers are experimenting with drugs, alcohol, and smoking cigarettes and marijuana than in the past (American Academy of Pediatrics [AAP], Committee on Child Health Financing and Committee on Substance Abuse, 2001). Marijuana smoking results in carbon monoxide levels five times higher than cigarette smoking, another factor that limits fetal growth and oxygenation (Chiriboga, 2003). Women under the influence of mind-altering substances are more likely to make poor choices and have an increased risk of engaging in unprotected sex resulting in an unplanned pregnancy.

Maternal alcohol ingestion during pregnancy can result in FAS. Incidence of FAS may be related to both environmental exposure and genetic susceptibility. Alcohol is believed to have a direct teratogenic effect that limits fetal growth and brain growth. According to the Substance Abuse and Mental Health Services Administration (SAMHSA), 10.8% of pregnant women between the ages of 15 and 44 report they currently use alcohol, 3.7% state they indulged in binge drinking, and 1.0% state they drank heavily (2011). The fetal effects of drinking are most pronounced if the fetus is exposed during the first trimester of pregnancy. The minimum amount of alcohol that is harmful to the fetal brain is not known. It is known that binge drinking (ingestion of more than five drinks at one occasion) leads to higher levels of blood alcohol. Binge drinking is a special concern in early pregnancy when the fetal brain is developing and women may not yet realize that they are even pregnant (Okah et al., 2005). Many pregnant women between the ages of 15 and 44 (10.1%) reported they were binge drinking during the first trimester of pregnancy (SAMHSA, 2011).

Illicit drug use in pregnant women ages 15 to 44 is estimated at 4.4% as compared to the rate of 10.9% in nonpregnant women. Illicit drug use rates are higher in pregnant women between the ages of 15 and 17 (16.2%) and 18 and 25 (7.4%) and lower in pregnant women aged 26 to 44 (1.9%) (SAMHSA, 2011). Pregnant women who abuse cocaine have higher levels of PTB, LBW, and SGA infants than nonusers of cocaine and are less likely to seek or receive adequate prenatal care (Gouin et al., 2011).

Nutrition

Adequate nutrition prior to conception and during pregnancy is important for maternal and fetal health. The pregnant woman needs to consume enough calories and nutrients to meet her own physiological needs as well as those of the developing fetus. Nutritional risks to consider include inadequate or excessive weight gain, medical conditions that complicate pregnancy such as hyperemesis gravidarum, dental conditions that compromise the ability to take in food, or inadequate resources to access food. Lack of adequate nutrients prior to or during early pregnancy can lead to birth defects. The importance for all women of childbearing age (between 15 and 45) to consume at least 400 mcg of folic acid daily to help prevent neural tube defects has been well established. The CDC (2013) estimates that 50% to 70% of all birth defects could be prevented by this simple measure!

Another important nutritional consideration is prevention of maternal anemia during pregnancy. Anemia is a serious problem affecting about half of pregnant women worldwide. It is more prevalent in nonindustrialized nations due to poor nutrition, iron deficient diets, presence of parasitic disease, and incidence of HIV/AIDS. Women who are anemic are less likely to withstand blood loss during delivery and have increased risks of perinatal death, LBW, stillbirths, and prematurity (WHO, 2005). Promoting adequate nutrition prior to pregnancy is a key to improving outcomes of pregnancy.

Inadequate nutrition may be another risk factor for prematurity, LBW, or pregnancy loss, especially in teenaged pregnancy or for women at risk for not eating due to food insufficiency or conditions such as anorexia nervosa or depression. Many teenaged girls do not eat an adequate diet, even when they may not be pregnant. They may not consume adequate trace elements or antioxidant micronutrients in their diet (i.e., selenium, copper, zinc, manganese, and vitamins C and E) during pregnancy which are essential in the promotion of adequate placental development, prevention of IUGR, preeclampsia, and prevention of fetal mortality and morbidity (Mistry & Williams, 2011). Young mothers who do not consume enough nutrients to maintain their own growth, as measured by gains in BMI or height, are more at risk to have LBW infants as compared to older mothers.

In countries where poor socioeconomic conditions contribute to chronic undernutrition in children, the outcomes of adolescent pregnancy may be worse. Girls are more at risk for nutritional deprivation in some countries due to girl gender bias. Prolonged periods of time without food can lead to increased maternal corticotropin-releasing hormone and can subsequently increase the risk for preterm delivery (Gennaro, 2005). Chronic undernutrition can delay menarche in young girls. In some cultures, especially rural, underdeveloped populations, early adolescent marriage and pregnancy are permissible. In a study conducted in India where many pregnant women experience chronic undernutrition, adolescent girls less than age 18 with low BMI of less than 18.5 kg/m^2 were found to be at increased risk for pregnancy wastage and prematurity as compared to those older than 18 with low BMI. Additionally, prematurity rates were significantly higher in girls who married prior to age 18, as compared with those who married after age 18. Pregnancy wastage was six times higher in mothers who conceived at less than 15.25 years as compared with those who conceived after 17.25 years. Factors including young age at conception and postmenarcheal stature growth due to chronic undernutrition negatively impacted pregnancy wastage and preterm delivery birth outcomes (Rao, Gokhale, Joshi, & Kanade, 2010). Food insecurity not only can increase risk for a LBW infant but can increase risks of birth defects. Food insecurity can also lead to changes in maternal mental health, including depression, anxiety, and low self-esteem (Ivers & Cullen, 2011). Interventions that can help improve nutritional status of pregnant women in food-insecure locations are also aimed at increasing infant birth weight which can markedly decrease infant mortality. Effective interventions include maternal supplementation with iron folate and micronutrients, calcium supplementation, iodized salt, reduction of indoor pollution and tobacco usage, deworming, intermittent preventative treatment for malaria, and use of insecticide-treated mosquito nets (Bhutta et al., 2008; Eisele et al., 2012).

Even in high- to moderate-income nations, some pregnant women living on low incomes do not get adequate nutrition. In the United States nutritional support during pregnancy along with nutritional education, and participation in programs such as the Special Supplemental Nutrition Program for Women, Infants, and Children have been demonstrated to increase the mean birth weight and reduce the odds for LBW for infants of low-income women on Medicaid. Implementation of similar programs for pregnant women in other countries where food supplies are insufficient could dramatically improve perinatal outcomes. Women who are depressed or stressed may also have poorer eating habits, leading to inadequate food intake. Women with social support have less stress and better eating habits (Fowles et al., 2011).

Maternal obesity is another nutritional concern for pregnancy. Infants of obese women (defined as BMI over 30.0 kg/m^2) have more than twice the risk for stillbirth and neonatal death after adjusting for other factors including smoking, alcohol, maternal age, parity, hypertension, and diabetes (Kristensen, Vestergaard, Wisborg, Kesmodel, & Secher, 2005). Obesity in pregnancy is not a risk factor for preterm birth (Aly et al., 2010).

Maternal foodborne illness or ingestion of toxic substances during pregnancy can be harmful to the fetus. *Listeria monocytogenes*, even though rare, is a special concern in pregnancy since about 30% of all cases occur in pregnant women. Women who ingest food contaminated with *Listeria* do not usually feel ill; however, the fetus can be significantly affected. Eating food contaminated by microorganisms like *Listeria* or substances like heavy metals can cause abortion, stillbirth, preterm delivery, neonatal infections, fetal brain or kidney problems, or even maternal death. While *Listeria* is found in many foods, teaching pregnant women simple basic precautions such as hand washing when preparing food, avoiding cross-contamination of meat dishes or other prepared foods, and avoiding nonpasteurized milk may help prevent infection (Janakiraman, 2008).

Pica is an interesting dietary practice seen during pregnancy in almost every culture. Substances like starch, ice, clay, or dirt are ingested as a craving in an attempt to possibly increase iron or calcium intake. Pica is not generally harmful to the fetus and may help alleviate gastrointestinal distress in pregnant women (Young et al., 2010). Women who practice pica tend to have lower hemoglobin and hematocrit levels, be more underweight at the start of their pregnancy, and smoke less than other women (Corbett, Ryan, & Weinrich, 2003; Young et al., 2010). One concern if the mother eats dirt is that it could possibly be contaminated with lead or heavy metals which could be harmful, cause anemia, or lead poisoning (Silbergeld & Patrick, 2005).

The influence of cultural dietary practices as potential risk factors can't be ignored and must be assessed. Asian women who ingest betel nuts which contain arecoline are at higher risk for spontaneous abortion, LBW, and PTB, placental changes, and neonatal withdrawal (Garcia-Algar et al., 2005). The health care practitioner must become familiar with the food and complementary medicine cultural practices of local ethnic groups, as they may affect pregnancy outcomes.

Over-the-Counter and Complementary Drugs

Drugs taken during pregnancy can have harmful effects on the fetus whether they are controlled substances or over-the-counter medications. Despite warnings that pregnant women should not take any medications without consulting with their health care provider, many pregnant women take over-the-counter or nonprescribed medications during pregnancy, including complementary therapies they might not consider to be harmful. Findings of a study on the prevalence of medication use by pregnant women between 2006 and 2008 reported that 70% to 80% of women said they used one or more medication during their pregnancy. About 50% said they used one or more prescription medications in the first trimester of pregnancy. Trends over the past 30 years indicate that the use of medications during the first trimester has increased by 60% with the number of pregnant women who use four or more medications in the first trimester tripling. Antidepressant use has dramatically increased over the past 30 years (Mitchell et al., 2011). Many women regularly take over-the-counter drugs such as cold remedies, aspirin, nonsteroidal anti-inflammatory drugs, or herbal teas. Some women might take medications that could be harmful to the fetus before they know that they are pregnant. Even vitamins and dietary supplements taken in excessive dosages can be harmful to the fetus. Pregnant women with preexisting medical problems such as asthma, arthritis, heart problems, diabetes, or epilepsy who have to continue to take their prescribed medications during pregnancy should check with their health care provider to determine if the prescribed medication will need to be changed to one that is less harmful to the fetus.

Health care providers must be cognizant of Food and Drug Administration (FDA) pregnancy categories and drugs that must be used with caution or that are contraindicated in pregnancy. One concern is that thalidomide received FDA approval for treatment of leprosy in 1998 and is currently being evaluated in clinical trials for treatment of renal cell cancer, AIDS, and tuberculosis (TB). Thalidomide was withdrawn from the market in the 1960s after it was linked to fetal limb shortening birth defects when it was used during pregnancy. Now there are stringent educational requirements, warnings about risks in pregnancy, and mandatory contraception for both men and women who use thalidomide. It is possible that pregnancy could occur despite these measures.

Environmental Influences

Every individual is conceived with a unique genetic makeup called a genotype. The phenotype, or the person's ultimate physiological and psychological makeup, is determined during the postconceptual period until after birth. The expression of the genetic inheritance (i.e., actual physiological and psychological makeup of the person) is the result of complex gene–gene interactions and environmental influences upon genes that occur at the molecular level. Exposure by the mother to environmental toxicants either before or during pregnancy can precipitate gene–environment interactions that can alter these molecular interactions, especially if the exposure to the harmful substance occurs at critical periods of fetal development. Two critical periods when gene–environmental interactions can be most harmful are during organogenesis (when fetal organs are being formed) and during the fetal period when there is rapid growth of all systems. Spina bifida is an example of a gene–environment interaction. At conception a fertilized egg might inherit the genes to have an intact neural tube. Neural tube defects occur when there is a lack of adequate folic acid at a critical stage of development while in utero. Exposure to teratogens, substances that are known to cause birth defects, during these times can result in birth defects or other adverse outcomes. Two pregnant women could be exposed to the same toxicants at the same point during pregnancy and could have infants with different outcomes. For example, two infants could inherit the genetic trait for sickle cell disease, yet when they are born they could have different expressions of the disease based upon other complex molecular interactions that happen within genes which could be influenced by the environment. It is now recognized that these factors continue to influence functional and developmental outcomes throughout the person's life (Mattison, 2010). The study of epigenetics is an evolving science that looks at factors such as genetic inheritance, imprinting, or nutritional factors that are hypothesized to mediate genetic interactions at the molecular level and that may one day provide more insight into these complex processes.

Environmental hazards are found in air, water, and food. These seemingly innocuous substances can contain high levels of contaminants such as pesticides, heavy metals, and solvents (Silbergeld & Patrick, 2005). Maternal exposure to air pollutants during the first trimester of pregnancy has been associated with decreased fetal birth weight (Gouveia, Bremner, & Novaes, 2004). Some ethnic variations in timing of prenatal exposure to air pollutants and fetal outcomes have been reported (Mattison, 2010). Poor or socially disadvantaged women, especially women of color, are more often exposed to environmental hazards because they tend to live in older sections of town or work in areas with high exposure. Their homes are usually older, increasing the risk for lead paint exposure. Poor parts of town are often located close to factories where pregnant women are exposed to incinerator emissions or other sources of air pollution. The poor are more likely to be exposed to agricultural pesticides or chemicals as they are more likely to work on farms or as migrant workers. Both maternal and paternal exposure to environmental toxins can be contributors to fetal risk. In fact, fetal congenital anomalies and death were noted in the offspring of male agricultural workers who worked where pesticides were used. More fetuses died in seasons when pesticide usage was highest (Regidor, Ronda, Garcia, & Dominguez, 2004). The disadvantaged might be more likely to reside on or near land that once served as a hazardous waste dumpsite (Silbergeld & Patrick, 2005). Cultural practices such as pica place some pregnant women at increased risk for exposure to environmental pollutants including heavy metals.

Another environmental influence that could possibly affect birth outcomes is the occurrence of natural or man-made disasters such as hurricanes, severe ice storms, earthquakes, chemical spills, or terrorism. The occurrence of a disaster can alter availability of food, water, or adequate prenatal care, which may increase risks for PTB. Increased maternal stress could cause mothers to use substances such as alcohol or tobacco for stress management. There have been some studies linking certain disasters with outcomes such as increased rates of spontaneous abortion, congenital anomalies, decreased fetal growth, and changes in maternal mental health status, although disasters do not seem to cause PTB. The severity and timing of maternal exposure to natural disasters relative to trimester of pregnancy need further study (Harville, Xiong, & Buekens, 2011).

Other Emerging Risk Factors

Other risk factors that may affect perinatal outcomes are constantly under investigation. Recently, obesity has been identified as an emerging risk factor for PTB. Obese and superobese women, defined as a BMI greater than 50%, are at increased risk for PTB. Because a higher percentage of pregnant Black women are obese, this group has the highest risk for PTB, followed by White, then Hispanic obese women (Salihu et al., 2009).

Severe maternal snoring and maternal sleep deprivation in the last trimester of pregnancy have been linked to an increased risk for fetal growth restriction or LBW. The suggested link between snoring and fetal growth restriction or LBW is possibly due to maternal hypoxemia while snoring, which leads to decreased delivery of oxygenation to the fetus. Maternal sleep deprivation in the last trimester of pregnancy has been linked to a twofold increased risk of premature birth. The link between sleep deprivation and preterm delivery may relate to an increase in proinflammatory serum cytokines in sleep-deprived women, triggering a systemic inflammatory response (Micheli et al., 2011).

MATERNAL MEDICAL AND OBSTETRIC CONDITIONS

Diabetes, hypertension, and bleeding disorders are some of the most common maternal complications of pregnancy worldwide (UNICEF, 2009). These complications can lead to preterm delivery, perinatal death, or can influence fetal morbidity. Risk of maternal complications of pregnancy increases with advanced maternal age (Yaniv et al., 2011).

Diabetes

Women with known pregestational diabetes should seek preconceptual care prior to getting pregnant. The preconceptual visit should include a complete physical examination with evaluation of blood glucose levels, cardiovascular and renal health, gastrointestinal system, an eye examination to check for diabetic retinopathy, and evaluation of the presence of neuropathy. A team approach with a diabetes nurse educator and dietician can teach the woman how to implement the dietary and lifestyle changes needed for a healthy pregnancy. Oral hypoglycemics should be discontinued and changed to human insulin or metformin prior to pregnancy. Metformin can be used safely in the preconceptual period and during pregnancy for type 2 diabetics (Chakraborti, 2012). Ideally, the woman with diabetes should maintain euglycemia for several months prior to pregnancy, as hyperglycemia in early pregnancy has been associated with increased risk for pregnancy loss and serious congenital defects (Kitzmiller et al., 2008). During pregnancy, regulation of blood glucose is sometimes difficult since pregnancy creates a state of insulin resistance and insulin needs change with each trimester. Glycosylated hemoglobin levels (HbA1c) should be maintained to as close to normal range as possible during pregnancy, especially during the period of fetal organogenesis. If blood glucose is greater than 200, the pregnant woman should check urine for ketones and notify the health care provider that ketones are present since diabetic ketoacidosis can cause fetal demise (Kitzmiller et al., 2008).

About 5% of pregnancies are complicated by gestational diabetes (American Diabetes Association [ADA], 2005). Worldwide prevalence of gestational diabetes mellitus (GDM) is difficult to establish since the parameters for screening and diagnosis of GDM vary across different countries. In the United States there are ethnic variations in prevalence of GDM, with Asian, Hispanic, and Native American women having higher rates than NHB and NHW women. The prevalence of gestational diabetes seems to be increasing (Hunt & Schuller, 2007). Identification and treatment of women with gestational diabetes is the key to promoting positive neonatal outcomes. The most important principle of diabetes management for all pregnant women with diabetes is to maintain tight glycemic control. Poor glycemic control increases the risks for miscarriage or stillbirth and the infant's risk for birth defects (i.e., cardiovascular, musculoskeletal, and central nervous system anomalies), hypoglycemia, hyperbilirubinemia, erythrocytosis, respiratory complications, and shoulder dystocia (Chakraborti, 2012; Langer, Yogev, Most, & Xenakis, 2005; Schaefer-Graf et al., 2000). Risks for birth defects are similar in gestational diabetics as compared with women with type 2 diabetes (Chakraborti, 2012; Schaefer-Graf et al., 2000).

All pregnant women should be screened for gestational diabetes through patient history, presence of clinical risk factors, or administration of a 50 g 1-hour oral glucose tolerance test (OGTT) between 24 and 28 weeks gestation (ACOG, 2011). The ADA recommends a 75-g OGTT at 24 to 28 weeks with blood glucose measurement when fasting, and at 1 and 2 hours after blood glucose administration. The diagnosis of gestational diabetes is based upon results of the blood glucose screening which exceed predetermined lab values for the test (ADA, 2005).

Diabetes during pregnancy is frequently accompanied by maternal vascular changes that can compromise uteroplacental circulation; therefore, fetal nonstress testing is recommended in the last trimester. If early delivery is indicated, amniocentesis can be done to determine fetal lung maturity; however, results of the lecithin sphingomyelin (L/S) ratio are often inaccurate for infants of mothers with diabetes. Infants of diabetic mothers generally have macrosomia. These large babies have increased risks for birth injuries due to shoulder dystocia, including fractured clavicles or nerve palsies. Large infants are more likely to be delivered by cesarean section. Infants of diabetic mothers should be closely monitored for hypoglycemia in the immediate postbirth period and until feeding is well established.

Hypertension in Pregnancy

Approximately 6% to 8% of pregnancies are complicated by hypertensive disorders. The National High Blood Pressure Education Working Group defined four categories of hypertension in pregnancy: chronic hypertension, gestational hypertension, preeclampsia, and preeclampsia superimposed on chronic hypertension. Chronic hypertension exists when there is a history of hypertension prior to the pregnancy, or it can also be diagnosed during pregnancy for the first time. About 20% of women with preexisting hypertension develop superimposed preeclampsia during their pregnancy (Seely & Solomon, 2003). Women with chronic hypertension who develop proteinuria are at increased risks for fetal complications, especially if serum creatinine levels are above 1.4 mg/dL at conception. They are also at increased risks for placental abruption. Gestational hypertension is diagnosed during pregnancy and usually disappears within 12 weeks after delivery. Preeclampsia is a pregnancy-specific disease that usually occurs after 20 weeks of pregnancy. It is characterized by hypertension and proteinuria. As the condition progressively worsens, maternal lab work indicates elevations in liver enzymes and low platelets. HELLP syndrome occurs in about 20% of pregnancies complicated by preeclampsia. It is characterized by hemolysis, elevated liver enzymes, and low platelets. Approximately half of women with HELLP syndrome are preterm.

Hypertension in pregnancy causes vasoconstriction with subsequent poor maternal circulatory and placental perfusion. Decreased uteroplacental circulation compromises the fetus; therefore, it is more likely to be growth restricted, SGA, or at increased risk for stillbirth. Women with PIH are also at increased risk for abruptio placenta. Delivery is the definitive treatment and is generally recommended if the fetus is 34 weeks gestation or more; however, it might not be appropriate if the fetus is immature. Early delivery will be based upon stability of the mother and outcomes of fetal testing. A serious risk for the preeclamptic mother is the possibility of eclamptic seizures due to cerebral edema and central nervous system excitability or progression to the HELLP syndrome. Seizures increase the risk for a placental abruption. Therefore, if the mother's condition worsens, early delivery will be elected; however, the ability of the fetus to survive must be considered. Corticosteroid administration is advised and may be beneficial if the fetus is between 24 and 34 weeks gestational age and if the mother has never had them (Leeman & Fontaine, 2008). Patients with preeclampsia tend to have infants with lower gestational ages at delivery and lower birth weights than do patients with gestational hypertension alone (Barton, O'Brien, Bergauer, Jacques, & Sibai, 2001). Women with severe gestational hypertension (defined as blood pressure > 160/110) without proteinuria tend to have higher rates of preterm delivery and are more likely to have a baby who is SGA as compared to mothers who are normotensive, have mild gestational hypertension or mild preeclampsia (Buchbinder et al., 2002). The earlier that hypertensive disease occurs in pregnancy, the more likely it is that proteinuria will develop. The development of proteinuria in women with gestational hypertension increases the chances for adverse maternal and neonatal outcomes (Barton et al., 2001).

If preeclampsia worsens, the pregnant woman is admitted to the hospital for stabilization and delivery. If the woman has a seizure, oxygen should be provided during and immediately following the seizure and the fetus should be monitored for signs of distress. Magnesium sulfate is the drug of choice to prevent central nervous system excitability from cerebral edema. Infants rarely have harmful effects from in utero exposure to magnesium sulfate prior to delivery, but should be monitored for signs of respiratory depression or hypotonia after birth.

Ethnic differences in the progression of hypertensive disorders in pregnancy have been noted. African American women were hospitalized earlier in the pregnancy for treatment of PIH. Their babies had lower gestational age and birth weight. African American women also had a higher incidence of abruptio placenta, stillbirths, and neonatal deaths than other ethnic groups. More Hispanic women developed proteinuria in pregnancy, and their disease was more likely to progress to severe preeclampsia (Barton, Barton, O'Brien, Bergauer, & Sibai, 2002).

PROM

PROM is a cause of preterm delivery and occurs in about 3% of all births. Once the membranes rupture, the fetus is at high risk for problems related to oligohydramnios, cord compression, chorioamnionitis, and abruptio placenta. Women with PROM may report that they are leaking fluid from the vagina or may have experienced a gush of fluid. Sterile speculum examination, nitrazine testing, and microscopic examination of fluid for ferning are methods to evaluate if membranes have ruptured. The decision of whether to deliver or to use expectant management must weigh the advantage of postponing delivery until gestational age increases against the risk for maternal or fetal sepsis. About 13% of pregnancies complicated with PROM develop chorioamnionitis (Ramsey, Lieman, Brumfield, & Carlo, 2005). Signs of intrauterine infection include fever greater than 100.4°F (38.0°C), uterine tenderness, and maternal or fetal tachycardia. Results of the white blood cell count tests should be used judiciously as indicator of infection, especially if steroids have been given within the previous 5 to 7 days.

Fetal outcomes after PROM are related to gestational age at time of membrane rupture and whether infant is delivered without complications of infection or asphyxia from cord compression or prolapse. Prior to 23 weeks gestation, if the fetus delivers after PROM it will not survive. As gestational age increases from 23 weeks to 32 weeks gestation, outcomes after PROM improve. Preterm PROM near term occurs between 32 and 36 weeks gestation, and infants who are delivered at this time are more likely to survive if they do not have other complications. Sometimes in the absence of other indications, a wait and see approach might be taken where delivery is not expedited. Maternal monitoring for signs of infection (i.e., fever, uterine tenderness, maternal and fetal tachycardia) and initiation of antibiotics have been shown to prolong the interval from PROM to delivery and improve fetal outcomes. A single course of corticosteroids should be administered to the mother to promote fetal lung maturity if PROM occurs prior to 32 weeks or up to 34 weeks if fetal immaturity is suspected (Mercer, 2003). If PROM occurs at earlier gestational ages the risk for chorioamnionitis increases. At delivery, infants of women with chorioamnionitis tend to be of younger gestational age and to weigh less than infants of women who do not have chorioamnionitis. Neonatal morbidity is increased when chorioamnionitis occurs as a complication of PROM. The use of prophylactic antibiotics given to the mother when chorioamnionitis is present does not prevent poor neonatal outcomes (Ramsey et al., 2005). However, antibiotic therapy has been demonstrated to lower the number of infants with respiratory distress syndrome, death, early sepsis, severe intraventricular hemorrhage, and severe necrotizing enterocolitis. Antibiotics also reduced the incidence of group B streptococcus sepsis, amnionitis, and pneumonia (Mercer, 2003).

Maternal Infections

Infections are a major risk factor for maternal and fetal health during pregnancy. Women may be infected prior to pregnancy or acquire the infection during pregnancy. Maternal infections can be transmitted to the infant while in utero across the placenta, during the birth process, or even during the postpartum period. Fetal infections can cause congenital anomalies, LBW, respiratory illness after birth, or even death. Infectious agents include protozoal infections, helminthic infections, sexually transmitted diseases (STDs), viruses, and bacterial organisms.

Three infectious diseases, HIV/AIDS, TB, and malaria, are the leading causes of perinatal morbidity and mortality, especially in sub-Saharan Africa and Asia. Interactions between these diseases during pregnancy can increase maternal risk of contracting other infectious diseases or can potentiate the existing diseases, making them more deadly. For example, malaria and TB infections can increase risk of vertical transmission of HIV to the fetus. Presence of maternal HIV infection can decrease maternal immunity, lowering resistance to TB or malaria (Ezechi, Petterson, & Byamugisha, 2012). People living with HIV have 34 times the risk of developing TB (WHO, 2011a). TB-infected women are more at risk to contract malaria or HIV. Tragically, many of these deaths could be prevented through use of low-cost interventions to prevent vertical transmission of HIV, intermittent prophylactic therapy, use of insecticide treated nets for malaria prevention, and infection control practices for TB (Ezechi et al., 2012). Only about 35% of pregnant women in low- and middle-income countries are tested for HIV status during pregnancy. An estimated 48% of pregnant women in low- and middle-income countries are receiving the most effective treatment regimens to prevent mother to child HIV transmission with lowest rates of coverage in North Africa and the Middle East (4%), East, South and Southeast Asia (16%), and Western and Central Africa (18%) (WHO, 2011b). In the United States about 150 to 250 infants a year contract HIV from their mother during the perinatal period (March of Dimes, 2009).

Vaccine-preventable infections kill more women and babies in low-income nations because basic immunization practices, such as tetanus or rubella vaccination, may be unavailable to them. Tetanus, a disease that can be easily prevented, accounts for about 7% of neonatal deaths in developing nations. Tetanus develops in newborns due to unclean cord-handling practices, including instrumentation and use of traditional cord salves that can cause infection. Once infected, the infant loses the ability to suck within a few days of exposure and progresses through stiffness, seizures, and death (Lawn, Cousens, & Zupan, 2005). About 110,000 babies are born each year with congenital rubella syndrome, although this number is most likely underreported (Reef, Strebel, Dabbagh, Gacic-Dobo, & Cochil, 2011; WHO, 2005).

MDG 6 focuses on combatting HIV/AIDS, malaria, TB, and other infectious diseases and on the prevention and treatment before and during pregnancy of infectious and noncommunicable diseases known to increase risk of PTB (WHO et al., 2012). Every pregnant woman must be screened for risk factors for infection. Early identification and treatment of women with infections will improve both maternal and neonatal outcomes.

Abruptio Placenta

Abruptio placenta, or premature separation of the placenta prior to delivery, is a leading cause of stillbirth and neonatal mortality. Placental separation is thought to be due to changes in placental vasculature, thrombosis, and reduced placental perfusion. A genetic basis for abruptio placenta has been speculated that causes these changes. Placental separation occurs in several ways. In marginal separation the edges of the placenta separate and bright red bleeding is present. Occult or hidden abruptio placenta occurs when the edges of the placenta are intact but the central part of the placenta detaches from the uterus, allowing blood loss to accumulate behind the placenta without any outward signs of bleeding. Complete abruptio placenta occurs when the placenta totally detaches, a situation that is incompatible with fetal survival. There is a four to six times higher risk of premature delivery when there is a diagnosis of abruption placenta. Premature delivery increases the risk for infant mortality. Risk of mortality due to abruptio placenta is 16.5 times higher than when abruptio placenta is not present (Ananth & VanderWeel, 2011). Infants of mothers with abruptio placenta who survive must be closely monitored for signs of blood loss and shock.

Risk factors for abruptio placenta include smoking, multiple pregnancy, and maternal age greater than 50. Increased risk in older women could be related to increased rates of chronic hypertensive disorders or aging of the uterine blood vessels. The risk of abruptio placenta increases with multiple pregnancy as the number of fetuses increases from singleton to triplet pregnancies. Perinatal death from abruptio placenta is higher for singletons than for multiples, possibly due to IUGR, chronic fetal compromise, LBW, or blood loss from the abruption, while in multiples a different etiology could be a factor (Salihu, Shumpert, Slay, Kirby, & Alexander, 2003).

POSTPARTUM RISK FACTORS

After birth, the five leading causes of infant death are complications of congenital anomalies, complications of prematurity and LBW, SIDS, result of maternal complications, and placental-cord complications. Congenital anomalies account for most neonatal deaths in the first month of life. Infants who are LBW are more likely to die from complications of prematurity (respiratory distress, infections, or anemia), maternal complications in pregnancy, or placenta/cord conditions. In addition to these leading causes of death, other risk factors could affect the health of the neonate or cause injury such as maternal smoking or drug usage. Providing information and anticipatory guidance to the parents to increase awareness of some of these factors might be enough to protect the infant and to promote positive outcomes.

Drugs Excreted in Maternal Milk

Maternal medications taken while lactating are a concern as they may alter the milk supply or cross to the infant though the milk supply. While many medications have been demonstrated to be safe, there are still others that have not been reported in the literature. Psychotropic drugs pose a special concern since there has been an increase in their use. These drugs and their metabolites have long half-lives and are detectable in infant tissues and the developing brain. The long-term consequences of this exposure have not been thoroughly studied. As new drugs are placed on the market, their safety for the infant must be evaluated. Some untoward effects on the infant from use of prescribed maternal drugs include possible immune suppression, neutropenia, skin rash, central nervous system changes including irritability, restlessness, sleepiness, lethargy, or convulsions, gastrointestinal effects such as feeding problems, vomiting, diarrhea, slow weight gain, blood in stool, jaundice, or dark urine. A comprehensive list of drugs, foods, and environmental agents that are excreted in human milk and that could be potentially harmful to neonates is available from the American Academy of Pediatrics (AAP).

The AAP, Committee on Drugs (2001) recommends that whenever drugs are prescribed for lactating women, the following factors be considered. When a medication is absolutely necessary, the baby's pediatrician and mother's physician should consult together to select the most appropriate drug for the mother, with minimal effects upon lactation and minimal transfer to the infant. Select the safest drug when there are several to choose from. Consider measuring the infant's blood concentration of the drug if there are potential risks from the drug for the infant. Advise the nursing mother to take the medication immediately after breastfeeding the infant or after a feeding that will be followed by an expected infant sleep period, to minimize infant drug exposure.

Sudden Infant Death Syndrome

SIDS is the leading cause of death in infants in the postneonatal period in the United States as well as other developed countries. Programs such as the AAP Back to Sleep campaign urged parents to place their infants on their backs instead of prone for sleeping. This change in recommended practice dramatically lowered infant deaths from SIDS. In the United States, the SIDS death rate was lowered by 50% between 1992 and 2001, from 1.2 to 0.56 per 1,000 live births (AAP, 2005). Despite these advances, disparities in SIDS rates exist. Infants born to Black or American Indian or Alaskan Native mothers have the highest rates of death from SIDS: twice the rate of infants of White mothers, three times the rate of infants of Hispanic mothers, and four times the rate of infants of Asian or Pacific Islander mothers who have the lowest rates (Hauck et al., 2011). Maternal risk factors include young, single mothers with a history of prenatal smoking or substance abuse. Infants of mothers with higher levels of education have lower rates of death from SIDS (Hauck et al., 2011).

Over 70 causes of SIDS have been proposed. SIDS has been blamed on environmental factors such as soft bedding, overheating, entanglement in blankets, immunizations, tobacco smoke exposure, or bed sharing with parents or siblings, especially if a bed partner consumes alcohol (AAP, 2005; Hunt, 2005). Genetic factors have also been blamed for findings. Prolonged QT interval has been found in up to 30% to 35% of SIDS cases. Possible structural defects in the brain that control cardiac and respiratory function might explain the diminished arousal response in infants with SIDS that precedes death. SIDS is not always sudden; some infants have evidence of chronic hypoxia upon autopsy (Burnett & Adler, 2011). In reality, the cause of SIDS is probably multifactorial. The triple risk theory proposes that multiple complex factors (including genetics, prenatal risk factors, and environmental risk factors) make some babies more vulnerable to environmental triggering events and unable to respond to these events through usual homeostatic mechanisms (AAP, 2005; Burnett & Adler, 2011).

Infants at risk for SIDS have many of the same risk factors seen with prematurity and LBW. Preterm or LBW infants and infants with a history of apnea are at increased risk for SIDS. The peak age at death from SIDS is between 2 and 4 months. SIDS is unusual after the age of 6 months. Term infants who have had apparent life-threatening events with apnea, cyanosis, choking, and gagging are at increased risk for SIDS (Burnett & Adler, 2011). No definitive link between SIDS and immunizations has been established.

Sleeping in the prone position has been highly associated with SIDS and is one reason the Back to Sleep campaign has been so successful in reducing SIDS death rates. The rate of SIDS increases for preterm infants who are placed in the prone position. Many parents of premature infants place their infant to sleep on their stomach or side once at home. It is possible that new parents are learning the practice of putting their baby in either the prone position or side-lying position by watching caregivers in the NICU. Neonatal care practices that place preterm infants in the prone or side-lying positions are providing poor role models for parents. Every time parents see their baby in a prone or side-lying position while in the hospital, they are getting reinforcement of a poor practice about how to provide care to their baby at home. Infants become habituated to the prone position for sleeping, especially if they have had a prolonged hospitalization, which makes it more difficult for parents to change the baby's sleeping position to the back-lying position (Burnett & Adler, 2011). Another concern is that about 20% of SIDS deaths occur while the infant is in the home of a childcare provider. Placing the infant in an unaccustomed prone position for sleep increases the risk for SIDS. Many childcare providers are not knowledgeable of newer recommendations for supine sleep positions. Nurses need to educate parents to share information with their childcare providers about placing the baby on the back to sleep (AAP, 2005). Neonatal nurses must continue to educate each parent about the risk factors for SIDS and remind parents that the safest place for a baby is in its own crib in the parents' room for the first 6 months.

Child Abuse

Child abuse in infants is sometimes difficult to identify. Parents of an injured infant arrive for emergency treatment and seem severely distraught and worried about their child's injuries. They often offer reasonable explanations for the injury that must be ruled out with medical tests. The victims, the babies, can't speak for themselves to describe what happened. New parents are subject to many stressors that could trigger child abuse such as lack of sleep, financial strain, and dealing with inconsolable infants. Health care providers have a legal and ethical duty to report cases of suspected child abuse to child protective services (Smith, 2003). Two forms of child abuse are discussed further: abusive head trauma (AHT), formerly called shaken baby syndrome (SBS), and Munchausen syndrome by proxy (MSBP).

Abusive Head Trauma/Shaken Baby Syndrome

AHT describes a serious form of head trauma caused by several mechanisms including abusive shaking of an infant causing a whiplash-type injury, blunt trauma, or a combination of both (Christian, Block, & The Committee on Child Abuse and Neglect, 2009). It is a public health issue and the leading cause of death due to child abuse. When the infant is shaken, the head flops back and forth causing rapid acceleration, deceleration, and/or rotational forces of the brain within the skull, causing stretching, shearing, and tearing of blood vessels of the brain. Infants are more at risk for severe injury from AHT/SBS because of their weak neck muscles, proportionately large head size with soft skull and open fontanels, and immaturity of brain development (King, MacKay, & Sirnick, 2003).

Several types of injuries occur with AHT/SBS. Intracranial injuries cause direct brain injury and damage to the axons. Shearing forces exerted on the veins that bridge from the dura to the brain cause intracranial bleeding. During shaking there is a lack of oxygen to the brain that is further compounded by chemical processes that occur within the damaged cells. These injuries lead to swelling of the brain and increased intracranial pressure that further compromises brain oxygenation. Most SBS children have retinal hemorrhages, but as many as 15% may not have any. Absence of retinal hemorrhages does not rule out child abuse (Levin, 2006). While external signs of injury to the face or head are uncommon, injuries or bruising of the long bones, thorax, or abdomen may occur as a result of firmly grasping the infant during the shaking episode (Reece, 2005).

AHT/SBS most often results when a parent becomes frustrated with their infant who is crying and inconsolable. Parents who are stressed with the parenting role, parents of premature infants, those who are sleep deprived, or parents who do not have support or help to care for their baby's needs may have low tolerance of infant crying. Poverty and stress are risk factors for abuse. In frustration they may pick up the baby and shake it to try to quiet the baby. Newborns are more susceptible to the forces of shaking and may sustain injury even if not shaken as roughly as an older child. Once parents shake their child and get a response, they might shake the child again over time causing the infant to be injured repeatedly. Because the intracranial bleeding can be slow initially, the child might not manifest symptoms until 48 to 72 hours after the injury.

When parents seek medical attention for the infant, the history of events that preceded the infant's symptoms is often vague. The father or boyfriend is more likely to be the person responsible for the injury, and the mother may be unaware that the shaking incident occurred (King et al., 2003). Signs of AHT/SBS vary based on extent of the injury and are sometimes subtle such as feeding difficulties, vomiting, lethargy, hypothermia, failure to thrive, and increased somnolence. More life-threatening signs include seizures, bulging fontanelle, apnea, coma, bradycardia, or complete cardiovascular collapse. Outcomes are poor for children who present with coma; approximately 60% will die. Survivors of coma may have severe neuromotor impairment, visual impairment, and developmental delay. They may require shunting for hydrocephalus. Long-term occupational therapy, physical therapy, and speech therapy will be needed to help the children achieve their maximum potential. Approximately 20% of infants might die as a result of the shaking abuse. A small percentage of children will have no outward ill effects from the shaking. The remaining children have long-term sequelae, including ongoing neurological injuries and visual impairment. A delay of 12 to 18 months might occur before symptoms are evident (King et al., 2003).

New parents need to be taught not to shake their infant at any time. Prior to discharge, time should be spent exploring parents' concerns about taking a newborn home, their sources of support, and their coping strategies under stress. Teach parents about normal infant crying patterns and how to handle their stress or frustration due to prolonged periods of infant crying. Referral for stress management techniques, anger management, and provision of a parenting hotline number might help prevent this devastating injury.

MSBP

MSBP is a rare form of child abuse where a parent, usually a mother, fabricates illness in a dependent child in order to draw attention to themselves as the parent of a sick child. Four criteria are required for a diagnosis: (a) a parent or guardian fabricates illness in the child, (b) the child is presented for medical care, (c) the perpetrator denies knowledge of the cause of the child's illness, and (d) the signs and symptoms subside if the child is separated from the perpetrator (Barber & Davis, 2002). The diagnosis of MSBP includes two diagnoses; one for the child and one for the parent. The parent response might range from fabricating illness of a child, exaggerating symptoms of the sick child, to actually inducing the symptoms in the child such as by attempts to suffocate or poison the child. About 200 new cases of MSBP occur each year, but this number may underestimate the actual prevalence (Abdulhamid & Pataki, 2011). Some of the most common types of fabrications include gastrointestinal (diarrhea), neurologic (seizures), infections (fevers), dermatologic (strange rashes), and cardiopulmonary (acute life-threatening events). Some children will die as a result of the parent's abuse or ministrations. Unwittingly, physicians or health care workers can be drawn into the situation attempting to help the child based upon parent's descriptions of what is occurring. Health care professionals might prescribe unnecessary diagnostic tests or treatments for the child (Yonge & Haase, 2004). Health care professionals need increased awareness of MSBP and should question cases where children are seen constantly for parental reported conditions not witnessed by anyone else or if siblings of the child have had similar hospitalizations or have died from SIDS or under suspicious circumstances. Cases where children who are not gaining weight begin to gain during hospitalization are also suspect. If the parent is approached and refuses to get psychological help, or, if the child has been subjected to a major illness because of the parent then the child may need to be placed into a protective environment. MSBP has long-term psychological implications for the child, including posttraumatic stress disorder, behavioral problems, and depression (Abdulhamid & Pataki, 2011).

PERINATAL CARE IN DEVELOPING NATIONS

Pregnant women in developing nations have many of the same risk factors for prematurity and LBW as women in the United States such as poor prepregnancy physical condition, inadequate spacing between pregnancies, inadequate nutrition, decreased weight gain during pregnancy, maternal anemia, and lack of access for perinatal care. They also have to contend with other risk factors not even seen in the United States such as diseases like malaria and or lack of sanitation or clean water. Poverty and lack of education about pregnancy health are sometimes compounded by lack of skilled care providers, lack of transportation to health care centers, problems of war, civil unrest, and low status of women (UNICEF, 2009).

Decreasing worldwide maternal and neonatal mortality rates is a priority of the United Nations MDGs. Maternal mortality rates have declined 34% since 1990 in response to global efforts toward achieving the MDGs. Partnership programs have developed in many countries to improve access to birth control and prenatal care. Management of chronic diseases such as HIV and malaria, efforts to assure a skilled attendant at delivery, and use of evidence-based practices are beginning to make a positive difference (United States Agency for International Development [USAID], 2011). However the numbers of maternal deaths are still too high; 358,000 mothers died worldwide due to complications of pregnancy and childbirth in 2008. Almost 99% of these deaths occurred in developing countries, with highest rates in Africa and South Asia (WHO, 2011c).

Globally the neonatal mortality rate is not declining (USAID, 2011). Neonatal mortality is on the rise and accounts for more than 40% of deaths in children younger than age 5 worldwide. Prevention of neonatal mortality will significantly improve death rates of children under age 5 (WHO et al., 2012). The worldwide average is 24 neonatal deaths per 1,000 live births, ranging from 4 neonatal deaths per 1,000 live births for high-income countries to 36 neonatal deaths per 1,000 live births in low-income countries. Stillbirth rates globally average 19 stillbirths per 1,000 live births, with a range from 3 per 1,000 live births in high-income to 26 per 1,000 in low-income countries (WHO, 2011c). Each year 3 million babies will die during the immediate neonatal period; most of these are from developing nations. Improved prenatal care, having a skilled attendant at delivery, improved use of hygienic practices for clamping and care of the umbilical cord, and concerted efforts to provide basic resuscitation equipment and training in neonatal resuscitation have had good results in some countries, but much work still needs to be done (USAID, 2011).

Many neonates worldwide have died from preventable conditions. Some congenital anomalies could have been prevented with maternal folic acid supplementation. Many newborns die from birth asphyxia, which might have been prevented through use of timely neonatal resuscitation at delivery. Some deaths from prematurity might have been prevented with adequate prenatal care or a system of basic neonatal care for premature infants. Some deaths from infections could have been prevented with use of hygienic practices at birth, patient teaching about cord care, immunizations, maternal screening for communicable disease risks, or treatment for HIV during pregnancy. Keys to making changes include creating funding partnerships, improving infrastructure, professional education, and implementation of culturally appropriate evidence-based care.

Four interventions are recommended to improve birth outcomes and decrease neonatal loss in developing nations. These perinatal programs can be tailored to meet the specific needs of each country. First, antenatal care should be implemented on a local level not only for screening for possible problems but also to educate women about how to promote a healthy pregnancy. Optimal timing and spacing of pregnancy is another important part of prenatal care to promote mothers who are in the best physical condition prior to conception. Prevention and control of infection are also important during the prenatal period. Proper medical treatment of women who are infected with STDs or HIV/AIDS during pregnancy will increase the infant's chances of healthy survival.

Antenatal screening alone can't predict or prevent most problems during pregnancy or delivery; therefore, the second intervention is that all pregnant women should be considered high risk and must have access to skilled birth attendants and timely emergency obstetric care. Nations with the highest rates of neonatal and maternal mortality are those that have the lowest number of births attended by a skilled birth attendant. In some countries access to medical care is difficult due to living in remote village locations, a lack of basic transportation, or poor infrastructure, making it difficult to transport women or infants with problems to specialized centers. Sometimes the policies of developing nations interfere with the provision of safe obstetric care. For example, some countries limit the type of health care providers who can perform cesarean sections or administer anesthesia, thereby limiting access to these services (Mavalankar & Rosenfield, 2005).

Third, basic training and equipment for infant resuscitation at birth will help prevent some of the poor birth outcomes related to birth asphyxia. Many facilities in developing nations are working with antiquated equipment as they attempt to provide care for neonates. Textbooks are often outdated or are not written in the native language of the health care provider. The AAP Neonatal Resuscitation Program (NRP) has been demonstrated to be an effective method to provide immediate resuscitative care to neonates. This program has been translated into at least 20 languages and is being taught in other countries through formally organized courses through the AAP or by independent efforts of NRP instructors (AAP, 2012a). The Helping Babies Breathe program is an evidence-based infant resuscitation program designed for settings where human or technology resources are limited. It is not designed to replace NRP but serves as an adjunct for training birth attendants in how to assess and stimulate breathing during the initial Golden Minute of life. It is estimated that as many as 1 million infants can be saved worldwide through implementation of these NRPs (AAP, 2012b). Neonatal mortality is lower when the mother has received professional care during the antenatal period and during childbirth.

The fourth recommendation is to provide postpartum care that includes parent teaching about infant care and family planning services to help prevent close intrapregnancy levels. Strategies for successful breastfeeding, proper cord care, recognition of signs of illness, and promotion of psychosocial well-being are all skills that parents need to have in order to promote optimal newborn health. Women of childbearing age need to learn the importance of being in optimal physical condition prior to and during pregnancy. Family planning services will help women become empowered to make choices about when to have children and will help prevent unnecessary abortions.

SUMMARY

This chapter has presented an overview of some of the many prenatal, intrapartum, and postpartum risk factors that influence neonatal health, especially in relation to prematurity and LBW. The perinatal nurse must be aware of potential risk factors in order to screen pregnant women and provide counseling and support. Presence of risk factors can raise suspicion that a baby might have problems after delivery; however, many more babies, even in the presence of multiple risk factors, will be born healthy. Anticipation of neonates at risk helps assure that adequate personnel and equipment are available at birth to manage problems should they occur. Patient education about modifiable risk factors and support for altering HCBs can help prevent some adverse neonatal outcomes.

There have been some inroads made to improve maternal and child health internationally. There are still many barriers for many nations, including creation of the infrastructure needed to support the WHO recommendations and training of adequate health care professionals to provide care. Some countries are beginning to see successes in reducing their maternal and infant mortality. A sustained worldwide effort is needed to continue to improve these outcomes.

CASE STUDY

■ Identification of the Problem. A 28-year-old woman arrives at the clinic reporting she had a positive home pregnancy test in the past week. Her LMP was 4 months ago. The nurse practitioner assesses the woman for potential antepartum risk factors during the first prenatal visit.

■ Assessment, History

- *Menstrual history*: Menarche at age 14. Reports her periods are regular every 30 days with duration of 4 to 5 days. LMP was five months ago on March 10.
- *Obstetric history*: G5T2P1A1L2—reports she had four previous pregnancies. The first pregnancy was a term vaginal delivery 7 years ago. The female infant weighed 2,500 g at birth and is in good health today. The second vaginal delivery a year later was a preterm male born at 30 weeks gestation after the mother went to the hospital with cramping and heavy bleeding. The infant expired from respiratory complications at 4 days old. The third vaginal delivery was a term female infant at 38 weeks gestation. The child is now 5 years old and reported to be in good health. The mother reports that she had a spontaneous abortion in the first trimester about 6 months ago. She had a dilatation and curettage after the spontaneous abortion. Estimated date of confinement is December 17.
- *Past gynecologic history*: Reports she uses no contraception because she does not believe in taking birth control pills. Reports having a history of multiple sexual partners, currently in monogamous relationship. Was treated for unspecified STD 2 years ago at a state health department clinic. HIV status is unknown. Reports blood type is O+.
- *Past medical history*: Reports she had gestational diabetes (GDM) when pregnant with her 5-year-old that was managed with diet. Reports she had mild hypertension in the last trimester of last pregnancy that was managed with bed rest.
- *Drug/substance abuse history*: Denies taking any prescription, over-the-counter, homeopathic, or street drugs. Has not taken prenatal vitamins. Smokes 20 cigarettes a day, occasional marijuana. Alcohol: consumes two to three beers a day. Reports occasional binge drinking. Denies alcohol use since she found out she was pregnant.
- *Family/social history*: Lives with boyfriend who is father of baby. Denies familial history of genetic problems. Employed part-time as a housekeeper in nursing home. Reports boyfriend yells at her a lot and has hit her a couple of times. Reports they are getting along great now.

■ Physical Examination

- NEUROLOGICAL: alert, oriented; pupils dilated, equal and reactive to light and accommodation; DTRs 2+ bilaterally without clonus
- HEAD AND NECK: neck supple, thyroid examination unremarkable; denies headache, blurred vision, flashing lights in eyes, or scotoma
- CARDIOVASCULAR: heart rate regular without murmur-denies palpitations, chest pain
- RESPIRATORY: lungs clear to auscultation-denies history of asthma, TB, or bronchitis; reports chronic smoker's cough, denies thick sputum
- ABDOMEN/GASTROINTESTINAL: gravid abdomen, distended, fundal height 20 cm, uterine fundus at umbilicus; bowel sounds present, active, denies problems with constipation or diarrhea; reports appetite is good, denies nausea or vomiting
- GENITOURINARY: denies vaginal spotting or cramping; reports urinary frequency during the day, denies burning with urination
- EXTREMITIES: varicosities on lower legs, 1+ edema noted in pretibial area. DTRs 2+
- OTHER: reports backache if standing for prolonged periods at work; reports breast tenderness, no colostrum noted

■ Diagnostic Tests

- Blood type: O+
- Hgb: 10.9; Hct: 34%
- HIV test: negative
- Vaginal cultures: + Chlamydia
- 100 g 3 hour glucose tolerance test (GTT) results
- Fasting: 130 mg/dL
- 1 hour: 190 mg/dL
- 2 hour: 155 mg/dL
- 3 hour: 138 mg/dL

■ Working Nursing Diagnoses

- Increased risk for prematurity due to previous history of previous PTB, smoking, and short interconceptual length.
- Increased risk for gestational diabetes due to previous history
- Increased risk for PIH due to previous history
- Increased risk for infection related to history of STDs
- Increased risk for injury due to anemia
- Increased risk for injury related to potential physical abuse from significant other
- Increased risk to fetus for FAS due to report of maternal binge drinking in early pregnancy and regular drinking
- Increased risk for SGA infant due to maternal smoking

■ Development of Management Plan

1. Counsel regarding alcohol use in pregnancy, consider outpatient treatment

2. Provide contact information for emergency women's shelter
3. Teach danger signs during pregnancy and symptoms of PTL and when to notify practitioner
4. HIV testing, screen/treat for STDs
5. Obtain GTT at 24 weeks, follow blood glucose closely
6. Dietary counseling for iron, diabetic diet
7. Promote breastfeeding
8. Serial ultrasounds to monitor infant growth
9. Offer progesterone therapy

■ **Implementation.** The patient and nurse discussed needed lifestyle modifications during pregnancy and developed a plan to support the patient counsel, refer to support group for smoking cessation. Mother agreed to attend smoking cessation group for pregnant women. Patient agreed to refrain from alcohol usage during pregnancy. HIV testing completed. Chlamydia treatment prescribed—erythromycin 500 mg QID X 7 days; negative follow-up culture. Completed GTT at 28 weeks and was referred for nutritional counseling for GDM and sources of iron in diet. Daily iron supplementation provided. Fetal growth was monitored with serial ultrasounds. Patient instructed in how to monitor daily fetal kick counts at 34 weeks. She was started on 100 mg progesterone vaginally daily starting at 22 weeks gestation which was discontinued at 36 weeks gestation.

■ **Evaluation of Effectiveness.** Patient attended smoking cessation group and reported that she cut down her smoking while pregnant to several cigarettes a day. She also reported she avoided partying and refrained from use of alcohol or other substances during remainder of pregnancy. GTT was positive for GDM, but she was able to maintain control of blood glucose with diet and exercise. She also developed mild hypertension and 3+ proteinuria during the last weeks of pregnancy that was managed with bed rest in the last 2 weeks of pregnancy.

■ **Outcome.** Patient went into spontaneous labor at 38 weeks gestation and delivered a 4,138 g (9 lb 2 oz) boy. His Apgar scores at 1 minute and 5 minutes were 7 and 9. Infant had mild transient hypoglycemia after birth. No signs of FAS noted on admission physical examination. The mother had a postpartum tubal ligation after delivery. Mother was discharged breastfeeding the infant and scheduled for follow-up postpartum visit in 6 weeks.

EVIDENCE-BASED PRACTICE BOX

Progesterone Supplementation in Pregnancy to Decrease PTB

PTL is a major problem worldwide. In the United States about 12% of births are preterm (March of Dimes, 2012). The current treatment regimen for women in PTL includes bed rest, hydration, antibiotics, and tocolytics. However, most of these treatments do not prolong pregnancy beyond 24 to 48 hours (Norwitz & Caughey, 2011). Prevention or delay of PTB allows the fetus a longer period to mature, which can result in decreased neonatal morbidity and mortality. Prevention of PTB could translate into significant savings or health care dollars spent on care of women in premature labor or care of preterm infants in the NICU.

Two factors that increase the risk of preterm delivery include: (a) previous history of an unexplained PTB and (b) a shortened cervical length. A shortened cervical length is an important predictor of PTL; as the cervical length shortens, the risk for PTL increases. Starting at the middle of the second trimester (about 24 weeks), if the cervical length is very thin (< 10% of expected cervical length for the gestational weeks), the risk of premature delivery before 35 weeks gestation is six times greater (Iams et al., 1996). It is thought that progesterone inhibits cervical ripening that precedes labor (DeFranco et al., 2007).

Review of Studies

Progesterone for Prevention of PTB in Women With Prior History PTB

A systematic review and meta-analysis assessed the role of progesterone in prevention of PTB (Dodd, Crowther, Cincotta, Flenady, & Robinson, 2005). Seven randomized controlled trials (RCTs) conducted between 1983 and 2005 were identified where either intramuscular (IM) progesterone (six studies) or vaginal progesterone (one study) were compared to either placebo or no medication in pregnant women with a prior history of preterm delivery or who were considered to be at risk for PTB. In total 1,020 women were included in the studies. Women who received progesterone were significantly less likely to give birth prior to 37 weeks in six of the studies.

Progesterone in Asymptomatic Pregnant Women With Singleton Pregnancy With Shortened Cervical Length

A systematic review and individual patient data meta-analysis of studies of asymptomatic women who had cervical shortening (≤ 25 mm) at mid-trimester diagnosed by sonogram

(*continued*)

who received either vaginal progesterone, placebo, or no treatment included five high-quality studies conducted between 2007 and 2011. Studies included women (n = 775) with singleton (n = 723) or twin (n = 52) pregnancy who did or did not have a history of prior preterm delivery. Treatment with vaginal progesterone significantly reduced risk of spontaneous PTB at less than 33 weeks gestation and less than 34 weeks gestation (Romero et al., 2012).

17-Hydroxyprogesterone Caproate in Prevention of PTB in Multiples

Four RCTs were identified that studied prophylactic use of progesterone, in either injectable or vaginal forms as compared with placebo, for prevention of PTB in mothers with multiple pregnancy. These studies with a combined sample of 1,409 women pregnant with multiples found no differences in premature birth rates in women who received progesterone (Combs et al., 2011; Durnwald et al., 2010; Lim et al., 2011; Rode et al., 2011). It is hypothesized that PTL in women pregnant with multiples may be due to a different mechanism than in singletons, such as uterine overdistention, which is not responsive to progesterone.

Outcomes of Infants of Mothers Who Received Progesterone

A systematic review by Dodd, Flenady, Cincotta, and Crowther (2006) reviewed the evidence for benefits or harms to infants of mothers who used progesterone for prevention of PTB as a secondary outcome. The authors located 11 RCTs, which included a total of 2,714 women and 3,452 infants. Infants whose mothers received progesterone had significantly less risk of birth weight less than 2,500 g (2 studies of 501 infants) and less incidence of necrotizing enterocolitis (2 studies of 1,070 infants) as compared with infants of mothers who were administered placebos. No significant differences in incidence of other infant outcomes were reported between progesterone and placebo groups, including perinatal death, intrauterine fetal death, neonatal death, respiratory distress syndrome, intraventricular hemorrhage (all grades and grade 3 or 4), retinopathy of prematurity, neonatal sepsis, or patent ductus arteriosus. Another systematic review of outcomes for infants (n = 827) indicated infants of mothers who received progesterone had a significantly lower risk of respiratory distress syndrome, lower composite neonatal morbidity and mortality, lower risk to weigh less than 1,500 g, and lower risk for admission to the NICU or to need for mechanical ventilation (Romero et al., 2012).

Recommendations

The ACOG (2008) recommend progesterone supplementation is offered to women with a single fetus and a prior history of PTB due to either spontaneous preterm birth (SPTB) or PROM. Progesterone therapy is not recommended for multiple pregnancies. Progesterone may also be used if short cervical length (< 15 mm) is incidentally identified; however, routine cervical length screening is not recommended. The ideal formulation of progesterone was not recommended.

The Society of Obstetricians and Gynaecologists of Canada (SOGC) state indications for progesterone therapy include previous PTB or short cervix (< 16 mm at 22–26 weeks) measured by transvaginal ultrasound. Progesterone should be started after 20 weeks gestation and continue until risk of prematurity is low (Farine et al., 2008).

Recommended dosage of progesterone based on RCTs and meta-analyses for prevention of PTL in women with previous history of PTL is 17 alpha-hydroxyprogesterone caproate 250 mg IM weekly or progesterone 100 mg daily vaginally. For women with short cervix less than 15 mm at 22 to 26 weeks detected by transvaginal ultrasound progesterone 200 mg vaginally daily (Farine et al., 2008).

SOGC recommends that women at risk for PTB should be encouraged to participate in studies on the role of progesterone in reducing risks of PTL (Farine et al., 2008).

References

American College of Obstetricians and Gynecologists. (2008). Use of progesterone to prevent preterm birth. ACOG committee Opinion no. 419. *Obstetrics & Gynecology, 112*, 963–965.

Combs, C., Garite, T., Maurel, K., Das, A., Porto, M., & Obstetrix Collaborative Research Network. (2011). 17-hydroxyprogesterone caproate for twin pregnancy: A double-blind, randomized clinical trial. *American Journal of Obstetrics & Gynecology, 204*(221), e1–e8.

DeFranco, E., O'Brien, J., Adair, C., Lewis, D., Hall, D., Fusey, S., & Creasy, G. (2007). Vaginal progesterone is associated with a decrease in risk for early preterm birth and improved neonatal outcome in women with a short cervix: A secondary analysis from a randomized, double-blind, placebo-controlled trial. *Ultrasound in Obstetrics & Gynecology, 30*(5), 697–705.

Dodd, J., Crowhter, C., Cincotta, R., Flenady, V., & Robinson, J. (2005). Progesterone supplementation for preventing preterm birth: A systematic review and meta-analysis. *Acta Obstetricia et Gynecologica Scandinavica, 84*(6), 526–533.

Dodd, J., Flenady, V., Cincotta, R., & Crowther, C. (2006). Prenatal administration of progesterone for preventing preterm birth in women considered to be at risk of preterm birth. *Cochrane Database of Systematic Reviews, (1), CD004947*. doi:10.1002/14651858.CD004947.pub2

Durnwald, C., Momirova, V., Rouse, D., Caritis, S., Peaceman, A., Sciscione, A., & Eunice Shriver National Institute for Child Health and Human Development Maternal-Fetal Medicine Units Network. (2010). Second trimester cervical length and risk of preterm birth in women with twin gestations treated with 17-α hydroxyprogesterone caproate. *The Journal of Maternal-Fetal and Neonatal Medicine, 23*(12), 1360–1364.

Farine, D., Mundle, W. R., Dodd, J., Basso, M., Delisle, M., Farine, D., . . . Maternal Fetal Medicine Committee, Society of Obstetricians and Gynaecologists of Canada. (2008). The

(*continued*)

use of progesterone for prevention of preterm birth. *Journal of Obstetrics & Gynaecology Canada, 30(1), 67–71.*

Iams, J., Goldenberg, R., Meis, P., Mercer, B., Moawad, A., Das, A., & Roberts, J. (1996). The length of the cervix and the risk of spontaneous premature delivery. National Institute of Child Health and Human Development Maternal Fetal Medicine Unit Network. *New England Journal of Medicine, 334*(9), 567–572.

Lim, A., *Schuit, E., Bloemenkamp, K., Bernardus, R.,* Duvekot, J., Jaap, J., & Bruinse, H. (2011). 17-hydroxyprogesterone caproate for the prevention of adverse neonatal outcome in multiple pregnancies: A randomized controlled trial. *Obstetrics & Gynecology, 118*(3), *513–520.*

March of Dimes. (2012). March of Dimes 2011 Premature Birth Report Card. Retrieved from http://www.marchofdimes.com/peristats/pdflib/998/US.pdf

Norwitz, E. R., & Caughey, A. B. (2011). Progesterone supplementation and the prevention of preterm birth. *Reviews in Obstetrics and Gynecology, 4*(2), *60–72.*

Rode, L., Klein, K., Nicolaides, K., Krampl-Bettleheim, E., Tabor, A., & Predict Group. (2011). Prevention of preterm delivery in twin gestations (PREDICT): A multicenter, randomized, placebo-controlled trial on the effect of vaginal micronized progesterone. *Ultrasound in Obstetrics & Gynecology, 38*(3), 272–280.

Romero, R., Nicolaides, K., Conde-Auudelo, A., Tabor, A., O'Brien, J., Cetingoz, E., Hassan, S. (2012). Vaginal progesterone in women with an asymptomatic sonographic short cervix in the midtrimester decreases preterm delivery and neonatal morbidity: A systematic review and meta-analysis of individual patient data. *American Journal of Obstetrics & Gynecology, 206*(124), e1–e19.

ONLINE RESOURCES

Born Too Soon: The Global Action Report on Preterm Birth
http://www.who.int/pmnch/media/news/2012/preterm_birth_report/en/index.html

CDC-Medications and Pregnancy
http://www.cdc.gov/ncbddd/pregnancy_gateway/meds/index.html

MedCalc: Ballard Maturational Assessment of Gestational Age
An interactive website for determining gestational age of the infant at birth
http://www.medcalc.com/ballard.html

National Center on Shaken Baby Syndrome
Website provides educational information about SBS
http://www.dontshake.org/sbs.php?topNavID=3 . . . subNavID=317

The MDG Monitor
Provides information about the MDGs, how they link to prematurity, and allows users to track global progress towards attaining the goals. Sponsored by United Nations
http://www.mdgmonitor.org/index.cfm

REFERENCES

Abdulhamid, I., & Pataki, C. (2011). Pediatric Munchausen syndrome by proxy. *Medscape Reference*. Retrieved from http://emedicine.medscape.com/article/917525-overview#a1

Ahn, Y. (2008). Assessment of gestational age using an extended new Ballard examination in Korean infants. *The Journal of Tropical Paediatrics, 54*(4), 278–281.

Alexander, G. (2007). Prematurity at birth: Determinants, consequences, and geographic variation in Institute of Medicine (US) Committee on understanding premature birth and assuring healthy outcomes. In R. E. Berhman & A. S. Butler (Eds.), *Preterm birth: Causes, consequences, and prevention* (pp. 604–643). Washington, DC: National Academies Press.

Aliyu, M. H., Salihu, H. M., Keith, L. G., Ehiri, J. E., Islam, M. A., & Jolly, P. E. (2005). High parity and fetal morbidity outcomes. *Obstetrics & Gynecology, 105*(5), 1045–1051.

Aly, H., Hammad, T., Nada, A., Mohamed, M., Bathgate, S., & El-Mohandes, A. (2010). Maternal obesity associated complications and risk of prematurity. *Journal of Perinatology, 30*(7), 447–451.

American Academy of Pediatrics. (2012a). *Neonatal resuscitation program: International NRP Abroad*. Retrieved from http://www2.aap.org/nrp/providers/intl/intl_abroad.html

American Academy of Pediatrics. (2012b). *Helping babies breathe: The golden minute*. Retrieved from http://www.helpingbabiesbreathe.org/index.html

American Academy of Pediatrics, Committee on Child Health Financing and Committee on Substance Abuse. (2001). Improving substance abuse prevention, assessment, and treatment financing for children and adolescents. *Pediatrics, 108*(4), 1025–1029.

American Academy of Pediatrics, Committee on Drugs. (2001). The transfer of drugs and other chemicals into human milk. *Pediatrics, 108*, 776–789.

American Academy of Pediatrics, Task Force on Sudden Infant Death Syndrome. (2005). The changing concept of sudden infant death syndrome: Diagnostic coding shifts, controversies regarding the sleeping environment, and new variables to consider in reducing risk. *Pediatrics, 116*(5), 1245–1255.

American College of Obstetricians and Gynecologists, Committee on Practice. (2004). Management of postterm pregnancy. ACOG practice bulletin: Clinical management guidelines for obstetrician-gynecologists. No. 55. *Obstetrics & Gynecology, 104*(3), 639–646.

American College of Obstetricians and Gynecologists. (2011). Screening and diagnosis of gestational diabetes mellitus. Committee Opinion No. 504. *Obstetrics & Gynecology, 118*, 751–753.

American Diabetes Association. (2005). Standards of medical care. *Diabetes Care, 28*, S4–S36.

Amina, P., Alio, A., Salihu, H., McIntosh, C., August, E., Weldeselasse, H., . . . Mbah, A. (2012). The effect of paternal age on fetal birth outcomes. *American Journal of Men's Health, 6*(5), 427–435.

Ananth, C., & VanderWeel, T. (2011). Placental abruption and perinatal mortality with preterm delivery as a mediator: Disentangling direct and indirect effects. *American Journal of Epidemiology, 174*(1), 99–108.

Ananth, C., Wilcox, A., Savitz, D., Bowes, W., & Luther, E. (1996). Effect of maternal age and parity on the risk of uteroplacental bleeding disorders in pregnancy. *Obstetrics & Gynecology, 88*(4 Pt. 1), 511–516.

Andersen, A., Wohlfahrt, J., Christens, P., Olsen, J., & Melbye, M. (2000). Maternal age and fetal loss: Population based register linkage study. *British Medical Journal, 320*(7251), 1708–1712.

Anderson, P., & Doyle, L. (2003). Neurobehavioral outcomes of school-age children born extremely low birth weight or very preterm in the 1990s. *Journal of the American Medical Association, 289*, 3264–3272.

Ballard, J., Khoury, J., Wedig, K., Wang, L., Eilers-Walsman, B., & Lipp, R. (1991). New Ballard score, expanded to include extremely premature infants. *Journal of Pediatrics, 119*(3), 417–423.

Barber, M., & Davis, P. (2002). Fits, faints, or fatal fantasy? Fabricated seizures and child abuse. *Archives in Disease in Childhood, 86*, 230–233.

Barker, D. (2006). Adult consequences of fetal growth restriction. *Clinical Obstetrics and Gynecology, 49*(2), 273–280.

Barton, C., Barton, J., O'Brien, J., Bergauer, N., & Sibai, B. (2002). Mild gestational hypertension: Differences in ethnicity are associated with altered outcomes in women who undergo outpatient treatment. *American Journal of Obstetrics & Gynecology, 186*(5), 896–898.

Barton, J., O'Brien, J., Bergauer, N., Jacques, D., & Sibai, B. (2001). Mild gestational hypertension remote from term: Progression and outcome. *American Journal of Obstetrics & Gynecology, 184*(5), 979–983.

Bhutta, Z., Ahmed, T., Black, R., Cousens, S., Dewey, K., Giugliani, E., & Shekar, M. (2008). What works? Interventions for maternal and child undernutrition and survival. *Lancet, 371*(9610), 417–440. doi:10.1016/S0140-6736(07) 61693-6

Blosky, M. A., Zhengmin, O., Wood, C., Betoni, J., Black, L., Wary, A., & Stewart, W. (2010). Premature birth, initial hospital length of stay and costs. *Clinical Medicine & Research, 8*(3–4), 184. doi:10.3121/cmr.2010.943.ps1-22

Braveman, P., & Barclay, C. (2009). Health disparities beginning in childhood: A life-course perspective. *Pediatrics, 124*, S163. doi:10.1542/peds.2009-1100D

Buchbinder, A., Sibai, B., Caritis, S., MacPherson, C., Hauth, J., Lindheimer, M., & Thurnau, G. (2002). Adverse perinatal outcomes are significantly higher in severe gestational hypertension than in mild preeclampsia. *American Journal of Obstetrics & Gynecology, 186*(1), 66–71.

Burnett, L., & Adler, J. (2011). Sudden infant death syndrome in emergency medicine. *Medscape Reference*. Retrieved from http://www.emedicine.com/emerg/topic407.htm#section~author_information

Caughey, A., Stotland, N., Washington, A., & Escobar, G. (2007). Maternal and obstetric complications of pregnancy are associated with increasing gestational age at term. *American Journal of Obstetrics and Gynecology, 196*(2), 155e1–155e6.

Caughey, A., Washington, A., & Laros, R. (2005). Neonatal complications of term pregnancy: Rates by gestational age increase in a continuous not threshold fashion. *American Journal of Obstetrics and Gynecology, 192*, 185–190.

Centers for Disease Control and Prevention. (2011). *What is assisted reproductive technology?* Retrieved from http://www.cdc.gov/ART/index.htm

Centers for Disease Control and Prevention. (2013). *Folic acid-data and statistics*. Retrieved from http://www.cdc.gov/ncbddd/folicacid/data.html

Central Intelligence Agency. (2012). *The world factbook 2012*. Washington, DC: Central Intelligence Agency. Retrieved from https://www.cia.gov/library/publications/the-world-factbook/fields/2091.html#xx

Chakraborti, I. (2012). Management of diabetes before, during and after pregnancy. *Prescriber, 23*(6), 28–34.

Chiriboga, C. (2003). Fetal alcohol and drug effects. *The Neurologist, 9*(6), 267–279.

Christian, C., Block, R., & The Committee on Child Abuse and Neglect. (2009). Abusive head trauma in infants and children. *Pediatrics, 123*(5), 1409–1411. doi:10.1542/peds.2009-0408

Class, Q. A., Lichtenstein, P., Langstrom, N., & D'Onofrio, B. (2011). Timing of prenatal maternal exposure to severe life events and adverse pregnancy outcomes: A population study of 2.6 million pregnancies. *Psychosomatic Medicine, 73*, 234–241. doi:10.1097/PSY.0b013e31820a62ce

Cleary-Goldman, J., Malone, F., Vidaver, J., Ball, R., Nyberg, D., Comstock, C., & D'Alton, M. (2005). Impact of maternal age on obstetric outcome. *Obstetrics & Gynecology, 105*(5), 983–990.

Corbett, R. W., Ryan, C., & Weinrich, S. (2003). Pica in pregnancy: Does it affect pregnancy outcomes? *MCN: The American Journal of Maternal/Child Nursing, 28*(3), 183–191.

Dunkel Schetter, C. (2011). Psychological science on pregnancy: Stress processes, biopsychosocial models, and emerging research issues. *The Annual Review of Psychology, 62*, 531–558. doi:10.1146/annurev.psych.031809.130727

Eisele, T., Larsen, D., Walker, N., Cibulskis, R., Yukich, J., Zikusooka, C., & Steketee, R. (2012). Estimates of child deaths prevented from malaria prevention scale-up in Africa 2001–2010. *Malaria Journal, 11*, 93. (Published online March 28, 2012). doi:10.1186/1475-2875-11-93

Ezechi, O., Petterson, K., & Byamugisha, J. (2012). HIV/AIDS, tuberculosis, and malaria in pregnancy. *Journal of Pregnancy*. doi:10.1155/2012/140826

Faraci, M., Renda, E., Santo, M., DiPrima, F., Valenti, O., DeDomenico, R., . . . Hyseni, E. (2011). Fetal growth restriction: Current perspectives. *Journal Prenatal Medicine, 5*(2), 31–33.

Fowles, E., Bryant, M., Kim, S. H., Walker, L., Ruiz, R., Timmerman, G., & Brown, A. (2011). Predictors of dietary quality in low-income pregnant women. *Nursing Research, 60*(5), 286–294.

Fraser, A. M., Brockert, J. E., & Ward, R. H. (1995). Association of young maternal age with adverse reproductive outcomes. *The New England Journal of Medicine, 332*(17), 1113–1118.

Fuentes-Afflick, E., & Hessol, N. A. (2000). Interpregnancy interval and the risk of premature infants. *Obstetrics & Gynecology, 95*(3), 383–390.

Garcia-Algar, O., Vall, O., Alameda, F., Puig, C., Pellegrini, M., Pacifici, R., & Pichini, S. (2005). Prenatal exposure to arecoline (areca nut alkaloid) and birth outcomes. *Archives of Disease in Childhood Fetal and Neonatal Edition, 90*(3), F276–F277.

Gennaro, S. (2005). Overview of current state of research on pregnancy outcomes in minority populations. *American Journal of Obstetrics and Gynecology, 192*(Suppl. 5), S3–S10.

Geronimus, A. (1992). The weathering hypothesis and the health of African-American women and infants: Evidence and speculations. *Ethnicity & Disease, 2*(3), 207–221.

Geronimus, A. (1996). Black/White differences in the relationship of maternal age to birthweight: A population-based test of the weathering hypothesis. *Social Science & Medicine, 43*(4), 589–597.

Giurgescu, C., McFarlin, B., Lomax, J., Craddock, C., & Albrecht, A. (2011). Racial discrimination and the black-white gap in adverse birth outcomes: A review. *Journal of Midwifery and Women's Health, 56*(4), 362–370.

Gleicher, N., Weghofer, A., & Barad, D. (2011). Defining ovarian reserve to better understand ovarian aging. *Reproductive Biology and Endocrinology, 9*, 23. doi:10.1186/1477-7827-9-23

Gouin, K., Murphy, K., Shah, P., Murphy, K., McDonald, S., Hutton, E., & Beyene, J. (2011). Effects of cocaine use during pregnancy on low birthweight and preterm birth: Systematic review and meta-analyses. *American Journal of Obstetrics & Gynecology, 204*(340), e1–e12.

Gould, J., Madan, A., Qin, C., & Chavez, G. (2003). Perinatal outcomes in two dissimilar immigrant populations in the United States: A dual epidemiologic paradox. *Pediatrics, 111*(6), 676–682.

Gouveia, N., Bremner, S., & Novaes, H. (2004). Association between ambient air pollution and birth weight in São Paulo, Brazil. *Journal of Epidemiology and Community Health, 58*(1), 11–17.

Green, N. (2004). Risks of birth defects and other adverse outcomes associated with assisted reproductive technology. *Pediatrics, 114*(1), 256–259.

Haas, J., Fuentes-Afflick, E., Stewart, A., Jackson, R., Dean, M., Brawarsky, P., & Escobar, G. (2005). Prepregnancy health status and the risk of preterm delivery. *Archives of Pediatrics and Adolescent Medicine, 159*(1), 58–63.

Hamilton, B., Martin, J., & Ventura, S. (2011). Births: Preliminary data for 2010. *National Vital Statistics Reports, 60*(2). Retrieved from http://www.cdc.gov/nchs/data/nvsr/nvsr60/nvsr60_02.pdf

Harville, E., Xiong, X., & Buekens, P. (2011). Disasters and perinatal health: A systematic review. *Obstetrical and Gynecological Survey, 65*(11), 713–728.

Hauck, F., Tanabe, K., & Moon, R. (2011). Racial and ethnic disparities in infant mortality. *Seminars in Perinatology, 35*(4), 209–220.

Heffner, L. (2004). Advanced maternal age—How old is too old? *New England Journal of Medicine, 351*(19), 1927–1929.

Hogue, C. R., & Bremner, J. D. (2005). Stress model for research into preterm delivery among black women. *American Journal of Obstetrics & Gynecology, 192*(Suppl. 5), S47–S55.

Hook, E., & Lindsjo, A. (1978). Down syndrome in live births by single year maternal age interval in a Swedish study: Comparison with results from a New York State study. *American Journal of Human Genetics, 30*(1), 19–27.

Hunt, C. E. (2005). Gene-environment interactions: Implications for sudden unexpected deaths in infancy. *Archives Disease in Childhood, 90*(1), 48–53.

Hunt, K., & Schuller, K. (2007). The increasing prevalence of diabetes in pregnancy. *Obstetrics and Gynecology Clinics of North America, 34*(2), 173, vii. doi:10.1016/j.ogc.2007.03.00

Institute of Medicine (U.S.) Committee on Understanding Premature Birth and Assuring Healthy Outcomes, Berhman, R. E., & Butler, A. S. (Eds.). (2007). *Preterm birth: Causes, consequences, and prevention*. Washington, DC: National Academies Press.

Ivers, L., & Cullen, K. (2011). Food insecurity: Special considerations for women. *American Journal of Clinical Nutrition, 94*(6), 1740S–1744S.

Janakiraman, V. (2008). Listeriosis in pregnancy: Diagnosis, treatment, and prevention. *Reviews in Obstetrics & Gynecology, 1*(4), 179–185.

Joss-Moore, L., & Lane, R. (2009). The developmental origins of adult disease. *Current Opinion in Pediatrics, 21*(2), 230–234.

Kanungo, J., James, A., McMillan, D., Lodha, A., Faucher, D., Lee, S., & Canadian Neonatal Network. (2011). Advanced maternal age and the outcomes of preterm neonates: A social paradox? *Obstetrics and Gynecology, 118*(4), 872–877.

Khashan, A., McNamee, R., Abel, K., Mortensen, P., Kenny, L., Pedersen, M., & Baker, P. (2009). Rates of preterm birth following antenatal maternal exposure to severe life events: A population-based cohort study. *Human Reproduction, 24*(2), 429–437.

King, W., MacKay, M., & Sirnick, A. (2003). Shaken baby syndrome in Canada: Clinical characteristics and outcomes of hospital cases. *Canadian Medical Association Journal, 168*(2), 155–159.

Kitzmiller, J., Block, J., Brown, F., Catalano, P., Conway, D., Coustan, D., & Kirkman, M. (2008). Managing preexisting diabetes for pregnancy: Summary of evidence and consensus recommendations for care. *Diabetes Care, 31*(5), 1060–1079. doi:10.2337/dc08-9020

Kongnyuy, E., Nana, P., Fomulu, N., Wiysonge, S., Kouam, L., & Doh, A. S. (2008). Adverse perinatal outcomes of adolescent pregnancies in Cameroon. *Maternal Child Health Journal, 12*, 149–154.

Kramer, K., & Lancaster, J. (2010). Teen motherhood in cross-cultural perspective. *Annals of Human Biology, 37*(5), 613–628.

Kristensen, J., Vestergaard, M., Wisborg, K., Kesmodel, U., & Secher, N. (2005). Pre-pregnancy weight and the risk of stillbirth and neonatal death. *BJOG: An International Journal of Obstetrics and Gynaecology, 112*(4), 403–408.

Langer, O., Yogev, Y., Most, O., & Xenakis, E. (2005). Gestational diabetes: The consequences of not treating. *American Journal of Obstetrics and Gynecology, 192*(4), 989–997.

Lawn, J., Cousens, S., & Zupan, J. (2005). 4 million neonatal deaths: When? where? why? *Lancet, 365*(9474), 1845.

Leeman, L., & Fontaine, P. (2008). Hypertensive disorders of pregnancy. *American Family Physician, 78*(1), 93–100.

Levin, A. (2006). Eye findings in shaken baby syndrome. National Center on Shaken Baby Syndrome. Retrieved from http://dontshake.org/sbs.php?topNavID=3 . . . subNavID=25 . . . navID=279

Lung, F., Shu, B., Chiang, T., & Lin, S. (2009). Twin–singleton influence on infant development: A national birth cohort study. *Child: Care, Health and Development, 35*(3), 409–418.

MacDorman, M., & Mathews, T. (2011). *Understanding racial and ethnic disparities in U.S. Infant mortality rates*. NCHS Data Brief, No. 74. Hyattsville, MD: National Center for Health Statistics. Retrieved from http://www.cdc.gov/nchs/data/databriefs/db74.htm

MacDorman, M., Mathews, T., National Center for Health Statistics, & Centers for Disease Control. (2011). Infant deaths United States-2000–2007. *Morbidity & Mortality Weekly Report-Supplements*, 60(01), 49–51. Retrieved from http://www.cdc.gov/mmwr/preview/mmwrhtml/su6001a9.htm?s_cid=su6001a9_w

MacIntosh, G., Olshan, A., & Baird, P. (1995). Paternal age and the risk of birth defects in offspring. *Epidemiology, 6*(6), 640–641.

Manipalviratn, S., DeCherney, A., & Segars, J. (2009). Imprinting disorders and assisted reproductive technology. *Fertility and Sterility, 91*(2), 305–315.

March of Dimes. (2009). HIV and AIDS in pregnancy: Professionals and researchers quick reference and fact sheet. Retrieved from http://www.milesforbabies.org/professionals/14332_1223.asp#head4

Margerison-Zilko, C., Catalano, R., Hubbard, A., & Ahern, J. (2011). Maternal exposure to unexpected economic contraction and birth weight for gestational age. *Epidemiology, 22*(6), 855–858.

Martens, P., Derksen, S., & Gupta, S. (2004). Predictors of hospital readmisson of Manitoba newborns within six weeks postbirth discharge: A population-based study. *Pediatrics, 114*(3), 708–713.

Martin, J., Hamilton, B., Sutton, P., Ventura, S., Menacker, M., Kirkmeyer, S., & Mathews, T. (2009). Births: Final data for 2006. *National Vital Statistics Reports, 57*(1), 1–104.

Mathews, T. J., & MacDorman, M. F. (2012). Infant mortality statistics from the 2008 period linked birth/infant death data set. *National Vital Statistics Reports, 60*(5), 1–49. Retrieved from http://www.cdc.gov/nchs/data/nvsr/nvsr60/nvsr60_05.pdf

Mathews, T., Miniño, A., Osterman, M., Strobino, D., & Guyer, B. (2011). Annual summary of vital statistics: 2008. *Pediatrics, 127*, 146–157.

Mattison, D. R. (2010). Environmental exposures and development. *Current Opinions in Pediatrics, 22*, 208–218. doi:10.1097/MOP.0b013e32833779bf

Mavalankar, D. V., & Rosenfield, A. (2005). Maternal mortality in resource-poor settings: Policy barriers to care. *American Journal of Public Health, 95*(2), 200–203.

Mercer, B. (2003). Preterm premature rupture of the membranes. *Obstetrics & Gynecology, 101*(1), 178–193.

Micheli, K., Komninos, I., Bagkeris, E., Roumeliotaki, T., Koutis, A., Kogevina, T., & Chatzi, L. (2011). Sleep patterns in late pregnancy and risk of preterm birth and fetal growth restriction. *Epidemiology, 22*, 738–744.

Mistry, H., & Williams, P. (2011). The importance of antioxidant micronutrients in pregnancy. *Oxidative Medicine and Cellular Longevity*. doi:10.1155/2011/841749

Mitchell, A., Gilboa, S., Werler, M., Kelley, K., Louik, C., & Hernández-Díaz, S. (2011). Medication use during pregnancy, with particular focus on prescription drugs: 1976–2008. *American Journal of Obstetrics & Gynecology, 205*(1), 51.e1–51.e8.

Morantz, C., & Torrey, B. (2004). Practice guideline briefs: Management of postterm pregnancy. *American Family Physician, 70*(9) [electronic version]. Retrieved from http://www.aafp.org/afp/2004/1101/p1808.html

Muglia, L., & Katz, M. (2010). The enigma of spontaneous preterm birth. *The New England Journal of Medicine, 362*, 529–535.

Murphy, S., Xu, J., & Kochanek, K. (2012). Deaths: Preliminary data for 2010. *National Vital Statistics Reports, 60*(4). Retrieved from http://www.cdc.gov/nchs/data/nvsr/nvsr60/nvsr60_04.pdf

Nahum, G., Talavera, F., Legro, R., Gaupp, F., & Smith, C. (2011). Estimation of fetal weight. *Medscape*. Retrieved from http://emedicine.medscape.com/article/262865-overview#aw2aab6b2

Norwitz, E., & Caughey, A. (2011). Progesterone supplementation and the prevention of preterm birth. *Reviews in Obstetrics & Gynecology, 4*(2), 60–72.

Norwitz, E., Snegovskikh, V., & Caughey, A. (2007). Prolonged pregnancy: When should we intervene? *Clinical Obstetrics & Gynecology, 50*(2), 547–557.

Nuru-Jeter, A., Dominguez, T., Hammon, W., Leu, J., Skaff, M., Egerter, S., & Braveman, P. (2009)."It's the skin you're in": African-American women talk about their experiences in racism. An exploratory study to develop measures of racism for birth outcomes studies. *Maternal Child Health Journal, 13*(1), 29–39. doi:10.1007/s10995-008-0357-x

Okah, F., Cai, J., & Hoff, G. (2005). Term-gestation low birth weight and health-compromising behaviors during pregnancy. *Obstetrics and Gynecology, 105*(3), 543–550.

Patrick, T., & Bryan, T. (2005). Research strategies for optimizing pregnancy outcomes in minority populations. *American Journal of Obstetrics & Gynecology, 192*, S64–S70.

Rao, S., Gokhale, M., Joshi, S., & Kanade, A. (2010). Early life undernutrition and adolescent pregnancy outcome in rural India. *Annals of Human Biology, 37*(4), 475–487. doi:10.3109/03014460903434941

Ramsey, P., Lieman, J., Brumfield, C., & Carlo, W. (2005). Chorioamnionitis increases neonatal morbidity in pregnancies complicated by preterm premature rupture of membranes. *American Journal of Obstetrics & Gynecology, 192*, 1162–1166.

Reece, R. (2005). *What the literature tells us about rib fractures in infancy.* National Center on Shaken Baby Syndrome. Retrieved from http://dontshake.org/sbs.php?topNavID=3 . . . subNavID=28 . . . navID=106

Reef, S., Strebel, P., Dabbagh, A., Gacic-Dobo, M., & Cochil, S. (2011). Progress toward control of rubella and prevention of congenital rubella syndrome—Worldwide, 2009. *The Journal of Infectious Diseases, 204*, S24–S27.

Regidor, E., Ronda, E., Garcia, A. M., & Dominguez, V. (2004). Paternal exposure to agricultural pesticides and cause specific fetal death. *Occupational and Environmental Medicine, 61*(4), 334–339.

Rich-Edwards, J. W., Buka, S., Brennan, R., & Earls, F. (2003). Diverging associations of maternal age with low birthweight for black and white mothers. *International Journal of Epidemiology, 32*(1), 83–90.

Rich-Edwards, J. W., & Grizzard, T. A. (2005). Psychosocial stress and neuroendocrine mechanisms in preterm delivery. *American Journal of Obstetrics and Gynecology, 192*(Suppl. 5), S30–S35.

Rosenthal, L., & Lobel, M. (2011). Explaining racial disparities in adverse birth outcomes: Unique sources of stress for Black American women. *Social Science & Medicine, 72*, 977–983. doi:10.1016/j.socimed.2011.01.013

Ross, M., Mansano, R., Talavera, F., & Smith, C. (2011). Fetal growth restriction. *Medscape*. Retrieved from http://emedicine.medscape.com/article/261226-overview

Rowbottom, S. (2007). *Giving girls today and tomorrow: Breaking the cycle of adolescent pregnancy*. New York, NY: United Nations Population Fund (UNFPA). Retrieved from http://www.unfpa.org/webdav/site/global/shared/documents/publications/2007/giving_girls.pdf

Ruiz-Mirazo, E., Lopez-Yarto, M., & McDonald, S. D. (2012). Group prenatal care versus individual prenatal care: A systematic review and meta-analyses. *Journal of Obstetrics and Gynaecology Canada, 34*(3), 223–229.

Salihu, H., Luke, S., Alio, A., Wathington, D., Mbah, A., Marty, P., & Whiteman, V. (2009). The superobese mother and ethnic disparities in preterm birth. *Journal of the National Medical Association, 101*(11), 1125–1131.

Salihu, H., Shumpert, M., Slay, M., Kirby, R., & Alexander, G. (2003). Childbearing beyond maternal age 50 and fetal outcomes in the United States. *Obstetrics and Gynecology, 102*, 1006–1014.

Salihu, H., Wilson, R., Alio, A., & Kirby, R. (2008). Advanced maternal age and risk of antepartum and intrapartum stillbirth. *Journal of Obstetrical and Gynaecological Research, 34*(5), 843–850.

Schaefer-Graf, U., Buchanan, T., Xiang, A., Songster, G., Montoro, M., & Kjos, S. (2000). Patterns of congenital anomalies and relationship to initial maternal fasting glucose levels in pregnancies complicated by type 2 and gestational diabetes. *American Journal of Obstetrics & Gynecology, 182*(2), 313–320.

Schempf, A., Branum, A., Lukacs, S., & Schoendorf, K. (2007). Maternal age and parity-associated risks of preterm birth: Differences by race/ethnicity. *Paediatric and Perinatal Epidemiology, 21*, 34–43.

Scifres, C., Stamilo, D., Macones, G., & Odibo, A. (2009). Predicting perinatal mortality in preterm intrauterine growth restriction. *American Journal of Perinatology, 26*(10), 723–728.

Seely, E., & Solomon, C. (2003). Insulin resistance and its potential role in pregnancy-induced hypertension. *The Journal of Clinical Endocrinology & Metabolism, 88*(6), 2393–2398.

Shah, P., Ohlsson, A., McDonald, S., Hutton, E., Shah, V., Beyene, J., & Allen, V. (2010). Paternal factors and low birthweight, preterm, and small for gestational age births: A systematic review. *American Journal of Obstetrics & Gynecology, 202*(2), 103–123.

Silbergeld, E., & Patrick, T. (2005). Environmental exposures, toxicologic mechanisms, and adverse pregnancy outcomes. *American Journal of Obstetrics & Gynecology, 192*(Suppl. 5), S11–S21.

Smith, J. (2003). Shaken baby syndrome. *Orthopaedic Nursing, 22*(3), 196–203.

Smith-Battle, L. (2006). Helping teen mothers succeed. *The Journal of School Nursing, 22*(3), 130–135.

Substance Abuse and Mental Health Services Administration. (2011). *Results from the 2010 national survey on drug use and health: Summary of national findings*, NSDUH Series H-41, HHS Publication No. (SMA) 11-4658. Rockville, MD.

Sunderam, S., Chang, J., Flowers, L., Kulkami, A., Sentelle, G., Jeng, G., . . . & National Center for Chronic Disease Prevention and Health Promotion. (2009). Assisted reproductive technologies surveillance-2009. *Morbidity and Mortality Weekly Report*, 58(SS-05), 1–25.

Swanson, J., Entringer, S., Buss, C., & Wadhwa, P. (2009). Developmental origins of health and disease: Environmental exposures and the DOHaD approach. *Seminars in Reproductive Medicine, 27*(5), 391–402.

Taylor, R., Denison, F., Beyai, S., & Owens, S. (2010). The external Ballard examination does not accurately assess the gestational age of infants born at home in a rural community of the Gambia. *Annals of Tropical Paediatrics, 30*(3), 197–204.

Tegethoff, M., Greene, N., Olsen, J., Schaffner, E., & Meinlschmidt, G. (2011). Stress during pregnancy and offspring pediatric disease: Discussion and conclusions. *Environmental Health Perspectives, 119*(11), 1647–1652.

Torche, F. (2011). The effect of maternal stress on birth outcomes: Exploiting a natural experiment. *Demography, 48*(4), 1473–1491.

United Nations Children's Fund. (2009). *The state of the world's children: Maternal and newborn health.* Retrieved from http://www.unicef.org/sowc09/report/report.php

United States Agency for International Development. (2011). *Global health and child survival: Progress report to Congress 2010–2011.* Retrieved from http://transition.usaid.gov/our_work/global_health/home/Publications/csh_2012.html

U.S. Department of Health and Human Services. (2010). *Rethinking MCH: The life course model as an organizing framework—A concept paper.* Health Resources and Services Administration, Maternal and Child Bureau. Retrieved from http://www.hrsa.gov/ourstories/mchb75th/images/rethinkingmch.pdf

Vintzileos, A., Ananth, C., Smulian, J., Scorza, W., & Knuppel, R. (2002). The impact of prenatal care on postneonatal deaths in the presence and absence of antenatal high-risk conditions. *American Journal of Obstetrics and Gynecology, 187*(5), 1258–1262.

Wadhwa, P., Entringer, S., Buss, C., & Lu, M. (2011). The contribution of maternal stress to preterm birth: Issues and considerations. *Clinical Perinatology, 38*, 351–384.

Williamson, D., Abe, K., Bean, C., Ferre, C., Henderson, Z., & Lackritz, E. (2008). Current research in preterm birth. *Journal of Women's Health, 17*(10), 1545–1549.

Wilson-Costello, D., Friedman, H., Minich, N., Fanaroff, A., & Hack, M. (2005). Improved survival rates with increased neurodevelopmental disability for extremely low birth weight infants in the 1990s. *Pediatrics, 115*(4), 997–1003.

Wong, A., & Grobman, W. (2011). Medically indicated-iatrogenic prematurity. *Clinical Perinatology, 38*, 423–439. doi:10.1016/j.clp.2011.06.002

World Health Organization. (2005). *The world health report 2005—Make every mother and child count.* Retrieved from http://www.who.int/whr/2005/whr2005_en.pdf

World Health Organization. (2011a). WHO warns of consequences of underfunding TB. *World Health Organization Media Centre.* Retrieved from http://www.who.int/mediacentre/news/releases/2011/tb_20111011/en/index.html

World Health Organization. (2011b). *Global HIV/AIDS response: Epidemic update and health sector progress towards universal goals.* Retrieved from http://www.who.int/hiv/pub/progress_report2011/summary_en.pdf

World Health Organization. (2011c). *World health statistic 2011.* Retrieved from http://www.who.int/whosis/whostat/2011/en/index.html

World Health Organization, Howson, C., Kinney, M., & Lawn, J. (Eds.). (2012). *Born Too Soon: The global action report.* Retrieved from http://www.who.int/pmnch/media/news/2012/201204_borntoosoon-report.pdf

Yaniv, S., Levy, A., Wiznitzer, A., Holcberg, G., Mazor, M., & Sheiner, E. (2011). A significant linear association exists between advanced maternal age and adverse perinatal outcomes. *Archives of Gynecology and Obstetrics, 283*, 755–759.

Yogev, Y., Melamed, N., Bardin, R., Tenenbaum-Gavish, K., Ben-Shitrit, G., & Ben-Haroush, H. (2010). Pregnancy outcome at extremely advanced maternal age. *American Journal of Obstetrics and Gynecology, 203*, 558.e1–558.e7.

Yonge, O., & Haase, M. (2004). Munchausen syndrome and Munchausen syndrome by proxy in a student nurse. *Nurse Educator, 29*(4), 166–169.

Young, S., Khalfan, S., Farag, T., Kavle, J., Ali, S., Hajji, H., & Stolzfus, R. (2010). Association of pica with anemia and gastrointestinal distress among pregnant women in Zanzibar, Tanzania. *The American Journal of Tropical Medicine and Hygiene, 83*(1), 144–151. doi:10.4269/ajtmh.2010.09-0442

Zhang, J., Merialdi, M., Platt, L., & Kramer, M. S. (2010). Defining normal and abnormal fetal growth: Promises and challenges. *American Journal of Obstetrics and Gynecology, 202*(6), 522–528. doi:10.1016/j.ajog.2009.10.889

Zhu, J., Basso, O., Obel, C., Bille, C., & Olsen, J. (2006). Infertility, infertility treatment, and congenital malformations: Danish national birth cohort. *British Medical Journal, 333*(7570), 679–681.

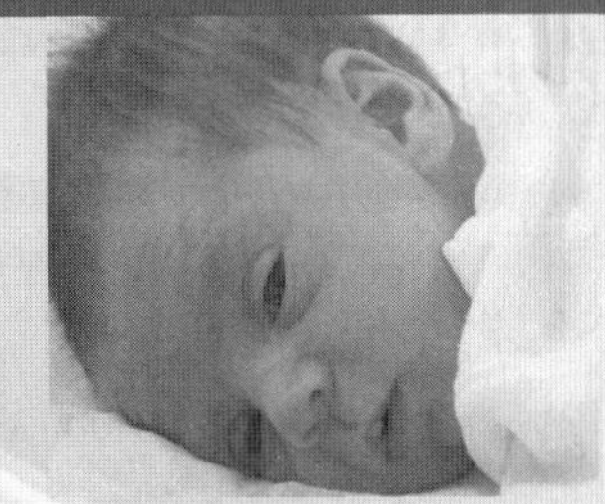

CHAPTER 3

Resuscitation and Stabilization of the Newborn and Infant

■ Gail A. Bagwell

The vulnerable and sick infant requires the health professional to quickly assess and take action when signs of cardiac or respiratory depression are present. This chapter begins with a discussion of risk factors that predispose the newborn to cardiorespiratory depression followed by a description of the actions to be taken to avoid this depression or to alleviate the symptoms and reverse a downward spiral and concludes with a short discussion on the stabilization of the ill neonate.

CAUSES OF CARDIORESPIRATORY DEPRESSION IN THE NEWBORN

The combined effects of numerous maternal, fetal, and intrauterine factors determine the condition of an infant at birth (some of these factors are listed in Table 3.1). Although some of these factors emerge only during labor and delivery (e.g., cord prolapse), most arise during gestation (e.g., placenta previa) or even before conception

TABLE 3.1

CONDITIONS ASSOCIATED WITH ASPHYXIATION OF NEWBORNS

Source of Problem	Conditions
Maternal	Amnionitis, anemia, gestational or insulin-dependent diabetes, gestational hypertension, preeclampsia or eclampsia, chronic maternal hypertension, maternal cardiac, pulmonary, renal, thyroid, neurologic or genetic disease, maternal deformities, hypotension, infection, polyhydramnios, oligohydramios, drug therapy such as magnesium sulfate, adrenergic agonists, maternal substance abuse, no prenatal care, mother older than 35 years of age, previous fetal or neonatal death
Uterine	Preterm labor, prolonged labor, premature rupture of membranes, multiple gestation, breech or other abnormal fetal presentation, precipitous delivery, uterine tachysystole with fetal heart rate changes
Placental	Placenta previa, abruption placentae, any second or third trimester bleeding, other significant intrapartum bleeding, placental insuffiency, postterm gestation
Umbilical	Cord prolapse, entanglement, compression, or rupture
Fetal	Category 2 or 3 fetal heart rate patterns, cephalopelvic disproportion, size date discrepancy, macrosomia, prematurity, intrauterine growth retardation, congenital abnormalities, fetal anemia or isoimmunization, erythroblastosis fetalis, intrauterine infection, decreased fetal activity, narcotics administered to the mother within 4 hours of delivery, meconium-stained fluid
Iatrogenic	Mechanical (difficult forceps or vacuum delivery), emergency C-section, drugs – general anesthesia

(e.g., maternal diabetes). Regardless of the site or time of origin, the influence of each of these problems can manifest as cardiorespiratory depression in the newborn.

To provide effective care, the nurse must be able not only to recognize potential risk factors but also to understand the ways in which they disrupt cardiorespiratory function. Ideally, the health professional determines that cardiorespiratory depression may occur and is thoroughly prepared to intervene. Although many risk factors come into play, the underlying pathogenic processes can be divided into six major categories. The mnemonic TAMMSS can be used as a simple but effective means of remembering these etiologic groups:

T Trauma
A Asphyxia (intrauterine)
M Medication
M Malformation
S Sepsis
S Shock (hypovolemia)

Trauma

Traumatic injury to the central or peripheral nervous system is an uncommon occurrence that can result in immediate or delayed respiratory depression. Because the skull is incompletely mineralized and has open sutures, it can undergo considerable distortion without fracture. However, the underlying membranes and vessels are much less resilient and are easily stretched or torn (subgaleal hemorrhage) if overly compressed, particularly if the pressure is abruptly applied. Similarly, forced traction or torsion of the neck during delivery may damage the spinal cord or the phrenic nerve, with consequent paralysis of the diaphragm. An unusually long and difficult delivery, multiple gestation, abnormal presentation (especially breech), cephalopelvic disproportion (secondary to macrosomia or a small or contracted pelvis), shoulder dystocia, or rapid extraction by forceps (as may be required for fetal distress) frequently are involved. Despite their generally low birth weight, premature infants also may be at risk because of the unusual compliance of their skulls.

Asphyxia (Intrauterine)

The most common cause of cardiorespiratory depression at birth is fetal hypoxia and asphyxia. Any condition that reduces oxygen delivery to the fetus may be the cause. Such conditions include maternal hypoxia (from hypoventilation and hyperventilation, respiratory or heart disease, anemia, postural hypotension); maternal vascular disease that results in placental insufficiency (from preexisting or pregnancy-induced diabetes, primary or pregnancy-induced hypertension); and accidents involving the umbilical cord (compression, entanglement, or prolapse). Postterm pregnancies also are at risk, perhaps because of placental aging and progressive placental insufficiency. An asphyxia episode occasionally may trigger the passage and aspiration of meconium in utero for term and postterm infants.

Medication

Pharmacologic agents given to the mother during labor and delivery as well as any medications including over the counter or herbs taken by the mother prior to the delivery may affect the fetus both directly and indirectly. Indirectly, these agents may cause maternal hypoventilation and hypotension or adversely affect placental perfusion. Hypnotic, analgesic, or anesthetic drugs may depress maternal respirations, resulting in reduced oxygen intake and delivery to the tissues and organs, including the uterus and placenta. Anesthetic agents, because of their effect on the sympathetic nervous system, may also cause peripheral vasodilation, diminished cardiac output, and hypotension with decreased placental perfusion. Narcotic analgesics, which rapidly cross the placenta, may directly depress the neonatal respiratory drive. Oxytocin (Pitocin), on the other hand, may cause uterine hyperstimulation and shorten placental perfusion time. Each of these conditions places the fetus at greater risk of fetal hypoxia and asphyxia. In addition, prescription and nonprescription medications and herbs that the mother may take prior to delivery may also affect the fetus. Many street drugs, especially opiate derivatives, are known to cause infants to deliver prematurely and may be associated with congenital anomalies, as well as cause infants to be depressed on delivery.

Malformation

Infants may have any of a vast array of congenital anomalies, but the ones that cause the most problems during the first few minutes of life are those associated with facial or upper airway deformities and conditions that lead to pulmonary hypoplasia. Many of these conditions can be diagnosed through antenatal ultrasonographic examinations and other screening techniques, but suspicion also should be raised if oligiohydramnios or polyhydramnios is reported.

Oligiohydramnios is seen with prolonged rupture or leakage of membranes and neonates with renal agenesis or dysplasia or urethral obstruction. If fluid is lost or diminished, the developing fetal structures may be compressed, leading to characteristic Potter facies (including micrognathia) or pulmonary hypoplasia. Polyhydramnios is seen in infants with impaired swallowing ability (as in anencephaly and neuromuscular disorders); in those with real or functional obstruction high in the gastrointestinal tract (as with esophageal atresia); and in those with profuse leakage of cerebrospinal fluid (as in neural tube defects), which contributes to the volume of amniotic fluid. Polyhydramnios is also noted with diaphragmatic hernia and hydrops fetalis.

Sepsis

The fetus may acquire bacterial or viral agents from infected amniotic fluid, from maternal blood crossing the placenta, or from direct contact on passage through the birth canal. An infant is especially susceptible to infection if born prematurely (because these infants are relatively immunocompromised) or if born to a mother who had a premature rupture of membranes or a history of infection or chorioamnionitis. If infection is acquired in utero, the lungs tend to be heavily involved, and the alveoli may be filled with exudate. The infant may be apneic at birth, may be slow to establish a spontaneous and regular breathing pattern, or may show frank signs of respiratory distress.

Shock (Hypovolemia)

Most of the blood lost during delivery is from the maternal side of the placenta and therefore is of no consequence to the newborn. However, blood loss from the fetal side of the placenta as a result of abruptio placenta or placenta previa can lead to acute hypovolemia and cardiovascular collapse. Normally the umbilical cord is unusually strong, but ruptures are possible if cord tension increases suddenly, as in a precipitous delivery, or if the vessels are superficially implanted in the placenta (velamentous insertions). In rare cases acute hypovolemia may occur without frank hemorrhage. With severe cord compression, for example, blood flow to the fetus is impeded. The umbilical arteries, however, are much more resistant to compression and continue to pump blood back to the placenta. In this case, the effects of hypovolemia and asphyxia may be superimposed. Infants with chronic blood loss (as in fetal-maternal hemorrhage or twin-to-twin transfusions) generally are asymptomatic immediately after delivery.

PREPARATION FOR DELIVERY

While the majority of deliveries will result in a healthy neonate that can go immediately to a mother's chest for skin-to-skin care, health care professionals must always be prepared for a problem to arise. The success of resuscitative efforts depends on multiple factors: (1) anticipation of the need, (2) the presence of trained personnel, (3) ready availability of necessary equipment and supplies, and (4) good communication and teamwork. The most competent personnel and the finest equipment are useless if they are not present in the delivery room. Frantic calls for assistance or a scavenger hunt for equipment should never occur; they needlessly delay intervention and can compromise the patient's outcome.

The antepartum and intrapartum history of each pregnant woman must be carefully reviewed to identify those at risk of delivering a depressed infant. Especially worrisome is a fetus that clinically demonstrates the effects of asphyxia (i.e., an indeterminate/abnormal fetal heart rate pattern, particularly bradycardia and persistently minimal or loss of fetal heart rate variability; acidosis, as determined by fetal scalp blood sampling; or meconium-stained amniotic fluid).

Personnel

Although most risk factors can be identified at some time during the pregnancy, many may not become apparent until birth. Delivery through meconium-stained amniotic fluid and unexpected diaphragmatic hernia are just two cases in point. Consequently, at least one person competent in neonatal resuscitation should be present at every delivery. Obviously, additional personnel should be made available if a depressed newborn is expected (Kattwinkel, 2011; Kattwinkel et al., 2010).

When a team is required, the role each member is to play in the resuscitative effort should be predetermined, including the head of the team. The head of the team, who has a complete set of resuscitation skills, will be the one to position the baby, open the airway and intubate the trachea if necessary, and evaluate and direct the resuscitation efforts. A second person will assist with positioning, suctioning, drying, as well as giving oxygen and positive pressure ventilation (PPV). A third person is responsible for monitoring the heart rate and for initiating chest compressions, if needed. If intravenous (IV) medications are required, two additional individuals are needed, one to catherize the umbilical vein and administer the drugs and the other to pass equipment and prepare the medications. The person who passes the equipment and prepares the medications may also be responsible for documenting the resuscitation process, but a sixth person is preferable to do this because minute-to-minute notations must be made. The individual delivering the baby is not considered part of this resuscitative team, as his or her main concern is the mother.

Equipment and Supplies

A newly born infant is predisposed to heat loss (particularly evaporative and radiant losses) and, if unprotected, can quickly become cold stressed. The consequences of such stress include hypoxemia, metabolic acidosis, and rapid depletion of glycogen stores with hypoglycemia. All are conditions that may exacerbate asphyxia and thus complicate resuscitation. Clearly, measures to prevent hypothermia must be part of any resuscitative effort. The delivery room should be kept warm, and the radiant bed should be preheated, if possible. Prewarming of linens, towels, and caps or other head coverings is also helpful.

For an extremely premature baby less than 28 weeks gestation, the use of a food-grade polyethylene bag or wrap up to the baby's neck, without drying, will reduce heat loss and help maintain the infant's body temperature in the delivery room. In addition, it has been found that a delivery room of at least 26°C assists with maintaining a premature infant's (<28 weeks gestation) body temperature in combination with the use of a polyethylene bag or wrap. Because of this finding, all delivery room temperatures should be at least 26°C or 78.8°F when delivering a baby less than 28 weeks gestation (Kattwinkel, 2011; Kattwinkel et al., 2010; Perlman et al., 2010).

Possible exposure to blood and body fluids is of particular concern in the delivery room. Gloves, gowns, masks, and protective eyewear should be worn during procedures that are likely to generate droplets or splashes of blood or other body fluids.

The additional equipment and supplies needed to carry out a full resuscitation (Box 3.1) should be checked as part of the daily routine. Small supplies should be organized according to frequency of use and may be displayed on a wall board, kept in the radiant warmer (if there is sufficient drawer space), and stored in a cart or specially designed tackle box. Breakaway security clips may be used to safeguard materials when they are not in use, but foolproof or locking closures that require a key are not appropriate in delivery rooms, birthing rooms, or nurseries. A bedside table or flat surface (other than the bed) should be within reach to provide space for catheter trays and medication preparation.

As the delivery nears, the team should double-check all supplies and make sure the equipment is in working order. Having an organized routine of checking the equipment will ensure that all equipment is present and in working order. Hospital infection control policies dictate how far in advance packaged supplies can be opened, connected to tubing, and otherwise prepared. A backup or duplicate set of materials should be maintained in case of equipment failure, contamination, or multiple births. All items used should be restocked as soon as possible after the resuscitation.

Good Communication and Teamwork

Communication and teamwork are behavior skills that are essential to a successful neonatal resuscitation. The best clinicians working together in resuscitation will not work effectively together, if they do not possess the skills to communicate and coordinate with each other. Learning to communicate and assign tasks is as essential to a neonatal resuscitation as the ability to perform bag/mask ventilation or cardiac compressions.

BOX 3.1

EQUIPMENT AND SUPPLIES NEEDED FOR FULL RESUSCITATION

Suction Equipment

Bulb syringe

Mechanical suction device and tubing

Suction catheters (5 or 6 French, 8 French, 10 French, 12 French, or 14 French)

8 French feeding tube and 20-mL syringe

Meconium aspirator

Bag and Mask Equipment

Device for delivering PPV, capable of delivering 90%–100% oxygen

Face masks, newborn and premature sizes (cushioned rim masks preferred)

Oxygen source

Compressed air source

Oxygen blender to mix oxygen and compressed air with flowmeter (flow rate up to 10 L/min) and tubing

Intubation Equipment

Laryngoscope with straight blades, No. 0 (preterm) and No. 1 (term)

Extra bulbs and batteries for laryngoscope

ET tubes—2.5, 3.0, 3.5, and 4.0 mm internal diameter

Stylet (optional)

Scissors

Tape or securing device for ET tube

Alcohol sponges

CO_2 detector or capnograph

LMA

Medications

Epinephrine 1:10,000 (0.1 mg.mL)—3-mL or 10-mL ampules

Isotonic crystalloid (normal saline or Ringer's lactate) for volume expansion—100 or 250 mL

Dextrose 10% (250 mL)

Normal saline (for flushes)

Umbilical Vessel Catheterization Supplies

Sterile gloves

Scalpel or scissors

Antiseptic prep solution

Umbilical tape

Umbilical catheters—3.5 French, 5 French

Three-way stopcock

Syringes—1, 3, 5, 10, 20, 50 mL

Needles—25, 21, 18 gauge—or puncture device for needleless system

Miscellaneous

Gloves and appropriate personal protection

Radiant warmer or other heat source

Firm, padded resuscitation surface

Clock with second hand (timer optional)

Warmed linens

Stethoscope (neonatal head preferred)

Tape, ½ or ¾ inch

Cardiac monitor and electrodes or pulse oximeter and probe (optional for delivery room)

Oropharyngeal airways—0, 00, 000 sizes or 30, 40, and 50 mm lengths

For Very Preterm Babies

Size 00 laryngoscope blade (optional)

Reclosable, food-grade plastic bag (1-gallon size) or plastic wrap

Chemically activated warming pad (optional)

Transport incubator to maintain baby's temperature during move to the nursery

Adapted from Kattwinkel (2011) (Lesson 1: Overview and Principles of Resuscitation).

GENERAL CONSIDERATIONS

The two goals of resuscitation are: (1) to remove or ameliorate the underlying cause of asphyxia and (2) to reverse or correct the associated chain of events (hypoxia, hypercarbia, acidosis, bradycardia, and hypotension). To achieve these ends, resuscitation management should be centered on attempts to expand, ventilate, and oxygenate the lungs, with cardiac assistance provided as necessary. However, intervention must be specific to each infant in extent and form and must be determined by appropriate assessment.

The Apgar score provides a shorthand description of the neonate's condition at specific intervals after birth and may be useful as a rough prognostic indicator of long-term outcome; however, it does have limitations. Although it is a quantitative tool, the scoring often is subjectively or retrospectively applied. It often is poorly correlated with other indicators of well-being, such as cord pH. Its usefulness is suspect with extremely preterm infants who may have poor respiratory drive and who may be relatively hyporeflexive and hypotonic because of immaturity rather than distress. Finally waiting until the first Apgar score is assigned at 1 minute of age causes unnecessary delay in care. For these reasons, the Apgar score should not be used to determine the need for or course of resuscitation (Kattwinkel, 2011).

As soon as the need for resuscitation is determined, the initiation and progression of resuscitation are based on three signs: respirations, heart rate, and oxygenation. Heart rate is the most sensitive indicator of resuscitation efforts, with auscultation being the most accurate. In the past several years there have been an increasing number of studies done showing that health care professionals are not reliable in judging a neonate's color in the delivery room as well as studies showing the use of a pulse oximeter in the delivery room to be accurate in measuring a heart rate and O_2 saturations after 90 seconds from birth (Altuncu, Ozek, Bilgen, Topuzoglu, & Kavuncuoglu, 2008; O'Donnell, Kamlin, Davis, Carlin, & Morley, 2007; O'Donnell, Kamlin, Davis, & Morley, 2005). Other studies on oxygenation of the neonate have shown that hyperoxia can be as detrimental to a neonate as hypoxia at the cellular and functional levels (Davis, Tan, O'Donnell, & Schulze, 2004; Rabi, Rabi, & Yee, 2007; Saugstad, Rootwelt, & Aalen, 1998; Vento et al., 2001; Wang et al., 2008). Because of these studies the use of color has been removed and the use of a pulse oximeter designed to reduce movement artifact and a neonatal probe is now recommended. When placing a pulse oximeter, place it on the neonate's right hand or wrist, as preductal values are higher than postductal values. Always place the probe on the neonate prior to connecting the probe to the machine to produce quicker and more reliable values (O'Donnell et al., 2005).

As soon as the infant has been positioned under a radiant warmer, thoroughly dried, airway cleared if necessary and stimulated, these signs are to be assessed at 30-second intervals and interventions are carried out as needed. The basics of neonatal resuscitation are as easy as ABCD: *airway, breathing, circulation, and drugs*. These are the critical elements of any resuscitative effort.

Airway Control

■ Positioning. Airway control is a fundamental prerequisite for effective oxygenation and ventilation. To achieve this, the infant should be placed in a flat supine or side-lying position. The practice of placing the infant in a slight head-down tilt (Trendelenburg position) has been abandoned. This maneuver historically was used under the presumption that fluids from the lower extremities would be redistributed to the intrathoracic compartment. Studies with healthy adults in the Trendelenburg position have demonstrated improvement, albeit transient (lasting <10 minutes), in the stroke volume of the heart, but they have also indicated that a tilt as slight as 10 degrees may cause blood to pool in the dependent cerebrovascular bed. Infants have only a limited ability to increase stroke volume but are at greater risk than older children and adults for intraventricular hemorrhages secondary to rupture of the vulnerable microvessels of the germinal matrix; consequently, the potential benefit, if any, of the head-down tilt position is not believed to be worth the risk.

Once the infant is in the supine position, the neck is placed in a neutral or slightly extended "sniffing" position which aligns the posterior pharynx, larynx, and trachea (Kattwinkel, 2011; Kattwinkel et al., 2010). Compared with the adult tongue, an infant's tongue is relatively large in proportion to the mouth, and this slight extension moves the tongue and epiglottis away from the posterior pharyngeal wall and opens the airway. However, care must be taken to avoid full extension, which reduces the circumference of the airway and increases airway resistance. The reasonably safe extension posture appears to be no more than 15 to 30 degrees from neutral. An oral airway should be placed if the tongue is unusually large (as in Beckwith-Wiedemann syndrome) or if the chin is unusually small, causing posterior displacement of the tongue (as in Pierre Robin sequence or Potter association). Because newborns also have a relatively large head in comparison with the chest and tend naturally to fall into a flexed position, a shoulder roll made of a blanket or small towel may be used to raise the chest and align the cervical vertebrae. This roll may be particularly helpful if the occiput is exaggerated in size by molding, edema, or prematurity. If these procedures fail to provide an unobstructed airway, the placement of a laryngeal mask airway (LMA) or intubation is indicated (Kattwinkel, 2011).

■ Suctioning. Routine suctioning of neonates on the perineum was a standard of care for all deliveries whether the amniotic fluid was clear or meconium stained. There is no evidence to support this practice (Gungor et al., 2006; Velaphi & Vidyasagar, 2008), so routine intrapartum oropharyngeal and nasopharyngeal suctioning for babies born with either clear or meconium-stained amniotic fluid is no longer recommended (Kattwinkel, 2011; Perlman et al., 2010). After delivery, the infant is placed on the warming bed, quickly dried and positioned, and the airway is cleared by wiping the nose and mouth with a towel or by suctioning with a bulb syringe, or suction catheter if necessary. Increasing amounts of evidence show that suctioning, either bulb or mechanical, of the nasopharynx can create bradycardia during resuscitation, so the 2010 recommendations for suctioning (including bulb suction) immediately following birth is to be reserved for those neonates who have an obvious obstruction to spontaneous breathing or for those babies requiring PPV (Kattwinkel, 2011). Because suctioning may cause inadvertent stimulation and gasping, the mouth should always be suctioned before the nose, "M" before "N." Mechanical suction often is mentioned as an alternative to the bulb syringe, but it generally should not be used immediately after delivery. If infants are suctioned vigorously within the first 5 minutes of life, apnea or arrhythmias may follow. These symptoms probably are due to vagal stimulation, with reflex bradycardia. If a bulb syringe can be used instead of a suction catheter, this situation usually can be avoided. If mechanical suction is required (i.e., for meconium removal), it should be applied for no longer than 5 seconds at a time with an 8 or 10 French suction catheter and with the equipment set to produce no more than 100 mmHg (136 cm H_2O) negative pressure (Kattwinkel, 2011). To assist with the removal of a large amount of secretions from the mouth, turn the baby's head to the side, which will allow for the secretions to pool in the baby's cheek where they will be more easily removed.

If meconium is present in the amniotic fluid and the baby is vigorous (strong respiratory effort, good muscle tone, and heart rate >100 beats per minute [bpm]), the baby should be treated as a nonmeconium baby. If meconium is present and the baby is nonvigorous (depressed respirations, decreased muscle tone, and/or a heart rate below 100 bpm), the baby will need direct suctioning of the trachea before beginning the steps of resuscitation to decrease the chance of the baby aspirating the meconium. To do this, insert a laryngoscope into the baby's mouth and use a 12 or 14 French suction catheter to clear the mouth and posterior pharynx so that the glottis can be visualized, then insert the endotracheal (ET) tube into the trachea, attach the tube to a meconium aspirator which is attached directly to the suction tubing, apply suction to the tube for 3 seconds, and withdraw the ET tube. Repeat as necessary until little or no meconium is removed or until the baby's heart rate indicates further resuscitation needs to begin. This suctioning is performed before the infant is dried or otherwise stimulated. There is some controversy over the benefit of ET suctioning when the meconium is thin versus thick; but there are no current studies that justify basing guidelines for suctioning on the consistency of the meconium. Techniques involving mouth suction should not be used because of the risk of exposure of personnel to blood and other body fluids. Also, passing a suction catheter through the ET tube or directly intubating the trachea with a suction catheter is an inadequate substitute for the ET tube, because the small bore of these catheters is easily clogged with the thick, tenacious meconium (Kattwinkel, 2011).

■ **Tactile Stimulation.** In a mildly depressed infant, drying and suctioning will usually be enough stimulation to induce effective respirations. If the respiratory rate and depth are nevertheless diminished, rubbing the back, trunk, or extremities as well as slapping or flicking the soles of the feet briefly will stimulate the infant to breathe. If the infant's reflexes are intact, 10 to 15 seconds of stimulation should be sufficient to elicit a response. Longer and more vigorous methods of stimulation should be avoided. Never spend more than 30 seconds to further stimulate an infant, as it is a waste of valuable time. Remember that the first 60 seconds after birth is now called the "Golden Minute," so if clearing the airway and stimulating the neonate to breathe does not result in improvement after 60 seconds, PPV should be started (Kattwinkel, 2011).

VENTILATION AND OXYGENATION

The most important and effective action in a neonatal resuscitation is effective ventilation of the compromised neonate. In fact, most infants who require resuscitation can be revived with ventilation and oxygen as needed, alone. Even when more aggressive therapies are required, they ultimately are undertaken to support oxygen delivery to the tissues, either by optimizing the airway (i.e., LMA or intubation) or by supporting the heart that "pushes" oxygen to the periphery (i.e., chest compressions, medications).

Free-Flow Administration of Oxygen

Blow-by of 100% oxygen given at delivery was a common intervention in the past, but as stated earlier increasing amounts of research show that increasing the neonate's oxygen saturations more quickly than a healthy term neonate can be toxic and detrimental to not only a preterm infant, but to term infants as well. Studies have shown that neonates that were given intermittent PPV with 100% oxygen showed no advantage to intermittent PPV with room air (RA) and actually delayed the time to first breathe and/or cry in term infants (Saugstad et al., 1998; Vento et al., 2001). Because of the increasing evidence on the detriments of hyperoxia, the use of RA at the beginning of resuscitation is now recommended. But if there is no improvement in heart rate or oxygenation by pulse oximetry despite adequate ventilation, then increasing the amount of oxygen the neonate is receiving should be considered (Kattwinkel, 2011; Kattwinkel et al., 2010; Perlman et al., 2010). An infant who is breathing spontaneously, but appears cyanotic or fails to maintain its SaO_2 within the range for the age of the infant, in room air (Table 3.2), needs supplemental oxygen. The oxygen can be provided directly from the end of the oxygen tube held

TABLE 3.2

TARGETED PREDUCTAL SpO_2 AFTER BIRTH

Age in Minutes	SpO_2 Range
1	60%–65%
2	65%–70%
3	70%–75%
4	75%–80%
5	80%–85%
10	85%–95%

Data from Kattwinkel (2011).

in a cupped hand, by a funnel or face mask attached to the tubing, by a flow-inflating ventilation bag, or by a T-piece resuscitator. The flow should be set to deliver at least 5L/min, and the tubing, funnel, or mask should be held close to the infant's face to maximize the inhaled concentration of oxygen (Kattwinkel, 2011).

During resuscitation, start with room air (21%) and then using the preductal pulse oximeter as your guide, increase your oxygen concentration as necessary to maintain the appropriate O_2 saturation for the infant's age in minutes after birth (Kattwinkel, 2011). Evidence to support resuscitations starting with room air, especially in the term infant, is mounting (Davis & Dawson, 2012). The Neonatal Resuscitation Program (NRP) Guidelines (Kattwinkel, 2011) have been changed since 2006 to reflect the use of room air initially even for preterm infants, yet these guidelines are not consistently followed. A Canadian team of researchers examined this issue and found great variations in practice regarding the implementation of Canadian NRP guidelines, including the use of room air (El-Naggar & McNamara, 2012). As more research is done to support resuscitation best practices, further examination of the actual implementation of these practices should be conducted.

Ventilation

If the infant fails to obtain a normal O_2 saturation with free-flow oxygen increased to 100% or shows other signs of cardiorespiratory decompensation (apnea or gasping respirations or a heart rate below 100 bpm), PPV should be instituted. Begin PPV with a pressure of 30 to 40 cm H_2O to inflate the lungs of term neonates and 20 to 25 cm H_2O for preterm neonates. You may need to adjust the pressure as needed to achieve a rising heart rate, chest expansion, and audible breath sounds. Occasionally the need to increase the positive pressure higher is necessary if no improvement occurs. Positive end expiratory pressure can be beneficial in preterm neonates that are apneic who require PPV, but should only be used if suitable equipment is available. A ventilation rate of 40 to 60 breaths/minute should be used when ventilating the newborn (Kattwinkel, 2011; Perlman et al., 2010).

Continuous Positive Airway Pressure

The use of continuous positive airway pressure (CPAP) in the delivery room for preterm babies is a common practice to assist them to breathe. Studies have been done to assess the outcomes of preterm neonates who had CPAP in the delivery room versus being intubated and given PPV. A study by Morley and Davis in 2008 showed that spontaneously breathing 25- to 28-week gestation infants given CPAP had reduced rates of mechanical ventilation and surfactant use when compared to infants of the same gestational age who were intubated and given PPV, though they also found in this study that the CPAP babies had an increased incidence of pneumothorax than the intubated babies. Another study of very preterm neonates that looked at a multifaceted intervention that included CPAP being started in the delivery room showed a reduced need for intubation and mechanical ventilation at 72 hours of age and decreased the incidence of bronchopulmonary dysplasia when compared to those very preterm neonates who had PPV with a face mask. When the comparison of very preterm neonates who received CPAP was made to historic controls of very preterm neonates who were given PPV, the CPAP neonates had decreased days of intubation, mechanical ventilation, and use of postnatal steroids (Lindener, Vossbeck, Hummler, & Pohlandt, 1999).

Taking the results of these and other studies into consideration, the recommendation now is that spontaneously breathing preterm neonates with respiratory distress may be supported with either CPAP or intubation and mechanical ventilation. The choice of what do is to be guided by the expertise and preference of the health care professional at the delivery.

Positive Pressure Devices

Three types of ventilation devices are available for neonatal use: the self-inflating bag, the flow-inflating bag, and the T-piece resuscitator. Whichever one is used, it should have the capability to deliver an oxygen concentration between 21% and 100%.

Self-inflating bags do not require gas flow but do require a reservoir to deliver high concentrations of oxygen. Traditionally, these bags have been fitted with a pressure-release "popoff" valve preset at 30 to 40 cm H_2O to prevent over-inflation of the lungs and the risk of pneumothorax. Most self-inflating bags must be squeezed to move gas through the circuit and are not capable of passive, free-flow oxygen delivery.

Flow-inflating bags, on the other hand, are closed systems and therefore must be connected to a compressed gas source. Although self-inflating bags have the advantages of being both easy to operate and gas flow independent, flow-inflating bags provide more reliable oxygen concentrations (particularly at low flow rates), better control of inspiratory times, and a greater range of peak inspiratory pressures, as well as providing free-flow oxygen.

T-piece resuscitator is a mechanical device that provides flow-controlled and pressure-limited breaths. Like the flow-inflating bag, it requires a compressed gas source to operate. The peak inspiratory pressure and end expiratory pressure are set manually with adjustable controls and the breaths are delivered manually when the operator alternately occludes and opens the aperture on the tubing attached to the mask, LMA or ET tube.

All three of the devices can be used to provide ventilation by mask, LMA, or ET tube. Both types of ventilation bags can be equipped with a manometer to monitor airway pressure as well. Though a manometer is important, visualization of the chest is equally, if not more, important. The degree of chest rise should simulate that seen when a normal newborn takes an easy breath. Excessive chest rise reflects overzealous delivery of tidal volume; if there is no movement, delivery is inadequate. A self-inflating or flow-inflating bag that has a regulatory valve with a minimum volume of 200 mL and a maximum volume of 750 mL should be used in resuscitating neonates. Term newborns require only 10 to 25 mL with each ventilation (4–6 mL/kg). A bag larger than this makes delivering the correct size breath difficult (Kattwinkel, 2011).

Methods of Ventilation

For mask ventilation, a face mask is used to provide an oxygen-enriched "microenvironment." An anatomically shaped mask with a cushioned rim is preferred for this purpose. Because masks are available in a variety of sizes, care must be taken to select one that covers the tip of the chin, the mouth, and the nose but not the eyes. Mask ventilation is a simple, noninvasive method of oxygen delivery that can be initiated without delay, but use of a mask has disadvantages. First, it may be difficult to obtain and maintain a good seal between the mask and the infant's face, particularly around the nose. Any leakage of air results in underventilation, which is aggravated if low lung compliance or high airway resistance is a factor. The seal should be "airtight" without excessive pressure applied. Second, the mask itself has a considerable amount of dead space. Consequently, a sufficient tidal volume must be delivered to prevent accumulation and rebreathing of carbon dioxide. Masks used for neonatal resuscitation ideally should have a dead space of less than 5 mL. Finally, prolonged bag and mask ventilation may produce gastric distention from swallowed gas, which in turn impedes diaphragmatic excursions and places the infant at risk of regurgitation and aspiration. However, this problem can be easily avoided by inserting an 8 French orogastric tube if mask ventilation continues beyond several minutes. The gastric contents should be suctioned and the tube left in place as a vent as long as mask ventilation is provided (Kattwinkel, 2011).

Mask ventilation suffices for most infants, but if it proves ineffective (as evidenced by poor chest rise or continuing bradycardia) or if prolonged ventilation is expected, an LMA or ET tube should be inserted. Premature infants (certainly those weighing < 1,000 g) who have diminished lung compliance, immature respiratory musculature, and decreased respiratory drive may also benefit from early intubation (Kattwinkel, 2011). In research comparing outcomes for very-low-birth-weight infants (those weighing < 1,500 g) who were selectively intubated at delivery or given a trial of spontaneous ventilation, the results showed that the infants who were immediately intubated had higher 5-minute Apgar scores, less acidosis, less hypoglycemia, and fewer pneumothoraces and required slower ventilatory rates.

Infants suspected of having a diaphragmatic hernia, hydrops fetalis, or certain airway or gastrointestinal abnormalities also benefit from immediate intubation. Uncuffed ET tubes with a uniform internal diameter should be used. The proper tube size and depth of insertion are determined by the infant's size by weight (Table 3.3). Most neonatal ET tubes have a black line (vocal cord guide) near the tip of the tube that serves as a guide for insertion. When this guide is placed at the level of the vocal cords, the tube should be properly positioned with its tip in the mid-trachea. As an alternative, the distance from the mid-trachea (tube tip) to the infant's upper lip may be estimated using the simple tip-to-lip formula:

TABLE 3.3

ENDOTRACHEAL TUBE SIZE AND PLACEMENT

Infant's Weight (kg)	Tube Size (mm)	Insertion Depth (cm)
< 1	2.5	< 7
1–2	3	7–8
2–3	3.5	8–9
> 3	3.5–4	> 9

Data from the American Heart Association Emergency Cardiac Care Committee and Subcommittees (1992) and Kattwinkel (2011).

$$\text{Weight}(\text{kg}) + 6 = \text{Tip-to-lip distance}$$

When the tube is properly situated, the centimeter marking on the side of the tube at the level of the upper lip should be at or near the tip-to-lip distance. For example, infants weighing 1 kg are intubated to a depth of 7 cm (1 + 6 = 7); those weighing 2 kg to a depth of 8 cm (2 + 6 = 8); and so on. Tubes with metallic markers or fiber-optic illumination at the tip may make it possible to determine the depth of the tube transdermally (i.e., by observing a circle of light on the skin or by hearing an audible signal from a transcutaneous locator instrument), but these modifications do not allow differentiation between ET intubation and esophageal intubation and therefore offer no advantage in an emergency situation (Heller & Heller, 1994). Similarly, capnometers used during resuscitation to measure end-tidal carbon dioxide and thus confirm tube placement in the trachea may be inaccurate when pulmonary blood flow is poor or absent (Bhende & Thompson, 1995).

Correct placement is best demonstrated by the tried and true methods: improved clinical signs (heart rate, improving oxygenation, and activity), symmetric chest rise, bilateral and equal breath sounds (as auscultated in the axillae), and fogging of the tube on exhalation. Air should not be heard entering the stomach, and the abdomen should not be distended. If any doubts exist, tube placement can be checked by repeated laryngoscopy; the tube should be clearly seen passing through the glottic opening (Kattwinkel, 2011).

ET intubation is the definitive technique for airway management and ventilation. However, agility and accuracy in placement require continual practice. Also, many hospital personnel are restricted by policy or statute from learning or using this skill. The LMA, which was approved by the U.S. Food and Drug Administration in 1991, has been enthusiastically accepted in some settings as an alternative that offers most of the advantages of intubation but does not require laryngoscopy for placement.

The LMA (Figure 3.1) is a relatively long tube with a bag connector and an inflation port at one end and an inflatable soft cuff at the other. The tube is blindly passed into

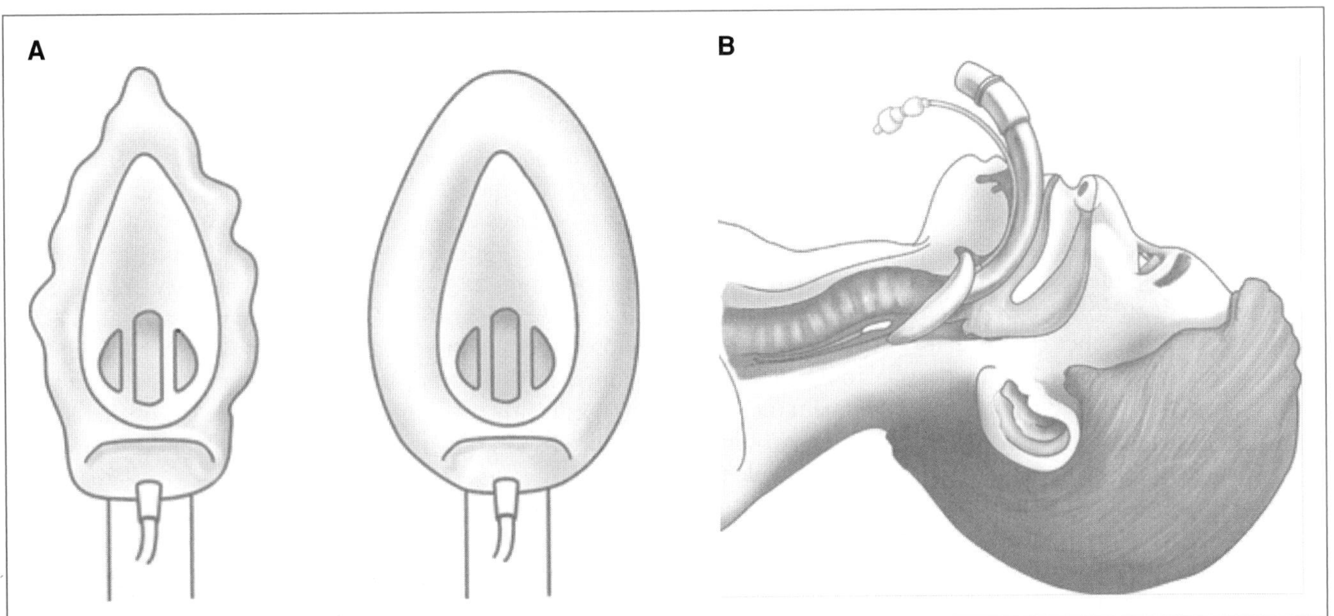

FIGURE 3.1 (A) LMA deflated for insertion *(left)* and with cuff inflated *(right)*. (B) LMA in position with cuff inflated around laryngeal inlet.
From Efrat et al. (1994).

the hypopharynx so that the tip of the cuff lodges in the esophageal opening. Inflated, the cuff creates a seal around the larynx. The tube then is connected to a bag that delivers oxygen by ventilation through the central aperture of the laryngeal mask.

Since the LMA was approved for use by the Food and Drug Administration, research has been done to assess the effectiveness in neonates. For ventilation purposes, the LMA is as effective as, but never more effective than, intubation. Placement of the LMA has been studied in neonates who are 34 weeks and older or who weigh more than 2,000 g, and case reports have been written that have shown LMAs to be an effective alternative when mask ventilation and intubation were unsuccessful. These studies also showed that effective ventilation was achieved quickly using an LMA (Gandini & Brimacombe, 1999; Trevisanuto et al., 2004; Zanardo, Simbi, Savio, Micaglio, & Trevisanuto, 2004). An advantage to an LMA is that it can be placed by an RN, respiratory therapist (RT), or MD, making providing an airway to neonates in distress easier in facilities where a physician might not be in-house 24 hours a day. Training health care professionals to place an LMA can be done using a mannequin. Studies have shown that the use of a mannequin for LMA training is an effective training tool (Gandini & Brimacombe, 2004; Murray, Vemeulen, Morrison, & Waite, 2002).

Situations where an LMA may be useful include when a neonate has a congenital anomaly of the mouth, lip or palate, anomalies of the head, neck, tongue, or pharynx, a small mandible or when ventilation with a mask is ineffective and intubation is not feasible. A disadvantage to a LMA is that even with successful placement, nearly a quarter of infants with a LMA subsequently develop airway obstruction, probably because of displacement during patient movement. The cuff provides only a low-pressure seal around the larynx, which limits the airway pressures that can be achieved during ventilation. The risks of gastric insufflation and regurgitation of gastric contents are reduced but not eliminated. Because of its size, the LMA currently is restricted to infants greater than 34 weeks gestation or 2.0 kg, although there have been anecdotal reports of successful use in very small infants (1–1.5 kg). The LMA also does not provide access to the lower airway and therefore is not suitable for meconium removal or drug administration, nor does it preserve the airway during laryngospasm. Its usefulness in neonates who require chest compressions and in those with oropharyngeal disease or diaphragmatic hernia has yet to be assessed (Kattwinkel, 2011; Kattwinkel et al., 2010; Perlman et al., 2010).

■ **Chest Compressions.** Chest compressions rarely are required for resuscitation in the delivery room. They are performed in only 1 of every 1,000 deliveries but probably are avoidable even in most of these cases. According to some authorities, approximately one third of the infants who received chest compressions have showed biochemical evidence of asphyxia (acidemia), but the remaining two thirds were found to have a malpositioned ET tube or inadequate ventilatory support (i.e., insufficient rate or pressure). Clearly, the airway should be reassessed, and respiratory support should be optimized before chest compressions are initiated. Assuming that these components are satisfactory, chest compressions are begun if the heart rate drops below 60 beats per minute after 30 seconds of *effective* ventilation (Kattwinkel, 2011).

Chest compressions provide temporary support for circulation and oxygen delivery. Pressing on the sternum has two effects: It compresses the heart against the vertebral column, and it increases intrathoracic pressure. Both effects cause blood to be pushed out of the heart into the arterial circulation. When the sternal pressure is released, the ventricles return to their original shape; intrathoracic pressure falls toward zero; and venous blood is pulled into the heart by a suction effect (Kattwinkel, 2011).

Either of two techniques may be used to perform chest compressions, but the thumb method is preferred by the American Academy of Pediatrics (AAP). For the thumb method, both hands encircle the chest; the fingers support the back, and the thumbs (pointing cephalad either side by side or one on top of the other, depending on the infant's size) are used to press the sternum downward. For the two-finger method, one hand supports the back from below while two fingers of the free hand are held perpendicular to the chest and the fingertips are used to apply downward pressure on the sternum. Comparative studies have shown that higher systolic blood pressure, higher diastolic blood pressure, higher mean arterial pressure, and higher coronary perfusion pressure are generated with less external compression force when the thumb method is used. This method also has had fewer reports of trauma to the liver and other abdominal organs. Moreover, the thumb method is perhaps easier and certainly less tiring to perform. The thumb method therefore is preferred, but the two-finger method may be necessary if the nurse's hands are too small to encircle the chest properly. If access to the umbilicus is needed to facilitate placement of an umbilical venous catheter (UVC) for administration of emergency drugs, the compressor should move to the head of the bed next to the person providing ventilation and continue compressing with the two-thumb method, though the thumbs will now be pointing caudally (Kattwinkel, 2011).

For both methods, the pressure is applied to the lower third of the sternum (just below the nipple line but above the xiphoid process) where the right ventricle lies closest to the sternum. Just enough force is used to depress the sternum one third of the anterior/posterior chest wall diameter (Kattwinkel, 2011). Research indicates that myocardial and cerebral blood flows are optimal when the downward stroke and release phases of the compression are equal in time (Niermeyer & Keenan, 2001). This equalization is best accomplished with a smooth stroke and release rhythm.

PPV with 100% oxygen must be given while chest compressions are performed. The most recent guidelines recommend interposing chest compressions with ventilations at a 3 to 1 ratio. Every fourth compression is dropped to allow delivery of a single, effective breath. During the course of a full minute, 90 compressions and 30 ventilations are given (Kattwinkel, 2011). In order to give an adequate number of compressions without doing simultaneous compression/ventilation, the ventilation rate is dropped to 30 from the 40 to 60 that were done with ventilation alone.

Faster rates were recommended in the past, but they only increase the chance of administering simultaneous compressions and ventilations. Most research indicates that simultaneous delivery increases the intrathoracic pressure to a level at which ventilation is impeded and coronary perfusion is reduced. Whether there is any effect on cerebral blood flow is equivocal, but there have been other reports of lower survival rates when simultaneous compression and ventilation was used.

Experimental techniques, such as external circulatory assist devices (e.g., mechanical "thumpers," pneumatic vests, and abdominal binders), counterpoint abdominal compressions (e.g., cough cardiopulmonary resuscitation), and active decompression (e.g., plumber's plunger), have shown promise in animal studies. However, few large-scale clinical trials have been done, and most of those used adults. Consequently, these methods cannot be advocated for neonatal resuscitation at this time.

Medications

■ **Epinephrine.** Epinephrine is a direct-acting catecholamine with both alpha-adrenergic and beta-adrenergic effects. These effects lead to peripheral vasoconstriction, acceleration of the heart rate, and an increase in the forcefulness of cardiac contractions. The net effect is a sharp rise in blood pressure (pressor effect) and an increase in cardiac output. The marked pressor effect combined with the increased aortic diastolic pressure increases the cerebral and myocardial perfusion pressures, maintaining blood flow to these critical organs during resuscitation. Epinephrine therefore is considered the drug of choice with asystole or persistent bradycardia (heart rate <60 beats/min) despite effective ventilation with 100% oxygen and chest compressions for 45 to 60 seconds. For newborns the recommended dosage is 0.1 to 0.3 mL/kg of 1:10,000 solution (0.01–0.03 mg/kg) intravenously (Kattwinkel, 2011; Perlman et al., 2010). The drug is rapidly inactivated by an enzymatically driven process known as sulfoconjugation, in which the active compound is conjugated with sulfate. The half-life of infused epinephrine is approximately 3 minutes. Consequently, the dose may be repeated every 3 to 5 minutes as clinically indicated.

Epinephrine ideally should be administered the IV/UVC route. Because IV/UVC placement may be difficult and time-consuming during resuscitation, an initial dose of epinephrine can be given by the ET tube. Unfortunately, absorption into the circulation from the pulmonary capillary bed may be highly variable because of the low-blood-flow state associated with resuscitation. In addition, much of the ET-instilled drug remains along the walls of the ET tube and in the conducting airways, with a relatively small amount finding its way into the deep absorptive surfaces of the alveoli. If epinephrine is given by the ET tube, a higher dose of 0.5 to 1 mL/kg of 1:10,000 solution (0.05–0.1 mg/kg) should be given (Kattwinkel, 2011; Perlman et al., 2010).

A number of steps can be taken to aid delivery when the ET route is necessary. First, to optimize blood flow to the lungs, every effort must be made to ensure that chest compressions are performed effectively. Second, epinephrine may be dispersed more quickly to deeper pulmonary tissues by following the instillation with a few forceful ventilations. When giving epinephrine via the ET tube you will be giving higher doses, which will lead to increased volume of fluid of up to 1 mL, so dilution is no longer needed (Kattwinkel, 2011). As an alternative, some individuals prefer to administer the drug through a 5 French feeding tube positioned through the ET tube, but a study done by Rehan and colleagues (2004) on epinephrine delivery methods showed that the direct ET tube method was more effective and less cumbersome than the catheter-inserted method for administering epinephrine during resuscitation.

Although higher doses of epinephrine administered by the ET route may have a role in exceptional situations, routine IV/UVC administration of high-dose epinephrine is not recommended in newborns. Studies with adults and older children have shown a dose-response relationship, with higher doses bringing about greater improvements in coronary and cerebral blood flow; in neonates, however, the efficacy and safety of high-dose IV/UVC epinephrine have not been adequately evaluated. Most of these studies have been done with patients with a history of coronary artery disease who demonstrate ventricular fibrillation. Neonates, however, more commonly have bradycardia caused by hypoxia. These pathophysiologic differences prevent extrapolation of findings. Furthermore, administration of high doses generally has been followed by a prolonged period of hypertension. Because the newborn, particularly the prematurely born, has a vascular germinal matrix, the risk may be greater for intraventricular hemorrhage. In fact, this area of the brain is most susceptible to hemorrhage when hypertension is preceded by hypotension, which is the case with resuscitation. For this reason, only the standard dose of epinephrine (0.1–0.3 mL/kg) should be given by the IV/UVC route.

■ **Volume Expanders.** Volume expanders are indicated with evidence or suspicion of acute blood loss with signs of hypovolemia. These signs include pallor despite oxygen therapy, hypotension with weak pulses despite a normal heart rate, delayed capillary refill, and failure to respond to resuscitation (Kattwinkel, 2011; Perlman et al., 2010). Low hematocrit and hemoglobin concentrations are diagnostic of blood loss, but the levels may be misleadingly normal immediately after acute loss. In general, it takes about 3 hours for a sufficient amount of fluid to shift from the interstitial to the intravascular space to produce the degree of compensatory hemodilution reflected by a fall in laboratory values.

The basic requirement for any replacement solution is that the electrolyte and protein composition be roughly equivalent to that which was lost. Otherwise, an osmotic pressure gradient is created, and fluids are driven out of the capillaries into the interstitial tissue. The expansion of circulatory volume is only transient, and the infant is put at risk for secondary problems, particularly pulmonary edema. Clearly, whole blood is the fluid of choice for volume replacement, and it offers the added benefit of oxygen-carrying capacity. Fresh O-negative blood cross-matched against the mother should be used. When blood is not readily available, isotonic fluids (normal saline or Ringer's lactate) may also be used (Kattwinkel, 2011). Glucose-containing fluids (e.g., D5W or D10W) should not be given by bolus because of the risk of profound hyperglycemia. Hyperglycemia with untreated asphyxia may aggravate metabolic acidosis.

For emergency treatment of hypovolemia, 10 mL/kg of volume expander is given slowly over 5 to 10 minutes by the IV/UVC route (Kattwinkel, 2011). Rapid infusion must be avoided, because abrupt changes in vascular pressure in the vulnerable germinal matrix capillaries place the infant (especially a preterm infant) at greater risk of intraventricular hemorrhage. The response usually is dramatic, with a prompt improvement in blood pressure, pulses, and color. If the signs of hypovolemia continue, however, a second volume replacement may be given. Persistent failure beyond this point probably indicates some degree of "pump failure," and further improvement is not likely until cardiac function is improved. In fact, excessive volume administration may so engorge the heart and overstretch the cardiac muscle fibers that the strength of contractions is actually diminished. In such cases, administration of sodium bicarbonate (to correct metabolic acidosis) or an inotropic agent (such as dopamine) should be considered (Kattwinkel, 2011).

■ **Sodium Bicarbonate.** Of the biochemical events that arise from asphyxia, the most significant is the conversion from aerobic to anaerobic metabolism with the production of lactic acid. As this strong acid accumulates, metabolic acidosis develops, myocardial contractility declines, hypotension worsens, and the cardiac response to catecholamines weakens. In such cases, the best treatment for acidosis is directed at its cause, hypoxemia. Immediate therapy includes ventilation with 100% oxygen and cardiac compressions to restore blood flow and tissue oxygenation. However, if the resuscitation is prolonged and the infant remains unresponsive, alkali therapy may be helpful. Sodium bicarbonate is the most frequently used alkalinizing agent, but its use remains controversial; therefore, it should be used only when no improvement is seen (Kattwinkel, 2011).

Sodium bicarbonate ($NaHCO_3$) is a physiologic buffer. When it is added to a solution of strong acid, such as hydrochloric acid (HCl), the bicarbonate anion (HCO_3^-) combines with the hydrogen ion (H^+) from the acid to form the weaker carbonic acid (H_2CO_3) and a neutral salt, such as sodium chloride (NaCl):

$$HCl + NaHCO_3 = H_2CO_3 + NaCl$$

The carbonic acid rapidly dissociates into water (H_2O) and carbon dioxide (CO_2), and the blood transports the dissolved carbon dioxide to the lungs, where it is eliminated:

$$H_2CO_3 = H_2O + CO_2$$

Although sodium bicarbonate historically was considered a pharmacologic mainstay of neonatal resuscitation, a growing body of research suggests that sodium bicarbonate administration may actually be counterproductive and possibly injurious. First and foremost, effective removal of carbon dioxide by the lungs depends on both ventilation and pulmonary blood flow. If either is inadequate (which frequently is the case during resuscitation), CO_2 accumulates, with a shift from metabolic to respiratory acidosis without any real resolution of acid–base imbalance. Second, CO_2 diffuses across cell membranes much more rapidly and easily than does bicarbonate. That is, CO_2 quickly moves out of the capillaries into cells, whereas bicarbonate lags behind in the intravascular space. The blood pH rises, but intracellular pH transiently falls. Therefore, when the cells of the heart are involved, intramyocardial acidosis worsens and cardiac performance declines further. Other possible consequences of sodium bicarbonate administration are intraventricular hemorrhage (as a result of rapid infusion of hypertonic solution) and hypernatremia.

Administration of sodium bicarbonate should not be undertaken lightly and is in fact discouraged for brief resuscitation or episodes of bradycardia. It should be reserved for prolonged arrest unresponsive to other therapy and then used only after effective ventilation and compressions have been established. The dosage currently recommended is 4 mL/kg of 4.2% solution (2 mEq/kg) by the IV/UVC route. This hypertonic solution contains 0.5 mEq/mL and therefore should be given slowly over at least 2 minutes (1 mEq/kg/min) (Kattwinkel, 2011). At the first opportunity, samples for blood gas analysis should be drawn from whatever site is available to confirm metabolic acidosis.

■ **Naloxone.** For the mother, narcotic analgesics are an effective means of pain control during labor. Unfortunately, these lipid-soluble drugs rapidly cross the placenta within 2 minutes of administration and can cause neonatal respiratory depression. Peak fetal narcotic levels occur 30 minutes to 2 hours after administration to the mother. The degree and duration of depression shown by the newborn depend on the dose, the route, and how soon before delivery the drug is given. Affected neonates show decreased respiratory effort and muscle tone but typically have a good heart rate and perfusion. In cases such as this, the administration of naloxone can be considered for neonates who demonstrate continued respiratory depression and have a history of maternal narcotic administration within the past 4 hours, which will temporarily reverse the effects of the narcotics. The routine administration of naloxone is no longer recommended as long as the neonate can be adequately ventilated (Kattwinkel, 2011).

Naloxone hydrochloride is a synthetic narcotic antagonist designed to reverse narcotic-induced respiratory depression. It acts by competing with narcotics for receptor sites in the central nervous system. As a pure competitive antagonist, it binds with but does not activate receptors. Consequently, in the absence of narcotics, naloxone exhibits essentially no pharmacologic activity. As always, ventilatory support is still the first defense against respiratory depression.

Naloxone is available in a variety of concentrations; however, the NRP currently recommends the use of the 1 mg/mL preparation. Neonatal naloxone (0.02 mg/mL) should not be used because of the fluid volume that would be given. The dosage is 0.1 mg/kg of the 1.0 mg/mL, which may be repeated every 2 to 3 minutes as needed. Administration by the IV/UVC is preferred, but the drug also can be given intramuscularly (IM), because affected newborns generally have good perfusion. The IV/UVC route provides the quickest onset of action (generally apparent within 2 minutes), but IM injection produces a more prolonged effect. Adequate ventilatory assistance must be provided until reversal is complete. Close monitoring should continue for 4 to 6 hours after administration. Because the liver rapidly metabolizes naloxone, its duration of effect may be shorter than that of some narcotics, and respiratory depression may recur. Although naloxone has no known short-term toxic effects, it is contraindicated in infants born to narcotic-dependent mothers. Because abrupt and complete reversal of narcotic effects may precipitate seizures (withdrawal reaction), assisted ventilation is provided in this circumstance until the respiratory drive is adequate (Kattwinkel, 2011).

Because several studies have suggested that hypoxia and acidosis stimulate the release of endogenous opiates (endorphins), it has been theorized that these endorphins might accentuate the depressing effect of hypoxemia on the cardiorespiratory system. However, clinical trials of naloxone administration to infants with 1-minute Apgar scores of 6 or lower have shown no effect on spontaneous respiratory frequency or heart rate.

■ **Other Drugs.** Dopamine, atropine, and calcium were at one time used routinely in the acute phases of neonatal resuscitation, but no longer are used as they are rarely very useful (Kattwinkel, 2011; Perlman et al., 2010). These drugs are more commonly used now in the postresuscitation period in the neonatal special care or intensive care unit.

■ **Special Circumstances.** For some infants, changes in or variations of the usual resuscitative measures are needed. Most of these infants are extremely premature, have congenital anomalies, structural defects, or conditions that compromise the cardiovascular system, such as neural tube defects, abdominal wall defects, diaphragmatic hernias, hydrops fetalis, esophageal atresia, pneumothorax, choanal atresia, and laryngeal anomalies. Resuscitative measures with these disorders are discussed in greater detail elsewhere in this text.

■ **Withholding or Discontinuing Resuscitation.** The law and its underlying ethical principles require that treatment be provided and continued as long as it is judged to be effective in ameliorating or correcting an underlying pathophysiologic process. Unfortunately, the data are insufficient to allow a general recommendation for how long resuscitation should be performed before continuation can be deemed futile and efforts are terminated. There is evidence that survival is unlikely at any birth weight if the Apgar score remains zero after 10 minutes of resuscitation that has effective ventilation, coordinated with chest compressions and administration of medication. The current NRP states that noninitiation of resuscitation would be appropriate for (1) confirmed gestational age of less than 23 weeks or a birth weight of less than 400 g, (2) anencephaly, (3) confirmed lethal genetic disorder or malformation, and (4) when data is available that supports an unacceptably high likelihood of death or severe disability (Kattwinkel, 2011).

Although many hospitals have guidelines for withholding full resuscitation for extremely-low-birth-weight infants and those with lethal anomalies, early and well-documented discussion with parents is recommended when such events are anticipated prenatally. If the event was not anticipated, great attention should be given to postmortem evaluation. Blood for chromosome examination and other pertinent laboratory work, radiographs, and an autopsy are important both for family counseling and for evaluation of the resuscitation process.

■ Postresuscitation Management. A successfully resuscitated neonate requires special consideration during stabilization. The goal of care after resuscitation is to reverse the causes of cell death and tissue injury (hypoxia, ischemia, and acidosis) and avoid or treat any exacerbating conditions (hypothermia, hypoglycemia, respiratory failure, infection). There are several postresuscitation programs, such as Perinatal Continuing Education Program and the S.T.A.B.L.E.® Program, that are available to assist health care professionals with learning the skills necessary to stabilize the successfully resuscitated neonate. Both programs cover fluid administration, maintenance of the glucose levels, temperature regulation, airway management, blood pressure stabilization, lab work needed, and antibiotic administration as well as parental support. All of these topics are discussed more fully in other sections of this text.

■ Documentation. No resuscitative event can go unrecorded. Unfortunately, the circumstances surrounding resuscitation are fraught with medicolegal hazards. Assessment of the infant generally is limited to the most basic measurements (respiratory rate, heart rate, and oxygenation). Immediate response may be affected by many factors unrelated to professional competence. Furthermore, the ultimate outcome may not become apparent for years. Even the best, most appropriate care can look "bad" in retrospect if documentation is incomplete or inaccurate. Yet no area of the hospital is perhaps less conducive to quality documentation than the delivery room, where a variety of professionals (nurses, physicians, and respiratory therapists) from different clinical areas (obstetrics, neonatology, anesthesiology), each with a unique perspective on the situation, are brought together in an emergency. Notes are jotted on bed linen, scrub clothes, paper towels, or anything at hand. More often than not, these brief notes are so hastily written that they are little more than a list of the medications given. When transcribed, the events may be documented in two totally separate charts, one for the mother and another for the infant. Great care must be taken with record keeping so that events and actions can be accurately reconstructed many years in the future.

Descriptive charting is most appropriate in this situation. The record should include the pertinent perinatal factors, the physical findings, the activities performed, and the infant's response, but definitive diagnoses should not be offered. It is particularly important that information concerning the pregnancy, labor, and delivery be based on fact and not hearsay. Terms such as "fetal distress" and "asphyxia" tend to take on a life of their own once they have been committed to paper, even if they are not supported by clinical evidence. It is best to record factual data, such as vital signs and blood gas determinations, without adding an interpretation. Ventilation, chest compressions, and administration of medications are essential items for documentation, but the basics should not be dismissed. It is just as important to note that attempts were made to keep the infant dry and warm.

Accurate timing of notes can be critical, because actions are judged by the minute-to-minute changes noted in the chart. A preprinted recording form not only helps in this regard but also can provide a structure for evaluation and decision making.

Care of the Family During Resuscitation and Stabilization

An ill neonate is a crisis for families as no one expects their baby to be born prematurely or ill. When risk factors are known that could result in a neonate needing to be resuscitated (i.e., extremely premature baby), the physician should discuss with the parents prior to the delivery, if time allows, the options available as well as survival rates of the diagnosed condition of the infant. Parents have a role in deciding the goals of the care to be delivered to their baby, but they cannot make an informed decision unless they have been presented complete and reliable information. Unfortunately, many times this type of information may not be available until after the initial resuscitation or many hours later.

During resuscitation and stabilization health care professionals should keep the parents informed of what is occurring to their newborn. Parents' wishes should be honored, if appropriate. Parents may wish to be present during resuscitation efforts. Research studies have supported this presence from both a health professional's and parent's point of view (Gold, Gorenflo, Schwenk, & Bratton, 2006). Some professionals are concerned about legal ramifications of the family's presence during cardiopulmonary resuscitation but the positives for both the family and health care team outweigh the negatives (Jones, Parker-Raley, Maxson, & Brown, 2011).

SUMMARY

Although most depressed infants respond to drying, warming, positioning, suctioning, and tactile stimulation, every obstetric and neonatal unit should be adequately equipped and well prepared to handle neonatal emergencies. To provide neonatal care effectively, nurses must understand the cardiorespiratory transition and must be able to identify factors that may interfere with successful transition, comprehend the principles of resuscitation, and intervene based on assessment of respirations, heart rate, and color.

CASE STUDY

A 32-year-old Caucasian female is admitted to your hospital labor and delivery unit via the emergency squad. She was brought in after she started to have heavy bleeding while at work. She is approximately 28 weeks gestation and actively bleeding. Fetal heart tones are audible with a Category III tracing. She is prepped for an emergency cesarean section.

What equipment, personnel, and medications are needed to prepare for the resuscitation of the infant?
Increase delivery room temperature to 76°F, preheat a radiant warmer, personnel protective equipment, assure stethoscope present, bulb syringe, suction catheter and tubing, wall suction set at 100 mmHg, a properly functioning laryngoscope with appropriate size blade, ET tubes, polyethylene bag, pulse oximeter, 1:10,000 epinephrine 0.5 to 1.0 mL/kg drawn up in a 3 mL syringe for ET administration and 0.1 to 0.3 mL/kg drawn up in 1 mL syringe for IV administration, normal saline – 10 mL/kg, umbilical vein catheter tray, umbilical vein catheters. Will need at least one other person besides you, as well as a person able to do intubation and UVC placement present or readily available.
The baby is born by cesarean section; he appears to be 28 weeks gestation and approximately 800 g and is handed to you blue, pale, limp and not breathing. There is no meconium present.

What are your initial steps?
Place on preheated radiant warmer in a polyethylene bag, place temperature probe on infant and switch to servo mode, place hat on baby's head, position head in a sniffing position, continue to stimulate, suction the infant's mouth, then nose, provide blow-by oxygen, place pulse oximeter on baby's right hand.
Your evaluation after doing the initial steps of resuscitation shows that the infant remains pale, apneic with a heart rate of 40 and a pulse oximeter reading of 50.

What do you do next?
Start bag/mask ventilation with oxygen between 30% and 40% concentrations at a rate of 40 to 60 breaths per minute. Reevaluate the infant in 30 seconds.

After 30 seconds of bag/mask ventilation, the infant remains pale and apneic; his heart rate remains at 40 bpm, pulse oximeter reading 50.

What are your next steps?
Check to assure that chest is rising and if not, do steps for correction per the Neonatal Resuscitation Program and continue bag/mask ventilation with oxygen at 100%; begin cardiac compressions at a ratio of 3 to 1. Prepare equipment for intubation.
The baby is intubated orally with a # 2.5 ET tube on the first attempt. There are no spontaneous respirations, and the heart rate continues to be 40 bpm and pulse oximeter 50.

What are your next steps?
Secure the ET tube, give 0.40 mL of 1:10,000 Epinephrine (0.5 mL/kg) via the ET tube, and prepare to place a UVC for IV epinephrine administration and normal saline bolus. Continue to bag with oxygen and compressions at a 3 to 1 ratio.
A # 3.5 umbilical vein catheter is placed at approximately 3 cm; a good blood return is obtained. Normal saline - 8 mL is given via the UVC over 5 minutes. The infant is pink, has no spontaneous respirations, and his heart rate increases to 80 bpm and pulse oximeter reading is now 70.

What would you do next?
Stop compressions, continue to bag the infant via the ET tube, and move the infant from the delivery room to the newborn unit.

What would your initial steps of stabilization be upon admission to the unit?
Place in a neutral thermal environment with 80% humidity
Obtain glucose
Start an IV of D10W at 80 mL/kg/d
Obtain a complete blood count with differential and platelets
Obtain a blood culture
Place infant on a ventilator: FiO2-100%, P/P - 20/5, IMV - 40, IT – 0.3
Obtain a blood gas
Surfactant – 4 mL/kg
Ampicillin – 100 mg/kg q 12 hours
Gentamicin – 5 mg/kg q 36 hours
PRBC – 15 mL/kg

EVIDENCE-BASED PRACTICE BOX

In recent years the use of 100% oxygen in neonatal resuscitation has been reevaluated to the point that the new AAP NRP advocates the starting of resuscitation for term infants in 21% oxygen and something greater than 21% but less than 100% for preterm infants. This change of philosophy in the use of oxygen is a result of multiple studies that show that there are no advantages to 100% oxygen versus 21% as well as the fact that many studies have shown the hyperoxia effects of oxygen to a neonate to be detrimental in the long term.

One set of studies (Cnattingius et al., 1995; Naumberg, Bellocco, Cnattingius, Jonzon, & Ekbom, 2002) that have shown the negative effects of oxygen use in the immediate postpartum period for the neonate shows an

(continued)

increase in childhood lymphatic leukemia. Both studies showed that infants resuscitated with 100% oxygen with a face mask immediately postpartum had an increased risk of developing childhood lymphatic leukemia, and if they received oxygen for greater than 3 minutes or more by manual ventilation the risks increased more.

Randomized controlled clinical studies have shown that there is no advantage to starting resuscitation with 100% oxygen over 21% oxygen and it actually takes longer for an infant to take its first breath or to cry. Two meta analyses by Davis et al. (2004) and Rabi et al. (2007) show that neonates resuscitated with 21% oxygen had slightly lower mortality rates than those resuscitated with 100% oxygen. Animal studies have shown potentially harmful damage at the cellular level from oxygen.

Research continues on the effects of oxygen on the developing neonate, and as more evidence continues to emerge, changes to how we resuscitate newborns will continue to evolve.

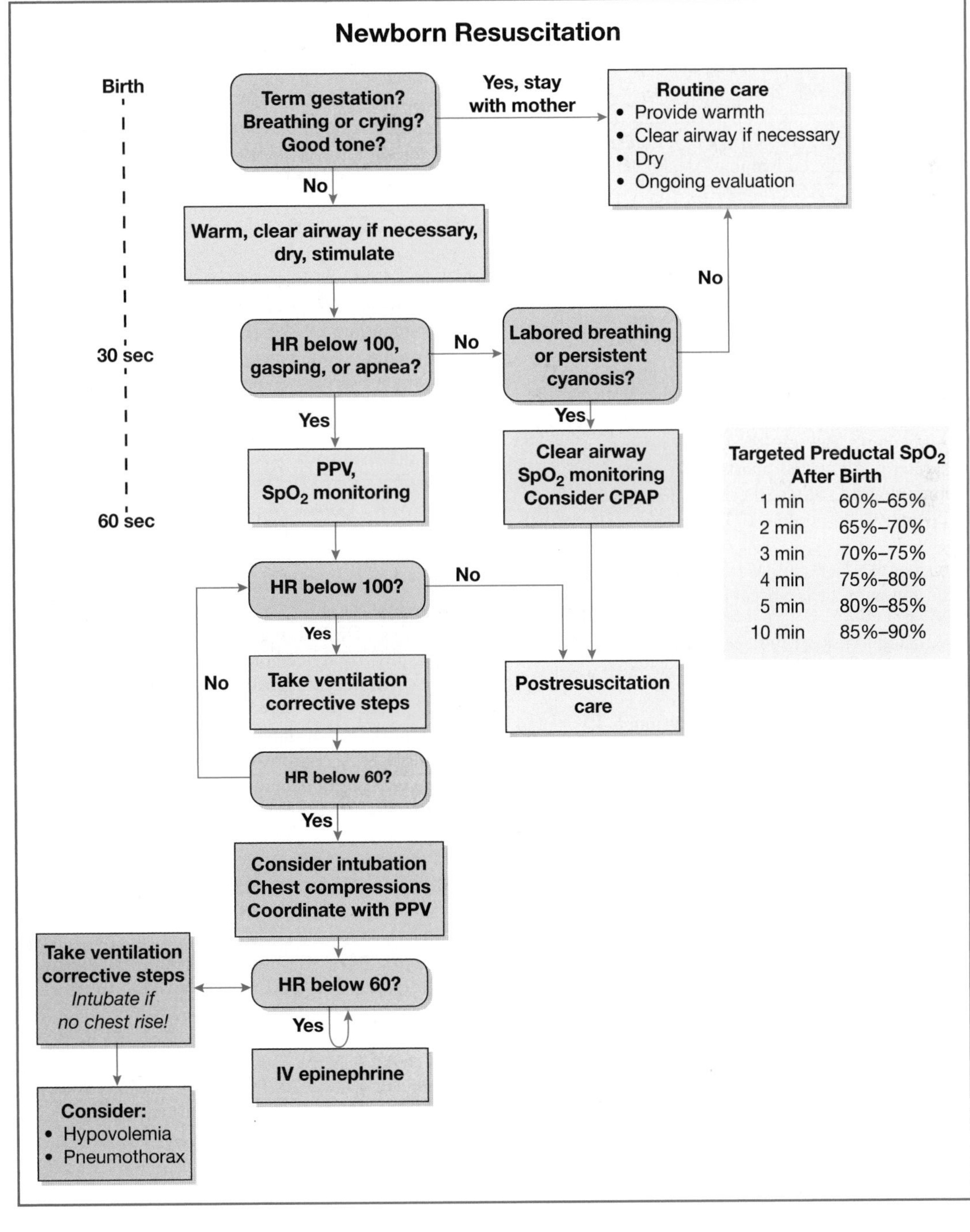

ONLINE RESOURCES

AAP NRP
http://www.aap.org/nrp
Perinatal Continuing Education Program
http://www.healthsystem.virginia.edu/internet/pcep
The S.T.A.B.L.E.® Program
http://www.thestableprogram.org

REFERENCES

Altuncu, E., Ozek, E., Bilgen, H., Topuzoglu, A., & Kavuncuoglu, S. (2008). Percentiles of oxygen saturations in healthy term newborns in the first minutes of life. *European Journal of Pediatrics, 167*, 687–688.

American Heart Association Emergency Cardiac Care Committee and Subcommittees (1992). Guidelines for cardiopulmonary resuscitation and emergency cardiac care. VII. Neonatal resuscitation. *Journal of the American Medical Association, 268*, 2276–2281.

Bhende, M. S., & Thompson, A. E. (1995). Evaluation of the end-tidal CO2 detector during pediatric cardiopulmonary resuscitation. *Pediatrics, 95*, 395–399.

Cnattingius, S., Zack, M. M., Ekbom, A., Gunnarskoq, J., Kreuger, A., Linet, M., & Adami, H. O. (1995, June 21). Prenatal and neonatal risk factor for childhood lymphatic leukemia. *Journal of National Cancer Institute, 87*(12), 908–914.

Davis, P. G., & Dawson, J. A. (2012). New concepts in neonatal resuscitation. *Current Opinion in Pediatrics, 24*(2), 147–153. doi:10.1097/MOP.0b013e3283504e11

Davis, P. G., Tan, A., O'Donell, C. P., & Schulze, A. (2004). Resuscitation of newborn infants with 100% oxygen or air: A systemic review and meta-analysis. *Lancet, 364*, 1329–1333.

Efrat, R., Kadari, A., & Katz, S. (1994). The LMA in pediatric anesthesia: Experience with 120 patients undergoing elective groin surgery. *Journal of Pediatric Surgery, 29*(1), 23–41; *29*(2), 206–208.

El-Naggar, W., & McNamara, P. J. (2012). Delivery room resuscitation of preterm infants in Canada: Current practice and views of neonatologists at level III centers. *Journal of Perinatology, 32*(7), 491–497. doi:10.1038/jp.2011.128 jp2011128

Gandini, D., & Brimacombe, J. (2004). Manikin training for neonatal resuscitation with the laryngeal mask airway. *Pediatric Anesthesia, 14*(6), 493–494.

Gandini, D., & Brimacombe, J. R. (1999). Neonatal resuscitation with the laryngeal mask airway in normal and low birth weight infants. *Anesthesia and Analgesia, 89*, 642–643.

Gold, K. J., Gorenflo, D. W., Schwenk, T. L., & Bratton, S. L. (2006). Physician experience with family presence during cardiopulmonary resuscitation in children. *Pediatric Critical Care Medicine, 7*(5), 428–433.

Gungor, S., Kurt, E., Teksoz, E., Goktolga, U., Ceyhan, T., & Baser, I. (2006). Oronasopharyngeal suction versus no suction in normal and term infants delivered by elective cesarean section: A prospective randomized controlled trial. *Gynecologic and Obstetric Investigation, 61*, 9–14.

Heller, R. M., & Heller, T. W. (1994). Experience with the illuminated endotracheal tube in the prevention of unsafe intubations in the premature and full term newborn. *Pediatrics, 93*, 389–391.

Jones, B. L., Parker-Raley, J., Maxson, T., & Brown, C. (2011). Understanding health care professionals' views of family presence during pediatric resuscitation. *American Journal of Critical Care, 20*(3), 199–207.

Kattwinkel, J. (Ed.). (2011). *Textbook of neonatal resuscitation* (6th ed.). Elk Grove, IL: American Academy of Pediatrics and American Heart Association.

Kattwinkel, J., Perlman, J. M., Aziz, K., Colby, C., Fairchild, K., Gallagher, J., . . . Zaichkin, J. (2010). Neonatal resuscitation: 2010 American heart association guidelines for cardiopulmonary resuscitation and emergency cardiovascular care. *Pediatrics, 126*, e 1400. doi:10.1542/peds. 2010–2972E (Originally published online 2010, October 18)

Lindener, W., Vossbeck, S., Hummler, H., & Pohlandt, F. (1999). Delivery room management of extremely low birth weight infants: Spontaneous breathing or intubation. *Pediatrics, 103*, 961–967.

Morley, C. J., & Davis, P. G. (2008, April). Continuous positive airway pressure: Scientific and clinical rationale. *Current Opinion in Pediatrics, 20*(2), 119–124. Review.

Murray, M. J., Vemeulen, M. J., Morrison, L. J., & Waite, T. (2002). Evaluation of pre-hospital insertion of the laryngeal mask airway by primary care paramedics with only classroom mannequin training. *Canadian Journal of Emergency Medicine, 5*, 338–343.

Naumberg, E., Bellocco, R., Cnattingius, S., Jonzon, A., & Ekbom, A. (2002). Supplementary oxygen and risk of childhood lymphatic leukemia. *Acta Pediactrica, 91*, 1328–1333.

Niermeyer, S., & Keenan, W. (2001). Resuscitation of the newborn infant. In M. G. Klaus & A. A. Fanaroff (Eds.), *Care of the high-risk neonate* (5th ed.). Philadelphia, PA: WB Saunders.

O'Donnell, C. P., Kamlin, C. O., Davis, P. G., Carlin, J. B., & Morley, C. J. (2007). Clinical assessment of infant colour at delivery. *Archives Diseases in Childhood. Fetal and Neonatal Edition, 92*(6), F465–F467. Epub. 2007, July 5.

O'Donnell, C. P., Kamlin, C. O., Davis, P. G., & Morley, C. G. (2005). Feasibility of and delay in obtaining pulse oximetry during neonatal resuscitation. *Journal of Pediatrics, 145*, 698–699.

Perlman, J. M., Wyllie, J., Kattwinkel, J., Atkins, D. L., Chameides, L., Goldsmith, J. P., . . . Velaphi, S. (2010). Neonatal resuscitation: 2010 International consensus on cardiopulmonary resuscitation and emergency cardiovascular care science with treatment recommendations. *Pediatrics, 126*, e1319. doi:10.1542/peds.2010–2972B (Originally published online October 18, 2010)

Rabi, Y., Rabi, D., & Yee, W. (2007). Room air resuscitation of the depressed newborn: A systematic review and meta-analysis. *Resuscitation, 72*, 353–363.

Rehan, V. K., Garcia, M., Kao, J., Tucker, C. M., & Patel, S. M. (2004). Epinephrine delivery during neonatal resuscitation: Comparison of direct endotracheal tube vs. catheter inserted into endotracheal tube administration. *Journal of Perinatology, 24*, 686–690.

Saugstad, O. D., Rootwelt, T., & Aalen, O. (1998). Resuscitation of asphyxiated newborn infants with room air or oxygen: An international controlled trial: The RESAIR2 study. *Pediatrics, 102*, e1.

Trevisanuto, D., Micaglio, M., Pitton, M., Magarotto, M., Piva, D., & Zanardo, V. (2004). Laryngeal mask airway: Is the management of neonates requiring positive pressure ventilation at birth changing? *Resuscitation, 62*, 151–157.

Velaphi, S., & Vidyasagar, D. (2008, December). The pros and cons of suctioning at the perineum (intrapartum) and post-delivery with and without meconium. *Seminars in Fetal and Neonatal Medicine, 13*(6), 375–382. Epub. 2008, May 13.

Vento, M., Asesni, M., Sastre, J., Garcia-Sala, F., Pallardo, F. V., & Vina, J. (2001). Resuscitation with room air instead of 100% oxygen prevents oxidative stress in moderately asphyxiated term neonates. *Pediatrics, 107*, 643–647.

Wang, C. L., Anderson, C., Leone, T. A., Rich, W., Govindaswami, B., & Finer, N. N. (2008). Resuscitation of preterm neonates by using room air or 100% oxygen. *Pediatrics, 121*, 1083–1089.

Zanardo, V., Simbi, A. K., Savio, V., Micaglio, M., & Trevisanuto, D. (2004). Neonatal resuscitation by laryngeal mask airway after elective cesarean section. *Fetal Diagnosis and Therapy, 19*, 228–231.

CHAPTER

4

Assessment of the Newborn and Infant

■ Terri A. Cavaliere and Debra A. Sansoucie

Assessment is a continuous process of evaluation throughout the course of routine care of the neonate and infant. However, periodically a more formalized, comprehensive examination must be undertaken to determine wellness or to evaluate a specific problem. The results of the comprehensive physical assessment serve as the database on which clinical judgments about diagnosis and treatment are based.

A comprehensive physical assessment is performed for various reasons. The assessment may be the initial examination at birth, assessment of extrauterine transition, determination of gestational age (GA), comprehensive assessment after transition, discharge examination, well-baby outpatient examination, or evaluation of an illness or injury. Although these assessments have many commonalities, each has a somewhat different purpose. The importance of a comprehensive physical assessment cannot be overstressed. While advances in technology have improved our ability to provide care to newborns there is no substitute for hands-on assessment. This chapter discusses various aspects of a comprehensive physical assessment.

FIRST NEONATAL ASSESSMENT AND THE APGAR SCORE

The initial neonatal assessment occurs immediately after delivery with the assignment of Apgar scores. These scores were devised in 1952 by Virginia Apgar as a means of assessing the clinical status of infants immediately after delivery (Apgar, 1953). The Apgar score consists of five components—heart rate, respiratory effort, muscle tone, reflex irritability, and color—and each component is given a score of zero, one, or two; the scores are then added to obtain a total score (Table 4.1). Although the total score originally was assigned at 1 minute after birth, the current recommendation is that it be assigned at 1 and 5 minutes. If the total score is below 7 at 5 minutes, the assessment is repeated every 5 minutes for 20 minutes or until a score above 7 has been achieved twice consecutively.

TABLE 4.1

APGAR SCORING SYSTEM

	Assigned Points		
Sign	**0**	**1**	**2**
Heart rate	Absent	Slow (<100 beats/min)	100 beats/min
Respirations	Absent	Weak cry; hypoventilation	Good, strong cry
Muscle tone	Limp	Some flexion	Active motion
Reflex irritability	No response	Grimace	Cough or sneeze
Color	Blue or pale	Body pink; extremities blue	Completely pink

Used with permission of American Academy of Pediatrics, Committee on the Fetus and Newborn and the American College of Obstetricians and Gynecologists Committee on Obstetrics (1996).

The value of the Apgar score has been challenged because of its misuse in the identification of birth asphyxia and prediction of neurologic outcome. It is important to recognize that elements of the Apgar score may be influenced by a variety of factors besides birth asphyxia, including, among others, preterm birth, administration of drugs to the mother, and congenital anomalies. A low 1-minute Apgar score does not correlate with the newborn's future outcome. The 5-minute Apgar score, especially the change in the score between 1 and 5 minutes, is a useful indicator of the effectiveness of resuscitation efforts. However, even a 5-minute score of 0 to 3, although possibly a result of hypoxia, is limited as an indicator of the severity of the problem and in and of itself correlates poorly with future neurologic outcome (Kattwinkel,

Zaichkin, McGowan, American Heart Association, & American Academy of Pediatrics, 2011; Stanley, 1994).

The Apgar score is not meant to be used to determine the need for resuscitation but to convey information about the newborn's response to resuscitation (Goldsmith, 2011). Values of components of the Apgar score are affected by resuscitation; therefore, the chart should reflect what measures, if any, are underway (Kattwinkel et al., 2011). The value of the Apgar score for the evaluation of extremely premature infants has also been questioned. Several components of the Apgar score, such as reflex irritability, muscle tone, and respiratory effort, are affected by the maturity of the infant; therefore, premature infants are unsurprisingly assigned lower Apgar scores than infants born at term (Als & Butler, 2011).

OTHER CONSIDERATIONS FOR THE INITIAL NEONATAL ASSESSMENT

A brief physical examination should be performed before the infant leaves the delivery area. Considerations for this assessment include inspection for birth injuries and major congenital anomalies and evaluation of pulmonary and cardiovascular adjustment to extrauterine life. Evaluation of early transition to extrauterine life includes observation of color for adequacy of perfusion and oxygenation, appraisal of respiratory effort, auscultation of breath sounds and heart sounds, and inspection of the amount, color, and consistency of secretions. The infant's tone, activity, and appropriateness of state should also be noted at this time. A cursory inspection of all external areas should be performed before the infant leaves the delivery area, including a general inspection of the external genitalia and, in males, palpation for testes in the scrotum. The entire examination should be performed under a radiant heat source to prevent significant heat loss from the infant.

Evaluation of Transition

Adaptation to both intrapartum and neonatal events is reflected in the transition from a fetal to an extrauterine environment. These events result in sympathetic activity that affects the infant's color, respiration, heart rate, behavioral state, gastrointestinal function, and temperature (Gardner & Hernandez, 2011). It is important to remember that the physiologic and biochemical changes peculiar to the period of transition to extrauterine life affect the physical findings of early examinations. The examination performed during transition is described separately because characteristics that are normal during transition may be abnormal if they appear at other times.

As the neonate's circulation converts from the fetal route, there may be a period in which pulmonary vascular resistance remains greater than systemic vascular resistance, resulting in a right to left shunt across the ductus arteriosus. Higher preductal oxygen saturation causes the neonate's face and upper body to appear pink while the lower body and legs appear pale or blue; this creates a visible demarcation across the chest. As the fetal circulation successfully converts to the neonatal pathway, this transitional differential cyanosis disappears (D'Harlingue & Durand, 2001).

Acrocyanosis is common during this period. To evaluate babies with deeper skin pigmentation, the nurse should observe the color of the mucous membranes. When the neonate is stimulated, the skin may appear blushed or bright red; this change in color is called erythema neonatorum, or generalized hyperemia, which develops a few hours after birth. It generally resolves within several minutes to an hour and rarely appears with the same intensity (Gomella, 2009). Erythema neonatorum is not synonymous with erythema toxicum neonatorum.

The neonatal heart rate may range from 160 to 180 beats/min in the first 15 minutes of life; it slowly falls to a baseline rate of 100 to 120 beats/min by 30 minutes of life. The heart rate is labile, and brief periods of asymptomatic, irregular heart rates are not pathologic. Murmurs are common, because the ductus arteriosus may still be patent. Respirations are also irregular during the first 15 minutes, with rates ranging from 60 to 100 breaths/min. Grunting, flaring, retractions, and brief periods of apnea may also be seen in the neonate. Crackles may be present on auscultation (Gardner & Hernandez, 2011).

Despite the changes in the heart and respiratory rates during the initial 15 to 30 minutes of life, healthy term infants are awake and alert. They may rest quietly, cry periodically, startle spontaneously, and breastfeed during this period. Full-term babies often show flexed posture with good muscle tone; preterm newborns, in comparison, have less flexion and tone (Sansoucie & Cavaliere, 2007). Temperature is decreased, and gastrointestinal activity includes the establishment of bowel sounds and the production of saliva. This first period of reactivity may be prolonged in infants who have experienced difficult labor and delivery, in sick term infants, and in well premature infants (Gardner & Hernandez, 2011).

After the first period of reactivity, the infant is relatively unresponsive or sleeping, and the heart rate drops to a baseline of 100 to 120 beats per minute. This interval, which lasts approximately 60 to 100 minutes, is followed by a second period of reactivity, which lasts anywhere from 10 minutes to several hours. During this time the infant may show rapid color changes, intermittent tachypnea and tachycardia, and changes in tone. A healthy infant may have periods during which the respiratory rate is considerably higher than 60 breaths/min; however, the infant does not appear distressed and can slow this rate enough to nipple feed successfully. Meconium often is passed during this period (Gardner & Hernandez, 2011). The chart in Figure 4.1 summarizes some of the physical changes seen during the transition period.

Newborn Examination

The comprehensive newborn examination generally is performed within the first 12 to 18 hours of life, after transition has been completed successfully. The examination should be initiated when the infant is quiet and should progress from assessments that are least likely to bother

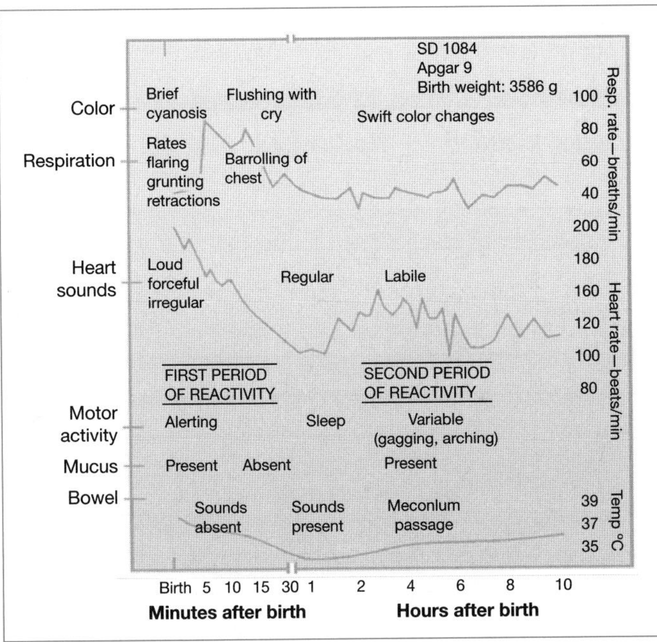

FIGURE 4.1 Normal transition period.
Based on Desmond, Rudolph, and Phitaksphraiwan (1966).

the infant to those that are most irritating. An examination sequence based on the infant's state is outlined in Table 4.2.

Discharge Examination

The purpose of the discharge examination is to assess the infant's ability to be cared for outside the controlled environment of the hospital. The focus of the assessment depends primarily on how long the infant has been hospitalized and for what reasons. The needs of a healthy, full-term infant being discharged home with the mother are different from those of a growing, preterm infant who has been hospitalized for weeks or months and who has significant sequelae. Evaluating the caretaker's capability to care for and observe changes in the infant is an important aspect of the discharge assessment and follow-up plan. Anticipatory guidance regarding feedings, sleeping position and environment, skin care, safety practices, and recognition of signs and symptoms of illness should be provided at this time.

Outpatient Examination

The focus of the first outpatient examination is the infant's adaptation to the home environment. This examination includes assessment of any issues highlighted at discharge. Some factors to be considered in the infant are temperature stability, ability and success at feeding and elimination, sleep patterns, normal color, drying of the umbilical cord, reassessment of hip stability, and normal state and behavior. Any areas that may have been relatively inaccessible during earlier examinations should be included, such as the eyes, ear canals, and eardrums (Fletcher, 1998).

The birth history, including the birth weight, GA, and any problems, should be reviewed. As part of the complete physical examination, height, weight, and head circumference should be plotted and developmental progress observed. The results of newborn metabolic screening and the infant's immunization status should be reviewed. For sick infants, general assessment assists in the establishment of priorities. For example, if a child is experiencing pronounced respiratory problems, assessment of this area is a priority. Anticipatory guidance issues include nutrition, elimination, sleep patterns, development and behavior, social and family relationships, and injury prevention (Hagan, Shaw, & Duncan, 2008). A more detailed description of health maintenance for high-risk infants during the first year of life is presented later in this chapter.

Environment

The routine neonatal assessment should take place in a quiet, warm environment. The room should be lighted well enough for appropriate observation, but the light should not be so strong that the infant is deterred from opening the eyes. Prevention of heat loss is critical to the infant's comfort and to the maintenance of thermal neutrality and glucose homeostasis. Most healthy term infants can tolerate being undressed in a reasonably warm room for the 5 to 10 minutes required to perform the physical assessment. If the environment is cool or drafty or if the infant is sick or preterm, an external heat source should be provided, such as a radiant warmer or heat lamps. If heat lamps are used, the infant's eyes should be shielded to prevent adverse effects from prolonged exposure of the infant's eyes to the bright light of the lamps. The examiner should warm the hands and examination equipment before beginning the assessment. This practice not only prevents heat loss but also avoids upsetting an otherwise quiet and cooperative infant.

The examination should be conducted in a quiet environment with a calm infant. A placid infant provides the best opportunity for gathering meaningful data. Extraneous environmental noise hampers auscultation and assessment of bodily sounds and may overwhelm a sick or immature infant, causing changes in state and cardiovascular status (Honeyfield, 2009). Handling the infant gently and speaking in a soothing voice may allow the examiner to complete most of the assessment without distressing the infant. Disturbing components of the examination, such as deep palpation of the abdomen and assessment of the hips, should be performed last.

Having one or both parents present during the routine neonatal assessment offers the opportunity to assess their competence in care giving and to educate them about the unique physical traits, behavior, and coping skills of their infant. The examiner may also use this time to build rapport and trust with the parents, to listen to their concerns, and to offer pertinent information. Some issues may require privacy for discussion; therefore, confidentiality should be considered when conversing with parents in the presence of others.

TABLE 4.2

EXAMINATION SEQUENCE BASED ON INFANT'S STATE

Assessment Technique	Required State	Arousing Maneuver	Equipment
Observe general appearance			
Observe color			
Observe resting posture	Quiet		
Observe spontaneous activity	Active		
Count respirations	Quiet		Clock
Count heartbeats	Quiet		Clock
Inspect facies at rest	Quiet		
Auscultate heart sounds	Quiet		Stethoscope
Auscultate breath sounds	Quiet		Stethoscope
Measure blood pressure	Quiet		Blood pressure cuff
Inspect head and neck region			
Stimulate response to sound	Quiet		Calibrated noise maker
Inspect trunk anteriorly			
Palpate abdomen, cardiac impulse	Quiet		
Feel pulses			
Examine genitalia			Lubricant for rectal examination
Inspect trunk posteriorly			
Inspect arms and hands			
Inspect legs and feet			
Assess passive tone			
Assess active tone	Active	X	
Elicit primitive reflexes	Active	X	
Assess muscle strength	Active	X	
Assess GA			
Test range in major joints		X	
Manipulate hips		X	
Measure temperature			Thermometer
Examine ears			Otoscope
Determine pupil response			Bright light
Examine fundi	Quiet	X	
Elicit tendon reflexes		X	Percussion hammer
Stimulate response to pain		X	
Weigh infant	Quiet	X	Scales, growth chart
Measure head circumference			Tape measure, growth chart
Measure chest and abdominal circumferences		X	Tape measure
Measure length			Tape measure, growth chart
Transilluminate head		X	High-intensity light
Percuss abdomen	Quiet		
Percuss lungs	Quiet		

Data from Fletcher (1998).

COMPONENTS OF A COMPREHENSIVE HISTORY

The neonatal history is very similar to that for an older child or adult, including information about the past medical history, the current condition, and the family. For a newly delivered infant, the initial neonatal assessment probably will be conducted before the nurse speaks to the parents. Basic information about the pregnancy and delivery should be available in the maternal records, but a complete history lays the foundation for the comprehensive newborn examination and should be elicited directly from the parents. Without a complete history, the examiner may lack adequate information to formulate an accurate impression.

The components of a complete history are the identifying data; chief complaint; interim neonatal history or history of presenting problem or illness; antepartum history; obstetric history; intrapartum history; and the maternal medical, family medical, and social histories (Table 4.3). After data collected from the complete history and physical assessment are organized and all expected and unexpected findings have been reviewed, areas of concern are identified and prioritized for further evaluation and attention. This forms the framework for the clinical diagnosis and plan of care.

Interviewing the Parents

The interview with the parents is a vital component of the health assessment of a newborn or an infant. This interview offers the nurse an excellent opportunity to develop a therapeutic partnership with the parents in the care of their baby. Ideally, the interview is conducted in a quiet, comfortable setting; if it takes place at the bedside in a busy intensive care unit, the parents may be distracted and overwhelmed by the sounds and sights customary to this environment. If the ideal setting is not possible, the nurse can provide a focal point of warmth and attention by using a conversational tone of voice, maintaining eye contact, and concentrating fully on the parents. However, this can be done only with a discipline that dispels both personal and professional distractions.

It is important that nurses introduce themselves and clearly state their names and roles in the baby's care. Nurses should make sure they understand the parents' names and should pronounce them correctly. They should ask the baby's name and use it often during the conversation. During this session, the purposes of the health interview and physical assessment should be clarified. Cooperation and sharing are more likely if the parents understand that the questions lead to better care for their infant.

TABLE 4.3

COMPONENTS OF A COMPREHENSIVE NEONATAL HISTORY

Component	Data Required
Identifying data	Infant's name, parents' names, parents' telephone numbers (home and work), infant's date of birth, gender, and race; source of referral (obstetric or pediatric provider) if any.
Chief complaint	Statement of initial known status (age, gender, birth and current weights, GA by dates and examination) and problems infant might have; for a newborn or well-baby examination, the statement simply reflects the current health status (e.g., "Full-term male infant, now 1 week of age, for well-baby follow-up").
Interim history/ history of	Chronologic record of newborn's history from time of delivery to present or, if older infant, presenting problem chronologic narrative of chief complaint. Narrative should answer questions related to where (location), what (quality, factors that aggravate or relieve symptoms), when (onset, duration, frequency), and how much (intensity, severity).
Antepartum history	Historical data about the pregnancy, including maternal age, gravidity, parity, last menstrual period, and estimated date of delivery. Date and GA at which prenatal care began, provider of care, and number of visits should be recorded here. Mother's health during pregnancy, infections, medications taken, use of illicit drugs or alcohol, abnormal bleeding, and results of prenatal screening tests also should be included.
Obstetric history	Significant history regarding previous pregnancies; neonatal problems or subsequent major medical problems of previous children and current age and health status of living children should be noted.
Intrapartum history	Duration of labor, whether it was spontaneous or induced, duration of rupture of membranes, type of delivery, complications; infant's birth weight, presentation at delivery, and Apgar scores; resuscitative measures if required and response to those measures.
Past medical history	Significant maternal history of chronic health problems or diseases treated in the past or during the pregnancy, including surgical procedures and hospitalizations before or during the pregnancy. For older infants, also obtain information about infant's history, including feeding, development, illness, and immunizations.
Family medical history	Significant family medical history of chronic disorders, disabilities, known hereditary diseases, or consanguinity.
Social history	Parents' marital status, paternal involvement, parents' occupations and educational level; sources of financial support, housing accommodations, and insurance status must be noted, as well as any support agencies involved. Family unit should be defined and religious and cultural affiliations noted, along with number of individuals living in the home. Plans for child care should be elicited, as well as any current family stressors (e.g., moving, death in the family).

The use of silence and listening, as well as allowing ample time for response to questions, is crucial to reassuring parents that what they say is worthwhile. Also, the parents can easily be shown that the interview is important and will not be rushed. Nurses should fix their attention on the parents and listen and should not interrupt unless necessary. They also should avoid asking the next questions before listening to the complete answer to the current question. They should indicate that they understand the responses and should request clarification if necessary. Nurses should take care to avoid overly technical language, medical jargon, and the tendency to inundate the parents with information. They should attempt to verify that the parents understand what has happened and what they have been told and that they seem to be coping. Nurses should always discuss and explain what the parents can expect to happen next; they should also bring up methods of keeping in touch, pertinent telephone numbers, and the visitation policy, if appropriate.

It is often difficult to approach parents about sensitive matters, such as drug or alcohol use or concerns about the death of their infant. Seidel, Ball, Dains, and Benedict (2003) have offered suggestions that may assist in the discussion of sensitive issues. Nurses should:

- Respect the individual's privacy
- Avoid discussing sensitive topics where the conversation might be overheard
- Begin the discussion with open-ended questions and ask the least threatening questions first
- Not be patronizing, but use language that is straightforward and understandable
- Take a direct and firm approach
- Avoid apologizing for asking a question (the nurse is doing nothing wrong)
- Avoid lecturing (the nurse is not there to pass judgment)
- Understand that defensive behavior might be the individual's way of coping
- Proceed slowly and take care not to demean the individual's behavior
- Offer feedback to ensure that the individual agrees that your interpretation is appropriate
- Provide an opportunity for the individual to ask relevant questions.

It is vital that, in communicating with parents from diverse cultures, nurses appreciate and respect differences in communication patterns and in childbearing and health practices. Knowledge of cultural variations in family and health practices assists nurses in developing sensitivity to differences; however, the family must be observed carefully for cues to family practices and relationships with children and one another.

Incorporation of a family history tool such as *My Family Health Portrait Tool* (http://www.hhs.gov/familyhistory) introduced by the former Surgeon General Richard Carmona, MD, RN, will give at least a three-generation history that may reveal genetic conditions. Some families will already have completed this information online. The tool takes very little time to complete and can be used in conjunction with the standard history questions.

Physical Assessment Techniques

The techniques used for physical assessment are inspection, palpation, percussion, and auscultation. Learning these skills requires patience and practice, and the inability of the newborn to provide verbal cues presents an additional challenge. With experience, the practitioner learns to process a multitude of observations while assessing individual systems and then to use these data to form a clinical impression and plan of care.

■ Inspection. Inspection is the simple yet intricate use of the auditory and visual senses to evaluate an infant's state, color, respiratory effort, posture, and activity, as well as the shape and symmetry of various body regions. It is a crucial skill in the physical assessment of neonates, but it is also a difficult one to master. The sense of smell may be used to note unusual odors. The impression obtained from methodical observation establishes priorities for the remainder of the systematic assessment. In the physical examination, thoughtful observation, rather than simple looking, is the most efficient means of detecting changes. Inspection should be used throughout the physical assessment and should continue as long as the infant remains in the nurse's care.

■ Auscultation. Auscultation is the process of listening for sounds made by the body. The bell of the stethoscope is used for low-pitched sounds (e.g., cardiovascular sounds) and the diaphragm for higher pitched sounds (e.g., lung and bowel sounds). The stethoscope should be placed lightly but firmly against the wall of the body part being assessed. A calm infant and quiet environment facilitate auscultation. Practice in recognizing normal body sounds is required before abnormal sounds can be identified accurately.

■ Palpation. With palpation, the examiner uses the sense of touch to determine hydration, texture, tension, pulsation, vibration, amplitude, and tenderness, as well as the depth, size, shape, and location of deep structures. The touch used for palpation must be gentle and is performed with the flats of the finger pads rather than the fingertips (Fletcher, 1998). To gather the most accurate information, the infant should be calm at the onset of the abdominal examination. Relaxing the abdominal musculature by flexing the infant's knees and hips with one hand facilitates palpation of the liver and spleen. Gentle pressure must be emphasized during palpation of sensitive organs (e.g., liver, spleen, and skin) that are at greater risk for injury and bleeding in neonates, particular preterm infants, or those that have hepatomegaly. Warming of the examiner's hands, use of a pacifier, and progression from superficial to deep palpation help maintain the infant's comfort throughout most of the examination. Tender areas should always be palpated last.

■ Percussion. Percussion is the use of tapping to produce sound waves that may be assessed according to intensity, pitch, duration, and quality (Table 4.4). Percussion may be direct or indirect. For direct percussion, the examiner directly strikes the body part to be assessed with the tip of

TABLE 4.4

PERCUSSION SOUNDS

Type of Sound	Intensity	Pitch	Duration	Quality	Common Locations
Tympany	Loud	High	Moderate	Drumlike	Gastric bubble; air-filled intestine (simulate by tapping puffed out cheeks)
Resonance	Moderate to loud	Low	Long	Hollow	Lungs
Hyperresonance	Very loud	Very low	Long	Booming	Lungs with trapped air; lungs of a young child
Dullness	Soft to moderate	High	Moderate	Thudlike	Liver, fluid-filled space (e.g., stomach)
Flatness	Soft	High	Short	Flat	Muscle

Data from Engel (2006).

the middle right finger. For indirect percussion, the examiner places the middle finger of the nondominant hand against the skin of the body part to be assessed and strikes the distal joint with the tip of the middle finger of the dominant hand. The wrist must make a snapping motion, creating a brisk thump with the tip of the right middle finger against the left middle finger's distal joint. Vibrations are transmitted from the bones of the finger joint touching the infant's body to the underlying tissue (Figure 4.2). Although percussion is rarely used in neonatal assessment, it may be a useful technique for examining the older infant or child.

Assessment of Size and Growth

Well-being in the fetal and neonatal periods is reflected by a normal growth pattern. Fetal and neonatal growth rates are predictable and can be measured by various methods. To determine if an individual infant's growth is adequate, an appropriate standard must be used with which the child's measurements can be compared. The growth curves used must match the patient as closely as possible in gender, race, GA, genetic potential, and environmental factors, such as altitude. A discussion of the techniques used to estimate and assess fetal growth is beyond the scope of this chapter and can be found elsewhere in this text. Two methods of evaluating adequacy of growth in the newborn are the GA assessment and the clinical assessment of nutritional status.

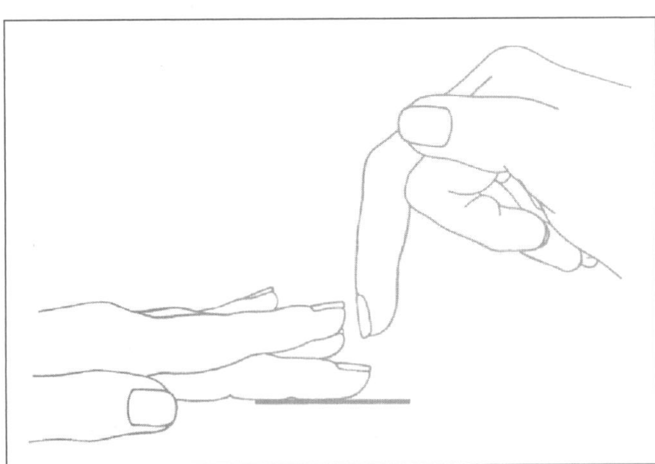

FIGURE 4.2 Percussion. Note the position of the fingers.
From Engel (2006).

One tool that may be used to assess nutritional status in the clinical setting is the CANSCORE developed by McLean and Usher (1970).

Assessment of GA

A determination of GA is part of the physical examination of every newborn. Classification of newborns by GA enables the health care provider to determine the neonatal mortality risk (Figure 4.3) and to identify possible disorders (Figure 4.4) and initiate intervention or screening (Gardner & Hernandez, 2011). Figure 4.5 shows the classification of newborns by intrauterine growth and GA. Table 4.5 presents terms used in GA assessment and in determining the adequacy of in utero growth.

As was previously mentioned, morbidity and mortality can be predicted from the GA assessment (see Figures 4.3 and 4.4). Neonates with the lowest risk of problems associated with morbidity and mortality are term infants who developmentally are appropriate for gestational age (AGA). Risks associated with categories of GA and intrauterine growth restriction are shown in Table 4.6.

After birth, GA is determined by the evaluation of physical, neurologic, and neuromuscular characteristics. A number of methods have been developed to assess GA in newborns. The New Ballard score (NBS) is a widely used assessment tool (Figure 4.6). It includes six neurologic and six physical criteria and permits assessment of extremely premature infants. Despite its advantages over the other scoring systems, the NBS is accurate only to within 2 weeks and tends toward overestimating the GA of extremely premature neonates (Lissauer, 2011). Performing the examination as soon as possible in the first 12 hours of life enhances its accuracy.

Although GA assessment is discussed separately, the components of the assessment should be performed as part of the infant's general physical examination. Table 4.7 presents the essentials of the NBS; each component is scored as shown in Figure 4.6. The total score is calculated, and the resulting GA is plotted on a graph (see Figure 4.5).

Clinical Assessment of Nutritional Status

GA assessment does not identify all infants with intrauterine malnutrition. Although the terms *small for gestational*

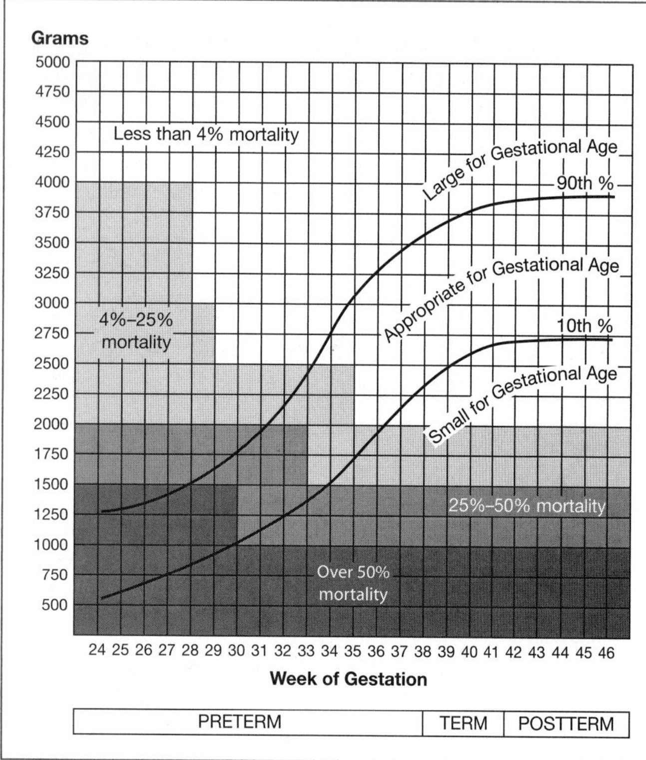

FIGURE 4.3 University of Colorado Medical Center classification of newborns by birth weight and GA and by neonatal mortality risk. From Battaglia and Lubchenco (1967).

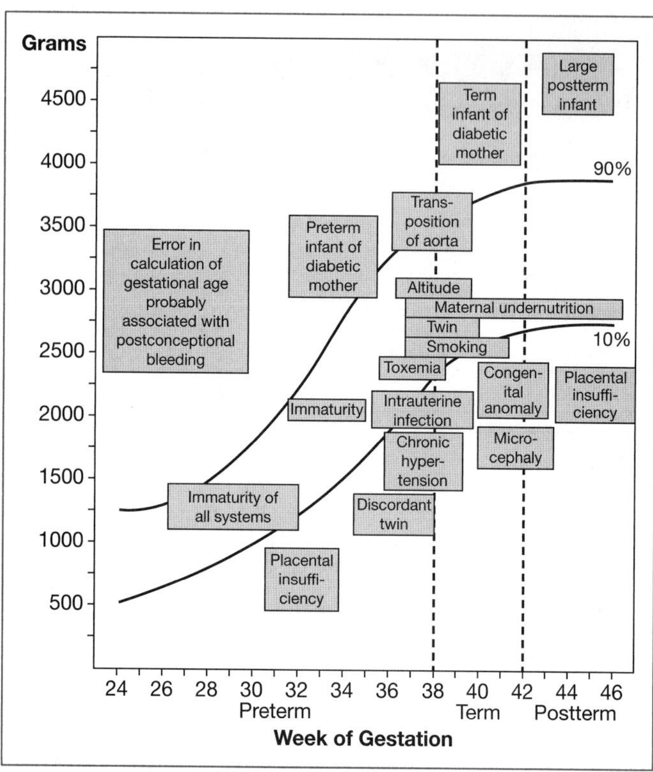

FIGURE 4.4 Deviations of intrauterine growth: Neonatal morbidity by birth weight and GA.
Modified from Lubchenco (1967).

age (SGA) and *intrauterine growth retardation/restriction* (IUGR) are related, they are not synonymous. IUGR represents a reduction in the expected fetal growth pattern, whereas SGA refers to an infant whose birth weight is less than population norms. Not all IUGR infants are SGA, and not all SGA infants are IUGR (Kliegman, 2011; Trotter, 2009).

Many but not all infants who are either SGA or IUGR are malnourished in utero. However, malnutrition can occur in neonates of any birth weight. Because malnutrition alters body composition and can prevent adequate brain growth, it is important to identify infants who have been affected in utero. These infants may be at risk for problems associated with aberrant growth (Kliegman, 2011).

McLean and Usher (1970) described physical findings that are suggestive of weight loss or poor nutrition. These physical characteristics form the basis of the CANSCORE that may be used in the clinical evaluation of nutritional status in newborns at term.

Measurement Techniques

For most infants the parameters of weight, length, and occipitofrontal circumference (OFC) are adequate for the basic physical assessment. These measurements are compared against standard growth curves. If the infant has any abnormalities in the size of a body component or if the infant shows disproportionate growth, the involved areas should be measured and compared with established norms (Fletcher, 1998).

■ **Weight and Length.** The infant should be weighed while unclothed and quiet. Weight can be falsely increased by a significant amount of infant motion (Fletcher, 1998). The weight of the average full-term that is AGA is 3.5 kg, with a range of 2,700 to 4,000 g (Grover, 2000a; Tappero, 2009). Generally African American, Hawaiian, and Asian neonates weigh less than Caucasian infants (Tappero, 2009).

The crown-to-heel length can be obtained using a measurement board or a standard tape measure. With the infant supine and legs extended, the nurse draws a line on the bed at the baby's head and another at the heels and then measures the distance between these two points (Figure 4.7). The average full-term newborn is 50 cm long with a range of 48 to 53 cm (Tappero, 2009). Other measurement techniques are described in the appropriate sections.

Physical Examination of the Neonate

The following sections describe the newborn examination beyond the transition period.

■ **Vital Signs.** Once transition is complete, the neonate has a respiratory rate between 40 and 60 breaths per minute, and the rate may be irregular. Respirations are easy and unlabored; breath sounds should be clear on auscultation. The heart rate varies from 100 to 160 beats per minute, depending on the infant's state and GA (Vargo, 2009). Premature neonates have a higher baseline heart rate. The resting heart rate is the most representative for any baby.

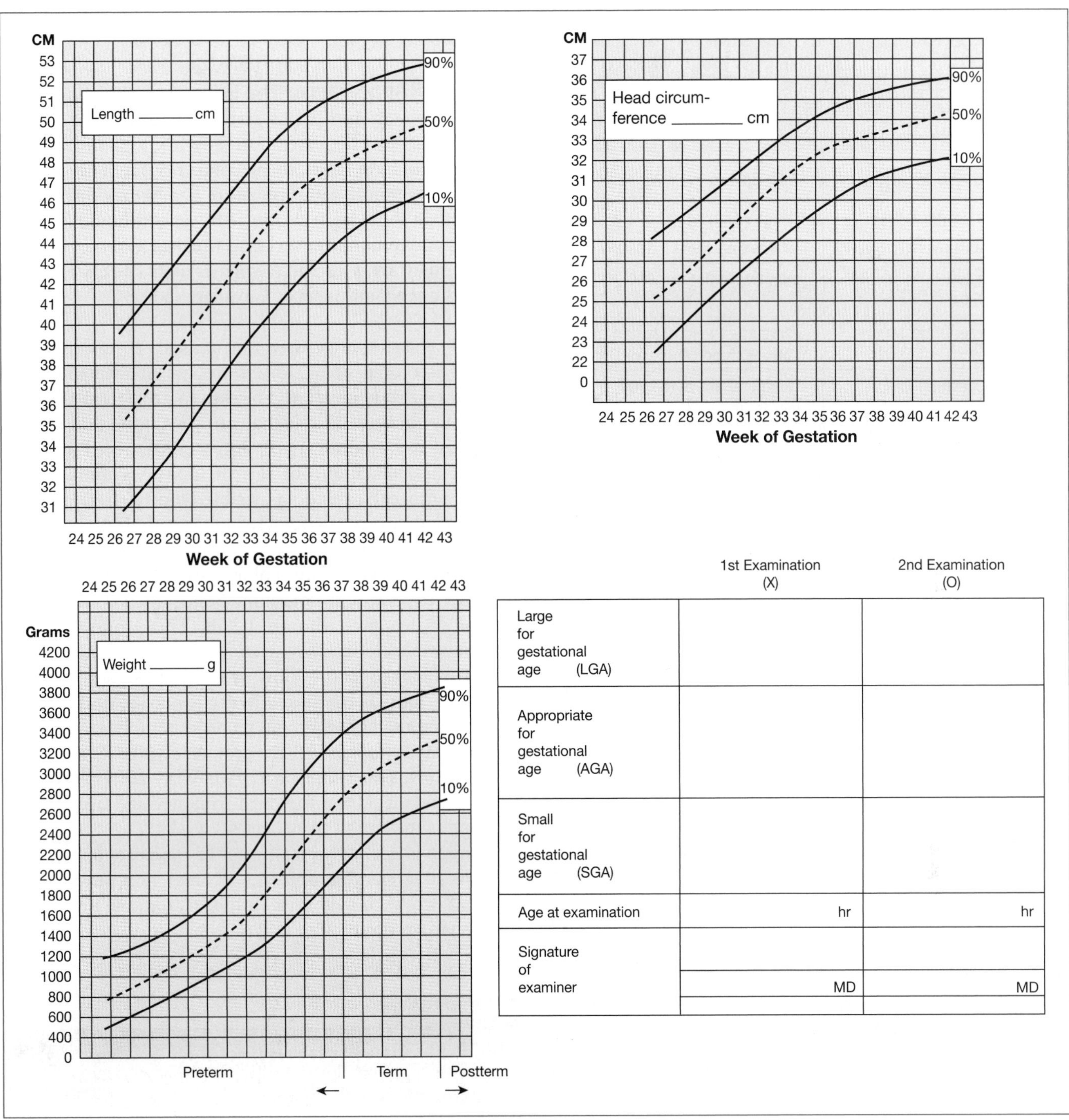

FIGURE 4.5 Estimating GA: Newborn classification based on maturity and intrauterine growth.
Modified from Lubchenco et al. (1966) and Battaglia and Lubchenco (1967).

Normal blood pressure ranges depend on gestational and chronologic ages and the methods used. Blood pressure in premature babies is proportional to size; therefore, normal values are lower than for term babies (Hegyi et al., 1994). Figures 4.8 and 4.9 and Tables 4.8 through 4.10 show normal blood pressure values over various time frames and GAs.

Temperature is determined by axillary measurement; acceptable values range from 35.5°C to 37.5°C (Brown & Landers, 2011).

■ Cardiovascular Values. The heart is assessed for rate, rhythm, character of heart sounds, and presence of murmurs. During infancy the position of the heart changes and the point of maximal impulse (PMI) shifts (Fletcher, 1998). In the first few days of life the PMI is located at the fourth intercostal space at or to the left of the midclavicular line. Auscultation should be performed at the second and fourth intercostal spaces, cardiac apex, and axilla (Vargo, 2009). Murmurs are commonly heard before the ductus arteriosus closes completely. However, murmurs that are persistent may not be normal and require evaluation. Brief asymptomatic irregularities in rate and rhythm are not uncommon, especially in the preterm baby. The most common benign dysrhythmias are sinus bradycardia

TABLE 4.5

TERMS AND ABBREVIATIONS USED IN ASSESSMENT OF GA AND ADEQUACY OF INTRAUTERINE GROWTH

Term and Abbreviation	Description
Low birth weight (LBW)	Infant weighing < 2,500 g[a]
Very low birth weight (VLBW)	Infant weighing < 1,500 g[a]
Extremely low birth weight (ELBW)	Infant weighing < 1,000 g[a]
Appropriate for gestational age (AGA)	Parameter (weight) within the 10th–90th percentile for GA
Large for gestational age (LGA)	Parameter above the 90th percentile for GA
Small for gestational age (SGA)	Parameter below the 10th percentile for GA
Intrauterine growth restriction (IUGR)	Slowing of intrauterine growth documented by ultrasound; a neonate may be IUGR without being SGA
Symmetric IUGR	Measurements for weight, length, and head circumference all within the same growth curve even if neonate is AGA, LGA, or SGA
Asymmetric IUGR	Measurements for weight, length, and head circumference in different growth curves
Term gestation	Neonate born between 37 and 42 weeks gestation
Preterm gestation	Neonate delivered before completion of week 37 of gestation
Postterm gestation	Neonate delivered after completion of week 42 of gestation

[a] Regardless of length of gestation.

or tachycardia and premature atrial or ventricular contractions (Vargo, 2009). An electrocardiogram (ECG) or heart monitor is needed to properly identify the abnormality. Exact identification of the abnormality cannot be made solely by auscultation.

A precordial impulse may be visible along the left sternal border during the first 6 hours (Fletcher, 1998; Vargo, 2009). In premature neonates, because of their thin skin and absence of subcutaneous fat, the precordial impulse may be visible for a longer period. Pulses are palpated for rate, strength, and synchrony.

Figure 4.10 shows the location of pulses in the neonate (Vargo, 2009). Radial or brachial pulses are compared for timing and intensity, and the same is then done for bilateral femoral pulses. Finally, the preductal and postductal pulses are examined.

The adequacy of the infant's perfusion is determined by checking the capillary refill. This is assessed by depressing the skin over the abdomen or on an extremity until the area blanches. The capillary refill time is the number of seconds that elapse until the color returns to the area. This should be less than 3 seconds.

■ **General Appearance.** The infant's general appearance is indicative of nutritional status, maturity, and overall well-being. Term neonates normally are well formed and rounded and have stores of subcutaneous fat. They assume the fetal position at rest. Premature babies may display less flexion than those born at term. Movement should be spontaneous and tremulous. Neonates range in mood from quiet to alert; they are consolable when crying. The cry is strong and sustained (Sansoucie & Cavaliere, 2007).

■ **Skin.** The skin is assessed for maturity, consistency, and color. Discolored areas, variations, or abnormalities are noted for size and location. The skin of a full-term newborn contains subcutaneous fat that provides insulation against heat loss. It is smooth, pink, and wrinkle free. Premature infants lack subcutaneous fat; their skin is thinner than that of term babies and has visible blood vessels over the chest and abdomen. Extremely immature babies often have a gelatinous appearance with transparent skin. They commonly have a red, ruddy color caused by underdevelopment of the stratum corneum. Subcutaneous fat also is lacking in neonates who are IUGR. This group of babies may have loose skin folds, particularly around the knees.

Vernix is the greasy yellow or white substance found on fetal skin, particularly in the axillary, nuchal, and inguinal folds. Composed of sebaceous gland secretions, lanugo, and desquamated epithelial cells, it protects against fluid loss and bacterial invasion (Charsha, 2010; Witt, 2009). Vernix is most abundant during the third trimester and decreases in amount as the fetus approaches 40 weeks.

Lanugo is fine, downy hair that first appears on the fetus at 19 to 20 weeks gestation and becomes most prominent at 27 to 28 weeks. It begins to disappear from the lower back and usually is not present at term.

TABLE 4.6

RISKS ASSOCIATED WITH GA AND INTRAUTERINE GROWTH RESTRICTION

Category	Risks
SGA, LGA, intrauterine growth retardation/ restriction (IUGR)	Perinatal and long-term problems
Preterm SGA	Problems associated with immaturity of body systems and placental insufficiency
Preterm	Problems associated with immaturity of body systems
Postterm	Problems associated with placental Insufficiency
Term LGA	Risks are greatest in perinatal period, but long-term problems can develop

Neuromuscular Maturity

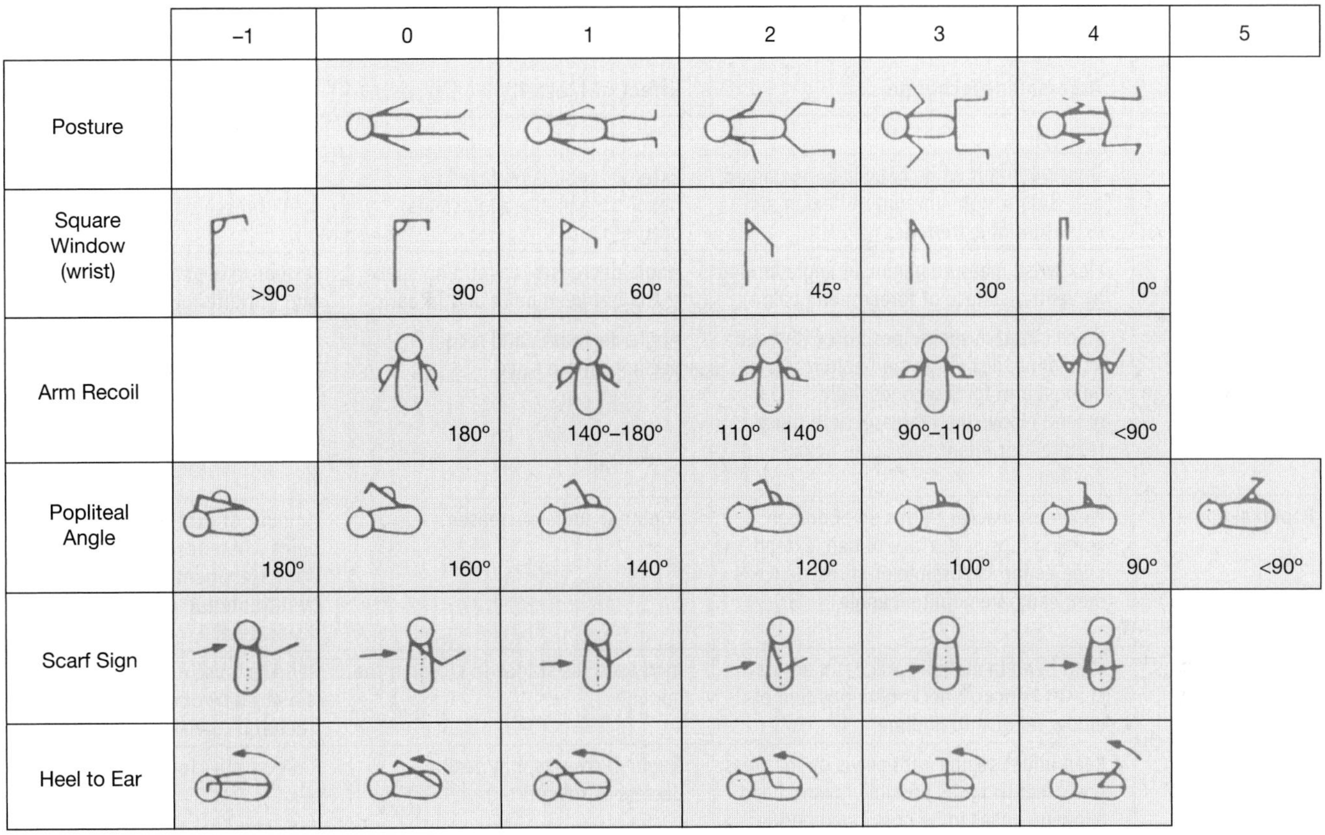

	−1	0	1	2	3	4	5
Posture							
Square Window (wrist)	>90°	90°	60°	45°	30°	0°	
Arm Recoil		180°	140°–180°	110° 140°	90°–110°	<90°	
Popliteal Angle	180°	160°	140°	120°	100°	90°	<90°
Scarf Sign							
Heel to Ear							

Physical Maturity

Skin	sticky friable transparent	gelatinous red, translucent	smooth pink, visible veins	superficial peeling &/ or rash few veins	cracking pale areas rare veins	parchment deep cracking no vessels	leathery cracked wrinkled
Lanugo	none	sparse	abundant	thinning	bald areas	mostly bald	
Plantar Surface	heel-toe 40–50 mm: −1 <40 mm: −2	>50 mm no crease	faint red marks	anterior transverse crease only	creases ant. 2/3	creases over entire sole	
Breast	imperceptible	barely perceptible	flat areola no bud	stippled areola 1–2 mm bud	raised areola 3–4 mm bud	full areola 5–10 mm bud	
Eye/Ear	lids fused loosely: −1 tightly: −2	lids open pinna flat stays folded	sl. curved pinna; soft; slow recoil	well-curved pinna; soft but ready recoil	formed & firm instant recoil	thick cartilage ear stiff	
Genitals (male)	scrotum flat smooth	scrotum empty faint rugae	testes in upper canal rare rugae	testes descending few rugae	testes down good rugae	testes pendulous deep rugae	
Genitals (female)	clitoris prominent labia flat	prominent clitoris small labia minora	prominent clitoris enlarging minora	majora & minora equally prominent	majora large minora small	majora cover clitoris & minora	

Maturity Rating

score	weeks
−10	20
−5	22
0	24
5	26
10	28
15	30
20	32
25	34
30	36
35	38
40	40
45	42
50	44

FIGURE 4.6 Maturational assessment of GA: New Ballard scoring system. From Ballard et al. (1991).

■ **Head.** The head is inspected for shape, symmetry, bruises, and lesions. Neonates delivered by cesarean section generally have a rounded head. Infants born vaginally in vertex position can have overriding sutures; this results in an irregularly shaped head that persists only for a few days in full-term neonates but may be evident for several weeks in premature

TABLE 4.7

NEW BALLARD SCORING SYSTEM

Component	Assessment Technique	Effect of Maturity	Comments
Neuromuscular Maturity			
Posture	Observe infant while baby is unrestrained and supine; note amount of flexion and extension of extremities	Extensor tone is replaced by flexor tone in a cephalocaudal progression	Knees may be hyperextended in a frank breech delivery
Square window	Flex wrist; measure minimum angle formed by ventral surface of forearm and palm	Angle decreases; at term no space exists between palm and forearm	Response depends on muscle tone and intrauterine position
Arm recoil	Place infant in supine position with head in midline; flex elbow and hold forearm against arm for 5 seconds; fully extend elbow, then release; note time required for infant to resume flexed position	Angle decreases and recoil becomes more rapid	
Popliteal angle	Flex hips, placing thighs on abdomen; keeping hips on surface of bed, extend knee as far as possible until resistance is met; estimate popliteal angle	Popliteal angle decreases	Amount of extension can be beyond point where resistance is first met; this assessment also is affected by intrauterine position and hip dislocation
Scarf sign	With head in midline, pull hand across chest to encircle neck; note position of elbow relative to midline	Increased resistance to crossing the midline	Reflects muscle tone; response is altered by obesity, hydrops, or fractured clavicle
Heel to ear	Keep infant supine with pelvis on mattress; press feet as far as possible toward head, allowing knees to be positioned beside abdomen; estimate angle created by arc from back of heel to mattress	Angle decreases; hip flexion decreases toward term	Reflects muscle tone
Physical Maturity			
Skin	Observe translucency of skin over abdominal wall	Skin becomes thicker and ultimately dry and peeling; pigmentation increases	Skin becomes drier hours after birth; phototherapy or sunlight enhances pigmentation
Lanugo	Assess for presence and length of hair over back	Lanugo emerges at 19–20 weeks and is most prominent at 27–28 weeks; then gradually disappears, first from the lower back and then from at least half of the back	The degree of pigmentation and quantity of hair are related to race, nutritional status
Plantar surface	Measure length of foot; determine presence or absence of true deep creases (not merely wrinkles)	Early in gestation, foot length correlates with fetal growth; creases develop from toes to heel, and absence of creases correlates with immaturity	Plantar creases also reflect intrauterine fetal activity; accelerated creasing is seen with oligohydramnios; diminished creasing suggests lack of activity in a mature fetus
Breast	Estimate diameter of breast bud; assess color and stippling of areola	Definition and stippling of areola and pigmentation are evident near term; bud size increases because of maternal hormones and fat accumulation	With intrauterine growth restriction, breast tissue may be diminished, but development of areola proceeds regardless of malnutrition
Ear cartilage	Fold top of auricle; observe speed of recoil	Cartilage becomes stiff, and auricle thickens	Compression in utero and absence or dysfunction of auricular muscles diminishes firmness
Eyelid opening	Without attempting to separate eyelids, evaluate degree of fusion	Opening begins at 22 weeks; lids are completely unfused by 28 weeks	Fused eyelids should not be considered a sign of nonviability; lids may be fused at term with anophthalmia

(*continued*)

TABLE 4.7

NEW BALLARD SCORING SYSTEM (CONTINUED)

Component	Assessment Technique	Effect of Maturity	Comments
External Genitalia			
Male	Palpate scrotum to assess degree of descent of testes; observe rugae and suspension (cryptorchidism)	At 27–28 weeks, testes begin to descend into scrotum; rugae formation of scrotum. begins at about 28 weeks; by term, rugae are well defined, and scrotum is pendulous	Rugae are decreased with scrotal edema; testes may be absent
Female	Assess size of labia minora and labia majora	Labia minora increase in size before labia majora; at term labia majora cover labia minora completely	Size of labia majora depends on amount of body fat; with malnutrition, size may be diminished; edema may increase size of labia majora

Data from Lissauer (2011) and Gardner and Hernandez (2011).

babies (Sansoucie & Cavaliere, 2007). The head circumference is measured in the occipitofrontal plane and is the largest diameter around the head. It is obtained with the tape measure placed snugly above the ears, the eyebrow ridges, and the occiput of the head. The average OFC in a full-term neonate is 35 cm, with a normal range of 31 to 38 cm (Sansoucie & Cavaliere, 2007). The major bones of the head, as well as sutures and fontanelles, are shown in Figure 4.11.

The head should be palpated to assess the firmness of bone and the size and configuration of fontanelles and sutures and also to detect swelling, masses, or bony defects. The amount of overlap of sutures may vary, depending on the extent of molding. Normally the sutures should move freely when gentle pressure is applied to the bones on opposite sides of the suture lines (Furdon & Clark, 2003). Directly after birth, it may be difficult to determine if the sutures are fused or merely overlapping. Reevaluation when molding and overlap have resolved may yield more reliable information about the presence of craniosynostosis (Fletcher, 1998).

The anterior fontanelle is 2 to 3 cm wide, 3 to 4 cm long, and diamond shaped (see Figure 4.11). It should be flat and soft; tense, bulging fontanelles may be reflective of intracranial pressure, while a sunken fontanelle can signify dehydration (Johnson, 2009). The posterior fontanelle is 1 to 2 cm wide and triangular. It may be difficult to palpate the fontanelles directly after birth because of cranial molding (Sansoucie & Cavaliere, 2007). Tension in the fontanelle should be assessed with the infant both recumbent and upright. Serial measurements of the width of the anterior fontanelle are more helpful than a single measurement because of wide variations in size and differences in measurement techniques (Fletcher, 1998).

Hair is evaluated for color, length, continuity, texture, quantity, position and number of hair whorls, and hairlines. Term newborns have fine hair with identifiable individual strands. Hair may appear disheveled for the first several weeks to months (Fletcher, 1998). In premature neonates the hair is more widely dispersed and is described as "fuzzy." Normally, hair color is fairly uniform, although some neonates have a blend of light and dark hair (Furdon & Clark, 2003). Sporadic patches of white hair may be a familial trait and is a benign finding, but a white forelock and other pigmentation defects in the eyes or skin may be associated with deafness or mental retardation (Fletcher, 1998; Waardenburg, 1951). The anterior hairline varies, with normal growth of pigmented hair onto the forehead of hirsute babies. The posterior hairline ends at the neck crease. Usually one off-center hair whorl is present in the parietal region (Furdon & Clark, 2003).

■ **Face and Neck.** The face should be inspected for shape, symmetry, and the presence of bruising or dysmorphic features. The overall facial configuration should be evaluated; the features should be proportional and symmetric. Unusual facial features may be familial or pathognomonic of a malformation syndrome. Gag, sucking, and rooting reflexes should be evaluated.

The newborn has a relatively short neck that should be palpated or observed for symmetry, appearance of the skin, range of motion, masses, and fistulous openings. The neck should be symmetric with the head, demonstrating full range of motion (Sansoucie & Cavaliere, 2007). In utero positioning can cause asymmetry of the neck. Redundant skin or webbing may be evident (Smith, 2012). The clavicles can be palpated at this time; they should be intact and without crepitus or swelling.

■ **Ears.** The ears are evaluated and compared for shape, configuration, position, amount of cartilage, and signs of trauma. The position of the ears at term should be similar bilaterally; approximately 30% of the pinna should lie above a line from the inner and outer canthi of the eye toward the occiput. The rotation of the ears should also be assessed; the long axis of the pinna should lie approximately 15 degrees posterior to the true vertical axis of the head (Fletcher, 1998) (Figure 4.12). Abnormalities of the external ear may be associated with syndromes, but often they represent minor structural variations and may be within the normal range (Johnson, 2009).

The presence and patency of the auditory canal can be documented by inspection. Otoscopic examination is not usually part of the examination in the newborn period because the ear canals are filled with vernix, amniotic debris, and blood. This condition clears in approximately 60% of term infants by 1 week of age but may persist for weeks. Less debris is seen in preterm babies, whose canals may clear more quickly.

Because infants frequently remain hospitalized beyond the neonatal period and because evaluation of the middle ear is part of a health maintenance examination, it is appropriate to include otoscopic examination in this section. The otoscope is used differently in young infants than in adults. In a neonate the ear lobe is pulled toward the chin, and the speculum is directed toward the face. The ear canals of preterm babies are prone to collapse because they are more pliable. Positive pressure applied through the pneumatic otoscope prevents the cartilaginous ear canal from obscuring the view (Fletcher, 1998). The neonatal tympanic membrane is thicker, grayer, and more vascular than that of an adult or older child (Figure 4.13).

Infants should also be assessed for behavioral response to noise stimuli. However, routine formal audiologic testing is becoming more common in the newborn period.

■ **Eyes.** The eyes should show spontaneous range of motion and conjugate movements. The lids should be symmetric in both horizontal and vertical placement, and the lashes should be directed outward in an orderly fashion. The eyes should be clear and should have an evenly colored iris, which may be dark gray, blue, or brown, depending on race. Pigmentation should be similar between the two eyes. Permanent eye color is not established for several months, but darker races may show permanent pigmentation in the first week of life. The surface of the conjunctiva should be smooth. During the first few days of life, the cornea may appear slightly hazy as a result of corneal edema, but thereafter the cornea should be clear and shiny. The sclerae normally are white, but a bluish coloration may be noted in premature and other small infants because their sclerae are thinner (Fletcher, 1998; Kaufman, Miller, & Gupta, 2011).

An ophthalmoscope is used to assess the pupillary and red reflexes. The light should be directed on the pupils from a distance of approximately 6 inches. The pupils should be round and equal in diameter and should constrict equally in response to light (pupils equal and reactive to light, or PERL) (Johnson, 2009). The beam of light illuminating the retina causes the red reflex. The retina (fundus) appears as a yellowish-white/gray or red background, depending on the amount of melanin in the pigment epithelium. The pigment varies with the complexion of the baby; in dark-skinned infants, the reflex will be pale or cloudy (Honeyfield, 2009; Wright, 1999).

■ **Nose.** The nose should be evaluated for shape and symmetry, patency of nares, skin lesions, or signs of trauma. The nasal mucosa should be pink and slightly moist; secretions should be thin, clear, and usually scanty (Fletcher, 1998). The nose should be midline. Immediately after birth the nose may be misshapen as a result of compression in utero, but this should correct spontaneously in a few days (Fletcher, 1998; Sansoucie & Cavaliere, 2007). Obstructions and deformities may denote anatomic malformations or congenital syndromes. The patency of the nares can be demonstrated by alternate occlusion of each naris using gentle pressure (Fletcher, 1998). Nasal flaring may be indicative of respiratory distress, but in an otherwise healthy newborn it does not indicate respiratory distress when it appears as the only symptom (Gardner & Hernandez, 2011; Fletcher, 1998).

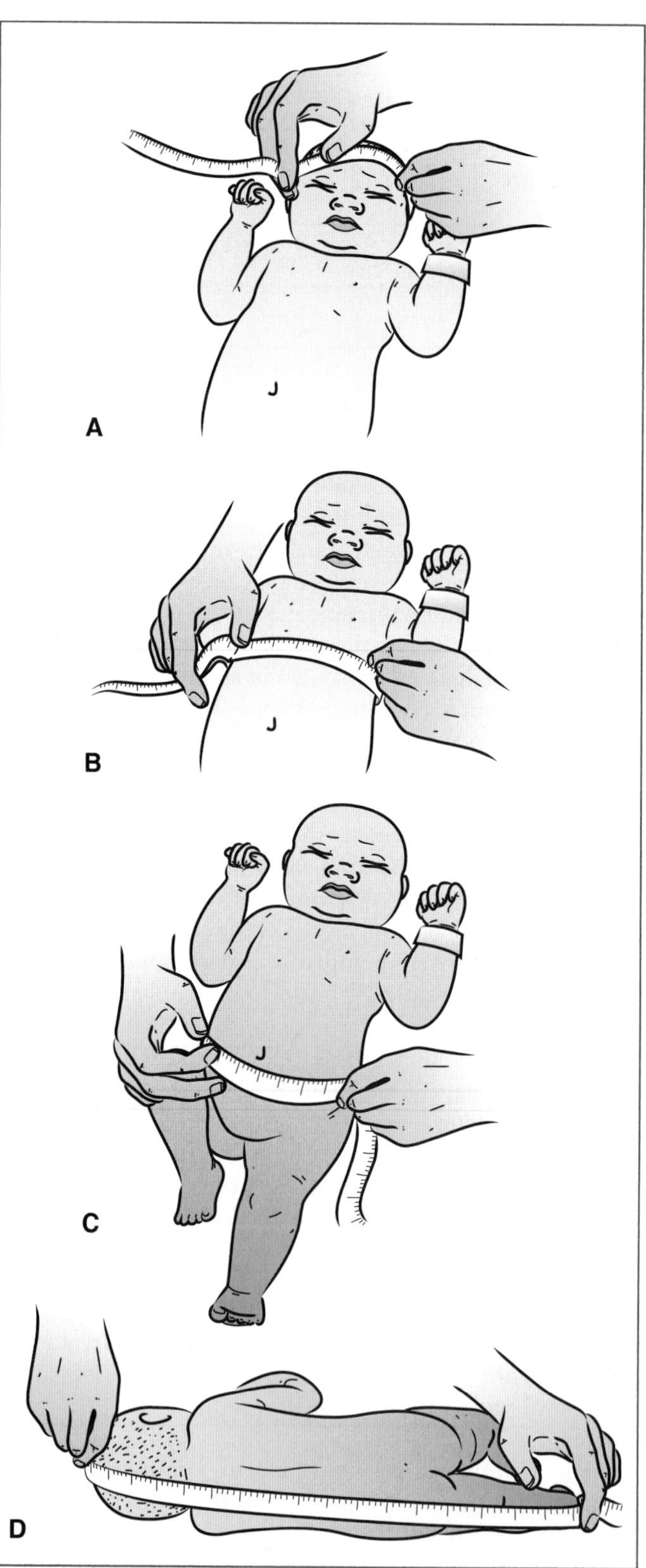

FIGURE 4.7 Newborn measurements: (A) circumference of head, (B) circumference of chest, (C) circumference of abdomen, (D) length, crown to rump. (Total length includes the length of the legs.) If the measurements are taken before the infant's first bath, the nurse must wear gloves.
Modified from Marjorie Pyle, RNC, Lifecircle, Costa Mesa, CA.

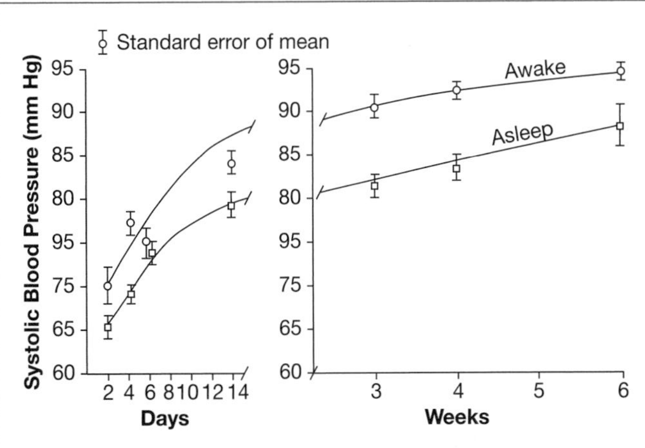

FIGURE 4.8 Increase in systolic blood pressure between ages 2 days and 6 weeks in infants awake and asleep (values obtained by cuff measurement).
Modified from Early et al. (1980).

TABLE 4.8

BLOOD PRESSURE VALUES ACCORDING TO SITE AND AGE

	Blood Pressure (mmHg)		
Site and Age	**Systolic**	**Diastolic**	**Mean**
Calf			
Less than 36 hours old	61.9 ± 7	39.6 ± 5.3	47.6 ± 6
Over 36 hours old	66.8 ± 10.1[a]	42.5 ± 7.3[a]	51.5 ± 9[a]
Total	63.6 ± 8.6	40.6 ± 6.3	49 ± 7.5

Values were obtained by blood pressure cuff measurement in 219 healthy term infants, 140 less than 36 hours old and 79 over 36 hours old. Values are given as means ± standard deviation.

[a] Significantly different from values in infants less than 36 hours old ($p < .05$).

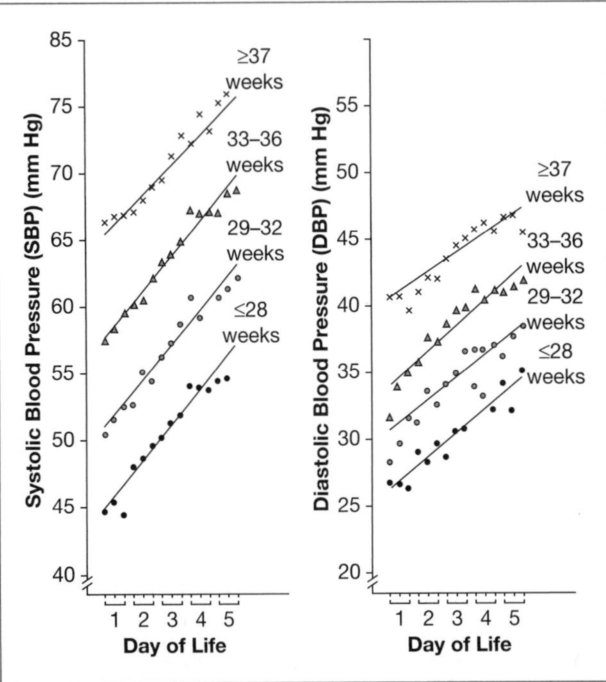

FIGURE 4.9 Systolic and diastolic blood pressures plotted for the first 5 days of life, with each day subdivided into 8-hour periods. Infants are categorized by GA into four groups: 28 weeks or younger (n = 33), 29 to 32 weeks (n = 73), 33 to 36 weeks (n = 100), and 37 weeks or older (n = 110).
Modified from Zubrow et al. (1995).

TABLE 4.9

BLOOD PRESSURE RANGES IN DIFFERENT WEIGHT GROUPS OF PREMATURE NEWBORNS

	Blood Pressure (mmHg)	
Birth Weight (g)	**Systolic**	**Diastolic**
501–750 (n = 18)	50–62	26–36
751–1,000 (n = 39)	48–59	23–36
1,001–1,250 (n = 30)	49–61	26–35
1,251–1,500 (n = 45)	46–56	23–33
1,501–1,750 (n = 51)	46–58	23–33
1,751–2,000 (n = 61)	48–61	24–35

Measurements were obtained by blood pressure cuff or umbilical artery transducer in the first 3 to 6 hours of life.
From Hegyi et al. (1994).

TABLE 4.10

OSCILLOMETRIC MEASUREMENTS: MEAN ARTERIAL BLOOD PRESSURE

	Mean Arterial Pressure ± Standard Deviation		
Birth Weight (g)	**Day 3**	**Day 17**	**Day 31**
501–750	38 ± 8	44 ± 8	46 ± 11
751–1,000	43 ± 8	45 ± 7	47 ± 9
1,001–1,250	43 ± 8	46 ± 9	48 ± 8
1,251–1,500	45 ± 8	47 ± 8	47 ± 9

From Fanaroff and Wright (1990).

■ **Mouth.** The mouth is inspected for size, shape, color, and presence of abnormal structures and masses. It should be evaluated both at rest and while the infant is crying. The speed of response and intensity of neonatal reflexes, such as rooting, gagging, and sucking, are also assessed. The mouth is a midline structure, symmetric in shape and movement. The mouth, chin, and tongue should be in proportion, with the lips fully formed (Sansoucie & Cavaliere, 2007).

The mucous membranes should be pink and moist, and oral secretions should be thin and clear. Excessive secretions or drooling suggests inability to swallow or esophageal or pharyngeal obstruction. Both the hard and soft palates should be inspected and palpated to rule out clefts. A high-arched palate may be seen in malformation syndromes, but it generally is insignificant if it appears as an isolated characteristic (Lissauer, 2011).

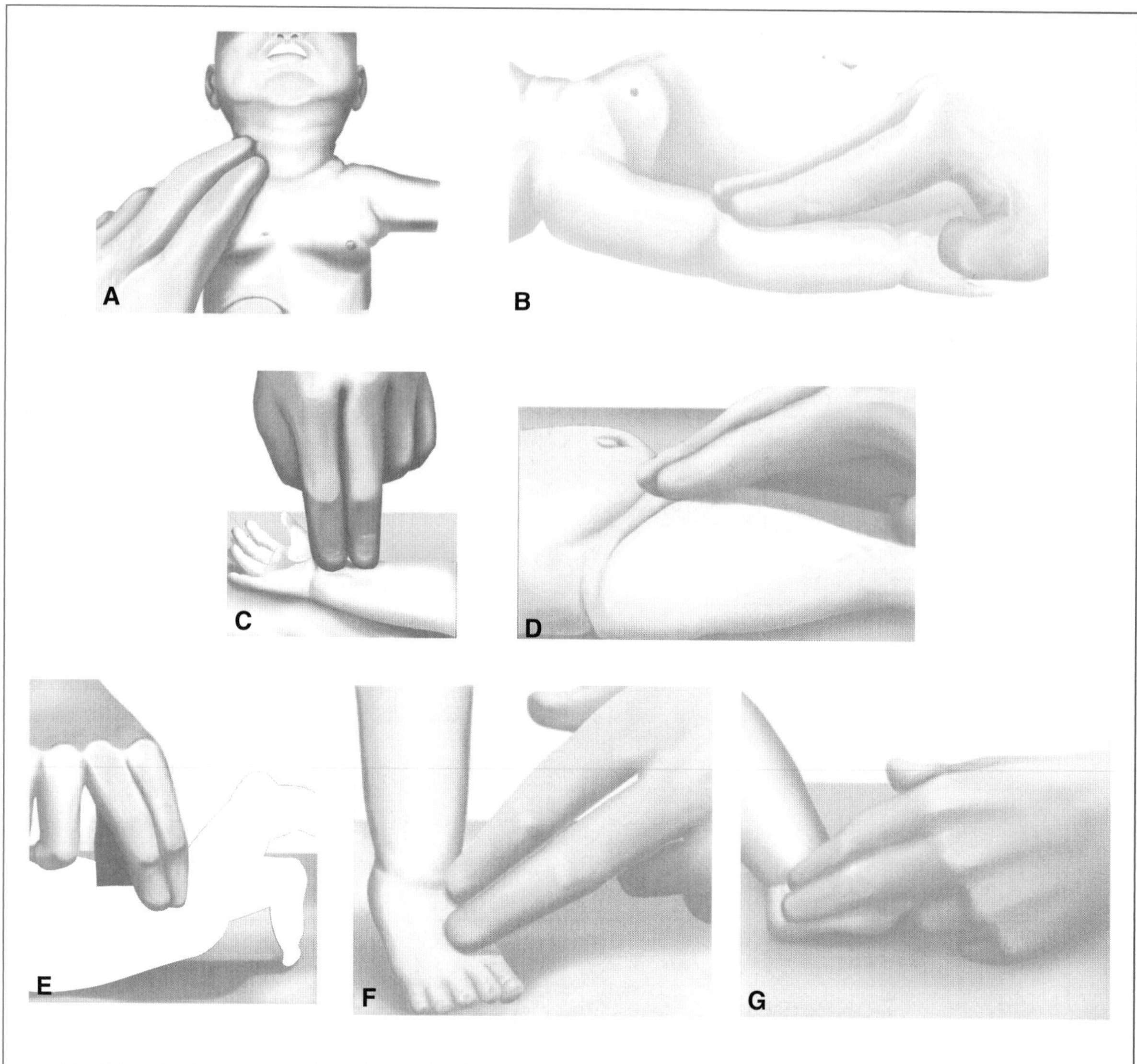

FIGURE 4.10 Palpation of arterial pulses: (A) carotid, (B) brachial, (C) radial, (D) femoral, (E) popliteal, (F) dorsalis pedis, and (G) posterior tibial.

The tongue should be smooth on all surfaces; the lingual frenulum may be short but not so short as to restrict tongue movement. Limitation of movement would be obvious on crying, when the tip of the tongue would form an inverted *V* (Fletcher, 1998).

■ **Thorax.** The chest is evaluated for size, symmetry, musculature, bony structure, number and location of nipples, and ease of respiration. It should be symmetric in shape and movements. Because the anteroposterior diameter is approximately equal to the transverse diameter, the chest appears round. The chest circumference of a term infant should be about 2 cm smaller than the head circumference (Askin, 2009). At all GAs, the chest measurement normally is smaller than the OFC (Fletcher, 1998).

Occasional mild subcostal retractions may be seen in healthy newborns because of decreased compliance of the ribs. A paradoxical breathing pattern is typical of newborns, especially during sleep. On inspiration the chest wall is drawn in and the abdomen protrudes; the reverse occurs on expiration (Fletcher, 1998).

The amount of breast tissue depends on the GA and birth weight, whereas areolar development reflects only GA. Two nipples should be present in equal alignment. The internipple distance varies by GA and chest circumference, but the ratio of internipple distance to chest circumference should be less than 0.28 (Fletcher, 1998). Widely spaced nipples are associated with a variety of congenital syndromes.

Newborn breast tissue may hypertrophy as a result of the influence of maternal hormones. A milky substance (witches' milk) may appear toward the end of the first week of life, and this discharge may persist for a few weeks to several months (Askin, 2009; Fletcher, 1998).

■ **Abdomen.** The abdomen is inspected for contour and size, symmetry, character of skin, and umbilical cord location and anatomy. Palpation yields information about muscle mass and tone of the abdominal wall, location and size of viscera, tenderness, and masses (Fletcher, 1998). Bowel sounds are detected on auscultation; they are relatively quiet in newborns until feedings are established. Compared with term babies, preterm neonates have less active bowel sounds. Evaluating changes in bowel sounds from the infant's baseline is more clinically useful than an isolated assessment (Fletcher, 1998).

The normal abdomen in an infant is round and soft and protrudes slightly. The umbilical cord should be bluish white, shiny, and moist and should have two arteries and one vein. To facilitate palpation, the knees and legs should be flexed toward the hips, which allow the abdominal muscles to relax. The edge of the liver can be palpated 1 to 2 cm below the right costal margin at the midclavicular line; this edge should be smooth, firm, and well defined (Goodwin, 2009). The tip of the spleen can be felt below the left costal margin in newborn infants. The size of the spleen depends on variables such as circulating blood volume, day of life, method of delivery, and type of therapy, which must be considered when interpreting the significance of mild enlargement (Fletcher, 1998).

The kidneys are located in the flanks. The lower pole of both kidneys should be palpable because of the reduced tone of neonatal abdominal muscles (Vogt & Dell, 2011). The kidneys should be smooth and firm to the touch. Enlarged kidneys are somewhat easy to detect, but normal-size neonatal kidneys may be somewhat more difficult to find. The presence of renal tissue is confirmed when voiding has occurred (Cavaliere, 2009).

■ **Anogenital Area.** The anogenital area should be examined with the infant supine. GA affects the appearance of the external genitalia. Maturational changes are described in Figure 4.6 and Table 4.7. The genitalia should be readily identifiable as male or female.

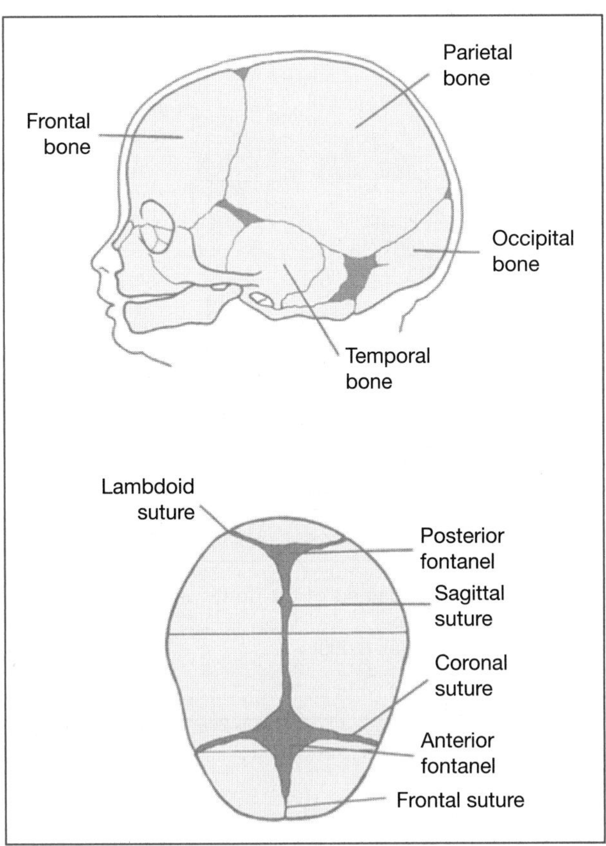

FIGURE 4.11 Major bones of the head in the newborn with sutures and fontanelles.
Modified from Fletcher (1998).

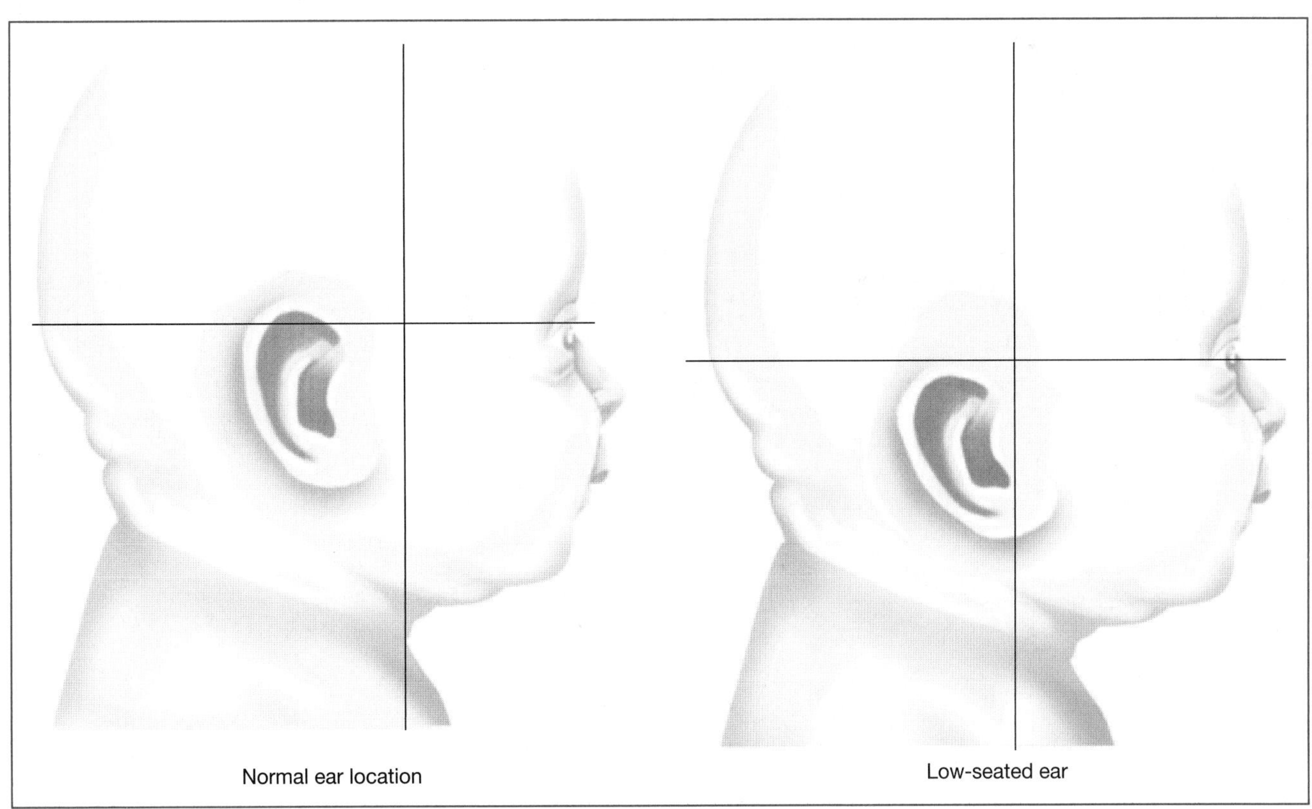

FIGURE 4.12 Ear position.

- *Males*: The normal length of the penis at term is 3.5 cm (plus or minus 0.7 cm) (Fletcher, 1998). Gentle traction is applied on the foreskin to visualize the urethral meatus; the opening should be at the central tip of the glans. Physiologic phimosis, a nonretractable foreskin, normally is seen in newborns. The opening in the prepuce should be large enough to allow urination. The urine stream should be forceful and straight. The inguinal area and scrotum should be palpated for masses, swelling, and the presence of testes. The testes should be firm, smooth, and comparatively equal in size. Testicular descent begins at approximately 27 weeks gestation. At term both testes should be in the scrotum, which should be fully rugated. The scrotum should be more deeply pigmented than the surrounding skin (Cavaliere, 2009).
- *Females*: The labial, inguinal, and suprapubic areas are inspected and palpated to detect masses, swelling, or bulges. The clitoris should be located superior to the vaginal opening. Hymenal tags and mucous/bloody vaginal discharges are benign, transient findings.

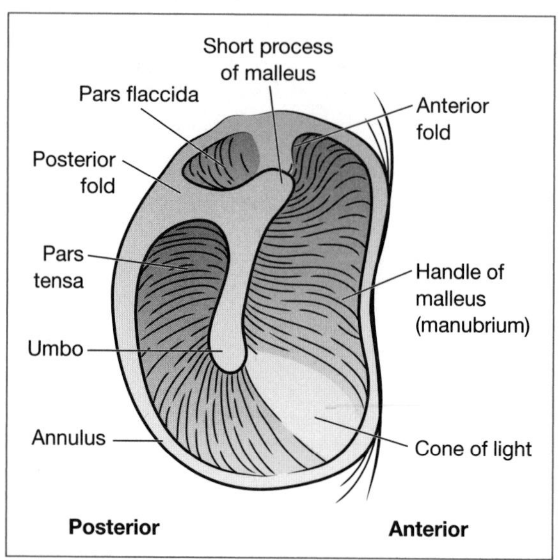

FIGURE 4.13 Normal landmarks of the right tympanic membrane as seen through an otoscope.
Modified from Lewis et al. (2000).

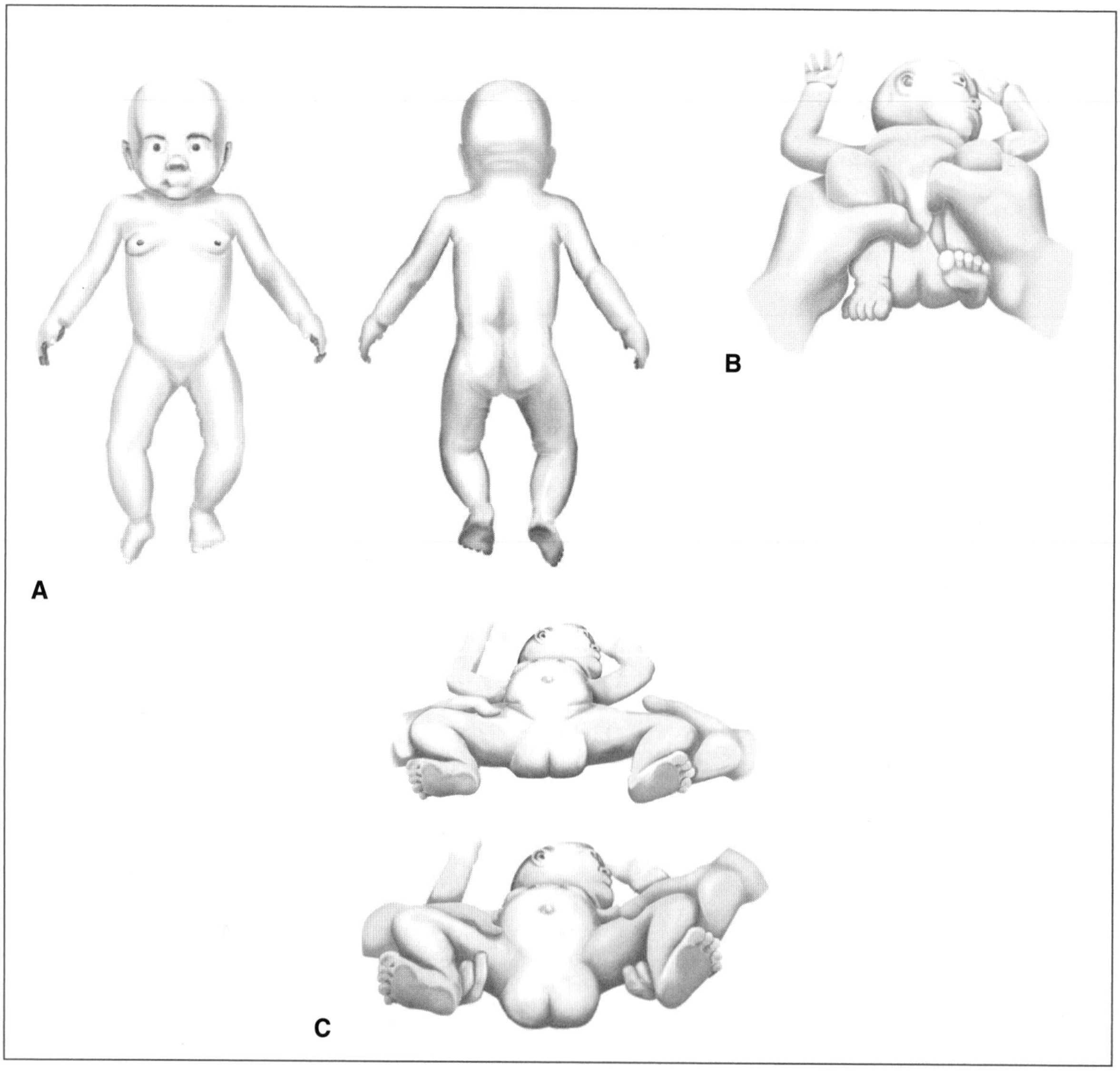

FIGURE 4.14 Signs of congenital dislocation of hip: (A) asymmetry of gluteal and thigh folds, (B) Barlow maneuver, and (C) Ortolani maneuver.
Redrawn from Wong (2003).

Edema of the genitalia is common in both sexes in breech deliveries. It may also be due to the effects of transplacentally acquired maternal hormones. The perineum should be smooth and should have no dimpling, fistulae, or discharges (Cavaliere, 2009; Gardner & Hernandez, 2011).

The anus is evaluated for patency and tone. Patency can be documented by gentle insertion of a soft rubber catheter. The passage of meconium does not confirm a patent anus, because meconium may be passed through a fistulous tract (Fletcher, 1998). Gentle stroking of the anal area should produce constriction of the sphincter, known as the anal wink (Sansoucie & Cavaliere, 2007).

■ **Back.** The infant should be placed in the prone position while the back is examined for curvature, patency, and presence of structural abnormalities. Vertebrae are palpated for enlargement and pain. Symmetry should be seen on both sides of the back and between the two scapulae. The spine should be straight and flexible and should have no visible defects, such as pits, hair tufts, or dimples (Sansoucie & Cavaliere, 2007).

■ **Extremities and Hips.** The extremities are observed for symmetry, degree of flexion, and presence of defects and fractures. Full range of motion should be present, and the extremities should move symmetrically. Although symmetry of gluteal skin folds suggests normal hips, the Ortolani and Barlow maneuvers should be performed to confirm the stability of the hips (Figure 4.14). The Ortolani maneuver reduces a dislocated femoral head into the acetabulum, and the Barlow maneuver reflects the ability of the femoral head to be dislocated (Fletcher, 1998; Tappero, 2009).

The limbs should be equal in length, and they should be in proportion to the body; they also should be straight and should have no edema or crepitus. Palpation or movement of the limbs should not produce a painful response. The digits should be equally spaced and have no webbing. The nails should extend to the end of the nail beds.

■ **Reflexes.** The most common neonatal reflexes are presented in Table 4.11.

Variations and Abnormal Findings on Physical Examination

Minor variations and abnormal findings of the physical examination are presented in Table 4.12.

TABLE 4.11

ASSESSMENT OF NEONATAL REFLEXES

Reflex	Technique	Response	Comments
Asymmetric tonic neck	With infant supine and in light sleep or quiet awake state, turn head to right until jaw is over shoulder; hold for 15 seconds, then release.	Occipital flexion and mental extension; right arm and leg are extended; left arm and leg are flexed. Premature neonates may lie at rest in this position for extended periods.	Reflex appears at 35 weeks gestation and disappears by 6–7 months of age.
Babinski	Using thumbnail, scratch sole of foot at lateral side from toes to heel.	Dorsal flexion of great toe with extension of other toes.	Care must be taken not to elicit plantar grasp by stimulating sole of foot. Reflex appears at 34–36 weeks gestation, is well established at 38 weeks, and disappears at 12 months of age.
Doll's eyes	Rotate head from side to side, observing eye movement.	As head is moved to right or left, eyes move in opposite direction.	Lack of eye movement with head rotation or movement of eyes in same direction as head may indicate brainstem or oculomotor nerve dysfunction. Reflex is well established and may even be exaggerated at 24–25 weeks gestation.
Galant (truncal incurvation)	Place infant prone, either lying on flat surface or in suspension; lightly stroke along either side of spinal column from shoulder to buttocks.	Normal response is strong incurvation of whole vertebral column toward stimulated side.	Reflex is first seen at 28 weeks gestation.
Glabellar	Hold head firmly and tap forehead just above nose.	Normal response is tighter closure of both eyes and wrinkling of brow.	Asymmetry, absent or exceptionally strong response (closure longer than 1 second), or generalized startle is abnormal.

(*continued*)

TABLE 4.11

ASSESSMENT OF NEONATAL REFLEXES (CONTINUED)

Reflex	Technique	Response	Comments
Moro	Hold infant suspended over mattress, supporting head with one hand and body with other hand; rapidly lower both hands 10–20 cm without flexing neck, but do not allow baby to drop back to mattress.	Symmetric abduction of arms and extension at elbows with hands open completely, followed by adduction of arms and flexion at elbows with curling of fingers; infant cries or grimaces at conclusion.	Response attenuates and ultimately disappears with repetition as habituation occurs. No response is seen at < 26 weeks gestation; extension only at 30 weeks; variable adduction at 34 weeks; complete response at 38 weeks. Reflex disappears at 6 months of age.
Palmar grasp	Stimulate palmar surface of hand with a finger.	Neonate grasps finger; grasp tightens with attempt to remove finger.	Reflex appears at 28 weeks gestation, is well established after 32 weeks, and disappears at 2 months of age.
Pupillary	Elicit in darkened environment by presenting bright, sharply focused light from periphery.	Pupils constrict equally.	Reflex is sluggish but present between 28 and 32 weeks gestation in healthy neonates; it is fully present after 34 weeks.
Rooting	Stroke cheek and corner of mouth.	Mouth opens and head turns toward stimulus.	Reflex appears at 28 weeks gestation, followed by long latency period beginning at 30 weeks; it is well established at 32–34 weeks and disappears by 3–4 months of age.
Stepping	Hold neonate upright and allow feet to touch flat surface.	Alternating stepping movements.	Reflex appears at 35–36 weeks gestation, is well established at 37 weeks, and disappears at 3–4 months of age.
Sucking	Touch or stroke lips.	Mouth opens, and neonate begins to suck.	Reflex appears at 28 weeks gestation, is well established by 32–34 weeks, and disappears at 12 months of age.

Data from Heaberlin (2009).

TABLE 4.12

ABNORMALITIES AND VARIATIONS FOUND ON PHYSICAL EXAMINATION OF NEWBORNS AND INFANTS

Finding	Definition/Description	Comments
Skin		
Color	Acrocyanosis (blue discoloration of the hands, feet, and perioral area), commonly seen in the first 6–24 hours of life.	Occurs when blood flow to an area is sluggish and all available oxygen has been extracted (Fletcher, 1998); exacerbated by cooling and diminished by warming; normal variation but abnormal if persists beyond the first 24 hours of life.
	Cutis marmorata (mottling of the skin in response to cold or other stressful stimuli); caused by dilation of capillaries, usually greatest on the extremities but may be seen on the trunk.	May be suggestive of other conditions (e.g., cardiovascular hypertension, hypothyroidism) if mottling is extensive, shows no improvement with warming, or persists beyond first few months (Fletcher, 1998).
	Cyanosis (blue discoloration of the skin, tongue, and mucous membranes).	Caused by excess of desaturated hemoglobin in the blood (cardiopulmonary disease) or a structural defect in the hemoglobin molecule (methemoglobin); always an abnormal finding.
	Jaundice (yellow coloring of the skin, mucous membranes, and sclerae).	Caused by deposition of bilirubin; may be physiologic.
	Pallor (absence of color or paleness of the skin).	Caused by a decrease in cardiac output, subcutaneous edema, anemia, or asphyxia (Lissauer, 2011).
	Plethora (ruddy skin coloration in the newborn).	Caused by high circulating red blood cell volume (abnormal finding).

(*continued*)

TABLE 4.12

ABNORMALITIES AND VARIATIONS FOUND ON PHYSICAL EXAMINATION OF NEWBORNS AND INFANTS (CONTINUED)

Finding	Definition/Description	Comments
Lesions	Café au lait spots (light tan or brown macules with well-defined borders, representing areas of increased epidermal melanosis); except for deeper pigmentation, appearance is not different from that of surrounding skin.	More common in normal infants of color. Six or more macules, regardless of spots' size or infant's race, may be pathologically significant, especially if located in the axilla.
	Cutis aplasia (localized or widespread foci of absence of some or all layers of skin); defect may be covered by a thin, translucent membrane or scar tissue, or area may be raw and ulcerated.	Occurs predominantly on the scalp and less frequently on the limbs and trunk.
	Ecchymosis (nonblanching purple or blue-black macule larger than 2 mm in diameter); represents extravasation of blood into subcutaneous tissue.	Results from trauma to underlying blood vessels or fragility of the vessel walls.
	Erythema toxicum (white or yellow papules on red macular base), commonly found on face, trunk, or proximal extremities but not on hands or feet.	Common, benign finding; vesicles are rare, sterile, and composed primarily of eosinophils. When vesicles are pronounced or coalescent, they may mimic postural infectious rash (Furdon & Clark, 2005).
	Harlequin fetus (most severe form of congenital ichthyosis; skin is completely covered with thick, horny scales resembling armor that are divided by deep red fissures).	Most such infants die of dehydration, infection, or respiratory insufficiency within a few hours or days.
	Harlequin sign (vascular phenomenon represented by distinct midline demarcation in side-lying infants; dependent half is deep red, upper half is pale).	Benign finding that lasts a few seconds to 30 minutes, occasionally reverses when position is changed. The physiologic basis is unidentified; without pathologic significance. Occurs most frequently in LBW neonates (Hoath & Narendran, 2011).
	Strawberry hemangioma (red, raised, circumscribed, soft, compressible, lobulated tumor; may occur anywhere on the body).	Benign tumor of the vascular endothelium that has a proliferative and an involutional phase; most involute spontaneously. Treatment is unnecessary unless vital functions are affected.
	Cavernous hemangioma (similar to strawberry hemangioma; involves dermis and subcutaneous tissue and is soft and compressible on palpation; overlying skin is bluish-red in color).	Cavernous lesions may cause thrombocytopenia (Kasabach-Merritt syndrome) or hypertrophy of bone and soft structures of extremities (Klippel-Trenaunay-Weber syndrome) (Hoath & Narendran, 2011; Witt, 2009).
	Mongolian spot (blue-black macule, lacking a sharp border, most frequently seen on sacrum, buttocks, flanks, or shoulders).	Benign lesion, common in dark-skinned neonates, resulting from delayed disappearance of dermal melanocytes; lesion gradually disappears during the first years of life (Witt, 2009).
	Milia (1 mm, pearly white or yellow papules without erythema; in the mouth these are called Epstein's pearls).	Epidermal inclusion cysts caused by blockage of sebaceous glands; a benign finding that resolves during the first weeks of life.
	Miliaria crystallina (1–2 mm, thin-walled vesicles with nonerythematous and nonpigmented base).	Lesions caused by blockage of sweat glands. They are exacerbated by a warm, humid environment and most frequently develop in intertriginous areas and over the face and scalp. They resolve when the environmental factors are eliminated.
	Miliaria rubra (small, erythematous, grouped papules [prickly heat]).	
	Miliaria pustulosis (nonerythematous pustules).	
	Neonatal pustular melanosis (small, superficial vesiculopustules with little or no surrounding erythema; crusted or scaly collarettes appear after vesicles rupture; lesions eventually resolve into hyperpigmented areas).	Transient and benign; frequently confused with infectious lesions. Smears of pustular material reveal predominantly neutrophils and no bacteria.

(continued)

TABLE 4.12

ABNORMALITIES AND VARIATIONS FOUND ON PHYSICAL EXAMINATION OF NEWBORNS AND INFANTS (CONTINUED)

Finding	Definition/Description	Comments
	Salmon patch (nevus; dull, pink-red, irregularly shaped macules that blanch on pressure; commonly found on nape of neck (stork bite), glabella, forehead, eyelids, and upper lip).	Benign finding; lesions are composed of distended, dilated capillaries, and most lesions (except those on the neck) disappear by 1 year of age.
	Port wine stain (nevus, macular lesion; present at birth but may be pale and hard to discern; initially pink in color with sharply delineated borders; progresses to dark red/purple; some develop small, angiomatous nodules).	Developmental vascular malformation that occurs mostly on the face; does not increase in size but grows with the infant; may occur alone or with structural anomalies (e.g., Sturge–Weber syndrome) (Hoath & Narendral, 2011; Witt, 2009).
	Petechiae (tiny red or purple, nonblanching macules that range from pinpoint to pin head size).	Caused by minute hemorrhages in the dermal or submucosal layers; may be benign and self-limiting or pathognomonic of serious underlying conditions. They are benign when found on presenting part and when localized areas appear at the same time; progressive, widespread areas require evaluation (Fletcher, 1998).
Redundant skin	More skin than is necessary or normally present in a particular area.	Seen in the neck after resolution of cystic hygroma or in the abdomen in a neonate with prune belly syndrome.
Sclerema neonatorum	Diffuse, stone-hard, nonpitting cutaneous induration; overlying skin appears pale and waxy; face has a mask-like appearance; joints are stiff.	Occurs in debilitated neonates; diffuse systemic process with grave prognosis (Hoath & Narendran, 2011).
Subcutaneous fat necrosis	Firm, nonpitting, poorly circumscribed, reddish violet lesions appearing in the first weeks of life on the face, arms, trunk, thighs, and buttocks. Affected areas may be slightly elevated above adjacent skin (Mangurten & Puppala, 2011).	Most often seen in areas where a fat pad is present. May occur secondary to cold or trauma and sometimes accompanied by hypercalcemia (Hoath & Narendran, 2011).
Head and Neck		
Acrocephaly	Congenital malformation of the skull caused by premature closure of the coronal and sagittal sutures; accelerated upward growth of the head gives it a long, narrow appearance with a conic shape at the top (also called oxycephaly).	May be associated with premature closure of sutures; found with certain syndromes (e.g., Crouzon's, Apert's) (Cohen, 2011).
Anencephaly	Failed closure of the anterior neural tube without skull formation; the brain is severely malformed, lacking definable structure, although a rudimentary brainstem usually is present.	Most affected neonates (75%) are stillborn; without intervention; the remainder die in the neonatal period (Gressens & Huppi, 2011).
Brachycephaly	Congenital malformation of the skull caused by premature closure of the coronal suture; excessive lateral growth of the head gives it a short, broad appearance.	Condition found with certain syndromes (e.g., trisomy 21, Apert's) (Cohen, 2011).
Bruit	Abnormal murmur-like sound heard on auscultation of an organ or gland that is caused by dilated, tortuous, or constricted vessels. The specific character of the bruit, its location, its association with other clinical findings, and the time of occurrence in a cycle of other sounds is of diagnostic importance.	Bruits heard over the fontanelle or lateral skull associated with signs of congestive heart failure may denote intracranial arteriovenous malformation (Heaberlin, 2009; Johnson, 2009).
Caput succedaneum	Vaguely demarcated pitting edema of the scalp that may extend across suture lines and can shift in response to gravity.	Benign finding that appears at birth (from pressure of the maternal cervix on the fetal skull) and resolves in a few days (Mangurten & Puppala, 2011).

(*continued*)

TABLE 4.12

ABNORMALITIES AND VARIATIONS FOUND ON PHYSICAL EXAMINATION OF NEWBORNS AND INFANTS (CONTINUED)

Finding	Definition/Description	Comments
Cephalohematoma	Extradural fluid collection caused by bleeding between the skull and periosteum; generally occurs over one or both parietal bones and does not cross the suture lines; has distinct margins and may be fluctuant or tense.	1. May form during labor and enlarges for the first 12–24 hours; most resolve spontaneously over several weeks to months (Johnson, 2009; Johnson & Cochran 2012). 2. Linear skull fracture is found in 5% of unilateral and 18% of bilateral lesions (Abdulhayoglu, 2012; Madan, Hamrick, & Ferriero, 2005). 3. May result in hyperbilirubinemia (Mangurten & Puppala, 2011).
Craniosynostosis	Premature closure of one or more cranial sutures, causing abnormal skull shape and possibly a palpable ridge along the suture line.	Head growth is restricted in the area perpendicular to the stenotic suture and is excessive in unrestricted areas. Most cases are isolated events, but the condition can occur in some syndromes (Cohen, 2011).
Craniotabes	Congenital thinness of bone at the top and back of the head. Bones may collapse with gentle pressure and recoil (ping-pong).	1. May be a normal variant if present to a mild degree near suture lines. May be caused by the pressure of the skull against the maternal pelvic brim; spontaneous resolution usually occurs in a few weeks (Fletcher, 1998). 2. May be associated with congenital syphilis and other congenital conditions (osteogenesis imperfecta); due to bone resorption or delay in ossification (Smith, 2012).
Dolichocephaly or scaphocephaly	Congenital malformation of the skull in which premature closure of the sagittal suture results in restricted lateral growth.	Long, narrow head (Cohen, 2011).
	Skull shape often seen in premature babies as a result of prolonged positioning with head turned to the side.	
Encephalocele	Protrusion of brain tissue through a congenital defect in the cranium; most often occurs in the occipital midline but may also be seen in the frontal, temporal, or parietal areas.	Other cranial defects, congenital anomalies (hydrocephalus, microcephaly, craniosynostosis), and autosomal recessive syndromes (Walker-Warburg) are frequently seen (Back, 2012; Gressens & Huppi, 2011).
Hair whorls	Two or more hair whorls, or abnormally placed whorls (other than parietal area).	May indicate brain anomaly; it has been postulated that the pattern of hair development correlates with underlying brain development (Furdon & Clark, 2003).
Macrocephaly	Excessive head size in relation to weight, length, and GA. OFC is over 90th percentile.	1. Familial; facial features usually are normal. 2. May reflect pathologic condition (e.g., hydrocephaly, hydrancephaly) or chromosomal or neuroendocrine disorder (Back, 2012).
Microcephaly	Abnormally small head size relative to weight, length, and GA. OFC is under 10th percentile.	Associated with either microcephaly (marked reduction in size of brain or cerebral hemispheres) or acquired brain atrophy (Back, 2012).
Molding	Process by which the head shape is altered as the fetus passes through the birth canal.	Benign finding; condition usually resolves during the first few postnatal days.
	The biparietal diameter becomes compressed, the head is elongated, and the skull bones may overlap at the suture lines.	
Neck masses	May be detected on palpation or inspection.	Most common neck mass; caused by development of sequestered lymph channels, which dilate into cysts (Lissauer, 2011; Johnson, 2009).

(continued)

TABLE 4.12

ABNORMALITIES AND VARIATIONS FOUND ON PHYSICAL EXAMINATION OF NEWBORNS AND INFANTS (CONTINUED)

Finding	Definition/Description	Comments
	Cystic hygroma (soft, fluctuant mass that is easily trans illuminated; usually laterally placed or over clavicles).	
	Goiter (anterior mass caused by hypothyroidism).	Rare in neonates (Johnson, 2009).
	Thyroglossal duct cyst/branchial cleft cyst; a mass may be found high in the neck.	Rare in neonates (Johnson, 2009).
Plagiocephaly	Asymmetry of the skull due to flattening of the occiput. Can be deformational (positional) or due to premature or irregular closure of the coronal or lambdoidal sutures.	1. Posterior plagiocephaly almost always due to mechanical forces (positional; "back to sleep"). 2. Anterior plagiocephaly most commonly due to premature fusion of the sutures (Cohen, 2011).
Subgaleal	Bleeding into the potential space between the epicranial aponeurosis and the periosteum of the skull; manifests as a firm to fluctuant scalp mass with poorly demarcated borders that may extend onto the face, forehead, or neck and may be accompanied by signs of hypovolemia.	May be a life-threatening condition; can be caused by hemorrhage coagulopathy, asphyxia, or vacuum extraction (Johnson & Cochran, 2012; Madan et al., 2005; Mangurten & Puppala, 2011).
Webbed neck	Redundant skin at posterolateral region of neck.	Found with Turner's, Noonan's, and Down syndromes (Bennet & Meier, 2009).
Face		
Asymmetry	Unequal appearance or movement of mouth and lips; unequal closure of eyes; uneven appearance of nasolabial folds.	Often caused by in utero positioning but may be due to facial nerve paresis; in mild cases may be evident only with crying (affected side fails to move or moves less when infant cries).
Ears		
Auricular appendage	Accessory tragi, most commonly in pretragal area; may occur within or behind the ear. These structures contain cartilage and are not truly skin tags.	Primarily of cosmetic significance unless accompanied by other diffuse malformations. Seen in certain congenital syndromes (e.g., Goldenhar's, Treacher Collins); hearing assessment is indicated when other anomalies are present (Parikh & Weisner, 2011; Spillman, 2002).
Auricular sinus	Narrow, fistulous tract most often located directly anterior to helix.	May be familial or may be associated with microtia, auricular appendage, facial cleft syndromes, and syndromic anomalies of the outer ear (Parikh & Weisner, 2011; Spillman, 2002).
Low-set ears	Superior attachment of pinna lies below imaginary line drawn between both inner canthi and extended posteriorly.	May be associated with chromosomal or renal anomalies (Spillman, 2002).
Microtia	Severely misshapen, dysplastic external ear.	Frequently associated with other malformations that result in conductive hearing loss (i.e., atresia of auditory meatus, abnormalities of middle ear) (Smith, 2012; Parikh & Wiesner, 2011).
Eyes		
Blepharophimosis	Narrow palpebral fissures in the horizontal measurement; also known as short palpebral fissures.	Usually caused by lateral displacement of the inner canthi; seen in certain dysmorphic or chromosomal syndromes (Fletcher, 1998; Kaufman et al., 2011).
Brushfield spots	Pinpoint white or light yellow spots on the iris.	Seen in 75% of neonates with Down syndrome but may also be a normal variant; not always visible at birth (Johnson, 2009).
Coloboma	Cleft-shaped defect in ocular tissue (eyelid, iris, ciliary body, retina, or optic nerve).	Result of incomplete embryologic closure of ocular structures; may be an isolated finding or part of a malformation syndrome (CHARGE, trisomies 13, 18, 22) (Madan & Good, 2005).

(*continued*)

TABLE 4.12

ABNORMALITIES AND VARIATIONS FOUND ON PHYSICAL EXAMINATION OF NEWBORNS AND INFANTS (CONTINUED)

Finding	Definition/Description	Comments
Ectropion	Eversion of the margin of the eyelid, which leaves the conjunctiva exposed.	Seen in facial nerve paralysis, in certain syndromes, and in harlequin fetus and collodion baby (Fletcher, 1998; Kaufman et al., 2011).
Entropion	Inversion of the eyelid; eyelashes may be in contact with the cornea and conjunctiva.	Congenital condition that usually resolves spontaneously without damage (Fletcher, 1998; Kaufman et al., 2011).
Epicanthal folds	Vertical fold of skin at the inner canthus on either side of the nose.	A feature of normal fetal development and may be present in normal infants. Characteristic of trisomy 21 but may occur in malformation syndromes, especially those with a flat nasal bridge; may also be a physical manifestation of in utero compression (Potter facies) (Parikh & Wiesner, 2011).
Exophthalmos	Abnormal displacement of the eye characterized by protrusion of the eyeball.	May be caused by increased volume of the orbit (tumor), swelling secondary to edema or hemorrhage, endocrine disorder (e.g., Graves' disease, hyperthyroidism); known as proptosis when accompanied by shallow orbits (Crouzon's disease) (Fletcher, 1998; Kaufman et al., 2011).
Hypertelorism	Increased distance between the orbits, observed clinically as a large interpupillary distance (see Telecanthus) (Parikh & Wiesner, 2011).	Frequently seen in craniofacial syndromes (Kaufman et al., 2011).
Hypotelorism	Decreased distance between the orbits, observed clinically as smaller than normal interpupillary distance (Parikh & Wiesner, 2011).	Frequently seen in trisomies 13 and 21 and in other syndromes (Kaufman et al., 2011).
Leukocoria	White pupil, denoting an abnormality of the lens, vitreous, or fundus; an indication for further evaluation (Kaufman et al., 2011).	May be seen on direct visualization, or as absence of a red reflex (Fletcher, 1998); most commonly seen in cataracts; also found in retinoblastoma, retinal detachment, and vitreous hemorrhage.
Microphthalmia	Small eye; diameter measures less than 2/3 of the normal 16 mm at birth (Kaufman et al., 2011).	Can be hereditary or caused by chromosomal anomalies and environmental influences during development. Associated with multisystem conditions or syndromes (e.g., CHARGE, trisomy 13, fetal rubella effects).
Nystagmus	Involuntary, rhythmic movements of the eye; may be horizontal, vertical, rotary, or mixed. Optokinetic nystagmus reflexive response to a moving target.	Occasional, intermittent nystagmus in an otherwise healthy newborn may be normal in the neonatal period; however, it must be evaluated if frequent or persistent (or both). Pathologic forms may be due to ocular, neurologic, or vestibular defects (Kaufman et al., 2011).
Ptosis (blepharoptosis)	Abnormal drooping of one or both upper eyelids; lid does not rise to normal level.	Caused by congenital or acquired weakness in the levator muscle or paralysis of the third cranial nerve; may be difficult to detect in neonates unless unilateral with asymmetry between the eyelids (Kaufman et al., 2011).
Strabismus	Misalignment of the visual axes: Esotropia—crossed eyes Exotropia—wall eye.	Refer for ophthalmologic evaluation if present by third month of age. Results from inheritance, paralysis of the lateral rectus muscle, or refractive errors; may be due to diseases that reduce visual acuity in one eye. Rare in neonates; usually does not appear until 1–2 years of age (Kaufman et al., 2011).

(*continued*)

TABLE 4.12

ABNORMALITIES AND VARIATIONS FOUND ON PHYSICAL EXAMINATION OF NEWBORNS AND INFANTS (CONTINUED)

Finding	Definition/Description	Comments
Subconjunctival hemorrhage	Bright red area on sclerae.	Caused by rupture of a capillary in the mucous membrane that lines the conjunctiva; commonly seen after vaginal delivery, does not reflect ocular trauma unless massive and associated with other findings; usually resolves in 7–10 days (Mangurten & Puppala, 2011).
Synophrys	Meeting of the eyebrows in the midline.	Seen in multisystem conditions or syndromes (e.g., Cornelia de Lange's, congenital hypertrichosis) (Kaufman et al., 2011).
Telecanthus	Lateral displacement of the inner canthi; eyes appear too widely set because of a disproportionate increase between the inner canthi; interorbital distance is appropriate (Parikh & Wiesner, 2011).	Evident in fetal alcohol syndrome and other syndromes; not synonymous with hypertelorism, although its presence can lead to a false impression of hypertelorism (Kaufman et al., 2011).
Nose		
Choanal atresia	Obstruction of posterior nasal passages.	Patency is assessed in the quiet state. If condition is bilateral, neonate is cyanotic at rest and pink when crying; if unilateral, baby is unable to breathe if mouth is held closed and unaffected naris is occluded with examiner's finger. Atresia/stenosis may be confirmed by passing a catheter.
Nasal deformation	May result from pressure in utero.	Benign condition that resolves in a few days.
	May be due to dislocation of the septal cartilage.	Attempts to restore normal anatomy are unsuccessful; nares remain asymmetric when tip of nose is compressed (Johnson, 2009; Mangurten & Puppala, 2011).
Mouth		
Cleft lip/palate	Failure of midline fusion during first trimester.	May occur alone or with other malformations.
Epstein's pearls	Small, white, pearl-like inclusion cysts that appear on the palate and gums.	Benign finding that disappears spontaneously by a few weeks of age (Johnson, 2009).
Micrognathia	Underdevelopment of the jaw, especially the mandible.	Dysmorphic feature seen in certain malformation syndromes (e.g., Pierre Robin sequence) (Bennett & Meier, 2009; Johnson, 2009).
Thorax/Chest		
Auscultation	Adventitious breath sounds	(Askin, 2009)
	Crackles	Discrete, noncontinuous bubbling sounds during inspiration; classified as fine, medium, or coarse. Previously called rales.
	Rhonchi	Continuous, nonmusical, low-pitched sounds occurring on inspiration and expiration; caused by secretions or aspirated matter in large airways.
	Stridor	Rough, harsh sounds caused by narrowing of upper airways; present during both phases of respiratory cycle but worse during inspiration; common with laryngomalacia, subglottic stenosis, and vascular ring.
	Wheezes	Musical, high-pitched sound generated by air passing at high velocity through a narrowed airway; heard most often on expiration but can be noted during both phases of respiratory cycle if airway diameter is restricted and fixed.
	Grunting	Sound produced by forceful expiration against a closed glottis; compensatory mechanism to prevent or reverse alveolar collapse.

(continued)

TABLE 4.12

ABNORMALITIES AND VARIATIONS FOUND ON PHYSICAL EXAMINATION OF NEWBORNS AND INFANTS (CONTINUED)

Finding	Definition/Description	Comments
	Murmur	Grades I through VI assigned depending on intensity and presence of thrill.
Asymmetry	May be unequal in shape or excursion.	1. Asymmetric shape caused by positioning in utero or presence of air trapping or space-occupying lesions. 2. Unequal excursion caused by diaphragmatic hernia, phrenic nerve damage, or air leakage or trapping (Askin, 2009).
Barrel chest	Increased anteroposterior diameter of the chest.	Result of air trapping in the pleural space (pneumothorax) or distal airways (aspiration or pneumonia), space-occupying lesions, or over distention from mechanical ventilation (Fletcher, 1998).
Heave	Diffuse, gradually rising impulse seen in the anterior chest overlying the ventricular area.	Usually indicates volume overload.
Pectus carinatum	Deformation of chest wall caused by protuberant sternum; also called pigeon chest.	May be associated with Marfan, Noonan's, and other syndromes (Askin, 2009).
Pectus excavatum	Deformation of chest wall caused by depressed sternum; also called funnel chest.	May be associated with Marfan, Noonan's, and other syndromes (Askin, 2009); may develop after birth in neonates with laryngomalacia.
Retractions	Drawing in of the soft tissues of the chest between and around the firmer tissue of the cartilaginous and bony ribs; seen in intercostal, subcostal, substernal, and suprasternal areas.	Mild subcostal retractions may be seen in healthy newborns; intercostal, substernal, and suprasternal retractions reflect increased work of breathing and suggest respiratory distress.
Supernumerary nipples (polythelia)	Extra nipples; may appear as slightly pigmented linear dimples or may be more defined, with palpable breast nodules.	Normal variant; nipples appear along the mammary line. Prospective studies have refuted the association with renal anomalies; no indication for further evaluation based solely on the presence of supernumerary nipples.
Abdomen		
Abdominal wall defects	Exstrophy of the bladder (protrusion and eversion of the bladder through an embryologic defect, resulting in absence of muscle and connective tissue on the anterior abdominal wall).	Often associated with other defects of the genitourinary (GU) and musculoskeletal systems and the gastrointestinal (GI) tract (Cavaliere, 2009; Zderic, 2005).
	Gastroschisis (protrusion of viscera through an abdominal wall defect arising outside the umbilical ring; the cord therefore is not inserted on the defect, and the herniated organs are not covered by peritoneum).	Defect usually is to the right of the umbilicus (Barksdale, Chwals, Magnuson, & Parry, 2011; Goodwin, 2009).
	Omphalocele (herniation of viscera through an abdominal wall defect within the umbilical ring; defect usually is covered by a translucent, avascular sac at the base of the umbilicus).	Umbilical cord always inserts into the sac; occasionally the sac may rupture. Defect usually is larger than 4 cm and may be associated with other congenital defects and chromosomal anomalies (Barksdale et al., 2011; Goodwin, 2009).
	Umbilical hernia (failure of the umbilical ring to contract, allowing protrusion of bowel or omentum through the abdominal wall).	Characterized by a fascial defect smaller than 4 cm and intact umbilical skin (Barksdale et al., 2011; Fletcher, 1998).
Bruit	See section under Head and Neck	Persistence after a position change may indicate abnormalities of the umbilical vein or hepatic vascular system, hepatic hemangioma, or renal artery stenosis (Goodwin, 2009).
Diastasis rectus	Midline bulge from xiphoid to umbilicus, seen when abdominal muscles are flexed.	Caused by separation of the two rectus muscles along the median line of the abdominal wall; a common benign finding in newborns that has no clinical significance; resolves without intervention (Goodwin, 2009).

(continued)

TABLE 4.12

ABNORMALITIES AND VARIATIONS FOUND ON PHYSICAL EXAMINATION OF NEWBORNS AND INFANTS (CONTINUED)

Finding	Definition/Description	Comments
Distention	Increase in abdominal girth caused by an increase in the volume of intraperitoneal, thoracic, or pelvic contents.	May be pathologic or benign. Pathologic causes include GI obstruction, ascites, abdominal mass, organomegaly, and depression of the diaphragm (tension pneumothorax). Benign causes include postprandial state, crying, swallowing of air with feedings, air leakage with mechanical ventilation, and administration of continuous positive airway pressure (CPAP).
Patent urachus	Postnatal persistence of communication between the urinary bladder and the umbilicus; may result in passage of urine from the umbilicus, which otherwise appears normal. Other signs are a large, edematous cord that fails to separate after the normal interval and retraction of the umbilical cord during urination.	Lower urinary tract obstruction should be considered (Cavaliere, 2009; Donlon & Furdon, 2002).
Prune belly syndrome	Congenital deficiency of abdominal musculature, characterized by a large, flaccid, wrinkled abdomen, cryptorchidism, and GU malformations.	Almost always seen in males (Vogt & Dell, 2011).
Scaphoid abdomen	Abdomen with a sunken anterior wall.	May be present with a diaphragmatic hernia or malnutrition.
Single umbilical artery		Seen in fewer than 1% of neonates; approximately 40% of affected newborns have other major congenital malformations. When condition occurs without other abnormalities, it usually is a benign finding (Lissauer, 2011).
Genitalia/Perineum		
Ambiguous	Presence of a phallic structure not discretely male or female, abnormally placed urethral meatus, and inability to palpate one or both gonads in a male.	May be associated with serious endocrine disorders; rapid evaluation and diagnosis are critical (Cavaliere, 2009; Schulman, Palmert, & Wherrett, 2011).
Anal atresia	Absence of an external anal opening; imperforate anus.	May be evident by inspection; infant may fail to pass meconium. However, meconium may be passed through a rectovaginal or rectovestibular fistula in a female or a rectoperineal or rectourethral fistula in a male (Goodwin, 2009).
Chordee	Ventral or dorsal curvature of the penis; most evident on erection.	May occur alone but often accompanies hypospadias (Cavaliere, 2009).
Clitoromegaly	The appearance of an enlarged clitoris, with no regard to cause (Schulman et al., 2011); it may be swollen, enlarged, widened, or merely prominent, as in premature females.	May be a normal finding in a premature female or may represent masculinization from exposure to excess androgens during fetal life (Schulman et al., 2011).
Cryptorchidism	Testis or testes in extrascrotal location (undescended testis or testes); characterized by empty, hypoplastic scrotal sac.	In most cases descent occurs spontaneously by 6–9 months of age; descent after 9 months is rare. Bilateral cryptorchidism occurs in up to 30% of patients; consider disorder of sexual differentiation until proven otherwise (Zderic, 2005).
Epispadias	Abnormal location of urethral meatus on the dorsal surface of the penis; abnormal urine stream may be seen.	Varies in severity from mild (glanular) to complete version seen in exstrophy of the bladder; all forms are associated with dorsal chordee; may require evaluation by a urologist before circumcision (Vogt & Dell, 2011; Zaontz & Packer, 1997).
Hydrocele	Nontender scrotal swelling caused by fluid collection; arises from passage of peritoneal fluid through patent processus vaginalis.	May be seen with inguinal hernia but can be distinguished from hernia because hydrocele appears translucent on transillumination; entire circumference of testis may be palpated; and it cannot be reduced (Cavaliere, 2009).
Hydrocolpos/ hydrometrocolpos	Manifests as suprapubic mass or protruding perineal mass as a result of accumulation of secretions in vagina or vagina and uterus.	Caused by excessive intrauterine stimulation by maternal estrogens, with obstruction of the genital tract by an intact hymen, hymenal bands, vaginal membrane, or vaginal atresia (Cavaliere, 2009; Fletcher, 1998).

(continued)

TABLE 4.12

ABNORMALITIES AND VARIATIONS FOUND ON PHYSICAL EXAMINATION OF NEWBORNS AND INFANTS (CONTINUED)

Finding	Definition/Description	Comments
Hypospadias	Abnormal location of urethral meatus on the ventral surface of the penis; caused by incomplete development of the anterior urethra; abnormal urine stream may be seen.	Urethral opening may be found on the glans, scrotum, or perineum. Infants with penoscrotal or perineal type or with glanular form and other genital anomalies or dysmorphic features should be evaluated to rule out disorders of sexual differentiation (Schulman et al., 2011). Evaluation by a urologist may be required before circumcision.
Hymenal tag	Redundant tissue manifesting as an annular tag protruding from the vagina.	Benign finding; most disappear during the first year of life.
Inguinal hernia	Scrotal mass caused by the presence of loops of intestines in the scrotal sac; arises from persistence of processus vaginalis, often associated with hydrocele.	On examination, the entire circumference of the testis is not palpable, and the scrotum cannot be transilluminated. Unless incarcerated, hernias are reducible (Benjamin, 2002; Cavaliere, 2009).
Micropenis/ microphallus	Abnormally short or thin penis.	Penis more than two standard deviations below the mean of length and width for age according to standard charts; frequently requires evaluation by an endocrinologist and a geneticist (Schulman et al., 2011).
Phimosis	Intractable foreskin.	Must be differentiated from physiologic phimosis, a nonretractable foreskin that is a normal finding in neonates (Cavaliere, 2009).
Priapism	Constantly erect penis.	Abnormal finding in neonate (Rozinski & Bloom, 1997).
Retractile testis	Normally descended testis that recedes into the inguinal canal because of activity of the cremaster muscle.	May not be seen in the newborn period because of lack of cremaster reflex in this age group; however, some newborns do demonstrate this response (Cavaliere, 2009; Cilento, Najjar, & Atala, 1994; Fletcher, 1998).
Testicular torsion	Twisting of the testis or testes on the spermatic cord; manifests as a swollen, red or bluish-red scrotum; may be painful, but this is not a universal symptom in the neonate.	Urgent evaluation and management are required, because the blood supply to the testis is compromised, which results in irreversible ischemic damage to the testis; condition may occur in utero (Zderic, 2005).
Musculoskeletal System		
Arachnodactyly	Unusually long, spiderlike digits.	Characteristic of, but not universally present in, Marfan syndrome and homocystinuria (Parikh & Wiesner, 2011).
Arthrogryposis	Persistent flexure or contracture of one or more joints.	May be associated with oligohydramnios or an underlying neuromuscular disorder (Parikh & Wiesner, 2011).
Brachydactyly	Shortening of one or more digits as a result of abnormal development of phalanges, metacarpals, or metatarsals.	Benign trait if an isolated finding; may be a component of skeletal dysplasias (achondroplasia) and syndromes (trisomy 21) (Parikh & Wiesner, 2011).
Calcaneus foot	Abduction of the forefoot with the heel in valgus position (turned outward).	Associated with external tibial torsion; often caused by in utero positioning (Furdon & Donlon, 2002).
Camptodactyly	Congenital flexion deformity of the finger; bent finger.	Usually involves the little finger; can be a minor variant, familial trait, or part of a syndrome (Parikh & Wiesner, 2011).
Clinodactyly	Lateral angulation deformity of a finger with either radial or ulnar deviation.	Usually involves the little finger; may be a benign finding if occurring alone but can be associated with congenital syndromes (Parikh & Wiesner, 2011).
Crepitus	Crackling sensation produced by the presence of air in tissues (subcutaneous emphysema) or the movement of bone fragments (clavicular fracture).	
Genu recurvatum	Abnormal hyperextensibility of the knee allowing the knee to bend backward.	May be due to trauma, prolonged intrauterine pressure, or general joint laxity. May be a feature of other disorders (Ehlers-Danlos, Marfan syndromes) (Smith, 2012).

(*continued*)

TABLE 4.12

ABNORMALITIES AND VARIATIONS FOUND ON PHYSICAL EXAMINATION OF NEWBORNS AND INFANTS (CONTINUED)

Finding	Definition/Description	Comments
Kyphosis	Round shoulder deformity; forward bending of the spine. Caused by congenital failure of formation of all or part of the vertebral body, with preservation of the posterior elements and failure of the anterior segmentation of the spine.	Severe deformities may be apparent at birth; less severe abnormalities may not appear until several years later; a progressive deformity can result in paraplegia (Parikh & Wiesner, 2011).
Lordosis	Exaggeration of the normal curvature in the cervical and lumbar spine.	Caused by a bony abnormality of the spine (Bennett & Meier, 2009).
Lymphedema	Puffiness of the dorsum of the hands or feet.	Characteristic of Noonan's or Turner's syndrome (Parikh & Wiesner, 2011).
Meningocele	Saclike protrusion of the spinal meninges through a congenital defect in the spinal column.	Herniated cyst is filled with cerebrospinal fluid but does not contain neural tissue; affected infants usually do not show neurologic deficits (Cohen & Walsh, 2011).
Metatarsus valgus	Congenital deformity of the foot in which the forepart rotates outward away from the midline and the heel remains straight.	Fixed deformity of the foot, which cannot be brought into neutral position; compare with metatarsus adductus, a functional deformity in which the foot can be brought into neutral position (Cooperman & Thompson, 2011; Grover, 2000b).
Metatarsus varus	Congenital bony abnormality of the foot in which the forepart rotates inward toward the midline and the heel remains straight.	Fixed deformity; the foot cannot be brought into neutral position. Compare with metatarsus adductus, a functional deformity in which the foot can be brought into neutral position (Cooperman & Thompson, 2011; Grover, 2000b).
Myelomeningocele	Defect identical to meningocele but with associated abnormalities in the structure and position of the spinal cord.	Affected infants usually show neurologic deficits below the level of the abnormality (Cohen & Walsh, 2011).
Polydactyly	Presence of more than the normal number of digits; there may be a complete extra digit (preaxial) that is normal in appearance, or a skin tag (postaxial).	May be an isolated finding, inherited as an autosomal dominant trait, or may occur in a variety of syndromes (trisomy 13, Meckel-Gruber syndrome) (Cooperman & Thompson, 2011; Parikh & Wiesner, 2011).
Rachischisis	Congenital fissure of the spinal cord in which the incompletely folded cord is splayed apart and exposed along the back.	Caused by incomplete neurulation; often accompanied by anencephaly (Fletcher, 1998; Gressens & Huppi, 2011).
Rocker bottom feet	Deformity of the foot in which the arch is disrupted, giving a rounded appearance (rocker bottom) to the sole.	Usually seen in conjunction with congenital syndromes (trisomies 13 and 18) (Parikh & Wiesner, 2011).
Scoliosis	Failure of formation or segmentation of the vertebrae; manifests as lateral (side to side) curvature of the spine.	May be congenital or acquired; may occur as part of another condition or may be idiopathic (Cooperman & Thompson, 2011; Fletcher, 1998).
Simian crease	Single transverse line in the palm.	May be benign, but when accompanied by other dysmorphic features (e.g., incurving fifth finger, epicanthal folds, low-set thumb), it may be a sign of trisomy 21 (Parikh & Wiesner, 2011).
Spinal dimple, dermal sinus	Pit or depression that occurs along the midline of the back, often at the base of the spinal cord in the lumbosacral area; may be accompanied by tufts of hair.	May be a benign finding, especially if the base of the defect can be visualized; however, defect can extend into the spinal cord, representing a neural tube defect and tethered spinal cord (Heaberlin, 2009).
Syndactyly	Fusion of two or more digits; may involve only soft tissue (simple) or may include bone or cartilage (complex).	May occur as an isolated defect or as part of a syndrome (e.g., Cornelia de Lange's, Smith-Lemli-Opitz) (Cooperman & Thompson, 2011).
Talipes equinovarus	Clubfoot; congenital deformity of the foot and lower leg marked by adduction of the forefoot (turned inward and pointed medially), varus position of the heel (turned inward), and downward pointing of the toes.	May be congenital (isolated deformity), teratologic (associated with underlying neuromuscular disorder), or positional (normal foot held in equinovarus position in utero) (Cooperman & Thompson, 2011).
Tibial torsion	Abnormal rotation of the feet while the knees are pointing forward; may be internal (toes in) or external (toes out).	Often caused by in utero positioning; resolves spontaneously (Cooperman & Thompson, 2011).

(*continued*)

TABLE 4.12

ABNORMALITIES AND VARIATIONS FOUND ON PHYSICAL EXAMINATION OF NEWBORNS AND INFANTS (CONTINUED)

Finding	Definition/Description	Comments
Torticollis	Shortening of the sternocleidomastoid muscle, resulting in head tilt toward the affected muscle and chin rotation toward the unaffected muscle; a palpable mass may appear during the first few weeks of life.	May be due to birth trauma, intrauterine malposition, muscle fibrosis, venous abnormalities in the muscle, or congenital cervical vertebral abnormalities (Cooperman & Thompson, 2011).
Neurological Examination		
Brachial plexus injuries	Peripheral damage to the network of spinal nerves supplying the arm, forearm, and hand.	Multifactorial etiology; interaction between characteristics of the brachial plexus, maternal and fetal risk factors, and birth trauma (Benjamin, 2005).
	Erb-Duchenne palsy (upper arm paralysis): Arm is adducted and internally rotated, with elbow extension, flexion of the wrist, and pronation of the forearm. The arm falls to the side of the body when passively abducted, and the Moro reflex is absent on the affected side but the grasp is intact.	Arises from injury to the fifth and sixth cervical roots; most common brachial plexus injury (Mangurten & Puppala, 2011).
	Klumpke palsy (lower arm paralysis): Hand is paralyzed, and voluntary movement of the wrist and grasp reflex are absent.	Rare; results from injury to the eighth cervical and first thoracic roots; usually Horner's syndrome (ptosis, miosis, and enophthalmos) is present on the affected side; delayed pigmentation of the iris may be seen (Mangurten & Puppala, 2011).
	Paralysis of the entire arm: Arm is completely motionless, flaccid, and powerless and hangs limply; all reflexes are absent, and sensory deficit may extend to the shoulder.	(Mangurten & Puppala, 2011)
Facial nerve palsy	Facial weakness or paralysis arising from compression of the seventh cranial nerve, caused by intrauterine position or forceps delivery; characterized by asymmetry of facial movement (most evident on crying), ptosis, and unequal nasolabial folds.	(Mangurten & Puppala, 2011)
Phrenic nerve injury	Cause of respiratory distress secondary to paralysis of the diaphragm; arises from upper brachial plexus injury.	Rarely occurs as an isolated phenomenon; accompanies signs and symptoms of Erb-Duchenne palsy (Cooperman & Thompson, 2011; Mangurten & Puppala, 2011).

HEALTH MAINTENANCE IN THE FIRST YEAR OF LIFE

The goal of health maintenance, or primary care, is to provide consistent preventive health care for the infant and education for the parents. In addition to the basic surveillance provided for all infants, high-risk infants have other needs that must be addressed. Primary care for these infants often requires a multidisciplinary approach, and the health care provider is responsible for coordinating medical, developmental, and social services. Because high-risk infants face the possibility of developmental delays, neurologic sequelae, and nutritional deficits, follow-up must include formal developmental, neurologic, and nutritional assessments in addition to routine screening tests. The health care provider may need to schedule longer and more frequent visits to evaluate the infant adequately and to assess the family's adjustment to caring for the child. The health care provider also is responsible for giving the parents comprehensive anticipatory guidance (American Academy of Pediatrics [AAP], 2002; Hagan et al., 2008; Sifuentes, 2000).

There are published guidelines for health supervision (AAP, 2002; Dunn, 2009). These guidelines indicate the elements that can be included in office visits for patients from birth to 21 years of age. The guidelines are intended to be used for those infants and children whose health needs are considered to be within the normal range (AAP, 2002; Dunn, 2009). Although the guidelines were intended to be flexible and easily modified for follow-up of high-risk infants, there are resources available for chronic and disabling conditions (Allen, 2004; Stewart & Joselow, 2012). The reader is encouraged to consult these resources for assistance in planning health maintenance for infants with special needs. Guidelines for health supervision for the first year of life are summarized in Box 4.1.

Immunizations

The AAP has published recommendations for routine childhood immunization through the first 18 years of age. These latest recommendations are presented in Figure 4.15.

BOX 4.1

GUIDELINES FOR HEALTH SUPERVISION OF INFANTS IN THE FIRST YEAR OF LIFE

Newborn

Health Assessment

- Visit may take place while the infant is still in the hospital
- Ask welcoming questions (e.g., "How is the baby?" "How are you doing?")

Physical Examination

- Examine the baby with the parents present and demonstrate all findings
- Observe parent–infant interactions
- Take measurements (length, weight, head circumference)

Testing

- Laboratory tests for mother
- Blood incompatibility
- Metabolic screening

Immunization

- Hepatitis B (dose 1) may be given

Anticipatory Guidance

Nutrition

- Discuss the feeding method the parents have chosen
- Discuss vitamin and fluoride supplementation if indicated

Sleep Patterns

- Discuss the infant's sleep position and surroundings

Skin Care

- Explain the care of the skin, cord, and circumcision

Signs and Symptoms That Need Follow-up

- Explain when to call the health care provider
- Discuss the reasons for breast engorgement and vaginal discharge
- Discuss the postpartum adjustment of the entire family

Social and Family Relationships

- Discuss the extent of visitation and individuality of the infant

Injury Prevention

- Discuss microwave do's and don'ts
- Discuss car seat safety
- Discuss crib safety
- Discuss siblings
- Discuss pets

Closing the Visit

- Ask the parents if they have any questions or concerns on discharge
- Comment on the parents' strength and capability

2 to 4 Weeks

Health Assessment

- Ask welcoming questions
- Inquire about changes in family life and if stressors have arisen
- Review the concerns discussed at the newborn visit if any

Examination of the Infant

- Review the birth history and complete a family history: diabetes, tuberculosis, anemia, emotional problems, other significant conditions, household composition, pets, use of cigarettes, alcohol, or other drugs

Physical Examination

- Take measurements (length, weight, head circumference)
- Check for red reflex, heart murmurs, abdominal masses, and hip dislocation
- Perform metabolic screening
- Review results of newborn metabolic screening

Immunizations

- Give hepatitis B (dose 1 if not given at birth; dose 2 if first dose was given at birth)

Anticipatory Guidance

Nutrition

- Answer questions about breastfeeding
- Discuss vitamin and fluoride supplementation if indicated

Sleep Patterns

- Suggest naps for the mother
- Discuss infant's sleeping position

Social Interaction With Family

- Suggest ways to encourage interaction with the infant

Injury Prevention

- Discuss car seat safety
- Discuss hot water heater temperature

Closing the Visit

- Review the problems discussed and devise a management plan
- Ask the parents if they have any questions or concerns
- Make positive statements about the baby's development
- Comment encouragingly on the parents' care giving skills

2 Months

Health Assessment

- Ask welcoming questions
- Ask if the parents have any concerns and ask about siblings and stress in the family
- Inquire about the mother's return to work
- Review the issues discussed at the previous visit
- Ask specific questions about the infant's nutrition, elimination, sleep pattern, behavior, and development

Physical Examination

- Take measurements (height, weight, head circumference) and perform a general physical examination

Observation of Behavior and Development

- Note developmental milestones
- Note temperament
- Note parent–infant interaction

Testing

- Draw blood for hematocrit/hemoglobin if infant was premature or LBW or had significant hemolysis or excessive blood loss

Immunizations

- Provide the family with vaccine information
- Give diphtheria-tetanus-pertussis (DTaP or DPT; dose 1); polio (dose 1); Haemophilus

(continued)

influenzae type b (Hib; dose 1); hepatitis B (dose 1 or dose 2)
- Recommend acetaminophen for fever or irritability

Anticipatory Guidance

Nutrition

- Discuss supplementation of vitamin D, iron, and fluoride if neccessary
- Advise the parents not to give the baby honey or corn syrup
- Recommend that no solids be given until the baby is 4 to 6 months old

Elimination

- Discuss normal patterns of elimination

Social and Family Relationships

- Urge the parents to talk to and cuddle with the baby
- Inquire about alternative care arrangements when both parents work
- Advise the parents to spend time alone with the other children
- Assess for signs of maternal depression

Injury Prevention

- Discuss the use of car seats
- Emphasize the hazard of the infant falling from the bed or table
- Stress the importance of a smoke-free environment
- Discuss gun safety

Closing the Visit

- Review the problems discussed and devise a management plan
- Ask the parents if they have any questions or concerns
- Schedule the next visit

4 Months

Health Assessment

- Ask welcoming questions
- Ask if parents have any concerns or questions
- Ask about stress
- Inquire about work and child-care issues
- Review the issues discussed at the previous visit
- Ask specific questions about the infant's nutrition, elimination, sleep pattern, behavior, and development, and family relationships

Physical Examination

- Take measurements (height, weight, head circumference) and perform a general physical examination

Observation of Behavior and Development

- Note developmental milestones
- Note parent–infant interactions
- Note temperament

Testing

- Draw blood for hematocrit/hemoglobin if necessary

Immunizations

- Provide the family with vaccine information
- Give DTaP or DPT (dose 2); polio (dose 2); Hib (dose 2); hepatitis B (dose 2 if not yet given)
- Recommend acetaminophen for fever or irritability

Anticipatory Guidance

Infections

- Advise the parents to expect about six upper respiratory tract infections a year; explain that antibiotics usually are ineffective against these infections and that unnecessary antibiotics can be harmful

Nutrition

- Recommend the gradule introduction of solid foods
- Advise not to give the baby honey or corn syrup until the infant is 1 year old
- Discuss iron supplementation

Elimination

- Ask about elimination patterns

Developmental Progress

- Consider investigation of persistent "colic"

Social and Family Relationships

- Urge the parents to talk to and cuddle with the baby
- Inquire about sibling rivalry
- Recommend that the parents plan "free time" for themselves

Injury Prevention

- Discuss car seat safety
- Explain how to choose safe toys
- Repeat warning about the danger of the infant falling from a bed or table
- Discuss the use of a microwave oven to heat the baby's food

Closing the Visit

- Review the problems discussed and devise a management plan
- Ask the parents if they have any questions or concerns
- Make positive statements about the baby's development and temperament
- Schedule the next appointment

6 Months

Health Assessment

- Ask welcoming questions
- Ask if there are issues to be discussed
- Ask about stress in the family
- Inquire about work and child care issues
- Review issues discussed at the previous visit
- Ask specific questions about the infant's nutrition, elimination, sleep pattern, behavior, and development, and about family relationships

Physical Examination

- Take measurements (height, weight, head circumference)
- Perform a general physical examination

Observation of Behavior and Development

- Note developmental milestones
- Note parent–infant interactions
- Note temperament

(*continued*)

Testing

- Draw blood for hematocrit/ hemoglobin (at 6–12 months)
- Test for sickle cell disease (as indicated)

Immunizations

- Provide vaccine information for the family; review the benefits and risks of vaccines
- Give DTaP or DPT (dose 3); polio (dose 3); Hib (dose 3); hepatitis B (dose 3 if due)
- Recommend acetaminophen for fever or irritability

Anticipatory Guidance

Nutrition

- Advise the introduction of solids (if not already started)
- Recommend offering the infant sips from a cup

Elimination

- Ask family about elimination patterns

Sleep Patterns

- Ask family about sleep patterns

Observation of Development and Behavior

- Note anxiety to strangers
- Note language development (advise parents to talk and read to the infant)

Injury Prevention

- Advise the parents about child-proofing the home (e.g., protecting the infant from hot surfaces)
- Provide the local poison control information
- Explain the use of ipecac
- Discourage the use of infant walkers
- Reinforce the proper use of microwave ovens in heating baby food
- Encourage the use of sunscreen
- Explain that swim classes are not recommended at this age

Closing the Visit

- Review the problems discussed and devise a management plan
- Ask the parents if they have other questions or concerns
- Make positive statements about the baby's development and temperament
- Schedule the next appointment

9 Months

Health Assessment

- Ask welcoming questions
- Ask if there are issues to be discussed at this visit
- Inquire about changes and stress in the family
- Inquire about the parents' approach to discipline
- Review issues discussed at the previous visit
- Ask specific questions about the infant's nutrition, elimination, sleep pattern, behavior, and development, and family relationships and injury prevention measures

Physical Examination

- Take measurements (height, weight, head circumference)
- Perform a general physical examination

Observation of Behavior and Development

- Note developmental milestones
- Note interactions with parents
- Note temperament

Testing

- Draw blood for hematocrit/ hemoglobin (at 6–12 months)
- Perform lead toxicity screening

Immunizations

- Review immunizations to see if the infant is up-to-date
- Give PPD (this is given at 9 months or at 1 year if the infant is at risk of exposure to tuberculosis)
- Give hepatitis B (dose 3 if due)

Anticipatory Guidance

Nutrition

- Encourage the parents to establish regular mealtimes
- Recommend the introduction of grownup foods and drinking from a cup

Elimination

- Recommend that parents delay toilet training until about 2 years of age or until the baby seems ready

Sleep Patterns

- Recommend that the parents establish a regular bedtime

Observation of Development and Behavior

- Note separation anxiety
- Note discipline
- Note language development
- Note intensified sibling rivalry

Injury Prevention

- Advise the parents on child-proof homes
- Advise the parents not to give the baby foods that can be aspirated; stress safety while eating
- Provide local poison control information
- Explain the use of ipecac
- Discourage the use of infant walkers
- Recommend changing from an infant to a toddler car seat

Closing the Visit

- Review the problems discussed and devise a management plan
- Ask the parents if they have other questions
- Make positive statements about the baby's development and temperament
- Schedule the next appointment

12 Months

Health Assessment

- Ask welcoming questions
- Ask what issues need to be discussed
- Inquire about changes or stress in the family
- Ask about the parents' approach to discipline
- Review issues discussed at the previous visit
- Ask specific questions about the infant's nutrition, elimination, sleep pattern, behavior, and development, and family relationships and injury prevention measures

(*continued*)

Physical Examination

- Take measurements (height, weight, head circumference)
- Perform a general physical examination

Observation of Behavior and Development

- Note developmental milestones
- Note interactions with parents
- Note temperament

Testing

- Draw blood for hematocrit/ hemoglobin (at 6–12 months)
- Perform lead toxicity screening
- Give PPD (if not administered at 9 months, if the infant is at risk of exposure to tuberculosis)

Immunizations

- Provide the family with vaccine information
- Review immunizations to see if the infant is up-to-date
- Give measles, mumps, and rubella (MMR) (per local regulations)
- Varicella vaccine may be administered

Anticipatory Guidance

Infections

- Advise the parents to expect about six upper respiratory tract infections a year; explain that antibiotics usually are ineffective for these infections and that unnecessary antibiotic use may be harmful

Nutrition

- Explain that, if the infant seems to have less of an appetite, do not to force food on the child
- Recommend weaning to a cup
- Recommend changing from baby food to all grownup foods

Elimination

- Advise the parents to delay toilet training until about 2 years of age or until the baby seems ready

Sleep Patterns

- Recommend that the parents establish a regular bedtime
- Advise the parents not to allow the baby to sleep with them unless this is a cultural practice

Observation of Development and Behavior

- Note infant's developing autonomy (explain this to the parents)
- Note discipline
- Note language development
- Note cognitive and motor skills

Injury Prevention

- Recommend ways to childproof homes
- Stress stair and bathtub safety
- Advise the parents not to give the baby foods that can be aspirated
- Provide local poison control information
- Explain the use of ipecac
- Discourage the use of infant walkers
- Stress the importance of using an appropriate car seat

Closing the Visit

- Review the problems discussed and devise a management plan
- Ask the parents if they have other concerns
- Make positive statements about the baby's development and temperament
- Schedule the next appointment

Modified from American Academy of Pediatrics, Committee on Psychosocial Aspects of Child and Family Health, *Guidelines for Health Supervision of Infants, Children, and Adolescents*, 3rd edition (2007).

HEALTH MAINTENANCE FOR HIGH-RISK INFANTS IN THE FIRST YEAR OF LIFE

History

It is important for the primary care provider to review the infant's medical history, including a complete family history and the record of the hospital course. Pertinent history to be reviewed is shown in Table 4.13. In addition to providing routine health care maintenance and anticipatory guidance to the parents, the primary care provider must monitor the status of associated medical conditions and developmental sequelae.

Growth and Nutrition

Expected increases in weight, length/height, and head circumference in the first year are summarized in Table 4.14. Weight, length/height, and OFC are measured and plotted on the appropriate graphs. The parameters for premature infants must be corrected for preterm birth. Adjustments generally are made until 2 to $2\frac{1}{2}$ years of age. Premature infants frequently show accelerated ("catch-up") growth, which first manifests in the head circumference. This may begin as early as 36 weeks postconceptional age or as late as 8 months adjusted age (Sifuentes, 2000). Increases in the OFC of more than 2 cm per week are worrisome and should be investigated, because they may signify a pathologic process (hydrocephalus) rather than catch-up growth (Allen & Lynch, 2004).

Weight gain is evaluated in grams per day. Many high-risk infants are placed on special diets (24 calories/ounce) or feeding regimens (feedings every 2 hours or continuous feedings). It is important to review the necessity of continuing or modifying the feeding plan according to the adequacy of growth. The need for dietary supplements (vitamins, minerals, human milk fortifier), medications (ranitidine, metoclopramide), and biochemical monitoring (e.g., for rickets or osteopenia) should also be addressed.

Physical Examination

A complete physical examination should be performed at each visit. Depending on the infant's history and needs,

Vaccine ▼ Age ►	Birth	1 month	2 months	4 months	6 months	9 months	12 months	15 months	18 months	19–23 months	2–3 years	4–6 years
Hepatitis B[1]	Hep B	HepB			HepB							
Rotavirus[2]			RV	RV	RV[2]							
Diphtheria, tetanus, pertussis[3]			DTaP	DTaP	DTaP		*see footnote[3]*	DTaP				DTaP
Haemophilus influenzae type b[4]			Hib	Hib	Hib[4]		Hib					
Pneumococcal[5]			PCV	PCV	PCV		PCV				PPSV	
Inactivated poliovirus[6]			IPV	IPV	IPV							IPV
Influenza[7]					Influenza (Yearly)							
Measles, mumps, rubella[8]							MMR			*see footnote[8]*		MMR
Varicella[9]							Varicella			*see footnote[9]*		Varicella
Hepatitis A[10]							Dose 1[10]				HepA Series	
Meningococcal[11]						MCV4 — see footnote [11]						

- Range of recommended ages for all children
- Range of recommended ages for certain high-risk groups
- Range of recommended ages for all children and certain high-risk groups

This schedule includes recommendations in effect as of December 23, 2011. Any dose not administered at the recommended age should be administered at a subsequent visit, when indicated and feasible. The use of a combination vaccine generally is preferred over separate injections of its equivalent component vaccines. Vaccination providers should consult the relevant Advisory Committee on Immunization Practices (ACIP) statement for detailed recommendations, available online at http://www.cdc.gov/vaccines/pubs/acip-list.htm. Clinically significant adverse events that follow vaccination should be reported to the Vaccine Adverse Event Reporting System (VAERS) online (http://www.vaers.hhs.gov) or by telephone (800-822-7967).

1. **Hepatitis B (HepB) vaccine.** (Minimum age: birth)
   At birth:
   - Administer monovalent HepB vaccine to all newborns before hospital discharge.
   - For infants born to hepatitis B surface antigen (HBsAg)–positive mothers, administer HepB vaccine and 0.5 mL of hepatitis B immune globulin (HBIG) within 12 hours of birth. These infants should be tested for HBsAg and antibody to HBsAg (anti-HBs) 1 to 2 months after completion of at least 3 doses of the HepB series, at age 9 through 18 months (generally at the next well-child visit).
   - If mother's HBsAg status is unknown, within 12 hours of birth administer HepB vaccine for infants weighing ≥2,000 grams, and HepB vaccine plus HBIG for infants weighing <2,000 grams. Determine mother's HBsAg status as soon as possible and, if she is HBsAg-positive, administer HBIG for infants weighing ≥2,000 grams (no later than age 1 week).

   Doses after the birth dose:
   - The second dose should be administered at age 1 to 2 months. Monovalent HepB vaccine should be used for doses administered before age 6 weeks.
   - Administration of a total of 4 doses of HepB vaccine is permissible when a combination vaccine containing HepB is administered after the birth dose.
   - Infants who did not receive a birth dose should receive 3 doses of a HepB-containing vaccine starting as soon as feasible (Figure 3).
   - The minimum interval between dose 1 and dose 2 is 4 weeks, and between dose 2 and 3 is 8 weeks. The final (third or fourth) dose in the HepB vaccine series should be administered no earlier than age 24 weeks and at least 16 weeks after the first dose.
2. **Rotavirus (RV) vaccines.** (Minimum age: 6 weeks for both RV-1 [Rotarix] and RV-5 [Rota Teq])
   - The maximum age for the first dose in the series is 14 weeks, 6 days; and 8 months, 0 days for the final dose in the series. Vaccination should not be initiated for infants aged 15 weeks, 0 days or older.
   - If RV-1 (Rotarix) is administered at ages 2 and 4 months, a dose at 6 months is not indicated.
3. **Diphtheria and tetanus toxoids and acellular pertussis (DTaP) vaccine.** (Minimum age: 6 weeks)
   - The fourth dose may be administered as early as age 12 months, provided at least 6 months have elapsed since the third dose.
4. ***Haemophilus influenzae* type b (Hib) conjugate vaccine.** (Minimum age: 6 weeks)
   - If PRP-OMP (PedvaxHIB or Comvax [HepB-Hib]) is administered at ages 2 and 4 months, a dose at age 6 months is not indicated.
   - Hiberix should only be used for the booster (final) dose in children aged 12 months through 4 years.
5. **Pneumococcal vaccines.** (Minimum age: 6 weeks for pneumococcal conjugate vaccine [PCV]; 2 years for pneumococcal polysaccharide vaccine [PPSV])
   - Administer 1 dose of PCV to all healthy children aged 24 through 59 months who are not completely vaccinated for their age.
   - For children who have received an age-appropriate series of 7-valent PCV (PCV7), a single supplemental dose of 13-valent PCV (PCV13) is recommended for:
     — All children aged 14 through 59 months
     — Children aged 60 through 71 months with underlying medical conditions.
   - Administer PPSV at least 8 weeks after last dose of PCV to children aged 2 years or older with certain underlying medical conditions, including a cochlear implant. See *MMWR* 2010:59(No. RR-11), available at http://www.cdc.gov/mmwr/pdf/rr/rr5911.pdf.
6. **Inactivated poliovirus vaccine (IPV).** (Minimum age: 6 weeks)
   - If 4 or more doses are administered before age 4 years, an additional dose should be administered at age 4 through 6 years.
   - The final dose in the series should be administered on or after the fourth birthday and at least 6 months after the previous dose.
7. **Influenza vaccines.** (Minimum age: 6 months for trivalent inactivated influenza vaccine [TIV]; 2 years for live, attenuated influenza vaccine [LAIV])
   - For most healthy children aged 2 years and older, either LAIV or TIV may be used. However, LAIV should not be administered to some children, including 1) children with asthma, 2) children 2 through 4 years who had wheezing in the past 12 months, or 3) children who have any other underlying medical conditions that predispose them to influenza complications. For all other contraindications to use of LAIV, see *MMWR* 2010;59(No. RR-8), available at http://www.cdc.gov/mmwr/pdf/rr/rr5908.pdf.
   - For children aged 6 months through 8 years:
     — For the 2011–12 season, administer 2 doses (separated by at least 4 weeks) to those who did not receive at least 1 dose of the 2010–11 vaccine. Those who received at least 1 dose of the 2010–11 vaccine require 1 dose for the 2011–12 season.
     — For the 2012–13 season, follow dosing guidelines in the 2012 ACIP influenza vaccine recommendations.
8. **Measles, mumps, and rubella (MMR) vaccine.** (Minimum age: 12 months)
   - The second dose may be administered before age 4 years, provided at least 4 weeks have elapsed since the first dose.
   - Administer MMR vaccine to infants aged 6 through 11 months who are traveling internationally. These children should be revaccinated with 2 doses of MMR vaccine, the first at ages 12 through 15 months and at least 4 weeks after the previous dose, and the second at ages 4 through 6 years.
9. **Varicella (VAR) vaccine.** (Minimum age: 12 months)
   - The second dose may be administered before age 4 years, provided at least 3 months have elapsed since the first dose.
   - For children aged 12 months through 12 years, the recommended minimum interval between doses is 3 months. However, if the second dose was administered at least 4 weeks after the first dose, it can be accepted as valid.
10. **Hepatitis A (HepA) vaccine.** (Minimum age: 12 months)
    - Administer the second (final) dose 6 to18 months after the first.
    - Unvaccinated children 24 months and older at high risk should be vaccinated. See *MMWR* 2006;55(No. RR-7), available at http://www.cdc.gov/mmwr/pdf/rr/rr5507.pdf.
    - A 2-dose HepA vaccine series is recommended for anyone aged 24 months and older, previously unvaccinated, for whom immunity against hepatitis A virus infection is desired.
11. **Meningococcal conjugate vaccines, quadrivalent (MCV4).** (Minimum age: 9 months for Menactra [MCV4-D], 2 years for Menveo [MCV4-CRM])
    - For children aged 9 through 23 months 1) with persistent complement component deficiency; 2) who are residents of or travelers to countries with hyperendemic or epidemic disease; or 3) who are present during outbreaks caused by a vaccine serogroup, administer 2 primary doses of MCV4-D, ideally at ages 9 months and 12 months or at least 8 weeks apart.
    - For children aged 24 months and older with 1) persistent complement component deficiency who have not been previously vaccinated; or 2) anatomic/functional asplenia, administer 2 primary doses of either MCV4 at least 8 weeks apart.
    - For children with anatomic/functional asplenia, if MCV4-D (Menactra) is used, administer at a minimum age of 2 years and at least 4 weeks after completion of all PCV doses.
    - See *MMWR* 2011;60:72–6, available at http://www.cdc.gov/mmwr/pdf/wk/mm6003. pdf, and Vaccines for Children Program resolution No. 6/11-1, available at http://www.cdc.gov/vaccines/programs/vfc/downloads/resolutions/06-11mening-mcv.pdf, and *MMWR* 2011;60:1391–2, available at http://www.cdc.gov/mmwr/pdf/wk/mm6040. pdf, for further guidance, including revaccination guidelines.

This schedule is approved by the Advisory Committee on Immunization Practices (http://www.cdc.gov/vaccines/recs/acip), the American Academy of Pediatrics (http://www.aap.org), and the American Academy of Family Physicians (http://www.aafp.org).
Department of Health and Human Services • Centers for Disease Control and Prevention

FIGURE 4.15 Recommended childhood and adolescent immunization schedule, by vaccine and age—United States, 2012. Adapted from American Academy of Pediatrics, Committee on Infectious Diseases (2012).

TABLE 4.13

RECORDED ELEMENTS OF THE HISTORY, MEDICAL COURSE, AND CURRENT NEEDS FOR NEONATES

Component	Elements
History	Prenatal and perinatal course Hospital course: Birth weight, gestation Illnesses, surgical procedures Radiographic studies Discharge examination Weight, head circumference, length
Nutrition information	Current diet and feeding schedule Feeding problems: Gastroesophageal (GE) reflux, feeding intolerance Dietary supplements: Vitamins, minerals, human milk fortifier Current deficiencies: Osteopenia/rickets, anemia
Medications	Doses Serum levels Oxygen requirements
Immunizations	Immunizations given in the hospital RSV prophylaxis
Laboratory data	Most recent values: Hemoglobin, hematocrit Bilirubin Pending laboratory studies Need for further testing Newborn screening results
Current problems and complications	ROP, ophthalmologic problems (e.g., strabismus) Hearing deficits Bronchopulmonary dysplasia (BPD)/chronic lung problems GE reflux Intraventricular hemorrhage (IVH) Developmental deficits Other

Data from Sifuentes (2000).

special attention may be required in certain areas, which are listed in Table 4.15.

Laboratory Tests and Monitoring Examinations

All standard screening tests required for healthy infants should be performed according to AAP recommendations. Other tests may be necessary for high-risk infants, such as periodic electrolyte determinations for babies receiving diuretics. Consideration should be given to measuring serum levels for such drugs as anticonvulsants, methylxanthines, and digoxin.

Repeat ophthalmologic examinations may be required to evaluate the extent and progression or regression of retinopathy of prematurity (ROP). Further follow-up may be indicated, because some infants are at risk for strabismus, myopia, amblyopia, glaucoma, and other visual deficits. The infant may need serial auditory evaluations (brainstem auditory evoked response [BAER] behavioral audiograms) and other studies, such as electroencephalography, electrocardiography, echocardiography, radiography, pneumography, and neuroradiologic imaging (computed tomography [CT] or magnetic resonance imaging [MRI]). Infants receiving supplemental oxygen often benefit from periodic pulse oximetry (Allen & Lynch, 2004; Sifuentes, 2000).

Immunizations

Vaccines are administered according to chronologic (postnatal) age, not GA. The standard doses and intervals are followed, as recommended by the AAP (see Box 4.1). Former premature infants have adequate serologic responses to immunizations without increased incidence of untoward effects. There is benefit derived from respiratory syncytial virus (RSV) prophylaxis for high-risk infants, especially premature infants with a history of respiratory distress syndrome (RDS) or RDS/BPD (RSD with bronchopulmonary dysplasia).

TABLE 4.14

EXPECTED INCREASES IN WEIGHT, LENGTH/HEIGHT, AND HEAD CIRCUMFERENCE IN THE FIRST YEAR OF LIFE

Parameter	Age (months)	Expected Increase
Weight	Birth to 3	25–35 g/d
	3–6	12–21 g/d
	6–12	10–13 g/d
Length/height	Birth to 12	25 cm/y
OFC	Birth to 3	2 cm/mo
	4–6	1 cm/mo
	7–12	0.5 cm/mo

Data from Grover (2000a) and Ditmyer (2004).

TABLE 4.15

MONITORING FOR SUBSEQUENT CONDITIONS IN HIGH-RISK INFANTS

System	Condition	Comments
Ocular	ROP, strabismus, visual abnormalities	
Oropharyngeal	Palatal groove, high-arched palate, abnormal tooth formation	May develop secondary to intubation or may be due to congenital abnormalities
	Discolored teeth	Caused by high bilirubin levels
Thoracic/respiratory	Retractions, wheezing, stridor, chest scars	Sequelae of chronic lung disease. Caused by chest tube placement
Cardiovascular	Hypertension	Blood pressure monitoring is especially important for an infant who had umbilical artery catheters in place
Abdominal	Hypoplastic umbilicus	Use of umbilical catheters and suturing frequently are the cause of this condition
Genitourinary	Hernias Cryptorchidism	Increased risk in preterm babies
Extremities	Developmental hip dysplasia Scars on heels or extremities	Sequelae of blood sampling, placement of intravenous (IV) lines, or extravasation of IV fluid
Neuromuscular	Abnormal tone, asymmetric movements and reflexes, persistence of primitive reflexes and fisting, sustained clonus, scissoring, poor suck-swallow coordination	Abnormalities must be identified as soon as possible and the patient and family referred to appropriate intervention services

Data from Sifuentes (2000) and Allen (2004).

Psychosocial Needs

Families of high-risk infants require a great deal of support and anticipatory guidance. Health care providers must seek to understand parental expectations and legitimize their fears while providing support and encouragement. Parents should be given consistent, honest information and realistic appraisals of their infant's status and prognosis.

NICU graduates may be at risk for vulnerable child syndrome (VCS) (Box 4.2). Because parents continue to perceive their child as vulnerable and fragile, abnormal parent-infant interactions develop. By assessing for early, subtle signs, health care providers may prevent progression of the disorder.

BOX 4.2

CHARACTERISTICS OF VCS

- Exaggerated separation anxiety (both infant and parent)
- Sleep difficulties
- Overprotectiveness
- Overindulgence
- Lack of appropriate discipline
- Excessive parental preoccupation with infant's health

SUMMARY

The comprehensive history and physical assessment create the framework for identifying problems and planning interventions. Assessment allows the nurse to gather information and to evaluate and integrate that information as care of the newborn proceeds. Although careful attention to the obvious is important, subtle findings detected by an experienced practitioner also may play a crucial role in the continuing care of the infant and family.

CASE STUDY

■ Identification of Patient Problem. You are assessing a full-term female infant who was born 15 minutes previously via vaginal delivery. You note a firm but fluctuant cranial mass with ill-defined borders swelling across the suture lines to the ear and neck. The pinna appears to be protuberant.

■ Assessment: History and Physical Examination

Obtain detailed history to include:

- Maternal medications used during pregnancy (aspirin, ibuprofen, phenytoin)
- History of placental insufficiency or fetal asphyxia during delivery
- Length of time spent pushing
- If delivery was vacuum assisted, number of attempts and length of application
- Presentation of fetus at delivery
- Infant's Apgar scores
- History of previous child with clotting or bleeding disorder
- Family history of bleeding or clotting disorders
- Detailed examination (to be performed on open warmer):
  Observe general appearance of infant including color of skin and mucous membranes, overall perfusion, size and symmetry of head and face, obvious deformities or evidence of birth trauma
  Monitor vital signs (VS)
  Assess state of alertness, tone, resting posture/position, and cry
- Note any arching or posturing with movement

■ Head

- Observe general appearance, size, and movement of head and neck
- Observe shape and symmetry of head, neck, pinna bilaterally
- Inspect and palpate sutures and fontanelles
- Measure head circumference
- Observe hair growth patterns and check for signs of birth trauma or other anomalies
- Auscultate fontanelles

■ Face

- Observe for symmetrical movement of facial features
- Assess eyes, pupillary response to light, red reflex and blink reflex in response to light
- Inspect for facial, head, neck edema, ecchymosis
- Assess gag, suck/rooting reflex, palate, color of mucous membranes, suck/swallow coordination, tongue, midline, moves freely, color, proportional size
- Observe for facial palsy

■ Ears

- Assess for any drainage or bleeding from the ear canals
- Inspect shape, placement, swelling, and position of ears
- Inspect ears for lesions, cysts, nodules
- Inspect nose: appearance, patency of nares

■ Neck

- Observe appearance, noting any abnormalities such as short, redundant skin, webbing
- Assess clavicles

■ Chest

- Assess color and perfusion prior to starting examination and note any changes throughout examination
- Palpate quality of pulses and compare upper to lower
- Observe for active precordium
- Assess capillary refill
- Auscultate lung sounds, noting any retractions, grunting, flaring, asymmetrical chest movement, or aeration
- Auscultate chest for murmurs, clicks, and rubs, PMI
- Assess for placement of breasts/nipples, presence of breast tissue, symmetry

■ Abdomen

- Observe color and size, shape, and symmetry of abdomen.
- Auscultate abdomen for bowel sounds
- Palpate for loops, noting any tenderness and guarding with examination
- Palpate for hepatosplenomegaly

■ Genitourinary

- Inspect external genitalia and inguinal area/suprapubic area
- Inspect labia, clitoris, urethral meatus, and any bleeding or discharge
- Inspect for any discoloration/bruising or other signs of birth trauma
- Assess anus for patency and placement

■ Musculoskeletal

- Observe for spontaneous, symmetrical movement in all four limbs

- Inspect entire body for ecchymosis and petechiae or other signs of bleeding with careful documentation (mark borders if necessary)

Neurologic

- Assess reflexes: tonic neck reflex, Moro reflex, grasp reflex, Babinski reflex, and trunk incurvation

Differential Diagnosis

- Caput succedaneum, cephalohematoma, skull fracture, subgaleal hematoma

Diagnostic Tests

- Continuous monitoring: heart rate, respiratory rate, blood pressure, and pulse oximetry
- Blood gas to assess for metabolic acidosis
- Hematocrit, platelets, clotting factors, to assess for blood loss and/or coagulopathy
- Liver function studies, blood glucose level
- Skull radiograph to assess for skull fracture
- Depending on the results of the neurologic examination, a head CT may be necessary

Working Diagnosis

- Subgaleal hemorrhage

Development of Management Plan

- Admit to NICU for close observation
- Monitor VS closely and continuously (HR, RR, BP); pulse oximetry, observing closely for signs of hypovolemic shock (tachycardia, hypotension, respiratory distress)
- Monitor neurologic VS closely for possible deterioration in level of consciousness
- Monitor intake and output strictly

Blood work to be done:

- Blood gas (for baseline respiratory function)
- Complete blood count (for baseline hematocrit)
- Coagulation factors (for potential indication of massive bleeding and coagulopathy)
- Bilirubin level (for baseline: during resolution the breakdown of the blood may cause hyperbilirubinemia requiring treatment; thus levels of bilirubin need to be followed closely as well)
- Blood urea nitrogen and creatinine (for baseline of kidney function and hydration)

- Keep the patient NPO for now
- Provide maintenance IV solution
- Blood products or NS boluses can be given as required for replacement of blood volume

Meet with parents: Careful preparation of the parents for the acute side effects and sequelae of subgaleal hemorrhage is important. Parents should be warned of the possibility of swelling and discoloration of the face, head, and neck. They should also know that spontaneous resolution usually occurs within 2 to 3 weeks and some infants require close long-term follow-up for sequelae.

Implementation and Evaluation of Effectiveness

Implement above plan with continuous monitoring for deterioration of infant's cardiovascular or neurologic status.

EVIDENCE-BASED PRACTICE BOX

Assessment

Although the 10-point Apgar score has been used to evaluate the physical condition of newly born infants since it was proposed by Virginia Apgar in 1952, its value has become controversial due to attempts to use it as a predictor of neurologic outcome. Casey, McIntire, and Leveno (2001) undertook to study whether the Apgar scoring system remains relevant as a prognosticator of survival during the neonatal period, an intent for which it was originally developed. A retrospective analysis was conducted of 151,891 live-born singleton infants delivered at 26 weeks gestation or later at an inner-city public hospital over a 10-year period. Apgar scores were compared to umbilical-artery blood pH values to assess which test best predicted neonatal death during the first 28 days after birth. The 5-minute Apgar score was found to be a better predictor of neonatal outcome than was measurement of umbilical-artery blood pH, even for newborn infants with severe academia. It was noted, however, that the combination of five-minute Apgar scores of 0 to 3 and umbilical-artery blood pH values of 7.0 or less increased the relative risk of death in both preterm and term infants. Based on their analysis, these investigators concluded that the Apgar system continues to be an important tool in the prediction of neonatal outcome.

Reference

Casey, B. M., McIntire, D. D., & Leveno, K. J. (2001). The continuing value of the Apgar score for the assessment of newborn infants. *The New England Journal of Medicine, 344*(7), 467–471.

ONLINE RESOURCES

Newborn Physical Assessment
http://www.youtube.com/watch?v=yAWEWfwyWBo

Physical Assessment of the Newborn
http://www.duq.edu/academics/schools/nursing/newborn-assessment

Physical Examination
http://www.youtube.com/watch?v=8gnO4Py0_08

REFERENCES

Abdulhayoglu, E. (2012). Birth trauma. In J. P. Cloherty, E. C. Eichenwald, A. R. Hansen, & A. R. Stark (Eds.), *Manual of neonatal care* (7th ed., pp. 63–73). Philadelphia, PA: Lippincott Williams & Wilkins.

Allen, P. J. (2004). The primary care provider and children with chronic conditions. In P. J. Allen & J. A. Judith (Eds.), *Primary care of the child with a chronic condition* (4th ed., pp. 3–22). St Louis, MO: Mosby.

Allen, P. J., & Lynch, M. E. (2004). Prematurity. In P. J. Allen & J. A. Vessey (Eds.), *Primary care of the child with a chronic condition* (4th ed., pp. 682–707). Philadelphia, PA: Mosby.

Als, H., & Butler, S. (2011). Neurobehavioral development of the preterm infant. In R. J. Martin, A. A. Fanaroff, & M. C. Walsh (Eds.), *Neonatal-perinatal medicine: Diseases of the fetus and infant* (9th ed., pp. 1057–1074). St Louis, MO: Mosby.

American Academy of Pediatrics, Committee on Infectious Diseases. (2012). Recommended childhood and adolescent immunization schedules—United States. *Pediatrics, 129*(2), 385–386. doi:10.1542/peds.2011-3630.

American Academy of Pediatrics, Committee on the Fetus and Newborn and the American College of Obstetricians and Gynecologists Committee on Obstetrics. (1996). Use and abuse of the Apgar score. *Pediatrics, 98*, 141–142.

American Academy of Pediatrics Committee on Psychosocial Aspects of Child and Family Health. (2002). *Guidelines for health supervision III*. Elk Grove Village, IL: American Academy of Pediatrics.

Apgar, V. A. (1953). A proposal for a new method of evaluation of the newborn infant. *Current Research in Anesthesiology and Analgesia, 32*, 260–267.

Askin, D. (2009). Chest and lungs assessment. In E. P. Tappero & M. E. Honeyfield (Eds.), *Physical assessment of the newborn* (4th ed., pp 75–87). Petaluma, CA: NICU Ink.

Back, S. (2012). Congenital malformations of the central nervous system. In H. W. Taeusch, R. A. Ballard, & C. A. Gleason (Eds.), *Avery's diseases of the newborn* (8th ed., pp. 938–963). Philadelphia, PA: Saunders.

Ballard, J. L., Khoury, J. C., Wedig, K., Wang, L., Eilers-Walsman, B. L., & Lipp, R. (1991). New Ballard score, expanded to include extremely premature infants. *Journal of Pediatrics, 119*, 417–423.

Barksdale, E. M., Chwals, W. J., Magnuson, D. K., & Parry, R. L. (2011). Selected gastrointestinal anomalies. In R. J. Martin, A. A. Fanaroff, & M. C. Walsh (Eds.), *Neonatal-perinatal medicine: Diseases of the fetus and infant* (9th ed., pp. 1400–1430). St Louis, MO: Mosby.

Battaglia, F. C., & Lubchenco, L. O. (1967). A practical classification of newborn infants by weight and gestational age. *Journal of Pediatrics, 71*, 159–163.

Benjamin, K. (2002). Scrotal and inguinal masses in the newborn period. *Advances in Neonatal Care, 2*(3), 140–148.

Benjamin, K. (2005). Part I. Injuries to the brachial plexus. *Advances in Neonatal Care, 5*(4), 181–189.

Bennett, M., & Meier, S. (2009). Assessment of the dysmorphic infant. In E. P. Tappero & M. E. Honeyfield (Eds.), *Physical assessment of the newborn* (4th ed., pp. 201–218). Petaluma, CA: NICU Ink.

Brown, V. D., & Landers, S. (2011). Heat balance. In S. L. Gardner, B. S. Carter, M. I. Enzman-Hines, & J. A. Hernandez (Eds.), *Handbook of neonatal intensive care* (7th ed., pp. 113–133). St Louis, MO: Mosby.

Cavaliere, T. A. (2009). Genitourinary assessment. In E. P. Tappero, & M. E. Honeyfield (Eds.), *Physical assessment of the newborn* (4th ed., pp. 115–133). Petaluma, CA: NICU Ink.

Charsha, D. S. (2010). Care of the extremely low birth weight infant. In M. T. Verklan & M. Walden (Eds.), *Core curriculum for neonatal intensive care nursing* (4th ed., pp. 434–446). St Louis, MO: Saunders.

Cilento, B. G., Najjar, S. S., & Atala, A. (1994). Cryptorchidism and testicular torsion. *Pediatric Clinics of North America, 40*, 1133–1149.

Cohen, A. R. (2011). Disorders in head shape and size. In R. J. Martin, A. A. Fanaroff, & M. C. Walsh (Eds.), *Neonatal-perinatal medicine: Diseases of the fetus and infant* (9th ed., pp. 1010–1034). St Louis, MO: Mosby.

Cooperman, D. R., & Thompson, G. H. (2011). Neonatal orthopedics. In R. J. Martin, A. A. Fanaroff, & M. C. Walsh (Eds.), *Neonatal-perinatal medicine: Diseases of the fetus and infant* (9th ed., pp. 1771–1801). St Louis, MO: Mosby.

D'Harlingue, A. E., & Durand, D. J. (2001). Recognition, stabilization, and transport of the high-risk newborn. In M. H. Klaus & A. A. Fanaroff (Eds.), *Care of the high risk neonate* (5th ed.). Philadelphia, PA: Saunders.

Ditmyer, S. (2004). Hydrocephalus. In P. J. Allen & J. A. Vessey (Eds.). *Primary care of the child with a chronic condition* (4th ed., pp. 543–560). Philadelphia, PA: Mosby.

Desmond, M. M., Rudolph, A. J., & Phitaksphraiwan, P. (1966). The transitional care nursery. A mechanism for preventive medicine in the newborn. *Pediatric Clinics of North America, 13*(3), 651–668.

Donlon, C. R., & Furdon, S. A. (2002). Part 2. Assessment of the umbilical cord outside of the delivery room. *Advances in Neonatal Care, 2*(1), 187–197.

Dunn, A. M. (2009). Health perception and health management patterns. In C. E. Burns, A. M. Dunn, M. A. Brady, N. B. Starr, & C. G. Blosser (Eds.), *Pediatric primary care* (4th ed., pp. 169–190). St Louis, MO: Saunders.

Early, A., Fayers, P., Ng, S., Shinebourne, E. A., & de Sweit, M. (1980). Blood pressure in the first six weeks of life. *Archives of Disease in Childhood, 55*, 755–757.

Engel, J. (2006). *Pocket guide to pediatric assessment* (5th ed.). St Louis, MO: Mosby.

Fanaroff, A. A., & Wright, E. (1990). Profiles of mean arterial blood pressure (MAP) for infants weighing 500–1500 grams. *Pediatric Research, 27*, 205A.

Fletcher, M. A. (1998). *Physical diagnosis in neonatology*. Philadelphia, PA: Lippincott-Raven.

Furdon, S. A., & Clark, D. A. (2003). Scalp hair characteristics in the newborn. *Advances in Neonatal Care, 3*(6), 286–298.

Furdon, S. A., & Clark, D. A. (2005). Discriminating between skin lesions in the newborn. *Advances in Neonatal Care, 1*(2), 84–90.

Furdon, S. A., & Donlon, C. R. (2002). Examination of the newborn foot. *Advances in Neonatal Care, 2*(5), 248–258.

Gardner, S. L., & Hernandez, J. A. (2011). Initial nursery care. In S. L. Gardner, B. S. Carter, M. I. Enzman-Hines, & J. A. Hernandez (Eds.), *Merenstein & Gardner's handbook of neonatal intensive care* (7th ed., pp. 78–112). St Louis, MO: Mosby.

Goldsmith, J. (2011). Delivery room resuscitation of the newborn. Overview and initial management. In R. J. Martin, A. A. Fanaroff, & M. C. Walsh (Eds.), *Neonatal-perinatal medicine: Diseases of the fetus and infant* (9th ed., pp. 449–458). St Louis, MO: Mosby.

Gomella, T. L. (2009). Newborn physical examination. In T. L. Gomella, M. D. Cunningham, & F. G. Eyal (Eds.), *Neonatology. Management, procedures, on all problems, diseases, & drugs* (6th ed., pp. 31–43). New York, NY: McGraw-Hill.

Goodwin, M. (2009). Abdomen assessment. In E. P. Tappero & M. E. Honeyfield (Eds.), *Physical assessment of the newborn* (4th ed., pp. 105–114). Petaluma, CA: NICU Ink.

Gressens, P., & Huppi, P. (2011). Normal and abnormal brain development. In R. J. Martin, A. A. Fanaroff, & M. C. Walsh (Eds.), *Neonatal-perinatal medicine: Diseases of the fetus and infant* (9th ed., pp. 887–917). St Louis, MO: Mosby.

Grover, G. (2000a). Nutritional needs. In C. D. Berkowitz (Ed.), *Pediatrics: A primary care approach* (2nd ed.). Philadelphia, PA: Saunders.

Grover, G. (2000b). Rotational problems of the lower extremities: In-toeing and out-toeing. In C. D. Berkowitz (Ed.), *Pediatrics: A primary care approach* (2nd ed.). Philadelphia, PA: Saunders.

Hagan, J. F., Shaw, J. S., & Duncan, P. (2008). *Bright futures. Guidelines for health supervision of infants, children and adolescents* (3rd ed.). Elk Grove, IL: AAP.

Heaberlin, P. D. (2009). Neurologic assessment. In E. P. Tappero & M. E. Honeyfield (Eds.), *Physical assessment of the newborn* (4th ed., pp. 159–184). Petaluma, CA: NICU Ink.

Hegyi, T., Carbone, M. T., Anwar, M., Ostfeld, B., Hiatt, M., Koons, A., . . . Paneth, N. (1994). Blood pressure ranges in premature infants. I. The first hours of life. *Journal of Pediatrics, 124*, 627–633.

Hoath, S. B., & Narendran, V. (2011). The skin. In R. J. Martin, A. A. Fanaroff, & M. C. Walsh (Eds.), *Neonatal-perinatal medicine: Diseases of the fetus and infant* (9th ed., pp. 1705–1736). St Louis, MO: Mosby.

Honeyfield, M. E. (2009). Principles of physical assessment. In E. P. Tappero & M. E. Honeyfield (Eds.), *Physical assessment of the newborn* (4th ed., pp. 1–8). Petaluma, CA: NICU Ink.

Johnson, L., & Cochran, W. D. (2012). Assessment of the newborn history and physical examination of the newborn. In J. P. Cloherty, E. C. Eichenwald, A. R. Hansen, & A. R. Stark (Eds.), *Manual of neonatal care* (7th ed., pp. 91–102). Philadelphia, PA: Lippincott Williams & Wilkins.

Johnson, P. J. (2009). Head, eyes, ears, nose, mouth, and neck assessment. In E. P. Tappero & M. E. Honeyfield (Eds.), *Physical assessment of the newborn* (4th ed., pp. 57–74). Petaluma, CA: NICU Ink.

Kattwinkel, J., Zaichkin, J., McGowan, J., American Heart Association, & American Academy of Pediatrics. (2011). *Neonatal resuscitation textbook* (6th ed.), AHA/AAP, Elk Grove, IL: AAP.

Kaufman, L. M., Miller, M. T., & Gupta, B. K. (2011). The eye: Examination and common problems. In R. J. Martin, A. A. Fanaroff, & M. C. Walsh (Eds.), *Neonatal-perinatal medicine: Diseases of the fetus and infant* (9th ed., pp. 1737–1763). St Louis, MO: Mosby.

Kliegman, R. M. (2011). Intrauterine growth restriction. In R. J. Martin, A. A. Fanaroff, & M. C. Walsh (Eds.), *Neonatal-perinatal medicine: Diseases of the fetus and infant* (9th ed., pp. 245–277). St Louis, MO: Mosby.

Lewis, S. M., et al. (2000). *Medical-surgical nursing: Assessment and management of clinical problems* (5th ed.). St Louis, MO: Mosby.

Lissauer, T. (2011). Physical examination of the newborn. In R. J. Martin, A. A. Fanaroff, & M. C. Walsh (Eds.), *Neonatal-perinatal medicine: Diseases of the fetus and infant* (9th ed., pp. 485–500). St Louis, MO: Mosby.

Lubchenco, L., et al. (1966). Intrauterine growth in length and head circumference as estimated from live births at gestational ages from 26 to 42 weeks. *Journal of Pediatrics, 37*, 403.

Lubchenco, L. O. (1967). *The high risk infant*. Philadelphia, PA: Saunders.

Madan, A., & Good, W. (2005). The eye. In H. W. Taeusch, R. A. Ballard, & C. A. Gleason (Eds.), *Avery's diseases of the newborn* (8th ed., pp. 1539–1555). Philadelphia, PA: Saunders.

Madan, A., Hamrick, S. E., & Ferriero, D. M. (2005). Central nervous system injury and neuroprotection. In H. W. Taeusch, R. A. Ballard, & C. A. Gleason (Eds.), *Avery's diseases of the newborn* (8th ed., pp. 965–992). Philadelphia, PA: Saunders.

Mangurten, H. M., & Puppila, B. L. (2011). Birth injuries. In R. J. Martin, A. A. Fanaroff, & M. C. Walsh (Eds.), *Neonatal-perinatal medicine: Diseases of the fetus and infant* (9th ed., pp. 501–529). St Louis, MO: Mosby.

McLean, F., & Usher, R. (1970). Measurements of liveborn fetal malnutrition infants compared with similar gestation and with similar birth weight normal controls. *Biology of the Neonate, 16*, 215–221.

Parikh, A. S., & Wiesner, G. L. (2011). Congenital anomalies. In R. J. Martin, A. A. Fanaroff, & M. C. Walsh (Eds.), *Neonatal-perinatal medicine: Diseases of the fetus and infant* (9th ed., pp. 531–552). St Louis, MO: Mosby.

Rozinski, T. A., & Bloom, D. A. (1997). Male genital tract. In K. T. Oldham, P. M. Colombani, R. P. Foglia (Eds.), *Surgery of infants and children: Scientific principles and practice* (pp. 1543–1558). Philadelphia, PA: Lippincott-Raven.

Sansoucie, D. A., & Cavaliere, T. A. (2007). Assessment of the newborn and infant. In C. Kenner & L. W. Lott (Eds.), *Comprehensive neonatal nursing: A physiologic perspective* (3rd ed., pp. 677–718). Philadelphia, PA: Saunders.

Schulman, R. M., Palmert, M. R., & Wherrett, D. K. (2011). Disorders of sex development. In R. J. Martin, A. A. Fanaroff, & M. C. Walsh (Eds.), *Neonatal-perinatal medicine: Diseases of the fetus and infant* (9th ed., pp. 1584–1620). St Louis, MO: Mosby.

Seidel, H. M., Ball, J. W., Dains, J. E., & Benedict, W. G. (2003). *Mosby's guide to physical examination* (5th ed.). St Louis, MO: Mosby.

Sifuentes, M. (2000). Well-child care for preterm infants. In C. D. Berkowitz (Ed.), *Pediatrics: A primary care approach* (2nd ed.). Philadelphia, PA: Saunders.

Smith, J. B. (2012). Initial evaluation: History and physical examination of the newborn. In C. A. Gleason & S. U. Devaskar (Eds.), *Avery's diseases of the newborn* (9th ed., pp. 328–340). Philadelphia, PA: Saunders.

Spillman, L. (2002). Examination of the external ear. *Advances in Neonatal Care, 2*(2), 72–80.

Stanley, F. J. (1994). Cerebral palsy trends: Implications for perinatal care. *Acta obstetricia et gynecologica Scandinavica (Copenhagen), 73*, 5–9.

Stewart, J. E., & Joselow, M. R. (2012). Follow up care of very preterm and very low birth weight infants. In J. P. Cloherty (Ed.), *Manual of neonatal care* (7th ed., pp. 185–191). Philadelphia, PA: Lippincott Williams & Wilkins.

Tappero, E. P. (2009). Musculoskeletal system assessment. In E. P. Tappero & M. E. Honeyfield (Eds.), *Physical assessment of the newborn* (4th ed., pp. 133–158). Petaluma, CA: NICU Ink.

Trotter, C. W. (2009). Gestational age assessment. In E. P. Tappero & M. E. Honeyfield (Eds.), *Physical assessment of the newborn* (4th ed., pp. 21–40). Petaluma, CA: NICU Ink.

Vargo, L. (2009). Cardiovascular assessment. In E. P. Tappero & M. E. Honeyfield (Eds.), *Physical assessment of the newborn* (4th ed., pp. 87–104). Petaluma, CA: NICU Ink.

Vogt, B. A., & Dell, K. M. (2011). The kidney and urinary tract. In R. J. Martin, A. A. Fanaroff, & M. C. Walsh (Eds.), *Neonatal-perinatal medicine: Diseases of the fetus and infant* (9th ed., pp. 1659–1703). St Louis, MO: Mosby.

Waardenburg, P. J. (1951). A new syndrome combining developmental anomalies of the eyelids, eyebrows, and nose root with pigmentary defects of the iris and head hair and with congenital deafness. *American Journal of Human Genetics, 3*, 195.

Witt, C. (2009). Skin assessment. In E. P. Tappero & M. E. Honeyfield (Eds.), *Physical assessment of the newborn* (4th ed., pp. 41–56). Petaluma, CA: NICU Ink.

Wong, D. L. (2003). *Wong's nursing care of infants and children* (7th ed.). St Louis, MO: Mosby.

Wright, K. W. (1999). *Pediatric ophthalmology for pediatrician*. Baltimore, MD: Williams & Wilkins.

Zaontz, M. R., & Packer, M. G. (1997). Abnormalities of the external genitalia. *Pediatric Clinics of North America, 44*(5), 1267–1297.

Zderic, S. A. (2005). Developmental abnormalities of the genitourinary system. In H. W. Taeusch, R. A. Ballard, & C. A. Gleason (Eds.), *Avery's diseases of the newborn* (8th ed., pp. 1287–1297). Philadelphia, PA: Saunders.

Zubrow, A. B., Hulman, S., Kushner, H., & Falkner, B. (1995). Determinants of blood pressure in infants admitted to neonatal intensive care units: A prospective multicenter study. Philadelphia Neonatal Blood Pressure Study Group. *Journal of Perinatology, 15*, 470.

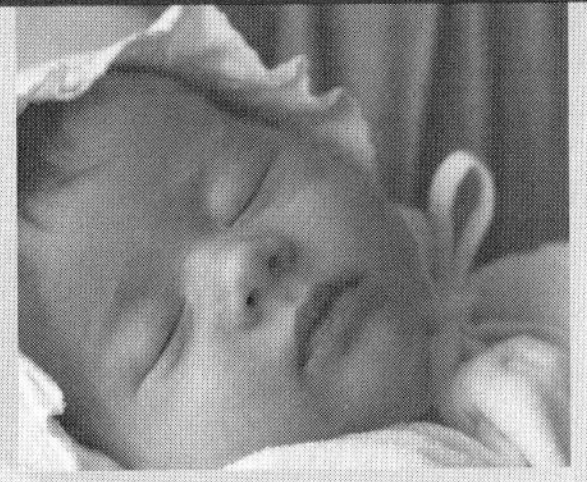

CHAPTER 5

Normal Term Newborn

■ Cheryl Riley, Becky Spencer, and Lyn S. Prater

The nurse caring for the newborn plays a unique role in not only providing care to the newborn but assisting in the integration of the baby into the family. Understanding of the newborn is optimized when information related to the mother and family is known. The information from the maternal history, which includes previous health issues, prenatal, intrapartum, and postpartum histories is critical for assessing adaptation to extrauterine life. This information gives insight into the environment from which the newborn has come and therefore helps determine the nurse's plan of care. Therefore, skills of assessment, analysis, planning, implementation, and evaluation of both mother and newborn are critical and must occur in synchrony for the nurse to assist the newborn's transition from birth to discharge. See Chapter 4 for a list of the components of a comprehensive maternal and neonatal history.

ADMISSION

Upon admission, the newborn infant is placed on a radiant warmer that provides warmth and an unobstructed view of the newborn infant. The admission nurse receives a comprehensive report from the labor and delivery nurse, which includes the maternal history and the delivery summary. Care of the infant is then assumed by the nursery nurse. Risk factors alerting the nurse for possible problems are identified, and a cursory visual assessment is done to assess for any signs of maladaption to extrauterine life.

Vital Signs

A complete physical assessment of the newborn is done on admission (see Chapter 4). Vital signs are taken during the initial physical assessment and are repeated periodically according to the institution's protocol. The vital signs include temperature, respiratory rate, heart rate, rhythm, the presence of thrills or murmur, and a four-point blood pressure (see Table 5.1).

The initial temperature gives the nurse a baseline from which to evaluate the thermoregulation ability of the newborn and is taken via the axillary route. The acceptable range of values are from 35.5°C to 37.5°C. The apical heart rate is counted for one full minute, and the acceptable range is from 100 to 160 beats per minute (bpm). The respiratory rate is also counted for one full minute, and the acceptable range of values is from 30 to 60 breaths per minute, although it is not uncommon to have respiratory rates as high as 80 to 100 breaths per minute within the first 20 minutes of life and most likely represents normal transition to extrauterine life. A four-point blood pressure is taken, and the acceptable range values are systolic 60 to 80 mmHg and diastolic from 40 to 50 mmHg. Pain is assessed as the fifth vital sign by using a pain scale (Raeside, 2011). Blood glucose should be obtained within the first 2 hours of life and after the first feeding in all newborns that are identified as high risk for the development of hypoglycemia or any newborn with signs and symptoms of hypoglycemia.

Medications

The administration of vitamin K is given as a prophylaxis for hemorrhagic disease of the newborn and is given by the intramuscular route using the vastus lateralis muscle.

As a prophylaxis against neonatal opthalmia due to organisms such as gonorrhea and chlamydia, erythromycin ointment is applied by placing a ribbon of medication into each eye from the inner to the outer canthus. This practice is mandated by state law and is required in all states (Mabry-Hernandez & Oliverio-Hoffman, 2010).

After signed consent at the parents' request, hepatitis B vaccine will be given intramuscularly. Hepatitis B is a serious viral disease that affects the liver. This virus is spread through contact with blood or other body fluids of an infected person. The vaccine can prevent hepatitis B and the serious complications associated with it that include liver cancer and cirrhosis. Routine hepatitis vaccination in

TABLE 5.1

NORMAL RANGE FOR VITAL SIGNS

Temperature	Respiratory Rate	Heart Rate	Blood Pressure Systolic	Blood Pressure Diastolic
35.5°C–37.5°C	30–60 breaths/min	100–160 beats/min	60–80 mmHg	40–50 mmHg

the United States began in 1991. Since then, the reported incidence of hepatitis B in children has dropped more than 95% and by 75% in all age groups (Centers for Disease Control and Prevention [CDC], 2007).

Measurements

Measurements of the newborn provide information for comparisons to normal growth curves and help the nurse identify potential risk factors. The newborn's length is measured from the crown of the head to the heel with the leg fully extended. The average newborn length is 50 cm. Head circumference is measured placing the tape measure around the fullest part of the occiput. The average head circumference is 35.5 cm. Chest circumference is measured using the nipple line as a reference point and crossing the lower border of the scapulae. The average chest circumference is 33 cm and is usually 2 to 3 cm smaller than the head. The abdominal circumference is measured at just above the umbilicus. All measurements are documented in the medical record. These measurements are plotted on a growth chart to determine if the newborn is small for gestation (SGA), appropriate for gestation (AGA), or large for gestation (LGA) (Kaneshiro, 2011).

The First Bath

The first bath is given after the newborn has achieved thermal and cardiorespiratory stability, which is usually 2 to 4 hours after birth. Prior to bathing, ensure that the bath equipment is disinfected and done before and after each use. The bath water should be approximately 38°C (100°F) and the room temperature should be between 26°C and 27°C (79°F–81°F) (Association of Women's Health, Obstetric and Neonatal Nurses [AWHONN], 2007). It is important to keep the duration of the bath to a minimum. A mild pH-neutral cleanser may be used to remove blood and amniotic fluid. Residual vernix does not have to be removed unless it is stained with blood or meconium. In that case gently remove the stained portion. Vernix has potential benefits that include: protection from infection, decreased skin permeability and decreased transepidermal water loss, moisturizing properties, pH development, and wound healing (AWHONN, 2007). Dry the newborn with prewarmed towels or blankets and place back on a preheated radiant warmer or in skin-to-skin contact with the mother if possible.

Cord Care

During the first bath clean the umbilical cord and surrounding skin to remove debris. Dry the cord with clean absorbent gauze and leave uncovered. Allow the cord to dry naturally. These means keep the umbilical cord area clean and dry without the routine use of topical agents. Keep the diaper folded down to leave the cord uncovered to help prevent contamination with urine and/or stool. The routine use of antimicrobial agents such as isopropyl alcohol, povidone-iodine, topical antibacterial agents, and triple dye is not recommended (AWHONN, 2007). If there is redness, swelling, or drainage, it may be a sign of infection and should be reported to the primary care provider.

SECURITY

Safety and security measures are important components of any environment that provides care to newborns. Institutions are required to have a safety and security system in place to ensure the infant's safety during their birth hospitalization. These systems also provide parents with the reassurance that their baby is safe, not only from internal threats, but from external ones as well.

Identification bracelets are placed at birth with a printed number on each of the bracelets, along with the identifying information of the mother, birth date, time, and gender. Typically two bracelets are placed on the baby: one on the wrist and one on the leg. Another bracelet is placed on the mother, and the fourth bracelet is placed on the father or significant other. Wearing the matching bracelet means that the person is allowed the privilege of receiving the baby from the nursery nurse or taking the baby from the nursery. These bracelets are also used to match the baby with mother every time the baby is brought to the room or taken from the nursery. This is an important policy that assures that the baby is always given to the correct mother.

Security sensors can be placed either on the umbilical cord via the cord clamp or on the leg with a strap. These sensors monitor the baby's location at all times and will send out a signal if the sensor passes too close to an open elevator or stairwell door. These tracking systems vary from institution to institution but are usually connected to the security systems of the hospital. Whenever the alarm is set off or activated, a "Code Pink" is broadcasted throughout the hospital and security personnel are deployed to that area of the hospital for follow-up. The security sensors are then removed prior to discharge.

An *ID Badge* with the health care employee's picture and name are now required by most institutions while the employee is on duty. Many institutions also use a color-coded badge to identify which health care workers are allowed to transport the baby from the mother's room to the newborn nursery and back. This safety measure is in place to assure that only qualified employees care for the newborn infants.

Passwords are used at many institutions as another form of security to identify employees who are allowed to transport newborns. These passwords are typically changed daily, and the parents will be given the new password at the beginning of the nursing shift. Parents are requested to ask anyone who attempts to take their baby out of their room for the password of the day. If the transporter cannot tell them the correct password for the day, the parents should call the newborn nursery for help before allowing the newborn to be taken.

Teaching the parents how to use the *bulb syringe* to clear oral or nasal secretions is an important aspect of the newborn nurse's initial visit, along with showing the parents how to use the *emergency call button*. Demonstrating how to use these two safety measures along with requesting the mother to repeat the demonstrations helps assure the newborn nurse that the baby is in a safe environment.

BACK TO SLEEP

Since 1994, when the National Institute of Child Health and Human Development along with America Academy of Pediatrics (AAP) launched the Back to Sleep campaign in an effort to reduce the risk of sudden infant death syndrome (SIDS), the U.S. SIDS rate has declined by an impressive 50%. However, the number of sleep-related infant deaths that are not attributed to SIDS has increased. Therefore, promoting a safe sleep environment has been emphasized to the general public which has led to the expanded Back to Sleep campaign scheduled to debut in 2012. The unsafe sleep environments contributing to the rise of infant deaths includes infants sleeping with their parents, co-bedding with siblings and sleeping on soft materials such as couches. A safe alternative is placing the baby on the back in a bassinet in the mother's or parent's room.

In the newborn nursery, infants are placed on their backs in the cribs, and this practice is taught to parents as a part of the initial safety teaching protocol. Studies show that parents take their cues from the nurses in the nursery regarding the handling and positioning of their infant. This role-modeling behavior of nurses is a critical way for information to be transferred to parents (Carrier, 2009). Teaching the parents about a safe sleep environment is important due to the direct correlation between increased infant mortality and where and how infants sleep (Ibarra & Goodstein, 2011).

DAILY CARE

The daily care of the newborn includes obtaining the weight every 24 hours and documenting the weight in the medical record. If the newborn has lost more than 7% of his or her birth weight, the primary care provider should be notified.

Vital signs are obtained and documented at every shift. Any abnormal value should be reported, and more frequent assessments of vital signs may be required.

Reviewing the intake and output is an important parameter to measure the nutritional status of the newborn. Many times this form is filled out by the parents and may require verification for any missing information.

The newborn should void within the first 24 hours of life and stool within the first 48 hours of life. If this does not occur, the primary care provider should be notified.

Lactation consults should be ordered for all breastfeeding mothers.

A physical examination is completed every shift and documented in the medical record. Any abnormalities should be reported to the primary care provider.

Discharge teaching begins at admission and continues throughout the birth hospitalization.

CIRCUMCISION

The issue of circumcision has long been debated as to its medical necessity, and the latest policy statement by the AAP in 1999 states "existing scientific evidence demonstrates potential benefits of newborn male circumcision; however, these data are not sufficient to recommend routine circumcision" (p. 686). While neonatal circumcision is cited as one of the most commonly performed procedures in the United States today (Ahmed & Ellsworth, 2012), it is a topic that health care providers must be able to discuss with their patients. Whether or not parents decide to have their male infants circumcised, the decision should be made only after appropriate counseling by their primary health care provider so that they may make an informed decision.

The nurse caring for the newborn who is to be circumcised must ensure that the proper consent form has been signed by the parent, assemble necessary equipment for the procedure, and then participate in the "time-out" surgical protocol before the care provider initiates the surgical procedure. Because circumcision is a painful procedure, pain management techniques must be implemented before, during, and after the procedure. Before the procedure, it is common for the care provider to order a topical analgesic cream which should be applied 20 to 30 minutes before the surgical procedure. Acetaminophen may also be ordered presurgery for pain control. During the procedure, the newborn is swaddled in blankets with only the groin area exposed while being strapped to the circumcision board. This swaddling provides for tactile comfort and warmth while being securely strapped to the board. Giving the newborn an oral sucrose solution along with nonnutritive sucking on either the nurse's finger or pacifier has also been shown to decrease the infant's pain during the circumcision (Hardcastle, 2010). Utilizing a dorsal penile block or ring block by the care provider in combination with the administration of sucrose provides the best pain relief for the newborn during circumcision (Razmus, Dalton, & Wilson, 2004). After the circumcision, it is important to monitor the newborn's pain response and treat with acetaminophen as necessary for the first 24 hours postprocedure. It is also imperative that the nurse monitor for bleeding at the site as well as preventing infection. Depending upon the type of circumcision device used, a petroleum jelly dressing should be applied to keep the wound from adhering to the diaper. This dressing should be changed after every void or stool to maintain cleanliness at the surgical site. Teaching the parents to care for the circumcised penis is important during hospitalization as well as in preparation for discharge. This should include cleansing the area with water at each diaper change, monitoring for signs and symptoms of infection, and refraining from tugging at the plastibell ring until it falls off on its own.

There are basically three types of circumcision devices used in the United States today: the Gomco or Yellen clamp, the plastibell, and the Mogen clamp. The type chosen by the care provider is usually determined by which device was in use during their medical training program. The most important factor is that the health care professional performing the procedure is familiar with the equipment or device he or she is using (Ellsworth, 2012). Whichever device is used, it is the nurse's responsibility to ensure that the equipment is sterile and in good working order and that appropriate sizes are available for use. "Clamps that are poorly serviced, fatigued from long use, or reassembled with mismatched components may break, slip, fall off during use, or fail to make a tight seal. The result can be excessive bleeding, lacerations or tears of the glans penis" (Swayze, 1999, p. 73).

NEONATAL THERMOREGULATION

Thermoregulation is the ability to balance heat production and heat loss in order to maintain normal body temperature. The infant loses heat by evaporation, convection, conduction, and radiation. Evaporation is heat loss that occurs by the evaporation of water from the skin and respiratory tract. Convection is heat loss from cooler surroundings such as the delivery room. Conduction is heat loss to cooler objects that are in direct contact with the infant such as a cold bed. In contrast with conduction, radiation is heat loss to cooler objects where there is no direct contact. Evaporation of amniotic fluid from the infant's skin in the delivery room is the main source of heat loss in the initial newborn period. Normal adaptation to extrauterine life requires minimizing all the mechanisms for heat loss. The goal of care is to maintain a neutral thermal environment for the infant in whom heat balance is maintained (Matthias et al., 2000).

Nonshivering Thermogenesis

A thermogenic response begins within the first few minutes of life. There are two mechanisms for heat production. First, there is an increase in cellular metabolic activity primarily in the brain, heart, and liver, and second, heat is produced by nonshivering thermogenesis (NST). NST is the primary source of heat production and is entirely dependent on brown adipose tissue. Brown adipose tissue is deposited after 28 weeks gestation and is primarily found around the scapulae, kidneys, adrenals, neck, and axilla. Heat is produced by uncoupling adenosine triphosphate synthesis via the oxidation of fatty acids in the mitochondria, utilizing uncoupled protein (Matthias et al., 2000). Brown fat has an increased vascular and nerve supply that other fats do not. Significant lipid metabolic activity in the brown fat can warm the infant by increasing heat production by 100%. Brown fat stores are usually present for several weeks after birth but are rapidly depleted in the presence of cold stress (McCall, Alderdice, Halliday, Jenkins, & Vohra, 2010).

Cold Stress

The presence of cold stress increases metabolic and physiologic demands on all infants. When an infant has cold stress, there is an increase in oxygen consumption and energy is shifted from maintaining normal function of vital organs to thermogenesis for survival. If adequate oxygen tension cannot be maintained there is vasoconstriction which can lead to increased pulmonary pressure. This causes a decrease in the partial pressure of arterial oxygen and blood pH. These changes may prevent the ductus arteriosus from closing and cause a right to left shunt. The basal metabolic rate also increases with cold stress and if it is prolonged it can lead to lactic acid production, which causes metabolic acidosis (McCall et al., 2010).

Management

In cases of mild hypothermia (36.0°C–36.4°C), the infant can be rewarmed by skin-to-skin contact in a warm room. This entails placing the infant with only a diaper on directly on the mother's bare chest and covering them both with a blanket with the infant's head exposed. With moderate hypothermia (32.0°C–35.9°C), the infant should be placed on a radiant warmer or a preheated isolette set at 35.0°C to 36.0°C. In cases of severe hypothermia (<32°C), the infant should be rewarmed on a radiant warmer over several hours. Feeding should be continued to provide calories and fluid to prevent hypoglycemia, which is common in infants experiencing hypothermia.

Hyperthermia

Hyperthermia is less common than hypothermia but does occur and needs to be corrected. Hyperthermia is defined as a body temperature greater than 37.5°C. The most common cause for hyperthermia is excess environmental heat. It is important to differentiate hyperthermia from fever which is a raised body temperature in response to infection and/or inflammation. Although it is not possible to distinguish between fever and hyperthermia based on the measurement of body temperature alone, infection should always be considered first. Assessment of the environmental factors such as the mode and temperature that the radiant warmer is set on and the number of blankets the infant is swaddled in is necessary. Steps should be taken to correct any environmental factors present. The clinical appearance of the infants often indicates the causative mechanism. Any signs and symptoms of infection should be reported to the health care provider.

GLUCOSE HOMEOSTASIS

The screening and management of hypoglycemia is based on identified risk factors that include late preterm infants born between 34 and 36 completed weeks of gestation, SGA, intrauterine growth restriction (IUGR), LGA, and infant of diabetic mother (IDM) of all types. An expert panel convened by the National Institutes of Health in 2008 concluded that there is not an evidenced-based definition for clinically significant neonatal hypoglycemia especially regarding how it relates to brain injury. Blood glucose concentrations as low as 30 mg/dL are common in healthy infants by 1 to 2 hours after birth and are usually transient, asymptomatic, and considered to be part of the normal adaptation to extrauterine life. Most infants will compensate for this physiologic hypoglycemia by producing alternate energy sources such as ketone bodies, which are released from fat. Clinically significant hypoglycemia on the other hand reflects an imbalance between the supply and use of glucose and alternative fuels (Adamkin, 2011).

Hypoglycemia is most common in infants that are SGA age, infants of diabetic mothers, and late preterm infants. It remains unclear if otherwise healthy infants that are LGA age are at risk for hypoglycemia because it is difficult to exclude maternal diabetes or maternal hyperglycemia with standard glucose-tolerance tests. Therefore screening should be reserved for at-risk infants, including SGA, IDM/LGA, and late preterm infants. Routine glucose screening is not necessary in healthy term newborns after a normal pregnancy and delivery. In any infant with signs and symptoms of hypoglycemia, blood glucose should be collected and sent to the lab as soon as possible. Breastfed infants have a lower concentration of serum glucose but a higher concentration of ketone bodies when compared to formula-fed infants. It is hypothesized that breastfed infants tolerate lower serum glucose concentrations without signs and symptoms because of the increased ketone levels (Adamkin, 2011).

Screening

Infants of mothers with diabetes may develop asymptomatic hypoglycemia as early as 1 hour after birth and up to 12 hours of age. While SGA or LGA infants may develop hypoglycemia as early as 3 hours of age, they may be at risk for up to 10 days. Because of this, decisions related to how often to obtain glucose levels need to be based on the infants' individual risk factors. Screening for the asymptomatic at risk infants should be performed within the first few hours of life and continue through several feedings. SGA infants should be fed every 2 to 3 hours and have their glucose checked prior to each feed for the first 24 hours. After that, if the glucose remains greater than 45 mg/dL, they may be discontinued. Due to the limitations of point of care monitoring, a blood or serum glucose must be confirmed by the laboratory. If there is a delay in processing the sample, it can give you a falsely low value due to the metabolism of glucose by the erythrocytes. Treatment of low point of care results should not be delayed while waiting on laboratory results (Adamkin, 2011).

Management

Signs and symptoms of hypoglycemia include jitteriness, cyanosis, seizures, apneic episodes, tachypnea, weak or high pitched cry, decreased tone, lethargy, poor feeding, and eye rolling. It is important to assess for underlying conditions such as sepsis. Coma and seizures may occur with prolonged and repetitive hypoglycemia, usually less than 10 mg/dL. Because of the risk of brain injury, special attention should be paid to neurologic signs and symptoms (Adamkin, 2011).

The recommendations shown in Figure 5.1 for the treatment of hypoglycemia are divided into two time periods that reflect the changing glucose levels within the first 12 hours of life. This algorithm provides a range of options for the treatment of hypoglycemia that include refeeding or giving intravenous glucose. The target glucose range is greater than or equal to 45 mg/dL prior to each feed. Infants that are at risk should be fed within the first hour of life and screened 30 minutes after the feeding. This recommendation is consistent with the World Health Organization (WHO). If the infant does not feed well, gavage feedings can be considered. LGA and infants of diabetic mothers should be screened prior to each feeding for 12 hours, with a goal of a glucose level greater than 40 mg/dL prior to each feed. SGA and late preterm infants should be screened for the first 24 hours. Glucose levels should be stable for a minimum of three feedings prior to discharge (Adamkin, 2011).

HYPERBILIRUBINEMIA

Jaundice is the most common clinical diagnosis affecting approximately 80% of all newborns in the United States (Bhutani, Vilms, & Hamerman-Johnson, 2010). Jaundice is caused by an elevation in unconjugated (indirect) and/or conjugated (direct) bilirubin levels. Bilirubin is an antioxidant in low levels and a potent neurotoxin in high levels. Elevations in bilirubin are either due to an increase in production (breakdown of heme containing proteins) and/or a delay in the elimination of bilirubin as well as the reabsorption of bilirubin through the enterohepatic pathway (Bhutani et al., 2010).

Seventy-five percent of bilirubin comes from the breakdown of red blood cells and 25% from ineffective erythropoiesis in the bone marrow and breakdown of tissue heme and heme proteins by the liver (Dennery, Seidman, & Stevenson, 2001). Heme is degraded by heme oxygenase, resulting in the release of iron and the formation of carbon monoxide and biliverdin. Biliverdin is then reduced to bilirubin by biliverdin reductase. The bilirubin that is formed is taken up by the liver bound to protein Y or ligandin and conjugated in the smooth endoplasmic reticulum with glucuronides to form bilirubin monoglucuronide in a reaction catalyzed by uridine dophosphate and monophosphate glucuronosyltransferase. The now water-soluble bilirubin glucuronide is excreted into the intestinal lumen to be eliminated in stool. The conjugated bilirubin can be deconjugated by the intestinal enzyme beta-glucuronidase and reabsorbed into circulation intestinal. This process is known as the enterohepatic pathway (Alkalay & Simmons, 2005; Bhutani et al., 2010; Dennery et al., 2001).

Physiologic Jaundice

Physiologic jaundice in the healthy term newborn follows a typical pattern and does not present within the first 24 hours of life. The average total serum bilirubin (TSB) usually peaks at 5 to 6 mg/dL on the third to fourth day of life, then declines over the first week of life. Bilirubin levels increase to 12 mg/dL in approximately 6.1% of healthy newborns and increase to 15 mg/dL in only 3% of healthy newborns (Bhutani et al., 2010; Blackwell, 2003). Factors that contribute to the development of hyperbilirubinemia include relative polycythemia, shortened erythrocyte life span, immature hepatic uptake and conjugation processes, and increased enterohepatic circulation. Additional risk factors that increase the risk of hyperbilirubinemia are having a previous sibling with jaundice, advanced maternal age, diabetics, first trimester bleeding, prematurity, male sex, and Asian, American Indian, and Greek ethnicity.

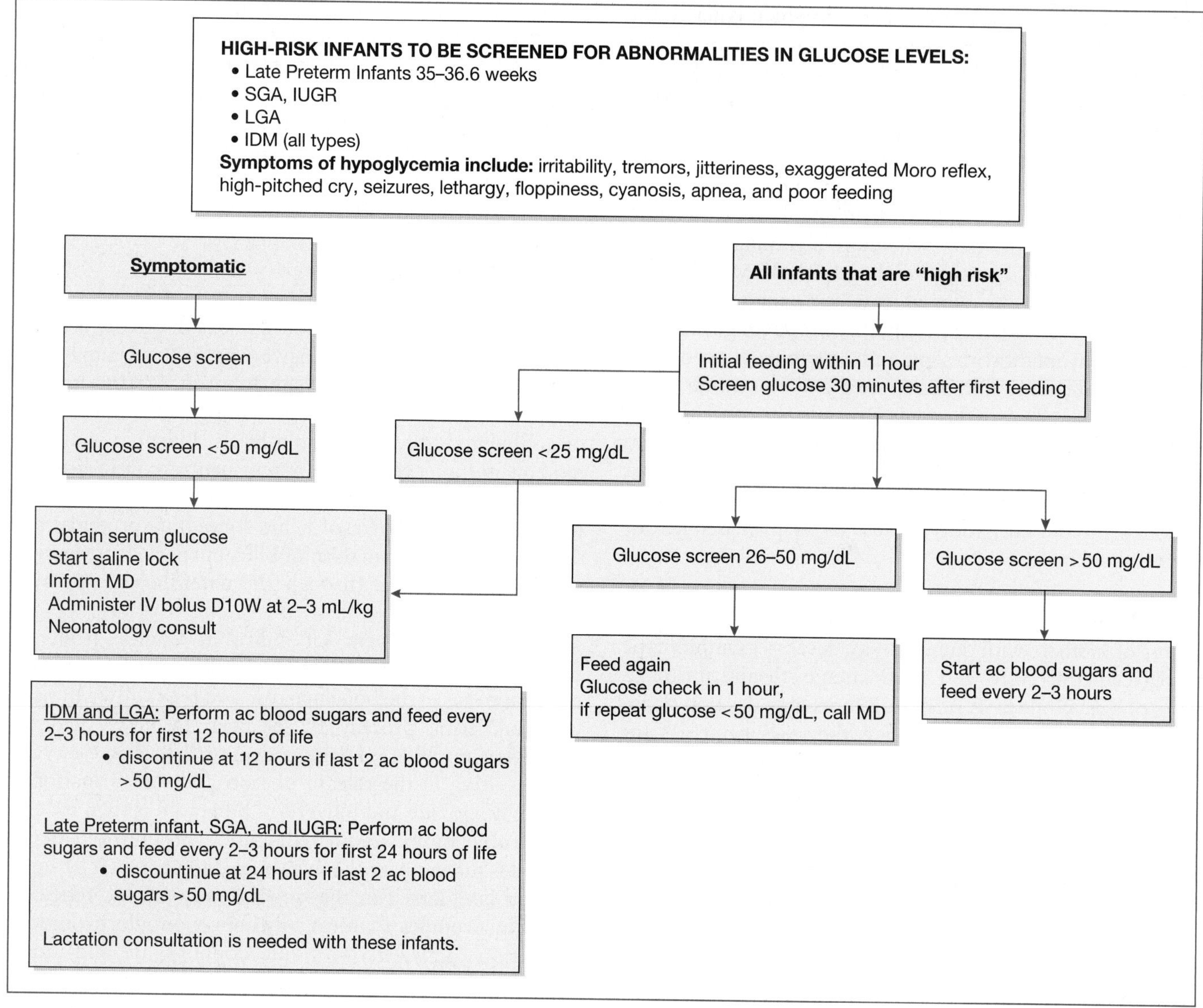

FIGURE 5.1 Screening and management of hypoglycemia.
From Adamkini (2011).

Breastfeeding Jaundice

Breastfed newborns may be at an increased risk for developing early-onset jaundice due to decreased volume and frequency of feeding which may result in mild dehydration and delayed passage of meconium. When compared to formula-fed newborns, breastfed newborns are 12% to 13% more likely to have peak serum bilirubin levels of 12 mg/dL. These newborns require frequent feeding, and mothers should be encouraged to breastfeed often. If there is significant (8%–10%) weight loss, decreased stooling, and decreased nutritional intake, supplementation with expressed breast milk or formula may be needed (Dennery et al., 2001).

Breast Milk Jaundice

Breast milk jaundice occurs later in the newborn period, and the incidence is 2% to 4% in term newborns. The bilirubin begins to rise around day of life 4 and continues to rise and may reach 20 mg/dL by day of life 14 and remain elevated for 2 weeks. The underlying cause of breast milk jaundice is unknown. The breast milk may have substances such as beta-glucuronidase and nonesterified fatty acids that may inhibit normal bilirubin metabolism. If breastfeeding is discontinued there will be a rapid decline in bilirubin within 48 hours, confirming the diagnosis. During this time it is important to encourage mothers to continue to pump their breast milk to enable continued breastfeeding. There is only a small increase in the bilirubin when breastfeeding is resumed. Mothers of newborns with breast milk jaundice have a 70% chance of this reoccurring with future pregnancies.

Pathologic Jaundice

Pathological jaundice in term infants is diagnosed if jaundice appears within the first 24 hours of life, after the first week of life, or lasts greater than 2 weeks. TSB that rises by greater than 5 mg/dL/d or TSB greater than 18 mg/dL is also considered pathologic. Term infants that show signs and symptoms of underlying illness need further evaluation. Some of the most common pathologic causes of pathologic jaundice are immune and nonimmune hemolytic anemia, G6PD deficiency, hematoma resorption, sepsis, and hypothyroidism (Alkalay & Simmons, 2005; Alkalay, Bresee, & Simmons, 2010). Approximately 5% to 11% of term infants will develop severe hyperbilirubinemia, which is defined as a TSB greater than the 95th percentile for age in hours and require phototherapy (Bhutani et al., 2010).

Acute Bilirubin Encephalopathy and Kernicterus

Acute bilirubin encephalopathy (ABE) and kernicterus is a preventable form of neonatal bilirubin-related brain injury. ABE is a clinical central nervous system finding that is caused by bilirubin toxicity to the basal ganglia and various brainstem nuclei that is seen in the first few weeks of life. In the early stage of ABE, the severely jaundiced infant will become lethargic and hypotonic and have a poor suck. The next stage is characterized by moderate stupor, irritability, and hypertonia. The infant may also develop a fever and/or a high-pitched cry that may alternate with hypotonia and drowsiness. The hypertonia may present with arching of the neck and trunk. There is evidence that an exchange transfusion at this stage can reverse the central nervous system changes. The advanced stage is characterized by probable permanent central nervous system damage, pronounced retrocollis-opisthotonos, shrill cry, inability to feed, apnea, fever, deep stupor to coma, seizures, and death (Alkalay & Simmons, 2005).

Kernicterus is the chronic form of ABE in surviving infants. It is characterized by some or all of the following: athetoid cerebral palsy, auditory dysfunction, dental-enamel dysplasia, paralysis of upward gaze, and occasional intellectual and other handicaps. The hallmark sign of kernicterus is the icteric staining of the basal ganglia, which is usually found at autopsy. Injury occurs when the TSB levels exceed the infant's neuroprotective defenses and results in neuronal damage. Risk factors for kernicterus are late preterm birth, plethora, hemolytic disease, and genetic abnormalities as well as complications from dehydration, sepsis, acidosis, poor feeding, and hypoalbuminemia (Bhutani et al., 2010).

Assessment

Assessment of hyperbilirubinemia should be done through diagnostic testing and screening and not by visual inspection alone. Screening tests for hyperbilirubinemia consist of assessing clinical risk factors and measuring bilirubin levels either by serum or transcutaneously (TcB), and plotting them on an age in hour specific bilirubin nomogram (see Figure 5.2). This range of TSB levels rather than one specific level provides the threshold for the onset of neurotoxicity. Predischarge assessment by either a TSB or TcB measurement that is plotted on an age in hour specific nomogram that identifies risk zones should be done on all infants. This provides a simple and accurate method of identifying the risk that a newborn will develop hyperbilirubinemia that requires treatment after discharge. The AAP (2004), Canadian Paediatric Society (2007), Joint Commission on Accreditation of Health Care Organizations (2004), and National Association of Neonatal Nurses (2011) recommend the following clinical practices:

- Successful breastfeeding should be promoted and supported to decrease the incidence of severe hyperbilirubinemia.

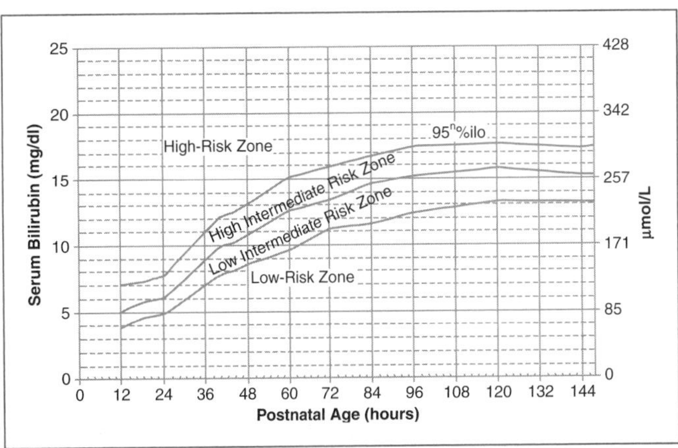

FIGURE 5.2 Homogram for designation of risk in 2,840 well newborns at 36 or more weeks gestational age with birth weight of 2,000 g or more or 35 or more weeks gestational age and birth weight of 2,500 g or more based on the hour-specific serum bilirubin values.
Adapted from Blackwell (2004).

- Nursery protocols for the identification and evaluation of hyperbilirubinemia should be established.
  - Hospitals should adapt facility-wide policies and procedures that maintain an adequate standard of care for all newborns in order to prevent ABE and kernicterus.
  - Bilirubin levels should be carefully monitored in infants found to be jaundiced in the first 24 hours of life.
  - Jaundice should be assessed regularly at least every 8 to 12 hours, and nurses should have independent authority to obtain a TSB or TcB level.
- Education for health care providers must emphasize that visual inspection is not reliable as the sole method for assessing jaundice.
- Bilirubin levels must be interpreted according to the infant's age in hours.
- Closer surveillance of infants with a gestational age of less than 38 weeks is necessary because of their higher risk for severe hyperbilirubinemia.
- All infants should be assessed for adequacy of breastfeeding and for the risk of severe hyperbilirubinemia before discharge. Universal discharge screening should be combined with an assessment of clinical risk factors (of which gestational age and exclusive breastfeeding are the most important) and a targeted follow-up.
- Parents should receive written and verbal information about jaundice.
- Follow-up care should be based on time of discharge and risk assessment.
- Phototherapy and exchange transfusion are to be used for treatment when indicated.
  - All nurseries should have the equipment to provide intensive phototherapy.
  - Breastfeeding should be encouraged for the infant receiving phototherapy or nutritional supplementation.
- Directive that bilirubin levels must be evaluated according to the infant's age in hours, not days.

- Underscoring of the increased risk of hyperbilirubinemia in infants less than 38 weeks gestation.
- Directive that risk assessment must be included in the evaluation of all newborns (Alkalay & Simmons, 2005; Bhutani et al., 2010).

Management

Phototherapy is used to decrease the TSB level and prevent the accumulation of bilirubin in the brain. The photoisomerization of bilirubin begins as soon as the light is turned on. The light causes the bilirubin molecules to undergo quick photochemical reactions that form nontoxic, excretable isomers. These isomers have different shapes when compared to the conjugated bilirubin. They can be excreted into the bile without conjugation or special transport carriers. This effective process has almost eliminated the need for exchange transfusions and is one of the most effective treatments to prevent severe hyperbilirubinemia (Stokowski, 2011).

Factors that affect the dose of phototherapy include the spectral qualities of the light source, the intensity of the light, the distance between the light and the infant, and the amount of surface area exposed. The blue, green, and turquoise lights are considered the most effective. With regard to the number of devices used, phototherapy can be ordered as single, double, triple, or quadruple. Fiberoptic blankets may also be used. The pad containing fiberoptic fibers can be placed against the skin and remains cool. Due to the spectral power of the pad alone, it is commonly used in combination with overhead lights (Stokowski, 2011).

Opaque eye shields are required during phototherapy to protect the eyes from retinal damage. During the assessment of the infant, the phototherapy lights should be turned off and the eye shields removed to assess the eyes for drainage, edema, and redness. Complications of eye shields include eye irritation, corneal abrasion, blocked tear ducts, and conjunctivitis. Eye care is important and should include cleaning the eyes with sterile water or saline. A separate cleaning pad should be used for each eye and should be cleaned from the inner canthus outward. Sterile gloves should be worn while providing eye care. Some phototherapy units produce heat, and the infant's temperature must be monitored to avoid overheating. Phototherapy can also cause diarrhea and water loss in stools. It is important to monitor for skin breakdown in the perianal area and use protective barriers if needed (Stokowski, 2011).

During phototherapy, the infant is separated from the mother and has the potential to interfere with lactation. As long as the hyperbilirubinemia is not severe, the phototherapy can be interrupted to allow for breastfeeding and skin-to-skin care. Eye shields can be removed during this time (Stokowski, 2011).

FEEDING THE HEALTHY NEWBORN

Human milk provides optimal nutrition for infants. The AAP *Policy Statement on Breastfeeding and the Use of Human Milk* (Eidelman & Schanler, 2012) recommends exclusive breastfeeding for 6 months and continued breastfeeding through the first year of life with the introduction of solids foods. Breastfeeding beyond 1 year of age is also supported if mother and baby so desire. The existing empirical evidence regarding the effects of breastfeeding on the health of infants and mothers was evaluated and synthesized in the meta-analysis by Ip et al. (2007) for the Agency for Health Care Research and Quality. Breastfeeding was found to be associated with:

- A significant reduction in acute otitis media, atopic dermatitis, gastrointestinal infection, lower respiratory infection, asthma, acute lymphocytic leukemia, acute myelogenous leukemia, and SIDS
- A decreased incidence of necrotizing enterocolitis in preterm infants
- Likelihood of fewer occurrences of obesity and type 2 diabetes later in life
- A reduced maternal risk for type 2 diabetes and breast and ovarian cancers (Ip et al., 2007)

Bartick and Reinhold (2010) conducted a breastfeeding cost analysis related to the following pediatric diseases: necrotizing enterocolitis, otitis media, gastroenteritis, hospitalization for lower respiratory tract infections, atopic dermatitis, SIDS, childhood asthma, childhood leukemia, type 1 diabetes, and childhood obesity. The authors calculated a $13 billion per year savings in health care costs if 90% of mothers would breastfeed their infants exclusively for 6 months.

All health care professionals who provide care to women of childbearing age and their children have an obligation to recommend, promote, and educate women and their support persons about breastfeeding. In 1991 the WHO and United Nations Children's Fund (UNICEF) created the Baby Friendly Hospital Initiative to offer recognition to hospitals and birthing centers worldwide that provide the optimal environments for breastfeeding initiation. Hospitals and birthing centers can receive the Baby Friendly designation when they fully implement and demonstrate the *Ten Steps to Successful Breastfeeding for Hospitals* as outlined by WHO/UNICEF (Table 5.2). As of March 2012 over 19,000 hospitals and birthing centers worldwide have achieved Baby Friendly designation. In the United States 140 hospitals and birthing centers are currently designated Baby Friendly (Baby-Friendly USA, 2012).

NURSING INTERVENTIONS THAT PROMOTE SUCCESSFUL BREASTFEEDING

Skin-to-Skin

Providing the optimal breastfeeding environment begins at birth. The healthy, stable newborn should be placed directly on the mother's bare chest immediately after birth. Initial nursing interventions after birth including drying the infant, initial assessment, and Apgar scoring should occur while baby is skin-to-skin with the mother. Nursing interventions including birth weight, vitamin K, and ophthalmic antibiotic administration should be delayed to allow at least 1 hour of uninterrupted skin-to-skin contact and breastfeeding

TABLE 5.2

WHO/UNICEF BABY-FRIENDLY HOSPITAL INITIATIVE

Ten Steps to Successful Breastfeeding for Hospitals in the United States
1. Have a written breastfeeding policy that is routinely communicated to all health care staff.
2. Train all health care staff in skills necessary to implement this policy.
3. Inform all pregnant women about the benefits and management of breastfeeding.
4. Help mothers initiate breastfeeding within 1 hour of birth.
5. Show mothers how to breastfeed and how to maintain lactation, even if they are separated from their infants.
6. Give newborn infants no food or drink other than breast milk, unless *medically* indicated.
7. Practice "rooming in"—allow mothers and infants to remain together 24 hours a day.
8. Encourage breastfeeding on demand.
9. Give no pacifiers or artificial nipples to breastfeeding infants.
10. Foster the establishment of breastfeeding support groups and refer mothers to them on discharge from the hospital or clinic.

attempts. Nurses should remain with the mother during this time and assist with breastfeeding positioning and latch. Berg and Hung (2011) demonstrated through a quality improvement project that skin-to-skin in the operating room after a cesarean can safely occur and promote exclusive breastfeeding.

The 2009 Cochrane review regarding early skin-to-skin contact of mothers and healthy infants revealed empirical evidence that early and frequent skin-to-skin contact "reduces crying, improves mother-baby interaction, keeps the baby warmer, and helps women breastfeed successfully" (Moore, Anderson, & Bergman, 2009, p. 2). Earlier onset of lactogenesis II (milk production) and increased milk production as a result of frequent skin-to-skin are also suggested in the literature (Chen, Nommsen-Rivers, Dewey, & Lonnerdal, 1998; De Carvalho, Klaus, & Merkatz, 1982). Frequent skin-to-skin contact between mother and baby should be encouraged throughout the postpartum hospital stay and after discharge to home. Infants should be undressed (diaper only) and placed directly on the mother's bare chest. Mother and baby should then be covered with a blanket with the infant's head exposed.

Maternal–Infant Separation Only When Medically Necessary

Health care professionals should recommend 10 to 12 feedings at breast per 24-hour period in the first 3 to 5 days after birth. Milk production is the result of lactogenesis I and II. Lactogenesis I begins around the 10th to 22nd week of pregnancy and is hormonally mediated. During lactogenesis I growth of glandular tissue occurs, and the mammary secretory cells, lactocytes, are formed. Lactogenesis II, the onset of milk production, begins with the separation of the placenta from the uterus at birth, which results in a drop in mother's serum progesterone. Lactogenesis II is dependent on frequent suckling at the breast. When the infant suckles at the breast, prolactin is released from the mother's anterior pituitary gland, and oxytocin is released from the posterior pituitary gland. Prolactin is responsible for milk production in the mammary gland, and oxytocin is responsible for the milk ejection reflex, which allows the release of the milk from the mammary gland to the milk ducts (Riordan & Wambach, 2010).

The more time the infant is separated from the mother in the hospital, the less opportunity for breastfeeding occurs. In the first few days after birth, several attempts at latching at the breast may be necessary before a good sustained latch is achieved; therefore, mothers need uninterrupted time together with their infants to learn to identify hunger cues and have adequate practice and assistance with breastfeeding. Parents need to be educated in the identification of their infant's hunger cues and to offer the breast when the infant expresses early rather than late hunger cues. Early hunger cues include movement of arms and legs, rooting, lip smacking, and fingers or fist to mouth movement. Early hunger cues may occur while the infant is in a light sleep state with eyes closed. Later hunger cues include restlessness, intermittent or full cry, and inconsolable screaming (Riordan & Wambach, 2010).

Mothers should be encouraged to room in (keep their infants with them continuously through the day and night) to promote quicker response to hunger cues and identification of infant needs. Infant assessments by all providers can and should occur in the mother's hospital room rather than in the nursery. Increased maternal sleep or perceived rest has not been substantiated in the literature when infants are separated from the mother or sent to the nursery (Keefe, 1987, 1988; Doan, Gardiner, Gay & Lee, 2007; Waldenström & Swenson, 1991). The breastfeeding mother–infant dyad should only be separated when medically necessary.

Pacifier Use

Pacifier use in the healthy term breastfed infant is a somewhat controversial topic. Pacifier use has been associated with shorter breastfeeding duration (Howard et al., 2003; Nelson, Yu, & Williams, 2005) and decreased exclusive breastfeeding (Vogel, Hutchison, & Mitchell, 2001). Long-term pacifier use beyond 6 months of age has been associated with increased risk of otitis media (Niemelä, Pihakari, Pokka,

& Uhari, 2000) and dental malocclusion (Peres, Barros, Peres, & Victora, 2007). As a result, WHO and UNICEF through the *Ten Steps to Successful Breastfeeding* recommend no use of pacifiers in breastfeeding infants.

However, the AAP has identified pacifier usage to potentially decrease the incidence of SIDS (Hauck, Omojokun, & Siadaty, 2005; Li et al., 2006) and serve as a method of effective pain control in combination with sucrose for infants undergoing painful procedures, for example, heel sticks or circumcision (Stevens, Yamada, & Ohlsson, 2010). The specific recommendations of the AAP regarding pacifier use and breastfeeding infants are to avoid pacifier use in the neonatal period until breastfeeding is well established. The AAP encourages pacifier use in infants undergoing painful procedures and during nap and sleep times as a potential protection against SIDS (Eidelman & Schanler, 2012). One further recommendation is to discourage the use of pacifiers to rule out hunger or delay a feeding; breastfeeding should occur before offering a pacifier. Parents must be educated on all the risks and benefits of pacifier use in the breastfed infant so they can make an informed decision that best suits their needs and parenting philosophy.

Adequacy of Breastfeeding

The three main indicators of adequate breastmilk transfer are audible swallowing by the infant, adequate urine and stool output, and weight gain. All health care professionals who care for breastfeeding mother–infant dyads in the neonatal period must demonstrate competence in assessing an adequate transfer of breastmilk. At least one complete breastfeed from latch to satiety should be observed, preferably once per shift after birth, but at least once before discharge. Mothers need education on positioning the infant during breastfeeding and how to achieve a deep latch. The football hold, cross-cradle hold, and the side-lying position are common ways to hold the infant to promote a deep latch. The mother should be taught to support the infant's head with one hand and her breast with the other hand during latching. The mother should hold her breast so that her fingers do not cover her areola. The mother should be taught to hand-express drops of breastmilk from her nipple and place on the infant's lips to entice a wide mouth gape. Once the infant has a wide mouth gape he should be brought quickly to the breast. The infant needs to feel the nipple on his palate to elicit the sucking reflex. The infant should take in most of the mother's areola, and lips should be flanged on the breast.

Once latched and sucking, the health care provider should listen for audible swallowing by the infant. In the first few days of breastfeeding the infant will take 5 to 10 sucks before a swallow will be heard as a soft "k" sound. As the mother's milk begins to come in, swallowing will become more frequent and more audible. An adequate breastfeed is sustained sucking and swallowing for at least 10 to 15 minutes on at least one breast. If the infant detaches from the first breast, the mother can continue feeding on the other breast. Encourage the mother to alternate which breast she starts on with each feeding. Length of feedings in minutes is a less important measure of adequate breastfeeding than sustained audible swallowing followed by signs of satiety, including slowing of sucking, falling asleep, and self-detaching (Riordan & Wambach, 2010). Several breastfeeding assessment tools have been developed and tested in an effort to measure the adequacy of breastfeeding in the early days after birth. The LATCH assessment tool by Jensen, Wallace, and Kelsay (1994) is one such tool that evaluates five different indicators of breastfeeding adequacy (Table 5.3). Each assessment is scored from 0 to 10, with a

TABLE 5.3

LATCH BREASTFEEDING ASSESSMENT TOOL

	0	1	2
Latch	Too sleepy or reluctant No latch achieved	Repeated attempts Hold nipple in mouth Stimulate suck	Grasps breast Tongue down Lips flanged Rhythmic sucking
Audible swallowing	None	A few with stimulation	Spontaneous and intermittent less than 24 hours old Spontaneous and frequent more than 24 hours old
Type of nipple	Inverted	Flat	Everted (with stimulation)
Comfort of mother	Engorged Cracked/bleeding/large blisters or bruises Severe discomfort	Filling Reddened/small blisters or bruises Mild/moderate discomfort	Soft Nontender
Hold or positioning	Full assist (staff holds infant at breast)	Minimal assist Teach one side; mother does other Staff holds and then mother takes over	No assist from staff Mother able to position/hold infant

From Jensen et al. (1994).

higher score indicating adequate latch and transfer of milk as well as relative comfort of the mother.

The second indicator of adequate breastfeeding is the amount of urine and stool output. Breastfed infants should have one wet diaper the first day of life and increase by one wet diaper for each day of life up to five to six wet diapers per day. Diapers should feel heavier when wet rather than just damp. The urine should be light in color and have slight to no odor. It is normal for breastfed neonates to have reddish colored urine in the first few days of life and is not an indicator of dehydration (Kernerman & Newman, 2009). Neonates should have at least one stool on the first and second days of life that is green to black and a tarry consistency. By the third and fourth day of life, the neonate should have one to three stools per day that begin to change to a green looser stool as the mother's milk begins to come in. By the fourth to seventh days of life, the neonate should have one to four stools per day that are yellow, loose, and seedy in consistency. By the end of the second week of life, the neonate should have three to five stools per day that are the same consistency, but the volume of the stool will increase as the volume of milk intake from the mother increases. It can be normal for infants to have no stool on an occasional day (Riordan & Wambach, 2010). If a neonate does not have adequate output as described above, the health care professional should assess a breastfeeding for adequate transfer of milk and frequency of breastfeedings, and assess the neonate for jaundice and signs and symptoms of dehydration. Health care professionals should refer mothers to a lactation consultant for breastfeeding difficulties.

The third indicator of adequate breastfeeding is weight gain. Some weight loss is expected in the healthy term neonate. A weight loss up to 5% of birth weight in the first 3 days is considered normal and can be partially attributed to evaporative loss after birth. At 7% weight loss, the health care provider should assess breastfeeding as described above and also assess urine and stool output. A neonate with a greater than 7% weight loss who is having adequate breastfeeding and output could have been fluid overloaded as a result of large quantities of intravenous fluids given to the mother during labor (Lawrence, 2010). If a 10% weight loss occurs in the first 3 days of life, intervention is necessary to assist the mother's body with lactogenesis II and to assist the baby in adequate transfer of milk. Mothers should be educated and encouraged to pump both breasts after a feeding with a hospital-grade breast pump for 10 to 15 minutes at least eight times per day. This will provide extra stimulation and assist with onset of milk. The mother should feed any expressed breastmilk to the baby via cup, finger feeding, or at breast. If the mother is unable to pump adequate volumes of breastmilk, the neonate's urine and stool output is not adequate, and the baby is unable to consistently transfer milk from the breast, then supplementation with formula may be necessary. Formula supplementation in the first 24 to 48 hours after birth should be limited to 10 to 15 mL per feeding given after a breastfeeding attempt (Riordan & Wambach, 2010). At greater than 48 hours of birth, formula supplementation should be limited to 30 mL per feeding and should be given after breastfeeding attempts. Supplementation should only continue until mother's milk is established.

Breastfeeding Follow-Up After Discharge

Breastfed neonates should be seen by a health care provider within 3 to 5 days after discharge from the hospital stay to assess breastfeeding adequacy, the onset of mother's milk, presence of jaundice or elevated bilirubin levels, and weight gain. Neonates with weight loss should gain back to birth weight by 14 days of age. Breastfeeding should be assessed at all subsequent infant health care provider visits to include not only the baby's health and growth, but also the mother's support systems and motivation to continue breastfeeding. Exclusive breastfeeding should be encouraged and promoted throughout the infant's first year of life and beyond if mother and infant desire, and formula supplementation should be avoided unless medically indicated.

Formula Feeding

If a mother chooses not to breastfeed or breastfeeding is contraindicated (maternal infection with HIV, active TB, human T-cell lymphotrophic virus, untreated brucellosis, or treatment with chemotherapeutic agents) and banked milk is not available or feasible, then formula feeding is the most available alternative (Eidelman & Schanler, 2012). Commercially prepared cow's milk-based formulas are all relatively similar in their composition of nutrients, vitamins, minerals, proteins, carbohydrates, and fat. Three other types of formula are soy-based formulas, casein or whey-hydrolysate formulas, and amino acid formulas. Soy formulas are generally recommended to mothers whose infants have a cow's milk intolerance, galactosemia, and heredity lactase deficiency. Casein or whey-hydrolysate formulas are recommended to children who cannot tolerate cow's milk or soy-based formulas.

Formulas come in many forms and concentrations, for example, concentrate, ready to feed, or powder. Parents and caregivers need to be educated on how to prepare the formula correctly according to product package instructions. Improperly prepared formula can lead to infant malnutrition, electrolyte imbalance, and even death (Walker, 1993). Formula or breast milk should never be heated in a microwave because of uneven heating and the potential for burns. Energy requirements for normal growth and activity of infants is ~108 kcal/kg/d from birth to 6 months of age and ~98 kcal/kg/d from 6 months to 12 months of age (Kleinman, 2008). Newborns receiving formula should be fed 1 to 2 ounces per feeding every 3 to 4 hours for the first week, and advance to 2 to 4 ounces per feeding around 1 week of age. A general volume recommendation is 2.5 ounces per pound, per day. For example, a 10-pound baby would receive 25 ounces of formula per day divided into approximately six to eight feedings (every 3–4 hours) of 3 to 4 ounces per bottle (Blum-Kemelor & Leonberg, 2009). Prepared formula cannot sit at room temperature for more than 2 hours. After 2 hours at room temperature bacteria growth begins to proliferate (WHO, 2007). Any formula that the baby does not consume from a bottle should be thrown away and not refrigerated. Prepared formula can be refrigerated for 24 hours prior to consumption.

DISCHARGE SCREENING

Hearing Screening

Hearing loss is one of the most common congenital anomalies, occurring in approximately 2 to 4 infants per 1,000 (Delaney et al., 2012). Prior to implementation of universal newborn screening (NBS), testing was only done on infants who met the criteria of the high-risk register. Unfortunately, about 50% of infants born with hearing loss have no known risk factors (Delaney et al., 2012).

The ability to hear during the first few years of life is critical for the development of speech, language, and cognition. Early identification and intervention can prevent severe psychosocial, educational, and linguistic repercussions. Infants who are not identified as having hearing loss by 6 months of age will likely have delays in speech and language development. Intervention at or before 6 months of age promotes the ability of a child with hearing loss to develop normal speech and language development (Delaney et al., 2012).

The two methods used in most universal hearing-screening programs are the otoacoustic emissions (OAEs) and automated auditory brainstem response (AABR). OAEs are used to assess cochlear integrity and are physiologic measurements of the response of the outer hair cells to acoustic stimuli. When using the OAE method, a probe is placed in the ear canal and click stimuli are delivered causing the OAEs to be generated by the cochlea, which is then measured with a microphone (Delaney et al., 2012). The presence of the OAE responses indicates that hearing is in the normal to near-normal range.

AABR is an electrophysiologic measurement that is used to assess auditory function from the eighth nerve through the auditory brainstem (Delaney et al., 2012). This method is done by placing disposable electrodes high on the forehead, on the mastoid, and on the nape of the neck. The click stimulus is delivered to the infant's ear with small disposable earphones. Most AABR systems compare an infant's waveform with a control that was developed from normal ABR infant data (Delaney et al., 2012). A pass or fail response is determined from this comparison. Infants who do not pass the universal hearing screening at birth should have follow-up testing within 1 month. This follow-up appointment allows for additional testing and medical diagnosis.

Newborn Screening

NBS tests the newborn for many hormonal, genetic, and metabolic disorders. This screening is done with a simple blood test and allows for early detection of preventable life-threatening disorders. There are 30 disorders that have been identified for routine screening. Current standards are determined at the state level, and most states screen for the majority of the recommended disorders, though there is some variation from state to state on the specific disorders tested (National Newborn Screening and Genetic Resource Center, 2009).

Without proper screening and treatment infants and children can suffer mental retardation, physical disability, or even death. With early treatment shortly after birth, many affected infants and children can lead normal healthy lives (AWHONN, 2011). There is a need for the development of national standards to ensure that all states are screening for all of the recommended disorders.

In April 2008, the Newborn Screening Saves Lives Act (Public Law 110 to 204, 2008) was signed into law, but this law recommends rather than mandates states to increase the number of disorders they test for.

In 1999, the AAP developed a task force that recommended greater uniformity among states. In response, the American College of Medical Genetics issued guidelines for state NBS programs that recommended all states test for a core panel of 29 disorders (AAP, 2008). Then, in 2010, the Advisory Committee for Heritable Disorders in Newborns and Children agreed to include the Severe Combined Immunodeficiency in the panel (AWHONN, 2011). The following is a complete list of the disorders:

Organic acid metabolism disorders

- Isovaleric acidemia
- Glutaric acidemia
- 3-OH 3-CH3 glutaric aciduria
- Multiple carboxylase deficiency
- Methylmalonic acidemia due to mutase deficiency
- Methylmalonic acidemia (Cbl A, B)
- 3-methylcrotonly-CoA carboxylase deficiency
- Propionic acidemia
- Beta-ketothiolase deficiency

Fatty acid oxidation disorders

- Medium-chain acyl-CoA dehydrogenase
- Very-long-chain acyl-CoA dehydrogenase deficiency
- Long-chain L-3-OH acyl-CoA dehydrogenase deficiency
- Trifunctional protein deficiency
- Carnitine uptake defect

Amino acid metabolism disorders

- Phenylketonuria
- Maple syrup urine disease
- Homocystinuria due to cystathionine beta synthase (CBS) deficiency
- Citrullinemia
- Argininosuccinic acidemia
- Tyrosinemia type 1

Hemoglobinopathies

- Sickle cell anemia (Hb SS)
- Hemoglobin S/beta-thalassemia (Hb S/Th)
- Hemoglobin S/C (Hb S/C)

Others

- Congenital hypothyroidism
- Biotinidase deficiency
- Congenital adrenal hyperplasia due to 21-hydroxylase deficiency
- Classic galactosemia
- Hearing loss
- Cystic fibrosis
- Severe combined immunodeficiency

March of Dimes Foundation (2012) developed a recommendation for all states to test for these 30 conditions, grouping them into five categories:

- Amino acid metabolism disorders
- Organic acid metabolism disorders
- Fatty acid oxidation disorders
- Hemoglobinopathies
- Others, please see http://www.milesforbabies.org/professionals/14332_15455.asp for more specific information

All states collect blood samples from newborns during their birth hospitalization; these samples are usually referred to as blood spots (see Figure 5.3). Some states discard the blood samples when the NBS is complete, and others store

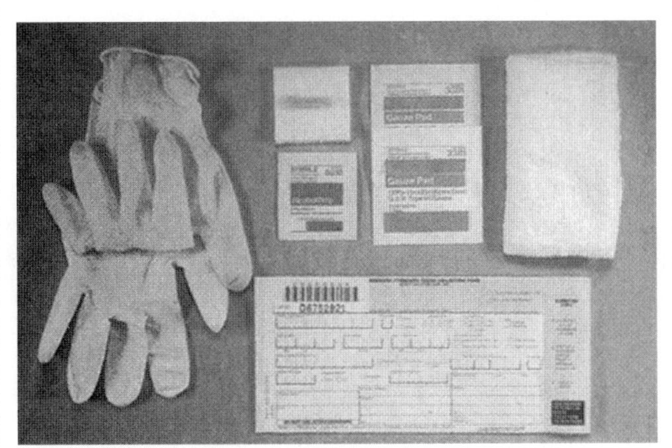

FIGURE 5.3 Newborn screen blood specimen collection and handling procedure.

1. Equipment: sterile lancet with tip less than 2.4 mm, sterile alcohol prep, sterile gauze pads, soft cloth, blood collection form, gloves.

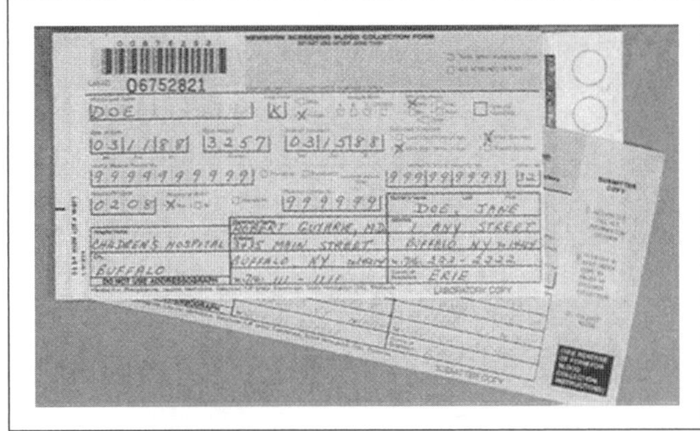

2. Complete *all* information. Do not contaminate filter paper circles by allowing the circles to come in contact with spillage or by touching before or after blood collection.

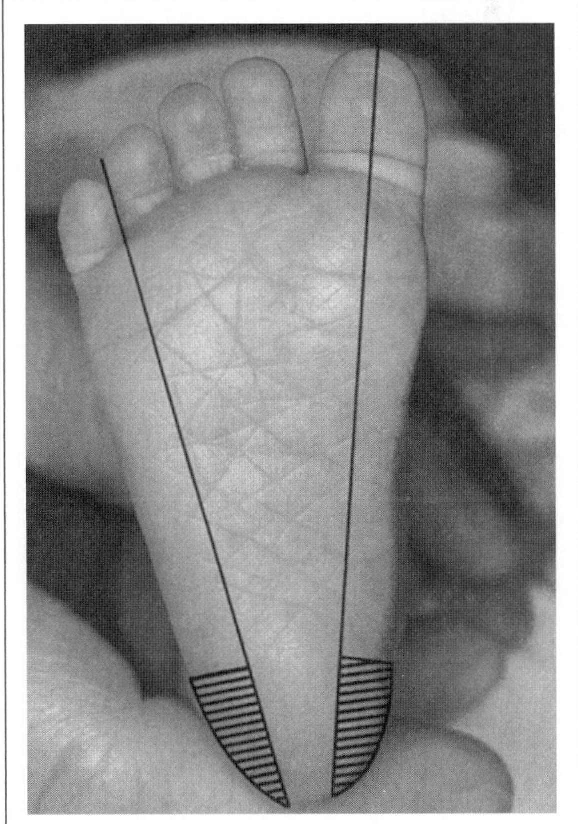

3. Hatched area indicates safe areas for puncture site.

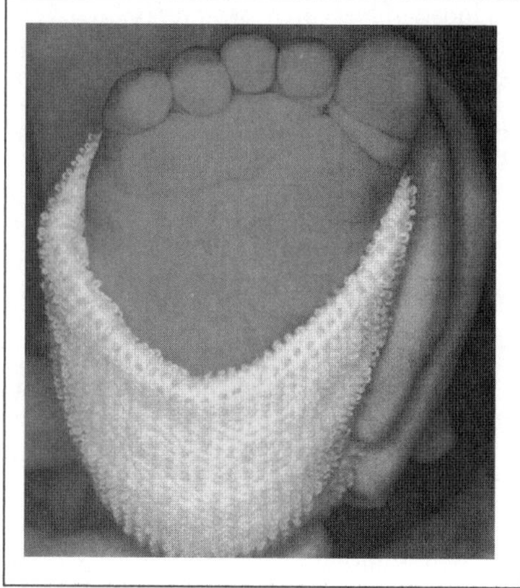

4. Warm site with soft cloth, moistened with warm water or a heel warmer for 3 to 5 minutes.

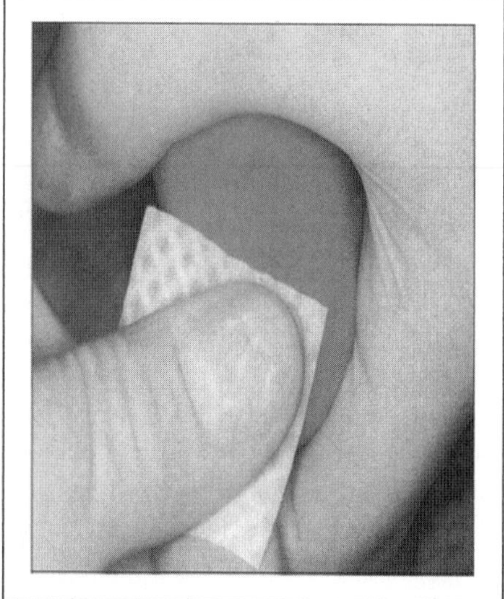

5. Cleanse site with alcohol prep. Wipe *dry* with sterile gauze pad.

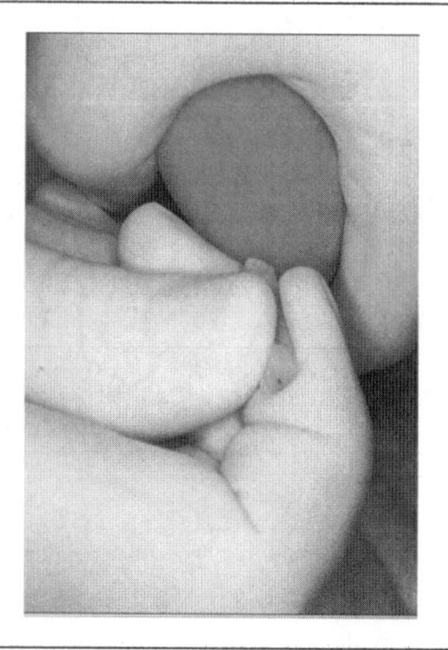

6. Puncture heel. Wipe away first blood drop with sterile gauze pad. Allow another *large* blood drop to form.

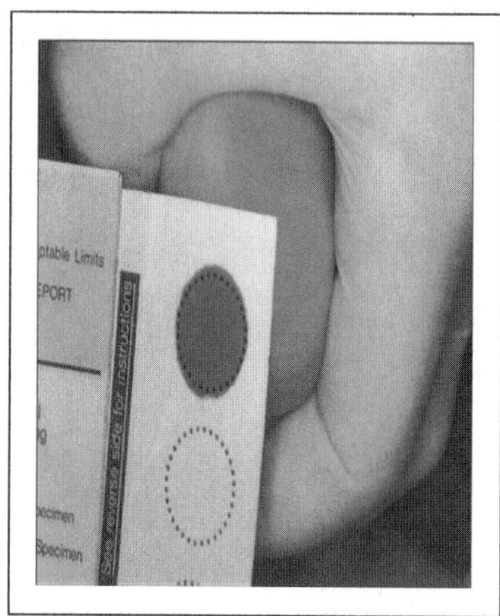

7. Lightly touch filter paper to *large* blood drop. Allow blood to soak through and completely fill circle with *single* application to *large* blood drop. (To enhance blood flow, *very gentle* intermittent pressure may be applied to area surrounding puncture site.) Apply blood to one side of filter paper only.

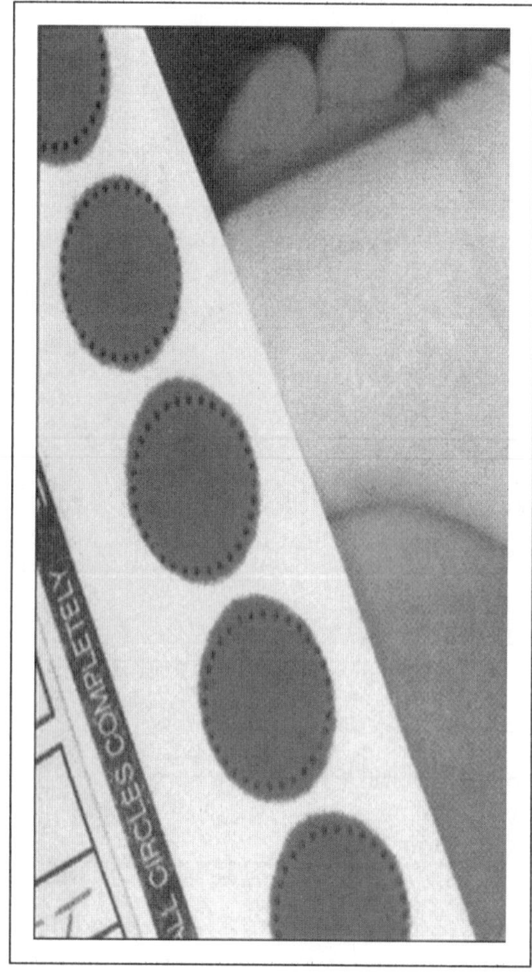

8. Fill remaining circles in the same manner as in step 7, with successive blood drops. If blood flow is diminished, repeat steps 5 through 7. Care of skin puncture site should be consistent with your institution's procedures.

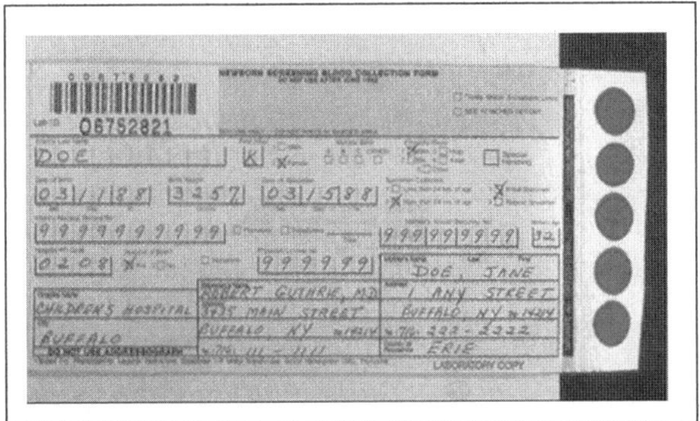

9. Dry blood spots on a dry, clean, flat nonabsorbent surface for a minimum of 4 hours.

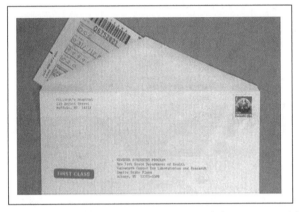

10. Mail completed form to testing laboratory within 24 hours of collection.

the blood spots for future research. Genetic privacy, parental consent, and security must be incorporated into any blood storage system and there needs to be a mechanism in place that addresses parent's rights with regard to storage and future uses with the blood spots (AWHONN, 2011).

EMERGING SCREENING

Pulse oximetry screening (POS) of the newborn for critical congenital heart disease is an effective, noninvasive, and inexpensive tool that is beneficial in detecting critical congenital heart disease (cCHD) in newborns (Riede et al., 2010). Congenital heart defects are the most common serious birth defect, affecting approximately 8 of every 1,000 newborns, and cCHDs affect 2 to 3 per 1,000 live births. The seven defects classified as critical congenital heart defects (cCHDs) are hypoplastic left heart syndrome, pulmonary atresia (with intact septum), tetralogy of Fallot, total anomalous pulmonary venous return, transposition of the great arteries, tricuspid atresia, and truncus arteriosus. Babies with one of these cCHDs are at significant risk for death or disability if their heart defect is not diagnosed and treated soon after birth. These seven cCHDs potentially can be detected using POS, which is a test to determine the amount of oxygen in the blood and pulse rate. Certain hospitals routinely screen all newborns using POS. However, POS is not currently included in NBS in most states (CDC, 2012). Prenatal ultrasound and physical examination alone can miss cCHDs because symptoms may not appear until after discharge when the ductus arteriousus closes. Heart murmurs may be absent or misleading due to underlying anatomy, prolonged decline of pulmonary vascular resistance, or reduced ventricular function (Riede et al., 2010). Diagnosis may be further complicated by trends to discharge early. It has been estimated that at least 280 infants with an unrecognized cCHD are discharged each year from newborn nurseries in the United States (CDC, 2012). These babies are at risk for having serious problems within the first few days or weeks of life and often require emergency care.

The first signs of acute cCHD may be circulatory collapse requiring the need for cardiopulmonary resuscitation or death. Delays in diagnosis have been associated with significant morbidity and mortality. The current incidence of serious compromise resulting for undiagnosed cCHD has been estimated to be 1 per 15,000 to 1 per 26,000 live births (Riede et al., 2010). These data have led to a broad consensus that screening for cCHD is warranted.

Pulse oximetry can detect mild hypoxemia, which is a sign for many types of cCHD that may not be recognized by physical examination. This was first reported in 1995, and since then many studies have shown that screening with pulse oximetry is an effective tool for the detection of cCHD (Riede et al., 2010). Once identified, babies with a cCHD can be seen by cardiologists and can receive specialized care and treatment that could prevent death or disability early in life. Treatment can include medications and/or surgery.

When to Screen

Screening is done when a baby is 24 to 48 hours of age. If the baby is to be discharged from the hospital before he or she is 24 hours of age, screening should be done as late as possible before discharge. If the results are "negative" (in-range result), it means that the baby's test results did not show signs of a cCHD. This type of screening test does not detect all cCHDs, so it is possible to still have a critical or other heart defect with a negative screening result. If the results are "positive" (out-of-range result), it means that the baby's test results showed low levels of oxygen in the blood. This can be a sign of a cCHD. This does not always mean that the baby has a cCHD. It just means that more testing such as an echocardiogram is needed. The algorithm in Figure 5.4 shows the steps on how to complete the screening.

A screen is considered positive if (1) any oxygen saturation measure is less than 90% (in the initial screen or in repeat screens); (2) oxygen saturation is less than 95% in the right hand and foot on three measures, each separated by 1 hour; or (3) a greater than 3% absolute difference exists in oxygen saturation between the right hand and foot on three measures, each separated by 1 hour. Any screening that is ≤95% in the right hand or foot with a ≤3% absolute difference in oxygen saturation between the right hand or foot is considered a negative screen, and screening would end.

Any infant with a positive screen should have a diagnostic echocardiogram, which would involve an echocardiogram within the hospital or birthing center, transport to another institution for the procedure, or use of telemedicine

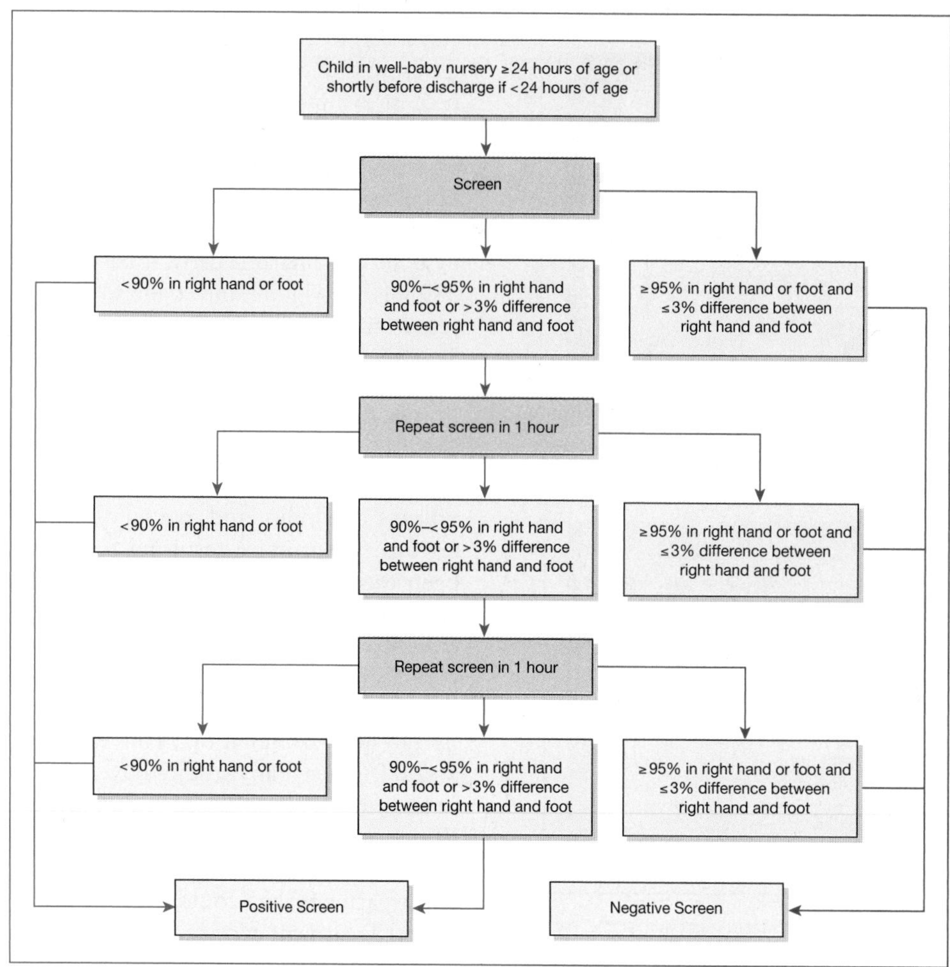

FIGURE 5.4 Percentages refer to oxygen saturation as measured by pulse oximeter.
Data from the Centers for Disease Control and Prevention (2012).

for remote evaluation. The infant's health care provider should be notified immediately, and the infant might need to be seen by a cardiologist for follow-up.

False positives are decreased if the infant is alert, and timing cCHD screening around the time of the newborn hearing screening improves efficiency. POS should not replace taking a complete family medical and pregnancy history and completing a physical examination, which sometimes can detect cCHD before the development of hypoxia.

DISCHARGE

Planning for discharge should begin at the time of admission. Every interaction with the parents should be a teaching moment. Discharge instructions for the parents should be given by both the nurse caring for the newborn and the primary care provider and should include early follow-up appointment with the pediatrician or primary care provider within 72 hours of discharge from the birth hospitalization, feeding schedules, routine bathing, home care needs, umbilical cord care, signs and symptoms of infection, when to call your primary care provider, voiding and stooling patterns, and infant safety.

SUMMARY

This chapter has outlined the basic information for assessing, managing, and discharging the normal newborn. There is growing evidence to support the need for neonatal nurses to have a better understanding of the normal newborn as they care for the sick and/or preterm infant.

CASE STUDY

■ **Identification of the Problem.** A term male infant presented at birth with 2 to 5 mm pustules covering his face, chest, trunk, and scrotum.

■ **Assessment: History and Physical Examination.** A term male infant, 39 + 4 weeks gestation, weighing 3.6 kg, was born via a cesarean section for failure to progress. Apgars were 8 and 9 at 1 and 5 minutes. The mother was a 33-year-old G1P0. The pregnancy was uncomplicated, mother's blood type is A+, syphilis screen was negative, hepatitis screen was negative, HIV screen was negative, and Rubella was immune. Group B strep culture was negative. Mother received prenatal care. Medications during the pregnancy included prenatal vitamins. Complications during labor included failure to progress, requiring a cesarean section.

■ Physical Examination on Admission to the Newborn Nursery

- GENERAL: AGA term male infant in no distress with pustules covering his body. On admission to the newborn nursery the infant was placed on a radiant warmer. Vital signs were stable: temp 98.2, heart rate 158, respirations 48, blood pressure 72/48 m = 52; blood sugar was 86.
- HEENT: mild caput, anterior fontanelle soft and flat, sutures approximated and mobile, palate intact, and ears appropriately placed; eyes normally spaced with red reflex bilaterally, pupils reactive, no hemorrhage noted. Ears with ready recoil and symmetrical
- RESP: bilateral breath sounds clear and equal, no grunting or retractions
- CV: regular rate and rhythm, good perfusion, brisk cap refill, normal pulses X 4 extremities, and no murmur
- ABDOMEN: soft, flat, and nontender. Active bowel sounds and no hepatomegaly
- GU: normal male genitalia, testes descended bilaterally, rugae present, and anus patent
- NEURO: awake and active, tone AGA. Good suck and gag reflex
- SPINE: spine straight and intact, no dimple and neck supple, no masses
- EXTREMITIES: moving all extremities well with symmetrical extremities; no hip clicks or clunks
- SKIN: warm and dry. Moderate nonerythematous pustule approximately between 1 and 4 mm on the face, chest, trunk, scrotum, and thighs. Vesicle appears to contain milky, purulent exudate. The pustules rupture easily. Some appear superficial and wiped off easily with vernix.

■ Differential Diagnosis

- Acropustulosis
- Candidiasis
- Erythema toxicum
- Herpes simplex virus infection
- Milia
- Miliaria
- Neonatal pustular melanosis
- *Staphylococcus aureus* infection

■ Diagnostic Tests. If the appearance is typical of transient neonatal pustular melanosis, no further workup is indicated. If appearance is not typical, potassium hydroxide preparation, Gram stain, and Wright-Giemsa stain can be obtained to support other diagnoses in the differential. Bacterial and viral cultures can be done from the pustule. If there is a clustering of pustules, a polymerase chain reaction to identify possible herpes simplex should be considered.

■ Working Diagnosis. Transient neonatal pustular melanosis.

This is a benign, self-limiting rash of unknown etiology. In the United States incidence has been reported to be 2.2% in White infants and as high as 4.4% in Black infants and infants with darker pigmentation.

The rash starts in utero, so eruptions are always present at birth but the clinical appearance can vary. At first the pustules appear as uniform, round, 2- to 4-mm nonerythematous pustules that rupture easily. There is a thin white scale that is left around the perimeter of each denuded pustule. After a few hours, a central pigmented brown macule appears. This is smooth and has distinct borders that look like a freckle. The hallmark of this rash is this hyperpigmented spot that remains after the pustule has resolved. They may be profuse or sparse and typically are found under the chin and on the neck, upper chest, back, and buttocks. Occasionally, the palms, soles, and scalp are affected.

■ Management. No treatment is indicated. Parents will be anxious when they see pustules covering their baby and will need reassurance that neonatal pustular melanosis is a benign finding and that it fades and disappears over a period of months.

EVIDENCE-BASED PRACTICE BOX

Early Skin-to-Skin Contact in the Healthy Term Newborn

Skin-to-skin contact (SSC) between mother and baby at birth has been associated with numerous physiological and psychological benefits, including temperature, heart rate, and respiratory rate stabilization of the newborn, less crying, and less incidence of hypoglycemia in the newborn (Bergman, Linley, & Fawcus, 2004; Christensson et al., 1992; Christensson et al., 1995; Nolan & Lawrence, 2009). Breastfeeding initiation and duration is also positively impacted by SSC. Mothers who engaged in SSC with their newborns at birth were more likely to have a successful breastfeed, postbirth, than mothers who did not engage in SSC (Carefoot, Williamson, & Dickson, 2004; Carefoot, Williamson, & Dickson, 2005; Khadivzadeh & Karimi, 2009). Mothers who engaged in SSC were also more likely to be exclusively breastfeeding at 3 and 6 months postbirth (Anderson et al., 2003; Gouchon et al., 2010; Vaidya, Sharma, & Dhungel, 2005). Mothers who engage in SSC also have reported less pain (Nolan & Lawrence), state less anxiety 3 days postbirth (Shiau, 1997), and report less postpartum

(*continued*)

depressive symptoms and physiological stress (Bigelow, Power, MacLellan-Peters, Alex, and McDonald, 2012).

Moore, Anderson, Bergman, and Dowswell (2012) conducted a meta-analysis of 34 randomized control trials regarding SSC and concluded that SSC was significantly associated with less crying in newborns and successful initiation and continuation of breastfeeding. The American Academy of Pediatrics (2012), the Academy of Breastfeeding Medicine (2010), the American Association of Women's Health, Obstetric, and Neonatal Nursing (Dabrowski, 2007), and the Baby Friendly Hospital Initiative (2010) all have position statements and recommendations for policy regarding the implementation of SSC at birth. All healthy term infants are recommended to be placed skin-to-skin immediately after delivery for at least 1 hour. Newborns should be placed naked or with diaper only, and prone on the mother's chest. Mother and baby should be covered with a warm blanket. From this position, the infant can be dried, Apgar scores assigned, initial assessment completed, and identification bracelets can be placed on mother and newborn. Newborn care and measurements/weight, length, including bathing, vitamin K, and erythromycin administration, should be delayed to allow uninterrupted SSC and optimal opportunity for the initial breastfeed within the first hour after birth.

Hung and Berg (2011) conducted a feasibility study exploring the implementation of SSC in the operating room (OR) after cesarean delivery. The authors not only concluded that SSC in the OR with healthy term newborns was feasible, but also that newborns who received SSC in the OR had lower rates of formula supplementation. While the evidence for SSC is strong, barriers to implementation do exist. Haxton, Doering, Gingras, and Kelly (2012) discussed challenges including overcoming staff concerns, modifying unit order sets, and adapting electronic medical records to allow for documentation and tracking of SSC. While overcoming these challenges took time and coordination, the authors express that the outcome of increasing breastfeeding initiation rates from 74% to 84% within a 6-month time frame was worth their effort.

ONLINE RESOURCES

Academy of Breastfeeding Medicine information on breastfeeding for health care professionals
http://www.bfmed.org

American Academy of Pediatrics Breastfeeding information for families and health care professionals
http://www2.aap.org/breastfeeding

Association of Women's Health, Obstetric, Gynecologic, and Neonatal Nursing policy statement on breastfeeding
http://www.awhonn.org/awhonn/content.do?name=02_PracticeResources/2C1_breastfeeding.htm

CDC Screening for Critical Congenital Heart Defects **http://www.cdc.gov/ncbddd/pediatricgenetics/pulse.html**

Clinical Report Postnatal Glucose Homeostasis in Late-Preterm and Term Infants
Pediatrics Vol. 127 No. 3 March 1, 2011 pp. 575–579 (doi: 10.1542/peds.2010-3851)
http://pediatrics.aappublications.org/content/127/3/575.full

La Leche League International resources for families and health care providers regarding breastfeeding
http://www.lalecheleague.org

Tools for Health Professionals—Kernicterus in Full-Term Infants
http://www.cdc.gov/ncbddd/jaundice/hcp.html

U.S. Department of Health and Human Services Office on Women's Health breastfeeding information site for families
http://www.womenshealth.gov/breastfeeding

REFERENCES

Academy of Breastfeeding Medicine. (2010). Clinical protocol #7: Model breastfeeding policy. Retrieved from http://www.bfmed.org/Resources/Protocols.aspx

Adamkin, D. H. (2011). Clinical report-postnatal glucose homeostasis in late-preterm and term infants. *Pediatrics, 127*(3), 575–579. doi:10.1542/peds.2010-3851

Ahmed, A., & Ellsworth, P. (2012). To circ or not: A reappraisal. *Urologic Nursing, 32*(1), 10–19.

Alkalay, A. L., Bresee, C. J., & Simmons, C. F. (2010). Decreased neonatal jaundice readmission rate after implementing hyperbilirubinezmia guidelines and universal screening for bilirubin. *Clinical Pediatrics, 49*(9), 830–833. Retrieved from http://ezproxy.baylor.edu/login?url=http://search.ebscohost.com/login.aspx?direct=true&db=cmedm&AN=20693521&site=ehost-live&scope=site

Alkalay, A. L., & Simmons, C. F. (2005). Hyperbilirubinemia guidelines in newborn infants. *Pediatrics, 115*(3), 824–825.

American Academy of Pediatrics, Newborn Screening Authoring Committee. (2008). Screening expands: Recommendations for pediatricians and medical homes, implications for the system. *Pediatrics, 121*, 192–217.

American Academy of Pediatrics, Subcommittee on Hyperbilirubinemia (2004). Management of hyperbilirubinemia in the newborn infant 35 or more weeks of gestation. *Pediatrics 114*, 297–316. Retrieved from http://ezproxy.baylor.edu/login?url=http://search.ebscohost.com/login.aspx?direct=true&db=c8h&AN=2005119313&site=ehost-live&scope=site

American Academy of Pediatrics Policy Statement. (2012). Breastfeeding and the use of human milk. *Pediatrics, 129*, e827–e841. doi:10.1542/peds.2011–3552

American Academy of Pediatrics, Task Force on Circumscision. (1999). Circumcision policy statement. *Pediatrics, 103*(3), 686–693.

Anderson, G.C., Chiu, S.H., Dombrowski, M.A., Swinth, J.Y., Albert, J.M., & Wada, N. (2009). Mother-newborn contact in a randomized trial of kangaroo (skin-to-skin) care. *Journal of Obstetric, Gynecologic, and Neonatal Nursing, 32*, 604–611.

Association of Women's Health, Obstetric and Neonatal Nurses. (2007). *Evidence-based clinical practice guideline: Neonatal skin care* (2nd ed., Vol. 8., p. 228).

Association of Women's Health, Obstetric and Neonatal Nurses. (2011). AWHONN position statement: Newborn screening. *JOGNN, 40*, 136–137.

Baby Friendly USA, Inc. (2012). *Ten steps to successful breastfeeding.* Retrieved from http://www.babyfriendlyusa.org/eng/index.html

Bartick, M., & Reinhold, A. (2010). The burden of suboptimal breastfeeding in the United States: A pediatric cost analysis. *Pediatrics, 125*(5), 1048–1056.

Berg, O., & Hung, K. J. (2011). Early skin-to-skin to improve breastfeeding after cesarean birth. *Journal of Obstetric, Gynecologic &*

Neonatal Nursing, 40, S18–S19. doi:10.1111/j.1552-6909.2011.01242_24.x

Bergman, N.J., Linley, L.L., & Fawcus, S.R. (2004). Randomized control trial of skin-to-skin contact from birth versus conventional incubator for physiological stabilization. *Acta Paediatrica*, 93, 779–785.

Bhutani, V. K., Vilms, R. J., & Hamerman-Johnson, L. (2010). Universal bilirubin screening for severe neonatal hyperbilirubinemia. *Journal of Perinatology: Official Journal of the California Perinatal Association, 30*(Suppl.), S6–S15. Retrieved from http://ezproxy.baylor.edu/login?url=http://search.ebscohost.com/login.aspx?direct=true&db=cmedm&AN=20877410&site=ehost-live&scope=site

Bigelow, A., Power, M., MacLellan-Peters, J., Alex, M., & McDonald, C. (2012). Effect of mother/infant skin-to-skin contact on postpartum depressive symptoms and maternal physiological stress. *Journal of Obstetric, Gynecologic, and Neonatal Nursing, 41*, 369–382. doi:10.1111/j.1552–6909.2012.01350.x

Blackwell, J. T. (2003). Clinical practice guidelines. Management of hyperbilirubinemia in the healthy term newborn. *Journal of the American Academy of Nurse Practitioners, 15*(5), 194–198. Retrieved from http://ezproxy.baylor.edu/login?url=http://search.ebscohost.com/login.aspx?direct=true&db=c8h&AN=2003093969&site=ehost-live&scope=site intervention, and parent counseling

Blum-Kemelor, D., & Leonberg, B. (2009). *Infant nutrition and feeding: A guide for use in the WIC and CSF programs* (FNS-288). Washington, DC: United States Department of Agriculture.

Canadian Paediatric Society. (2007). Guidelines for detection, management and prevention of hyperbilirubinemia in term and late preterm newborn infants (35 or more weeks gestation). *Paediatrics and Child Health, 12*(5), 1B–12B.

Carefoot, S., Williamson, P.R., & Dickson, R. (2004). The value of a pilot study in breastfeeding research. *Midwifery*, 20, 188–193.

Carefoot, S., Williamson, P.R., & Dickson, R. (2005). A randomized control trial in the north of England examining the effects of skin-to-skin care on breastfeeding. *Midwifery*, 21, 71–79.

Carrier, C. (2009). Back to sleep: A culture change to improve practice. *Newborn and Infant Nursing Reviews, 9*(3), 163–168.

Centers for Disease Control and Prevention. (2007). *Hepatitis B vaccine: What you need to know*. Retrieved from http://www.cdc.gov/vaccines/pubs/vis/downloads/vis/hep-b.pdf

Centers for Disease Control and Prevention (2012). *Pulse oximetry screening for critical congenital heart defects*. Screening for critical congenital heart defects. Retrieved from http://www.cdc.gov/ncbddd/pediatricgenetics/pulse.html

Chen, D. C., Nommsen-Rivers, L., Dewey, K. G., & Lonnerdal, B. (1998). Stress during labor and delivery and early lactation performance. *The American Journal of Clinical Nutrition, 68*, 335–344.

Christensson, K., Cabrera, T. Christensson, E., Unvas Moberg, K., & Winberg, J. (1995). Separation distress call in the human neonate in the absence of maternal body contact. *Acta Paediatrica, 84*, 468–473.

Christensson, K. Siles, C., Moreno, L., Belaustequi, A., De La Fuente, P., Lagercrantz, H., … Winberg, J. (1992). Temperature, metabolic adaption, and crying in healthy full-term newborns cared for skin-to-skin or in a cot. *Acta Paediatrica, 81*, 488–493.

Dabrowski, G.A. (2007). Skin-to-skin contact: Giving birth back to mothers and babies. *Nursing for Women's Health, 11*, 64–71. doi:10.1111/j.1751-486X.2007.00119.x

De Carvalho, M., Klaus, M. H., & Merkatz, R. B. (1982). Frequency of breastfeeding and serum bilirubin concentration. *American Journal of Diseases of Children, 136*, 737–738.

Delaney, A., Meyers, A., Roger, R., Russell, F., Talavera, F., Roland, P., & Slack, C. (2012). *Newborn hearing screening*. Retrieved from http://emedicine.medscape.com/article/836646-overview#a1

Dennery, P. A., Seidman, D. S., & Stevenson, D. K. (2001). Neonatal hyperbilirubinemia. *New England Journal of Medicine, 344*(8), 581–590. doi:10.1056/NEJM200102223440807

Doan, T., Gardiner, A., Gay, C. L., & Lee, K. A. (2007). Breast-feeding increases sleep duration of new parents. *Journal of Perinatal and Neonatal Nursing, 21*, 200–206.

Eidelman, A. I., & Schanler, R. J. (2012). Breastfeeding and the use of human milk: Policy statement of the American Academy of Pediatrics. *Pediatrics, 129*, e827–e841.

Ellsworth, P. (2012). Circumcision devices. *Medscape Reference. Drugs, Diseases and Procedures*. Retrieved from http://emedicine.medscape.com/article/2069034-overview

Gouchon, S., Gregori, D., Picotto, A., Patrucco, G., Nangeroni, M., & Di Giulio, P. (2010). Skin-to-skin after cesarean delivery: An experimental study. *Nursing Research, 59*(2), 78–84.

Hardcastle, T. (2010). Sucrose has been shown to have analgesic properties when administered to neonates and infants: Is there the potential for its use in post-operative pain management? *Journal of Perioperative Practice, 20*(1), 19–22.

Hauck, F. R., Omojokun, O. O., & Siadaty, M. S. (2005). Do pacifiers reduce the risk of sudden infant death syndrome? A meta-analysis. *Pediatrics, 116*, e715–e724.

Haxton, D., Doering, J., Gingras, L., & Kelly, L. (2012). Implementing skin-to-skin contact at birth using the Iowa model. *Nursing for Women's Health, 16*, 222–230. doi:10.1111/j.1751–486x.2012.01733.x

Howard, C. R., Howard, F. M., Lanphear, B., Eberly, S., deBliek, E. A., Oakes, D., & Lawrence, R. (2003). Randomized clinical trial of pacifier use and bottle-feeding or cupfeeding and their effect on breastfeeding. *Pediatrics, 111*, 511–518.

Ibarra, B., & Goodstein, M. (2011). A parent's guide to a safe sleep environment. *Advances in Neonatal Care, 11*(1), 27–28.

Ip, S., Chung, M., Raman, G., Chew, P., Magula, N., DeVine, D., . . . Lau, J. (2007). *Breastfeeding and maternal and infant outcomes in developed countries* (AHRQ publication no. 07-E007). Rockville, MD: Agency for Health care Research and Quality.

Jensen, D., Wallace, S., & Kelsay, P. (1994). LATCH: A breastfeeding charting system and documentation tool. *Journal of Obstetric, Gynecologic, and Neonatal Nursing, 23*, 27–32.

Joint Commission on Accreditation of Healthcare Organizations. (2004). Revised guidance to help prevent kernicterus. *Sentinel Event Alert*. Retrieved from www.jointcommission.org/SentinelEvent/SentinelEventAlert/sea_31.htm

Kaneshiro, N. (2011). Appropriate for gestational age (AGA). *MedlinePlus*. Retrieved from http://www.nlm.nih.gov/medlineplus/ency/article/002225.htm

Keefe, M. R. (1987). Comparison of neonatal nighttime sleep-wake patterns in nursery versus rooming-in environments. *Nursing Research, 36*(3), 140–144.

Keefe, M. R. (1988). The impact of infant rooming-in on maternal sleep at night. *Journal of Obstetric, Gynecologic, and Neonatal Nursing, 17*(2), 122–126.

Kernerman, E., & Newman, J. (2009). *Breastfeeding Inc.: Is my baby getting enough food?* Retrieved from http://www.breastfeedinginc.ca/content.php?pagename=doc-IMB

Khadivzadeh, T., & Karimi, A. (2009). The effects of post-birth mother–infant skin-to-skin contact on first breastfeeding. *International Journal of Nurse Midwifery Research, 14*, 111–116.

Kleinman, R. E. (Ed.). (2008). *American academy of pediatrics: Pediatric nutrition handbook* (6th ed.). Elk Grove Village, IL: American Academy of Pediatrics.

Lawrence, R. A. (2010). *Breastfeeding: A guide for the medical profession* (7th ed.). Maryland Heights, MO: Elsevier Mosby.

Li, D. K., Willinger, M., Petitti, D. B., Odouli, R., Liu, L., & Hoffman, H. J. (2006). Use of a dummy (pacifier) during sleep and risk of sudden infant death syndrome (SIDS): Population based case-control study. *British Medical Journal, 332*(7532), 18–22.

Mabry-Hernandez, I., & Oliverio-Hoffman, R. (2010). *Ocular prophylaxis for gonococcal ophthalmia neonatorum evidence update for the U.S. preventive services task force reaffirmation recommendation statement.* AHRQ Publication No. 10–05146. Rockville, MD: Agency for Healthcare Research and Quality.

March of Dimes Foundation. (2012). *Recommended newborn screening tests: 30 disorders.* Retrieved from http://www.milesforbabies.org/professionals/14332_15455.asp

Matthias, A., Ohlson, K., Fredriksson, J., Jacobsson, A., Nedergaard, J., & Cannon, B. (2000). Thermogenic responses in brown fat cells are fully UCP1-dependent. UCP2 or UCP3 do not substitute for UCP1 in adrenergically or fatty acid-induced thermogenesis. *Journal of Biological Chemistry, 275*(33), 25073–25081.

McCall, E. M., Alderdice, F., Halliday, H. L., Jenkins, J. G., & Vohra, S. (2010). Interventions to prevent hypothermia at birth in preterm and/or low birthweight infants. *Cochrane Database of Systematic Reviews, 3.* Art. No.: CD004210. doi:10.1002/14651858.CD004210.pub4

Moore, E. R., Anderson, G. C., & Bergman, N. (2009). Early skin-to-skin contact for mothers and their healthy newborn infants. *The Cochrane Database of Systematic Reviews, 18,* CD003519.

NANN Board of Directors. (2011). Prevention of acute bilirubin encephalopathy and kernicterus in newborns, Position Statement # 3049. *Advances in Neonatal Care, 11*(5S), S3–S9.

National Newborn Screening and Genetics Resource Center. (2009). *National screening status report.* Retrieved from http://genes-r-us.uthscsa.edu/nbsdisorders.pdf

Nelson, E. A. S., Yu, L., & Williams, S. (2005). International child care practices study: Breastfeeding and pacifier use. *Journal of Human Lactation, 21,* 289–295.

Niemelä, M., Pihakari, O., Pokka, T., & Uhari, M. (2000). Pacifier as a risk for acute otitis media: A randomized controlled trial of parental counseling. *Pediatrics, 106,* 483–488.

Nolan, A., & Lawrence, C. (2009). A pilot study of a nursing intervention protocol to minimize maternal–infant separation after cesarean birth. *Journal of Obstetric, Gynecologic, and Neonatal Nursing, 38,* 430–442.

Peres, K. G., Barros, A. J. D., Peres, M. A., & Victora, C. G. (2007). Effects of breastfeeding and sucking habits on malocclusion in a birth cohort study. *Revisita De Saúde Pública* (Revisit Public Health), *41,* 343–350.

Public Law 110–204. (2008). *Newborn screening saves lives act of 2007.* Retrieved from http://www.govtrack.us/congress/billtext.xpd?bill=s110-1858

Raeside, L. (2011). Physiological measures of assessing infant pain: A literature review. *British Journal of Nursing, 20*(21), 1370–1376.

Razmus, I., Dalton, M., & Wilson, D. (2004). Pain management for newborn circumcision. *Pediatric Nursing, 30*(5), 414–417, 427.

Riede, F., Wörner, C., Dähnert, I., Möckel, A., Kostelka, M., & Schneider, P. (2010). Effectiveness of neonatal pulse oximetry screening for detection of critical congenital heart disease in daily clinical routine—Results from a prospective multicenter study. *European Journal of Pediatrics, 169*(8), 975–981. Retrieved from http://ezproxy.baylor.edu/login?url=http://search.ebscohost.com/login.aspx?direct=true&db=eoah&AN=20793031&site=ehost-live&scope=site

Riordan, J., & Wambach, K. (Eds.). (2010). *Breastfeeding and human lactation* (4th ed.). Sudbury, MA: Jones and Bartlett Publishers.

Shiau, S.-H.H. (1997). Randomized control trial of kangaroo care with full-term infants: Effects on maternal anxiety, breast milk maturation, breast engorgement, and breastfeeding status. (Doctoral dissertation). Retrieved from Proquest Dissertations and Theses. (9810943).

Stevens, B., Yamada, J., & Ohlsson, A. (2010). Sucrose for analgesia in newborn infants undergoing painful procedures [Review]. *Cochrane Database of Systematic Reviews, 1,* CD001069.

Stokowski, L. (2011). Fundamentals of phototherapy for neonatal jaundice. *Advances in Neonatal Care, 11*(5S), 10–21.

Swayze, S. (1999). Clamping down on circumcision. *Nursing, 29*(9), 73.

Vaidya, K., Sharma, A., & Dhungel, S. (2005). Effect of early mother–baby close contact over the duration of exclusive breastfeeding. *Nepal Medical College Journal, 7,* 138–140.

Vogel, A. M., Hutchison, B. L., & Mitchell, E. A., (2001). The impact of pacifier use on breastfeeding: A prospective cohort study. *Journal of Paediatrics and Child Health, 37,* 58–63.

Waldenström, U., & Swenson, A. (1991). Rooming-in at night in the postpartum ward. *Midwifery, 7*(2), 82–89.

Walker, M. (1993). A fresh look at the risks of artificial infant feeding. *Journal of Human Lactation, 9*(2), 97–107.

World Health Organization. (2007). *Safe preparation, storage, and handling of powdered infant Formula guidelines.* Geneva, Switzerland: World Health Organization (Joint publication with the Food and Agriculture Organization of the United Nations).

UNIT III: SYSTEMS ASSESSMENT AND MANAGEMENT OF DISORDERS

CHAPTER

6

Respiratory System

■ Thomas D. Soltau and Waldemar A. Carlo

The mechanisms that bring about normal pulmonary function are complex. The clinician must fully comprehend the physiologic processes associated with various respiratory diseases of the neonate. Only through advanced knowledge can the clinician efficiently assess and evaluate the newborn's respiratory status. Systematic use of these assessment skills allows the clinician, as part of the collaborative team, to positively affect patient outcome.

EMBRYOLOGIC DEVELOPMENT OF THE LUNG

Pulmonary development of the embryo proceeds along a predetermined sequence throughout gestation (Greenough & Milner, 2005). Pulmonary development begins with the formation of an outpouching of the embryonic foregut during the fourth week of gestation. Sequential branching of the lung bud, which appears at about 4 weeks and is complete by the sixth week, marks the embryonic phase of lung development. Weeks 6 to 16 are marked by the formation of conducting airways by branching of the aforementioned lung buds. This phase, the pseudoglandular phase ends with completion of the conducting airways. The canalicular phase follows through week 28, when gas-exchange units, known as acini, develop. Surfactant producing type II alveolar cells begin to form during the latter part of this phase. Mature, vascularized gas-exchange sites form during the saccular phase, which spans the 29th through 35th weeks. During this phase, the interstitial space between alveoli thins, so respiratory epithelial cells tightly contact developing capillaries. The alveolar development phase, marked by expansion of the gas-exchange surface area, begins at 36 weeks and extends into the postnatal period. Additional alveoli continue to develop well into childhood, perhaps as late as the seventh year of life (Table 6.1). The alveolar wall and interstitial spaces become very thin, and the single capillary network comes into close proximity to the alveolar membrane. No firm boundaries separate these phases, and gas exchange, albeit inefficient, is possible relatively early in gestation, even before mature, vascularized gas-exchange sites form. Lung development is a continuum that is marked by rapid structural changes. Interference at any time by premature birth or by disease introduces the possibility of inducing lung injury through intervention.

NEWBORN PULMONARY PHYSIOLOGY AND THE ONSET OF BREATHING

The fetal lung is fluid filled, underperfused, and dormant with regard to gas exchange. The fetal lung receives only approximately 10% of the cardiac output (CO). Because the placenta is the gas-exchange organ in fetal life, high blood flow is preferentially directed toward it rather than to the lungs. The pulmonary vasculature maintains a high vascular resistance. Consequently, most of the right ventricular output is shunted from the pulmonary artery across the ductus arteriosus into the aorta, bypassing the pulmonary circulation.

Within moments after the umbilical cord is clamped, the newborn undergoes a transformation from a fetus floating in amniotic fluid to an air-breathing neonate. When the normal onset of breathing occurs, the ensuing chain of events converts the fetal circulation to the circulation pattern of an adult. The lung fluid is absorbed and replaced with air, thus establishing lung volume and allowing for normal neonatal pulmonary function. The process of fetal lung fluid absorption begins before birth when the rate of alveolar fluid secretion declines. Reabsorption speeds up during labor. Animal data suggest that as much as two thirds of the total clearance of lung fluid occurs during labor. This clearance probably results from the cessation of active chloride secretion into the alveolar space. Perinatal fluid clearance is also related to epithelial sodium channels induced by the increase in serum cortisol after delivery (Janér, Pitkänen, Helve, & Andersson, 2011). Oncotic pressure favors the movement of water from the air space back into the interstitium and into the vascular space. With the onset of breathing and lung expansion, water moves rapidly from the air spaces into the interstitium and is removed from the lung by lymphatic and pulmonary blood vessels. Because a large portion of the clearance of lung fluid occurs during the labor process, neonates born without labor after a scheduled cesarean

TABLE 6.1

STAGES OF NORMAL LUNG GROWTH

Phase	Timing	Major Event
Embryonic	Weeks 4–6	Formation of proximal airway
Pseudoglandular	Weeks 7–16	Formation of conducting airways
Canalicular	Weeks 17–28	Formation of acini
Saccular	Weeks 29–35	Development of gas-exchange sites
Alveolar	Weeks 36 through postnatal life	Expansion of surface area

section are at particularly high risk for delayed absorption of fetal lung fluid and thus for transient tachypnea of the newborn. Birth prior to 38 weeks by elective scheduled cesarean section is especially associated with an increased risk of respiratory disorders and an increase in mortality risk (Tita et al., 2009).

Several cardiac changes must take place to complete the process of transition from the intrauterine to extrauterine environment. With the onset of breathing, highly negative intrathoracic pressures are generated with inspiratory efforts, filling the alveoli with air. Replacing alveolar fluid with air causes a precipitous decrease in hydrostatic pressure in the lung, leading to a decrease in pulmonary artery pressure. These cause a decrease in right atrial pressure and an increase in pulmonary blood flow, resulting in increases in alveolar oxygen tension (PaO_2) and constriction of the ductus arteriosus, which normally shunts right ventricular blood away from the lungs. By clamping the cord, the large, low-resistance, placental surface area is removed from the circulation. This change in resistance causes an abrupt increase in systemic arterial pressure, reflected all the way back to the left atrium. As left atrial pressure rises, its flap valve closes the opening between the atria, known as the foramen ovale. This closure prevents blood from bypassing the lungs by eliminating the shunt across the foramen ovale from the right atrium to the left atrium. As a result of this closure of the ductus arteriosus and the foramen ovale and the decrease in pulmonary vascular resistance, systemic pressure becomes greater than pulmonary artery pressure. The infant successfully converts from the pattern of fetal circulation to neonatal circulation when blood coming from the right ventricle flows in its new path of least resistance (lower pressure) to the lungs, instead of shunting across the foramen ovale to the left atrium or across the ductus arteriosus from the pulmonary artery to the aorta.

Understanding ventilation enables the clinician to assess the infant in respiratory distress and devise strategies for management. The respiratory system is composed of the following: (1) the pumping system (the chest-wall muscles, diaphragm, and accessory muscles of respiration), which moves free gas into the lungs; (2) the bony rib cage, which provides structural support for the respiratory muscles and limits lung deflation; (3) the conducting airways, which connect gas-exchanging units with the outside but offer resistance to gas flow; (4) an elastic element, which offers some resistance to gas flow but provides pumping force for moving stale gas out of the system; (5) air–liquid interfaces, which generate surface tension that opposes lung expansion on inspiration but supports lung deflation on expiration; and (6) the abdominal muscles, which aid exhalation by active contraction.

Limitations in the respiratory system predispose the newborn to respiratory difficulty. The circular, poorly ossified rib cage, with a flat instead of angular insertion of the diaphragm, is less efficient at generating negative intrathoracic pressure to move air into the system. The highly compliant chest wall often moves in a contrary manner to the desired flow of air. Small muscles and a relative paucity of type I muscle fibers hinder the strength and endurance of respiratory muscles. The newborn has a relatively low functional residual capacity (lung volume at the end of exhalation) because the comparatively floppy chest wall offers little resistance to collapse, even when a normal amount of functional surfactant is present.

Surface tension is the force that arises from the interaction among the molecules of a liquid. Molecules in the interior of the liquid bulk are attracted to each other, but molecules on the surface of the liquid are attracted to other molecules in the interior of the liquid, which results in the movement of the surface molecule toward the bulk of the liquid. This explains why a droplet of water over a surface tends to adopt a given size and not continuously expand. If we think of the alveolus as a soap bubble, the molecules of the wall of the bubble are attracted to each other, which tend to collapse the bubble. The pressures across the wall of the bubble act against the surface tension and avoid the collapse of the bubble. The relationship between the surface tension and the distending pressures and the pressure across the wall of the bubble are described by Laplace's law, as shown in the following equation:

$$P = \frac{2ST}{r}$$

P is pressure, ST is surface tension, and r is radius of the alveolus. It is difficult to inflate a small or collapsed alveolus because it has a very small diameter. As its volume increases, the pressure needed to continue inflation becomes progressively less—that is, compliance of the alveolus and thus compliance of the lung have improved. Coating the alveoli with an agent that decreases surface tension reduces the effort required to inflate the lungs from a low volume.

An alveolar cell known as the type II pneumocyte produces pulmonary surfactant. Surfactant is a mixture of proteins and phospholipids that naturally coats the mature alveoli, preventing alveolar collapse and loss of lung volume during expiration—that is, as expiration ensues and the lung deflates, the alveolar diameter becomes smaller.

Surfactant coating of the alveolus reduces surface tension so that collapse is prevented and less pressure is required to reinflate it with the next inspiration. Neonates with respiratory distress syndrome (RDS) have surfactant deficiency. In the absence of surfactant, surface tension is high, and the tendency is toward collapse of alveoli at end expiration and resulting micro atelectasis.

Compliance is the elasticity, or distensibility, of the lung. It is expressed as the change in volume caused by a change in pressure as follows:

$$CL = \frac{V}{P}$$

CL is compliance of the lung; V is volume; and P is pressure. The higher the compliance, the larger the volume delivered to the alveoli per unit of applied inspiratory pressure. Surface tension and compliance are particularly important in the preterm infant with RDS. Surface tension is a force that opposes lung expansion. Surfactant deficiency leads to increased surface tension in the alveoli. Lungs with higher surface tension are more difficult to inflate. During expiration, some alveoli collapse. This results in a decreased lung volume at the end of expiration (low functional residual capacity). Clinically, the presence of retractions and other signs of respiratory distress manifest the effects of this increased surface tension. Respiratory muscles contract to inflate the lungs against the surface tension that acts in the opposite direction. The negative pleural pressure easily deforms the floppy thoracic wall of the preterm infant. When a preterm infant with RDS is intubated, a high peak inspiratory pressure (PIP) is required to expand the thorax (i.e., tidal volume is obtained only with a high change in pressure). After surfactant is administered, chest expansion increases with the same PIP. This effect (increased compliance) is due to a decrease in surface tension (i.e., a smaller force opposing lung distention). Thus the tidal volume obtained with the same PIP is increased. Before surfactant is administered, it is very difficult to inflate the lung because compliance is low. After surfactant is administered, surface tension decreases, and it becomes easier to inflate the lung (i.e., compliance is improved).

Resistance is a term used to describe characteristics of gas flow through the airways and pulmonary tissues. Resistance can be thought of as the capacity of the lung to resist airflow. The principal component of resistance is determined by the small airways. Pressure is required to force gas through the airways (airway resistance) and to overcome the forces of the lung and chest wall, which work to deflate the respiratory system (tissue resistance). At a specific flow rate, resistance is described by the following equation:

$$R = \frac{P1 - P2}{\dot{V}}$$

P1 and P2 are pressures at opposite ends of the airway, and $\dot{V}$ is the flow rate of gas (volume per unit of time). Resistance increases as airway diameter decreases. Because the infant has airways of relatively small radius, the resistance to gas flow through those airways is high. Poiseuille's law recognizes that resistance to flow through a cylindrical object is inversely proportional to the fourth power of the radius.

$$R = \frac{8\eta L}{2\pi r^4}$$

In other words, if the radius of the airway is decreased by half, the resulting resistance to flow through the airway is increased 16-fold.

The time constant is the time necessary for airway pressure to partially equilibrate throughout the respiratory system and equals the mathematic product of compliance and resistance. In other words, the time constant is a measure of how quickly the lungs can inhale or exhale. The time constant (Kt) is directly related to both compliance (C) and resistance (R). This relationship is described by the following equation:

$$Kt = C \times R$$

An infant with RDS has decreased compliance, so the time constant of the respiratory system is relatively short. In such an infant, little time is required for pressure to equilibrate between the proximal airway and alveoli, so short inspiratory and expiratory times may be appropriate during mechanical ventilation. This allows the child with RDS to be ventilated with higher rates than would commonly be tolerated in most other populations. When compliance improves (increases), however, the time constant becomes longer. If sufficient time is not allowed for expiration, the alveoli may become overdistended, and an air leak may result.

Blood Gas Analysis and Acid–Base Balance

Oxygen diffuses across the alveolar-capillary membrane, moved by the difference in oxygen pressure between the alveoli and the blood. In the blood, oxygen dissolves in the plasma and binds to hemoglobin. Thus arterial oxygen content (CaO_2) is the sum of dissolved and hemoglobin-bound oxygen, as is shown by the following equation:

$$CaO_2 = (1.37 \times Hb \times SaO_2)\ (0.003 \times PaO_2)$$

CaO_2 is arterial oxygen content (mL/100 mL of blood); 1.37 is the milliliters of oxygen bound to 1 g of hemoglobin at 100% saturation; Hb is hemoglobin concentration per 100 mL of blood (g/100 mL); SaO_2 is the percentage of hemoglobin bound to oxygen (%); 0.003 is the solubility factor of oxygen in plasma (mL/mmHg); and PaO_2 is oxygen partial pressure in arterial blood (mmHg).

In the equation for arterial oxygen content, the first term—($1.37 \times Hb \times SaO_2$)—is the amount of oxygen bound to hemoglobin. The second term—($0.003 \times PaO_2$)—is the amount of oxygen dissolved in plasma. Most of the oxygen in the blood is carried by hemoglobin. For example, if a premature infant has a PaO_2 of 60 mmHg, an SaO_2 of 92%, and a hemoglobin concentration of

14 g/100 mL, then CaO_2 is the sum of oxygen bound to hemoglobin (1.37 × 14 × 0.92) = 17.6 mL, plus the oxygen dissolved in plasma (0.003 × 60) = 0.1 mL. In this typical example, only less than 1% of oxygen in blood is dissolved in plasma; more than 99% is carried by hemoglobin. If the infant has a sudden decrease in the hemoglobin concentration to 10.5g/dL but PaO_2 and SaO_2 remain the same, then CaO_2 (1.37 × 10.5 × 0.92) + (0.003 × 60) equals 13.4 mL/100 mL of blood. Thus, without any change in PaO_2 or SaO_2, a 25% decrease in hemoglobin concentration (from 14 to 10.5g/dL) reduces the amount of oxygen in arterial blood by 24% (from 17.6 to 13.4 mL/100 mL of blood). This is an important concept for clinicians who care for patients with respiratory disease. SaO_2 and hemoglobin should be monitored and, if low, corrected to keep an adequate level of tissue oxygenation. Besides SaO_2 and hemoglobin, CO is the other major determination of oxygen delivery to the tissues.

The force that loads hemoglobin with oxygen in the lungs and unloads it in the tissues is the difference in partial pressure of oxygen. In the lungs, alveolar oxygen partial pressure is higher than capillary oxygen partial pressure, so that oxygen moves to the capillaries and binds to the hemoglobin. Tissue partial pressure of oxygen is lower than that of the blood, so oxygen moves from hemoglobin to the tissues. The relationship between partial pressure of oxygen and hemoglobin is better understood with the oxyhemoglobin dissociation curve (Figure 6.1). Several factors can affect the affinity of hemoglobin for oxygen. Alkalosis, hypothermia, hypocapnia, and decreased levels of 2,3-diphosphoglycerate (2,3-DPG) increase the affinity of hemoglobin for oxygen (as shown in Figure 6.1 by a left shift of the curve). Acidosis, hyperthermia, hypercapnia, and increased 2,3-DPG have the opposite effect, decreasing the affinity of hemoglobin for oxygen, so that the hemoglobin dissociation curve shifts to the right. This characteristic of hemoglobin facilitates oxygen loading in the lung and unloading in the tissue, where the pH is lower and alveolar carbon dioxide tension ($PaCO_2$) is higher. Fetal hemoglobin, which has a higher affinity for oxygen than adult hemoglobin, is more fully oxygen-saturated at lower PaO_2 values. This is represented by a leftward shift on the hemoglobin oxygen dissociation curve.

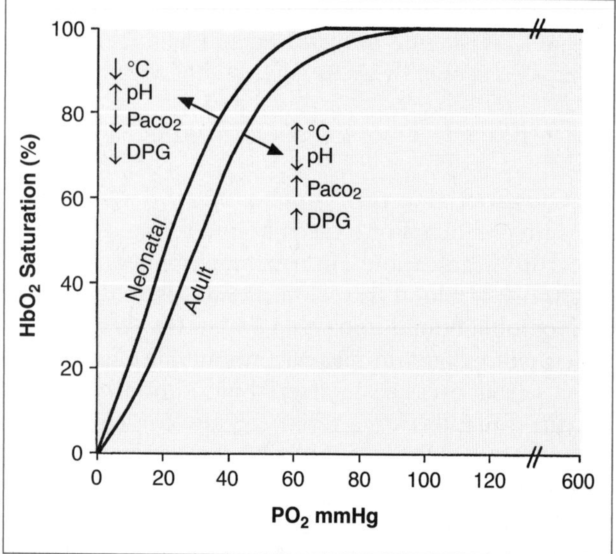

FIGURE 6.1 Oxyhemoglobin equilibrium curves of blood from term infants at birth and from adults (at pH 7.40).

Once loaded with oxygen, the blood should reach the tissues to transfer oxygen to the cells. Oxygen delivery to the tissue depends on CO and CaO_2, as described in the following equation:

$$\text{Oxygen delivery} = \text{CO} \times \text{CaO}_2$$

In the case of the infant discussed previously, increased CO compensates for the decrease in CaO_2 that result from anemia. The key concept is that when a patient's oxygenation is assessed, more information than just PaO_2 and SaO_2 should be considered. PaO_2 and SaO_2 may be normal, but, if hemoglobin concentration is low or CO is decreased, oxygen delivery to the tissues is decreased. With this approach, the clinician should be able to better plan the interventions needed to improve oxygenation.

As in the adult, the acid–base balance in the neonate is maintained within narrow limits by complex interactions between the pulmonary system (which eliminates carbon dioxide) and the kidneys (which conserve carbon dioxide and eliminate metabolic acids). Carbon dioxide elimination, which is more efficient than oxygenation across the alveolar-capillary membrane, is usually not as problematic as oxygenation. Carbon dioxide has a high solubility coefficient, so cellular diffusion is efficient and no measurable partial pressure gradient exists between venous blood and the tissues. Therefore elevated carbon dioxide tension (PCO_2) values in arterial blood samples nearly always indicate ventilatory dysfunction. Dissolved carbon dioxide moves rapidly across cell membranes of peripheral chemoreceptors, thereby making them sensitive to changes in ventilation. Increased intracellular PCO_2 elevates the cellular hydrogen ion concentration as carbon dioxide combines with water to form carbonic acid. This stimulates neural impulses to the medulla, which in turn stimulates respiration. However, excessively high PCO_2 levels can depress ventilation. Acid–base balance is controlled by homeostatic mechanisms and is expressed by the Henderson-Hasselbalch equilibrium equation:

$$\text{pH} = 6.1 + \frac{\log \text{HCO}_3^-}{0.03 \times \text{PCO}_2}$$

It can be seen from this mathematical relationship that acid–base balance depends on the interplay of bicarbonate ion (HCO_3^-) and carbon dioxide (CO_2). Low pH (in other words, acidosis) can contribute to vasoconstriction and can result in worsening hypoxemia caused by extrapulmonary shunt across the ductus or foramen ovale. A pH of less than 7.0 is not well tolerated and is associated with a poor survival rate in these patients.

If $PaCO_2$ rises above normal, as in hypoventilation, pH declines and the patient suffers from respiratory acidosis. The patient with a chronic respiratory acidosis may retain bicarbonate, thus self-inducing a compensatory metabolic alkalosis. A patient who is hyperventilated with a low $PaCO_2$ has respiratory alkalosis. Depressed bicarbonate ion concentration (less than approximately 20 mmol/L in plasma) is called metabolic acidosis and can be associated with any cause of anaerobic metabolism, such as poor CO from congenital heart disease—for example, hypoplastic left heart syndrome or severe aortic coarctation—or from myocardial ischemia, myocardiopathy, myocarditis, hypoxia, or septic shock. Metabolic acidosis that results from renal bicarbonate wasting commonly develops in extremely premature infants. Less common causes for prolonged and severe metabolic acidosis are the inborn errors of metabolism, including urea-cycle defects and aminoacidopathies.

The clinician should become proficient at interpreting blood gas data. With knowledge of the accepted normal values and definitions of the simple blood gas disorders and their compensatory mechanisms, the clinician can examine data in light of the disease process and interpret blood gas values in a fairly straightforward manner. Normally, the body does not overcompensate for a pH above or below the normal range. Therefore, when presented with an abnormal pH, the clinician should rapidly determine whether acidosis (Figure 6.2, A) or alkalosis (Figure 6.2, B) exists. An examination of $PaCO_2$ and HCO_3^- determines whether the process is respiratory, metabolic, or mixed. The clinician should determine which derangement occurred first. For example, an acidotic, acutely ill hypoxemic infant with a high $PaCO_2$ and depressed HCO_3^- is usually hypoventilating and suffering metabolic acidosis secondary to anaerobic metabolism. The infant with a low $PaCO_2$ is hyperventilating, either spontaneously or secondary to overzealous mechanical ventilation. A concomitantly low pH and low $PaCO_2$ indicate that the infant is compensating for metabolic acidosis with hyperventilation in an effort to normalize the pH. A pure metabolic alkalosis with high

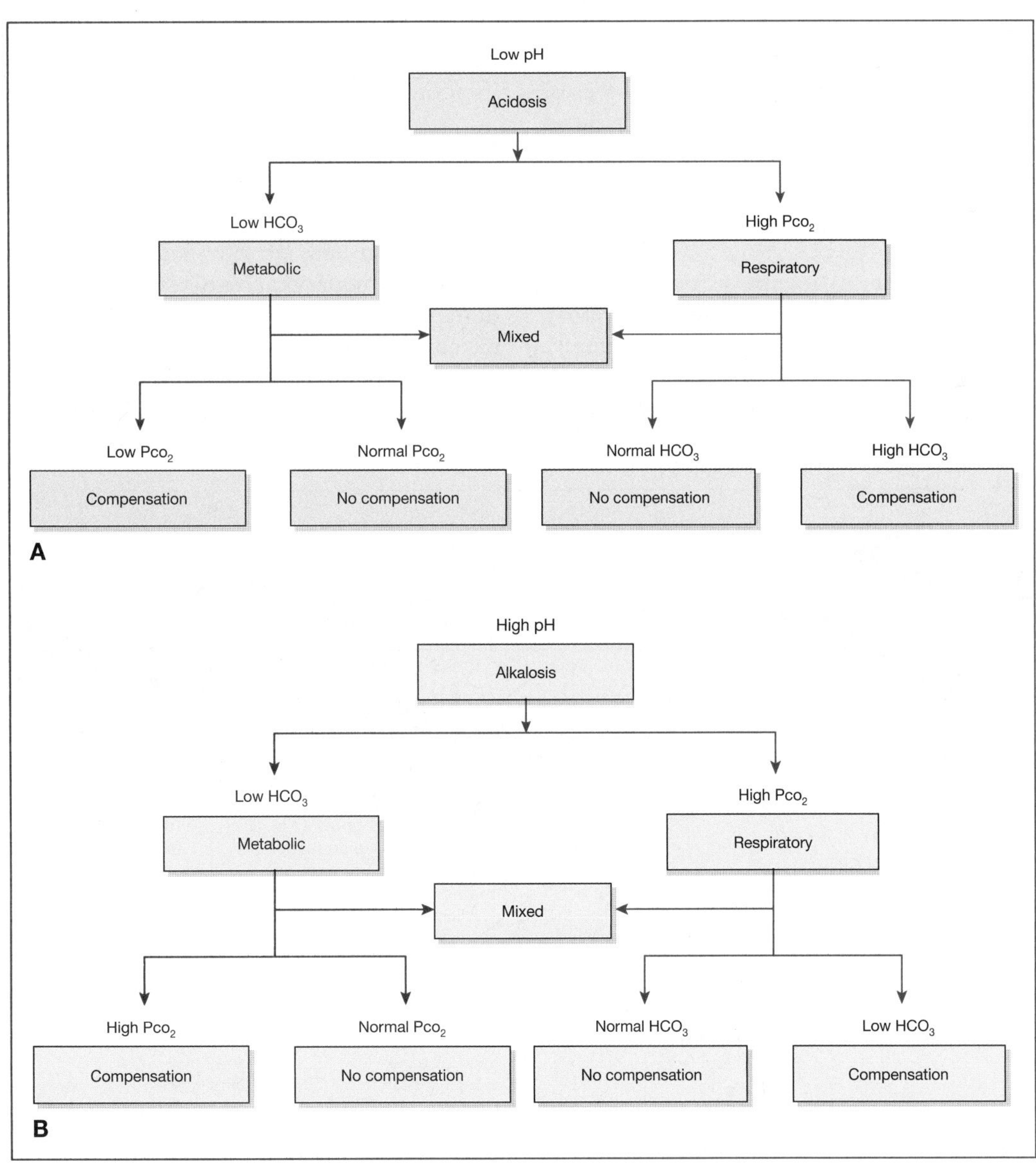

FIGURE 6.2 Acid–base balance: diagnostic approach. (A) low pH; (B) high pH.

pH can be caused by bicarbonate administration or gastric losses due to pyloric stenosis or gastric suctioning. Infants with bronchopulmonary dysplasia (BPD) usually have a compensated respiratory acidosis, with an elevated $PaCO_2$ and concomitantly elevated HCO_3^-. The pH may be in the normal range or slightly acidotic. A severely depressed pH usually indicates acute decompensation.

ASSESSMENT OF THE NEONATE WITH RESPIRATORY DISTRESS

The assessment of a neonate with respiratory distress should always begin with the compilation of a detailed perinatal history. In some cases, the history is difficult to obtain, especially when the infant has been transferred from one center to another, often with incomplete records. Even so, every effort should be made to obtain as much pertinent information as possible. The clinician is often able to gain important supplemental information from the father or visiting relatives at the bedside. A review of the maternal-perinatal history and a complete physical examination, combined with a limited laboratory and radiologic evaluation, leads to a timely diagnosis in most circumstances. Many neonatal diseases, including many with nonpulmonary origins, may manifest with signs of respiratory distress. Therefore a comprehensive differential diagnosis must be considered (Figure 6.3).

History

In most situations, data from a patient's history can direct the clinician to the correct diagnosis of neonatal respiratory distress. The prenatal record should be reviewed carefully for possible causes of the infant's difficulties. The mother's age, gravidity, parity, blood type, and Rh status should be recorded. The obstetrician's best estimate of gestational age should be documented as determined by first-trimester ultrasound or last menstrual period. Ultrasonography often provides information related to anomalies, which is useful in the anticipation of required support at birth. Historical information such as previous preterm birth is relevant, as it is often associated with an increased risk of premature delivery in subsequent pregnancies. Because excessive maternal weight gain occurs with diabetes, multiple gestation, or polyhydramnios, prepregnancy weight and total gain should be noted. The clinician is often alerted to the possibility of gestational diabetes with abnormal glucose tolerance screening results, which again should be reflected in the prenatal record.

The duration of membrane rupture, the presence of maternal fever with or without accompanying chorioamnionitis, and the presence of meconium-stained amniotic fluid are important pieces of information that may help in the differential diagnosis of a newborn with respiratory distress. Additionally, antepartum and intrapartum administration of certain medications may affect respiratory outcomes. Administration of steroids to the mother reduces the likelihood that RDS will develop in the infant; administration of narcotics to the mother close to delivery may result in poor respiratory effort by an otherwise normal infant.

Physical Examination of the Respiratory System

One or more of the major signs of respiratory difficulty (e.g., cyanosis, tachypnea, grunting, retractions, and nasal flaring) are usually present in neonates with both pulmonary and nonpulmonary causes of respiratory distress. Observation of the distressed infant with the unaided eye and ear is the clinician's first step in the physical assessment. Cyanosis may be central, as caused by pulmonary disease and cyanotic heart disease, or peripheral, as occurs in conditions with impaired

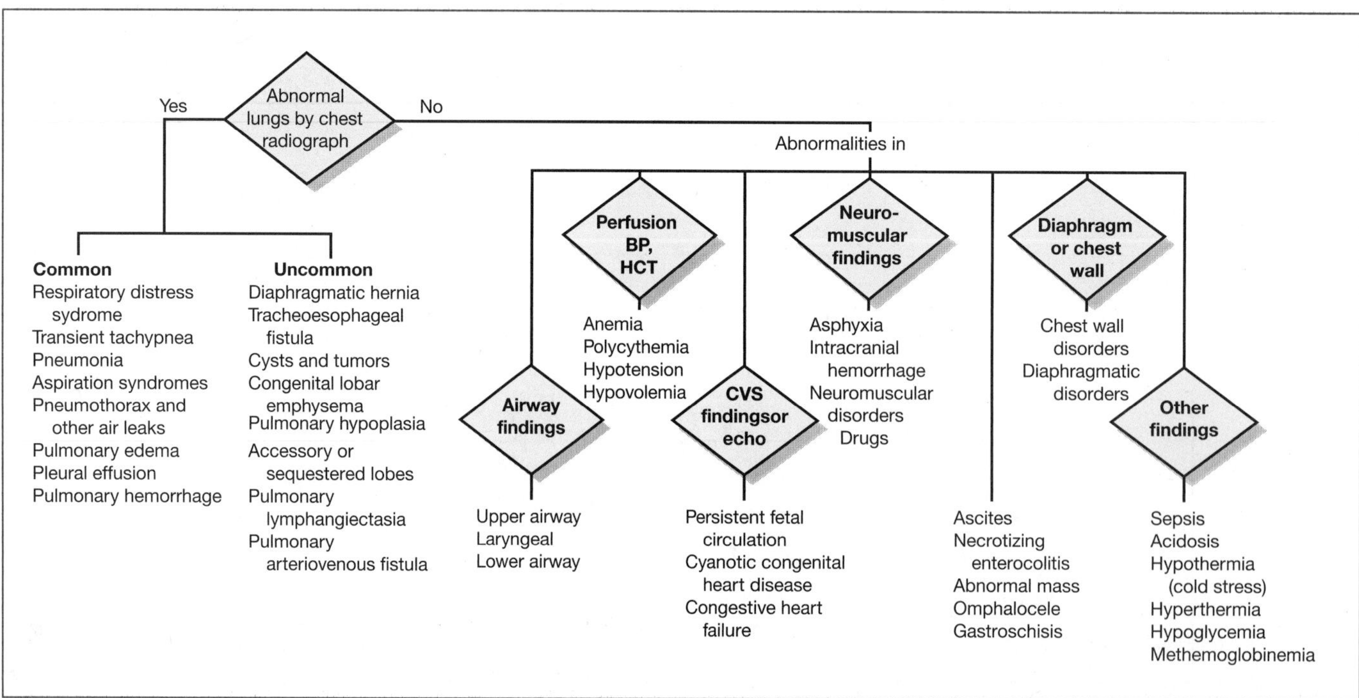

FIGURE 6.3 Neonate with acute respiratory distress.

CO. Tachypnea typically manifests in infants with decreased lung compliance, such as RDS, whereas patients with high airway resistance (e.g., airway obstruction) usually have deep but slow breathing. Grunting is produced by an adduction of vocal cords during expiration. Grunting holds gas in the lungs throughout expiration, which helps maintain lung volume and avoid alveolar collapse. At the end of expiration the gas is released and rapidly propelled, causing an audible grunt. Grunting is more typical of infants with decreased functional residual capacity, such as preterm infants with RDS. Chest wall retractions occur more often in very premature infants because of the highly compliant chest wall (Carlo & Di Fiore, 2011). When the infant is intubated, observation of the chest gives important information. Careful observation of chest wall excursions produced by the ventilator allows the clinician to adjust the magnitude of the ventilator pressure so that optimal gas exchange is achieved while risk of volutrauma is minimized. The chest of an intubated infant should move the same or only slightly less than that of a healthy spontaneously breathing infant. The clinician should assess the appropriateness of the magnitude of the chest expansion in ventilated patients. A reported abrupt decrease in the chest rise may indicate atelectasis, a plugged endotracheal tube, a pneumothorax, or ventilator failure. Slow decreases in the chest rise over hours may indicate a deteriorating lung compliance or gas trapping. An overinflated thorax, as determined from radiographs, is a sign of gas trapping. In the intubated infant, this observation should prompt the clinician to adjust the positive end-expiratory pressure (PEEP) or expiratory time so that gas trapping and air leakage are prevented. An anguished intubated infant with cyanosis and gasping efforts may have endotracheal tube obstruction.

Careful attention should be given to the sounds that emanate from the respiratory tract, as variations in quality often aid in localization of the source of respiratory distress. Stridor is common in neonates with upper airway and laryngeal lesions. Inspiratory stridor occurs most often with upper airway and laryngeal lesions, whereas expiratory stridor suggests lower airway problems. Hoarseness is a common sign of laryngeal disorders. Forced inspiratory efforts may indicate upper airway or laryngeal involvement, whereas expiratory wheezes suggest a lower airway disease. Congenital airway disorders that may cause respiratory distress in the neonate are included in Figure 6.3.

Auscultation of the chest further aids the examiner. Because infants with RDS have low lung volumes, breath sounds are faint, usually without rales. In comparison, the infant with pneumonia may have rales indicative of alveolar filling. Auscultation allows the clinician to detect the presence of secretions in the airway and to evaluate the response to physiotherapy and suctioning. Rhonchi may be heard in neonates with airway disease, such as meconium aspiration syndrome (MAS). Unequal breath sounds may be due to a pneumothorax or to one of the many causes of diminished ventilation to a lung lobe (e.g., atelectasis, main-stem bronchial intubation, and pleural effusion). A shift of the apex of the heart can occur with a pneumothorax, diaphragmatic hernia, unilateral pulmonary interstitial emphysema, pleural effusion, dextrocardia, or atelectasis, which may be differentiated by transillumination of the chest and chest imaging. Dullness to percussion may be due to a pleural effusion or solid mass. Muffled heart tones suggest a pneumopericardium or a pericardial effusion. Respiratory distress may occur in many chest wall disorders that restrict rib-cage movements. Increased oral secretions and choking with feedings are common in neonates with a tracheoesophageal fistula. Because newborns are obligate nasal breathers, those with choanal atresia typically improve with crying and have worsening respiratory distress at rest or with feeding. Characteristic Potter facies and other compression deformities and contractures may be present in neonates with hypoplastic lungs secondary to oligohydramnios.

Examination of the cardiovascular system and assessment of peripheral perfusion yield many clues toward a diagnosis. Pallor and poor perfusion may indicate anemia, hypotension, or hypovolemia. Polycythemia with plethora may also cause respiratory distress. Cardiovascular signs of congestive failure (e.g., hyperactive precordium, tachycardia, and hepatomegaly), poor CO, pathologic murmurs, decreased femoral pulses, and nonsinus rhythm suggest a primary cardiac cause for the respiratory distress.

When hypotonia, muscle weakness, or areflexia accompanies respiratory distress, a neuromuscular cause should be considered (Box 6.1). In such cases, an accompanying history of less frequent fetal movement often is involved. Sometimes a history of muscular disease exists in the family. Brachial plexus injury or fracture of a clavicle may accompany phrenic nerve injury and diaphragm paralysis.

Abnormalities found on abdominal examination enlighten the examiner to other causes of respiratory difficulty. Abdominal distention that results from causes such as ascites, necrotizing enterocolitis, abdominal mass, ileus, or tracheoesophageal fistula can cause respiratory distress, whereas a scaphoid configuration of the abdomen suggests a diaphragmatic hernia.

Other nonpulmonary disorders such as sepsis, metabolic acidosis, hypothermia, hyperthermia, hypoglycemia, and methemoglobinemia may also cause respiratory distress in the neonate.

■ **Radiographic and Laboratory Investigation.** Radiographic examination is often the most useful part of the laboratory evaluation and may serve to narrow the

BOX 6.1

NEUROMUSCULAR DISORDERS THAT MAY CAUSE RESPIRATORY DISTRESS IN THE NEONATE

Myopathies
Myasthenia gravis
Werdnig Hoffman (spinal muscular atrophy)
Spinal cord disorder
Poliomyelitis
Others

Adapted from Battista and Carlo (1992).

differential diagnosis. An anteroposterior view is usually sufficient, but a lateral chest radiograph may be useful when fluid, masses, or pneumothorax is suspected. Other diagnostic imaging techniques (ultrasonography, fluoroscopy, computed tomography, or magnetic resonance imaging) may be helpful in selected patients. Bronchoscopy allows direct visualization of the upper airway. This technique, albeit invasive and technically difficult, may in selected cases be a great aid in the differential diagnosis and treatment of patients with a suspected airway lesion.

Much can be learned from a relatively small battery of laboratory tests. In the neonatal intensive care unit (NICU) setting, the clinician is often required to collect specimens for and interpret the results of physiologic testing. Considerable skill is required in sampling both venous and arterial blood from small patients who are at substantial risk for iatrogenic anemia and vascular damage. Ideally, the hospital laboratory is equipped to do most routine tests on microliter quantities of blood. The clinician must monitor total quantities of blood sampled from the infant and be alert to the development of iatrogenic anemia.

Analysis of arterial blood for pH and gas tensions is perhaps one of the most common tasks of the clinicians caring for the infant with respiratory illness. Noninvasive methods to assess gas exchange, such as transcutaneous blood gas measurements or oxygen saturation, are very useful. Because oxygen delivery to the tissues so intimately depends on circulating red blood cell volume, a hematocrit should be performed.

COMMON DISORDERS OF THE RESPIRATORY SYSTEM

There are a large variety of respiratory disorders that occur in neonates. The most common disorders are discussed here. Figure 6.3 lists both pulmonary and nonpulmonary disorders that cause respiratory symptoms in the newborn infant. There are also several diseases that have their roots in the neonatal period and extend into infancy (Box 6.2). The most common is BPD, a chronic lung disease that affects newborns, mainly premature infants exposed to mechanical ventilation for RDS or other respiratory problems.

RDS

RDS, formerly known as hyaline membrane disease (the term *hyaline membrane disease* originated from the histological observation of alveolar space lined by an eosinophilic membrane formed by cellular debris), is the most common cause of respiratory distress in premature neonates (Hamvas, 2011). RDS is common in preterm infants. A recent cohort of infants born at National Institute of Child Health and Development (NICHD) Neonatal Research Network Centers showed that most children born extremely premature have RDS. The incidence decreased from 98% at 23 weeks to 86% at 28 weeks. Approximately 97% of 23 week infants are treated with surfactant. This decreases to 65% at 28 weeks (Stoll et al., 2010). In rare cases, RDS develops in full-term infants born to mothers with diabetes or in full-term infants who have experienced asphyxia. RDS is progressively more common the lower the infant's gestational age.

BOX 6.2

CAUSES OF LATE RESPIRATORY DISTRESS IN THE NEONATE

BPD
Pneumonia (bacterial, viral, or fungal)
Congestive heart failure
Recurrent pneumonitis or aspiration
Upper airway obstruction
Wilson-Mikity syndrome
Idiopathic pulmonary fibrosis (Hamman-Rich syndrome)
Pulmonary lymphangiectasia
Cystic fibrosis
Immature lungs

■ **Antenatal Steroids.** Acceleration of lung maturation with antenatal steroids is now the standard of care in women with preterm labor of up to 34 weeks. Antenatal corticosteroid therapy to the mothers of preterm fetuses of up to 34 weeks significantly reduces the incidence of RDS with odds ratios of around 0.5 and decreases mortality, with odds ratios of around 0.6. Subgroup analyses confirm that these benefits occur regardless of race and gender. No adverse effects have been reported with the usual single course of antenatal steroids. There are also other nonrespiratory benefits of steroid administration to mothers, including reductions in intraventricular hemorrhage and necrotizing enterocolitis. The current guidelines are to provide steroids to mothers between 24 and 34 weeks of gestation; however, emerging data at the limits of viability show benefits to giving steroids to infants as early as 22 weeks (Carlo et al., 2011).

■ **Treatment.** The lungs of infants with RDS are deficient in pulmonary surfactant, the surface tension–reducing agent that prevents alveolar collapse and loss of lung volume at end expiration. Treatment with surfactant is quite effective. Progressive atelectasis leads to intrapulmonary shunting, owing to perfusion of unventilated lung, and subsequent hypoxemia. The radiograph displays a characteristic ground glass, reticulogranular appearance with air bronchograms. When the lung inflation is poor, the arterial blood gas analysis usually reveals respiratory acidemia as well as hypoxemia.

Therapy is directed toward improving oxygenation as well as maintaining optimal lung volume. Continuous positive airway pressure (CPAP) or PEEP is applied to prevent volume loss during expiration. In severe cases, mechanical ventilation via tracheal tube is required. Exogenous surfactants (artificial and natural), which are available for intratracheal instillation, improve survival and reduce some of the associated morbidity of RDS. Earlier clinical trials indicated that prophylactic surfactant administration to extremely premature infants in the delivery room is more effective than waiting for the treatment after development of RDS (Soll & Morley, 2001). However, several recent trials, including the large SUPPORT trial in which prophylactic surfactant was compared to CPAP started at birth with rescue surfactant, showed equivalence, though many of the infants in the early

CPAP arm ultimately required surfactant administration (Finer et al., 2010). The most recent Cochrane review of the topic did not recommend routine administration of prophylactic surfactant administration, as there was less risk of BPD or death at 36 weeks when using early CPAP with selective surfactant administration for infants requiring intubation (Rojas-Reyes, Morley, & Soll, 2012). Prophylactic high-frequency ventilation for treatment of RDS has mixed results, but these modes of ventilation should be considered as alternatives to conventional mechanical ventilation in specific circumstances, such as in infants with air leaks as interstitial emphysema or bronchopleural fistula. Infants greater than 34 weeks who have RDS and respiratory failure unresponsive to ventilatory management have responded favorably to extracorporeal membrane oxygenation (ECMO) (Thome, Carlo, & Pohlandt, 2005).

Nursing care for infants with RDS is demanding; the most unstable infants often require a one to one, nurse to patient ratio. The nurse must monitor the quality of respirations and observe the degree of difficulty that the infant is experiencing. Worsening retractions may signal progressive volume loss and impending respiratory failure. Arterial blood gas tensions and pH should be measured frequently, and continuous noninvasive monitoring of oxygenation may allow early identification of gas-exchange problems. The risk of pneumothorax and right main-stem intubation is high, and the symmetry of breath sounds must be verified regularly. A crying infant loses airway pressure when the mouth is open and therefore must be kept calm when receiving nasal CPAP. The intubated infant must be monitored for appropriate endotracheal tube position and patency. Suctioning of the airway should be done carefully. The suction catheter should be passed only as far as the end of the endotracheal tube because overzealous suctioning can denude the tracheal epithelium (Cordero, Sananes, & Ayers, 2000). Lung volume can be lost during prolonged disconnection from the ventilator. Rapid loss of lung volume can precipitate hypoxemia, so disconnection time should be minimized. Any sudden decompensation should alert the nurse to investigate for ventilator failure, pneumothorax, or tracheal tube plugging (Figure 6.4). The infant also should be closely monitored for changes in pulmonary compliance, especially after surfactant administration.

BPD is a common outcome in tiny infants with RDS. BPD generally refers to a chronic pulmonary disorder characterized by pulmonary fibrosis, bronchiolar metaplasia, emphysema, and interstitial edema. It is most commonly seen in survivors of extreme prematurity who were diagnosed with RDS, but extremely-low-birth-weight infants may develop BPD without history of RDS. According to the National Institute of Child Health and Human Development consensus, infants with mild BPD are those who continue to require oxygen supplementation for a total of at least 28 days, while those with moderate or severe BPD require oxygen supplementation and/or ventilatory support at 36 weeks of postmenstrual age and for more than 28 days (Jobe & Bancalari, 2001). The incidence of BPD increases as gestational age decreases. Of the infants less than or equal to 1,000 g at birth, 77% develop mild BPD, while 46% develop moderate BPD and 16% develop severe BPD (Ehrenkranz et al., 2005). The incidence of BPD also increases with decreasing gestational age. Of survivors to 36 weeks corrected gestational age, 85% of infants born at 22 weeks had an oxygen requirement as opposed to 22% for infants born at 28 weeks (Stoll et al., 2010). Pulmonary morbidities and adverse neurodevelopmental outcomes at 18 to 22 months were more prevalent within an increased severity of BPD.

■ **Air Leaks.** Air leaks frequently complicate RDS and other neonatal respiratory disorders. Air leaks are characterized by air in an ectopic location (Box 6.3). Many air-leak syndromes begin with at least some degree of pulmonary interstitial emphysema, which is the result of alveolar rupture from overdistention, usually concomitant with mechanical ventilation or continuous distending airway pressure. Pulmonary interstitial emphysema occurs most commonly in preterm infants but may be seen in infants of any gestational age. Lung compliance is nonuniform, and areas of poor aeration and alveolar collapse exist. Interspersed are alveoli of normal or near-normal compliance, which become overdistended. The more normal lung units (those with better compliance) become overdistended and eventually rupture. Air is forced

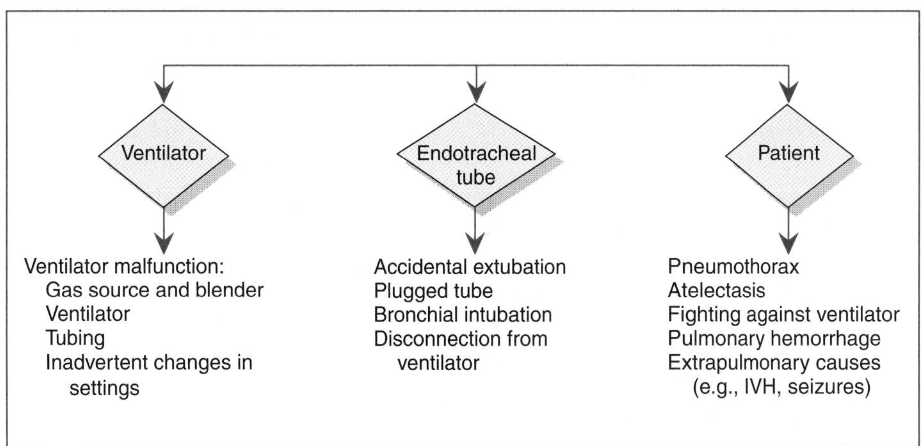

FIGURE 6.4 Acute deterioration in a ventilated patient.

BOX 6.3

AIR LEAK PHENOMENA IN THE NEONATE

Pneumothorax
Pulmonary interstitial emphysema
Pneumomediastinum
Pneumopericardium
Pneumoperitoneum
Pulmonary venous air embolism
Subcutaneous emphysema
Pseudocyst

From Battista and Carlo (1992).

from the alveolus into the loose tissue of the interstitial space and dissects toward the hilum of the lung, where it may track into the mediastinum—causing a pneumomediastinum—or into the pericardium—causing a pneumopericardium. The astute clinician may notice that an infant's chest becomes barrel-shaped with overdistention and that breath sounds become distant on the affected side. In contrast, the infant who suffers a pneumothorax usually becomes unstable, with development of cyanosis, oxygen desaturation, and carbon dioxide retention. The infant may become hypotensive and bradycardic because the high intrathoracic pressure impedes venous return. A tension pneumothorax, in which the free pleural air compresses the lung, is a medical emergency, and prompt relief by thoracentesis or tube thoracostomy is indicated. There are infants who are medically stable with a pneumothorax who can be managed expectantly without decompression (Litmanovitz & Carlo, 2008). However, it is important to ensure that these infants truly are medically stable and if they deteriorate, to intervene when needed to relieve the pneumothorax.

Transient Tachypnea of the Newborn

Transient tachypnea of the newborn occurs typically in infants born by cesarean section, particularly in the absence of labor or in those infants born vaginally but who delivered precipitously. The cause of the disorder is thought to be transient pulmonary edema that results from decreased absorption of pulmonary alveolar fluid. The chest radiograph may show increased perihilar interstitial markings and small pleural fluid collections, especially in the minor fissure. In contrast to the infants with RDS, infants with transient tachypnea tend to have a normal or low PCO_2. Oxygenation can usually be maintained by supplementing oxygen with a hood, although some infants benefit from a short course of positive pressure support. The infant usually recovers in 24 to 48 hours.

Pneumonia

Pneumonia may be of bacterial, viral, or other infectious origin (Table 6.2). Pneumonia may be transmitted transplacentally, as has been shown with group B streptococcus, or via an ascending bacterial invasion associated with maternal chorioamnionitis and prolonged rupture of the membranes. The usual causative organisms of pneumonia are group B *streptococcus*, *Escherichia coli*, *Haemophilus influenzae*, and, less commonly, *Streptococcus viridans*, *Listeria monocytogenes*, and anaerobes.

A strong association exists between bacterial pneumonias and premature birth, which may be due to a developmental deficiency of bacteriostatic factors in the amniotic fluid. Alternatively, the infection may be a precipitating factor in preterm labor. Chorioamnionitis can occur even in the presence of intact membranes. Blood cultures and other diagnostic tests are necessary to help direct specific antimicrobial therapy. The clinician should be attuned to the labor history. Were membranes ruptured for more than 12 to 24 hours? Did the mother have fever before delivery? Did the mother receive intrapartum antibiotics if risk factors for group B streptococcus sepsis were present? The full-term infant who exhibits tachypnea, grunting, retractions, or temperature instability should be evaluated carefully. Blood counts may be helpful, and the neutropenic infant in particular should be carefully monitored. Infection should be considered in any newborn with respiratory distress or more than transient oxygen requirements. Tracheal aspirates obtained within 8 hours of birth and that show both bacteria and white blood cells on Wright's stain are highly predictive of pneumonia.

Pending culture results, treatment is usually begun with broad-spectrum antibiotics, typically a penicillin and aminoglycoside or cephalosporin. A lumbar puncture may be undertaken or may be postponed until results of blood culture are obtained. When cultures result in the identification of the organism, the study of antibiotic sensitivity allows the clinician to identify the most effective antibiotic or combination of antibiotics for the causative agent. Antibiotic treatment for up to 10 to 14 days may be necessary.

Persistent Pulmonary Hypertension of the Newborn

Persistent pulmonary hypertension of the newborn (PPHN), or persistent fetal circulation, is a term applied to the combination of pulmonary hypertension (high pressure in the pulmonary artery), subsequent right-to-left shunting through fetal channels (the foramen ovale or ductus arteriosus) away from the pulmonary vascular bed, and a structurally normal heart. The syndrome may be idiopathic or, more commonly, secondary to another disorder—such as MAS, congenital diaphragmatic hernia (CDH), RDS, asphyxia, sepsis, pneumonia, hyperviscosity of the blood, or hypoglycemia (Walsh-Sukys et al., 2000). Idiopathic causes may be related to maternal late trimester nonsteroidal anti-inflammatory drug use or maternal use of selective serotonin reuptake inhibitors (Dhillon, 2011).

The neonatal pulmonary vasculature is sensitive to changes in PaO_2 and pH and, during stress, can become even hyperreactive and constrict to cause increased pressure against which the neonatal heart cannot force blood flow to the lungs. If the pulmonary artery pressure is higher than systemic pressure, blood flows through the path of least resistance, away from the lungs through the foramen ovale and the ductus arteriosus. The infant becomes progressively hypoxemic and acidemic, leading to further cycles of increased pulmonary vascular resistance.

Management of infants with PPHN demands high vigilance. Because the pulmonary vasculature is unstable, almost any event can precipitate severe hypoxemia, including

TABLE 6.2

CAUSES OF PNEUMONIA

Bacterial	Viral	Other
Group B streptococcus	Cytomegalovirus	*Candida* and other fungi
Escherichia coli	Adenovirus	*Ureaplasma*
Klebsiella	Rhinovirus	*Chlamydia*
Staphylococcus aureus	Respiratory syncytial virus	Syphilis
Listeria monocytogenes	Parainfluenza	*Pneumocystis jeroveci*
Enterobacter	Enterovirus	Tuberculosis
Haemophilus influenzae	Rubella	
Streptococcus pneumonia		
Pseudomonas		
Bacteroides		
Others		

Adapted from Battista and Carlo (1992).

routine procedures such as endotracheal tube suctioning, weighing, positioning, and diaper changes. Under these circumstances, minimal stimulation is usually practiced.

Occasionally, sedation, and even muscle paralysis, is necessary to prevent spontaneous episodes of hypoxemia or deterioration associated with procedures (e.g., suctioning and position changes). Mild alkalosis—either with bicarbonate infusion or by mild hyperventilation—often relaxes the pulmonary vascular bed and allows better pulmonary perfusion and thus oxygenation. The approach to therapy should be directed toward preventing hypoxemia and acidosis. The critical pH necessary for overcoming pulmonary vasoconstriction seems to be unique to the individual. High applied ventilator pressures predispose the lung to air-leak syndromes, further increasing the risk of sudden destabilization. Vasopressor therapy with dopamine and dobutamine is often used in conjunction with hyperventilation, but controlled data are not available. Presumably, they act both to improve contractility of the stressed myocardium, which improves CO, and to raise systemic arterial pressure above pulmonary artery pressure to reduce right-to-left shunting.

When conventional therapies fail, high-frequency ventilation may be attempted. Approximately 30% to 60% of patients who fail conventional mechanical ventilation respond to high-frequency ventilation. However, the exact role of high-frequency ventilation in mortality or in preventing the need for ECMO needs further evaluation. Since the early 1990s, inhalation of nitric oxide—alone and in association with high-frequency ventilation—has been shown to be an effective therapy for PPHN (Davidson et al., 1998; Finer & Barrington, 2006; The Neonatal Inhaled Nitric Oxide Study Group, 1997).

When oxygenation cannot be accomplished despite the use of conventional mechanical ventilation, high-frequency ventilation, or nitric oxide, ECMO has proven to be an effective therapy (UK Collaborative ECMO Trial Group, 1996). Neonatologists disagree about the exact indications for ECMO, and some centers report impressive survival statistics without the use of ECMO (Mok, Yates, & Tasker, 1999). However, ECMO often is the only treatment that improves the outcome of some infants who fail less invasive therapies.

MAS

MAS is the most common aspiration syndrome that causes respiratory distress in neonates. The role of meconium in the pathophysiology of aspiration pneumonia has become controversial. It is unclear whether the material itself causes pneumonitis severe enough to lead to hypoxemia, acidosis, and pulmonary hypertension or whether the presence of meconium in the amniotic fluid is merely a marker for other events that may have predisposed the fetus to severe pulmonary disease. The severely ill infant with MAS typically comes from a stressed labor and has depressed cord pH from metabolic acidosis. These infants are often postmature and exhibit classic signs of weight loss, skin peeling, and deep staining of the nails and umbilical cord.

Pharyngeal suctioning at the time of birth does not reduce MAS (Vain et al., 2004). The nonvigorous infant with meconium-stained fluid should receive rapid intubation under direct laryngoscopy to allow for suctioning of the airway (Zaichkin & Weiner, 2011). Endotracheal suctioning at birth is used to prevent MAS in the newly born with meconium-stained fluid but is not necessary if the infant is vigorous at birth (Wiswell et al., 2000). Vigorousness in a newborn infant implies that the infant is spontaneously breathing well, has a heart rate greater than 100 bpm, and has normal active tone.

Pulmonary disease in infants with MAS arises from chemical pneumonitis, interstitial edema, and small-airway obstruction and from concomitant persistent pulmonary hypertension. The infant may have uneven pulmonary ventilation with hyperinflation of some areas and atelectasis of others, leading to ventilation-perfusion mismatching and subsequent hypoxemia. The hypoxemia may then exacerbate pulmonary vasoconstriction, leading to deeper hypoxemia and acidosis. Infants with MAS may have evidence of lung overinflation with a barrel-chested appearance. Auscultation reveals rales and rhonchi. The radiograph shows patchy or streaky areas of atelectasis and other areas of overinflation.

As with other cases of pulmonary hypertension, nursing care of infants with MAS centers on maintenance of adequate oxygenation and acid–base balance and on the avoidance of cold stress, which contributes to acidosis. A high incidence of air leaks exists in these infants, and positive pressure ventilation is best avoided if the patient can be adequately oxygenated, even at very high-inspired oxygen concentrations. Antibiotics are often used, particularly in desperately ill infants, at least until a bacterial infection is ruled out, but antibiotic therapy may not be necessary. The infant is often exquisitely sensitive to environmental stimuli and should be treated in as quiet an environment as possible. Interventions should be preplanned to maximize efficiency of handling the infant. Infants with very severe respiratory failure and MAS improve with the administration of exogenous surfactant (El Shahed, Dargaville, Ohlsson, & Soll, 2007).

Although aspiration of meconium is most common, the neonate may become symptomatic as a result of the aspiration of blood, amniotic fluid, or gastrointestinal contents. The history is important in the differential diagnosis because radiographs are nondiagnostic.

Pulmonary Hemorrhage

Pulmonary hemorrhage is rarely an isolated condition and usually occurs in an otherwise sick infant. RDS, asphyxia, congenital heart disease, aspiration of gastric content or maternal blood, and disseminated intravascular coagulation and other bleeding disorders may play a role in the cause of pulmonary hemorrhage. The risk for pulmonary hemorrhage is increased by approximately 5% in infants receiving either natural or artificial surfactant. Massive bleeding may also occur as a complication of airway suction secondary to direct trauma of the respiratory epithelium.

Pulmonary hemorrhage is manifested by the presence of bloody fluid from the trachea. When massive, it may be heralded by a sudden deterioration with pallor, shock, cyanosis, or bradycardia. Attention must be given to maintenance of a patent airway because an obstructed endotracheal tube requires emergency replacement. However, replacing an occluded airway in the context of a massive pulmonary hemorrhage should be undertaken with caution as the bleeding can make visualization of the trachea difficult. Suctioning must be done with great care to avoid precipitation of further bleeding. Clotting factors can be consumed rapidly, and the nurse should be alert to signs of generalized bleeding.

Pleural Effusions

Pleural effusions may be caused by accumulation of fluid between the parietal pleura of the chest wall and the visceral pleura enveloping the lung. A pleural effusion may also be due to chylothorax (lymphatic fluid) or hemothorax (blood). Lymphatics drain fluid that filters into the pleural space. Fluid accumulates in the pleural space as a result of either increased filtration or decreased absorption. An increase in filtration pressure, as seen with increased venous pressure in hydrops fetalis or congestive heart failure, leads to pleural effusion. The rate of filtration into the pleural space also increases if the pleural membrane becomes more permeable to water and protein, as occurs with infection.

Pleural effusion with high glucose content in an infant who is receiving parenteral nutrition via a central venous catheter should raise the suspicion of catheter perforation into the pleural space. If the infant is also receiving lipid infusion, the fluid may appear milky and be confused with chylothorax.

Chylothorax may be either congenital or acquired. Congenital chylothorax frequently presents at delivery or shortly after with respiratory distress. Chylothorax can also be acquired as a surgical complication of repair of diaphragmatic hernia, tracheoesophageal fistula, or congenital heart defect. Congenital chylothorax may be suspected in the infant who cannot be ventilated in the delivery room. Breath sounds are difficult to hear, and chest movement with ventilation is minimal. Bilateral thoracenteses may be lifesaving. The typical pleural fluid in a chylothorax—opalescent and rich in fat—is present only if the infant has been fed. Therefore the fluid aspirated in the delivery room or shortly after birth in a child with congenital chylothorax often has a low triglyceride level.

Pleural effusions that impede respiratory function typically require drainage by thoracentesis or tube thoracostomy. It may be necessary for chest tubes placed for chylothorax and thoracic duct injury to remain in place for extended periods while the infant is given total parenteral nutrition, receiving nothing by mouth, thus minimizing thoracic duct flow.

Apnea

Apnea is the common end product of a myriad of neonatal physiologic events. Hypoxemia, infection, anemia, thermal instability, metabolic derangement, drugs, and intracranial disease can cause apnea. These causes should be considered before idiopathic apnea of prematurity is diagnosed.

Apnea is observed in more than half of surviving premature infants who weigh less than 1.5 kg at birth. The respiratory control mechanism and central responsiveness to carbon dioxide is progressively less mature the lower the gestational age. In contrast to adults, infants respond to hypoxemia with only a brief hyperpneic response followed by hypoventilation or apnea. In any infant who has apnea, hypoxemia should always be ruled out before the clinician embarks on any other workup or institutes therapy.

Care of the infant experiencing apneic episodes requires close observation. Obstructive apnea cannot be detected with the impedance respiratory monitor because normal or pronounced respiratory excursions of the chest wall exist. Prompt tactile stimulation for mild "spells" is often sufficient to abort the episode of apnea, obviating the need for further therapy. Infants with apneic episodes accompanied by profound bradycardia need prompt attention to their immediate needs as well as more aggressive diagnostic and therapeutic intervention.

Sensory stimulation with waterbeds or other means can sometimes be used to manage these infants, particularly those with mild apnea. Many apneic neonates respond to nasal CPAP at low pressures because the apnea may be due to airway obstruction or intermittent hypoxemia. Pressure support may also stimulate pulmonary stretch receptors, thus stimulating respiration. Nursing care that is directed toward promoting a neutral thermal environment, normoxia, optimal airway maintenance, and prevention of aspiration is essential in the care of neonates at risk for apnea.

Use of methylxanthines, such as caffeine and aminophylline, has markedly simplified the treatment of apnea in some premature infants. Xanthines appear to exert a central stimulatory effect on brainstem respiratory neurons and often markedly decrease the frequency and severity of apneic episodes. The clinician must be attuned to the toxicities of xanthines, including tachycardia, excessive diuresis, and vomiting, which may precede neurologic toxicity at inadvertently high blood drug levels. Caffeine may be associated with a lower risk of adverse effects (Schmidt et al., 2006).

CONGENITAL ANOMALIES THAT AFFECT RESPIRATORY FUNCTION

Diaphragmatic Hernia

CDH occurs at a frequency of 1 in 2,500 live births and may be unsuspected until birth. Herniation of abdominal contents into the chest cavity early in gestation is accompanied by ipsilateral pulmonary hypoplasia. By mechanisms that are not well understood, there is often some degree of pulmonary hypoplasia on the contralateral side as well. Most infants are symptomatic at birth, with severe respiratory distress in the delivery room. The affected newborn's abdomen is usually scaphoid, and breath sounds are absent on the side of the defect (a left-sided defect occurs in 90% of cases). Bowel sounds may be heard in the chest, and heart sounds may be heard on the right side because the herniated abdominal contents push the mediastinum to the right.

As soon as the diagnosis is suspected, bag and mask ventilation should be avoided because it fills the herniated intestinal contents with gas which can lead to further lung compression and worsening ventilation. When CDH has been diagnosed prenatally, the infant should be intubated and mechanical ventilation should be initiated immediately after birth. An orogastric tube should be placed to aid in decompression of the herniated abdominal viscera. Ventilation should be attempted with a rapid rate and low inflation pressure and tolerating hypercapnia. Symptomatic neonates often have pulmonary hypertension and progressive right-to-left shunting. Hypotension is common, and, when adequate intravascular volume is established, dopamine infusion may be helpful. Studies of inhaled nitric oxide have shown limited evidence for effectiveness in the treatment of diaphragmatic hernia (Finer & Barrington, 2006). Although evidence of surfactant deficiency in these newborns exists, surfactant administration does not appear to improve their clinical course or outcome (Colby et al., 2004).

Survival rates are poor in infants who are symptomatic at birth, and ECMO commonly is required, often to no avail. Surgery to repair the defect is indicated. Controversy regarding the urgency of the procedure exists among pediatric surgeons, and some prefer to stabilize the patient with mechanical ventilation, vasopressors, and correction of acidosis before undertaking surgical intervention; others perform surgical repair while the patient is maintained on ECMO.

Congenital Heart Disease

Congenital heart disease commonly manifests with signs of respiratory distress. Neonates with congenital heart disease who demonstrate right-to-left shunting and decreased pulmonary blood flow (e.g., tetralogy of Fallot, pulmonary valve atresia, and tricuspid valve atresia or stenosis) usually present with profound cyanosis unresponsive to oxygen supplementation. Neonates with congenital heart disease who demonstrate increased pulmonary blood flow or obstruction to the left outflow tract (e.g., transposition of the great vessels, total anomalous pulmonary venous return, atrioventricular canal, hypoplastic left heart syndrome, and critical coarctation of the aorta) may transiently improve with oxygen supplementation. However, oxygen supplementation in some conditions such as hypoplastic left heart syndrome can worsen systemic flow and make the child worse. Neonates with noncyanotic lesions such as patent ductus arteriosus and ventricular septal defect may present with signs of congestive heart failure (see Chapter 7).

Choanal Atresia

Choanal atresia causes upper airway obstruction in the neonate. The choanae, or nasal passages, are separated from the nasopharynx by a structure known as the bucconasal membrane, which normally perforates during gestation. Failure of this developmental event results in an obstructed airway, occurring bilaterally in 50% of cases. Most affected infants are female and half of affected infants have associated anomalies such as CHARGE (coloboma, heart defects, atresia of the choanae, retardation of growth and development, genital and urinary abnormalities, and ear abnormalities and/or hearing loss) syndrome. Because newborns are obligate nasal breathers, they have chest retractions and severe cyanosis (particularly during feeding), and paradoxically turn pink when crying. Emergency treatment consists of tracheal intubation or placement of an oral airway. Surgical correction is indicated, though the ideal surgical intervention remains unclear (Cedin, Atallah, Andriolo, Cruz, & Pignatari, 2012).

Cystic Hygroma

A variety of space-occupying lesions can impose on the airway of the newborn (Box 6.4). Most are derived from embryonic tissues. Cystic hygroma, derived from lymphatic tissue, is the most common lateral neck mass in the newborn. It is multilobular, is multicystic, and, when large, obstructs the airway. Surgery is curative, although it is sometimes technically difficult. The clinician must always be mindful of the airway and its patency. Many of these lesions are of great cosmetic concern and cause great distress in the parents. A care plan should address these parental concerns. It is sometimes helpful to facilitate contact with parents of other children with similar problems who can share similar experiences.

Pierre Robin Sequence

The major feature of Pierre Robin sequence is micrognathia (a small mandible). The tongue is posteriorly displaced into the oropharynx, thus obstructing the airway. Sixty percent of affected patients also have a cleft palate. Obstructive respiratory distress and cyanosis are common and may be severe. In an emergency, as with all airway obstructions (obstructive apnea), tracheal intubation should be undertaken. Infants with Pierre Robin sequence are nursed in the prone position to prevent the tongue from falling backward. Nasogastric tube feedings are usually required in the neonatal period. With good care, the infant has a good prognosis for survival; the mandible usually grows; and the problem resolves by 6 to 12 months of age.

BOX 6.4

THORACIC CYSTS AND TUMORS THAT MAY CAUSE RESPIRATORY DISTRESS IN THE NEONATE

Teratoma
Cystic hygroma

- Neurogenic tumor
- Neuroblastoma
- Ganglioneuroma
- Neurofibroma

Bronchial or bronchogenic cyst
Intrapulmonary cyst
Gastrogenic cyst
Hemangioma
Angiosarcoma
Mediastinal goiter
Thymoma
Mesenchymoma
Lipoma
Cystic adenomatous malformation

Adapted from Battista and Carlo (1992).

COLLABORATIVE MANAGEMENT OF INFANTS WITH RESPIRATORY DISORDERS

Supportive Care

Supportive care of the infant in respiratory distress requires attention to detail. The clinicians' primary goals are to minimize oxygen consumption and carbon dioxide production. These goals are accomplished by maintaining a neutral thermal environment. The nurse must be skilled in physical assessment to interpret signs and symptoms, such as cyanosis, gasping, tachypnea, grunting, nasal flaring, and retractions. By understanding the pathophysiology of breathing, the nurse knows that the infant with retractions has decreased lung compliance and that the cyanotic infant has poor tissue oxygenation.

Excellent communication is needed between the neonatal nurse and the rest of the neonatal team. Acutely ill neonates with respiratory disease are often unstable and their condition can deteriorate rapidly, so astute observation skills are necessary. Assessment is a continuous process, and effective communication among nurses, respiratory therapists, physicians, and support staff is necessary for proper delivery of intensive care. The nurse, who is the primary bedside caregiver, is the gatekeeper for all interactions between the patient and the environment. The nurse who is caring for an unstable patient should be the patient's advocate, whether such a role involves regulating the timing of a physical examination by the physician or venipuncture for laboratory investigation.

Technical competence is an important facet of the nurse's repertoire. The nurse is responsible for maintaining intravenous lines and tracheal tube patency, accurately measuring volumes of intravenous intake as well as urinary output, and operating advanced electronic machinery. Moreover, the nurse must also be adept at interpreting arterial blood gas and laboratory data in order to communicate these to the rest of the care team and to develop a cogent management plan. Many functions are shared to some degree with respiratory therapists. Whether nurses or respiratory therapists make ventilator changes, the nurse should become familiar with the effects of ventilator setting changes on blood gases. $PaCO_2$ is affected by changes in ventilator rate and tidal volume. Tidal volume depends on the difference between PIP and PEEP. Thus, to decrease $PaCO_2$, either rate or inspiratory pressure should be increased. PaO_2 depends on the fraction of inspired oxygen concentration (FiO_2) and mean airway pressure (MAP). MAP depends on PIP, PEEP, inspiratory to expiratory time ratio, and gas flow. To improve PaO_2, the most effective changes are to increase MAP by increasing PIP or PEEP or to increase FiO_2. The nurse should also be familiar with ventilator functioning so that malfunctions can be detected promptly. The nurse should always be prepared to bag-ventilate an intubated neonate in the event that decompensation occurs while the status of the ventilatory apparatus is checked. Nurses and therapists often share such functions as airway suctioning, monitoring and recording of inspired oxygen concentration, and delivery of chest physical therapy.

The delivery of oxygen therapy should always be carefully monitored. Desired oxygenation parameters should be recorded in the nurse's notes and followed up with measurement of arterial blood gases or by noninvasive means. The acutely ill infant should have FiO_2 measured continuously and recorded frequently. The goal for oxygenation depends on the patient's diagnosis and condition. For example, in infants with PPHN, an apparently acceptable saturation may occur despite marked right-to-left shunting. In preterm infants oxygen saturation should be kept in the low 90s, thus avoiding the risks associated with hyperoxia or hypoxemia. Recent large randomized controlled trials (Carlo et al., 2010; Stenson et al., 2011) indicate that targeting lower oxygen saturations (85%–89%) versus higher saturations (91%–95%) decreases the rates of retinopathy of prematurity but increases mortality.

Airway suctioning is a procedure that may be associated with cardiopulmonary derangement, hypoxemia, bradycardia, and hypertension. Various techniques to perform airway suctioning exist—including preoxygenation (increase in FiO_2 before the procedure), normal saline instillation before the suctioning to improve secretion aspiration, and the use of a closed system to avoid disconnection from the ventilator. The nurse should become familiar with the techniques used in the NICU and be aware of the associated complications.

The sudden decompensation of a ventilated infant should alert the nurse to assess disconnection of the ventilator, pulmonary air leak, ventilator failure, or obstructed tracheal tube (see Figure 6.4). The very small infant who suddenly decompensates may have experienced a severe intracranial hemorrhage.

Care of the infant who is receiving CPAP can be particularly challenging. These infants should be kept calm and swaddled if necessary. Crying releases pressure through the mouth; thus lung volume is lost. Nasal CPAP can be effective, but particular attention must be given to maintaining patency of the nose, the nasal prongs, and the pharynx. The infant's nares and nasal septum should be guarded from pressure necrosis from inappropriately applied prongs. The infant who requires mechanical ventilation must be constantly assessed for airway patency. If the infant is unable to grunt against a closed glottis and maintain positive airway pressure, the condition may worsen if airway pressure is not maintained properly. Suctioning of the airway should be done only as often as necessary to remove pulmonary secretions that could occlude the airway. The suction catheter should be passed no further than the end of the tracheal tube because epithelium is easily damaged. Vibration and percussion should be used judiciously in the infant with pulmonary secretions to loosen them and allow removal via suction. There is perhaps little need to vigorously suction the intubated infant with RDS in the first days after birth because secretions are minimal and lung volume is lost with every disconnection of the ventilator circuit.

ASSESSMENT AND MONITORING

The most important aspect in monitoring patients with respiratory disease is the close and continuous observation of signs and symptoms. The color of the patient gives important clues. An infant with pink lips and oral mucosa has good oxygenation and perfusion; a cyanotic patient has poor tissue oxygenation. If the hemoglobin concentration is too low, the patient can be hypoxemic, but because the concentration of deoxyhemoglobin is low, there may be no cyanosis. An infant with tachypnea and retraction usually has decreased lung compliance. A patient with a barrel-shaped thorax, taking deep breaths, and with a normal or low respiratory rate probably has an increased airway resistance and gas trapping. Observation of the intubated patient is especially important. An anguished infant, who is cyanotic and breathing deeply, may have an obstructed endotracheal tube. An infant with RDS and increased chest expansion over time, despite no change in ventilatory pressure, is experiencing improvement in lung compliance. The same infant with later asymmetry in chest and sudden deterioration of oxygenation may have a pneumothorax. Cardiac beats, easily seen through the thoracic wall, may be caused by the presence of a symptomatic patent ductus arteriosus. A recently extubated infant, in whom increased retractions and inspiratory stridor develop, probably has upper airway obstruction. Auscultation helps in the diagnosis of increased airway resistance or the presence of secretions. It also allows the clinician to assess the response to different treatment maneuvers, such as suctioning, chest physiotherapy, and bronchodilation. Asymmetries in auscultation suggest mainstream bronchial intubation, atelectasis, pneumothorax, or pleural effusion.

Great progress has been made in noninvasive monitoring of blood gas tensions, but blood sampling is still necessary for pH determination and arterial samples are preferable. Capillary specimens are undependable, especially for PO_2. If peripheral perfusion is adequate, capillary blood approximates arterial values of pH and PCO_2. However, capillary blood PO_2 values do not reliably reflect arterial oxygenation.

Neonatal care has changed dramatically with the advent and widespread use of transcutaneous monitoring of PaO_2, $PaCO_2$, and SaO_2. The neonatal intensive care team should become familiar with the devices used in noninvasive gas monitoring. Knowing the basis for their functioning as well as how to interpret the information they provide and being aware of clinical situations in which the information provided is not reliable or needs to be complemented before any management decisions are made is essential.

Transcutaneous PO_2 ($TcPO_2$) is measured with an electrode that is applied over the skin and heated to 42°C to 44°C. The electrode measures skin PO_2, not arterial PO_2. Skin PO_2 measurement depends on skin perfusion and on oxygen diffusion across the epidermis. Warming the skin to 42°C to 44°C under the electrode increases skin perfusion so that $TcPO_2$ correlates better with arterial PO_2.

For initiation of $TcPO_2$ monitoring, 10 to 15 minutes are needed to obtain a stable reading. After that, $TcPO_2$ reflects changes on FiO_2 with a 10- to 20-second delay. After 4 to 6 hours, the method becomes unreliable because of changes in skin secondary to hyperthermia, so the electrode position should be changed. In premature infants with more labile skin, the electrode placement should be changed even more frequently to avoid skin burns. The nurse should be aware of situations that make $TcPO_2$ lose its reliability. Overestimation of oxygenation occurs when an air bubble or leak between the electrode and the skin occurs or when the calibration is improper. Underestimation occurs with skin hypoperfusion, in older infants (increased thickness of the skin), with insufficient heating of the electrodes, or with improper calibration.

$TcPO_2$ monitoring has been largely supplanted by continuous pulse oximetry. Arterial oxygen saturation is computed from absorption of emitted low-intensity red or infrared light. The probe is attached to a finger or toe in large infants or to a hand or foot in small premature infants. Pulse oximetry offers the following advantages over transcutaneous oxygen monitoring: (1) avoidance of heating the skin and the risk of burns; (2) elimination of a delay period for transducer equilibration; (3) accurate measurement regardless of presence of edema or patient age; (4) in vitro calibration not required; and (5) frequent position changes not required. However, the nurse should be aware that SaO_2 higher than 97% may be associated with PaO_2 higher than 100 mmHg. This is important in premature infants who are at risk for retinopathy of prematurity. SaO_2 between 85% and 95% probably is associated with a safe range of PaO_2. With SaO_2 over 95% to 97% and especially when it is 100%, the clinician cannot predict a patient's PaO_2. When the saturation is 100%, the PaO_2 can be approximately 100 mmHg or much higher (see Figure 6.1). This situation is particularly important in infants with PPHN because the decision whether to wean ventilator settings depends on PaO_2. In these patients, the simultaneous use of $TcPO_2$ and pulse oximetry is a useful alternative.

A common problem of pulse oximetry is the presence of motion artifact, an altered signal caused by movement of the part of the body where the sensor is applied. Because the pulse waveform is not detected, this movement is recognized by the loss of correlation between the oximeter pulse rate and the electrical monitor heart rate. With current technology the motion artifacts have been minimized (Malviya et al., 2000). Peripheral pulse oximetry may not detect pulse signals in patients with hypotension and poor perfusion. $TcPO_2$ may also give false readings in this situation. The clinician should be aware that pressure of the probe over the skin can produce skin pressure necrosis. This consideration is particularly important in the premature infant. Phototherapy may interfere with accuracy of SaO_2 monitoring, but this problem can be avoided by covering the sensor with an opaque material (e.g., a diaper).

$TcPO_2$ monitoring and pulse oximetry are useful in several clinical situations. They may be used in neonates with mild respiratory distress, such as transient tachypnea, to assess the oxygen requirement and to allow weaning without placement of an arterial catheter. In infants receiving mechanical ventilation, $TcPO_2$ or pulse oximetry helps to assess the effects of ventilator setting changes, thus reducing the need for arterial blood sampling. Continuous oxygenation monitoring reduces the risk of hyperoxemia or hypoxemia during interventions such as airway suctioning, position change, lumbar puncture, or venous cannulation. This monitoring is particularly helpful in the care of infants who do not tolerate excessive stimulation, such as those with PPHN. $TcPO_2$ and pulse-oximetry monitoring are also useful in caring for patients with PPHN because simultaneous monitoring of preductal (head, right arm, right upper chest) and postductal (left arm, abdomen, legs) $TcPO_2$ or SaO_2 allows assessment of the magnitude of ductal shunting or the response to therapies such as vasodilation or alkalinization.

Transcutaneously measured PCO_2 is accomplished with a glass electrode that is pH-sensitive. Transcutaneous PCO_2 response is slower than that of $TcPO_2$, and the value measured must be corrected for skin production of carbon dioxide. Thus transcutaneously measured values are approximately 1.3 to 1.4 times higher than arterial PCO_2 values. Most modern monitors display an electronically corrected value to $TcPO_2$. This modality is especially useful for monitoring chronically ventilated patients without indwelling catheters. Blood gas values during arterial puncture or vigorous crying during the procedure are often affected by breath holding and shunting and thus may be misleading.

ENVIRONMENTAL CONSIDERATIONS

Maintenance of the therapeutic environment is an important nursing function. Much attention has been given recently to the effects of sensory stimulation on the infant with respiratory distress. The sick newborn often has unstable pulmonary vasculature and may be particularly prone to hypoxic vasoconstriction. This phenomenon may be triggered in some individuals by excess stimulation, such as loud noise, handling, or venipuncture. It has been shown that the agitated neonate has more difficulty with oxygenation and that a quiet, minimally stimulating environment allows for more stable oxygenation (Als, 1998). The nurse should develop a care plan that allows the baby long periods of undisturbed rest by clustering interventions into short periods whenever possible. Positioning the infant in the flexed or fetal position or "nesting" may help in calming some infants. Always watch for stress cues to see how the infant is tolerating the care. Clustering of care only works if the infant tolerates a longer period of care rather than episodic care. Either way the infant needs undisturbed periods where rest and recovery can occur.

FAMILY CARE

Neonates with respiratory distress frequently require multiple instrumentations. They may have endotracheal tubes, umbilical catheters, oximeter probes, chest leads, and other paraphernalia attached or applied to the skin. All of these interventions can give parents a feeling of increased separation from the infant. The nurse should explain the equipment surrounding the bedside as well as the function of invasive catheters, monitoring leads, and tracheal tubes. Terminology appropriate to the parents' level of understanding should be used. Even the most astute parents may be bewildered, and repetition is necessary. Staff should maintain consistent terminology so that the parents do not become confused between "respirators" and "ventilators." Whenever possible, the use of frightening or inaccurate terms should be avoided. Imagine the fear engendered by the phrase, "We paralyzed your baby last night."

Parents should be involved in developing and implementing the plan of care as much as possible. The mother who plans to breastfeed can be assisted in pumping her breasts and freezing the milk, even if enteral feedings are delayed for some time. This pumping may be the only thing that she alone can do for her baby.

Often lost in the bustle of critical care is the need for privacy. The perceptive nurse senses this need and backs away from the bedside when appropriate, allowing the parent some time with the infant. Care of the neonate requires a team—a coordinate team and that includes the parents!

SUMMARY

Most infants admitted to the NICU present with breathing difficulty. Nursing care of these infants requires a broad knowledge of newborn physiology and practical skills in the application of therapies that are directed toward solving the many problems that sick infants can have. The nurse often must anticipate these problems. While managing the nursing care for several patients, the neonatal nurse must also care for the sickest of infants. Parents and family of all infants in the NICU require special attention not only to achieve an understanding of the complex issues surrounding the infant's illness but also to calm fears and guilt that are often experienced. The rewards of being part of the accomplishments in the NICU may be overlooked as they are usually slowly achieved. But, when they are recognized, the victories surpass the greatest of expectations.

CASE STUDY

■ Identification of the Problem. A term infant was admitted to the NICU. The infant developed respiratory distress soon after birth. Birth weight was 4,000 g. Since birth, the infant had an increasing oxygen requirement and because of a recent desaturation episode, he is now receiving 100% oxygen on a ventilator. The ventilatory settings are PIP of 25 cm H_2O, PEEP of 5 cm H_2O, ventilator rate 60 per minute, and inspiratory time 0.4 seconds. A recent blood gas showed a pH of 7.35 $pC0_2$ of 42, pO_2 of 60, and bicarbonate of 22.

■ Assessment: History and Physical Examination. The infant was born by emergency C-section because of late decelerations and thick meconium-stained fluid. No signs of infection were observed. His mother had gestational diabetes and was maintained on insulin. The infant was not vigorous at birth and was intubated and received endotracheal suction. No meconium was aspirated from below the vocal cords. Blow-by oxygen was given and the infant responded well, initially weaned to 40% oxygen. However, after transfer to the NICU, he had increasing oxygen requirements.

The physical examination is now pertinent for excellent chest rise, equal breath sounds, central cyanosis with oxygen saturations in the mid-80s, good color and perfusion, and normal tone and reflexes.

■ Differential Diagnosis. Many conditions should be considered in the differential diagnosis in this patient.

1. Persistent pulmonary hypertension of the neonate. This is likely, given the severity and persistence of the very abnormal alveolar to arterial oxygen gradient ($AaDO_2$). Pulmonary hypertension may be associated with MAS. It is important to consider that right-to-left shunting can occur associated with disorders such as myocardial dysfunction, sepsis, metabolic abnormalities, and others.
2. MAS. MAS with intrapulmonary (ventilation-perfusion mismatch) or extrapulmonary shunting (atrial or ductal shunting with pulmonary hypertension) may lead to desaturation despite high oxygen supplementation.
3. Pneumothorax. Infants with MAS are at high risk for pneumothorax. A pneumothorax can cause severe desaturation.
4. Gas trapping. Because this infant has a large tidal volume for the given pressure gradient (PIP minus PEEP) and thus high compliance, a long-time constant of the respiratory system leading to gas trapping at a borderline high ventilator rate should be considered.
5. Other causes. There are other less frequent causes in the differential diagnosis.

■ Diagnostic Tests. The chest radiograph was obtained, repeat blood gases were followed, and pre- and postductal pulse oximetry and transcutaneous measurements of gases were monitored continuously. In addition, a complete blood count (CBC) and blood culture were obtained. Four extremity blood pressures and an echocardiogram were obtained.

■ Working Diagnosis. The chest radiograph showed bilateral gas trapping. The CBC and the blood cultures were negative. The echocardiogram was consistent with persistent pulmonary hypertension.

■ Development of Management Plan. The infant was given surfactant, and initial improvement was seen. However, during the next 24 hours there were episodes of repeated intracardiac and ductal shunting, which led to the initiation of nitric oxide.

■ Implementation and Evaluation of Effectiveness Nitric oxide resulted in a marked reduction of the shunting episodes. The infant was gradually weaned off FiO_2 and subsequently weaned off nitric oxide before extubation. He was entirely weaned off the ventilator and FiO_2 over the subsequent 3 days.

EVIDENCE-BASED PRACTICE BOX

RDS is the most common cause of respiratory distress in preterm neonates (Hamvas, 2011). Most children that are born extremely premature develop RDS in the first hours after birth. The incidence of RDS is progressively more common the lower the infant's gestational age. Up to 98% of infants born at 23 weeks and 86% of infants born at 28 weeks develop RDS (Stoll et al., 2010). Many of these are treated with surfactant (Stoll et al., 2010). RDS can develop in term infants born to mothers with diabetes or in term infants who have experienced asphyxia, but it is substantially less frequent than in premature infants.

Antenatal steroids accelerate lung maturation. Present recommendations are to give steroids to all mothers between 24 and 34 weeks gestational age with threatened delivery. Antenatal steroids significantly reduce the incidence of RDS in premature infants. Antenatal steroids also decrease mortality, intraventricular hemorrhage, necrotizing enterocolitis, and neurodevelopmental impairment (Carlo et al., 2011; Schmidt et al., 2006). Adverse effects have not been reported with the usual single course of antenatal steroids (Carlo et al., 2011; Schmidt et al., 2006). Data at the limits of viability (i.e., <25 weeks) show benefits to giving steroids to infants as early as 22 weeks (Carlo et al., 2011).

The hallmark of RDS is deficiency of pulmonary surfactant. Surfactant reduces the alveolar surface tension thus preventing alveolar collapse. Therapy is directed toward improving oxygenation as well as maintaining optimal lung volume. CPAP can be used to prevent volume loss during expiration. Exogenous surfactants are also quite effective at treating RDS but require endotracheal intubation and exposure to mechanical ventilation. Early clinical trials indicated that prophylactic surfactant administration to extremely premature infants in the delivery room is more effective than waiting for the treatment after development of RDS (Soll & Morley, 2001). However, more recent trials show equivalence between prophylactic surfactant administration and early CPAP with rescue surfactant (Finer et al., 2010). The most recent Cochrane review of the topic did not recommend routine administration of prophylactic surfactant administration as there was less risk of BPD death at 36 weeks when using early CPAP with selective surfactant administration for infants requiring intubation (Rojas-Reyes et al., 2012).

ONLINE RESOURCES

Association of Women's Health, Obstetric and Neonatal Nurses (AWHONN)
http://www.awhonn.org

National Association of Neonatal Nurses (NANN)
http://www.nann.org

Neonatology on the web
http://www.neonatology.org

NICHD calculators (NICHD gestational age calculator; mortality calculator; survival calculator; extreme prematurity calculator; neonatal outcomes calculator, preemie calculator)

NICHD Neonatal Research Network (NRN): Extremely Preterm Birth Outcome Data
http://www.nichd.nih.gov/about/org/cdbpm/pp/prog_epbo/epbo_case.cfm
http://www.nichd.nih.gov/neonatalestimate

The NICHD Cochrane Neonatal Collaborative
http://www.nichd.nih.gov/cochrane

REFERENCES

Als, H. (1998). Developmental care in the newborn intensive care unit. *Current Opinion in Pediatrics, 10*, 138–142.

Battista, M. A., & Carlo, W. A. (1992). Differential diagnosis of acute respiratory distress in the neonate. *Tufts University School of Medicine and Floating Hospital for Children Reports on Neonatal Respiratory Diseases, 2*(3), 1–4, 9–11.

Carlo, W. A., & Di Fiore, J. M. (2011). The respiratory system: Part 2 assessment of pulmonary function. In A. A. Fanaroff & R. J. Martin (Eds.), *Neonatal-perinatal medicine: Diseases of the fetus and infant* (9th ed.). St Louis, MO: Mosby.

Carlo, W. A., Finer, N. N., Walsh, M. C., Rich, W., Gantz, M. G., Laptook, A. R., . . . SUPPORT Study Group of the Eunice Kennedy Shriver NICHD Neonatal Research Network. (2010). Target ranges of oxygen saturation in extremely preterm infants. *New England Journal of Medicine, 362*, 1959–1969.

Carlo, W. A., McDonald, S. A., Fanaroff, A. A., Vohr, B. R., Stoll, B. J., Ehrenkranz, R. A., . . . Eunice Kennedy Shriver National Institute of Child Health and Human Development Neonatal Research Network. (2011). Association of antenatal corticosteroids with mortality and neurodevelopmental outcomes among infants born at 22 to 25 weeks' gestation. *Journal of the American Medical Association, 306*, 2348–2358.

Cedin, A. C., Atallah, A. N., Andriolo, R. B., Cruz, O. L., & Pignatari, S. N. (2012). Surgery for congenital choanal atresia. *Cochrane Database of Systematic Reviews*, (2), CD008993.

Colby, C. E., Lally, K. P., Hintz, S. R., Lally, P. A., Tibboel, D., Moya, F. R., . . . Congenital Diaphragmatic Hernia Study Group. (2004). Surfactant replacement therapy on ECMO does not improve outcome in neonates with congenital diaphragmatic hernia. *Journal of Pediatric Surgery, 39*, 1632–1637.

Cordero, L., Sananes, M., & Ayers, L. W. (2000). Comparison of a closed (trach care MAC) with an open endotracheal suction system in small premature infants. *Journal of Perinatology, 20*, 151–156.

Davidson, D., Barefield, E. S., Kattwinkel, J., Dudell, G., Damask, M., Straube, R., . . . Chang, C. T. (1998). Inhaled nitric oxide for the early treatment of persistent pulmonary hypertension of the term newborn: A randomized, double-masked, placebo-controlled, dose-response multicenter study. *Pediatrics, 101*, 325–334.

Dhillon, R. (2011, January 30). The management of neonatal pulmonary hypertension. *Archives of Disease in Childhood Fetal and Neonatal Edition, 97* (3).

Ehrenkranz, R. A., Walsh, M. C., Vohr, B. R., Jobe, A. H., Wright, L. L., Fanaroff, A. A., . . . National Institutes of Child Health and Human Development Neonatal Research Network. (2005). Validation of the National Institutes of Health consensus definition of bronchopulmonary dysplasia. *Pediatrics, 116*, 1353–1360.

El Shahed, A. I., Dargaville, P., Ohlsson, A., & Soll, R. F. (2007). Surfactant for meconium aspiration syndrome in full term/near term infants. *Cochrane Database of Systematic Reviews*, (3), CD002054.

Finer, N. N., & Barrington, K. J. (2006). Nitric oxide for respiratory failure in infants born at or near term. *Cochrane Database of Systematic Reviews*, (4), CD000399.

Finer, N. N., Carlo, W. A., Walsh, M. C., Rich, W., Gantz, M. G., Laptook, A. R., . . . SUPPORT Study Group of the Eunice Kennedy Shriver NICHD Neonatal Research Network. (2010, May 27). Early CPAP versus surfactant in extremely preterm infants. *New England Journal of Medicine, 362*(21), 1970–1979.

Greenough, A., & Milner, A. D. (2005). Pulmonary disease of the newborn. In J. M. Rennie (Ed.), *Roberton's textbook of neonatology* (4th ed.). London, England: Churchill Livingstone.

Hamvas, A. (2011). The respiratory system: Part 3 pathophysiology and management of Respiratory Distress Syndrome. In A. A. Fanaroff & R. J. Martin (Eds.), *Neonatal-perinatal medicine: Diseases of the fetus and infant* (9th ed.). St Louis, MO: Mosby.

Janér, C., Pitkänen, O. M., Helve, O., & Andersson, S. (2011, July 18). Airway expression of the epithelial sodium channel α-subunit correlates with cortisol in term newborns. *Pediatrics, 128*, e414.

Jobe, A. H., & Bancalari, E. (2001). Bronchopulmonary dysplasia. *American Journal of Respiratory Critical Care Medicine, 163*, 1723–1729.

Litmanovitz, I., & Carlo, W. A. (2008). Expectant management of pneumothorax in ventilated neonates. *Pediatrics, 122*, e975–e979.

Malviya, S., Reynolds, P. I., Voepel-Lewis, T., Siewert, M., Watson, D., Tait, A. R., & Tremper, K. (2000). False alarms and sensitivity of conventional pulse oximetry versus the Masimo SET technology in the pediatric post anesthesia care unit. *Anesthesia and Analgesia, 90*(6), 1336–1340.

Mok, Q., Yates, R., & Tasker, R. C. (1999). Persistent pulmonary hypertension of the term neonate: A strategy for management. *European Journal of Pediatrics, 158*, 825–827.

Roberts, D., & Dalziel, S. (2007). Antenatal steroids for accelerating fetal lung maturation for women at risk of preterm birth (Review). The Cochrane Collaboration. Hoboken, NJ: John Wiley & Sons, Ltd.

Rojas-Reyes, M. X., Morley, C. J., & Soll, R. (2012). Prophylactic versus selective use of surfactant in preventing morbidity and mortality in preterm infants. *Cochrane Database of Systematic Reviews*, (3), CD000510.

Schmidt, B., Roberts, R. S., Davis, P., Doyle, L. W., Barrington, K. J., Ohlsson, A., . . . Caffeine for Apnea of Prematurity Trial Group. (2006). Caffeine therapy for apnea of prematurity. *New England Journal of Medicine, 354*(20), 2179–2180.

Soll, R. F., & Morley, C. J. (2001). Prophylactic versus selective use of surfactant for preventing morbidity and mortality in preterm infants. *Cochrane Database of Systematic Reviews*, (2), CD000510.

Stenson, B., Brocklehurst, P., Tarnow-Mordi, W., U.K. BOOST II trial, Australian BOOST II Trial & New Zealand BOOST II Trial. (2011). Increased 36-week survival with high oxygen saturation target in extremely preterm infants. *New England Journal of Medicine, 364*, 1680–1682.

Stoll, B. J., Hansen, N. I., Bell, E. F., Shankaran, S., Laptook, A. R., Walsh, M. C., . . . Eunice Kennedy Shriver National Institute of Child Health and Human Development Neonatal Research Network. (2010). Neonatal outcomes of extremely preterm infants from the NICHD Neonatal Research Network. *Pediatrics, 26*, 443–456.

The Neonatal Inhaled Nitric Oxide Study Group. (1997). Inhaled nitric oxide in full-term and nearly full-term infants with hypoxic respiratory failure. *New England Journal of Medicine, 336*(9), 597–604.

Thome, U. H., Carlo, W. A., & Pohlandt, F. (2005). Ventilation strategies and outcome in randomized trials of high frequency ventilation. *Archives of Disease in Childhood: Fetal and Neonatal Edition, 90*, F466–F473.

Tita, A. T., Landon, M. B., Spong, C. Y., Lai, Y., Leveno, K. J., Varner, M. W., . . . Eunice Kennedy Shriver NICHD Maternal-Fetal Medicine Units Network. (2009). Timing of elective repeat cesarean delivery at term and neonatal outcomes. *New England Journal of Medicine, 360*(2), 111–120.

UK Collaborative ECMO Trial Group. (1996). UK collaborative randomised trial of neonatal extracorporeal membrane oxygenation. *Lancet, 348*(9020), 75–82.

Vain, N. E., Szyld, E. G., Prudent, L. M., Wiswell, T. E., Aguilar, A. M., & Vivas, N. I. (2004). Oropharyngeal and nasopharyngeal suctioning of meconium-stained neonates before delivery of their shoulders: Multicentre, randomised controlled trial. *Lancet, 364*, 597–602.

Walsh-Sukys, M. C., Tyson, J. E., Wright, L. L., Bauer, C. R., Korones, S. B., Stevenson, D. K., . . . Fanaroff, A. A. (2000). Persistent pulmonary hypertension of the newborn in the era before nitric oxide: Practice variation and outcomes. *Pediatrics, 105*, 14–20.

Wiswell, T. E., Gannon, C. M., Jacob, J., Goldsmith, L., Szyld, E., Weiss, K., . . . Padula, M. (2000). Delivery room management of the apparently vigorous meconium-stained neonate: Results of the multicenter, international collaborative trial. *Pediatrics, 105*, 1–7.

Zaichkin, J., & Weiner, G. M. (2011, February). Neonatal Resuscitation Program (NRP) 2011: New science, new strategies. *Advances in Neonatal Care, 11*(1), 43–51.

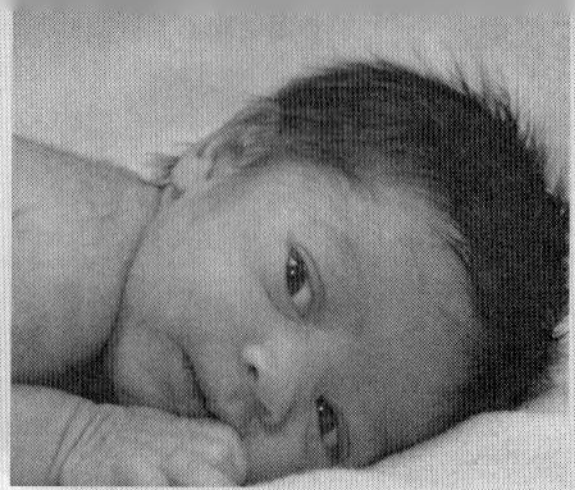

CHAPTER

7

Cardiovascular System

■ Judy Wright Lott

This chapter presents the physiology of normal cardiac function, including fetal circulatory patterns and the changes that occur during transition to extrauterine life. The most common congenital heart defects (CHDs) and cardiac complications are described. Information about incidence, hemodynamics, manifestations, diagnosis, and medical and surgical management is included. Because some CHDs are not identified during the neonatal period, information about presentation of some defects in older infants is included. The chapter concludes with a discussion about the support of the family of an infant with a CHD. A case study is used to illustrate the complex care infants and families of infants with cardiac disorders require.

CARDIOVASCULAR ADAPTATION

Fetal Circulation

Knowledge of the normal route of fetal blood flow is essential for understanding the circulatory changes that occur in the newborn at delivery. The pattern of fetal circulation is illustrated in Figure 7.1. Fetal circulation involves four unique anatomic features.

In fetal life, the placenta serves as the exchange organ for oxygen and carbon dioxide and for nutrients and wastes. The ductus venosus (DV) is a shunt that permits the majority of blood from the placenta to bypass the liver and enter the inferior vena cava (IVC). The foramen ovale (FO), an opening in the septum between the atria, permits a portion of the blood to flow from the right atrium directly to the left atrium; this reduces pulmonary blood flow. The patent ductus arteriosus (PDA) is a tubular communication between the pulmonary artery and the descending aorta that allows blood to flow from the right ventricle through the pulmonary artery to the descending aorta. This further decreases the amount of blood circulation through the fetal lungs (Park, 2007; Webb, Smallhorn, Therrien, & Reddington, 2011).

Oxygen diffuses into the fetal circulation from the maternal uterine arteries in the placenta. From the placenta, the oxygenated blood flows through the umbilical vein to the fetus. The fetal circulation divides at the liver; about half of the blood enters the liver. The remainder bypasses the liver and enters the IVC through the DV. In the IVC, the blood with lower oxygen content coming from the gastrointestinal tract, legs, and liver mixes with the blood of higher oxygen content. The mixed blood enters the right atrium (Park, 2007; Webb et al., 2011).

From this point, the blood from the right atrium flows directly to the left atrium through the FO. From the left atrium, the blood goes to the left ventricle and then to the head and neck through the ascending aorta. This circulatory pattern ensures that the fetal brain constantly receives well-oxygenated blood (Park, 2007; Webb et al., 2011).

The blood returns from the head and neck through the superior vena cava (SVC) to the right atrium, then into the right ventricle. From the right ventricle, the blood enters the pulmonary arteries. Only a small portion of this blood enters the pulmonary circuit to perfuse the lungs; most of the blood is shunted through the *ductus arteriosus* (DA) into the aorta to supply oxygen and nutrients to the trunk and lower extremities (Park, 2007; Webb et al., 2011).

The majority of the blood flow from the lower extremities rejoins the fetal circulation through the internal iliac arteries via the umbilical cord to the placenta, where it is reoxygenated and recirculated. A small amount of the blood from the lower extremities passes back into the ascending vena cava, mixed with fresh blood from the umbilical vein, and recirculated without reoxygenation. Fetal circulation consists of two parallel circuits rather than the serial circuit present in extrauterine life (Park, 2007; Webb et al., 2011).

Extrauterine Circulation

The cardiac and pulmonary systems undergo drastic changes at birth; these changes usually occur functionally immediately upon onset of respirations. The most significant change

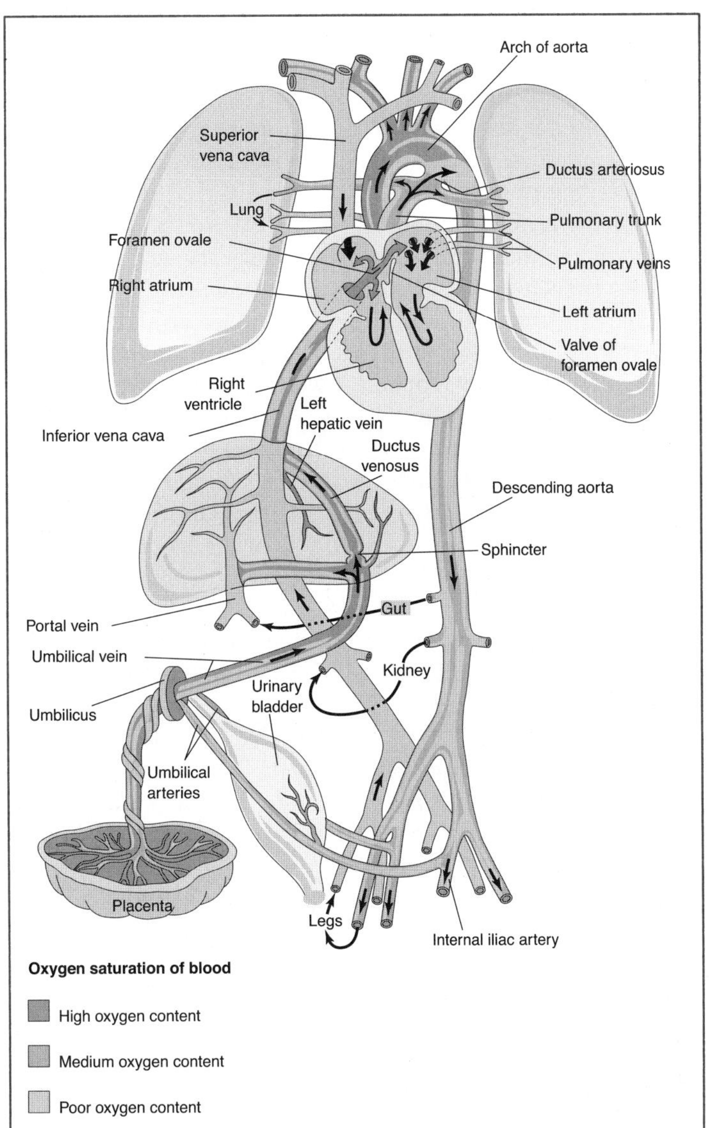

FIGURE 7.1 Fetal circulation.
Adapted and modified from Ross Laboratories, Columbus, OH, Clinical Education Aid, 1985.

is that the lungs assume the role of primary oxygenation. Clamping of the umbilical cord removes the placenta, and subsequently effects immediate circulatory changes in the newborn. With the first breath and occlusion of the umbilical cord, the newborn's systemic resistance is elevated, which decreases the amount of blood flow through the DA. Cord occlusion causes an increase in blood pressure and a corresponding stimulation of the aortic baroreceptors and the sympathetic nervous system. The onset of respirations and consequent lung expansion causes a decrease in pulmonary vascular resistance secondary to the direct effect of oxygen and carbon dioxide on the blood vessels. Pulmonary vascular resistance decreases as arterial oxygen increases and arterial carbon dioxide decreases (Park, 2007; Webb et al., 2011).

Most of the right ventricular output flows through the lungs and increases the pulmonary venous return to the left atrium. The increased amount of blood in the lungs and the heart causes pressure in the left atrium of the heart. The increased pressure in the left atrium, combined with the increased systemic vascular resistance, functionally closes the FO.

The DA generally closes within 15 to 24 hours postbirth in response to increased arterial oxygen content caused by pulmonary respiratory effort of the newborn and the effects of sympathomimetic amines and prostaglandins. The DA is anatomically obliterated by constriction by 3 to 4 weeks of age. Clamping of the umbilical cord causes the cessation of blood flow through the DV; it is anatomically obliterated by approximately 1 to 2 weeks postbirth. After birth, the umbilical vein and arteries no longer transport blood and are obliterated.

Functional closure refers to the cessation of flow through the structure caused by changes in pressure. *Anatomic closure* refers to obliteration of the structure by constriction or growth of tissue.

Because anatomic closure of the fetal pathways lags behind functional closure, the shunts may open and close intermittently before anatomic closure, resulting in transient functional murmurs.

Pulmonary artery pressure remains high for several hours after delivery. As the pulmonary vascular resistance decreases, the direction of blood flow through the DA reverses. Initially bidirectional, the flow becomes entirely left to right; it is functionally insignificant by approximately 15 hours after birth. Intermittent or functional murmurs do not cause any cardiovascular compromise for the newborn and are not clinically significant. Conditions that cause transient opening of fetal shunts, allowing un-oxygenated blood to shunt from the right side of the heart to the left, thereby bypassing the pulmonary circuit, produce transient cyanosis. Any murmur or cyanosis in the newborn should be carefully evaluated and monitored to detect cardiovascular abnormalities (Jones, 2005; Park, 2007; Webb et al., 2011). Hypoxemia can cause a constricted DA to reopen and may reestablish increased pulmonary vascular resistance, leading to persistent pulmonary hypertension of the newborn (PPHN). The DA responds to hypoxemia by opening, whereas the pulmonary arterioles respond by constricting (Park, 2007; Webb et al., 2011).

NORMAL CARDIAC FUNCTION

The normal anatomy of the heart is shown in Figure 7.2.

Cardiac Valves

Blood flow through the heart is directed through two sets of one-way valves. The *semilunar valves* consist of the *pulmonary valve* and the *aortic valve*. The pulmonary valve connects the right ventricle and the pulmonary artery.

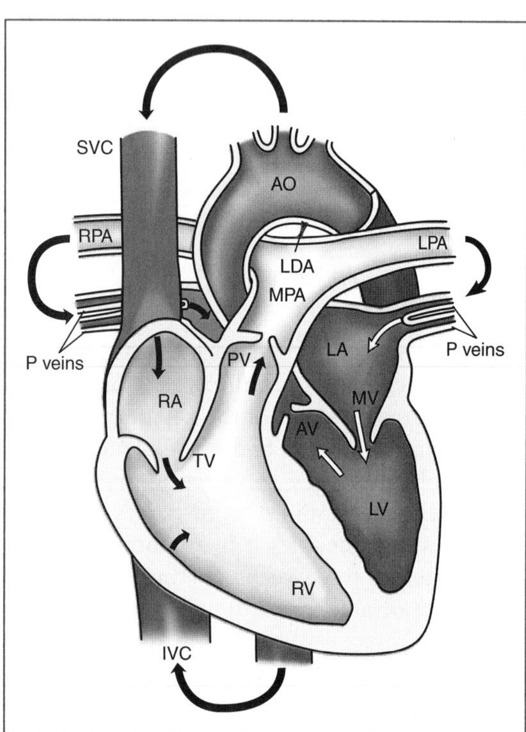

FIGURE 7.2 Normal cardiac anatomy and circulation. AO, aorta; AV, aortic valve; IVC, inferior vena cava; LA, left atrium; LDA, ligamentum ductus arteriosus; LPA, left pulmonary artery; LV, left ventricle; MPA, main pulmonary artery; MV, mitral valve; PV, pulmonary valve; P VEINS, pulmonary veins; RA, right atrium; RPA, right pulmonary artery; RV, right ventricle; SVC, superior vena cava; TV, tricuspid valve.
Adapted and modified from Ross Laboratories, Columbus, OH, Clinical Education Aid, 1985.

The aortic valve connects the left ventricle and the aorta. The *atrioventricular valves* (AVs) consist of the *tricuspid valve* and the *mitral valve*. The tricuspid valve connects the right atrium and the right ventricle. The mitral valve connects the left atrium and the left ventricle.

Cardiac Cycle

Normal cardiac function involves two stages: *systole* and *diastole*. During systole, contraction of the ventricle causes the pressure inside the ventricle to increase to approximately 70 mmHg in newborns (compared to 120 mmHg in adults). When sufficient pressure is generated, the aortic and pulmonary valves open and blood is ejected from the ventricles. As the blood flows from the ventricles, the pressure decreases, causing the aortic and pulmonary valves to close.

During diastole, the mitral and tricuspid valves open and 70% of the blood in the atria enters the ventricles. A small portion of the blood flows back into the aorta and enters the coronary arteries to perfuse the heart. At the end of diastole, a small atrial contraction occurs (4–6 mmHg on the right side; 7–8 mmHg on the left side), and the mitral and tricuspid valves close. Metabolism of the heart is decreased during diastole. The average newborn's cardiac cycle is approximately 0.4 second, with 0.2 second for diastole and 0.2 second for systole (based on a heart rate [HR] of approximately 150 beats per minute [bpm]) (Opie & Hasenfuss, 2012).

Cardiac Output

Cardiac output (CO) is the amount of blood pumped by the left ventricle in 1 minute. CO is equal to the stroke volume (SV) times the HR (CO = SV × HR). The SV is the volume of blood pumped per beat from each ventricle. The higher the SV, the greater the volume of blood in the systemic circulation. An increase in CO increases systole and decreases diastole. CO is influenced by changes in HR, pulmonary vascular resistance, and systemic resistance to flow.

CO is influenced by the amount of blood returned to the heart, as explained by the Frank–Starling law, which states that within physiologic limits, the heart pumps all the blood that enters it without allowing excessive accumulation of blood in the veins. Venous return is determined by the passive movement of blood through the veins, the thoracic pump, and the venous muscle pump. Normally, when increased volume enters the heart, contractility is increased as a response to stimulation of stretch receptors in the heart muscle. The newborn's heart has fewer fibers and is unable to stretch sufficiently to accommodate increased volume; therefore, increased HR is the only effective mechanism by which the newborn can respond to increased volume (Mann, 2012; Opie & Hasenfuss, 2012).

Cardiac failure occurs when the volume exceeds the ability of the heart to pump. Local factors that affect venous return to the heart include hypoxia, acidosis, hypercarbia, hyperthermia, increased metabolic demand, and increased metabolites (potassium, adenosine triphosphate, and lactic acid).

Vascular pressure and resistance also influence CO. Pressure and resistance are inversely related: if pressure in the arterial bed is increased, resistance is decreased and flow is improved. The size (radius) of vessels influences resistance: the greater the radius of a vessel, the lower the resistance. Vessels obstructed by thromboses or constriction have greater resistance to vascular flow (Mann, 2012; Opie & Hasenfuss, 2012).

Autonomic Cardiac Control

Cardiovascular function is modulated by the autonomic nervous system (ANS). Baroreceptors and chemoreceptors in the aorta and carotid sinus provide feedback to the ANS. Feedback from these receptors stimulates the parasympathetic or sympathetic nervous system.

The parasympathetic nervous system is less powerful than the sympathetic system. Stimulation of the parasympathetic and sympathetic nervous systems results in vagal nerve stimulation and decreased HR. Most parasympathetic and sympathetic nervous system effects are on the atria, but decreased ventricular contractility may also occur. Right vagal stimulation affects the sinoatrial (SA) node, and left vagal stimulation affects the AV node. Acetylcholine is the active neurotransmitter for the parasympathetic and sympathetic nervous systems (Colucci & Braunwald, 2011; Opie & Hasenfuss, 2012).

Stimulation of the sympathetic nervous system through the ganglionic chain releases norepinephrine and epinephrine, which act on the SA node, the AV node, the atria, and the ventricles. Maximal stimulation of the sympathetic nervous system can increase HR to 250 to 300 bpm. Contractility can be improved by approximately 100%. Alpha-adrenergic and beta-adrenergic receptors are stimulated. Alpha-receptors cause increased contractility (inotropic) and increased rate (chronotropic); β_2 receptors cause vasodilation, bronchodilatation, and smooth muscle relaxation (Kaplan, 2011).

Term newborns have a decreased number of receptors but are capable of normal cardiovascular system function. The preterm newborn is not able to smoothly maintain autonomic function, and energy expenditure is increased. Hence, the cardiovascular signs such as color changes and bradycardia may occur as a result of excessive demand for ANS function.

CARDIAC ASSESSMENT

Early recognition of signs and symptoms of CHD leads to earlier diagnosis and treatment and may improve outcome (Meberg et al., 2008). Careful newborn assessment is a crucial component of newborn care. Cardiac assessment includes history taking, physical assessment, and interpretation of diagnostic tests. Review of the maternal, fetal, and neonatal history is helpful in cardiac evaluation of the newborn. Associated with CHDs are (1) maternal infections, especially viral and protozoal infections early in pregnancy; (2) maternal use of tobacco, alcohol, or drugs; and (3) maternal diseases. Table 7.1 lists heart defects commonly associated with maternal history. Birth weight may also aid in the identification of a CHD. Macrosomia is associated with maternal diabetes and transposition of the great

TABLE 7.1

MATERNAL CONDITION AND ASSOCIATED CONGENITAL HEART DEFECTS

Condition	Defect
Maternal Disease	
Diabetes mellitus	Cardiomyopathy, TGA, VSD, PDA
Lupus erythematosus	Congenital heart block
Collagen disease	Congenital heart block
Congenital heart defect	Increased risk for congenital heart defect (3%–4%)
Viral Disease	
Rubella	
First trimester	PDA, pulmonary artery branch stenosis
Later	Various cardiac and other defects
Cytomegalovirus	Various cardiac and other defects
Herpesvirus	Various cardiac and other defects
Coxsackievirus B	Cardiomyopathy
Drugs	
Amphetamines	VSD, PDA, ASD, TGA
Phenytoin	PS, AS, COA, PDA
Trimethadione	TGA, TOF, HLHS
Progesterone/estrogen	VSD, TOF, TGA
Alcohol	VSD, PDA, ASD, TOF

AS, aortic stenosis; ASD, atrial septal defect; COA, coarctation of the aorta; HLHS, hypoplastic left heart syndrome; PDA, patent ductus arteriosus; PS, pulmonary stenosis; TGA, transposition of the great arteries; TOF, tetralogy of Fallot; VSD, ventricular septal defect.
Data from Hazinski (1984) and Park (1988).

arteries (TGA), whereas infants of mothers with viral diseases are frequently small for gestational age (SGA) (Park, 2007; Webb et al., 2011).

Methods of Assessment

Assessment for evidence of a cardiovascular disorder begins with a careful history, followed by a thorough physical examination. Family history of hereditary diseases, CHD, or rheumatic fever is significant. Certain hereditary diseases have a CHD as part of the expression (Table 7.2).

The overall incidence of CHDs is approximately 1%, or 8 per 1,000 live births, excluding persistent PDA in preterm newborns. If the mother had a CHD, however, the incidence increases in the offspring to approximately 3% to 4% (Park, 2007; Siedman, Pyeritz, & Siedman, 2011).

A neonatal history of cyanosis, tachypnea without pulmonary disease, sweating, poor feeding, edema, or, in older infants, failure to gain weight is suggestive of CHD. Careful evaluation of the maternal, fetal, and neonatal history, in conjunction with a thorough physical assessment helps identify infants for whom further diagnostic testing is indicated.

Physical examination of the newborn with a suspected cardiovascular dysfunction includes inspection, palpation, and auscultation (Park, 2007).

Inspection

Valuable information about the cardiovascular system of the newborn can be obtained by observation of the infant's general appearance before examination. The following states of the newborn should be observed: sleeping or awake, alert or lethargic, anxious or relaxed. Respiratory effort, including signs of respiratory distress such as nasal flaring, expiratory grunting, stridor, retractions, or paradoxical respirations, should be noted. Tachypnea and tachycardia are early signs of left ventricular failure. Severe left ventricular failure also causes dyspnea and retractions (Park, 2007).

The color of the neonate should be observed. Cyanosis is the bluish color of the skin, mucous membranes, and nail beds that occurs when there is at least 5 g/100 mL of deoxygenated hemoglobin in the circulation. If cyanosis is present, note whether it is peripheral or central cyanosis and whether it improves, does not change, or becomes worse with crying. Cyanosis can result from pulmonary, hematologic, CNS, or metabolic diseases, as well as from cardiac defects. Pulmonary and cardiac defects are the two most common causes of central cyanosis in the newborn.

Pallor may indicate vasoconstriction resulting from congestive heart failure (CHF) or circulatory shock caused by severe anemia. Prolonged physiologic jaundice may occur in infants with CHF or congenital hypothyroidism, which is associated with PDA and pulmonary stenosis (PS). A ruddy or plethoric appearance is often seen in polycythemia. These infants may appear cyanotic without significant arterial desaturation.

The presence of sweating is very suggestive of a CHD in the newborn. The cause of sweating is sympathetic overactivity as a compensatory mechanism for decreased CO. Precordial activity is a reliable parameter of cardiac dysfunction. Precordial bulging is suggestive of chronic cardiac enlargement. Precordial activity without bulging may be associated with acute onset of cardiac dysfunction. Pectus excavatum may cause a pulmonary systolic ejection murmur (SEM) or a large cardiac silhouette on an anteroposterior (AP) chest radiograph because of the decreased AP chest diameter. Pectus excavatum does not cause cardiac dysfunction (Park, 2007).

Palpation

Palpation includes the palpation of the precordium and peripheral pulses. Palpation of the precordium detects hyperactivity, thrill, and the point of maximal impulse (PMI). Irregularities or inequalities of rate or volume can be detected by counting the peripheral pulse rate. Evaluation of the carotid, brachial, femoral, and pedal pulses detects differences between sides and upper and lower extremities. If pulses are unequal, four extremity blood pressures should be measured. Weak leg pulses with strong arm pulses suggest coarctation of the aorta (COA). If the right brachial pulse is stronger than the left, supravalvular aortic

TABLE 7.2

CONGENITAL HEART DEFECTS ASSOCIATED WITH SPECIFIC GENETIC OR CHROMOSOMAL ABNORMALITIES

Disease or Syndrome	Defect
Trisomy 13, 18	PDA, VSD
Trisomy 21	ECD, VSD, PDA
Turner's syndrome	COA
Marfan syndrome	AS, MVS, aortic aneurysms, TAPVR
Williams syndrome or elfin facies	AS, PPAS
DiGeorge syndrome	Interrupted aortic arch
Neurofibromatosis	PVS

AS, aortic stenosis; COA, coarctation of the aorta; ECD, endocardial cushion defect; MVS, mitral valve stenosis; PDA, patent ductus arteriosus; PPAS, peripheral pulmonic arterial stenosis; PVS, pulmonic valvular stenosis; TAPVR, total anomalous pulmonary venous return; VSD, ventricular septal defect.
Data from Park (1988).

stenosis (AS) or coarctation proximal to or near the origin of the left subclavian artery, may be present (Park, 2007).

Heart defects that lead to "aortic runoff," such as PDA, aortic insufficiency, large arteriovenous fistula, or persistent truncus arteriosus (PTA), cause bounding pulses. Preterm newborns frequently have a bounding pulse secondary to relatively decreased subcutaneous tissue. Preterm infants frequently have PDA secondary to their prematurity. Cardiac failure or circulatory shock causes weak or thready pulses (Park, 2007).

The hyperactive precordium indicates a heart defect with increased volume, such as CHDs with large left-to-right shunts (e.g., PDA, ventricular septal defect [VSD]) or heart disease with valvular regurgitation (e.g., aortic regurgitation or mitral regurgitation). The location of the PMI depends upon whether the right or left ventricle is dominant. With right ventricular dominance, the PMI is at the lower left sternal border (LLSB). Left ventricular dominance places the PMI at the apex. A diffuse, slow-rising PMI is called a *heave* and is associated with volume overload. A sharp, fast-rising PMI is called a *tap* and is associated with pressure overload. The normal newborn has a right ventricular dominance (Park, 2007).

The apical impulse of the newborn is normally felt in the fourth intercostal space to the left of the midclavicular line. Lateral or downward displacement of the apical impulse may indicate cardiac enlargement (Park, 2007).

The presence and location of a thrill provides important diagnostic information. The palms of the hands, rather than the fingertips, should be used to feel for a thrill, except in the suprasternal notch and carotid arteries. The examiner should palpate for the presence of thrills in the upper left, upper right, and lower left sternal border, in the suprasternal notch, and over the carotid arteries. A thrill in the upper left sternal border is derived from the pulmonary valve or pulmonary artery. Thrills in the LLSB suggest PS, pulmonary artery atresia, or, occasionally, PDA. A thrill felt in the upper right sternal border signifies aortic origin, usually AS or, less frequently, PS, PDA, or coarcation of the aorta (COA). A thrill over the carotid arteries along with a thrill in the suprasternal notch suggests COA or AS, or other defects of the aorta or aortic valve (Park, 2007).

Palpation of the abdomen is performed to determine the size, consistency, and location of the liver and spleen. Increased liver size is a frequent finding with CHF (Park, 2007).

Auscultation

Careful auscultation by a skilled evaluator is an essential component of any cardiovascular assessment. Auscultation includes HR and regularity, heart sounds, systolic and diastolic sounds, and heart murmurs. The skillful evaluation of cardiac sounds requires systematic auscultation and much practice.

Identification of Heart Sounds

Individual heart sounds should be identified and evaluated before evaluation of cardiac murmurs is attempted. There are four individual heart sounds: S_1, S_2, S_3, and S_4. However, S_3 and S_4 are rarely heard in the newborn. S_1 is the sound resulting from closure of the mitral and tricuspid valves following atrial systole and is best heard at the apex or LLSB. S_1 is the beginning of ventricular systole. Splitting of S_1 is infrequently heard in newborns. Wide splitting of S_1 is heard in right bundle branch block or Ebstein's anomaly (Park, 2007).

S_2 is the sound created by closure of the aortic and pulmonary valves, which marks the end of systole and the beginning of ventricular diastole. S_2 is best heard in the upper left sternal border or pulmonic area. Evaluation of the splitting of S_2 is important diagnostically. The timing of the closure of the aortic and pulmonary valves is determined by the volume of blood ejected from the aorta and pulmonary artery and the resistance against which the ventricles must pump. In the immediate newborn period, there may be no appreciable splitting of S_2. Because the right and left ventricles pump similar quantities of blood and the pulmonary pressure is close to the aortic pressure, these valves close almost simultaneously. Thus, S_2 is heard as a single sound. As the pulmonary vascular resistance decreases, the pulmonary resistance decreases and becomes lower than the aortic pressure, causing a splitting of S_2 as the valve leaflets on the left side of the heart (aortic valve) close before those on the right (pulmonary valve). By 72 hours of life, S_2 should be split. The absence of a split S_2 or the presence of a widely split S_2 usually indicates an abnormality. A fixed, widely split S_2 occurs in conditions that prolong right ventricular ejection time or shorten left ventricular ejection time. It occurs in (1) atrial septal defect (ASD) and partial anomalous pulmonary venous return (PAPVR) (amount of blood ejected by right ventricle is increased, resulting in volume overload), (2) PS (stenosis delays right ventricular ejection time, resulting in pressure overload), (3) right bundle branch block (delayed electrical activation of right ventricle), (4) mitral regurgitation (decreased forward output, decreased left ventricular ejection time), and (5) idiopathic dilated main pulmonary artery (increased capacity of main pulmonary artery produces less recoil to close the valves, delaying closure) (Park, 2007).

A narrowly split S_2 occurs when there is early closure of the pulmonary valve (pulmonary hypertension) or a delay in aortic closure. A single S_2 is significant because it could represent the presence of only one semilunar valve (e.g., aortic or pulmonary atresia [PA] and truncus arteriosus [TA]). A single S_2 may also occur with a critical PS, TGA, or tetralogy of Fallot (TOF), in which the pulmonary closure is not audible. Severe AS may also cause a single S_2 because aortic closure is delayed. Severe pulmonary hypertension may cause early closure of the pulmonary valve, thus causing a single S_2.

The relative intensity of the aortic and pulmonary components of S_2 must be assessed. In the pulmonary area (upper left sternal border), the aortic component is usually louder than the pulmonary component. Increased intensity of the pulmonary component, compared with the aortic component, occurs with pulmonary hypertension. Conditions that cause decreased diastolic pressure of the pulmonary artery (e.g., critical PS, TOF, tricuspid atresia) may cause decreased intensity of the pulmonary component. Evaluation of intensity is difficult, requiring frequent practice listening to heart sounds (Park, 2007).

As discussed, S_3 and S_4 are rarely heard in the neonatal period; their presence denotes pathologic origin. Likewise, a gallop rhythm, the result of a loud S_3 and S_4, and tachycardia are abnormal.

After evaluation of individual heart sounds, the systolic and diastolic sounds are evaluated. The ejection sound, or click, occurs after S_1 and may sound like splitting of S_1. The ejection click is best heard at the upper left or right sternal border or base. The pulmonary click can best be heard at the second or third left intercostal space and is louder with expiration. The aortic click, best heard at the second right intercostal space, does not change in intensity with change in respiration. Ejection clicks are associated with pulmonary or AS or with the dilated great arteries seen in systemic or pulmonary hypertension, idiopathic dilation of the main pulmonary artery, TOF, or TA (Park, 2007).

CARDIAC MURMURS

Cardiac murmurs should be evaluated for intensity (grades 1–6), timing (systolic or diastolic), location, transmission, and quality (musical, vibratory, or blowing).

The grade scale for murmurs is as follows:

Grade 1: barely audible
Grade 2: soft but easily audible
Grade 3: moderately loud, no thrill
Grade 4: loud, thrill present
Grade 5: loud, audible with stethoscope barely on chest
Grade 6: loud, audible with stethoscope near chest

The murmur grade is recorded as 1/6, 2/6, and so on. Again, practice in auscultation improves the listener's evaluation skills. The intensity of the murmur is affected by CO; anything that increases CO (e.g., anemia, fever, exercise) increases the intensity of the murmur (Park, 2007).

The next step in evaluating a murmur is its classification in relation to S_1 and S_2. There are three types of murmurs: systolic, diastolic, and continuous.

Systolic Murmurs

Most heart murmurs are systolic, occurring between S_1 and S_2. Systolic murmurs are either ejection or regurgitation murmurs. Ejection murmurs occur after S_1 and end before S_2. Ejection murmurs are caused by flow of blood through narrowed or deformed semilunar valves or increased flow through normal semilunar valves. SEMs are best heard at the second left or right intercostal space. Regurgitant systolic murmurs begin with S_1, with no interval between S_1 and the beginning of the murmur. Regurgitation murmurs generally continue throughout systole (pansystolic or holosystolic). Regurgitation systolic murmurs are caused by flow of blood from a chamber at a higher pressure throughout systole than the receiving chamber. Regurgitation systolic murmurs are associated with only three conditions: (1) VSD, (2) mitral regurgitation, and (3) tricuspid regurgitation (Park, 2007).

Location

The location of the maximal intensity of the murmur is helpful in evaluation of the cardiac murmur. Figure 7.3 shows the locations at which various systolic murmurs can be heard.

Related to the location is the transmission of the murmur. Knowledge of transmission can assist in determining the origin of the murmur. A SEM that transmits well to the neck is usually aortic in origin, whereas one that transmits to the back is usually pulmonary in origin. An apical systolic murmur that transmits well to the left axilla and lower back is characteristic of mitral regurgitation, but one that transmits to the upper right sternal border and neck is likely to be aortic in nature (Park, 2007).

Quality

Murmurs are described as musical, vibratory, or blowing (Park, 2007). VSDs or mitral regurgitation murmurs have a high-pitched, blowing quality. AS and pulmonary valve stenosis (PVS) murmurs have a rough, grating quality. Establishing the quality of the murmur is subjective, and expertise is gained only after extensive practice.

Diastolic Murmurs

Diastolic murmurs occur between S_1 and S_2. Diastolic murmurs are classified according to their timing in relation to heart sounds as early diastolic, middiastolic, or presystolic.

Early diastolic (proto-diastolic) murmurs occur early in diastole, right after S_2, caused by incompetence of the

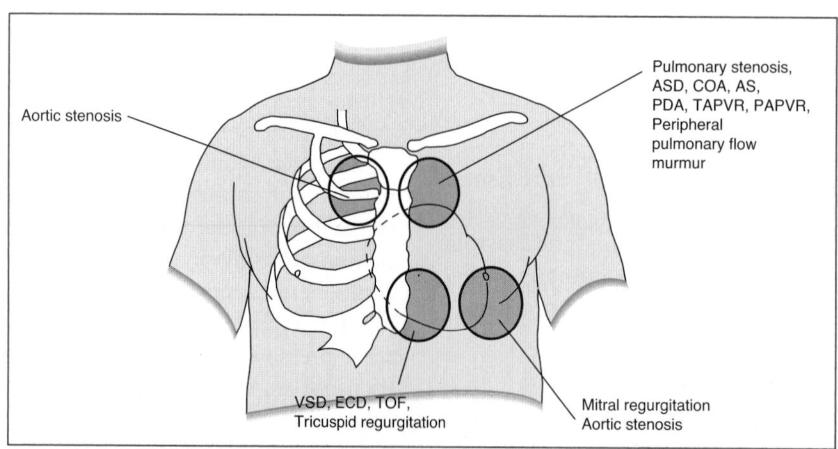

FIGURE 7.3 Location of systolic murmurs. AS, aortic stenosis; ASD, atrial septal defect; COA, coarctation of the aorta; ECD, endocardial cushion defect; PAPVR, partial anomalous pulmonary venous return; PDA, patent ductus arteriosus; TAPVR, total anomalous pulmonary venous return; TOF, tetralogy of Fallot; VSD, ventricular septal defect.

aortic or pulmonary valve. Aortic regurgitation murmurs are high-pitched and are best heard with the diaphragm of the stethoscope at the third left intercostal space. Aortic regurgitation murmurs radiate to the apex. Bounding pulses are present with significant regurgitation. Aortic regurgitation murmurs occur with bicuspid aortic valve, sub-AS, and sub-arterial infundibular VSD. Pulmonary regurgitation murmurs are medium-pitched unless pulmonary hypertension is present, in which case they are high-pitched. Diastolic regurgitation murmurs are heard best at the second left intercostal space, radiating along the left sternal border. Pulmonary regurgitation murmurs occur with postoperative TOF, pulmonary hypertension, postoperative pulmonary valvotomy for PS, or other deformity of the pulmonary valve (Park, 2007).

Middiastolic murmurs result from abnormal ventricular filling. These murmurs are low-pitched and can best be heard with the bell of the stethoscope placed lightly on the chest wall. The murmur results from turbulent flow caused by stenosis of the tricuspid or mitral valve. Mitral middiastolic murmurs are best heard at the apex and are referred to as *apical rumbles*. Mitral middiastolic murmurs are associated with mitral stenosis or large VSDs with a large left-to-right shunt or PDA, producing relative mitral stenosis secondary to increased flow across the normal-sized mitral valve. Tricuspid middiastolic murmurs can best be heard along the LLSB and are associated with ASD, total or PAPVR, endocardial cushion defects (ECDs), or abnormal stenosis of the tricuspid valve. Presystolic or late diastolic murmurs result from flow through AV valves during ventricular diastole as a result of active atrial contraction ejecting blood into the ventricle. These are low-frequency murmurs found with true mitral or tricuspid valve stenosis (Park, 2007).

Continuous Murmurs

Continuous murmurs begin in systole and continue throughout S_2 into all or part of diastole. Continuous murmurs are caused by (1) aorticopulmonary or AV connection (e.g., PDA, AV fistula, or PTA), (2) disturbances of flow in veins (e.g., venous hum), and (3) disturbances of flow in arteries (e.g., COA or pulmonary artery stenosis) (Park, 2007).

PDA is the most commonly heard continuous murmur in the newborn. The PDA murmur is described as a machinery murmur, louder during systole, peaking at S_2, and decreased in diastole. PDA murmurs are loudest in the left infraclavicular area or the upper left sternal border (Park, 2007).

Other Murmurs

Functional or innocent cardiac murmurs are common in children and can occur in newborns. Innocent murmurs occur in the absence of abnormal cardiac structures. Functional murmurs are asymptomatic. The presence of any unusual or abnormal finding warrants consultation. Findings such as cyanosis, enlarged heart size on examination or enlarged cardiac silhouette on radiograph, abnormal electrocardiogram (ECG), diastolic murmur, grade 3/6 systolic murmur or a less intense murmur with a thrill, weak or bounding pulses, or other abnormal heart sounds have pathologic origins and must be investigated (Park, 2007).

The pulmonary flow murmur is commonly found in low-birth-weight infants. Infants with a pulmonary flow murmur have relative hypoplastic right and left pulmonary arteries at birth, which are a result of the small amount of blood flow during fetal life. The increased flow after birth creates turbulence in the small vessels, which is transmitted along the smaller branches of the pulmonary arteries. This murmur is best heard at the upper left sternal border. The pulmonary flow murmur has a grade of 1/6 to 2/6 intensity, but is transmitted to the right and left chest, both axillae, and back. There are no other significant cardiac findings. It usually disappears by 3 to 6 months postbirth. Persistence beyond this period should lead to further evaluation for anatomic pulmonary artery stenosis (Park, 2007).

CONGENITAL HEART DEFECTS

Etiology

Cardiac development occurs during the first 7 weeks of gestation. Major structural defects can occur if there is an interference with the maternal-placental-fetal unit during this critical period. Causes of CHDs are classified as chromosomal (10%–12%), genetic (1%–2%), maternal or environmental (1%–2%), or multifactorial (85%) (Wernovsky & Gruber, 2005).

Many chromosomal abnormalities are associated with structural heart defects. Thirty to fifty percent of infants with trisomy 21 (Down syndrome) have a structural heart defect. In one study of 243 children with Trisomy 21, 44% had associated CHDs. The most common CHDs with trisomy 21 are ECD; the most common ECD was an ASD and VSD (Freeman et al., 2008). Specific genetic abnormalities account for only a small percentage of CHDs. Marfan syndrome is associated with defects of the aorta, such as aortic insufficiency or an aortic aneurysm (Park, 2007).

Maternal or environmental factors include maternal illness and drug ingestion. Maternal rubella during the first 7 weeks of pregnancy carries a 50% risk of congenital rubella syndrome (CRS) with major defects of multiple organ systems. Heart defects seen with CRS include PDA and pulmonary artery branch stenosis. Other viral diseases, such as cytomegalovirus, or protozoal diseases, such as toxoplasmosis, are also associated with CHDs. The diagnosis of a CHD calls for a careful maternal history to identify viral-like illnesses that may have been unrecognized or unreported at the time of occurrence and careful examination to rule out the presence of other congenital defects (Park, 2007; Siedman et al., 2011).

Maternal drug use may also cause cardiac malformations. Fifty percent of newborns with fetal alcohol syndrome (FAS) have a CHD. Only a few drugs are proven teratogens (e.g., thalidomide); however, *no* drugs are known to be completely safe. The threat of environmental hazards to fetal development has only recently been recognized.

Metabolic disease of the mother increases the risk for CHDs. Infants of diabetic mothers have a 10% risk of having a CHD. TGA, VSD, or generalized hypertrophic cardiomyopathy are the most common types of defects found in infants of diabetic mothers (Park, 2007).

Most CHDs are considered to be of multifactorial origin; these defects are probably the result of an interaction effect of the other causes. Research into genetic causes of cardiac defects may identify specific genetic causes for some heart defects that are currently thought to have multifactorial origin. Infants with other congenital defects often have associated CHDs. Multiple defects affect the development of structures that are forming at the time of the interference with normal development.

Incidence

Estimates of incidence of CHD vary from 4.05 to 10.2 per 1,000 live births. The overall incidence of CHD is slightly less than 1%, or 8 per 1,000 live births, excluding PDA in the preterm newborn (Nouri, 1997; Park, 2007; Webb et al., 2011). CHDs are the single largest factor for infant mortality due to all birth defects, with hypoplastic left heart syndrome (HLHS) being the largest specific cause of CHD (Kochanek & Smith, 2004). Recent reviews of the incidence of CHDs have demonstrated an overall prevalence of CHDs. It is surmised that some of the increase can be attributed to better diagnosis and reporting; however, changes in the distribution of risk factors may account for actual increases. Prevalence of VSDs, TOF, atrioventricular septal defects, and PS increased from 1968 through 1997. The prevalence of TGA decreased during that same time period (Nembhard, Wang, Loscalzo, & Salemi, 2010). Because the overall incidence of CHD is approximately 1% of all live births and because the incidence of individual defects is less than 1%, the incidence of individual defects is usually given as a percent of total CHDs. The incidence of a specific defect within the overall incidence of CHDs is included in the discussion of that defect. Identification of cardiovascular abnormalities and prompt institution of appropriate therapy are extremely important in the care of newborns, as approximately 95% of CHDs can be partially or fully corrected (Cooley, 1997).

Some CHDs are not detected in the neonatal period; others are identified, but are initially managed medically. Thus, the following discussion of CHDs extends beyond the neonatal period. Table 7.3 is an overview of the diagnosis of CHDs.

The discussion of defects is based on the common pathophysiologic features. CHDs can be classified in numerous ways. The simplest classification is based on whether the defect produces cyanosis, a method described by Dr. Taussig in 1947. Cyanosis is the bluish discoloration of the skin that occurs when there is approximately 5 g/100 mL of desaturated hemoglobin in the circulating

TABLE 7.3

DIAGNOSIS OF CONGENITAL HEART DEFECTS

Defect	Chest Radiograph	ECG	Echocardiogram	Catheterization	Lab Tests
PDA	Increased pulmonary vascularity; cardiac enlargement; left aortic arch	Left atrial and ventricular enlargement; abnormal QRS axis for age	LA:AO ratio >1.3 (term), 1.0 (preterm); increased left atrium and ventricle (2D)	Increased O_2 saturation in pulmonary artery; increased right ventricular and pulmonary artery pressure (with pulmonary hypertension)	NA
ASD	Mild heart enlargement; prominent main pulmonary artery; increased pulmonary vascularity	Right axis deviation; incomplete right bundle branch block; right ventricular hypertrophy	Dilated right ventricle; paradoxical movement of ventricular septum	Increased O_2 in right atrium; normal right side atrium; normal right side pressure; 10%: PAPVR	NA
AS	Normal heart size; slight prominence of left ventricle and aorta	Normal or mild left ventricular hypertrophy; inverted T waves	Prominent septal thickening; abnormal mitral valve motions	Anatomic and physiologic alterations in cardiac function	NA
VSD	Enlarged heart; increased pulmonary markings	Left and right ventricular hypertrophy	Large left atrium (M-mode); presence or absence of other defects (2D)	Increased O_2 in right ventricle; increased systolic pressure in right ventricle and pulmonary artery	NA
ECD	Cardiomegaly; increased pulmonary vascularity	Left axis deviation; prolonged P-R interval; right and left atrial enlargement; right ventricular hypertrophy; incomplete right bundle branch block	Ventricular dilation; abnormal mitral and tricuspid valves	Increased O_2 in right atrium; increased right ventricular and/or pulmonary artery pressure; with angiography, a "goose neck" deformity of ventricular outflow area	NA

(continued)

TABLE 7.3

DIAGNOSIS OF CONGENITAL HEART DEFECTS (CONTINUED)

Defect	Chest Radiograph	ECG	Echocardiogram	Catheterization	Lab Tests
TOF	Normal heart size; boot-shaped contour; decreased pulmonary markings; prominent aorta; right aortic arch in 13 cases	Right axis deviation; right ventricular hypertrophy	Large VSD, aortic dextroposition, and PS; size of main, right, and left pulmonary arteries (2D)	Demonstrates anatomy of right ventricular outflow region; microcytic anemia	Increased Hgb and HCT clotting time
PS	Normal heart size; normal pulmonary vascularity; enlarged pulmonary artery; right ventricle filling (lateral)	Right axis deviation; right atrial enlargement; right ventricular hypertrophy	Decreased valve leaflet motion; small changes in right ventricular wall thickness	Elevated right ventricular pressure; normal or slightly lowered pulmonary artery pressure	NA
TA	Cardiomegaly; absence of main pulmonary artery segment; large aorta; increased pulmonary vascularity	Right and/or left ventricular hypertrophy	Absence of two semilunar valves	Left-to-right shunt at level of ventricle; pressure equal in ventricles, truncus, and pulmonary arteries	Increased Hgb and HCT
TGA	Enlarged heart with narrow base; enlarged ventricles; increased pulmonary vascularity	Right axis deviation; right ventricular hypertrophy	Abnormal origin of great vessels	Increased right ventricular pressure; catheter can enter aorta from right ventricle; pulmonary artery can be entered only through PDA or ASD	Increased Hgb and HCT; polycythemia
COA	Cardiomegaly; postcoarctation dilation (by age 5 years); notching of ribs from collateral vessels	Left ventricular hypertrophy; inverted T waves in left precordial leads; right ventricular hypertrophy (severe)	Visualization of narrowed aorta and location of associated defects; allows evaluation of aortic valve movement, structure, and function and left ventricular size and function	Performed to determine exact location and evaluation	NA
HLHS	Cardiomegaly; increased pulmonary vascularity; interstitial emphysema	Prominent right ventricular forces; decreased left ventricular forces	Small left ventricle	Performed for evaluation for surgical intervention or if echocardiogram is inconclusive	NA
TAPVR	Cardiac enlargement; large pulmonary artery; increased pulmonary flow	Right ventricular hypertrophy; right axis deviation; right atrial hypertrophy (after 1 month)	Presence of right atrial enlargement; patent foramen ovale; inability to demonstrate continuity between the pulmonary veins and left atrium (2D)	Higher O_2 saturation in right atrium; angiography reveals opacification of pulmonary arterial circulation, pulmonary venous circulation, and abnormal circulation	NA

AS, aortic stenosis; ASD, atrial septal defect; COA, coarctation of the aorta; ECG, electrocardiogram; HCT, hematocrit; Hgb, hemoglobin; HLHS, hypoplastic left heart syndrome; LA:AO, left atrium to aortic root; Lab, laboratory; NA, not applicable; PAPVR, partial anomalous pulmonary venous return; PDA, patent ductus arteriosus; PS, pulmonary stenosis; TA, truncus arteriosus; TAPVR, total anomalous pulmonary venous return; TGA, transposition of the great arteries; TOF, tetralogy of Fallot; VSD, ventricular septal defect.

volume (Taussig, 1947). Thus, the appearance of cyanosis depends on the hemoglobin concentration. An infant with low hemoglobin may be hypoxic but may not appear cyanotic; thus low hemoglobin cannot be the sole criterion for determining pathologic origin. Cyanosis in the extremities, or acrocyanosis, is frequently seen in newborns because of reduced blood flow through the small capillaries. Oxygen is extracted from the hemoglobin in the capillaries, giving the skin a blue appearance. This blue appearance is a normal phenomenon in the newborn. Differentiation of central cyanosis from peripheral or acrocyanosis is essential.

The presence or absence of cyanosis depends upon whether or not deoxygenated blood is oxygenated by going through the lungs. CHDs that allow the blood to go through the lungs and then shunt from the left side of the heart and back to the right side of the heart are generally acyanotic. Defects that shunt deoxygenated blood directly to the left side of the heart, bypassing the lungs are cyanotic heart defects. Some defects have mixed anatomic or functional features and do not fit into this schema, or there is overlap between the classifications. For this discussion, the following categories will be used: (1) defects with communication between the systemic and pulmonary circulations, that is, those with a left-to-right shunt or acyanotic; (2) defects that have obstructions of the vascular system or valvular systems, with or without right-to-left shunt; and (3) defects with abnormalities in the origin of the pulmonary arteries or veins.

Defects With Communication Between the Systemic and Pulmonary Circulations With Left-to-Right Shunt (Acyanotic Defects)

Typically, these defects do not produce cyanosis because there is sufficient oxygenated blood in the circulation. The left-to-right shunts produce increased pulmonary blood flow and increased workload on the heart. The acyanotic heart defects discussed here are PDA, VSD, ASD, ECD, and PTA.

Patent Ductus Arteriosus

The DA is a wide muscular connection between the pulmonary artery and the aorta. The DA originates from the left pulmonary artery and enters the aorta below the subclavian artery; it allows oxygenated blood from the placenta to bypass the lungs and enter the circulation. The DA closes functionally by about 15 hours postbirth. During the first 24 hours postbirth, there may be some shunting of blood, but the ductal opening must be greater than 2 mm for significant shunting to occur.

Closure of the DA occurs in response to increased arterial oxygen concentration after the initiation of pulmonary function. Other factors that contribute to closure of the DA include a decrease in prostaglandin E (PGE) and an increase in acetylcholine and bradykinin (Park, 2007). Closure of the DA occurs within 48 hours in 80% of newborns and close to 100% close within 96 hours. PDA in the preterm newborn presents a different clinical problem and is discussed separately from PDA in the term newborn (Park, 2007; Webb et al., 2011).

Patent Ductus Arteriosus in the Term Newborn

■ Incidence. PDA accounts for approximately 5% to 10% of all CHDs, excluding those in preterm newborns. There is a higher ratio of PDA in females (about 3:1). CHDs are more common with infants with Down syndrome or those whose mothers had rubella during pregnancy (Park, 2007).

■ Hemodynamics. In extrauterine life, the flow of blood through the DA is reversed. The PDA allows blood to flow from left-to-right, thereby reentering the pulmonary circuit and increasing pulmonary blood flow. The amount of blood flow through the PDA and the effects of the ductal flow depend on the difference between systemic and pulmonary vascular resistance and the diameter and length of the ductus. High pulmonary blood flow causes increased pulmonary vascular resistance, pulmonary hypertension, and right ventricular hypertrophy. Figure 7.4 depicts the hemodynamics of PDA.

■ Manifestations. A small PDA may be asymptomatic. A large PDA with significant shunting may cause signs of CHF including tachypnea, dyspnea, and hoarse cry. Frequent lower respiratory tract infections, coughing, and poor weight gain are common in older infants with PDA.

■ Diagnosis. The diagnosis of PDA is based upon history and physical examination findings, radiograph, and echocardiogram. Characteristic findings on physical examination include bounding peripheral pulses, widened pulse pressure (>25), and a hyperactive precordium. A systolic thrill may be felt at the upper left sternal border. A grade 1/6 to 4/6 continuous "machinery" murmur is audible at the upper left sternal border or left infraclavicular area. The murmur is heard throughout the entire cardiac cycle because of the pressure gradient between the aorta and the pulmonary artery in both systole and diastole. In severe PDA with large shunt, the S_2 may be accentuated because of pulmonary hypertension (Park, 2007; Webb et al., 2011).

A small PDA may not be distinguishable on radiograph. With more severe shunting, there may be cardiomegaly and increased pulmonary vascularity. ECG may show left atrial and ventricular enlargement and an abnormal QRS axis for age. The definitive diagnosis is made by echocardiogram.

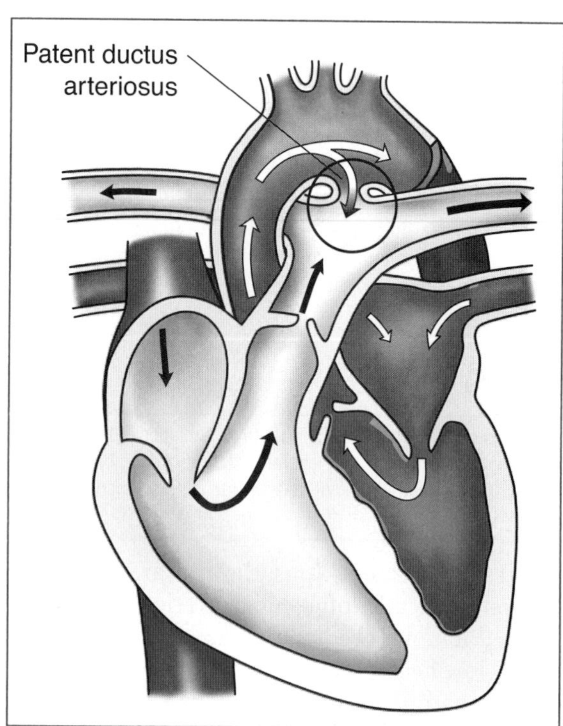

FIGURE 7.4 Patent ductus arteriosus is a communication between the pulmonary artery and the aorta.
Adapted and modified from Ross Laboratories, Columbus, OH, Clinical Education Aid, 1985.

With two-dimensional echocardiogram, a PDA can be directly visualized. A ductus is considered to be hemodynamically significant if the left atrium to aortic root ratio (LA : AO) is greater than 1:3 in term newborns or greater than 1:0 in preterm newborns (Park, 2007; Webb et al., 2011).

■ **Management.** The treatment of the clinically significant PDA is medical or surgical closure. However, there is no absolute agreement on the criteria for determining clinical significance in the term newborn. If the term newborn's signs and symptoms are not affecting growth or development, a conservative approach to management may be used because the ductus may close on its own. Conservative treatment includes fluid management, antibacterial administration to prevent endocardial bacteriosus, and close observation to assure that the baby is growing. The incidence of spontaneous closure decreases as the infant becomes older. If the newborn exhibits signs of increased pulmonary blood flow, such as respiratory distress or inability to feed, closure of the PDA is indicated. Medical management includes the administration of medications to cause the constriction of the DA. Indomethacin or ibuprofen are the two medications that can be used. These medications are discussed more fully in the section on preterm neonates with PDA, because it is more common in preterm newborns. Closure by medications is generally not effective after the newborn period; this method is not recommended for older infants. If the noninvasive methods do not work, or if they are contraindicated because of potential side effects, closure may be effected through a cardiac catheterization procedure in which a coil or device is placed into the patent ductus to obstruct the flow.

Surgical ligation through a posterolateral thoracotomy is the preferred method of closure in cases of very large PDAs or if there are structural challenges due to anatomical variations. The mortality rate is less than 1% (excluding preterm newborns). The prognosis is excellent, and complications are rare (Park, 2007; Webb et al., 2011).

Patent Ductus Arteriosus in the Preterm Newborn

PDA is a common complicating factor in the care of preterm newborns. As the newborn recovers from respiratory distress, pulmonary vascular resistance decreases as oxygenation improves. The ductus ateriosus in the preterm newborn is not as responsive (compared to term newborns) to increased oxygen content and does not close. Decreased pulmonary vascular resistance causes blood to shunt from left to right and reenter the pulmonary circuit, leading to increased pulmonary venous congestion, which decreases lung compliance and stiff lungs. Consequences of large shunts include symptoms of CHF, inability to wean ventilatory support, or increased oxygen requirement.

Clinical findings indicative of PDA include bounding peripheral pulses, hyperactive precordium, widened pulse pressures (>25), and a continuous murmur, best heard at the upper left and middle sternal border. Radiographic findings include increased pulmonary vascularity and cardiomegaly. PDA can be directly visualized by two-dimensional echocardiogram and Doppler flow studies (Park, 2007; Webb et al., 2011).

Management of PDA depends on the severity of the symptoms. In asymptomatic or mildly symptomatic newborns, conservative management may be elected to allow for spontaneous closure of the DA. A study by Koch and colleagues (2006) found that one third of ELBW neonates underwent spontaneous closure. Conservative management consists of fluid restriction, diuretic therapy, and careful monitoring (Park, 2007).

In symptomatic newborns or in preterm newborns or in ventilated newborns, closure of the DA may improve oxygenation and has been associated with decreased complications of prematurity (Koch et al., 2006). Two medications can be used to promote ductal closure. Indomethacin is a prostaglandin synthetase inhibitor. PGE_2 is produced in the walls of the DA to prevent closure during fetal life. Indomethacin inhibits the production of PGE_2 and promotes ductal closure. Smaller babies may require a higher dose to obtain effective plasma levels. Indomethacin is highly nephrotoxic, so the blood urea nitrogen (BUN) and creatinine levels must be followed to monitor renal function. Contraindications to using indomethacin include renal failure, low platelet count, bleeding disorders, necrotizing enterocolitis (NEC), and hyperbilirubinemia (Park, 2007; Webb et al., 2011). Ibuprofen is an alternative to indomethacin for closure of the DA in preterm infants. Both medications are equally effective in closure of PDA and have similar adverse effects on renal function (Kushnir & Pinheiro, 2011; Sekar & Corff, 2008). Surgical ligation is reserved for cases in which indomethacin or ibuprofen fails or are contraindicated. Mortality from surgical ligation is highest in the more preterm, sicker infants, especially if pulmonary hypertension has developed (Park, 2007; Webb et al., 2011). Associated complications of short- and long-term outcomes of ligation, such as neurodevelopmental outcomes, must be considered in the selection of management of PDA.

Ventricular Septal Defect

A VSD is a defect or opening in the ventricular septum that results from imperfect ventricular division during early fetal development. The defect can occur anywhere in the muscular or membranous ventricular septum. The size of the defect and the degree of pulmonary vascular resistance are more important in determining the severity than the location. With a small defect, there is a large resistance to the left-to-right shunt at the defect, and the shunt is not dependent on the pulmonary vascular resistance. With a large VSD, there is little resistance at the defect and the amount of left-to-right shunt is dependent on the level of pulmonary vascular resistance (Park, 2007; Turner, Hunter, & Wyllie, 1999; Webb et al., 2011).

■ **Incidence.** VSD is the most common CHD. It accounts for approximately 20% to 25% of all CHDs.

■ **Hemodynamics.** The hemodynamic consequences of a VSD depend on its size: small, moderate, or large.

Small VSD. Small VSDs produce minimal shunting and may not be symptomatic. Chest radiograph and ECG are generally normal. A loud, harsh pansystolic heart murmur may be best heard in the third and fourth left intercostal space at the sternal border (Park, 2007; Turner et al., 1999; Webb et al., 2011). Figure 7.5 shows a VSD.

Moderate VSD. With moderate-sized VSDs, the blood is shunted from the left to right ventricle because of higher pressure in the left ventricle and higher systemic vascular resistance. The shunt of blood occurs during systole, when the right ventricle contracts, so that the blood enters the pulmonary artery rather than remaining in the right ventricle. This prevents the development of right ventricular hypertrophy.

Large VSD. With large VSDs, blood is shunted from the left to right ventricle. The volume of blood shunted is related to the size of the VSD. The larger the VSD, the greater the volume of blood shunted, and the higher the pressure in the right ventricle and pulmonary artery. If pulmonary artery pressure is significantly increased, thickening of the walls of the pulmonary arterioles may develop, and the increased resistance may decrease the left-to-right shunt. Pulmonary vascular disease can lead to right-to-left shunting and cyanosis.

■ **Manifestations.** Manifestations of VSD depend on the degree of shunting. Small VSDs may produce no hemodynamic compromise and be asymptomatic. Larger defects are associated with decreased exertional tolerance, recurrent pulmonary infections, poor growth, and symptoms of CHF. With severe VSD, there may be pulmonary hypertension and cyanosis.

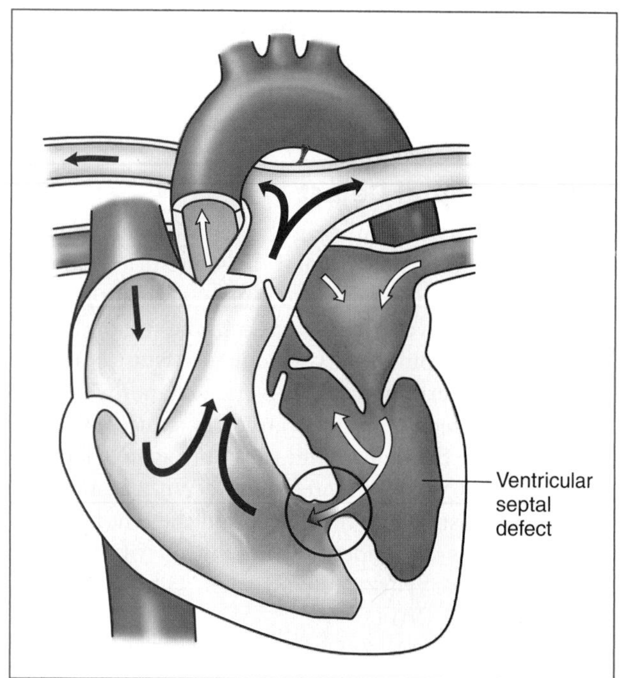

FIGURE 7.5 Ventricular septal defect is a communication between the right and left ventricles.
Adapted and modified from Ross Laboratories, Columbus, OH, Clinical Education Aid, 1985.

■ **Diagnosis.** In VSD, a systolic thrill may be palpated at the LLSB. There may be a precordial bulge with very large VSDs. A grade 2/6 to 5/6 regurgitant systolic murmur is heard at the LLSB. There may also be an apical diastolic rumble and the pulmonary heart sound may be loud.

X-ray can be of benefit in detecting intermediate to large VSD (Danford, Gumbiner, Martin, & Fletcher, 2000). Radiographs show cardiomegaly involving the left atrium, left ventricle, and possibly the right ventricle, as well as increased pulmonary vascularity. ECG may reveal left ventricular hypertrophy. Right ventricular hypertrophy may also be present in severe cases. Echocardiogram (M-mode) shows a large left atrium. Two-dimensional echocardiogram shows other defects and the size and location of the VSD (Park, 2007; Webb et al., 2011). Magnetic resonance imaging (MRI) is used to determine the amount of blood flow to the lungs.

Physical examination of infants with a large VSD not detected in the neonatal period may reveal inadequate weight gain, cyanosis, and clubbing of the digits.

■ **Management.** Treatment of the VSD depends upon the severity of the defect and the symptoms produced. Spontaneous closure of the VSD can occur, so that defects that cause no compromise may be observed to allow time for spontaneous closure to occur. Small VSDs generally spontaneously close by approximately 6 years of age. Muscular VSDs have a higher spontaneous closure rate than do perimembraneous VSDs (29% vs. 69%) (Turner et al., 1999).

Initial management of the hemodynamically significant VSD includes monitoring for signs of CHF and prompt initiation of therapy. CHF in the older infant is treated with diuretics and digitalis. Unless there is pulmonary hypertension, there is no need to restrict activities. Prophylaxis against bacterial endocarditis is indicated.

Surgical management involves direct closure of the VSD. Cardiopulmonary bypass is required for the surgical correction. The timing of the surgery depends on the severity of the circulatory and pulmonary compromise. Infants with significant left-to-right shunting with evidence of severe compromise require surgery. Signs of CHF that do not respond to conservative medical management or increasing pulmonary vascular resistance are indications for surgical correction. Asymptomatic children with a moderate VSD usually have surgical correction between 2 and 4 years of age. Thomson, Gibbs, and Van Doorn (2000) reported using a cardiac catheter across a muscular VSD to aid closure, a technique that allowed improved visualization of the defect from the right side of the heart and minimized the size of the surgical incision of the left ventricle.

The mortality rate for VSD correction is approximately 5%. The mortality rate is higher among smaller infants, those with other defects, and those with multiple VSDs.

Atrial Septal Defect

An ASD is a defect or opening in the atrial septum that develops as a result of improper septal formation early in fetal cardiac development.

There are three types of ASDs (Park, 2007; Webb et al., 2011).

1. Ostium secundum, commonly associated with mitral valve
2. Ostium primum, an ECD associated with anomalies of one or both AV valves
3. Sinus venosus, often associated with partial anomalous pulmonary venous connection

■ **Incidence.** ASDs account for 5% to 10% of all CHDs.

■ **Hemodynamics.** An ASD usually does not produce symptoms until pulmonary vascular resistance begins to decrease and right ventricular end-diastolic and right atrial pressures decline. All types of ASDs produce some blood flow alterations. With an ASD, blood shunts from left to right across the defect because the right ventricle offers less resistance to filling because it is more compliant than the left. Any factors that decrease right ventricular distensibility or obstruct flow into the right ventricle (e.g., PS or tricuspid stenosis) can reduce or reverse the shunt direction (Massin, Derkenne, & von Bernuth, 1998). The left-to-right shunt increases right ventricular volume, but pulmonary vascular resistance decreases, so pulmonary artery pressure is almost normal. The large pulmonary blood flow gradually leads to increased pulmonary artery pressures. Figure 7.6 shows an ASD.

■ **Manifestations.** Newborns with ASDs are usually asymptomatic, although there may be a grade 2/6 to 3/6 SEM, which can best be heard at the upper left sternal border. S_2 may be widely split and fixed. With a large ASD, there may be a middiastolic rumble caused by the relative tricuspid stenosis audible at the LLSB (Park, 2007; Webb et al., 2011). On chest radiograph, the heart is enlarged, with a prominent main pulmonary artery segment and increased pulmonary vascularity. ECG enhances detection of ASD, showing right axis deviation and mild right ventricular hypertrophy. There may be incomplete right bundle branch block (Danford et al., 2000; Park, 2007).

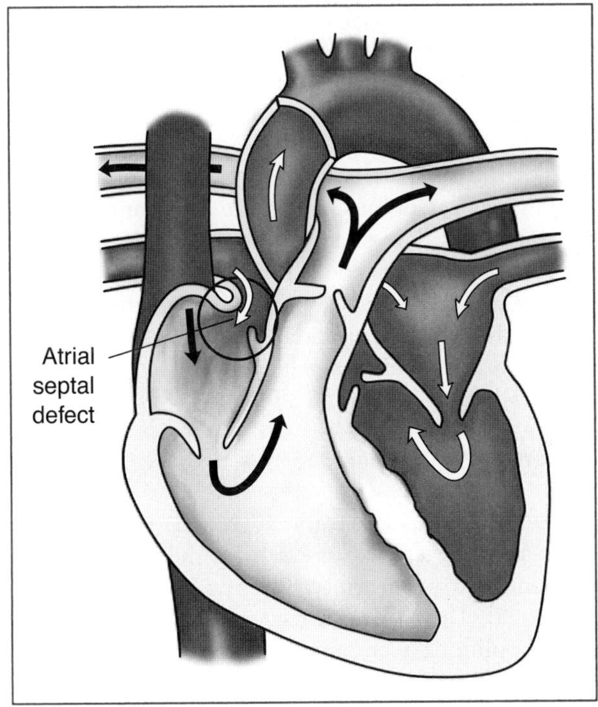

FIGURE 7.6 Atrial septal defect is a communication between the right and left atria.
Adapted and modified from Ross Laboratories, Columbus, OH, Clinical Education Aid, 1985.

Echocardiogram shows increased right ventricular dimension and paradoxical movement of the ventricular septum. Diagnosis can be made by two-dimensional echocardiogram, which shows the location and size of the defect. Children with ASDs are usually thin and may be easily fatigued. By late infancy, there may be a precordial bulge caused by enlargement of the right side of the heart.

■ **Management.** Untreated ASD can lead to CHF, pulmonary hypertension, and atrial dysrhythmias in adults. Spontaneous closure of ASDs occurs in the first 5 years of age in up to 40% of children (Park, 2007). Medical management of ASD consists of prevention or treatment of CHF. There is no need to limit activity. Closure of the ASD may be accomplished through the insertion of a device that covers the ASD and is attached to the atrial septum during cardiac catheterization. This approach does not require cardiopulmonary bypass, is less invasive, less traumatic for the patient and family, and does not cause scarring.

Surgical correction is reserved for infants for whom the transcatheter approach is contraindicated or unsuccessful. Surgical correction is accomplished by a simple patch or with direct closure during open-heart surgery using cardiopulmonary bypass. Timing of surgery depends on the severity of the defect. The presence of a significant left-to-right shunt is an indication for surgical correction. Surgery is performed when the patient is between 2 and 5 years of age. The surgery is not performed in infants unless there is CHF that is unresponsive to medical management. The mortality rate of the surgery is less than 1%. The highest risk is for small infants with CHF or increased pulmonary vascular resistance (Park, 2007; Webb et al., 2011).

Endocardial Cushion Defects

ECDs result from inappropriate fusion of the endocardial cushions during fetal development. ECDs produce abnormalities of the atrial septum (ostium primum), ventricular septum, and AV valves. ECDs take many forms and are characterized by downward displacement of the AV valves as a result of deficiency in ventricular septal tissue and an elongation of the left ventricular outflow tract. The term *complete AV canal* describes the large opening in the center of the heart between the atria and the ventricles. The following defects can occur in the AV canal: (1) an ostium primum ASD, (2) a VSD in the inlet portion of the ventricular septum, (3) a cleft in the anterior mitral valve leaflet, and (4) a cleft in the septal leaflet of the tricuspid valve, which results in common anterior and posterior cusps of the AV valve (Park, 2007).

■ **Incidence.** ECDs account for 2% of all CHDs. Thirty percent of ECDs present in infants with Down syndrome. Ten percent of infants with ECDs also have PDA, and 10% have TOF (Park, 2007).

■ **Hemodynamics.** The hemodynamic consequences of ECDs depend on the type and severity. There may be interatrial and interventricular shunts, left ventricle to right atrium shunts, or AV valve regurgitation. Figure 7.7 shows an ECD.

■ **Manifestations.** The manifestations of ECDs result from the increased pulmonary blood flow caused by the abnormal connection between both ventricles and the atria and by absent or malformed AV valves. The newborn may have respiratory distress, signs of CHF, tachycardia, and a cardiac murmur. The mitral regurgitation may be heard as a grade 3/6 to 4/6 holosystolic regurgitant murmur audible at the LLSB, which transmits to the left back and may be audible at the apex. There is also a middiastolic rumble at the LLSB or at the apex caused by the relative stenosis of tricuspid and mitral valves. S_1 is accentuated, and S_2 is narrowly split. The sound of the pulmonary closure is increased in intensity (Freedom, Yoo, & Coles, 2007; Park, 2007).

Chest radiograph reveals generalized cardiomegaly with increased pulmonary vascularity and a prominent main pulmonary artery segment. ECG shows left axis deviation with a prolonged P-R interval, right and left atrial enlargement, right ventricular hypertrophy, and incomplete right bundle branch block. An infant with an ECD may demonstrate signs of CHF, recurrent respiratory infections, and failure to thrive. Physical examination of an untreated infant with ECD reveals a poorly nourished infant with signs of respiratory distress and tachycardia (Freedom et al., 2007; McElhinney, Paridon, & Spray, 2000; Park, 2007).

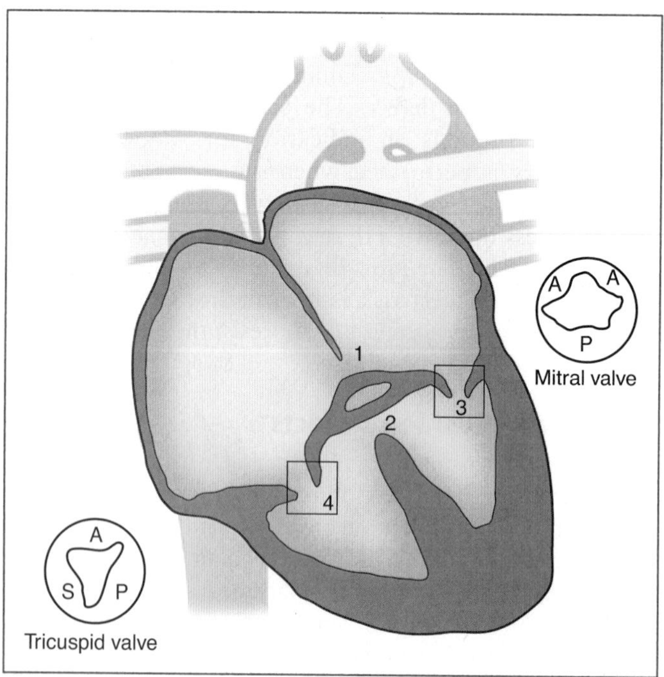

FIGURE 7.7 Endocardial cushion defect. *1*, ostium primum atrial septal defect; *2*, a ventricular septal defect in the inlet portion of ventricular septum; *3*, cleft in anterior mitral valve leaflet; *4*, cleft in septal leaflet of the tricuspid valve, resulting in common anterior and posterior cusps of the atrioventricular valve. A, anterior; S, septal; P, posterior.

■ **Management.** Initial medical management is aimed at preventing or treating CHF with diuretics and digitalis. Prophylaxis against bacterial endocarditis is required before and after surgical correction. Definitive management consists of surgical closure of the ASD and VSD, with reconstruction of AV valves under cardiopulmonary bypass, deep hypothermia, or both. Rarely, pulmonary artery banding may be performed as a temporizing palliative procedure as part of a two-staged surgical correction. The double staged repair carries a slightly higher mortality risk than when primary surgical repair is performed.

Surgery is indicated when there is CHF unresponsive to medical therapy, recurrent pneumonia, failure to thrive, or a large shunt with development of pulmonary hypertension and increasing pulmonary vascular resistance. The repair is performed in patients aged approximately 6 months to 2 years. The mortality rate has declined in recent years to approximately 5% to 10%. The mortality rate for patients who undergo pulmonary banding is approximately 15%. Factors that increase the risks of ECD surgical repair include (1) very young age, (2) severe AV valve incompetence, (3) hypoplastic left ventricle, and (4) severe symptoms before surgery (Park, 2007).

Persistent Truncus Arteriosus

The truncus artery is a large vessel located in front of the developing fetal heart. The truncus artery gives rise to the coronary and pulmonary arteries and the aorta. The persistence of the TA results from inadequate division of the common great vessel into a separate aorta and pulmonary artery during fetal cardiac development. A single, large great vessel arises from the ventricles and gives rise to the systemic, pulmonary, and coronary circulations. Inadequate closure of the conal ventricular septum results in a VSD. Four types of this defect have been described; see Table 7.4 for the classifications (Park, 2007).

■ **Incidence.** PTA accounts for less than 1% of all CHDs.

■ **Hemodynamics.** Desaturated blood from the right ventricle and oxygenated blood from the left ventricle are received in the truncus artery. The pressures of both ventricles are equal. The truncus artery supplies blood to the systemic and pulmonary circuits. The amount of flow depends on the resistance of the two circulations. Pulmonary vascular resistance is high at birth, so pulmonary and systemic flow is relatively equal initially. Pulmonary resistance gradually decreases, causing increased pulmonary blood flow. CHF may develop as a result of increased pulmonary blood

TABLE 7.4

FOUR MAJOR TYPES OF TRUNCUS ARTERIOSUS

Type	Incidence (%)	Description
I	60	Main pulmonary artery arises from truncus and divides into left and right pulmonary artery; results in increased pulmonary blood flow
II	20	Pulmonary artery arises from posterior portion of truncus arteriosus; pulmonary blood flow is normal
III	10	Pulmonary artery arises from sides of truncus arteriosus; pulmonary blood flow is normal
IV	10	Bronchial arteries arise from descending aorta to supply lungs; pulmonary blood flow is decreased

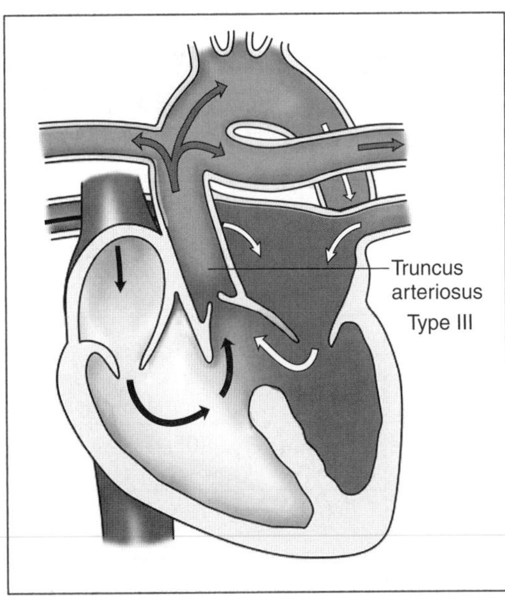

FIGURE 7.8 The truncus arteriosus is a single arterial vessel that gives rise to the coronary arteries, pulmonary arteries, and aorta.
Adapted and modified from Ross Laboratories, Columbus, OH, Clinical Education Aid, 1985.

flow. If not corrected, pulmonary vascular disease develops in response to high pressure and increased pulmonary blood flow, subsequently decreasing pulmonary blood flow. These changes, although compensatory initially, complicate the hemodynamics after surgical correction. The volume overload is compounded by incompetent truncal valves, which allow regurgitation of blood into the ventricles. TA is illustrated in Figure 7.8.

■ **Manifestations.** The presence of cyanosis depends on the amount of pulmonary blood flow. Signs of CHF may be the first indication of PTA. On auscultation, there may be a systolic click at the apex and upper left sternal border. The VSD may produce a harsh, grade 2/6 to 4/6 systolic murmur heard along the lower sternal border. Increased pulmonary blood flow may produce an atrial rumble. Truncal valve insufficiency produces a high-pitched, early diastolic decrescendo murmur. There may be bounding arterial pulses and a widened pulse pressure. S_2 is single. If TA is not detected in the newborn period, symptoms of poor feeding, failure to thrive, frequent respiratory infections, and signs of CHF appear.

■ **Diagnosis.** On x-ray the heart size is increased and pulmonary blood flow may be increased. Fifty percent of cases have a right aortic arch (Park, 2007). Electrocardiography reveals a normal QRS axis and ventricular hypertrophy. Echocardiography demonstrates the presence of the TA overriding a VSD and the absence of the pulmonary valve (Park, 2007).

■ **Management.** Medical management consists primarily of treatment of CHF and prophylaxis with antimicrobials. Current surgical correction consists of complete primary repair, with closure of the VSD, committing the common arterial trunk to the left ventricle, and reconstruction of the right ventricular outflow tract (Park, 2007). The definitive surgical correction is Rastelli's procedure (see Table 7.5 for a description of common surgical procedures). Surgery is performed in infants because there is a high mortality rate for uncorrected TA. The mortality rate associated with surgery has decreased to approximately 10% in newborns undergoing early correction. Delayed surgical correction has a higher mortality rate. Repeated surgery may be required to enlarge the conduit as growth occurs (Park, 2007).

Defects That Have Obstructions of the Vascular or Valvular Systems, With or Without Right-to-Left Shunt

These are CHDs resulting from a defect of either the vascular or the valvular system with a consequent obstruction of blood flow with a right-to-left shunt with either reduced or increased pulmonary blood flow. The defects described in this section include AS, TOF, pulmonary valve atresia (PVA) or PVS, HLHS, and COA.

Aortic Stenosis

AS is one of a group of defects that produce obstruction to ventricular outflow. AS may be valvular, subvalvular, or supravalvular. Valvular stenosis is the most common, and supravalvular is the least common (Park, 2007).

In valvular stenosis, there is usually a bicuspid valve. Subvalvular stenosis can involve either a simple diaphragm or a long tunnel-like ventricular outflow tract. Idiopathic hypertrophic subaortic stenosis is a form of subvalvular stenosis that presents as a cardiomyopathy. Supravalvular stenosis is associated with Williams syndrome, or elfin facies, characterized by mental retardation, short palpebral fissures, and thick lips (Park, 2007).

TABLE 7.5

COMMON CARDIAC SURGICAL PROCEDURES

Procedure	Type	Defect	Description
Blalock–Hanlon	Palliative	TGA	Surgical creation of an ASD: rarely used; still useful for complex TGA or mitral atresia and single ventricle
Blalock–Taussig	Palliative	TOF, PA, PS, VSD	Anastomosis of the subclavian artery and pulmonary artery to improve pulmonary blood flow
Brock	Corrective	PVA	Blind pulmonary valvotomy incision of PV
Fontan	Corrective	HLHS (stage 2), tricuspid atresia, tricuspid stenosis	Bypass of the right ventricle by connection of the right atrium to pulmonary artery
Gore-Tex shunt	Palliative	TOF	Interposition of Gore-Tex between subclavian artery and ipsilateral pulmonary artery
Jatene	Corrective	TGA	Switching of transposed great arteries to their anatomically correct position
Mustard	Corrective	TGA	Use of a pericardial or synthetic baffle in the atria so that venous blood is shunted across the right atrium to the left ventricle and into the pulmonary artery. Systemic blood is shunted across the left atrium to the right ventricle, which delivers blood to the aorta.
Norwood	Palliative	HLHS (stage 1)	1. Main pulmonary artery is divided, and the proximal stump is anastomosed to the descending aorta; distal main pulmonary artery is closed 2. Right-sided Gore-Tex shunt is performed to increase pulmonary blood flow 3. Excision of atrial septum to allow interatrial mixing
Potts	Palliative	TOF	Surgical creation of a window between descending aorta and left pulmonary artery; difficult to take down; rarely used
Pulmonary artery banding	Palliative	VSD, single ventricle	Placement of a band around the pulmonary artery to decrease the blood flow to the lungs
Rashkind	Corrective	PA, TGA	Atrial septostomy created at cardiac catheterization by passing a balloon-tipped catheter through the patent foramen ovale, inflating the balloon, and snapping it back through the patent foramen
Rastelli	Corrective	TGA, TOF, PA, TA	Commonly applied to all valved conduits from the right ventricle to pulmonary artery
Senning	Corrective	TGA	Creation of an intra-atrial baffle, using atrial tissue, to shunt blood from the vena cava to the left ventricle and from the pulmonary veins to the right ventricle
Waterston		TOF	Window created between the ascending aorta and the pulmonary artery, improving oxygenation of systemic blood; rarely used because of the distortion and/or obstruction of pulmonary artery

ASD, atrial septal defect; HLHS, hypoplastic left heart syndrome; PA, pulmonary artery; PS, pulmonary stenosis; PV, pulmonary valve; PVA, pulmonic valve atresia; TA, truncus arteriosus; TGA, transposition of the great arteries; TOF, tetralogy of Fallot; VSD, ventricular septal defect.

■ **Incidence.** AS accounts for 5% of all CHDs. It is four times more common in males.

■ **Hemodynamics.** AS causes increased pressure load on the left ventricle, leading to left ventricular hypertrophy. The resistance to blood flow through the stenosis gradually causes a pressure gradient between the ventricle and the aorta and coronary blood flow decreases. AS is illustrated in Figure 7.9.

■ **Manifestations.** Symptoms depend on the severity of the defect. Mild AS may be asymptomatic, with more severe defects; there is activity intolerance, chest pain, or syncope. With severe defects, CHF develops.

■ **Diagnosis.** Physical examination reveals normal development without cyanosis. There may be a narrow pulse pressure and a higher systolic pressure in the right arm with severe supravalvular AS. There is a systolic murmur of approximately grade 2/6 to 4/6, best heard at the second right or left intercostal space with transmission to the neck. With valvular AS, there may be an ejection click. With severe AS, there may be paradoxical splitting of S_2. Aortic insufficiency may cause a high-pitched, early diastolic decrescendo murmur if there is bicuspid aortic valve or subvalvular stenosis (Park, 2007).

Chest radiographs may be normal or may show a dilated ascending aorta or, in the case of valvular stenosis, a prominent aortic "knob" caused by poststenotic

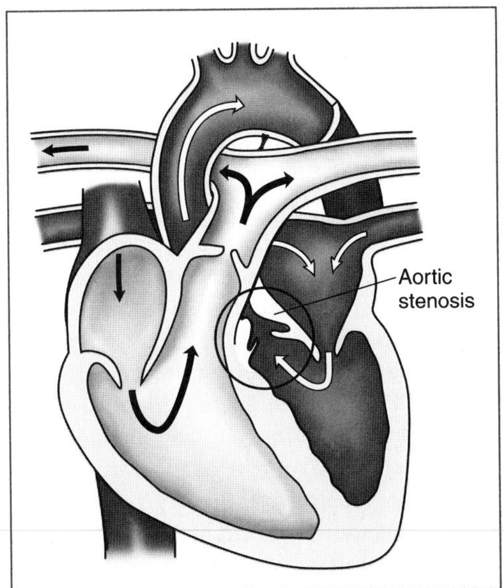

FIGURE 7.9 Aortic stenosis is a narrowing or thickening of the aortic valvular region.
Adapted and modified from Ross Laboratories, Columbus, OH, Clinical Education Aid, 1985.

dilation (Park, 2007). Cardiomegaly is present if there is CHF or severe aortic regurgitation. ECG may be normal or may show mild left ventricular hypertrophy and inverted T waves. Echocardiogram shows prominent thickening of the septum and abnormal mitral valve motions. Two-dimensional echocardiogram shows the anatomy of the aortic valve (bicuspid, tricuspid, or unicuspid) and that of subvalvular and supravalvular AS. Cardiac catheterization may be performed to identify the exact anatomy and to analyze pressure gradients.

■ Management. Management is aimed at preventing or treating the CHF with fluid restriction, diuretics, and digitalis. In children with moderate to severe AS, activity is restricted to prevent increased demand on the heart. Balloon valvuloplasty is sometimes performed at the time of cardiac catheterization to improve circulation. In critical AS, maintenance of the patency of the DA with PGE_1 at a dose of 0.01 to 0.1 mcg/kg/min is administered to prevent hypoxia.

The type of surgical correction depends on the exact location and severity of the defect. The procedure may consist of aortic valve commissurotomy or valve replacement with a prosthetic valve or a graft. The placement of prosthetic valves is usually deferred until adult-sized prosthetic valves can be inserted. The timing of the surgery depends on the severity of the defect. Infants with critical AS with CHF must have corrective surgery. Surgery is performed on children when there is a peak systolic pressure gradient greater than 80 mmHg or when there are symptoms of chest pain.

The mortality risk for infants and small children is 15% to 20%. As in all cases, the sicker, smaller infants have the highest mortality rate. The mortality rate in older children is approximately 1% to 2% (Park, 2007).

Tetralogy of Fallot (TOF)

TOF was first described in 1888. TOF develops as a result of lack of development of the subpulmonary conus during fetal life. TOF consists of a large VSD, PS or other right ventricular outflow tract obstruction, overriding aorta, and hypertrophied right ventricle. The right ventricle may not be hypertrophied initially. In the most severe form, there is PVA.

■ Incidence. TOF accounts for 10% of all CHDs. Because complete repair is generally not carried out in the first year of life, TOF is the most common cyanotic heart defect beyond infancy.

■ Hemodynamics. In TOF, the VSD causes equalization of pressure in the ventricles. Unsaturated blood flows through the VSD into the aorta because of the obstruction to blood flow from the right ventricle into the pulmonary artery. TOF is illustrated in Figure 7.10.

■ Manifestations. Cyanosis, hypoxia, and dyspnea are the cardinal signs of TOF. Newborns can present with just a loud murmur, or they may be cyanotic. Severe decompensation or "tet" spells are common in infants or children but can also occur in neonates. Children instinctively assume a squatting position, which traps venous blood in the legs and decreases systemic venous return to the heart. Chronic arterial desaturation stimulates erythropoiesis, causing polycythemia. Increased viscosity of the blood caused by the increased red blood cells and microcytic anemia may lead to cerebrovascular accident (stroke). Brain abscesses may also occur as a result of bacteremia and compromised cerebral flow in the microcirculation. The chronic hypoxemia and polycythemia cause (1) an increased risk of hemorrhagic diathesis because decreased platelet survival time and reduced platelet aggregation cause thrombocytopenia and (2) impaired synthesis of vitamin K–dependent clotting factors.

■ Diagnosis. Neonates with TOF exhibit varying degrees of cyanosis, depending on the severity of the obstruction of blood flow through the right ventricular outflow tract. A long, loud, grade 3/6 to 5/6 SEM is heard at the middle and upper left sternal border. There may also be a ventricular tap along the LLSB and a systolic thrill at the lower and middle left sternal border. A PDA murmur may also be heard in severe TOF (Park, 2007).

Chest radiograph demonstrates decreased or normal heart size with decreased pulmonary vascularity. The contour of the heart may be boot-shaped due to the concave main pulmonary artery segment with upturned apex. There may also be right atrial enlargement and a right aortic arch.

Echocardiography shows a large VSD and overriding aorta. The anatomy of the right ventricular outflow tract and pulmonary valve can be identified by two-dimensional echocardiogram.

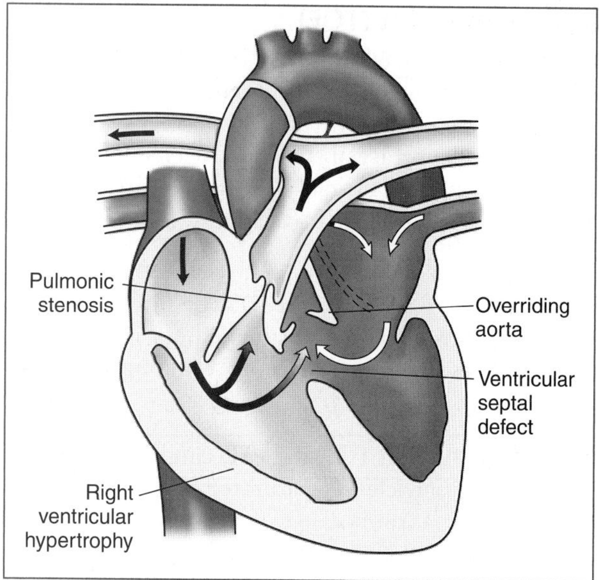

FIGURE 7.10 Tetralogy of Fallot consists of pulmonary stenosis, ventricular septal defect, overriding aorta, and hypertrophy of the right ventricle.
Adapted and modified from Ross Laboratories, Columbus, OH, Clinical Education Aid, 1985.

In addition to the manifestations present in the neonate, clubbing of the fingers may be present in the infant or child with TOF.

■ **Management.** The definitive therapy for TOF is surgical repair under cardiopulmonary bypass. The surgical correction can sometimes be delayed with careful medical management. Neonates with only mild cyanosis improve when the pulmonary vascular resistance decreases. Medical management is aimed at prevention or treatment of hypoxemia, polycythemia, infection, and microcytic hypochromic anemia. Careful follow-up is essential to detect signs of clinical deterioration. Parents need adequate education and support for home management (Dipchand, Giuffre, & Freedom, 1999; Park, 2007).

Dehydration must be avoided to prevent increased risk of cerebral infarcts caused by hemoconcentration. Polycythemia develops as a compensatory mechanism to increase the oxygen-carrying capacity of the blood. In the presence of decreased volume, however, the increased viscosity of the blood may further impede cerebral circulation.

Parents must be taught how to recognize the early signs and symptoms of decompensation. They must also be taught to recognize and treat hypercyanotic or "tet" spells (Table 7.6). Tet spells are precipitated by events that lower the systemic vascular resistance, producing a large right-to-left ventricular shunt. Increased activity, crying, nursing, or defecation may trigger a hypoxemic episode. The right-to-left shunt causes a decreased PO_2, increased PCO_2, and decreased pH, which stimulates the respiratory center, causing increased rate and depth of respirations (hyperpnea). The hyperpnea causes increased systemic venous return by increasing the efficiency of the thoracic pump. The right ventricular outflow tract obstruction prevents the increased blood flow from entering the pulmonary artery, so the increased flow is shunted through the aorta, which further decreases the arterial PO_2. Severe, uninterrupted hypercyanotic spells lead to loss of consciousness, hypoxemia, seizures, and death.

Surgical treatment is indicated in the presence of hypercyantoic spells (tet spells) that result in increased hypoxemia, metabolic acidosis, inadequate systemic perfusion, increased cyanosis, or polycythemia. Systemic perfusion can be evaluated by observing peripheral pulse intensity, urine output, capillary filling time, blood pressure, or peripheral vasoconstriction.

Surgical management can be either palliative or corrective. Palliative procedures are undertaken to improve pulmonary blood flow by creating a pathway between the systemic and pulmonary circulation. In addition, these procedures allow time for the right and left pulmonary arteries to grow. Palliative procedures are indicated for newborns with TOF and PA, severely cyanotic infants younger than 6 months, infants with medically unmanageable tet spells, or children with a hypoplastic pulmonary artery, in whom corrective surgery is difficult (Park, 2007). Common surgical procedures are listed in Table 7.5.

TABLE 7.6

RECOGNITION AND TREATMENT OF TET SPELLS

Manifestations	Treatment	Rationale
Irritability, crying, hyperpnea	Knee to chest or squatting position	Traps blood in lower extremities to decrease systemic venous return; increases pulmonary blood flow
Cyanosis	Oxygen administration	Improves arterial oxygen saturation
Diaphoresis, loss of consciousness	Morphine sulfate (0.1–0.2 mg/kg/dose)	Suppresses respiratory center to decrease hyperpnea
Seizures	Bicarbonate	Corrects acidosis and eliminates stimulation of respiratory center
Decreased murmur	Propranolol (Inderal) (0.15–0.25 mg/kg/dose)	May decrease spasm of right ventricular outflow tract or may act peripherally to stabilize

Surgical correction is performed under cardiopulmonary bypass after the infant is 6 months old. Surgery may be delayed until age 2 to 4 years in asymptomatic children or in children who undergo palliative procedures. The defect is repaired by patch closure of the VSD and resection and widening of the right ventricular outflow tract. Postoperative care of the newborn requires careful assessment and monitoring so that complications can be prevented or quickly identified and treated (Russo & Russo, 2005). Complications of cardiac surgery are listed in Tables 7.7 and 7.8. The mortality rate for TOF varies with the severity of the circulatory compromise caused by the defect. The postoperative mortality rate is 5% to 10% in the first 2 years for uncomplicated TOF. More severe cases have a higher mortality rate, exhibit residual pulmonary outflow tract obstruction, and may require further surgery. Because myocardial damage may occur from the restriction of the right ventricular blood flow during the surgery, cardiac support is needed to ensure adequate myocardial perfusion. Extracorporeal membrane oxygenation (ECMO) is being used by some centers to support the cardiovascular perfusion. ECMO is also being attempted after surgical procedures for TGA and total anomalous pulmonary venous return (TAPVR), but infants with TOF make up the largest group of patients who benefit from its use. Many of these infants experience pulmonary hypertension secondary to the cardiac problem or the surgical correction. With ECMO, management of cases can focus on decreasing pulmonary vascular resistance and diminishing right-to-left shunting during the immediate postoperative period.

TABLE 7.7

COMPLICATIONS OF CARDIAC SURGERY

Low Cardiac Output	Low cardiac output
Hypovolemia	Pulmonary hypertension
Hemorrhage	Inadequate ventilatory support
Diuresis	Ineffective pleural drainage
Inadequate fluid volume	Hypoventilation secondary to pain
Tamponade	***Renal Dysfunction or Failure***
Mediastinal bleeding	Poor systemic and renal perfusion
Inadequate mediastinal drainage	Intravascular hemolysis
Decreased cardiac contractility	Thromboembolus
Hypervolemia	Nephrotoxic drugs
Electrolyte imbalance	***Electrolyte Imbalance***
Cardiac dysfunction	Effects of cardiopulmonary bypass
Increased systemic vascular resistance	Diuretics
Increased pulmonary vascular resistance	Stress response
Arrhythmias	Fluid administration
Hypothermia	Blood administration
Congestive Heart Failure	Renal failure
Uncorrected CHD (after palliative procedure)	***Neurologic Abnormalities***
Corrected CHD, causing alterations in ventricular preload, contractility, and afterload	Hypoxia
Hypervolemia	Acidosis
Electrolyte imbalance	Poor systemic perfusion
Arrhythmias	Thromboembolism
Respiratory Distress	Electrolyte imbalance
Atelectasis	***Infection***
Pneumothorax	Surgery
Hemothorax	Prosthetic material
Pleural effusion	Invasive monitoring and/or procedures
Chylothorax	Inadequate nutrition
Congestive heart failure	

CHD, congenital heart defect.

TABLE 7.8

COMPLICATIONS OF CARDIAC SURGERY: POSTOPERATIVE SYNDROMES

	Causes	Manifestations	Treatment
Postcoarctectomy syndrome	Results from changes in pressure and flow	Severe intermittent abdominal pain, fever, and leukocytosis; abdominal distention, melena, and ascites with gangrenous bowel; rebound systemic hypertension	Monitor blood pressure; prevent hypertension; delay postoperative feeding
Postpericardiotomy syndrome	Immunologic syndrome in response to blood in the pericardial sac	Fever, chest pain, pericardial and pleural effusions, hepatomegaly, leukocytosis, left shift, increased ESR, persistent ST and T wave changes on ECG; rare in children younger than 2 years of age	Rest, aspirin for pain, corticosteroids in severe cases, pericardiocentesis if tamponade develops, diuretics
Postperfusion syndrome	Cytomegalovirus	Onset 3–6 weeks after surgery; fever, splenomegaly, atypical lymphocytosis	Supportive care; self-limiting disease process
Hemolytic anemia syndrome	Trauma of RBCs or autoimmune action	Onset 1–2 weeks postoperatively; fever, jaundice, hepatomegaly, reticulocytosis	Iron supplementation or blood transfusions, correction of turbulent flow

ECG, electrocardiogram; ESR, erythrocyte sedimentation rate; RBC, red blood cell.

Pulmonary Atresia

PA results in the absence of communication between the right ventricle and the pulmonary artery. The atresia can be at the level of the main pulmonary artery or the pulmonary valve. Atresia of the pulmonary valve, with a diaphragm-like membrane, is the most common type. The right ventricle is usually hypoplastic, with thick ventricular walls. Less frequently, the right ventricle is of normal size with tricuspid regurgitation. The presence of a PDA, ASD, or patent foramen ovale (PFO) to allow mixing of blood is crucial for survival.

■ **Incidence.** PA accounts for less than 1% of all CHDs (Park, 2007).

■ **Hemodynamics.** PA with ASD results in a small, hypoplastic right heart. The absence of a right ventricular outflow tract results in high right ventricular end-diastolic pressures. Tricuspid insufficiency occurs and right atrial pressures increase, causing systemic venous blood to shunt from the right to the left atrium through the PFO or ASD. Mixed venous blood flows into the left ventricle and aorta. The PDA produces the only pulmonary blood flow. Closure of the PDA causes severe cyanosis, hypoxemia, and acidosis.

In the presence of a VSD, right ventricular size is usually adequate. Systemic venous blood shunts from the right ventricle through the VSD to the left ventricle and enters the aorta. The PDA still provides the only pulmonary blood flow. PA is shown in Figure 7.11.

■ **Manifestations.** PA usually is seen with cyanosis at birth. Tachypnea is present, but there is no obvious respiratory distress. S_2 is single, and a soft systolic PDA murmur can be heard in the upper left sternal border. Tricuspid insufficiency may produce a harsh systolic murmur along the lower right and left sternal border (Park, 2007).

Heart size may be normal or enlarged on radiograph. The main pulmonary artery segment is concave and similar to the radiographic appearance of tricuspid atresia. Pulmonary vascular markings are decreased and continue to decrease as the PDA closes.

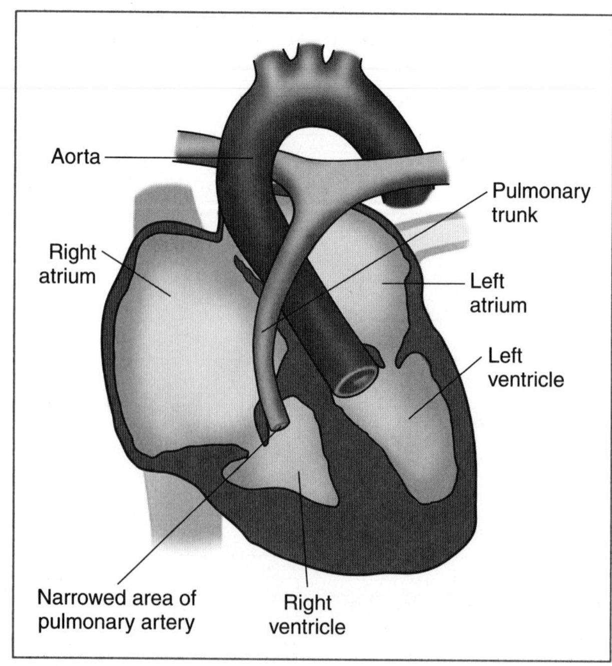

FIGURE 7.11 Pulmonary atresia.

ECG may reveal a normal QRS axis, left ventricular hypertrophy (type I), or, less frequently, right ventricular hypertrophy (type II). Right atrial hypertrophy is seen in approximately 70% of cases (Park, 2007). Two-dimensional echocardiogram reveals the atretic pulmonary valve and the hypoplastic right ventricular cavity and tricuspid valve. The location and size of the atrial communication are estimated by echocardiogram.

■ **Management.** Immediate management of PA is administration of prostaglandin to maintain ductal patency. PGE_1 (Prostin) is given as a continuous intravenous infusion. The initial dose is started at 0.1 µg/kg/min. When the desired effect is achieved, the dose is incrementally decreased to a maintenance dose of 0.01 µg/kg/min. Careful attention to the site of the infusion is important.

A balloon atrial septostomy is performed at cardiac catheterization to promote better mixing of systemic and pulmonary venous blood in the atria. As soon as the newborn is stabilized, surgical correction is performed. Initially, a systemic-pulmonary artery shunt using Gore-Tex between the left subclavian artery and the left pulmonary artery (Blalock–Taussig procedure) is performed. If PVA is present, a closed heart pulmonary valvotomy (Brock's procedure) may be performed. The mortality rate for these procedures varies from 10% to 25%, depending upon the severity of the defect, the alterations in blood flow, and other associated complications

If the initial systemic-pulmonary shunt is not effective, a second shunt is attempted in another location. Right ventricular outflow tract reconstruction can be attempted if the right ventricle size is adequate. This procedure has a mortality rate of 25%. The Fontan procedure is attempted in the presence of a hypoplastic right ventricle in late childhood. The mortality rate for this procedure can be as high as 40%.

The prognosis for PA depends on the size of the pulmonary outflow tract established through surgery and the degree of fibrosis of the right ventricle. If severe fibrosis and significant outflow tract obstruction are present, there is an increased risk of development of dysrhythmias and right ventricular dysfunction (Park, 2007).

Pulmonary Stenosis

PS is caused by abnormal formation of the pulmonary valve leaflets during fetal cardiac development. PS can be valvular, subvalvular (infundibular), or supravalvular. Valvular PS is the most common, accounting for 90% of cases. PS is frequently seen in Noonan syndrome. It is one of the four defects found in TOF. Isolated infundibular PS is uncommon.

■ **Incidence.** PS makes up 5% to 8% of all CHDs. It is often associated with other defects.

■ **Hemodynamics.** PS results in obstruction to blood flow from the right ventricle to the pulmonary artery. The right ventricle hypertrophies in response to the increased pressure caused by the obstruction to outflow. Pulmonary blood flow volume is normal in the absence of intracardiac shunting. PS is shown in Figure 7.12.

■ **Manifestations.** Pulmonary stenosis may be asymptomatic if it is mild. Moderate PS may cause easy tiring. Severe or critical PS causes CHF.

■ **Diagnosis.** The findings of PS depend on the severity of the defect. A pulmonary systolic ejection click can be heard at the upper left sternal border. S_2 may be widely split, and the pulmonary component may be soft and delayed. A SEM (grade 2/6–5/6) is audible at the upper left sternal border and transmits across the back. The severity of the PS is directly related to the loudness and duration of the murmur. A systolic thrill can sometimes be felt at the upper left sternal border. Hepatosplenomegaly may be present along with CHF.

The ECG is normal in mild PS. There may be right axis deviation and right ventricular hypertrophy with moderate stenosis. Right atrial hypertrophy and right ventricular strain occur with severe PS.

Radiographically, the heart size is normal, with a prominent main pulmonary artery segment. In mild to moderate PS, pulmonary markings are normal. The critical type of PS causes decreased pulmonary markings. CHF results in increased heart size. Echocardiogram demonstrates decreased motion of the pulmonary valve leaflets and poststenotic dilation of the main pulmonary artery segment (Danford, Salaymeb, Martin, Fletcher, & Gumbiner, 1999; Park, 2007).

■ **Management.** Management of PS is determined by the severity of the obstruction to flow. The mild type generally requires no therapy except antimicrobial prophylaxis against subacute infective endocarditis (SAIE). Moderate PS is treated

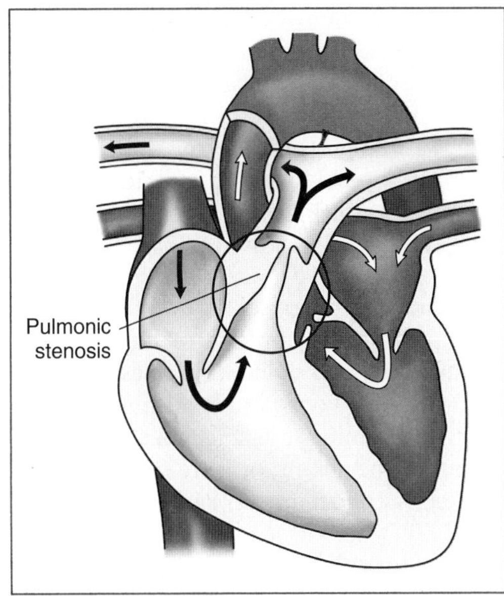

FIGURE 7.12 Pulmonary stenosis.

through balloon valvuloplasty during cardiac catheterization. Surgical correction is performed in children when the right ventricular pressure measures 80 to 100 mmHg and balloon valvuloplasty is not successful or when the PS is infundibular in origin. Infants with critical PS and CHF require PGE_1 infusion to maintain ductal patency until surgery is performed (Park, 2007). Careful fluid and electrolyte management requires balancing the need for fluids against the prevention of further expansion of the extracellular fluid volume and consequent strain on the heart (Agras et al., 2005).

The overall prognosis for PS is excellent. The mortality rate is less than 1% in older infants. The mortality rate is higher in newborns with critical PS and CHF (Park, 2007).

Hypoplastic Left Heart Syndrome

HLHS consists of a group of cardiac defects, including a small aorta, aortic and mitral valve stenosis or atresia, and a small left atrium and ventricle. The great vessels are usually normally related.

■ Incidence. HLHS accounts for 1% to 2% of all CHDs, but it accounts for 7% to 8% of heart defects, producing symptoms in the first year of life; it is the leading cause of death from CHDs in the first month of life. HLHS is not associated with abnormalities in other organ systems.

■ Hemodynamics. Left ventricular output is greatly reduced or eliminated secondary to the valvular obstruction and small size of the left ventricle. Left atrial and pulmonary venous pressures are elevated, and there is pulmonary edema and pulmonary hypertension. With a PDA, blood shunts from the pulmonary artery into the aorta, providing the only CO because there is little or no flow across the aortic valve. Retrograde flow through the aortic arch supplies the head, upper extremities, and coronary arteries.

Although circulation is abnormal in utero, the high pulmonary vascular resistance and the low systemic vascular resistance make survival possible. The right ventricle maintains normal perfusion pressure in the descending aorta by a right-to-left ductal shunt. At birth, the onset of pulmonary ventilation causes decreased pulmonary vascular resistance. The systemic vascular resistance increases because the placenta is eliminated. Closure of the DA further decreases systemic CO and aortic pressure, leading to metabolic acidosis and circulatory shock. Increased pulmonary blood flow causes increased left atrial pressure and pulmonary edema (Park, 2007). Figure 7.13 shows HLHS.

■ Manifestations. Progressive cyanosis, pallor, and mottling are presenting symptoms of HLHS. Tachycardia, tachypnea, dyspnea, and pulmonary rales are present. The S_2 is loud and single. Poor peripheral pulses and vasoconstriction of the extremities are noted on examination. A cardiac murmur may be absent, or there may be a grade 1/6 to 3/6 nonspecific systolic murmur (Park, 2007).

■ Diagnosis. On radiographic study of HLHS, there is mild to moderate heart enlargement and pulmonary venous congestion or pulmonary edema. Metabolic acidosis occurs as a result of decreased CO. Right ventricular hypertrophy is the characteristic finding on ECG. Echocardiography is usually diagnostic. Findings demonstrate the components of the small left-sided heart structures and the dilated or hypertrophied right-sided heart structures. Findings include a small left ventricle, small ascending aorta and aortic root, absent or abnormal mitral valve, and enlarged right ventricle. An abnormal left-ventricle-to-right-ventricle end-diastolic ratio is present (Park, 2007).

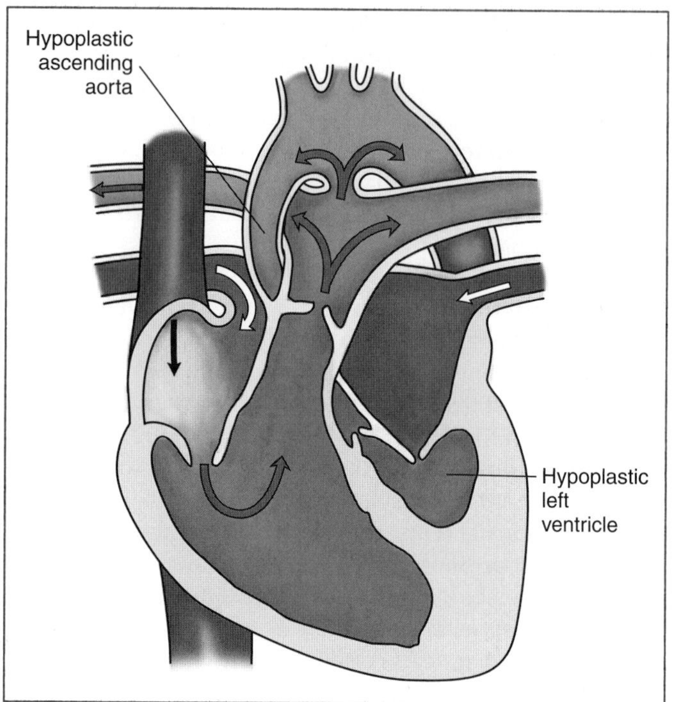

FIGURE 7.13 Hypoplastic left heart syndrome.

■ Management. Medical management of HLHS is aimed at prevention of hypoxemia and correction of metabolic acidosis. PGE_1 is administered through continuous infusion to maintain ductal patency. Balloon atrial septostomy may be performed to decompress the left atrium.

Surgical correction of the HLHS is complex and has a high mortality rate; however, HLHS was once considered 100% fatal. Surgical correction is performed in stages. The first stage, the modified Norwood procedure, is performed in the neonatal period to maintain pulmonary blood flow and create interatrial mixing of blood. The second stage, a modified Fontan procedure, is performed in patients at 6 months to 2 years of age. This procedure is named for the cardiac surgeon who developed and first performed this type of surgery (Norwood, Lang, & Hansen, 1983). The first stage closes the Gore-Tex shunt, closes the atrial communication, and forms a direct anastomosis of the right atrium and pulmonary artery. See Table 7.5 for a description of these procedures (Park, 2007).

The mortality rate for HLHS remains high. The first-stage surgical repair has a mortality rate of nearly 25%. For the survivors, there is a 50% mortality rate with the second-stage operation (Park, 2007). Nursing care is focused on assessment of homeostasis and pulmonary blood flow during the immediate postoperative period. Attention to nutritional status is important for the long-term recovery. Postoperative care requires close monitoring of vital signs, chest tube output, platelet counts, liver function tests, guaiac tests, and pulmonary and circulatory status.

Use of dopamine at 5 to 10 μg/kg/min may be needed to decrease pulmonary vasoconstriction. Dobutamine or isoproterenol are avoided because they dilate the pulmonary arterioles, making the situation worse. Fentanyl may be used to balance pulmonary vascular resistance. Diuretics or peritoneal dialysis may be necessary to maintain fluid balance. High-frequency ventilation (HFV) is sometimes used to support pulmonary function when there are acidosis and stiff lungs. ECMO has also been used to maintain oxygenation and ventilation.

Nutritional support is provided through total parenteral nutrition (TPN). Monitoring of daily weights, of urine for ketones, glucose, and protein, and of serum levels of electrolytes and trace minerals is necessary to adjust the parenteral fluids. Enteral feedings may be started in the first 2 weeks postoperatively if the infant is stable, after the greatest danger of NEC is past.

Pericardial effusion may occur several days or weeks after the Fontan procedure; this can cause alterations in tissue perfusion and changes in systemic blood flow return. An alternative treatment option for HLHS is cardiac transplantation. Further information about cardiac transplantation is found in Chapter 27. It is essential that parents be informed of all available treatments, including risks and prognosis if surgical intervention is an option.

Coarctation of the Aorta

COA is a narrowing or constriction of the aorta in the aortic arch segment. The most common location is below the origin of the left subclavian artery. COA may occur as a single lesion due to improper development of the aorta or may occur secondary to constriction of the DA. The severity of the circulatory compromise depends on the location and degree of constriction. COA proximal to the DA (preductal COA) has associated defects in 40% of cases. Associated defects include VSD, TGA, and PDA. Collateral circulation is poorly developed with preductal COA. Postductal COA is usually not associated with other defects, and collateral circulation is more effective. Infants with postductal COA may be asymptomatic. More than half of infants with COA have a bicuspid aortic valve (Park, 2007).

■ **Incidence.** COA accounts for 8% of all CHDs. Coarctation occurs twice as often in males. COA is found in 30% of infants with Turner syndrome (Park, 2007).

■ **Hemodynamics.** COA causes obstruction to flow, which leads to varying pressure across the aortic segment. The portion of aorta proximal to the constriction has an elevated pressure, which leads to increased left ventricular pressure. The increased left ventricular pressure results in left ventricular hypertrophy and dilation. Collateral circulation develops from the proximal to distal arteries, bypassing the constricted segment of the aorta. This is a compensatory mechanism to increase flow to the lower extremities and abdomen, producing lower pulses in the lower extremities. COA is shown in Figure 7.14 (Park, 2007).

■ **Manifestations.** The severity and time of appearance of symptoms of COA depend on the location and degree of constriction, as well as the presence of associated cardiac defects. Symptoms of COA include signs of CHF and absent, weak, or delayed pulses in the lower extremities, with bounding pulses in the upper extremities. In the presence of CHF, however, all pulses may be weak. With severe COA, S_2 is loud and single. A systolic thrill may be felt in the suprasternal notch. An ejection click may be audible at the apex if there is a bicuspid aortic valve or if systemic hypertension is present. A SEM of grade 2/6 to 3/6 can be heard at the upper right and middle or lower left sternal border, and at the left interscapular area in the infant's back; however, no murmur is heard in more than half of infants with COA (Park, 2007).

■ **Diagnosis.** Diagnosis of COA is based on history, physical findings, radiograph, ECG, and echocardiographic data. In asymptomatic infants and children, radiographs may show a normal or slightly enlarged heart. Dilation of the ascending aorta may be evident. The "E" sign on barium swallow is characteristic but is usually not evident until at least 4 months of age. The "E" appearance is due to the large proximal aortic segment or prominent subclavian artery above and the poststenotic dilation of the descending aorta below the constricted segment (Park, 2007). In symptomatic infants and children, radiographs show cardiomegaly and increased pulmonary venous congestion.

The ECG of asymptomatic children may show left axis deviation of the QRS and left ventricular hypertrophy. In symptomatic children, the ECG reveals normal or right axis

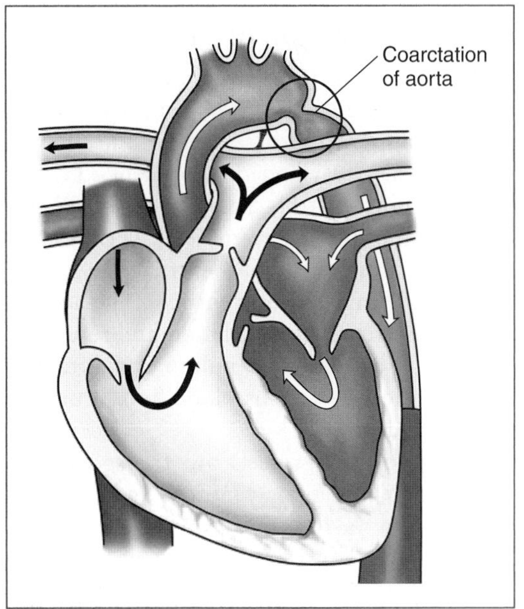

FIGURE 7.14 Coarctation of the aorta is a narrowing or constriction of the aorta near the ductus arteriosus.
Adapted and modified from Ross Laboratories, Columbus, OH, Clinical Education Aid, 1985.

deviation of the QRS. Right ventricular hypertrophy or right bundle branch block is present in infants, whereas left ventricular hypertrophy is present in older children (Park, 2007). Two-dimensional echocardiogram demonstrates the location and degree of the constriction and the presence of associated defects.

■ **Management.** Surgical correction of COA is the definitive treatment. Critically symptomatic newborns require immediate surgery. Surgery may be delayed until age 3 to 5 years if signs and symptoms can be medically controlled. Medical management is aimed at providing adequate oxygenation, preventing or treating CHF, and preventing SAIE. PGE_1 may be needed to maintain ductal patency if the constricted segment is at the level of the DA (Park, 2007).

Surgical intervention of COA involves the excision of the constricted segment of the aorta with end-to-end anastomosis, patch graft, bypass tube graft, or Dacron graft (Park, 2007). Alternatively, a subclavian flap aortoplasty may be performed. Surgery is indicated in the presence of CHF with or without circulatory shock. The mortality rate for surgical corrections is less than 5%. Postoperative complications include renal failure and recoarctation, which occurs in almost 20% of newborns.

Defects With Abnormalities in the Origin of the Pulmonary Arteries or Veins

These defects arise from a defect in the bending and rotation of the heart as it grows and elongates during fetal development. The result is abnormal alignment of the heart vessels and resulting cyanosis.

Transposition Defects

Transposition defects include a group of malformations that have in common an abnormal anatomical relationship between the cardiac chambers and the great arteries.

Complete Transposition of the Great Arteries or Vessels

Transposition of the great arteries (TGA) or vessels is the result of inappropriate septation and migration of the TA during fetal cardiac development. TGA may be dextrotransposition of the great arteries (D-TGA) or levotransposition of the great arteries (L-TGA). In D-TGA, the aorta arises from the right ventricle, and the pulmonary artery arises from the left ventricle. The aorta receives un-oxygenated systemic venous blood and returns it to the systemic arterial circuit. The pulmonary artery receives oxygenated pulmonary venous blood and returns it to the pulmonary circulation.

In L-TGA, the great vessels are transposed, with the aorta arising from the right ventricle and the pulmonary artery arising from the left ventricle. The aorta is to the left and anterior to the pulmonary artery. This type of transposition is called *corrected* because functionally the hemodynamics are normal. The oxygenated blood comes into the left atrium, enters the right ventricle, and goes through the aorta to the systemic circulation. However, frequently there are other associated cardiac defects (Park, 2007).

■ **Incidence.** TGA accounts for 5% of all CHDs. It is more common in males (3:1). D-TGA is the most common cyanotic heart defect in newborns.

■ **Hemodynamics.** Hemodynamically, two separate parallel circulations result from complete D-TGA. Oxygenated blood from the lungs is returned to the left atrium, enters the left ventricle, and goes through the pulmonary artery to the lungs again. Desaturated blood from the systemic circulation enters the right atrium, goes to the right ventricle, enters the aorta, and is directed back into the systemic circulation. The end result is that the heart and brain and other vital tissues are perfused with desaturated blood. This defect is incompatible with life. A communication between the two circulations must exist to allow mixing of the oxygenated and desaturated blood. This communication can be at the ductal, atrial, or ventricular level. The best mixing occurs with a large VSD. Figure 7.15 shows TGA (Park, 2007).

■ **Manifestations.** Marked cyanosis is the prominent sign of TGA. The degree of cyanosis varies with the amount of communication between the two circulations. Signs of CHF are present. S_2 is loud and single. If a VSD is present, there is a loud, harsh systolic murmur of variable intensity. Hypoglycemia, hypocalcemia, and metabolic acidosis are frequently present.

■ **Diagnosis.** On radiographic study of TGA, the heart is enlarged and has a narrow base because the aorta is over the pulmonary artery. The heart is described as egg-shaped (Park, 2007). Pulmonary blood flow is increased. On ECG, there is right axis deviation of the QRS and right ventricular hypertrophy. Echocardiography reveals the abnormal origin of the great arteries from the ventricles. Associated defects can also be visualized by echocardiography.

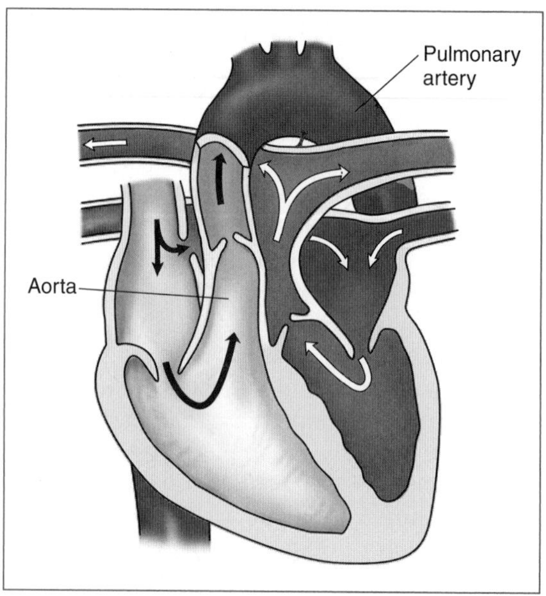

FIGURE 7.15 Transposition of the great arteries or vessels is a condition in which the aorta arises from the right ventricle and the pulmonary artery arises from the left ventricle. The result is two distinct circulatory (parallel) pathways.

■ **Management.** TGA is a cardiac emergency. Immediate medical management includes correction of acidosis, hypoglycemia, and hypocalcemia and administration of oxygen and infusion of PGE_1, and treatment of CHF. A cardiac catheterization is performed and a balloon atrial septostomy is carried out to promote mixing of oxygenated and desaturated blood in the atria. If the septostomy and PGE_1 infusion do not sufficiently improve oxygenation, surgical excision of the posterior aspect of the atrial septum (Blalock–Hanlon procedure) is performed without cardiopulmonary bypass as a palliative measure. This procedure is associated with a relatively higher mortality rate (10%–25%) because of the severe hemodynamic abnormalities (Park, 2007).

Definitive surgical correction is achieved through an arterial switch, which consists of switching the right- and left-sided structures at the ventricular level (Rastelli's procedure), the artery level (Jatene's procedure), or the atrial level (Senning's or Mustard's procedure). See Table 7.5 for a description of these procedures.

The prognosis for TGA without surgical intervention is poor; 90% of patients die within the first year of life. The surgical procedures have high mortality rates and are associated with significant postoperative complications (e.g., dysrhythmias, obstruction to systemic or pulmonary venous return, and right ventricular dysfunction). Jatene's procedure is newer but seems to minimize many complications associated with the intra-atrial repair operations. The type and timing of surgical correction depend on the condition of the patient and the anatomic defect, so each case must be decided individually. A typical management approach is presented in the flow diagram in Figure 7.16.

Total Anomalous Pulmonary Venous Return (TAPVR)

With TAPVR, the pulmonary veins drain into the right atrium (rather than the left atrium) directly or through connection with the systemic veins. There is no direct connection between the pulmonary veins and the left atrium. Four types of TAPVR have been identified (Park, 2007).

■ **Incidence.** TAPVR accounts for 1% of all CHDs. There is a 1:1 male to female ratio of occurrence.

■ **Hemodynamics.** If there is an ASD or PFO in TAPVR, a portion of the mixed blood from the right atrium can cross into the left atrium, into the left ventricle, and on into the systemic circulation. The direction of the blood flow and the amount that crosses the atrial communication into the left atrium or that enters the left ventricle are determined by the compliance of the ventricles.

Two clinical hemodynamic states exist with TAPVR. If pulmonary blood flow is not obstructed, pulmonary flow is greatly increased. The result is highly saturated blood in the right atrium and mild cyanosis. If there is

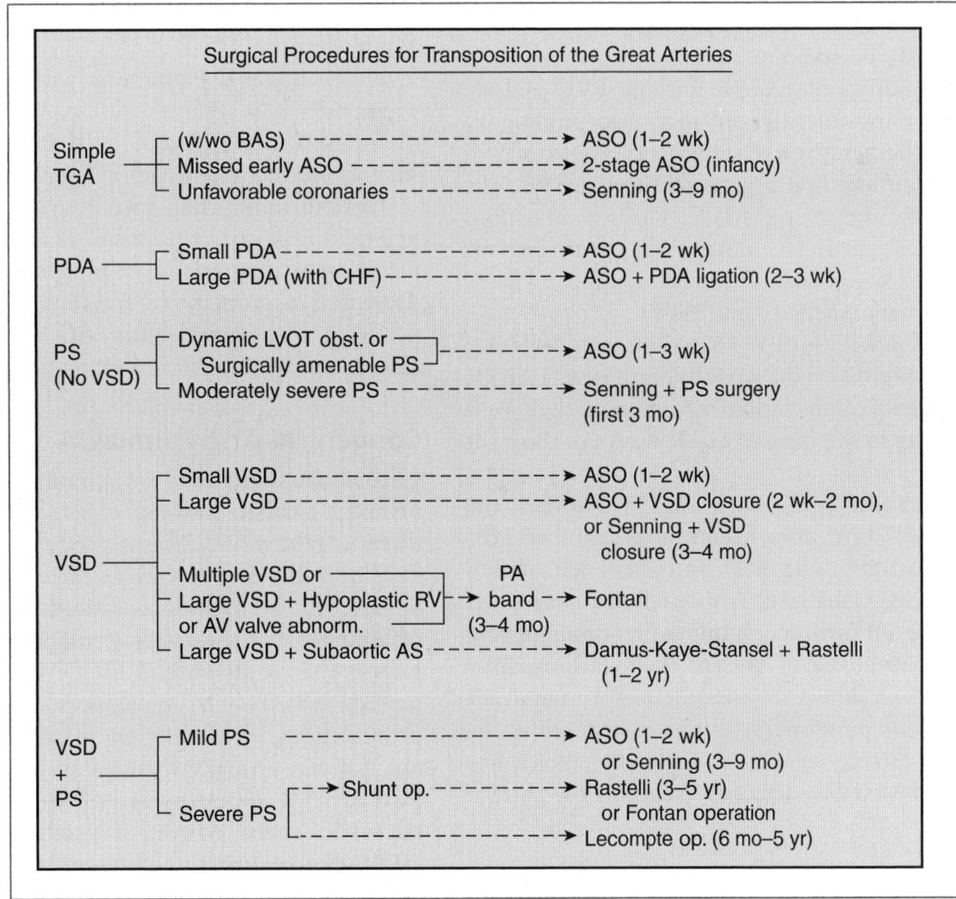

FIGURE 7.16 Management of transposition of the great arteries: flow diagram. *Senning is used to represent an intra-atrial repair, either the Senning operation or the Mustard operation.
Adapted from Park (1988).

obstruction to pulmonary blood flow, the volume of flow is decreased and cyanosis is severe. Pulmonary edema often occurs secondary to elevated pulmonary venous pressure. Obstruction to pulmonary blood flow is a common occurrence when the TAPVR is below the diaphragm (Park, 2007).

■ Manifestations. The manifestations of TAPVR depend on the presence of pulmonary venous obstruction (PVO). TAPVR without PVO includes a history of mild cyanosis, frequent pulmonary infections, poor growth, and CHF. TAPVR with PVO causes severe cyanosis and respiratory distress in the neonatal period, with progressive growth failure. Feeding is associated with increased cyanosis secondary to the compression of the common pulmonary vein by the filled esophagus (Park, 2007). Signs and symptoms of CHF are also present.

■ Diagnosis. TAPVR without PVO produces a precordial bulge with hyperactive right ventricular impulse. The PMI is at the xiphoid process or LLSB. S_2 is widely split and fixed; the pulmonic sound may be pronounced. A grade 2/6 to 3/6 SEM can be heard at the upper left sternal border, and there is always a middiastolic rumble at the LLSB. The rhythm is a quadruple or quintuple gallop (Park, 2007).

TAPVR with PVO may produce minimal cardiac findings. S_2 is loud and single, and there is a gallop rhythm. There may be a faint SEM at the upper left sternal border. Pulmonary rales may be audible.

Radiographic findings of TAPVR without PVO include mild to moderate cardiomegaly and increased pulmonary markings. The characteristic "snowman" sign occurs because of the anatomic appearance of the left SVC, the left innominate vein, and the right SVC. This sign is seldom visible before the patient is 4 months of age. With TAPVR with PVO, the heart size is normal on radiograph, and there are signs of pulmonary edema (Park, 2007).

On ECG, TAPVR without PVO has right axis deviation of the QRS and sometimes right atrial hypertrophy. TAPVR with PVO has right axis deviation for age and right ventricular hypertrophy in the form of tall R waves in the right precordial leads.

Echocardiography of TAPVR without PVO reveals the pulmonary veins draining into a common chamber posterior to the left atrium. The ASD and small left atrium and left ventricle are visualized. A dilated coronary sinus protruding into the left atrium or a dilated innominate vein and SVC can be visualized, if present. Echocardiography of TAPVR with PVO shows the small left atrium and left ventricle. Anomalous pulmonary venous return below the diaphragm can be directly visualized. Color Doppler echocardiography can be used to detect the venous flow pattern (Park, 2007).

■ Management. Management of TAPVR is surgical, and surgery is emergent when PVO is below the diaphragm. Medical management is aimed at preventing or treating CHF and preventing hypoxemia until surgical correction. Diuretics may be required to manage pulmonary edema. Balloon atrial septostomy at cardiac catheterization is performed to enlarge the interatrial communication and promote better mixing of blood. Surgery may be delayed when response to medical management is good, but it is usually performed when the patients are infants (Park, 2007).

The surgical procedure depends on the site of the anomalous drainage. Cardiopulmonary bypass is required. Surgery involves the anastomosis of the pulmonary veins to the left atrium, closure of the ASD, and division of the anomalous connection. The overall mortality rate for TAPVR with surgical correction has improved percentage, but it is lower than with medical management alone. The highest mortality rate is with the infracardiac type (Russo & Russo, 2005).

Postoperative Treatments

As discussed, morbidity and mortality rates remain high after surgery in many of the cardiac defects. Life-threatening complications can occur during the postoperative period. Treatment is aimed at decreasing pulmonary vascular resistance, decreasing pulmonary hypertension, improving CO, and reducing systemic inflammation. Methods such as extracorporeal membraneous oxygenation (ECMO) or extracorporeal life support (ECLS), high-frequency jet ventilation, inhaled nitric oxide (iNO), and modified ultrafiltration may ameliorate some of the postoperative complications.

iNO is a selective pulmonary dilator that acts directly on pulmonary and systemic vascular resistance. iNO is sometimes used after procedures that require cardiac bypass, such as bidirection Glenn or Fontan procedures.

Ultrafiltration after open heart surgery can help reverse hemodilution and decrease tissue edema. This results in improved pulmonary and left ventricular function, decreased postoperative bleeding, and may decrease the occurrence of pleural effusions. Ultrafiltration is still considered an experimental therapy (Park, 2007).

Congenital Arrhythmias

Cardiac arrhythmias in infants generally arise from primary cardiac lesions, generally from abnormal conduction pathways. Alternatively, cardiac arrhythmias can develop following corrective cardiac surgery. It is not clear whether the arrhythmia is caused by the surgical procedure or whether it is the result of the initial heart defect. Other factors that contribute to the development of arrhythmias include electrolyte imbalances, neurologic conditions, or infections. Generally in infants, rhythm disturbances are not the primary manifestation of a cardiac problem; instead CHF or cyanosis is present before dysrhythmias occur (Sacchetti, Moyer, Baricella, Cameron, & Moakes, 1999). Some conditions present with rhythm disturbances in the newborn period. The most commonly-occurring include congenital complete heart block (CCHB) and supraventricular tachycardia (SVT). These two dysrhythmias will be discussed.

Congenital Complete Heart Block

The AV node and the bundle of His arise as separate structures that join together. Congenital heart block is a result of a discontinuity between the atrial musculature and the AV node or the bundle of His and the AV node. For the majority of cases, the exact cause of the discontinuity is unknown, and the remainder of the heart anatomy is normal. Certain antibodies passed from mothers with systemic lupus erythematosus (SLE) are associated with congenital heart block. Congenital heart block can be a manifestation of CHDs, including congenitally corrected TGA.

CCHB can be diagnosed by detection of consistent fetal bradycardia (HR of 40–80 bpm) by auscultation, fetal echocardiography, or electronic monitoring. A newborn with a ventricular rate less than 50 bpm and an atrial rate greater than 150 bpm is at significant risk. If the newborn has an associated heart defect, the risk for mortality is higher.

■ Treatment. Asymptomatic infants do not require treatment. If the infant is in CHF, digitalization is generally the first line of treatment. Insertion of a pacemaker is necessary for infants in CHF that does not respond to digitalization. Children with pacemakers implanted need close follow-up due to complications or adverse effects of the pacemakers (Massimo et al., 2006; Webb et al., 2011).

Supraventricular Tachycardia

SVT can arise in utero or in the neonatal period. The most common arrhythmias that produce signs are paroxysmal SVT with or without ventricular pre-excitation, atrial flutter, and junctional tachycardia. If the SVT occurs in utero, it can lead to heart failure and hydrops fetalis. SVT in the fetus is treated through maternal administration of digitalis. If digitalization is not successful, propranolol, quinidine, felcainide, or amiodarone is used. The fetus is delivered if there is evidence of fetal lung maturity.

In most cases of SVT, no cause is found. Long-acting thyroid stimulators and immune gamma-2-globulin from hyperthyroid mothers, hypoglycemia, and Ebstein anomaly of the tricuspid valve can be the cause in other cases. Ten to fifty percent of infants with SVT have Wolfe–Parkinson–White (WPW) syndrome in which the atrial impulse activates the whole or some part of the ventricle, or the ventricular impulse activates the whole or some part of the atrium earlier than would be expected if the impulse traveled via the normal pathway. WPW is characterized by a normal QRS, regular rhythm, ventricular rates of 150 to 200 bpm, sudden onset, and sudden termination (Olgin & Zipes, 2011).

Symptoms produced by the SVT after birth are subtle and often are undetected until signs of CHF have been present for 24 to 36 hours. Treatment with digitalis or adenosine, cardioversion, transesophogeal atrial pacing, or a elicitation of a diving reflex by covering the face with a cold washcloth for 4 to 5 seconds generally is successful in establishing normal sinus rhythm. After conversion, digitalis is continued for 9 to 12 months. Therapy is discontinued abruptly, without weaning dosages.

Recurrence in patients with WPW is more likely and is treated with the above drugs, alone or in combination. Recurrence decreases between ages 2 and 10 years of age. Prognosis for SVT is good (Webb et al., 2011).

Congestive Heart Failure

CHF is a condition in which the blood supply to the body is insufficient to meet the metabolic requirements of the organs. CHF is a manifestation of an underlying disease or defect, rather than a disease itself. Before development of CHF, compensatory mechanisms are activated to maintain adequate CO (Park, 2007; Wernovsky & Gruber, 2005). Normal mechanisms for regulation of CO are listed in Box 7.1. CHF is classified according to the cause. Box 7.2 shows common causes of CHF in newborns.

Increased volume may be caused by fluid overload or fluid retention. In the normally functioning myocardium, fluid retention does not cause CHF; however, fluid retention complicates CHF from other causes. In neonates, the most common cause of increased volume is CHD or altered hemodynamics, as in PDA.

CHF caused by obstruction to outflow occurs when the normal myocardium pumps against increased resistance. This increased resistance may be caused by structural defects, such as valvular stenosis or COA, or by pulmonary disease or pulmonary hypertension. CHF caused by pulmonary disease is called *cor pulmonale*. Severe systemic hypertension can also cause increased resistance.

CHF in the neonate usually results from abnormal stresses placed on the heart rather than from an ineffective myocardium. However, electrolyte imbalances, acidosis, and myocardial ischemia affect the ability of the heart to function effectively. Conditions such as rheumatic fever, infectious myocarditis, Kawasaki disease, and anomalous origin of the left coronary artery reduce the effectiveness of the heart.

Dysrhythmias that may produce CHF include complete AV block or sustained primary tachycardia. AV block results in a severe bradycardia that prohibits adequate circulation of blood. Tachycardia causes insufficient time for ventricular filling, decreasing CO.

Severe anemia can cause CHF because of excessive demand for CO. Because the oxygen-carrying capacity of the blood is diminished, the heart must pump more blood per minute to meet the tissue oxygenation requirements. If the heart cannot meet the excessive demand, CHF develops (Park, 2007).

Compensatory mechanisms function to meet the body's increased demand for CO. These mechanisms are regulated by the sympathetic nervous system and mechanical factors. The compensatory mechanisms can sustain adequate CO for only a short period of time. If the underlying condition is not corrected, CHF develops.

■ Sympathetic Nervous System Compensatory Mechanisms. Decreased blood pressure stimulates vascular stretch receptors and baroreceptors in the aorta and carotid arteries, which trigger the sympathetic nervous system. Decreased systemic blood pressure inactivates baroreceptors, causing (1) increased sympathetic stimulation, (2) increased HR, (3) increased cardiac contractility, and

BOX 7.1

MECHANISMS OF CARDIAC OUTPUT REGULATION

Sympathetic nervous system activated by:
- Vasomotor center through peripheral sympathetic fibers
- Secretion of norepinephrine from adrenal medullary "fight or flight" response
- Characterized by tachycardia, increased contractility, peripheral vasoconstriction, pupil dilation
- Parasympathetic nervous system activated by vagal fibers
- Atrial stimulation causes decreased heart rate
- Ventricles stimulation causes decreased contractility
- Baroreceptor reflexes
- Located in walls of carotid sinuses and in aortic arch
- Pressure receptors stimulated by blood pressure
- Stimulation causes inhibition of the sympathetic portion of the vasomotor center and stimulation of the parasympathetic (vagal) center; decreased arterial blood pressure

(4) increased arterial blood pressure. Catecholamine release and b-receptor stimulation increase the rate and force of myocardial contraction. Catecholamines also increase venous tone, so that blood is returned to the heart more effectively. Circulation to the skin, kidneys, extremities, and splanchnic bed is decreased, allowing better circulation to the brain, heart, and lungs. Decreased renal blood flow stimulates the release of renin, angiotensin, and aldosterone. This release causes retention of sodium and fluid, resulting in increased circulating volume. The increased volume puts additional work on the heart.

■ **Mechanical Compensatory Mechanisms.** The heart muscle thickens to increase myocardial pressure. The hypertrophy is effective in the early stages, but as soon as the muscle mass increases, compliance decreases. This change in compliance requires greater filling pressure for adequate CO. The hypertrophied heart eventually becomes ischemic because it does not receive adequate circulation to meet its metabolic needs. Ventricular dilation occurs as myocardial fibers stretch to accommodate heart volume. Initially, this increases the force of the contraction, but it, too, fails after a point.

BOX 7.2

CAUSES OF CONGESTIVE HEART FAILURE IN THE NEWBORN

Increased volume
Obstruction to flow
Ineffective myocardial function
Arrhythmias
Excessive demand for cardiac output

Congenital heart defects
Hypoplastic left heart syndrome
Interrupted aortic arch
Coarctation of the aorta
Total anomalous pulmonary venous return with obstruction
Arteriovenous malformation (cranial or hepatic)
Transposition of the great arteries
Patent ductus arteriosus (in preterm infants)

Acquired heart defects
Myocardial dysfunction
Anemia
Polycythemia or hyperviscosity
Tachyarrhythmias
Myocarditis

■ **Effects of Congestive Heart Failure.** When the right ventricle is unable to pump blood into the pulmonary artery, less blood is oxygenated by the lungs, there is increased pressure in the right atrium and systemic venous circulation, and edema occurs in the extremities and viscera. When the left ventricle is unable to pump blood into the systemic circulation, there is increased pressure in the left atrium and pulmonary veins. The lungs become congested with blood, causing elevated pulmonary pressures and pulmonary edema.

The end effects of CHF include decreased CO, decreased renal perfusion, systemic venous engorgement, and pulmonary venous engorgement and their consequent effects. Decreased CO stimulates the sympathetic nervous system, causing tachycardia, increased contractility, increased vasomotor tone, peripheral vasoconstriction, and diaphoresis. Decreased renal perfusion stimulates the renin–angiotensin–aldosterone mechanism, causing sodium and water retention. Systemic venous engorgement leads to hepatomegaly, jugular venous distention, periorbital and facial edema, and, occasionally, ascites and dependent edema. Pulmonary venous engorgement results in tachypnea, decreased tidal volume, decreased lung compliance, increased airway resistance, early closure of the small airways with air trapping, increased work of breathing, and increased respiratory effort, grunting, and rales. Stimulation of the j-receptors in the lung causes the infant to become apprehensive and irritable.

■ **Diagnosis.** The diagnosis of CHF is based on clinical signs and symptoms, laboratory data, and chest radiography. In contrast to infants with cyanotic heart disease, infants with CHF usually have significant respiratory distress with tachypnea, grunting, and retractions.

They exhibit peripheral pallor, appearing to be ashen or gray in color. The precordium is active, and there are usually loud murmurs heard throughout systole and diastole. Pulses are usually full, but there may be a difference between the upper and the lower extremities. Hepatomegaly is common. The infants demonstrate signs of irritability because of the increased effort of breathing and air hunger.

In addition to demonstrating hypoxemia, arterial blood gas may reveal a metabolic acidosis resulting from the decreased systemic blood flow. If acidosis is severe, there may be concurrent respiratory acidosis because of the pulmonary edema caused by left-sided heart failure. Pulmonary ventilation–perfusion mismatch may cause hypoxemia. Hypocalcemia is often present in infants with CHF because they have an inappropriate response to stress. In addition, infants with DiGeorge syndrome may have hypocalcemia because of absent parathyroids. Aortic arch abnormalities (e.g., interrupted aortic arch, hypoplastic left heart, and COA) are commonly associated with DiGeorge syndrome (Park, 2007).

Hypoglycemia may be present in infants with severe CHF. The myocardium is dependent on glucose; decreased glucose levels diminish the ability of the heart to compensate for CHF. On chest radiograph, the heart is enlarged and there is increased pulmonary congestion. ECG is not generally diagnostic, unless the CHF is caused by an arrhythmia. There may be nonspecific changes in the T waves, changes in the ST segment, and an increase in the height of the P wave.

Electrolyte imbalances usually include relative hyponatremia, which is due to the increase in free water. Hypochloremia and increased bicarbonate may result from respiratory acidemia and the use of loop diuretics. Hyperkalemia results from the release of intracellular cations, which is related to poor tissue perfusion. Elevated lactic acid levels are also indicative of tissue hypoxia. Atrial natriuretic factor (ANF), a peptide hormone, may be important in the regulation of volume and blood pressure. ANF is released from the atria when they are distended. ANF release causes natriuresis, diuresis, and vasodilation. ANF acts with other volume regulators, such as renin, aldosterone, and vasopressin. An increased ANF level may be found when there is increased pulmonary blood flow, increased left atrial pressure, or pulmonary hypertension.

Children with corrected or noncorrected CHDs frequently have abnormal homeostasis, suggesting a chronic compensated disseminated intravascular coagulopathy, with reduced synthesis of clotting factors and/or deranged platelet aggregation that can lead to bleeding problems (Goel, Shome, Singh, Bhattacharjee, & Khalil, 2000).

■ Treatment. The goal of management of CHF is to improve cardiac function while identifying and correcting the underlying cause. General measures that decrease the demand on the heart are helpful; however, pharmacologic intervention is the most efficacious therapy.

General Measures. General measures to manage CHF include the administration of oxygen to improve ventilation and perfusion at the alveolar level. Ventilation with positive end-expiratory pressure at 6 to 10 cm/H_2O may relieve the effects of CHF by reducing pulmonary edema.

Fluid restriction may decrease the circulating volume. Careful monitoring of serum electrolytes, intake and output, and weight is essential. It is imperative that *all* fluid be counted in the total daily fluid volume. Infants with CHF do not usually feed well and may require caloric supplementation with hyperalimentation or gavage feedings (Park, 2007).

Infants with CHF are irritable and agitated, which further complicates their status. Sedation with continuous infusions of morphine sulfate or fentanyl may improve the infant's comfort and oxygenation. Other measures that reduce cardiac demand include maintenance of a normal hematocrit, maintenance of the thermoneutral environment, and minimal stimulation. Cautious use of sedation may reduce anxiety and agitation, increasing comfort and decreasing the demand for oxygen (Verklan & Walden, 2004).

Pharmacologic Interventions. Table 7.9 lists the medications most commonly used in the management of cardiac conditions. The mainstay of management of CHF *beyond* the neonatal period is digitalis (digoxin). Digoxin slows conduction through the AV node, prolongs the refractory period, and slows the HR through vagal effects on the SA node.

The use of digoxin in preterm or term neonates is controversial. The preterm newborn is at risk for digitalis toxicity because of the narrow range between therapeutic and toxic drug levels. The preterm infant requires a lower maintenance dose because of limited renal excretion of the drug (Table 7.10). If digoxin is used, the neonate must be carefully monitored for signs and symptoms of digitalis toxicity. Lead II ECGs should be obtained before each dose for the first 3 days; the dose should be withheld if the P-R interval is greater than 0.16 second or if there is an arrhythmia present. Digoxin levels should be monitored and should be less than 2.0 ng/mL (Park, 2007). Blood samples for digoxin levels should be drawn after the drug has achieved equilibrium in the body, approximately 6 to 8 hours after administration.

Other inotropic agents can be used to improve CO. Dopamine, a norepinephrine precursor, has direct and indirect beta-adrenergic effects that are dose dependent. At low doses (2–5 µg/kg/min), there is increased renal blood flow with minimal effect on HR, blood pressure, or contractility. Medium doses (5–10 µg/kg/min) increase renal blood flow, HR, blood pressure, and contractility. Pulmonary artery pressure may be increased; peripheral resistance is not affected. High doses (10–20 µg/kg/min) cause a effects, resulting in peripheral vasoconstriction, increased cardiac rate, and increased contractility (Park, 2007).

TABLE 7.9

DRUGS USED IN THE MANAGEMENT OF CONGENITAL HEART DEFECTS

Drug	Dosage	Action	Onset	Comments
Diuretics				
Furosemide (Lasix)	1 mg/kg/dose IV	Loop diuretic; inhibits sodium and chloride reabsorption in proximal tubule	15–30 minutes	Associated with increased PDA; calcium loss
	1–3 mg/kg/dose		30–60 minutes	
Spironolactone (Aldactone)	1.5–3.0 mg/kg/d PO	Competitive antagonist of aldosterone	3–5 days	Potassium sparing
Chlorothiazide	20–40 mg/kg/d PO	Inhibits sodium and chloride reabsorption along the distal tubules	1–2 hours	
Inotropic Agents				
Dopamine	Low: 2–5 μg/kg/min	Increased renal blood flow; beta-adrenergic effects		Monitor ECG; BP
	Mod: 5–10 μg/kg/min	Increased renal blood flow; heart rate, BP, and contractility		
	High: 10–20 μg/kg/min	Peripheral vasoconstriction, increased heart rate, and contractility		
Dobutamine	2–10 μg/kg/min	Increased renal blood flow; increased contractility	Rapid	Decreased systemic vascular resistance; increased pulmonary wedge pressure
Isoproterenol	0.05–0.5 mg/kg/min	Increased venous return to heart and decreased pulmonary vascular resistance		Tachycardia, dysrhythmias, decreased renal perfusion
Vasodilators				
Sodium nitroprusside (Nipride)	0.5–6 μg/kg/min	Directly relaxes smooth muscles in arteriolar and venous walls; increases cardiac output if the decrease is secondary to myocardial dysfunction	Seconds	Monitor BP and thiocyanate levels; light sensitive; monitor heart rate
Prostaglandins				
PGE_1	0.05–0.1 mg/kg/min	Produces vasodilation and smooth muscle relaxation of ductus arteriosus and pulmonary and systemic circulations; increased arterial saturation by 25%–100%	Rapid	Monitor BP; vasopressors may be required; apnea, flush, fever, seizure-like activity; decreased heart rate
Prostaglandin Synthetase Inhibitors				
Indomethacin	0.2 mg/kg IV (1st) q 24 hr	Promotes ductal closure by inhibition of PGE_2 in the walls of the ductus	12–24 hours	Monitor renal function, bilirubin, electrolytes, glucose, platelets, bleeding
	0.1 mg/kg IV (2nd and 3rd)			
	>48 hr and <14 d: 0.3 mg/kg IV and 3 doses q 24 hr			
	>14 d and <6 wk: 0.2–0.3 mg/kg q 12 hr			

BP, blood pressure; ECG, electrocardiogram; IV, intravenously; PDA, patent ductus arteriosus; PO, by mouth; q, every.

Dobutamine is a synthetic catecholamine that acts on beta- and alpha-adrenergic receptors. Dobutamine (2–10 μg/min) has decreased effects on the HR and rhythm and causes less peripheral vasoconstriction.

Isoproterenol (Isuprel), a synthetic epinephrine-like substance, has β_1- and β_2-adrenergic effects. The usefulness of Isuprel in the neonate is limited because it produces increased HR, arrhythmias, and decreased systemic vascular resistance, which may worsen the hypotension (Park, 2007).

Diuretics. Diuretics are useful in the treatment of CHF to decrease sodium and water retention. The primary

TABLE 7.10

DIGOXIN PRESCRIPTION INFORMATION

	Total Digitalizing Dose (TDD)	Maintenance Dose
Preterm	0.025–0.05 mg/kg	0.008–0.012 mg/kg/d
Term	0.04–0.08 mg/kg	0.01–0.02 mg/kg/d (1/8 TDD)

To digitalize:
1. Give 1/2 TDD
2. 6 to 8 hours later, give 1/4 TDD
3. 6 to 8 hours later, get a rhythm strip; if normal, give 1/4 TDD
4. Give maintenance dose (1/8 TDD) 12 hours after last digitalizing dose and then every 12 hours

Slow digitalization, with decreased risk of toxicity, can be achieved by starting with the maintenance dose

goal is to increase renal perfusion (with inotropic agents or vasodilators) and to increase sodium delivery to distal diluting sites of the renal tubules. Diuretic agents increase the renal excretion of sodium and other anions by inhibition of tubular reabsorption of sodium (Park, 2007).

Furosemide (Lasix), a loop diuretic, blocks sodium and chloride reabsorption in the ascending limb of the loop of Henle. Loop diuretics interfere with the formation of free water and free water reabsorption by preventing the transport of sodium, potassium, and chloride into the medullary interstitium. Loop diuretics cause increased excretion of potassium by delivering increased quantities of sodium to sites in the distal nephron where potassium can be excreted. Furosemide also increases excretion of calcium but does not affect the ability of the kidney to regulate acid–base balance.

An aldosterone antagonist such as spironolactone (Aldactone) may be used because it is a potassium-sparing diuretic. Spironolactone works by binding to the cytoplasmic receptor sites and blocking aldosterone action, thus impairing the reabsorption of sodium and the secretion of potassium and hydrogen ion. Spironolactone has no effect on free water production and absorption. Thiazide diuretics (chlorothiazide and hydrochlorothiazide) inhibit sodium and chloride reabsorption along the distal tubules. They are not as effective as the loop diuretics and are infrequently used (Park, 2007).

■ **Complications of Diuretic Therapy.** Diuretic therapy can cause severe electrolyte imbalances if not monitored carefully. The complications of diuretic therapy include (1) volume contraction, (2) hyponatremia, (3) metabolic alkalemia or acidemia, and (4) hypokalemia or hyperkalemia. When using diuretics, fluid and electrolyte balance must be maintained by the administration of water and electrolytes. The adequacy of the volume can be determined by monitoring serum electrolytes, BUN, creatinine, urinary output, weight, specific gravity, and skin turgor.

The increased renal losses of sodium can lead to hyponatremia, unless adequate amounts of sodium are provided. There may also be increased antidiuretic hormone (ADH) release secondary to changes in the osmoreceptors or inhibition of ADH action. This can best be managed by decreasing the amount of total water and improving the CO, thus increasing renal perfusion.

Metabolic alkalosis can result from administration of loop diuretics that interfere with sodium- and potassium-dependent chloride reabsorption. Hypochloremia results in a greater aldosterone production and an increase in bicarbonate concentration. Hypokalemia is a frequent complication of loop diuretic therapy. An increased ratio of intracellular to extracellular potassium results in the clinical signs and symptoms of hypokalemia. Hypokalemia increases the risk for digoxin toxicity. In contrast, hyperkalemia may result when CO is low and tissue perfusion is severely compromised. Other complications of diuretic therapy include increased calcium excretion, hyperuricemia, and glucose intolerance.

Vasodilators may be used in severe CHF to reduce the right and left ventricular preload and afterload to improve cardiac function. Vasodilators cause arterial and venous dilation, resulting in decreased systemic and pulmonary vascular resistance. Sodium nitroprusside (Nipride) is a smooth muscle relaxant that decreases ventricular afterload by decreasing pulmonary and systemic vascular resistance and decreases venous return and ventricular preload. This leads to decreased ventricular end-diastolic volume, increased ejection fraction, increased HR and cardiac index, and decreased pulmonary and systemic resistance. Sodium nitroprusside is sensitive to light and must be stored in dark containers. Side effects are cyanide toxicity and decreased platelet function (Park, 2007). The prognosis for CHF depends on the severity of the underlying condition and on the degree of CHF.

Subacute Bacterial Infective Endocarditis

Subacute bacterial infective endocarditis (SBIE or SBE) can be a complication of CHD. Two factors are important in the development of SBIE: (1) structural abnormalities that create turbulent flow or pressure gradients and (2) bacteremia. All cardiac defects that produce turbulent flow or have a significant pressure gradient predispose the patient to bacterial invasion of the cardiac endothelium. The turbulent flow damages the endothelial lining and platelet–fibrin thrombus formation. Prevention of bacterial SBIE requires scrupulous daily oral care as well as prophylactic antimicrobials for dental procedures (Park, 2007). All CHDs, except secundum-type ASDs, predispose the patient to SBIE. VSDs, TOF, and AS are the CHDs most commonly associated with SBIE (Park, 2007).

Vegetation of SBIE is usually on the low pressure side of the defect, where endothelial damage is established by the jet effect of the defect. More than 90% of SBIE cases are caused by *Streptococcus viridans, Streptococcus faecalis* (enterococcus), and *Staphylococcus aureus*. Other organisms include *Haemophilus influenzae, Pseudomonas, Escherichia coli, Proteus, Aerobacter*, and *Listeria. Candida* may infect infants who have been on long-term antimicrobial or steroid therapy.

Prevention. Procedures for which SBIE prophylaxis is indicated include (1) all dental procedures, (2) tonsillectomy or adenoidectomy, (3) surgical procedures involving the respiratory mucosa, (4) bronchoscopy, (5) incision and drainage of infected tissue, and (6) gastrointestinal or genitourinary procedures.

For complete prescribing and dosing information, refer to the Committee on Rheumatic Fever and Infective Endocarditis of the Council on Cardiovascular Diseases in the Young. The recommendations for children are listed in Table 7.11.

Family Support

Families of infants who are critically ill or have congenital defects generally experience confusion, guilt, anger, and fear. The family must cope with short- and long-term consequences of the CHD. Severity of the defect, availability of treatment, and prognosis influence the amount and kind of support required. Parents may be overwhelmed by the knowledge of their infant's heart defect, regardless of the severity. With treatment now available, over 95% of CHDs can be partially or fully corrected through a combination of medical and surgical management (Cooley, 1997). However, residual defects or cardiovascular sequelae after surgical correction are common (Meberg, Otterstad, Froland, Lindberg, & Sorland, 2000). Parents need to be able to discuss quality of life issues with the health care professionals in order to assure that parents can make informed decisions about possible treatment options (Moyen et al., 1997). All options must be explained and described objectively. The impact of the cardiac defect on other systems must also be included when giving parents information, as the parents may not be aware of the associated complications, such as respiratory problems, that often accompany cardiac defects (Lubica, 1996). Although often overlooked, neurological prognosis is a key factor in determining the overall quality of life of a child with a CHD. Pediatric neurologists can be integrated into the health care team to assist parents in assessing the neurological prognosis of their child as well as begin early intervention programs to facilitate the best outcomes (Shevell, 1999). Parents need frequent contact with members of the health care team. Caretakers should speak with the parents routinely, not just when there are major changes in the infant's condition.

Although the majority of CHDs do not have an identifiable genetic pattern, genetic counseling should be offered to all parents with a newborn with a CHD. Parents will want answers to questions about the cause of the defect, the likelihood of a recurrence in future pregnancies, and if there may be associated defects (Welch & Brown, 2000; Wolf & Basson, 2010). In addition, future innovation may

TABLE 7.11

ANTIMICROBIAL PROPHYLAXIS TO PREVENT SUBACUTE INFECTIVE ENDOCARDITIS IN CHILDREN WITH CARDIAC DEFECTS

I. Dental procedures and oral respiratory tract surgery

- A. Standard regimen
  1. Amoxicillin 50 mg/kg 1 hour before procedure, followed by 25 mg/kg 6 hours after procedure
- B. Alternative regimens
  1. Allergic to penicillin and/or amoxicillin: erythromycin ethylsuccinate or erythromycin stearate 20 mg/kg orally 2 hours before procedure, followed by erythromycin 10 mg/kg 6 hours after initial dose
  2. Children unable to take oral medications: ampicillin 50 mg/kg IV or IM 30 minutes before procedure, followed by ampicillin 25 mg/kg IV or IM 6 hours after initial dose
  3. Allergic to penicillin and/or amoxicillin and unable to take oral medications: clindamycin 10 mg/kg IV 30 minutes before procedure, followed by clindamycin 5 mg/kg IV 6 hours after initial dose
  4. High-risk children not candidates for standard regimen: ampicillin 50 mg/kg IV or IM plus gentamicin 2.0 mg/kg IV or IM 30 minutes before procedure, followed by amoxicillin 25 mg/kg orally 6 hours after initial dose or a repeat of the ampicillin plus gentamicin regimen
  5. High-risk children allergic to ampicillin, amoxicillin, or penicillin: vancomycin 20 mg/kg IV over 1 hour, starting 1 hour before procedure. No repeat dose necessary

(*continued*)

TABLE 7.11

ANTIMICROBIAL PROPHYLAXIS TO PREVENT SUBACUTE INFECTIVE ENDOCARDITIS IN CHILDREN WITH CARDIAC DEFECTS (CONTINUED)

II. Gastrointestinal or genitourinary procedure
A. Standard regimen
1. Ampicillin 50 mg/kg plus gentamicin 2.0 mg/kg IV or IM 30 minutes before procedure, followed by amoxicillin 25 mg/kg 6 hours after initial dose; or repeat ampicillin plus gentamicin regimen 8 hours after initial dose
B. Alternative regimens
1. Ampicillin/amoxicillin/penicillin-allergic children: vancomycin 20 mg/kg IV over 1 hour plus gentamicin 2.0 mg/kg IV or IM 1 hour before procedure; repeat the vancomycin plus gentamicin regimen 8 hours after initial dose
2. Low-risk patient alternative regimen: amoxicillin 50 mg/kg orally 1 hour before procedure, followed by amoxicillin 25 mg/kg 6 hours after initial dose

From Dajani et al. (1997).

greatly improve the ability to diagnose CHDs prenatally (Bakiler et al., 2007; Landis et al., 2012), thus increasing the opportunity for fetal surgery for correction of some defects, improved immediate management at birth, or in some cases, termination of the pregnancy. The majority of CHDs can be identified through targeted transvaginal or transabdominal ultrasound; however, they evolve in utero at different stages; thus a single sonogram may not be sufficient to detect all CHDs (Yagel et al., 1997). Health care professionals must be keenly aware of all options to assure that parents receive the most up-to-date information on which to base decisions.

Family members should be given an accurate description of the defect; diagrams and models illustrating the defect should be used. Parents need frequent reassurance and repetition of information. Parents of infants who do not require immediate surgery but who will eventually require surgical correction must be educated about all aspects of the infant's care, including signs and symptoms of deterioration, medication administration, activity limitations, and normal development. Because growth failure with a cardiac defect is common, efforts to maximize nutrition are important; extra support is needed if the mother planned to breastfeed her baby (Barbas & Kelleher, 2004; Varan, Tokel, & Yilmaz, 1999). Careful follow-up is important to prevent complications.

Identification of support persons for the family is extremely valuable. Parents may be encouraged to talk to other parents of newborns with the same or similar defects. Many neonatal intensive care units (NICUs) have active support groups consisting of parents of patients. Care should be taken in selection of supporters. Parents with a term newborn with a CHD may not be able to relate to parents of a preterm neonate. Other family members or friends should not be overlooked; they can become valuable support persons if they are provided appropriate guidance and education. The needs of siblings should also be assessed. Siblings need support, education, and guidance appropriate for their age and comprehension of the situation. Parents may not recognize their needs because of the overwhelming situation. Health care providers can facilitate the parent–child relationship during the initial period and throughout the course of the management.

Financial resources should be addressed because preoperative, operative, and postoperative care is expensive. Many parents need assistance in obtaining aid to which they are entitled. Even the most knowledgeable of parents may not be aware of resources available to them. If experimental surgery is contemplated, parents may need assistance in speaking with private insurance companies regarding coverage. Referrals to appropriate local, state, federal, or private organizations that pertain to the CHD should be made for the parents. These include the Department of Family and Children Services, the March of Dimes, and Children's Medical Services. The family may qualify for the Special Supplemental Nutrition Program for Women, Infants, and Children (WIC).

Discharge planning must be comprehensive for the neonate who will receive medical management for a CHD before corrective surgery. A thorough assessment of the home may be needed before discharge. Contact with the primary care provider who will perform the routine management of the infant is imperative. Initial contact by telephone should be followed up with a copy of the complete medical record and discharge summary. If the infant requires any special equipment for home care, the equipment should be obtained before discharge so that the parents can be taught how to use it. Also, practical details such as whether there are enough electrical outlets in the infant's room must be determined. Notification of local emergency medical services, power companies, and other relevant companies should be completed before discharge.

CONCLUSION

The most common CHDs were described based on the effects on cardiovascular circulation. The most common dysrhythmic disorders seen in the newborn were discussed. The diagnosis and management of the most frequent complications of CHDs, CHF, and SBIE was included. Parental support of families with newborns and children with CHDs was discussed.

CASE STUDY

The NICU in a large women's and children's hospital received a call for assistance on the adjacent mother and baby unit to evaluate an infant for cyanosis. Nurse Johnson responded to the call and discovered that Baby Johanna was pale, cyanotic, and tachypneic. Nurse Johnson positioned the baby for optimal oxygenation and supplied oxygen via blow-by. Baby Johanna responded to the blow-by oxygen with improved color and tone. Nurse Johnson told the mother that she would take the baby to the NICU for further evaluation and would update her as soon as possible. In the NICU, the baby's pediatrician was called and the birth history was obtained from the medical record, supplied by the Mother and Baby Unit personnel. Baby Johanna was put in an Oxyhood, and vital signs were obtained. The baby was now pink, HR was 164, respiratory rate was 76, and the mean blood pressure was 58.

Johanna was born to a Gravida 1, para 0 (now 1), 24-year-old mother with uncomplicated pregnancy and delivery. Birth weight was 3.3 kg, and Apgar scores were 8/9 (–1 color, –1 tone; –1 color). Johanna showed no distress, and the pediatrician's examination at 3 hours postbirth was within normal limits, with some slight acrocyanosis of the hands and feet present. Johanna had been in the Mother/Baby unit and the mom was nursing. At this feeding, the mother had offered the baby a bottle following nursing. She called the floor nurse because the baby seemed to turn blue during the feeding.

Upon auscultation, a soft ejection-type murmur was noted at the left upper sternal border. Right radial arterial blood gas showed a partially compensated metabolic acidosis on 70% FiO_2 per hood. The pulse oximeter registered an oxygen saturation of 58% on arms and legs. A hyperoxia test using 100% FiO_2 showed no improvement in arterial oxygenation. The cardiac murmur had increased and was determined to be systolic in origin and probably, tricuspid regurgitation. Chest x-ray showed a normal heart size and decreased pulmonary markings. A stat cardiac echocardiogram was ordered to determine whether a cardiac defect was present.

1. What other intervention should be initiated while the definitive diagnosis is being obtained?
2. What are the most likely cardiac defects with this presentation?
3. How does the timing of the episode influence the differential diagnosis?

Echocardiography revealed presence of PA with intact intraventricular septum, reverse flow into the pulmonary system through a PDA, maintained by the continuous infusion of PGE_1 started after the chest x-ray was obtained.

4. What is the general management for PA?
5. What information should be shared with the parents regarding short- and long-term treatment and prognosis?

EVIDENCE-BASED PRACTICE BOX

Screening for Critical Congenital Heart Defects With Pulse Oximetry

The overall incidence of CHD is slightly less than 1%, or 8 per 1,000 live births, excluding PDA in the preterm newborn which is the single largest factor for infant mortality due to all birth defects. CHDs that usually cause hypoxia in the newborn period and are associated with the highest mortality are categorized as *critical congenital heart defects* (CCHDs). Newborns with CCHDs require immediate intervention to prevent death or disability.

Seven cardiac defects make up the CCHDs: HLHS, PA (with intact septum), TOF, TAPVR, TGA, tricuspid atresia, and TA. Approximately 4,800 babies are born each year in the United States with one of these seven CCHDs.

Delayed diagnosis of any of these defects significantly increases the risk for morbidity or mortality. Currently, diagnosis depends on prenatal ultrasound identification or physical examination of the newborn. This approach does not identify all defects, and so it leads to late diagnosis and increased morbidity. Methods that allow earlier identification of these cardiac defects would lead to quicker diagnosis, implementation of treatment, and improved outcome.

Routine screening of newborns with pulse oximetry was proposed as one method to improve early diagnosis of CCHDs. Pulse oximetry is a noninvasive, painless, relatively inexpensive, and readily available method that measures blood oxygen saturation. The CCHDs are associated with hypoxia, and thus this screening could identify newborns with one of these defects. Numerous studies were conducted in the United States and in other countries, including Sweden and Germany to determine whether routine pulse oximetry measurements on newborns improved the detection of CCHDs.

The U.S. Health and Human Services Secretary convened a group of experts to examine evidence of the effectiveness of pulse oximetry screening. The group consisted of members recommended by the Secretary's Advisory Committee on Heritable Diseases in Newborns and Children, the American Academy of Pediatrics, the American College of Cardiology Foundation, and the

(*continued*)

American Heart Association. The work group found sufficient evidence to recommend routine screening with pulse oximetry monitoring to identify low blood oxygen saturation in newborns in well-infant and intermediate nurseries. They recommended further study for screening of special populations, such as in high altitudes.

Based on this review of the evidence, Secretary of Health and Human Services Kathleen Sebelius recommended the addition of screening for CCHD in newborns in 2011. This recommendation was officially endorsed by the American Academy of Pediatrics (AAP). Some hospitals have adopted this screening method; however, there are differences in the screening process and in the number and type of conditions that are screened for in each state. Some states have introduced or passed legislation to add the pulse oximetry screening to the current newborn screening. Go to this website to see the status of legislation in your state: http://www.cchdscreeningmap.com.

Some hospitals have implemented the screening process voluntarily. This is an example of evidence-based practice change.

ONLINE RESOURCES

Alabama Department of Public Health; Hospital Guidelines for Implementing Pulse Oximetry Screening for Critical Congenital Heart Disease
http://www.adph.org/newbornscreening/assets/FHS.NBS.CCHDGuidelines.0312.na.pdf

CDC—Screening for Critical Congenital Heart Defects
http://www.cdc.gov/ncbddd/pediatricgenetics/pulse.html

Pulse oximetry screening for CCHDs in asymptomatic newborn babies: A systematic review and meta-analysis
http://www.thelancet.com/journals/lancet/article/PIIS0140-6736%2812%2960107-X/abstract

Role of Pulse Oximetry in Examining Newborns for Congenital Heart Disease: A Scientific Statement from the AHA and AAP
http://pediatrics.aappublications.org/content/124/2/823.short

Screening for Critical Congenital Heart Disease: A Federal Agency Plan of Action
http://www.hrsa.gov/advisorycommittees/mchbadvisory/heritabledisorders/recommendations/correspondence/cyanoticheartsecre09212011.pdf

REFERENCES

Agras, P. I., Derbent, M., Ozcay, F., Baskin, E., Turkoglu, S., Aldemir, D., Tokel, K., & Saatci, U. (2005). Effect of congenital heart disease on renal function in childhood. *Nephron Physiology, 99*(1), 10–15.

Bakiler, A. R., Ozer, E. A., Kanik, A., Kanit, H., & Aktas, F. N. (2007). Accuracy of prenatal diagnosis of congenital heart disease with fetal echocardiography. *Fetal Diagnostic Therapy, 22*(4), 241–244.

Barbas, K. H., & Kelleher, D. K. (2004). Breastfeeding success among infants with congenital heart disease. *Pediatric Nursing, 30*(4), 285–289.

Cooley, D. A. (1997). Early development of congenital heart surgery: Open heart procedures. *The Annals of Thoracic Surgery, 64*(5), 1544–1548.

Dajani, A. S., Taubert, K. A., Wilson, W., Bolger, A. F., Bayer, A., Ferrieri, P., . . . Zuccaro, G. (1997). *Prevention of bacterial endocarditis*. Recommendations by the American Heart Association. Dallas, TX: AHA.

Danford, D. A., Gumbiner, C. H., Martin, A. B., & Fletcher, S. E. (2000). Effects of electrocardiography and chest radiography on the accuracy of preliminary diagnosis of common congenital cardiac defects. *Pediatric Cardiology, 21*(4), 334–340.

Danford, D. A., Salaymeb, K. J., Martin, A. B., Fletcher, S. E., & Gumbiner, C. H. (1999). Pulmonary stenosis: Defect-specific diagnostic accuracy of heart murmurs in children. *Journal of Pediatrics, 134*(1), 76–81.

Dipchand, A. I., Giuffre, M., & Freedom, R. M. (1999). Tetralogy of Fallot with non-confluent pulmonary arteries and aortopulmonary septal defect. *Cardiology in the Young, 9*(1), 75–77.

Freedom, R. M., Yoo, S. -J., & Coles, J. G. (2007). Atrioventricular septal defect. In R. M. Freedom, S.-J. Yoo, H. Mikailian, & W. G. Williams (Eds.), *The natural and modifed history of congenital heart disease*. Elmsford, NY: Blackwell Publishing. doi:10.1002/9780470986905.ch5

Freeman, S. B., Bean, L. H., Allen, E. G., Tinker, S. W., Locke, A. E., Druschel, C., . . . Sherman, S. L. (2008). Ethnicity, sex, and the incidence of congenital heart defects: A report from the National Down Syndrome Project. *Genetics in Medicine, 10*, 173–180.

Goel, M., Shome, D. K., Singh, Z. N., Bhattacharjee, J., & Khalil, A. (2000). Haemostatic changes in children with cyanotic and acyanotic congenital heart disease. *International Health care Journal (IHJ), 52*(5), 559–563.

Hazinski, M. F. (1984). Cardiovascular disorders. In M. F. Hazinski (Ed.), *Nursing care of the critically ill child* (pp. 63–252). St. Louis: C. V. Mosby.

Jones, K. (2005). *Smith's recognizable patterns of human malformation* (6th ed.). Philadelphia, PA: Saunders.

Kaplan, N. M. (2011). Systemic hypertension therapy. In R. Bonow, D. Mann, D. P. Zipes, P. Libby, & E. Braunwald (Eds.), *Braunwald's Heart disease: A textbook of cardiovascular medicine* (pp. 955–975). Philadelphia, PA: WB Saunders.

Koch, J., Hensley, G., Roy, L., Brown, S., Ramaciotti, C., & Rosenfeld, C. (2006). Prevalence of spontaneous closure of the ductus arteriosus in neonates at a birth weight of 1000 grams or less. *Pediatrics, 117*(4), 1113–1121.

Kochanek, K. D., & Smith, B. L. (2004). *Deaths: Preliminary data for 2002* (National vital statistics reports; Vol. 52, No. 13). Hyattsville, MD: National Center for Health Statistics.

Kushnir, A., & Pinheiro, J. M. (2011). Comparison of renal effects of ibuprofen versus indomethacin during treatment of patent ductus arteriosus in contiguous historical cohorts. *BMC Clinical Pharmacology*. http:/www.biomedcentral.com/1472–6904/11/8

Lambert, J. M., & Watters N. E. (1998). Breastfeeding the infant/child with a cardiac defect: An informal survey. *Journal of Human Lactation, 14*(3), 205–206.

Landis, B. J., Levey, A., Levasseur, S. M., Glickstein, J. S., Kleinman, C. S., Simpson, L. L., & Williams, I. A. (2013). Prenatal diagnosis of congenital heart disease and birth outcomes. *Pediatric Cardiology, 34*(3), 597–605. doi: 10.1007/s00246-012-0504-4. Epub 2012 Oct 6

Lubica, H. (1996). Pathologic lung function in children and adolescents with congenital heart defects. *Pediatric Cardiology, 17*(5), 314–315.

Mann, D. (2012). Pathophysiology of heart failure. In R. O. Bonow, D. Mann, D. P. Zipes, P. Libby, & E. Braunwald (Eds.), *Braunwald's heart disease: A textbook of cardiovascular medicine* (pp. 487–504). Philadelphia, PA: W.B. Saunders.

Massimo, S. S., Drago, F., Grutter, G., De Santis, A., Di Ciommo, V., & Rava, L. (2006). Twenty years of paediatric cardiac pacing: 515 pacemakers and 480 leads implanted in 292 patients. *Europace, 8*(7), 530–536.

Massin, M. M., Derkenne, B., & von Bernuth, G. (1998). Heart rate behavior in children with atrial septal defect. *Cardiology, 90*(4), 269–270.

McElhinney, D. B., Paridon, S., & Spray, T. L. (2000). Aortopulmonary window associated with complete atrioventricular septal defect. *The Journal of Thoracic and Cardiovascular Surgery, 119*(6), 1284–1285.

Meberg, A., Brügmann-Pieper, S., Due, R., Jr., Eskedal, L., Fagerli, I., Farstad, T., . . . Silberg, I. E. (2008). First day of life pulse oximetry screening to detect congenital heart defects. *Journal of Pediatrics, 152*(6), 761–765.

Meberg, A., Otterstad, J. E., Froland, G., Lindberg, H., & Sorland, S. J. (2000). Outcome of congenital heart defects—A population-based study. *Acta Paediatrica, 89*(11), 1344–1351.

Moyen, L. K., Meberg, A., Otterstad, J. E., Froland, G., Sorland, S., Lindstrom, B., & Erickson, B. (1997). Quality of life in children with congenital heart defects. *Acta Paediatrica, 86*(9), 975–980.

Nembhard, W. N., Wang, T., Loscalzo, M. L., & Salemi, J. L. (2010). Variation in the prevalence of congenital heart defects by maternal race/ethnicity and infant sex. *Journal of Pediatrics, 156*(2), 259–264.

Norwood, W. I., Lang, P., & Hansen, D. D. (1983). Physiologic repair of aortic atresia—Hypoplastic left heart syndrome. *New England Journal of Medicine, 308*(1), 3–26.

Nouri, S. (1997). Congenital heart defects: Cyanotic and acyanotic. *Pediatric Annals, 26*(2), 95–98.

Olgin, J. E., & Zipes, D. P. (2012). Specific arrhythmias: Diagnosis and treatment. In R. Bonow, D. Mann, D. P. Zipes, P. Libby, & E. Braunwald (Eds.), *Braunwald's heart disease: A textbook of cardiovascular medicine* (9th ed., chap 39). St. Louis, MO: WB Saunders.

Opie, L. H., & Hasenfuss, G. (2012). Mechanisms of cardiac contraction and relaxation. In R. Bonow, D. Mann, D. P. Zipes, P. Libby, & E. Braunwald (Eds.), *Braunwald's heart disease: A textbook of cardiovascular medicine* (pp. 459–486). Philadelphia, PA: WB Saunders.

Park, M. K. (1988). *Pediatric cardiology for practitioners*. Chicago, IL: Mosby–Year Book.

Park, M. K. (2007). *Pediatric cardiology for practitioners*. Chicago, IL: Mosby.

Pierpoint, T., Thomas, B., Judd, A., Brugha, R., Taylor-Robinson, D., & Renton A. (2000). Prevalence of Chlamydia trachomatis in young men in northwest London. *Sexually Transmitted Infections, 76*, 273–276.

Sacchetti, A., Moyer, V., Baricella, R., Cameron, J., & Moakes, M. E. (1999). Primary cardiac arrhythmias in children. *Pediatric Emergency Care, 15*(2), 95–98.

Seidman, J. G., Pyeritz, R., & Seidman, C. (2011). Inherited causes of cardiovascular disease. In R. Bonow, D. Mann, D. P. Zipes, P. Libby, & E. Braunwald (Eds.), *Braunwald's heart disease: A textbook of cardiovascular medicine* (pp. 70–80). Philadelphia, PA: WB Saunders.

Sekar, K. C., & Corff, K. E. (2008). Treatment of patent ductus arteriosus: Indomethacin or ibuprofen? *Journal of Perinatology, 28*(Suppl. 1), S60–S62.

Shevell, M. I. (1999). The role of the pediatric neurologist in the management of children with congenital heart defects: A commentary. *Seminars in Pediatric Neurology, 6*(1), 64–66.

Russo, P., & Russo, J. G. (2005). Congenital heart defects in newborns and infants: Cardiothoracic repair. In A. R. Spitzer (Ed.), *Intensive care of the fetus & neonate* (2nd ed., pp. 939–953). Philadelphia, PA: Elsevier.

Taussig, W. B. (1947). *Cyanosis in congenital malformations of the heart*. New York, NY: Oxford University Press.

Thomson, J. D., Gibbs, J. L., & Van Doorn, C. (2000). Cardiac catheter guided surgical closure of an apical ventricular septal defect. *The Annals of Thoracic Surgery, 70*(4), 1402–1404.

Turner, S. W., Hunter, S., & Wyllie, J. P. (1999). The natural history of ventricular septal defects. *Archives of Disease in Childhood, 81*(5), 413–416.

Varan, B., Tokel, K., & Yilmaz, G. (1999). Malnutrition and growth failure in cyanotic and acyanotic congenital heart disease with and without pulmonary hypertension. *Archives of Disease in Children, 81*(1), 49–52.

Verklan, M. T., & Walden, M. (2004). *Core curriculum for neonatal intensive care nursing*. St. Louis, MO: Elsevier Saunders.

Webb, G., Smallhorn, J., Therrien, J., & Reddington, A. (2011). Congenital heart disease. In R. Bonow, D. Mann, D. P. Zipes, P. Libby, & E. Braunwald (Eds.), *Braunwald's heart disease: A textbook of cardiovascular medicine* (pp. 1411–1467). Philadelphia, PA: WB. Saunders.

Welch, K. K., & Brown, S. A. (2000). The role of genetic counseling in the management of prenatally detected congenital heart defects. *Seminars in Perinatology, 24*(5), 373–379.

Wernovsky, G., & Gruber, P. J. (2005). Common congenital heart disease: Presentation, management, and outcomes. In H. W. Taeusch, R. A. Ballard, & C. A. Gleason (Eds.), *Avery's diseases of the newborn* (8th ed., pp. 827–871). Philadelphia, PA: Elsevier.

Wolf, M., & Basson, C. (2010). The molecular genetics of congenital heart disease: A review of recent developments. *Current Opinion Cardiology, 25*(3), 192–197.

Yagel, S., Weissman, A., Rotstein, Z., Manor, M., Hegesh, J., Anteby, E., . . . Achiron, R. (1997). Congenital heart defects natural course and in utero development. *Circulation, 96*(2), 550–555.

CHAPTER

8

Gastrointestinal System

■ Sheryl J. Montrowl

The intake and digestion of food and the elimination of waste products are critical to long-term survival. Although many complex metabolic processes are involved, the ability to maintain adequate nutrition ultimately requires that the gastrointestinal (GI) tract be patent and structurally intact. With only a few exceptions, the vast majority of conditions causing GI dysfunction are the result of congenital anatomic malformations. The discovery and management of GI dysfunction requires knowledge of both embryogenesis and normal anatomy. External defects are immediately apparent, but most causes of dysfunction have few initial symptoms unless allowed to progress to serious pathophysiologic changes resulting in major threat to life. The input and support of a variety of nursing, medical, and other specialists are required for the optimal outcomes of the infant's physiologic well-being and the parents' psychosocial stability. Visible defects, especially those involving the face, appear to be particularly difficult for parents to accept. GI malformations, often associated with other congenital anomalies and prematurity, and the need for transport to a distant center where corrective surgery can be accomplished place additional demands on parental coping.

Parents' emotional needs and their ability to work through the grief process over the loss of the expected "perfect" child cannot be underestimated.

The GI tract is the site of the many complex transport and enzymatic mechanisms required for the biologic absorption and digestion of nutrients. The successful intake and assimilation of these nutrients, however, rests on the ability of the gut to act as a conduit for ingestion, digestion, and elimination. Congenital malformations, particularly those involving anatomic or functional obstruction, clearly hinder this process. Even when structurally intact, the supporting gastric and intestinal musculature of the newborn is relatively deficient, increasing the tendency toward distention as a result of infrequent and irregular peristaltic movements. Transport of materials through the tract is further diminished in premature infants who may have poor sucking and swallowing abilities; small gastric capacity; and an incompetent cardioesophageal sphincter. Debilitated, hypotonic infants may similarly exhibit poor sucking and swallowing and decreased motility. In addition, the bowel seems particularly susceptible to ischemic conditions in which blood flow is preferentially directed away from the GI tract, the kidneys, and the peripheral vascular bed toward the brain and heart.

Untoward effects of drugs commonly used in the nursery may further compromise intestinal function or integrity. Morphine, for example, in addition to its desired analgesic effect, also slows gastric emptying and reduces propulsive peristalsis. Conversely, erythromycin has been shown to accelerate gastric emptying. Ulceration of the GI tract with possible bleeding and perforation are reported side effects of tolazoline, dexamethasone, and indomethacin (Zenk, Sills, & Koeppel, 2003). Mydriatics administered for ophthalmologic examination in the preterm infant decrease duodenal activity and gastric emptying (James, 2002). Xanthines may cause or exacerbate gastroesophageal reflux (Jadcherla, 2002). The major purposes of this chapter are to discuss the embryologic development and normal anatomic structure of the GI tract and to describe common causes of neonatal dysfunction and their implications for care.

EMBRYOLOGY OF THE GI TRACT

Formation of the GI tract is largely dependent on the folding of the embryo during the first month of development. At the beginning of the third week of gestation as a result of the neural plate development, the flat, trilaminar embryonic disc begins to fold in both a cephalic-caudal and a ventral direction, invaginating the dorsal portion of the yolk sac. By the fourth week this folding is complete, resulting in a horseshoe-shaped cylinder. This hollow tube is divided into three sections corresponding to the foregut, the midgut, and the hindgut.

Foregut

The foregut forms part of the mouth, esophagus, stomach, proximal duodenum, pancreas, liver, and extra hepatic biliary system as well as the lower respiratory system. The most cranial area of the foregut is often known as the pharyngeal gut. Early in the fourth week of fetal life, a depression appears on the ventral surface of the head called the stomodeum or primitive mouth. Oval thickenings, the nasal placodes, develop above and on either side of the primitive mouth, eventually becoming the nostrils. These nasal elevations and the area above the stomodeum merge to form the philtrum. By the eighth week a continuous ridge forming the upper lip has developed from maxillary processes on either side of the stomodeum fusing with the nasal pits and philtrum. The lower lip and jaw are formed when two mandibular processes below the stomodeum grow and fuse. Beginning in the fifth week, the primary palate begins to form from a wedge-shaped extension of the maxillary processes, thus separating the future nostrils from the upper lip. Lateral palatine processes also form on each side of the tongue and fuse with the nasal septum, anteriorly progressing posteriorly to form the secondary palate during the ninth to twelfth week of development.

At the same time that the mouth is formed, the rest of the foregut is also developing. During the fourth and fifth weeks of gestation an esophagotracheal septum is formed dividing the proximal foregut into the anterior trachea and posterior esophagus. Initially short, the esophagus elongates over a 2- to 3-week period to allow the development of the lungs, heart, and neck. The stomach, first appearing as a dilation of the foregut, begins to grow with the dorsal aspect outpacing the ventral aspect, thus forming the greater curvature. As the esophagus grows, the stomach initially in the region of the neck descends and rotates 90° on its longitudinal axis until it reaches its final position.

The duodenum develops from the caudal portion of the foregut as well as the cranial portion of the midgut. Around the fifth or sixth week, villi grow and temporarily occlude the lumen until the ninth or tenth week of gestation. Several other buds on the foregut also form the liver, gallbladder, bile ducts, and pancreas.

Midgut

The midgut consists of the distal duodenum, jejunum, ileum, cecum, appendix, ascending colon, and the right two thirds of the transverse colon. Blood is supplied by the superior mesenteric artery. Although initially in tandem, the lengthening of the tubular intestine outpaces the overall elongation of the embryo. By the sixth week of gestation, the rate of growth causes the tube to bend ventrally. Simultaneously, rapid growth of the liver quickly limits space within the abdominal cavity. Consequently, around 7 weeks gestation, loops of intestine begin to protrude into the umbilical cord. As the midgut herniates, it rotates in a counterclockwise fashion approximately 90° around an axis formed by the superior mesenteric artery. At around 10 weeks, when the abdominal cavity has expanded sufficiently and the growth of the liver has slowed, reduction of the midgut herniation occurs. As the loops of intestine are retracted into the abdomen they rotate another 180°, resulting in a full rotation of 270°. This counterclockwise rotation allows the transverse colon to pass in front of the duodenum and places the cecum and appendix in the right lower quadrant of the abdomen. Once the intestine has rotated into proper placement, the mesentery attaches to the posterior abdominal wall.

Hindgut

The GI components of the hindgut include the left one-third of the transverse colon, the descending colon, ascending colon, sigmoid colon, rectum, and superior portion of the anal canal. Blood is supplied from the inferior mesenteric artery. The major developmental changes occur in the terminal hindgut known as the cloaca and involve formation of the anus. The hindgut initially ends at the cloacal membrane, which separates it from the anal pit or proctodeum. Around the fourth week of gestation, the urorectal septum forms and by the sixth week divides the cloaca into a ventral urogenital sinus and a dorsal anorectal canal. By the eighth week of gestation, the anal membrane has moved inferior and is found at the bottom of the proctodeum. In the ninth week this membrane ruptures, completing patency of the GI tract.

PHYSIOLOGY OF THE GI TRACT

The major function of the GI tract is to transfer food and water from the external to the internal environment, where they can be digested, absorbed, and distributed to the cells of the body by the circulatory system. While these processes are occurring, contractions of the smooth muscle lining the walls of the intestine move the contents through the lumen, releasing any material not digested and absorbed during transit back into the external environment. Although some end products, such as the breakdown products of hemoglobin, are contained in the stool, most metabolic end products are actually eliminated by the kidneys and lungs.

Structure

The GI tract consists of a tube of varying diameter with the same general structure throughout most of its length. Moving from the outside inward toward the lumen, six concentric layers can be identified in the wall of the intestine (Figure 8.1). The outermost layer is composed of connective tissue. In the esophagus, where the connective layer is continuous with the deep fascia, it is called the adventitia. In all other portions of the gut, the connective tissue layer is covered with peritoneal epithelial cells and is called the serosa. The second and third layers are made up of smooth muscle in which each exhibits a different orientation of its muscle fibers. The muscle fibers of the outer muscle layer run longitudinally along the gut while the inner muscle layer circles the gut. The fourth layer, the submucosa, is composed primarily of connective tissue as well as a few exocrine gland cells, blood vessels, and lymphatics. The fifth

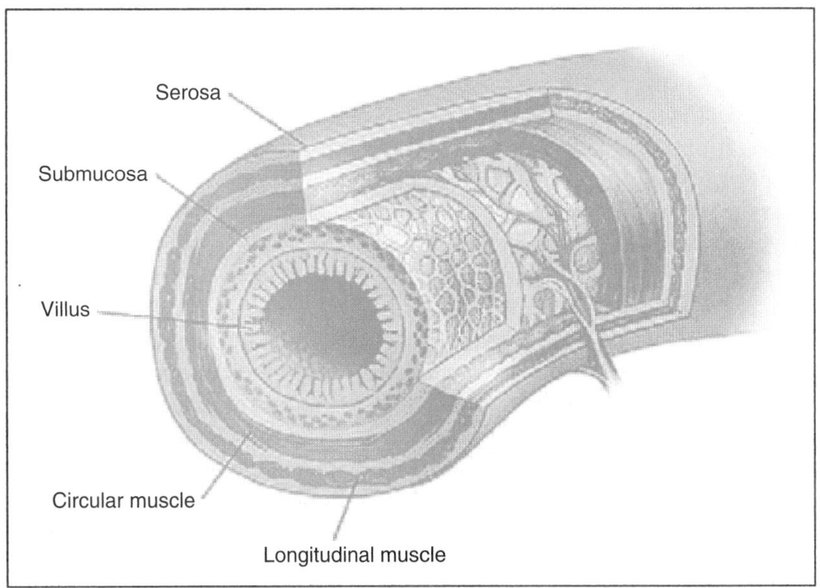

FIGURE 8.1 Anatomy of the intestinal wall.
Adapted from WebMD (2013).

layer is again composed of smooth muscle but is of mixed orientation with both longitudinal and circular fibers. The last layer, which actually lines the lumen of the gut, is known as the mucosa and contains most of the exocrine gland cells as well as epithelial cells. The mucosal surface is highly convoluted in the small intestine, with many ridges and valleys giving it a larger surface area for absorption compared with a smoother surface elsewhere. In addition to these six structural layers, two major nerve plexuses regulating the contraction of the smooth muscle are found in the gut wall. The myenteric plexus lies between the longitudinal and circular layers of muscle and is largely motor in function. The submucosal plexus, as its name implies, is located in the submucosa and is mainly sensory. Synaptic connections between the two nerve networks allow one plexus to stimulate the other and vice versa, leading to activity that is conducted both up and down the length of the gut.

Circulation

After birth, the intestine is a site for intense metabolic activity. Blood flow significantly increases from days 1 to 3, then plateaus until day 12, and declines progressively until day 30. Introduction of feedings causes vasodilation and increased oxygen delivery (postprandial hyperemic response) from capillary to cell to meet increased demand for digestion. Changes in flow are mediated by nitric oxide (NO), a vasodilator, myogenic response, and endothelin (ET-1), which provide vasoconstriction. Infants have altered capacity to respond to systemic circulatory problems such as decreased arterial pressure and hypoxemia (Reber, Nankervis, & Nowicki, 2002).

Motility

Once food enters the esophagus, it is moved along by peristaltic waves initiated by impulses from autonomic nerves, specifically the enteric nervous system (ENS), and coordinated by the swallowing center in the medulla. The ENS is regulated by a series of genes that influence receptor sites, transcription, and translation of neuronal signals (Bates, Dunagan, Welch, Kaul, & Harvey, 2006). As the contractions begin, the gastroesophageal sphincter temporarily relaxes to allow the bolus to enter the stomach. Although this sphincter is anatomically indistinct from the remainder of the esophagus, it normally remains contracted so that the contents of the stomach, which are under relatively higher internal pressure in relation to that experienced in the esophagus, do not reflux.

Peristaltic waves spread across the stomach as it fills with food toward the small intestine. These contractions are no longer mediated by the medulla but by the nerve plexuses and the effect of smooth muscle stretching. The muscle layers of the stomach are thicker in the distal portion (antrum) in comparison with the relatively thin layer surrounding the upper portion (fundus), resulting in the most powerful and intense contractions in the antrum. These strong antral contractions are the primary force acting to break up the gastric contents and mix them with enzymes to form a semifluid mixture called chyme. In addition, they force the chyme past the pyloric sphincter into the duodenum. Although the rate of gastric emptying is normally controlled by the chemical composition and amount of chyme, gastric motility may actually be decreased by stomach distention, increased caloric density, or high loads of carbohydrate, fat, or acid, to provide more time for digestion and absorption in the small intestine. In general, formula empties more slowly than breast milk. Right lateral positioning increases gastric emptying, but is associated with increased occurrence of gastric esophageal reflux (GER) as compared to left lateral positioning (Omari et al., 2004).

The strong stomach contractions become more oscillatory in nature in the small intestine, promoting the digestive and absorptive processes. Pancreatic secretions and bile secreted by the liver into the duodenum, just below the stomach, assist in the process. Muscular activity becomes progressively slower in the small intestine as chyme passes from the duodenum to the jejunum to the ileum, but is sufficient to move the contents slowly downward toward the colon. Distention and luminal injury may cause muscular activity to cease.

Interruption of normal peristaltic activity results in overgrowth of anaerobic bacteria in the small intestines and malabsorption of nutrients. The coordination of peristalsis may not be developed fully until late in the third trimester, around 34 to 35 weeks gestation (Neu & Bernstein, 2002).

The colon functions primarily as a storage area and is structurally different from the small intestine in several major ways. No digestive enzymes are secreted, the lumen is no longer convoluted, and it lacks villi, as only a small amount of the total intestinal content is absorbed here. In addition, the longitudinal smooth muscle layer is incomplete leading to segmental, not propulsive, movements. When the luminal contents enter the colon through the ileocecal sphincter, they are merely concentrated (through the reabsorption of water) until distention of the rectum initiates the defecation reflex and the fecal matter is expelled.

Immunity

The neonatal gut is constantly exposed to bacteria and antigens. Complex immune and nonimmune host defenses are present in the newborn and serve to enhance the neonate's immune response.

Motility, as discussed earlier, is important to decrease time for colonization in the lumen of the gut. The release of gastric acid and pancreaticobiliary secretions inhibits bacterial growth and activates proteolysis, altering antigen structure. Unfed infants have a decreased release of these secretions, which may impair the host defense. The mucus lining of the gut provides a protective physical barrier to larger molecules.

Epithelial cells, goblet cells, M cells, and subepithelial cells provide innate immune defense by retarding cellular penetration of large macromolecules and delivering foreign molecules and microorganisms to lymphoid tissue. T cells, B cells, and macrophages are present in the fetal intestine by 20 weeks gestation, but antigenic stimulation of lymphoid tissue is not demonstrated until 46 weeks (Berseth, 2005a; Burrin & Stoll, 2002; Neu & Bernstein, 2002).

Cytokines are soluble proteins that are important in stimulating chemotaxis of neutrophils, promotion of IgA expression, and epithelial cell proliferation after mucosal injury. Several nutrients (immunonutrients) may play a role in the immune defenses of the neonate, including glutamine, arginine, short-chain fatty acids, long-chain fatty acids, nucleotides, probiotics, and prebiotics. Glutamine helps in maintaining epithelial cell integrity, cell growth, and mounting inflammatory response. Probiotics are live microbes that improve intestinal microbial balance. Prebiotics are nondigestible food ingredients that enhance growth of nonpathogenic organisms. Manipulation of the microenvironment of the newborn intestine may provide a way for improving outcomes (Berseth, 2005a; Burrin & Stoll, 2002; Neu & Bernstein, 2002).

MATURATION OF GI FUNCTION

Anatomic structures of the GI tract are well formed by the second trimester. However, many GI functions are still immature in the term infant at birth as functional maturation occurs later (Berseth, 2005a).

The gross anatomy of the supporting musculature and the functional development of GI motility have not been as well studied as the development of the secretory and absorptive capabilities of the bowel. These supporting structures are relatively thinner in the newborn, especially in the premature newborn, than in the adult. The muscular layers of the stomach are somewhat deficient, with the longitudinal muscle layer being especially thin over the greater curvature. Similarly, the musculature of the intestine is also relatively thin, constituting approximately 50% of the bowel wall in the newborn, as compared with approximately 60% in the adult.

Under normal circumstances little propulsive peristaltic muscle activity appears to occur until late in gestation, and this activity is still irregular and slowed at term gestation in comparison to the adult. The presence of lanugo and squamous cells in meconium, however, indicates that at least some movement of materials from swallowed amniotic fluid occurs. Measurable duodenal contractions have been demonstrated by indwelling intraluminal manometry in the infant born as early as the 26th week of gestation, although they occur infrequently (mean of 1.9 contractions per minute) and are relatively weak (mean of 6.3 mmHg at peak pressure). Between 29 and 32 weeks of gestation, motility spontaneously and significantly improves, with contractions occurring at an average rate of 6.5 per minute and an average force of 17.1 mmHg. The timing of this narrow maturational window does not appear to be affected by postnatal age, type of enteral feed given (breast milk vs. formula), or mode of feeding (instillation by orogastric vs. transpyloric tube) (Morriss, Moore, Weisbrodt, & West, 1986). Evidence does point to a somewhat enhanced maturation in infants who receive early enteral feedings with volumes as small as 10 to 20 mL/kg/d for 4 to 7 days (Schanler, 2005). Use of diluted formula for these early feedings is controversial because the onset, strength, and duration of motor activity appear to be inversely related to the concentration of formula. Manometric studies indicate that the routine use of diluted formula (even one-third strength) may not provide an optimal stimulus for gut motility (Koenig, Amarnath, Hench, & Berseth, 1995). Antenatal corticosteroid treatment to initiate production of pulmonary surfactant does appear to promote gut maturation, but maturation appears to be delayed in infants affected with significant central nervous system insult or abnormality such as asphyxia and hydrocephalus. After 32 weeks gestation, duodenal function steadily improves and by term has a contraction frequency similar to but less than the fasting adults (10 vs. 11 contractions per minute). Furthermore, the number of contractions that occur in a burst or rapid sequence is often fewer than that measured in adults.

The motor mechanism of the colon also appears to be affected by maturation and illness. Although virtually all healthy, full-term newborns (99.8%) and a majority of preterm infants pass meconium within 48 hours of delivery, the first passage of stool can be delayed in premature infants without underlying GI disease. Infants weighing less than 1,250 g at birth had a median age of 43 hours for first passage of meconium, although the 75th percentile was 10 days. Low-birth-weight infants who are ill, especially those with severe respiratory distress syndrome, in whom enteral feedings are consequently delayed, may experience further delay (Baldassarre et al., 2010; Meetze et al., 1993).

Bacterial Colonization

After birth, bacteria are introduced to the GI tract through feedings and invasive procedures. The once sterile gut rapidly changes, depending on the timing and type of feeding. Lactobacillus is passed to the infant through breast milk and assists with lactose reduction. Secretory IgA and bactericidal enzymes are also passed on to breastfed infants, thus affecting the bacterial growth in the gut. Aerobic organisms appear within a few hours and anaerobic organisms by 24 hours. The organisms are important in metabolizing bile acids, nonabsorbed proteins, lipids, and carbohydrates (Berseth, 2005a). The colonization is disrupted by the introduction of medications that change the normal flora, especially antibiotics. Profound intestinal dysfunction can occur when the gut flora is altered (Neu & Walker, 2011).

Delayed Transit

The relatively deficient supporting musculature and immature motor mechanisms of the newborn, particularly the premature newborn, results in irregular peristaltic activity that occurs in disorganized patterns. This infrequent and irregular activity increases the tendency toward distention in the ill or premature infant, thus increasing the likelihood of delayed transit and stooling. Complete and thorough assessment of the GI tract therefore becomes essential to distinguish the expected physiologic deficiencies of the newborn from pathologic causes of dysfunction.

ASSESSMENT OF THE GI TRACT

History

Assessment of the newborn infant ideally begins during the prenatal period as each infant has a history dating to the time of conception. Consequently, historical antecedents to birth may serve as an indicator of increased likelihood of dysfunction of a specific organ system such as the GI tract. Although most cases of isolated abdominal and GI defects occur sporadically, some (such as cleft lip or palate, or both, and pyloric stenosis) may exhibit familial recurrence patterns, thus suggesting at least some degree of genetic influence mediated by environmental factors. Therefore, any initial history should include questioning parents to identify siblings and/or other family members with a history of genetic or congenital anomaly. Major syndromes that have frequently associated GI anomalies are listed in Table 8.1.

Although a certain degree of risk may be established through genetic screening, the best evidence of fetal GI anomalies is obtained through prenatal ultrasonography. The fetal abdomen can be identified as early as 10 weeks from the last menstrual period, and the stomach can be visualized at 13 weeks gestation. The transient herniation of the intestine into the umbilical cord has even been documented by ultrasonography. However, because the fetus is still undergoing embryogenesis at this time, first-trimester diagnosis of defects, particularly small ones, is exceptionally difficult. It is generally not until the second and third trimesters, when the GI structures are established, that reliable visualization becomes possible. Ultrasound at that point would include a survey of the abdominal wall, insertion of the umbilical cord, visualization of the fluid-filled stomach, and a search for bowel dilation or abnormal echolucencies resembling cysts that might indicate collection of fluid within the bowel secondary to obstruction. Prenatal echogenic bowel has been associated with cystic

TABLE 8.1

MAJOR SYNDROMES ASSOCIATED WITH GASTROINTESTINAL DYSFUNCTION

Syndrome	Gastrointestinal Component
Apert	Narrow palate with or without cleft
	Palate or bifid uvula
	Pyloric stenosis
	Ectopic anus
Beckwith–Weidemann	Omphalocele
Fetal hydantoin	Cleft lip and palate
	Pyloric stenosis
	Duodenal atresia
	Anal atresia
Meckel–Gruber	Cleft palate with or without cleft lip
	Bile duct proliferation, fibrosis, cysts
	Omphalocele
	Malrotation
	Imperforate anus
Sirenomelia (mermaid syndrome)	Imperforate anus
	Esophageal atresia with
	Tracheoesophageal fistula
Trisomy 13	Cleft lip with or without cleft palate
	Omphalocele
	Malrotation
Trisomy 18	Cleft lip with or without cleft palate
	Pyloric stenosis
	Biliary atresia
	Omphalocele
	Malrotation
	Imperforate anus
Trisomy 21	Short palate
	Tracheoesophageal fistula
	Duodenal atresia
	VATER association
	Imperforate anus with or without fistula
	Anular pancreas
	Hirschsprung disease

Adapted from Jones (2006).

fibrosis, chromosomal abnormalities, congenital infections, uteroplacental insufficiency, meconium peritonitis, and various causes of intestinal obstruction (Cass & Wesson, 2002). Abnormal facial features such as clefting may be identified if examination is targeted for that area and fetal position allows. The presence of polyhydramnios may provide an additional clue to defects high in the GI tract. In utero the fetus normally swallows, absorbs, and metabolizes amniotic fluid. Polyhydramnios results when the fetus is unable to swallow effectively because of a GI obstruction.

Postnatally, three cardinal signs point to the possibility of GI obstruction, whether structural or functional: (1) persistent vomiting, especially if it is bile stained; (2) abdominal distention; and (3) failure to pass meconium within the first 48 hours after birth in the term infant.

Vomiting, as differentiated from reflux, indicates an attempt by an irritated or overdistended bowel to rid itself of its contents. Although vomiting may be initiated by distention or irritative stimuli at any point along the length of the gut, the stomach and duodenum appear to be the most sensitive to these stimuli. Consequently, vomiting is most often considered an indicator of defects high in the GI tract. The presence of bile further indicates that the point of obstruction is distal to the ampulla of Vater, where bile is emptied from the common bile duct into the duodenum. Conversely, nonbilious vomiting would be noted if obstruction were proximal to the ampulla. Because the mechanism for vomiting requires expulsion of the offending contents up through the esophagus, a patent esophagus is required for true vomiting to occur.

Abdominal distention related to obstruction occurs when large amounts of swallowed air and fluid collect in the bowel and cannot pass through the gut. Abdominal distention worsens as digestive fluids and electrolytes continue to be secreted and proteins are lost from the circulation into the intestinal lumen leading to a progressively edematous bowel. The stomach is shielded by the rib cage; therefore distention is generally observed when obstruction occurs in the lower small intestine or colon.

Most normal full-term infants pass their first stool by 48 hours of age. Failure to pass meconium within the first 2 days of life therefore generally indicates obstruction of the large intestine, unless such delay can be attributed to an oversedated, debilitated, or premature infant.

Physical Assessment

A systematic approach to assessment of the newborn GI tract includes inspection, auscultation, and palpation. Percussion is unreliable and difficult to perform in the infant because the internal abdominal organs are small and close together. Consequently, the examiner tends to rely on radiography and other diagnostic procedures instead of percussion.

■ **Inspection.** Inspection is a fundamental part of the assessment as many GI defects are grossly apparent. The mouth is observed for its position, shape, size, and symmetry, and the lips, palate, and uvula are evaluated for clefts. Although complete separation of the lip extending up into the nasal area is obvious, close attention must also be paid for any niche in the lip that might easily be overlooked. Abundant oral secretions or saliva provide an early clue to esophageal atresia (EA), particularly when a history of polyhydramnios has been reported.

The abdomen is next inspected for contour, symmetry, and integrity. Distention of the abdomen, which is normally slightly rounded, serves as a hallmark of obstruction. Although the decreased muscle tone in a premature infant may allow visualization of peristalsis, such movement is not normally observed, and when noted in the presence of vomiting or distention, suggests the possibility of obstruction. The character of the umbilical cord and site of insertion are checked. Although most cases of omphalocele are obvious, an abnormal thickness to the stump or cord itself should raise suspicion of a single herniated loop of intestine. Any such enlargement must be differentiated from a Wharton's jelly cyst or umbilical hernia through the lax rectus muscles. The anus is examined for position, and the perineal area is inspected for fistulas. The muscle tone of the anal sphincter can be determined by stroking the anal area with a gloved finger and observing for the contraction "wink" that normally occurs around the anal opening. If clinically indicated, the examiner can assess for anal patency by digital examination using the gloved little finger. Insertion of a rectal thermometer presents the risk of perforating the rectum and should not be performed for assessment purposes.

■ **Auscultation.** Although initially absent, bowel sounds generally become audible within the first 15 to 30 minutes of life as the bowel fills with swallowed air and peristaltic activity is activated by the parasympathetic nervous system. Normally these sounds should be of a metallic tinkling quality and occur approximately two to five times per minute. Sounds may be hyperactive, absent, or even normal in the case of neonatal obstruction. The presence and intensity of bowel sounds must be interpreted in relation to other pertinent historical and clinical findings. Hyperdynamic sounds in a recently fed infant with a benign history and otherwise insignificant examination should be considered normal. Hyperdynamic bowel sounds found in an infant with concurrent findings of distention and vomiting should be concerning. More often than not, however, the abdomen is misleadingly silent.

■ **Palpation.** Abdominal palpation is best performed with the infant quiet in a supine position, preferably during the first 24 hours of life, when the abdominal musculature is lax. Holding the infant's knees and hips in a flexed position also helps to relax the abdominal musculature. The liver, spleen, and kidneys should be felt with a warm hand using the pads of the fingers applying slow, gentle pressure. Care to perform abdominal palpation in as gentle a manner as possible cannot be overemphasized. The multiple maneuvers involved are often distressing to the newborn, and the pressure applied even during a routine examination may result in significant, although transient, elevations in both systolic and diastolic blood pressures.

The liver is found by placing the index finger just above and to the right of the groin and slowly advancing upward until the edge of the liver can be felt beneath the pad of the finger. Normally the organ is firm, but not hard, with a sharp edge that extends 1 to 2 cm below the right costal margin and can be followed across the abdomen into the left upper quadrant. The spleen is found on the left side in a similar manner, but generally only the tip of the organ is felt at the left costal margin, although it may be entirely unpalpable. The kidneys are located in the flank areas above the level of the umbilicus and are normally 4.5 to 5 cm in length in the term infant. Palpation may be performed bimanually (with one hand supporting and stabilizing the flank posteriorly while the thumb or a finger of the free hand is moved anteriorly over the same area), or a single hand may be used (with the fingers of the hand supporting the flank posteriorly while the free thumb of the same hand explores the flank anteriorly). Although the overlying liver may obscure the upper position of the right kidney, the entire left kidney should be felt easily. The remainder of the abdominal examination consists of a gentle search for pathologic masses. Although most masses found are of renal origin, it may be possible to detect stool-filled bowel, particularly in the case of meconium ileus.

Related Findings

Prenatal ultrasonography and direct postnatal visualization of external defects are diagnostic of GI anomalies. In the absence of these obvious signs, a history of maternal polyhydramnios, vomiting, distention, and failure to pass stool are most indicative of GI dysfunction. Other relatively subtle and nonspecific signs may also be noted.

Respiratory difficulty may arise as the result of an inability to handle the abundant oral secretions commonly found in EA or may develop as a result of aspiration of gastric contents by way of an associated tracheoesophageal fistula (TEF). Abdominal distention may also decrease ventilation by impeding diaphragmatic excursions. Frank airway obstruction may even occur in the case of cleft palate, if the negative inspiratory pressure pulls the tongue into the hypopharynx.

Jaundice may occur if the excretion of bilirubin is hampered. In the case of biliary atresia, the conjugated bilirubin, which is a normal component of bile, is unable to pass into the duodenum for excretion in the stool. In cases of intestinal atresias, meconium ileus, and Hirschsprung disease, the enterohepatic circulation becomes exaggerated as stasis of the luminal contents promotes intestinal reabsorption of the bilirubin that is present. Systemic hypertension may be an additional, though rare, subtle sign. This increase in blood pressure may be appreciated in situations in which masses or distention significantly increases intra-abdominal pressure.

Risk Factors

Maternal, neonatal, and other risk factors associated with GI dysfunction are discussed in the sections outlining the management of specific problems.

Once the family history has been obtained, it may be clear that a genetic history is important. Some GI disorders are related to chromosomal and single-gene defects, or as part of multisystem syndromes (see Table 8.1). For example, omphalocele, duodenal atresia, and stenosis have a high association with trisomy disorders. At least 95% of cases of meconium ileus occur in infants with cystic fibrosis (Merenstein & Gardner, 2006). A family history of cystic fibrosis may or may not exist, as it is inherited as an autosomal recessive disease. Pyloric stenosis has an 87% inheritance rate (Krogh et al., 2010). Genetic consultation is suggested for infants with these disorders to provide additional counseling to parents regarding the risk of recurrence. Chromosomal studies should be performed if additional physical findings associated with GI anomaly are found.

Diagnostic Procedures

■ **Radiologic Examination.** Air in the GI tract serves as a naturally occurring contrast medium that makes radiologic evaluation of the abdomen a useful tool in the diagnosis of obstruction. At birth, the gut is fluid-filled, but as the infant swallows air after delivery, the radiolucent gas may be followed radiographically as it passes through the bowel. Within the first 30 minutes of life, air should be present in the stomach. By 3 to 4 hours, gas should be seen in the small bowel. After 6 to 8 hours, the entire gut including the colon and rectum should be filled with air. This normal progression of gas through the GI tract cannot occur if obstruction is present and the intestine distal to the obstruction is generally airless. Nevertheless, air continues to be swallowed so that the alimentary tract that lies proximal to the obstruction can become quite distended and is demonstrated on radiograph by often-dramatic radiolucent (black) bubbles. Flat and upright radiographic studies of the chest and abdomen may suffice for identifying esophageal or intestinal atresias. Cross-table lateral radiographs may be helpful by identifying air in the rectum of infants suspected of having intestinal obstruction. A left lateral decubitus film may determine the presence of free air in the peritoneal cavity.

An upper GI series is often used to diagnose GER, pyloric stenosis, and malrotation. Contrast material, such as barium or Gastrograffin, is swallowed or administered by nasogastric tube and observed by fluoroscopy as it passes through the digestive tract. Gastrograffin, meglumine diatrizoate, is preferred if perforation is suspected because it is a water-soluble solution (Kee, 2001). The procedure may last 30 minutes to 4 hours, depending on the rate of small intestine motility. The patient is usually placed on a nothing by mouth status 4 to 6 hours before the examination but may continue feedings after the examination.

Contrast enema is used for examination of the large intestine after barium or Gastrograffin is instilled through the rectum. It may be diagnostic in cases of malrotation, suspected Hirschsprung disease, meconium ileus, and meconium plug syndrome. The procedure should be performed prior to any planned upper GI examination because contrast material from the upper GI tract may take several days to clear. No special preparation is necessary before the study. Gentle saline enemas may be helpful in clearing barium and trapped air after the contrast procedure. If barium is allowed to harden and form concretions that become impacted, more aggressive procedures may be required for evacuation.

■ **Ultrasonography.** Ultrasonography may be diagnostic in cases of pyloric stenosis, enteric duplication, or biliary atresia if the intrahepatic or proximal extrahepatic tracts are dilated. Conducting gel is placed on the abdomen, and the transducer is placed against the gel on the abdomen. The computer transforms reflected sound waves from tissues into scans, graphs, or audible sound (Kee, 2001).

■ **Gastric Aspirate.** A gastric aspirate may be obtained to measure the pH of the gastric contents. A premeasured feeding tube is passed into the stomach. At least 1 mL of gastric contents is gently aspirated into a syringe, and the feeding tube is withdrawn. The syringe is capped, labeled, and sent for testing.

■ **Apt Test.** The Apt test may be used to determine the origin of blood in vomitus or stool by differentiating neonatal GI blood loss from swallowed maternal blood. Bloody aspirate or bloody stool is centrifuged in 5 mL water. One part 0.25% sodium hydroxide is added to five parts supernatant. The fluid remains pink in the presence of fetal blood but turns brown in the presence of maternal blood.

■ **Stool Culture.** A stool culture may differentiate between an intestinal lining insult and an infection as the cause of bloody diarrhea. A stool sample is taken from a diaper, placed in a specimen container, labeled, and sent for testing.

■ **Stool Hematest.** A stool Hematest is a rapid and convenient method for detection of fecal occult blood which is a possible indication of GI disease. The test is based on the oxidation of guaiac by hydrogen peroxide, thus resulting in a blue compound. A thin smear of stool is placed on guaiac paper. Developer is applied over the smear. Results are read in 60 seconds. Any blue colorization on or at the edge of the smear indicates a positive occult blood result. Fecal samples need not be tested if hematuria or obvious rectal bleeding is present. Drugs that influence positive results include iron preparations, indomethacin, potassium preparations, salicylates, and steroids. Large amounts of ascorbic acid may cause a false-negative result (Kee, 2001).

■ **Stool-Reducing Substances.** Carbohydrate intolerance is detected by the presence of reducing substances in the stool. A stool sample is placed in a specimen container and sent for testing. If the stool is watery, the liquid portion of stool, which can be collected in a diaper, is aspirated into a syringe. A 1 to 2 ratio of stool to water is obtained. Fifteen drops of this supernatant are placed in a clean test tube, and a Clinitest (test for urinary glucose) tablet is added. After 15 seconds, the test tube is shaken gently, and the color of the liquid is compared with the color chart provided with the Clinitest tablets. More than 0.5% glucose in the stool indicates an abnormal amount of sugar.

■ **pH Probe Test.** The 24-hour pH probe test is considered the gold standard for the diagnosis of GER. A thin, flexible, pH-sensitive electrode is placed into the distal esophagus. The study is scored by determining the amount of time the esophagus is exposed to an acidic pH level, which is usually less than 4 minutes. Scoring for abnormal results is based on frequency of reflux, number of episodes greater than 4 minutes duration, time of longest episode, and the percentage of time in reflux. A dual sensor may be used, which places an electrode in the distal esophagus and another in the pharyngeal area of the esophagus.

The use of formula feedings may obscure episodes of reflux by buffering the gastric acid. Many clinicians use acidic feedings, such as apple juice, to better estimate the true amount of gastric reflux in the esophagus. Interpretation of the data is complex due to confounding factors such as position, activity, frequency and composition of feeding, and medication. Nursing responsibilities include recording the time of feedings and describing the activity level of the infant throughout the test.

■ **Scintigraphy.** Gastroesophageal scintigraphy, by feeding radionucleotide-tagged formula to the infant, may be used to measure gastric emptying, aspiration with swallowing, and reflux with aspiration. A technetium radioisotope is used because it has relatively low radiation and is easily added to formula.

■ **Endoscopy.** Flexible endoscopy with biopsy of the distal esophagus is used to diagnose esophagitis. Biopsy findings suggestive of esophagitis include basal cell hyperplasia, increased stromal papillary length, and demonstration of intraepithelial eosinophils.

■ **Fecal Fat.** A fecal fat test may be helpful to screen for malabsorption. Fecal fat content of greater than 6 g/24 hr is predictive of malabsorption syndrome. A very small stool sample can cause false test results.

COLLABORATIVE MANAGEMENT

General Principles

To decrease the likelihood of a poor outcome, early recognition accompanied by medical or surgical intervention is necessary for infants with GI obstructions or alterations. General nursing care considerations in management of GI system alterations include GI decompression, fluid and electrolyte balance, thermoregulation, positioning, prevention of infection, nutrition, and pain management.

Gastric Decompression

Gastric decompression is extremely important to prevent aspiration, respiratory compromise, or gastric perforation. If the intestinal obstruction is not relieved, abdominal distention may become severe and the upward pressure on the diaphragm may compromise respirations. Connection of an orogastric or nasogastric tube to low intermittent suction minimizes the risk of aspiration and prevents distention from swallowed air. Tube patency is essential if gastric decompression is to be maintained. An 8 or 10 French red rubber Robinson tube or a 10 French soft vinyl, double-lumen gastric sump tube provides sufficient decompression for most infants. Irrigating the tube every 2 to 4 hours with 2 mL air helps ensure that the tube remains open and functioning.

Fluid and Electrolytes

Large amounts of extracellular fluid pass into and out of the GI tract as part of the normal digestive process. Intestinal obstruction causes the fluids that are normally reabsorbed by the intestine to become trapped. Additionally, infants with obstruction often experience "third-spacing," with a shift of fluid from the vascular bed into the interstitial compartment. This third-spacing is also referred to as capillary leak syndrome. If severe, this loss of intravascular volume can result in relative hypovolemia and hypoperfusion with all their attendant risks. Furthermore, vomiting, diarrhea, and gastric suction can cause excessive volume depletion and electrolyte abnormalities, especially losses of sodium, potassium, and chloride.

The goal of collaborative management is to maintain fluid and electrolyte balance. Maintenance fluids are usually run at 60 to 80 mL/kg for the first 24 hours of life and are increased by 10 mL/kg/d or as needed to 120 to 160 mL/kg/d (Zenk et al., 2003). A rate should be maintained at which urine output is at least 1 to 2 mL/kg/hr, and a specific gravity of 1.005 to 1.012 is sustained. Sodium is provided at a rate of 2 to 3 mEq/kg/d and potassium at 2 mEq/kg/d, as serum electrolytes indicate.

For the infant who is receiving gastric suction, the amount of gastric loss is determined by measuring drainage every 4 to 8 hours. The total volume of gastric output should be replaced every 4 to 8 hours with one half normal saline with potassium chloride 10 to 20 mEq/L. The replacement fluids are given in addition to maintenance fluids. Fluid volume deficit and electrolyte imbalances may occur if replacement therapy is inadequate. The adequacy for fluid replacement is assessed by changes in vital signs, amount of urinary output, urine specific gravity, levels of electrolytes, blood urea nitrogen, and hematocrit values.

Metabolic alkalosis may occur with pyloric stenosis or high jejunal obstruction because of loss of acidic gastric juice. In obstructions in the distal segment of the small intestine, larger quantities of alkaline fluids than acidic fluids may be lost, thus resulting in metabolic acidosis. If the obstruction is below the proximal colon, acid–base balance may be maintained because most of the GI fluids are absorbed before reaching the obstruction. Respiratory acidosis may develop in patients with abdominal distention because of carbon dioxide retention from hypoventilation.

Thermoregulation

Thermoregulation is vital in the care of all newborns and becomes more critical for the stressed neonate. Cold stress dramatically increases oxygen requirements and predisposes the infant to hypoglycemia, hypoxia, and metabolic acidosis. An appropriate heat source and monitoring must be ensured for any infant with GI dysfunction. Gastroschisis and omphalocele in particular cause profound heat loss from exposed bowel. Preoperative nursing intervention includes provision of an external heat source and head covering, hourly monitoring of temperature, and in the case of exposed bowel, use of warm saline soaks over the defect, with a bowel bag or plastic wrap from the feet to the axilla.

Positioning

Head-up positioning accomplishes two management goals in the infant with GI dysfunction. In suspected GER, a 30° prone position or left lateral position has been shown to be the most effective position to decrease reflux. For the infant with tracheal esophageal fistula, elevating the head of the bed 30° to 40° helps to avoid reflux of gastric contents into the trachea via a distal fistula. In the case of an isolated EA, a flat or head-down position may assist gravity drainage from an overflowing esophageal pouch.

Prevention of Infection

Newborn infants are uniquely at risk for infections acquired prenatally, intrapartally, and postnatally. Infants who require specialized care as the result of medical or surgical problems have an increased susceptibility for infection. Broad-spectrum antibiotics are administered immediately in presumed neonatal infections. Many institutions administer antibiotics preoperatively to prevent infection.

Pain Management

Infants with GI disorders are at high risk for pain preoperatively and postoperatively. It is important to assess the infant's risk for pain and constantly monitor the infant's physiologic and behavioral cues to pain. Both nonpharmacologic and pharmacologic therapies are used in pain management. Containment and positioning strategies are utilized as well as a quiet and dimly lit environment. Opioids, particularly morphine and fentanyl, are the most commonly used agents for analgesia.

Postoperatively, it may be useful to implement analgesia every 2 to 4 hours around the clock in anticipation of expected pain. Pain levels must be assessed and reassessed at regular intervals. Pain scores, intervention, and responses are critical to evaluate for effective relief.

Nutrition

Meeting the caloric and metabolic needs postoperatively in the infant with GI dysfunction is challenging. Enteral feedings are often delayed after surgery of the alimentary tract, necessitating the use of hyperalimentation to supply metabolic needs. Peripherally inserted central catheters or surgically placed central catheters are needed in order to manage the nutritional needs of most infants with GI disorders. When the infant is ready to begin enteral feedings, clear liquids are begun and may progress to elemental feedings such as Pregestimil (protein hydrolysate formula). Bowel loss or severity of the defect influences the infant's tolerance to feedings. Small, frequent, or continuous-drip feedings, initially supplemented with intravenous hyperalimentation, are gradually advanced. Advancement of feeding should be stopped if signs of intolerance, such as diarrhea, vomiting, abdominal distention, or presence of reducing substances in stool appear (Zenk et al., 2003).

GENERAL PREOPERATIVE MANAGEMENT

Surgery presents an additional stress that the baby with GI dysfunction is often ill-equipped to tolerate. The principles of preoperative management revolve around the prevention or minimization of identified stressors. Replacement of fluid losses, decompressing the distended bowel, and supporting failing organ systems by means of assisted ventilation, radiant heating, parenteral nutrition, and pain management should be implemented as needed. Appropriate fluid and electrolyte balance is challenging due to third-space losses in the infant with bowel obstruction or necrotizing enterocolitis (NEC). The third-space fluid losses are isotonic and have an electrolyte composition like that of serum. Fluid losses from the GI tract due to vomiting or nasogastric suction additionally contribute to negative fluid balance and electrolyte depletion. Gastric fluid losses need to be replaced at full volume using one-half normal saline with potassium chloride at 10 to 20 mEq/L. Careful monitoring of the clinical status, which includes the heart rate, blood pressure, perfusion, capillary refill, and urine output, helps guide the rate of fluid replacement. Laboratory monitoring for potential abnormalities is essential.

Antibiotics should be started early in the neonate with bowel dysfunction, until the etiology is clear. Antibiotic regimens usually include combining a penicillin and an aminoglycoside, such as ampicillin and gentamicin. Clindamycin or metronidazole may be added to cover anaerobic infection, especially in the presence of bowel perforation.

GENERAL POSTOPERATIVE MANAGEMENT

Hydration, maintenance of electrolyte balance, gastric decompression, fluid loss replacement, and pain management are continued postoperatively, along with respiratory and other therapy that the individual case warrants. Most patients will have extraneous tubes or devices such as gastrostomy tubes, chest tubes, or drains as well as incision sites. Meticulous care is needed to maintain skin integrity. Skin must be kept dry as much as possible. When tape or adhesive has been placed directly on the skin, gentle and careful removal is mandatory. Pectin-based skin barriers can be used to protect the skin from tape. If enteral feedings are expected to be delayed beyond 3 to 5 days, total parenteral nutrition should be instituted to prevent excessive catabolism. Feedings are generally started when bowel sounds are present, stools are passed normally, and the gastric drainage clears and lessens in amount.

Ostomy Care

Infants with ostomies require special management. The primary diagnoses leading to fecal diversion in infants are NEC, imperforate anus, and Hirschsprung disease. A colostomy/ileostomy/jejunostomy is formed surgically by opening part of the bowel to the outside of the abdomen for the evacuation of feces. It may be temporary or permanent, depending on the indication for surgery. The opening is called a stoma, which is made from the innermost lining of the intestine. Stomas are insensate (no sensory nerves) and incontinent (no sphincter control) and usually shrink for the first 6 to 8 weeks after surgery. If there is more than one stoma, the proximal stoma is the functioning one and any distal stomas are called mucous fistulas. If two stomas are close, they may both be pouched together. If not, the distal stomas can be covered with dry gauze.

The primary goal in ostomy care is to keep stool off of the skin. The area around the stoma is washed with warm water, rinsed well, and dried. Soap is not used because it may irritate the skin. The skin and stomas are observed for swelling, change in color, or bleeding. Pouching of the stomas is necessary when drainage begins, usually 1 to 2 days postoperatively. A pattern is drawn for the pectin-based skin-barrier wafer and pouch, to be used for further pouch changes. The opening of the pouch is cut out so that it fits up close to the stoma with no peristomal skin exposed to stool. If the hole is cut too large, stool will leak out and irritate skin or cause the wafer to lose its seal. If the pattern size is too small, the pouch's wafer will sit on the wet stoma, and the pouch will not stick. The hole in the wafer should not be more than one-eighth inch larger than the stoma, and the hole in the pouch should be about one quarter inch larger than the hole in the wafer. The wafer is applied to the skin, and the pouch is applied to the top of the wafer. The bottom of the pouch is folded and tied with a rubber band. The length of time that the pouch stays adhered depends on how active the baby is, how liquid the stool is, and how "budded" the stoma is. Usually an infant pouch will stay on 2 to 4 days. To improve the pouch's seal, the peristomal skin needs to be dry before applying the pouch, and the pouch needs to be held in place for 5 minutes after applying. The bag is emptied as needed, usually when it is a third to half full. If it gets too full, it may break the seal of the wafer and cause the pouch to come off.

Complications

Complications are inherent in postoperative surgical patients and may include infection, respiratory distress, fluid and electrolyte imbalances, third spacing of fluids, oliguria, pain management issues, skin breakdown around surgical sites and tubes, and intestinal obstruction related to adhesions, strictures, or volvulus.

Short-bowel syndrome (SBS) is an unfortunate complication of many neonatal surgeries that involve extensive resection of the GI tract. The loss of considerable absorptive surface results in a complex malabsorptive problem with episodic diarrhea, steatorrhea, and dehydration, which, if allowed to progress, may cause metabolic derangements and ultimately poor growth and development.

Peritonitis, chemical or bacterial, is a concerning complication of infants with GI disorders, with a mortality rate of 33% to 80%. Meconium peritonitis can result from intestinal perforation related to meconium ileus, intussusception, volvulus, incarcerated internal hernia, imperforate anus, and meconium plugs (Berseth, 2005b). Infectious peritonitis is usually caused by mixed anaerobic and aerobic organisms associated with NEC, appendicitis, biliary tract disease, rupture of visceral abscess, or infection of indwelling foreign objects. Candida is also associated with approximately 10% of cases of peritonitis, seen primarily in extremely premature infants, extended use of umbilical arterial catheters, prolonged intubation, or prolonged use of antibiotics (Berseth, 2005b). Treatment includes surgical drainage and administration of antibiotics or antifungal agents.

CONSIDERATION OF ETHICAL ISSUES

Congenital malformations often have associated organ defects. When another defect or organ system dysfunction represents a major threat to life, decisions regarding the timing of surgical intervention must be made. For example, repair of a serious heart lesion may precede repair of EA, but the resection of necrotic bowel must precede both conditions. Such scheduling decisions are made difficult when it is recognized that some conditions may be improved only at the expense of others. Even when surgical correction of GI dysfunction can be achieved successfully, in the face of multiple malformations (which may not be equally amenable to operative treatment or may result in early demise), the appropriateness of intervention must be evaluated. Each affected newborn deserves individual consideration. The wishes of the parents and the opinion of each member of the management team must be considered.

MANAGEMENT OF PROBLEMS WITH INGESTION

Cleft Lip and Palate

■ Anatomy. In general, cleft lip is the term that signifies a congenital fissure in the upper lip, whereas cleft palate indicates a congenital fissure in either the soft palate alone or in both the hard and soft palates. The two conditions may occur in isolation or together. Isolated cleft lip may be either unilateral or bilateral and range in severity from a slight notch in the lip to a complete cleft into the nostril. Isolated cleft palate may also be unilateral or bilateral and as mild as a submucous cleft characterized by a notch at the posterior edge of the hard palate, an imperfect muscle union across the palate, a thin mucosal surface, and a bifid uvula. In this mild form, the diagnosis may never be made. Combined clefts of the lip and palate are the most severe form of the defect, particularly if they are bilateral.

■ Pathophysiology. Although cleft lip and palate are often associated, these defects are embryologically distinct disorders. Cleft lip occurs when the maxillary process fails to merge with the medial nasal elevation on one or both sides. Cleft palate occurs when the lateral palatine processes fail to meet and fuse with each other, the primary palate, or the nasal septum. When both cleft lip and palate occur together, the failure of the secondary palate to close may be a developmental consequence of the abnormalities in the primary palate associated with the cleft lip, rather than an intrinsic defect in the secondary palate. It is possible that isolated cleft lip and cleft lip with an associated cleft palate represent varying degrees of the same embryologic defect.

Rates of cleft lip with or without an associated cleft palate have been reported to be 1/700 in different populations, depending on geographic location, ethnic group, and socioeconomic conditions (Vieira, 2008). The defects appear in both syndromic and nonsyndromic forms. Rates are higher in males than in females and in Asians than in Whites. Isolated cleft palate has a lower incidence rate, occurring more frequently in females, and has no clear racial variation. Approximately 70% of infants with unilateral cleft lip and 85% of infants with a bilateral cleft lip will also have a cleft palate (Merritt, 2005a). These defects are usually isolated, but 10% of infants with cleft lip and cleft palate will have an associated syndrome. When a parent has cleft lip/palate, there is a 3% to 5% risk of having an affected child. Recurrence rate for parents with one affected child rises to 40% for another affected child (Merritt, 2005a). No single gene has been identified to explain clefts, but various mutations of at least 14 genes have been associated. MSX1 mutations are found in 2% of cases of clefting and would warrant genetic counseling in families with dental anomalies associated with clefting phenotypes (Jezewski et al., 2003). In addition, IRF6, FGF, and PVRL1 genes have also been associated (Teitelbaum, 2008; Vieira, 2008). Although genetic factors are often involved, environmental factors also appear to contribute in some way, indicating a multifactorial mode of inheritance.

Maternal medications during the first trimester, especially benzodiazepines, phenytoin, opiates, penicillin, salicylates, cortisone, and high doses of vitamin A, have been associated with clefting. Occurrence of fever and influenza during the first trimester has also been demonstrated as a potential cause. However, it is questionable if this is attributed to the viral agent or the therapeutic drugs. Threatened abortion in the first and second trimesters and premature delivery of neonates with clefts have also been reported, but it is uncertain whether this indicates an unfavorable intrauterine environment or simply a symptom of an already malformed fetus (e.g., Pierre Robin syndrome or sequence). An association between clefting and variables such as maternal smoking, maternal alcohol use, maternal diabetes, hypovitaminosis, and hypervitaminosis, especially vitamin A, has also been supported (Spritz, 2001). There appears to be a one third reduction in risk of orofacial clefts in mothers taking folic acid (Wilcox et al., 2007).

Clearly, cleft lip, cleft palate, or both can have multiple causes and may represent a malformation, a disruption, or a deformation. When the defect is the result of an inherently abnormal developmental process, as in the case of genetic derangement, it is appropriately called a malformation. Pits within the lower lip that lead to a cleft associated with Van der Woude syndrome, an autosomal dominant condition; holoprosencephaly associated with a median cleft lip; and Smith–Lemli–Opitz syndrome, a condition that has deviations along the palatal ridges and can result in a cleft palate, are examples. When the developmental process is originally normal but goes awry because of extrinsic factors, as in the case of teratogenic exposure, it is called a disruption. Deformation results when mechanical forces interfere with normal development, as in the case of Pierre Robin syndrome or sequence in which mandibular hypoplasia causes the tongue to be posteriorly displaced, thus interfering with the fusion of the lateral palatine shelves.

■ Treatment. Effective management of an individual born with a cleft defect requires the services of a multidisciplinary team including pediatrician, plastic surgeon, audiologist, speech pathologist, dental specialist, geneticist, social worker, and nursing personnel at various levels.

Emotional preparation of the parents is frequently the most immediate and demanding nursing problem encountered. The birth of a defective child comes as both a shock and a disappointment to the parents. Information and reassurance are desperately needed at this critical time. Nurses can also provide a role model to influence the parents' attitude toward the child positively and to provide guidance and support as the family copes with the reactions of others. "About Face USA" (http://www.aboutfaceUSA.org) is an organization that provides information, emotional support, and educational programs to patients and families experiencing facial differences.

Understanding the etiology of the defect is assisted through the familial history, antenatal exposure to potential teratogens, chromosomal analysis, and thorough systematic physical exam (Merritt, 2005b).

Surgical repair is a priority not only to achieve closure of the defect but also to minimize maxillary growth retardation, to limit dental deformity, and to allow normal speech development. If the infant is healthy and no complications are expected, a cleft lip can be repaired at about 3 months of age. Repair of an associated cleft palate is generally postponed until a later time to allow medial movement of the palatal shelves, which appears to be initiated by lip closure. Depending on the involvement, palate closure may occur as a two-step process, with the hard palate being corrected at 14 to 16 months of age, followed by soft palate repair by 18 months of age. The timing of repair is controversial, and some surgeons perform the correction in the neonatal period. If additional repair of the lip or nose is required for aesthetic purposes, it is postponed until sufficient structural growth has been achieved, generally after 12 years of age (Teitelbaum, 2008).

Feeding is another important aspect in the care of an infant with cleft lip or palate and requires a great deal of patience and attention to technique. Infants with cleft palates may find it difficult to hold the nipple in their mouth and be unable to create the vacuum necessary for adequate sucking. The bottle should be held securely and the cheeks grasped so that the cleft is pushed closed. Frequent burping should be performed as large amounts of air may still be swallowed. These infants also benefit from an upright or semi-upright position to avoid choking, and the flow of milk should be directed to the side of the mouth. Use of a "preemie" nipple or a special cleft palate nipple and squeeze bottle may also be helpful. Frequent, small feedings help in preventing fatigue and frustration. Although easier to use than rigid bottles, there is no evidence supporting improved growth outcomes of infants fed with a squeeze bottle (Bessell et al., 2011). Breastfeeding is certainly possible, although considerable creativity may be required. A pillow placed between the infant's back and the mother's arm can maintain the infant in an upright position. Because the cleft areas easily become encrusted with milk and are therefore prone to excoriation and infection, a small amount of sterile water should be offered after each feeding. Some craniofacial centers design a prosthetic device to occlude the cleft. This device made of hard or soft plastic and molded to the shape of the infant's mouth is thought to help in feeding and speech development until repair is possible. The device is removed and rinsed with water after each feeding (Merritt, 2005b).

The major condition that requires differential diagnosis is Van der Woude syndrome, which is inherited as an autosomal dominant trait. This syndrome ranges in appearance from a single, barely visible lower lip depression to frank pits or fistulas usually occurring in pairs on the vermilion of the lower lips, with clefting of the lip with or without palate involvement (Merritt, 2005a).

Although an excellent prognosis for survival can be expected, an individual born with a cleft defect is faced with more than just a cosmetic problem. Language and speech tend to be delayed in affected individuals. This retardation is further compounded by a higher incidence of hearing impairment. Olfactory defects have also been demonstrated in people with cleft palate; however, males seem more affected than females. Dental problems, such as malocclusion, irregularity of the teeth, and increased frequency of caries, may also be encountered in affected individuals. Although the majority of cases of cleft lip, cleft palate or both are not associated with any recognizable syndrome there are more than 300 syndromes that include cleft lip or palate, or both, as a feature (Merritt, 2005a). Associated anomalies might not be recognized initially but diagnosed by the first year of life (Rittler et al., 2011). The prognosis in such cases varies with the associated anomalies involved.

Esophageal Atresia/TEF

■ Anatomy. EA is defined as a complete interruption in the continuity of the esophagus. TEF is a congenital fistulous connection of the proximal and/or distal esophagus and the airway. They can exist as separate congenital anomalies, but most patients will have both EA and TEF.

■ Pathophysiology. EA and TEF occur when the trachea fails to differentiate and separate from the esophagus. The atresia is most likely the result of either a spontaneous posterior deviation of the esophagotracheal septum or some mechanical force that pushes the dorsal wall of the foregut in an anterior direction. A fistula occurs when the lateral ridges of the septum fail to close completely in their normal zipper-like fashion so that a communication is left between the foregut and the primitive respiratory tree.

The infant with EA may appear well at birth, but oral secretions and saliva collect in the upper esophageal pouch and appear in the mouth and around the lips because effective swallowing is not possible. Secretions are more visible due to inability to swallow rather than increased production. Respiratory difficulties may be encountered when the secretions and mucus fill the esophageal pouch and overflow into the upper airway or leak into the trachea through a proximal fistula. Any attempts at feeding are generally accompanied by coughing, choking, and cyanosis. If a distal fistula is present, crying may force air into the stomach, where it collects and causes progressive distention. This gastric distention may impede diaphragmatic excursion, thus leading to worsening respiratory status or a reflux of gastric contents back up through the fistula into the trachea. If there is no distal fistula, the abdomen is more likely to appear scaphoid secondary to the lack of swallowed air. True vomiting is not possible (except in the case of an isolated TEF) because the esophagus and stomach are not connected. Maternal polyhydramnios in combination with excessive secretions, reflux, and respiratory distress are highly suggestive of EA and require investigation. The clinical presentation may vary slightly, depending on the specific type of anomaly found (Figure 8.2). There are five major pathologic types of EA with or without TEF; however, approximately 100 subtypes have been described.

EA with or without TEF occurs approximately once in every 2,400 to 4,500 live births (Cass & Wesson, 2002; Kovesi & Rubin, 2004). Isolated TEF occurs 5% in the absence of EA. Symptoms include coughing, cyanosis, choking with feedings, and recurring pneumonia. Although rare cases of familial occurrence have been reported, most cases represent an accident of embryology. A history of maternal polyhydramnios is reported in 14% to 90% of cases of EA. The higher rates are found with isolated EA; the lower rates are found when a fistula allows passage of swallowed amniotic fluid around the obstruction. Associated malformations are present in 30% to 70% of infants. Congenital heart disease is reported most frequently (25%–40%), with ventricular and atrial septal defects being the most common lesions. Other associated anomalies include vertebral malformations (13%), atresias of the small intestine (5%), imperforate anus (10%–20%), and genitourinary anomalies (10%–24%). Congenital lung anomalies such as pulmonary and lobar agenesis, horseshoe lung, and pulmonary hypoplasia have been reported in infants with EA/TEF (Kovesi & Rubin, 2004).

Approximately 25% present as part of the VATER association. This acronym represents a complex of V, vertebral and ventricular septal defects; A, anal atresia; tracheoesophageal (TE), TEF with E, EA; and RR, radial and renal anomalies (Spoon, 2003). Some experts describe the same cluster of symptoms but use the VACTERL association. The C stands for congenital heart defects, and the L is for limb deformities. Overall, 20% to 30% of these infants are premature or small for gestational age, but in isolated EA, the incidence of prematurity approaches 50%. EA/TEF has also been associated in patients with DiGeorge syndrome, Down syndrome, Pierre Robin syndrome, and CHARGE association (Jones, 2006).

■ **Treatment.** Diagnosis of EA is confirmed by attempting to pass a radiopaque catheter from the nares through the esophagus into the stomach. If the esophagus is atretic, the catheter cannot be advanced further than a depth of approximately 9 to 12 cm before meeting resistance, and any contents that are aspirated are alkaline rather than acidic. A chest radiograph shows the tube ending or coiling in the upper esophageal pouch. Air in the bowel indicates the presence of a distal TEF. If the abdomen is airless, no such fistula is present. Contrast studies are generally contraindicated owing to the danger of aspiration but may become necessary in the diagnosis of an isolated or H-type TEF. In these cases, which are more difficult to diagnose, bronchoscopy or endoscopy may be required to allow direct visualization of the fistulous site.

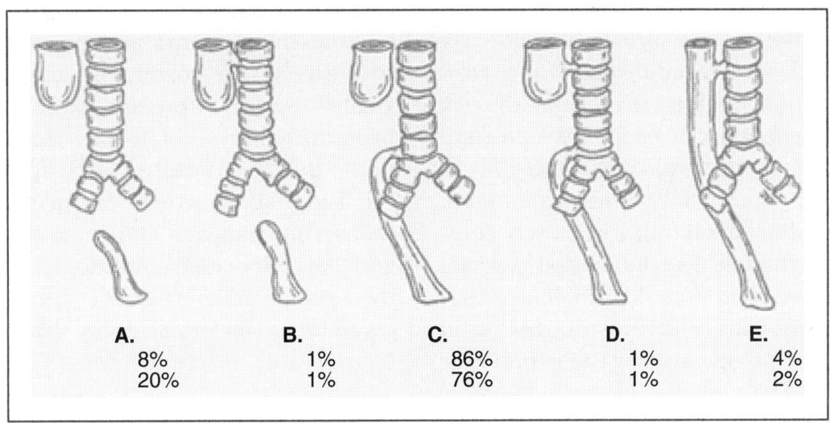

FIGURE 8.2 Diagram of the main types of EA with or without a tracheoesophageal fistula (TEF). Type A is EA without a TEF and is often called pure EA. Shown are the blind upper and lower esophageal pouches next to the ringed windpipe (trachea) and the branches (bronchi) which lead to each lung. Type B has a connection (fistula) between the upper pouch and the trachea (a TEF). Type C is by far the most common form of EA and has a fistula between the lower esophagus and the trachea (one form of TEF) with a blind upper pouch. A rare form (1%) is type D with two TEFs, one between both the upper and lower esophageal segments and the trachea. Type E has only a TEF and no EA. This is usually referred to as an H- or N-shaped fistula and may be 2% to 4% of this group. The H-fistulas are divided surgically, and nothing further needs to be done to the esophagus, which is intact and reaches normally to the stomach.

Surgical correction involves esophageal anastomosis (esophagoesophagostomy) and obliteration of any fistula that is present. The procedure may be done thoracically or laparoscopically. Generally, repair is performed through an incision at the base of the neck, but if the lesion is exceptionally low within the chest, a thoracic approach may be used, thus necessitating chest tube placement. The exact technique varies with the type of defect present, but if a great distance separates the two ends of the esophagus, the repair is more difficult and must often be staged. In this case, the ends may be brought into closer approximation either preoperatively by stretching the upper esophageal pouch daily with a bougie to produce progressive elongation or intraoperatively by performing multiple circular myotomies so that the upper esophageal segment can be lengthened in a telescoping fashion. Alternatively, a combination of the two methods may be used. If these procedures are ineffective or if the gap is particularly large, a segment of the small or large intestine or an inverted tube of gastric tissue may be used for esophageal replacement. Such an involved procedure is generally delayed until 1 year of age. If primary repair of the gap is impossible, the upper esophageal pouch can be brought to the surface as a cervical esophagostomy ("spit fistula") to allow the drainage of saliva, with gastrostomy performed for feeding. In these protracted cases, sham feeding may be attempted. Orally fed milk is collected with saliva in the ostomy bag attached to the esophagostomy stoma and refed through the gastrostomy tube into the stomach.

Preoperative care is focused primarily on the reduction of symptoms. To prevent overflow of secretions, a sump catheter (Replogle tube) is placed in the upper esophageal pouch and connected to low continuous suction. The tube lumen becomes easily occluded by tenacious secretions and should therefore be changed daily. Periodic catheter irrigations are usually required to maintain patency. If the secretions are particularly thick, humidified air may assist in liquefying them for easier removal. Elevating the head 30° to 40° helps avoid reflux of gastric secretions into the trachea via a distal fistula. Comfort measures to prevent crying reduce the amount of air swallowed through the fistula, thus limiting gastric distention and further reducing the risk of reflux. If no TEF is present, a flat or head-down position may be preferable to avoid gravity drainage of saliva from an overflowing esophageal pouch. Intravenous fluids are used for hydration. Electrolytes are monitored closely. Supplemental oxygen and intubation may be needed if respiratory distress occurs. However, use of positive-pressure ventilation increases the propensity for gastric distention and may even necessitate preoperative gastrostomy for decompression.

Boston Children's Hospital uses the Foker process for surgical treatment. This technique was developed by Dr. John Foker. It involves use of traction sutures placed at each end of the esophagus. Each day these sutures are tightened to bring the two distant esophageal ends together. This traction is done until the two ends are adjacent in close enough proximity to suture them together. For the long gaps this will take time, but the process has been used successfully and fosters the move to solid foods more rapidly than most other procedures. For more information and a demonstration of this technique, please see http://www.childrenshospital.org/clinicalservices/Site2807/mainpageS2807P0.html?_vsignck&_vsrefdom=EAT.

Postoperatively, vital signs are monitored closely, and assessment of the anastomotic site for leaks should be done frequently. If a chest tube has been placed, such leakage presents as persistent or increased drainage. The endotracheal tube is generally left in place for at least 24 hours to allow full recovery from anesthesia and relaxants. For suctioning of the airway, the catheter should be well marked and inserted to a predetermined depth above the surgical site to avoid disruption or trauma. The quantity and appearance of secretions and any respiratory difficulties are reported. Oral feeds are generally withheld for 5 to 10 days to ensure healing, but gastrostomy feeds may be started within 48 hours. Gastroesophageal reflux occurs in 40% to 70% of infants because of the upward pull on the lower esophageal pouch and stomach and generally poor peristalsis. Management of GER will be discussed in the next section. Other postoperative complications that are frequently seen arising over time include anastomotic leak (17%), stricture of the anastomosis (40%–50%), recurrence of the fistula (5%–12%), and abnormal esophageal peristalsis (75%–100%) (Berseth & Poenaru, 2005c; Kovesi & Rubin, 2004).

With early diagnosis and efforts to prevent aspiration pneumonia, most full-term infants do well, with a survival rate of 97%. However, mortality dramatically increases when prematurity or associated major anomalies coexist. When birth weight is less than 1,500 g or major cardiac disease is present, survival is approximately 85%. Morbidity and mortality rates depend on coexisting conditions such as syndromes or associations. In premature infants with coexisting conditions, mortality is about 50% (Kovesi & Rubin, 2004; Teitelbaum, 2008). Support and communication are the cornerstones of parental care throughout hospitalization. Encouraging mothers to hold their infants and providing skin-to-skin (kangaroo care) help foster the maternal–child relationship. Centers such as Boston Children's Hospital now have programs that specialize in the treatment of this condition. Boston Children's Hospital's program is called the Esophageal Atresia Treatment (EAT) Program that focuses on patients and their families with EA and TEF and the associated conditions. For more information on this program, please see http://www.childrenshospital.org/clinicalservices/Site2807/mainpageS2807P0.html?_vsignck&_vsrefdom=EAT.

Gastroesophageal Reflux

■ **Anatomy.** Gastroesophageal reflux (GER) is the effortless retrograde passage of acidic gastric contents from the stomach into the esophagus. The term *chalasia* refers to an abnormal relaxation of the gastroesophageal junction. Infants are at greater risk for GER because of altered esophageal motility and peristalsis; lower esophageal sphincter (LES) position and immaturity; limited gastric volume; delayed gastric emptying; and impaired intestinal motility.

In adults, the upper portion of the esophagus lies in the thorax, the middle section at the diaphragm, and the lower segment in the abdomen. This segment of terminal esophagus has a higher pressure than that of the stomach below or the esophagus above and helps prevent retrograde flow of gastric contents into the esophagus. LES tone normally increases in response to abdominal pressure, thus protecting against reflux. In infants, this protective mechanism is less effective because the LES is primarily above the diaphragm and subjected to intrathoracic pressure. An immature LES in the preterm infant may not allow effective pressure to be generated and may cause inappropriate relaxation of the muscle. LES pressure remains low for the initial 2 weeks of life and increases markedly between 2 and 4 weeks. By 18 to 24 months, the esophagus has grown such that the LES is below the diaphragm. Conditions delaying or altering the maturation of this valve may cause reflux of stomach contents. In addition, the angle from the esophagus to stomach (the angle of His) is obtuse in infants, allowing stomach contents to more easily reflux. This angle lessens with growth, providing a natural barrier to reflux.

■ **Pathophysiology.** Approximately 50% to 70% of healthy infants between the ages of birth and 6 months may have symptomatic reflux. Regurgitation peaks at 3 months of age and usually resolves by 6 to 12 months of age (Rudolph & Hassall, 2008). The resting LES pressure at birth is 2 to 3 mmHg and increases to adult levels on average by 2 months of age (Barksdale, Chwals, Magnuson, & Parry, 2011). Medical intervention is often not warranted, but parents will need support and reassurance to cope with the frustrations. Symptomatic GER has been reported in 3% to 10% of very-low-birth-weight infants (VLBW < 1,500 g). GER in infants that interferes with growth or results in respiratory impairment is termed gastroesophageal reflux disease.

GER may be asymptomatic, present with nonspecific symptoms such as inconsolability, irritability, sleep disturbance, food refusal, and failure to thrive, or present with more obvious symptoms of postprandial regurgitation or vomiting. It has also been implicated in the pathogenesis of apnea, hoarse cry, stridor, reactive airway disease, recurrent bronchopulmonary infections, bronchopulmonary dysplasia (BPD), chronic lung disease, and ventilator dependence. Persistent vomiting due to GER often leads to failure to thrive. Such infants tend to be pale, thin, hypoactive, listless, and underweight and may be misdiagnosed with a nutritional deficiency. The most commonly recognized pulmonary symptom associated with GER is recurrent aspiration pneumonia, characterized by fever, cough, poor appetite, and typical findings on radiography.

Apneic spells, most commonly seen in the early weeks of life, may be caused by reflux. Gastroesophageal reflux is capable of causing laryngospasm, with cardiac slowing or arrest. Acid in the esophagus can lead to apnea or bronchospasm with wheezing or stridor. Worsening of chronic lung disease or BPD has also been associated with GER. Near sudden infant death syndrome episodes have been linked with GER, although the association is unclear. Well-documented recurrent apneic spells have been completely eliminated in many cases after antireflux surgery. Asthma or asthma-like symptoms related to reflux are rare during the first year of life but have been seen occasionally in infants. Although generally not seen in the early months of life, infants who suffer from esophagitis caused by GER are usually fussy, irritable, and colicky. Frank bleeding is rare but may be present with anemia and guaiac-positive stools.

Healthy premature infants often demonstrate behavior that in symptomatic older infants is associated with acid reflux but in the preterm infant is not reflux. Reflux-specific behavior such as irritability, crying, or grimacing established in older term infants may be inappropriate as diagnostic criteria for GER in preterm infants and may lead to unnecessary use of antireflux medications.

Infants with high bowel obstructions have delayed maturation of the valve mechanism and are at risk for chalasia resulting from structural weakness. Most infants with congenital diaphragmatic hernia experience reflux after repair likely caused by deviation of the esophagus to the affected side, malposition of the stomach, increased intra-abdominal pressure, gastric dysmotility, or a combination of these factors. Additionally, infants who have undergone operative repair of TEF or EA have extremely high incidence of GER, as do infants with congenital abdominal wall defects. A high percentage of infants with neurologic damage exhibit GER, possibly due to reduced swallowing frequency and weaker esophageal sphincter control. Some medications such as diazepam, calcium-channel blockers, theophylline, caffeine, and anticholinergics may worsen GER (Jadcherla, 2002; Khalaf, Porat, Brodsky, & Bhandari, 2001).

■ **Treatment.** Most infants can be safely treated medically for 3 months before it may be judged that conservative therapy has failed. Seventy-five percent recover when treated medically, 10% to 15% require prolonged medical management, and 10% to 15% require surgery. When symptoms are controlled by medical means, reflux ceases by 15 months of age and therapy can be discontinued. Surgical long-term results are good, with a positive result reported 76% to 91% of the time as assessed at check-ups after 10 years or more (Salminen, Hurme, & Ovaska, 2012). Adverse side effects, including mild gas bloating, slow eating, and nability to burp or vomit, are seen in approximately one third of surgically treated patients.

Careful history and clinical evaluation are needed to rule out other diseases that present with emesis. Included in the differential diagnosis are distal outlet obstruction as in pyloric stenosis or antral web; volvulus; intussusception; meconium ileus/plug; Hirschsprung disease; sepsis; abnormalities of amino acid metabolism, such as urea cycle defects; galactosemia; congenital adrenal hyperplasia; increased intracranial pressure; NEC; gastroenteritis; formula intolerance; pancreatitis; cholecystitis; pyelonephritis; hydronephrosis; rumination; and drug toxicity.

A barium swallow is a poor test for diagnosing GER, but is useful to confirm normal esophageal, gastric, and intestinal anatomy. The 24-hour pH probe test is considered the gold standard for the diagnosis of GER. This may be misleading in premature infants as the majority of reflux episodes are nonacidic in nature. The study is scored by determining the amount of time the esophagus is exposed to an acid pH level. Scoring for abnormal results is based on frequency of reflux, number of episodes greater than 4 minutes in duration, time of longest episode, and percentage of time in reflux. Interpretation of the data is complex because of confounding factors such as position; activity; frequency and composition of feeding; and medication. Nursing responsibilities include recording the time of feedings and describing the activity level of the infant throughout the test. Newer techniques combine pH probe studies with electrical esophageal electric impedance monitoring, also known as multichannel intraesophageal impedance but are not clinically useful at present secondary to the cost and technical expertise needed to perform and interpret this test. Technetium scintigraphy may be used to measure gastric emptying, aspiration with swallowing, and reflux with aspiration. A technetium radioisotope is used because it has relatively low radiation and is easily added to formula. Flexible endoscopy with biopsy of the distal esophagus is used to diagnose esophagitis. Laryngoscopy and bronchoscopy can be helpful in assessing vocal cord erosion or inflammation or identifying milk-laden macrophages (Rudolph & Hassall, 2008).

A multidisciplinary approach in the assessment of the infant with GER and its related problems is important in the diagnostic process. The history, physical examination, and results of the upper gastroesophgeal (GE) series or pH probe testing confirm or deny the diagnosis. A clinical distinction must be made as to whether the GER is physiologic or pathologic based on the infant's ability to thrive. In the face of pathologic GER, nursing and medical collaboration is necessary to assess the effectiveness of conservative treatment modalities. These methods include positioning, thickening of feedings, monitoring for apnea, pharmacologic management, and parental support.

Prone or left lateral positioning after feedings has been shown to decrease GER episodes (Corvaglia et al., 2007). Infants placed in infant seats have 50% more reflux episodes that last twice as long as those that occur in the prone position. Slouching increases pressure on the stomach and the risk of reflux. When infants are positioned in infant seats or car seats, their trunks must be supported to minimize abdominal compression. Kangaroo care has been anecdotally reported to help as infants are held in a prone elevated position. Positioning the infant at a 45° to 60° angle during feedings has been shown to reduce reflux.

Thickened feedings with one tablespoon of rice cereal added to 1 to 2 ounces of formula may reduce vomiting and crying and increase sleep time after feedings for some infants. Thickened feedings have not been shown to reduce reflux during concurrent pH probe studies unless the infants were also in an elevated prone position. For some infants, thickened feedings increase the length of reflux episodes, thus causing increased coughing and pulmonary complications.

Apneic episodes and recurrent aspiration pneumonia have been associated with GER. Infants suspected of and documented as having clinically significant reflux should therefore undergo continuous respiratory monitoring especially when xanthines are used to treat the apnea. Although xanthines are used to improve respiratory function and reduce apnea, they also increase gastric acid secretion and decrease LES pressure, which may further increase GER (Zenk et al., 2003).

Histamine-2 antagonists (famotidine or ranitidine) are used to reduce acidity and associated esophageal pain and damage from acid reflux. Omeprazole, pantoprazole, lansoprazole, and rabeprazole are proton pump antagonists, blocking acid production. They have been used in infants with severe esophagitis who do not respond to other agents. Several studies have questioned the practice of acid reduction, as an association with NEC and late-onset sepsis has been shown (Bianconi et al., 2007; Gulliet et al., 2006; Orenstein, Hassall, Furmaga-Jablonska, Atkinson, & Raanan, 2009). Antacids such as aluminum hydroxide and magnesium hydroxide are rarely used due to side effects of constipation and diarrhea (Bell, 2003). The pharmacologic mainstay of treatment for GER has been the prokinetic drug metoclopramide, a dopamine receptor antagonist, which decreases gastric emptying time and enhances LES pressure. It has a narrow therapeutic range with onset of 30 to 34 minutes. Extrapyramidal side effects sometimes include restlessness, lethargy, and abnormal posturing. Less commonly seen side effects include nausea, vomiting, and diarrhea. A systematic review of the literature, however, states that the evidence is insufficient to support the use of metoclopramide in infants (Hibbs & Lorch, 2006). Erythromycin, a macrolide antibiotic, with prokinetic effects is used rarely to treat GER in the infant because of cardiac and GI side effects (Malcolm & Cotten, 2012). Cisapride, a prokinetic agent that enhances gastric motility, was widely used in the 1980s and 1990s to manage GER in infants. Concern about its use in preterm infants due to prolonged QT intervals on electrocardiographs prompted warning from the Food and Drug Administration and the subsequent discontinuance of use.

If medical management fails to control life-threatening complications, surgical intervention is indicated. Although many procedures have been devised, the Nissen fundoplication is most widely used in the neonate. In this procedure, the proximal stomach is wrapped around the distal esophagus, creating a junction that is effective in preventing reflux. Laparoscopic techniques have been successful in even the smallest of infants. Complication rates are comparable, and there appears to be less mortality, less postoperative sepsis, and shorter hospital stay (Rhee et al., 2011). Infants may have a temporary gastrostomy placed to vent swallowed air and decrease bloating. The tube is usually removed after 3 to 6 weeks. Rate of revision of the fundoplication has been reported to be 5% to 19%; the highest failure occurs in infants with associated anomalies such as TEF, lung abnormalities, congenital diaphragmatic hernia (CDH), and neurologic disorders (Kubiak, Spitz, Kiely, Drake, & Pierro, 1999). Parental support is essential in nursing management of the infant with GER. The nurse can help parents to identify feeding, positioning, and soothing techniques. Parents need to learn the etiology and course of GER as well as interventions, including medication administration. Parents can also be referred to local support groups or Pediatric and Adolescent Gastroesophageal Reflux (PAGER) at http://www.reflux.org, for additional information and support.

Pyloric Stenosis

■ Anatomy. Although many cases of pyloric stenosis may be acquired postnatally, this disorder is properly referred to as congenital hypertrophic pyloric stenosis. The pathologic picture consists of marked hypertrophy of the pylorus with spasm of the muscular coat, creating a tumor-like nodule, resulting in a partial gastric outlet obstruction.

■ Pathophysiology. The infant typically appears healthy for the first 2 weeks of life and then begins nonbilious vomiting, which worsens to frequent projectile vomiting. The infant may be anxious, irritable, excessively hungry, have decreased frequency of stool, and lose weight. Vomiting may cause dehydration, metabolic alkalosis, hypochloremia, and hypokalemia. The level of indirect bilirubin can be significantly elevated in affected infants but resolves when stenosis is corrected.

The cause is poorly understood but is influenced not only by genetic factors but also environmental factors. The prevalence rate typically ranges from 1 to 2 per 1,000, with higher rates in Whites than in Blacks. More males have the disease than do females with a 4 to 1 increase. Associated factors include maternal stress and anxiety, sleep position, feeding practices, and antenatal exposure to thalidomide, hydantoins, and trimethadione (Krogh et al., 2010; Rannells, Carver, & Kirby, 2011).

■ Treatment. Medical and nursing assessment of the infant is critical throughout the process of management. Diagnosis of pyloric stenosis may be made by palpation of the hypertrophied pylorus, an olive-like mass in the deep right upper quadrant of the abdomen. Most surgeons are not comfortable with palpatory findings alone and request confirmatory ultrasound before surgical intervention (Berseth & Poenaru, 2005c).

There is no effective medical treatment, although the use of atropine has been reported. The treatment of choice is repair by pyloromyotomy. A simple incision is made in the hypertrophied longitudinal and circular muscles of the pylorus, thus releasing the obstruction. Laparoscopic pyloromyotomy, introduced in 1991, is an alternative, leaving essentially no scar, and may reduce postoperative pain and the duration of gastric ileus (Harmon, 2011, Rannells et al., 2011).

Preoperatively, fluid and electrolyte management is paramount. A nasogastric tube connected to low intermittent suction is maintained to prevent distention and vomiting and to decrease the risk of aspiration. Thermoregulation is maintained to prevent exacerbation of symptoms. Infants with severe dehydration and electrolyte imbalances should be corrected prior to surgery.

Postoperatively, intravenous hydration and electrolyte balance must be maintained. Nasogastric suction is continued for 4 to 24 hours. The tube may be removed when the infant is fully awake and bowel sounds are present. Assessment of the suture line is made for signs of infection or skin breakdown. Feedings are begun 4 to 24 hours after surgery when the baby is fully awake.

Once diagnosed and surgically treated, the prognosis for pyloric stenosis is excellent, with complete relief of symptoms. The mortality rate is low, provided that the infant has not become too dehydrated and malnourished.

MANAGEMENT OF PROBLEMS WITH DIGESTION

Biliary Atresia

■ Anatomy. Biliary atresia is the complete obstruction of bile flow due to fibrosis of the extrahepatic ducts. Infants appear normal at birth and pass stools with appropriate pigmentation. Clinical signs are subtle, with jaundice persisting after the first week of life. The direct bilirubin level slowly increases and results in a greenish bronze appearance of the skin. Gradually stools become yellowish tan to pale clay-colored, and the urine becomes dark as the result of bile excretion. Over a 2- to 3-month period, the liver becomes cirrhotic. Portal hypertension is a major complication. The reverse blood flow results in enlargement of esophageal, umbilical, and rectal veins, manifested as splenomegaly, hemorrhoids, enlarged abdominal veins, ascites, and blood in the stools. Additional complications include decreased clotting ability, anemia, and ineffective metabolism of nutrients. End-stage liver disease may lead to rupture of veins in the esophagus and stomach or hepatic coma with eventual death from liver failure.

■ Pathophysiology. Biliary atresia is the most common form of ductal cholestasis and occurs in approximately 1 in every 15,000 births, with a female predominance. Biliary atresia is categorized into three types depending on the level of obstruction. Type 1 obstruction is at the common bile duct, type 2 at the common hepatic duct, and type 3, the most prevalent, is seen at the porta hepatis (Hartley, Davenport, & Kelly, 2009). Pathologically, the obstruction of the common bile duct prevents bile from entering the duodenum. Obstruction leads to bile accumulation in the ducts and gallbladder and causes distention of these structures. Consequently, digestion and absorption of fat are impaired, thus leading to deficiencies in fat-soluble vitamins, especially vitamin K, which affects bleeding tendencies. The atresia appears to progress to the intrahepatic ducts, leading to biliary cirrhosis and ultimately death if the bile flow is not established.

Etiology remains unclear. Some clinicians theorize that the obstruction is due to injured bile ducts leading to atresia, others describe an inflammatory process, whereas still others propose an intrauterine insult from environmental factors or failure of ducts to recanalize. Regardless of the mechanism, most clinicians agree that the cause is multifactorial combining genetic and environmental factors.

Associated congenital defects, found in 15% of reported cases, include congenital heart disease, polysplenic syndrome, small bowel atresia, bronchobiliary atresia, and trisomies 17 and 18. Teratogenic factors include ionizing radiation, drugs, ischemic episode, and viruses such as reovirus type 3, cytomegalovirus, rubella, and hepatitis A and B (Hartley et al., 2009).

■ Treatment. Medical, surgical, and nursing staff must work together to facilitate a timely diagnosis and ultimate treatment. Multiple causes of cholestasis in the infant exist and must be considered in the presence of conjugated hyperbilirubinemia. The differential diagnosis includes neonatal hepatitis, choledochal cyst, errors of metabolism, trisomies 18 and 21, α_1-antitrypsin deficiency, neonatal hypopituitarism, cystic fibrosis, TORCH infectious agents, bacterial sepsis, drug-induced cholestasis, and cholestasis associated with parenteral nutrition. Nurses take an active role in the complex task of diagnosis and treatment of the infant with biliary atresia. Risk of portal hypertension and bleeding tendencies require careful monitoring of vital signs and blood pressure. Collection of multiple blood samples is required for tests, including liver function tests, α_1-antitrypsin, gamma-glutamyltransferase, cholesterol determinations, prothrombin time, complete blood count, reticulocyte count, Coombs' test, measurement of platelets, red blood cell morphologic features, thyroxine, thyroid-stimulating hormone, glucose determinations, cultures, and TORCH titers. Urine is collected for urinalysis, culture, and metabolic screens. Radiography, ultrasonography, liver biopsy, and radioisotope excretion hepatobiliary scan can be done to aid in diagnosis. The last is used to determine adequacy of the liver function. If diagnosis is still unclear, an endoscopic retrograde cholangiopancreatography may be necessary. Magnetic resonance imaging can also be done, but interpretation is difficult secondary to technical limitations (Hartley et al., 2009).

Surgical intervention involves a hepatic portoenterostomy, the Kasai procedure, which consists of dissection and resection of the extrahepatic bile duct. The porta hepatis, where the ducts normally occur, is cut and a loop of bowel is brought up to permit bile drainage from the liver surface to the GI tract. If the Kasai procedure is unsuccessful, the only alternative for treatment is transplantation.

Survival in untreated cases of biliary atresia is less than 2 years. Approximately 20% of patients with a Kasai portoenterostomy will survive more than 20 years without liver transplantation (Sokol et al., 2007). One third of the patients drain bile but develop complications of cirrhosis and require liver transplantation before the age of 10. The remaining third of patients have bile flow that is inadequate after the Kasai procedure and develop fibrosis and cirrhosis. The overall survival rate after the Kasai procedure and transplantation is greater than 90% (Pakarinen & Rintala, 2011). Sequential surgical treatment of Kasai portoenterostomy in infancy followed by selective liver transplantation for children with progressive hepatic deterioration yields improved overall survival. Limited donor availability and increased complications after liver transplantation in infants less than 1 year of age support the use of a Kasai procedure as the primary treatment of biliary atresia.

Predictors of poor outcome after portoenterostomy include operative age greater than 2 months of age, presence of cirrhosis at first biopsy, total nonpatency of extrahepatic ducts, absence of bile ducts at transected liver hilus, and subsequent development of varices or ascites.

Affects on metabolism make it difficult to meet nutritional requirements. The infant needs one and one-half to two times the normal caloric requirements, yet ascites and pressure on the stomach make it difficult for the child to eat. Formulas must contain medium-chain triglycerides for easier absorption. Supplementation with fat-soluble vitamins is required because of impaired absorption. Parenteral nutrition is often given to provide adequate calories. Phenobarbital, Actigall, and cholestyramine may be an ongoing therapy to stimulate bile flow. Vitamin K may be given for coagulopathy. Consultation and follow-up care by a gastroenterologist provide guidance for feeding and drug therapy modalities.

The entire family requires comprehensive psychosocial support. Family and work life is disrupted by lengthy, repeated hospitalizations. The emotional and physical toll is high because of complex care demands and dealing with the suffering of the child. Social support systems need to be explored to assist families in coping with the long-term health crisis of an infant with biliary atresia. Parents of these infants can benefit from social services, chaplains, or support counseling sources.

Duodenal Atresia

■ Anatomy. Approximately half of all atresias occur in the duodenum (Barksdale et al., 2011). Although atresias may be located at any point along the duodenum, most obstructions (80%–90%) are situated below the ampulla of Vater (Kimura & Loening-Baucke, 2000). Consequently, bilious vomiting is a common presenting sign, and failure to pass meconium is noted in approximately 70% of patients. Both the onset of vomiting and the ability to pass stool are related to the site of obstruction. Proximal duodenal obstructions tend to present with vomiting within a few hours of birth, although stool may be passed normally. Distal obstructions tend to present with a later onset of vomiting and failure to pass stool. Abdominal distention, generally not noted, when present is confined to the upper abdomen, resulting in an almost scaphoid appearance of the lower abdomen in contrast.

■ Pathophysiology. Duodenal atresia occurs as the result of incomplete recanalization of the intestinal lumen. The mechanism by which recanalization is prevented is not known but most likely occurs when the proliferative villi adhere abnormally to one another. The result is the formation of a transverse diaphragm of tissue that completely obstructs the lumen. Polyhydramnios has been identified as a significant risk factor that occurs in one quarter to one half of women who deliver affected infants. Overall occurrence is approximately 1 in every 5,000 to 10,000 live births with a male predominance. Over one quarter of these cases are related to Trisomy 21 (Kimura & Loening-Baucke, 2000; Mustafawi & Hassan, 2008). Associated anomalies, present in 60% to 70% of patients, are numerous and include trisomy 21, malrotation, TE anomalies, imperforate anus, congenital heart disease, VATER or VACTERL association, and renal anomalies. An annular pancreas resulting from the failure of the two pancreatic buds to fuse normally, allowing the deformed pancreas to encircle the duodenum, is rare but can cause duodenal obstruction. Patients with annular pancreas tend to be more premature (Barksdale et al., 2011; Escobar et al., 2004).

■ Treatment. Radiographic examination provides confirmation of duodenal atresia with the classic finding of a "double bubble." These bubbles reflect the localization of swallowed air in the stomach and in the distended portion of the duodenum lying above the obstruction with the remainder of the bowel totally gasless. If gas is present elsewhere, other anomalies causing partial obstruction must be presumed. An upper GI series may be helpful in identifying incomplete obstructions such as duodenal stenosis, duodenal web, or annular pancreas or in ruling out associated malrotation.

Surgical treatment involves excision of the atretic site (unless the area so closely approximates the pancreatic and bile ducts that injury to these structures is risked) and side-to-side anastomosis of the free ends. Duodenoduodenostomy is the procedure of choice, but the level of the obstruction determines whether a duodenojejunostomy needs to be performed instead (Escobar et al., 2004). Tapering of a distended duodenum may be done to reduce future duodenal dysmotility. A gastrostomy may also be performed for decompression to avoid trauma to the anastomotic site. A combined nursing and medical approach facilitates both preoperative stabilization and postoperative recuperation.

Preoperative care is directed toward hydration and gastric decompression. Intermittent gastric suction by use of a sump tube reduces the risk of aspiration or perforation due to overdistention. Vital signs, fluid intake and output, urine specific gravity, and serum electrolytes must be closely monitored, and fluids, electrolytes, and crystalloid must be provided as needed. Antibiotics may be instituted for preoperative prophylaxis or when perforation or sepsis is suspected.

Continued decompression and nutrition are the major postoperative concerns. Total parenteral nutrition is given initially. Oral feedings are generally begun at 10 to 14 days with an oral electrolyte solution and advanced to low-osmolality formulas such as Nutramigen or Pregestimil (protein hydrolysate formulas) before advancing to regular formula.

Late complications such as peptic ulcers, adhesions, and need for revision of correction have been reported in 12% of patients. A 95% survival rate is reported, with deaths attributed to associated cardiac or renal anomalies or to infectious or respiratory complications (Barksdale et al., 2011; Escobar et al., 2004).

Jejunal/Ileal Atresia

■ Anatomy. Thirty-nine percent of intestinal atresias occur in the jejunum or ileum where there is complete obstruction of the intestinal lumen (Wax et al., 2006). These atresias can often be associated with other intestinal processes, including intussusception, volvulus, and abdominal wall defects. Signs and symptoms generally present at 1 or 2 days of age and are virtually the same for all types of jejunoileal atresia. Presentation includes bilious vomiting, failure to pass stool, and generalized abdominal distention.

■ Pathophysiology. Typically, atresias of the jejunum and ileum were thought to result from mesenteric vascular compromise with necrosis and eventual resorption of the involved area. Newer research in animals suggests that atresias are more likely caused by disruption in the endoderm, with the vascular compromise occurring later (Nichol, Reeder, & Botham, 2011). The presence of bile, meconium, epithelial cells, and lanugo distal to the atresia indicates that this ischemic injury occurs relatively late in utero, possibly as late as 3 to 6 months gestation. A single atresia is present in approximately 90% of cases (Barksdale et al., 2011). The occurrence rate is 1 in 3,000 to 5,000 live births, with an apparently equal distribution of atresias between the jejunum and the ileum (Wax et al., 2006). There is no linkage to gender and the development of this form of atresia (Berseth & Poenaru, 2005c).

Maternal polyhydramnios can be present in jejunal atresia but generally does not present in ileal atresia. Associated anomalies are rare and are primarily restricted to the GI tract, with malrotation and meconium ileus being most common. Between 25% and 30% of patients experience hyperbilirubinemia, and 25% to 38% are born prematurely. Of the different types of jejunoileal atresia that have been identified only the "apple peel" or "Christmas tree" type is typically familial, thus indicating that this one form alone may involve some autosomal recessive or multifactorial type of inheritance. Although it is the rarest form of jejunoileal atresia, it carries the highest mortality rate and higher rates of prematurity and malrotation in comparison with the more conventional types.

■ Treatment. Abdominal radiographs show multiple bubbles that reflect dilation and collection of swallowed air proximal to the obstruction and a gasless abdomen distal to the obstruction. Intraperitoneal calcifications are present in 12% of patients, which indicates antenatal intestinal perforation with resultant meconium peritonitis (Barksdale et al., 2011). The peritonitis in this case is due to chemical irritation (there is no infection because the bowel and meconium are sterile before birth), thus causing fibrosis, granuloma formation, and ultimately calcifications. The perforated site usually heals spontaneously before delivery and leaves no evidence other than the residual calcifications. The airless, unused distal portion of the gut is generally contracted and of a much smaller caliber than normal. A limited upper GI contrast study to rule out malrotation or a contrast enema to eliminate the diagnosis of meconium ileus may be necessary.

Surgical management begins with resection of the dilated proximal gut and atretic, bulbous ending, and a search for multiple distal atresias. Primary closure by end-to-end or side-to-end anastomosis generally follows, but preliminary tapering of the distended distal segment may be required; as a third alternative, an end-to-oblique closure may be performed. Ostomy formation is avoided if possible but may be needed if it is not possible to perform a primary repair secondary to bowel ischemia or inflammation. Once surgical correction is complete, collaboration with the nutritional support team is essential.

The principles of preoperative care involve bowel decompression and intravenous hydration with the correction of any electrolyte imbalance that may occur as the result of vomiting or third-spacing-capillary leak syndrome. Antibiotics may be given prophylactically or therapeutically in the case of peritonitis. Recovery of bowel peristalsis and enzymatic integrity may be delayed, thus necessitating parenteral nutrition. When started, initial feedings are of a clear electrolyte solution and progress serially to elemental formulas such as Nutramigen or Pregestimil (protein hydrolysate formulas) until standard formula can be tolerated. The nurses should diligently assess for evidence of SBS, commonly seen with atresias that are multiple or of the "apple peel" variety, which necessitated excision of an extensive length of bowel.

With the availability of parenteral alimentation, survival rates have risen to as high as 84% (Dalla Vecchia et al., 1998). Deaths are generally the result of prematurity, postoperative SBS, or infectious complications.

Omphalocele

■ **Anatomy.** Omphalocele is generally an immediately apparent anomaly and ranges between 2 and 15 cm in size. However, the small defects that involve perhaps a single loop of intestine may be easily overlooked unless the physical examination is carried out in an unhurried fashion and the umbilical ring is clearly absent on palpation. The larger defects generally contain the intestine and possibly the liver, spleen, stomach, bladder, ovaries and tubes, or testicles. These two extremes most likely reflect the difference in the time at which normal embryogenesis is interrupted. If the interruption is early, around the 3- to 4-week window when infolding is in its last stages, the defect is large. If the interruption occurs later, at about 9 to 10 weeks when migration is generally completed, the defect is smaller. However, in both cases, the intestine and possibly other abdominal organs herniate into the umbilical cord. A thin, transparent membrane composed of peritoneum and amnion covers the viscera, and the visible bowel has a normal appearance. The abdominal cavity is often relatively small and underdeveloped, having never held the growing intestine. Although a membrane generally covers omphaloceles, intrauterine rupture of that membrane occurs in 10% to 18% of patients (Somme & Langer, 2006). As a consequence of prolonged exposure to the amniotic fluid, the bowel becomes matted and edematous in appearance and difficult to differentiate from gastroschisis. Closer examination may reveal the sac remnants, but if not noted, one need only look to the base of the cord. In gastroschisis, the umbilical cord is intact, inserted normally at the abdominal wall, and separated from the defect by a small amount of skin.

■ **Pathophysiology.** Omphalocele is an abdominal wall defect usually at the level of the umbilicus. It results from failure of the umbilical ring to close with subsequent herniation of the intestines. Whether the herniation is a failure of the intestine to undergo normal rotation and return to the abdominal cavity or herniation secondary to abnormal abdominal wall musculature is unclear. Defects that occur above the umibilicus are part of the pentalogy of Cantrell deformity. Pentalogy of Cantrell is a constellation of anomalies involving the sternum, diaphragm, pericardium, as well as the upper abdominal omphalocele and ectopic cordis. Herniation below the umbilicus often involves bladder or cloacal exstrophy (Barksdale et al., 2011).

Omphalocele occurs in roughly 1 of every 3,000 to 6,000 live births, with a male predominance. Mothers tend to be younger (93% <29 years old). Multiple and often life-threatening syndromes and anomalies occur greater than 50% of the time and include trisomy 13, trisomy 18, Beckwith–Wiedemann syndrome, pentalogy syndrome, congenital heart defects, diaphragmatic and upper midline defects, malrotation, intestinal atresia, and genitourinary anomalies. Additionally, 30% to 33% of affected infants are premature, and approximately 19% are small for gestational age (P. Hwang & Kousseff, 2004).

■ **Treatment.** With the advancement in prenatal diagnosis, most incidences of abdominal wall defects are known well in advance of delivery. This knowledge allows preparation of the family and of the fetus. Ideally, maternal transport to a tertiary center avoids the emergency situation of transporting an infant with such a defect. With the improved diagnostics, karyotyping can also be done to determine whether life-threatening chromosomal conditions exist. Omphalocele is often used as an indicator for cesarean section, yet studies have shown no significant difference in morbidity and mortality according to delivery mode (Heider, Strauss, & Kuller, 2004).

The definitive surgical treatment is return of the viscera into the abdominal cavity and closure of the defect. This can be done via skin-flap closure or staged reduction. The procedure employed varies with the size of the defect. Typically, primary closure has been the preferred method, but a trend toward staged reduction has been reported (Marven & Owen, 2008). Larger defects (>5 cm) may require a staged repair with a preformed or custom silo used to suspend the viscera above the patient. Reduction maneuvers are carried out daily to return the suspended organs into the relatively small abdominal cavity. A forceful return and closure under pressure would risk compression of the inferior vena cava, with reduced filling of the heart and decreased cardiac output and impedance of the diaphragmatic excursions, thus resulting in respiratory compromise. A gastrostomy to provide decompression and an appendectomy to avoid atypically presenting appendicitis later in life may be carried out with both primary and staged procedures, depending on the preferences of the surgical team. If a staged repair is performed, complete return of the organs into the abdominal cavity is generally achieved over a period of 7 to 10 days. At that time, the infant is returned to surgery for final closure of the abdominal wall. If surgery is contraindicated because of coexisting chromosomal or other syndromes, the defect may be treated medically by repeatedly painting the sac with silver sulfadiazine mercurochrome. Topical agents promote eschar formation and epithelialization with complete coverage by skin within 6 to 8 weeks. Should the patient survive, a later repair of the muscle wall becomes necessary (Barksdale et al., 2011). Biologic dressings have also been used to provide temporary protection. In some cases porcine and human skin grafts are also used.

These children often require aggressive postoperative respiratory management followed by prolonged total parenteral nutrition. Early psychosocial support of parents must be provided to promote their involvement in what is commonly an extended hospital stay. Genetic counseling may also be warranted.

The cornerstones of preoperative management include protection of the eviscerated organs, decompression of the gut, and hydration (Berseth & Poenaru, 2005a). Thermoregulation is a particular concern because massive evaporative and radiant heat losses may occur through the exposed defect. Care directed in these four areas may overlap, but all are necessary. The first step is to loosely apply sterile, warmed, saline-soaked gauze in a turban style around the defect, wrapping the ends around the body. Great care must be taken to prevent tight application, which might create pressure; two fingers should fit easily between the trunk and the encircling gauze. Some clinicians suggest that an outer, dry sterile dressing also be applied. The dressing is then covered with plastic wrap. As an alternative, sterile bowel bags may be used. Both wrapping and bag techniques provide protection to the defect from trauma and infection and help limit the loss of fluids and body heat. Sterile gloves must be worn during the necessary manipulation of the bowel. If the defect is small, the infant may be positioned on the back, but if the defect is large, it may be best to place the infant on the side. In the side-lying position, a small blanket or diaper may be slipped between the covered viscera and the bed surface so that no traction is placed on the bowel, which might cause physical injury to the gut or impede circulation. A gastric tube should be passed and set to low intermittent suction for decompression. Appropriate comfort measures to reduce or prevent crying with concomitant air swallowing should also be employed. Intravenous fluids should be started immediately to counteract direct fluid losses from exposure of the defect and the loss of fluids from the circulation caused by inflammation and third-spacing. Potential for vena cava compression resulting in poor venous return from the lower extremities is also a concern. Hydration status, fluid intake and output, and vital signs should be monitored closely for tachycardia, thready pulses, hypotension, poor perfusion, and decreased urine output, with increased specific gravity suggesting hypovolemia. Umbilical catheterization for venous access is contraindicated because of the nature and site of the defect. Prophylactic antibiotic administration should also be started.

Postoperative support varies slightly according to the repair procedure used, but both methods should generally include measures of hydration, decompression, and a search for evidence of increased intra-abdominal pressure. Third-spacing, or capillary leak syndrome, may continue to be a problem and may actually be exacerbated by the trauma of surgical manipulation of the bowel. Assessment for signs of hypovolemia should be documented. Serum electrolytes, albumin, and total serum protein values should also be followed, with fluid and other replacements made as necessary. Decompression by gastric tube or gastrostomy is generally required for a considerable time until peristaltic activity returns. Ileus and cholestasis are common following repair, so enteral feedings may be delayed, and parenteral alimentation is provided during the interval. When feedings are begun, an elemental formula may be used initially. Respiratory support with increased pressures may be required to achieve adequate ventilation if diaphragmatic movements are hampered. Inspection of the lower extremities and palpation of pedal pulses are helpful in assessing for impaired circulation. Elevating the extremities may promote venous return to the heart. In addition to these measures, if a staged repair is undertaken, particular attention must be paid to the infant's tolerance of daily reduction attempts. Furthermore, the silo provides an open port for bacterial invasion. Povidone-iodine or silver sulfadiazine (Silvadene) ointment may be applied with dressing changes, and antibiotic therapy is continued postoperatively.

The overall mortality rate is reported as 5% to 80% depending on the size of the defect, associated chromosomal and other anomalies, early detection, and coincidental prematurity or low birth weight (Boyd, Bhattacharjee, Gould, Manning, & Chamberlain, 1998; P. Hwang & Kousseff, 2004). Malrotation with the resultant danger of volvulus, ischemia, and necrosis is common. Antenatal membrane rupture may also add the dimension of potential sepsis.

Gastroschisis

■ Anatomy. Gastroschisis is a full-thickness defect in the abdominal wall through which the uncovered intestines protrude. Although often confused with a ruptured omphalocele, in gastroschisis the umbilical cord is inserted normally. The defect is next to rather than in the umbilical cord, and there is no protective sac, nor remnants thereof.

The liver and other solid organs generally remain in the abdominal cavity, although evisceration is possible. The defect is usually small (2–5 cm) and located to the right of the umbilicus, from which it is separated by a narrow margin of skin. The bowel is uncovered and, as a consequence of chemical peritonitis caused by long exposure to the amniotic fluid, appears as an edematous and matted mass with no identifiable loops. The abdominal cavity is small and underdeveloped.

■ Pathophysiology. Gastroschisis is generally thought to arise as the result of incomplete lateral infolding of the embryonic disk. As a result of this primary failure, the abdominal wall is incompletely formed, allowing herniation of the gut. Three other accepted theories have also been offered. The first suggests that the umbilical coelom (cavity) fails to form, so normal herniation of the midgut into the cord cannot occur. Consequently, during its rapid growth phase the intestine ruptures through the embryonic body wall. Another view considers that a vascular accident occurring in utero leads to occlusion of the omphalomesenteric artery. With its circulation removed, the base of the cord becomes necrotic, leaving an opening through which the intestine can eviscerate. The last theory proposes that gastroschisis may simply be a variant of omphalocele, with early intrauterine rupture of its membranous covering. The membrane remnants are subsequently reabsorbed, and the umbilical cord is reformed around the offset umbilical vessels (Feldkamp, Carey, & Sadler, 2007). For the last two theories, the gap between the evisceration and cord base is presumably filled in by skin.

Prematurity (60%) and low birth weight are extremely common. Malrotation is found in all affected infants, and a few may exhibit intestinal atresia, but anomalies of systems other than the GI tract are infrequent and relatively minor (Holland, Walker, & Badawi, 2010). The overall incidence of gastroschisis has been steadily rising over the past several decades with incidence of approximately 3 to 5 per 10,000 live births. Males are affected 1.2 times more often than females. It appears to be more common in mothers less than 20 years of age and rarely occurs in women over 30 years old. Nutritional alterations, maternal smoking, and use of vasoactive drugs have been associated with an increased incidence (Alvarez & Burd, 2007; David, Tan, & Curry, 2008).

■ Treatment. Cesarean section is often chosen for delivery to avoid injury to exposed bowel. A systematic review of the literature could not document an advantage to cesarean delivery in the absence of obstetrical indications (Segel, Marder, Parry, & Macones, 2001). Several studies have shown no difference in mortality or morbidity for infants born vaginally or by cesarean section. Some clinicians have proposed premature delivery when there is evidence of bowel compromise. Routine preterm delivery of infants with gastroschisis is not recommended because of inherent risk factors of prematurity and the reversibility of most intestinal damage (King & Askin, 2003; Salihu, Boos, & Schmidt, 2004).

A primary closure is the preferred surgical technique; however, the majority of defects are closed by staged repair using a fabricated spring-loaded silo that can be inserted at the bedside. This gradual approach to closure has shown fewer ventilation days, decreased time to full feeds, and shorter hospital days (Cass & Wesson, 2002; Schlatter, 2003). Although gastroschisis is a smaller defect than omphalocele, the distortion of the viscera with typical thickening and edema of the bowel make primary closure more difficult. Often the defect must be surgically enlarged to allow thorough inspection of the entire length of the GI tract and to avoid restricting the passage of the eviscerated intestine back into the abdominal cavity. All display some degree of malrotation, predisposing them to both intestinal atresias and infarction. Bowel resection and anastomosis are often necessary; however, primary anastomosis is contraindicated in the face of peritonitis or inflammation. In such situations, an enterostomy is performed away from the defect, with anastomosis delayed until final closure of the abdominal wall. The visceral mass is returned to the abdominal cavity as a whole. Because of the potential for bowel injury and blood loss, no attempt is made to unravel the adherent loops of bowel.

Preoperative nutritional and respiratory support is essential. Consultation with social services is helpful in providing parental support and establishing healthy parent–child relationships. The care of patients with gastroschisis is much like that for omphalocele. The intestines should be covered to protect them from injury and to reduce the loss of fluids and heat. Preoperative care is rounded out by use of gastric decompression, fluid resuscitation, and antibiotic prophylaxis.

Following surgery, the major concerns are venous stasis, respiratory compromise, infection, and nutrition. Edema and cyanosis of the lower extremities and evidence of decreased cardiac output should be reported immediately. Intensive respiratory support is provided, and oxygenation and ventilation are monitored closely. Infection is prevented by careful aseptic dressing changes, daily applications of bacteriostatic solutions or ointments, and systemic administration of antibiotics. Total parenteral nutrition is generally continued for several weeks until intestinal function returns. Feedings are usually begun with elemental formula, eventually progressing to standard formula, with diligent assessment for evidence of intestinal obstruction during the process.

A mortality rate of less than 8% is reported for uncomplicated gastroschisis, but the rate can rise to 90% when complicated by bowel atresia, necrosis, and volvulus (David et al., 2008; Marven & Owen, 2008). Early deaths are largely attributable to a combination of shock, sepsis (associated with perforation or contamination of the exposed bowel), and hypothermia. Profound hypothermia (temperature lower than 35°C [95°F]) can occur. Late deaths come as a result of sepsis, respiratory failure, and the inability of the bowel to sustain nutrition.

Malrotation With Volvulus

■ **Anatomy.** Malrotation is an anomaly of intestinal rotation and fixation where the base of the mesentery becomes short. It is this malfixation that is concerning, placing the small bowel at risk of volvulus and ischemia. Of all the affected infants, only about half will present with symptoms in the first week of life. In those who do, the symptoms are generally intermittent or recurrent, indicating that most of these obstructions are partial rather than complete. Most infants demonstrate progressive bilious vomiting. When a previously well infant presents with sudden bilious vomiting, a malrotation with volvulus should be first in the differential diagnosis. In the case of volvulus, the abdomen may become distended, and the stools may be bloody. Bleeding occurs when twisting is severe enough to interfere with venous return from the bowel, thus causing the vessels to become engorged and leak blood into the gut.

■ **Pathophysiology.** The abnormality most likely arises between the 8th and 10th week of gestation as the intestine rotates around the axis of the superior mesenteric artery during its entry into and movement from the umbilical cord. Once returned to the abdominal cavity, the intestinal mesentery lies along and eventually adheres to the posterior abdominal wall, thus fixing the intestine in place. The normal 270° counterclockwise rotation can be interrupted or deviated at any time, and consequently a variety of rotation and fixation anomalies are possible.

The major danger with malrotation is that the intestinal loops may become kinked, knotted, or otherwise obstructed. This knotting and twisting of the bowel is called a volvulus. This occlusion of the intestinal tract or its blood supply can lead to widespread ischemia and necrosis. Over 50% of patients with malrotation present within the first month of life and another 25% by one year of age; the other 25% present as children or adults (Barksdale et al., 2011). Nearly two thirds of all cases of malrotation are complicated by volvulus, with the incidence varying with age at the onset of symptoms, but 80% occurring in the neonatal period (Berseth & Poenaru, 2005c). Intestinal rotational anomalies occur in approximately 1 in 6,000 live births (Barksdale et al., 2011). The anomaly does appear to predominate in males with no specific cause identified.

Almost all cases of omphalocele, gastroschisis, and diaphragmatic hernia entail some component of malrotation. The frequency is in fact so high that many clinicians do not consider malrotation an anomaly associated with these conditions but rather an expected component of them. Associated anomalies such as intestinal atresias, annular pancreas, Meckel's diverticulum, and urinary tract malformation as well as congenital heart disease are found in patients with malrotation.

■ **Treatment.** On plain radiograph, the stomach and upper small intestine are generally distended with air and may mimic the characteristic "double-bubble" of duodenal atresia. However, the presence of small amounts of gas in the distal positions of the gut is more reflective of a partial obstruction by malrotation than of an atresia in the jejunum or ileum. A contrast enema can be given to locate the position of the cecum under fluoroscopy. If a misplaced colon is seen, the diagnosis of malrotation is confirmed. However, some malrotations (notably reverse rotation) may not be demonstrated. An upper GI series is diagnostic in all cases and allows the exact position of the duodenum to be seen. When volvulus is present, the contrast column is noted to end with a peculiar "beaking" effect that is caused by the twisting of the bowel into a sharp point. Ultrasound has been used to assess position of the superior mesenteric vein in relation to the artery but does not always provide a definite diagnosis.

The goals for surgical management are the release of obstruction and counterclockwise rotational reduction of the bowel. The volvulus is relieved by counterclockwise rotation, and the viability of the bowel is determined with necrotic sections removed. When necrosis is not expected, successful laparoscopic surgery for repair has been reported (Hsiao & Langer, 2011). If the necrosis is extensive, rather than perform massive bowel resection, the abdomen may be closed. A return "second look" surgery is performed in 24 to 48 hours, at which time it becomes mandatory to remove any diseased, infarcted bowel. If the bowel appears viable, the Ladd bands (if present) are divided, and the entrapped duodenum is freed. The entire length of the bowel is then inspected for patency and associated defects and returned to the abdominal cavity; the small intestine is placed on the right and the colon on the left side of the abdominal cavity. Suture fixation of the replaced bowel generally is not necessary. Appendectomy and gastrostomy may be performed as well.

The major postoperative complication is SBS, which results from the excision of major portions of the gut. The complex malabsorption problems and prolonged hospitalization with total parenteral nutrition call for consultation and close collaboration with members of the nutritional support team and social services. Wound problems and prolonged ileus may also be noted.

The principles of preoperative stabilization include gastric decompression and correction of fluid and electrolyte deficits. The presence of volvulus places the infant at particular risk for both hypovolemia and metabolic acidosis. Hypovolemia occurs as a result of fluid accumulation in the bowel wall, which effectively reduces the circulating blood volume. Clinically, as the infant worsens, the abdomen becomes distended, erythematous, and tender, and blood is passed into the stool. The heart rate quickens in an attempt to maintain cardiac output, and the infant's color may become ashen. This state constitutes a true surgical emergency.

The same principles of decompression and fluid and electrolyte resuscitation apply postoperatively. Total parenteral nutrition is instituted and continued, often for months in the case of SBS, until the intestine has had an opportunity to recover and grow. When feedings are begun, elemental or dilute formula is given initially; the volume and then the concentration are gradually increased until a normal amount of full-strength formula can be tolerated. This feeding progression is often a tedious process fraught with many setbacks that are frustrating to both the nurse and the parents.

When the condition is uncomplicated by infarction or associated anomalies, the survival rate is excellent and may be as high as 97%. However, in the presence of necrosis, survival is decreased. An increased risk of dying is also noted with younger age (< 3 months) at the time of surgery.

MANAGEMENT OF PROBLEMS WITH ELIMINATION

Hirschsprung Disease

■ **Anatomy.** Hirschsprung disease (also known as congenital megacolon or aganglionic megacolon), an abnormality of the colon marked by the congenital absence of ganglion cells (aganglionosis) is the most common cause of obstruction in the neonate. The signs and symptoms of Hirschsprung disease in the newborn are primarily those of intestinal obstruction, including bilious vomiting, distention, and failure to pass meconium. The rectum is empty of stool unless the aganglionic segment is very short, in which case rectal examination with the gloved little finger may cause explosive release of gas and evacuation of meconium. If the disease goes undiagnosed, fecal stagnation may lead to increased intraluminal pressures, reduced colonic blood flow, and bacterial overgrowth with resultant enterocolitis. This severe bowel irritation and inflammation may cause "overflow" diarrhea, with complicating dehydration, hypoproteinemia, electrolyte imbalance, and sometimes perforation and shock.

■ **Pathophysiology.** Failure of the neural crest cells to migrate in their usual craniocaudal fashion results in aberrant bowel innervation and interrupted neuromuscular conduction of the messages that promote peristalsis of the anal sphincter. This local failure of relaxation results in functional intestinal obstruction. Fecal matter accumulates in the normally innervated proximal bowel, producing dilation (megacolon) and hypertrophy of the muscular wall as normal peristaltic activity works against the obstruction. The distal, aganglionic segment is unused and may appear narrowed in relation to the proximal dilation, but it is in fact of normal caliber. Between the ganglionic proximal section and the distal aganglionic section is a "transition zone" of tapered bowel. The rectum is always involved, and more than 75% involve the sigmoid colon as well. Total colonic aganglionosis may be found in 8% of cases (Barksdale et al., 2011). Atypical forms of Hirschsprung disease, in which areas of normal innervation are found between aganglionic areas, have also been described, but the presence of such "skip areas" is extremely rare.

The cause of the interrupted migration of ganglion cells is not known, but anoxia is often cited. The theory is that local anoxemia, because of an interference with the source of oxygen to the site, may lead to ischemia, atrophy, and regression of the cells. There is increasing evidence that Hirschsprung disease is linked to a genetic defect in neural crest stem cell function. RET mutations have been found in 30% to 50% of patients with familial Hirschsprung disease, and EDNRB mutations in 20% (Iwashita, Kruger, Pardal, Kiel, & Morrison, 2003; Kenny, Tam, & Garcia-Barcelo, 2010; Puri & Shinkai, 2004).

The incidence of Hirschsprung disease is 1 in 5,000 live births with a 4 to 1 male to female predominance. Associated anomalies are relatively infrequent but include trisomy 21, Waardenburg syndrome, Smith–Lemli–Opitz syndrome, central hypoventilation syndrome, and asymptomatic urologic anomalies. The ganglionic plexuses of the bowel are derived from the same craniocervical neural crest as are the oral, facial, and cranial ganglia. Consequently, a limited number of infants may also exhibit congenital deafness and ocular neurocristopathies, most commonly in association with Waardenburg syndrome. Approximately 5% have associated neurologic abnormalities ranging from developmental delay to mental retardation or cerebral palsy (Kenny et al., 2010).

■ **Treatment.** Hirschsprung disease may be clinically indistinguishable from jejunoileal atresia, meconium ileus, meconium plug syndrome, and small left colon syndrome. Plain radiographic examination offers little or no help in differentiation. All conditions show large gas-filled loops of bowel consistent with intestinal obstruction. The rectum may or may not contain air, but when air is present, it generally is of a reduced amount consistent with partial or functional obstruction.

Barium contrast studies may be indicated to determine the caliber of the distal colon. Microcolon is typically found with jejunoileal atresia and meconium ileus, but if the colon is of normal size or somewhat enlarged, the obstruction may be the result of Hirschsprung disease, meconium plug syndrome, or small left colon syndrome. In about 60% of studies, barium enema demonstrates the "pigtail" or "funnel" sign characteristic of Hirschsprung disease. This sign is simply a demonstration of the tapering transition zone lying between the dilated, innervated proximal segment and the normal-caliber, aganglionic distal bowel. When the sign is present, usually in infants older than 2 months of age, it highly suggests Hirschsprung disease, but it may also be found in small left colon syndrome. The margins of the distal colon generally have a sawtooth appearance in Hirschsprung disease, whereas smooth margins are typically described with small left colon syndrome. Although suggestive of Hirschsprung disease, retention of contrast material or barium noted on follow-up film 24 hours later may also be noted in its absence.

Anorectal manometry has been used as an alternative diagnostic tool but is not recommended for patients less than 1 year of age. The test is performed to determine the ability of the internal sphincter to relax. Findings should not be considered conclusive but only suggestive in neonates (Noviello, Cobellis, Romano, Amici, & Martino, 2009). Further tests must be done to confirm the diagnosis. Definitive diagnosis is made only by suction or punch rectal biopsy through the anus and histologic examination of the specimen obtained. No anesthesia is required, but sedation and pain management are used. The procedure can easily be performed in the nursery. If ganglionic bowel is obtained, either meconium plug syndrome or small left colon syndrome is possible. The absence of ganglionic cells in the submucosal plexus firmly establishes the diagnosis of Hirschsprung disease. Should questions regarding diagnosis persist, a full-thickness operative biopsy under general anesthesia may be performed to collect deeper nerve plexuses, but this is rarely needed.

Although older children with mild symptoms of Hirschsprung disease may be managed medically with a daily colonic lavage of normal saline to evacuate the bowel, such conservative therapy is inappropriate in the neonatal period secondary to the risk of fatal enterocolitis with perforation, peritonitis, and septicemia.

The surgical goal is to bring normal bowel down to the anus. In the past this was done in a two- to three-stage pull-through procedure with a preliminary stoma. There has been a gradual transition to primary repair with endorectal pull-through. The laparoscopic approach has been established as the standard surgical approach in many centers. This technique is less invasive, but relies heavily on accurate biopsy location of normal ganglionic cells. In a two-stage procedure, a temporary colostomy is placed proximal to the aganglionic segment, to decompress the bowel and divert the fecal contents. The definitive repair is carried out between 6 and 12 months of age and involves resection of the affected, aganglionic bowel and anastomosis of the normal bowel to the anus.

One of several surgical procedures may be performed; the Swenson procedure: abdominoperineal sphincter-saving proctectomy and end-to-end anastomosis in the rectal area; the Duhamel procedure: oblique end-to-side anastomosis between the proximal ganglionic colon and the anterior aganglionic anorectal wall, thus forming a new rectum, with the posterior portion pulled through the intestine and making a sleeve of good tissue; and the Soave procedure: an endorectal mucosal dissection in the area of the rectum where the muscular tissue is preserved and a sleeve of good, innervated tissue is pulled through to create a viable bowel surface (Barksdale et al., 2011).

No matter what the surgical procedure, the initial nursing care is directed toward abdominal decompression, return of fluid and electrolyte balance, and the treatment of sepsis. A gastric tube is set to low intermittent suction, and all drainage is measured. Fluids with appropriate electrolytes for the maintenance and replacement of gastric losses should be provided. Actions to combat the fluid shifts that are common following contrast studies with hyperosmolar media may also be necessary. Prophylactic antibiotic therapy is initiated because of the high risk of enterocolitis. If enterocolitis is present, aggressive therapy with fluids, blood, or plasma may be required. The infant should be monitored closely after rectal biopsy. Bleeding can usually be controlled with digital pressure.

A preoperative colonic lavage or enema may be given to evacuate and prepare the bowel for surgery. Only isotonic solutions such as normal saline should be used to avoid water intoxication and resultant hyponatremia. Following colostomy, the infant must be assessed frequently for respiratory compromise, abdominal distention, hemorrhage, wound dehiscence, and infection. The stomal perfusion and appearance should also be noted and appropriate skin care provided. Intravenous fluids and/or parenteral nutrition are continued until oral feedings can be started. Involvement of the enterostomal therapist may be necessary as the infant becomes ready for discharge. The focus of care shifts to readying the parents for home management of the colostomy. Family teaching should include skin care, normal stomal appearance and stool output, and the construction and application of appliances.

The mortality rate for Hirschsprung disease is generally low with most deaths attributable to delayed diagnosis or development of enterocolitis. Good surgical results can be expected in the vast majority of patients, but diarrhea, constipation with distention, and intermittent colitis may occur as the result of residual aganglionosis, postoperative stricture formation, overactivity of the sphincter, or motility disorders. Delayed toilet training is frequently reported, with the actual rate varying in direct proportion to the length of the aganglionic segment.

Small Left Colon

■ **Anatomy.** Neonatal small left colon syndrome is a condition of functional immaturity of the large bowel in which the left colon is uniformly narrowed from the anus to the splenic flexure. The proximal colon above the flexure is dilated and distended with meconium. A cone-shaped transition zone lies between the dilated and narrowed distal segments.

Presenting signs and symptoms are those associated with low intestinal obstruction. These manifestations include bile-stained vomitus, abdominal distention, and failure to pass meconium spontaneously. Rectal examination may be followed by the passage of very small amounts of meconium in approximately a third of patients.

■ **Pathophysiology.** The cause of small left colon syndrome is unclear, but is generally thought to involve the myenteric plexuses that innervate the GI tract in a cephalocaudal direction between 5 and 12 weeks gestation. Once the plexuses are in position, their maturation and function are largely determined by gestational age. The impression that this condition results from intramural immaturity is supported by histologic findings of increased numbers of small, immature neuronal elements in contrast to the larger, multipolar ganglion cells that normally predominate at term. The neuronal plexuses are present but immature; morphologically, they resemble the structure expected at approximately, 32 weeks gestation. The syndrome might therefore be best described as a disease of decreased intestinal motility.

Approximately 40% of those with small left colon syndrome are the infants of mothers with diabetes. Fifty percent of asymptomatic infants of mothers with diabetes have shown a demonstrable narrowed colonic configuration in the absence of frank symptoms. Variable degrees of hypoglycemia, hypocalcemia, and hyperbilirubinemia have also been reported, but these findings may simply reflect the predisposition for hyperinsulinemia and polycythemia in the general population of infants of mothers with diabetes (Philippart & Georgeson, 1975).

■ **Treatment.** On clinical presentation and with plain radiographic studies, this condition is indistinguishable from Hirschsprung disease and meconium plug syndrome. Multiple gas-filled loops of bowel are seen proximally, with decreased air noted distally. Barium enema shows the uniformly small left colon with a zone of transition at the splenic flexure. Although a zone of transition may also be noted with Hirschsprung disease, the margins of the distal colon generally appear smooth with small left colon syndrome rather than jagged or serrated as described in Hirschsprung disease. Perhaps more distinguishing from Hirschsprung disease is the incidental finding that following contrast studies, the majority of infants with small left colon syndrome promptly evacuate the barium and begin passing stools spontaneously. As a consequence, the signs and symptoms of low intestinal obstruction disappear. The meconium rarely contains a significant rubbery plug.

Rectal biopsy for the presence of ganglion cells, although they may appear atypically immature in small left colon syndrome, may ultimately be required to differentiate this syndrome from Hirschsprung disease. If the possibility of meconium plug persists, a follow-up contrast examination should be performed. Despite the passage of meconium, the transition zone persists in infants suffering from small left colon syndrome.

Management is generally conservative. The diagnostic barium enema is generally curative. Only in the rare case of significant intermittent obstruction or cecal perforation is a colostomy required.

As with all intestinal obstructions, initial management involves decompression, intravenous fluids for hydration, and the treatment of electrolyte imbalance. Symptoms generally resolve following barium enema, and oral feeding may be instituted gradually. The nurse must be diligent in looking for evidence of persistent or recurrent obstruction and report abnormal findings accordingly. Although the initial presentation may be dramatic, many cases are apparently asymptomatic and go undiagnosed. In either case, the condition spontaneously resolves within the neonatal period with no subsequent stooling problems encountered. Late intermittent obstruction with or without cecal perforation is reported rarely.

Meconium Ileus

■ Anatomy. Meconium ileus is an obstruction of the distal ileum due to an accumulation of abnormally thick, tarry meconium. Meconium ileus generally presents first with progressive abdominal distention (within 12 to 24 hours of birth), followed by bilious vomiting and failure to pass meconium. On physical examination the meconium mass may be palpated as a movable, doughy or putty-like ball; smaller pellet-like concretions of inspissated meconium may be felt distally. Rectal examination should produce no meconium, but normal sphincter tone should be felt.

■ Pathophysiology. Historically 90% of children with meconium ileus were thought to have cystic fibrosis (CF), although only a small proportion (10%–15%) of infants with CF present with meconium ileus. Several studies, however, have found between 30% and 50% of children presenting with meconium ileus do not have CF. Prematurity and low birth weight were also noted to be associated with non-CF patients (Gorter, Karimi, Sleeboom, Kneepkens, & Heji, 2010; Olsen, Luck, Lloyd-Still, & Raffensperger, 1982; Steiner, Mogilner, Siplovich, & Eldar, 1997).

In CF patients the condition is a result of pancreatic insufficiency. Pancreatic hydrolytic enzymes are normally responsible for the metabolism of fat and protein. Consequently, if these enzymes are absent, the meconium has an unusually high protein content and abnormal mucous glycoprotein, which makes it more viscid than usual. The resultant thick, tenacious material literally becomes impacted within the ileal lumen, thus producing a functional obstruction. The cause of these findings in non-CF patients is not known but is thought to be related to genetic and pathological abnormalities. Meconium ileus can be divided into simple and complex. Complex cases are associated with GI complications such as atresias, necrosis, and perforation. Complex meconium ileus was found in 80% of non-CF patients as opposed to 39% with CF (Gorter et al., 2010).

■ Treatment. Plain abdominal films show distended loops proximal to the point of obstruction, but unlike the uniformly lucent areas seen in jejunoileal atresia, the dilated areas typical of meconium ileus are of varying sizes and have a "soap-bubble" or "ground-glass" appearance. This appearance reflects the mixture of trapped air and meconium. Calcifications that are the result of antenatal intestinal perforation and consequent meconium peritonitis may also be noted. Contrast enema demonstrates a distally unused microcolon, thus differentiating this condition from Hirschsprung disease. The smaller pellet-like masses of meconium may also be noted in the distal segment. A history of cystic fibrosis in siblings virtually ensures the diagnosis of meconium ileus. An immunoreactive trypsin test using a dry blood spot provides a screen for cystic fibrosis, with confirmation by sweat test and DNA analysis for cystic fibrosis mutations.

In the case of uncomplicated meconium ileus, the bowel can generally be evacuated using a hyperosmolar contrast enema such as meglumine diatrizoate. Because of the hyperosmolarity of the contrast, fluid is drawn from the interstitial and intravascular spaces into the intestinal lumen, softening the impacted meconium and allowing it to pull away from the intestinal wall. The mass can then be evacuated by normal peristalsis.

If repeated enemas are not productive, or if meconium ileus is complicated by bowel ischemia, sepsis, or hypovolemic shock, the obstructing meconium may be surgically removed. A temporary ileostomy may be established. Such an ileostomy is irrigated daily with dilute acetylcysteine until any residual meconium is softened and evacuated. Chest physiotherapy, acetylcysteine sodium aerosols (Mucomyst, New York: Bristol-Myers, Squibb), and extra humidity may be helpful in preventing postoperative pulmonary complications (such as atelectasis and pneumonia), to which infants with cystic fibrosis are particularly prone.

All infants with meconium ileus need to be evaluated for cystic fibrosis. Genetic counseling should be provided to parents of affected children, with appropriate referral to a geneticist or genetic counselor. A social worker or other mental health professional may help parents explore their feelings concerning their child's prognosis and their future reproductive plans. Extensive parent teaching of pulmonary toilet and enzyme supplementation is needed. Respiratory therapy personnel and the nutritional support team should be included in parent teaching. Many larger communities have special follow-up clinics for cystic fibrosis patients that may be used to ensure continuity and coordination of care after discharge.

Immediate stabilization of the child with meconium ileus requires decompression with gastric suction and the correction of fluid and electrolyte imbalances. Hydration is particularly important in patients being treated medically with hyperosmolar enemas. Fluids drawn into the intestinal lumen to allow softening and evacuation of the meconium are by default removed from the effective circulation, thus placing the infant at risk for severe hypovolemia and vascular collapse. The extracted fluids should be replaced accordingly. Generally, 4 mL of one-half normal saline solution is given for every 1 mL of retained enema. Fluids and suction are continued until the meconium is evacuated and the clinical manifestations of obstruction resolve. When intestinal function is deemed adequate, elemental formula feedings may be started, together with a pancreatic enzyme if CF is present. If the obstruction is not relieved, decompression, fluids, and electrolytes are continued until surgical treatment can be carried out. Postoperatively, ostomy care becomes a part of nursing management, along with assistance in providing pulmonary toilet. The infant's respiratory status should be monitored closely. If adhesions secondary to meconium peritonitis or surgical manipulation are noted or if the meconium is incompletely removed, signs of obstruction may recur. These signs of persistent or recurrent obstruction must be reported immediately to allow early intervention and reoperation as needed. Feedings are delayed until the obstruction is relieved, the ileostomy is functioning, and bowel activity has returned. Many of these infants feed quite poorly, however, and total parenteral nutrition may be required for an extended period of time.

Cystic fibrosis is a condition of delayed mortality, with a mean survival of 40 to 50 years (Dodge, Lewis, Stanton, & Wilsher, 2007). At this age, death comes as a result of obstructive pulmonary disease and infection. The intervening period is marked by poor growth and chronic respiratory and GI dysfunction. One year survival in simple and complex meconium ileus is 92% and 89%, respectively (Hajivassiliou, 2003).

Meconium Plug

■ Anatomy. Meconium plug syndrome is a condition in which intestinal obstruction (generally of the lower colon and rectum) occurs as the result of unusually thick meconium in the absence of demonstrable enzymatic deficiency. The signs are low intestinal obstruction with failure to stool, followed by abdominal distention and bilious vomiting. Hyperactive bowel sounds are often noted on auscultation, and normal sphincter tone is generally felt on rectal examination. The meconium plug and flatus are often passed after digital examination or contrast enema (Keckler et al., 2008).

■ Pathophysiology. The syndrome is most likely the result of abnormal gut motility associated with immaturity or hypotonia. Ganglion deficiency associated with Hirschsprung disease is found in approximately 13% of patients (Keckler et al., 2008). The plug is formed primarily from mucus and secretions and therefore appears yellowish white and is gelatinous in consistency, lacking the usual flow properties of normal meconium.

Premature infants are especially prone to meconium plug syndrome; however, the condition may also be found in hypotonic infants with central nervous system damage and in some infants of diabetic mothers. In the latter case, meconium plug syndrome is considered to be a variant of small left colon syndrome. Treatment of the mother with magnesium sulfate is an additional risk factor that has been noted by some clinicians. Meconium plugs are found in about 1 of every 500 to 1,000 newborns (Loening-Baucke & Kimura, 1999).

■ Treatment. Plain radiographs with a low intestinal obstruction with multiple distended loops of proximal bowel indicate a number of possible conditions, including jejunoileal atresia, meconium ileus, Hirschsprung disease, small left colon syndrome, or meconium plug syndrome. On barium enema examination, the colon is generally described as being of normal caliber with no evidence of microcolon, thus eliminating the diagnosis of jejunoileal atresia or meconium ileus. The presence of normal ganglion cells on rectal biopsy removes Hirschsprung disease from the differential diagnosis.

Small enemas of warm saline, meglumine diatrizoate, or acetylcysteine are usually all that are needed to dislodge the obstructing meconium plug if it has not already been expelled following rectal examination. Normal stooling patterns should follow. Surgical intervention is rarely needed (Loening-Baucke & Kimura, 1999).

Decompression, hydration, and electrolyte balance are the immediate concerns. Once the plug is evacuated, symptoms have resolved, and normal intestinal function has returned, feedings can be started. Complete recovery should follow. If continued stooling problems occur, infants should be evaluated for Hirchsprung disease.

Anorectal Agenesis

■ Anatomy. Anorectal agenesis (imperforate anus) refers to a group of congenital malformations that involve the anus or rectum or the junction between the two structures. If the urorectal septum deviates during its growth, the cloaca is abnormally or incompletely partitioned, thus resulting in rectal stenosis or atresia. Rectourethral and rectovaginal fistulas occur in 95% of patients with these defects. If the anal membrane fails to rupture, the result is a membranous anal atresia.

For intervention and long-term outcome predictions, defects should be classified according to anatomical location. For ease of understanding they are generally classified into four major types. Presenting signs and symptoms vary slightly with the particular type of defect present. For the majority (those with type III agenesis), the anus is clearly imperforate. With the high incidence of fistulas, meconium may be passed in the urine (in males), or its presence may be noted at the vaginal outlet (in females). With anal stenosis (type I), the anus and rectal vaults are patent but narrowed so that the pasty stools of the newborn may be passed. The stenosis is generally suspected by the microscopic appearance of the anus and is confirmed on rectal examination. With the remaining two types, the anus may appear misleadingly normal on first inspection. In the membranous type (type II), the anal membrane may become visible within 24 to 48 hours as meconium bulges from beneath the thin epithelial covering, but by then the signs of low intestinal obstruction (distention, bilious vomiting, and failure to pass stool) are also becoming apparent. The atretic type (type IV) is rare and generally presents with the full-blown manifestations of obstruction.

■ Pathophysiology. Anorectal agenesis occurs in 1 of every 5,000 live births with a slight male predominance. Greater than 50% of all affected infants have an associated anomaly (Berseth & Poenaru, 2005c). The incidence increases to 1 in 100 for siblings of affected individuals. The cause of deviated or arrested anorectal development is not known, but both environmental and genetic factors are involved. Considering its common origin from the cloaca, it is not surprising that genitourinary tract abnormalities are found most frequently (20%–50%). Congenital heart disease (10%) and EA (5%) are also reported occasionally, and when the latter is found, the VATER and VACTERL associations should be considered. Twenty-five percent of affected patients will have a tethered cord (Barksdale et al., 2011).

■ Treatment. The treatment of anorectal anomalies varies with the nature of the defect. The higher the lesion, the more technically complicated the repair becomes. Reconstruction can be done using a posterior sagittal or laparoscopic approach. Laparoscopy minimizes trauma to surrounding tissue, but a recent review of the literature found no clear advantage to one approach over the other in terms of functional outcome (Bischoff, Levitt, & Pena 2011; Sydorak & Albanese, 2002). The specific technique used should be based on the anatomical location of the defect. Careful perineal examination is generally diagnostic. In the presence of a fistula, the urine may also be examined for meconium epithelial cells.

An inverted lateral radiograph (upside-down Wangensteen–Rice technique) or cross-table prone film may demonstrate air collected in the blind-ending upper rectal pouch, but is generally unreliable for determining the level of obstruction, secondary to the considerable time required for swallowed air to reach this portion of the gut. Even when sufficient time is given, air may be prevented by meconium from reaching the end of the pouch. If a fistula is present, air may be seen in the bladder or vagina on the plain film. An abdominal ultrasound, echocardiogram, and skeletal films are needed to rule out associated defects.

The treatment of anal stenosis (type I defect) consists of repeated dilation using Hegar dilators. If the infant is otherwise stable and the anus is sufficiently enlarged, the patient is discharged with daily digital dilation (using the little finger) to be performed by the parents. Membranous defects (type II) require minimal surgical therapy. The membrane is simply punctured with a hemostat or excised using a scalpel. Repeated dilation is performed as needed.

Low agenesis (translevator, type III lesion) is corrected by perineal anoplasty. After locating the position of the superficial external sphincter using a nerve stimulator, the rectal pouch is brought down through the sphincter to the opening on the anal skin. The fistulous connection, if present, is removed. Gentle irrigations help facilitate stooling and keep the anastomotic site clean until daily dilations can be started, generally between 10 and 14 days postoperatively.

High agenesis (intermediate or high supralevator, type III lesions) and atresia (supralevator, type IV lesions) generally are treated in two phases. The first step is immediate placement of a colostomy for decompression and diversion of fecal contents. If present, the urethrorectal fistula is generally closed or excised to avoid "spill-over" fecal contamination with resultant urinary tract infection. The definitive repair is generally delayed 3 to 12 months to allow growth and pelvic enlargement. At that time, an abdominal-perineal pull-through procedure is performed in which the rectal pouch is literally pulled through the levator sling and anchored to the skin. The colostomy is left intact until healing is complete.

Nonemergent cases (typically stenosis) usually require little in the way of stabilization other than replacement and correction of fluid and electrolyte imbalance. If a fistula is present, these infants are at risk for the development of hyperchloremic acidosis as a result of the absorption of urine from the colon. Gastric suction for decompression is instituted prophylactically (in the case of agenesis when the defect is obvious on inspection) or therapeutically (when membranous and atretic types begin to display symptoms of obstruction).

Postoperatively, wound care and monitoring for postoperative complications are added to the regimen. If anoplasty is performed, the site should be inspected (as allowed by the surgical team) for mucosal prolapse, which may occur if there is inadequate sphincter preservation. Mineral oil may be used to clean meconium gently from the anal area. A colostomy placed for higher defects should receive the standard care and monitoring. The surgeon initially carries out dilatory procedures, but when digital dilation becomes possible, the nurse may assume this task, making sure to provide bedside parent teaching. Throughout recuperation, the urine (or vaginal outlet) should be closely observed for the presence of meconium, which would indicate a recurrent fistula. If such a fistula is suspected, electrolyte and acid–base status should also be monitored for hyperchloremic acidosis. Otherwise, feeding may begin when the colostomy or anoplasty is sufficiently healed and intestinal function resumes. Stool-softening agents may be required.

The outcome for infants with anorectal anomalies largely depends on the type of defect and on the level of the upper rectal pouch in relation to the puborectal muscle, which is the main muscle of sphincter function and continence. This muscle is a central component of the levator ani muscle, which spans the pelvis much like a sling to support the lower end of the rectum. On radiography, the position of this muscle can be estimated by drawing an imaginary line between the symphysis pubis and the developing coccyx. Based on the relation of the pouch to this pubococcygeal line, anorectal anomalies can be classified into three groups that indicate low, high, or intermediate level defect. In low (translevator) types, the rectum descends through and is surrounded by the puborectalis and levator ani muscles so that the sensorimotor mechanisms are generally intact. With high (supralevator) defects, the rectal pouch ends above the puborectalis and levator ani muscles so that the neurologic and muscular mechanisms of continence may be impaired. In intermediate types (supralevator), the rectum again ends above the puborectalis, but the pouch is cradled in the muscular hammock formed by the levator ani so that neuromuscular function is variable and repair more complicated.

The overall mortality rate is approximately 15%, with death largely a reflection of the nature of the defect and the presence of associated anomalies (Mirza, Ijaz, Saleem, Sharif, & Sheikh, 2011). For survivors, the main criterion for outcome is fecal continence. When anorectal anomalies are reviewed as a whole, 75% of patients can be expected to have good results, with normal anal function and control of defecation (Barksdale et al., 2011).

Intussusception

■ Anatomy. Intussusception is an acquired obstruction in which a part of the intestine prolapses into the lumen of an adjoining distal intestinal segment. This luminal prolapse may occur at any site in the GI tract, but typically there are four varieties: (1) enteric intussusception, in which the small intestine prolapses into itself; (2) colic intussusception, in which the large intestine prolapses into itself; (3) ileocecal intussusception, in which the ileocecal valve is inverted and pushed into the cecum, pulling a segment of ileum with it; and (4) ileocolic intussusception, in which the ileocecal valve remains in place but the ileum prolapses through it into the colon. Rarely, a retrograde intussusception may occur in which a distal intestinal segment prolapses upward into a proximal part. In the neonate, the majority of cases are of the ileocecal type.

Regardless of the site, the intussusception results in two problems. First, it causes a simple mechanical obstruction as the result of the blockage of the distal intestinal lumen by the prolapsed proximal segment. Second, as the intestinal walls are telescoped into one another, the mucosal blood vessels become compressed, congested, and prone to ischemia or infarction. Thus the symptoms of intussusception typically include vomiting, colicky pain, and bloody stools or red "currant jelly" stools. In premature infants, however, intussusception can mimic signs of NEC and go unnoticed initially. These infants are typically not as unstable as infants with NEC until intestinal perforation has occurred.

■ Pathophysiology. Although intussusception in the neonatal period is rare, representing only 3% of all intestinal obstructions, it is the most common cause of intestinal obstruction in children. It can present at any age but typically presents between 3 months and 9 months of age, peaking around 6 months. Incidence is 2 to 5 per 100,000 births in the first 2 months of life (Tate et al., 2008; N. L. Wang et al., 1998). Intussusception is an acquired condition and therefore not easily explained by any one causative factor. A small proportion of cases appear to have a "lead point," a demonstrable anatomic lesion or defect that may have been the cause of intussusception. Such lead points may include Meckel's diverticula, duplication defects, polyps, hematomas, and lymphomas. The viscid stool common in cystic fibrosis may even be a potential cause. Most cases of intussusception are idiopathic; however, there is often a history of preceding upper respiratory infection or gastroenteritis, especially adenovirus. The role played by infection in the phenomenon of intussusception has not yet been determined. The inflammatory response of the intestine to infection may possibly cause an abnormal hyperplasia of lymphoid tissue. The hyperplastic site might then serve as a lead point for intussusception.

■ Treatment. Plain radiographs may not be helpful in the diagnosis, with 20% to 30% showing only a general picture of intestinal obstruction with dilated proximal loops and an airless distal bowel. On ultrasonography, the affected area often appears as a "doughnut sign" on cross section. Definitive diagnosis is by barium enema, with the contrast media outlining the gut and ending proximally in a characteristic "coiled-spring" pattern. In older children and adults, an attempt is first made to reduce the intussusception by using the hydrostatic pressure produced by a barium enema. Barium is injected into the rectum and allowed to flow distally until the "coiled-spring" pattern appears. A balloon-tipped catheter is then inserted into the rectum. The balloon is inflated with air, and gentle traction is applied until the balloon is pulled back against the muscular sling of the levatores, thus preventing any outflow of barium. The administration of barium is restarted, which causes the intraluminal pressure to rise slowly as more and more contrast medium is added without an avenue for escape. The pressure is maintained until the intussusception is pushed distally and freed. If the intussusception is fully reduced, the barium is seen suddenly to flow freely into the proximal bowel, and the clinical status of the patient should immediately improve. Unfortunately, in infants, full reduction is generally not accomplished, and surgical reduction is required.

Surgical intervention involves a manual reduction of the intussusception using a "milking" motion on the proximal bowel. The pressure and squeezing are continued until the loop is freed; traction and pulling should never be applied. The bowel is carefully inspected. Any necrotic tissue is removed and lead points are resected.

The major concerns before reduction are sepsis and shock. In light of the strong association with adenovirus and the frequent history of gastroenteritis or respiratory infection, sepsis should be expected. Antibiotic therapy is initiated pending culture results. Fluid lost into the wall of the trapped intestine or blood lost from congested vessels into the lumen of the intestine, or a combination of both, predisposes to shock and should be appropriately managed with fluid resuscitation and volume expansion. Decompression by gastric suction is also recommended.

Postoperative care is fairly routine. Fluids, electrolytes, and decompression are provided as needed. The recurrence risk is more common following hydrostatic reduction (11%–16%) than after surgical reduction (0%–3%) (Niramis et al., 2010). Consequently, even though the intussusception has presumably been resolved, the nurse must be alert for the return of associated signs and symptoms.

The overall mortality for intussusception has declined over the years and is 2.1 per 1 million live births with the peak age of death at 5 months (Desai, Curns, Patel, & Parashar, 2012). The higher mortality in young infants may be related to the lack of classic signs, thereby delaying diagnosis.

NEC

■ Anatomy. NEC is an acquired disorder characterized by hemorrhage, ischemia, and often necrosis of the mucosal and submucosal layers of the intestinal tract. Any portion of the bowel including the entire GI tract can be affected but the disease most often occurs in the ileocecal area. NEC is the most common GI disorder seen in the neonatal intensive care unit (NICU), affecting approximately 7% of infants weighing less than 1,500 g (Holman et al., 2006). NEC not only increases mortality and morbidity, it significantly increases both length of hospitalization and cost of care. Length of hospitalization is prolonged by 22 to 60 days, and hospital costs increased by $73,700 to $186,000 depending on whether the infant requires surgical intervention (Bisquera, Cooper, & Berseth, 2002).

■ Pathophysiology. Age of onset of disease is typically dependent on gestational age, with the more immature infants presenting at a later chronological age (Neu, 2005). Initial symptoms include abdominal distention, increased gastric residuals, emesis, and bloody stools. Nonspecific signs of sepsis are often present, including lethargy, temperature instability, apnea, and poor feeding. Laboratory findings include metabolic and respiratory acidosis, electrolyte abnormalities, neutropenia or neutrophilia, and thrombocytopenia. Infants may become acutely ill with hypotension, respiratory failure, and disseminating intravascular coagulation. Peritonitis may be evident by the presence of erythema, edema, and tenderness of the abdominal wall (Hsueh et al., 2002).

Radiologic evidence includes the presence of pneumotosis intestinalis where gas dissects beneath the serosal and submucosal layers of the intestine. This is appreciated on radiograph as radiolucent linear streaks or small bubbles in the lumen of the intestine. If the gas ruptures into the mesenteric vascular bed, it can distribute through the systemic vessels into the venous system of the liver forming portal venous gas seen as branching vessels in the liver. Finally if the intestines rupture, a pneumoperitonium or gas outside the bowel wall can be seen. Assessment of a pneumoperitonium is often done with a left lateral decubitus radiograph where gas can be appreciated between the liver and the right lateral abdominal wall. Removal of electrode wires, temperature probes, and so forth from the abdomen prior to decubitus radiograph is an important nursing consideration to allow optimal evaluation of the abdomen.

A staging system for NEC developed by Bell in 1978 and later adapted is used to determine the severity of the disease (Walsh & Kliegman, 1986). Stage I consists of nonspecific abdominal symptoms and signs of sepsis. Stage II signifies a more advanced disease with continued nonspecific symptoms and radiographic findings, including pneumotosis intestinalis. Stage III is the most severe stage, with perforation and peritonitis in a critically ill infant.

The etiology and pathogenesis of NEC have been the focus of extensive debate and research for the past 30 years. Historically, the etiology was comprised of hypoxia/hypotension, feeding, and the presence of bacteria. Unfortunately, the etiology is multifactorial and much more complicated. Currently, the most prevalent theory regarding the etiology includes three distinctive events: intestinal mucosal injury, intestinal mucosal inflammation, and pathogenic bacterial colonization of the intestinal tract (Schmolzer et al., 2006).

Initial injury to the intestinal mucosa may be caused by hypoxia, ischemia, intestinal inflammation, and/or bacterial infection (Hsueh et al., 2002). The premature infant is susceptible to intestinal injury due to intestinal immaturity, including decreased motility and absorption and decreased intestinal and systemic immune function (Martin & Walker, 2006).

Intestinal ischemia, enteral feedings (especially formula feedings), and bacterial invasion of the bowel wall can result in intestinal mucosal inflammation and subsequent activation of the inflammatory cascade (Nanthakumar, Fusunyan, Sanderson, & Walker, 2000). This may be particularly important due to the premature infant's overactive inflammatory response (Neu & Walker, 2011). The presence of intestinal inflammation further damages the intestinal wall, potentially causing bacterial translocation (Taylor, Basile, Ebeling, & Wagner, 2009). Bacterial translocation, the passage of pathogenic bacteria across the intestinal barrier, is common in premature infants due to a weakened intestinal barrier and increased intraluminal bacterial overgrowth. Bacterial translocation activates the inflammatory cascade, promoting further damage to the intestinal mucosa (Annand, Leaphart, Mollen, & Hacken, 2007). Activation of the inflammatory cascade results in the release of several important chemical mediators including platelet activating factor, interleukin 1 to 6, tumor necrotizing factor, and NO (Annand et al., 2007; Emani et al., 2009). These chemical mediators cause further damage to intestinal epithelial cells, leading to necrosis and impairment of intestinal integrity (Claud & Walker, 2001).

Colonization of the intestinal tract with pathologic bacteria is also important in the pathogenesis of NEC. Normal intestinal colonization in premature infants is disrupted because of administration of antibiotics, delay of enteral feedings, and exposure to abnormal and antibiotic-resistant organisms (Caicedo, Schanler, Li, & Neu, 2005). Premature infants are therefore colonized with increased numbers of pathogenic bacteria potentially activating the inflammatory cascade resulting in intestinal damage.

Colonization with beneficial bacteria may protect against NEC through prevention of bacterial translocation, promotion of a protective intestinal barrier, and maintenance of intestinal integrity (Emani et al., 2009). An association between NEC and infective agents is supported by the epidemic nature of NEC, especially during times of nursery crowding (Berseth & Poenaru, 2005b).

Although NEC occasionally presents in term infants, prematurity is by far the predominate risk factor partly due to immaturity of the GI and immune system. Ninety percent of infants affected with NEC are born prematurely, and the incidence is inversely related to gestational age and birth weight (Fanaroff et al., 2007; Maayan-Metzger, Itzchak, Mazkereth, & Kuint, 2004). GI immaturity decreases intestinal motility and absorption of nutrients (Boston, 2006). Impaired intestinal motility prevents movement of feeds through the intestinal tract, resulting in stasis and possible bacterial overgrowth (Neu, 2007). Impaired nutritional absorption can cause carbohydrate fermentations, leading to gaseous intestinal distention which can damage the intestinal epithelium and promote bacterial invasion of the intestinal wall (Kliegman, 2003). Premature infants also have an immature immune system as evidenced by deficient antibacterial properties and altered immune cellular production that may predispose them to sepsis and NEC (Emani et al., 2009). Feeding, especially formula feeding, and intrauterine growth are also risks, in addition to other less well established factors (Manogura et al., 2008).

NEC is associated with significant increases in both mortality and morbidity. The mortality rate for NEC is estimated to be 30%, with those infants undergoing surgical therapy having the highest rate of mortality (Fitzgibbons et al., 2009). Other poor prognostic indicators include persistent acidosis, severe pneumatosis intestinalis, and presence of portal venous gas (Berseth & Poenaru, 2005b). Intestinal strictures (mostly colonic) occur in approximately 10% to 30% of survivors due to structural changes in nonperforated, healed ischemic sites (Yeh, Chang, & Kao, 2004). Surgical resection of the stricture is required to optimize bowel motility. When extensive resection of the intestines is necessary, infants have severe complications related to SBS. Survivors of NEC have also been shown to have an increased risk of neurodevelopmental delay (Bedrick, 2004).

■ **Treatment.** Medical management of NEC includes discontinuation of all enteral nutrition and decompression of the stomach by low intermittent suction through a large-bore orogastric tube. Close monitoring and adjustment of fluids and electrolytes is imperative, with infants often requiring additional fluids due to loss of fluid through the damaged intestinal wall. Total parenteral nutrition should be initiated as soon as possible, and a central venous line inserted when the infant has negative blood cultures. Serial abdominal radiographs should be ordered every 6 to 8 hours during the acute phase of the illness to monitor progression of the disease and to evaluate for intestinal perforation. Broad spectrum antibiotic therapy should be initiated after blood cultures have been obtained and continued for 7 to 14 days. An antifungal should also be added if perforation is highly suspected or confirmed on radiograph. Antibiotics effective against anaerobic bacteria should be added if intestinal perforation, intestinal necrosis, or severe disease is present (Berman & Moss, 2011).

Further management is highly dependent on the severity of the illness as progression of the disease can rapidly occur. Critically ill infants may require intubation and ventilation, management of acid–base derangements, and vasopressors to maintain blood pressure and perfusion. Intubation and ventilation are frequently required for severe apnea and increasing respiratory distress due to compression of the diaphragm from the distended abdomen. Infants may require frequent blood gas monitoring to evaluate oxygen and acid–base status. Administration of sodium bicarbonate may be indicated for metabolic acidosis. Hematologic studies should be performed to assess for anemia, thrombocytopenia, and abnormal coagulation. Platelets, packed red blood cells, fresh frozen plasma, and cryoprecipitate should be administered as indicated.

Surgical intervention is required in approximately 25% to 50% of infants affected with NEC (Sharma et al., 2006). Criteria for surgery are somewhat controversial and are often dependent on individual surgeon preference and institution familiarity. Absolute indications are pneumoperitoneum or confirmation of intestinal gangrene by positive paracentesis. Nonspecific but supportive findings of clinical deterioration include metabolic acidosis, respiratory failure, thrombocytopenia, white blood cell abnormalities, oliguria, portal venous air, erythema of the abdominal wall, or a persistently dilated and fixed loop of bowel in spite of vigorous clinical management.

Currently, surgical intervention performed on infants with NEC includes laporatomy or placement of a peritoneal drain (Berman & Moss, 2011). During a laparotomy, resection of necrotic bowel is performed, and the ends of the ligated intestines are brought to the surface to create an ostomy. If the viability of extensive portions of the intestine is uncertain, resection may be deferred, with a subsequent operation in 24 to 48 hours to assess the overall intestinal viability.

Placement of a peritoneal drain can be used as either a temporary or definitive treatment. Placement involves making a right lower quadrant incision under local anesthesia and the insertion of a Penrose drain. Peritoneal drains are less invasive and do not require general anesthesia (Berman & Moss, 2011). The outcome of peritoneal drain placement for treatment of NEC is controversial. While some studies have shown no difference in mortality or short-term complications (Rees et al., 2008), others show an increased mortality and long-term morbidity in infants treated with a peritoneal drain (Sola, Tepas, & Koniaris, 2010). In addition, infants often ultimately require a laparotomy even after placement of the peritoneal drain.

Postoperatively, the infant may continue to require ongoing fluid resuscitation, blood pressure, and respiratory support. Feedings are generally reinitiated after bowel function has recovered; however, this may be significantly delayed in infants with significant intestinal resection. See section on SBS for additional information. Following initiation, feedings are gradually and carefully advanced, depending on tolerance of feeds and if a stoma is present, amount of ostomy output.

Due to the poorly understood pathophysiology of NEC, few advances have been made in our ability to prevent this devastating disease. Few measures have consistently been shown to decrease the incidence of NEC. Antenatal steroids have been associated with a decrease in the risk of NEC through enhancement of intestinal maturation, improved intestinal mucosal function, promotion of less pathogenic intestinal colonization, and reduction of bacterial translocation (Roberts & Dalziel, 2006; Shulman et al., 1998). Several studies have reported an association between human milk feedings and a decreased incidence and severity of NEC (Sisk, Lovelady, Dillard, Gruber, & O'Shea, 2007). These protective effects appear to be dose-dependent, with infants receiving a greater proportion of breast milk demonstrating the lowest incidence of NEC (Meinzen-Derr et al., 2009).

Recently there has been considerable interest in the prophylactic use of probiotics to decrease the incidence of NEC. Probiotics may limit the number of intestinal pathogenic bacteria through competition for binding sites and nutrition, production of an acidic environment, and fortification of the intestinal mucosal barrier (Mattar, Drongowski, Coran, & Hartmon, 2001). Probiotics may also enhance intestinal mobility and maturation, alleviate intestinal inflammation, and produce specific protective agents such as arginine, glutamine, and short-chain fatty acids (Schanler, 2006).

Administration of probiotics has been shown in infants to reduce the incidence and severity of NEC (Alfaleh, Anabrees, Bassler, & Al-Kharfi, 2011; Deshpande, Rao, Patole, & Bulsara, 2010). While some feel sufficient evidence exists to support the routine use of probiotics in premature infants, others feel additional research is necessary to determine optimal dose, most appropriate strain for use, frequency of dose, and length of treatment. Additional studies to determine the incidence of complications are also necessary.

Nurses, as the main caregivers of premature infants in the NICU, are often the first to recognize the early symptoms of NEC, including abdominal distention, subtle signs of sepsis, and emesis. Following a diagnosis of NEC, circulatory status must be evaluated frequently by monitoring perfusion, vital signs, and urinary output. Gentle reexamination of the abdomen should be carried out every 6 to 8 hours for the first 48 to 72 hours to evaluate for progression of the disease and presence of tenderness, increased distention, or erythema possibly indicating peritonitis.

OTHER GI DISORDERS

The majority of GI disorders are categorized as problems of ingestion, digestion, or elimination. Additional disorders that overlap or do not fit these categories are presented, including short-bowel or short-gut syndrome, spontaneous bowel and gastric perforation, peptic ulcer, umbilical hernia, and lactobezoars.

Short-Bowel Syndrome

■ **Anatomy.** SBS (short-gut) is an unfortunate complication of many neonatal surgeries that involve extensive resection of the GI tract. SBS can be defined by residual length of bowel, serum citrulline level, or need for parenteral nutrition greater than 3 months. No matter how it is defined, SBS is characterized by malabsorption, diarrhea, and failure to thrive. The loss of considerable absorptive surface results in a complex malabsorptive problem with episodic diarrhea, steatorrhea, and dehydration. If allowed to progress, metabolic derangements and ultimately poor growth and development may occur. In the presence of SBS, the prolonged hospitalizations of even 1 to 2 years may not be unusual. The duration of initial hospitalization and length of dependence on parenteral nutrition are both inversely related to the length of bowel that remains after resection. The median length of small intestine in a term infant is 250 cm (Barksdale et al., 2011). Infants with as little as 10 cm and an intact ileocecal valve have survived. If the ileocecal valve is removed, then a minimum of 25 cm is necessary. The ileocecal valve delays transit time and allows for increased digestion and absorption. Additionally, it acts as a barrier to prevent overgrowth of colonic bacteria in the small intestine (Lilja, Finkel, Paulsson, & Lucas, 2011).

■ **Pathophysiology.** SBS is a complication of surgeries involving extensive resection of the GI tract, from disease processes such as NEC, gastroschisis, megacystic microcolon, intestinal atresia, Hirschsprung disease, and volvulus. Congenital short bowel is extremely rare, but has been reported in about 30 patients (Hasosah, Lemberg, Skarsgard, & Schreiber, 2008; S. T. Hwang & Shulman, 2002). Overall incidence of SBS is 21 per 1,000 NICU admissions and 24.5 per 100,000 live births. Incidence is higher is preterm infants (Wales et al., 2004).

Most infants eventually experience progressive small bowel adaptation especially in the premature infant as the small bowel normally doubles in size during the third trimester (Gutierrez, Kang, & Jaksic, 2011). Bowel adaptation begins within 48 hours of resection and continues for 12 to 18 months. As the surgically shortened intestine grows the mucosal wall hypertrophies and the villi become hyperplastic so that the absorptive area is increased. Enteral feeds assist in this process. Blood flow to the residual intestine and the proportion of the villus that is enzymatically active are both initially increased but gradually decline as the surface area and length continue to increase with time (Bhatia, Gates, & Parish, 2010; Neu & Bernstein, 2002). However, completely normal absorption may never be achieved in cases of extensive resection in which less than 75 cm of the bowel remains, especially if the ileocecal valve is removed.

In addition, strategies to avoid intestinal failure-associated liver disease (ILFAD) and catheter-related infections must be instituted to improve morbidity and mortality. The duration of initial hospitalization and length of dependence on parenteral nutrition are both inversely related to the length of remaining bowel (S. T. Hwang & Shulman, 2002).

■ **Treatment.** Treatment of SBS is challenging. Infants postoperatively often fail to tolerate even small amounts of enteral nutrition and exhibit diarrhea and malabsorption as intestinal adaptation is a lengthy process. Parenteral nutrition is initiated soon after surgery and continues throughout the period of refeeding. Elemental formula is often required usually by continuous infusion and is very gradually increased. Small oral feeds should be introduced to prevent oral aversion. Refeeding ostomy drainage into the distal bowel has been shown to improve weight gain and decrease parenteral nutrition usage (Gardner, Walton, & Chessell, 2003). Medications such as loperamide, diphenoxylate, phenothiazines, ocreotide, and dietary fiber have been used in individual patients to help control diarrhea. Cholestyramine may be used to help bind bile acid and thereby decrease diarrhea. Trimethoprim-sulfamethoxazole and metronidazole are used in the treatment of bacterial overgrowth. New intralipid preparations with omega 3 fatty acids to prevent ILFAD are being investigated. Gastroenterology consultation is essential for guidance in feeding practices, medication therapies, vitamin supplementation, and referral for transplantation if needed.

Infants who show no adaptive response after months of feeding attempts may have radical surgery to slow intestinal transit (e.g., intestinal valves, reversed segment, colon interposition, intestinal pacing, intestinal lengthening, tapering enteroplasty, or neomucosa). Small-bowel transplantation presents a lifesaving option for these patients. Results of intestinal transplantation continue to improve, with survival rates of 85% at 1 year to 42% by 10 years posttransplant (Abu-Elmagd et al., 2009).

Nursing care of the infant with SBS includes collaborative management with team members to monitor fluid, electrolyte, acid–base balance, and nutritional status. Prevention of skin breakdown due to diarrhea and infection are critical. Parents must be involved in their infants' care, and every effort must be made to stimulate normal growth and development.

Infant survival after massive bowel resection is related to the maturity of the infant at the time of resection, length of the remaining intestine, presence of distal small intestine, presence of the ileocecal valve, presence of an intact colon, intactness of pancreatic and liver function, and absence of other complicating congenital anomalies. Patients with SBS with chronic dependence on total parenteral nutrition (TPN) usually have poor quality of life and numerous readmissions for abdominal surgeries, central venous catheter-related infections, dislodgement of central line catheters and/or feeding tubes, wound infections and dehiscence, developmental delay, and TPN-associated liver failure.

Gastric Perforations

■ **Anatomy.** Gastric perforations result in free air into the peritoneum. The infant becomes symptomatic usually in the first week of life, most commonly on the third or fourth day. There is marked abdominal distention that is tender to the touch and respiratory distress that worsens as the distention increases. There may or may not be vomiting. If the perforation has progressed, hypovolemic shock is possible. This condition is considered a neonatal surgical emergency.

■ **Pathophysiology.** Gastric perforations classified as traumatic, ischemic, or spontaneous are the most common cause of pneumopertioneum in the first week of life. Incidence is 1 per 2,900 live births, and mortality has been reported to be as high as 62% and 26% in preterm and term infants, respectively. Etiology is unknown but has been associated with prematurity, perinatal stress, NEC, bowel ischemia, invasive procedures such as gastric intubation or nasogastric tube placement, and steroid therapy. Isolated intestinal perforation is seen in very-low-birth-weight infants, usually before feedings have been initiated, associated with patent ductus arteriosus and indomethacin therapy. Although indomethacin has been minimally associated with isolated bowel perforation, the incidence markedly increases when coupled with stress doses of glucocorticoids (Clyman, 2005). Premature infants do not have pneumatosis intestinalis, but develop a distended abdomen with blue-gray discoloration from the perforation. These infants usually have better outcomes than infants with perforation caused by NEC (Neu & Bernstein, 2002).

■ **Treatment.** Radiographic studies will confirm perforations with the presence of free air. The initial treatment is abdominal decompression by paracentesis. Fluid resuscitation, insertion of a nasogastric tube for decompression, and broad-spectrum antibiotic administration are required. Surgery is performed to remove any torn tissue and to close the perforation.

Postoperative care centers on maintenance of fluids and electrolytes, blood volume, gastric suction, and broad-spectrum antibiotics. The prognosis is directly related to how quickly the situation is recognized, the age of the infant (maturity), and the severity of the perforation. Early recognition and treatment are associated with high survival rates (Jawad et al., 2002).

Peptic Ulcer

■ **Anatomy.** Ulceration may occur in the gastric or duodenal mucosa. Ulcers are rare in newborns and are usually related to underlying systemic disorders.

■ **Pathophysiology.** The cause of ulcers in newborns is probably multifactorial, including genetic, dietary, and environmental factors; the amount of hydrochloric acid; and local tissue resistance. Drugs such as indomethacin or conditions such as acidosis and shock may precipitate mucosal destruction and ulcer formation (Berseth & Poenaru, 2005c).

■ **Treatment.** Bloody emesis may be acute with considerable blood loss, or there may be gradual bleeding seen as "coffee ground" emesis or occult blood in the stools. Fibroscopic endoscopy is effective in diagnosing gastric ulcers.

The treatment is aimed at prompt replacement of blood loss. A normal saline lavage is used to evacuate bloody residue. Antacids and/or histamine H_2 receptor antagonists are administered for up to 6 to 8 weeks. Sucralfate has been effective when used for a short term after gastric bleeding (Zenk et al., 2003). Feedings can be resumed after 24 hours if there is no further bleeding (Berseth & Poenaru, 2005c).

Umbilical Hernia

■ **Anatomy.** Umbilical hernias are an outpouching of intestines through the umbilical ring. The defect size ranges from 1 to 4 cm in diameter (Berseth & Poenaru, 2005a).

■ **Pathophysiology.** Umbilical hernias occur because of failure of closure of the umbilical ring. The hernia contains a loop of bowel that is easily reduced. The occurrence rate is 10% to 30% in White children increasing to as high as 85% in African American children and low-birth-weight infants. It is more common in low-birth-weight infants and infants with Down syndrome. There is a familial association. Approximately 90% of hernias spontaneously close by 3 to 4 years of age (Zendejas et al., 2011).

■ **Treatment.** In the absence of clinical symptoms, no treatment is necessary. Surgical closure is indicated in large defects in children more than 4 years of age or when there are signs of incarceration.

Lactobezoars

■ **Anatomy.** Lactobezoars are a mixture of undigested milk curds and mucus that form a compact mass usually in the stomach. Thought to be an adverse effect of high-caloric feedings or use of casein protein, lactobezoars have been reported in infants receiving breast milk and older children. They are firm balls of fat that form in the infant's intestinal tract about 3 to 12 days after enteral feedings have started (Dubose, Southgate, & Hill, 2001; Singer, 1988; Usmann & Levenbrown, 1989). The most common symptoms are those associated with an intestinal obstruction including abdominal distention, vomiting, diarrhea, and increasing gastric aspirates. The infant may or may not have guaiac-positive stools, depending on how long the bezoar has been present and the amount of pressure it is exerting on the intestinal wall.

■ **Pathophysiology.** Prematurity, low birth weight, and the introduction of high-calorie, highly dense formulas are the most common risk factors. They may be secondary to delayed gastric emptying, but in most cases there is no known etiology.

■ **Treatment.** The diagnosis can be made either by palpation of a firm ball or mass usually in the upper left quadrant or by radiographic studies. Contrast studies following injection of a small amount of air into the gastric area can also help with the diagnostic evaluation, as the mass will appear on a radiograph (Barksdale et al., 2011).

The treatment is aimed at relief of the intestinal obstruction and usually involves discontinuing feeds for 24 to 48 hours and initiating gastric lavage. Gastric decompression may or may not be needed to relieve the distention. Although rare, the patient should be evaluated for the possibility of gastric perforation. The prognosis is good and most cases resolve with minimal complications.

SUPPORT OF FAMILY WITH AN INFANT WITH A GI SYSTEM DISORDER

The birth of an infant with a congenital anomaly or who is acutely ill elicits feelings of loss, guilt, and confusion for parents. Nurses and other health professionals must expect grief reactions and be prepared to help the family cope with the crisis. Strategies to cope include support for early contact between parents and infant and open lines of communication to provide factual information of the infant's condition and plan of care. Health care providers also need to patiently reinforce information on an ongoing basis as the family begins to process and accept the diagnosis. Understanding of the disease process is essential for parents to cope with the prognosis and ongoing health care needs. Encourage the parents to hold their infants; to provide skin-to-skin (kangaroo care) as early as possible. Encourage them to express their concerns before they are discharged home.

SUMMARY

The GI system is vital to human growth and development and ultimately long-term survival. The vast majority of conditions that cause GI dysfunction in the infant are the result of congenital anatomic malformations. Additionally, any condition or situation that leads to ischemia and bacterial overgrowth places an infant at risk of NEC and resultant long-term sequelae. The input and support of a variety of nursing, medical, and other specialists are required for optimal outcomes of the infant's physiologic well-being and the parents' psychosocial stability. The major purposes of this chapter were to present the embryologic development of the GI tract and resultant anatomic structure and to describe common causes of neonatal dysfunction with implications for care.

CASE STUDY

Identification of the Problem. An 18-day-old, 38-week gestation male infant who presented to the ER with history of poor feeding, poor stooling pattern, abdominal distention, listlessness. He was admitted with a diagnosis of failure to thrive and had an orogastric tube placed and Pedialyte started. He was transferred to a tertiary care NICU for inability to establish IV access.

Assessment: History and Physical Examination

- 38-week gestation male infant born by NSVD (normal spontaneous vaginal delivery) to a 28-year-old, G4, P3003 mother who had an unremarkable pregnancy. Serologies negative, BW 3,220 g and Apgar scores of 8 at 1 minute and 9 at 5 minutes of life.
- At birth admission infant required observation in the hospital for failure to stool. A contrast enema on DOL 2 showed movable stool in the colon and no anatomical problems. He was discharged to home on DOL 4 after passing two stools.
- On DOL 16 his mother brought him to the hospital because he was irritable, lethargic, and feeding poorly. He was evaluated and sent home.
- On DOL 18 he presented to the ER with listlessness and abdominal distention and was admitted for failure to thrive. Weight at admission was 2,930 g. Unable to secure IV access, he was transferred to an NICU.
- Vital signs: Temp 37, HR 147, RR (respiratory rate) 40, BP 86/55 67, CRT 2 seconds, abd girth 36 cm

Physical examination on admission to the NICU:

- GENERAL: irritable active infant with good perfusion, slightly pale, OG tube in place
- HEENT: anterior fontanel soft, flat with sutures approximated, eyes clear with + red reflex
- CV: RRR, no murmur noted, pulses 2+ and equal
- RESP: on room air with bilateral clear breath sounds
- ABD: grossly distended, tender to the touch, BS audible, anus is patent and normally placed
- GU: normal male genitalia
- NEURO: lethargic, irritable

Evaluation after transfer to NICU included lab work with electrolytes, CBC/diff, C-reactive protein (CRP), blood culture. Peripheral IV placed and parenteral nutrition and antibiotics were started. A Replogle tube was placed to low constant wall suction.

Differential Diagnosis

- Hirschsprung disease
- Jejunoileal atresia
- Meconium ileus
- Meconium plug syndrome
- Small left colon syndrome

Diagnostic Tests

Laboratory tests:

- CBC/differential: WBC 7.5, segmented cells 10, bands 24, hematocrit 45, platelet 326,000/mm^3
- CRP: 11.7
- Electrolytes WNL
- Blood cultures remained negative

Imaging tests:

- Contrast enema DOL 2: showed movable stool in the colon and no anatomical problems
- Abdominal radiographs: revealed extremely gaseous, distended bowel with no air in the rectum
- Contrast enema (repeated secondary to no rectal air): normal caliber colon with a transition zone noted at the level of the mid- to distal descending colon
- Rectal biopsy: absence of ganglion cells

Hirschsprung disease presents similarly to jejunoileal atresia, meconium ileus, meconium plug syndrome, and small left colon syndrome. A contrast enema can be helpful in diagnosing the disease by determining the caliber of the colon. Microcolon is typically seen with jejunoileal atresia and meconium ileus. Normal or enlarged colon is seen with Hirschsprung disease, meconium plug, and small left colon syndrome. Retention of contrast material 24 hours after exam is suggestive of Hirschsprung disease. Final diagnosis can be made by rectal biopsy through the anus with histologic examination of the specimen. Absence of ganglion cells in the submucosa confirms the diagnosis of Hirschsprung disease.

Working Diagnosis

- Term infant with Hirschsprung disease: based on absence of ganglion cells
- Colitis due to tender abdomen
- Clinical sepsis due to elevated CRP, shifted CBC, and lethargy

Development of Management Plan

- Gastric decompression
- Maintenance fluid support
- Continuous monitoring of vital signs and abdominal girths every 6 hours
- Antibiotics
- Surgical consult

Implementation and Evaluation of Effectiveness

Implementation of management plan:

- Gastric decompression was initiated immediately
- IV access was obtained on admission
- Parenteral nutrition started for total fluid volume ~140 mL/kg/d to 150 mL/kg/d, 3 g/kg/d of AA, IL at 3 g/kg/d
- Labs work sent for sepsis w/u and electrolytes
- Ampicillin, gentamicin, and flagyl were started
- Abdominal radiograph was obtained

- Electrolytes were obtained daily until stable, then every 2 to 3 days
- CBC/diff obtained daily until WNL, then PRN
- Pediatric surgery consulted and performed normal saline enemas until surgery could be performed
- After diagnostic workup complete decision made to attempt colon endorectal pull-through, although family was informed that a colostomy may be necessary if sequential histologic examinations made during surgery showed higher colonic involvement
- Social work services consulted to provide support to family

Effectiveness of management plan:

- Abdominal girth improved within 2 hours
- A laparoscopic subtotal protocolectomy–right colon endorectal pull-through was successfully performed
- Ventilated 3 days postoperatively and then successfully extubated to room air
- Ampicillin and gentamicin were discontinued postoperatively
- Treated with rocephin and flagyl for 5 days postop and will be discharged home on flagyl for 1 to 2 months
- Pain was controlled with morphine and Ativan prn
- Parenteral nutrition was provided at 140 mL/kg/d with 3 g/kg/d protein and intralipids at 3 g/kg/d
- Enteral feeds were begun on the fifth postoperative day and advanced slowly with full feeds reached in 4 days.

■ **Outcome.** He was discharged to home in room air, on full feedings, and Flagyl. Follow-up was with his pediatrician in 1 week and pediatric surgeon in 2 weeks after discharge.

EVIDENCE-BASED PRACTICE BOX

NEC is an acquired disorder characterized by hemorrhage, ischemia, and often necrosis of the mucosal and submucosal layers of the intestinal tract. NEC is the most common GI disorder seen in the NICU, affecting approximately 7% of infants weighing less than 1,500 g (Holman et al., 2006). NEC not only increases mortality and morbidity, it significantly increases both length of hospitalization and cost of care. The etiology and pathogenesis of NEC as well as potential preventative strategies have been the focus of extensive debate and research for the past 30 years. One area of research that has garnered significant attention in the last several years has been the use of probiotics.

Probiotics, living nonpathogenic organisms introduced into the GI tract, are believed to enhance intestinal mucus function, increase anti-inflammatory cytokines, and decrease pathogenic overgrowth by competing for binding sites. A recent meta-analysis by Q. Wang, Dong, and Zhu (2012) of 20 original randomized controlled trials stated that the use of probiotics was beneficial in reducing the incidence and severity of NEC. A total of 3,816 patients less than 34 weeks gestation and less than 1,500 g were included in the review. Based on this review, many researchers believe the widespread use of probiotics should be instituted. Other researchers, however, are more cautious, as these studies used varying strains and doses of probiotics. Additional concerns regarding long-term effects on development, cross contamination in the nursery, the potential to change the normal pathologic flora of NICUs, and the possibility of sepsis with the introduction of live organisms into immunocompromised patients have also been raised. Further studies are necessary, and currently a multicenter, randomized double-blinded, placebo-controlled trial of 1,100 preterm infants at less than 32 weeks gestation and less than 1,500 g investigating a probiotic combination is underway (Garland et al., 2011).

ONLINE RESOURCES

About Face
http:// www.aboutfaceUSA.org

Boston Children's Hospital EAT Program (Esophageal Atresia Treatment Program)
http://www.childrenshospital.org/clinicalservices/Site2807/mainpageS2807P0.html?_vsignck&_vsrefdom=EAT

Foker Process
http://www.youtube.com/watch?v=bD3GTO3BiiY

Gastro Kids
http://www.gastrokids.org

Necrotizing Enterocolitis
http://www.emedicine.medscape.com/article/977956-overview

PAGER
http://www.reflux.org

Pediatric Imaging Online
http://www.pediatricimagingonline.com (free website but does require an account set up)

REFERENCES

Abu-Elmagd, K. M., Costa, G., Bond, G. J., Soltys, K., Sindhi, R., Wu, T., & Mazariegos, G. (2009). Five hundred intestinal and multiviseral transplantations at a single center: Major advance with new challenges. *Annals of Surgery, 250*(4), 567–581.

Alfaleh, K., Anabrees, J., Bassler, D., & Al-Kharfi, T. (2011). Probiotics for prevention of necrotizing enterocolitis in preterm infants. *Cochrane Database Systematic Review*, CD005496.

Alvarez, S. M., & Burd, R. S. (2007). Increasing prevalence of gastrochisis repairs in the United States: 1996-2003. *Journal of Pediatric Surgery, 42*(6), 943–946.

Annand, R. J., Leaphart, C. L., Mollen, K. P., & Hackam, D. J. (2007). The role of the intestinal barrier in the pathogenesis of NEC. *Shock, 27*, 124–133.

Baldassarre, M. E., Laneve, A., Fanelli, M., Russo, F., Varsalone, F., Sportelli, F., . . . Laforgia, N. (2010). Duration of meconium passage in preterm and term infants. *Archives of Disease in Childhood. Fetal and Neonatal Edition, 95*(1), F74–F75.

Barksdale, E., Chwals, W. J., Magnuson, D. K., & Parry, R. L. (2011). Selected gastrointestinal anomalies. In A. A. Fanaroff & R. J. Martin (Eds.), *Neonatal perinatal medicine: Diseases of the fetus and infant* (9th ed., pp. 1400–1430). St. Louis, MO: Mosby.

Bates, M. D., Dunagan, D. T., Welch, L. C., Kaul, A., & Harvey, R. P. (2006). The Hlx homeobox transcription factor is required early in enteric nervous system development. *BMC Development Biology, 6*, 33.

Bedrick, A. D. (2004). Necrotizing enterocolitis: Neurodevelopment "risky business." *Journal of Perinatology, 24*, 351–353.

Bell, S. G. (2003). Gastroesophageal reflux and histamine2 antagonists. *Neonatal Network, 22*(2), 53–57.

Berman, L., & Moss, R. L. (2011). Necrotizing enterocolitis: An update. *Seminars in Fetal & Neonatal Medicine, 16*, 145–150.

Berseth, C. L. (2005a). Developmental anatomy and physiology of the gastrointestinal tract. In H. W. Taeusch & D. Brodsky (Eds.), *Avery's diseases of the newborn* (8th ed., pp. 1071–1085). Philadelphia, PA: Saunders.

Berseth, C. L. (2005b). Physiologic and inflammatory abnormalities of the gastrointestinal tract. In H. W. Taeusch & D. Brodsky (Eds.), *Avery's diseases of the newborn* (8th ed., pp. 1103–1112). Philadelphia, PA: Saunders.

Berseth, C. L., & Poenaru, D. (2005a). Abdominal wall problems. In H. W. Taeusch & D. Brodsky (Eds.), *Avery's diseases of the newborn* (8th ed., pp. 1113–1122). Philadelphia, PA: Saunders.

Berseth, C. L., & Poenaru, D. (2005b). Necrotizing enterocolitis and short bowel syndrome. In H. W. Taeusch & D. Brodsky (Eds.), *Avery's diseases of the newborn* (8th ed., pp. 1123–1133). Philadelphia, PA: Saunders.

Berseth, C. L., & Poenaru, D. (2005c). Structural anomalies of the gastrointestinal tract. In H. W. Taeusch & D. Brodsky (Eds.), *Avery's diseases of the newborn* (8th ed., pp. 1086–1102). Philadelphia, PA: Saunders.

Bessell, A., Hooper, L., Shaw, W. C., Reilly, S., Reid, J., & Glenny, A. M. (2011). Feeding interventions for growth and development in infants with cleft lip, cleft palate or cleft lip and palate. *Cochrane Database of Systematic Reviews*, CD003315. doi:10.1002/1465185

Bhatia, J., Gates, A., & Parish, A. (2010). Medical management of short gut syndrome. *Journal of Perinatology, 30*(Suppl.), S2–S5.

Bianconi, S., Gudavalli, M., Sutija, V. G., Lopez, A. L., Barillas-Arias, L., & Ron, N. J. (2007). Ranitidine and late-onset sepsis in the neonatal intensive care unit. *Journal of Perinatal Medicine, 35*(2), 147–150.

Bischoff, A., Levitt, M. A., & Pena, A. (2011). Laparaoscopy and its use in the repair of anorectal malformations. *Journal of Pediatric Surgery, 46*(8), 1609–1717.

Bisquera, J. A., Cooper, T. R., & Berseth, C. L. (2002). Impact of necrotizing enterocolitis on length of stay and hospital charges in very low birth weight infants. *Pediatrics, 109*(3), 423–428.

Boston, V. E. (2006). Necrotizing enterocolitis and localized intestinal perforation: Different diseases or ends of a spectrum of pathology. *Pediatric Surgery International, 22*, 477–484.

Boyd, P. A., Bhattacharjee, A., Gould, S., Manning, N., & Chamberlain, P. (1998). Outcome of prenatally diagnosed anterior abdominal wall defects. *Archives of Disease in Childhood. Fetal and Neonatal Edition, 78*(3), F209–F213.

Burrin, D. G., & Stoll, B. (2002). Key nutrients and growth factors for the neonatal gastrointestinal tract. In C. L. Berseth (Ed.), *Clinics in perinatology: Recent advances in neonatal gastroenterology* (pp. 65–96). Philadelphia, PA: Saunders.

Caicedo, R., Schanler, R., Li, N., & Neu, J. (2005). The developing intestinal ecosystem: Implications for the neonate. *Pediatric Research, 58*, 625–629.

Cass, D. L., & Wesson, D. E. (2002). Advances in fetal and neonatal surgery for gastrointestinal anomalies and disease. In C. L. Berseth (Ed.), *Clinics in perinatology: Recent advances in neonatal gastroenterology* (pp. 1–22). Philadelphia, PA: Saunders.

Claud, E., & Walker, W. (2001). Hypothesis: Inappropriate colonization of the premature intestine can cause neonatal NEC. *FASEB Journal, 15*, 1398–1403.

Clyman, R. I. (2005). Patent ductus arteriosus in the preterm infant. In H. W. Taeusch & D. Brodsky (Eds.), *Avery's diseases of the newborn* (8th ed., pp. 816–826). Philadelphia, PA: Saunders.

Corvaglia, L., Rotatori, R., Ferlini, M., Aceti, A., Ancora, G., & Faldella, G. (2007). The effect of body positioning on gastroesophageal reflux in premature infants: Evaluation by combined impedance and pH monitoring. *Journal of Pediatrics, 151*(6), 591–596.

Dalla Vecchia, L. K., Grosfield, J. L., West, K. W., Rescorla, F. J., Scherer, L. R., & Engum, S. A. (1998). Intestinal atresia and stenosis: A 25 year experience with 277 cases. *Archives of Surgery, 133*(5), 490–496.

David, A. L., Tan, A., & Curry, J. (2008). Gastrochisis: Sonographic diagnosis, associations, management and outcome. *Prenatal Diagnosis, 28*, 663–644.

Desai, R., Curns, A. T., Patel, M. M., & Parashar, U. D. (2012). Trends in intussuseption-associated deaths among U.S. infants from 1979–2007. *Journal of Pediatrics, 160*(3), 456–460.

Deshpande, G., Rao, S., Patole, S., & Bulsara, M. (2010). Updated meta-analysis of probiotics for preventing necrotizing enterocolitis in preterm neonates. *Pediatrics, 125*(5), 921–930.

Dodge, J. A., Lewis, P. A., Stanton, M., & Wilsher, J. (2007). Cystic fibrosis mortality and survival in the UK: 1947-2003. *European Respiratory Journal, 29*(3), 522–526.

Dubose, T. M., Southgate, W. M., & Hill, J. G. (2001). Lactobezoars: A patient series and literature review. *Clinical Pediatrics, 40*(11), 603–606.

Emani, C. N., Petrosyan, M., Guiliani, S., Williams, M., Hunter, C., Prasadarao, N. V., & Ford, H. R. (2009). Role of the host defense system and intestinal microbial flora in the pathogenesis of necrotizing entercolitis. *Surgical Infections, 10*(5), 407–417.

Escobar, M. A., Ladd, A. P., Grosfield, J. L., West, K. W., Rescorla, F. J., Scherer, L. R., . . . Billmire, D. F. (2004). Duodenal atresia and stenosis: Long-term follow-up over 30 years. *Journal of Pediatric Surgery, 39*(6), 867–871.

Fanaroff, A. A., Stoll, B. J., Wright, L. L., Carlo, W. A., Ehernkranz, R. A., Stark, A. R., . . . NICHD Neonatal Rresearch Network. (2007). Trends in neonatal morbidity and mortality for very low birthweight infants. *American Journal of Obstetrics and Gynecology, 196*(2), e1–e8.

Feldkamp, M. L., Carey, J. C., & Sadler, T. W. (2007). Development of gastrochisis: Review of hypotheses, a novel hypotheses, and implications for research. *American Journal of Medical Genetics. Part A, 143*(7), 639–652.

Fitzgibbons, S. C., Ching, Y., Yu, D., Carpenter, J., Kenny, M., Weldon, C., . . . Jaksic, T. (2009). Mortality of necrotizing enterocolitis expressed by birth weight categories. *Journal of Pediatric Surgery, 44*, 1072–1075.

Gardner, V. A., Walton, J. M., & Chessell, L. (2003). A case study utilizing an enteral refedding technique in a premature infant with short bowel syndrome. *Advances in Neonatal Care, 3*(6), 258–271.

Garland, S. M., Tobin, J. M., Pirotta, M., Tabrizi, S. N., Opie, G., Donath, S., . . . Jacobs, S. E. (2011). The ProPrems trial:

Investigating the effects of probiotics on late onset sepsis in very preterm infants. *BMC Infectious Diseases, 11*, 210.

Gorter, R. R., Karimi, A., Sleeboom, C., Kneepkens, C. M., & Heij, H. A. (2010). Clinical and genetic characteristics of meconium ileus in newborns with and without cystic fibrosis. *Journal of Pediatric Gastroenterology and Nutrition, 50*(5), 569–572.

Gulliet, R., Stoll, B. J., Cotton, C. M., Gantz, M., McDonald, S., Poole, W. K., & Phelps, D. L. (2006). Association of H2-blocker therapy and higher incidence of necrotizing enterocolitis in very low birth weight infants. *Pediatrics, 117*(2), 137–142.

Gutierrez, I. M., Kang, K. H., & Jaksic, T. (2011). Neonatal short bowel syndrome. *Seminars in Fetal & Neonatal Medicine, 16*(3), 157–163.

Hajivassiliou, C. A. (2003). Intestinal obstruction in neonatal/pediatric surgery. *Seminars in Pediatric Surgery, 12*(4), 241–253.

Harmon, C. M. (2011). Single-site umbilical larparoscopic pyloromyotomy. *Seminars in Pediatric Surgery, 20*(4), 208–211.

Hartley, J. L., Davenport, M., & Kelly, D. A. (2009). Biliary atresia. *Lancet, 374*(9702), 1704–1713.

Hasosah, M., Lemberg, D. A., Skarsgard, E., & Schreiber, R. (2008). Congenital short bowel syndrome: A case report and review of the literature. *Canadian Journal of Gastroenterology, 22*(1), 37–46.

Heider, A. L., Strauss, R. A., & Kuller, J. A. (2004). Omphalocele: Clinical outcomes in cases with normal karyotypes. *American Journal of Obstetrics and Gynecology, 190*(1), 135–141.

Hibbs, A. M., & Lorch, S. A. (2006). Metaclopramide for the treatment of gastroesophageal reflux disease in infants: A systematic review. *Pediatrics, 118*(2), 746–752.

Holland, A. J., Walker, K., & Badawi, N. (2010). Gastroschisis: An update. *Pediatric Surgery International, 26*(9), 871–878.

Holman, R. C., Stoll, B. J., Curns, A. T., Yorika, K. L., Steiner, C. A., & Schonberger, L. B. (2006). Necrotizing enterocolits hospitalizations among neonates in the United States. *Paediatric and Perinatal Epidemiology, 20*, 498–506.

Hsiao, M., & Langer, J. C. (2011). Value of laparoscopy in children with a suspected rotation abnormality on imaging. *Journal of Pediatric Surgery, 46*(7), 1347–1352.

Hsueh, W., Caplan, M., Qu, X., Tan, X., De Plaen, I., & Gonzalez-Crussi, F. (2002). Neonatal NEC: Clinical considerations and pathogenetic concepts. *Pediatric and Development Pathology, 6*, 6–23.

Hwang, P., & Kousseff, B. G. (2004). Omphalocele and gastroschisis: An 18 year review study. *Genetics in Medicine, 6*(4), 232–236.

Hwang, S. T., & Shulman, R. J. (2002). Update on management and treatment of short gut. In C. L. Berseth (Ed.), *Clinics in perinatology: Recent advances in neonatal gastroenterology* (pp. 181–194). Philadelphia, PA: Saunders.

Iwashita, T., Kruger, G. M., Pardal, R., Kiel, M. J., & Morrison, S. J. (2003). Hirschsprung disease is linked to defects in neural crest stem cell function. *Science, 301*(5635), 972–976.

Jadcherla, S. R. (2002). Gastroesophageal reflux in the neonate. In C. L. Berseth (Ed.), *Clinics in perinatology: Recent advances in neonatal gastroenterology* (pp. 135–158). Philadelphia, PA: Saunders.

James, L. P. (2002). Pharmacology for the gastrointestinal tract. In C. L. Berseth (Ed.), *Clinics in perinatology: Recent advances in neonatal gastroenterology* (pp. 115–134). Philadelphia, PA: Saunders.

Jawad, A. J., Al-Rabie, A., Hadi, A., Al-Sowailem, A., Al-Rawaf, A., Abu-Touk, B., . . . Al-Sammarai, A. (2002). Spontaneous neonatal gastric perforation. *Pediatric Surgery International, 18*(5–6), 396–399.

Jezewski, P. A., Vieira, A. R., Nishimura, C., Ludwig, B., Johnson, M., O'Brien, S. E., . . . Murray, J. C. (2003). Complete sequencing shows a role for MSX1 in non-syndromic cleft lip and palate. *Journal of Medical Genetics, 40*(6), 399–407.

Jones, K. L. (2006). *Smith's recognizable patterns of human malformation* (6th ed.). Philadelphia, PA: Elsevier Saunders.

Keckler, S. J., St Peter, S. D., Spilde, T. L., Tsao, K., Ostllie, D. J., Holcomb, G. W., & Synder, C. L. (2008). Current significance of meconium plug syndrome. *Journal of Pediatric Surgery, 43*(5), 896–898.

Kee, J. L. (2001). *Laboratory and diagnostic tests with nursing implications* (4th ed.). Upper Saddle River, NJ: Prentice Hall.

Kenny, S. E., Tam, P. K., & Garcia-Barcelo, M. (2010). Hirschsprung's disease. *Seminars in Pediatric Surgery, 19*(3), 194–200.

Khalaf, M. N., Porat, R., Brodsky, N. L., & Bhandari, V. (2001). Clinical correlations in infants in the neonatal intensive care unit with vaying severity of gastroesophageal reflux. *Journal of Pediatric Gastroenterology and Nutrition, 32*(1), 45–49.

Kimura, K., & Loening-Baucke, V. (2000). Bilious vomiting in the newborn: Rapid diagnosis of intestinal obstruction. *American Family Physician, 61*, 2791–2798.

King, J., & Askin, D. F. (2003). Gastrochisis: Etiology, diagnosis, delivery options and care. *Neonatal Network, 22*(4), 7–12.

Kliegman, R. (2003). The relationship of neonatal feeding practices and the pathogenesis and prevention of NEC. *Pediatrics, 117*, S52–S58.

Koenig, W. J., Amarnath, R. P., Hench, V., & Berseth, C. L. (1995). Manometrics for preterm and term infants: A new tool for old questions. *Pediatrics, 95*(2), 203–206.

Kovesi, T., & Rubin, S. (2004). Long-term complications of congenital esophageal atresia and/or tracheoesophageal fistula. *Chest, 126*(3), 915–926.

Krogh, C., Fischer, T. K., Skotte, L., Biggar, R. J., Oyen, N., Skytthe, A., . . . Melbye, M. (2010). Familial aggregation and heritability of pyloric stenosis. *JAMA, 303*(23), 2393–2399.

Kubiak, R., Spitz, L., Kiely, E. M., Drake, D., & Pierro, A. (1999). Effectiveness of fundoplication in early infancy. *Journal of Pediatric Surgery, 34*(2), 295–299.

Lilja, H. E., Finkel, Y., Paulsson, M., & Lucas, S. (2011). Prevention and reversal of intestinal failure-associated liver disease in premature infants with short bowel syndrome using intravenous fish oil in combination with omega-6/9 lipid emulsions. *Journal of Pediatric Surgery, 46*(7), 1361–1367.

Loening-Baucke, V., & Kimura, K. (1999). Failure to pass meconium: Diagnosing neonatal intestinal obstruction. *American Family Physician, 60*(7), 2043–2050.

Maayan-Metzger, A., Itzchak, A., Mazkereth, R., & Kuint, J. (2004). Necrotizing enterocolitis in full-term infants: Case-control study and review of the literature. *Journal of Perinatology, 24*(8), 494–499.

Malcolm, W. F., & Cotton, C. M. (2012). Metaclopromide, H2 blockers, and proton pump inhibitors: Pharmocotherapy for gastroesophageal reflux in neonates. *Clinics in Perinatology, 39*(1), pp. 99–109.

Manogura, A. C., Turan, O., Kush, M. L., Berg, C., Bhide, A., Turan, S., . . . Baschat, A. A. (2008). Predictors necrotizing enterocolits in preterm growth-restricted neonates. *American Journal of Obstetrics and Gynecology, 198*, 638e1–645e1.

Martin, C. R., & Walker, W. A. (2006). Intestinal immune defenses and the inflammatory response in necrotizing enterocolitis. *Seminars in Fetal and Neonatal Medicine, 11*, 369–377.

Marven, S., & Owen, A. (2008). Contemporary postnatal surgical management strategies for congenital abdominal wall defects. *Seminars in Pediatric Surgery, 17*(4), 222–235.

Mattar, A. F., Drongowski, R. A., Coran, A. G., & Harmon, C. M. (2001). Effects of probiotics on enterocyte bacterial translocation in vitro. *Pediatric Surgery International, 17*(4), 265–268.

Meetze, W. H., Palazzolo, V. L., Bowling, D., Behnke, M., Burchfield, D. J., & Neu, J. (1993). Meconium passage in very-low-birth-weight infants. *Journal of Parenteral and Enteral Nutrition, 17*(6), 537–540.

Meinzen-Derr, J., Morrow, A. L., Hornung, R. W., Donovan, E. F., Dietrich, K. N., & Succop, P. A. (2009). Epidemiology of necrotizing enterocolitis temporal clustering in two neonatology practices. *Journal of Pediatrics, 154*(5), 656–661.

Merenstein, G. B., & Gardner, S. L. (2006). *Handbook of neonatal intensive care* (6th ed.). St Louis, MO: Mosby.

Merritt, L. (2005a). Part 1: Understanding the embryology and genetics of cleft lip and palate. *Advances in Neonatal Care, 5*(2), 64–71.

Merritt, L. (2005b). Part 2: Physical assessment of the infant with cleft lip and/or palate. *Advances in Neonatal Care, 5*(3), 125–134.

Mirza, B., Ijaz, L., Saleem, M., Sharif, M., & Sheikh, A. (2011). Anorectal malformations in neonates. *African Journal of Paediatric Surgery, 8*(2), 151–154.

Morriss, F. H., Moore, M., Weisbrodt, N. W., & West, M. S. (1986). Ontogenic development of gastrointestinal motility: IV. Duodenal contractions in preterm infants. *Pediatrics, 78*(6), 1106–1113.

Mustafawi, A. R., & Hassan, M. E. (2008). Congenital duodenal obstruction in children: A decade's experience. *European Journal of Pediatric Surgery, 18*(2), 93–97.

Nanthakumar, N. N., Fusunyan, R. D., Sanderson, I., & Walker, W. A. (2000). Inflammation in the developing human intestine: A possible pathophysiologic contribution to necrotizing enterocolitis. *Proceedings of the National Academy of Sciences of the USA, 97*, 6043–6048.

Neu, J. (2005). Neonatal necrotizing enterocolits: An update. *Acta Paediatrica Supplementum, 94*, 100–105.

Neu, J. (2007). Gastrointestinal development and meeting the nutritional needs of premature infants. *American Journal of Clinical Nutrition, 85*(Suppl.), 629S–634S.

Neu, J., & Bernstein, H. (2002). Update on host defense and immunonutrients. In C. L. Berseth (Ed.), *Clinics in perinatology: Recent advances in neonatal gastroenterology* (pp. 41–64). Philadelphia, PA: Saunders.

Neu, J., & Walker, W. A. (2011). Necrotizing enterocolitis. *New England Journal of Medicine, 364*(3), 255–264.

Nichol, P. F., Reeder, A., & Botham, R. (2011). Humans, mice, and mechanisms of intestinal atresias: A window into understanding early intestinal development. *Journal of Gastrointestinal Surgery, 15*(4), 694–700.

Niramis, R., Watanatittan, S., Kruatrachue, A., Annutkosol, M., Buranakitjaroen, V., Rattanasuwan, T., . . . Tongsin, A. (2010). Management of recurrent intussusception: Nonoperative or operative reduction. *Journal of Pediatric Surgery, 45*(11), 2175–2180.

Noviello, C., Cobellis, G., Romano, M., Amici, G., & Martino, A. (2010). Diagnosis of Hirschsprung's disease: An age-related approach in children below or above one year. *Colorectal Disease, 12*(10), 1044–1048.

Olsen, M. M., Luck, S. R., Lloyd-Still, J., & Raffensperger, J. G. (1982). The spectrum of meconium disease in infancy. *Journal of Pediatric Surgery, 17*(5), 479–481.

Omari, T. I., Rommel, N., Staunton, E., Lontis, R., Goodchild, L., Haslam, R. R., . . . Davidson, G. P. (2004). Paradoxical impact of body positioning on gastroesophageal reflux and gastric emptying in the premature neonate. *Journal of Pediatrics, 145*(2), 194–200.

Orenstein, S. R., Hassall, E., Furmaga-Jablonska, W., Atkinson, S., & Raanan, M. (2009). Multicenter, double-blind, randomized, placebo-controlled trial assessing the efficacy and safety of proton pump inhibitor lansoprazole in infants with symptoms of gastroesophageal reflux disease. *Journal of Pediatrics, 154*(4), 514–520.

Pakarinen, M. P., & Rintala, R. J. (2011). Surgery of biliary atresia. *Scandinavian Journal of Surgery, 100*(1), 49–53.

Philippart, A. I., & Georgeson, K. E. (1975). Neonatal small left colon syndrome: Intramural not intraluminal obstruction. *Journal of Pediatric Surgery, 10*(5), 733–740.

Puri, P., & Shinkai, T. (2004). Pathogenesis of Hirschsprung's disease and its variants: Recent progress. *Seminars in Pediatric Surgery, 13*(1), 18–24.

Rannells, J. D., Carver, J. K., & Kirby, R. S. (2011). Infantile hypertrophic pyloric stenosis: Epidemiology, genetics, and clinical update. *Advances in Pediatrics, 58*(1), 195–206.

Reber, K. M., Nankervis, C. A., & Nowicki, P. T. (2002). Newborn intestinal circulation: Physiology and pathophysiology. In C. L. Berseth (Ed.), *Clinics in perinatology: Recent advances in neonatal gastroenterology* (pp. 23–40). Philadelphia, PA: Saunders.

Rees, C. M., Eaton, S., Kiely, E. M., Wade, A. M., McHugh, K., & Pierro, A. (2008). Peritoneal drainage or laparotomy for neonatal bowel peforation? A randomized controlled trial. *Annals of Surgery, 248*, 44–51.

Rhee, D., Zhang, Y., Chang, D. C., Arnold, M. A., Salazar-Osuna, J. H., Chrouser, K., . . . Abdullah, F. (2011). Population-based comparison of open vs laparoscopic esophagogastric fundoplication in children: Application of the Agency for Health care Research and Quality pediatric quality indicators. *Journal of Pediatric Surgery, 46*(4), 648–654.

Rittler, M., Cosentino, V., Lopez-Camelo, J. S., Murray, J. C., Wehby, G., & Castilla, E. E. (2011). Associated anomalies among infants with oral clefts at birth and during a 1-year follow-up. *American Journal of Medical Genetics Part A, 155A*(7), 1588–1596.

Roberts, D., & Dalziel, S. (2006). Antenatal corticosteroids for accelerating fetal lung maturation for women at risk of preterm birth. *Cochrane Database Systematic Review*, CD004454.

Rudolph, C. D., & Hassall, E. (2008). Gastroesophageal reflux. In R. Kleinman, O. Goulet, G. Mieli-Vergani, I. R. Sanderson, P. Sherman & B. L. Shneider (Eds.), *Walker's pediatric gastrointestinal disease: Physiology, diagnosis, management* (5th ed., pp. 59–71). Hamilton, Ontario: B.C. Decker.

Salihu, H. M., Boos, R., & Schmidt, W. (2004). Mode of delivery and neonatal survival of infants with isolated gastroschisis. *Journal of Obstetrics & Gynecology, 104*(4), 678–683.

Salminen, P., Hurme, S., & Ovaska, J. (2012). Fifteen-year outcome of laproscopic and open nissen fundoplication: A randomized clinical trial. *Annals of Thoracic Surgery, 93*(1), 228–233.

Schanler, R. J. (2005). Enteral nutrition for the high-risk neonate. In H. W. Taeusch & D. Brodsky (Eds.), *Avery's diseases of the newborn* (8th ed., pp. 1043–1060). Philadelphia, PA: Saunders.

Schanler, R. J. (2006). Probiotics and necrotising enterocolitis in premature infants. *Archives of Disease in Childhood. Fetal and Neonatal Edition, 91*(6), F395–F397.

Schlatter, M. (2003). Preformed silos in the management of gastrschisis: New progress with an old idea. *Current Opinion in Pediatrics, 15*(3), 239–242.

Schmolzer, G., Urlesberger, B., Haim, M., Kutschera, J., Pichler, G., Ritschi, E., . . . Muller, W. (2006). Multi-modal approach to prophylaxis of necrotizing enterocolitis: Clinical report and review of literature. *Pediatric Surgery International, 22*, 573–580.

Segel, S. Y., Marder, S. J., Parry, S., & Macones, G. A. (2001). Fetal abdominal wall defects and mode of delivery: A systematic review. *Obstetrics and Gynecology, 98*(5 Pt. 1), 867–873.

Sharma, R., Hudak, M. L., Tepas, J. J. III, Wludyka, P. S., Marvin, W. J., Bradshaw, J. A., & Pieper, P. (2006). Impact of gestational age on the clinical presentation and surgical outcome of necrotizing enterocolits. *Journal of Perinatology, 26*(6), 342–327.

Shulman, R. J., Schanler, R. J., Lau, C., Heitkemper, M., Ou, C. N., & Smith, E. O. (1998). Early feeding, antenatal glucocorticoids, and human milk decreases intestinal permeability in preterm infants. *Pediatric Research, 44*, 519–523.

Singer, J. I. (1988). Lactobezoar causing an abdominal triad of colicky pain, emesis, and mass. *Pediatric Emergency Care, 4*(3), 194–196.

Sisk, P. M., Lovelady, C. A., Dillard, R. G., Gruber, K. J., & O'Shea, T. M. (2007). Early human milk feeding is associated with a lower risk of necrotizing enterocolitis in very low birth weight infants. *Journal of Perinatology, 27*(7), 428–433.

Sokol, R. J., Shepherd, R. W., Superina, R., Bezerra, J. A., Robuck, P., & Hoffnagle, J. H. (2007). Screening and outcomes in biliary atresia: Summary of a National Institutes of Health workshop. *JH Hepatology, 46*(2), 566–581.

Sola, J. B., Tepas, J. J. III & Koniaris, L. G. (2010). Peritoneal drainage versus laparotomy for necrotizing enterocolits and intestinal perforation: A meta-analysis. *Journal of Surgical Research, 161*, 95–100.

Somme, S., & Langer, J. C. (2006). Omphalocele. In P. Puri & M. Hollwarth (Eds.), *Pediatric surgery* (pp. 153–160). New York, NY: Springer.

Spoon, J. M. (2003). VATER association. *Neonatal Network, 22*(3), 71–75.

Spritz, R. (2001). The genetics and epigenetics of orofacial cleft. *Current Opinion in Pediatrics, 13*(6), 556–560.

Steiner, Z., Mogilner, J., Siplovich, L., & Eldar, S. (1997). T-tubes in the management of meconium ileus. *Pediatric Surgery International, 12*(2/3), 140–141.

Sydorak, R. M., & Albanese, C. T. (2002). Laparoscopic repair of high imperforate anus. *Seminars in Pediatric Surgery, 11*(4), 217–225.

Tate, J. E., Simonsen, L., Viboud, C., Steiner, C., Patel, M. M., Curns, A. T., & Parashar, U. D. (2008). Trends in intussusception hospitalizations among U.S. infants, 1993-2004: Implications for monitoring the safety of the new rotavirus vaccination program. *Pediatrics, 121*(5), 1125–1132.

Taylor, S. N., Basile, L. A., Ebeling, M., & Wagner, C. L. (2009). Intestinal permeability in preterm infants by feeding type: Mother's milk versus formula. *Breastfeeding Medicine, 4*(1), 11–15.

Teitelbaum, J. (2008). Congenital anomalies. In R. Kleinman, O. Goulet, G. Mieli-Vergani, I. R. Sanderson, P. Sherman & B. L. Shneider (Eds.), *Walker's pediatric gastrointestinal disease: Physiology, diagnosis, management* (5th ed., pp. 7–18). Hamilton, Ontario: B.C. Decker.

Usmann, S. S., & Levenbrown, J. (1989). Lactobezoar in a full-term breast-fed infant. *American Journal of Gastroenterology, 84*(6), 647–649.

Vieira, A. R. (2008). Unraveling human cleft lip and palate research. *Journal of Dental Research, 87*(2), 119–125.

Wales, P. W., de Silva, N., Kim, J., Leece, L., To, T., & Moore, A. (2004). Neonatal short bowel syndrome: Population-based estimates of incidence and mortality rates. *Journal of Pediatric Surgery, 39*(5), 690–695.

Walsh, M. C., & Kleigman, R. M. (1986). Necrotizing enterocolitis: Treatment based on staging criteria. *Pediatric Clinics of North America, 33*, 179–201.

Wang, N. L., Yeh, M. L., Chang, P. Y., Sheu, J. C., Chen, C. C., Lee, H. C., . . . Hsu, C. H. (1998). Prenatal and neonatal intussusception. *Pediatric Surgery International, 13*(4), 232–236.

Wang, Q., Dong, J., & Zhu, Y. (2012). Probiotic supplement reduces risk of necrotizing enterocolitis and mortality in preterm very low-birth-weight infants: An updated meta-analysis of 20 randomized controlled trials. *Journal of Pediatric Surgery, 47*(1), 241–248.

Wax, J. R., Hamilton, T., Cartin, A., Dudley, J., Pinette, M. G., & Blackstone, J. (2006). Congenital jejunal and ileal atresia: Natural prenatal songographic history and association with neonatal outcome. *Journal of Ultrasound in Medicine, 25*(3), 337–342.

Wilcox, A. J., Lie, R. T., Solvoll, K., Taylor, J., McConnaughey, D. R., Abyholm, F., . . . Drevon, C. A. (2007). Folic acid supplements and risk of facial clefts: National population based case control study. *British Medical Journal, 25*(3), 334–464.

Yeh, T. C., Chang, J. H., & Kao, H. A. (2004). Necrotizing enterocolitis in infants: Clinical outcome and influence on growth and neurodevelopment. *Journal of the Formosan Medical Association, 103*, 761–766.

Zendejas, B., Kuchena, A., Onkendi, E. O., Lohse, C. M., Moir, C. R., Ishitani, M. B., . . . Zarroug, A. E. (2011). Fifty-three-year experience with pediatric umbilical hernia repairs. *Journal of Pediatric Surgery, 46*(11), 2151–2156.

Zenk, K. E., Sills, J. H., & Koeppel, R. M. (2003). *Neonatal medications and nutrition: A comprehensive guide* (3rd ed.). Santa Rosa, CA: NICU Ink.

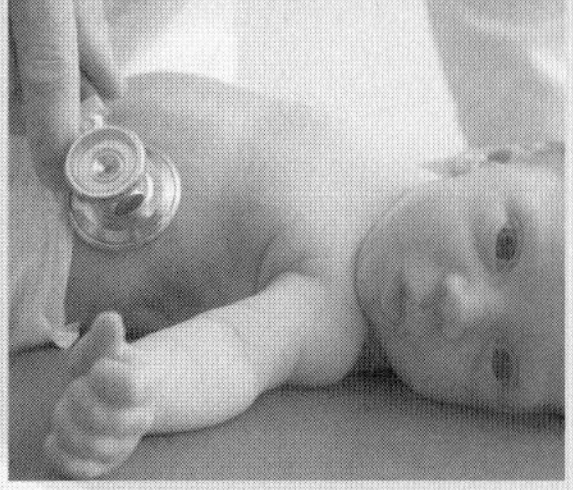

CHAPTER

9

Metabolic System

■ Laura A. Stokowski

Metabolic disorders, or inborn errors of metabolism (IEMs), encompass a group of disorders in which gene mutations cause clinically significant blocks in metabolic pathways. Most IEMs are inherited in an autosomal recessive fashion; a few are X-linked. The major categories are disorders of amino acid metabolism, organic acidemias, fatty acid oxidation disorders (FAODs), congenital lactic acidoses, disorders of carbohydrate metabolism, lysosomal disorders, peroxisomal disorders, cholesterol biosynthetic disorders, and disorders of metal metabolism. Into these categories fall hundreds of individual disorders of metabolism, many of which have their onset in the neonatal period. The inherited metabolic disorders manifesting in the early neonatal period will be the focus of this chapter.

GENERAL PRINCIPLES: THE NEONATE WITH A METABOLIC DISORDER

Pathophysiology of IEMs

The genetic mechanisms through which biochemical disease is inherited include autosomal dominant, autosomal recessive, sex-linked recessive, or a mutation in mitochondrial DNA (Cederbaum, 2012). The genetic mutation leads to an absent or defective gene product or enzyme, causing either an accumulation of precursors before a blocked step in a metabolic pathway, a deficiency of a critical metabolic product, or both. In disorders involving the intermediary metabolism of small molecules (such as maple syrup urine disease [MSUD]), the accumulated molecules give rise to an "intoxication syndrome" because of the profoundly toxic nature of these substances and their effect on the central nervous system (CNS). Disorders involving energy metabolism (such as pyruvate dehydrogenase [PDH] deficiency) lead to a failure of energy production or utilization with a broad range of symptoms and physiologic consequences. Other disorders, such as lysosomal storage diseases, involve complex molecules, and symptoms that arise from these disorders are permanent, progressive, and independent of intercurrent events.

Clinical Manifestations of IEMs

Most neonates who are eventually diagnosed with IEMs appear essentially normal at birth and have no history of antepartum or intrapartum complications. The placenta and maternal circulation protect the fetus from the damaging effects of toxins. Birth is followed by a symptom-free interval of variable duration. Some metabolic disorders are unmasked by the ingestion of formula, milk, or fructose. Others are unrelated to feeding or may be brought on by fasting, infection, or stress.

Metabolic disease in the newborn can be clinically silent, indolent, or acute (Cederbaum, 2012). Five common presentations have been described (Leonard & Morris, 2010):

- Neurological presentation—acute encephalopathy, seizures, lethargy
- Hypoglycemia
- Acid–base abnormalities—particularly metabolic acidosis and respiratory alkalosis
- Cardiomyopathy and cardiac arrhythmias
- Acute liver disease

In the neonate, nonspecific clinical findings such as feeding problems (poor intake, vomiting) or respiratory distress can be indicators of metabolic disease. The presentation might be consistent with neonatal sepsis, because the neonate has a limited repertoire of responses to severe illness. The infant with underlying metabolic disease often deteriorates rapidly and does not respond to symptomatic therapy.

A complete family history should be obtained to determine if other individuals in the family have had similar symptoms or the same disorder, or if there is a history of unexplained infant death, sudden infant death syndrome (SIDS), mental retardation, or consanguinity (Leonard & Morris, 2010).

Diagnosis of IEMs

The trigger for a metabolic work-up varies with the situation. In infants initially suspected of having sepsis, a metabolic workup might be initiated when laboratory results to investigate infection fail to confirm infection. Persistent metabolic acidosis with an increased anion gap, hypoglycemia, significant hyperammonemia, unexplained hepatic dysfunction, or ketonuria should always raise suspicion of IEM (Leonard & Morris, 2010). Although only a minority of IEMs are associated with dysmorphism, the possibility of metabolic disease should not be discounted in the neonate with congenital malformations or unusual features.

The initial laboratory investigation of a suspected error of metabolism includes a broad range of tests of both blood and urine (Box 9.1). Nonspecific screening tests do not provide a diagnosis; at best they will support a strong suspicion of a metabolic disorder and suggest a specific category of disease (e.g., organic acidemia, FAOD). Interpretation of results can be tricky. Conditions of sampling can profoundly affect results. Blood and urine samples must be obtained prior to the initiation of therapy, and whenever possible, both should be collected when the infant is symptomatic (S. A. Berry, Nathan, Hoffman, & Sarafoglou, 2009). Extra blood and urine samples should be obtained and frozen for later testing.

Secondary metabolic derangements can interfere with test interpretation, and biochemical abnormalities might be present only during acute episodes. Laboratory abnormalities can also be transient; a result within the reference range does not necessarily rule out a metabolic disorder. Studies may need to be repeated at specific times. Clinicians might be falsely reassured by screening tests that are inadequate to exclude certain conditions. Therefore, consultation with a metabolic specialist is recommended. Furthermore, a clinical history and as much information as possible about the infant's symptoms and the suspected diagnosis should be provided to the referral laboratory to improve the accuracy of testing and interpretation of results.

■ Postmortem Diagnosis. If a neonate with a possible metabolic disorder dies suddenly, it is of great importance to continue to try to establish the proper diagnosis for purposes of genetic counseling and future antenatal diagnosis. In addition to standard blood and urine samples, a sample of cerebrospinal fluid (CSF) should be obtained if possible, and whole blood and bile should be collected on filter paper. The routine state newborn screening card should be completed and sent. If the family declines a full autopsy, tissue biopsies should be obtained. Tissue samples of value are skin, liver, kidney, and muscle.

BOX 9.1

GENERAL SCREENING TESTS FOR ERRORS OF METABOLISM

Blood Tests

Glucose

CBC with differential

Blood gases

Electrolytes (and anion gap[a])

Liver function tests

BUN and creatinine

Total and direct bilirubin

Prothrombin time (PT) and partial thromboplastin time (PTT)

Uric acid

Ammonia

Lactate

Pyruvate

Amino acids

Free fatty acids

Ketones (3OH-butyrate, acetoacetate)

Creatinine phosphokinase (CPK)

Newborn metabolic screen/blood acylcarnitine analysis

CSF glycine (to rule out nonketotic hyperglycinemia)

Urine Tests

Glucose

Ketones

pH

Reducing substances

Ferric chloride reaction

Dinitrophenylhydrazine reaction

Amino acids

Organic acids

Odor

Orotic acid (if blood NH_4 elevated)

[a] Anion gap is (sodium – [chloride + bicarbonate]). Normal is less than 15 mEq/L.

■ Neonatal Screening. The development of tandem mass spectrometry (MS/MS) has greatly improved the presymptomatic detection of a large number of errors of metabolism. With MS/MS, it is possible to measure 30 or 40 different metabolites in less than 2 or 3 minutes, using a single dried blood spot. MS/MS works by applying a charge to the compounds in solution, sending them through an electromagnetic field, and sorting them out and weighing them according to their mass-to-charge ratio. Expanded newborn screening using MS/MS is mandated in some states as part of the routine newborn screening program. It is also available to parents who wish to purchase it from a number of private laboratories at a nominal cost. Currently, MS/MS screens only for disorders of intermediary metabolism, including amino acid disorders, organic acid disorders, and FAODs. A normal neonatal screen, even an expanded newborn screen by MS/MS, does not rule out an error of metabolism in a suspicious clinical setting. If newborn screening tests are still pending when a neonate manifests potential signs and symptoms of metabolic disease, clinicians should contact the screening laboratory promptly to determine whether a diagnosis can be provided or to expedite results (Summar, 2009).

Management of the Newborn With an IEM. As soon as it becomes apparent that the infant has some type of metabolic disorder, it is important to consult a metabolic specialist/geneticist. In addition to general supportive measures as indicated by the infant's symptoms, both general and specific treatments should be initiated. Oral feedings and amino acid solutions (all protein sources) are withheld, and 10% glucose solution with electrolytes is administered temporarily until the precise diagnosis is ascertained. A glucose infusion rate of at least 5 mg/kg/min (and higher if tolerated, aiming for 120 to 150 kcal/kg/d), is administered because many metabolic disorders are exacerbated by tissue catabolism (Cederbaum, 2012). Intralipids are withheld until disorders of fatty acid oxidation have been ruled out. Acute hypoglycemia, metabolic acidosis, dehydration, hypovolemia, and electrolyte imbalances are corrected as part of the overall supportive management of a metabolic disorder. If the infant is to be transferred to a referral center, reliable vascular access should be secured prior to transport. Hemodialysis or extracorporeal membrane oxygenation (ECMO) may be required for emergency management of some IEMs. Liver transplantation can be life-saving in some IEMs. Many disorders with rapid neonatal or prenatal onset are lethal, and all that can be offered are palliative and symptomatic care.

Interactions with parents and other family members are critically important, not only at the time of diagnosis, but throughout the course of care. IEMs occur in newborn infants with a broad range of racial/ethnic backgrounds. It is important to provide culturally sensitive care, which includes access to interpreter services, exploration of the family's sociocultural background, and bidirectional communication and decision making in the best interest of the child (Stockler, Moeslinger, Herle, Wimmer, & Ipsiroglu, 2012).

UREA CYCLE DISORDERS

Urea cycle disorders (UCDs) are caused by inherited defects in genes encoding enzymes or membrane transporters involved in ureagenesis. All are transmitted as autosomal recessive traits except ornithine transcarbamylase (OTC) deficiency, which is X-linked, and the most common of the primary defects. In aggregate, the prevalence of UCDs is believed to be approximately 1 per 10,000 live births, if partial defects are included.

Pathophysiology of UCDs

The hepatic urea cycle is the mechanism used by the body to detoxify and eliminate ammonia generated from nitrogen waste. Five enzymatic reactions make up the urea cycle, leading to the incorporation of ammonia into urea and enabling its excretion in the urine (Figure 9.1). The first two steps, the carbamyl phosphate synthetase (CPS) and OTC reactions take place in the mitochondria and lead to the synthesis of citrulline. In a subsequent cytosolic reaction, citrulline is converted to argininosuccinate, which is hydrolyzed to arginine and fumarate. Arginine is then hydrolyzed to urea and ornithine is regenerated.

A block of the urea cycle can result from a deficiency of any one of the first five enzymes in the urea cycle pathway: carbamyl phosphate synthetase I (CPSI deficiency), OTC deficiency, argininosuccinic acid synthetase (citrullinemia), argininosuccinic acid lyase (argininosuccinic aciduria), a cofactor producer, N-acetylglutamate synthase (NAGS deficiency), or a transport protein (Summar, 2009). The outcome of a block in the urea cycle is an accumulation of precursor metabolites, including ammonia, which have no effective alternate clearance pathway. The neonate, with an immature liver and tendency toward catabolism, is poorly equipped to handle the excess metabolites and rapidly succumbs to the neurotoxic effects of high ammonia levels. Hyperammonemic encephalopathy results from osmotic swelling in the brain caused by glutamine accumulation in cerebral astrocytes, where glutamine synthesis is increased in response to high ammonia levels. The developing brain is much more susceptible to the deleterious effects of excess ammonia than the adult brain, leading to irreversible cortical atrophy, ventricular enlargement, demyelination, or gray and white matter hypodensities in survivors, the extent of which depends on the magnitude and duration of ammonia exposure and the degree of brain maturation (Braissant, 2010).

Clinical Manifestations of UCDs

Infants with complete urea cycle enzyme defects such as OTC and CPSI deficiency are usually born at term, with no prenatal complications, because the maternal circulation prevents a buildup of toxic ammonia (Summar, 2009). Affected newborns are initially healthy, but shortly after receiving their first protein feedings, they begin to show signs of clinical decompensation and hyperammonemic encephalopathy. The earliest signs of ammonia toxicity are irritability, hypotonia, hypothermia, lethargy, poor feeding, vomiting, and hyperventilation. A mild respiratory alkalosis with tachypnea is a common early finding that should prompt measurement of a plasma ammonia level. Neurologic deterioration is

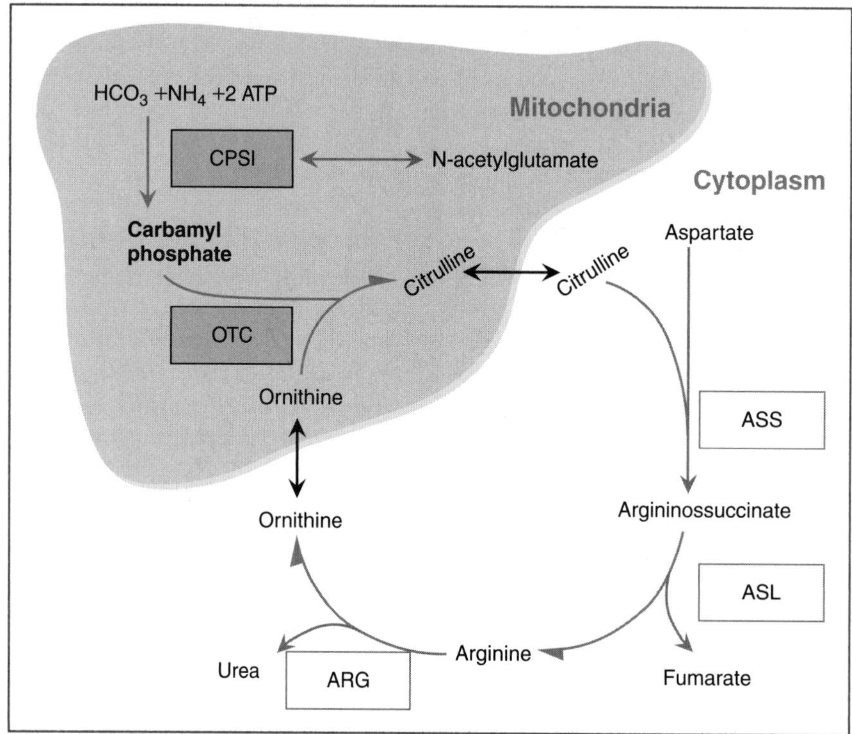

FIGURE 9.1 The urea cycle and alternative pathways of nitrogen excretion. Nitrogen is converted to ammonia (NH_4) and transported to the liver where it is processed via the urea cycle, composed of five enzymes in the direct pathway: (1) carbamyl phosphate synthetase I (CPSI); (2) OTC; (3) argininosuccinic acid synthetase (ASS); (4) argininosuccinic acid lyase (ASL); (5) arginase (ARG).
From GeneReviews: Genetic Disease Online Reviews, Pagon et al. (2013).

progressive, with loss of tone and reflexes, eventually leading to respiratory failure and coma. Hepatomegaly may also be present. Without treatment, most infants will die from complications such as cerebral, pulmonary hemorrhage, or neurologic or cardiac problems.

Diagnosis of UCDs

The hallmark of a UCD is an elevated blood ammonia level. A plasma ammonia level of 150 µmol/L (>260 mcg/dL) or higher in neonates, with a normal anion gap and a normal blood glucose level, is a strong indicator of a urea cycle defect (Summar, 2009). The exception is arginase (ARG) deficiency, which does not typically cause a rapid rise in plasma ammonia level. A normal ammonia level in a healthy infant is less than 65 mcmol/L. Blood sampling and handling techniques can affect results. Blood for ammonia levels should be collected by arterial or venous sampling and kept on ice, and plasma should be separated within 15 minutes of collection. Hemolysis, delayed processing, and exposure to room air can falsely elevate ammonia levels. Blood taken by capillary puncture is not appropriate for measurement of blood ammonia levels because of hemolysis (Leonard & Morris, 2010). If the ammonia level of a newborn with a suspected UCD is only modestly elevated, it should be repeated after several hours because the level can rise rapidly.

Blood gases, electrolytes, glucose, and other routine clinical laboratory tests should be obtained. Metabolic acidosis with a normal anion gap is sometimes present in UCDs, but not as often as in disorders of organic acid metabolism. Blood urea nitrogen (BUN) is low, but this is not specific or sensitive for UCDs. Liver function tests are important to rule out possible causes of hyperammonemia related to liver disorders or dysfunction (Cederbaum & Berry, 2012).

To arrive at a more precise diagnosis, quantitative plasma and urinary amino acids are necessary. Plasma glutamine, alanine, and asparagine, which serve as waste storage forms of nitrogen, may all be elevated. Plasma arginine is low in all UCDs of neonatal onset. The amounts of citrulline, *argininosuccinic acid*, and arginine in plasma and orotic acid in urine are usually sufficient to differentiate among UCDs. Measuring enzyme activity in tissue (liver, cultured skin fibroblasts, or RBCs) at a later point in time provides a definitive diagnosis that may be desirable for genetic counseling or future prenatal testing. Molecular genetic testing using linkage analysis or mutation scanning is available for OTC and CPSI deficiencies as well as citrullinemia, allowing for diagnostic confirmation, carrier detection, and prenatal diagnosis. Three UCDs (citrullinemia, argininosuccinate lyase deficiency, and ARG deficiency) can also be detected by the amino acid panels of expanded newborn screening programs employing MS/MS.

■ Differential Diagnosis of Hyperammonemia

Several other errors of metabolism can cause hyperammonemia in the newborn, notably the organic acidemias propionic, methylmalonic acidemia (MMA) and the

FAODs medium-chain acyl-CoA dehydrogenase deficiency (MCAD), systemic carnitine deficiency, and long-chain FAODs, although the last group is also associated with hypoglycemia. Hyperammonemia is also a feature of pyruvate carboxylase deficiency (PCD) and PDH deficiency. In transient hyperammonemia of the newborn (THAN), very high plasma ammonia levels, often matching those of UCDs, exist for which no underlying cause can be found. THAN is usually associated with prematurity and has no genetic basis, nor does it recur in infants who survive the initial episode (Cederbaum & Berry, 2012). A simple algorithm can be useful to determine the cause of hyperammonemia (Figure 9.2).

Currently, only two UCDs (ASA lyase and citrullinemia) are included on the list of core conditions for the uniform newborn screening panel (U.S. Department of HHS, 2011). To date, no screening is available for OTC, CPS1, or NAGS deficiency.

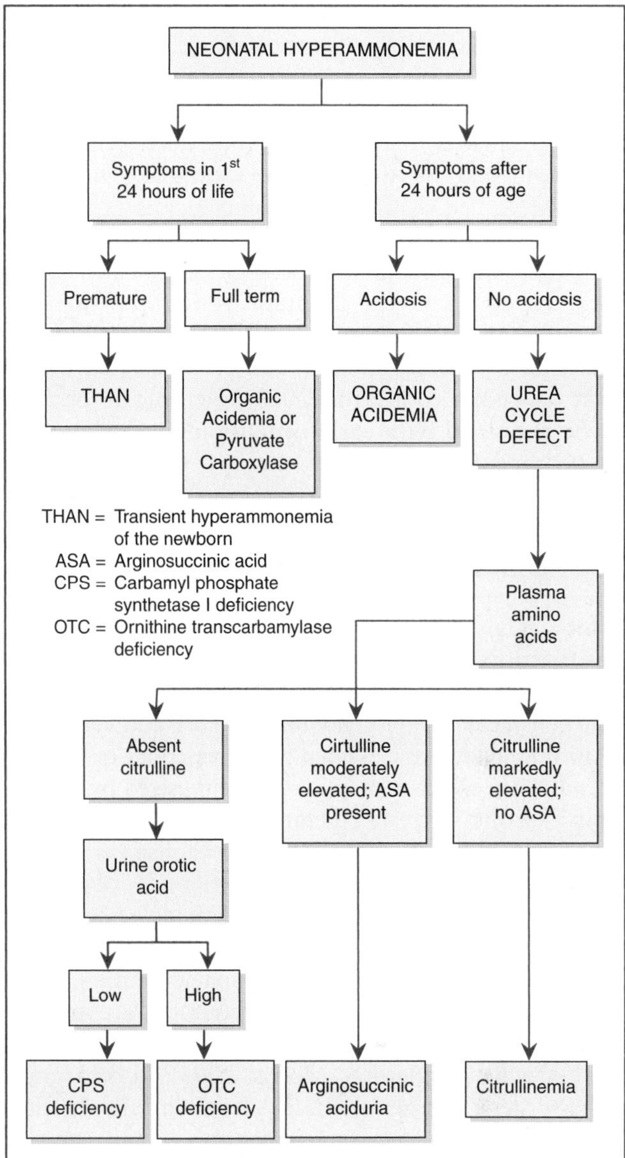

FIGURE 9.2 Algorithm to differentiate among conditions that produce neonatal hyperammonemia.
Redrawn from Burton (2000).

Management of UCDs

The emergency treatment of an infant with a suspected UCD has three simultaneous requirements: (1) physical removal of ammonia from the circulation; (2) reversal of catabolism; and (3) scavenging of excess nitrogen (Summar, 2009). Dietary protein intake should cease and be replaced by high-energy intake with a protein-free formula or by intravenous glucose and lipid infusion started, if enteral feeding cannot be tolerated. Protein intake is stopped only temporarily, however, because failure to supply essential amino acids will eventually result in catabolism and further ammonia production. Within 48 hours, 1 to 1.5 g/kg/d of protein should be restarted, with 50% as essential amino acids. Fever, if present, must be aggressively treated. The kidneys remove ammonia poorly, so plasma ammonia levels are monitored closely and ammonia concentrations greater than 500 mcmol/L must be reduced promptly with hemodialysis, or hemofiltration. Peritoneal dialysis is much less effective in clearing ammonia from the body. For this reason, it is recommended that neonates with symptomatic hyperammonemia be transferred without delay to a neonatal facility capable of providing effective toxin removal.

Compounds that conjugate to amino acids, providing an alternate route for the excretion of nitrogen, can be given to lower the nitrogen burden, and therefore the ammonia burden, of an infant with a UCD. These agents (called "scavenger drugs" or diversion therapy) include N-carbamylglutamate (which activates carbamoyl phosphate synthase I and stimulates ureagenesis), sodium benzoate (which is conjugated with glycine to form hippurate), and sodium phenylbutyrate (which is oxidized in the liver to phenylacetate and then with glutamine and excreted in the urine). N-carbamylglutamate has been effectively used to treat NAGS deficiency (Daniotti, laMarca, Fiorini, & Filippi, 2011). Serum potassium levels must be monitored closely when these drugs are used. A preparation combining both sodium phenylbutyrate and sodium benzoate is also available. In babies with citrullinemia and argininosuccinic aciduria, nitrogen can be excreted by increasing losses of citrulline and argininosuccinic acid, respectively. Arginine supplementation enhances the excretion of these metabolites by replenishing the supply of ornithine. However, high doses of the intravenous preparation l-arginine-HCl can cause metabolic acidosis and must be administered via central line because it can cause tissue necrosis if extravasation occurs.

A neonate in acute hyperammonemic coma caused by a suspected UCD should be given loading doses followed by continuous infusions of the ammonia-scavenging drugs (l-arginine-HCl, N-carbamylglutamate, sodium benzoate, and sodium phenylacetate), and drug levels should be monitored to reduce the risk for toxicity. Dietary protein is reintroduced in low amounts (0.5 g/kg/d) to encourage an anabolic state, while continuing diversion therapy to control ammonia levels. Alternative therapies that have been used with variable success for neonatal UCDs include liver and hepatocyte transplantation.

■ **Prognosis.** Even with the most vigorous intervention, UCDs of neonatal onset are often fatal, and the few survivors have a high rate of neurologic disability (Braissant, 2010). In a recent series, a mortality rate of 32% was found in infants with UCDs who were symptomatic within the first 30 days of life (Summar, Dobbelaere, Brusilow, & Lee, 2008). OTC deficiency is typically the most severe and lethal defect, particularly among males. The extent of permanent neurologic impairment in survivors is related to the duration of the hyperammonemic coma, plasma ammonia level at diagnosis, and other unidentified factors. Neonatal onset is associated with the worst prognosis (Braissant, 2010). Neurologic outcomes can be improved with early orthotopic liver transplantation (Campeau et al., 2010).

DISORDERS OF AMINO ACID METABOLISM

Amino acids play a role in literally all metabolic and cellular functions. As the constituents of protein, amino acids are used for the synthesis of new protein and as a source of carbon skeletons for generating glucose and ketone bodies. Amino acids are classified as nonessential or essential, depending on whether they can be synthesized by the body or must be obtained from dietary sources.

The disorders of amino acid metabolism, also called aminoacidopathies, arise from deficiencies of enzymes required to metabolize specific amino acids or amino acid transporters. The effects of the aberrant metabolism are highly disease-specific. In some aminoacidopathies, clinical symptoms are caused by the relatively rapid accumulation of toxic metabolites that are substrates for the dysfunctional enzyme (Leonard & Morris, 2006). In other amino acid disorders, damaging effects of the enzyme deficiency are more gradual and chronic in nature.

The most well-known disorder of amino acid metabolism, perhaps of all the errors of metabolism, is phenylketonuria (PKU). The clinically and biochemically heterogeneous disorders of amino acid metabolism are inherited primarily as autosomal recessive traits.

Nonketotic Hyperglycinemia (NKH)

■ **Pathophysiology.** NKH (also known as glycine encephalopathy) is a disorder of glycine metabolism that is generally fatal in its neonatal form. Glycine, a glucogenic amino acid, is normally metabolized by a complex of enzymes known as the glycine cleavage complex, consisting of four proteins encoded on four different chromosomes. A defect in any of these enzymes interferes with the cleavage of glycine, resulting in a steep rise in glycine concentration in the blood and CSF. The exact pathophysiology of NKH is not known, but it is believed to be related to glycine's role as a neurotransmitter (Hyland, Gibson, Sharma, vanHove, & Hoffman, 2009).

■ **Clinical Manifestations.** In classic neonatal NKH, symptoms usually start soon after birth and are not related to feedings. The clinical picture is dominated by neurologic decompensation: rapidly increasing stupor, lethargy, unresponsiveness, apnea, and sustained seizures that are difficult to control (Hyland et al., 2009). Myoclonic jerking and hiccupping (from diaphragmatic spasms) are also common. Within 1 to 3 days, the infant becomes comatose and death ensues. Babies who survive have intractable seizures and uniformly poor neurologic outcomes.

■ **Diagnosis.** Glycine is elevated in plasma, urine, and CSF. The CSF-to-plasma glycine concentration ratio of affected infants is greater than 0.09 (normal is <0.04). The diagnostic workup fails to find evidence such as metabolic acidosis, ketosis, hyperammonemia, or abnormal organic acids in blood or urine suggestive of another IEM. Electroencephalographic (EEG) tracings typically show a burst suppression pattern with hypsarrhythmia (random, high-voltage slow waves and spikes that arise from multiple foci and spread to all cortical areas). Confirmation of the exact enzyme deficiency is made by enzyme assay of a liver sample or by molecular analysis.

■ **Management.** No consistently effective therapy has been discovered for classic neonatal onset NKH. Attempts to reduce plasma glycine levels with sodium benzoate, and manage seizures with anticonvulsants have not changed the poor neurodevelopmental outcomes of NKH (Hyland et al., 2009).

Hereditary Tyrosinemia

Hereditary tyrosinemia type I, also called hepatorenal tyrosinemia or fumarylacetoacetate hydrolase (FAH) deficiency, is a severe autosomal recessive metabolic disorder affecting the liver, kidney, and nervous system.

■ **Pathophysiology.** Tyrosine is derived from the metabolism of dietary phenylalanine, and from catabolic processes. Tyrosine degradation requires a series of enzymes, the last of which is FAH. A deficiency of this enzyme characterizes tyrosinemia type I (Leonard & Morris, 2009). The offending compounds in tyrosinemia type I are fumarylacetoacetate and maleylacetoacetate, both of which accumulate in the cells of the liver and kidney and cause cell death by apoptosis. Although hepatocytes are quickly regenerated, liver function can deteriorate rapidly in babies with tyrosinemia type I (Cederbaum, 2012).

■ **Clinical Manifestations.** Patients with hereditary tyrosinemia type I may come to clinical attention in the newborn period or within the first 3 weeks of life. Newborns present with evidence of liver dysfunction including firm hepatomegaly, splenomegaly, bleeding from coagulation defects, jaundice, and ascites (Leonard & Morris, 2009). Renal tubular dysfunction and hypophosphatemic rickets are common.

■ **Diagnosis.** The diagnostic workup includes liver function tests, which typically show elevated transaminases, and prolonged PT and PTT. Plasma tyrosine, phenylalanine, methionine, bilirubin, and serum alphafeto protein (AFP) may be elevated. The urine organic acid analysis reveals increased excretion of succinylacetone. The diagnosis can be confirmed by enzyme analysis of cultured skin fibroblasts or molecular studies. Hereditary tyrosinemia is included on the recommended uniform newborn screening panel (U.S. Department of HHS, 2011).

■ **Management.** Hereditary tyrosinemia type I is now treated with nitisinone, a potent inhibitor of 4-hydroxyphenylpyruvate dioxygenase (Leonard & Morris, 2009). The response is monitored with urine succinylacetone, liver function tests, clotting studies, renal tubular function, and serum AFP. Most patients respond within a week with improved liver and renal function.

Dietary management involves feeding the infant a phenylalanine- and tyrosine-free formula, or breastfeeding, with phenylalanine supplementation sparingly, if needed (Leonard & Morris, 2009). Some infants will require a liver transplant to avoid the development of hepatocellular carcinoma.

Transient Tyrosinemia

Transient tyrosinemia in the newborn is the most common disorder of tyrosine metabolism.

■ **Pathophysiology.** Transient tyrosinemia is most likely caused by immaturity of 4-hydroxyphenylpyruvic acid dioxygenase (4HPPD), a vitamin C–dependent enzyme in the tyrosine degradation pathway. Risk factors include prematurity (hepatic immaturity), low vitamin C intake, and excessive protein intake. In some infants, transient tyrosinemia may be precipitated by endogenous catabolism. Tyrosinemia peaks in the first 14 days of life and resolves by 1 month of life (Leonard & Morris, 2009).

■ **Clinical Manifestations.** Lethargy and poor feeding may be seen in neonates with hypertyrosinemia, particularly in preterm infants.

■ **Diagnosis.** Transient hypertyrosinemia is identified by positive newborn metabolic screen.

■ **Management.** All infants with an elevated tyrosine on initial newborn screen should have a repeat screen done; with confirmatory testing for those who remain abnormal (see Hereditary Tyrosinemia). This is usually a self-limited disorder that does not require therapy. Therapies include a low protein diet and supplemental vitamin C as a cofactor to increase the activity of 4HPPD and accelerate the fall in tyrosine concentration.

PKU

Classical PKU is an autosomal recessive disorder caused by mutations in both alleles of the gene for phenylalanine hydroxylase, found on chromosome 12. Classic PKU occurs in about 1 in 10,000 to 13,000 live births (Hertzberg, Hinton, Therrell, & Shapira, 2011). Although PKU rarely manifests clinically in the newborn period, it will be discussed here because it is important for neonatal caregivers to be able to provide accurate information to parents about key genetic conditions for which their newborn infants are being screened.

■ **Pathophysiology.** The effect of the inactive phenylalanine hydroxylase enzyme is an inability to metabolize phenylalanine, resulting in hyperphenylalaninemia. Following ingestion of adequate amounts of breast milk or formula, blood phenylalanine levels gradually increase. Phenylketonuric compounds are excreted in the urine, one of which (phenylacetic acid) imparts the musty or mousy odor characteristic of PKU. If dietary therapy is not implemented at birth, mental retardation can occur.

■ **Clinical Manifestations.** Biochemical manifestations of PKU are present in the newborn, but there are no outward clinical signs or symptoms. A musty odor may be detectable in the infant's urine around the end of the first week of life, if plasma phenylalanine levels reach 10 to 15 mg/dL.

■ **Diagnosis.** Early diagnosis is critical because PKU is a preventable cause of mental retardation. Plasma phenylalanine in the normal infant is less than 2 mg/dL. In infants with PKU, the plasma phenylalanine level usually exceeds 4 mg/dL by 24 hours of age and is 20 to 40 mg/dL by the end of the first week of life. PKU is a pioneer among metabolic disorders: It was the first disorder for which a screening test was developed in 1961 (the Guthrie test, a bacterial inhibition assay), and the first disorder to be screened for using MS/MS. MS/MS has dramatically decreased the number of false positive screening results, as well as further clarifying the prevalence of variants of hyperphenylalaninemia in the population.

■ **Management.** PKU is currently treated with a low-phenylalanine diet; however, compliance can be a long-term problem and dietary treatment can be associated with other nutritional deficiencies. Enzyme substitution with recombinant phenylalanine ammonia lyase is being explored as an alternative form of therapy (Cleary, 2010).

DISORDERS OF ORGANIC ACID METABOLISM

The organic acid disorders are disorders of intermediary metabolism resulting from a deficient enzyme or transport protein, the lack of which causes a block in a metabolic pathway. The block occurs in a step after deamination of the amino acid, and the resulting metabolites are organic acid derivatives. An organic acid is distinguished from an amino acid in that it contains no nitrogen. Because these disorders lead to an accumulation of organic acids in the urine, they are often referred to as "organic acidurias."

MSUD

MSUD, a branched-chain organic aciduria, is a disorder resulting from one or more mutations in the gene encoding the enzymes that catalyze the branched-chain amino acids (BCAA) leucine, isoleucine, and valine. The name maple syrup urine disease refers to the intensely sweet, maple sugar odor of the cerumen, skin, and urine that accompanies the disorder (Box 9.2). The incidence of MSUD is about 1 in 200,000 in the general population, but in the Old Order Mennonites of southeastern Pennsylvania the frequency is 1 in 358 births (Puffenberger, 2003).

■ **Pathophysiology.** The second common step in the degradation of a BCAA involves the enzyme branched-chain ketoacid dehydrogenase (BCKAD) complex. This enzyme catalyzes the conversion of the 3-ketoacid derivatives of the BCAA into their decarboxylated coenzyme metabolites within the mitochondria (Hoffman & Schulze, 2009). A deficiency of BCKAD results in an accumulation of the three BCAAs and their metabolites.

The neurotoxicity of MSUD is secondary to the accumulation of the ketoacid of leucine, 2-oxoisocaproic acid, in the plasma and organs. Leucine intoxication impairs the volume-regulating mechanisms in the brain, liver, muscle, and pancreatic cells. A fall in serum sodium precipitates a redistribution of water in the intracellular spaces of the brain, causing cerebral edema. The brains of newborns with MSUD exhibit severe cytotoxic edema with involvement of myelinated white matter on MRI (Kilicarslan, Alkan, Demirkol, Toprak, & Sharifov, 2012).

■ **Clinical Manifestations.** The neonate with classical MSUD is usually born at term after an uncomplicated pregnancy and delivery. A short symptom-free interval occurs after birth. During this time, the usual postnatal endogenous protein catabolism causes a progressive rise in BCAA levels, with concomitant metabolic acidosis.

By about 48 hours of age, the untreated infant begins to show signs of the disorder. The earliest and most specific sign is the unique maple syrup odor of the cerumen. Other early signs and symptoms of MSUD are feeding difficulties, irritability, lethargy, and dystonia. Over the ensuing hours, neurologic deterioration predominates, as drowsiness and lethargy progress to coma. Periods of lethargy and hypotonia alternate with muscular rigidity, hypertonia, and seizures. Opisthotonic posturing is a characteristic feature of classic MSUD (Hoffmann & Schulze, 2009).

BOX 9.2

UNUSUAL ODORS ASSOCIATED WITH IEMs

Disorder	Odor
MSUD	Maple syrup—burnt sugar
Tyrosinemia type I	Cabbage or rancid butter
Multiple acyl-CoA dehydrogenase deficiency	Sweaty socks—rancid cheese
Phenylketonuria	Mousy—musty
PA	Cat urine
Isovaleric acidemia	Sweaty socks—rancid cheese
Ketoaciduria	Fruity
3-Methylglutaconic aciduria	Tomcat urine
Trimethylaminuria	Fish

■ **Diagnosis.** Early diagnosis and management are essential to prevent permanent brain damage. MSUD is diagnosed by plasma amino acid assay. An elevated leucine level and a high leucine-to-alanine ratio are diagnostic of MSUD. A dinitrophenylhydrazine (DNPH) test of the urine, which screens for the presence of a-ketoacids, will be positive. Urine should also be tested for ketones, which are typically present. Ketonuria is never normal in the neonate and should always suggest the possibility of an IEM. Urinary organic acid analysis should also be performed.

By the time of diagnosis on clinical grounds, many infants with MSUD are severely encephalopathic and require emergency therapy to lower the BCAA levels. Newborn screening by tandem MS allows for detection of elevated BCAA concentrations in blood in patients with classical MSUD before the onset of severe encephalopathy. All states include MSUD on their newborn screening panels. Unfortunately, these specimens are often collected after 24 hours of age, and results are not reported until infants are 6 to 10 days of age. An infant with classic MSUD would already be seriously ill by this time.

■ **Management.** The aims of treatment of MSUD are to rapidly lower the plasma leucine level and achieve stable, long-term metabolic control with a carefully monitored low-BCAA diet. Hemodialysis, hemofiltration, or ECMO are used to remove toxins. High-energy enteral or parenteral nutrition, with close monitoring of BCAA levels, is the dietary therapy used in the newborn period to augment toxin removal. Even after the infant is in good metabolic control, however, common infections and injuries can rapidly induce biochemical disturbances requiring prompt changes in management to prevent a metabolic crisis (Cederbaum, 2012).

Isovaleric Acidemia

Isovaleric acidemia (IVA) is a disorder of leucine metabolism caused by mutations in the gene encoding the enzyme isovaleryl-CoA dehydrogenase, mapped to chromosome 15. IVA has an incidence of about 1 in 67,000 live births (Ensenauer et al., 2011). The disorder has both an acute and chronic form; the acute form manifests in the neonatal period as catastrophic disease.

■ **Pathophysiology.** Isovaleryl-CoA dehydrogenase catalyzes the third step in the catabolism of the BCAA leucine in the inner mitochondrial matrix (Grünert et al., 2012). A deficiency of isovaleryl-CoA dehydrogenase leads to accumulations of highly toxic free isovaleric acid, 3-hydroxyvaleric acid, and N-isovalerylglycine. Excess organic acids in the bloodstream inhibit gluconeogenesis and ureagenesis, predisposing the infant to both hypoglycemia and hyperammonemia, and causing fulminant metabolic acidosis (Grunert et al., 2012). Hypoglycemia stimulates the release of free fatty acids, which are transported into the mitochondria where they are oxidized to produce ketones, the source of ketosis in infants with IVA and other organic acidemias. These organic acids also arrest maturation of hematopoietic precursors, leading to leukopenia and thrombocytopenia (Hoffmann & Schulze, 2009; Wicken, 2010).

■ **Clinical Manifestations.** Infants with IVA become extremely ill in the first week of life. Early symptoms are poor feeding, vomiting, lethargy, and hypothermia. Clinical evidence of dehydration is often present. Untreated infants progress to coma, and less than half survive the initial metabolic crisis. IVA can be recognized by the unpleasant "sweaty feet" or "rancid cheese" odor of body fluids. Hepatomegaly is present in some infants.

■ **Diagnosis.** The diagnosis of IVA is based on the presence of isovalerylglycine and its metabolites in urine, and of isovalerylcarnitine in plasma. Plasma organic acid analysis also reveals markedly elevated N-isovalerylglycine and 3-hydroxyvaleric acid. A secondary carnitine deficiency can develop. Both ketosis and metabolic acidosis, with an elevated anion gap, are present. Secondary derangements include hyperammonemia, thrombocytopenia, neutropenia, and anemia. IVA can be detected by MS/MS using filter-paper bloodspot samples and is included on the recommended uniform newborn screening panel (U.S. Department of HHS, 2011).

■ **Management.** Infants who are extremely ill as a result of accumulation of isovaleric acid will need exogenous toxin removal with hemodialysis, hemofiltration, or ECMO (Cederbaum, 2012). Supplementation with l-glycine is also effective for IVA. Glycine promotes the formation of isovalerylglycine, which is excreted more efficiently than free isovaleric acid. l-Carnitine is given to replace lost carnitine and to provide substrate for the formation of isovalerylcarnitine, a nontoxic by-product that can be excreted in the urine (Cederbaum, 2012). If metabolic acidosis is severe, bicarbonate therapy is indicated. Adequate fluids are mandatory to promote excretion of isovaleric acid because the primary route of elimination is the kidney. Urine output must be carefully monitored. Initially, until the diagnosis is confirmed, protein is removed from the diet and a high-energy intake of glucose and intralipid is administered. Nutritional support is subsequently provided in the form of leucine-free amino acid mixtures followed by a reduced leucine diet. It is important to reintroduce a balanced nutritional intake, including protein, as soon as possible to promote an anabolic state in these infants.

Propionic Acidemia

Propionic acidemia (PA) is a severe autosomal recessive disorder caused by mutations in the genes that encode the two nonidentical subunits (alpha and beta) of the propionyl-CoA carboxylase enzyme. Its estimated incidence is less than 1 in 100,000 births.

■ **Pathophysiology.** Propionyl-CoA carboxylase is involved in the metabolism of BCAA, odd-chain fatty acids, and cholesterol (Daniotti et al., 2011). Propionyl-CoA carboxylase is necessary for the synthesis of nicotinamide adenine dinucleotide, the main substrate of the mitochondrial respiratory chain (Romano et al., 2010). Propionate is a product of catabolism of amino acids (isoleucine, valine, threonine, and methionine), oxidation of odd-chain fatty acids, and gut bacterial activity. A deficiency of propionyl-CoA carboxylase results in an accumulation of toxic organic acid metabolites in the mitochondria causing severe ketoacidosis (see also Isovaleric Acidemia).

■ **Clinical Manifestations.** The clinical features of PA typically manifest shortly after birth, beginning with poor feeding, vomiting, lethargy, and hypotonia (Chapman et al., 2012). Ketonuria and metabolic acidosis develop in most infants, and severe intracellular dehydration may develop. Seizures often follow. Hepatomegaly may stem from steatosis. Infants with PA are susceptible to bacterial infections as a result of neutropenia and thrombocytopenia. The odor imparted to body fluids by propionic acid has been likened to "cat urine." Cardiomyopathy of uncertain pathogenesis is associated with PA (Romano et al., 2010) and may be associated with rapid deterioration and death in infants with this disorder. Magnetic resonance spectroscopy confirms compromised aerobic metabolism within brain tissue during acute metabolic decompensation (Davison et al., 2011). Neurologic sequelae of PA include encephalopathy, hypotonia, seizures, extrapyramidal symptoms, optic nerve atrophy, and stroke-like episodes (Johnson, Le, & Palacios, 2009).

■ **Diagnosis.** In most cases, there is a marked elevation of free propionate in the blood and urine. However, these findings are occasionally absent, and in those cases, significant elevations of other propionate metabolites, such as propionyl-carnitine, beta-hydroxypropionate, and methylcitrate, help to establish the diagnosis. However, propionyl-carnitine is not specific for PA; it can be elevated in MMA and disorders of vitamin B_{12} transport and synthesis (Chapman et al., 2012). Plasma glycine is also increased, but plasma carnitine is low. The diagnosis of PA can be confirmed either with analysis of enzyme activity in leukocytes or fibroblasts, or with specific mutation analysis. PA can be detected by MS/MS using filter-paper blood-spot samples and is included on the recommended uniform newborn screening panel (U.S. Department of HHS, 2011), allowing presymptomatic diagnosis for some infants (Chapman et al., 2012).

■ **Management.** PA is unique in that the urinary excretion of the toxin, propionic acid, is negligible, and no alternate route can adequately remove the toxin from affected newborns. Emergency treatment to remove toxins using hemodialysis or hemofiltration is imperative. Initially, protein intake is stopped and a high-calorie intake of glucose and intralipid or nonprotein formula is substituted to suppress catabolism. Protein is reintroduced in small quantities after a few days of protein restriction. Secondary hyperammonemia may respond to administration of N-carbamylglutamate (Ah Mew et al., 2010; Kasapkara et al., 2011) sodium benzoate, sodium phenylacetate, or a combined preparation to provide an alternate route for excretion of nitrogen. In some cases, dramatic response to N-carbamylglutamate has obviated the need for hemodialysis (Fillippi et al., 2010). Blood ammonia levels should be followed closely. Carnitine supplementation, to prevent carnitine deficiency and to augment excretion of propionate, has also been used in the early management of infants with PA. In addition, because propionyl-CoA is a biotin-containing enzyme, biotin and cobalamin are given to evaluate for a vitamin-responsive disorder.

Antimicrobial therapy with oral broad-spectrum antibiotics, such as metronidazole or neomycin, inhibits anaerobic colonic flora, thereby suppressing propionate production in the gut. Infants with PA are immune-compromised and easily susceptible to infection; therefore, strict measures to avoid exposure to microbes must be observed. Laboratory indicators of infection must be monitored closely. Infants with PA should also be assessed for evidence of cardiac failure secondary to cardiomyopathy. Long-term dietary management consists of a low-protein, high-energy diet centered on the proportion of valine, a direct precursor to propionyl-CoA. Discharge teaching should include the importance of seeking medical attention immediately for any sign of illness or infection, because even a minor illness can lead to rapid deterioration in an infant with PA.

MMA

MMA is really a group of disorders representing inherited deficiencies of the activity of methylmalonyl-CoA mutase, a vitamin B_{12}–dependent enzyme. MMA is one of the more common organic acidemias, occurring in about 1 in 25,000 to 48,000 infants. About half of the mutations causing MMA are in the genes encoding this enzyme; other mutations can occur in genes required for provision of cobalamin cofactors. In the most severe form of MMA, enzyme activity is completely absent.

■ **Pathophysiology.** Methylmalonyl-CoA mutase is normally responsible for the conversion of methylmalonyl-CoA to succinyl-CoA, a Krebs cycle intermediate. The lack of methylmalonyl-CoA mutase activity results in an intracellular accumulation of methylmalonic acid, impairing mitochondrial oxidative metabolism. A secondary inhibition of propionyl-CoA results in an accumulation of propionic acid and its metabolites. These compounds have inhibitory effects on many intermediary metabolic pathways, leading to hypoglycemia, hyperammonemia, and hyperglycinemia. Conjugation with carnitine results in a relative carnitine deficiency.

■ **Clinical Manifestations.** Most infants with MMA begin showing symptoms before the end of the first week of life. Lethargy, hypotonia, and vomiting with signs of dehydration are followed by respiratory distress, acute encephalopathy, and eventual coma. Untreated infants develop hypoglycemia, hyperammonemia, anion gap metabolic acidosis, and ketosis. MMA is similar to PA in that many infants become neutropenic and thrombocytopenic.

■ **Diagnosis.** Plasma methylmalonic acid and propionylcarnitine are increased in MMA. The presence of C4-dicarboxylic acylcarnitine distinguishes MMA from PA. Urine organic acid analysis demonstrates greatly increased methylmalonic acid and its precursors, methylcitric acid and beta-hydroxypropionate. MMA is detected by MS/MS in states that have adopted the recommended uniform newborn screening panel (U.S. Department of HHS, 2011). Among the many other nonspecific laboratory findings in MMA are metabolic acidosis, hyperammonemia, hyperglycinemia, leukopenia, anemia, thrombocytopenia, and ketonuria. Molecular genetic testing is available for prenatal diagnosis.

■ **Management.** Infants who are severely moribund and those with extreme hyperammonemia (>600 mcmol/L) are likely to have very high levels of toxic organic acids that must be removed expeditiously with hemodialysis or hemofiltration. Severe hyperammonemia can also be treated with N-carbamylglutamate (Tuchman et al., 2008), sodium benzoate, or sodium phenylacetate or a combined preparation to provide an alternate pathway for nitrogen removal. The acute metabolic crisis of MMA is further managed with protein restriction and administration of IV glucose and intralipid. Adequate fluid intake will enhance the elimination of methylmalonic acid, which is relatively efficiently removed from the body by the kidneys. Blood gases should be monitored to evaluate the degree of metabolic acidosis, and sodium bicarbonate may be required to control severe metabolic acidosis. In the event that the infant has a cofactor-responsive disease, pharmacologic doses of vitamin B_{12} are given. Because excess propionate is also a problem in MMA, broad-spectrum antibiotics are given to inhibit anaerobic flora and reduce intestinal propionate production. Supplemental carnitine is used to replace carnitine depletion and promote urinary propionylcarnitine elimination.

Like infants with PA, those with MMA are at high risk for infection owing to compromised immunity reflected by neutropenia and thrombocytopenia. Close monitoring of clinical and laboratory indicators of infection is warranted. These infants must also be monitored for evidence of cardiac failure related to cardiomyopathy. The discharge planning needs of infants with MMA are similar to those of infants with PA. Parents or other caretakers must be aware that even a minor illness or infection in their baby with MMA can represent a potential metabolic crisis and requires prompt medical attention.

FAODs

FAODs are a subset of organic acid disorders that are among the most common of the known inherited disorders of metabolism. The population frequency of FAODs is estimated to be 1 in 8,000 to 16,000, although a number of neonates die before the diagnosis is made. An FAOD can be caused by a deficiency of any of the enzymes involved in cellular uptake, transport, and mitochondrial oxidation of fatty acids. To date, more than 20 defects and their gene mutations have been discovered (Rector & Ibdah, 2010). The most common is MCAD. Short-, long-, and very-long-chain forms of this enzyme deficiency also exist (SCAD, LCAD, very long-chain acyl-CoA dehydrogenase [VLCAD]), as well as carnitine transporter defects, and deficiencies of the mitochondrial trifunctional protein (MTP) complex. The FAODs are considered treatable, and the prognosis for many FAODs has improved in recent years (Wilckin, 2010).

Pathophysiology of FAODs

The fatty acids are the largest source of energy in the body and are the preferred fuels of the liver, heart, and skeletal muscles. Neonatal brown fat uses fatty acids to sustain nonshivering thermogenesis. When glucose levels are low during long periods between feedings, glucagon secreted by the pancreas stimulates adipose cell lipase to liberate free fatty acids. These fatty acids are oxidized to provide energy through the mitochondrial beta-oxidation pathway. Fatty acid oxidation also provides the substrate for hepatic ketogenesis. Fatty acids as a source of energy are particularly critical for the neonate who has limited stores of glycogen and a high metabolic rate; thus, any perturbation in the fatty acid oxidation pathway can rapidly lead to metabolic decompensation.

■ **Fatty Acid Oxidation.** Three subsystems are required for the production of energy in the normal fat oxidation process (Figure 9.3): (1) the carnitine cycle, (2) the mitochondrial inner membrane system, and (3) the

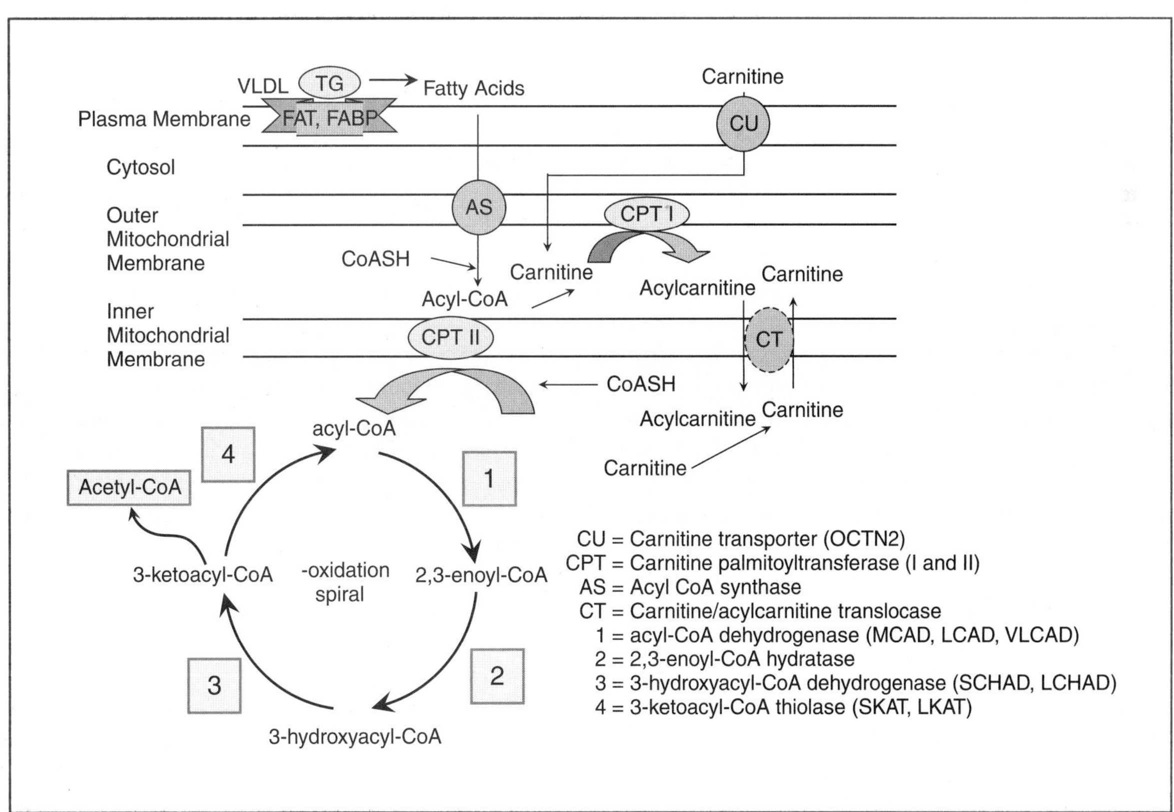

FIGURE 9.3 The mitochondrial fatty acid oxidation pathway. This schematic representation shows the uptake of fatty acids and carnitine into the cell, transfer of fatty acid from the cytosol into mitochondria, and the fatty acid beta-oxidation spiral.
Adapted from Shekhawat et al. (2003).

mitochondrial matrix system (Strauss, Andresen, & Bennett, 2009). In the first step, l-carnitine and fatty acids are taken up by the cell, and fatty acids are conjugated to fatty acyl-CoAs in the cytoplasm by enzymes of the outer mitochondrial membrane. Medium- and short-chain fatty acids can penetrate the inner mitochondrial membrane for beta-oxidation, but longer-chain fatty acids of dietary fat (those with carbon lengths of 14 to 20) must be actively transported into the matrix via the carnitine cycle. Activated acyl-CoAs are converted to carnitine esters by carnitine palmitoyltransferase I (CPT I), transported across the mitochondrial membrane by carnitine-acylcarnitine translocase, and reactivated by carnitine palmitoyltransferase II (CPT II).

Within the mitochondrion, long-chain acyl-CoAs are degraded by enzymes in the inner membrane system in a recurring cyclic sequence of four reactions (Strauss et al., 2009). These are catalyzed by VLCAD and the MTP complex encompassing the three enzymes required for a single cycle of beta oxidation: enoyl-CoA hydratase, l to 3-hydroxy acyl-CoA dehydrogenase (LCHAD), and thiolase. In each full cycle, the fatty acid is progressively shortened by two carbons from long, to medium, and finally to short-chain acyl-CoAs. The final system, the mitochondrial matrix, oxidizes shorter chain length fatty acids resulting from the enzymatic steps in the inner membrane system. l-Carnitine is not required for the latter process. The result of the beta-oxidation system is generation of acetyl-CoA, used by the liver to produce ketone bodies and as a major source of cellular ATP.

■ Defective Fatty Acid Oxidation

Inborn errors of fatty acid oxidation result in a buildup of toxic metabolites both proximal and distal to the block, and an insufficient yield of substrate for energy production. A deficiency of any of the enzymes required for fatty acid transport or metabolism can result in a failure of fatty acid oxidation. The primary physiologic consequence is inadequate ATP and ketone body generation, and a failure of energy production. This becomes apparent during periods of increased energy demand, such as a prolonged period of fasting, fever, or other illness. Under normal circumstances, when glycogen stores are depleted in the newborn, free fatty acids are released as a source of energy. However, the neonate with an FAOD is unable to use fatty acids for fuel and rapidly becomes hypoglycemic. As a result of hypoketogenesis, the brain is without an alternate fuel source. Without early treatment, neurologic morbidity and mortality are high. A second consequence of FAODs is the accumulation of fatty acids and their derivatives, which can have toxic effects. When their oxidation is blocked, fatty acids are stored in the cytosol as triglycerides, resulting in muscular, hepatic, and cardiac lipidoses. Skeletal muscle tissue begins to break down (rhabdomyolysis), causing a skeletal myopathy characterized by muscle weakness. In defects downstream from CPT-I in the carnitine cycle, the acylcarnitine that accumulates has detergent-like properties that may disrupt the integrity of muscle membranes. In the heart muscle, accumulated long-chain fatty acyl-CoAs can produce electrophysiologic abnormalities, including arrhythmias and cardiac arrest.

Clinical Manifestations of FAODs

Affected neonates are almost always born at term. A fasting stress sufficient to reveal the disorder can result with early breastfeeding, especially in infants who do not nurse well (Jameson & Walter, 2010). Mitochondrial FAODs in the neonate present with three clinical phenotypes that, depending on the disorder, can be seen individually or in combination: hypoketotic hypoglycemia, cardiomyopathy, and skeletal myopathy (Rector & Ibdah, 2010). Neonates with MCAD the most common of the FAODs usually present with glucose instability, but there have been reports of acute life-threatening episodes and even sudden death (Rector & Ibdah, 2010).

Neonates with VLCAD are similarly intolerant to fasting and develop hypoglycemia without ketosis. Moreover, VLCAD can be associated with evidence of cardiomyopathy, including cardiomegaly, ventricular arrhythmias, or unexplained cardiac arrest. Other physical findings that have been reported in neonates with disorders of fatty acid oxidation include hypotonia, seizures, irritability or lethargy (mimicking acute encephalopathy), hepatomegaly, and associated congenital malformations, such as cystic renal dysplasia.

Diagnosis of FAODs

An FAOD must be considered in any infant with an unexplained nonketotic hypoglycemia, hepatic dysfunction, isolated arrhythmia, or cardiomegaly. The initial screen for FAOD includes urine organic acid analysis, and plasma and urine free and total carnitine, collected during a period of acute decompensation. A strong clue to an FAOD is urinary excretion of dicarboxylic acids, compounds not normally found in the urine (Rector & Ibdah, 2010). Plasma carnitine levels will be markedly reduced.

To reach a specific diagnosis of mitochondrial fat oxidation, a plasma acylcarnitine profile must be obtained (Rector & Ibdah, 2010). Using whole blood samples on filter paper and MS/MS, the acylcarnitine intermediates formed as a result of the enzymatic block somewhere in the fat oxidation cycle can be quantified. A plasma acylcarnitine profile reveals accumulation of acyl-CoA conjugates proximal to the defect. When MS/MS screening is not available, the most useful indirect laboratory tests in neonates with suspected FAODs are glucose, electrolytes, BUN, creatinine, lactate, ammonia, transaminases, and creatine kinase. Elevated creatine kinase and myoglobinuria reflect rhabdomyolysis. Plasma carnitine levels are markedly reduced, except in CPT-1 deficiency (Strauss et al., 2009). Additional laboratory results may show hyperammonemia, metabolic acidosis, and increased uric acid and transaminases. A liver biopsy performed during the acute phase usually reveals microvesicular and macrovesicular fatty infiltration.

Family and perinatal history can be particularly important to the diagnosis of an FAOD. Many infants diagnosed with an FAOD have a history of a sibling who died of sudden infant death. In addition, an association has been found between acute fatty liver of pregnancy (AFLP) or HELLP (hemolysis, elevated liver enzymes, low platelets) syndrome in the mother and fetal deficiency of long-chain 3-hydroxyacyl coenzyme A dehydrogenase (LCHAD), one of the enzymes in the MTP complex. When a woman is carrying an affected fetus, the placenta and fetus are unable to oxidize fatty acids, leading to transfer of accumulated fatty acid intermediates to the maternal circulation. For unclear reasons, in some women these fatty acids overwhelm the maternal liver and contribute to HELLP syndrome and maternal hepatic fat deposition (AFLP).

The newborn infants of women with AFLP or mothers who are known carriers for FAODs should be evaluated immediately after birth with blood-spot acylcarnitine profiles, and treated as if they have an FAOD until test results are known.

■ **Neonatal Screening and Confirmatory Testing for FAOD.** The key to preventing the morbidity and mortality associated with FAOD is through presymptomatic diagnosis, allowing early treatment and avoidance of metabolic crisis. Neonatal screening for FAODs by MS/MS analyzes acylcarnitines from dried blood spots and can identify 22 different abnormalities. However, an abnormal acylcarnitine profile can represent more than one FAOD, so more specific testing is required. Using cultured skin fibroblasts (or amniocytes) that have been incubated with deuterium-labeled fatty acid precursors and excess l-carnitine, MS/MS can rapidly detect any enzyme defect from translocase through SCAD. This method is possible because the enzymes of fatty acid oxidation are also expressed in the skin and other cells. Mutational analysis, if available, can also provide a definitive diagnosis (Strauss et al., 2009).

Management of FAODs

The primary goal is to provide nutrition that will control endogenous lipolysis and prevent tissue catabolism. This involves a high-carbohydrate, low-fat diet. The newborn should feed every 3 to 4 hours, with close monitoring of blood sugar level. Breastfeeding mothers should receive lactation assistance to ensure successful breastfeeding with evidence of milk transfer. If hypoglycemia persists or the infant is unable to tolerate enteral feeding, glucose should be administered intravenously. Closely monitor for cardiac conduction disturbances.

The nurse is in a key position to prevent stressors, such as hypothermia or pain, that could precipitate a metabolic crisis, and to assess the infant for signs of intercurrent illness that might require additional therapy. Discharge teaching should emphasize the need to avoid prolonged periods of fasting and to seek medical attention if the infant shows signs of illness (fever, vomiting, diarrhea, refusal to eat, lethargy, or any other change in normal behavior). A consult should be made with a neonatal nutritionist or dietary specialist to arrange teaching for the family about the infant's postdischarge dietary regimen. The infant's diet will continue to be high in carbohydrate and restricted in fat. Supplementation with l-carnitine has not been shown to be beneficial (Spiekerkoetter et al., 2010; Wilcken, 2011).

Multiple Acyl-CoA Dehydrogenase Deficiency (Glutaric Aciduria Type II)

■ **Pathophysiology.** Multiple acyl-CoA dehydrogenase deficiency (MADD), formerly known as glutaric aciduria type II, is a disorder caused by a defective electron transfer flavoprotein (ETF) or electron transfer flavoprotein dehydrogenase (ETF-QO). MADD impairs both fatty acid oxidation and oxidation of branched amino acids lysine and glutaric acid. The heart, liver, and kidneys become infiltrated with fat.

■ **Clinical Manifestations.** Two different neonatal presentations have been described for MADD; both involve overwhelming illness with rapid progression to coma and death (Strauss et al., 2009). One presentation is a neonate, often preterm, with dysmorphic facial features, polycystic kidneys, and hepatomegaly. Within the first 24 to 48 hours of life the infant develops hypotonia, metabolic acidosis, severe nonketotic hypoglycemia, and a distinctive "sweaty feet" odor of body fluids. The alternate neonatal presentation is the infant without congenital anomalies, but with similar symptoms and metabolic aberrations. Neither group lives longer than a few weeks; the few babies who survive generally succumb at a few months of age to cardiac failure.

■ **Diagnosis.** Tandem MS rapidly detects elevated acylcarnitines (C4, C5, C8, C10, and C16). Quantitative urine organic acid analysis usually reveals a pattern of elevated organic acids: lactic, glutaric, 2-hydroxyglutaric, ethylmalonic, adipic, suberic, sebacic, and other acids, some in very high amounts. The same organic acids are increased in the plasma. Volatile acid (isovaleric, acetic, isobutyric, propionic, butyric) concentrations in plasma are excessive, accounting for the characteristic odor associated with the disorder. Plasma carnitine may be low. Mutations have been identified in the genes for flavoproteins ETF and ETF-QO.

■ **Management.** There is no effective treatment other than supportive care (fluids, glucose, sodium bicarbonate) for the rapid-onset, severe neonatal presentation. For the rare infant who survives the initial crisis, management involves frequent feedings with avoidance of fasting, and a diet low in fat and protein and high in carbohydrates. Some patients also respond to riboflavin.

CONGENITAL LACTIC ACIDOSES

The congenital lactic acidoses (also called primary lactic acidoses) are a group of disorders of lactate metabolism caused by defects in the mitochondrial respiratory or electron transport chain, the tricarboxylic acid (Krebs) cycle, or in pyruvate metabolism.

Lactic acid is the major end product of anaerobic glycolysis, accumulating when production of pyruvate exceeds utilization. The brain's dependence on oxidative metabolism makes it particularly susceptible to damage in disorders of oxidation that lead to lactic acidosis.

PDH Deficiency

PDH complex disorders are the most common inborn errors of pyruvate metabolism. Most cases of PDH are caused by mutations in the X-linked *PDHA1* gene, which encodes the E1 alpha subunit of the PDH enzyme complex (Brown, 2012).

■ **Pathophysiology.** PDH complex efficiently and irreversibly converts pyruvate, a product of glucose metabolism, to acetyl-CoA. Acetyl-CoA is one of two essential substrates needed to generate citrate for the energy-producing tricarboxylic acid cycle (also called the citric acid cycle or Krebs cycle). Thus PDH provides the link between glycolysis and the tricarboxylic acid cycle. PDH complex activity is regulated primarily by reversible phosphorylation (inactivation) of the enzyme's E1 alpha subunit. A deficiency in the PDH complex limits the production of acetyl-CoA, and in turn the production of citrate, blocking the tricarboxylic acid cycle and creating an energy deficit. Persistent glycolysis without pyruvate oxidation leads to the accumulation of lactate because excess pyruvate is reduced to lactate in the cytoplasm. Tissues with high energy requirements, such as those of central nervous system, are vulnerable to injury when cellular energy production is impaired.

■ **Clinical Manifestations.** The nonspecific early signs and symptoms of PDH deficiency develop soon after birth and are similar to those of other metabolic disorders. Poor feeding, lethargy, and tachypnea are followed by progressive neurologic deterioration, apnea, seizures, and coma. Fulminant lactic acidosis is present in infants with profound deficiencies of the PDH complex, and these patients often die early in the neonatal period. Infants with severe disease may have prenatal onset leading to structural brain abnormalities including microcephaly. MRI may show ventricular dilatation, cerebral atrophy, hydrancephaly, partial or complete absence of the corpus callosum, and periventricular leukomalacia (Sharma, Sharrard, Connolly, & Mordekar, 2012). Patients with PDH complex deficiency can also present with Leigh syndrome.

■ **Diagnosis.** Lactic acidosis is an important biochemical marker for mitochondrial dysfunction. Hyperlactatemia, with an elevated lactate:pyruvate ratio, is predictive of early demise (Patel, O'Brien, Subramony, Shuster, & Stacpoole, 2012). Lactate and pyruvate are also often elevated in the CSF of babies with this disorder. Plasma and urine amino acid analysis reveal hyperalaninemia. A definitive diagnosis of enzyme activity requires testing of leukocytes, fibroblasts, or tissue samples; or DNA analysis.

■ **Collaborative Management.** No effective treatment has been found to date for any of the PDH complex defects that manifest in the neonatal period. Therapies include alternate dietary regimens or vitamins such as thiamine that might stimulate residual enzyme activity or circumvent the enzyme defect. Because infants with PDH complex deficiency oxidize carbohydrates poorly, a ketogenic (high-fat, low-carbohydrate) diet has been used to provide an alternate energy source for acetyl-CoA production (Patel et al., 2012). These diets may reduce hyperlactatemia and improve short-term neuromuscular function in infants with PDH complex deficiency. Cofactor supplementation with thiamine, carnitine, and lipoic acid is another facet of the management of these infants.

Recently, dichloroacetate (DCA) has been used to treat PDH complex deficiency. DCA is believed to activate PDH complex activity by inhibiting PDH kinase. PDH complex is thereby "locked" in its unphosphorylated, catalytically active form (Patel et al., 2012).

PCD

PCD is a disorder of energy metabolism that exists in three different forms. The most severe of these is a neonatal-onset form known as type B, a disorder with a high mortality rate. All forms of PCD have a frequency of about 1 in 250,000 live births and are recessively inherited.

■ **Pathophysiology.** Pyruvate carboxylase is a biotin-containing mitochondrial enzyme responsible for the ATP-dependent carboxylation of pyruvate. This enzyme also catalyzes the conversion of pyruvate to oxaloacetate, an essential substrate in gluconeogenesis, glycogen synthesis, lipogenesis, and other metabolic pathways (Marin-Valencia, Roe, & Pascual, 2010). The absence of pyruvate carboxylase activity results in malfunction of the citric acid cycle and gluconeogenesis, thereby disrupting energy metabolism in the brain. A deficiency of aspartic acid, derived from oxaloacetate, disrupts the urea cycle as well, leading to a simultaneous failure of nitrogen excretion.

■ **Clinical Manifestations.** In PCD of neonatal onset, the earliest signs and symptoms begin at 72 hours and include severe truncal hypotonia and tachypnea associated with profound metabolic acidosis. Seizures, abnormal eye movements, and coma can occur. Hyperammonemia, hypoglycemia, ketosis, and ketonuria are frequent findings. Renal tubular acidosis can also accompany PCD.

■ **Diagnosis.** The diagnosis of PCD is based on the measurement of urinary organic acids and blood acylcarnitine profile. In type B PCD, the lactate/pyruvate ratio may be high (≥25). Plasma citrulline and lysine are elevated along with the ammonia level. Serum transaminases may also be elevated. The diagnosis can be confirmed by enzyme analysis of hepatic cells or leukocytes.

■ **Management.** PCD is a progressive disorder with no specific therapy. Some infants have biotin-responsive disease, so pharmacologic doses of biotin are administered and the response is evaluated. Therapeutic options that involve replenishment of citric acid cycle intermediates to interrupt the hyperactive catabolic cascade associated with the disorder and enhance ATP production are being explored (Marin-Valencia, Roe, & Pascual, 2010).

DISORDERS OF CARBOHYDRATE METABOLISM

Galactosemia

Galactosemia is an inherited disorder of carbohydrate metabolism caused by a deficiency in one of the three enzymes of the galactose metabolic pathway: galactose-1-phosphate uridyl transferase (GALT), galactokinase (GALK), or UDP-galactose-4-epimerase (GALE). GALT deficiency, affecting the second step in the galactose metabolism, accounts for more than 95% of galactosemias; thus it has become synonymous with classical galactosemia.

Galactosemia has an estimated prevalence of 1 in 40,000 to 60,000 live births (G. T. Berry, 2012). At least 24 different mutations have been identified to date in the human GALT gene, located on chromosome 9.

■ **Pathophysiology.** Infants with galactosemia are unable to metabolize the sugar galactose, derived from the disaccharide lactose, the major carbohydrate of mammalian milk. In normal galactose metabolism, galactose is first converted to galactose-1-phosphate by GALK, which is in turn converted by the GALT enzyme to uridyl diphosphate (UDP) glucose. The severe form of galactosemia features near total deficiency of GALT enzyme activity in all cells of the body. In the absence of GALT, ingestion of lactose-containing substances produces toxic levels of galactose-1-phosphate within cells. Surplus galactose is reduced to galactitol or oxidized to galactonate, metabolites that also have a direct toxic effect on the liver and other organs.

■ **Clinical Manifestations.** Most patients present in the neonatal period or in the first week or two of life. After ingestion of galactose (either cow's milk–based formula or breast milk), vomiting, diarrhea, poor weight gain, jaundice, hepatomegaly, and hypoglycemia become evident. In some infants, CNS symptoms, such as lethargy and hypotonia, predominate. Untreated infants will go on to develop cataracts secondary to the accumulation of galactitol. Sepsis, usually caused by *Escherichia coli*, is often the presenting problem, owing to low neutrophil bactericidal activity. Liver dysfunction is progressive, and many infants die during the first week of life from liver failure. In those who do survive, neurologic complications are frequent.

Two related disorders of galactose metabolism are GALK and GALE. In GALK deficiency, galactose cannot be phosphorylated into galactose-1-phosphate. The chief clinical finding in GALK deficiency is cataract formation. In GALE deficiency, most patients are asymptomatic and have normal growth and development.

■ **Diagnosis.** A galactose assay, measuring blood galactose, RBC galactose- 1-phosphate, and GALT enzyme activity is used to diagnose classic galactosemia. GALT activity is low or absent. Galactose and galactose-1-phosphate are elevated. DNA analysis for the common mutations associated with GALT deficiency can also be done. Urine is positive for reducing substances. Galactosemia is included on all routine state newborn screening panels, allowing presymptomatic diagnosis.

■ **Management.** Galactosemia is treated by feeding a soy-based formula, containing no galactose. Breastfeeding is not permitted. Other sources of galactose, including medications containing galactose, must also be avoided. Dietary restriction of galactose in the newborn will reverse the hepatic, renal, brain, and immune dysfunction and reduce the accumulated galactose metabolites. Additional measures include monitoring for and treating sepsis and coagulopathy. Despite dietary treatment, long-term neurodevelopmental outcomes have not been uniformly favorable. An important part of discharge education is dietary teaching to assist the family to maintain dietary control as the infant grows and develops and help them identify occult sources of galactose in foods and other substances.

Hereditary Fructose Intolerance

Hereditary fructose intolerance (HFI) is an inherited inability to digest fructose (fruit sugar) or its precursors (sugar, sorbitol, and brown sugar). This autosomal recessive disorder has a frequency of approximately 1 in 22,000 births.

■ **Pathophysiology.** Fructose is a naturally occurring sugar that is used as a sweetener in many foods, including many baby foods. A deficiency of activity of the enzyme fructose-1-phosphate aldolase impairs the body's ability to convert fructose-1-phosphate to glyceraldehyde and dihydroxyacetone phosphate. The outcome is an accumulation of fructose-1-phosphate in the liver, kidney, and small intestine, which inhibits glycogen breakdown and glucose synthesis and causes severe hypoglycemia following ingestion of fructose. This disorder can be life threatening to infants.

■ **Clinical Manifestations.** In the neonate, the onset of clinical symptoms follows ingestion of cow's milk formula and resembles that for galactosemia. Signs and symptoms include pallor, lethargy, poor feeding, irritability, vomiting, and hypoglycemia. Jaundice, hepatomegaly, and evidence of progressive liver disease may follow. In exclusively breastfed infants, symptoms will be delayed until the time of weaning to fruits and vegetables.

■ Diagnosis. The diagnosis of HFI is usually now by molecular analysis, rather than enzyme analysis or fructose tolerance testing (Cederbaum & Berry, 2012). Urine is positive for reducing substances.

■ Management. Management of HFI centers on removal of all sources of fructose and sucrose from the diet. All intravenous solutions and other medications must also be free of fructose, corn syrup, and sorbitol. Supportive care includes management of liver failure, kidney dysfunction, and coagulopathy, if present. The infant's parents will benefit from consultation with a dietary specialist to learn about long-term dietary management.

Fructose-1,6-Bisphosphatase Deficiency

Fructose-1,6-biphosphatase deficiency is a rare disorder of carbohydrate metabolism.

■ Pathophysiology. Fructose-1,6-bisphosphatase catalyzes the irreversible splitting of fructose-1,6-biphosphate into fructose-6-phosphate and inorganic phosphate. The enzyme's activity is highest in gluconeogenic tissues such as the liver and kidney. Fructose-1,6-biphosphatase deficiency is, therefore, a disorder of gluconeogenesis, resulting in glucose deprivation to the central nervous system.

■ Clinical Manifestations. In fructose-1,6-biphosphatase deficiency, hypoglycemia is precipitated by fasting, not by fructose ingestion (Cederbaum & Berry, 2012). Lactic acidosis and ketosis result from accumulating lactic, 3-hydroxybutyric, and acetoacetic acids. Hyperventilation followed by apnea may result from profound acidosis. Although the acidosis and hypoglycemia may be treated and the infant recovers from the acute attack, if the underlying disorder is not recognized, the infant can have many acute metabolic attacks and develop hepatomegaly and failure-to-thrive before the diagnosis is finally made.

■ Diagnosis. Definitive diagnosis is made by liver biopsy and assay of hepatic enzymes. Mutational analysis is available and can be used instead of biopsy.

■ Management. Acute management involves glucose administration with IV solutions and correction of acidosis with sodium bicarbonate. Frequent feedings and avoidance of fasting, with limitation of fructose and sucrose in the diet, usually prevent further episodes. Dietary restriction includes the many prescription and over-the-counter medications with a syrup base containing sucrose. Stress management (e.g., during times of fever, infection, or vomiting) is critical because illness can induce a metabolic attack.

Glycogen Storage Disease

Glycogen storage disease (GSD) is a group of inherited enzyme defects that affect the glycogen synthesis and degradation cycle. Liver and muscle, having the most abundant quantities of glycogen, are usually the most severely affected tissues (Hendriksz & Gissen, 2010). More than 10 different types of GSD have been identified with a collective incidence of about 1 in 20,000 births. Glycogen storage disease type I (GSD-I, also known as von Gierke's disease), the disorder most likely to have neonatal onset, occurs in about 1 in 100,000 births and has two main subtypes (Ia, Ib). GSD-II, known as Pompe's disease, is classified as a lysosomal storage disease.

■ Pathophysiology. GSD-Ia, the most common subtype, is the result of a deficiency of the hepatic enzyme glucose-6-phosphatase (G6Pase), an enzyme situated in the endoplasmic reticulum of the cell. Normally, G6Pase hydrolyzes glucose-6-phosphate to glucose and phosphate. An accumulation of glycogen in the liver, kidney, and intestines results from a deficiency of G6Pase. In the normal neonate, blood glucose falls during the first postnatal hours as the neonate uses circulating glucose obtained from the mother, but then rises as endogenous glucose production begins. In the neonate with GSD-I, blood glucose continues to decline because endogenous glucose production is severely compromised. Instead, the phosphorylated intermediate compounds of glycolysis produce an excess of lactate, resulting in hyperlacticacidemia. Secondary metabolic derangements typical of GSD-I include hyperuricemia and hyperlipidemia.

■ Clinical Manifestations. The neonate with GSD-I cannot cope with the normal postnatal drop in blood sugar. Despite a plentiful supply of glycogen, the neonate is unable to mobilize free glucose and becomes hypoglycemic. The abdomen may appear distended from birth as a result of an enlarged liver. Acute, nonspecific clinical deterioration is related to the buildup of lactic acid in the body.

■ Diagnosis. Definitive diagnosis of GSD-I is accomplished with molecular genetic testing. Typical laboratory findings in GSD-I include increased plasma lactate and metabolic acidosis with an increased anion gap. Ketosis and ketonuria will be found during hypoglycemia. Other routine tests that should be obtained are liver function tests, plasma uric acid, triglycerides, creatinine, coagulation studies, and complete blood count (CBC) with differential. Abdominal ultrasonography is performed to determine liver and kidney size.

■ Management. The goals of treatment of GSD-I are to prevent hypoglycemia and correct secondary biochemical abnormalities. Frequent feedings or continuous gastric feedings may be necessary to maintain normoglycemia and supply the brain with a steady source of glucose, even during the night. Blood glucose levels must be monitored closely. Pharmacologic therapy to address hyperuricemia and prevent the development of gout may be necessary. Very severely affected infants will require a liver transplant. Parent teaching about long-term nutritional management, prevention of hypoglycemia, and special considerations during stress or other illnesses is critically important.

PEROXISOMAL DISORDERS

Peroxisomal disorders are complex developmental and metabolic disorders caused by defects in peroxisome biosynthesis. Two of the better known disorders, Zellweger syndrome (ZS) and neonatal adrenoleukodystrophy (NALD), are now recognized as belonging to a continuous spectrum of disorders, of which ZS is the most severe. ZS has a reported incidence of about 1 in 25,000 to 50,000 births.

Pathophysiology

Peroxisomes are subcellular organelles that synthesize bile acids, cholesterol, and plasmalogens (a type of phospholipid found in myelin sheaths of nerve fibers). Peroxisomes are also critical in the beta-oxidation of very long-chain fatty acids. Peroxisomal disorders arise from either a defect in peroxisomal biosynthesis or a single peroxisomal enzyme or protein (Scott & Olpin, 2010). Individuals with peroxisome biogenesis defects such as ZS and NALD synthesize peroxisomes normally but display defects in the import of peroxisomal enzymes into the lumen of the organelle (Cederbaum & Berry, 2012). Biochemical abnormalities include impaired degradation of peroxide, very long-chain fatty acids, pipecolic acid, and phytanic acid and impaired synthesis of plasmalogens, bile acids, cholesterol, and docosahexaenoic acid. In ZS, the extent of progressive multisystemic disease is profound; in NALD the systemic involvement is milder, but the cerebral demyelination is more pronounced.

Clinical Manifestations

Infants with ZS present with characteristic facial dysmorphism including a high forehead, hypoplastic supraorbital ridges, flat occiput, low and broad nasal bridge, epicanthal folds, high arched palate, small nose with anteverted nares, micrognathia, large fontanelles, wide sutures, and eye abnormalities (Scott & Olpin, 2010). Typically, they have profound hypotonia, an absence of neonatal reflexes, and seizures. The disease affects every organ of the body, particularly the liver, kidney, and brain, resulting in hepatomegaly, renal cysts, white-matter abnormalities, and neuronal migration defects.

Diagnosis

Diagnosis of peroxisomal biosynthesis defects is based on indirect evidence of the defect. Initial tests for an infant with a suspected peroxisomal disorder include plasma very long-chain fatty acids, and plasmalogens in erythrocytes. Affected infants have elevated transaminases, bile acid intermediates, hypercholesterolemia, and increased iron and transferrin concentrations and are often hypoglycemic. A suspected peroxisomal disorder is confirmed by molecular studies if possible (Scott & Olpin, 2010).

Management

Currently, no successful treatment for the peroxisomal disorders is available. Management is supportive care and symptomatic therapy. The median life expectancy of ZS patients is less than 1 year. Milder forms of peroxisome disorders may respond to dietary therapy.

LYSOSOMAL DISORDERS

The lysosomal disorders are a diverse group of inherited conditions caused by dysfunctions in enzymes (called hydrolases) responsible for the degradation of complex macromolecules, such as glycogen, sphingolipids, glycoproteins, and glycosaminoglycans (Wraith, 2010). In these disorders, a complex substrate that is normally degraded by a series of lysosomal enzymes fails to undergo degradation owing to a deficiency or malfunction of one of these enzymes (Figure 9.4). Catabolism of the substrate into soluble end products is incomplete, and insoluble intermediates that are unable to escape from the organelle accumulate within the lysosome (Wraith, 2010). More than 50 lysosomal disorders are recognized, with a collective incidence of 1 in 7,000 to 10,000 births.

Niemann-Pick Type C

■ Pathophysiology. Niemann-Pick type C (NP-C) is a disorder of intracellular cholesterol transport that leads to an accumulation of unesterified cholesterol in lysosomes (Thomas, Greene, & Berry, 2012). Unesterified cholesterol, sphingomyelin, phospholipids, and glycolipids are stored in excess in the liver and spleen, and glycolipids are increased in the brain.

■ Clinical Manifestations. Neonatal-onset NP-C is characterized by conjugated hyperbilirubinemia, ascites, hepatosplenomegaly, and hypotonia (Thomas et al., 2012).

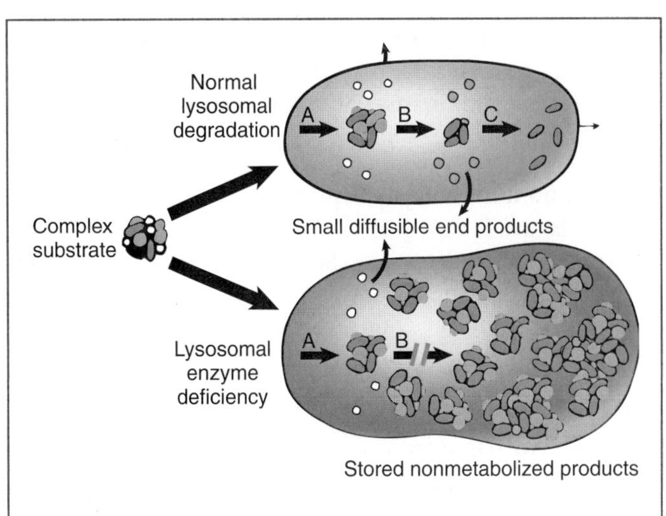

FIGURE 9.4 The pathogenesis of lysosomal storage diseases. A complex substrate is normally degraded by lysosomal enzymes A, B, and C into soluble end products. If these enzymes are deficient, catabolism is incomplete and nonmetabolized products accumulate in the lysosomes.
From Kumar, Abbas, Fausto, and Aster (2009).

Hydrops fetalis is a rare presentation. Respiratory failure can occur owing to lipid infiltration of the lungs (Wraith, 2010).

■ Diagnosis. The diagnosis of NP-C requires specialized testing that must be coordinated with a metabolic laboratory. In general, the diagnosis is made on the basis of filipin staining of cultured fibroblasts and cholesterol esterification studies (Wraith, 2010). Filipin is a fluorescent probe that detects unesterified cholesterol. Biliary atresia and congenital viral infection are the chief differential diagnoses.

■ Management. There is no definitive or consistently effective therapy for NP-C to date. Splenectomy is sometimes necessary if anemia and thrombocytopenia are severe. Liver transplantation corrects the hepatic dysfunction but not the neurodegenerative disease.

Gaucher Disease

■ Pathophysiology. Gaucher disease, the most common of the lysosomal storage diseases, is an inborn error of glycosphingolipid metabolism caused by the deficient activity of the lysosomal enzyme acid beta-glucosidase. Widespread accumulation of glucosylceramide-laden macrophages results from the enzyme deficiency. These accumulated compounds are toxic to various tissues in the body. There are three types of Gaucher disease. Type I is the most common (95%). A subset of type II, a neuronopathic form of Gaucher disease, is the only one with neonatal onset.

■ Clinical Manifestations. Neonates with type II Gaucher disease can present with congenital ichthyosis or a collodion membrane (hyperkeratotic scale), hepatosplenomegaly, and/or nonimmune hydrops fetalis, hypertonicity, seizures, and other evidence of neurologic deterioration.

■ Diagnosis. Diagnosis is made by analysis of acid beta-glucosidase activity in white blood cells or DNA analysis. Characteristic Gaucher cells (large, lipid-laden macrophages with foamy cytoplasm) can be seen in a bone marrow aspirate.

■ Management. Enzyme replacement therapy for Gaucher disease is available, but has not been very effective for patients with type II disease. Splenectomy may be necessary to manage severe anemia and thrombocytopenia. Death from respiratory insufficiency or severe neurologic disease usually occurs shortly after birth or within the first year of life.

GM1 Gangliosidosis

■ Pathophysiology. Gangliosides are normal components of cell membranes, particularly neurons. GM1 gangliosidosis is a devastating lysosomal storage disease caused by a deficiency of the enzyme acid beta-galactosidase, resulting in a generalized accumulation of GM1 gangliosides, oligosaccharides, and the mucopolysaccharide keratan sulfate in both the brain and viscera.

■ Clinical Manifestations. Affected infants may have coarse facial features known as a "Hurler phenotype" (frontal bossing, depressed nasal bridge, maxillary hyperplasia, large ears, wide upper lip, macroglossia, and gingival hyperplasia), hirsutism of forehead and neck, macular cherry-red spots, and corneal clouding (Figure 9.5). The dysmorphic features might not be obvious in the neonate (Thomas et al., 2012). Facial edema, pitting edema of the extremities, or ascites may also be apparent, and the neonate may present with hydrops fetalis and placental evidence of vacuolated cells. Neurologic examination reveals hypotonia and hypoactivity. The liver and spleen are both enlarged upon palpation.

■ Diagnosis. Diagnosis is made by demonstrating lack of beta-galactosidase activity in white blood cells. Galactose-containing oligosaccharides can also be measured in the urine.

■ Management. Currently there is no effective therapy for infants with GM1 gangliosidosis. Enzyme therapy and gene therapy are being studied as potential treatments for this lethal disorder.

Mucopolysaccharidoses

■ Pathophysiology. The mucopolysaccharidoses (MPS) are a family of seven disorders caused by deficiency of lysosomal enzymes required for the stepwise degradation of glycosaminoglycans (polysaccharides that make up an important component of connective tissue). The undegraded glycosaminoglycans are stored in lysosomes, causing cell, tissue, and organ dysfunction. MPS VII, the type with the most prominent neonatal presentation, is caused by a deficiency of the enzyme beta-glucuronidase.

■ Clinical Manifestations. MPS VII (Sly disease) has a well-recognized neonatal presentation with nonimmune hydrops fetalis, hepatosplenomegaly, ascites, pitting edema, hernias, skeletal abnormalities (dystosis multiplex), and corneal clouding. In the most severely affected patients, MPS I (Hurler syndrome) can present in the neonatal period with

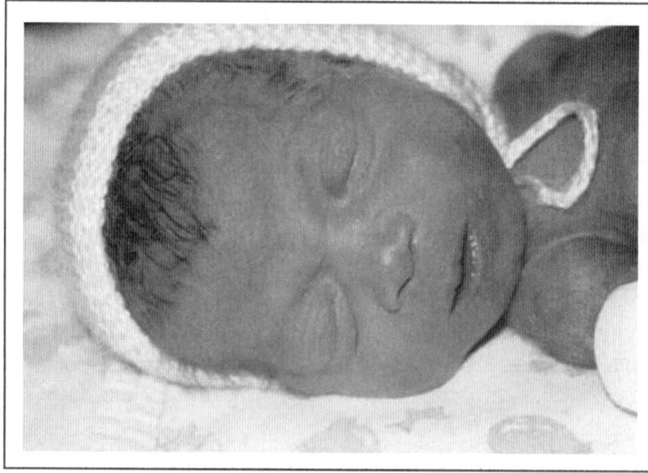

FIGURE 9.5 The "Hurler phenotype" seen in some neonates with lysosomal storage disorders.
From Wraith (2002).

an umbilical or inguinal hernia or an excess of mongolian spots. Hearing loss is common. Clinical evidence of heart disease is present in most patients with MPS.

■ **Diagnosis.** MPS VII is diagnosed by evaluating the activity of beta-glucuronidase in white blood cells. Urine glycosaminoglycans can also be quantitated.

■ **Management.** Management is primarily supportive care and treatment of complications. Range-of-motion exercises are important to preserve joint function and prevent joint stiffness. Recurrent pneumonia is a frequent complication of MPS VII. Development of hydrocephalus often necessitates the insertion of a ventriculoperitoneal shunt. An ophthalmologic examination should be performed to evaluate for corneal clouding and the development of glaucoma.

Glycogen Storage Disease Type II (Pompe's Disease)

■ **Pathophysiology.** Glycogen storage disease type II (GSD II), also called acid maltase deficiency or Pompe's disease, is an inherited disorder of glycogen metabolism resulting from defects in activity of the lysosomal hydrolase acid alpha-glucosidase in all tissues of the body. This enzyme is required for the degradation of a portion of the body's glycogen. Without it, excessive glycogen accumulates within the lysosomes, eventually causing cellular injury and enlarging and hindering the function of the entire organ, such as the heart. Energy production is not affected, and hypoglycemia does not occur. Pompe's disease has a worldwide incidence of about 1 in 40,000 births (Chien et al., 2009).

■ **Clinical Manifestations.** A prominent finding in infants is cardiomyopathy, progressive cardiomegaly and left ventricular thickening that eventually lead to outflow tract obstruction. Characteristic findings on ECG are large QRS complexes coupled with abnormally short PR interval. The QRS complex is the combination of the Q wave, R wave, and S wave and represents ventricular depolarization. The PR interval is the interval between the beginning of the P wave and the beginning of the QRS complex of an electrocardiogram that represents the time between the beginning of the contraction of the atria and the beginning of the contraction of the ventricles. Other manifestations are hepatomegaly, striking hypotonia, macroglossia, feeding difficulties, and respiratory distress complicated by pulmonary infection.

■ **Diagnosis.** Definitive diagnosis requires the measurement of acid alpha-glucosidase activity in cultured skin fibroblasts or white blood cells. Serum creatinine kinase (CK) is elevated (up to 10 times normal). Hepatic enzymes may also be elevated. Newborn screening for Pompe's disease is under study with the hope that presymptomatic diagnosis would permit earlier therapeutic intervention (before extensive muscle damage), leading to better outcomes (Chien et al., 2009).

■ **Management.** Until recently, no effective treatment was available for Pompe's disease, and these infants usually succumbed to cardiopulmonary failure. A recombinant version of human alpha-glucosidase, a glycoprotein enzyme needed for breakdown of glycogen in cell lysosomes, has now been developed for treatment of Pompe's disease.

DISORDERS OF CHOLESTEROL SYNTHESIS

Smith-Lemli-Opitz Syndrome

Smith-Lemli-Opitz (SLO) syndrome is a multiple congenital anomalies/mental retardation syndrome caused by an inherited defect in cholesterol biosynthesis. SLO syndrome has an estimated incidence of 1 in 10,000 to 60,000 births (Haas, Kelley, & Hoffmann, 2009).

■ **Pathophysiology.** The underlying biochemical defect in SLO syndrome is a lack of the microsomal enzyme 3 beta-hydroxysterol-delta 7 reductase (DHCR7), the final enzyme in the sterol biosynthetic pathway that converts 7-dehydrocholesterol (7DHC) to cholesterol. In the absence of DHCR7, the precursor 7DHC accumulates to potentially toxic levels, and insufficient cholesterol is produced. Because cholesterol is required for the development of cell membranes and myelin, and the production of steroid hormones and bile acids, a severe deficiency of cholesterol during morphogenesis is believed to contribute to the abnormalities associated with SLO syndrome. SLO syndrome is different from other disorders of intermediary metabolism, from which the fetus is protected until after birth. Without endogenous cholesterol, the growing embryo depends on maternal cholesterol, which may not be transported across the placenta in sufficient amounts. Thus, the fetus with SLO syndrome suffers systemic and cerebral malformations in proportion to the severity of the deficiency of cholesterol biosynthesis (Quélin et al., 2012).

■ **Clinical Manifestations.** Common findings at birth are intrauterine growth restriction, microcephaly, and hypotonia. Facial dysmorphism may feature epicanthic folds, ptosis, anteverted nares, broad nasal tip, micrognathia, and low-set ears. Associated anomalies include syndactyly of the second and third toes (>98%), postaxial polydactyly, small abnormally positioned thumbs, Hirschsprung's disease, and cataracts, and in males, hypospadias, cryptorchidism, and a hypoplastic scrotum. Common clinical manifestations in the newborn include severe hypotonia, feeding difficulties with poor suck and vomiting, and excessive sleepiness with poor responsiveness (Haas et al., 2009). A severe, lethal form of SLO syndrome presents with microcephaly, lethal cardiac and brain anomalies, and ambiguous genitalia (Quélin et al., 2012). These infants expire during the first week of life from multisystem organ failure.

■ **Diagnosis.** SLO syndrome is often recognized by its distinctive clinical features. Confirmation is made by finding elevated blood levels of its direct precursor, 7DHC. Plasma cholesterol may be normal or low. Some fetuses with SLO syndrome are identified by anomalies detected prior to birth by ultrasonography, and confirmation can be made by amniotic fluid or chorionic villus sample analysis.

■ Management. Immediate management is directed toward raising body cholesterol and removing toxic precursors. Providing exogenous cholesterol not only restores low cholesterol levels but suppresses the infant's endogenous cholesterol synthesis, decreasing the production of 7DHC (Haas et al., 2009).

DISORDERS OF METAL METABOLISM

Inborn errors of metal metabolism are genetic biochemical disorders in the way that metals are processed by the body: their synthesis, transport, absorption, storage, or utilization.

Molybdenum Cofactor Deficiency

■ Pathophysiology. The molybdenum cofactor is an essential component of a large family of enzymes involved in important transformations in carbon, nitrogen, and sulfur metabolism. Molybdenum cofactor deficiency is an autosomal recessive, fatal neurologic disorder, characterized by the combined deficiency of sulfite oxidase, xanthine dehydrogenase, and aldehyde oxidase.

■ Clinical Manifestations. Affected neonates are usually born after an uneventful pregnancy and normal delivery. Soon after birth, feeding difficulties and neurologic symptoms develop. The neurologic picture includes intractable tonic/clonic seizures, axial hypotonia, and peripheral hypertonicity (Koeller, 2009). Typical facial features include puffy cheeks, a long philtrum, and a small nose. The neuropathologic findings are consistent with a toxic insult to the brain that causes severe neuronal loss, demyelination of white matter, reactive astrogliosis, and spongiosis. Ectopia lentis (displacement of the lens) may be noted on ophthalmologic examination.

■ Diagnosis. Molybdenum cofactor deficiency can be difficult to diagnose because there are no clues on routine laboratory studies. A positive sulfite dipstick of fresh urine is suggestive of the disorder; however, a negative test does not rule it out. Urinary S-sulfocysteine, thiosulfate, urothion, xanthine, and hypoxanthine levels aid in the diagnosis of molybdenum cofactor deficiency (Koeller, 2009). Plasma uric acid is typically low.

■ Management. Substitution therapy with purified cyclic pyranopterin monophosphate (cPMP) has been described in the successful treatment of a 6-day-old infant with molybdenum cofactor deficiency (Veldman et al., 2010). No other therapy is currently available for molybdenum cofactor deficiency. One measure that has proved helpful is to limit the intake of sulfur-containing amino acids (cysteine and methionine). Seizures are often difficult to control.

SUMMARY

The number of known inherited disorders of metabolism has risen steadily in recent years and is likely to continue to do so. Although not all will manifest in the neonatal period, many disorders with neonatal onset are rapidly lethal if not recognized and treated without delay. Expanded newborn screening programs have saved many lives through presymptomatic diagnosis, but these programs currently screen for only a fraction of the hundreds of possible metabolic disorders. Neonatal health professionals must be vigilant and consider the diagnosis of an inborn error of metabolism in a neonate presenting with clinical manifestations resembling sepsis, or in an infant becoming ill after one or more days of normal health, particularly when the laboratory data do not fit the clinical picture. Although many neonatal metabolic disorders are not yet amenable to therapy, an exact diagnosis is important for genetic counseling and prenatal diagnostic procedures that the family may desire for future pregnancies.

CASE STUDY

■ Identification of the Problem. A newborn infant, just over 48 hours of age, was rooming with his mother, who noted him to be jaundiced and unusually sleepy. His mother could not awaken him to breastfeed and she notified the nurse, who took him to the nursery to check his bilirubin level. His total serum bilirubin was 10.4. However, the infant made no response to having his heel lanced for the blood draw, and the nurse was unable to awaken him to feed. She placed a call to the infant's pediatrician, and a CBC with differential and a blood culture were ordered. The infant was then transferred to the NICU for further evaluation. An IV of D10W at 100 mL/kg/d was begun, and ampicillin and gentamicin were given. However, the CBC, differential, and C-reactive protein (CRP) were all within normal limits, and subsequently, the blood culture was negative as well.

■ Assessment: History and Physical Examination The infant, a boy, was born by cesarean section to a 33-year-old G3, P2 group B streptococcus (GBS)–negative, insulin-dependent gestational diabetic mother, in satisfactory glucose control during the last trimester of pregnancy. Family history was significant for a maternal brother who died on the third day of life from unknown causes. Siblings of this infant were two healthy girls. This infant's Apgar scores were 8 and 9. Birth weight was 3,790 g. The infant's blood sugar levels on day 1 were all within normal limits; he appeared healthy and roomed in with his mother, breastfeeding on demand with occasional formula supplementation. He was voiding and stooling normally.

On examination his color was pale pink with mild jaundice in room air. Respirations were regular and rapid, but there were no retractions, grunting, or flaring. His axillary temperature was 97°F, heart rate 122, respiratory rate 80, blood pressure 60/36 (mean 44). Glucose screen (point of care) was 52. An arterial blood gas was obtained, and the results were pH 7.32, pO2 71, pCO2 30, base deficit −2. Capillary refill was 2 to 3 seconds, pulses were equal, and there was no murmur. His abdomen was rounded with mild hepatomegaly. He did not react to stimulation of any type and could not be aroused. His overall tone was decreased, he did not suck, and no Moro reflex was noted. Within 24 hours, he began having seizures requiring treatment with phenobarbital. Severe apnea and respiratory failure led to intubation and mechanical ventilation.

■ Differential Diagnosis. The chief differential diagnosis for a full-term infant becoming ill at about 48 hours of age is neonatal sepsis, although this mother was GBS negative, and the infant's laboratory data did not support this diagnosis. His serum bilirubin was not high enough to explain his somnolence and lethargy as stemming from bilirubin encephalopathy. Transient tachypnea of the newborn was unlikely because he did not appear to be in any significant respiratory distress other than his rapid respiratory rate, and the clinical picture was more consistent with a neurologic insult. The history did not suggest an etiology for neonatal encephalopathy. The next most likely diagnostic possibilities would be inborn errors of intermediary metabolism that present with an "intoxication" syndrome and without hypoglycemia, following a symptom-free interval: organic acid disorders, amino acid disorders, and UCDs.

■ Diagnostic Tests. To start differentiating between the most likely categories of metabolic disorders, a blood ammonia level is needed. Depending on this result, other important diagnostic tests might include electrolytes, BUN, creatinine, quantitative plasma and urine amino acids, urine organic acids, and urine orotic acid.

■ Working Diagnosis. The infant's blood ammonia level was 1,901 mcmol/L. This suggests a working diagnosis of a urea cycle defect. Additional testing revealed the following:

Plasma amino acids: Glutamine 1,632 mcmol/L (reference range 376 to 709 mcmol/L)

Citrulline trace (reference range 10 to 45 mcmol/L)

Urine orotic acid: 852 mmol/mol creatinine (reference range 0.12 to 3.07 mmol/mol creatinine)

Following the algorithm for neonatal hyperammonemia (see Figure 9.2), these findings point to a working diagnosis of OTC deficiency. In support of this diagnosis, the infant's symptoms began after 24 hours of age, and he had no significant acidosis.

■ Development of Management Plan. The most urgent priority was reduction of the baby's toxic blood ammonia level. In addition, all protein intake had to be stopped temporarily until the blood ammonia level was normalized, so the baby was made NPO and no amino acids were added to the IV solution. Protein would be reintroduced within 48 hours in small yet sufficient amounts to prevent catabolism. While preparations were being made for hemodialysis, an umbilical venous catheter was inserted for administration of "scavenger drugs," or agents that supply alternatives to urea for elimination of waste nitrogen.

■ Implementation and Evaluation of Effectiveness A loading dose of sodium phenylacetate plus sodium benzoate 2.5 mL/kg was given via central catheter over 90 minutes (Ammonul, Ucyclyd Pharma, Scottsdale, AZ). In addition, a dose of arginine HCl 10% (2.0 mL/kg) was administered. Hemodialysis was initiated, and after about 36 hours the infant's ammonia level was successfully reduced to less than 70 mcmol/L. He showed rapid improvement in neurologic status and was extubated. Amino acids were reintroduced to the intravenous solution after another 24 hours, and feedings were restarted shortly thereafter with citrulline supplementation. Following discharge, he was maintained on this regimen, plus pharmacologic diversion therapy, and he had two metabolic crises requiring hospitalization before receiving a liver transplant. An MRI of his brain at 1 year of age revealed that the neurologic prognosis remains guarded. The family also underwent genetic counseling regarding recurrence risks and prenatal genetic diagnosis for future pregnancies.

EVIDENCE-BASED PRACTICE BOX

Hyperammonia (plasma ammonium level > 150 μmol/L or > 260 mcg/dL) is a metabolic disturbance that is a characteristic feature of many different IEMs, including disorders of organic acids, fatty acid oxidation, and the urea cycle. Ammonia, a product of protein metabolism, is a neurotoxin that can accumulate in the brain along with glutamine, resulting in osmotic swelling, brain edema, and permanent brain damage.

Many areas of the developing brain are vulnerable to the effects of excess ammonia, and the neurologic sequelae are correlated with the duration and magnitude of hyperammonemia (Braissant, 2010). Therefore, the prevention or reversal of hyperammonemic coma is of prime concern in a suspected metabolic disorder. The initial management of ammonia encephalopathy must often proceed in the absence of a definitive diagnosis (Westrope, Morris, Burford, & Morrison, 2010). The kidneys clear ammonia poorly, so removal of ammonia from the body must be expedited by another method. Two means of accomplishing this are diversion therapy using ammonia-scavenging drugs, and physical removal of ammonia from the circulation with dialysis or hemofiltration.

Although the efficacy of dialysis or hemofiltration in the clearance of serum ammonia has been established, the optimal treatment modality has not. Few published studies have shown associations between specific dialysis modalities and survival rates. Owing to the rarity of the IEMs, randomized controlled trials to compare these therapies do not exist. The evidence is largely retrospective and observational, from single case reports and case series.

Expert consensus suggests that first-line treatment of hyperammonemia should involve stopping protein intake, suppressing protein catabolism, and administering agents that combine with ammonia to form compounds with high renal clearance. Many case reports describe successful medical treatment of newborns with various IEMs using N-carbamylglutamate (Filippi et al., 2010; Gessler et al., 2010; Kasapkara et al., 2011), sodium benzoate, and sodium phenylbutyrate. When plasma ammonia levels decline within 4 hours of treatment, the need for dialysis may be averted (Picca et al., 2001). During this 4-hour window, however, preparations should be underway to institute a more aggressive route of ammonia clearance in neonates who do not respond to medical treatment (Picca, Bartuli, & Dionisi-Vici, 2008).

If detoxification with ammonia-scavenging drugs fails to reduce the plasma ammonia level within a few hours, another method of clearance must be initiated without delay. Options include hemodialysis, continuous venovenous hemofiltration (CVVHF), continuous venovenous hemodialysis (CVVHD), and peritoneal dialysis. Methods that provide continuous renal replacement (hemodialysis or hemofiltration) are preferred over peritoneal dialysis, although evidence is scant. Picca et al. (2001) reported their experience using three different extracorporeal methods of clearing ammonia (continuous arteriovenous hemodialysis, CVVHD, and hemodialysis). They found that CVVHD was the most effective method to promptly lower ammonia levels. However, they also found that the most relevant indicator of prognosis was not how quickly the plasma ammonia level was reduced, but the duration of hyperammonemic coma before the initiation of dialysis (Picca et al., 2001). In particular, coma duration longer than 30 hours before dialysis initiation negatively affects the outcome (Picca et al., 2001). Therefore, they recommend that infants with rising ammonia levels should be transferred without delay to a facility capable of providing extracorporeal dialysis if medical therapy fails.

In a 10-year experience with CVVHF to treat hyperammonemia, Westrope et al. (2010) found this method to be safe, effective, and efficient in lowering plasma ammonia levels. However, neither the pretreatment ammonia level nor the speed of ammonia removal was associated with outcome (Westrope et al., 2010). This study suggests that the pretreatment status of the neonate may be the main determinant of outcome, reinforcing the need to initiate medical treatment and to proceed with continuous renal replacement therapy without delay.

In another series of 21 children (15 neonates), investigators retrospectively analyzed outcomes for patients receiving CVVHD or peritoneal dialysis (Arbeiter et al., 2010). A 50% reduction in serum ammonia levels was achieved significantly faster with CVVHD than with peritoneal dialysis. In neonatal patients, survival and survival without mental retardation were both better following CVVHD, although the sample sizes were small and the duration of pretreatment encephalopathy was not known. Of interest, these investigators documented the best outcomes in patients with neonatal-onset citrullinemia.

Although it would be desirable to have randomized, controlled trial evidence of the superiority of one method of treating hyperammonemia over another, the trend toward presymptomatic detection of metabolic disorders could, in future, lead to preventive treatments that will obviate the need for such aggressive approaches to hyperammonemia. In the meantime, clinicians should continue to collect data on the few patients encountered with these disorders to inform best practice and improve outcomes.

References

Arbeiter, A. K., Dranz, B., Wingen, A. M., Bonzel, K. E., Dohna-Schwake, C., Hanssle, L., Neudorf, U., Hoyer, P. F., & Büscher, R. (2010). Continuous venovenous haemodialysis (CVVHD) and continuous peritoneal dialysis (CPD) in the acute management of 21 children with inborn errors of metabolism. *Nephrology Dialysis and Transplantation*, *25*, 1257–1265.

Filippi, L., Gozini, E., Fiorini, P., Malvagia, S., la Marca, G., & Donati, M. A. (2010). N-carbamylglutamate in emergency management of hyperammonemia in neonatal acute onset propionic and methylmalonic aciduria. *Neonatology, 97*, 286–290.

Gessler, P., Buchal, P., Schwenk, H. U., & Wermuth, B. (2010). Favourable long-term outcome after immediate treatment of neonatal hyperammonemia due to N-acetyl glutamate synthase deficiency. *European Journal of Pediatrics, 169*, 197–199.

Kasapkara, C. S., Ezgu, F. S., Okur, I., Tumer, L., Biberoglu, G., & Hasanoglu, A. (2011). N-carbamylglutamate treatment for acute neonatal hyperammonemia in isovaleric acidemia. *European Journal of Pediatrics, 270*, 799–801.

Picca, S., Bartuli, A., & Dionisi-Vici, C. (2008). Medical management and dialysis therapy for the infant with an inborn error of metabolism. *Seminars in Nephrology, 28*, 477–480.

Picca, S., Dionisi-Vici, C., Abeni, D., Pastore, A., Rizzo, C., Orzalesi, M., . . . Bartuli, A. (2001). Extracorporeal dialysis in neonatal hyperammonemia: Modalities and prognostic indicators. *Pediatric Nephrology, 16*, 862–867.

Westrope, C., Morris, K., Burford, D., & Morrison, G. (2010). Continuous hemofiltration in the control of neonatal hyperammonemia: A 10-year experience. *Pediatric Nephrology, 25*, 1725–1730.

ONLINE RESOURCES

National for Advancing Translational Sciences-Office of Rare Diseases Research
http://www.rarediseases.info.nih.gov

National Newborn Screening and Genetics Resource Center
http://www.genes-r-us.uthscsa.edu/Office of Rare Diseases

Orphanet
http://www.orpha.net/consor/cgi-bin/index.php

REFERENCES

Ah Mew, N., McCarter, R., Daikhin, Y., Nissim, I., Yudkoff, M., & Tuchman, M. (2010). N-carbamylglutamate augments ureagenesis and reduces ammonia and glutamine in propionic acidemia. *Pediatrics, 126*, e208–e214.

Berry, G. T. (2012, March 21). Galactosemia: When is it a newborn screening emergency? *Molecular Genetics and Metabolism*. [Epub ahead of print].

Berry, S. A., Nathan, B., Hoffmann, G. F., & Sarafoglou, K. (2009). Emergency assessment and management of suspected inborn errors of metabolism and endocrine disorders. In K. Sarafoglou (Ed.), *Pediatric endocrinology and inborn errors of metabolism* (pp. 3–16). New York, NY: McGraw Hill.

Braissant, O. (2010). Current concepts in the pathogenesis of urea cycle disorders. *Molecular Genetics and Metabolism, 100*, S3–S12.

Brown, G. (2012). Pyruvate dehydrogenase deficiency and the brain. *Developmental Medicine and Child Neurology, 54*, 395–396.

Burton, B. K. (2000). Urea cycle disorders. *Clinics in Liver Disease, 4*:815–830.

Campeau, P. M., Pivalizza, P. J., Miller, G., McBride, K., Karpen, S., Goss, J. & Lee, B. H. (2010). Early orthotopic liver transplantation in urea cycle defects: Follow up of a developmental outcome study. *Molecular Genetics and Metabolism, 100*, S85–S87.

Cederbaum, S. (2012). Introduction to metabolic and biochemical genetic disease. In S. U. Devaskar & C. A. Gleason (Eds.), *Avery's diseases of the newborn* (9th ed., pp. 209–214). Philadelphia, PA: Elsevier.

Cederbaum, S. & Berry, G. T. (2012). Inborn errors of carbohydrate, ammonia, amino acid, and organic acid metabolism. In S. U. Devaskar & C. A. Gleason (Eds.), *Avery's diseases of the newborn* (9th ed., pp. 215–238). Philadelphia, PA: Elsevier.

Chapman, K. A., Gropman, A., MacLeod, E., Stagni, K., Summar, M. L., Ueda, K., . . . Chakrapani, A. (2012). Acute management of priopionic acidemia. *Molecular Genetics and Metabolism, 105*, 16–25.

Chien, Y. H., Lee, N. C., Thurberg, B. L., Chiang, S. C., Zhang, X. K., Keutzer, J., . . . Hwu, W. L. (2009). Pompe disease in infants: Improving the prognosis by newborn screening and early treatment. *Pediatrics, 124*, e1116–e1125.

Cleary, M. A. (2010). Phenylketonuria. *Paediatrics and Child Health, 12*, 2.

Daniotti, M., la Marca, G., Fiorini, P., & Filippi, L. (2011). New developments in the treatment of hyperammonemia: Emerging use of carglumic acid. *International Journal of Genetics in Medicine, 4*, 21–28.

Davison, J. E., Davies, N. P., Wilson, M., Sun, Y., Chakrapani, A. & McKiernan, P. J., . . . Peet, A. C. (2011). MR spectroscopy-based brain metabolite profiling in propionic acidaemia: Metabolic changes in the basal ganglia during acute decompensation and effect of liver transplantation. *Orphanet Journal of Rare Diseases, 9*, 19.

Ensenauer, R., Fingerhut, R., Maier, E. M., Polanetz, R., Olgemoller, B., Roschinger, W., & Muntau, A. C. (2011). Newborn screening for isovaleric acidemia using tandem mass spectrometry: Data from 1.6 million newborns. *Clinical Chemistry, 57*, 623–626.

Gessler, P., Buchal, P., Schwenk, H.U., & Wermuth, B. (2010). Favourable long-term outcome after immediate treatment of neonatal hyperammonemia due to N-acetyl glutamate synthase deficiency. *European Journal of Pediatrics, 169*, 197–199.

Grünert, S., Wendel, U., Lindner, M., Leichsenring, M., Schwab, O., & Vockley, J. (2012). Clinical and neurocognitive outcome in symptomatic isovaleric acidemia. *Orphanet Journal of Rare Diseases, 7*, 9.

Haas, D., Kelley, D. I., & Hoffmann, G. F. (2009). Defects of cholesterol biosynthesis. In K. Sarafoglou (Ed.), *Pediatric endocrinology and inborn errors of metabolism* (pp. 313–321). New York, NY: McGraw Hill.

Hendriksz, C. J., & Gissen, P. (2010). Glycogen storage disease. *Paediatrics and Child Health, 12*, 2.

Hertzberg, V. S., Hinton, C. F., Therrell, B. L., & Shapira, S. K. (2011). Birth prevalence rates of newborn screening disorders in relation to screening practices in the United States. *Journal of Pediatrics, 159*, 555–560.

Hoffmann, G. F., & Schulze, A. (2009). Organic acidurias. In K. Sarafoglou (Ed.), *Pediatric endocrinology and inborn errors of metabolism* (pp. 83–118). New York, NY: McGraw Hill.

Hyland, K., Gibson, K. M., Sharma, R., vanHove, J. L. K., & Hoffman, G. F. (2009). Neurotransmitter disorders. In K. Sarafoglou (Ed.), *Pediatric endocrinology and inborn errors of metabolism* (pp. 789–819). New York, NY: McGraw Hill.

Jameson, E., & Walter, J. H. (2010). Medium-chain acyl-CoA dehydrogenase deficiency - a review. *Paediatrics and Child Health*, *21*, 2.

Johnson, J. A., Le, K. L., & Palacios, E. (2009). Propionic acidemia: Case report and review of neurologic sequelae. *Pediatric Neurology, 40*, 317–320.

Kasapkara, C. S., Ezgu, F. S., Okur, I., Tumer, L., Biberoglu, G., & Hasanoglu, A. (2011). N-carbamylglutamate treatment for acute neonatal hyperammonemia in isovaleric acidemia. *European Journal of Pediatrics*, *170*, 799–801.

Kilicarslan, R., Alkan, A., Demirkol, D., Toprak, H., & Sharifov, R. (2012, April 3). Maple syrup urine disease: Diffusion-weighted MRI findings during acute metabolic encephalopathic crisis. *Japanese Journal of Radiology*. [Epub ahead of print].

Koeller, D. M. (2009). Disorders of mineral metabolism (iron, copper, zinc, and molybdenum). In K. Sarafoglou (Ed.), *Pediatric endocrinology and inborn errors of metabolism* (pp. 674–675). New York, NY: McGraw-Hill.

Kumar, V., Abbas, A. K., Fausto, N., & Aster, J. (2009). *Robbins and Cotran: pathologic basis of disease* (8th ed.). Philadelphia, PA: Elsevier.

Leonard, J. V., & Morris, A. A. (2006). Diagnosis and early management of inborn errors of metabolism presenting around the time of birth. *Acta Paediatrica*, *95*, 6–14.

Leonard, J. V., & Morris, A. M. M. (2009). Tyrosinemia and other disorders of tyrosine degradation. In K. Sarafoglou (Ed.), *Pediatric endocrinology and inborn errors of metabolism* (pp. 177–184). New York, NY: McGraw-Hill.

Leonard, J. V., & Morris, A. M. M. (2010). The investigation and initial management of children with suspected metabolic disease. *Paediatrics and Child Health, 21*, 51–55.

Marin-Valencia, I., Roe, C. R., & Pascual, J. M. (2010). Pyruvate carboxylase deficiency: Mechanisms, mimics, and anaplerosis. *Molecular Genetics and Metabolism*, *101*, 9–17.

Pagon, R. A., Adam, M. P., Bird, T. D. et al., editors. GeneReviews™ [Internet]. Seattle (WA): University of Washington, Seattle; 1993–2013. Available from http://www.ncbi.nlm.nih.gov/books/NBK1116

Patel, K. P., O'Brien, T. W., Subramony, S. H., Shuster, J., & Stacpoole, P. W. (2012). The spectrum of pyruvate dehydrogenase complex deficiency: Clinical, biochemical and genetic features in 371 patients. *Molecular Genetics and Metabolism, 105*, 34–43.

Puffenberger, E. G. (2003). Genetic heritage of the old order Mennonites of southeastern Pennsylvania. *American Journal of Medical Genetics Part C: Seminars in Medical Genetics, 121C*, 18–31.

Quélin, C., Loget, P., Verloes, A., Bazin, A., Bessières, B., Laquerrière, A., . . . Gonzales, M. (2012). Phenotypic spectrum of fetal Smith-Lemli-Opitz syndrome. *European Journal of Medical Genetics*, *55*, 81–90.

Rector, R. S., & Ibdah, J. A. (2010). Fatty acid oxidation disorders: Maternal health and neonatal outcomes. *Seminars in Fetal and Neonatal Medicine*, *15*, 122–128.

Romano, S., Valayannopoulos, V., Touati, G., Jais, J. P., Rabier, D., de Keyzer, Y., . . . de Lonlay, P. (2010). Cardiomyopathies in propionic aciduria are reversible after liver transplantation. *Journal of Pediatrics*, *156*, 128–134.

Scott, C., & Olpin, S. (2010). Peroxisomal disorders. *Paediatrics and Child Health*, *21*, 71–75.

Sharma, R., Sharrard, M. J., Connolly, D. J., & Mordekar, S. R. (2012). Unilateral periventricular leukomalacia in association with pyruvate dehydrogenase deficiency. *Developmental Medicine and Child Neurology*, *54*, 469–471.

Shekhawat, P., Bennett, M. J., Sadovsky, Y., Nelson, D. M., Rakheja, D., and Strauss, A. W. (2003). Human placenta metabolizes fatty acids: implications for fetal acid oxidation disorders and maternal liver diseases. *American Journal of Physiology, Endocrinology & Metabolism*, *284*, E1098–E1105.

Spiekerkoetter, U., Bastin, J., Gillingham, M., Morris, A., Wijburg, F., & Wilcken, B. (2010). Current issues regarding treatment of mitochondrial fatty acid oxidation disorders. *Journal of Inherited Metabolic Disease*, *33*, 555–561.

Stockler, S., Moeslinger, D., Herle, M., Wimmer, B., & Ipsiroglu, O. S. (2012, February 23). Cultural aspects in the management of inborn errors of metabolism. *Journal of Inherited Metabolic Disease*. [Epub ahead of print] doi:10.1007/s10545-012-9455-4

Strauss, A. W., Andresen, B. S., & Bennett, M. J. (2009). Mitochondrial fatty acid oxidation disorders. In K. Sarafoglou (Ed.), *Pediatric endocrinology and inborn errors of metabolism* (pp. 51–70). New York, NY: McGraw-Hill.

Summar, M. L. (2009). Urea cycle disorders. In K. Sarafoglou (Ed.), *Pediatric endocrinology and inborn errors of metabolism* (pp. 141–152). New York, NY: McGraw-Hill.

Summar, M. L., Dobbelaere, D., Brusilow, S., & Lee, B. (2008). Diagnosis, symptoms, frequency, and mortality of 260 patients with urea cycle disorders from a 21-year multicentre study of acute hyperammonaemic episodes. *Acta Paediatrica*, *97*, 1420–1425.

Thomas, J. A., Greene, C. L., & Berry, G. T. (2012). Lysosomal storage, peroxisomal and glycosylation disorders and Smith-Lemli-Opitz syndrome in the neonate. In S. U. Devaskar & C. A. Gleason (Eds.), *Avery's diseases of the newborn* (9th ed., pp. 239–257). Philadelphia, PA: Elsevier.

Tuchman, M., Caldovic, L., Daikhin, Y., Horryn, O., Nissim I, . . . Yudkoff, M. (2008). *N*-carbamylglutamate markedly enhances ureagenesis in *N*-acetylglutamate deficiency and propionic acidemia as measured by isotopic incorporation and blood biomarkers. *Pediatric Research*, *64*, 213–217.

U.S. Department of Health and Human Services. (2011, December). *Recommended uniform screening panel of the secretary's advisory committee on heritable disorders in newborns and children*. Retrieved from http://www.hrsa.gov/advisorycommittees/mchbadvisory/heritabledisorders/recommendedpanel/index.html

Veldman, A., Santamaria-Araujo, J. A., Sollazzo, S., Pitt, J., Gianello, R., Yaplito-Lee, J., . . . Schwarz, G. (2010). Successful treatment of molybdenum cofactor deficiency type A with cPMP. *Pediatrics*, *125*, e1249–e1254.

Wilcken, B. (2010). Fatty acid oxidation disorders: Outcome and long-term prognosis. *Journal of Inherited Metabolic Diseases*, *33*, 501–506.

Wraith, J. E. (2002). Lysosomal disorders. *Seminars in Neonatology, 7*, 81.

Wraith, J. E. (2010). Lysosomal disorders. *Paediatrics and Child Health*, *21*, 76–79.

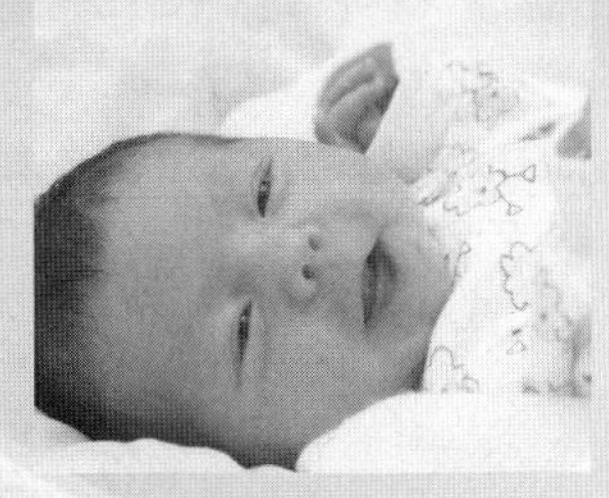

CHAPTER

10

Endocrine System

■ Laura A. Stokowski

Our understanding of endocrine disorders in the neonate advances to the molecular level in parallel with discoveries in genetics and cell biology. Endocrine processes are fundamental to growth and development of the fetus and newborn. Prompt recognition of endocrine disorders in the neonate is the chief prerequisite in our ability to institute life-saving treatment and minimize long-term morbidity. This chapter provides an overview of the clinical endocrine disorders that may be seen in the neonatal period.

THE ENDOCRINE SYSTEM

The word *endocrine*, from the Greek words *endo* (within) and *krinein* (to separate), describes a diverse group of ductless organs that secrete hormones directly into the bloodstream. The classic endocrine glands are the hypothalamus, pineal, pituitary, thyroid, parathyroid, thymus, pancreatic islet cells, adrenals, ovaries, and testes, although the heart, kidneys, and intestines also secrete and regulate hormones. Among the many functions of the endocrine system are coordination and regulation of metabolism and energy, the internal environment, growth and development, and sexual differentiation and reproduction. Maintenance of homeostasis (the metabolic milieu of the body in a steady state) is considered the most important function of the endocrine system (Bethin & Fuqua, 2010).

The endocrine glands synthesize, store, and secrete hormones, the chemical messengers, or signals, of the endocrine system, that are responsible for tight regulation of diverse physiologic functions. Hormones are peptides, amines, or steroids and are further classified as either regulatory or effector hormones (Bethin & Fuqua, 2010). Secreted into the blood or extracellular fluid, hormones exert their actions on specific cells, either locally or in distant tissues called target cells. Target cells respond to hormones that contain receptors for those precise hormones. Hormones must first bind to these receptor sites before exerting physiologic actions. Some hormones, such as insulin, are fully active on release into the circulatory system, whereas others, such as T4, require activation to produce their biologic effects. Hormones that must be modified to active hormone after synthesis are known as prepro- or prohormones.

Many hormones are insoluble in water and must be bound to carrier proteins to be transported in the circulatory system. These protein-bound hormones exist in rapid equilibrium with minute quantities of hormone that remain in the aqueous plasma. This "free" fraction of the circulating hormone is taken up by the cell and represents the active hormone concentration that provides feedback to regulate synthesis of the new hormone.

Target hormone levels also serve as powerful negative feedback regulators of their own production via suppression of trophic hormones and hypothalamic releasing hormones. As the target hormone level rises, a message is sent to the anterior pituitary to reduce production of the respective trophic hormone, and also to the hypothalamus to slow production of the respective releasing hormone. Endocrine disease has traditionally been classified as hormone excess, hormone deficiency, or altered tissue responses to hormones (e.g., hormone resistance). Clinical endocrine abnormalities can also be driven by deviations in the feedback systems that control hormone levels. An explosion of new data from molecular genetic studies is redefining "endocrine disease" as a broad array of mutations and alterations in expression of thousands of genes, that result in either "loss of function" or "gain of function," in other words, hyposecretory or hypersecretory disorders (Tenore & Driul, 2009).

Development of the fetal endocrine system is more or less independent of maternal endocrine influences (Rubin, 2012). The placenta blocks the entry of most maternal hormones into the fetal circulation, but the minute quantities that do achieve transplacental passage can have profound effects. Some of these prenatal exposures are essential to fetal growth and development; others may contribute to fetal and neonatal endocrine dysfunction.

FETAL ORIGINS OF ADULT DISEASE

The intrauterine endocrine milieu can have powerful effects on growth and development of the fetal endocrine system. When exposed to a variety of different stressors (maternal undernutrition, uteroplacental insufficiency, or psychologic stress) the fetus releases glucocorticoids and catecholamines that, during critical periods of development, affect the development of the fetal hypothalamic–pituitary–adrenal (HPA) axis. Chronic stress can also induce intrauterine growth restriction, or the so-called thrifty phenotype, in the fetus, an adaptation to the limited supply of nutrients (Rubin, 2012). The way in which the fetus adapts, a concept known as programming, is believed to permanently alter physiology and metabolism. Permanent alterations in fetal metabolic programming contribute to endocrine, metabolic, and cardiovascular disease in adult life (Seki, Williams, Vuguin, & Charron, 2012).

NEONATAL ENDOCRINE DISORDERS

Many neonatal endocrine disorders originate in developmental defects of, or injury to, the endocrine glands (Bethin & Fuqua, 2010). Endocrinopathy in the newborn can be caused by a mutation in a single gene or by genomic imprinting, when the expression of the gene depends on which parent passed on that particular gene (Rubin, 2012). In addition to well-described neonatal endocrine disorders such as hypothyroidism and congenital adrenal hyperplasia (CAH), endocrine dysfunction can affect the preterm infant in a variety of ways as a function of maturation. Exposure to various exogenous agents in the environment, known as "endocrine disruptors" can have deleterious effects on the development of the endocrine system. Numerous chemicals have known estrogenic or antiandrogenic properties and have been shown to disturb sexual differentiation in animals (Rubin, 2012). The extent to which endocrine disruptors are responsible for increases in hypospadias and testicular dysgenesis syndrome in humans that have been reported in some parts of the world is unknown.

PITUITARY GLAND AND HYPOTHALAMUS

The pituitary gland has two distinct structures, the anterior and posterior pituitary, with different embryologic origins. The anterior pituitary develops from oral ectoderm, a diverticulum called Rathke's pouch, and its cells differentiate into specific hormone-secreting cells. The posterior pituitary develops from neuroectoderm evaginating ventrally from the developing brain. The two tissues grow together into a single gland but remain functionally separate.

The hypothalamus, located just above the pituitary gland, secretes the releasing and inhibiting hormones that in turn influence the production of anterior pituitary hormones. Hypothalamic hormones are carried to the anterior pituitary via hypothalamic-hypophyseal portal veins where they bind to receptors on the anterior pituitary cells. The anterior pituitary regulates growth, differentiation, and homeostasis and produces growth hormone, prolactin, adrenocorticotropic hormone (ACTH), thyroid-stimulating hormone (TSH), follicle-stimulating hormone (FSH), and luteinizing hormone (LH). Hormones secreted by the posterior pituitary include oxytocin and hypothalamic-produced vasopressin (antidiuretic hormone, ADH). The hypothalamus is the interface between the endocrine and autonomic nervous systems.

DISORDERS OF THE ANTERIOR PITUITARY

Congenital Hypopituitarism

Congenital hypopituitarism, although rare in the newborn, has a number of possible etiologies. Some cases of congenital hypopituitarism are attributed to mutations in genes encoding transcription factors involved in pituitary gland development (Alatzoglu & Dattani, 2009). Congenital hypopituitarism can be an isolated defect, or associated with malformations including holoprosencephaly, septo-optic dysplasia, and other midline cerebral anomalies, the same developmental defects of the embryonic brain that lead to hypothalamic dysfunction. Infection and hypovolemic shock stemming from birth-related complications such as placenta previa and abruptio placentae are additional etiologies.

■ **Pathophysiology.** Complete absence of the pituitary gland (pituitary agenesis) and other pituitary lesions can produce deficiencies of one or all pituitary hormones. Panhypopituitarism is a deficiency of all pituitary hormones. In the newborn, the foremost effect of congenital hypopituitarism is hypoglycemia. Owing to the absence of growth hormone, and possibly cortisol as well, insulin is unopposed, placing the neonate at risk for hypoglycemia. Deficiency of growth hormone, and often gonadotropin, combine to stunt penile growth in utero; this is usually referred to as hypogonadotropic hypogonadism. Although fetal pituitary growth hormone is not the primary stimulus for fetal growth, growth hormone does make an important contribution to birth size.

■ **Clinical Manifestations.** Neonates with congenital hypopituitarism can initially be asymptomatic, with evidence of pituitary hormone deficiencies developing over time (Alatzoglu & Dattani, 2009). Neonates with hypopituitary syndromes can present with midline craniofacial defects such as cleft lip, cleft palate, or bifid uvula. Males may have a micropenis, defined as a normally formed and proportioned penis with a stretched penile length more than two standard deviations below the mean for age. Average penile length for preterm infants 30 weeks of age or older is 2.5 + 0.4 cm and for term infants 3.5 + 0.4 cm. For preterm infants 24 to 26 weeks gestation, the following formula can be used: penile length in centimeters = 2.27 + 0.16 ∞ (gestational age in weeks) (Tuladhar, Davis, Batch, & Doyle, 1998). Hypoglycemia can be mild or severe and persistent. Later in the neonatal period infants may present with prolonged jaundice and direct hyperbilirubinemia, or evidence of other endocrinopathy, such as diabetes insipidus (DI) (high urine output, dehydration, hypernatremia).

■ **Diagnosis.** A pediatric endocrinologist usually coordinates the diagnostic testing and interpretation for these infants. The aim of laboratory testing is to determine which hormone deficiencies are present. Measurement of growth hormone, thyroid hormone, and cortisol is essential. Magnetic resonance imaging (MRI) of the brain is used to define the anatomy and look for a structural cause of hypopituitarism. For infants with suspected septo-optic dysplasia, an ophthalmologic examination is indicated.

■ **Management.** The immediate goals of management are to stabilize the neonate's blood sugar and ensure that the neonate is not at risk for life-threatening cortisol insufficiency. Hypoglycemia might not resolve without growth hormone replacement. Further treatment is geared toward correcting specific hormonal deficiencies. The infant will require follow-up management by the pediatric endocrinologist throughout hospitalization and after discharge.

DISORDERS OF THE POSTERIOR PITUITARY

Diabetes Insipidus

DI is a deficiency of ADH (vasopressin). In neonates, central or neurogenic DI can be associated with congenital midline anatomic defects (septo-optic dysplasia, holoprosencephaly), central nervous system (CNS) injury such as intracranial hemorrhage or hypoxia, neoplasms, or it can be idiopathic. As many as 90% of neonates with inherited nephrogenic DI are boys with an X-linked form caused by mutations in the *arginine vasopressin receptor 2* (*AVP2R*) gene, a condition that can be diagnosed prenatally (Copelovitch & Kaplan, 2012).

■ **Pathophysiology.** Normally, ADH secretion is triggered by changes in osmolality detected by supraoptic and paraventricular osmosensors in the brain. Increased osmolality stimulates the posterior pituitary to release ADH, which in turn increases the permeability of the renal collecting tubules to water, reducing urinary water loss. Damage to the osmosensors, the posterior pituitary gland, or the hypothalamic–hypophyseal axis results in a deficiency of ADH and increased urinary free water loss.

■ **Clinical Manifestations.** Neonates with DI may suck vigorously during feeding but vomit immediately afterward, resulting in poor growth. Urine output is high, in excess of 5 mL/kg/hr, with low specific gravity (<1.010). Irritability and fever may accompany evidence of dehydration (poor skin turgor, depressed anterior fontanelle, sunken eyes, mottled skin, weak pulses, low blood pressure, and constipation).

■ **Diagnosis.** Serum electrolytes, osmolality, and plasma ADH levels are the primary laboratory tests used to diagnose DI. Plasma ADH is normally elevated in the newborn following delivery, playing a role in the low urine output that is typical on the first day of life. In neonates with DL, hypernatremia may result in levels as high as 180 mEq/L with elevated serum osmolality. Urinalysis reveals inappropriately dilute urine (low urine osmolality and low specific gravity). MRI is used to visualize the pituitary gland and stalk to delineate the possible cause of DI.

■ **Management.** DI in neonates requires very careful fluid management. Severe dehydration and hypernatremia are corrected primarily with intravenous fluids. Insensible water losses should be minimized. Serum electrolytes and osmolality, blood glucose, accurate intake and output, and the evidence of dehydration (weight loss, blood pressure, pulses, skin turgor, etc.) should be closely monitored during treatment. Infants with severe hypernatremia must be observed for possible seizure activity. Although it is expected that serum sodium will decline, very rapid shifts in serum sodium should be avoided. During therapy to correct serum sodium, the infant's neurologic status must be monitored closely for signs and symptoms of cerebral edema. Hyperglycemia must be avoided as this may lead to glycosuria and exaggerate the diuresis. If possible, DI in the neonate should be managed with fluid therapy alone, preferably breast milk or formula with a whey-to-casein ratio of 60 to 40, supplemented with free water if necessary (Srivatsa, Majzoub, & Kappy, 2010). If it is not possible to manage DI with fluids alone, the agent of choice for pharmacologic treatment is desmopressin (DDAVP), a long-acting synthetic analogue of pituitary ADH. Intranasal DDAVP can be diluted with normal saline for administration to the neonate. Subcutaneous and oral formulations of DDAVP are also available, as well as short-acting intravenous aqueous pitressin for emergency treatment of severe dehydration. Caution must be observed when using vasopressin and high fluid intake to manage DI in the neonate because this combination can result in severe hyponatremia (Srivatsa et al., 2010).

Syndrome of Inappropriate Antidiuretic Hormone

Syndrome of inappropriate antidiuretic hormone (SIADH) is an impairment of free water clearance associated with inappropriately raised secretion of ADH. SIADH is believed to be associated with CNS infection and injury (birth asphyxia, intracranial hemorrhage, meningitis), pain, and maternal substance abuse (Modi, 2012).

■ **Pathophysiology.** An uncontrolled release of ADH can occur in sick preterm and term infants, resulting in renal free water retention that is inappropriate to the level of serum osmolality. The infant becomes hyponatremic, not because of true sodium depletion, but because of a dilutional effect from the fluid that is retained. ADH levels can become elevated in infants born after fetal distress, or those with severe pulmonary disease, undergoing surgery, or experiencing pain. Raised ADH levels are common in acutely ill neonates (Modi, 2012).

■ **Clinical Manifestations.** Signs and symptoms of SIADH are oliguria, hyponatremia, low serum osmolality (<275 mOsm/L), weight gain, and edema. Patients with SIADH are euvolemic or hypervolemic.

■ Diagnosis. The diagnosis of SIADH should be made only when hyponatremia exists with normovolemia, normal blood pressure, normal renal and cardiac function, evidence of continuing sodium excretion, and urine that is not maximally dilute (Modi, 2012). True SIADH fulfilling all diagnostic criteria is probably uncommon in the neonate. Apparent SIADH may be due to hypovolemia-induced baroreceptor-driven ADH secretion, a normal response to reduced blood volume in the sick neonate (Modi, 2012).

■ Collaborative Management. Fluid restriction, with close monitoring of intake, output, serum electrolytes, blood glucose, accurate daily weights, evidence of increasing edema, and measures of hydration are the essentials of management. It can be difficult to restrict fluids because infants receive all of their nutrition in liquid form. Diuretics are sometimes used to promote free water excretion. Comparison of intake and output is important. A careful neurologic assessment should be performed, noting changes in relation to fluid or sodium balance.

THYROID GLAND

The thyroid gland is a butterfly-shaped structure made up of two lateral lobes connected by a thin band of tissue called the isthmus. Composed of densely packed follicular cells containing colloid, the thyroid gland also contains parafollicular cells (C-cells) that produce the calcium-lowering hormone calcitonin.

The thyroid hormones thyroxine (T4) and triiodothyronine (T3) are produced from the amino acid tyrosine. Essential to this process is the trapping and storage of iodide, a trace element required for thyroid hormone synthesis. Thyroglobulin (Tg), a thyroid hormone precursor, is synthesized in the follicular cell. Iodine is taken up by the Tg molecule, incorporated into its tyrosine residues, and returned to the colloid, where a coupling reaction takes place. This step, called organification, is catalyzed by the enzyme thyroid peroxidase (TPO). The coupling of two tyrosine residues produces T4, whereas the coupling of diiodotyrosine (DIT) with monoiodotyrosine (MIT) produces T3. These are stored in the follicular lumens until TSH stimulates their release into the circulation.

The thyroid gland produces mostly T4, which serves as a storage pool for T3. T3 is the most biologically active thyroid hormone, with greater affinity for the thyroid receptor. Circulating T4 is metabolized by outer ring 5′ monodeiodination to T3 in the peripheral tissues. Inner ring 5′ monodeiodination of T4 produces reverse T3 (rT3), an inactive metabolite. T4 and T3 circulate in plasma bound to thyroid-binding globulin (TBG), leaving just a small fraction in equilibrium as free hormone. It is possible for TBG, which is synthesized in the liver, to be deficient even though the free hormone levels are normal. It is the free hormone that is available to the tissues, with the bound hormone acting as a circulating reservoir. The concentration of free hormone determines the individual's metabolic state.

The hypothalamic–pituitary–thyroid (HPT) axis controls thyroid hormone secretion (Figure 10.1). The hypothalamus synthesizes thyrotropin, stimulating release of TSH from the anterior pituitary. In turn, TSH stimulates uptake of iodine by the thyroid, thyroid hormone synthesis and release, and increased size and vascularity of the thyroid gland itself. The feedback loop is responsive to changes in free hormone concentration, and TSH secretion adjusts accordingly.

Fetal and Neonatal Thyroid Development

The thyroid gland is the first endocrine organ to develop in the human embryo. Concurrent with development of the fetal thyroid are growth and maturation of the hypothalamus and pituitary glands, which are required for thyroid function. At about 10 to 12 weeks gestation, the hypothalamus begins synthesizing TRH, the pituitary gland begins secreting TSH, and TBG is detectable in fetal serum. Maternal thyroxine is measurable in amniotic fluid before the onset of fetal thyroid function. Before 20 weeks gestation, transplacental passage of maternal T4 largely provides for fetal thyroidal needs and is critical for normal development. Maternal hypothyroidism during early gestation can impair CNS development in the fetus. By the start of the second trimester, however, the fetal contribution to circulating thyroid hormones is significant. The capacity of the fetal thyroid gland to trap and store iodide and synthesize thyroid hormones begins at about 11 weeks gestation, but hormone production is limited until 18 to 20 weeks, when iodine uptake increases markedly. The only source of iodide for the fetus is transplacental passage from the maternal circulation and placenta.

As pregnancy progresses, the placenta becomes less permeable to maternal thyroid hormone. Permeability is likely to be highest during the first trimester because

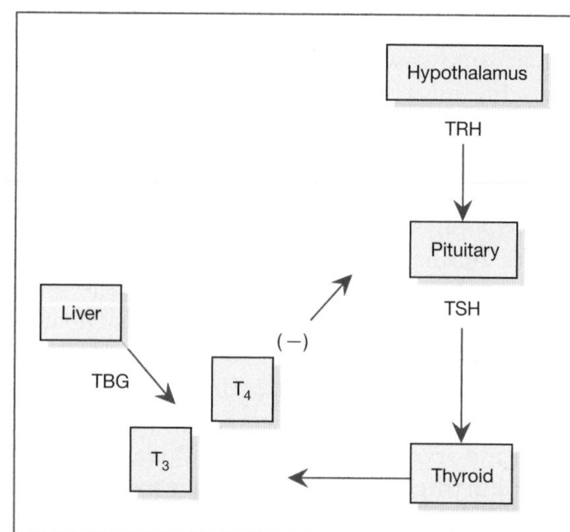

FIGURE 10.1 The hypothalamic–pituitary–thyroid (HPT) axis. Thyroid hormone levels are regulated by a system of feedback inhibition operating along the HPT axis. The hypothalamus secretes thyrotropin-releasing hormone (TRH), which stimulates the pituitary to secrete thyroid-stimulating hormone (TSH). TSH, in turn, stimulates the thyroid gland to produce and secrete thyroid hormones (T4 and T3) into the circulation, which circulate bound to thyroid-binding globulin (TBG) synthesized by the liver. Once levels of T4 and T3 are adequate, further production of TSH is suppressed.

thyroid hormone is critical to fetal neurodevelopment, and no other source is available to the fetus during this period. The fetal HPT axis develops from mid-gestation through 4 weeks post birth. In infants born before term, maturation of the HPT axis is disrupted (Simpser & Rapaport, 2010). In the last trimester, the fetus is less dependent on maternally derived thyroid hormone. Although thyroid hormone is required for CNS maturation, it is not needed for metabolism, growth, or generation of heat. An excess of bioactive T3 could be harmful to fetal development. For this reason, the concentration of T3 is tightly controlled in the tissues (van Wassenaer & Kok, 2004). This is accomplished by preferential conversion of excess fetal T4 to the bioinactive reverse T3 by type III deiodinase. In the event of T4 deficiency, as in fetal hypothyroidism, T4 is shunted to the brain where it is deiodinated to T3 to provide a critical source of intracellular T3 to the developing brain.

Birth represents a temporary state of hyperthyroidism for the newborn. In response to sudden exposure to a cold environment, the pituitary releases a surge of TSH that peaks at 70 to 100 munits/mL at 30 minutes after birth. This cold-stimulated TSH surge provokes rises in serum T4, T3, and free T4, all of which peak at about 48 hours. T4 increases in most infants to a level of 6.5 mcg/dL or higher. The rise in T4 causes the TSH to decline to 20 munits/mL or less (the cutoff used in most screening programs for congenital hypothyroidism [CH]) because of feedback inhibition. Free and total T4 and T3 gradually decrease over the next 1 to 2 months.

Congenital Hypothyroidism

CH is a deficiency of thyroid function present at the time of birth. With an incidence of 1 in 2,000 to 4,000 births (Rastogi & LaFranchi, 2010), it is the most common congenital endocrine disorder (Polak & Van Vliet, 2009). CH is classified as either permanent or transient, depending on the underlying etiology. Early diagnosis and appropriate treatment are essential to prevent permanent neurologic damage. Because most affected infants are asymptomatic at birth, neonatal screening for hypothyroidism is now mandated so infants with CH are promptly identified and treated.

Thyroid Dysgenesis

The most common cause (85%) of permanent CH is thyroid dysgenesis, which includes thyroidal ectopy, hypoplasia, and complete thyroid agenesis. The severity of thyroid dysfunction is variable, depending on the amount of functional thyroid tissue present. Thyroidal ectopy accounts for two-thirds of neonates with thyroid dysgenesis. Ectopic thyroid tissue (lingual, sublingual, subhyoid) provides adequate amounts of thyroid hormone in some infants. Occasionally, ectopias are associated with thyroglossal duct cysts. Most of these infants have a thyroid remnant, usually found midline at the base of the tongue, as a result of failure of the gland to descend normally during embryologic development.

Thyroid dysgenesis occurs in 1 in 4,000 live births; however, the incidence in Black infants is 1 in 32,000 live births and in Hispanic infants, 1 in 2,000. The disorder has a female to male ratio of 2 to 1. Only 3% of thyroid dysgenesis is due to mutations in the homeobox genes that control thyroid differentiation (TTF-2, NKX2.1, NKX2.5, or PAX-8) (Tenore & Driul, 2009). Down syndrome is associated with an increased prevalence of thyroid dysgenesis, and extrathyroidal abnormalities (cardiac, gastrointestinal, CNS and eyes) are also more common. No serum Tg is measurable in thyroid agenesis, distinguishing it from functional thyroid tissue, which is associated with measurable serum Tg concentrations.

Thyroid Dyshormonogenesis

About 10% to 20% of infants with CH have inborn defects of thyroid hormone metabolism. Mutations in genes coding for proteins involved in thyroid hormone synthesis, secretion, or transport, result in failure of one of the steps in this process, leading to thyroid insufficiency. These biochemical defects are usually inherited as autosomal recessive traits and include TSH hormone resistance, iodide organification defects, iodide transport defects, iodotyrosine deiodinase defects, and thyroglobulin deficiency. Deficient activity of the enzyme TPO is one of the most common disorders of thyroid synthesis, caused by mutations of THOX1 or THOX2 (Bollepalli & Rose, 2012). Although dyshormonogenesis eventually results in a compensatory goiter, it is not typically apparent during the neonatal period.

Thyroid-Binding Globulin Deficiency

Infants born with congenital TBG deficiency have low TBG and total T4 but normal TSH concentrations and are normal with respect to thyroid function. Familial congenital TBG deficiency, transmitted as an X-linked trait, occurs in 1 in 9,000 newborns (Simpser & Rapaport, 2010). The defect can be complete or partial and is frequently an incidental finding on neonatal screening. A TBG level can be measured to confirm the diagnosis for the purpose of parental counseling, but no treatment is recommended.

Hypothalamic-Pituitary Hypothyroidism

Five to ten percent of infants with CH can be accounted for by what is called "secondary-tertiary" or "central" hypothyroidism. A deficiency of hypothalamic TRH or pituitary TSH can occur as a consequence of a developmental defect of the pituitary or hypothalamus. Central hypothyroidism is generally associated with other anomalies of the midbrain (such as absence of the septum pellucidum or other midline defects), hypopituitarism, pituitary stalk interruption, or empty sella syndrome, all of which lead to typical laboratory findings of low serum T4 and low or inappropriately normal serum TSH.

Thyroid Hormone Resistance

An increasing number of patients are being found with resistance to the actions of endogenous and exogenous T4 and triiodothyronine (T3), a form of "peripheral hypothyroidism." At least 90% of these cases are caused by a mutation in the genes encoding for thyroid hormone receptor β (Rastogi & LaFranchi, 2010). Most patients have goiter, and levels of T4, T3, free T4, and free T3 are elevated. These findings have often led to the erroneous diagnosis of Graves' disease, although most affected patients are clinically euthyroid. The unresponsiveness to thyroid hormone may vary among tissues.

Clinical Manifestations of Congenital Hypothyroidism

Few neonates are diagnosed with CH solely on clinical grounds. Signs and symptoms of CH can be slow to develop owing to persistence of maternal thyroid hormone. When present, signs and symptoms of CH in the neonate are subtle and nonspecific; thus they are not immediately linked with hypothyroidism. Early diagnosis is critical, however, to ensure prompt treatment that will reduce the risk for mental retardation. The signs and symptoms of hypothyroidism in the neonate reflect the wide-ranging actions of thyroid hormones on metabolism, intestinal motility, cardiac function, temperature regulation, neurologic function, and skeletal maturation (Box 10.1). The possibility of CH must be considered in infants presenting with birth weight in excess of the 90th percentile, prolonged jaundice, hypothermia and cold mottled skin, an enlarged (> 1 cm) posterior fontanelle, umbilical hernia, and failure to feed well (Rastogi & LaFranchi, 2010).

Other features traditionally associated with hypothyroidism (macroglossia, dry skin, lethargy, hypotonia, hoarse cry, coarse hair, and constipation) evolve over the first weeks of life. A palpable, enlarged thyroid gland (also called a goiter) can be associated with impaired thyroid hormone synthesis and hypothyroidism. Hyperplasia of the thyroid gland results from hypersecretion of TSH in response to low T3 and T4 levels. Infants with suspected central hypothyroidism may present with midline or cranial defects or other signs of pituitary deficiency. Central hypothyroidism should be suspected in infants presenting with septo-optic dysplasia, hypoglycemia, micropenis, or cleft lip/palate.

Diagnosis of Congenital Hypothyroidism

■ Neonatal Screening. Because even severe CH can be clinically silent, universal newborn screening for CH is widely practiced. Routine screening of all newborn infants for CH has greatly improved early detection and treatment of the disorder, preventing much of the mental retardation that was previously associated with CH. The incidence of CH, as detected through newborn screening, is approximately 1 per 3,000 to 4,000. Screening all newborns for CH is mandated in all U.S. states and throughout Canada. Recent increases in the incidence of CH reported by some screening programs could be the result of increased detection of mild hypothyroidism and preterm infants with delayed TSH rise (Mitchell, Hsu, & Sahai, 2011).

Some screening programs in North America measure the TSH directly from blood samples collected on filter paper. Other programs initially measure T4 on all specimens, followed by TSH measurement only if T4 is low. Owing to the physiologic surge in TSH in the first hours of life as the newborn adapts to the extrauterine environment, the screening specimen must be collected when the infant is at least 24 hours of age, and preferably between 2 and 4 days of age. If blood is collected earlier, particularly in the first 3 hours of life, a false positive result can occur. In those instances, a repeat specimen must be collected within the first 7 days of life, regardless of prior test results. Protein intake is not required prior to screening for CH.

False negatives can also occur with screening. When only T4 testing is done, as many as 8% of infants with central CH can be missed (Bollepalli & Rose, 2012) Their initial T4 levels are in the normal range (Bollepalli & Rose, 2012). A similar problem can occur with infants who have hypothyroxinemia with delayed TSH elevation and those with residual thyroid tissue (such as an ectopic thyroid gland), because their initial T4 levels are also in the normal range. All of these infants would be detected by repeat screening at 2 to 6 weeks of age.

Certain infants are at risk for a missed or delayed diagnosis, including those born at home, those who are extremely ill in the neonatal period, and those who are transferred between hospitals at an early age. Screening errors, including incorrect specimen collection, or improper storage and transport can result in a false negative test. Thyroid medications taken by the mother during pregnancy can also produce false negative results. Blood transfusions can alter test results. Preservatives (EDTA or citrate) in blood-collection containers can result in false negative or false positive screening results.

When a low T4 and elevated TSH level (>40 munits/L) are encountered, the neonate should be presumed to have primary hypothyroidism until proven otherwise. A thorough examination for signs and symptoms of CH is indicated, along with confirmatory serum testing. Treatment with l-thyroxine should be initiated while awaiting the results of further testing.

■ Laboratory Testing. Low serum total and free T4 and T3, along with elevated TSH levels, confirm CH in the neonate. Permanent congenital CH is highly likely in a full-term neonate with a serum T4 less than 6 mcg/dL and a serum TSH greater than 50 munits/L. A normal T4 (e.g., >10 mcg/dL) in combination with elevated TSH suggests that the infant has enough functional thyroid tissue to respond to excess TSH stimulation, the pattern seen in a subgroup of infants with

BOX 10.1

SIGNS AND SYMPTOMS OF HYPOTHYROIDISM IN THE NEONATE

- Birth weight greater than 4 kg, gestation longer than 42 weeks
- Large, open posterior fontanelle (> 1 cm)
- Umbilical hernia
- Abdominal distention
- Poor feeding
- Hypothermia, cool extremities
- Prolonged jaundice
- Bradycardia
- Poor muscle tone
- Mottled skin
- Delayed skeletal maturation

compensated or subclinical hypothyroidism. Age-related reference norms, for both gestational age and hours of age, should be used when interpreting all thyroid test results. If maternal antibody-mediated hypothyroidism is suspected, maternal antithyroid (TSH receptor blocking, TRBAb) antibody testing should be done. Other thyroid autoantibodies that can produce hypothyroidism include thyroglobulin (TGAb) and thyroperoxidase antibodies (TPOAb). TBG levels can be measured to rule out TBG deficiency. Thyroglobulin levels in infants with possible CH can help to differentiate between thyroid agenesis and dyshormonogenesis, as an adjunct to thyroid imaging. Genetic studies have already helped to identify the etiology of CH in some infants.

■ **Imaging Studies.** Infants with biochemical evidence of CH usually undergo scintigraphy with iodine-123 (^{123}I) or pertechnetate ($^{99m}T_cO_4$) which is trapped by the thyroid gland and like iodine (Polak & Van Vliet, 2009) aids in detection of an ectopic (lingual or sublingual) or missing gland. A normal or enlarged gland suggests a defect in thyroxine synthesis as the source of CH. Thyroid ultrasound can also be useful initially to demonstrate presence or absence of a gland. Lateral radiographs of the knee and foot reveal bone age, indicating the degree of intrauterine hypothyroidism experienced by the fetus. Ossification of the distal femoral epiphysis usually appears at 36 weeks gestation; its absence in a term or post term infant suggests delayed bone maturation from long-standing hypothyroidism.

Management of Hypothyroidism

Early, adequate treatment of permanent CH is critical for optimal neurologic development. The goal of hormone replacement therapy is to rapidly normalize the infant's serum T4 level and maintain it in the upper half of the normal range, which should result in a TSH of 0.5 to 4 mU/L (Bollepalli & Rose, 2012). The agent of choice is sodium-l-thyroxine (NaT4) because it is substantially converted to T3 within the brain. Tablets are crushed and given in a small amount of liquid. One method is to instruct parents to crush the tablet and place it on the baby's tongue just before feeding (Polak & Van Vliet, 2009). The tablet should not be diluted in the entire volume of the baby's bottle because if the bottle is not finished, the baby will not receive the full dose needed. Parents should be counseled about the importance of consistent administration of the medication, and instructed on actions to take if a dose is missed or the infant vomits after a dose is given.

Infants receiving thyroid replacement therapy must be monitored closely for adequacy of treatment and evidence of thyrotoxicosis (irritability, tachycardia, poor weight gain). Serum T4 should normalize in 1 to 2 weeks; serum TSH can take longer to normalize.

TRANSIENT DISORDERS OF THYROID FUNCTION

Transient Hypothyroxinemia of Prematurity

Preterm infants have the same incidence of permanent CH as full-term infants (Srinivasan, Harigopal, Turner, & Cheetham, 2012). In addition, about 50% of infants born at less than 30 weeks gestation exhibit transiently low thyroxine levels when compared with their full-term counterparts. This relative hypothyroxinemia is primarily a function of HPT axis immaturity, a physiologically normal stage of thyroid system development. However, many other factors influence thyroid function, particularly in the extremely preterm infant (Hyman, Novoa, & Holzman, 2011). The abrupt cessation of maternal T4 supply, occurring at the time of birth when demand for thyroid hormone is high, contributes to low thyroid hormone levels. Other factors include immature ability to concentrate iodine and to synthesize and iodinate thyroglobulin. Preterm infants may also suffer from insufficient iodine intake during the early weeks after birth before full enteral feeding is established. In addition, iodine excess related to the use of iodine-containing antiseptics and radiopaque agents can interfere with thyroid function by blocking thyroid hormone release from the thyroid gland.

■ **Pathophysiology.** The postnatal TSH surge of the preterm infant is similar, yet quantitatively lower, than that of the more mature infant. Likewise, the corresponding rise in T4 that occurs in preterm infants is blunted in comparison to term infants. It takes approximately 4 to 8 weeks, depending on the gestational age at birth, for normal term hormone levels to be reached. The more premature the infant, the more severe the hypothyroxinemia is. Infants with transiently low thyroxine need follow-up testing to ensure that the low T4 levels rise into the normal range over time.

Extremely preterm infants (24 to 27 weeks gestation) are at an even greater disadvantage, having a distinct and more ineffective pattern of postnatal thyroid function. The TSH surge of these very immature infants is significantly attenuated, and TSH levels continue to fall after birth to less than cord blood values by 7 hours of age. Such very low TSH levels fail to stimulate a postnatal rise in T4 at all. T4 levels in extremely immature infants remain quite low after birth and are even slightly lower than cord blood values at 24 hours of age.

■ **Clinical Manifestations.** Hypothyroxinemia of prematurity is a subtle condition, with no overt signs or symptoms of hypothyroidism. Many classic signs and symptoms of hypothyroidism are common clinical findings in the preterm infant (slow intestinal motility, distention, prolonged jaundice, low muscle tone, mottled skin, etc.). Thyroid hormones are critical to brain development, so a prolonged low thyroxine level while the brain is still undeveloped could be a factor in poor neurocognitive outcomes in these infants.

■ **Diagnosis.** Hypothyroxinemia of prematurity is identified by routine newborn screening. T4 and free T4 are low, but TSH is not elevated above the cutoff of 20 munits/L. This is the critical difference between transient hypothyroxinemia of prematurity and CH. A repeat test is conducted after several weeks to recheck T4 and monitor for a possible delayed rise in TSH.

■ **Management.** The bothersome fact about hypothyroxinemia of prematurity is that it is associated with higher mortality and neurodevelopmental deficits, yet cumulative evidence to date has not been able to demonstrate clear benefits of routinely supplementing these infants with thyroxine during early life. It has been suggested that using a continuous dose of 4 μg/kg/d, rather than a single daily supplement, would be a more physiologic way to raise thyroxine levels and maintain biologic euthyroidism in very low gestational age infants (La Gamma et al., 2009). However, long-term studies to show the neurocognitive benefit of this approach are lacking. A recent *Cochrane Database of Systematic Reviews* did not support the use of prophylactic thyroid hormones in preterm infants to reduce neonatal mortality and neonatal morbidity or improve neurodevelopmental outcomes (Osborn & Hunt, 2007). The exception is the infant with an elevated TSH level; these infants require treatment. Thyroid function tests should be followed carefully in preterm infants at risk for hypothyroxinemia, and treatment should be instituted promptly if indicated by elevated TSH. It is a good idea to flag or highlight the low thyroid results from the initial newborn screen to ensure that repeat thyroid testing is not overlooked.

However, we should not assume that just because studies to date haven't been able to demonstrate the benefits of treating hypothyroxinemia of prematurity this condition isn't significant. The persisting neurodevelopmental deficits in extremely low gestational age neonates could be, in part, related to their thyroid status during critical periods of CNS development (LaGamma & Paneth, 2012).

Nonthyroidal Illness

In some ill preterm infants, T4 is preferentially converted to rT3 instead of T3, possibly as an adaptive response to lower the metabolic rate during times of severe illness. The outcome is low serum concentrations of both T4 and T3. Reverse T3 is elevated and TSH is normal. This condition, also known as "low T3 syndrome" or "euthyroid sick syndrome," occurs in infants who have immature lungs or infections, because the cytokines produced in response to illness or inflammation are believed to inhibit thyroid function, metabolism, or action (van Wassanaer & Kok, 2004). The low T4 from nonthyroidal illness reverses spontaneously when the infant's condition improves. No treatment is required. Similar effects are seen in infants who are receiving dopamine or glucocorticoids, both of which can lower serum T4 concentrations.

Transient Primary Hypothyroidism

Hypothyroidism is defined as transient when a low T4 and elevated TSH in apparently healthy full-term infants revert to normal spontaneously or after several months of thyroxine supplementation. About 5% to 10% of the infants identified by newborn screening programs as having CH eventually are recognized as having a transient condition. Initial management is the same as for CH.

Transplacental Passage of Drugs or Antibodies

Transient hypothyroidism in the newborn can be precipitated by transplacental passage of antithyroid agents taken during pregnancy for the treatment of maternal Graves' disease. Medications such as propylthiouracil (PTU), methimazole, radioiodine, and amiodarone can inhibit fetal thyroid production. A similar inhibitory effect can occur if the fetus is exposed to excess iodine in utero. If the mother has a history of autoimmune thyroid disease, maternal TSH receptor–blocking antibodies (TRBAb, also termed thyrotropin binding inhibitor immunoglobulin, or TBII) readily cross the placenta and block the fetal thyroid, producing hypothyroidism. These TRBAbs can persist in the infant's circulation for 2 to 3 months after birth before they are completely metabolized and disappear. However, it can be difficult to predict the effects of these antibodies because some mothers will simultaneously produce TSH-receptor stimulating antibodies that will offset the effects of the TRBAbs.

■ **Clinical Manifestations.** Like CH, transient hypothyroidism is usually asymptomatic in the newborn. If present, the signs and symptoms are the same as for CH. Transient hypothyroidism caused by antithyroid drugs (goitrogens) can cause a goiter in the neonate. Iodine deficiency or excess has a similar effect.

■ **Diagnosis.** Transient hypothyroidism is typically detected by routine neonatal screening or is based on maternal history. The neonate displays the thyroid profile of low T4 and elevated TSH that is characteristic of hypothyroidism. When the maternal history is positive for autoimmune thyroid disease, TRBAb and TRSAb levels (as indicated) are also obtained for baseline purposes. Thyroid imaging tests may also be conducted.

■ **Management.** Transient hypothyroidism caused by maternal antithyroid medication will resolve spontaneously when the medication is cleared from the infant's circulation, usually within a day or two after birth. The infant's serum T4 and TSH should be monitored to ensure that they return to normal. Supplementation with l-thyroxine is not usually necessary. Transplacentally acquired TSH receptor– blocking antibodies can be slow to degrade completely; therefore most infants will require supplementation for several months. TRBAb levels in the infant can be monitored to determine when to discontinue therapy. Breastfeeding is not contraindicated in neonates whose mothers continue their antithyroid medication in the postpartum period, as very little passes into the breast milk.

Hyperthyroidism (Neonatal Graves' Disease)

■ **Pathophysiology.** The transient condition neonatal Graves' disease occurs in infants born to mothers with active or inactive Graves' disease, to those who have undergone thyroidectomy or radioiodine ablation of the thyroid gland, and to women taking antithyroid drugs. Maternal TRSAbs cross the placenta readily and stimulate the fetal thyroid gland, causing an overproduction of thyroid hormone and in some cases, development of a goiter. Usually the higher the TRSAb level in the mother, the more severely affected the infant. Hyperthyroidism in the neonate is typically transient, lasting approximately 3 to 12 weeks. The clinical course varies depending on characteristics of the mother's disease and treatment. The onset of hyperthyroidism may be delayed for a week or longer in neonates whose mothers produce not only TRSAb but TSH receptor–blocking antibodies as well. Similarly, if the mother took antithyroid medication during pregnancy, the neonate might not exhibit evidence of hyperthyroidism for several days until the drugs are metabolized (and, in fact, some infants are hypothyroid during that time). Occasionally, the hyperthyroidism persists beyond the expected recovery period and becomes true, permanent Graves' disease.

■ **Clinical Manifestations.** Neonates may be born preterm, often with evidence of intrauterine growth restriction. Common clinical signs of thyrotoxicosis include tachycardia, arrhythmias, hypertension, tachypnea, poor feeding, vomiting, sweating, hyperthermia, flushing, diarrhea, restlessness, tremors, irritability, and hyperalertness. In severe cases of untreated maternal Graves' disease, advanced bone age, craniosynostosis, and microcephaly are evident in both the fetus and newborn. The infant should be examined for a goiter, which can be very small or large enough to compress the trachea and cause respiratory distress in the newborn. A goiter is a symmetrical, smooth enlargement of the gland and can be recognized as a swelling in the anterior neck of the neonate (Figure 10.2). To examine the neonate for goiter, place the infant supine and elevate the trunk while allowing the head to fall back gently (LynShue & Witchel, 2007). It is important to appreciate that a goiter can increase in size during the early neonatal period.

■ **Diagnosis.** Serum T4, free T4, and T3 are elevated, and serum TSH is low, all relative to age-appropriate norms. A TRSAb titer in the neonate will give an indication of the expected severity of the disease course. Infants at risk (e.g., high maternal titer of TRSAb) for severe thyrotoxicosis require frequent monitoring of free T4 and TSH. A good maternal history is essential (e.g., history of radioablation therapy, antithyroid drugs taken during pregnancy and when they were taken, and maternal symptoms, if any).

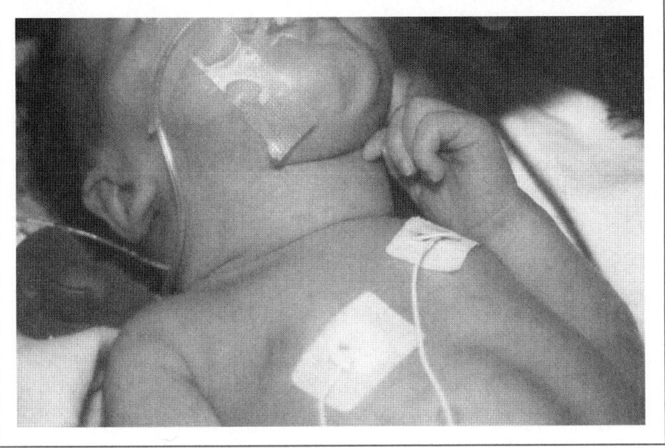

FIGURE 10.2 Newborn infant presenting at birth with goiter.

■ **Management.** The mainstays of treatment of hyperthyroidism in the neonate are iodine, antithyroid medication, sedation, and β-adrenergic blockers, if needed. Treatment is tailored to the severity of the infant's symptoms. Lugol's iodine solution (potassium iodide), given in a single drop three times daily, acutely inhibits the release of thyroxine from the thyroid gland. Other preparations include iodine-based contrast agents (ipodate), PTU, and methimazole. Propranolol can be used to manage cardiovascular symptoms. The infant's serum T4 must be followed closely during treatment for possible iatrogenic hypothyroidism. TRSAb levels are also followed to monitor the infant's recovery and aid in determining the appropriate time for weaning antithyroid medication.

ADRENAL GLAND

The highly vascular adrenal glands are located at the superior poles of the kidneys. Each gland is composed of two distinct, independently functioning organs: the outer cortex, which produces steroid hormones (mineralocorticoids, glucocorticoids, and androgens), and the inner medulla, which produces catecholamines. Adrenal steroid production and regulation require a functional HPA axis. Cortisol is also released in response to stress, hypoglycemia, surgery, extreme heat or cold, hypoxia, infection, or injury.

Aldosterone, the most important mineralocorticoid, regulates renal sodium and water retention and potassium excretion. Aldosterone influences not only electrolyte balance but blood pressure and intravascular volume as well. Aldosterone is regulated by the plasma renin-angiotensin system.

Adrenal androgens include dehydroepiandrosterone (DHEA), DHEA sulfate, and androstenedione and are regulated by ACTH. These steroids have minimal androgenic activity but are converted in the peripheral tissues to two more potent androgens, testosterone and dihydrotestosterone (DHT), required for normal sexual differentiation.

FETAL ADRENAL GLAND

The fetal adrenal gland is evident from 6 to 8 weeks gestation and rapidly increases in size. Fetal cortisol is secreted at 8 weeks gestation. Early in gestation, the fetal adrenal cortex differentiates into three regions: an inner prominent fetal zone, an outer definitive zone, and a transitional zone. After birth, the fetal zone involutes and the definitive zone is transformed into the mature gland. Cortisol maintains intrauterine homeostasis and influences the development of a wide variety of fetal tissues. Cortisol is essential for prenatal maturation of organ systems, including lungs, GI tract, liver, and the CNS, which are vital for neonatal survival.

The fetal adrenal gland and the placenta are an integrated endocrine system known as the fetoplacental unit. The fetal zone of the developing adrenal gland produces DHEA and DHEA sulfate, precursors for placental estrogen, which is critical to maintenance of the pregnancy and fetal well-being. In turn, the placenta regulates fetal exposure to maternal cortisol by oxidizing cortisol to the biologically inactive cortisone, protecting the fetus from excessive cortisol levels. The placenta also releases corticotropin-releasing hormone (CRH), which heightens activity of the fetal HPA axis and stimulates fetal cortisol production. All of this contributes to the prenatal cortisol surge that prepares the fetus for the stress of birth and adaptation to the extrauterine environment.

NEONATAL ADRENOCORTICAL FUNCTION

Plasma cortisol levels are elevated at the time of birth but decline in the first few days of life. In term infants, a nadir is seen on day 4 of life. Likewise, levels of cortisol precursors such as 17-hydroxyprogesterone (17-OHP) are high at birth but decrease to normal neonatal levels by 12 to 24 hours of age. Cortisol is regulated by pituitary ACTH, which in turn is controlled by hypothalamic CRH via a negative feedback loop. Cortisol in the newborn plays a key role in response to stress and illness, and is important in the maintenance of blood pressure (Ng, 2011).

Aldosterone and plasma renin activity (PRA) are elevated in neonates compared with values for older infants, allowing for positive sodium balance until the kidneys fully mature. The hyponatremia and urinary sodium losses often seen in preterm infants during the early postnatal weeks are due to a relative mineralocorticoid deficiency as a consequence of immaturity of both the kidneys and the adrenal glands.

ADRENAL DISORDERS IN THE NEONATE

Transient Adrenocortical Insufficiency of Prematurity

A limited ability of the adrenal glands to maintain cortisol homeostasis in the early days of life has been observed in some preterm newborns. Manifestations are a low serum cortisol, normal or exaggerated pituitary response, and good recovery of adrenal function by day 14 of life (Ng, 2011). A proportion of very-low-birth-weight infants with inotrope and volume-resistant hypotension show an inadequate adrenal response to stress in the immediate postnatal period (Ng, 2011). Whether a relative adrenal insufficiency contributes to hemodynamic instability and hypotension in critically ill infants is still under debate (Nimkarn & New, 2012).

Adrenal Hemorrhage

Adrenal hemorrhage in the neonate can be precipitated by traumatic delivery, breech presentation, macrosomia, or disseminated intravascular coagulation. The large size and vascularity of the fetal adrenal gland predisposes the gland to injury and rupture during the birth process. Although often asymptomatic, classic findings include jaundice, pallor, a flank mass on either side (although hemorrhage is more common on the right) with discoloration and purpura of the overlying skin and discoloration of the scrotum (Mutlu, Karaguzel, Aslan, Cansu, & Okten, 2011). In severe cases, the infant may exhibit signs of adrenal insufficiency. Small hemorrhages can be initially undetected, but eventually manifest in anemia and persistent jaundice (Janjua & Batisky, 2012). Adrenal hemorrhage can be visualized on ultrasound and usually resolves in 4 to 16 weeks (Mutlu et al., 2011).

Congenital Adrenal Hyperplasia

CAH is a spectrum of autosomal recessive disorders resulting from a deficiency of one of the five enzymes required to synthesize cortisol from cholesterol in the adrenal cortex. Each enzyme is encoded by its own gene, and mutations in the 21-hydroxylase (21-OHD) gene, *CYP21A2*, are the most frequent. To date, 127 different mutations of *CYP2A12* have been described, ranging from complete loss of enzyme function to partial enzyme activity (Witchell & Azziz, 2011). The severity of the disease correlates with *CYP21A2* allelic variation (Speiser et al., 2010). 21-OHD deficiency accounts for 95% of CAH and is the most common cause of ambiguous genitalia of the neonate.

■ **Pathophysiology.** A lack of 21-OHD prevents conversion of progesterone to its two end products: cortisol and aldosterone (Figure 10.3). By reduced negative feedback regulation, the absence of cortisol causes oversecretion of ACTH, which chronically stimulates the adrenal cortex, resulting in hyperplasia of the gland. The precursor steroids proximal to the blocked step accumulate and are shunted into other metabolic pathways such as androgen biosynthesis. In a female fetus, these superfluous yet potent systemic androgens cause virilization of the developing external genitalia. Also important may be the effects of this androgen exposure on the developing CNS. Internal reproductive organs (ovaries, fallopian tubes, and uterus) are not affected by androgen exposure and develop normally.

Classic 21-OHD has a worldwide incidence of about 1 in 5,000 to 1 in 15,000 live births (Witchell & Azziz, 2011). Two thirds of those have a severe form known as salt-wasting or salt-losing in which there is a concurrent inability to produce aldosterone. High sodium excretion leads to profound hyponatremia, dehydration, and hyperkalemia. Glucocorticoid deficiency impairs carbohydrate metabolism, resulting in hypoglycemia and leading to hypotension, shock, and cardiovascular collapse from adrenal insufficiency. The remaining one third has a simple virilizing form. These infants have an incomplete enzymatic block, with enough aldosterone biosynthesis to maintain fluid and electrolyte homeostasis.

■ **Clinical Manifestations.** Affected female infants are usually recognized at birth by their nontypical genitals, a cardinal feature of CAH. A range of findings is possible, including clitoromegaly, posterior fusion of the labia majora with rugae, and a single perineal orifice instead of separate urethral and vaginal openings (Witchel & Azziz, 2011). In the last instance, the vagina joins the urethra above the perineum, forming a single urogenital. In severe cases, clitoral hypertrophy is so marked that it resembles a penile urethra (Figure 10.4). These infants can be mistaken for boys with bilateral cryptorchidism and hypospadias. There may also be hyperpigmentation of the genital skin resulting from excessive pituitary ACTH secretion. Male infants with 21-OHD are phenotypically normal and may not be identified in the immediate neonatal period, because the onset of adrenal symptoms is delayed until 7 to 14 days of life. Undetected infants may present to the emergency room

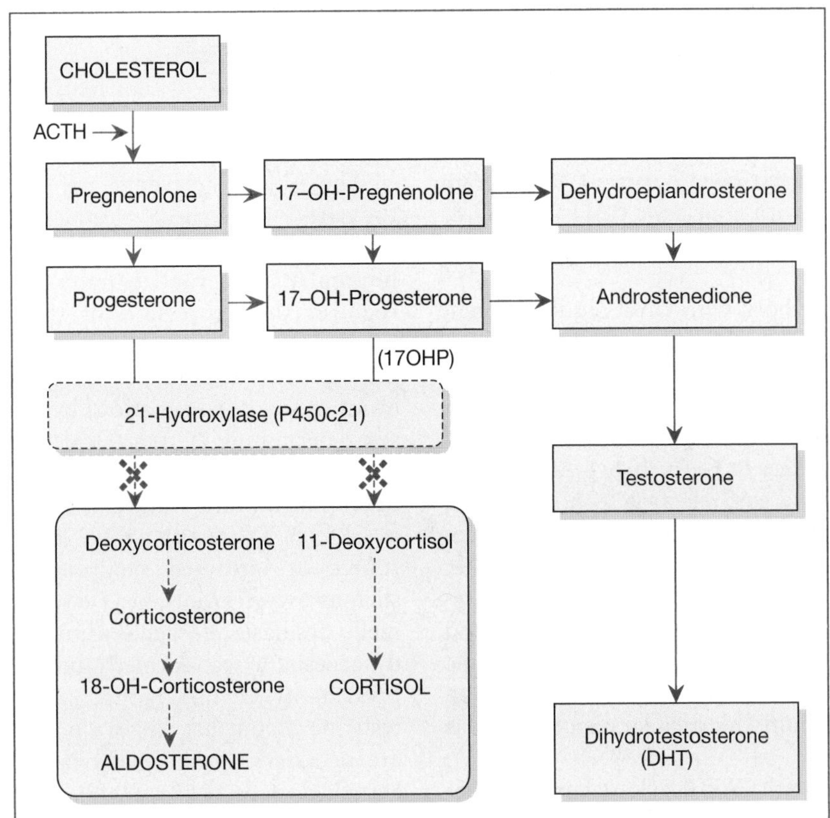

FIGURE 10.3 Pathophysiology of congenital adrenal hyperplasia caused by 21-hydroxylase (21-OHD) deficiency. A deficiency of the enzyme 21-OHD prevents the normal conversion of cholesterol to aldosterone and cortisol. Precursor steroids including 17-hydroxyprogesterone proximal to the blocked step are shunted into the androgen synthesis pathway, resulting in an excess production of androgens.

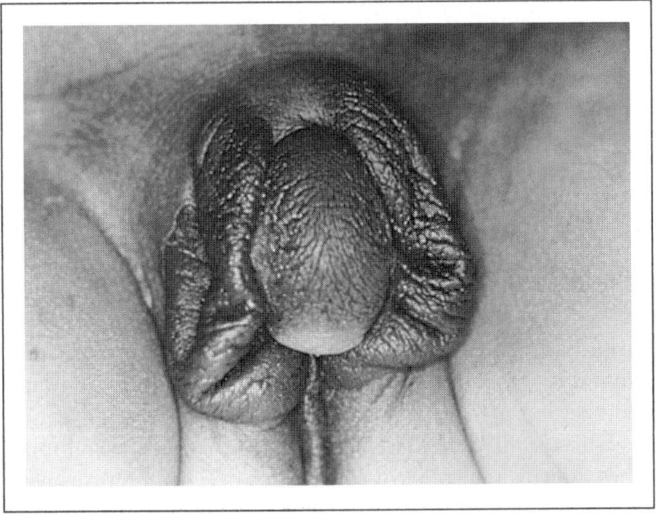

FIGURE 10.4 External genitalia of 46XX neonate with congenital adrenal hyperplasia. Note clitoromegaly with rugosed, hyperpigmented, and partly fused labioscrotal folds.
From Stokowski (2004).

with signs and symptoms of impending adrenal collapse: vomiting, weight loss, lethargy, dehydration, hyponatremia, hyperkalemia, hypoglycemia, hypovolemia, and shock. Infants of either sex who are untreated will undergo rapid postnatal growth and sexual precocity; those with severe enzyme deficiencies can develop salt loss and die (Speiser et al., 2010).

■ **Diagnosis.** A markedly elevated 17-OHP level is diagnostic for classic 21-OHD deficiency. Random 17-OHP levels in affected infants can reach 10,000 ng/dL (normal is < 100 ng/dL). However, such high 17-OHP levels may not be reached until the second or third day of life, so a specimen drawn too early could lead to false reassurance that the infant does not have CAH. Prenatal or postnatal steroids can suppress the 17-OHP level and produce a false negative result as well. Biochemical support for the diagnosis of CAH also includes elevated serum DHEA and androstenedione levels in males and females, and elevated serum testosterone in females. Molecular genetic analysis is not usually essential for the diagnosis but may be helpful to confirm the exact type of defect and to aid in genetic counseling.

Part of the evaluation of every newborn with ambiguous genitalia is a karyotype or FISH test for sex chromosome material, and this is also true when the suspected diagnosis is CAH. Imaging studies, including pelvic and abdominal ultrasound, will determine the presence or absence of a uterus, evaluate adrenal size, and more rapidly identify the gender of the infant.

The increased serum 17-OHP levels in affected infants permit screening for the disorder using blood filter specimens on routine newborn screening panels. The major objectives of newborn screening for CAH are the presymptomatic identification of infants at risk for the development of life-threatening adrenal crises and prevention of incorrect sex assignment of affected female infants with ambiguous genitalia. The former is particularly important for affected boys whose initial manifestation may be adrenal crisis. All 50 states now screen newborns for CAH. False positives occur in about 1% of all tests, and can also occur in preterm infants or sick infants, both of whom have higher levels of 17-OHP (Speiser et al., 2010). The higher 17-OHP concentrations of preterm infants, sick infants, and heterozygotic carriers can overlap the levels typical of babies with nonclassic CAH (Witchel & Azziz, 2011).

■ **Management.** The newborn with CAH requires urgent expert medical attention. When the diagnosis of CAH is confirmed, physiologic replacement dosing of cortisol is initiated to overcome cortisol deficiency and to suppress ACTH and androgen overproduction, without completely suppressing the HPA axis (Pass & Neto, 2011). Aldosterone replacement maintains fluid and electrolyte homeostasis. Agents of choice in the newborn are hydrocortisone, a glucocorticoid, plus fludrocortisone, a mineralocorticoid. Further clinical management is guided by daily weights, adrenal steroid concentrations, PRA, electrolytes, blood glucose, and other data. PRA should be compared against age-specific norms, because basal PRA is higher in the newborn than in older infants. Dietary sodium chloride supplementation is often necessary.

Most 46XX individuals with CAH develop a female gender identity, regardless of the degree of genital virilization present at birth, according to currently available evidence (Houk & Lee, 2012). Therefore, even in cases where babies are initially "misassigned" as boys, it is still generally recommended that these genetic females with CAH be raised as females (Brown & Warne, 2005), although some experts maintain that in extensively virilized infants, a male sex assignment should be considered (Houk & Lee, 2012). Hypertrophy of the clitoris will gradually abate with medical therapy; however, severe virilization will not be reversed. Parents of virilized female infants may have many questions about possible genital surgery. Although such surgery is not usually performed until the infant is 2 to 6 months of age, it is helpful for the parents to meet with the pediatric endocrinologist and pediatric urologic surgeon during the initial hospitalization or shortly afterward to discuss available options, one of which is to delay surgery performed for cosmetic purposes until the child is old enough to participate in the decision (Auchus et al., 2010; ISNA, 2006). The goals of genital surgery for virilized girls with CAH are to achieve genital appearance compatible with gender, unobstructed urinary emptying without incontinence or infections, and good adult sexual and reproductive function. After discharge, infants with CAH must be closely followed by a pediatric endocrinologist for assessments of hormone levels, blood sugar, blood pressure, growth, skeletal maturation, and other parameters necessary to guard against over- or undertreatment.

AMBIGUOUS GENITALIA

Sexual Development in the Fetus

Sexual differentiation is a sequential process with three stages: (1) fertilization (determination of chromosomal sex), (2) gonadal differentiation, and (3) differentiation of phenotypic sex (internal ductal system and external genitalia (Lin-Su & New, 2012).

At the time of conception, the sex chromosome complement of the fertilizing sperm determines the chromosomal sex.

The following events are directed by genes. During the early weeks of development, all embryos have bipotential gonads and structures for both male and female internal and external genitalia. Male-specific development requires the expression of the testis-determining gene (*SRY*) located on the short arm of the Y chromosome. This directs the gonad to differentiate to a testis, the key event in sex determination, by downstream regulation of sex-determining factors (Ocal, 2011).

Numerous other genes are required for normal gonadal development, and mutations in many of these genes (such as *SRY, WT1, SOX9, DAX-1, DMRT1* and *SF1*) are the source of identified syndromes of gonadal dysgenesis, such as Swyer syndrome, Denys–Drash syndrome, campomelic dysplasia, dosage-sensitive sex reversal, and gonadal dysgenesis. It was formerly believed that the ovary developed as a "default" gonad (in the absence of genes for testis development), but we now know that specific genes are necessary for normal ovarian differentiation (Vilain, Seragloglou, & Yehya, 2009).

Internal Genitalia

The next events in sexual development are hormonally mediated, predicated on the established gonadal sex (Lin-Su & New, 2012). By 7 weeks gestation, the fetus has two sets of primitive ducts that will become the internal reproductive tracts: the Müllerian (female) and Wolffian (male). In the XY fetus, the testis differentiates by the end of week 7. The embryonic testis develops two types of hormone-producing cells: the Sertoli and the Leydig cells. The Sertoli cells begin secreting Müllerian-inhibiting factor (MIF), causing the Müllerian ducts to regress. By the ninth week, testicular Leydig cells are secreting the androgens necessary for further virilization of the male fetus.

Testosterone, the major androgen produced by the testes, acts locally in high concentrations to induce development of the Wolffian ducts into the epididymis, vas deferens, and seminal vesicles. In the absence of testosterone, the Wolffian ducts regress at 11 weeks gestation. Müllerian ducts require no ovarian hormonal inducement to develop into Fallopian tubes, uterus, and upper vagina. This occurs in fetuses with a normal ovary or on any side lacking a gonad.

External Genitalia

The primitive external genital structures are identical in both sexes (Figure 10.5). In this indifferent stage, a genital tubercle forms and elongates to form a phallus and urogenital sinus, surrounded by inner urogenital folds and labioscrotal swellings. Between the 8th and 14th weeks gestation, male differentiation of the external genitalia takes place. Central to this development is availability of DHT, a potent metabolite produced from testosterone by the enzyme 5 alpha-reductase-2 (5-ARD-2). With 10 times the binding affinity of testosterone, DHT binds to androgen receptors in the genital tissues, stimulating fusion of the urethral folds to form the penile shaft, and the labioscrotal swellings to form the scrotum. The urogenital sinus becomes the urethra. Penile growth continues throughout gestation, and migration of the testes from the abdominal cavity to the scrotum is a late event, at 25 to 35 weeks gestation. Androgen exposure after about 14 weeks contributes to further phallic enlargement (Lin-Su & New, 2012).

In the absence of DHT, feminization of the external genitalia occurs. The phallus becomes a clitoris, and the labioscrotal swellings remain unfused to form the labia majora and minora. The urogenital sinus develops into the lower vagina and urethra. Feminine external genital development is complete by 11 weeks gestation. Androgen exposure after this critical period can promote growth of the clitoris but does not cause labial fusion or the development of a penile urethra (Lin-Su & New, 2012).

Disorders of Sexual Development

A disorder of sexual development (DSD) is a misalignment, and therefore incongruence, between molecular, gonadal, and phenotypic sex (Houk & Lee, 2012). Most DSDs result from one of two events: either a failure in one of the steps of the male sexual developmental pathway, or the exposure of an XX fetus to androgens during a sensitive period of development. Less frequent are DSDs resulting from gonadal differentiation, chromosomal disorders, and syndromes associated with ambiguous genitalia (Lin-Su & New, 2012). The genes and multigenic factors responsible for DSDs are just beginning to be understood, but this information has yet to prove beneficial in terms of clinical management.

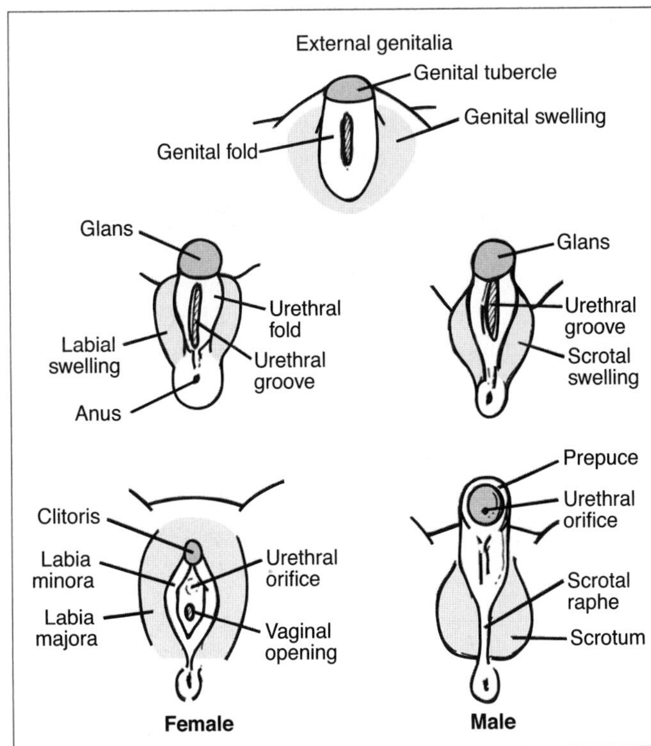

FIGURE 10.5 Development of the external genitalia. From Houk (2005).

46XX DSD Trimester

The most frequently encountered DSD in the neonate is the virilized female, or the 46XX infant with ambiguous external genitalia but normal female internal structures. The most common etiology is CAH, caused by 21-OHD deficiency. This enzyme deficiency results in an overproduction of androgens at a critical stage of development, causing masculinization of the external, but not the internal (ovaries, uterus, fallopian tubes), genitalia. In the most severe cases, the excess androgens also prevent the vagina from fully descending into the perineum, leaving a common urogenital canal (see previous section, Adrenal Disorders).

Other possible, yet rare, causes of virilization of external genitalia in the 46XX infant are placental aromatase deficiency, maternal androgen-producing or adrenal tumors, and maternal medications with androgenic action taken during pregnancy.

46XY DSD

The combination of a 46XY karyotype with ambiguous genitalia results from a failure in one of the steps involved in the synthesis or response to testosterone during sexual differentiation and penile growth. These infants have bilateral testicular development, but incomplete virilization of the internal or external genitalia. This results in an external phenotype ranging from completely female to isolated hypospadias or cryptorchidism. Another condition associated with incomplete virilization in the XY male is cloacal exstrophy, a defect of embryogenesis involving exstrophy of the bladder. Although not a DSD, significant ambiguity of external genitalia may be present. In most cases of 46 XY DSD, it has not been possible to determine the causative genetic mutation (Houk & Lee, 2012).

Androgen Insensitivity Syndrome

■ **Pathophysiology.** Androgen insensitivity syndrome (AIS) is caused by a loss-of-function mutation in the androgen receptor gene located on the long arm of the X chromosome. More than 300 different mutations have been identified (Lin-Su & New, 2012). Both testosterone and its target tissue metabolite, DHT, must bind to androgen receptors to masculinize the genital tissues. When androgen receptor activity is impaired, androgen binding is insufficient. One variant of AIS is receptor negative: Cytosol receptors are incapable of binding DHT. Another variant is receptor positive: Receptors are able to bind DHT, but this does not result in normal differentiation. Both internal Wolffian structures and external genitalia fail to respond to high levels of testosterone and DHT. There are partial and complete forms of the disorder, resulting in different degrees of undervirilization. In partial androgen insensitivity syndrome (PAIS) the clinical phenotype varies considerably and often parallels the severity of androgen resistance, but genotype-phenotype correlations have not been found.

■ **Clinical Manifestations.** Infants with PAIS have undervirilization ranging from simple hypospadias to microphallus with a labia majora-like bifid scrotum, undescended testes, and a urogenital sinus. No visible features distinguish PAIS from other causes of incomplete masculinization. Infants with complete androgen insensitivity (CAIS) are born with apparently female genitalia. However, these neonates may have palpable inguinal or labial masses, which further testing will reveal to be testes. Some may also have a short, blind-ending vagina.

■ **Diagnosis.** The diagnosis of CAIS is missed in the newborn period unless the infant presents with bilateral masses in the labia or inguinal canals or a boy was expected based on a prenatal karyotype. CAIS might also be discovered at the time of inguinal hernia repair, or there may be a history of similarly affected family members. Important investigations include a karyotype, levels of testosterone, DHT, and LH. In PAIS, the ratio of androstenedione to testosterone is normal. Testosterone, estradiol, and LH are normal or high: FSH is usually normal.

Androgen receptor binding assays are not always helpful, because normal ligand binding does not rule out androgen insensitivity caused by mutations in other domains of the androgen receptor (Lin-Su & New, 2012). Less than half of infants with suspected PAIS have abnormal androgen binding; those with normal binding may have a defect in DNA binding or transcriptional activation (Misra & Lee, 2005). A test for direct sequencing of the AR for mutational analysis is commercially available, but AR mutations are not always found in PAIS (Lin-Su & New, 2012). Imaging studies reveal the absence of female internal reproductive structures (uterus, fallopian tubes). Two normal testes are present.

■ **Management.** Infants with CAIS have unambiguously female external anatomy and are raised in the female gender. Testes are removed (usually after puberty) to prevent later malignancy. The gender assignment of infants with PAIS can be more complex and is often based on the severity of the phenotype (Misra & Lee, 2005). When the phenotype is predominantly male, a male sex rearing is recommended. However, no consensus exists for the management of infants with severe perineoscrotal hypospadias and microphallus. The detection of somatic mutations in AIS is of importance for correct sex assignment because the presence of a functional wild-type AR receptor can induce virilization at puberty (Kohler et al., 2005). When a male sex of rearing is contemplated, a therapeutic trial with pharmacologic doses of androgen, especially in those with an identified AR mutation, is often used to predict potential androgen responsiveness at puberty. If the phallus does not grow in response to testosterone, some experts would recommend consideration of a female gender assignment. However, many experts now believe that, given the putative influence of prenatal androgen exposure on the developing CNS, and the possibility that the child will develop a male gender identity, it is more prudent to raise these infants as boys.

Testosterone Biosynthetic Defects

■ **Pathophysiology.** Defects in the chain of steroidogenic enzymes involved in the testosterone biosynthesis pathway result in insufficient androgen concentrations during fetal development. Disorders include congenital lipoid adrenal hyperplasia (CLAH), 3 beta-HDD, 17 alpha-hydroxylase/17,20 lyase deficiency, and 17 beta-hydroxysteroid dehydrogenase deficiency (17 beta-HSD). CLAH is caused by a defect in the steroidogenic acute regulatory (StAR) protein, responsible for transporting cholesterol to the inner membrane of the mitochondria. Insufficient testosterone in affected males leads to underdeveloped Wolffian duct structures and external male anatomy. Müllerian structures are absent because there is normal testicular MIF production.

■ **Clinical Manifestations.** Male infants with CLAH present with complete adrenal insufficiency: vomiting, weight loss, and hypotension. Genital appearance is primarily female. Infants with 3 beta-HDD can present with varying degrees of genital ambiguity and evidence of salt-losing crisis (see 21-OHD). Infants with 17 alpha-hydroxylase/17,20 lyase deficiency have genital ambiguity, whereas patients with primary 17 alpha-hydroxylase deficiency also have hypertension. Male infants with 17 beta-HSD present with what appear to be external female genitalia that may include mild clitoral enlargement. An inguinal hernia may be present, possibly the only finding that will bring the infant to medical attention.

■ **Diagnosis.** General laboratory investigations in suspected testosterone biosynthetic defects include chromosomes, baseline levels of testosterone, androgen precursors and DHT, and levels of steroids and steroid precursors. An hCG stimulation test can be performed to measure the ratio of androstenedione to testosterone; an elevated ratio suggests 17 beta-HSD deficiency. In CLAH, ultrasound, CT or MRI may show enlarged, lipid-laden adrenal glands (Lin-Su & New, 2012).

■ **Management.** Acute management of these disorders requires full steroid replacement with both glucocorticoids and mineralocorticoids. In CLAH and 3 beta-HDD, general supportive measures may be necessary, as severe adrenal insufficiency can cause rapid metabolic decompensation if the disorder is not recognized at birth (Misra & Lee, 2005). Genetic XY infants with CLAH are raised in the female gender. Children with 17 beta-HSD often virilize significantly at puberty owing to increased peripheral conversion of androstenedione to testosterone by 17 beta-HSD isoenzymes, making gender assignment of those diagnosed as neonates a less straightforward decision.

5α-Reductase-2 Deficiency

■ **Pathophysiology.** 5-ARD-2 deficiency is an autosomal recessive disorder caused by more than 20 different mutations of the 5-ARD gene. 5-ARD-2 is an enzyme found in the genital skin and fibroblasts of the developing fetus, without which testosterone is not converted to DHT, and fetal external genitalia do not virilize. Development of the internal structures is unaffected because DHT is not required, so the Wolffian ducts differentiate normally in response to testosterone and the Müllerian ducts regress. At puberty, the external genitalia become virilized and fertility is possible (Misra & Lee, 2005).

■ Clinical Manifestations. The spectrum of findings ranges from mild (isolated micropenis or hypospadias) to severe (a female phenotype with clitoromegaly, mild rugation, or pigmentation) undervirilization (Figure 10.6). Testes are intact and are found in the inguinal canals or labioscrotal folds, or are retained in the abdomen. The uterus and fallopian tubes regress because of normal secretion of MIS. Wolffian duct differentiation is not affected because DHT is not required. Male internal ducts terminate either in a blind pseudovaginal pouch or on the perineum.

■ Diagnosis. Diagnosis is made by assessing the ratio of testosterone to DHT following an hCG stimulation test. A normal T/DHT ratio is less than 4 to 1. In 5-ARD-2 deficiency, this ratio is elevated to higher than 14 to 1 (Lin-Su & New, 2012). The hCG stimulation test also rules out other causes of undervirilization, such as Leydig cell hypoplasia and testosterone biosynthetic defects. Analysis of 5-ARD-2 activity in genital skin fibroblasts provides a definitive diagnosis.

■ Management. Boys with 5-ARD-2 respond to endogenous testosterone and undergo virilization and penile growth at puberty. The mechanism behind this late virilization may be extraglandular DHT formation due to peripheral conversion of increased testicular testosterone by unaffected isoenzymes. For this reason, it is recommended that when the diagnosis is made in the newborn period, a male sex assignment is usually made.

Gonadal Dysgenesis

This group of disorders is usually associated with chromosomal anomalies or mutations or deletions of genes responsible for sexual differentiation. Karyotypes producing gonadal dysgenesis include 46XY, 46XX, 46XY/46X, and mosaic forms including the Y chromosome. Gonadal dysgenesis can occur as an isolated condition or as part of a complex syndrome such as Fraser, Denys–Drash, or campomelic dysplasia (Brown & Warne, 2005).

■ Pathophysiology. A dysgenetic testis either fails to produce testosterone at all or produces insufficient testosterone, resulting in varying degrees of undervirilization of the fetus. Gonadal dysgenesis is considered partial or incomplete when the testes are dysgenetic or incompletely formed, and complete when the gonads are streaks containing only stromal tissue. Mixed gonadal dysgenesis occurs when one gonad is a streak and the other is a well-formed testis. The internal ducts correlate with the ipsilateral gonad. On the side of a streak gonad, a fallopian tube and a hemiuterus will develop, and on the side of a normal testis, the vas deferens and epididymis will form.

■ Clinical Manifestations. The external genitalia are highly variable depending on how much testosterone is produced. In mixed gonadal dysgenesis, the external genitalia are asymmetric, appearing male on one side and female on the other. A vagina and uterine cavity may be present. Complete (or pure) gonadal dysgenesis is a form of sex reversal that results in unambiguously female genitalia with features of Turner's syndrome. These infants might not be identified in the newborn period unless a discrepancy is noted between a prenatal karyotype (46XY) and appearance of the genitals.

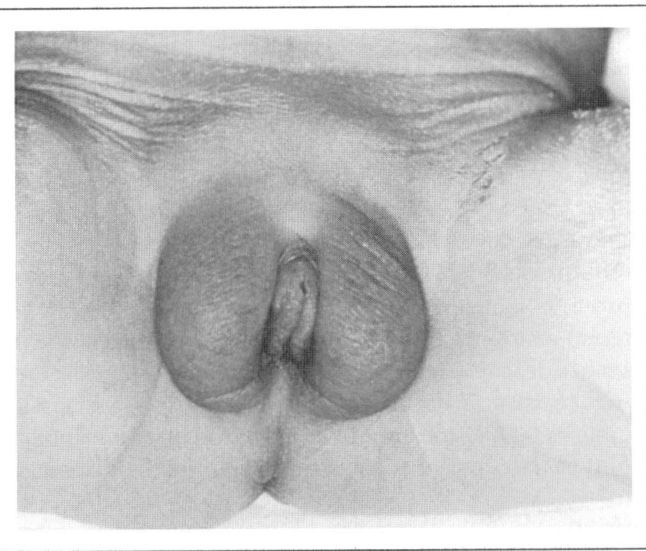

FIGURE 10.6 External genitalia of 46XY neonate with 5 α-reductase deficiency. Undervirilization is so severe in this infant that the phenotype is almost completely female, with labia majora–like bifid scrotum and severe microphallus.
From Stokowski (2004).

■ Diagnosis. Determining the sex chromosome complement by FISH testing is the most important diagnostic test. Imaging studies, genitography, or laparoscopy are used to define the internal anatomy. Gonadal histologic analysis is necessary to differentiate gonadal dysgenesis from ovotesticular DSD, a condition wherein elements of both testes and ovaries are present in the same individual (see later discussion).

■ Management. Determining the sex of rearing for the infant with partial or mixed gonadal dysgenesis can be a difficult decision, one that is typically based on the degree of virilization and details of the internal anatomy. When a uterus is present, the female sex assignment may be preferred. Most infants with complete gonadal dysgenesis are raised as females.

Ovotesticular DSD

In ovotesticular DSDs both ovarian and testicular components are present in the same individual. Possible combinations include an ovary on one side and a testis on the other, an ovary or testis with an ovotestis, or two ovotestes. More than half of affected babies will have an XX karyotype. This condition was formerly known as true hermaphroditism, a label that is considered outdated.

■ Pathophysiology. The amount of testosterone produced by the testicular tissue that is present determines the degree of differentiation of Wolffian ducts, regression of Müllerian ducts, and virilization of external genitalia. The internal ducts usually parallel the ipsilateral gonadal histology. Ovarian tissue can be normal.

■ Clinical Manifestations. Asymmetry of the external genitalia is a hallmark of ovotesticular DSD. Genital ambiguity ranges from a female phenotype with slight clitoromegaly to a mildly undervirilized male phenotype. The most common presentation is marked genital ambiguity: microphallus with penoscrotal or perineoscrotal hypospadias, fusion of labioscrotal folds, and cryptorchidism (Misra & Lee, 2005).

■ Diagnosis. FISH testing is used to determine the sex chromosome complement. Imaging studies are used to define the internal anatomy. To diagnose ovotesticular dysgenesis, the presence of functional ovarian tissue containing follicles and testicular tissue with distinct seminiferous tubules must be established (Misra & Lee, 2005). Laparoscopy with gonadal biopsy is necessary at some point to confirm the diagnosis.

■ Management. Principles of management for infants with true ovotesticular DSD are similar to those of gonadal dysgenesis.

General Principles of Management of DSDs

The fact that doctors and nurses are not quite sure if one's long-awaited newborn baby is a boy or a girl must surely be one of the most incomprehensible things that parents can hear in the delivery room. This situation requires a high degree of sensitivity and tact. Many infants are identified prenatally following ultrasound recognition of genital ambiguity or a karyotype/phenotype discordance, and these families will be prepared, to some degree, for the experience of having a baby of uncertain sex. Others will be taken completely by surprise. In spite of the family's desire for a quick answer, no attempt should be made by medical professionals at the time of birth to guess the sex of the baby (Ogilvy-Stuart & Brain, 2004). The extreme phenotypic heterogeneity seen in DSDs makes it impossible to accurately predict either the diagnosis or the karyotype from a brief genital examination (Houk & Lee, 2005). Neonates who do not have health concerns requiring intensive care monitoring or treatment should not be transferred to the neonatal intensive care unit (NICU). Admission to the NICU heightens the parents' anxiety unnecessarily and impairs parent–infant bonding (ISNA, 2006).

The Lawson Wilkins Pediatric Society and the European Society for Paediatric Endocrinology recently established an International Consensus Conference on Intersex. The result was a consensus statement on management of DSDs (Lee, Houk, Ahmed, Hughes, & International Consensus Conference on Intersex organized by the Lawson Wilkins Pediatric Endocrine Society and the European Society for Paediatric Endocrinology, 2006). That document represents the first agreed-on set of guiding principles for approaching and managing the newborn with a DSD.

■ Clinical Manifestations. Essential to the evaluation of the neonate with genital ambiguity is obtaining a detailed family history. Any of the following might suggest a congenital or inherited DSD: maternal virilization or ingestion of hormones or oral contraceptives during pregnancy; consanguinity; history of urologic abnormalities, infertility, or genital ambiguity in other family members; or previous neonatal deaths that might suggest an undiagnosed adrenal crisis. Dysmorphic features suggest the possibility of a syndrome.

A detailed assessment of the genitalia should be conducted. This and all subsequent examinations should respect the privacy of the infant and the family as much as possible, avoiding overexposure of the infant even for educational purposes (Auchus et al., 2010). Because of considerable overlap in the genital anatomy among DSDs, the physical assessment alone does not permit a firm diagnosis (Lin-su & New, 2012). However, some assessment findings can provide clues to the underlying pathophysiology and guide the diagnostic process in one direction or another. A precise description of the anatomy is more useful than simple staging classifications. If preferred, however, the degree of virilization can be documented by Prader staging from a phenotypic female with mild clitoromegaly (Prader stage II) to phenotypic male with glandular hypospadias (Prader stage V) (Figure 10.7). Look for symmetry or asymmetry of the genitalia, which provides an important clue. The presence of a uterus can be determined by digital rectal examination as an anterior midline cordlike structure.

■ Gonads. Determine whether gonads are palpable. The presence or absence of palpable gonads helps to differentiate the major categories of DSDs. An apparent male infant with bilateral or a single impalpable testis with hypospadias should be considered as having a potential DSD until proven otherwise. A palpable gonad excludes the diagnosis of virilized genetic female (46XX) with CAH. A gonad palpated below the external inguinal ring is presumed to contain testicular tissue. Because ovaries are rarely palpable, a unilateral gonad is usually a testis or occasionally an ovotestis. To palpate testes, place finger flat from internal ring and milk down into the labioscrotal folds. Gonads may be situated high in the inguinal canal, requiring a careful examination. Sweep the fingers down along the line of the inguinal canal on each side, beginning well above the site of the internal inguinal ring. A gonad milked down by this maneuver is gently grasped by the other hand and its size and consistency are noted. Ovotestes are softer and less homogeneous than testes (Brown & Warne, 2005). Bilateral absence of the testes is known as cryptorchidism.

■ Phallus. Phallic size should be measured with a straight-edge ruler, depressing the fat pad and measuring the stretched length from pubic tubercle to tip of penis, not including the foreskin. Both length and mid-shaft diameter of the penis should be noted. Chordee, ventral curvature of the penis caused by residual urethral tissue that tethers the phallus to the perineum, should be noted because it can reduce the apparent length of the penis (Lin-Su & New, 2012). The actual position of the urethral meatus and the severity of hypospadias, if present, should be determined.

Clitoral size should also be measured when clitoromegaly is present. Clitoral length greater than 9 mm in term infants is considered excessive. Clitoral size often appears large in preterm infants because breadth remains constant from 27 weeks onward. A prominent, but not truly enlarged, clitoris, or a normally sized penis concealed by an abundance of prepubic fat are two normal assessment findings that sometimes prompt referrals for genital ambiguity (Houk & Lee, 2005).

■ Labioscrotal Folds. Labial fullness, a benign finding, is another feature occasionally mistaken for genital ambiguity. The labioscrotal folds are examined for fusion, which starts posteriorly and moves anteriorly, increasing the anogenital distance. The perineum is inspected by gently separating the labia and using an exam light to confirm the presence of separate urethral and vaginal openings or a single urogenital orifice (an opening connected to both urinary and genital systems). Visualization of voiding is helpful. If skin tags with slightly bluish hue are seen, a hymen and vagina are present. Note rugosity or hyperpigmentation of the labioscrotal fold, signifying hypersecretion of ACTH associated with CAH. Other variations include a bifid scrotum (a deep midline cleft) or a shawl scrotum (scrotum surrounds the penis like a shawl).

■ Diagnostic Studies. DSDs are diagnosed with a combination of biochemical, hormonal, imaging, and molecular testing. Many diagnostic algorithms have been published, but no single algorithm is perfect for all circumstances. (Lee et al., 2006) The principal aim of an initial investigation is to rule out a life-threatening illness such as CAH, which can precipitate an adrenal crisis. Such testing includes serum 17-OHP level (after 24–48 hours of age), electrolytes, glucose, baseline levels of testosterone, DHT, and other steroid precursors (progesterone, DHEA, Δ4-androstenedione, and 17 alpha-hydroxypregnenolone). A karyotype with X- and Y-specific probe detection is obtained from all infants, even if a prenatal karyotype is available (Allen, 2009).

A urinary steroid profile is helpful in the diagnosis of disorders of steroid biosynthesis. Other investigations that may be warranted include ACTH stimulation test, PRA, and serum MIF, LH, and FSH. An hCG stimulation test is undertaken to delineate a block in testosterone biosynthesis from androstenedione (17 beta-hydroxysteroid dehydrogenase deficiency) or conversion of testosterone to DHT (5 alpha-reductase deficiency). An hCG test involves measuring baseline levels of testosterone and its precursors DHEA or DHEA sulfate and androstenedione and its metabolite DHT. One to three intramuscular injections of high-dose hCG are given at 24-hour intervals, and repeat testosterone levels are drawn at 72 or 24 hours after the last injection (Ogilvy-Stuart & Brain, 2004).

Imaging studies include abdomino-pelvic ultrasound (to determine the presence or absence of a uterus, to visualize the presence or absence of gonads in the inguinal region, and to assess the Müllerian anatomy), genitourethrogram (to delineate the anatomy of the vagina and urethra, and where the vagina opens into the urogenital sinus), and pelvic MRI. Laparoscopic exploration with gonadal biopsy may be necessary to evaluate gonadal histology. Finally, molecular analysis may be required to arrive at a definitive diagnosis for some disorders, although molecular diagnosis continues to be limited by cost, accessibility, and quality control (Lee et al., 2006).

■ Interpretation of Findings. The most common cause of genital ambiguity in the newborn is 21-OHD deficiency. This form of CAH, responsible for over 90% of cases of ambiguous genitalia, presents with a virilized XX (female) infant and should be suspected in the presence of a virilized infant with a uterus and no palpable gonads (Ocal, 2011).

Among the remainder of cases of ambiguous genitalia, the most common diagnoses are gonadal dysgenesis, followed by PAIS, and testosterone biosynthetic disorders. Symmetrical external genitalia, with or without palpable gonads, and no uterus, suggests an undervirilized male (Ocal, 2011). A micropenis should prompt investigation for hypopituitarism or growth hormone deficiency, particularly in the presence of hypoglycemia (Lin-Su & New, 2012).

It is not always possible to reach a diagnosis in the undervirilized male infant. In a study of 67 XY infants with external sexual ambiguity, testicular tissue, and/or a XY karyotype, in 52% of cases, no diagnosis could be reached, despite an exhaustive clinical and laboratory workup, including sequencing of the androgen receptor (Morel et al., 2002). Provisional diagnostic groupings can be determined based on the presence or absence of a uterus, symmetry of

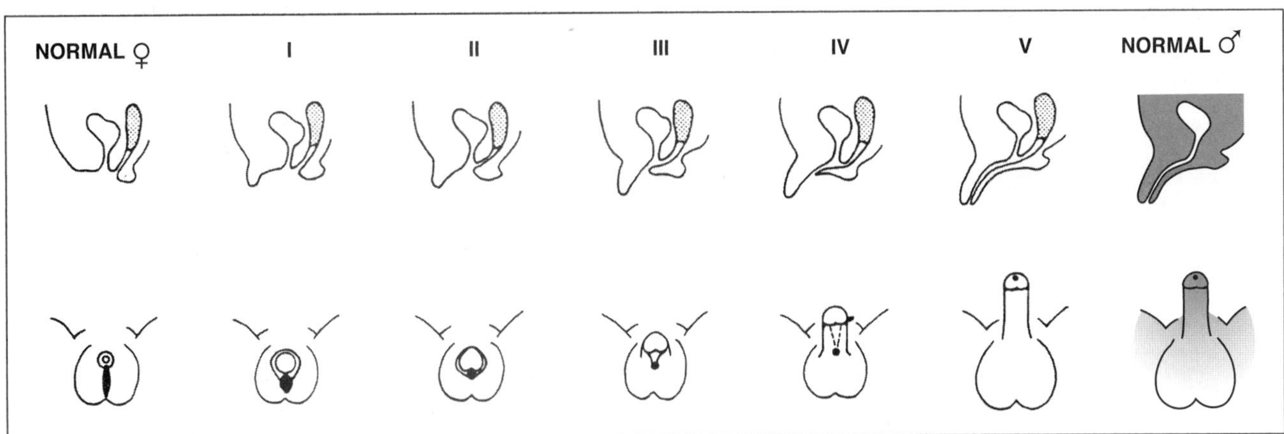

FIGURE 10.7 Degrees of genital virilization according to the stages of Prader. The upper panel shows sagittal view and the lower panel shows perineal view.
From Sperling (2006).

the external genitalia, and presence of gonads (Table 10.1), providing a basis for more focused additional investigations (Brown & Warne, 2005).

■ Talking With Families. Optimal care of the infant with a DSD involves a well-coordinated team approach. The team comprises at minimum the attending neonatologist, neonatal nurse, endocrinologist, pediatric surgeon/pediatric urologic surgeon, social worker, counselor or other mental health professional, and in some instances, geneticist. The initial contact with parents of a newborn with a DSD is extremely important. This interaction should emphasize that a DSD is not a shameful condition and does not preclude the child from becoming a well-adjusted, functional adult, who can be expected to lead a fulfilling life (Houk & Lee, 2012). A single person should be identified to communicate diagnostic findings and plans with the family. When discussing possible diagnoses with the family, language must be carefully chosen. The terms "hermaphrodite" and "pseudohermaphrodite" are outdated, confusing, and perceived as distasteful by many (Lee et al., 2006). These words should not be used, and instead, accurate, informative terms that describe the infant's diagnosis should be used. A clear explanation of sexual development in the fetus will help parents understand how an infant can be born with atypical genitalia, an important component of parental coping (Houk & Lee, 2005). It is helpful to explain that the appearance of the external genitalia is determined by prenatal androgen exposure, and not the molecular sex (Witchel & Azziz, 2011).

It is the parents who have the responsibility to make or defer decisions about care for their infant with a DSD, including gender-of-rearing (Houk & Lee, 2005). The role of the health care team is to provide information, to share and explain all diagnostic findings, to inform parents of all available options, and to support the parents in the decision-making process. The approach should be family-centered as well as culturally sensitive (Thyen, Richter-Appelt, Wiesemann, Holterhus, & Hiort, 2005). Family concerns must be respected and addressed in strict confidence (Auchus et al., 2010). A relationship of trust is paramount, and this requires open and honest communication and full disclosure of available information (Lin-Su & New, 2012), including candid discussion of the controversies and dilemmas concerning gender assignment and early genital surgery. Parental acceptance of the child with a DSD and condition are key determinants of a favorable outcome (Houk & Lee, 2012). Health care professionals must also recognize and respect the cultural and psychosocial influences on parents' decisions about care for their infant (Lin-Su & New, 2012).

■ Gender Assignment. Parents are naturally anxious to find out their baby's gender so that they can name the baby and announce the birth to family and friends. Nevertheless, it must be sensitively communicated that although their distress is acknowledged, when gender is in doubt, a gender-of-rearing decision is one with lifelong implications and cannot be made in haste. Gender assignment must be deferred until expert evaluation of the newborn takes place and sufficient data are available for a fully informed decision (Lee et al., 2006; Lin-Su & New, 2012).

Unfortunately, some tests required for evaluation of a DSD must be sent out to referral laboratories, and the long wait for results can be frustrating for the parents. It is helpful if an experienced mental health professional can meet very early with the parents to help them formulate what to tell family and friends in the interim (Ogilvy-Stuart & Brain, 2004). All infants should receive a gender assignment as soon as the best course is reasonably determined (Lee et al., 2006). Questions about the infant's future management and treatment needs, gender identity/gender role development, and potential long-term outcomes should be addressed by clinicians who have extensive experience with DSDs.

Pancreas

The pancreas is both an exocrine and endocrine gland. The endocrine pancreas is responsible for hormonal regulation of blood glucose levels. The endocrine functions are performed by clusters of cells called islets of Langerhans that include alpha, beta, and delta cells. Hormones secreted by the endocrine pancreas include glucagon, insulin, amylin, and somatostatin.

Fetal insulin, present by 8 to 10 weeks gestation, is secreted in response to both glucose and amino acids. The fetus is critically dependent for growth on its own supply of insulin, which does not cross the placenta. Insulin stimulates uptake of glucose by muscle and adipose tissue. The fetal pancreas becomes progressively more responsive to glucose late in gestation and beta-cell mass increases markedly. At birth, when maternal glucose supply ceases, the neonate's blood glucose level declines, along with plasma insulin. A concomitant surge in the counter-regulatory hormones

TABLE 10.1

DIAGNOSTIC GROUPING SUGGESTED BY ASSESSMENT FINDINGS

Diagnostic Grouping	Assessment Finding		
	Uterus	Gonads	External Genitalia
CAH (21-ODH) virilized female	Present	Not palpable	Symmetrical hyperpigmented
Undervirilized male (PAIS or testosterone biosynthetic defect)	Absent	Palpable	Symmetrical
Gonadal dysgenesis (with Y chromosome) ovotesticular DSD	Present	Palpable	Asymmetrical

epinephrine and glucagon sets in motion the production of glucose that will sustain the neonate until milk feeding is established.

The exocrine portion of the pancreas constitutes 80% of the total gland. Acinar cells secrete digestive enzymes including trypsin, lipase, and amylase into the duodenum. Epithelial cells along the pancreatic ducts secrete bicarbonate and water that neutralize gastric acid.

Disorders of the Pancreas

Rare pancreatic disorders in the newborn include congenital anomalies such as pancreatic agenesis, pancreatic hypoplasia, and annular pancreas. Disorders of the endocrine pancreas include neonatal diabetes mellitus (NDM) and hyperinsulinism, as well as the developmental disorder of the pancreas seen in the infant of the diabetic mother (IDM). The most common newborn disorder of the exocrine pancreas is cystic fibrosis (CF).

Infant of a Diabetic Mother

Diabetes in pregnancy is on the rise, paralleling the marked increase in people with type 2 diabetes and prediabetes (Homko, 2010). More newborns will be at risk for the problems associated with glucose intolerance and abnormal glucose regulation during pregnancy if this epidemic does not abate.

■ **Pathophysiology.** If maternal glycemic control is poor in the third trimester, high circulating maternal glucose levels chronically stimulate the fetal pancreas to release insulin, leading to fetal fat deposition. Maternal glucose homeostasis is a key determinant of fetal size (Walsh, Mahoney, Byrne, Foley, & McAuliffe, 2011). Fetal macrosomia is more likely to occur in women whose hyperglycemia occurs episodically, particularly after a meal, and from the transfer of lipids from mother to fetus (Hay, 2012). At birth, the neonatal beta-cells take time to adjust to the lower circulating glucose level, and continue to secrete insulin, preventing the mobilization of glycogen and fat as sources of glucose. This failure of normal metabolic adaptation places the baby at risk of hypoglycemia. Hyperinsulinemia, regardless of whether the mother had type 1 or type 2 diabetes, can result in increased glucose utilization, decreased glucose production, and reduced availability of alternate substrates in the newborn (Hay, 2012).

Excess fetal insulin may also be the cause of delayed maturation of type II alveolar cells and pulmonary surfactant deficiency seen in some IDMs. Transient functional anomalies of the heart, including cardiomyopathy and intraventricular septal hypertrophy, begin in utero with glycogen loading of the septum. A delayed adaptation in parathyroid regulation after birth is the source of hypocalcemia and hypomagnesemia of the IDM. An increase in fetal erythropoiesis leading to polycythemia in the IDM is common, but its etiology is unknown. Hyperbilirubinemia results from the presence of an excess hemoglobin, in turn, resulting in a larger than normal bilirubin load.

The higher rate of congenital anomalies associated with diabetic pregnancy is related to maternal glycemic control at the time of conception and during early gestation, when organogenesis is taking place. Congenital malformations associated with maternal diabetes include those of the CNS (anencephaly, meningomyelocele, encephalocele, caudal dysplasia), the heart (transposition of the great vessels, coarctation of the aorta, ventricular septal defects, atrial septal defects), the kidneys (hydronephrosis, renal agenesis), and the gastrointestinal tract (duodenal atresia, small left colon syndrome).

■ **Clinical Manifestations.** As a result of fat accumulation in late gestation, affected fetuses can develop macrosomia, with birth weights that are not in proportion with their length and head circumference measurements. Intrauterine growth restriction is a less common presentation, seen in advanced maternal diabetic vascular disease. Skin tones may be ruddy with sluggish capillary refill. The neonate may present in respiratory distress. If there is a history of difficult vaginal delivery with shoulder dystocia, the infant may present with musculoskeletal or peripheral nerve findings, suggesting fractured clavicle or humerus or brachial plexus palsy. With the latter condition, the affected arm is held limply at the side, and movements, including Moro responses, are asymmetric. Deep tendon reflexes are absent. Crepitus may be palpated along the clavicle if a fracture is present.

■ **Diagnosis.** Macrosomia at birth is a good marker for detecting the infant at risk for neonatal morbidities related to maternal diabetes. In spite of the IDM's size, it is also important to determine gestational age to assess the risk of problems related to prematurity. The IDM must be monitored for hypoglycemia, which usually occurs within an hour or two of birth. Objective measurements of blood and plasma glucose should be used rather than relying on symptoms of hypoglycemia, because the latter are nonspecific and unreliable. Point-of-care blood glucose test results indicating hypoglycemia (<40 mg/dL in the newborn) should be verified with a serum laboratory glucose; however, treatment should not be delayed while awaiting the results of the laboratory test. If no treatment is initiated and the serum glucose confirms hypoglycemia, valuable time is wasted, but if treatment is begun and the serum glucose is actually higher than the point-of-care glucose, the treatment is relatively benign.

Additional testing required for the IDM is a serum calcium concentration and, if this is low, a serum magnesium. Hemoglobin level should be measured with a venous, rather than a capillary, blood sample. Additional diagnostic tests will depend on findings of the initial physical examination.

■ **Management.** Close consultation between maternal and infant caregivers, particularly at the time of labor and delivery, is a necessary ingredient for successful management of the IDM (Hawdon, 2011). Unless life-threatening complications, such as perinatal asphyxia, are present, prevention of hypoglycemia is typically the primary concern in the early management of the IDM. Early, frequent milk feedings in stable infants are ideal, if tolerated. Infants born preterm may display immature feeding skills, despite their large size, and require gavage feedings. Severe or persistent hypoglycemia is managed with intravenous glucose boluses, followed by continuous glucose infusion starting at 6 to 8 mg/kg/min.

Glucose infusions must be weaned slowly, with close monitoring of blood glucose levels, as the neonate acquires the ability to sustain a normal blood sugar level between feedings.

Neonatal Diabetes Mellitus

NDM is a rare disorder manifested by persistent, insulin-sensitive hyperglycemia occurring as early as the first week of life and lasting more than 2 weeks. About half of all cases of NDM are of the transient form (TNDM), and half the permanent form (PNDM). Recent data suggest that the frequency of NDM is 1 in 100,000 live births (Grulich-Henn et al., 2010).

■ **Pathophysiology.** The fundamental problem in NDM is a failure of the pancreas to release sufficient insulin in response to high blood glucose levels. NDM is unrelated to the presence of anti-insulin or anti-islet cell antibodies. In TNDM, diabetes develops within days of birth and resolves again within weeks or months, before recurring, in a milder form, in late childhood. PNDM develops within days to months after birth and persists throughout life. Most cases of PNDM are caused by transcription factors involved in beta-cell development and in insulin secretion, the glucose-sensing enzyme glucokinase, and a gene-regulating immune response. About half of affected neonates have activating mutations of the KATP channel—KCNJ11 and ABCC8 (Edghill, Flanagan, & Ellard, 2010). Most cases of TNDM are caused by one of three genetic mechanisms: a paternal uniparental isodisomy of chromosome 6, a paternally inherited duplication of 6q24, or a maternal methylation defect within the same region (Sperling, 2006).

■ **Clinical Manifestations.** A common feature of NDM is intrauterine growth restriction, a result of insufficient insulin secretion and subsequent failure to thrive in utero. Intrauterine growth restriction in infants with deficient insulin secretion in utero highlights the importance of insulin as a growth hormone. In addition to being small for gestational age, infants with NDM exhibit hyperglycemia, glycosuria, osmotic polyuria, dehydration, and minimal ketoacidosis.

■ **Diagnosis.** The diagnosis is made by demonstrating hyperglycemia with low levels of insulin, insulin-like growth factor-1, and C-peptide. The hyperglycemia responds to insulin infusion. Antibodies to insulin or islet cells are absent. If there are signs and symptoms of malabsorption, pancreatic agenesis should be ruled out by abdominal ultrasound. TNDM and PNDM cannot be differentiated, based on clinical course, in the neonatal period; genetic testing for chromosome 6 anomalies is required. A genetic diagnosis is worth the expense in infants with NDM (Greeley et al., 2011). If the neonate is shown to have a mutation of the KATP channel, treatment with oral sulfonylureas, rather than insulin, is possible, which is tremendously beneficial to the child's glucose control and quality of life.

■ **Management.** Insulin therapy is necessary in some affected infants to manage hyperglycemia and achieve adequate growth, initially by continuous drip and transitioning to subcutaneous injection of an intermediate-acting insulin preparation when condition permits. A high caloric intake can be difficult to maintain. In some infants, insulin therapy can be withdrawn after a period of time when it is observed that exogenous insulin induces hypoglycemia. The course of disease in NDM is highly variable. Some infants with TNDM will have spontaneous recovery with no further disease recurrence, whereas others will have apparent remission with recurrence of permanent disease in late childhood. Infants with PNDM have no remission of their disease.

The opportunity for parents to speak with the pediatric endocrinologist and geneticist should be provided, if possible, for information and guidance about both the cause of NDM and the plans for continuing care for their infant. Close follow-up is essential even if the diabetes has resolved because of the high rate of recurrence later in childhood.

Congenital Hyperinsulinism

Congenital hyperinsulinism is not a single disorder, but a group of disorders with the common feature of hyperinsulinemic hypoglycemia, secondary to inappropriate secretion of insulin (Arnoux et al., 2011). It is the most frequent cause of severe, persistent hypoglycemia in the newborn, with an incidence of 1 in 30,000 to 50,000 live births (Jain, Chen, & Menon, 2012). Several different genetic forms have been described. Between 10% and 15% of congenital hyperinsulinism is transient and will spontaneously resolve at 1 month of age. Beckwith–Wiedemann syndrome is a congenital overgrowth syndrome, with hyperinsulinism caused by beta-cell hyperplasia.

■ **Pathophysiology.** Hyperinsulinism is due to unregulated insulin release from either the entire pancreas (diffuse beta-cell hyperfunction) or confined areas of the pancreas (focal adenomatous islet-cell hyperplasia). Insulin lowers circulating glucose, suppressing lipolysis and ketogenesis and decreasing the availability of free fatty acids and ketone bodies. Since these are alternative energy substrates for the brain during hypoglycemia, hyperinsulinemia places the infant at risk of severe neurologic dysfunction and seizures as consequences of neuroglycopenia.

■ **Clinical Manifestations.** Most infants with congenital hyperinsulinism present within the first postnatal days. Generally, they are born at term and are normal or large for gestational age. Many are macrosomic with a characteristic facial appearance. Neonates with Beckwith–Wiedemann syndrome present with a constellation of findings including macroglossia, abdominal wall defects, Wilms' tumors, renal abnormalities, and facial nevus.

■ **Diagnosis.** Congenital hyperinsulinism is recognized by severe hypoglycemia with an insulin level that is inappropriate to the level of blood glucose that is present (e.g., an insulin level >5 μunits/mL with a plasma glucose level <50 mg/dL).

Diagnostic criteria are a high glucose requirement (>6–8 m/kg/min) needed to maintain normoglycemia, low serum blood glucose by laboratory analysis, measurable insulin, raised C-peptide, low free fatty acids, and low ketone body concentrations. Blood sampling must take place during hypoglycemia to be of diagnostic value (Jain et al., 2012). The administration of glucagon during hypoglycemia results in a glycemic response.

■ Management. The cornerstones of management are a high caloric intake and pharmacologic therapy to inhibit insulin secretion by the pancreas. A central venous catheter is required for reliable and safe administration of high glucose infusates during the acute phase. Glucose infusion rates of 10 to 15 mg/kg/min or higher may be required, and the rate of glucose necessary to maintain normoglycemia (fasting blood glucose >70 mg/dL) is an indicator of the severity of the disease (Arnoux et al., 2011). Drugs include diazoxide, which inhibits insulin secretion by blocking the sulfonylurea receptor of the beta-cell, and octreotide, which is a somatostatin analogue. Diazoxide must be used with caution in the presence of hyperbilirubinemia because it is highly protein bound and will displace bilirubin from albumin binding sites. Glucagon to mobilize hepatic glucose can be added if needed as a short-term adjunct to therapy (Arnoux et al., 2011).

Unfortunately, the responsiveness of infants with hyperinsulinism to these agents is inconsistent and variable. Babies who do not show an adequate and immediate response may require pancreatectomy to prevent recurrent neuroglycopenia. Preoperative localization procedures and intraoperative biopsies will determine the exact nature of the lesion and how much of the pancreas must be removed. Focal disease may require only a partial pancreatectomy, but a near-total (>95%) removal of the pancreas is indicated for diffuse congenital hyperinsulinism. Loss of the pancreas can pose additional risks such as pancreatic insufficiency and diabetes mellitus.

Cystic Fibrosis

CF is an autosomal recessive disorder caused by mutations in the gene encoding for the CF transmembrane conductance regulator (CFTR) protein, of which more than 1,500 have been identified (O'Sullivan & Freedman, 2009). Data from newborn screening programs in the United States reveal that CF occurs in 1 in 3,000 White and 1 in 15,000 to 20,000 Blacks (Walters & Mehta, 2007).

■ Pathophysiology. Mutations in the *CFTR* gene affect the cyclic adenosine-5'-monophosphate (AMP)-mediated signals that stimulate chloride conductance in the epithelial cells of the exocrine ducts. Deficient chloride transport and the associated water transport abnormalities result in the production of abnormally viscid mucus. Nearly all organs and systems of the body are affected, including the lungs and upper respiratory tract, gastrointestinal tract, pancreas, liver, sweat glands, and genitourinary tract. In the neonate, hyperviscous secretions in the intestines and a deficiency of pancreatic enzymes can combine to create a sticky plug of meconium, a condition known as meconium ileus. The meconium has a higher protein and lower carbohydrate concentration, making it more viscid than normal meconium.

■ Clinical Manifestations. Without a family history or prenatal screening, CF is not recognized at the time of birth in most affected neonates unless a meconium ileus is present. A simple meconium ileus is usually identified at 24 to 48 hours of age (occasionally earlier) when there are signs of intestinal obstruction: abdominal distention, bilious vomiting, and either failure to pass meconium or passage of gray-colored stools. On examination, the dilated loops of bowel have a doughy character that indent on palpation. A complicated meconium ileus has a more dramatic presentation with severe abdominal distention, signs of peritonitis such as tenderness, erythema, and clinical evidence of sepsis. The neonate may be acutely ill and require urgent surgical attention. Although not always present in the neonatal period, most patients with CF have pancreatic enzyme insufficiency and present with digestive symptoms or failure to thrive early in life. Other neonatal signs and symptoms include intestinal atresia, prolonged jaundice, and abdominal or scrotal calcifications (O'Sullivan & Freedman, 2009).

■ Diagnosis. The possibility of CF is raised in the neonate with meconium ileus, and the diagnosis can be confirmed with DNA testing. A sweat test can also be performed after the first 48 hours of life, if the infant is not edematous. A sweat test uses electrical-chemical stimulation of the skin to induce sweat, which is collected and analyzed for chloride content. Newborn screening for CF can be accomplished by measuring immunoreactive trypsinogen in dried blood samples. Screening for CF is now universally conducted in all 50 states and the District of Columbia (Wagener, Zemanick, & Sontag, 2012). Sometimes a meconium ileus is identified on prenatal ultrasound as a hyperechoic mass in the terminal ileum, representing inspissated meconium, and dilated bowel loops. Postnatal abdominal radiographs show unevenly dilated bowel and, occasionally, a characteristic "soap bubble" pattern, or small bubbles of gas that are caused by air mixing with the tenacious meconium.

■ Management. A meconium ileus requires prompt attention to prevent complications such as volvulus, bowel necrosis, or intestinal perforation. Treatment for simple meconium ileus is a therapeutic Gastrograffin (meglumine diatrizoate) enema performed under fluoroscopy. Gastrograffin is a hyperosmolar, radiopaque solution that evacuates the inspissated meconium from the intestine. Gastrograffin is not used in infants with evidence of volvulus, gangrene, perforation, peritonitis, or atresia of the small bowel. The risks of the procedure are ischemia, hypovolemic shock, and perforation. It is essential to provide adequate hydration to compensate for the rapid fluid losses that can occur with the Gastrograffin enema. It usually takes 24 to 48 hours to evacuate the softened meconium, and serial radiographs are usually ordered to monitor the evacuation. Feedings are started when signs of obstruction have subsided. An infant who has undergone a Gastrograffin enema should be observed closely for at least 48 hours for signs and symptoms of perforation of the bowel; late perforation is a rare but possible complication as long as 48 hours after the procedure.

CF is also managed with a diet high in energy and fat to compensate for malabsorption and the increased energy demand of chronic inflammation. In addition to vitamin and mineral supplementation, a hydrolyzed protein formula containing medium-chain triglycerides is used. Medium-chain triglycerides do not require digestion by pancreatic enzymes for absorption. Pancreatic enzyme supplements are also needed to improve fat absorption. Meticulous care of the perianal area must be taken because these enzymes can cause severe perianal dermatitis. Breastfeeding has been shown to have significant benefits for infants with CF, although growth might be slightly slower, and should be encouraged (Wagener et al., 2012).

Infants can also develop early pulmonary infections with *Staphylococcus aureus* followed often by *Pseudomonas aeruginosa* (Wagener et al., 2012). Newer, promising therapies for the pulmonary complications of CF are currently under study. One of these is inhaled hypertonic saline, which draws water into the airways, rehydrating the periciliary layer, and improving mucociliary clearance (O'Sullivan & Freedman, 2009).

Finally, of utmost importance, the care of the neonate with CF requires a team approach, in order to provide the family with the necessary resources and anticipatory guidance to manage this disorder and prevent complications for the best possible outcome.

SUMMARY

Some neonatal endocrine disorders are quite rare, and recognizing them requires a high index of suspicion. In recent years, neonatal screening programs have permitted the presymptomatic diagnosis of some of these disorders. This has led to earlier treatment and reduced morbidity, although most endocrine disorders still imply lifelong therapy for the affected infant.

CASE STUDY

■ **Identification of the Problem.** A 34-week gestation, 1.33-kg male infant was admitted to the NICU for small size and prematurity. Admission vital signs were HR 128, RR 72, BP 42/23 (mean 30), axillary temperature 97.4°F. Blood glucose screen (point of care) was 104.

A peripheral IV was started with D10W at 80 mL/kg/d (GIR 5.5 mg/kg/min), and the infant was made NPO. A repeat blood glucose screen on D10W was 545. In the belief that this was an error, it was repeated, and the result was 550. A serum glucose level was drawn, and the IV fluids were changed to D5W. The serum glucose was 535. The initial D10W fluid bag was sent to the lab for analysis.

A repeat blood glucose screen on D5W was 550 (serum 632). IV fluids were changed to normal saline, and the repeat blood glucose was 443 (serum 635). An insulin drip was started at 0.05 units/kg/hr and titrated to maintain blood glucose level less than 250.

■ **Assessment: History and Physical Examination.** The infant was born by cesarean section to a 25-year-old G1P0 mother following a pregnancy complicated by oligohydramnios. Apgar scores were 7 and 9 and the arterial cord pH was 7.27. Length was 38.5 cm, and head circumference 28 cm, placing him below the 10th percentile for all growth parameters.

Arterial blood gas taken in room air: pH 7.30, pCO2 35, PO2 128, base excess –7.7

Following this, 10 mL/kg of normal saline was given for metabolic acidosis.

Examination revealed a small but healthy-appearing male infant, without evidence of respiratory distress.

■ **Differential Diagnosis.** The initial suspected "diagnosis" for the extremely elevated blood glucose in this case was operator error; when the same result was obtained with a repeat specimen and confirmed by serum glucose, it was still viewed with a high degree of suspicion and the intravenous fluids were sent to the laboratory for analysis. The differential diagnosis of hyperglycemia in neonates includes iatrogenic causes, poor insulin sensitivity of the very-low-birth-weight or growth-restricted infant, sepsis, pancreatic agenesis, insulin resistance, TNDM or PNDM, and side effects of medications such as glucocorticoids and theophylline. Several of these were ruled out as they did not apply (the infant was not extremely premature, nor had he received any medications known to cause blood glucose elevation). Furthermore, the problem persisted after changing the IV fluids, ruling out an iatrogenic cause. Insulin resistance was ruled out because the infant responded promptly to an infusion of insulin. He did show evidence of intrauterine growth restriction but it was believed more likely that this was a consequence, rather than a cause, of his primary problem.

■ **Diagnostic Tests.** The following tests were ordered to further hone in on the cause of hyperglycemia:

- CBC: Hct 42%; WBC 4.4; Segs 20; Bands 8; platelets 274,000
- Blood cultures were negative at 24 and 48 hours
- Abdominal ultrasound (to rule out pancreatic agenesis): the organ appeared normal
- Insulin autoantibodies were negative; the insulin drip was stopped for 2 hours and insulin and C-peptide levels were drawn
- RESULTS: insulin level less than 2 µIU/mL
- C-peptide less than 0.5 ng/mL (reference range 0.8–3.1 ng/mL)
- Concurrent plasma glucose was 412

■ **Working Diagnosis.** The infant's presentation at birth and clinical course were most consistent with a diagnosis of NDM. He was intrauterine growth restricted, indicating a prenatal onset of the condition, and he had a mild metabolic acidosis. He had no evidence of autoimmune or structural pancreatic disease. He did not have septicemia or evidence of other infection. Furthermore, his laboratory studies revealed severe insulinopenia. The low level of C-peptide, a single-chain amino acid normally released with insulin in equal amounts, supports this diagnosis. It was not known whether his NDM was transient or permanent; this would require molecular genetic analysis, a test that was not done during the initial hospitalization.

Development of Management Plan. The management plan was to reintroduce glucose while continuing the insulin infusion, advancing to total parental nutrition as tolerated. Glucose levels would be monitored at least every 2 hours, with the goal of keeping the blood glucose less than 250. The plan included the introduction of feedings as early as feasible to improve control of blood glucose. Continuous insulin would be weaned as tolerated. If his diabetes showed no signs of resolution, subcutaneous insulin would be started for long-term management. The infant would continue to be followed by the pediatric endocrinologist.

Implementation and Evaluation of Effectiveness Over the first few days, stabilization of the blood glucose level proved difficult. On total parenteral nutrition (TPN), the infant fluctuated between hyperglycemia and hypoglycemia. Feedings were introduced and this provided a measure of stability, although weight gain remained slow. The infant was eventually successfully managed with and discharged on subcutaneous insulin.

EVIDENCE-BASED PRACTICE BOX

Upon newborn screening, at least one of two extremely low gestational age neonates (24 to 28 weeks gestation) is found to have low serum thyroxine (T_4) levels. This condition is known as hypothyroxinemia of prematurity and is believed to be a transient maladaptation of physiology that reflects both immaturity and the effects of illness and treatments for other neonatal problems (La Gamma & Paneth, 2012). Both researchers and clinicians, however, have been uncertain about whether to treat hypothyroxinemia in these infants, or adopt a "watchful waiting" approach.

The concern about not treating these low T4 levels is that thyroid hormones are known to be critical to normal brain development. With the loss of maternal sources of thyroid hormone, low T4 levels exist at a vulnerable period of brain development. Evidence suggests that hypothyroxinemia of prematurity is associated with both cognitive and neurological delays (La Gamma, 2008). Therefore, studies have attempted to determine whether thyroid hormone supplementation would improve neurodevelopmental outcomes in low gestational age neonates. One such study, the largest interventional trial to date, tested the effects of a daily dose of 8 mg/kg of T4 for 42 days, compared with placebo (van Wassenaer et al., 1997). On follow-up testing, an 18-point improvement in IQ scores was found in mental development at 2 years of age, and there was an improvement in neurological outcomes in a subgroup of the most immature infants, less than 27 weeks gestation. At 5.5 and 10 years of follow-up, the benefits of T4 supplementation continued for this subgroup, but for more mature infants, the reverse was true (Briët et al., 2001; van Wassenaer, Westera, Houtzager, & Kok, 2005).

Against a backdrop of this evidence, researchers undertook a study of four different thyroid regimens for neonates less than 28 weeks gestation diagnosed with hypothyroxinemia of prematurity (La Gamma et al., 2009). The key difference between this and previous trials was that this study aimed to maintain "biochemical euthyroidism" by reducing suppression of TSH. In previous trials, thyroid supplementation had resulted in a suppression of TSH levels. La Gamma and colleagues found evidence of clinical benefit (shorter duration of mechanical ventilation, lower rates of retinopathy of prematurity and less necrotizing enterocolitis) with a *continuous* regimen of 4 μg/kg/d for 42 days rather than a single daily supplement. This regimen raised total T4 levels with only modest suppression of TSH.

As a result of this trial, study authors recommend T4 replacement of 4 μg/kg/d for 42 days, to achieve "biochemical euthyroidism," defined as a minimum free T4 level of 1.5 ng/dL, a minimum total T4 level of 6 mg/dL, a minimum total T3 level of 52 ng/dL, and minimal suppression of TSH level (< 0.4 mIU/L) (La Gamma et al., 2009). Continuous infusion of T4 is believed to more closely approximate normal physiology by achieving a sustained elevation in total T4. Iodide supplementation (30 mg/kg/d orally) is also essential. Only a randomized, placebo-controlled clinical trial can provide evidence of long-term neurodevelopmental improvement associated with this regimen. In the absence of such evidence, clinicians may remain reluctant to adopt a new standard of care.

References

Briët, J. M., van Wassenaer, A. G., Dekker, F. W., de Vijlder, J. J., van Baar, A., & Kok, J. H. (2001). Neonatal thyroxine supplementation in very preterm children: Developmental outcome evaluated at early school age. *Pediatrics, 107*, 712–718.

La Gamma, E. F. (2008).Transient hypothyroxinemia of prematurity: 10 reports from our group. *Seminars in Perinatology, 32*, 377–446.

La Gamma, E. F., & Paneth, N. (2012). Clinical importance of hypothyroxinemia in the preterm infant and a discussion of treatment concerns. *Current Opinion in Pediatrics, 24*, 172–180.

La Gamma, E. F., van Wassenaer, A. G., Ares, S., Golombek, S. G., Kok, J. H., Quero, J., . . . Paneth, N. (2009). Phase 1 trial of 4 thyroid hormone regimens for transient hypothyroxinemia in neonates of < 28 weeks' gestation. *Pediatrics, 124*, e258–e268.

(*continued*)

van Wassenaer, A. G., Kok, J. H., de Vijlder, J. J., Briët, J. M., Smit, B. J., Tamminga, P., . . . Vulsma, T. (1997). Effects of thyroxine supplementation on neurologic development in infants born at less than 30 weeks' gestation. *New England Journal of Medicine, 336*, 21–26.

van Wassenaer, A. G., Westera, J., Houtzager, B. A., & Kok, J. H. (2005). Ten-year follow-up of children born at < 30 weeks' gestational age supplemented with thyroxine in the neonatal period in a randomized, controlled trial. *Pediatrics, 116*, e613–e618.

ONLINE RESOURCES

The Endocrine Society
http://www.endo-society.org

National Newborn Screening and Genetics Resource Center
http://genes-r-us.uthscsa.edu

Orphanet
http://www.orpha.net/consor/cgi-bin/index.php

Pediatric Endocrine Society
http://www.lwpes.org

REFERENCES

Alatzoglou, K. S., & Dattani, M. T. (2009). Genetic forms of hypopituitarism and their manifestation in the neonatal period. *Early Human Development, 85*, 705–712.

Allen, L. (2009). Disorders of sexual development. *Obstetrics and Gynecological Clinics of North America, 36*, 25–45.

Arnoux, J. B., Verkarre, V., Saint-Martin, C., Montravers, F., Brassier, A., Valayannopoulos, V., . . . de Lonlay, P. (2011). Congenital hyperinsulinism: Current trends in diagnosis and therapy. *Orphanet Journal of Rare Diseases, 3*, 63.

Auchus, R. H., Witchel, S. F., Leight, K. R., Aisenberg, J., Azziz, R., Bachega, T. A., . . . Zuckerman, A. E. (2010). Guidelines for the development of comprehensive care centers for congenital adrenal hyperplasia: Guidance from the CARES Foundation Initiative. *International Journal of Pediatric Endocrinology, 2010*, 275–213.

Bethin, K., & Fuqua, J. S. (2010). General concepts and physiology. In M. S. Kappy, D. B. Allen, & M. E. Geffner (Eds.), *Pediatric practice: Endocrinology* (pp. 1–18). New York, NY: McGraw-Hill.

Bollepalli, S., & Rose, S. R. (2012). Disorders of the thyroid gland. In C. A. Gleason & S. U. Devaskar (Eds.), *Avery's diseases of the newborn* (9th ed., pp. 1307–1319). Philadelphia, PA: Elsevier Saunders.

Brown, J., & Warne, G. (2005). Practical management of the intersex infant. *Journal of Pediatric Endocrinology & Metabolism, 18*, 3–23.

Copelovitch, L., & Kaplan, B. S. (2012). Glomerulonephropathies and disorders of tubular function. In S. U. Devaskar & C. A. Gleason (Eds.), *Avery's diseases of the newborn* (9th ed., pp. 1222–1227). Philadelphia, PA: Elsevier.

Edghill, E. L., Flanagan, S. E., & Ellard, S. (2010). Permanent neonatal diabetes due to activating mutations in ABCC8 and KCNJ11. *Reviews in Endocrine and Metabolic Disorders, 11*, 193–198.

Greeley, S. A., John, P. M., Winn, A. N., Ornelas, J., Lipton, R. B., Philipson, L. H., . . . Huang, E. S. (2011). The cost-effectiveness of personalized genetic medicine: The case of genetic testing in neonatal diabetes. *Diabetes Care, 34*, 622–627.

Grulich-Henn, J., Wagner, V., Thon, A., Schober, E., Marg, W., Kapellen, T. M., . . . Holl, R. W. (2010). Entities and frequency of neonatal diabetes: Data from the diabetes documentation and quality management system (DVP). *Diabetic Medicine, 27*, 709–712.

Hawdon, J. M. (2011). Babies born after diabetes in pregnancy: What are the short- and long-term risks and how can we minimise them? *Best Practice and Research Clinical Obstetrics and Gynaecology, 25*, 91–104.

Hay, W. W., Jr. (2012). Care of the infant of the diabetic mother. *Current Diabetes Reports, 12*, 4–15.

Homko, C. J. (2010). Gestational diabetes mellitus: Can we reach consensus? *Current Diabetes Reports, 10*, 252–254.

Houk, C. P., & Lee, P. A. (2005). Intersexed states: Diagnosis and management. *Endocrinology and Metabolism Clinics of North America, 34*, 791–810.

Houk, C. P., & Lee, P. A. (2012). Update on disorders of sex development. *Current Opinion in Endocrinology, Diabetes, and Obesity, 19*, 28–32.

Hyman, S. J., Novoa, Y., & Holzman, I. (2011). Perinatal endocrinology: Common endocrine disorders in the sick and premature newborn. *Pediatric Clinics of North America, 58*, 1083–1098.

Intersex Society of North America (ISNA) Consortium on the Management of Disorders of Sex Development. (2006). *Clinical guidelines for the management of disorders of sex development in childhood.* Retrieved from http://www.dsdguidelines.org/files/clinical.pdf

Jain, V., Chen, M., & Menon, R. K. (2012). Disorders of carbohydrate metabolism. In S. U. Devaskar & C. A. Gleason (Eds.), *Avery's diseases of the newborn* (9th ed.). Philadelphia, PA: Elsevier.

Janjua, H. S., & Batisky, D. L. (2012). Renal vascular disease in the newborn. In S. U. Devaskar & C. A. Gleason (Eds.), *Avery's diseases of the newborn* (9th ed.). Philadelphia, PA: Elsevier.

Kohler, B., Lumbroso, S., Leger, J., Audran, F., Grau, E. S., Kurtz, F., . . . Sultan, C. (2005). Androgen insensitivity syndrome: Somatic mosaicism of the androgen receptor in seven families and consequences for sex assignment and genetic counseling. *Journal of Clinical Endocrinology & Metabolism, 90*, 106–111.

La Gamma, E. F., & Paneth, N. (2012). Clinical importance of hypothyroxinemia in the preterm infant and a discussion of treatment concerns. *Current Opinion in Pediatrics, 2*, 172–180.

La Gamma, E. F., van Wassenaer, A. G., Ares, S., Golombek, S. G., Kok, J. H., Quero, J., . . . Paneth, N. (2009). Phase 1 trial of 4 thyroid hormone regimens for transient hypothyroxinemia in neonates of < 28 weeks' gestation. *Pediatrics, 124*, e258–e268.

Lee, P. A., Houk, C. P., Ahmed, S. F., Hughes, I. A., & International Consensus Conference on Intersex organized by the Lawson Wilkins Pediatric Endocrine Society and the European Society for Paediatric Endocrinology. (2006). Consensus statement on management of intersex disorders. *Pediatrics, 118*, e488–e500.

Lin-Su, K., & New, M. I. (2012). Ambiguous genitalia in the newborn. In S. U. Devaskar & C. A. Gleason (Eds.), *Avery's diseases of the newborn* (9th ed.). Philadelphia, PA: Elsevier.

LynShue, K. A., & Witchel, S. F. (2007). Endocrinology. In B. J. Zitelli & H. W. Davis (Eds.), *Atlas of pediatric physical diagnosis*. Philadelphia, PA: Elsevier.

Misra, M., & Lee, M. M. (2005). Intersex disorders. In T. Moshang (Ed.), *Pediatric endocrinology*. St Louis, MO: Elsevier.

Mitchell, M. L., Hsu, H. W., Sahai, I., & Massachusetts Pediatric Endocrine Workgroup. (2011). The increased incidence of congenital hypothyroidism: Fact or fancy? *Clinical Endocrinology, 75*, 806–810.

Modi, N. (2012). Fluids, electrolytes, renal function, and acid–base balance. In A. Y. Elzouki, F. B. Stapleton, R. J. Whitley, W. OH, H. A. Harfi, & H. Nazer (Eds.), *Textbook of clinical pediatrics* (p. 256). Berlin, Germany: Springer Verlag.

Morel, Y., Rey, R., Teinturier, C., Nicolino, M., Michel-Calemard, L., Mowszowicz, I., . . . Josso, N. (2002). Aetiological diagnosis of male sex ambiguity: A collaborative study. *European Journal of Pediatrics, 161*, 49–59.

Mutlu, M., Karaguzel, G., Aslan, Y., Cansu, A., & Okten, A. (2011). Adrenal hemorrhage in newborns: A retrospective study. *World Journal of Pediatrics, 7*, 355–357.

Ng, P. C. (2011). Effect of stress on the hypothalamic-pituitary-adrenal axis in the fetus and newborn. *Journal of Pediatrics, 158*(Suppl. 2), e41–e43.

Nimkarn, S., & New, M. I. (2012). Disorders of the adrenal gland. In S. U. Devaskar & C. A. Gleason (Eds.), *Avery's diseases of the newborn* (9th ed.). Philadelphia, PA: Elsevier.

Ocal, G. (2011). Current concepts in disorders of sexual development. *Journal of Clinical Research in Pediatric Endocrinology, 3*, 105–114.

Ogilvy-Stuart, A. L., & Brain, C. E. (2004). Early assessment of ambiguous genitalia. *Archives of Disease in Childhood, 89*, 401–407.

Osborn, D. A., & Hunt, R. W. (2007). Prophylactic postnatal thyroid hormones for prevention of morbidity and mortality in preterm infants. *Cochrane Database of Systematic Reviews, 24*, CD005948.

O'Sullivan, B. P., & Freedman, S. D. (2009). Cystic fibrosis. *Lancet, 373*, 1891–1904.

Pass, K. A., & Neto, E. C. (2011). Update: Newborn screening for endocrinopathies. *Endocrinology and Metabolism Clinics of North America, 38*, 827–837.

Polak, M., & Van Vliet, G. (2009). Disorders of the thyroid gland. In K. Sarafoglou (Ed.), *Pediatric endocrinology and inborn errors of metabolism*. New York, NY: McGraw-Hill.

Rastogi, M. V., & LaFranchi, S. H. (2010). Congenital hypothyroidism. *Orphanet Journal of Rare Diseases, 5*, 17.

Rubin, L. P. (2012). Embryology, developmental biology, and anatomy of the endocrine system. In S. U. Devaskar & C. A. Gleason (Eds.), *Avery's diseases of the newborn* (9th ed., p. 1245). Philadelphia, PA: Elsevier.

Seki, Y., Williams, L., Vuguin, P. M., Charron, M. J. (2012). Minireview: Epigenetic programming of diabetes and obesity: Animal models. *Endocrinology, 153*, 1031–1038.

Simpser, T., & Rapaport, R. (2010). Update on some aspects of neonatal thyroid disease. *Journal of Clinical Research in Pediatric Endocrinology, 2*, 95–99.

Speiser, P. W., Azziz, R., Baskin, L. S., Ghizzoni, L., Hensle, T. W., Merke, D. P., . . . White, P. C. (2010). Congenital adrenal hyperplasia due to steroid 21-hydroxylase deficiency: An Endocrine Society clinical practice guideline. *Journal of Clinical Endocrinology and Metabolism, 95*, 4133–4160.

Sperling, M. A. (2006). The genetic basis of neonatal diabetes mellitus. *Pediatric Endocrinology, 4*(Suppl. 1), 71–75.

Srinivasan, R., Harigopal, S., Turner, S., & Cheetham, T. (2012). Permanent and transient congenital hypothyroidism in preterm infants. *Acta Paediatrica, 101*, e179–e182.

Srivatsa, A., Majzoub, J. A., & Kappy, M. S. (2010). Posterior pituitary and disorders of water metabolism. In M. S. Kappy, D. B. Allen, & M. E. Geffner (Eds.), *Pediatric practice: Endocrinology* (pp. 77–105). New York, NY: McGraw-Hill.

Stokowski, L. (2004). Endocrine disorders. In M. T. Verklan & M. Walden (Eds.), *Core curriculum for neonatal intensive care nursing* (p. 723). Philadelphia, PA: Elsevier.

Tenore, A., & Driul, D. (2009). Genomics in pediatric endocrinology—genetic disorders and new techniques. *Endocrinology and Metabolism Clinics of North America, 38*, 471–490.

Thyen, U., Richter-Appelt, H., Wiesemann, C., Holterhus, P. M., & Hiort, O. (2005). Deciding on gender in children with intersex conditions. *Treatments in Endocrinology, 4*, 1–8.

Tuladhar, R., Davis, P. G., Batch, J., & Doyle, L. W. (1998). Establishment of a normal range of penile length in preterm infants. *Journal of Paediatric and Child Health, 35*, 471–473.

van Wassenaer, A. G., & Kok, J. H. (2004). Hypothyroxinaemia and thyroid function after preterm birth. *Seminars in Neonatology, 9*, 3–11.

Vilain, E., Seragloglou, K., & Yehya, N. (2009). Disorders of sex development. In S. U. Devaskar & C. A. Gleason (Eds.), *Avery's diseases of the newborn* (9th ed., pp. 527–555). Philadelphia, PA: Elsevier.

Wagener, J. S., Zemanick, E. T., & Sontag, M. K. (2012). Newborn screening for cystic fibrosis. *Current Opinion in Pediatrics*. doi:10.1097/MOP.0b013e328353489a

Walsh, J. M., Mahony, R., Byrne, J., Foley, M., & McAuliffe, F. M. (2011). The association of maternal and fetal glucose homeostasis with fetal adiposity and birthweight. *European Journal of Obstetrics, Gynecology and Reproductive Biology, 159*, 338–341.

Walters, S., & Mehta, A. (2007). Epidemiology of cystic fibrosis. In M. Hodson, D. M. Geddes, & A. Bush (Eds.), *Cystic fibrosis* (3rd ed., pp. 21–45). London, UK: Edward Arnold Ltd.

Witchel, S. F., & Azziz, R. (2011). Congenital adrenal hyperplasia. *Journal of Pediatric and Adolescent Gynecology, 24*, 116–126.

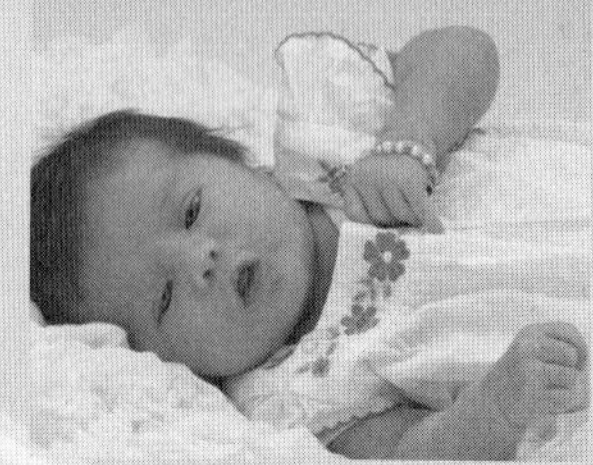

CHAPTER 11

Immune System

■ Mary Beth Bodin

The intact uterine environment protects the fetus from a variety of pathogens such as bacteria, viruses, fungi, protozoa, and parasites. The birth canal is not a sterile environment; therefore, the newborn is exposed to a wide variety of microorganisms during labor and delivery and in the event of ruptured membranes. The extrauterine environment exposes the infant to even more potential pathogens. Host defense mechanisms begin to develop early in gestation; however, they remain immature and often do not function efficiently even in the term newborn. The development of the immune system in the fetus and newborn cannot be studied in isolation from maternal influences. The ability of the mother's body to tolerate the fetus during pregnancy, rather than rejecting it as a foreign body, is not well understood. It is well documented that maternal blood with immunocompetent T-lymphocytes circulates in contact with fetal cells, that both fetal and maternal cells are exchanged through the placenta, and that humoral and cellular immunity to fetal antigens develops in the mother. The predominant transfer of antibody occurs by way of passage of immunoglobulin G (IgG) from the maternal to the fetal circulation by an active transport process. Such immunity is transient; nevertheless, it may provide protection during a vulnerable time of life. Although this passive antibody may protect the newborn, this process may interfere with active antibody synthesis after immunization. Secretory IgA in breast milk may also interfere with successful immunization, particularly with live poliovirus, by neutralization of virus by antibody in the gastrointestinal tract (Lewis & Wilson, 2011). Although the neonate's immune system is not fully developed, the newborn is able to respond to the environment, resulting in certain markers that can be detected in lab studies such as the complete blood count (CBC) and the C-reactive protein (CRP). Even so, the infant's immature immune system is easily overwhelmed. The immaturity of the immune system is responsible for the relatively high prevalence of infectious disease during the neonatal period, as well as the occurrence of neonatal infection from microorganisms that do not generally cause infection in older individuals (Kapur et al., 2002). The susceptibility to infectious processes and the associated high morbidity and mortality make early identification and treatment of infection in a newborn, a critical component of care.

ASSESSMENT AND MANAGEMENT OF THE INFANT WITH SUSPECTED OR PROVEN INFECTION

Identifying and caring for a newborn with an infection can be one of the greatest challenges in nursing. Nurses are often the first to recognize that there is something "wrong" with an infant, and this often leads to investigation of the signs. Generally, treatment is begun once a presumptive diagnosis of infection is made because the benefits of early treatment outweigh the risks of unnecessary treatment. This chapter will describe assessment parameters for evaluating the infant with suspected and culture-proven infection as well as diagnostic measures and treatment of the most common causes of newborn infection.

Incidence of Neonatal Infection

The incidence of infection varies according to the level of perinatal care available, economic standards, and other perinatal risk factors in term newborns. In the United States, the incidence in term newborns has been approximately 2% to 4% per 1,000 live births since 1980. Recent global data reflect that 36% of all neonatal deaths are attributable to serious infection. In those settings with the highest mortality (developing countries), neonatal infections may account for up to 50% of all neonatal deaths (Darmstadt, Zaidi, & Stoll, 2011). The highest prevalence of neonatal infection occurs in males and low-birth-weight infants. The lower the birth weight, and consequent lower gestational age, the higher the risk for infection (Baltimore, 2003). Improved knowledge and technology to care for less mature and smaller newborns have led to an increased population of newborns at higher risk for bacterial infection. Major complications of infection include respiratory distress, shock, acidosis, disseminated intravascular coagulation (DIC), and meningitis. Long-term morbidity remains a concerning consequence of neonatal infections.

Clinical Signs of Infection

Signs and symptoms of infection are listed in Box 11.1. Temperature instability or hypothermia, the inability of the neonate to maintain temperature in the normal range (usually between 96.8°F and 99°F axillary), is a frequent indication of serious infection (Nizet & Klein, 2011). Newborns traditionally do not have well-developed febrile mechanisms; therefore, the absence of fever does not indicate the absence of infection. Premature infants more often present with a low body temperature. Hyperthermia may occur in term newborns, with rectal temperatures of greater than 100.4°F (Nizet & Klein, 2011), but this is relatively rare in preterm infants. An infected infant may present with lethargy, poor feeding, decreased reflexes, abdominal distention, and delayed gastric emptying time, and perhaps diarrhea or loose green or brown stools. Hypoglycemia or hyperglycemia, as well as glycosuria, may result from the inability to maintain normal metabolic processes and impaired glucose metabolism.

Vascular perfusion is typically decreased; the infected neonate may appear gray, mottled, or ashen in color with poor perfusion, prolonged capillary filling time, and hypotension. Skin changes include cyanosis and petechiae. Thrombocytopenia is often present. Infections can cause DIC, resulting in altered prothrombin time, partial thromboplastin time, and split fibrin product laboratory values. Hemolytic anemia may occur as a part of the inflammatory process and this can significantly decrease oxygen-carrying capacity, especially in the preterm infant. Cardiovascular shock can be a sudden clinical sign of fulminant infection that requires immediate and aggressive intervention to restore adequate circulation. Unexplained bradycardia, sclerema, and sudden purpura, rash, or petechiae are other signs of systemic infection.

Apnea in a term (nonsedated) newborn in the first few hours of life should be considered a serious sign of inability to regulate the brain's respiratory center. Apnea in the first 24 hours of life in a preterm newborn is a common

BOX 11.1

SIGNS AND SYMPTOMS OF NEONATAL INFECTION

Clinical

- General
- Poor feeding
- Irritability
- Lethargy
- Temperature instability

Skin

- Petechiae
- Pustulosis
- Sclerema
- Edema
- Jaundice

Respiratory

- Grunting
- Nasal flaring
- Intercostal retractions
- Tachypnea/apnea

Gastrointestinal

- Diarrhea
- Hematochezia
- Abdominal distention
- Emesis
- Aspirates

CNS

- Hypotonia
- Seizures
- Poor spontaneous movement

Circulatory

- Bradycardia/tachycardia
- Hypotension
- Cyanosis
- Decreased perfusion

Laboratory Values:

White blood cell count

- Neutrophils

  <5000cells/mm3, neutropenia
  >25,000cells/mm3, neutrophilia
- Absolute neutrophil count (neutrophil and bands)

  <1800cells/mm3 (during first week)
- Immature: total neutrophil ratio

  0:2
- Platelet count

  <100,000, thrombocytopenia

Cerebrospinal fluid

- Protein

  150 to 200mg/L (term)
  300mg/L (preterm)
- Glucose

  50% to 60% or more of blood glucose level

Adapted with permission from Lott and Kilb (1992).

sign of infection. Respiratory distress can be an early sign of pneumonia and must be considered carefully.

Jaundice, hepatosplenomegaly, and irritability may also be found in infants with infection. The wide variability of signs of infection warrants inclusion of infection as part of the differential diagnosis in any ill infant.

Risk Factors

Prematurity is the most prevalent risk factor for infection, for these premature infants are far more susceptible to the invasion of foreign microorganisms. Preterm infants have decreased maternal antibodies (passive immunity). The maternal antibodies, developed by exposure to antigens and subsequent creation of an antibody defense system, provide temporary protection to the newborn, but preterm newborns are born before the majority of maternal antibodies are transferred from the maternal circulation. Also, the cellular immune system is not well developed in the preterm newborn, thus there is decreased phagocytic cellular defenses.

Prolonged rupture of the fetal membranes (PROM) is a well-known risk factor for the development of infection. The fetus is at increased risk because the break in the amniotic sac provides a pathway for the migration of microorganisms up the vaginal vault to the fetus. Delaying delivery in a pregnancy in a mother with PROM and a preterm fetus until pulmonary maturity is achieved creates the potential environment for bacterial proliferation and subsequent newborn infection. The benefit in promoting maturity of the immature lungs is weighed against the risk of overwhelming infection in the baby. Development of pulmonary hypoplasia is another serious concern when delivery is delayed after premature prolonged rupture of membranes (Gagnon & Gibbs, 2011). PROM lasting longer than 24 hours is considered a risk factor in the evaluation of infants for potential for infection.

Although the most common cause of maternal fever in labor is dehydration, a fever may indicate maternal infection. A mother with an infection before or during delivery may transmit it to the infant. If maternal temperature is greater than or equal to 100.4°F during labor, evaluation for infection in the newborn is warranted (Gagnon & Gibbs, 2011). Maternal cervical or amniotic fluid cultures may identify the causative microorganism. If the maternal illness suggests viral infection, newborn viral cultures should be obtained. Early identification of causative agents in the mother may help in the management of the newborn by allowing faster identification of the microorganism and initiation of appropriate antimicrobial therapy.

Foul-smelling amniotic fluid is an indication for newborn antimicrobial therapy in symptomatic infants. Routine blood cultures and a CBC with differential are indicated as a screen for newborn infection. Under these circumstances, the placenta should be sent for pathologic evaluation. Other risk factors associated with newborn infection are antenatal or intrapartal asphyxia, iatrogenic complications of treatment, and invasive procedures.

Stress inhibits the ability to fight infection by increasing the metabolic rate, which requires more oxygen and energy. A severely compromised hypoxemic newborn may have regional tissue damage. Ischemic or necrotic areas in the lungs, heart, brain, or gastrointestinal system promote colonization and overgrowth of normal bacterial flora. This overgrowth of bacteria is one of the most common sources of newborn infection. Tissue damage can be prevented or repaired only if the infectious process is reversed and adequate tissue perfusion is restored.

There are several known maternal factors associated with newborn infection: low socioeconomic status, malnutrition, inadequate prenatal care, substance abuse, premature or prolonged rupture of membranes, presence of a urinary tract infection at delivery, peripartum infection, clinical amnionitis, and general bacterial colonization. Newborn risk factors include antenatal stress, intrapartal stress (perinatal asphyxia), congenital anomalies, male sex, multiple gestations, concurrent neonatal disease processes, prematurity, immaturity of the immune system, invasive admission procedures, and antimicrobial therapies.

Diagnostic Work-Up

A high index of suspicion of infection, early identification of the microorganism, and institution of appropriate therapy provide the best outcome. Early and accurate diagnosis of infection in the newborn is a difficult task and is often complicated by the nonspecificity of the signs associated with sepsis exhibited by the newborn (Gerdes & Polin, 1998). The evaluation for infection in the newborn often depends on whether early-onset sepsis (EOS) or late-onset sepsis (LOS) is suspected. EOS is most often defined as sepsis that presents within the first 72 hours of life; however, many infections include sepsis that occurs within the first 6 days of life. LOS is, therefore, sepsis that presents after the first week of life (Nizet & Klein, 2011). The perfect screen for neonatal sepsis has not been determined, although some laboratory aids have been found to be very helpful in diagnosing neonatal sepsis. A CBC is often the first step in identifying infection. The CBC of an infected infant may reveal leukopenia, especially neutropenia with a cell count of polymorphonuclear (mature) leukocytes less than 5,000 cells/mm^3, or the infant may have a large number of immature leukocytes (>25,000 cells/mm^3), in particular, bands (immature neutrophil), with the immature-to-mature cell ratio greater than 0.2. Use of the CRP has added a level of confidence in excluding serious infection and in evaluating the infant's response to treatment and in determining length of therapy. Serial CRPs have been found to be more reliable than a single level. In the presence of sepsis, CRP levels may be normal at the onset of symptoms but are typically elevated by 24 hours of age and remain elevated during the acute phase of infection or inflammation (Weinberg & D'Angio, 2011). If signs of central nervous system (CNS) involvement are present, a lumbar puncture (LP) for cerebrospinal fluid (CSF) cultures is indicated, whether EOS or LOS is suspected. Since urinary tract infections are extremely uncommon during the first few days of life, a urine culture is not indicated for EOS (Polin & the Committee on Fetus and Newborn, 2012). Gram stain of the CSF or urine can give an early indication of the type of microorganism responsible for the infection. Cell count and protein and glucose levels of the CSF may also indicate the presence of infection. A chest radiograph can identify the presence of pneumonia. Other tests that may be useful include latex agglutination (LA) or counter-immunoelectrophoresis (CIE) of urine or CSF or other body cavity fluids, erythrocyte sedimentation rate (ESR).

Differential Diagnosis

The microorganisms responsible for newborn infection have changed over the past 60 years, and there are marked regional variations. Organisms responsible for EOS differ from those responsible for LOS; therefore, the antimicrobial agents of choice differ based on the timing of symptoms. Even with the implementation of prophylactic use of intrapartum antibiotics, group B streptococcus (GDS) remains the leading cause of EOS followed by *Escherichia coli* (Stroll et al., 2011). Some microorganisms, including *E. coli,* groups A and B streptococci, and *Listeria monocytogenes,* are often implicated in EOS and LOS. Other organisms, including *Staphylococcus aureus*, CoNS, and *Pseudomonas aeruginosa,* are typically associated with LOS (Nizet & Klein, 2011). After day 7, nosocomial microorganisms should be considered. These microorganisms include *Staphylococcus epidermidis*, particularly when invasive medical devices have been used; *S. aureus* (common skin contaminant); and the spectrum of gram-negative enteric rods, including *Klebsiella, Pseudomonas, Serratia*, and *E. coli*. Hospitalized preterm newborns are often affected by repeated episodes of infection. Many of these episodes are termed presumed, suspected, or clinical infection because no microorganism is recovered and cultured, despite clinical evidence of infection that responds to antimicrobial agent therapy.

Prognosis

The introduction of broad-spectrum antimicrobial agents dramatically improved the prognosis for infection, and there has been a decline in infection-associated neonatal and infant deaths in the United States. However, infection still accounts for significant morbidity and mortality in the neonatal period. Consequences of bacterial infection include prolonged hospitalization, increased hospital costs, and increased mortality. Term infants who are promptly and adequately treated for sepsis rarely have long-term sepsis-associated health problems; however, residual neurological sequelae are seen in 15% to 30% of infants with septic meningitis (Anderson-Berry, Bellig, & Ohnig, 2012). Preterm infants with sepsis are more likely to experience long-term neurologic damage, especially if shock is present (Volpe, 2008).

Management

Management of a newborn with an infection is aimed at the traditional "ABCs": airway, breathing, circulation, including oxygen, ventilation, correction of acidosis, volume expansion, respiratory support if indicated, antimicrobial agents, and consideration of immune therapy. The exact management plan is based on an assessment of clinical signs, careful history, and appropriate laboratory findings with consideration of the most likely microorganisms. Treatment should begin as soon as sepsis is suspected due to the newborn's state of immunosuppression. Antimicrobial agents should be started as soon as relevant diagnostic tests have been completed (Anderson-Berry et al., 2012).

Antimicrobial Agents

The selection of antimicrobial agents is based on identification of the microorganism and the infant's response to therapy. Infectious microorganisms are divided into two broad classes, based on Gram-stain results: gram-positive and gram-negative. The shape of the microorganism categorizes it as either a coccus or a rod. Generally, the gram-positive organisms respond to broad-spectrum antibiotics, such as penicillin analogues and first-generation cephalosporins (beta-lactamases), and the beta-lactamase penicillins. The gram-negative microorganisms are most often susceptible to aminoglycosides and cephalosporins. Tests must be run to determine the specific sensitivity of a microorganism to the antimicrobial agent selected to ensure that the appropriate agent is prescribed. In the United States and Canada, EOS sepsis is generally treated with a combined approach such as IV ampicillin and gentamicin. This approach provides coverage for the most likely organisms, which include gram-positive organisms such as GBS and gram-negative bacteria such as *E. coli*. If LOS is suspected, antibiotic choices should be those that are effective against known hospital-acquired infections such as *S. aureus, S. epidermidis,* and *Pseudomonas* species (Anderson-Berry et al., 2012).

Generally speaking, antimicrobial choices are based on organisms known to be present in the local nursery. Gram-positive cocci generally respond to penicillin, unless the microorganism produces beta-lactamase (or penicillinase). The beta-lactamase destroys the penicillin. *S. aureus* is a beta-lactamase-producing microorganism and is therefore not responsive to penicillin. A group of semisynthetic penicillins with added side chains are used for treatment of *S. aureus* infection. Of this group, nafcillin and oxacillin are most often used. Other similar drugs are methicillin, dicloxacillin, and cloxacillin. First-generation cephalosporins, such as cefazolin, cephalexin, and cephalothin, are also resistant to beta-lactamase. *S. epidermidis* and *S. aureus* strains may be resistant to penicillin, semisynthetic penicillins, and cephalosporins. Methicillin-resistant *S. aureus* is unresponsive to the semisynthetic penicillins. In this case, vancomycin is the drug of choice. It may also be used for *S. epidermidis* and infection related to foreign bodies or invasive procedures. The emergence of resistant strains to available antimicrobial agents is an increasing problem, due to the lack of other safe and effective antimicrobial agents to treat the infection.

Third-generation cephalosporins are used to treat gram-negative cocci that are penicillin and methicillin-resistant.

L. monocytogenes, a gram-positive rod, generally responds to ampicillin therapy. Aminoglycosides or third-generation cephalosporins are the drugs of choice for gram-negative enteric rods. Some gram-negative rods are classified according to their lactose fermentation ability. The lactose fermenters, *E. coli* and *Klebsiella*, are sensitive to aminoglycosides and third-generation cephalosporins. *Shigella* and *Salmonella* are non–lactose fermenters, which respond well to ampicillin and third-generation cephalosporins. *Haemophilus influenzae* is usually sensitive to ampicillin and third-generation cephalosporins, although some strains are ampicillin resistant. *Pseudomonas* requires the following combination therapy: aminoglycoside and an antipseudomonas penicillin such as azlocillin, carbenicillin, imipenem, mezlocillin, piperacillin, and ticarcillin.

Two anaerobic microorganisms, *Bacteroides fragilis* (gram-negative) and *Clostridium* (gram-positive), are sometimes the cause of newborn infections. *B. fragilis* is susceptible to metronidazole (Flagyl), clindamycin, chloramphenicol, and some of the newer beta-lactamases, such as imipenem and ampicillin with sulbactam. Clostridium is usually susceptible to penicillin.

A combination of ampicillin or penicillin and gentamicin is useful for antibacterial action against *Streptococcus*, *L. monocytogenes*, and gram-negative enteric rods. This combination of antimicrobial agents has a synergistic effect (in vitro), increasing the efficacy of either drug therapy used alone. Additional therapy or selection of other agents is necessary if staphylococcal infection is suspected, if *Pseudomonas* or *Bacteroides* (most often iatrogenically acquired) is present, if there is an outbreak of resistant organisms, or if prolonged ampicillin and gentamicin therapy has been used. Antimicrobial agents must be reevaluated after completion of cultures and sensitivity testing. Tables 11.1 and 11.2 show generally recommended antimicrobial choices for infections caused by gram-positive and gram-negative microorganisms.

TABLE 11.1

GENERAL ANTIMICROBIAL SELECTION GUIDELINES FOR GRAM-POSITIVE MICROORGANISMS

Microorganism	Antimicrobial
Streptococcus	Penicillin or ampicillin
Staphylococcus aureus	Semisynthetic penicillins, such as methicillin (or methicillin-type) nafcillin, oxacillin, dicloxicillin, cephalin, cephalothin
Methicillin-resistant *Staphylococcus aureus* (MRSA)	Vancomycin
Staphylococcus epidermidis	Vancomycin
Listeria monocytogenes	Ampicillin
Clostridium difficile	Penicillin

TABLE 11.2

GENERAL ANTIMICROBIAL SELECTION GUIDELINES FOR GRAM-NEGATIVE MICROORGANISMS

Microorganism	Antimicrobial
Escherichia coli	Aminoglycosides or third-generation cephalosporins
Klebsiella	Aminoglycosides or third-generation cephalosporins
Shigella	Ampicillin and third-generation cephalosporins
Salmonella	Ampicillin and third-generation cephalosporins
Haemophilus influenzae	Ampicillin and third-generation cephalosporins; some strains are ampicillin-resistant
Pseudomonas	Aminoglycoside plus an antipseudomonas penicillin
Bacteroides fragilis	Metronidazole, clindamycin, some beta-lactamases such as imipenum and ampicillin with sulbactim; and chloramphenicol

TYPES OF NEONATAL INFECTION

This section briefly describes the types of microorganisms that typically cause neonatal infection and their clinical manifestations, diagnosis, and collaborative management. The discussion includes both congenitally acquired and nosocomially acquired infections caused by bacterial, viral, fungal, and protozoal organisms.

Bacterial Infections

■ Group B Streptococcus. Group B β-hemolytic streptococci were unknown to the perinatal scene until the early 1970s when they replaced *E. coli* as the single most common agent associated with bacterial meningitis during the first 2 months of life. Since the implementation of intrapartum antibiotic prophylaxis for prevention of neonatal GBS disease, rates of EOS with GBS have declined; however, GBS sepsis continues to be the most common pathogen in term infants (Stroll et al., 2011). The number of newborn deaths associated with either early onset or late onset GBS continues to be high, particularly in high-risk urban centers. Potential for permanent neurologic sequelae for infant survivors of meningeal infections is approximately 15% (Edwards, Nizet, & Baker, 2005). The mortality rate of infected newborns varies according to time of onset. Early-onset infection (within the first week of life) has a mortality rate between 5% and 50%; late-onset (after first week of life) mortality is approximately 2% to 6% (Marcy, Baker, & Palazzi, 2005).

Pathophysiology. Streptococcus is a gram-positive diplococcus with an ultrastructure similar to that of other gram-positive cocci. It was classified as hemolytic because of its double zone of hemolysis surrounding colonies on blood agar plates. Culture of body fluids, such as blood, urine, CSF, and other secretions, is the most common method of identifying group B streptococci. Counterelectrophoresis and LA are rapid assays that enable a presumptive diagnosis before cultures are returned. Rapid identification of the GBS organism is important in treating colonized pregnant women and in the early diagnosis and treatment of infection in the sick, unstable septic infant. To accurately predict maternal colonization with group B streptococci, both vaginal and rectal areas should be cultured on more than one occasion (Adair et al., 2003; Benedetto et al., 2004). Newer techniques using the LightCycler Strep B analyte-specific reagents (Roche Diagnostics Corp, Indianapolis, IN) give results more rapidly than traditional cultures, thus decreasing time to diagnosis (Uhl et al., 2005).

Clinical Manifestations. GBS has been identified as a relatively common cause of mid-gestational fetal loss in women who experience vaginal hemorrhage, PROM, fetal membrane infection, and spontaneous abortion. The rate of stillbirth is reported to be as high as 61% in association with these bacteria. Early-onset neonatal infections with GBS can be asymptomatic or can manifest with severe symptoms of respiratory distress and shock, which can rapidly progress to death (Edwards et al., 2005).

Early-Onset Group B Streptococcus. Early-onset GBS infection usually appears within the first 24 hours of life and is most common in premature infants. Congenital pneumonia is a more common presentation sign in infants who weigh 1,000 g or less. The most common presentations are pneumonia and meningitis. Signs of respiratory distress, apnea, grunting, tachypnea, and cyanosis are common. Hypotension is found in 25% of newborns with GBS infection; these infants are at risk for cardiopulmonary collapse. Nonspecific signs of infection include lethargy, poor feeding, temperature instability, abdominal distention, pallor, tachycardia, and jaundice. Experienced nurses may observe that the neonate "just doesn't look right," which is sometimes a critical point for early detection and implementation of therapy. Overwhelming GBS septicemia is often compounded by meningitis. LP and examination of the CSF are the only way to exclude meningeal involvement and therefore represent an important part of the work-up. Seizures may occur in infants with GBS meningitis. Low-birth-weight infants have been identified as particularly vulnerable, but a study in Texas revealed a high incidence of infection in term newborns. These infants had no risk factors for infection; therefore, there was a delay in identification and treatment. The mortality rate in these term newborns was 14% (Edwards et al., 2005).

Late-Onset GBS Infection. Late-onset infection with GBS usually occurs in term newborns 7 days to 12 weeks of age. The fatality rate is less than that with early-onset infection, but meningitis may lead to permanent neurologic damage, varying in severity from mild handicaps to severe impairment. Complications include global or profound mental retardation, spastic quadriplegia, cortical blindness, deafness, uncontrolled seizures, hydrocephalus, and diabetes insipidus. Thus, early treatment is an important part of the prevention of long-term serious sequelae. An infant with a positive blood culture can often be asymptomatic initially. The diagnosis of GBS infection is complicated because signs and symptoms of neonatal infection are not specific and symptoms may represent other conditions of the neonate. For example, apnea may be a symptom of CNS immaturity in the preterm neonate, but it is also associated with infection. The caregiver must have a high index of suspicion for infection in all conditions involving the neonate. Infection should be considered in the differential diagnosis of most newborn illnesses. Screening tests, such as CBC with differential, are often used to identify the need for further evaluation for infection. Abnormal results indicate the necessity for definitive testing and implementation of antimicrobial therapy.

Management. Regional and hospital differences in infectious agents must be considered in the selection of antimicrobial therapy. Before culture results are returned, administration of a broad-spectrum penicillin and an aminoglycoside provides coverage for the most prevalent microorganisms. Generally, ampicillin and gentamicin are selected until culture results and sensitivities are available. GBS is generally very sensitive to penicillin G, and, in many institutions, penicillin G is substituted for ampicillin once the diagnosis is made. Therapy is maintained for 7 to 10 days for infection and 14 to 21 days for meningitis. The LP may be repeated midway or at the end of therapy to ensure that there are no microorganisms remaining in the CSF. Fluid management, volume expansion, and appropriate antimicrobial therapy are the key components of nursing care. Infants with GBS infection are often very labile and do not tolerate frequent interventions. Minimal handling is sometimes required for their care.

Edwards et al. (2005) suggest that the most potentially lasting method for prevention of early- and late-onset infections, as well as maternal morbidity associated with GBS, is the active immunization of all women of childbearing age, either before pregnancy or late in pregnancy (at approximately 7 months gestation). Passive transmission of antibodies to the newborn occurs via the placenta; however, women often deliver infants prematurely, before the successful transmission of appropriate protective antibodies. Edwards et al. state that because 65% to 85% of all infants with GBS disease are born at term, vaccines given to women early in the third trimester could prevent up to 95% of these infections. The cost of developing a suitable vaccine would probably be less than the cost of the care required by the critically ill newborn and the chronically ill, debilitated, severely handicapped newborn.

■ ***Staphylococcus.*** From the 1950s to the 1970s, coagulase-positive *S. aureus* was the main organism identified as a pathogen in hospitals. In the 1980s, coagulase-negative organisms, in particular *S. epidermidis*, were discovered to be equally important. These organisms have caused many serious and even fatal infections in newborns. Critically ill and preterm newborns are already immunocompromised and therefore are especially vulnerable to infections. Open skin lesions, surgical incisions, or puncture wounds caused by diagnostic tests or procedures are conducive to bacterial growth, especially *S. aureus* or *S. epidermidis* (Orschein et al., 2005). Nosocomial infections may also be transmitted to the neonate through contaminated articles or from the hands of health care providers. Overgrowth of *S. epidermidis* may occur in nurseries where an attempt has been made to reduce colonization of *S. aureus*. Development of resistant organisms is a risk for critically ill or preterm infants who require extensive invasive treatments. Coagulase-negative staphylococci or methicillin-resistant *S. aureus* have a potential for causing rapid decompensation (Healy, Palazzi, Edwards, Campbell, & Baker, 2004). Staphylococci release endotoxins that have systemic effects, including the alteration of the skin's protective layer. Scalded skin syndrome is one of the most common examples of this effect.

Management. Management and supportive therapy for staphylococcal infection are initially the same as for infection with group B streptococci. Antimicrobial therapy begins with ampicillin and gentamicin. Once definitive cultures and sensitivities are available and if the organism is ampicillin resistant, the drug of choice is one of the synthetic penicillins: oxacillin, methicillin, cloxacillin, dicloxacillin, or nafcillin. If the organism is methicillin resistant, the best available drug is vancomycin. It is essential that the choice of antimicrobial agent be carefully made and reconsidered when culture results are available.

■ ***Escherichia Coli.*** *E. coli* is second to GBS as the most common cause of EOS and is the most common cause of gram-negative infection in the newborn. Coliform organisms are common organisms in the maternal birth canal causing a high incidence of colonization in the lower gastrointestinal or respiratory tract of newborns at delivery (Nizet & Klein, 2011).

■ ***Listeria Monocytogenes.*** *L. monocytogenes* has been recognized as a cause of perinatal complications since the early 1900s. It is found in birds and mammals, including domestic and farm animals, and in unpasteurized milk, soil, and fecal material. *Listeria* infection appears to be underdiagnosed and an underreported cause of congenital infection. A study done at the University of Southern California looked at 20 mother–infant pairs from whom *Listeria* was isolated in the prior 10 years. Antepartum factors, such as high maternal leukocyte count, fetal tachycardia, decreased fetal heart rate variability, and absence of intrapartum fetal heart rate accelerations, were identified in the history of the newborns diagnosed with congenital *Listeria* infection. The reported incidence of listeriosis is between 2 and 13 per 100,000 live births. It is estimated that the true incidence is probably much higher due to the suspicion that spontaneous abortion and stillbirths attributable to *Listeria* are under reported (Bortolussi & Mailman, 2011).

Clinical Manifestations. A mother infected with *Listeria* commonly has flulike symptoms, including malaise, fever, chills, diarrhea, and back pain. It is also possible to contract the infection and remain asymptomatic or have only minor symptoms. If contracted between 17 and 28 weeks gestation, *Listeria* can cause fetal death or premature birth of an acutely ill newborn who may die hours later. However, early maternal treatment with intravenous ampicillin and gentamicin has been associated with normal newborn outcome (Bortolussi & Mailman, 2011). Infection late in pregnancy may cause the infant to be born with a congenital infection, usually pneumonia. Mortality rates are high but are usually related to the amount of prematurity. Late-onset listeriosis, which can occur up to 4 weeks after delivery, can easily result in meningitis. A term newborn with listeriosis has less chance of dying but often suffers complications of hydrocephalus and mental retardation. However, in either preterm or term neonates in whom meningitis develops, there is a 70% mortality rate if treatment is delayed (Bortolussi & Mailman, 2011). Newborns infected with *Listeria* may be born prematurely and be meconium stained, exhibit apnea and flaccidity, have a papular erythematous skin rash and hepatosplenomegaly, and be poor feeders. Preterm birth associated with meconium staining should always be considered suspicious for listeriosis.

Management. Intrapartum administration of antibiotics may decrease fetal morbidity and mortality rates. Ampicillin in combination with an aminoglycoside is the most common treatment. Investigators have shown that newborn survival rates are significantly different if the mother as well as the infant receives treatment (71% versus 29%) (Bortolussi & Mailman, 2011). Careful hand washing is a very important aspect of caring for the infant infected with *Listeria*. Institutional policy may require that the infant be isolated for the first 24 hours of life, until the antibiotics are on board. The mother's urine, stool, and lochia should be cultured, and if positive, she should be given ampicillin. Listeriosis often presents suddenly in the last trimester of pregnancy, precipitating an unexpected preterm delivery. Extensive emotional support may be necessary for the mother and family.

Neonatal Meningitis

■ **Pathophysiology.** Meningitis is commonly associated with newborn infection. The incidence of meningitis associated with newborn infection is thought to be approximately 25% of those presenting with infection. Meningitis is more common as a complication of late-onset infection. The morbidity rate is higher for preterm infants than for term infants. Morbidity of survivors of infection with gram-negative bacilli or Group B streptococci approaches 20% to 50%. These complications include mental and motor problems, seizure disorders, hydrocephalus, hearing loss, blindness, and abnormal speech patterns (Marcy, Baker, & Palazzi, 2005). In most cases, meningitis results from bacteremia. Thus, an inoculation of organisms may pass the blood–brain barrier and infect the CSF. Cytologic tests on the CSF can identify the presence of an inflammatory response. A Gram stain of the CSF fluid should be prepared and other appropriate cultures obtained. High CSF protein and low glucose levels are also indicators of meningitis. As with all procedures in the neonate, the LP presents risks, which must be weighed against the benefit of having a CSF culture. Often the preterm infant may be considered so critically unstable that the LP is deferred. Stoll et al. (2004) evaluated the epidemiology of meningitis in very-low-birth-weight infants and compared the CSF and blood culture results. In their review of 9,641 infant records, they found that one-third of the infants who had meningitis had negative blood cultures. They cautioned that the discordance in the CSF and blood culture results could lead to underdiagnosis of meningitis in low-birth-weight infants.

■ **Clinical Manifestations.** Initially, the infant with meningitis presents with signs and symptoms of generalized infection. In addition, the meningeal irritation results in increased irritability, crying, increased intracranial pressure leading to bulging fontanelles, lethargy, tremors or twitching, seizure activity, vomiting, alterations in consciousness, and diminished muscle tone. Focal signs include hemiparesis, horizontal deviation of the eyes, and some cranial nerve involvement (Marcy, Baker, & Palazzi, 2005).

■ Risk Factors. About one fourth of infants with infection will develop meningitis. Although the overall incidence of bacterial meningitis in newborns is less than 1%, the incidence is much higher in preterm newborns (Marcy, Baker, & Palazzi, 2005). Male infants are more vulnerable to infection and, consequently, meningitis. Female infants have lower rates of respiratory distress syndrome and lower rates of most congenital infections. Geography and socioeconomic factors are influential in patterns of neonatal disease. These differences probably reflect populations served, including unique cultural activities and sexual practices, as well as local customs. It probably also reflects different treatment patterns in local nurseries and variations of antimicrobial selections.

■ Prognosis. Brain abscess is associated with a poor prognosis; approximately 50% of affected patients die. Destruction of brain tissues, hemorrhages, and infarcts causing necrosis to vital brain cells may cause extensive brain damage, leading to death or poor neurologic outcomes. With the introduction of ultrasonography and computerized tomography, brain abscesses are being identified earlier.

■ Management. The selection of antimicrobial therapy for meningitis is based on the causative microorganism. Supportive therapy is necessary for the newborn with meningitis. Acute observation and monitoring of vital signs and activity level are crucial. Infants who become critically ill with meningitis may deteriorate quickly and need rapid, acute interventions. Infants often require long-term antibiotic therapy, and often, venous access is a problem. Placement of a percutaneous line for parenteral nutrition may be necessary. Families need educational and emotional support during the long-term hospitalizations, particularly if complications develop.

Congenital Infections

The microorganisms most often responsible for congenitally acquired infections have been grouped together as the TORCH infections. These include toxoplasmosis, others, rubella, cytomegalovirus (CMV), and herpes. The "others" category includes various microorganisms that have been responsible for congenital infections. However, the list of microorganisms implicated in congenital infections has grown, so the acronym is no longer inclusive. A more appropriate acronym, ToRCHES CLAP, is suggested by Maldonado, Nizet, Klein, Remington, and Wilson (2011). This new acronym includes: **To**, *Toxoplasma gondii*; **R**, rubella; **C**, CMV; **H**, herpes synplex virus (HSV); **E**, enteroviruses; **S**, syphilis (*Treponema pallidum*); **C**, chickenpox (varicella-zoster virus); **L**, Lyme disease (*Borrelia burgdorferi*); **A**, acquired immunodeficiency syndrome (AIDS/HIV); and **P**, parvovirus B9.

■ Toxoplasmosis. The importance of the parasite *T. gondii* was discovered by perinatal health care workers in the 1980s. Toxoplasma is a pathogen that is ever-present in nature. Perinatal transmission takes place when the mother contracts the protozoa and the subsequent protozoemia transmits the organism transplacentally to the fetus. The microorganisms then invade and multiply within the placenta and eventually enter the fetal circulation. The life cycle of Toxoplasma is complicated. The predominant host of this organism is the ordinary house cat; however, other animals, such as camels in the Middle East, can serve as hosts. There are significant differences in the prevalence rates of this microorganism throughout the world (Remington, McCleod, Wilson, & Desmont, 2011). The tissue cyst form of the microorganism persists in the flesh of animals, such as cattle and sheep. The oocyte form of the parasite persists in soil contaminated by cat feces. Thus, congenital toxoplasmosis is transmitted from undercooked meat or food or from fomites in cat feces. In the United States, approximately 20% to 70% of the population has been exposed to this protozoan. There is wide variability of the prevalence of seropositive women of childbearing age among countries, geographic regions of the same country, and ethnic origin; different cultural practices regarding food are probably the major cause of this difference. Since meat is the main vector for transmission, areas where there is less *T. gondii* present in meat because of improved methods for processing or cooking meat have lower prevalence rates. The greatest risk is when a nonimmune pregnant woman is exposed to *T. gondii* during fetal organogenesis (weeks 4–8 of gestation), when the risk for congenital anomalies is high (Remington et al., 2011).

Clinical Manifestations. Acute toxoplasmosis in a pregnant woman often goes undetected and undiagnosed because the signs and symptoms are not severe. Clinical questioning after the identification of an infected newborn or infant often leads to reflection and memories of a period of enlarged lymph nodes and fatigue without fever. Women sometimes report a mononucleosis-like or flulike syndrome that may have a febrile course, with malaise, headache, fatigue, sore throat, and sore muscles. These symptoms may persist up to 6 months; however, that duration is unusual. A newborn with congenital toxoplasmosis can present with hydrocephalus, chorioretinitis, and intracranial calcifications. There is a wide variety of clinical signs in the scope of the disease. The newborn can appear normal at birth, or exhibit severe erythroblastosis, hydrops fetalis, and other clinical signs (Remington et al., 2011). Neurologic signs similar to encephalitis (e.g., convulsions, bulging fontanelles, nystagmus, and increased head circumference) may be the only significant presentation of this clinical problem. If the newborn receives treatment, signs may disappear, allowing normal cerebral growth and development, if there was no permanent neurologic damage.

Mild cases of the disease may not be recognized in the newborn period. Signs of delayed onset of disease in premature newborns include severe CNS or eye lesions appearing at 3 months of age. In term newborns, delayed disease may occur in the first 2 months of life and is usually mild. Clinical signs include generalized infection, enlarged liver and spleen, late-onset jaundice, enlarged lymph nodes, or late-onset CNS problems, including hydrocephalus and eye lesions. Infants with congenital toxoplasmosis may have new lesions appearing until age 5 years (Remington et al., 2011).

Management. The best and most effective treatments are prevention and early recognition. The cost effectiveness of pregnancy serology screening depends on the costs of the tests and the estimated cost of treating the infection, if identified early. At present in the United States, screening is done erratically and there are no particular screening standards. Counseling education for the prevention of toxoplasmosis should focus on avoidance of raw meat and use of gloves during feline litter box handling and during gardening in what may be contaminated soil. Toxoplasmosis cannot be contracted by merely handling or being around a cat, so it is not necessary for the family cat to be banished. Pregnant women who are seronegative should exercise caution to avoid the risk of contracting *T. gondii* during pregnancy by avoiding cat litter, digging in the soil, and handling or eating undercooked meat. They should inform their health care provider if they experience any signs that could be attributed to *T. gondii* infection.

Treatment for congenital toxoplasmosis is pyrimethamine plus sulfonamides. The suggested dose is 2 mg/kg/d orally for 2 days followed by 1 mg/kg/d for 2 or 6 months, then 1 mg/kg/d every Monday, Wednesday, and Friday for 1 year. The medication is given in doses of 100 mg/kg/d in two divided oral doses for 1 year. Leucovorin 10 mg is given three times weekly during and for 1 week after pyrimethamine therapy. These drugs are potentially toxic and need close monitoring. Corticosteroids are given in the form of prednisone at 1 mg/kg/d in two divided doses until there is resolution of elevated protein in CSF or active chorioretinitis (Remington et al., 2011). Toxoplasmosis is one of the most common causes of deafness. The Collaborative Perinatal Project found a doubling in the frequency of deafness in infants of mothers with the antibody for toxoplasmosis. There was a 60% increase in microcephaly and a 30% increase in low intelligence quotients (< 70) in relation to high antibody levels in mothers (Remington et al., 2011).

Nursing Management. Nursing management is supportive and dependent on the severity of the infection. Neurologic impairment at birth can be significant, requiring ventilation and seizure control. Transmission of toxoplasmosis in humans occurs only from mother to child; therefore, the risk to health care personal is negligible. There is a theoretical risk of infection from contaminated urine, however.

■ **Rubella.** In 1941, N. McAlister Gregg described 78 patients with congenital cataracts. These patients were small for gestational age and had feeding difficulties and congenital heart problems. A history of German measles during pregnancy was found in 68 of the cases (87%). Much of the current knowledge about the effects of congenital rubella was established by Gregg's report on these patients (Gregg, 1941). It has been further established that the rubella virus can be responsible for other abnormalities. The most important consequences of rubella are the miscarriages, stillbirths, fetal anomalies, and therapeutic abortions that result when rubella infection occurs during early pregnancy, especially during the first trimester. Rubella virus transmission has been eliminated in the Americas; however, cases do still exist. Between 2005 and 2009, 4 to 16 cases were reported annually. Approximately 30% of these cases were attributable to travel from foreign countries (McLean & Reef, 2012). In 1989, a second dose of rubella vaccine was added to the immunization schedule to be given prior to school entry or in the prepubertal period (Plotkin, Reef, Cooper, & Alford, 2011).

In the United States, surveillance for CRS relies on a passive system. Consequently, the reported annual totals of CRS are regarded as minimum figures, representing an estimated 40% to 70% of all cases. Failure to immunize many young children has resulted in an increase in rubella incidence. Therefore, despite a national immunization program, at least 10% of women of childbearing age are vulnerable to the virus, particularly the wild virus, because either they have not been immunized or they have not acquired immunity from the infection themselves. Small rubella outbreaks have been reported all over the United States. Although there has been a change in the epidemiology of the infection over the past 25 years and a significant decrease in the incidence, rubella has not been eradicated. Prevention of rubella in postpubertal women and CRS continues to be a major goal of the CDC (Plotkin et al., 2011).

Clinical Manifestations. The abnormalities most commonly associated with CRS are auditory (e.g., sensorineural deafness), ophthalmic (e.g., cataracts, microphthalmia, glaucoma, chorioretinitis), cardiac (e.g., patent ductus arteriosus, peripheral pulmonary artery stenosis, atrial or ventricular septal defects), and neurologic (e.g., microcephaly, meningoencephalitis, mental retardation). In addition, infants with CRS frequently exhibit both intrauterine and postnatal growth restriction. Other conditions sometimes observed among babies who have CRS include radiolucent bone defects, hepatosplenomegaly, thrombocytopenia, and purpuric skin lesions. Newborns who are moderately or severely affected by CRS are readily recognizable at birth, but mild CRS (e.g., slight cardiac involvement or deafness) may be detected months or years after birth, or not at all (Plotkin et al., 2011). Although CRS has been estimated to occur among 20% to 25% of infants born to women who acquire rubella during the first 20 weeks of pregnancy, this figure may underestimate the risk for fetal infection and birth defects. When infants born to mothers who were infected during the first 8 weeks of gestation were followed for 4 years, 85% were found to be affected. The risk for a defect decreases to about 52% for infections that occur during the 9th to 12th weeks of gestation. Infection after the 20th week of gestation rarely causes defects. Subclinical maternal rubella infection can also cause congenital malformations. Fetal infection without clinical signs of CRS can occur during any stage of pregnancy (Plotkin et al., 2011).

The typical presentation of the rubella virus is mild, with malaise, low-grade fever, headache, and conjunctivitis.

In 1 to 5 days, a macular rash appears on the face and usually disappears after 3 to 4 days. Natural viremia is necessary for placental and fetal rubella infection. Most cases occur following primary disease. Frequently, skin rashes that resemble rubella may occur as a result of adenovirus, enterovirus, or other respiratory virus infections. Laboratory titers are recommended to confirm the diagnosis of rubella infection (Plotkin et al., 2011).

A fetus infected with rubella often has cardiac defects and deafness. The CNS seems particularly vulnerable to the rubella virus, especially if the virus is acquired before the first 16 weeks of gestation. Congenital rubella syndrome is described by the CDC as hearing loss, mental retardation, cardiac malformations, and eye defects.

The rubella virus can slow cell replication. This causes intrauterine growth restriction and a failure of cell differentiation during fetal organ formation. Tissue damage also seems to occur from the inflammatory response to the infection or is even possibly an autoimmune reaction. Myocarditis, pneumonitis, hepatosplenomegaly, and vascular stenosis can also be present because of these processes. As is seen with other severe congenital infections, signs and symptoms may continue to develop until the patient is 10 to 20 years of age. Late clinical signs of this disease include insulin-dependent diabetes, thyroid abnormalities, hypoadrenalism, hearing loss, and eye damage (Plotkin et al., 2011).

Differential Diagnosis. The possibility of subclinical infection with rubella highlights the need for laboratory confirmation. Clinical confirmation of rubella isolation is obtainable in approximately 4 to 6 weeks. The detection of rubella antibody confirms the presence of the infection. Rubella-specific IgG persists for life and can be detected by enzyme immunoassay. With confirmed serologic results, the risk of fetal damage after 16 weeks gestation appears to be small. Demonstration of rubella-specific IgM in fetal blood obtained by cordocentesis has been used to establish diagnosis in utero. Chorionic villus sampling has also demonstrated recovery of the virus during the first trimester (Plotkin et al., 2011).

Management. Infants should be vaccinated against rubella at 15 months of age and again prior to school entry. Women who do not have detectable IgG rubella antibody and are of childbearing age (and not pregnant) should be immunized. They should avoid pregnancy for at least 3 months after immunization to decrease the risk for development of rubella syndrome in the fetus. Health care workers who may be inadvertently exposed to rubella should be immunized if they do not have immune titers. If a woman receives a rubella vaccine and has recently received blood products or RhoGAM (RhIG), the vaccine may not trigger an immune response because blood products and RhoGAM have pooled sera that may contain antibodies against rubella. Thus, the woman's body does not produce antibodies. These women should have titers drawn 6 weeks after vaccination or at most 3 months after vaccination (McLean & Reef, 2012; Plotkin et al., 2011). In more than 500 women who were accidentally immunized against rubella while pregnant, there were no cases of congenital rubella syndrome. Rubella vaccination is not recommended during pregnancy, yet the risks to the fetus have been determined to be negligible and an inadvertent rubella vaccination by itself is not considered an indication for termination of pregnancy. Currently, treatment of the rubella-infected infant in the nursery is rare. Therapy for identified problems, such as respiratory, cardiac, or neurologic deficits, is supportive and there is no specific recommended therapy. Caretakers should have known immune titers and not be pregnant. Rubella-specific IgM can usually accurately identify these infants. Persistent shedding of the virus may last until 1 year of life; thus, pregnant women should avoid contact with these patients. Follow-up care for surgical corrections of heart defects and cataracts as well as special schooling may be needed for these infants.

■ Cytomegalovirus. Infection with CMV, a member of the herpes family, is common. CMV is a DNA virus covered with a glycoprotein coat that closely resembles the herpes and varicella-zoster viruses. By adulthood, most people have been exposed to CMV, and antibodies have developed to it. CMV infection is more prevalent in lower socioeconomic groups and is especially common in developing countries. In the United States, women of childbearing age from lower socioeconomic groups have an incidence of infection of approximately 6%, whereas those from higher socioeconomic groups have an incidence of approximately 2%. CMV may lie dormant, with periods of exacerbation followed by remission. During remission, the patient is asymptomatic, but the virus is shed (Britt, 2011). The virus is usually transmitted person to person through body fluids and secretions. Blood, urine, breast milk, cervical mucus, semen, and saliva harbor CMV. The virus can cause an infectious mononucleosis–like syndrome, with general malaise, liver complications, fever, and general fatigue. Perinatal transmission can occur within 2 to 3 days of infection by transplacental crossing of the organism. The fetus can also contract the virus intrapartally from infected maternal cervical secretions while descending through the birth canal. CMV can also be transmitted through infected breast milk (Britt, 2011).

Clinical Manifestations. More damage occurs to the fetus when the exposure to and acquisition of CMV occur from a primary lesion. Congenital CMV occurs in approximately 0.2% to 2.2% of all newborn infants. Primary lesions cause intrauterine growth restriction, microcephaly, periventricular calcifications, deafness, blindness, congenital cataracts, profound mental retardation, hepatosplenomegaly, and jaundice. A characteristic pattern of petechiae, called "blueberry muffin" syndrome, is associated with congenital CMV. Approximately 26% of severely infected infants die. Severe complications at birth are seen in approximately 5% of congenital infections. Sequelae develop in 5% to 15% of asymptomatic infected infants and in 90% of symptomatic infected infants. Recurrent CMV infections are not as severe because of partial antibody protection from previous exposure. The incidence of neonatal complications is reported to be from 5% to 10% of hearing loss, 2% for chorioretinitis, and less than 1% for mental retardation (Britt, 2011).

Diagnosis. Suspicious clinical findings or obstetric history warrant further investigation for CMV infection. Urine culture for CMV is the most rapid and sensitive indicator of infection. IgG and IgM antibody titers should also be measured. Elevated IgM levels alone denote exposure to CMV but are not diagnostic because there is no method to determine the timing of the exposure. Elevated neonatal IgG titers indicate perinatally acquired CMV infection. A negative maternal IgG titer and a positive neonatal IgG titer indicate postnatal transmission. Experimentally, elevated rheumatoid factors may provide evidence to support the diagnosis of CMV in subclinical cases (Britt, 2011).

Prevention. Transmission of CMV via infected blood products has been significantly decreased through the use of CMV-negative donors or irradiation of blood products. Premature and low-birth-weight infants are especially vulnerable to the infusion of this virus in blood products. The best method of prevention is the institution of universal precautions, including good hand washing techniques.

Management. Newborns infected with CMV display a wide range of signs. General supportive therapy is based on the presence of these clinical manifestations. Specific therapy for CMV is still in the experimental stage but includes immunoglobulin therapy, vaccines, and chemotherapy. Intravenous immunoglobulin therapy provides passive immunity to at-risk infants but not to those already infected. Two live attenuated vaccines for CMV have been developed and tested on renal transplant patients. Theoretically, these vaccines would be useful preconceptionally or perinatally to prevent vertical transmission; however, only limited research has been done with this population. Chemotherapy offers the most promise for treatment of neonatal CMV infection; however, clinically, it has not been shown to be effective in improving long-term outcome (Britt, 2011).

Hospital workers who are of childbearing age are often concerned about their risk for contracting CMV from their virus shedding patients. Generally, this risk is dependent on the prevalence of CMV secretion, the susceptibility of the worker, and the degree of exposure. Since implementation of universal precautions, the risk of nosocomial transmission of the virus has been very low and is considered lower than the risk of acquiring the infection in the community (Britt, 2011).

■ **Syphilis.** The microorganism *T. pallidum* has persisted as a threat to perinatal patients for over 400 years. The World Health Organization reports that one million pregnancies are complicated by syphilis annually and approximately half of those pregnancies end in abortion or perinatal mortality (Kollman & Dobson, 2011). Many women do not receive adequate treatment for primary or secondary infections, despite the availability of effective therapy for more than 40 years. The virus can be dormant for years, much like the herpes family of viruses. The incidence of syphilis is increasing because of increased substance abuse, sexual practices involving multiple partners, and increased numbers of human immunodeficiency virus (HIV)-positive immunocompromised individuals, who act as reservoirs for *T. pallidum*. Consequently, there has been a resurgence of congenital infections. Recent worldwide concern regarding the role of genital ulcers in conjunction with HIV infection has created great concern for eradication of sexually transmitted diseases (Kollman & Dobson, 2011). The diagnosis of antepartum syphilis is most often made by screening at the first prenatal visit. Screening usually involves the use of the Venereal Disease Research Laboratory (VDRL) test or rapid plasma reagin (RPR) test, each of which measures anticardiolipin antibody. These tests are reactive in almost 80% of patients with secondary or early latent (< 1-year duration) primary syphilis. A definitive diagnosis can be made with an elevated VDRL or RPR accompanied by a positive *T. pallidum* fluoroantibody test or a reactive serologic test for *T. pallidum* in the CSF. Condylomata lata, bony changes, or snuffles in the presence of a positive serologic test are diagnostic (Kollman & Dobson, 2011). Untreated syphilis adversely affects pregnancy outcome. Vertical transmission of treponemas can occur at any time during pregnancy. The microorganisms can cause preterm labor, PROM, stillbirth, congenital infection, or neonatal death. Current untreated secondary infection causes the greatest risk of damage to the fetus, particularly if infection occurs during the period of organogenesis. Late untreated syphilis in the mother usually results in delivery of an asymptomatic infant who needs treatment in the newborn nursery. Reports state that, between 1983 and 1985, 437 infants in the United States were delivered with congenital syphilis. The mean age of acquiring prenatal care was 22 weeks gestation, and at least half of the cases were preventable because they were results of failure of initial or third-trimester screening (Kollman & Dobson, 2011). A study by Ogunyemi and Hernández-Loera (2004) found that maternal use of cocaine led to a greater risk for untreated maternal syphilis and consequent congenital syphilis.

Clinical Manifestations. When newborns acquire syphilis from hematogenous spread across the placenta, the effects are on the major organ systems of the fetus, especially the CNS. Common presentations of the infected infant are hepatosplenomegaly, jaundice, low birth weight, intrauterine growth restriction, anemia, and osteochondritis. There is often a bilateral superficial peeling of the skin (desquamation) on the neonatal palms and soles. Nonimmune hydrops is a common presentation in congenital syphilis. The symptoms of perinatal syphilis are similar to those of any other viral infection that spreads hematogenously from the mother to the placenta and on to the developing fetus (Kollman & Dobson, 2011).

Differential Diagnosis. An LP for CSF analysis and radiographs of the long bones facilitate the definitive diagnosis of syphilis in the neonate. Congenital neurosyphilis is always a consideration, and the CSF should be examined for the presence of spirochetes. Radiologic changes such as osteochondritis (a blurring of the epiphyseal borders) demonstrate recent fetal infection (within 5 weeks), and periostitis represents prolonged involvement, probably within 16 weeks or second-trimester infection.

Stillborn infants should be examined by whole-body radiographic study and autopsy if possible. Spirochetes can be visualized by special staining techniques (Kollman & Dobson, 2011). Interpretation of serologic tests for syphilis on serum obtained from cord blood is complicated because of the transplacental transfer of maternal IgG antibody. VDRL titers at least two dilutions higher than maternal VDRL titers indicate probable fetal infection.

Prognosis. Infants with syphilis should receive the same amount of follow-up as normal infants. Serologic measurements can be made at follow-up visits at 1, 2, 3, 6, and 12 months of age. The infection can be effectively treated, but the physiologic and developmental prognosis depends on the degree of organ damage sustained during fetal development.

Management. The recommended treatment for a newborn presumed to be infected with congenital syphilis is aqueous penicillin G. In many perinatal centers, the presence of a positive VDRL in a neonate dictates treatment as if positive for syphilis. If neonatal clinical manifestations are highly suspicious for syphilis and there is a positive VDRL but the titer is not significantly higher than the maternal titer, syphilis treatment should be instituted. A newborn with an antibody titer four or more times higher than the maternal level should be treated as if a definitive diagnosis has been obtained. To prevent neurosyphilis, the infant should be given aqueous penicillin G, 100,000 to 150,000 units/kg intravenously in two or three divided doses for at least 10 to 14 days, or 50,000 units/kg/d of procaine penicillin in a daily dose for 10 to 14 days. For asymptomatic infants whose mothers were treated adequately during pregnancy, treatment is not necessary unless follow-up cannot be ensured. Some clinicians recommend a single dose of benzathine penicillin: 50,000 units/kg intramuscularly, if the infant is not likely to be followed up on. If maternal treatment did not include penicillin and if neonatal follow-up is likely to be unreliable, the neonate is given a full 10-day course (Kollmann & Dobson, 2011). Isolation of an infant with suspicious symptoms may be necessary until appropriate treatment is given. There is a definite role for nursing education and support in the treatment of an infant exposed to syphilis. The 10- to 14-day course of penicillin treatment may lead to the establishment of a trusting relationship between the nurse and family, thus providing an opportunity to give more information regarding sexual risk factors. Families often need encouragement and support to get treatment for other sexual partners and to obtain other necessary medical evaluations (such as HIV screening or drug counseling).

■ **Herpes Simplex Virus.** Herpes simplex virus (HSV) is a member of a family of large DNA viruses. They contain linear, double strands of DNA. The herpes family also includes CMV, varicella-zoster, and Epstein–Barr virus. HSV possesses the quality of "latency," whereby the virus can persist in a latent state for a period of time and then be reactivated by certain stimuli. A strand of the viral DNA persists in an infected individual for a lifetime; thus, the virus maintains a "foothold" in its host. Clinical experiences demonstrate that, after primary HSV infection, at the site of the infection (perhaps an oral or genital site) the microorganism invades the sensory nerve endings and remains there. The more severe the primary infection, as determined by the size and extent of the skin lesion, the more likely are frequent recurrences. Potential stimuli for HSV reactivation include periods of stress, emotional trauma, and prolonged exposure to the sun. Maintenance of the latency state and recurrence of the virus are topics of intense current research. There are many unanswered questions about what triggers latency and about the cofactors for reactivation of the virus.

Maternal HSV is usually the source of neonatal infection. The risk of neonatal infection is estimated to be 5% if it is recurrent herpes and higher if it is a primary infection (Gutierrez, Whitley, & Arvin, 2011; Langlet et al., 2003). Recurrent infections are the most common problem in pregnancy. Transmission of the infection to the fetus can be caused by passage through infected genital secretions in the intrapartum period or by ascending infection from the vaginal vault via ruptured (or not) membranes. Many women can be asymptomatic and still be shedding HSV. Although primary infection is less common, it causes the most severe neonatal disease, most likely including CNS problems, disseminated disease into other organ systems, and probable death. The incidence of intrapartum transmission with a primary infection is approximately 40% to 50%. Many neonatal complications such as prematurity, intrauterine restriction, and respiratory distress syndrome can potentiate the neonate's illness, limiting the ability to fight off HSV. There is a broad range of severity of neonatal infection, from severe to benign and asymptomatic. In the United States, there are from 11 to 33 cases of neonatal herpes infection per 100,000 live births. With approximately 4 million deliveries per year in the United States, that results in from 520 to 1,320 neonates with HSV (Gutierrez et al., 2011). Susceptibility of the newborn to HSV is increased because there is a lack of passively acquired maternal antibody in some infants.

Clinical Manifestations. Acquisition of HSV in utero can result in spontaneous abortion, preterm birth, or a normal baby. Manifestations of the disease are broad; the clinical presentation of the congenital acquisition of the infection includes skin vesicles or scarring, hypopigmentation, chorioretinitis, microcephaly, and hydranencephaly. There are three categories of neonatal patients. The first category includes patients with localized infections of the skin, eyes, or mouth. The second category includes patients with encephalitis. In this group, neurologic sequelae occur in approximately 50%. Approximately one third of these patients do not have skin vesicles, and they are identified by history alone. CSF is positive for the virus in 25% to 40% of these cases. Presence of cells and increased protein are very common in the CSF of patients with encephalitis, and they die if not treated. The third category of neonatal patients includes those with disseminated disease characterized by irritability, seizures, respiratory distress, jaundice, DIC, shock, and other symptoms of viral and bacterial infection. All major neonatal organs may be involved.

Liver and the adrenals are the most common reservoirs for the virus. The CNS is involved in 70% to 90% of affected neonates. In more than 20% of the newborns with disseminated disease, skin vesicles do not develop, making identification of positive infants more difficult (Gutierrez et al., 2011).

Differential Diagnosis. Laboratory tests can differentiate HSV infection from other bacterial and viral infections. The most rapid method employs cytologic examination. Routine cultures should be obtained from any vesicle on the skin, oropharyngeal or eye secretions, or stool. Viral typing is done for epidemiologic purposes only. HSV types I and II are the most commonly known. Type I has been most closely associated with any herpes found outside the genital area; type II is commonly referred to as genital herpes. However, either type can occur almost anywhere in the body. Treatment does not differ for these different viral types (Gutierrez et al., 2011).

Risk Factors. Intrapartal transmission is more likely to occur in the presence of ruptured membranes. Other risk factors include intrauterine fetal monitoring and fetal scalp sampling. It is not recommended that women infected with HSV be monitored by these methods. Transmission from mother to infant from an infected breast lesion has been reported. Transmission has also been documented from oral lesions.

Prevention. Presence of maternal active HSV genital lesions is a contraindication to vaginal delivery. If the membranes have been ruptured 4 hours or longer, cesarean section may or may not prevent transmission to the neonate. Postnatal nosocomial transmission is greatly reduced with good hand washing techniques and universal precautions.

Management. The most recent methods of treatment include the antiviral drugs acyclovir and vidarabine. The results of these methods of therapy and treatment are reported in the National Institute of Allergy and Infectious Diseases (NIAID) Joint Collaborative Antiviral Study. These drugs have potentially influenced neonatal morbidity and mortality from disseminated disease and encephalitis. Vidarabine is usually given intravenously in dosages of 15 to 30 mg/kg/d over a 12-hour period for 10 to 14 days. It has been reported that newborns receiving the higher doses of 30 mg/kg/d seem to progress to less serious forms of the disease. In some circumstances, longer periods of treatment may be necessary because infants can have either a clinical recurrence or a clinical progression of the disease (Gutierrez et al., 2011). Acyclovir, a relatively new antiviral agent undergoing clinical study, is the recommended mode of therapy at this writing. Acyclovir appears to be very helpful in decreasing the frequency of the reactivation of the virus, particularly in the treatment of herpes simplex encephalitis. Acyclovir is a selective inhibitor of viral replication and thus has few side effects. The recommended dosage is 30 mg/kg/d intravenously divided over 8 hours. Duration of therapy is 10 to 14 days (Gutierrez et al., 2011).

Early identification and intervention are essential, because early institution of antiviral therapy has been shown to improve outcome and decrease sequelae (Gutierrez et al., 2011). Newborns with eye involvement should be given topical antiviral agents such as trifluridine, one drop every 2 hours, as well as intravenous therapy. Vidarabine and acyclovir are potent drugs with a potential for toxicity. Neonatal therapeutic ranges for these drugs have not been established. Monitoring of the infant's physiologic status is necessary to detect potential side effects. Infected infants must be isolated because viral shedding provides a reservoir for infecting other infants in the nursery.

HSV continues to be a life-threatening neonatal infection in the United States. There is growing concern about transmission of the virus to unborn children with the concomitant increase in genital herpes as a sexually transmitted disease. It is important for all health care providers in the perinatal arena to maintain a high index of suspicion in infants whose symptoms may be compatible with HSV infection. Early identification allows prompt treatment or necessary continued observation, or both. Continued research may produce a more rapid method of virus identification and perhaps a safe and effective vaccine. Prevention of neonatal HSV depends on improved knowledge regarding the factors of virus transmission between mother and infant. Appropriate use of cesarean section in women with active genital herpes is an important management step (Gutierrez et al., 2011).

Primary nursing responsibilities in the management of a family with HSV infection are education and support. Mothers should be educated as to the mode, methods, and possible origins of the HSV, and concerns should be addressed regarding potential transmission to newborns. Nurses are often the first to document a mother's comment that she "had a small bump or blister and fever" right before her infant was born. Careful history taking and thorough questioning can often identify potentially infected patients early. With the diagnosis of genital herpes and subsequent monitoring procedures, families often feel stigmatized as well as anxious. Parents and responsible family members need education and support. Mothers with a history of genital HSV should be investigated for findings of active infection during the prepartum period. The definition of an active lesion includes one of the following at birth:

1. Positive viral culture of a lesion
2. Positive fluorescent antibody test
3. Presence of skin vesicles or lesions
4. Cytologic screen with identified HSV markers

All family members with active lesions anywhere on the body should be taught careful hand washing techniques to use before handling the baby. Any person with an oral HSV infection who handles the infant must wash well, wear a mask, and not kiss the infant anywhere until the lesions are completely crusted over and healed (Gutierrez et al., 2011).

A common nursery issue that arises when a mother has active genital herpes is whether isolation is required and what form of isolation is indicated. Transmission occurs through direct contact with the infected lesion. There must be thorough hand washing before handling the infant and after touching the genital area. The risks for transmission are unknown, but they are low. Hospital personnel usually gown and glove until viral status is known. Positive cultures at birth may just reflect colonization; cultures should be repeated at 24 to 48 hours. If cultures are positive, the infant is considered to be infected. Breastfeeding is contraindicated if the mother has a lesion on her breast. Infants are not isolated unless they themselves are infected. Many nurseries have guidelines regarding a 24- to 48-hour observation period to check cultures on an infant who was delivered vaginally through an infected genital area. An uninfected child does not require prolonged hospitalization, and, on discharge, the family needs information and education. Families should be informed that immediate medical consultation should be obtained with the development of major findings, including malaise, irritability, fever, temperature instability, respiratory distress, apnea, large abdomen or liver, sudden changes in skin color, new skin vesicles, lesions on the mucous membranes, or conjunctivitis. Sudden onset of systemic disease in a small, recovering preterm infant can include DIC and shock. Skin lesions are often absent in these severe cases, which may delay diagnosis (Gutierrez et al., 2011; Langlet et al., 2003).

■ Varicella. Varicella is the member of the herpes virus family that commonly causes chickenpox as well as varicella zoster. Most women of childbearing age in the United States have been exposed to or have contracted this virus, yet women from other parts of the world may not be seropositive. Incidence of this virus in pregnant women is very low, approximately in the range of 0.5 in 10,000 pregnancies (Gershon, 2011). Symptoms of varicella are usually present 10 to 20 days after exposure and include fever, malaise, and an itchy rash. The maculopapular rash eventually forms vesicles and crusts over.

Potential complications include pneumonia, encephalitis, arthritis, and bacterial cellulitis. If the virus is contracted early in pregnancy, the damage is likely to be cutaneous, musculoskeletal, neurologic, and ocular. Infants can have intrauterine growth restriction, microcephaly, cerebellar and cortical atrophy, cataracts, limb malformations, and chorioretinitis (Gershon, 2011). Viral infection in the last 3 weeks of pregnancy affects one in four newborns. The severity of neonatal disease is determined by the timing of the exposure. Infections are generally severe if contracted within 4 days before and 2 days after delivery. Severe viral respiratory distress with significantly depleted maternal passive antibody transmission puts the infant at an even greater risk for other complications. When maternal varicella infection occurs 5 to 21 days before delivery, the newborn has a much milder course of the disease and appears more capable of fighting the infection. This milder course is probably due to passive immunity transmitted to the infant via maternally derived antibodies (Gershon, 2011).

The diagnosis of varicella is made by isolation of HSV. Strict isolation of identified infants or of those whose symptoms are highly suspicious for infection is necessary. Vidarabine or acyclovir can be used for treatment of severe disease in newborns. Varicella-zoster immune globulin (VZIG) can be given to newborns to decrease the severity of infection in those exposed (Gershon, 2011). Typically, if a mother has contracted varicella infection late in pregnancy, other persons, such as health care workers, family members, or other newborns, may have been exposed. Exposed susceptible persons should be protected with VZIG. A live attenuated varicella vaccine approved by the Food and Drug Administration is produced by Merck & Co. Inc., Whitehouse Station, NJ (Gershon, 2011).

■ Gonorrhea. *Neisseria gonorrhoeae* is a species of small gram-negative diploid bacteria. They are diploid because they grow in pairs. Infection with this organism is seen most frequently in young adults aged 15 to 24 years. There are approximately 1 million new cases of gonorrhea each year. In females, infection is asymptomatic, which compromises detection of the disease. The organism is easily transmitted by infected tissue and secretions from the cervix, pharynx, urethra, or rectum. The incubation period is approximately 2 to 7 days. Pelvic inflammatory disease is often caused by the organism (Embree, 2011).

Clinical Manifestations. Gonorrhea infections are often mild but often cause blockage of the fallopian tubes. Perhaps 50% of women are asymptomatic with an infected cervix. In a pregnant woman, gonorrheal colonization of the cervix can cause inflammation and weakening of the fetal membranes and early rupture. Chorioamnionitis with *N. gonorrhoeae* as the causative organism can occur in the antepartum period and during labor and delivery; it is also related to increased risk of postpartum endometritis (Embree, 2011). Disseminated gonococcal infection may present during pregnancy, causing arthritis, tendinitis, general aching, fever, and malaise. A previous history of gonorrhea presents a strong possibility that it may recur during pregnancy. Sexual partners should be screened and given treatment, because reinfection after treatment is common (Embree, 2011).

Gonococcal conjunctivitis in the newborn has historically been a risk from transmission via the birth canal. Prophylaxis has been mandated by law in the United States, and silver nitrate 1% solution or erythromycin is administered in both eyes of the neonate at birth. Fetal scalp electrodes have been identified as a potential method of organism transmission to the fetus. *N. gonorrhoeae* has been isolated from scalp abscesses, gastric and pharyngeal aspirates, conjunctival aspirates, and other blood and body fluids. Maternal and neonatal risks from exposure to the gonorrheal microorganism are significant and make it particularly important to screen for gonorrhea during pregnancy. Infected women have a higher incidence of premature labor, PROM, and infectious complications (Embree, 2011).

Prevention. Use of silver nitrate solution or erythromycin for the prevention of gonococcal ophthalmia neonatorum is one of the early achievements in preventive medicine. Routine prophylaxis is mandated by law in the United States and has made a significant difference in the treatment of ocular disease. Chlamydia conjunctivitis has become far more common than gonococcal conjunctivitis in the neonate because of the continual screening for gonorrhea and the routine use of silver nitrate. Erythromycin ointment in both eyes is a more common prophylactic practice because it covers both gonococcal and chlamydial organisms (Embree, 2011).

Management: Mother. The appropriate treatment for a pregnant woman includes ceftriaxone, 250 mg intramuscularly once, plus erythromycin, 500 mg orally four times a day for 7 days. If gastrointestinal side effects are too severe, amoxicillin can be used. Follow-up, per the CDC, requires that cervical and rectal cultures for *N. gonorrhoeae* be obtained 4 to 7 days after treatment. Ideally, pregnant women should also receive treatment for chlamydia infection. In the nonpregnant woman, treatment with doxycycline, ofloxacin, and azithromycin is effective, but their use in pregnancy is not advised. Azithromycin has not been tested in pregnant women, but, if proven safe, only one dose would be required for effective treatment (Embree, 2011).

Management: Neonate. Infants who are delivered by an infected, untreated mother are usually given a complete infection work-up, including an LP, and placed on ampicillin and gentamicin therapy. If cultures confirm the presence of the microorganism and resistance is an issue, then infants should be treated with ceftriaxone, 25 to 50 mg/kg/d intravenously or intramuscularly in single doses, or cefotaxime, 25 mg/kg intravenously or intramuscularly every 12 hours (Embree, 2011). Education and support regarding the origin of the infectious agent are important in the treatment of gonorrhea. Sexual partners of infected persons should be encouraged to seek testing and appropriate antibiotic treatment for chlamydia as well as gonorrhea (Embree, 2011).

■ Hepatitis B Virus. The hepatitis B virus (HBV) is fairly large, approximately 42 nm in diameter. It is a double-stranded DNA–containing virus. Exposure to infected blood and body fluids, percutaneous introduction of blood, and administration of infected blood products are the principal routes of transmission. Contamination or infection of wounds can easily transmit the disease. The virus is fairly strong and is able to live on inanimate objects or fomites. Deactivation requires at least 1 minute in boiling water and extended autoclaving time. In the adult, HBV infection produces systemic illness with general malaise, jaundice, anorexia, and nausea. Early stages of the disease may include fever, rash, and sore joints. Health care workers have historically been particularly vulnerable to this virus because of their repeated exposure to contaminated blood and body fluids and needle sticks. A carrier state of HBV can precipitate chronic liver disease (Karnsakul & Schwarz, 2011). In certain areas of the world, such as Africa, Southeast Asia, and the Pacific Rim, the virus is considered endemic. In these areas, carrier rates are estimated to be 35%. Approximately 40% of these carriers have been identified as having been perinatally infected (Karnsakul & Schwarz, 2011).

Hepatitis B surface antigen (HBsAg) is an important test in assessing a woman's risk of transmitting HBV to her unborn child. The presence of HBsAg and hepatitis Be antigen (HBeAg) is the best indication of infectiousness. It is currently recommended that all pregnant women be screened at their first prenatal visit for HBsAg and HBeAg to prevent prenatal transmission (Karnsakul & Schwarz, 2011). Infection early in pregnancy with HBV causes a 50% risk of neonatal HBV infection. Ninety percent of infants born to women who are positive for both HBsAg and HBeAg are at risk for development of HBV infection by their first birthday if they are not given treatment. Infants born to women who are positive for HBsAg but negative for HBeAg have lower rates of perinatal infection (20%). Infants who do not receive treatment are likely to become carriers, which may eventually lead to primary hepatocellular carcinoma. Treatment for these infants should be HBV vaccine along with hepatitis B immunoglobulin. For neonates whose mothers are HBsAg positive or exposed, HBV vaccine, 0.5 mL (10 mcg/mL), should be given intramuscularly in the anterolateral thigh at or within 24 hours of birth. Immunoglobulin (0.5 mL) should be given concurrently at a separate site. Vaccination should be repeated at 1 and 6 months: 0.5 mL; booster injections are suggested at 12 months and may need repeating at 5-year intervals. The vaccine can be used in infants who have been exposed to HIV. There is usually an immune response in these infants despite an altered CD4 count. The response does appear to be somewhat diminished (Karnsakul & Schwarz, 2011).

Vertical transmission of HBV may occur during vaginal delivery. The sharing of bodily secretions during sexual intercourse can also result in disease transmission. HBV has a long incubation period—50 to 190 days with the average being 90 days. Current recommendations are for all pregnant women to be screened initially and again before delivery. Screening is essential to identify a potential risk for perinatal transmission and for protection of those who are exposed to antigen-positive blood. Family clustering of HBV has been identified and spread via household contact (Karnsakul & Schwarz, 2011).

Clinical Manifestations. Prematurity, low birth weight, and hyperbilirubinemia are clinical signs of HBV infection. Hepatosplenomegaly is also a common presenting symptom in an infant infected with a virus. An infant infected with HBV can be asymptomatic or present with a picture of fulminant infection (Karnsakul & Schwarz, 2011).

Risk Factors. Pregnant women in high-risk categories (i.e., they are known to have sexual contact with HBV-infected persons) should be screened so that appropriate follow-up can be provided. Persons in certain ethnic groups, such as Asians (Taiwanese especially) and Australian aborigines; intravenous drug users; and health professionals are at risk for the development of HBV. Individuals living in poor sanitary conditions are also at risk (Karnsakul & Schwarz, 2011).

Management and Prevention. Vaccination is recommended for individuals who are at risk for exposure to HBV, including health care workers, family members of chronic carriers, persons with large numbers of heterosexual partners, and intravenous drug users. HbsAg protein is administered to the deltoid muscle once and then again 1 and 6 months later. If the mother's antigen status is unknown at delivery, titers should be drawn and the woman should be vaccinated if the result is HbsAg positive. If the test results are unavailable or cannot be obtained, the neonate should be treated as if the mother were positive.

Proper and prompt identification of women in high-risk groups and knowledge of HBV status are important in the delivery room to determine whether the infant is at risk for infection. In accordance with universal infection control measures, appropriate barriers are used to protect health care workers from blood and body secretions. Delivery room and nursery personnel should always wear gloves when handling any new infant. The infant of a mother with confirmed HBV infection should be bathed with soap and water immediately, with special attention to removing all blood and secretions present on the skin and hair. The infant may be breastfed (unless the mother's nipples are cracked) and cared for routinely.

■ **Chlamydia.** Chlamydia is a genus of bacteria that grows between cells. Chlamydial infection is the most common sexually transmitted disease. Probably 50% of infected women of childbearing age are asymptomatic. Studies have shown that the infected population comprises sexually active women between 18 and 35 years of age having a high school education or less and three or more sexual partners in the previous 3 months. The infection can present as cervicitis, salpingitis, urethritis, or pelvic inflammatory disease. Chlamydia trachomatis infection has been identified as causing a significant increase in the incidence of PROM, the number of low-birth-weight babies, and the rate of infant mortality (Darville, 2011; Miller, 2004). Thus, screening pregnant women for chlamydia is important. Treatment with erythromycin or clindamycin may prevent transmission to the newborn.

Clinical Manifestations. Chlamydia conjunctivitis can present in the newborn with a very watery discharge that may progress to purulent exudate. Application of erythromycin ointment at birth for ocular prophylaxis successfully treats both chlamydial and gonococcal conjunctivitis. Pneumonia can occur in newborns who have contracted chlamydia from their mother's genital tract. The incubation period is anywhere from 5 days to 3 to 4 months. Typical presentation is tachypnea, barrel chest, and an increased oxygen requirement. The infant may have interstitial infiltrations, hepatosplenomegaly, and increased eosinophils. In a prospective study of chlamydia, there was a 16% incidence of pneumonia in infants identified as being at risk for chlamydial infection (Darville, 2011; Miller, 2004).

Diagnosis of chlamydial infections is based on physical and laboratory examination; in cases of conjunctivitis, Giemsa-stained conjunctival scrapings provide a method of direct fluorescent antibody testing. The definitive diagnosis for chlamydial pneumonia is made by culture of the respiratory tract or identification of high levels of IgM antibodies to chlamydia.

Management and Prevention. Treatment of chlamydia infection in the newborn is usually with ampicillin and gentamicin if the infant's work-up is for generic infection. Once the chlamydia organism is identified, more specific treatment is with erythromycin for 10 to 14 days. If chlamydia is confirmed in a pregnant woman and treated, her sexual partners also require treatment. Rapid screening and diagnosis can be made using monoclonal antibodies. Education and counseling regarding the method of transmission of chlamydia are important. This organism may be present for many years in the female genital tract and produce no symptoms. The organism does not respond to partial treatment; an infected woman and all her sexual partners must receive full treatment as soon as possible. Men should wear condoms during sexual relations to prevent transmission. Without treatment, the severe complications for the woman include pelvic inflammatory disease, ectopic pregnancy, and endometritis. The common newborn complication is pneumonia. Supportive ventilation in the newborn is usually necessary.

■ **Respiratory Syncytial Virus.** Respiratory syncytial virus (RSV) is an infection usually found in older infants. Most infants will have experienced RSV infection by 2 years of age. Between 0.5% and 2% of infants with initial infection will require hospitalization, with most of these less than 6 months of age (American Academy of Pediatrics, 2009). It is thought that maternal antibodies protect infants for the first few weeks of life, but as passive immunity diminishes, these infants become more susceptible (Maldonado, 2011).

Clinical Manifestations. An infant who is infected with RSV before 4 weeks of age may be asymptomatic or may have an upper respiratory infection with fever, bronchiolitis, apnea, or pneumonia. There may be a definite need for assisted ventilation, and deaths have occurred in rapidly fulminating disease, for which there is little available treatment. Small preterm infants who are already in significant pulmonary and cardiac jeopardy with respiratory distress syndrome or bronchopulmonary dysplasia are especially susceptible to the development of severe infections. Nosocomial transmission of the virus between caretakers is possible; such transmission appears to result in less severe infection. The first clinical signs of transmission include a clear nasal discharge at approximately 10 to 52 days of life, followed by cough and wheezing. Radiologic changes compatible with pneumonia may also be found (Leader & Kohlhase, 2002; Maldonado, 2011).

Treatment and Prevention. Good hand washing is extremely important in the prevention of transmission of RSV between critically ill patients. It has been shown that RSV-infected secretions can remain viable for up to 6 hours on countertops, 45 minutes on cloth gowns and paper tissues, and 20 minutes on skin. Thus, all infected infants should be cared for in cohort. Caretakers should be consistently assigned to decrease transmission rates. Gown and glove precautions can significantly reduce nosocomial transmission of RSV (Leader & Kohlhase, 2002; Maldonado, 2011).

Any infant with a runny nose, nasal congestion, or unexplained apnea should be considered for isolation and investigated for RSV infection. Attention should be specific for those infants older than 4 weeks of corrected age. Specific cultures and screens should be performed because specific treatment is available if RSV is found.

RSV prophylaxis with Palivizumab, a monoclonal antibody, is recommended for certain "at risk" infants. It is given intramuscularly once a month during RSV season, which is usually November through March in most parts of the United States. Palivizumab prophylaxis has been very successful in preventing hospitalizations in these infants who were born premature or had significant respiratory complications after birth (AAP, 2010; Maldonado, 2011).

Management. RSV infection is often self-limited, resolving by 10 to 14 days in uncomplicated cases. When hospitalization is required, the main focus is on prevention of dehydration and respiratory management. With severe or unusually complicated cases, mechanical ventilation may be required. Antibiotics are not effective against RSV.

Ribavirin is occasionally used in cases of complicated RSV pneumonia. Ribavirin administration should be closely monitored by those who have been trained appropriately (Leader & Kohlhase, 2003; Maldonado, 2011). Ribavirin can be administered safely to infants receiving mechanical ventilation and to infants in an oxygen hood. Specific safety precautions should be taken to protect the caretaker, because ribavirin has been identified as being potentially teratogenic. Protective measures include wearing a gown, gloves, and mask when in direct contact with the particles or mist containing ribavirin. Ideally, no pregnant woman would take care of an infant with RSV who is receiving ribavirin. Close monitoring of the pulmonary status, including the use of oxygen and mechanical ventilation, may be necessary. Isolation of the infected infant from other infants who could potentially be infected is important; the usual method for isolation is to minimize risk of the spread of the airborne virus and ribavirin particles.

Fungal Agents

■ ***Candida Albicans.*** *Candida* species is a fungus that is frequently found in humans, and *C. albicans* is the most prevalent form in neonates. *Candida* organisms are oval, yeast-like cells that can bud to reproduce. *C. albicans* produces endotoxins, hemolysis, pyrogens, and proteolytic enzymes that are damaging to tissues (Bendel, 2011). Early recognition and treatment of fungal infection are imperative to prevent severe CNS complications and death. Prolonged broad-spectrum antibiotic treatment for small premature infants may predispose infants to *Candida* overgrowth in the gastrointestinal tract. This overgrowth may predispose the infant to disseminated fungemia. Administration of hyperalimentation, frequent use of indwelling venous lines, and invasive procedures may also predispose the infant to *C. albicans* infection. One study has identified previous antibiotic therapy and assisted ventilation as the major factors that correlate to *Candida* infection (Bendel, 2011).

Clinical Manifestations. The newborn infected with *C. albicans* presents a picture similar to that of any septic infant. These newborns present with serious clinical signs of infection, often worsening with no presence of positive cultures. The infant is typically 20 to 30 days of age, has difficulties with oral feeds, depends on hyperalimentation, and has been given multiple courses of antibiotics. The infant may have respiratory distress, abdominal distention, guaiac-positive stools, carbohydrate intolerance, candiduria, temperature instability, and hypotension (Bendel, 2011).

Differential Diagnosis. A positive *Candida* culture should never be considered a contaminated specimen. Intermittently positive cultures may reflect transient candidemia, and, usually, removal of any indwelling catheters and lines and changing of antibiotic therapy may be indicated. In symptomatic low-birth-weight infants with positive systemic cultures, treatment should begin pending culture results.

Collaborative Management. The most effective drug for treatment of *C. albicans* infection is amphotericin B. This toxic, potent antifungal agent must be used cautiously. The initial dose is 0.1 to 0.3 mg/kg given intravenously over a period of 2 to 6 hours. The maintenance dosage is 0.5 to 1.0 mg/kg/d over 2 to 6 hours. Lower doses are started until higher doses can be tolerated. Increments of 0.1 mg/kg/d are used to increase the daily dose slowly. Many infants tolerate a total dose of 20 mg/kg if titrated over approximately 1 month. Often, if organ involvement is minimal, infants can be successfully given lower doses. If meningitis is suspected, 5-fluorouracil (5-FU) may be used. This antifungal agent acts to inhibit DNA synthesis so that *Candida* replication cannot occur.

Kidney toxicity is a major side effect of amphotericin B therapy because it causes renal vasoconstriction and decreases both renal blood flow and glomerular filtration rate. This damage can result in hyponatremia, hypokalemia, increased blood urea nitrogen, and increased creatinine, as well as acidosis. If the medication makes the patient oliguric, most physicians recommend stopping the drug until the next day. Thrombocytopenia, granulocytopenia, fever, nausea, and vomiting are the common side effects associated with amphotericin B. One major side effect of 5-FU is bone marrow depression, resulting in a decreased platelet count (Bendel, 2011).

Because of the insidious onset of candidiasis, the septic infant who is not responding to traditional antibiotic treatment may have *Candida*. Catheter tips at intravenous sites and percutaneous lines should be changed and cultured. Urine can easily be cultured for the presence of *Candida*. Thrush and monilial rashes are indicative of candidiasis. These can easily be treated with oral and local antifungal agents. Monitoring of infants receiving amphotericin B is challenging, because infants may have reactions to this medication. Blood pressure should be monitored every half hour, and urine output should be followed up closely. Vital signs and laboratory work, including liver enzyme tests, should be followed up daily to detect early signs of neonatal toxicity (Bendel, 2011).

Nosocomial Infections

Both colonization and infection are nosocomial events, meaning "of or related to a hospital." The common meaning of the term *nosocomial* is "hospital acquired." Nursery-acquired infections are reported to the Centers for Disease Control and Prevention, which has a National Nosocomial Infections Surveillance System. The incidence of nosocomial infections in NICUs is 5% to 25% (Heath & Zerr, 2005). Critically ill infants who remain in a pathogen-filled environment are often in jeopardy because of their prolonged length of stay in the hospital. The mortality rate associated with these infections is between 5% and 20%, depending on the geographic area and specific birth-weight groups (Heath & Zerr, 2005).

Coagulase-negative staphylococcus has been identified as a major cause of nosocomial infections. Low birth weight, multiple gestation, and prolonged hospitalization are significant factors for nosocomial infection. Yeast infections often occur if previous antibiotic therapy has been given. This infection is also associated with colonization of vascular catheters, assisted ventilation, and necrotizing enterocolitis (Maldonado et al., 2011).

Nursery epidemics can be caused by gram-negative and gram-positive or viral organisms because they have (1) the ability to colonize or infect human skin or the gastrointestinal tract, (2) the ability to be carried from person to person by hand contact, and (3) characteristics that allow existence on hands of personnel or in fluids or on inanimate objects, including intravenous fluids, respiratory support equipment, solutions used for medications, disinfectants, and banked breast milk (Maldonado et al., 2011).

Resistance to antibiotics is a serious problem in many NICUs, particularly with gram-negative enteric pathogens. Aminoglycoside resistance is a problem in many urban nurseries, as are colonization and infection with methicillin-resistant *S. aureus*. Respiratory infections with RSV, influenza virus, parainfluenza virus, rhinovirus, and echovirus occur in many nurseries. These are more difficult to identify and thus more difficult to report. CMV infection has been reported as a transfusion-related problem in low-birth-weight infants, thus prompting the current policy of using CMV-screened blood donors.

Hepatitis A infection has also been reported as a transfusion-related problem that may develop in infants and staff in NICUs (Britt, 2011). Hepatitis C has been linked to use of immunoglobulins such as Gammagard by Baxter Laboratories, Deerfield, IL (Lindenbach et al., 2005). Almost any organism given the right environment and support can become a nosocomially transmitted infection.

INFECTION CONTROL POLICIES

Policies and procedures in nurseries should be set up by the hospital infection control committee based on the recommendations of the American Academy of Pediatrics and the CDC. The significance of these policies to newborns should be detailed in a hospital policy book. The following topics should be covered: (1) ocular prophylaxis, (2) skin and cord care, (3) nursery staff, (4) nursery design and environment, (5) hand washing, (6) staff apparel, (7) isolation, (8) visitors, (9) employee health, and (10) epidemic control (Maldonado et al., 2011). The simplest, most effective weapon for preventing infection is the liberal use of soap and water!

SUMMARY

Many factors place the neonate at high risk for infection. The nurse is in a unique role to implement methods for prevention of infection in nurseries, to detect early signs and symptoms of infection, and to participate in infection control. A better understanding of the neonatal immune system, methods of perinatal acquisition of organisms, common microorganisms, signs and symptoms of infections, and appropriate therapy provides the nurse with a sound basis for management of care as well as the development of hospital infection control policies for the NICU.

CASE STUDY

■ **Identification of the Problem.** Term, female infant admitted to Well Baby Nursery following repeat C-section. Presented with grunting respirations, nasal flaring, and retractions (GFR) by 15 minutes of age.

■ **Assessment: History.** Baby S was delivered via repeat C-section under spinal anesthesia to a G2P1001 female with EGA of 39 weeks. Maternal labs: Blood type A$^+$, GBS negative at 35 weeks. RPR nonreactive, Hep B negative, HIV negative, and Rubella immune. Perinatal history: mother reports a UTI at 36 weeks gestation, which was treated with Macrodantin. No other problems were noted. Other than this treatment, only prenatal vitamins were taken during pregnancy. Membranes ruptured at delivery with clear amniotic fluid. Apgars: 8 at 1 minute and 9 at 5 minutes. The infant only required drying and stimulation at delivery. She was admitted to the WBN at 10 minutes of age for usual newborn care. The NNP was called to evaluate the infant at 15 minutes of age for GFR. An ABG, CBC with diff, and CRP were obtained. The ABG results were: pH 7.223 $PaCO_2$ 66 PaO_2 44. CBC and CRP results pending. The infant was transferred to the NICU with blow-by O_2 for further evaluation and treatment.

■ Physical Examination on Admission to the NICU

- GENERAL: term female infant with marked acrocyanosis. Resting supine with marked grunting, nasal flaring, and subcostal retractions; SpO_2 91% with blow-by O_2 at 5 L/min
- HEENT: normocephalic, AF soft and slightly concave; bilateral red reflexes and pupils equally reactive to light; ears normally placed; nares patent
- RESP: BBS clear to auscultation; marked GFR; RR 40
- CV: HR regular with normal sinus rhythm; HR 170; no murmur noted; brachial and femoral pulses 2+; capillary refill 4 seconds; BP: 76/35; mean BP: 37
- ABD: abdomen soft and nontender with no hepatosplenomegaly or masses palpable; three-vessel cord
- GI/GU: normal female infant genitalia; patent anus; anal wink present
- NEURO: decreased responses, with eyes open and unblinking; muscle tone markedly decreased
- SKIN: pale pink with mottling; no bruises or "birthmarks" noted
- EXTREMITIES: good passive ROM with 10 fingers and toes each extremity; no hip clunks noted

■ Differential Diagnoses

- Transient tachypnea of the newborn
- Pneumothorax
- Sepsis
- Pneumonia
- Shock

Diagnostic Tests

Laboratory tests:

- CBC/differenteral: WBC: 4.7 Hgb: 14.2 Hct: 45.2 Platelet count: 105,000 Segs: 35 Bands: 21 Metas: 2 Myelos: 1
- CRP: 6.8
- Repeat ABG: pH 7.12 $PaCO_2$ 71 PaO_2 49
- Blood cultures X 2. Endotracheal secretion culture. Blood cultures positive at 12 hours for gram-positive cocci; MIC pending

Imaging tests:

- Chest x-ray: Good expansion with mild reticulogranular appearance; no pneumothorax

Working Diagnosis. GBS sepsis with possible GBS pneumonia (based on preliminary BC report and chest x-ray appearance).

Development of Management Plan

- Respiratory support with mechanical ventilation as needed
- UAC and UVC placement for monitoring, sampling, and fluid management
- Continuous monitoring of arterial blood pressure, vital signs and neurologic status, every 2 to 4 hours
- CBC/diff and CRP every a.m.
- BMP at 12 hours of life and every a.m.
- ABG every 3 to 4 hours as needed for ventilator management
- Maintenance fluid support; fluid boluses to support intravascular volume
- Vasopressors to maintain adequate blood pressure and cerebral blood flow
- Ampicillin and gentamicin IV
- CSF cultures when stable

Implementation and Evaluation of Effectiveness

- Implementation of management plan (immediately after initial assessment in the NICU):
  - Infant intubated within the first 30 minutes of life and placed on mechanical ventilation with following settings: SIMV: 40 PIP: 24 Peep: 4 PSV: 12 FiO_2 50% (adjusted to keep SpO_2 90%–97%)
  - Chest x-ray to verify ETT placement
  - UAC and UVC placed; abdominal x-ray to verify umbilical line placement
  - Dopamine 10 mcg/kg/min initiated by 1 hour of life; weaned to 5 mcg/kg/min by 36 hours
- Effectiveness of management plan:
  - Despite maximum ventilatory support, Baby S developed severe PPHN and was transferred to a Children's Hospital for possible ECMO on day 3 of life
  - Blood cultures and ETT cultures were positive for Group B strep
  - CSF cultures were negative
  - GBS sepsis and GBS pneumonia were successfully treated with antibiotics

Outcome. The infant did well at the receiving hospital and did not require ECMO. She was treated with iNO for 3 days and was extubated by day 9 of life. Follow-up blood cultures were negative after 14 days of IV antibiotics. She was discharged home at 3 weeks of age and is developmentally appropriate at 3 years of age.

Discussion. Although the incidence of GBS sepsis is decreasing, it still remains the #1 cause of EOS in the newborn (Committee on Infectious Diseases and Committee on Fetus and Newborn, 2011). In the case presented, a high level of suspicion for sepsis was based on the history of the UTI in the mother. Although a woman's GBS screen is negative at the time it is tested, she may become positive later or the test may reveal a false negative—depending on the technique used (Pulver et al., 2009). Early recognition and rapid treatment can mean the difference between a poor outcome and a good outcome.

References

Committee on Infections Diseases and Committee on Fetus and Newborn. (2011). Policy statement: Recommendations for the prevention of perinatal group b streptococcal (GBS) disease. *Pediatrics, 128*(3), 1–5. doi:10.1542/peds.2011–1466. Retrieved from http://pediatrics.aappublications.org/content/early/20011/07/28/peds.2011–1466

Pulver, L. S., Hopfenbeck, M. M., Young, P. C., Stoddard, G. J., Korgenski, K., Daly, J., & Byington, C. L. (2009). Continued early onset group B streptococcal infections in the era of intrapartum prophylaxis. *Journal of Perinatology, 29*(1), 20–25.

EVIDENCE-BASED PRACTICE BOX

One of the most successful evidence-based practice changes in recent history has been the implementation of a Group B beta hemolytic streptococcus (GBS) prophylaxis protocol for the prevention of GBS sepsis in the newborn. During the 1970s, GBS sepsis exceeded *E. coli* as the leading cause of sepsis and meningitis in newborns (Edwards, Nizet, & Baker, 2005). Cases of GBS sepsis continued to increase over the next two decades. In 1996, the CDC published the first guidelines for the prevention of perinatal group B streptococcal disease, which were based on case reports and clinical trials demonstrating the effectiveness of intrapartum administration of antibiotics to women who were considered at risk for transmitting GBS to their newborns. These guidelines offered two prevention methods, a risk-based approach or a culture-based approach. Although there was a decrease in cases, GBS disease remained a leading

(*continued*)

cause of neonatal sepsis. Further studies comparing the two strategies revealed data that supported the culture-based method as the most effective strategy in preventing neonatal GBS disease. Therefore, in 2002, the CDC replaced the 1996 guidelines with recommendations that all pregnant women be screened for GBS between 35 and 37 weeks gestation with the use of intrapartum antibiotic administration during labor for culture positive women.

Significant declines in incidence of GBS disease occurred after the implementation of the 1996 guidelines, but a more dramatic decrease occurred after the updated guidelines in 2002. The CDC and other organizations continued to collect data and the guidelines were updated again in 2010. Few changes were made except for information related to testing methods and recommendations for antibiotics for women with penicillin allergy (CDC, 2010). Due to these recommendations, the incidence of neonatal GBS disease has decreased from 1.7 cases per 1,000 live births before the first guidelines to less than 0.4 cases per 1,000 live births in 2005 (Phares et al., 2008). Current data demonstrate a continued decline. Despite these dramatic results, GBS disease remains the leading cause of disease-related morbidity and mortality among newborns. It is important that we continue to evaluate our practices and make changes that are based on current evidence.

References

CDC. (2010). Prevention of perinatal group B streptococcal disease: Recommendations and Reports. *MMWR, 59*(RR10), 1–32.

Edwards, M. S., Nizet, V., & Baker, C. J. (2005). Group B streptococcal infections. In J. S. Remington & J. O. Klein (Eds.), *Infectious diseases of the fetus and newborn* (6th ed., pp. 385–392).

Phares, C. R., Lynfield, R., Farley, M. M., Mohle-Boetani, J., Harrison, L. H., Petit, S., ... Active Bacterial Core surveillance/ Emerging Infections Program Network. (2008). Epidemiology of invasive group B streptococcal disease in the Unites States, 1999–2005. *Journal of the American Medical Association, 299*(17), 2056–2065.

ACKNOWLEDGMENT

The author is indebted to Carole Kenner and Judy Wright Lott, whose previous contributions to this chapter and tables provided the strong baseline framework and inspiration for the current version.

ONLINE RESOURCES

Immunity of the newborn
http://www.uptodate.com/contents/immunity-of-the-newborn

Neonatal immunity
http://www.immunopaedia.org.za/index.php?id=617

Streptococcal infections
http://www.nhs.uk/conditions/Streptococcal-infections/Pages/Introduction.aspx

REFERENCES

Adair, C. E., Kowalsky, L., Quon, H., Ma, D., Stoffman, J., McGeer, A., ... Davies, H. D. (2003). Risk factors for early-onset group B streptococcal disease in neonates: A population-based case-control study. *Canadian Medical Association Journal, 169*, 198.

American Academy of Pediatrics. (2009). Respiratory syncytial virus. In L. K. Pickering, C. J. Baker, D. W. Kimberlin & S. S. Long (Eds.), *Red book: 2009 report of the Committee on Infectious Diseases* (28th ed.). Elk Grove Village, IL: American Academy of Pediatrics.

Anderson-Berry, A. L., Bellig, L. L., & Ohnig, B. L. (2012) Neonatal sepsis. In T. Rosenkrantz, D. A. Clark, S. S. MacGilvray & M. L. Windle (Eds.), *Medscape reference: Drugs, diseases & procedures*. Retrieved July 12, 2012, from http://emedicine.medscape.com/article/978352-overview

Baltimore, R. S. (2003). Neonatal infection epidemiology and management. *Pediatric Drugs, 5*(1), 723–740.

Bendel, C. M. (2011). Candidiasis. In J. S. Remington, J. O. Klein, C. B. Wilson, V. Nizet, & Y. A. Maldonado (Eds.), *Infectious diseases of the fetus and newborn* (7th ed., pp. 2505–2557). Philadelphia, PA: Elsevier.

Benedetto, C., Tibaldi, C., Marozio, L., Marini, S., Masuelli, G., Pelissetto, S., ... Latino, M. A. (2004). Cervicovaginal infections during pregnancy: Epidemiological and microbiological aspects. *Journal of Maternal-Fetal and Neonatal Medicine, 16*, 9–12.

Bortolussi, R., & Mailman, T. L. (2011). Listeriosis. In J. S. Remington, J. O. Klein, C. B. Wilson, V. Nizet & Y. A. Maldonado (Eds.), *Infectious diseases of the fetus and newborn* (7th ed., pp. 1166–1215). Philadelphia, PA: Elsevier.

Britt, W. (2011). Cytomegalovirus. In J. S. Remington, J. O. Klein, C. B. Wilson, V. Nizet & Y. A. Maldonado (Eds.), *Infectious diseases of the fetus and newborn* (7th ed., pp. 1729–1842). Philadelphia, PA: Elsevier.

Darmstadt, G. L., Zaidi, A. K. M., & B. J. Stoll. (2011). Neonatal infections. In J. S. Remington, J. O. Klein, C. B. Wilson, V. Nizet & Y. A. Maldonado (Eds.), *Infectious diseases of the fetus and newborn* (7th ed., pp. 67–133). Philadelphia, PA: Elsevier.

Darville, T. (2011). *Chlamydia* infections. In J. S. Remington, J. O. Klein, C. B. Wilson, V. Nizet & Y. A. Maldonado (Eds.), *Infectious diseases of the fetus and newborn* (7th ed., pp. 1492–1508). Philadelphia, PA: Elsevier.

Edwards, M. S., Nizet, V., & Baker, C. J. (2005). Group B streptococcal infections. In J. S. Remington & J. O. Klein (Eds.), *Infectious diseases of the fetus and newborn infant* (6th ed., pp. 406–464). Philadelphia, PA: Saunders.

Embree, J. E. (2011). Gonococcal infections. In J. S. Remington, J. O. Klein, C. B. Wilson, V. Nizet & Y. A. Maldonado (Eds.), *Infectious diseases of the fetus and newborn* (7th ed., pp. 1282–1302). Philadelphia, PA: Elsevier.

Gagnon, A. J., & Gibbs, R. S. (2011). Obstetric factors associated with infections of the fetus and newborn. In J. S. Remington, J. O. Klein, C. B. Wilson, V. Nizet & Y. A. Maldonado (Eds.), *Infectious diseases of the fetus and newborn* (7th ed., pp. 134–202). Philadelphia, PA: Elsevier.

Gerdes, J. S., & Polin, R. (1998). Early diagnosis and treatment of neonatal sepsis. *Indian Journal of Pediatrics, 65*, 63–78.

Gershon, A. A. (2011). Chickenpox, measles, and mumps. In J. S. Remington, J. O. Klein, C. B. Wilson, V. Nizet & Y. A. Maldonado (Eds.), *Infectious diseases of the fetus and newborn* (7th ed., pp. 1625–1728). Philadelphia, PA: Elsevier.

Gregg, N. M. (1941). Congenital cataract following German measles in the mother. *Transactions of the Ophthalmological Society of Australia, 3*, 35.

Gutierrez, K. M., Whitley, R. J., & Arvin, A. M. (2011). Herpes simplex virus infections. In J. S. Remington, J. O. Klein, C. B. Wilson, V. Nizet & Y. A. Maldonado (Eds.), *Infectious diseases of the fetus and newborn* (7th ed., pp. 1970–2014). Philadelphia, PA: Elsevier.

Healy, C. M., Palazzi, D. L., Edwards, M. S., Campbell, J. R., & Baker, C. J. (2004). Features of invasive staphylococcal disease in neonates. *Pediatrics, 114*, 953–961.

Heath, J. A., & Zerr, D. M. (2005). Infections acquired in the nursery: Epidemiology and control. In J. S. Remington & J. O. Klein (Eds.), *Infectious diseases of the fetus and newborn infant* (6th ed., pp. 1179–1206). Philadelphia, PA: Saunders.

Kapur, R., Yoder, M. C., & Polin, R. A. (2002). Developmental immunology. In A. A. Fanaroff & R. J. Martin (Eds.), *Neonatal-perinatal medicine: Diseases of the fetus and infant* (7th ed.). St Louis, MO: Mosby.

Karnsakul, W., & Schwarz, K. B. (2011). In J. S. Remington, J. O. Klein, C. B. Wilson, V. Nizet & Y. A. Maldonado (Eds.), *Infectious diseases of the fetus and newborn* (7th ed., pp. 1939–1969). Philadelphia, PA: Elsevier.

Kollman, T. R., & Dobson, S. (2011). Syphilis. In J. S. Remington, J. O. Klein, C. B. Wilson, V. Nizet & Y. A. Maldonado (Eds.), *Infectious diseases of the fetus and newborn* (7th ed., pp. 1303–1401). Philadelphia, PA: Elsevier.

Langlet, C., Gaugler, C., Castaing, M., Astruc, D., Falkenrodt, A., Neuville, A., & Messer, J. (2003). An uncommon case of disseminated neonatal herpes simplex infection presenting with pneumonia and pleural effusions. *European Journal of Pediatrics, 162*, 532–533.

Leader, S., & Kohlhase, K. (2002). Respiratory syncytial virus-coded pediatric hospitalizations, 1997 to 1999. *Pediatric Infectious Diseases Journal, 21*, 629–632.

Lewis, D. B., & Wilson, C. B. (2011). Developmental immunology and role of host defenses in fetal and neonatal susceptibility to infection. In J. S. Remington, J. O. Klein, C. B. Wilson, V. Nizet & Y. A. Maldonado (Eds.), *Infectious diseases of the fetus and newborn* (7th ed., pp. 203–452). Philadelphia, PA: Elsevier.

Lindenbach, B. D., Evans, M. J., Syder, A. J., Wölk, B., Tellinghuisen, T. L., Liu, C. C., ... Rice, C. M. (2005). Complete replication of hepatitis C virus in cell culture. *Science, 309*(5734), 623–626.

Lott, J. W., & Kilb, J. R. (1992). The selection of antibacterial agents for treatment of neonatal infection. *Neonatal Pharmacy Quarterly, 1*(1), 19–29.

Maldonado, Y. A. (2011). Less common viral infections. In J. S. Remington, J. O. Klein, C. B. Wilson, V. Nizet & Y. A. Maldonado (Eds.), *Infectious diseases of the fetus and newborn* (7th ed., pp. 2187–2217). Philadelphia, PA: Elsevier.

Maldonado, Y. A., Nizet, V., Klein, J. O., Remington, J. S., & Wilson, C. B. (2011). Current concepts of infections of the fetus and newborn infant. In J. S. Remington, J. O. Klein, C. B. Wilson, V. Nizet & Y. A. Maldonado (Eds.), *Infectious diseases of the fetus and newborn* (7th ed., pp. 23–67). Philadelphia, PA: Elsevier.

Marcy, S. M., Baker, C. & Palazzi, D. L. (2005). Bacterial sepsis and meningitis. In J. S. Remington & J. O. Klein (Eds.), *Infectious diseases of the fetus and newborn infant* (6th ed., pp. 247–296). Philadelphia, PA: Saunders.

McLean, H., & Reef, S. E. (2012). Chapter 3: Infectious diseases related to travel. In Centers for Disease Control and Prevention (Ed.), *CDC information for international travel*. Atlanta, GA: CDC.

Miller, K. E. (2004). Chlamydia trachomatis exposure in newborns. *American Family Physician, 69*, 727–730.

Nizet, V., & Klein, J. O. (2011). Bacterial sepsis and meningitis. In J. S. Remington, J. O. Klein, C. B. Wilson, V. Nizet & Y. A. Maldonado (Eds.), *Infectious diseases of the fetus and newborn* (7th ed., pp. 526–656). Philadelphia, PA: Elsevier.

Ogunyemi, D., & Hernández-Loera, G. E. (2004). The impact of antenatal cocaine use on maternal characteristics and neonatal outcomes. *Journal of Maternal-Fetal and Neonatal Medicine, 15*, 253–257.

Orschein, R. C., Shinefield, H. R., & St. Geme III, J. W. (2005). Staphylococcal infections. In J. S. Remington & J. O. Klein (Eds.), *Infectious diseases of the fetus and newborn infant* (6th ed., pp 513–544). Philadelphia, PA: Saunders.

Plotkin, S. A., Reef, S. E., Cooper, L. Z., & Alford, C. A. (2011). Rubella. In J. S. Remington, J. O. Klein, C. B. Wilson, V. Nizet & Y. A. Maldonado (Eds.), *Infectious diseases of the fetus and newborn* (7th ed., pp. 2080–2172). Philadelphia, PA: Elsevier.

Polin, R. A., & the Committee on Fetus and Newborn. (2012). Management of neonates with suspected or proven early-onset bacterial sepsis. *Pediatrics, 129*(5), 1006–1015.

Remington, J. S., McCleod, R., Wilson, C. B., & Desmont, G. (2011). Toxoplasmosis. In J. S. Remington, J. O. Klein, C. B. Wilson, V. Nizet & Y. A. Maldonado (Eds.), *Infectious diseases of the fetus and newborn* (7th ed., pp. 2219–2468). Philadelphia, PA: Elsevier.

Stoll, B. J., Hansen, N., Fanaroff, A. A., Wright, L. L., Carlo, W. A., Ehrenkranz, R. A., ... Poole, W. K. (2004). To tap or not to tap: High likelihood of meningitis without infection among very low birth weight infants. *Pediatrics, 113*, 1181–1186.

Stoll, B. J., Hansen, N. I., Sánchez, P. J., Faix, R. G., Poindexter, B. B., Van Meurs, K. P., ... Eunice Kennedy Shriver National Institute of Child Health and Human Development Neonatal Research Network. (2011). Early onset neonatal sepsis: The burden of Group B streptococcal and *E. coli* disease continues. *Pediatrics, 127*(5), 817–826.

Uhl, J. R., Vetter, E. A., Boldt, K. L., Johnston, B. W., Ramin, K. D., Adams, M. J., ... Cockerill, F. R., 3rd. (2005). Use of the Roche LightCycler Strep B assay for detection of group B streptococcus from vaginal and rectal swabs. *Journal of Clinical Microbiology, 43*(8), 4046–4051.

Volpe, J. J. (2008). Postnatal sepsis, necrotizing entercolitis, and the critical role of systemic inflammation in white matter injury in premature infants. (Editorial). *Journal of Pediatrics, 153*, 160–163. doi:10.1016/j.jpeds.2008.04.057

Weinberg, G. A., & D'Angio, C. T. (2011) Laboratory aids for diagnosis of neonatal sepsis. In J. S. Remington, J. O. Klein, C. B. Wilson, V. Nizet & Y. A. Maldonado (Eds.), *Infectious diseases of the fetus and newborn* (7th ed., pp. 2720–2760). Philadelphia, PA: Elsevier.

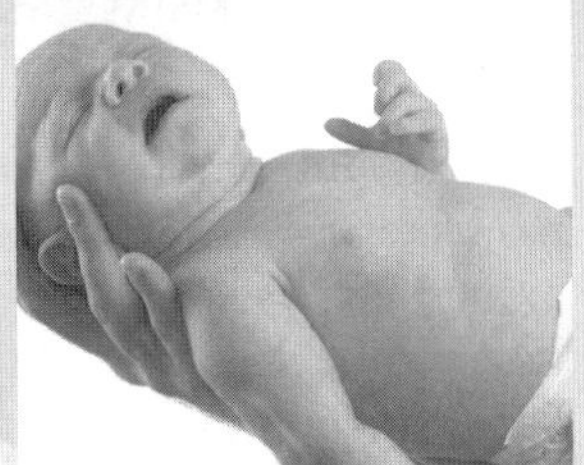

CHAPTER 12

Integumentary System

■ Carolyn Houska Lund and Joanne McManus Kuller

Skin phenomena, along with other examination findings, are used to assess maturity, duration of pregnancy, and neonatal vitality. The skin of a preterm infant makes up 13% of the body weight, compared with 3% in adults. This large organ provides a barrier against infection, protects internal organs, contributes to temperature regulation and prevention of insensible water loss (ISWL), stores fats, excretes electrolytes and water, and provides tactile sensory input. The sensations of touch, pressure, temperature, pain, and itch are received by millions of microscopic dermal nerve endings. The skin is instrumental in early establishment of the mother–infant relationship in that the quality of touch and stimulation that an infant receives is responsible for the infant's later responses to other people and to the environment. Thus, the skin fulfills a task of vital importance, particularly in the area of maternal–child nursing.

Care practices that affect the fragile, underdeveloped skin of the premature infant present major concerns as well as dilemmas for care providers. Life support and monitoring equipment must be securely attached and frequently removed or replaced; this practice can cause trauma to the skin. Necessary invasive procedures, such as vascular access, blood sampling, and chest tube insertion, invade the skin's barrier. Trauma to skin can result in the diversion of an excessive proportion of caloric intake to tissue repair. Other effects of trauma to premature skin include the energy demands of electrolyte imbalances and increased evaporative heat loss through damaged or immature skin and the risk of toxicity when substances are applied to the skin surface.

Trauma to the skin creates portals of entry for bacteria and fungus in an already immune-compromised host. Significant morbidity and mortality can be attributed to practices that cause either trauma to skin or alterations in normal skin function. Iatrogenically caused skin problems—including burns and caustic lesions from isopropyl alcohol and erythema and skin craters from transcutaneous oxygen monitoring—have been reported. Increased skin permeability and percutaneous toxicity from drugs and chemicals have also been documented in neonates.

This chapter covers the development and structure of skin, the normal physiologic variations in newborn skin, and dermatologic diseases. This information is then incorporated into the management of the neonatal skin.

SKIN STRUCTURE AND FUNCTION

Skin consists of three anatomically distinct layers: the epidermis, the dermis, and the subcutaneous tissue. The uppermost layer of the epidermis is the stratum corneum, primarily composed of nonliving cells made of protein, with layers of lipids that bind them; this has been described as similar to the "bricks and mortar of a wall." These cells, once exfoliated in utero, form part of the vernix caseosa, the cheese-like substance that covers and protects fetal skin. The bottom, living basal layer contain keratinocytes, which constantly replace the keratin cells in the stratum corneum; it takes approximately 26 days for keratinocytes to migrate up to the stratum corneum. Approximately 20% of an adult's protein requirement is needed for this purpose. Keratin-forming cells—which cornify the outer layer of the epidermis—and melanocytes are contained in the lower levels of the epidermis. Melanocytes begin producing melanin, or pigment, before birth and distribute it to the epidermal cells. Active pigmentary activity can be observed before birth in the epidermis of infants of dark-skinned races, but little evidence of such activity exists in white fetuses (Moore & Persaud, 2008).

The dermis lies directly under the epidermis and is 2 to 4 mm thick at birth. It is a closely woven layer of collagen, a fibrous protein, and elastin fibers. This fibrous complex provides mechanical strength as well as elasticity and allows the skin to withstand frictional stress while extending easily over joints. At term, the dermis is well organized but is thinner and has a higher water content compared to the adult dermis (Loomis, Koss, & Chu, 2008). Many nerves and a rich supply of blood vessels are contained there. They nourish the skin cells and act as carriers of the sensations of heat, touch, pressure, and pain from the skin to the brain.

Hair originates from deep in the dermis. Down-growths, called epidermal ridges, which extend into the developing dermis, result from a proliferation of cells in the basal layer. These ridges are permanently established by 17 weeks gestation and produce ridges and grooves on the surface of the palms including the fingers, and on the soles of the feet including the toes.

Determined genetically, this type of pattern constitutes the basis for the use of fingerprints in criminal investigations and medical genetics. Dermatoglyphics is the study of the pattern of these epidermal ridges. The presence of abnormal chromosome complements affects the development of the ridge-patterns. For example, infants with Down syndrome exhibit distinctive hand and feet patterns that are of diagnostic value (Moore & Persaud, 2008).

The major component of the subcutaneous layer is fatty connective tissue. The subcutaneous fat functions as a heat insulator, a shock absorber, and a calorie reserve area. Fat accumulation occurs predominantly in the last trimester. Sebaceous glands are found in both the dermis and the subcutaneous layer. Well-developed and potentially functional at birth, these glands have only minimal function until puberty. Sweat glands are also found in the dermis and the subcutaneous layer and are affected directly by external environmental temperature. In premature infants, sweat gland maturation occurs between 21 and 33 days of age. In term infants, this maturation occurs at about 5 days of age. Poor sweat production in the premature infant is caused by sweat gland immaturity. However, adult function is not achieved until the second or third year of life.

Term infant skin is soft, wrinkled, velvety, and covered with vernix caseosa (Visscher et al., 2005). Transformation of the fetal circulation is evident soon after the cord is cut, as the skin develops the intense red coloration characteristic of the newborn. This color may remain for hours. A blue, blotchy appearance may occur if the infant is exposed to a cool environment.

The insulating layer of vernix is usually lost during the first few days of life through traditional newborn skin care. This results in a loss of insulation for the stratum corneum, which then peels off, thus resulting in skin with a grayish-white or yellowish hue. Visible desquamation of newborn skin comes to an end after about 7 days. Vernix may provide bactericidal protection and contributes to the development of epidermal barrier function, heat flux, and surface electrical activities (Hoath, Narendran, & Visscher, 2001; Hoath & Pickins, 2003).

In comparison with the skin of the term infant, the premature infant's skin is more transparent, gelatinous, and unwrinkled. Lanugo, which has been lost in the full-term infant, may be present in varying degrees and is one criterion used to estimate gestational age. Additionally, subcutaneous edema may be present and is clinical evidence of a cutaneous excess of water and sodium. This edema decreases within the first few days of life, and the skin then lies loosely over the infant's entire body. The immaturity of the infant's skin is linked to the premature newborn's difficulty maintaining body temperature. A poorly developed fat supply and a large body surface area in relation to body weight add to temperature instability.

The premature infant has been shown to have a less well-developed stratum corneum; at less than 30 weeks gestation there may be only two to three layers of stratum corneum (Figure 12.1). This immaturity results in the premature infant's decreased capacity to resist particles, viruses, parasites, and bacteria in the external environment, thus leaving the infant readily susceptible to infection and irritation of the skin.

Transferring from the intrauterine aquatic environment to the external atmospheric environment stimulates and accelerates maturation of skin function. Embryologic skin development is described in Box 12.1.

Developmental Variations

Several factors are responsible for the functional differences between premature and term infants' skin. These differences subside with increasing gestational and postnatal age (Table 12.1).

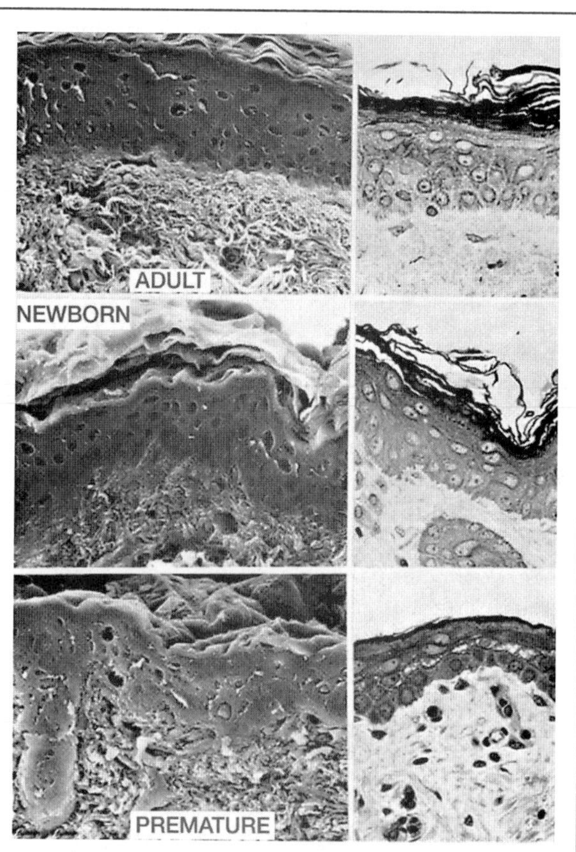

FIGURE 12.1 Photomicrograph of stratum corneum in an adult, in a full-term newborn, and in a premature infant of 28 weeks gestation.
Reprinted with permission from Holbrook (1982).

BOX 12.1

EMBRYOLOGIC DEVELOPMENT OF SKIN

The skin consists of two morphologically different layers, derived from two different germ layers. The epithelial structures (epidermis, pilosebaceous-apocrine unit, eccrine unit, and nails) are ectodermal derivatives. The ectoderm also gives rise to the hair, the teeth, and the sense organs of smell, taste, hearing, vision, and touch—everything involved with events that occur outside the organism. Mesenchymal structures (collagen, reticular, and elastic fibers; blood vessels; muscles; and fat) originate from the mesoderm. These developments are outlined in Table 12.2.

The epidermis, which develops from the surface ectoderm, consists of one layer of undifferentiated cells in a 3-week-old embryo. By 4 weeks gestational age, it has an inner germinative layer of cuboidal cells with dark, compact nuclei and an outer layer of slightly flatter cells covered by microvilli. About the middle of the second month of gestation, some of the cells begin to be crowded to the surface and form a thin, protective layer of flattened cells known as the periderm. The cells of this layer continually undergo keratinization and desquamation and are replaced by cells arising from the basal layer. The periderm is often called the epitrichial ("upon the hair") layer of the epidermis because the hairs that later grow up from the deeper layers are said not to penetrate this thin surface layer but to push it up on their growing tips, thus causing it to be cast off if it has not already disappeared. These exfoliated cells form part of the vernix caseosa.

During the later part of the second month, the epithelium tends to become thicker. This occurs (at first) by a staggering of the nuclei and the beginning of cell rearrangement, which leads rapidly to the formation of an intermediate layer between the flattened cells of the epitrichial layer and the basal layer adjacent to the underlying dermis. The cells of this intermediate layer tend to become enlarged and show a high degree of vacuolation. The basal layer of the epidermis is later called the stratum germinativum (Moore & Persaud, 2008).

At the end of the second month of gestation, the cutaneous nerves, which are detectable in embryonic dermis about the fifth week of gestation, appear to be functional, although the skin is primitive by comparison with that of an adult.

At about 10 weeks gestation, fingernail development begins at the tips of the digits. A thickened area of epithelium on the dorsum of each digit is the first sign of nail formation. Our nails are adaptations of the epidermis, homologous to the claws and hoofs of lower mammals, and are formed by a modified process of keratinization. Development of the fingernails is begun and completed (30–34 weeks) before that of the toenails (35–38 weeks).

By about 11 weeks gestation, collagen and elastic connective tissue fibers begin to develop in the dermis. The epidermal-dermal junction, which has been smooth up to this time, now becomes wavy as epidermal thickenings grow down into the dermis of the palm and the soles of the feet. Dermal papillae develop in these dermal projections. Capillary loops develop in some dermal papillae, and Meissner's corpuscles, which are the sensory nerve endings of touch, form in others (Moore & Persaud, 2008). These epidermal ridges produce ridges and grooves in a genetically determined pattern and are the basis for fingerprinting and footprinting. The development of these ridges can be distinctly affected by the presence of abnormal chromosome complements (e.g., as occurs in Down syndrome). These ridges are permanently established by about 17 weeks gestation.

During the third to fourth month of gestation, the stratum germinativum differentiates from the rest of the epithelium. These cells are termed the germinative layer because they undergo the repeated cell divisions that are responsible for the growth of the epidermis.

During the fourth month of gestation, the epithelium starts to become many cells thick, and keratin begins to accumulate in the cells above the stratum germinativum layer. Daughter cells from the basal layer are crowded upward and undergo progressive changes in each layer and finalize in cornification. The thin stratum granulosum epidermidis, which contains keratohyalin granules, is the layer directly above the stratum germinativum. The next higher layer is the thin and clear stratum lucidum epidermidis, the content of which is a fluid—eleidin—that replaces the granules. Above that is the keratinized multilayered stratum corneum epidermidis (Moore & Persaud, 2008). As the keratin accumulates in these cells, they become more and more sluggish and finally die, so that the surface layer of the epidermis is made up of tough, scale-like, dead cells that form a relatively impermeable membrane.

In areas such as the soles of the feet and the palms of the hands, where the skin is subjected to more than ordinary wear, the keratinization of the outer layer is much heavier than in the general body surface. Of interest, however, is that the greater thickness of palmar and plantar epidermis becomes evident in the embryo long before it is possible for these areas to have been subjected to any more wear than other parts of the skin. When the aforementioned layers are all completely differentiated, the structure of fetal epidermis resembles that of adult epidermis.

During the early fetal period, neural crest cells migrate into the dermis and differentiate into melanoblasts. At about 17 to 20 weeks of gestation, these melanoblasts differentiate into melanocytes, migrate to the epidermal–dermal border, and begin to produce melanin. Fetal melanocytes in white races contain little or no pigment, whereas in dark-skinned races, they produce melanin granules. The skin of Black newborns is only a little darker than that of white newborns. The skin at the bases of the fingernails and toenails is often noticeably darker, however.

(*continued*)

The skin of Black infants continues to darken after birth as increased melanin production occurs in response to light. When melanocytes remain behind in the dermis, they appear bluish through the overlying cutaneous tissue and are called mongolian spots. Some believe that it is not the number of melanocytes present that is important but rather their activity level. The hormone secreted by the pituitary gland that controls the clumping or dispersion of the melanin granules is melanocyte-stimulating hormone.

Around 20 weeks gestation, the eyebrows, upper lip, and chin hair are first recognizable. On the general body surface, the hair makes its appearance about a month later. These fine hairs are called lanugo. The emergence of this hair breaks off the periderm, and the periderm becomes one component of the vernix caseosa. The other components of vernix are sebum from the sebaceous glands, fetal hair, and desquamated cells from the amnion (Moore & Persaud, 2008). Vernix protects the epidermis against a macerating influence that would be exerted by the amniotic fluid and acts as a lubricant to prevent chafing injuries from the amnion as the growing fetus becomes progressively confined in its fluid-filled sac.

Between 21 and 24 weeks gestation, the fetus's skin is wrinkled, translucent, and pinkish-red because blood in the capillaries has become visible. Head and lanugo hair are well developed in a 26- to 29-week fetus. At this same time, eccrine sweat glands are anatomically developed and are found over the entire body. Their function, however, is somewhat immature in the perinatal period.

Brown adipose tissue cells begin to differentiate in the seventh month of gestation, and the accumulation of subcutaneous fat begins to smooth out the many skin wrinkles. Between the 30th and 34th week of gestation, the skin is pink and smooth, and the lanugo is beginning to shed. The fingernails reach the fingertips, but the distal part of the nail is still thin and soft (Moore & Persaud, 2008). During the last trimester of pregnancy, subcutaneous fat accumulates, and the fetus acquires a plump appearance. The composition of amniotic fluid tested at this time reflects skin function. The number of anucleated cells and keratinized lipid-containing skin flakes increases.

TABLE 12.1

STRUCTURAL DIFFERENCES BETWEEN INFANT AND ADULT SKIN

	Premature	Full Term	Adult
Epidermis	Thinner cells compressed Fewer desmosomes Fewer layers of stratum corneum Melanin production low	Stratum corneum appears as adherent cell layers Melanin production low	Good resistance to penetration
Dermoepidermal junction	Fewer hemidesmosomes Less cohesion between layers		
Dermis	Fewer elastin fibers Thinner than in the adult	Fewer elastin fibers Thinner than in the adult	Full complement of elastin fibers
Eccrine glands	May be more typical of fetus than adult Ducts patent Secretory cells undifferentiated	Equivalent in structure to adult Denser distribution	Distribution less dense than in infant
Hair	Lanugo hair may be present Hair growth synchronous	Vellus hair characteristic Hair growth synchronous	Both vellus and terminal hairs Hair growth dyssynchronous
Sebaceous glands	Large and active	Large and active but diminishing rapidly in both size and activity for several weeks after birth	Large and active
Nerve and vascular system	Not fully organized Most nerves are small in diameter, unmyelinated, sensory, and autonomic	Vascular system not fully organized until 3 months Cutaneous nerve network not fully developed; may continue to develop until puberty	Adult pattern

(*continued*)

TABLE 12.1

STRUCTURAL DIFFERENCES BETWEEN INFANT AND ADULT SKIN (CONTINUED)

	Premature	Full Term	Adult
	Unmyelinated nerves are typically fetal in structure Meissner's touch receptors not fully formed	Most nerves are small in diameter, unmyelinated, sensory, and autonomic Meissner's touch receptors not fully formed Good resistance to penetration	
Permeability	Highly permeable Higher penetrability of fat-soluble substances Greater absorption because of higher skin surface: body weight ratio	Good resistance to penetration Higher penetrability of fat-soluble substances Greater absorption because of higher skin surface: body weight ratio	
Eccrine sweating	Reduced sweating capability, especially for first 13 to 24 days	Reduced sweating capability, especially for first 2 to 5 days	Full sweating capability
Photosensitivity	Melanin production low; will sunburn readily	Melanin production low; will sunburn readily	Sensitivity to sun depends on skin type
Related conditions	Reduced ability to ward off infection because of deficient immune system Low reactivity to allergens	Reduced ability to ward off infection Low reactivity to allergens	Readily sensitized to allergens

Adapted from Shalita (1981).

Thickness of the Stratum Corneum and Permeability

The stratum corneum layer provides the barrier properties of the skin. This barrier is composed of keratinocytes coated by intercellular lipids. The stratum corneum begins to develop in the fetus after 21 weeks estimated gestational age (EGA). The stratum corneum in infants of 28 weeks gestation consists of only a few cell layers and is markedly thinner than that of term infants (see Figure 12.1). These findings correlate with the immaturity of barrier function of the stratum corneum and is characterized by increased permeability and increased transepidermal water loss (TEWL). By 32 to 34 weeks EGA, the stratum corneum has developed sufficiently to offer some protection.

The full-term infant has a fully functional stratum corneum. The stratum corneum, the nonliving layer of the epidermis, contains 10 to 20 layers in adults and term infants. The stratum corneum of term newborns has been shown to have lower TEWL and stratum corneum hydration (SCH) than that of adult skin, with the lowest levels seen on the first day of life. This suggests that the barrier is relatively impermeable to water to protect from maceration in utero and that a gradual drying process occurs over the first few days of life. In addition, the TEWL in different areas—such as the forehead, palms, and soles—is lower in newborns, whereas levels are higher on the forearm region (Yosipovitch, Maayan-Metzger, Merlob, & Sirota, 2000).

Despite reports of normal barrier function at birth, studies indicate that infant skin is prone to higher percutaneous absorption and exhibits a greater tendency to irritant and allergic contact dermatitis, prompting some to say that barrier function is not fully developed at birth (Hoeger & Enzmann, 2002; Nikolovski, Stamatas, Kollias, & Wiegand, 2008). In addition, infant stratum corneum is 30% thinner than adult, with the overall epidermis 20% to 30% smaller. Keratinocyte cells are smaller, with higher cell turnover rate that may explain observations of faster wound healing in infant skin (Nikolovski et al., 2008; Stamatas, Nikolovski, Mack, & Kollias, 2011).

The stratum corneum of premature infants was once thought to rapidly mature and reach adult barrier function within approximately 2 weeks after birth. However, this has been shown to be a slower process in premature infants less than 27 weeks gestation; rates of TEWL are nearly double adult levels, even at 28 days of life (Hammarlund & Sedin, 1979). In infants of 23 to 25 weeks gestation, skin barrier function reaches mature levels much more slowly (Agren, Sjors, & Sedin, 1998), as long as 8 weeks after birth in a 23-week gestation infant (Kalia, Nonato, Lund, & Guy, 1998). The undeveloped stratum corneum of the premature

TABLE 12.2

EMBRYONIC AND FETAL DEVELOPMENT OF SKIN[a]

Weeks of Gestation	Development
3	Epidermis, which develops from surface ectoderm, consists of one layer of cells
5	Cutaneous nerves are detectable in embryonic dermis
6–7	Periderm, a thin, protective layer of flattened cells, is formed
11	Collagen and elastic fibers are developing in the dermis Epidermal ridges (fingerprints) are forming Nails begin to develop at the tips of the digits
13–16	Scalp hair patterning is determined
17–20	Melanocytes migrate to the epidermal-dermal junction and begin to produce melanin Skin is covered with vernix caseosa and lanugo Keratin is accumulating in the epidermis
21–25	Skin is wrinkled, translucent, and pink to red because blood in the capillaries has become visible
26–29	Subcutaneous fat begins to be deposited and starts to smooth out the many wrinkles in the skin Eccrine sweat glands are anatomically developed and found over the entire body; their function, however, is somewhat immature in the perinatal period
30–34	Skin is pink and smooth Fingernails reach fingertips Lanugo begins to shed
35–38	Fetuses are usually plump Skin is usually white or bluish-pink Toenails reach toe tips

[a]Embryonic period: undoubtedly the most important period of human development because the beginnings of all major external and internal structures develop. Fetal period (ninth week to birth): primarily concerned with growth and differentiation of tissue and organs that started to develop during the embryonic period.
Adapted from Ackerman (1985).

infant's skin results in increased TEWL and evaporative heat loss, and contributes to the difficulty the premature newborn experiences in maintaining fluid balance and body temperature.

Neonatal skin is 40% to 60% thinner than adult skin, and the body surface/weight ratio is nearly five times greater, placing the newborn at risk for toxicity from topically applied substances (Mancini, 2004; Siegfried, 2008). The skin of a premature infant is remarkably permeable; permeability correlates inversely with gestational age. Sekkat, Kalia, and Guy (2004) have developed an in vitro model to examine the biophysical characteristics of TEWL in premature infants. This model will help clinicians understand how procedures coupled with gestational age can affect skin integrity, permeability, and TEWL.

Toxicity due to topically applied substances secondary to the increased permeability of both preterm and term infants' skin has been reported in numerous cases (Siegfried, 2008). All topical solutions during the first month of life should be carefully evaluated as to potential benefits, risks, and effectiveness.

Dermal Instability

Collagen in the dermis increases with gestational age as the tendency toward water fixation and edema decreases. The other component of the dermis, the elastin fibers, is formed mostly after birth and may not become fully mature until 3 years of age. Protection from pressure and ischemic injury includes routine turning and repositioning on surfaces such as gelled pads or water mattresses (Association of Women's Health, Obstetric, and Neonatal Nurses [AWHONN], 2007).

Diminished Cohesion

Another variation in the premature infant's skin structure and function is the diminished cohesion between the dermis and the epidermis. The junction of the epidermis and the dermis, which is normally connected by numerous fibrils, has fewer and more widely spaced fibrils in the premature infant than in term infants or adults (Figure 12.2). These fibrils become stronger with increasing gestational and postnatal age. Because care of the premature infant in the neonatal intensive care unit (NICU) often requires intravenous lines, cardiorespiratory electrodes, endotracheal

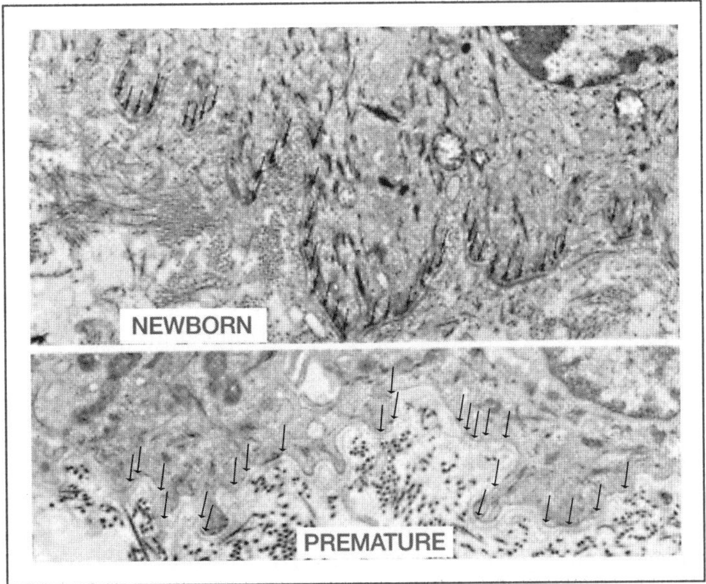

FIGURE 12.2 Arrows indicate anchoring fibrils at dermoepidermal junction in a full-term and a premature infant. Reprinted with permission from Holbrook (1982).

tubes, and umbilical artery catheters, the premature infant is at higher risk for blistering and stripping of the epidermis when adhesives that are used to secure these devices and monitors are removed. The cohesion between many of the currently used adhesives and the stratum corneum may be stronger than the bond between the dermis and the epidermis.

Skin pH

Another developmental variation of infant skin resides in the functional capacity of the skin to form a surface pH of less than 5.0, which is the acid mantle. A skin surface pH of less than 5.0 is ordinarily seen in both children and adults.

Full-term newborns' skin was found to have a mean pH of 6.34 immediately after birth. Within 4 days, the pH decreased to a mean of 4.95, and between 7 and 30 days it further decreased to 4.7. In a later study of 127 low-birth-weight infants, these authors documented that the mean pH decreased from 6.7 (day 1) to 5.04 (day 9). However, a different technique for measuring pH was used than in the previous study; thus the absolute values for pH may not be comparable. They concluded that acidification of the skin is independent of gestational age (Fox, Nelson, & Wareham, 1998).

An acidic skin surface is credited with having bactericidal qualities against some pathogens and serves in the defense against microorganisms. This acid mantle contributes to the stratum corneum's innate immune function by inhibiting the growth of pathogenic bacteria (Larson & Dinulos, 2005; Visscher et al., 2011). The retention of vernix caseosa has been shown to assist in earlier acidification of the newborn skin and may help to facilitate colonization by normal flora after birth (Tollin et al., 2005), while an increased pH may reduce stratum corneum integrity and enhance susceptibility to mechanical damage (Visscher et al., 2011).

Melanin Production

One of the primary functions of melanin is to screen the skin from the sun's harmful rays by absorbing their radiant energy. Although melanin production—and therefore pigmentation—are lower during the neonatal period than later in life, certain areas—such as the linea alba, the areola, and the scrotum—are often deeply pigmented as a result of high circulating levels of maternal and placental hormones. Melanin production in premature infants is even less than in term infants, thus placing them at greater risk for damage from sunlight and ultraviolet light (Williams, 2008).

Assessment and Physiologic Variations

Acrocyanosis, or peripheral cyanosis involving the hands, feet, and circumoral area is a common finding in the newborn. It occurs because of sluggish blood flow in the feet and hands that results from limited development of the peripheral capillary circulation. Acrocyanosis usually resolves within the first few days of life but may reappear with cold stress (Gardner & Hernandez, 2011).

Pallor is most commonly a sign of anemia, hypoxia, or poor peripheral perfusion that results from hypotension or infection. Meconium staining is caused by the passage of meconium in utero and usually requires at least 6 hours of meconium contact to stain the skin.

Jaundice, which occurs in 50% to 70% of newborns, is a yellowing of the skin and develops because of the presence of indirect bilirubin in the blood formed from the body's normal breakdown of red blood cells. Bilirubin is normally processed by the liver and is eliminated in the urine and feces. In newborns, the body cannot eliminate bilirubin as fast as it is produced.

For visible staining of the skin and sclera, a bilirubin level of at least 5 mg/100 mL is required. The predictable head-to-toe progression of jaundice over the body gives a crude estimate of the level of bilirubin. Typically, the bilirubin level is highest at 3 to 5 days (Bromiker et al., 2012).

Risk factors for high bilirubin levels or kernicterus, a neurologically damaging condition caused by hyperbilirubinemia, are: bruising at birth, prematurity, breastfeeding and poor feeding, glucose-6-phosphate dehydrogenase deficiency (G6PD), East Asian or Mediterranean descent, jaundice prior to 24 hours, and a prior sibling with jaundice (AWHONN, 2009).

Linea nigra is a line of increased pigmentation from the umbilicus to the genitals. This area of benign pigmentation may become less noticeable as the infant's skin darkens. Mongolian spots are collections of melanocytes located in the dermis that are most frequently seen at birth. They are slate blue, gray, or black, shaped as irregular, bruise-like spots that are seen primarily over the sacrum and the buttocks but may extend over the back and shoulders. Most commonly seen in newborns with darkly pigmented skin, they are found in 96% of African American, 86% of Asian, and 13% of Caucasian infants (Lucky, 2008). Although they look like bruises, they are harmless and resolve over several years.

Lanugo is the fine downy hair that is most commonly seen over the back, shoulders, and facial areas of a premature newborn. It is shed at the seventh to eighth month of gestation and is one criterion used to estimate gestational age.

Milia are common papules that occur primarily on the face but may also occur in other locations. They are seen as small, white, pinhead-sized bumps that are scattered over the chin, cheeks, noses, and forehead of 25% to 40% of full-term babies (Margileth, 2005). They spontaneously resolve within the first month of life. Mothers should be instructed not to squeeze or prick these pimple-like spots. Milia can develop on the foreskin of infant boys; these are called epidermal inclusion cysts. When they occur on the palate, they are called Epstein's pearls.

Miliaria is a general term for describing obstructions of the eccrine duct. The cause is retention of sweat as a result of edema of the stratum corneum; this edema blocks eccrine pores, thus resulting in four types of miliaria: rubra (prickly heat), crystallina, pustulosa, and profunda.

Miliaria pustulosa and miliaria profunda are rarely seen in temperate climates. Miliaria rubra is commonly observed in infants exposed to excessive environmental temperatures with humidity. It appears as pink or white pimples with a little redness around them. They resolve when the infant is moved to cooler temperatures. Miliaria crystallina presents as clear, 1- to 2-mm superficial water blisters without inflammation (Margileth, 2005). The distribution and grouping of vesicles that contain no eosinophils help to differentiate them from erythema toxicum neonatorum.

Harlequin color change is a dramatic but benign phenomenon in which the color on the dependent half of an infant in a side-lying position turns deep red while the upper half is pale. The color reverses when the infant is turned. Attributed to a temporary imbalance in the autonomic regulatory mechanism of the cutaneous vessels, this phenomenon is more common in low-birth-weight infants—whether well or sick.

Vernix caseosa is a grayish-white cheesy substance that is a mixture of 80% water, protein, lipids, and desquamating cells (Tollin et al., 2005). This covering is protective to the fetal skin while the fetus is in utero and helps the infant slide through the birth canal. Vernix production begins at the end of the second trimester and accumulates in a cephalocaudal manner (Haubrich, 2003.) The vernix covering diminishes as pulmonary surfactant rises and the fetus reaches term (Moraille, Pickens, Visscher, & Hoath, 2005). Surface distribution is dependent on gestational age, type of delivery, birth weight, race, gender, and the presence of meconium (Visscher et al., 2005). The World Health Organization (WHO) (2009) recommends leaving residual vernix in place, after initial drying, to wear off with normal care and handling.

In clinical care, vernix has been thought of as an unwanted soil from intrauterine life, but recent research has revealed that vernix has many functions and potential benefits for the newborn. These functions and potential benefits include: protection against infection (Akinbi, Narendran, Passs, Markart, & Hoath, 2004), decreased skin permeability and TEWL (Yoshio, Lagercrantz, Gudmundsson, & Agerberth, 2004), skin cleansing (Moraille et al., 2005), moisturization of the skin surface (Tansirikongkol, Visscher, & Wickett, 2007), pH development (Visscher et al., 2005), wound healing, and temperature regulation.

Cutis marmorata, or mottling, is a normal physiologic vascular response to cool air. This generalized mottling reflects the infant's vasomotor instability. The marbling disappears with rewarming and is uncommon after several months of age. Mottling is often prominent in infants with Cornelia de Lange syndrome and Down syndrome (Trisomy 21).

Erythema toxicum neonatorum, the most common rash of newborns, usually occurs within 5 days of birth and affects approximately half of term infants, although it is almost never seen in premature infants or those weighing less than 2,500 g. It appears as small, firm, white, or pale yellow pustules with an erythematous margin. Lesions may first appear on the face and spread to the trunk and extremities, but may appear anywhere on the body, except the soles and palms (Lucky, 2008). A smear and Wright's stain of the pustules reveal numerous infiltrates of eosinophils that are devoid of bacteria. The differential diagnosis includes transient neonatal pustular melanosis, candidiasis, staphylococcal pyoderma, and miliaria. No treatment is necessary.

Neonatal and infantile acne are two distinct conditions distinguished by the time of onset and clinical features. Neonatal acne involves inflammatory, erythematous papules, and pustules located primarily on the cheeks, often scattered over the face and extending into the scalp.

A hypothesis that neonatal acne may be an inflammatory response to Malassezia species of fungus has been proposed (Niamba et al., 1998; Rapelanoro, Mortureux, Couprie, Maleville, & Taieb, 1996). Other experts suggest that neonatal acne is related to sebum excretion rate while the infantile form is related to high androgen levels, but both have genetic influences (Herane & Ando, 2003). Infantile acne is considered to result in hyperplasia of sebaceous activity. It is found primarily on the face. Neonatal acne generally resolves without treatment. Infantile acne may be more persistent and even cause scarring. It may benefit from treatment with topical benzyl alcohol peroxide or erythromycin (Lucky, 2008). Some success has been reported with oral isotretinoin (Torrelo, Pastor, & Zambrano, 2005).

Transient neonatal pustular melanosis is a lesion that is similar to miliaria but is present at birth, usually causing the infant to be unnecessarily isolated. It occurs most commonly on the face, the palms of the hands, and the soles of the feet. It is most commonly seen in Black infants. The differential diagnosis includes erythema toxicum neonatorum, staphylococcal impetigo, neonatal candidiasis, miliaria crystallina or rubra, and acropustulosis of infancy. If the lesions are ruptured, smeared on a slide, and stained, the contents are found to be amorphous debris. The lesion is neither infectious nor contagious. It is self-limiting and requires no treatment.

Sucking blisters that contain sterile, serous fluid may be seen on the thumb, index finger, or lip. Presumably, they are the result of vigorous sucking in utero, are seen in approximately 1 in every 250 live births, and resolve without treatment (Howard & Frieden, 2008).

Pigmentary Lesions

Hyperpigmented lesions may be present at birth or during the first weeks of life. Some pigmentary problems are benign, such as mongolian spots, whereas others can be signs of a systemic or genetic disorder. Some of the more common are included in this section.

Café au lait spots are irregularly shaped, oval lesions. Their color resembles coffee to which milk has been added. They should be noted on the newborn's initial physical examination, and if they are larger than 4 to 6 cm or if more than six are present, a diagnosis of neurofibromatosis should be considered (Landau & Krafchik, 1999).

Hyperpigmentation that presents in a diffuse pattern is unusual in the newborn. When present, it may be caused by congenital Addison's disease, hepatic or biliary atresia, metabolic disease (Hartnup disease, porphyria), nutritional disorders (pellagra, sprue), hereditary disorders (lentiginosis, melanism), or unknown causes (the bronze discoloration seen in Niemann–Pick disease). Hyperpigmentation of the labial folds with clitoral hypertrophy may result from the transplacental passage of androgens (Margileth, 2005).

Hypopigmentation that presents as a diffuse or localized loss of pigment in the neonate may stem from metabolic (phenylketonuria), endocrine (Addison's disease), genetic (vitiligo, piebaldism, tuberous sclerosis, albinism), traumatic, or postinflammatory causes (Margileth, 2005).

Partial albinism (piebaldism) is an autosomal dominant disorder that is present at birth and is easily detected in the dark-skinned infant. Off-white macules are seen on the scalp, widow's peak, and forehead and extend to the base of the nose, trunk, and extremities. Differential diagnoses are Klein–Waardenburg syndrome, vitiligo, nevus anemicus, Addison's disease, and white macules of tuberous sclerosis. When illuminated with a Wood light, the amelanotic areas of piebaldism exhibit a brilliant whiteness (Margileth, 2005). Albinism refers to a group of genetic disorders involving abnormal melanin synthesis. It may occur in any race, with the incidence approximately 1 in 20,000, with a slightly higher rate in African Americans (Sethi, Schwartz, & Janniger, 1996). An autosomal recessive gene usually causes it, but rare cases of autosomal dominant inheritance have occurred (Margileth, 2005).

White leaf macules are the earliest cutaneous manifestations of tuberous sclerosis, an autosomal dominant neurocutaneous syndrome. They vary in size and shape but most often resemble a mountain ash leaflet. They may be difficult to see in a newborn infant and may be more readily observed by examination with a Wood lamp, which heightens the contrast between the macule and normal skin. Normal infants occasionally have a single lesion, but the presence of one or more of these macules in an infant with neurologic problems strongly suggests the diagnosis of tuberous sclerosis. Skin biopsy is nondiagnostic. A careful family history, physical examination, and, when appropriate, additional diagnostic studies are indicated in infants with these lesions.

Lesions Related to the Birth Process

Caput succedaneum is a diffuse, generalized edema of the scalp that is caused by local pressure and trauma during labor. The borders are not well defined, and the swelling crosses suture lines. Cephalohematoma is a subperiosteal hemorrhage caused by the trauma of labor and delivery. The margins of the suture lines are clearly demarcated, and the swelling never crosses suture lines. Sclerema neonatorum may have the same cause and adipose tissue abnormality in the subcutaneous tissues as those noted in fat necrosis. However, sclerema more commonly affects the premature or debilitated infant. It is a diffuse hardening of the subcutaneous tissue that results in cold, nonpitting skin. Low environmental temperature alone can produce this injury. The extremities may be involved at first, but generalized involvement occurs within 3 to 4 days. Infants with this disorder are usually critically ill, but if they survive, the sclerodermatous changes rarely last beyond 2 weeks. Treatment is based on therapy for the underlying systemic disease, restoration of body temperature, and adequate nutrition.

Forceps marks are identified by their rounded contours and position. The bruised area should be checked for underlying tissue and nerve damage. Scalp lacerations can occur in many ways. A laceration can be caused by the placement of an internal monitoring lead or by the artificial rupture of membranes. A circular red or ecchymotic area may be caused by the use of a vacuum extractor. Any abraded area may serve as a portal of entry for infection; therefore a scalp laceration should be carefully and continuously assessed for the presence of infection. Lacerations can also occur to other body surfaces from scalpel injuries during cesarean birth; an incidence of 1.9% was noted in a series of 896 cesarean section deliveries.

Subcutaneous fat necrosis is an uncommon disorder that occurs primarily in full-term infants. It has been associated with birth trauma, shock, asphyxia, hypothermia, seizures, preeclampsia, meconium aspiration, and intrapartum medications. One or several indurated, violet or red plaques or sharply defined subcutaneous nodules on the buttocks, thighs, trunk, face, or arms may appear (Cohen, 2008). Most areas of subcutaneous fat necrosis gradually reabsorb over weeks to months if left alone. Residual atrophy or scarring is unusual.

Internal fetal monitoring sites are at risk for infection, owing to the introduction of the maternal vaginal flora directly into the subcutaneous tissue of the fetus. Scalp abscesses caused by implantation of a fetal electrode are generally benign, self-limited occurrences. Rare instances of major complications have been reported, however—including significant areas of cellulitis, osteomyelitis, and sepsis.

Dermatologic Diseases

Diseases of the skin in newborns often present patterns that are different from the presentation of the same disease in adults. Therefore a careful physical examination of the skin is necessary for an accurate dermatologic diagnosis to be made. All lesions should be described and their location and pattern noted.

Lesions can be classified as either primary or secondary. Primary lesions are described as the initial or principal lesion that is identified when the disease begins. Primary lesions are classified as macule, patch, papule, plaque, nodule, tumor, vesicle, bulla, wheal, pustule, or abscess. Secondary lesions are brought about by the modification of a primary lesion. The secondary lesion may be called a crust, scale, erosion, ulcer, fissure, lichenification, atrophy, or scar.

■ **Terminology.** Ecchymoses appear as black and blue bruises of varying sizes anywhere over the body. Primarily seen over the presenting part in a difficult vertex delivery or a vaginal breech delivery, ecchymosis is most frequently due to trauma associated with labor and delivery. It occurs more commonly in the fragile premature infant. This bruising, however, can be indicative of serious infection or bleeding disorders.

Petechiae are pinpoint hemorrhagic areas, less than 1 mm in diameter, scattered over the upper trunk and face as a result of pressure during the descent and rotation of birth. Their incidence is increased when the umbilical cord has been around the neck or when the cervix clamps down after delivery of the head. They usually fade within 24 to 48 hours. If they continue to develop or are unusually numerous, a complete workup for infection or bleeding disorders should be performed.

Intracutaneous hemorrhage may be caused by thrombocytopenia, inherited disorders of coagulation, transient deficiency of vitamin K, disseminated intravascular coagulation (DIC), and trauma.

DIC should be suspected in an acutely ill infant who has an intracutaneous hemorrhage. Thrombocytopenia and disorders of coagulation may occur in infants who seem well otherwise. Thrombocytopenia should be suspected when the infant presents with general cutaneous petechiae. It frequently accompanies neonatal infections and is most commonly associated with the TORCH diseases (toxoplasmosis, others, rubella, cytomegalovirus [CMV], and herpes simplex).

Ecchymoses and petechiae are purple discolorations caused by hemorrhage into the superficial skin layers. They do not disappear with blanching because the blood is contained in the tissues. Macules are nonpalpable, nonraised lesions less than 1 cm in diameter that are identified only by color change. They are seen in measles, rubella, scarlet fever, roseola, typhoid fever, and drug reactions.

Papules are superficial elevated solid lesions less than 1 cm in diameter. They are firm and not fluid-filled. They may follow the macular stage in many eruptive diseases. Vesicles are skin elevations that contain serous fluid (blisters). They are commonly seen with herpes simplex, insect bites, and poison ivy.

Pustules are localized accumulations of pus in or just beneath the epidermis. They are often centered around appendageal structures (e.g., hair follicles) and are usually caused by bacterial infections or skin abscesses. When a pustule breaks, the degree of crusting is more marked than occurs with the rupture of a vesicle.

Nodules are deep solid lesions larger than 1 cm in diameter. Nodules are similar to papules but are larger. Because of their size, they are more likely to have a dermal component than are papules.

■ **Developmental Vascular Abnormalities.** The following two major groups of vascular birthmarks are seen:

1. Vascular malformations composed of dysplastic vessels
2. Vascular tumors that demonstrate cellular hyperplasia

Vascular malformations have various subcategories determined by the anomalous vessels involved—including capillary, venous, arteriovenous, or lymphatic. Hemangiomas or vascular nevi are the most common cutaneous congenital malformations seen during early infancy. They may be either involuting or noninvoluting vascular lesions, as well as flat (telangiectatic) or raised (hemangiomatous). The common involuting types include salmon patch, spider nevi (telangiectases), and strawberry and cavernous hemangiomas. Noninvoluting lesions, which are seen less commonly in newborns, are the port-wine stain and, rarely, the pyogenic granuloma (Enjolras & Garzon, 2008).

■ **Pigmented Nevus.** Pigmented nevi are benign tumors of the skin that contain nevus cells. Nevus cells can produce melanin and are closely related to melanocytes. In contrast to melanocytes, they tend to lie in groups or nests. Congenital pigmented nevi are different from pigmented nevi that arise later in that they are usually larger and more extensive. As the infant grows, the area becomes thicker and darker (Margileth, 2005).

Flat, junctional nevi are seen in about 1% of newborns. They are brown or black, and their size varies from one to several centimeters. When they are present at birth, they may be associated with neurofibromatosis, tuberous sclerosis, or bathing trunk nevi. Therapy is rarely needed, but lesions larger than 3 cm should be removed.

■ **Giant Hairy Nevus.** A giant hairy nevus is characterized by a pigmented, hairy, and softly infiltrated area. The color varies from pale brown to black. When the nevi are large, they tend to have a dermatomic distribution, and their location and size give them their name (e.g., bathing trunk nevus, vest nevus, shoulder stole nevus) (Figure 12.3). On histologic examination of a biopsy specimen, the nevus cells are seen penetrating deeply into the dermis and subcutaneous tissue.

When a giant nevus is situated on the head or neck, it may be associated with mental retardation, epilepsy, or hydrocephalus. Spina bifida or meningocele may occur when this nevus is present over the spine (Margileth, 2005). Other abnormalities that are sometimes associated with a giant pigmented nevus are clubfoot, hypertrophy or hypotrophy of the affected limb, and von Recklinghausen's disease (neurofibromatosis). Besides being a cosmetic problem, the giant nevus is associated with a higher incidence of malignancy. Malignant melanomas develop in as many as 15% of these patients. Management involves surgical excision of the entire lesion at or near puberty to prevent the development of skin cancer in the lesion. Plastic surgical reconstruction may be needed if the excision is extensive.

■ **Hemangiomas.** Hemangioma of infancy is an angiomatous disorder characterized by the proliferation of capillary endothelium and multilamination of the basement membrane and accumulation of mast cells, fibroblasts, and macrophages. Hemangiomas appear on 1% to 3% of infants at birth and develop on another 10%, usually within the first 3 to 4 weeks of life. The incidence is 22% in preterm babies who weigh less than 1,000 g and 15% in infants with birth weights of 1,000 to 1,500 g. When examined microscopically, hemangiomas are one of two kinds: capillary or cavernous. They most often appear in the skin as a single tumor, but multiple cutaneous lesions also occur, often with involvement of other organ systems.

The natural history of the hemangioma is characterized by their appearance during the first few weeks of life, rapid postnatal growth for 8 to 18 months (proliferative phase), which is followed by very slow but inevitable regression for the next 5 to 8 years (involutive phase). Hemangiomas completely resolve in more than 50% of children by 5 years of age and in more than 70% by 7 years of age, and continued improvement occurs in the remaining children until 10 to 12 years of age. The rate of regression does not seem to be related to the sex or age of the infant or to the site, size, or appearance of the hemangioma or the duration of the proliferative phase.

Strawberry hemangiomas consist of a dilated mass of capillaries in the dermal and subdermal layers that protrude above the skin surface. They are bright red, soft, compressible tumors that can appear anywhere on the body (Figure 12.4). They will generally increase in size for approximately 6 months and then gradually begin to regress or involute spontaneously. Complete involution may take several years to occur. These marks require no treatment, and no permanent scars occur if the marks are left alone. However, when these lesions interfere with vital functions such as vision, feeding, and respiration, intervention is required (Enjolras & Garzon, 2008).

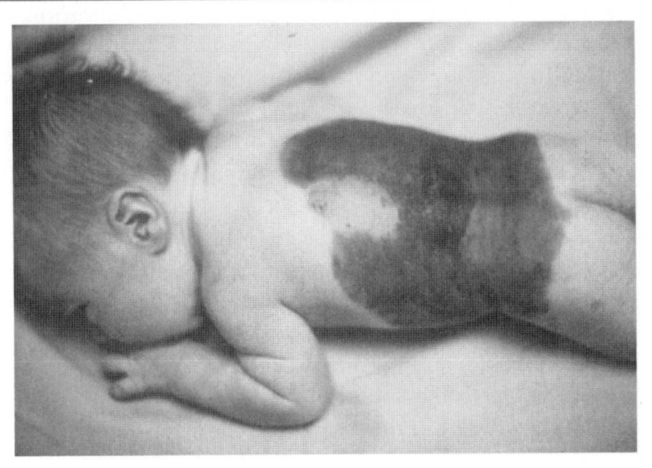

FIGURE 12.3 The giant pigmented hairy nevus of this infant involves the thorax, abdomen, and back and is commonly called a "bathing trunk" nevus. It is raised with fleshy elements and has a somewhat leathery texture.
Reprinted with permission from Clark and Thompson (1986). Copyright © Wyeth-Ayerst Labs.

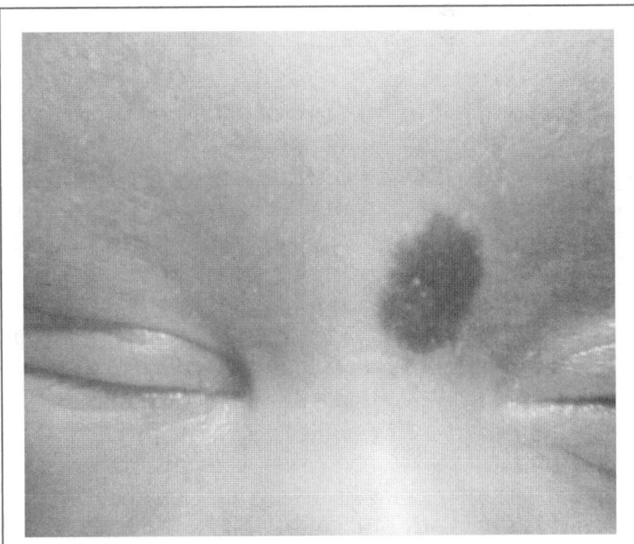

FIGURE 12.4 This photograph shows the early hemangioma in a 28-weeks gestation premature infant. Approximately 5 weeks after birth the first area of discoloration appeared. The irregular surface with sharp demarcation is typical of strawberry hemangioma, which eventually enlarges to twice the size it appears in this photograph before involution.
Reprinted with permission from Clark and Thompson (1986). Copyright © Wyeth-Ayerst Labs.

Cavernous hemangiomas are more deeply situated in the skin than are strawberry hemangiomas. They are bluish-red and feel spongy when touched. Most hemangiomas are small, harmless birthmarks that involute to leave either normal or slightly blemished skin. However, even a small hemangioma can obstruct the airway or impair vision. A large hemangioma in the liver or an extensive cutaneous hemangioma can divert a considerable volume of blood through its extensive labyrinth of capillaries and produce high-output heart failure. The increased capillary endothelial surface that characterizes a giant hemangioma can also trap platelets and may cause thrombocytopenic coagulopathy (Kasabach–Merritt syndrome).

A few hemangiomas grow to an alarming size or proliferate simultaneously in several organs and cause life-endangering conditions, such as soft-tissue destruction, deformation or obstruction of vital structures, serious bleeding, congestive heart failure, and sepsis. Large lesions can expand the skin, and even after they regress, they can result in excess slack skin, pigment changes, and a fibro-fatty residuum.

Visceral hemangiomas may arise in many organs, most commonly in the liver and larynx, with or without cutaneous involvement; a single lesion or multiple hemangiomas may occur. Flow through extensive hemangiomas increases the total blood volume, causes hemodeviation, and disturbs the hemodynamic equilibrium. The hyperdynamic cardiovascular state of the hemangiomas decreases or shunts blood away from other tissues, thus resulting in hypoperfusion of other tissues. This hypoperfusion may cause brain hypoxia and acidosis and predispose to seizures, as seen in some cases. Close surveillance of the cardiovascular system is necessary to determine the proper time to begin digitalization.

■ Management. Management of both strawberry and cavernous hemangiomas consists of a detailed history; close scrutiny of the lesion or lesions, including three-dimensional measurements; and evaluation of the growth pattern of the hemangioma. As involution progresses, the color gradually changes from grayish-pink to white or pink, and the tension of the lesion decreases. Ulcerated hemangiomas should be treated with topical antibiotics to prevent infection.

While the cutaneous lesions are being monitored, the infant's clinical course and physical development must be closely observed for poor growth, altered cry, stridor, dyspnea, cyanosis, feeding difficulties, or swallowing impairment. If any abnormal sign or symptoms appear—such as tachycardia, heart murmur, hepatomegaly, or bruit that can be heard over the liver—the infant should be examined for evidence of heart failure. Ultrasonography, echocardiography, and computed tomography may be needed.

In general, management consists of planned neglect, which is essential in avoiding disfiguring scars. Complications of therapy may be significant, but residual scarring after complete involution is uncommon. Hemangiomas located in exposed areas often cause great parental anxiety, which increases as the hemangioma grows. This anxiety often puts pressure on the physician to do something. However, the hemangioma should be left to regress spontaneously, and preconceived notions about birthmarks should be discussed with the family.

Treatment of hemangiomas may be needed. The following indications for treatment have been proposed: life-threatening or function-threatening hemangiomas, including those that cause impairment of vision, respiratory compromise, or congestive heart failure; hemangiomas occurring in certain anatomic locations such as the nose, lip, glabellar areas, and ear that may cause permanent deformity or scars; large facial hemangiomas, especially those with a large dermal component; and ulcerated hemangiomas (Enjolras & Garzon, 2008).

Alarming hemangiomas is a term used to categorize lesions that impair vital functions or cause life-threatening complications. A vascular mark was present at birth in 68% of these infants. Visceral hemangiomas are associated with cervicocephalic hemangiomas or with small hemangiomas scattered over the body. About a third of these life-threatening hemangiomas respond to treatment with corticosteroids, but for the others, no safe and effective treatment exists. The mortality rate can be as high as 54% for life-threatening visceral or hepatic hemangiomas and may be up to 30% to 40% with platelet-consumptive coagulopathy, despite the administration of steroids.

High-dose corticosteroid therapy is the primary means of controlling hemangiomas pharmacologically. These agents inhibit the activators of fibrinolysis in vessel walls, decrease plasminogen activator content of endothelium, and increase sensitivity to vasoactive amines, thus causing constriction of arterioles. When steroids fail, less conventional modalities, such as embolization, operative excision, pulsed dye laser, interferon-alpha, and sclerotherapy have been used (Smolinski & Yan, 2005).

Subcutaneous interferon-alpha-2a (2 million units per square meter of body surface area) has been used with life-threatening or vision-threatening hemangiomas that failed to respond to corticosteroid therapy. Their mechanisms of action include inhibition of motility and proliferation of endothelial cells and interference with new capillary vessel formation, thereby preventing platelet trapping. These daily injections seemed to reduce the local and systemic complications and appeared to shorten the length of time to involution in some infants. Sustained therapy for 9 to 14 months appeared to be desirable because earlier withdrawal was followed by regrowth of the lesion that was halted and reversed by reintroduction of the drug. Interferon alpha therapy was not found to have toxic effects.

Tranexamic acid, a fibrinolytic inhibitor that exerts its effect through inhibition of plasminogen activator and plasmin and through inhibition of tumor vessel proliferation, has been used in the treatment of giant hemangiomas. One of the infants had a measurable response in the size of the hemangioma and the extent of the coagulopathy. The other two had progression of their lesions. It appears that tranexamic acid is an additional agent for treatment of giant hemangiomas, but its efficacy is limited. Further study of this treatment is needed to determine which patients may respond best. Surgical therapy involving either laser removal or surgical excision is also a treatment option. Excision is usually done once the hemangioma has involuted, so as to remove residual tissue and redundant skin. Early excision is generally not recommended.

Propranolol appears to be an effective treatment for infantile hemangioma in the nonproliferative phase after the first year of life. Adverse effects that are potentially harmful include hypoglycemia, bronchospasm, and hypotension (de Graaf et al., 2011).

■ **Port-Wine Stain.** Port-wine stain is a capillary angioma consisting of dilated and congested capillaries lying directly beneath the epidermis. It appears in approximately 3 out of 1,000 newborns. This birthmark appears pink at birth but gradually darkens to purple. Most commonly found on the face and neck, it is a permanent developmental defect. Although a port-wine stain is primarily a cosmetic problem, it is occasionally an indicator of a multisystem disorder, such as Sturge–Weber syndrome or Klippel–Trenaunay–Weber syndrome. The presence of seizures, mental retardation, hemiplegia, or intracortical calcification suggests the presence of Sturge–Weber syndrome. An ophthalmologic examination is extremely important in these infants. Gradual thickening and nodule formation can occur with port-wine stain and thus support the need for early treatment in infancy and childhood. Recent advances in laser therapy techniques are shown to be more effective in previously resistant lesions. Although the timing of intervention is somewhat controversial, many dermatologists now advise laser treatment as early as possible in infancy to decrease the stigma associated with this lesion and to prevent skin thickening (Enjolras & Garzon, 2008). Pulsed dye laser is the gold standard for treatment of port-wine stain birthmarks, but multiple treatments are required and complete resolution is often not achieved (Tremaine et al., 2012).

Blistering Diseases

■ **Epidermolysis Bullosa.** Epidermolysis bullosa (EB) is a group of rare congenital blistering disorders, all of which are inherited. They are considered mechanobullous diseases, meaning that trauma to or friction on the skin induces blister formation. EB is caused by defects in the complex meshwork of proteins in the epidermis, dermis, and dermoepidermal junction that allow the skin to adhere in the presence of frictional stress. The underlying defect appears to be a lack of cellular glue in squamous epithelium, which is responsible for the maintenance of cellular integrity. Diagnostic studies should include a skin biopsy for light and electron microscopy.

EB is classified by the clinical extent and ultrastructural level of blistering, by inheritance pattern, and by specific molecular defect (Fine, Bauer, McGuire, & Moshell, 1999; Fine et al., 2000; Marinkovich, 1999). Although some subtypes of EB are severe in the neonatal period and milder later, others can be fatal in the first weeks as a result of severe generalized blistering and complications that arise from this. EB can be nonscarring or scarring. Inheritance may be either autosomal dominant or autosomal recessive.

EB simplex is the mildest form of EB. Most cases are autosomal dominant. The lesions occur at the basal layer of epidermis and do not lead to scarring and hyperkeratosis. Usually present at birth, the vesicles and bullae appear over the joints and the bony protuberances and at sites subjected to repeated trauma. The differential diagnosis may be aided by the absence of milia, which are commonly seen in the dystrophic types of EB. Little or no scarring is seen with EB simplex.

Junctional EB is the least common type of EB with autosomal recessive inheritance. In junctional EB, severe generalized blistering is present at birth, with subsequent extensive denudation. Marked mucosal blistering occurs, and erosions of the larynx, respiratory, gastrointestinal, and urinary tract may also be present. It may be fatal in a few days to a few months because of fluid loss or sepsis. Histopathologically, a separation occurs between the plasma membrane of the basal cells and the basal lamina. In junctional EB, healing is poor, and scarring is extensive.

Dystrophic EB results in blistering that occurs below the dermoepidermal junction and has either dominant or recessive inheritance. In the recessive form, blistering is severe, begins at birth, and can lead to marked scarring and joint contractures.

The dominant form of dystrophic EB is milder, with moderately severe blisters seen on the distal extremities and bony protuberances (Figure 12.5). Some scar formation occurs, and the nails may be mildly dystrophic. Atrophy may occur with healing. The external skin layer can be easily rubbed off by slight friction or injury. Milia, due to a functional disorder of the sweat glands, are found on the rims of the ears, the dorsa of the hands, and the extensor surfaces of the arms and legs. The oral, anal, and esophageal mucosa are frequently involved. Complications include infections and hemolytic, nutritional, orthopedic, gastrointestinal, and psychiatric sequelae. These vary according to the severity of the disease.

■ **Management.** EB can be a great challenge in the newborn period, particularly with the more severe forms.

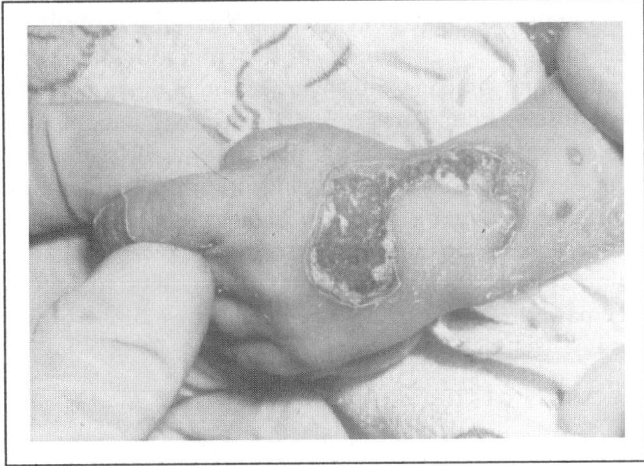

FIGURE 12.5 This photograph of epidermolysis bullosa shows the scaling, broken bullae with underlying erythroderma. Reprinted with permission from Clark and Thompson (1986). Copyright © Wyeth-Ayerst Labs.

Nursing care centers around three main issues: (1) skin breakdown, (2) prevention of infection, and (3) dysphagia. Many of the techniques used to protect the skin of very premature infants are useful with EB patients. Avoiding the use of tape and preventing traumatic injuries is important. Clean, soft dressings may be helpful over bony pressure points. Wound care involves providing a moist healing environment by covering open lesions with a thick coating of petrolatum-based emollients combined with topical antibiotic ointments and covering with nonstick dressings.

Many dermatologists will rotate topical antibiotics every few months to prevent resistance and may use wound cultures to guide selection of agents. Nonstick dressings include petrolatum gauze, Exu-dry, or silicone-based products such as Mepitel (Direct Medical Inc., Houston, TX). After this layer, the wound is further protected by wrapping with nonadhesive cotton gauze; some practitioners prefer cotton mesh, and others use Coban (3M, Indianapolis, IN), a wrap that adheres to itself without adhesives. When blisters are tense and fluid filled, they should be "unroofed" to prevent extension. This procedure is done with sharp, clean scissors, leaving the blister roof in place. Dressings are changed daily and removed gently; some prefer to remove dressings during immersion bathing.

From birth to 6 months of age, the environment is easy to control through the use of sheepskin, loose-fitting clothes, and mittens for the infant's hands and feet. Cloth diapers softened with fabric softener are preferred over rougher, disposable diapers. Any person handling the infant should avoid wearing jewelry. Protection of the infant becomes more difficult once the infant is mobile.

The infant should always wear long pants and foam rubber pads sewn into the knees help avoid trauma during crawling. Contractures may form quickly as scarring begins to occur. The pathologic increase in elastic skin fiber adds to this process. Gentle range-of-motion exercises lessen contracture formation.

Dysphagia can occur from facial and pharyngeal scarring, which is secondary to erosions on the buccal mucosa, tongue, palate, esophagus, and pharynx. Feedings should be performed slowly and carefully to avoid aspiration and to maintain adequate nutrition. The metabolic needs of these infants are high because of the continuous sloughing of epithelium, which results in large protein, fluid, and electrolyte losses. Adding more puncture holes to a nipple may help prevent oral mucosal trauma. If oral ulcerations do occur, several weeks of hyperalimentation and high-dose steroid therapy are instituted. Gavage feedings are discouraged because of the possibility of trauma. It is essential that the family receives genetic counseling regarding the inheritance pattern associated with EB; a negative family history does not exclude its occurrence.

Infections of the Skin

Previously, it was thought that after vaginal birth the skin colonization with microorganisms reflected the mother's vaginal flora, and after cesarean section birth without rupture of the amniotic membranes the skin was sterile. Recent research using DNA sequencing has begun to reveal that the skin microbiome begins in utero (Gregory, 2011). Some report that the skin microbiome of vaginally born infants does appear similar to the mother's vaginal flora but that the skin of cesarean section births resembles the mother's skin flora (Dominguez-Bello et al., 2010). Although the clinical significance of this difference has yet to be determined, it is likely that the skin and its normal flora are natural defense mechanisms against invading pathogens.

In the newborn, an immature immune system, prematurity, stress, and medical and surgical problems contribute to vulnerability and infection. Additionally, most infants in the NICU require a variety of invasive monitoring and diagnostic procedures that allow for breaks in the normally intact physical barrier of the skin, providing direct access to blood and deep tissues. The origin of skin infections and skin manifestations of systemic infection can be bacterial, viral, or fungal.

■ Bacterial. Bacterial skin infections can vary in initial clinical findings and potential for systemic symptoms and sequelae. The pathogen involved and the route of inoculation are two factors that affect the course of bacterial cutaneous infection (Dinulos & Pace, 2008). Types of bacterial skin infections include bullous and nonbullous impetigo, omphalitis, abscesses, and cellulitis. Severe dermatologic findings are also seen when endotoxins are released from bacteria, as in the case of staphylococcal scalded skin syndrome.

Staphylococcus Aureus. Infections resulting from *Staphylococcus aureus* are seen in newborns and can result in two types of skin lesions. Nonbullous impetigo is a superficial infection localized to the epidermis and is characterized by erythematous, honey-colored, crusted plaques. Bullous impetigo of the newborn involves blisters that originate in the subcorneal portion of the epidermis and are filled with clear or straw-colored fluid. Bullous impetigo often presents during the first 2 weeks of life. Few or many blisters may be dispersed widely over all areas of the body and may rupture easily, thus leaving denuded areas of skin. Bullous impetigo is predominantly caused by *S. aureus*, although some cases are caused by other bacteria such as *Streptococcus pyogenes*. If the bacteria is later spread via the bloodstream, the infection may result in osteomyelitis, septic arthritis, or septicemia in neonates (Dinulos & Pace, 2008). Isolation of hospitalized neonates is initiated and intravenous antibiotics are generally recommended in neonates after initial cultures are obtained. Treatment is then tailored to the specific organism when the antibiotic susceptibility profile is known.

Management. Medical and nursing management is focused on treatment of the affected infant and on prevention of the spread of infection to other infants, because this condition is highly contagious. Systemic antibiotics are administered parenterally initially and may be followed by oral treatment once the infection begins to subside. Antibiotics include oxacillin, nafcillin, or methicillin; vancomycin is used if the culture indicated methicillin-resistant *S. aureus*. Topical antibiotics are not indicated for treatment of bullous impetigo (Dinulos & Pace, 2008). Fluid and electrolyte monitoring is necessary if the denuded areas cover a large surface or if the infant is of low birth weight. Isolation of the affected infant is necessary to prevent the spread of the infection throughout the nursery.

Scalded Skin Syndrome. Staphylococcal scalded skin syndrome is an endotoxin-mediated disease with superficial, widespread blistering often leading to desquamation (Figure 12.6). Multiple sites are cultured when this disease is suspected, including any bullous lesions, blood, cerebrospinal fluid, nasopharynx, urine, and umbilicus in an effort to recover an organism.

Skin will appear bright red, like a burn, followed by the development of large, loose blisters that quickly progress to sheets of skin being shed. During the course of this disease, the entire epidermis may be shed. Emollients, together with semiocclusive dressings, provide gentle lubrication and pain relief.

Management. Medical and nursing management also involves administration of the appropriate antibiotic regimen and supportive measures in terms of fluid and electrolytic replacement, prevention of secondary infection through the damaged epidermis, and comfort. Applying local antibiotic solutions or ointments is not recommended; cleansing open skin areas with gentle irrigation using half normal saline promotes healing and prevents secondary infection. The infant may be more comfortable in an incubator rather than in a radiant warmer because the incubator is a convective heat source that does not have a direct cutaneous effect, whereas the radiant heat source heats directly through the skin. In addition, the radiant heat source may further increase the degree of ISWL through the damaged epidermis. Usually, a flaking process is observed on the skin during the healing process. Emollients may be helpful in treating dry skin at this point.

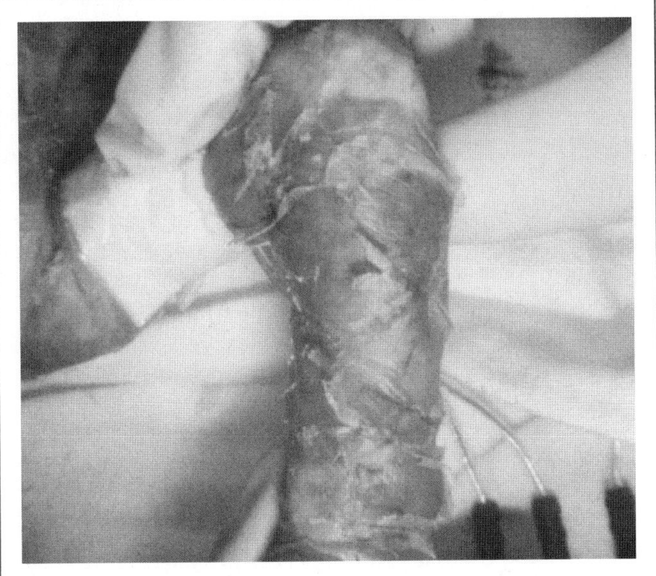

FIGURE 12.6 The peeling, scaling skin of this premature infant had an acute onset at approximately 2 weeks of age. This is the scalded skin syndrome that results from *Staphylococcus aureus*.
Reprinted with permission from Clark and Thompson (1986). Copyright © Wyeth-Ayerst Labs.

Listeria Monocytogenes. Another bacterial skin disease is listeriosis, caused by *Listeria monocytogenes*. This organism, which can cause severe systemic disease, can also result in a disseminated miliary granulomatosis in neonates (Hoath & Narendran, 2011). In some cases, miliary abscesses can occur, and occasionally, more generalized erythema or petechiae may be present. Systemic listeriosis is a severe infection that causes blood hemolysis and a high mortality rate. Prompt recognition and treatment with intravenous penicillin or ampicillin are indicated for the best prognosis. No direct skin therapy has been described as being necessary in this disease.

Syphilis. Congenital syphilis is another bacterial infection that has skin manifestations. If the infant with congenital syphilis is not treated after birth, a maculopapular or bullous skin eruption develops between 2 and 6 weeks of age (Margileth, 2005). Sometimes the bullous lesions may be observed at birth on the palms or the soles, thus signifying the presence of more severe disease. Fluid contained in the blisters contains spirochetes.

The lesions most commonly seen in congenital syphilis are copper-colored and maculopapular and are located on the soles and palms. In addition, open lesions may be present around the mouth, anus, or genitals, and a highly contagious nasal discharge is occasionally seen. If the syphilis remains untreated, the lesions regress in 1 to 3 months, leaving areas on the skin with either hyperpigmentation or hypopigmentation.

Management. Medical and nursing management for the infant with congenital syphilis involves prompt, consistent administration of penicillin—usually a 10-day course. Titers are obtained over the next year at 3-month intervals, and a negative serologic finding is expected at 1 year. Care of the skin lesions is primarily directed toward preventing the spread of infection during the active phase of the illness, especially when bullous lesions or open areas are apparent. No direct topical therapies have been advocated in the literature.

■ Viral. Viral infections can display a broad range of cutaneous manifestations in the neonate and can occur in utero, perinatally, or postnatally. Skin manifestations can be a direct result of skin infection or be a consequence of viral infection in other tissues. Viral infections that result in cutaneous manifestations include herpes simplex virus, CMV, rubella, varicella, enterovirus, parvovirus, and human immunodeficiency virus. Some of these have very specific cutaneous presentations (such as the classic "blueberry muffin" appearance of infants infected with rubella and cytomegalic virus), vesicles (as with herpes simplex), or nonspecific lesions. Toxoplasmosis, which has cutaneous manifestations and is caused by a parasite, is also discussed in this section.

Herpes Simplex. Herpes simplex virus types 1 and 2 are serious pathogens in newborns. The majority of newborns acquire infections from infectious vaginal secretions at the time of delivery. Vesicles that occur on the skin with this disease vary; a few faint scars may be present, or actual vesicle formations may be present with either one large swelling or discrete groups of vesicles. Vesicles may recede and then recur over months.

Herpes simplex virus, type 1 and 2, is one of the most serious viral infections to affect the newborn and can appear as disseminated infection, central nervous system infection, and infection localized to the skin, eyes, or mouth. Disseminated infection is the most devastating presentation, with a mortality rate of up to 75% without antiviral therapy, and about 50% if antiviral therapy is used (Friedlander & Bradley, 2008). Vesicle formations may present with either one large swelling or smaller groups of vesicles that crust over rapidly and then recede. Absence of vesicles does not rule out the disease. Management consists of early recognition and treatment with antiviral agents, such as acyclovir, along with isolation from other infants. If encephalitis develops, the prognosis is extremely poor with either a high risk of death or severe mental retardation.

Management. Medical and nursing management is centered primarily on early recognition and treatment with the antiviral medication acyclovir. The prognosis of systemic herpes simplex is extremely poor if encephalitis develops, with a high risk of either death or severe mental retardation. An important consideration in the care of infants with known or suspected herpes simplex infection is isolation from other patients to prevent transmission.

Varicella. Another viral infection with manifestation in the skin is varicella. Varicella infection is rare, but when it occurs in the first 10 days of life, it is generally thought to have been acquired in utero. The vesicular eruptions are the same as those in chickenpox acquired at any age. A mortality rate of 20% is associated with varicella infection in newborns, and certainly this infection poses a significant risk for the immunocompromised infants in premature and intensive care nurseries. No systemic medication or topical treatment is required for these lesions. Occasionally scarring can occur. Strict isolation is absolutely necessary to protect other infants from exposure because this virus is airborne. Passive immunization of infants exposed to the affected infant may also be necessary.

Toxoplasmosis. Toxoplasmosis, which is caused by an intracellular parasite (*Toxoplasma gondii*), can be transmitted transplacentally and can result in systemic infection. Some infants may have a generalized maculopapular rash as well as hepatosplenomegaly, jaundice, fever, and anemia. The rash may progress to desquamation and hypopigmentation in very severe cases. Direct topical therapy is not reported to be necessary or efficacious; systemic therapy may be considered.

Cytomegalovirus and Rubella. Both CMV and rubella have symptoms that are manifested in the skin. Petechial lesions can occur with both infections. These are the result of thrombocytopenia and dermal erythropoiesis and usually disappear in 2 to 6 weeks. In severe rubella infection, and very rarely in CMV, bluish-red papules that are 2 to 8 mm in diameter can occur on the head, trunk, and extremities (Figure 12.7), resulting in the description "blueberry muffin" syndrome. Neither of these lesions requires topical therapy (for a complete discussion of infections, see Chapter 26).

■ **Fungal.** *Candida albicans* infection is the primary fungal infection with cutaneous manifestations, although other species—such as *Candida parapsilosis*, *Candida tropicalis*, *Candida lusitaniae*, *Candida glabrata*, and *Malassezia furfur*—can also potentially colonize the skin of term and preterm newborns, particularly those who are hospitalized in an intensive care nursery. Clinical symptoms of this type of infection can range from diaper dermatitis to other mucous membranes or localized skin eruptions to systemic candidiasis, resulting in significant morbidity and mortality. *Candida* is not normally found on the skin of the newborn. The primary reservoir for this organism is the gastrointestinal tract, but the skin can be colonized at birth during passage through a contaminated birth canal. The incidence of *Candida* colonization is also increased with the frequent use of broad-spectrum antibiotics that alter normal skin flora in infants after delivery. Nursing assessment of the

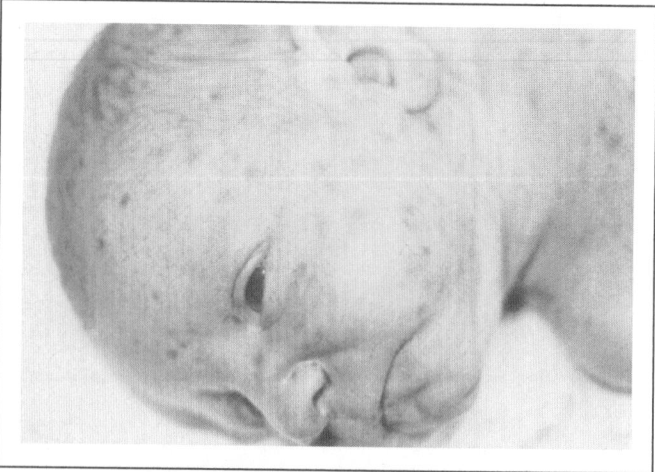

FIGURE 12.7 This is an example of the "blueberry muffin" syndrome, seen in an infant with congenital cytomegalovirus infection. The infant has multiple petechiae and purpura from thrombocytopenia in this systemic infection.
Reprinted with permission from Clark and Thompson (1986). Copyright © Wyeth-Ayerst Labs.

low-birth-weight infant should include the observation of a monilial diaper rash or a diffuse burn-like dermatitis affecting large areas of the lower back, buttocks, chest, and abdomen (Baley & Silverman, 1988). Although rare, cutaneous fungal infections in VLBW infants have also been reported due to aspergillosis (Woodruff & Herbert, 2002).

Premature neonates with systemic candidiasis may demonstrate cutaneous involvement. This cutaneous pattern may be a diffuse burn-like dermatitis that affects large areas on the lower back, buttocks, chest, and abdomen. In a few infants, the axilla and groin are affected. Scaling follows the erythematous macular patches, and in severe cases desquamation develops in a manner similar to that seen in staphylococcal scalded skin syndrome. These infants do not always have the satellite papules and pustules normally seen with *Candida* diaper dermatitis. The onset of the generalized rash often occurs within the first 3 days of life, but it can appear later. Erosive crusting lesions in a cohort of extremely premature infants as an invasive fungal dermatitis, leading also to systemic disease, were reported (Rowen, Atkins, Levy, Baer, & Baker, 1995). Skin biopsies performed on patients with this condition revealed fungal invasion that extended beyond the epidermis into the dermis. The onset is several days after birth, and associated factors included maternal colonization with vaginal birth, steroid administration, hyperglycemia, and skin trauma from adhesive removal.

Another important cause of necrotic and purpuric lesions in neonates with ecchymoses and crust-like plaques is cutaneous infection with mold species, such as *Aspergillus*, *Fusarium*, *Rhozopus*, and *Mucor* (Hook & Eichenfield, 2011). Biopsy is often part of the evaluation, particularly if surface cultures are not conclusive, and cutaneous debridement along with systemic antifungal agents may improve outcomes for these rare cases.

Management. Medical and nursing management of infants with systemic or local *Candida* infection involves therapy with systemic antifungal medications and antifungal ointments and creams. Cutaneous *Candida* in the extremely premature infant less than a week of age requires aggressive monitoring for systemic infection and may warrant parenteral antifungal agents to prevent dissemination of the fungal infection. Yeast is sometimes difficult to culture; techniques include obtaining urine to look for hyphae or budding yeast, blood cultures, and skin scrapings prepared with potassium hydroxide (KOH) obtained from the margins of the affected areas since this is the area of active growth, and examined for pseudohyphae (Cunningham & Wagner, 2008). Nursing observation in low-birth-weight infants for evidence of the diffuse burn-like dermatitis or a spreading monilial diaper rash is essential and may expedite the initiation of parenteral antifungal therapy with amphotericin B for systemic candidiasis.

Treatment for *Candida* diaper dermatitis consists of keeping the area clean and dry and applying an antifungal ointment or cream several times a day. Thrush, an oral fungal infection, appears as patches of white material scattered over the tongue that cannot be scraped off. It is treated with an oral form of nystatin.

Scaling Disorders

A scaly appearance in the skin of a newborn can have a range of causes, from relatively benign to long term and potentially life threatening. In this section, scaly skin due to postmaturity, essential fatty acid deficiency, congenital ichthyosis, and eczema is discussed, and areas of nursing management are determined.

■ **Postmaturity.** Many term infants born between 40 and 42 weeks gestation experience a period of shedding, or desquamation that is considered to be a normal physiologic process. Postmature infants born after 42 weeks gestation may also have this appearance, but other characteristics are different. The postmature infant may have a lean appearance, with little subcutaneous fat; the weight is low in relationship to length. The skin resembles parchment paper and may literally peel off in sheets. Fingernails may be stained with meconium and may be long. Long hair may also be present.

Skin care is not the major problem, nor is it the focus of medical or nursing management. Eventually, the skin underneath the peeling layers predominates; even during the period of desquamation, the skin functions well as a barrier because these infants have all the layers of stratum corneum of a term infant or adult. Aside from bathing with a mild soap initially, moisturizing with a petrolatum-based ointment may be appropriate. More careful attention is paid to the more compelling problems associated with postmaturity, such as hypoglycemia and meconium aspiration.

■ **Essential Fatty Acid Deficiency.** In newborns unable to receive an adequate diet because of other illnesses or surgical conditions, scaly dry skin may signify the development of essential fatty acid deficiency syndrome. Infants may be more prone to the development of this syndrome, especially if they are premature or postmature because of the decreased fat stores available. It may also occur in infants with severe fat malabsorption, such as those with cystic fibrosis.

The skin appearance in essential fatty acid deficiency includes a superficial scaling and, in some cases, desquamation. Later presentation may involve oozing and irritation in the neck, groin, or perianal region.

This syndrome is sometimes confused with other conditions that cause scaling or other skin disruptions, including ichthyosis, acrodermatitis enteropathica, and candidal infection. Laboratory findings that confirm this diagnosis are decreased serum essential fatty acid levels, possibly in conjunction with thrombocytopenia and impaired platelet aggregation, because essential fatty acids are necessary to ensure platelet function.

Management. Medical and nursing management consists of replacement of essential fatty acids through the administration of intravenous lipid solutions or diet. Human breast milk and most infant formulas contain more than adequate amounts of essential fatty acids. However, if the gastrointestinal system is not functioning well in the digestion and absorption of nutrients, intravenous therapy is required.

Once skin symptoms are present, administration of intravenous lipid solution can reverse the process in 1 to 2 weeks. Dietary replacement takes longer and is effective only in the presence of healthy gastrointestinal function.

Prevention of essential fatty acid deficiency is possible and should be the goal. The development of essential fatty acid deficiency can be prevented by the early administration of intravenous lipid solutions in the first weeks of life in a dose as low as 0.5 g/kg/d.

■ **Ichthyosis.** The most serious cause of scaly skin in the newborn is ichthyosis dermatosis. Four major types of ichthyosis exist: (1) X-linked ichthyosis; (2) lamellar ichthyosis; (3) bullous congenital ichthyosiform erythroderma, which is present at birth; and (4) ichthyosis vulgaris, which usually appears after the third month of life. Terms commonly used to describe infants with ichthyosis may include harlequin fetus and collodion baby, but these terms do not define which form of ichthyosis is present.

In the X-linked type of ichthyosis, males are affected. Some female heterozygotes may exhibit mild scaling of the arms and lower extremities. Affected male newborns have large yellow or brown plaques that cover the whole body, except the palms, soles, and midface, and over joints. At birth, some affected males may appear scaly, whereas others are often called collodion babies.

Lamellar ichthyosis, formerly called nonbullous congenital ichthyosiform erythroderma, is an autosomal recessive disorder. Initially, affected newborns may have a bright red appearance that rapidly progresses to desquamation; rarely is a collodion-baby appearance present at birth. Later, scales develop that are yellow to brown and that may eventually become thick, horny plates. Although the prognosis is usually good, infants who are severely affected—the so-called harlequin fetuses—may die of sepsis or require extensive plastic surgery (Figure 12.8).

In bullous congenital ichthyosiform erythroderma, autosomal dominance is the mode of heredity; thus several family members may be affected. Large bullae are initially seen, as are erythema and dry scaly skin; the blistering that recurs throughout childhood differentiates this form from the lamellar type. Extensive denuded areas of the skin can present a problem in the newborn as the blisters burst because secondary infections with *Streptococcus* or *Staphylococcus* can occur and are life threatening.

Management. Medical and nursing management of all forms of ichthyosis involves the continual use of topical therapies and prescription bathing techniques and the prevention of infection. Bathing is performed with a water-dispersible bath oil, and soaps that are excessively drying or irritating should be avoided. Collodion babies should be placed in a high-humidity incubator to increase hydration. Emollients that preserve moisturization such as Aquaphor ointment (Beiersdorf, Inc., Wilton, CT) should be applied several times daily.

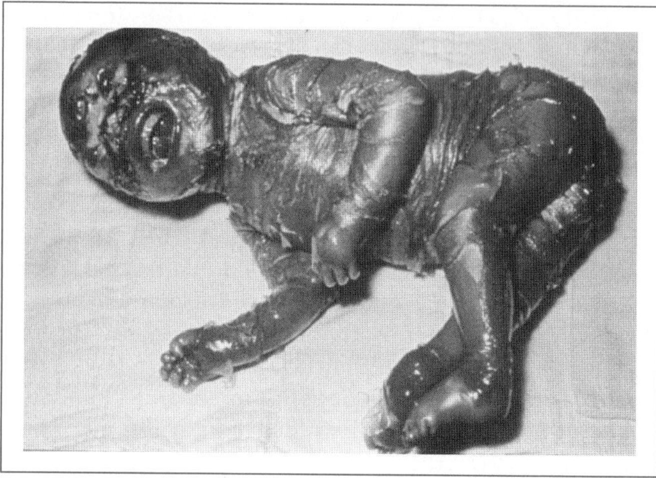

FIGURE 12.8 This harlequin infant is an example of the most severely affected ichthyotic infant. The skin is hard and thick, with deep crevices. The lack of elasticity of the skin results in fleshy deformities of joints and limbs.
Reprinted with permission from Clark and Thompson (1986). Copyright © Wyeth-Ayerst Labs.

Infants with severe skin involvement from ichthyosis may require protective isolation if they receive care in an intensive care nursery because of the higher risk of contact with nosocomial infections. Incubators provide a barrier to infection. Use of sterile linen and sterile gloves and other measures are needed if larger areas of denuded skin are present.

Comfort is another key nursing concern in the care of the infant who is significantly affected with ichthyosis. Fussy, irritable agitation may be seen and is related to pruritus or inflammation. Some form of analgesia may help, although the topical therapies prescribed have the most direct effect. Some authors describe the use of diphenhydramine (Benadryl, Pfizer, Morris Plains, NJ) if severe pruritus exists, but this would be hard to determine in a neonate, who lacks verbal or fine motor skills to communicate this symptom. A trial of this medication with careful observation might be helpful in the case of a frantic or irritable infant when other measures (e.g., topical treatment, pacifiers, feeding) are unsuccessful.

Working with the parents of an infant with ichthyosis has many facets. The appearance of the infant, especially if he or she is severely affected, could be shocking and traumatic to the parents and could require careful interventions. As with parents of infants with other congenital abnormalities, a period of shock, denial, and grief occurs over the loss of a perfect baby. In addition, the genetic nature of this disorder and the implications for future children must be comprehended. Parents of these infants need genetic counseling, support, and education as they come to terms with this disease.

■ **Eczema.** Eczema, which is a skin disorder that causes several degrees of skin irritation and has multiple causes, is rarely seen in the newborn period. It is more commonly seen after 2 months of age and involves an eruption that proceeds to the development of microvesicles and oozing, which later turns into scaling of the epidermis. The scaling is due to an attempt of the skin layer to regenerate rapidly. Lichenification, or thickening of the skin, which occurs in adult skin with eczema, is not seen in infants. Primary irritants—such as saliva, feces, and some soaps or skin preparations—rather than allergies are the usual causes of eczema in infants. It is important to have a good history of all products that have been applied to the skin to determine the cause. If external agents have been ruled out, other diagnoses are considered, such as seborrheic dermatitis and Leiner's disease, which involves a total exfoliation of the entire body.

Management. Medical and nursing treatment of eczema involves prevention by avoiding the primary irritant source, if it has been identified, or protection, as in the use of zinc oxide paste to the perianal area to prevent contact with feces. For more generalized eruptions, short-term therapy with topical steroids may be used. Bathing should be carried out in tepid water with water-dispersible oil; use of irritating or drying soaps should be avoided. If large areas of skin are involved, thermoregulation may be a concern, especially in dry climates. Humidification may be desirable in some climates, especially during the summer months. Air conditioning may also be necessary during the summer months. Discomfort is a significant concern because infants with eczema may experience considerable pruritus. Topical therapy is generally the first consideration, followed by the judicious use of diphenhydramine in severe cases.

SKIN CARE PRACTICES

The most basic aspects of skin care for newborns include daily bath; moisturizing with emollients; skin preparation with disinfectant solutions; and use of adhesives for life-support devices, monitoring of vital signs, and oxygenation, if the newborns are hospitalized. During all these practices, the skin of the newborn has the potential for trauma or alterations in normal barrier function and pH. The literature is reviewed to determine what is currently known about these and other common nursing practices and the impact on the skin of newborns.

Bathing

The purpose of bathing newborns includes providing overall hygiene, aesthetics, and protection of health care workers by removing blood and body fluids. However, bathing is not an innocuous procedure and during the immediate postbirth period can result in hypothermia, increased oxygen consumption, and respiratory distress. The first bath should be delayed until the infant's temperature has been stabilized in the normal range for 1 to 4 hours (Penny-MacGillivray, 1996; Varda & Behnke, 2000). Bathing has also been shown to destabilize vital signs and temperature in premature infants.

Bathing with antiseptic soaps and cleansers is still practiced in some nurseries. Studies have shown that although hexachlorophene reduced the number of *S. aureus* strains, toxicity was reported, especially in premature infants, and was associated with absorption through the skin; thus it should not be used (American Academy of Pediatrics, 1997). Both povidone-iodine and chlorhexidine are sometimes used for the initial bath in newborn nurseries, although the effect on bacterial colonization is transient.

Chlorhexidine has proven effective in reducing colonization for up to 4 hours but can also be absorbed. Although toxicity from chlorhexidine has not been identified, many nurseries do not use chlorhexidine for routine bathing because of the potential risk. No guidelines from the Centers for Disease Control (CDC, 2006) or the American Academy of Pediatrics recommend the use of antimicrobial cleansers for the newborn's first or subsequent baths (AAP & ACOG, 2007).

Products used in bathing include soaps made with lye and animal fats that are alkaline (pH > 7.0) and cleansing bars and liquids made with synthetic detergents that are formulated to a more neutral pH of 5.5 to 7.0. All soaps and cleansers are at least mildly irritating and drying to skin surfaces. Study of bathing with soap, cleansing liquid, or cleansing bar in infants ages 2 weeks to 16 months showed alterations in fat content, hydration, and skin surface pH—most significantly with alkaline soap (Gfatter, Hackl, & Braun, 1997). In addition, the degree to which the skin is irritated also depends on the length of contact and the frequency of bathing.

Selecting cleansers that have a neutral pH and minimal dyes and perfumes to reduce risk of future sensitization to these products and bathing only two to three times per week is the best course to follow. Reducing the frequency of bathing even to 4-day intervals did not increase colonization with pathogens or result in infections in a study of healthy premature infants (Franck, Quinn, & Zahr, 2000). For extremely premature infants, skin surfaces should be cleaned with warm water for the first week, with soft materials such as cotton balls or cloth. A rinsing technique is best during cleansing because rubbing is irritating to immature skin and is potentially uncomfortable. If areas of skin breakdown are evident, use warm sterile water.

Immersion bathing may be beneficial, when clinically possible, from a developmental perspective (Anderson, Lane, & Chang, 1995). Immersion bathing places the infant's entire body, except the head and neck, into warm water (100.4°F), deep enough to cover the shoulders. Stable premature infants (after umbilical catheters are removed) and term infants with umbilical clamp in place can safely be bathed in this way (AWHONN Guideline, 2007). A study of immersion versus sponge bathing in 102 newborns for their first and subsequent baths showed that the immersion-bathed infants had significantly less temperature drop, appeared more content, and their mothers reported more pleasure with the bath; there was no difference in cord healing scores with either immersion or sponge bathing (Bryanton, Walsh, Barrett, & Gaudet, 2004). Bathing is also an excellent time to educate parents about how to physically care for their babies and may also integrate information about their children's neurobehavioral status and social characteristics (Karl, 1999).

Emollients

The skin surface of term newborns is drier than that of adults but becomes gradually better hydrated as the eccrine sweat glands mature during the first year of life. Maintaining the hydration of the stratum corneum is necessary for an intact skin surface and normal barrier function. Skin that is dry, scaly, or cracking not only is uncomfortable but also can be a portal of entry for microorganisms.

Treatments for dry skin are called moisturizers or emollients. Emollients are classified as oil-in-water (ointments) or water-in-oil emulsions (creams, lotions). Ointments do not require a preservative, whereas creams and lotions do require preservatives due to the higher water content (Hoath & Narendran, 2000).

Several studies have evaluated emollient use in premature infants. Premature infants 29 to 36 weeks gestation were treated with a cream moisturizer twice daily and had less visible dermatitis but no change in skin barrier function (Lane & Drost, 1993). A randomized controlled trial of younger gestation premature infants receiving twice daily applications of a petrolatum ointment versus routine skin care reported improvements in skin barrier function (lower TEWL) and less visible dermatitis (Nopper et al., 1996). No increases in skin temperature or redness were seen if the infants were receiving phototherapy or cared for under radiant warmers, and no increase in bacterial or fungal cultures was reported. In addition, although there were not enough subjects to verify this outcome, the treated infants had fewer positive blood or cerebrospinal fluid cultures.

A large randomized controlled trial of 1,191 extremely-low-birth-weight infants (510–1,000 g) was undertaken to determine if the twice daily prophylactic application of petrolatum-based ointment would reduce the combined outcomes of mortality and sepsis (Edwards, Conner, & Soll, 2004). No effect was seen in these combined outcomes, although skin integrity appeared improved in the treated infants. It is important to note that in the less than 750 g group of infants, the incidence of bloodstream infections with coagulase-negative staphylococcus was increased in the group with prophylactic use of the emollient, although the mechanism and relationship to routine emollient use are not clearly understood. The control infants in this study also received emollients on an "as needed" basis for skin dryness.

A Cochrane review evaluated randomized controlled trials of emollient use in the NICU and concluded that the prophylactic application of topical ointment increases the risk of coagulase-negative staphylococcus infection, as well as other nosocomial infections. The routine use of emollients in preterm infants is not recommended (Conner, Soll, & Edwards, 2004).

The benefits of emollient use in premature infants must be carefully weighed against the risk of infection. In general, emollients can be safely used in this population to treat skin with excessive drying, skin cracking, and fissures. They may also be beneficial in reducing TEWL and evaporative heat loss, although other methods, such as using a high-humidity environment or transparent adhesive dressings, are also available for this purpose (AWHONN Guideline, 2007). Small tubes or jars for single patient use are recommended to prevent contamination with microorganisms.

The role of routine emollient use in healthy newborns is not clear. Benefits of emollient use for infants with eczema (atopic dermatitis) are known, and whether routine emollient use for newborns and infants with a strong family history of atopic dermatitis is beneficial has yet to be proven.

Disinfectants

Use of skin disinfectants prior to invasive procedures such as inserting intravenous lines, venipuncture, arterial puncture, umbilical catheter placement, and chest tube placement is commonly seen in neonatal nurseries. Skin antisepsis practices such as cord care regimens and application of antimicrobial washes before invasive procedures were adopted in attempts to control nursery epidemics of streptococcal and staphylococcal infections. Concerns with disinfection practices include the effects of absorption of disinfectants and skin injury resulting from topical skin preparation with these agents, which must be weighed against the effectiveness in preventing infection.

Disinfectants that are used in newborns include 70% isopropyl alcohol, 10% povidone-iodine, and chlorhexidine gluconate, in varying concentrations as both an aqueous solution and one combined with 70% isopropyl alcohol. There have been anecdotal reports of skin blistering, burns, and sloughing from isopropyl alcohol (Harpin & Rutter, 1982; Schick & Milstein, 1981) and chlorhexidine gluconate products (Andersen, Hart, Vemgal, & Harrison, 2005; Mannan, Chow, Lissauer, & Godambe, 2007; Reynolds, Banerjee, & Meek, 2005) in premature infants (Figure 12.9). Several prospective studies of routine povidone-iodine use in NICUs (Linder et al., 1997; Parravicini et al., 1996) found elevated urinary iodine levels and alterations in thyroid function in premature infants as a result of iodine absorption though the skin. Studies conducted in the United States have shown variable effects on thyroid function. AvRuskin, Greenfield, Prasad, Greig, and Juan (1994) found lower T3 and T4 levels in premature infants 26 to 30 weeks gestation, but no rise in thyroid-stimulating hormone (TSH) levels. Gordon, Rowitch, Mitchell, and Kohane (1995) reported no alterations in thyroid function levels (T3, T4, and TSH) despite measurable excretion of urinary iodine, although a single sample at 10 days of life may have been insufficient to capture this effect.

In addition to skin irritation and toxicity, the efficacy of these solutions is another important consideration. As a skin preparation prior to blood culture samples in children and adults, povidone-iodine was superior to isopropyl alcohol in decontaminating the skin surface (Choudhuri, McQueen, Inoue, & Gordon, 1990). A large study comparing chlorhexidine gluconate to povidone-iodine for blood cultures in adults found fewer contaminated cultures with chlorhexi-

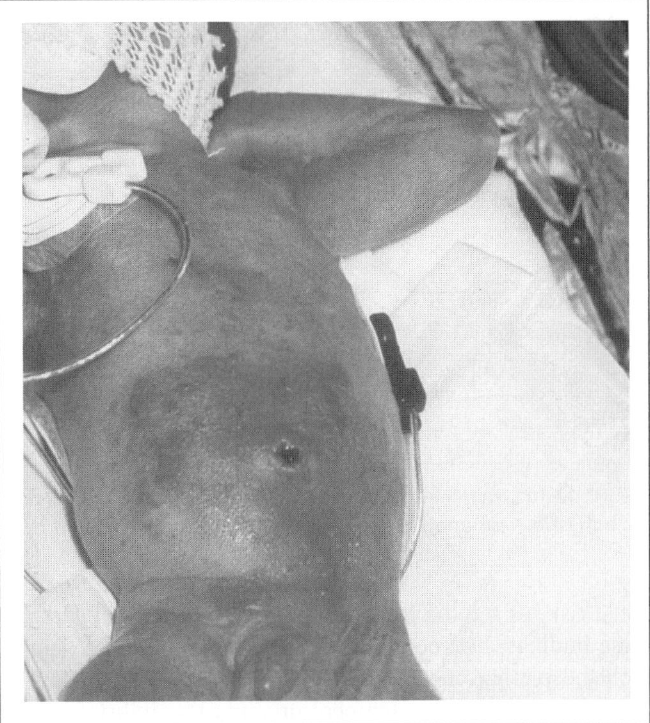

FIGURE 12.9 Skin injury resulting from skin disinfectant.

dine compared to povidone-iodine (Mimoz et al., 1999). A retrospective, quasi-experimental study of blood cultures in a pediatric emergency room population ages 2 to 36 months found contamination rates significantly lower when chlorhexidine gluconate (3.15% in 70% isopropyl alcohol) was used for skin antisepsis compared to povidone-iodine (Marlowe et al., 2010).

A number of studies support the efficacy of chlorhexidine-containing solutions in preventing colonization and infections in adults with central venous catheters (Chaiyakunapruk, Veenstra, Lipsky, & Saint, 2002). Large studies determining the best disinfectants for neonates with central venous catheters are not available. Chlorhexidine gluconate disinfection has been shown to reduce colonization with microorganisms in peripheral intravenous catheters in a large number of neonates (Garland et al., 1995). A pilot study of 47 infants comparing 2% CHG/isopropyl alcohol to povidone-iodine for percutaneously inserted central catheters in infants greater than 1,500 g, and greater than 7 days old found no difference in bloodstream infection, sepsis evaluations, and skin irritancy, but was terminated by the sponsor and was not powered to look at colonization rates (Garland et al., 2009).

The selection of appropriate disinfectants in neonates remains a dilemma. Chlorhexidine-containing products in the United States are limited to a 2% aqueous surgical scrub solution available only in 4-ounce bottles, and a 2% and 3.15% chlorhexidine solution in 70% isopropyl alcohol available in single-use packaging. The U. S. Food and Drug Administration states that chlorhexidine-containing disinfectants should be used with care around premature infants or infants less than 2 months of age, as these may cause skin irritation and chemical burns. Povidone-iodine continues to be used in many nurseries to avoid the above complications, although the issues of thyroid toxicity remain a concern.

Technique of application is another consideration. Chlorhexidine gluconate is applied in two consecutive wipings or for a 30-second scrub; aqueous chlorhexidine gluconate will not dry, but can be wiped off with sterile gauze after application. Povidone-iodine is applied with two consecutive applications and allowed to dry for 30 seconds. Isopropyl alcohol does evaporate after application, but due to the poor efficacy and potential skin damage, it is not recommended (AWHONN, 2007). Although the removal of disinfectants with sterile water or saline after the procedure is complete has been advocated (AWHONN, 2007), the manufacturer of the 2% CHG in isopropyl alcohol product advises that removal not be attempted, as the residual effect of the disinfectant on the skin may be beneficial. However, it is not known whether this feature may contribute to skin irritancy in newborns and premature infants.

Chlorhexidine should not be used as preoperative skin disinfection on the face or head because misuse has been reported to result in injury if it remains in contact with either the eye or ear during surgical procedures. However, careful use before scalp intravenous or central-line insertion is acceptable, providing that splashing or using excessive amounts of chlorhexidine is acceptable (AWHONN, 2007). In addition, there is no clinical data to discourage the use of chlorhexidine gluconate products prior to lumbar puncture or epidural catheter placement, as this is considered skin antisepsis (Milstone, Passaretti, & Perl, 2008).

The use of antibiotic ointments and skin antiseptics to the umbilical cord can prolong the time to cord separation and seems to have no beneficial effect on the frequency of infection (Zupan & Garner, 2000). A study of 1,811 newborns randomized to receive either routine isopropyl alcohol with each diaper change or natural drying found no umbilical infections in either group, and time to cord separation was reduced from 9.8 days in the alcohol-treated group to 8.16 days in the natural drying group (Dore et al., 1998). Another study randomized 766 newborns to receive either triple dye applied to the umbilical cord immediately after delivery followed by twice daily applications of isopropyl alcohol, or "dry care" without any treatment. Infants in the dry care group were more likely to be colonized with bacteria than the treatment group, and one infant in the dry care group developed omphalitis on the third day of life. The days to cord separation were not reported (Janssen, Selwood, Dobson, Peacock, & Thiessen, 2003). The development of omphalitis is not necessarily related to cord disinfection, as it also occurs in infants who have received topical disinfectants. However, vigilant attention to the signs and symptoms is necessary by health professionals, and parents need guidance about how to manage the umbilical cord and when to consult their health care provider (AWHONN, 2007).

Adhesives

Hospitalized full-term and premature newborns require the routine use of adhesives to secure life support and monitoring equipment such as endotracheal tubes, intravenous devices, oxygen saturation sensors, and electrodes. The evidence-based practice project involved in the development of the Neonatal Skin Care Guideline, which included skin and environment assessments for 2,820 premature and full-term newborns, found that adhesives were the primary cause of skin breakdown (Lund et al., 2001a). It is known that functional changes in adult skin, including altered skin barrier function (measured as increases in TEWL), are seen after 10 consecutive applications and removals of adhesive tape (Lo, Oriba, Maibach, & Bailin, 1990), and after one application/removal in premature infants (Harpin & Rutter, 1983; Lund et al., 1997).

Solvents are sometimes selected to reduce pain and skin irritation from adhesive removal. These products contain hydrocarbon derivatives, petrolatum distillates, or isopropyl alcohol with potential or proven systemic and topical toxicities. A case report of a premature infant developing a severe dermatologic reaction to an adhesive remover, including blistering and hemorrhage, suggest the lack of safety with these products in a NICU (Ittmann & Bozynski, 1993). Mineral oil or petrolatum ointment can facilitate the removal of adhesives but leave an oily residue that will interfere with later adhesive application. Removing adhesives with water-soaked cotton balls can be helpful, as well as gently pulling the adhesive parallel to the skin surface while holding the skin firmly during removal (Lund & Tucker, 2003).

Bonding agents promote the adherence of adhesives. These products are effective in securing tape strips used to close incisions in plastic surgery, for example, and facilitate the attachment to avoid dislodgment. However, when used on newborn skin, bonding agents may create a stronger bond to the epidermis than that between epidermis and dermis due to the fragile fibrils that connect these skin layers. Removal can result in epidermal stripping (Figure 12.9) and should be avoided. Plastic polymer skin protectants are available to protect skin from adhesives and not increase adhesive aggressiveness (Irving, 2001). Products that do not contain isopropyl alcohol are preferred, since the alcohol can also irritate newborn skin.

Hydrogel adhesives are available as electrodes for heart rate monitoring and as skin temperature probe covers. This type of adhesive cannot be used when adherence is critical, as they are easily dislodged and do not adhere well in high humidity environments; but they have been shown to reduce trauma associated with electrode removal (Lund et al., 1997; Webster & McCosker, 1994).

Skin barriers made from pectin and hydrocolloids are used to protect skin in ostomy patients and have been adapted for use as a "platform" between adhesives and skin in newborns (Figure 12.10) with less visible skin trauma when the adhesive was removed (Dollison & Beckstrand, 1995). A controlled trial of a pectin barrier, plastic perforated tape, and hydrogel adhesive found significant skin disruption, measured by elevated TEWL and visual inspection, following a single application and removal of both the pectin product and plastic tape (Lund et al., 1997). Significant changes were seen in all three weight groups studied (<1,000, 1,000–1,500 g, and 1,500–3,000 g), suggesting that more mature newborns are at risk for trauma from adhesive removal as well. Despite these findings, hydrocolloid products continue to be helpful in the hospitalized newborn due to improved adherence as the product warms to skin temperature, and the ability to mold to surfaces better than many other products. These adhesives do require care upon removal, similar to adhesive tapes.

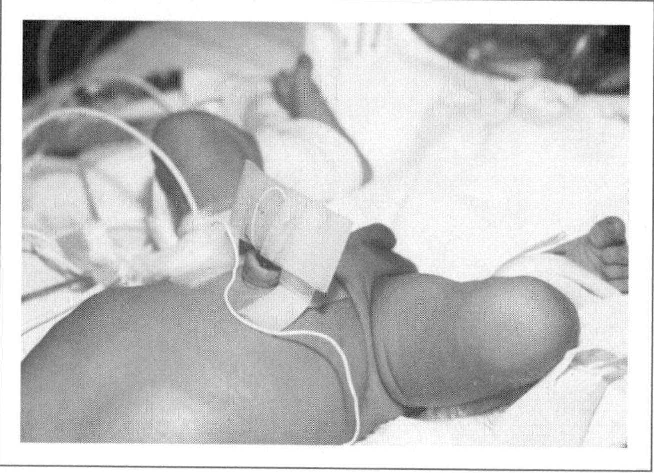

FIGURE 12.10 Skin in newborns with less visible skin trauma when the adhesive was removed.

Semipermeable dressings have proven to be very beneficial for selective taping procedures, such as intravenous and central venous catheter dressings, nasogastric tubes, and chest tubes. The potential for skin damage when removed is similar to other adhesive tapes.

Strategies to reduce skin injury from adhesives include using adhesives sparingly, avoiding the routine use of bandages after drawing blood samples, choosing adhesive products tailored to a specific task (i.e., endotracheal tube holders), using nonadhesive products when possible such as soft wraps, selective use of skin protectants to replace bonding agents, and "double-backing" tapes or deactivating tape with cotton when appropriate. Silicone-based adhesives developed for use in wound care products (Figure 12.11) are now available as silicone tapes, and have been shown to improve adherence to wounds and reduce discomfort when removed (Dykes, Heggie, & Hill, 2001; Gotschall, Morrison, & Eichelberger, 1998). This technology holds promise for developing future adhesive products for newborns.

Transepidermal Water Loss

Because of the poorly keratinized stratum corneum that provides minimal resistance to the diffusion of water, the preterm infant is subjected to TEWL and heat loss via evaporation that results in low body temperatures during the first few days after birth. Characteristic skin factors that predispose premature infants to excessive water loss include reduced skin barrier function from fewer layers of stratum corneum and thinner epidermis, larger surface area in relation to body weight, increased water content, increased permeability, and increased blood supply that is closer to the skin surface.

TEWL is directly correlated to gestational age and degree of maturation of the epidermal stratum corneum. Mature keratin, which is a major component of the tough, nonliving

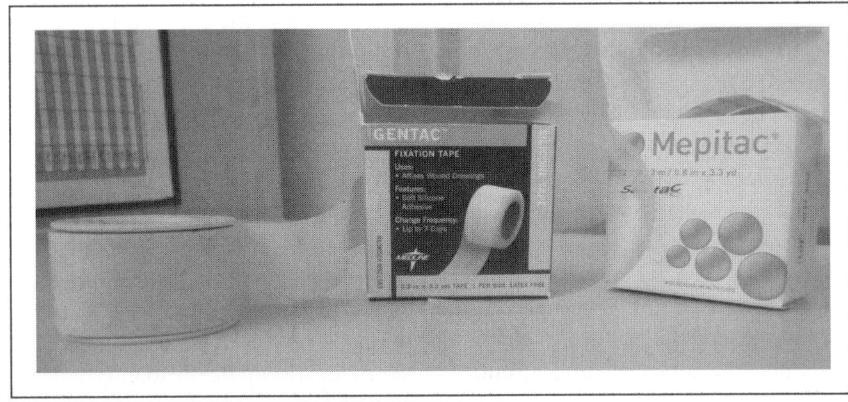

FIGURE 12.11 Silicone-based adhesives developed for use in wound care products are now available as silicone tapes, and have been shown to improve adherence to wounds and reduce discomfort when removed.

outer layer of the epidermis, is relatively water impermeable. Because keratin formation is directly related to gestational age, the extremely premature infant is at increased risk for increased evaporative losses. Water easily diffuses across the permeable skin barrier and evaporates. TEWL is influenced by many factors: ambient humidity, gestational age at birth, postnatal age, ambient temperature, weight, activity, and body temperature. Term infants have been shown to have lower TEWL levels compared to adults, with the exception of the antecubital region (Yosipovitch et al., 2000). Infants who are small for gestational age have a lower TEWL in the first day after birth than that of infants of the same gestational age whose weight is appropriate for gestational age.

The highest TEWL levels are seen in extremely premature infants. Water losses of 130 to 160 mL/kg/d have been measured in infants of 23 to 25 weeks gestation (Agren et al., 1998). Mature barrier function—at one time thought to advance rapidly over a 2-week period in premature infants less than 30 weeks gestation—has been shown to take longer in extremely premature infants of 23 to 24 weeks gestation and occurs when the infant reaches approximately 30 to 31 weeks postconceptional age (Kalia et al., 1998).

Several techniques that have been shown to reduce evaporative heat and TEWL in very-low-birth-weight infants include the use of double-walled incubators, increased ambient humidity, transparent adhesive dressings, and coating the skin with petrolatum-based emollients.

For the past two decades it has been known that ISWL is greater under radiant warmers than in incubators without shields. The addition of the heat shield reduces ISWL in the incubator but not under the radiant warmer. A plastic blanket under a radiant warmer reduces oxygen consumption, ISWL, and radiant-warmer demands. In 1995, Kjartansson, Arsan, Hammarlund, Sjors, and Sedin (1995) measured the rate of evaporation from the skin of 12 full-term and 16 preterm infants (gestational age of 25–34 weeks), both during incubator care and in care under a radiant warmer. They concluded that the evaporative water loss from the skin depends on the ambient water vapor pressure, irrespective of whether the infant is nursed under a radiant warmer or in an incubator. The higher rate of evaporation during care under a radiant warmer is due to the lower ambient water vapor pressure and not to any direct effect of the nonionizing radiation on the skin. Regardless of the device being used, the "microclimate" of the infant needs to be assessed. This assessment should consider the temperature and relative humidity (RH). A RH below 40% is drying to the skin and leads to excessive TEWL in the extremely premature infant.

Plastic wraps and transparent adhesive dressings have also been shown to reduce TEWL and evaporative heat loss. Immediately after delivery, infants greater than 28 weeks gestation wrapped with occlusive polyethylene bags covering their torso and extremities had significantly better temperatures than infants who received drying and radiant heat in the delivery room due to significantly reduced evaporative heat and water loss; the wrapping was removed upon admission to the NICU. Mortality also significantly decreased in the infants who were wrapped (Knobel, Wimmer, & Holbert, 2005; Vohra, Frent, Campbell, Abbott, & Whyte, 1999; Vohra, Roberts, Zhang, Janes, & Schmidt, 2004).

Transparent adhesive dressings applied to large areas of skin surfaces reduce TEWL (Bustamante & Steslow, 1989; Knauth, Gordin, McNelis, & Baumgart, 1989; Mancini, Sookdeo-Drost, Madison, Smoller, & Lane, 1994; Vernon, Lane, Wischerath, Davis, & Menegus, 1990). However, in a prospective study there was no difference in fluid intake or elevated serum sodium levels in infants treated with transparent adhesive dressings compared to controls (Donahue, Phelps, Richter, & Davis, 1996). Although a retrospective study reported improved fluid and sodium balance (Bhandari, Brodsky, & Porat, 2005), the deleterious effect of removal of these dressings similar to other adhesives has led to decreased interest in this technique for management of TEWL.

High humidity (>70% RH) added to the incubator has been shown to effectively reduce evaporative heat loss and TEWL; the rate of TEWL has been shown to decrease by half when the RH increases from 20% to 60% (Hammarlund & Sedin, 1979). High humidity reduced fluid requirements and serum sodium abnormalities in a cohort of premature infants compared to historical controls (Gaylord, Wright, Lorch, Lorch, & Walker, 2001). The use of humidified "hybrid" incubators in premature infants less than 1,000 g, capable of providing high humidity in a convectively heated incubator and also radiant heat for procedures and emergencies, resulted in positive effects on fluid balance, electrolyte stability, and growth velocity. However, the incidence of both gram-positive and gram-negative infection was higher in the humidified incubator group, although this was not found to be statistically significant (Kim, Lee, Chen, & Ringer, 2010). This study utilized high levels of humidity (70%–80%) for the first week of life, and reduced the humidity levels to 50% to 60% from the second week until the infant reached 30 to 32 weeks postconceptual age (Kim et al., 2010). The rationale for reducing the humidity level in this fashion was based on an earlier study that demonstrated improved skin barrier function and maturity when humidity levels were reduced to 50% compared to 75% in the second week of life (Agren et al., 2006).

Servo-controlled, actively generated heating and humidification systems do not cause airborne aerosols that can be contaminated with microorganisms. These can also be set for precise control of humidity and recovery of humidity levels because of continually added water vapor (Figure 12.12) (Drucker & Marshall, 1995; Marshall, 1997).

Application of petrolatum-based emollients every 6 to 12 hours also reduces TEWL and can be used on infants on radiant warmers or under phototherapy without temperature increases or burns (Nopper et al., 1996). A novel use of a protective barrier film was also shown to reduce TEWL compared to petrolatum ointment in premature infants less than 33 weeks gestation (Brandon, Coe, Hudson-Barr, Oliver, & Landerman, 2010). However, due to the concerns raised in a large randomized control trial of infants less than 1,000 g regarding increased coagulase negative staphylococcus infects with prophylactic use of this agent (Edwards et al., 2004), these approaches are not recommended without further study.

Although each of three techniques has been shown to be effective, none have been compared; thus it is not clear which is most effective with the fewest side effects. However, addressing the important area of reducing excessive heat loss and TEWL is necessary in the care of the small premature neonate with lung disease to maintain adequate hydration without excessive fluid intake. The goal of maintaining hydration and normal serum sodium levels on an intake of less than 150 mL/kg/d is optimal and achievable using one of these preventive strategies.

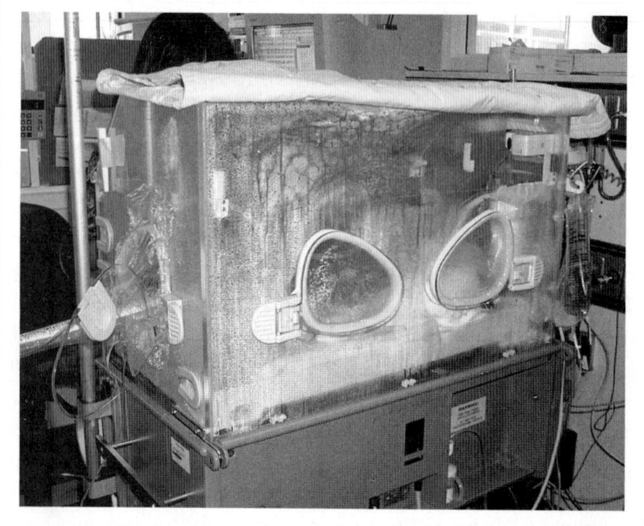

FIGURE 12.12 Incubator with more than 70% RH; humidity is generated by a heating system that is separate from circulating convective heat to prevent contamination with microorganisms.

MANAGEMENT OF SKIN CARE PROBLEMS

The stratum corneum can be traumatized by a variety of insults, including epidermal stripping from removal of adhesives; burns from transcutaneous oxygen electrodes; pressure sores; infection; nutritional inadequacies, such as zinc and essential fatty acid deficiency; extravasation of intravenous fluids; and diaper dermatitis. The goal of all skin care for neonates should be the maintenance of skin integrity; however, even with meticulous care, skin breakdown can occur.

Skin Assessment

A thorough examination of all skin surfaces on a daily basis will reveal the state of skin integrity in critically ill or extremely premature infants in the NICU. Early signs of skin abrasions or small excoriations may call for either diagnostic or treatment procedures. A skin assessment tool such as the Neonatal Skin Condition Score (NSCS) (Box 12.2, Figure 12.13), used in the AWHONN/National Association of Neonatal Nurses (NANN) research-based practice project may be beneficial when assessing skin conditions (Lund et al., 2001a, b). The NSCS was found to have both interrater and intrarater reliability, and validity was confirmed by the relationship of the skin scores with birth weight, number of observations over time, and prevalence of infection (Lund & Osborne, 2004). Identifying risk factors for skin injury in individual patients may include gestational age less than 32 weeks, use of paralytic medications and vasopressors, multiple tubes and lines, numerous monitors and probes, surgical wounds, ostomies, and technologies that limit patient movement such as high-frequency ventilation and extracorporeal membrane oxygenation. Other scoring tools such as the Braden Q and Starkid Scale that assess risk for pressure sores have been suggested (Curley, Razmus, Roberts, & Wypij, 2003; Suddaby, Barnett, & Facteau, 2005). However in these studies the number of neonates is not indicated, patients from ages 0 to 12 months are evaluated as a single group, and no premature infants were included so the applicability of these tools to a NICU population has not been demonstrated.

Skin Excoriations

When a skin excoriation is noted, the first step is to identify the cause of the injury before determining a treatment strategy. In cases in which no trauma has been known to occur, ruling out infectious causes—such as staphylococcal scalded skin syndrome and cutaneous candidiasis—is especially important because these conditions may require culturing and either systemic or topical antimicrobial treatment.

Ointments are sometimes used because of their antibacterial or antifungal properties and also because covering the wound with a semiocclusive layer promotes healing by facilitating the migration of epithelial cells across the surface. Petrolatum-based emollients and ointments are used to cover wounds and provide a semiocclusive layer that facilitates the migration of epithelial cells across the surface and may actually become

BOX 12.2

NEONATAL SKIN CONDITION SCORE

Dryness

1 = Normal, no sign of dry skin

2 = Dry skin, visible scaling

3 = Very dry skin, cracking/fissures

Erythema

1 = No evidence of erythema

2 = Visible erythema over less than 50% of the body's surface

3 = Visible erythema on more than 50% of the body's surface

Breakdown/Excoriation

1 = None evident

2 = Small localized areas

3 = Extensive

Perfect score = 3; worst score = 9

Adapted from the Association of Women's Health, Obstetric, and Neonatal Nurses (AWHONN) and the National Association of Neonatal Nurses, Skin Care Utilization Project. Copyright © 2001, AWHONN.

part of the stratum corneum layer during the healing process. Antibacterial ointments such as Polysporin, Bacitracin, or Bactroban are useful to treat gram-positive colonized surfaces, but can actually promote the growth of gram-negative organisms (Smack et al., 1996). Many dermatologists recommend against the use of Neosporin because of the potential for developing later sensitization to this ointment, although sensitization to Bacitracin is being reported with increasing frequency (Marks et al., 1995). If fungal infection is suspected, nystatin ointment is used and can also be applied to surrounding intact skin to prevent extension of the infection. In general, ointments are preferable to creams in this application because of better adherence and healing properties.

Transparent adhesive dressings made from a polyurethane film are backed with an adhesive that is impermeable to water and bacteria, but allows airflow. There must be a rim of intact skin around the wound to attach the dressing. Uses include wound care, dressings for IV devices—including central venous lines and percutaneous silicone catheters—and prevention of friction injuries to areas such as the knees or sacrum. When used for wound care, a transparent adhesive dressing promotes "moist healing" that allows the rapid migration of epithelial cells across the site. These dressings should only be used on "clean wounds" (uninfected) because bacteria and fungus can proliferate under the dressing. When placed over a clean wound, a serous or milky exudate often forms and is composed of leukocytes that actually aid in the prevention of infection. The dressings can be left in place for days at a time or until they become loose. Removing and reattaching the dressings on a daily basis is not recommended because the adhesive can injure the intact skin around the wound and further impede healing.

Some of the skin excoriations seen in the patient in the NICU cannot be easily covered with transparent adhesive dressings if no rim of intact skin exists around the site or if it is located in close proximity to other skin that cannot be separated or folds over the excoriation, such as the neck folds and the groin. Treatment of excoriations includes irrigating with sterile normal or half-normal saline every 4 to 6 hours and is effective in keeping the excoriation clean and moist. Dressings used in wound management include polyurethane films, hydrogel, hydrocolloid, and silicone dressings that promote moist healing (Baharestani, 2007; Fox, 2011). Silicone and hydrogel dressings can be used after irrigation of the wound and in conjunction with either antibacterial or antifungal ointment if the wound is infected. These dressings must be changed every 8 to 12 hours because they can dry out. It is best to avoid placing hydrogel dressings on intact skin surfaces because they can macerate the skin and actually reduce barrier function. Hydrocolloid dressings are used over uninfected wounds and can be left in place for 5 to 7 days while healing takes place (Sawatzky-Dickson & Bodnaryk, 2006). Surgical wounds that open or dehisce are infrequent but require expert wound management. Nutrition is often a part of the process in getting these wounds to heal, as is the prevention of infection. Often the surgeon or enterostomal therapist will design the appropriate wound management program for these situations.

Nutritional Deficiencies

Zinc is an essential trace element—essential because it is crucial for growth and development and a trace element because it is present in humans in quantities equal to or less than the quantities in which iron is present. Zinc is a cofactor in the reaction of more than 15 enzymes in many areas of metabolism. It is essential for lymphocyte transformation and is important for the metabolism of proteins, nucleic acids, and mucopolysaccharides of the skin and subcutaneous tissues. It is also an essential part of the enzyme structure of alkaline phosphatase (Prasad, 1995). In addition, zinc is required for normal taste, smell, and wound healing.

Zinc deficiency can result from inadequate intake, malabsorption, excessive loss, or a combination of factors (Coelho et al., 2006). Absorption and excretion of zinc occur primarily through the gastrointestinal tract. Deficiencies are related to abnormal losses of zinc in stool or urine, poor stores, or increased demands, as occur during rapid growth phases or stress. Total body zinc doubles between 32 and 40 weeks gestation, with two thirds of the maternal–fetal transport occurring during the last 10 weeks of gestation. Premature infants are at special risk for developing a zinc deficiency. Because they have trouble absorbing zinc and have not received adequate stores before birth, they may be in negative zinc balance for several weeks after birth. Other infants at risk for zinc deficiency include those with gastrointestinal pathology, chronic diarrhea, short-gut or short-bowel syndrome with jejunoileal bypass, necrotizing enterocolitis, or an ileostomy.

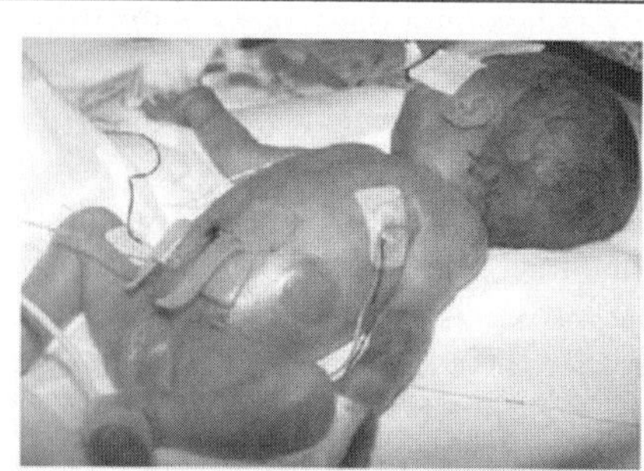

Dryness: 1 = normal, no sign of dry skin
Erythema: 2 = visible erythema <50% body surface
Breakdown: 3 = extensive

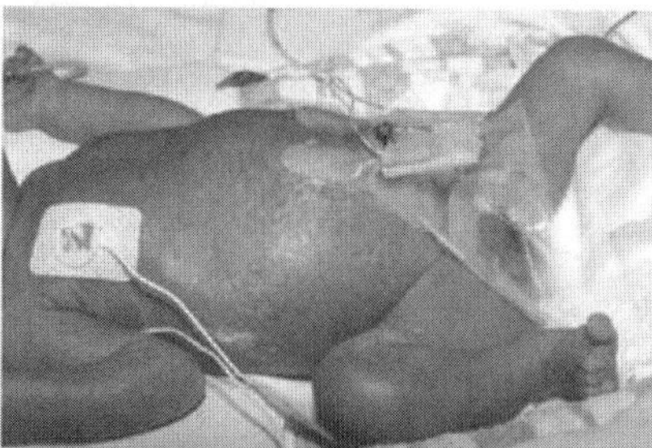

Dryness: 2 = dry skin, visible scaling
Erythema: 1 = no evidence of erythema
Breakdown: 1 = none evident

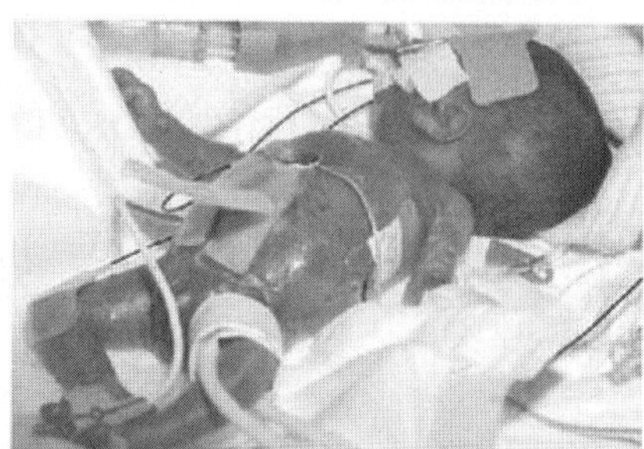

Dryness: 2 = dry skin, visible scaling
Erythema: 3 = visible erythema >50% body surface
Breakdown: 3 = extensive

FIGURE 12.13 Examples of skin assessments in three infants using the Neonatal Skin Condition Score (NSCS).

The clinical manifestations of zinc deficiency include lethargy, growth retardation, skin lesions, alopecia, and diarrhea; the striking sign of zinc deficiency, however, is some form of skin lesions. Common sites of involvement are the groin and perianal area, the neck folds, and the face, particularly the angles of the mouth and the cheeks. Lesions have also been noted at sites of trauma, such as endotracheal and cardiac monitor tape sites. The skin lesions are reddened, scaly, and moist. The skin eruption of zinc deficiency strongly resembles acrodermatitis enteropathica, a rare autosomal recessive disorder of zinc malabsorption and deficiency, in its morphologic features and distribution.

Zinc deficiency can result from inadequate intake of zinc. The routine supplementation of trace minerals in parenteral nutrition solutions has eliminated much of the zinc deficiency seen in the past. It is still seen in some premature infants who are exclusively breastfed. For infants receiving total parenteral nutrition, recommended zinc supplementation is 250 mcg/kg/d for term infants under 3 months of age and 400 mcg/kg/d for premature infants (Zenk, 1999). Oral supplementation with zinc sulfate ranges from 1 to 3 mg/kg/d. Recovery from zinc deficiency is dramatic once adequate zinc supplementation has begun. In general, skin conditions caused by nutritional deficiencies are often confused with infections and other irritants but do not respond until the deficiency itself is treated.

Intravenous Extravasations

The extravasation of intravenous fluids and medications can result in skin injury and, in some cases, deep-tissue injury to muscle and nerves (Figure 12.14). Neonates are at high risk for developing extravasation injuries because of their immature skin and the small size of their blood vessels. The most serious extravasation injuries are iatrogenic complications that can lead to pain, prolonged hospitalization, and increased morbidity, such as infection. Extravasation injuries can also result in increased hospital costs and the potential for legal action. Nursing actions such as the monitoring of intravenous sites and other preventive strategies as well as immediate interventions that can reduce the extent of tissue injury are important considerations for all nurseries that care for newborns with intravenous devices for fluid administration and medications. Some of the risk factors for tissue injury from intravenous extravasations in NICU patients are listed in Box 12.3.

Another risk factor is compromised perfusion to the skin, as evidenced by the poor capillary refill exhibited by the most critically ill neonates or by the obstructed venous circulations seen with taping methods that constrict the extremities in which the intravenous device is placed.

Prevention of skin injury after infiltration is the first important consideration. Strategies include ensuring that the insertion site is clearly visible by using transparent adhesive dressing or clear tape to secure the device and observing the site with appropriate documentation every hour. In addition, the tape should be carefully placed on the extremity to avoid obstruction of venous return. Tape placed loosely over a bony prominence, such as the knee or elbow, permits

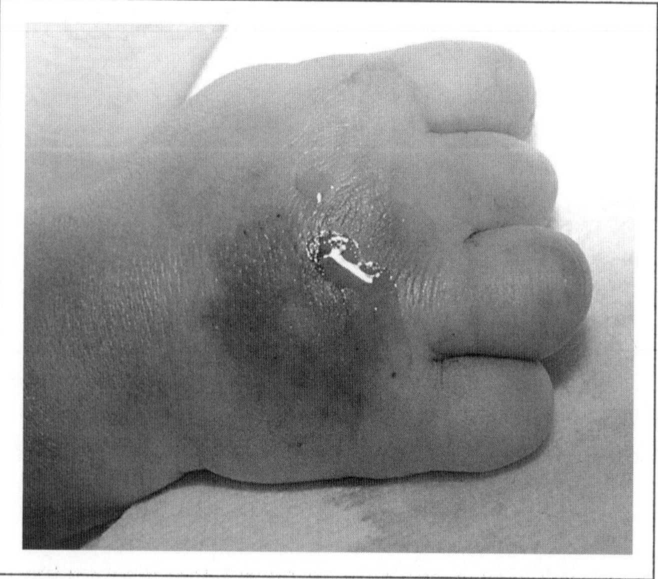

FIGURE 12.14 IV extravasation injury with swelling, discoloration, and leaking of fluid.

Box 12.3

RISKS FOR TISSUE INJURY FROM INTRAVENOUS EXTRAVASATIONS

Some of the factors known to increase the risk of tissue injury include:

- The length of exposure after extravasation occurs, especially when the patients are unable to verbalize the discomfort of pain or pressure
- The nature of the drug or solution; hypertonic solutions with high concentrations of calcium, potassium, glucose, or amino acids; and medications such as nafcillin have been identified as high risk for causing injury
- The mechanical compression caused by electronic infusion pumps

extravasated fluids and medications to disperse over a larger surface area and thus reduce the risk of injury, compared with extravasation that is limited to a small surface area. Avoiding extremities with poor perfusion in favor of better-perfused scalp veins (except, of course, those on the forehead) may also be prudent; in some cases, the wiser choice may be the placement of central venous lines for access. Nursery policies that limit the glucose (<12.5%), amino acid (<2%), and calcium (10%) concentrations are also strategies to reduce the risk of tissue injury from the extravasation of intravenous fluids and medications.

Once an intravenous extravasation has been identified, immediate measures to reduce injury are instituted (Thigpen, 2007). The device should be carefully removed, and the extremity should be elevated (if it is an arm or leg). Treatment with heat or moisture is not recommended because the delicate tissue could be further injured by a burn or the effects of maceration. Hyaluronidase is an enzyme that facilitates diffusion of the extravasated fluids by temporarily dissolving the normal interstitial barriers, reducing tissue damage (Banta & Noerr, 1992; Laurie, Wilson, Kernahan, Bauer, & Vistnes, 1984; Raszka, Kueser, Smith, & Bass, 1990). An alternative to intervention with hyaluronidase includes making multiple puncture holes over the area of greatest swelling and squeezing or allowing the fluid to leak out of the tissue to release the infiltrated fluid and potentially prevent skin injury (Chandavasu, Garrow, Valda, Alsheikh, & Dela Vega, 1986; Sawatzky-Dickson & Bodnaryk, 2006). Saline washout has also been described (Casanova, Bardot, & Magalon, 2001; Davies, Gault, & Buchdahl, 1994). Combinations of these steps may also prove beneficial.

If tissue damage results despite the immediate care measures, the use of topical wound care treatments is necessary. In the most severe cases of deep-tissue necrosis after extravasation injury, a surgical or plastic surgery consultation may be necessary (Figure 12.15).

Diaper Dermatitis

A common skin disruption that occurs in neonates and infants is diaper dermatitis (diaper rash). This term encompasses a range of processes that affect the perineum, groin, thighs, buttocks, and anal area of infants who are incontinent and wear some covering to collect urine and feces. Diaper dermatitis can be caused by many different mechanisms, but the condition of the skin has a direct role in the progression of skin injury. Review articles provide an excellent background for current evidence-based care in the prevention and treatment for diaper dermatitis (Adam, 2008; Heimall, Storey, Stellar, & Davis, 2012).

The pathogenesis of diaper dermatitis is partly related to the degree of wetness of the skin. Skin that is moist and macerated becomes more permeable and susceptible to injury because wetness increases friction. In addition, moisture-laden skin is more likely to contain microorganisms than dry skin is.

Another component in the process of skin injury from diaper dermatitis is the effect of an alkaline pH. The normal skin pH is acidic—ranging between 4.0 and 5.5—but can become alkaline when it is diapered (Visscher, Chatterjee, Ebel, LaRuffa, & Hoath, 2002; Visscher, Chatterjee, Munson, Pickens, & Hoath, 2000). It is the resulting increased pH of the skin that increases its vulnerability to injury and penetration by microorganisms. Another problem associated with increased pH of the skin is that it stimulates fecal enzyme activity. Specifically, both protease and lipase, which are found in stool, can injure the skin, which is made up of protein and fat components. These enzymes can cause significant injury to the epidermis fairly quickly and are responsible for the contact irritant diaper dermatitis that is commonly seen.

Once the epidermis has been impaired or becomes a less efficient barrier because of one of the aforementioned

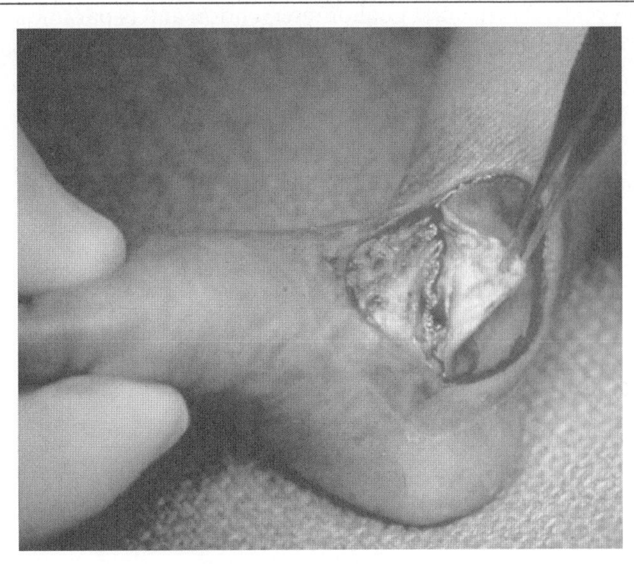

FIGURE 12.15 This IV extravasation injury will require plastic surgery.

mechanisms, invasion by bacteria or fungus can occur. Thus, a contact irritant diaper dermatitis can turn into a staphylococcal or fungal rash if this progression occurs. *S. aureus* can be found in large numbers on the skin surface, especially if it is inflamed or impaired, and can result in secondary infection. The classic presentation for *S. aureus* is pustule formation at the site of hair follicles, although the overall incidence of *S. aureus*-complicated diaper dermatitis is quite low.

Fungal rashes, primarily those caused by *C. albicans*, may have different mechanisms of invasion. Many researchers have identified *C. albicans* as a secondary invader of skin that has been injured by other mechanisms, whereas others suggest that *C. albicans* is a primary causative factor in diaper dermatitis. This theory is based on the ability of *C. albicans* to penetrate the stratum corneum, especially in a warm and moist environment, such as that found under an occlusive diaper. The resulting intense inflammation is significant and appears as brightly erythematous, sharply marginated dermatitis that involves the inguinal folds as well as the buttocks, thighs, abdomen, and genitalia, characteristically with satellite lesions that may extend the rash over the trunk (Figure 12.16). The gastrointestinal tract is often the reservoir for *C. albicans*, and it can frequently be recovered in stool. Oral therapy may be indicated, especially if evidence of oral infection, such as thrush, is apparent.

Diaper dermatitis can be the result of a primary dermatologic condition, such as psoriasis, eczema, and seborrheic dermatitis. Significant family history of these skin conditions may identify infants who are especially vulnerable to developing severe reactions to inflammation in the diaper area. The role of allergens has also been implicated in some cases of diaper dermatitis, and should be considered when treatment strategies fail (Smith & Jacob, 2009).

Management

Prevention is the first goal of intervention and is paramount in breaking the cycle of diaper dermatitis. Frequent diaper changes result in skin that is drier with a more normal pH and more normal functional barrier of the skin. Strategies to keep the skin dry also include the use of highly absorbent gelled diapers that act to "wick" moisture away from the skin. Use of talcum powders has been discouraged because of the risk of inhalation of silicone particles into the respiratory tract.

The use of commercially available diaper wipes, although in widespread use, has variable support in the literature with reports of contact allergens and concerns with product ingredients (Ehretsmann, Schaefer, & Adam, 2001; Fields, Nelson, & Powell, 2006; Smith & Jacob, 2009). A carefully controlled study of one brand of wipes compared to cloth and water for skin cleansing in the diaper area of premature infants showed improved skin pH and TEWL with the diaper wipe (Visscher et al., 2009). However, these findings are not generalizable to other products with different formulations.

Once diaper dermatitis occurs—and it is not completely avoidable in most infants—protection of injured skin during healing is the primary goal. Use of a generous layer of protective skin barriers that contain zinc oxide prevents further trauma and allows impaired skin to heal (Figure 12.17). Opening the skin to light and air is not effective if the fecal contents are allowed to have direct contact with already injured areas. Because protective skin barriers tend to adhere well to the skin, it is neither necessary nor desirable to completely remove them during diaper changes before more cream is applied. It is best to generously apply more cream to the site to protect the area from further injury.

Multiple products are used in the care of diaper dermatitis—including topical emollients, diaper rash balms, and wipes—but product selection is often affected by myth and tradition rather than science. A damp diaper covered with a plastic coating enhances the risk of irritation and percutaneous absorption. The risk of absorption is even greater in newborns and premature infants because of their

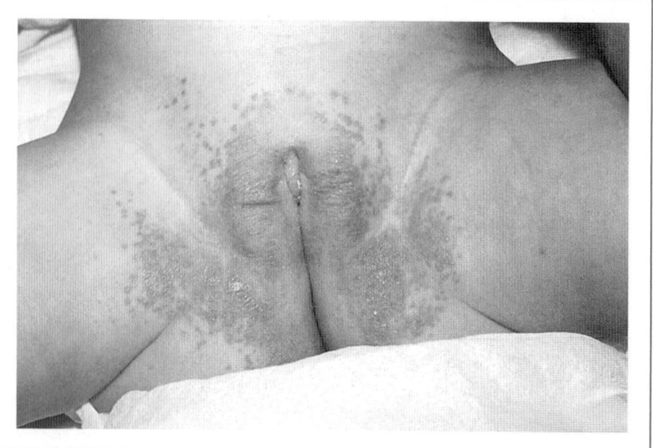

FIGURE 12.16 *Candida* diaper dermatitis involving labia and inguinal folds with characteristic satellite lesions.

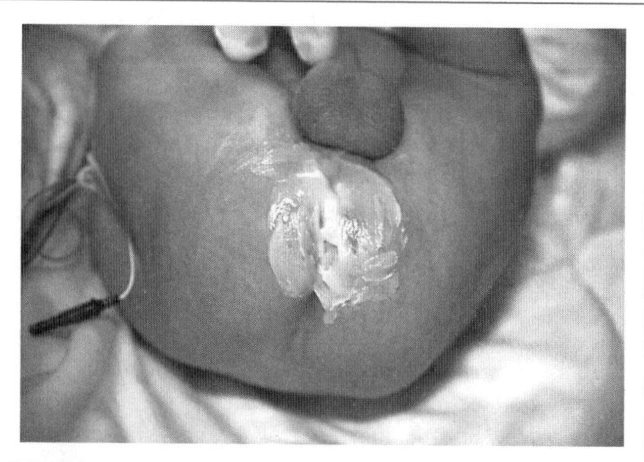

FIGURE 12.17 Use of thick layer of a skin barrier such as zinc oxide or pectin paste will prevent reinjury of skin damage in diaper dermatitis.

large surface area to body weight ratio and immature skin. The various compounds and numerous chemicals used have been described extensively (Siegfried & Shah, 1999; Gilliam & Williams, 2008), with concerns raised about potential toxicity, irritancy, and later sensitization. Simple, inexpensive products such as zinc oxide ointment are recommended over more complex compounds.

Treatment of diaper dermatitis that is solely due to invasion with *C. albicans* requires the use of antifungal creams or ointments. Some of the antifungal preparations include nystatin, miconazole, and clotrimazole. If the diaper dermatitis involves both fungus and a contact irritant component, alternating applications of the topical creams or ointments is effective.

Severe diaper dermatitis with deep excoriations can be seen in infants with malabsorption syndrome secondary to intestinal resection or mucosal injury. In these cases, the stool is extremely caustic and contains a higher level of enzyme activity, a lower pH as the result of rapid transit through the intestine, and significant amounts of undigested carbohydrates. In the case of opiate withdrawal, stool frequency is often greatly increased. Other infants at risk for severe diaper dermatitis include those with spina bifida, exstrophy of the bladder, and infants with decreased anal sphincter tone due to early pull-through procedures for Hirschprung's disease. In cases of loss of sphincter tone, fecal material constantly dribbles to the perianal area.

Although skin disruption frequently becomes the focus of nursing interventions, this symptom may be a significant indication of more serious physiologic concerns. These infants' stools should be carefully monitored by documentation of number and volume. The infants must be observed for the dehydration caused by extensive water losses in diarrhea. Once dietary manipulations and hydration have stabilized the general physiologic status, a program of skin protection is imperative because some level of chronic diarrhea may be ongoing for many weeks or months. Products such as pectin-based powders or pectin-containing pastes without alcohol may be better barriers to the caustic, constant fecal irritation if traditional zinc oxide creams do not work adequately. If yeast is present, antifungal creams may be applied in conjunction with protective barriers.

EVIDENCE-BASED SKIN CARE GUIDELINE

Many intensive care and newborn nurseries have written protocols for various aspects of neonatal skin care. The AWHONN and the NANN collaborated in the development of a comprehensive evidence-based neonatal skin care guideline. An extensive review of the scientific basis for neonatal skin care was undertaken by a team including advanced practice nurses and a pediatric dermatologist (Lund, Kuller, Lane, Lott, & Raines, 1999), and a neonatal skin guideline was written to address 11 aspects of skin care (Box 12.4). An evaluation project involving 51 nurseries was undertaken to evaluate the effect of using this guideline. The project involved identifying coordinators at each site who were willing to collect baseline information about the skin condition of infants in their units, implement the practice guideline in their respective units, and then collect skin condition information again once the guideline had been introduced. Issues of safety and feasibility were important, as was the evaluation of the impact of evidence-based practice on skin condition.

More than 11,000 skin observations using the NSCS were performed on 2,820 newborns of varying gestational ages and weights. An improvement in skin condition was observed after implementation of the guideline, as evidenced by overall lower scores on the NSCS during the observation period. Initial scores were similar in both the preguideline and postguideline groups but improved more rapidly after the guideline had been implemented. The results were more dramatic in the low-birth-weight infants, but improvement was seen in the "well-baby" sample as well.

The Neonatal Skin Care Guideline was revised in 2007, with the addition of a section on vernix caseosa due to the availability of numerous studies that were published on this topic. A third revision is planned for 2013.

Box 12.4

ELEMENTS OF THE AWHONN/NANN EVIDENCE-BASED PRACTICE GUIDELINE: NEONATAL SKIN CARE

1. Newborn skin assessment
2. Bathing, including first bath, routine, and immersion bathing
3. Cord care
4. Circumcision care
5. Disinfectants
6. Diaper dermatitis
7. Adhesives
8. Transepidermal water loss
9. Skin breakdown
10. IV infiltration
11. Vernix caseosa

Adapted from the Association of Women's Health, Obstetric, and Neonatal Nurses (AWHONN) Neonatal Skin Care Evidence-Based Clinical Practice Guideline. Copyright © 2007, AWHONN.

CASE STUDY

■ Identification of the Problem. This extremely premature infant was admitted to the NICU 3 days ago with respiratory distress syndrome; birth weight 650 g, gestational age 24 0/7 weeks. He has an endotracheal tube and is receiving assisted ventilation; catheters are inserted in both the umbilical artery and vein for blood sampling, blood pressure monitoring, and administration of IV fluids. An area of skin breakdown is noted on the abdomen where a temperature probe had been placed and removed on the first day of life. By day 3 the area is erythematous and oozing a yellow-tinged fluid. Surrounding areas are also quite red.

■ Assessment: History and Physical Examination. The infant, a baby boy, was born via vaginal delivery to a 30-year-old G1P1 mother. The pregnancy was complicated by preterm labor starting at 20 weeks, and a cervical cerclage was performed. A month later the mother was again hospitalized with prolonged rupture of membrane (PROM) and preterm labor. This time the efforts to stop labor were unsuccessful, and the infant was delivered vaginally 48 hours after a single course of betamethasone was administered.

The infant's Apgar scores were 4 and 7. The infant was intubated in the delivery room due to poor respiratory effort, and an initial dose of surfactant was administered. The infant was placed immediately into a polyurethane bag for reduction of evaporative heat and fluid loss in the delivery room. Upon arrival in the NICU, the infant was placed on a combination radiant warmer/incubator table for insertion of umbilical catheters. The skin was prepared with a disinfectant (2% chlorhexidine in 70% isopropyl alcohol) prior to placing umbilical catheters. After catheters were placed and position was confirmed with a radiograph, the disinfectant was wiped away using normal saline. At this time, the top of the heating device was lowered and converted to a convectively heated incubator with RH set at 80%.

The infant's skin was very moist and fragile in appearance. After placement of the umbilical catheters, although the periumbilical skin was cleansed with sterile water to remove the skin disinfectant, the skin was noted to be more erythematous than prior to insertion. A temperature probe was attached to the abdomen with a hydrogel electrode, which promptly slid off as a result of the high humidity in the environment. An adhesive-backed foil probe cover was used to secure the catheter.

■ Differential Diagnosis. The chief differential diagnoses for an extremely premature infant with skin breakdown includes trauma from adhesive removal, chemical burn from disinfectant used for periumbilical skin preparation, and infection. Although the original problem may be trauma, the wound can also be infected by microorganisms on the skin surface.

■ Diagnostic Tests. A skin culture with Gram stain and KOH prep is obtained from the area of breakdown. A CBC is obtained, as well as a blood culture. Although a catheter urine culture is requested, this is not obtained due to the extremely small size of the infant's penis and urethra; a "clean" bag specimen is collected instead.

■ Working Diagnosis. The Gram stain and KOH prep show budding yeast within 24 hours. The skin culture later shows a heavy growth of *C. albicans*. The blood and urine show no growth of microorganisms after 72 hours. The white blood cell remains unchanged from the first sample sent on the day of admission, but the platelet count has dropped from 100,000 to 60,000.

■ Development of Management Plan. After the Gram stain and KOH prep report, the area of breakdown appeared more extensive and the skin over the abdomen erythematous. The excoriated skin was gently debrided using a 30 mL syringe with warmed, one-half normal saline gently squirted through a 20-gauge Teflon catheter. Antifungal ointment, rather than cream or powder, was selected for topical treatment because of the potential healing benefits of ointments.

Because of the proximity of the excoriation to the umbilical catheter insertions, a decision was made to place a percutaneously inserted central line and peripheral arterial line so that the umbilical catheters could be discontinued.

■ Implementation and Evaluation of Effectiveness After receiving the preliminary culture report and noting the drop in platelet count, it was determined that further evaluation for systemic illness would be necessary. A subsequent platelet count was 45,000, and this, coupled with the need for dopamine infusion for hypotension, prompted the medical decision to initiate systemic antifungal treatment. Fluconazole infusion was begun, and a platelet transfusion was also administered.

After a second platelet transfusion, the platelet count had stabilized at 90,000 by the fifth day of treatment with Fluconazole.

Despite having no growth of *C. albicans* from blood or urine samples, fungal infections in extremely premature infants can initially be cutaneous infections. If not treated early, this can quickly progress to disseminated *Candida* infections involving the blood, urinary tract, cerebrospinal fluid, or other organs.

Factors associated with cutaneous fungal infections in the first week of life are instrumentation procedures, such as cerclage placement, and PROMs. The infant can be colonized from maternal fungal or bacterial flora. Additional risk factors are skin breakdown from trauma or irritation and glucosuria. Several authors recommend early, aggressive management of cutaneous manifestations of fungal infection to prevent further dissemination and systemic complications.

EVIDENCE-BASED PRACTICE BOX

Skin Care Guideline

Many intensive care and newborn nurseries have written protocols for various aspects of neonatal skin care. In 2001, two national nursing organizations, the AWHONN and the NANN, collaborated in the development of a comprehensive evidence-based neonatal skin care guideline. An extensive review of the scientific basis for neonatal skin care was undertaken by a team including advanced practice nurses and a pediatric dermatologist (Lund et al., 1999), and a neonatal skin guideline was written to address 11 aspects of skin care (Box 12.4). An evaluation project involving 51 nurseries was undertaken to evaluate the effect of using this guideline. The project involved identifying coordinators at each site who were willing to collect baseline information about the skin condition of infants in their units, implement the practice guideline in their respective units, and then collect skin condition information again once the guideline had been introduced. Issues of safety and feasibility were important, as was the evaluation of the impact of evidence-based practice on skin condition.

More than 11,000 skin observations using the NSCS were performed on 2,820 newborns of varying gestational ages and weights. An improvement in skin condition was observed after implementation of the guideline, as evidenced by overall lower scores on the NSCS during the observation period. Initial scores were similar in both the preguideline and postguideline groups but improved more rapidly after the guideline had been implemented. The results were more dramatic in the low-birth-weight infants, but improvement was seen in the "well-baby" sample as well.

The Neonatal Skin Care Guideline was revised in 2007. In addition to updated evidence-based information in all areas, a section on vernix caseosa was added. A third edition of the AWHONN Guideline will be published in 2013. New sections added to this edition include product selection principles, atopic dermatitis, parent education, and some of the emerging information on the skin microbiome.

SUMMARY

Neonatal skin management is a complex problem that requires a collaborative approach. Some research has been conducted in this area, but a lot remains to be done regarding the use of routine NICU equipment and its impact on neonatal skin, the use of skin barriers for protection, and the effect of a consistent approach to skin care on the integrity of neonatal skin. This chapter has outlined the development and structure of the skin. It has addressed differences in the skin based on gestational age variations. Normal physiologic as well as common dermatologic abnormalities have been presented. Evidence-based neonatal skin care is recommended and has proven to be feasible and safe and to result in improvement in skin condition for newborns.

ONLINE RESOURCES

Healthychildren.org
http://www2.kumc.edu/instruction/nursing/nrsg856/articles/NeonatalSkinCare.pdf
http://www.medscape.org/viewarticle/465017
http://www.livestrong.com/article/224401-skin-care-for-premature-infants
http://www.babycenter.com/baby-body-care
http://www.whattoexpect.com/first-year/gentle-care-for-newborn-skin.aspx
http://www.whattoexpect.com/first-year/gentle-care-for-newborn-skin.aspx
http://www.johnsonsbaby.com/newborn-skin-care
http://www.hcplive.com/conferences/napnap-2012/NAPNAP-2012-Newborn-Skin-Care-What-the-Evidence-Shows

REFERENCES

Ackerman, A (1985). Structure and function of the skin. In S. Moschella & H. Hurley (Eds.), *Dermatology* (2nd ed., Vol. 2). Philadelphia, PA: Saunders.

Adam, R. (2008). Skin care of the diaper area. *Pediatric Dermatology, 25*(4), 427–433.

Agren, J., Sjors, G., & Sedin, G. (1998). Transepidermal water loss in infants born at 24 and 25 weeks of gestation. *Acta Paediatrica, 87*(11), 1185–1190.

Agren J., Sjors G., & Sedin G. (2006). Ambient humidity influences the rate of skin barrier maturation in extremely preterm infants. *The Journal of Pediatrics, 148*, 613–617.

Akinbi, H. T., Narendran, V., Pass, A. K., Markart, P., & Hoath, S. B. (2004). Host defense proteins in vernix caseosa and amniotic fluid. *American Journal Obstetrics Gynecology, 191*(6), 2090–2096.

American Academy of Pediatrics. (1997). *Red book: Report of the committee on infectious diseases* (24th ed.). Elk Grove Village, IL: Author.

American Academy of Pediatrics, The American College of Obstetrics and Gynecologists. (2007). *Guidelines for perinatal care* (6th ed.). Elk Grove Village, IL: American Academy of Pediatrics; Washington, DC: American College of Obstetrics and Gynecologists.

Andersen, C., Hart, J., Vemgal, P., & Harrison, C. (2005). Prospective evaluation of a multi-factorial prevention strategy on the impact of nosocomial infection in very-low-birthweight infants. *Journal Hospital Infection, 61*(2), 162–167.

Anderson, G. C., Lane, A. E., & Chang, H. P. (1995). Axillary temperature in transitional newborn infants before and after tub bath. *Applied Nursing Research, 8*(3), 123–128.

Association of Women's Health, Obstetric, and Neonatal Nurses. (2007). *Evidence-based clinical practice guideline: Neonatal skin care*. Washington, DC: Author.

Association of Women's Health, Obstetric and Neonatal Nurses. (2009). *Universal screening for hyperbilirubinemia: AWHONN position statement*. Washington, DC: Author.

AvRuskin, T. W., Greenfield, E., Prasad, V., Greig, F., & Juan, C. S. (1994). Decreased t3 and t4 levels following topical application of povidone-iodine in premature neonates. *Journal of Pediatric Endocrinology, 7*(3), 205–209.

Baharestani, M. M. (2007). An overview of neonatal and pediatric wound care knowledge and considerations. *Ostomy Wound Manage, 53*(6), 34–55.

Baley, J. E., & Silverman, R. A. (1988). Systemic candidiasis: Cutaneous manifestations in low birth weight infants. *Pediatrics, 82*(2), 211–215.

Banta, C., & Noerr, B. (1992). Hyaluronidase. *Neonatal Network, 11*(6), 103–105.

Bhandari, V., Brodsky, N., & Porat, R. (2005). Improved outcome of extremely low birth weight infants with tegaderm application to skin. *Journal of Perinatology, 25*(4), 276–281.

Brandon, D. H., Coe, K., Hudson-Barr, D., Oliver, T., & Landerman, L. R. (2010). Effectiveness of no-sting skin protectant and aquaphor on water loss and skin integrity in premature infants. *Journal of Perinatology, 30*(6), 414–419.

Bromiker, Bin-Nun, Schimmel, Hammerman, C., & Kaplan, M. (2012). Neonatal hyperbilirubinemia in the low-intermediate–risk category on the bilirubin nomogram. *Pediatrics, 130*(3), e470–e475.

Bryanton, J., Walsh, D., Barrett, M., & Gaudet, D. (2004). Tub bathing versus traditional sponge bathing for the newborn. *Journal Obstetric Gynecology Neonatal Nursing, 33*(6), 704–712.

Bustamante, S. A., & Steslow, J. (1989). Use of a transparent adhesive dressing in very low birthweight infants. *Journal of Perinatology, 9*(2), 165–169.

Casanova, D., Bardot, J., & Magalon, G. (2001). Emergency treatment of accidental infusion leakage in the newborn: Report of 14 cases. *British Journal of Plastic Surgery, 54*(5), 396–399.

Centers for Disease Control and Prevention. (2006). Leads from the MMWR. Update: Universal precautions for preventions of transmission of human immunodeficiency virus, hepatitis B virus, and other bloodborne pathogens in health care settings. *Journal of the American Medical Association, 260*, 462–465.

Chaiyakunapruk, N., Veenstra, D. L., Lipsky, B. A., & Saint, S. (2002). Chlorhexidine compared with povidone-iodine solution for vascular catheter-site care: A meta-analysis. *Annals of Internal Medicine, 136*(11), 792–801.

Chandavasu, O., Garrow, E., Valda, V., Alsheikh, S., & Dela Vega, S. (1986). A new method for the prevention of skin sloughs and necrosis secondary to intravenous infiltration. *American Journal of Perinatology, 3*(1), 4–5.

Choudhuri, M., McQueen, R., Inoue, S., & Gordon, R. C. (1990). Efficiency of skin sterilization for a venipuncture with the use of commercially available alcohol or iodine pads. *American Journal of Infection Control, 18*(2), 82–85.

Clark, D., & Thompson, J. (1986). Dermatology of the newborn. Parts 1 and 2. In *Pathology of the neonate slide series* (Vol. 3., No. 4). Philadelphia, PA: Wyeth-Ayerst Laboratories.

Coelho, S., Fernandes, B., Rodrigues, F., Reis, J. P., Moreno, A., & Figueiredo, A. (2006). Transient zinc deficiency in a breast fed, premature infant. *European Journal of Dermatology, 16*(2), 193–195.

Cohen, B. A. (2008). Disorders of the subcutaneous tissue. In L. A. Eichenfield, I. J. Frieden, & N. B. Esterly (Eds.), *Neonatal dermatology* (2nd ed.). Philadelphia, PA: Saunders Elsevier.

Conner, J. M., Soll, R. F., & Edwards, W. H. (2004). Topical ointment for preventing infection in preterm infants. *Cochrane Database System Review,* (1), CD001150.

Cunningham, B. B., & Wagner, A. M. (2008). Diagnostic and therapeutic procedures. In L. A. Eichenfield, I. J. Frieden, & N. B. Esterly (Eds.), *Neonatal dermatology* (2nd ed.). Philadelphia, PA: Saunders Elsevier.

Curley, M. A., Razmus, I. S., Roberts, K. E., & Wypij, D. (2003). Predicting pressure ulcer risk in pediatric patients: The braden q scale. *Nursing Research, 52*(1), 22–33.

Davies, J., Gault, D., & Buchdahl, R. (1994). Preventing the scars of neonatal intensive care. *Archives of Disease in Childhood Fetal and Neonatal Editions, 70*(1), F50–F51.

de Graaf, M., Breur, J. M., Raphael, M. F., Vos, M., Breugem, C. C., & Pasmans, S. G. (2011). Adverse effects of propranolol when used in the treatment of hemangiomas: A case series of 28 infants. *Journal American Academy Dermatology, 65*(2), 320–327.

Dinulos, J. G., & Pace, N. C. (2008). Bacterial infections. In L. A. Eichenfield, I. J. Frieden, & N. B. Esterly (Eds.), *Neonatal dermatology* (2nd ed.). Philadelphia, PA: Saunders Elsevier.

Dollison, E. J., & Beckstrand, J. (1995). Adhesive tape vs pectin-based barrier use in preterm infants. *Neonatal Network, 14*(4), 35–39.

Dominguez-Bello, M. G., Costello, E. K., Contreras, M., Magris, M., Hidalgo, G., Fierer, N., & Knight, R. (2010). Delivery mode shapes the acquisition and structure of the initial microbiota across multiple body habitats in newborns. *Proceedings of the National Academy of Sciences of the United States of America, 107*(26), 11971–11975.

Donahue, M. L., Phelps, D. L., Richter, S. E., & Davis, J. M. (1996). A semipermeable skin dressing for extremely low birth weight infants. *Journal of Perinatology, 16*(1), 20–26.

Dore, S., Buchan, D., Coulas, S., Hamber, L., Stewart, M., Cowan, D., & Jamieson, L. (1998). Alcohol versus natural drying for newborn cord care. *Journal of Obstetrics, Gynecology and Neonatal Nursing, 27*(6), 621–627.

Drucker, D. A., & Marshall, N. (1995). Humidification without risk of infection in the Draeger Incubator 8000. *Neonatal Intensive Care, 8*, 44–46.

Dykes, P. J., Heggie, R., & Hill, S. A. (2001). Effects of adhesive dressings on the stratum corneum of the skin. *Journal of Wound Care, 10*(2), 7–10.

Edwards, W. H., Conner, J. M., & Soll, R. F. (2004). The effect of prophylactic ointment therapy on nosocomial sepsis rates and skin integrity in infants with birth weights of 501 to 1000 g. *Pediatrics, 113*(5), 1195–1203.

Ehretsmann, C., Schaefer, P., & Adam, R. (2001). Cutaneous tolerance of baby wipes by infants with atopic dermatitis, and comparison of the mildness of baby wipe and water in infant skin. *Journal of the European Academy of Dermatology Venereology, 15*(Suppl. 1), 16–21.

Enjolras, O., & Garzon, M. C. (2008). Vascular stains, malformations, and tumors. In L. A. Eichenfield, I. J. Frieden, & N. B. Esterly (Eds.), *Neonatal dermatology* (2nd ed.). Philadelphia, PA: Saunders Elsevier.

Fields, K. S., Nelson, T., & Powell, D. (2006). Contact dermatitis caused by baby wipes. *Journal of the American Academy Dermatology, 54*(5), S230–S232.

Fine, J. D., Bauer, E. A., McGuire, J., & Moshell, A. (1999). *Epidermolysi sbullosa: Clinical, epidemiologic, and laboratory advances and the findings of the national epidermolysis bullosa registry*. Baltimore, MD: Johns Hopkins University Press.

Fine, J. D., Eady, R. A., Bauer, E. A., Briggaman, R. A., Bruckner-Tuderman, L., Christiano, A., . . . Uitto, J. (2000). Revised classification system for inherited epidermolysis bullosa: Report of the second international consensus meeting on diagnosis and classification of epidermolysis bullosa. *Journal American Academy Dermatology, 42*(6), 1051–1066.

Fox, C., Nelson, D., & Wareham, J. (1998). The timing of skin acidification in very low birth weight infants. *Journal of Perinatology, 18*(4), 272–275.

Fox, M. D. (2011). Wound care in the neonatal intensive care unit. *Neonatal Network, 30*(5), 291–303.

Franck, L. S., Quinn, D., & Zahr, L. (2000). Effect of less frequent bathing of preterm infants on skin flora and pathogen colonization. *Journal Obstetrics Gynecology Neonatal Nursing, 29*(6), 584–589.

Friedlander, S. F., & Bradley, J. S. (2008). Viral infections. In L. A. Eichenfield, I. J. Frieden, & N. B. Esterly (Eds.), *Neonatal dermatology* (2nd ed.). Philadelphia, PA: Saunders Elsevier.

Gardner, S., Hernandez, J. (2011). Initial nursery care. In S. Gardner, B. S. Carter, M. E. Enzman-Hines, & J. Hernandez (Eds.), *Merenstein & Gardner's handbook of neonatal intensive care* (7th ed.). St. Louis, MO: Mosby.

Garland, J. S., Alex, C. P., Uhing, M. R., Peterside, I. E., Rentz, A., & Harris, M. C. (2009). Pilot trial to compare tolerance of chlorhexidine gluconate to povidone-iodine antisepsis for central venous catheter placement in neonates. *Journal of Perinatology, 29*(12), 808–813.

Garland, J. S., Buck, R. K., Maloney, P., Durkin, D. M., Toth-Lloyd, S., Duffy, M., . . . Goldmann, D. (1995). Comparison of 10% povidone-iodine and 0.5% chlorhexidine gluconate for the prevention of peripheral intravenous catheter colonization in neonates: A prospective trial. *Pediatric Infectious Disease Journal, 14*(6), 510–516.

Gaylord, M. S., Wright, K., Lorch, K., Lorch, V., & Walker, E. (2001). Improved fluid management utilizing humidified incubators in extremely low birth weight infants. *Journal of Perinatology, 21*(7), 438–443.

Gfatter, R., Hackl, P., & Braun, F. (1997). Effects of soap and detergents on skin surface ph, stratum corneum hydration and fat content in infants. *Dermatology, 195*(3), 258–262.

Gilliam, A. E., & Williams, M. L. (2008). Skin of the premature infant. In L. A. Eichenfield, I. J. Frieden, & N. B. Esterly (Eds.), *Neonatal dermatology* (2nd ed.). Philadelphia, PA: Saunders Elsevier.

Gordon, C. M., Rowitch, D. H., Mitchell, M. L., & Kohane, I. S. (1995). Topical iodine and neonatal hypothyroidism. *Archive Pediatric and Adolescent Medicine, 149*(12), 1336–1339.

Gotschall, C. S., Morrison, M. I., & Eichelberger, M. R. (1998). Prospective, randomized study of the efficacy of mepitel on children with partial-thickness scalds. *Journal of Burn Care Rehabilitation, 19*(4), 279–283.

Gregory, K. E. (2011). Microbiome aspects of perinatal and neonatal health. *Journal of Perinatal Neonatal Nursing, 25*(2), 158–162.

Hammarlund, K., & Sedin, G. (1979). Transepidermal water loss in newborn infants. III. Relation to gestational age. *Acta paediatrica Scandinavica, 68*(6), 795–801.

Harpin, V. A., & Rutter, N. (1982). Percutaneous alcohol absorption and skin necrosis in a preterm infant. *Archives Disease Childhood, 57*(6), 477–479.

Harpin, V. A., & Rutter, N. (1983). Barrier properties of the newborn infant's skin. *Journal Pediatrics, 102*(3), 419–425.

Haubrich, K. A. (2003). Role of vernix caseosa in the neonate: Potential application in the adult population. *AACN Clinical Issues, 14*(4), 457–464.

Heimall, L. M., Storey, B., Stellar, J. J., & Davis, K. F. (2012). Beginning at the bottom: Evidence-based care of diaper dermatitis. *MCN The American Journal of maternal Child Nursing, 37*(1), 10–16.

Herane, M. I., & Ando, I. (2003). Acne in infancy and acne genetics. *Dermatology, 206*(1), 24–28.

Hoath, S. B., & Narendran, V. (2000). Adhesives and emollients in the preterm infant. *Seminars in Neonatology, 5*(4), 289–296.

Hoath, S. B., & Narendran, V. (2011). The skin. In R. J. Martin, A. A. Fanaroff, & M. C. Walsh (Eds.), *Neonatal-perinatal medicine: Diseases of the fetus and infant* (9th ed.). St Louis, MO: Elsevier Mosby.

Hoath, S. B., Narendran, V., & Visscher, M. O. (2001). The biology and role of vernix. *Newborn and Infant Nursing Reviews, 1*(1), 53–58.

Hoath, S. B., & Pickins, W. L. (2003). The biology and role of vernix. In S. B. Hoath & H. I. Maibach (Eds.), *Neonatal skin: Structure and function* (2nd ed.). New York, NY: Marcel Dekker.

Hoeger, P. H., & Enzmann, C. C. (2002). Skin physiology of the neonate and young infant: A prospective study of functional skin parameters during early infancy. *Pediatric Dermatology, 19*(3), 256–262.

Holbrook, K. A. (1982). A histological comparison of infant and adult skin. In H. I. Maibach & E. K. Boisits (Eds.), *Neonatal skin: Structure and function*. New York, NY: Marcel Dekker.

Hook, K. P., & Eichenfield, L. F. (2011). Approach to the neonate with ecchymoses and crusts. *Dermatologic Therapy, 24*(2), 240–248.

Howard, R., & Frieden, I. J. (2008). Vesicles, pustules, bullae, erosions, and ulcerations. In L. A. Eichenfield, I. J. Frieden, & N. B. Esterly (Eds.), *Neonatal dermatology* (2nd ed.). Philadelphia, PA: Saunders Elsevier.

Irving, V. (2001). Reducing the risk of epidermal stripping in the neonatal population: An evaluation of an alcohol free barrier film. *Journal of Neonatal Nursing, 7*, 5–8.

Ittmann, P. I., & Bozynski, M. E. (1993). Toxic epidermal necrolysis in a newborn infant after exposure to adhesive remover. *Journal of Perinatology, 13*(6), 476–477.

Janssen, P. A., Selwood, B. L., Dobson, S. R., Peacock, D., & Thiessen, P. N. (2003). To dye or not to dye: A randomized, clinical trial of a triple dye/alcohol regime versus dry cord care. *Pediatrics, 111*(1), 15–20.

Kalia, Y. N., Nonato, L. B., Lund, C. H., & Guy, R. H. (1998). Development of skin barrier function in premature infants. *Journal of Investigative Dermatology, 111*(2), 320–326.

Karl, D. J. (1999). The interactive newborn bath. *American Journal maternal Child Nursing, 24*(6), 280–286.

Kim, S. M., Lee, E. Y., Chen, J., & Ringer, S. A. (2010). Improved care and growth outcomes by using hybrid humidified incubators in very preterm infants. *Pediatrics, 125* (1), e137–e145.

Kjartansson, S., Arsan, S., Hammarlund, K., Sjors, G., & Sedin, G. (1995). Water loss from the skin of term and preterm infants nursed under a radiant heater. *Pediatric Research, 37* (2), 233–238.

Knauth, A., Gordin, M., McNelis, W., & Baumgart, S. (1989). Semipermeable polyurethane membrane as an artificial skin for the premature neonate. *Pediatrics, 83*(6), 945–950.

Knobel, R. B., Wimmer, J. E., Jr., & Holbert, D. (2005). Heat loss prevention for preterm infants in the delivery room. *Journal of Perinatology, 25*(5), 304–308.

Landau, M., & Krafchik, B. R. (1999). The diagnostic value of cafe-au-lait macules. *Journal of American Academy of Dermatology, 40*(6), 877–890.

Lane, A. T., & Drost, S. S. (1993). Effects of repeated application of emollient cream to premature neonates' skin. *Pediatrics, 92*(3), 415–419.

Larson, A. A., & Dinulos, J. G. (2005). Cutaneous bacterial infections in the newborn. *Current Opinion Pediatrics, 17*(4), 481–485.

Laurie, S. W., Wilson, K. L., Kernahan, D. A., Bauer, B. S., & Vistnes, L. M. (1984). Intravenous extravasation injuries: The effectiveness of hyaluronidase in their treatment. *Annals of Plastic Surgery, 13*(3), 191–194.

Linder, N., Davidovitch, N., Reichman, B., Kuint, J., Lubin, D., Meyerovitch, J., . . . Sack, J. (1997). Topical iodine-containing antiseptics and subclinical hypothyroidism in preterm infants. *Journal of Pediatrics, 131*(3), 434–439.

Lo, J. S., Oriba, H. A., Maibach, H. I., & Bailin, P. L. (1990). Transepidermal potassium ion, chloride ion, and water flux across delipidized and cellophane tape-stripped skin. *Dermatologica, 180*(2), 66–68.

Loomis, C. A., Koss, T., & Chu, D., (2008). Fetal skin development. In L. A. Eichenfield, I. J. Frieden, & N. B. Esterly (Eds.), *Neonatal dermatology* (2nd ed.). Philadelphia, PA: Saunders Elsevier.

Lucky, A. W. (2008). Transient benign cutaneous lesions in the newborn. In L. A. Eichenfield, I. J. Frieden, & N. B. Esterly (Eds.), *Neonatal dermatology* (2nd ed.). Philadelphia, PA: Saunders Elsevier.

Lund, C., Kuller, J., Lane, A., Lott, J. W., & Raines, D. A. (1999). Neonatal skin care: The scientific basis for practice. *Journal of Obstetrics, Gynecology, and Neonatal Nursing, 28*(3), 241–254.

Lund, C., & Tucker, J. (2003). Skin adhesion. In S. B. Hoath & H. I. Maibach (Eds.), *Neonatal skin: Structure and function* (2nd ed.). New York, NY: Marcel Dekker.

Lund, C. H., Kuller, J., Lane, A. T., Lott, J. W., Raines, D. A., & Thomas, K. K. (2001a). Neonatal skin care: Evaluation of the AWHONN/NANN research-based practice project on knowledge and skin care practices. Association of women's health, obstetric and neonatal nurses/national association of neonatal nurses. *Journal of Obstetrics, Gynecology and Neonatal Nursing, 30*(1), 30–40.

Lund, C. H., Nonato, L. B., Kuller, J. M., Franck, L. S., Cullander, C., & Durand, D. J. (1997). Disruption of barrier function in neonatal skin associated with adhesive removal. *Journal of Pediatrics, 131*(3), 367–372.

Lund, C. H., & Osborne, J. W. (2004). Validity and reliability of the neonatal skin condition score. *Journal of Obstetrics, Gynecology and Neonatal Nursing, 33*(3), 320–327.

Lund, C. H., Osborne, J. W., Kuller, J., Lane, A. T., Lott, J. W., & Raines, D. A. (2001b). Neonatal skin care: Clinical outcomes of the AWHONN/NANN evidence-based clinical practice guideline. Association of women's health, obstetric and neonatal nurses and the national association of neonatal nurses. *Journal of Obstetrics, Gynecology, and Neonatal Nursing, 30*(1), 41–51.

Mancini, A. J. (2004). Skin. *Pediatrics, 113*(4), 1114–1119.

Mancini, A. J., Sookdeo-Drost, S., Madison, K. C., Smoller, B. R., & Lane, A. T. (1994). Semipermeable dressings improve epidermal barrier function in premature infants. *Pediatric Research, 36*(3), 306–314.

Mannan, K., Chow, P., Lissauer, T., & Godambe, S. (2007). Mistaken identity of skin cleansing solution leading to extensive chemical burns in an extremely preterm infant. *Acta Paediatrica, 96*(10), 1536–1537.

Margileth, A. M. (2005). Dermatologic conditions. In M. G. MacDonald, M. D. Mullett, & M. K. Seshia (Eds.), *Avery's neonatology: Pathophysiology and management of the newborn* (6th ed.). Philadelphia, PA: Lippincott.

Marinkovich, M. P. (1999). Update on inherited bullous dermatoses. *Dermatology Clinics, 17*(3), 473–485.

Marks, J. G., Belsito, D. V., DeLeo, V. A., Fowler, J. F., Fransway, A. F., Maibach, H. I., . . . Taylor, J. S. (1995). North American Contact Dermatitis Group standard tray patch test results. *American Journal of Contact Dermatitis, 6*(3), 160–165.

Marlowe, L., Mistry, R. D., Coffin, S., Leckerman, K. H., McGowan, K. L., Dai, D., . . . Zaoutis, T. (2010). Blood culture contamination rates after skin antisepsis with chlorhexidine gluconate versus povidone-iodine in a pediatric emergency department. *Infection Control and Hospital Epidemiology, 31*(2), 171–176.

Marshall, A. (1997). Humidifying the environment for the premature neonate: Maintenance of a thermoneutral environment. *Journal of Neonatal Nursing, 3*, 32–36.

Milstone, A. M., Passaretti, C. L., & Perl, T. M. (2008). Chlorhexidine: Expanding the armamentarium for infection control and prevention. *Clinical Infectious Diseases, 46*(2), 274–281.

Mimoz, O., Karim, A., Mercat, A., Cosseron, M., Falissard, B., Parker, F., . . . Nordmann, P. (1999). Chlorhexidine compared with povidone-iodine as skin preparation before blood culture. A randomized, controlled trial. *Annals of Internal Medicine, 131*(11), 834–837.

Moore, K. L., & Persaud, T. V. N. (2008). *The developing human: Clinically oriented embryology* (8th ed.). Philadelphia, PA: Saunders Elsevier.

Moraille, R., Pickens, W. L., Visscher, M. O., & Hoath, S. B. (2005). A novel role for vernix caseosa as a skin cleanser. *Biology of the Neonate, 87*(1), 8–14.

Niamba, P., Weill, F. X., Sarlangue, J., Labreze, C., Couprie, B., & Taieh, A. (1998). Is common neonatal cephalic pustulosis (neonatal acne) triggered by malassezia sympodialis? *Archives of Dermatology, 134*(8), 995–998.

Nikolovski, J., Stamatas, G. N., Kollias, N., & Wiegand, B. C. (2008). Barrier function and water-holding and transport properties of infant stratum corneum are different from adult and continue to develop through the first year of life. *Journal of Investigative Dermatology, 128*(7), 1728–1736.

Nopper, A. J., Horii, K. A., Sookdeo-Drost, S., Wang, T. H., Mancini, A. J., & Lane, A. T. (1996). Topical ointment therapy benefits premature infants. *Journal of Pediatrics, 128*(5), 660–669.

Parravicini, E., Fontana, C., Paterlini, G. L., Tagliabue, P., Rovelli, F., Leung, K., & Stark, R. I. (1996). Iodine, thyroid function, and very low birth weight infants. *Pediatrics, 98*(4), 730–734.

Penny-MacGillivray, T. (1996). A newborn's first bath: When? *Journal Obstetrics Gynecology Neonatal Nursing, 25*(6), 481–487.

Prasad, A. S. (1995). Zinc: An overview. *Nutrition, 11*(1), 93–99.

Rapelanoro, R., Mortureux, P., Couprie, B., Maleville, J., & Taieb, A. (1996). Neonatal malassezia furfur pustulosis. *Archives of Dermatology, 132*(2), 190–193.

Raszka, W. V., Jr., Kueser, T. K., Smith, F. R., & Bass, J. W. (1990). The use of hyaluronidase in the treatment of intravenous extravasation injuries. *Journal of Perinatology, 10*(2), 146–149.

Reynolds, P. R., Banerjee, S., & Meek, J. H. (2005). Alcohol burns in extremely low birthweight infants: Still occurring. *Archives Disease Child Fetal and Neonatal Edition, 90*(1), F10.

Rowen, J. L., Atkins, J. T., Levy, M. L., Baer, S. C., & Baker, C. J. (1995). Invasive fungal dermatitis in the < or = 1000-gram neonate. *Pediatrics, 95*(5), 682–687.

Sawatzky-Dickson, D., & Bodnaryk, K. (2006). Neonatal intravenous extravasation injuries: Evaluation of a wound care protocol. *Neonatal Network, 25*(1), 13–19.

Schick, J. B., & Milstein, J. M. (1981). Burn hazard of isopropyl alcohol in the neonate. *Pediatrics, 68*(4), 587–588.

Sekkat, N., Kalia, Y. N., & Guy, R. H. (2004). Development of an in vitro model for premature neonatal skin: Biophysical characterization using transepidermal water loss. *Journal of Pharmacological Sciences, 93*(12), 2936–2940.

Sethi, R., Schwartz, R. A., & Janniger, C. K. (1996). Oculocutaneous albinism. *Cutis, 57*(6), 397–401.

Shalita, A. (1981). *Principles of infant skin care*. Skillman, NJ: Johnson & Johnson Baby Products.

Siegfried, E. C., & Shah, P. Y. (1999). Skin care practices in the neonatal nursery: A clinical survey. *Journal of Perinatology, 19*(1), 31–39.

Siegfried, E. G. (2008). Neonatal skin care and toxicology. In L. A. Eichenfield, I. J. Frieden, & N. B. Esterly (Eds.), *Neonatal dermatology* (2nd ed.). Philadelphia, PA: Saunders Elsevier.

Smack, D. P., Harrington, A. C., Dunn, C., Howard, R. S., Szkutnik, A. J., Krivda, S. J., . . . James, W. D. (1996). Infection and allergy incidence in ambulatory surgery patients using white petrolatum vs bacitracin ointment. A randomized controlled trial. *Journal of American Medical Association, 276*(12), 972–977.

Smith, W. J., & Jacob, S. E. (2009). The role of allergic contact dermatitis in diaper dermatitis. *Pediatric Dermatology, 26*(3), 369–370.

Smolinski, K. N., & Yan, A. C. (2005). Hemangiomas of infancy: Clinical and biological characteristics. *Clinical Pediatrics, 44*(9), 747–766.

Stamatas, G. N., Nikolovski, J., Mack, M. C., & Kollias, N. (2011). Infant skin physiology and development during the first years of life: A review of recent findings based on in vivo studies. *International Journal of Cosmetic Science, 33*(1), 17–24.

Suddaby, E. C., Barnett, S., & Facteau, L. (2005). Skin breakdown in acute care pediatrics. *Pediatric Nursing, 31*(2), 132–138, 148.

Tansirikongkol, A., Visscher, M. O., & Wickett, R. R. (2007). Water-handling properties of vernix caseosa and a synthetic analogue. *Journal of Cosmetic Science, 58*(6), 651–662.

Thigpen, J. L. (2007). Peripheral intravenous extravasation: Nursing procedure for initial treatment. *Neonatal Network, 26*(6), 379–384.

Tollin, M., Bergsson, G., Kai-Larsen, Y., Lengqvist, J., Sjovall, J., Griffiths, W., . . . Agerberth, B. (2005). Vernix caseosa as a multi-component defence system based on polypeptides, lipids and their interactions. *Cellular & Molecular Life Sciences, 62*(19–20), 2390–2399.

Torrelo, A., Pastor, M. A., & Zambrano, A. (2005). Severe acne infantum successfully treated with isotretinoin. *Pediatric Dermatology, 22*(4), 357–359.

Tremaine, A. M., Armstrong, J., Huang, Y. C., Elkeeb, L., Ortiz, A., Harris, R., . . . Kelly, K. M. (2012). Enhanced port-wine stain lightening achieved with combined treatment of selective photothermolysis and imiquimod. *Journal American Academy Dermatology, 66*(4), 634–641.

Varda, K. E., & Behnke, R. S. (2000). The effect of timing of initial bath on newborn's temperature. *Journal Obstetrics Gynecology Neonatal Nursing, 29*(1), 27–32.

Vernon, H. J., Lane, A. T., Wischerath, L. J., Davis, J. M., & Menegus, M. A. (1990). Semipermeable dressing and transepidermal water loss in premature infants. *Pediatrics, 86*(3), 357–362.

Visscher, M. O., Chatterjee, R., Ebel, J. P., LaRuffa, A. A., & Hoath, S. B. (2002). Biomedical assessment and instrumental evaluation of healthy infant skin. *Pediatric Dermatology, 19*(6), 473–481.

Visscher, M. O., Chatterjee, R., Munson, K. A., Pickens, W. L., & Hoath, S. B. (2000). Changes in diapered and nondiapered infant skin over the first month of life. *Pediatric Dermatology, 17*(1), 45–51.

Visscher, M. O., Narendran, V., Pickens, W. L., LaRuffa, A. A., Meinzen-Derr, J., Allen, K., & Hoath, S. B. (2005). Vernix caseosa in neonatal adaptation. *Journal of Perinatology, 25*(7), 440–446.

Visscher, M., Odio, M., Taylor, T., White, T., Sargent, S., Sluder, L., . . . Bondurant, P. (2009). Skin care in the NICU patient: Effects of wipes versus cloth and water on stratum corneum integrity. *Neonatology, 96*(4), 226–234.

Visscher, M. O., Utturkar, R., Pickens, W. L., LaRuffa, A. A., Robinson, M., Wickett, R. R., . . . Hoath, S. B. (2011). Neonatal skin maturation—Vernix caseosa and free amino acids. *Pediatric Dermatology, 28*(2), 122–132.

Vohra, S., Frent, G., Campbell, V., Abbott, M., & Whyte, R. (1999). Effect of polyethylene occlusive skin wrapping on heat loss in very low birth weight infants at delivery: A randomized trial. *Journal of Pediatrics, 134*(5), 547–551.

Vohra, S., Roberts, R. S., Zhang, B., Janes, M., & Schmidt, B. (2004). Heat loss prevention (help) in the delivery room: A randomized controlled trial of polyethylene occlusive skin wrapping in very preterm infants. *Journal of Pediatrics, 145*(6), 750–753.

Webster, J., & McCosker, H. (1994). Cardiac monitoring in the neonatal intensive care unit: An evaluation of electrodes. *Neonatal Network, 13*(2), 51–54.

Williams, M. L. (2008). Skin of the premature. In L. A. Eichenfield, I. J. Frieden, & N. B. Esterly (Eds.), *Neonatal dermatology* (2nd ed.). Philadelphia, PA: Saunders Elsevier.

Woodruff, C. A., & Hebert, A. A. (2002). Neonatal primary cutaneous aspergillosis: Case report and review of the literature. *Pediatric Dermatology, 19*(5), 439–444.

World Health Organization. (2009). *Pregnancy, childbirth, postpartum and newborn care: A guide for essential practice.* Geneva, Switzerland: Author.

Yoshio, H., Lagercrantz, H., Gudmundsson, G. H., & Agerberth, B. (2004). First line of defense in early human life. *Seminars Perinatology, 28*(4), 304–311.

Yosipovitch, G., Maayan-Metzger, A., Merlob, P., & Sirota, L. (2000). Skin barrier properties in different body areas in neonates. *Pediatrics, 106*, 105–108.

Zenk, K. (1999). *Neonatal medications and nutrition: A comprehensive guide*. Santa Rosa, CA: NICU Ink.

Zupan, J., & Garner, P. (2000). Topical umbilical cord care at birth. *The Cochrane Database of Systematic Reviews* (2), CD001057.

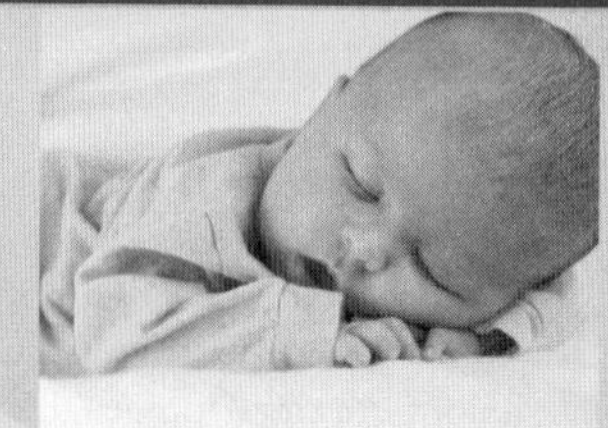

CHAPTER 13

Hematologic System

■ Gail A. Bagwell

The hematologic system is probably one of the least understood body systems of the neonate by the neonatal nurse. But in order to provide the utmost care to the neonate, a thorough and complete understanding of the hematologic system and its components is necessary. The knowledge of how the blood cells develop and function as well as how the hemostatic system functions is essential in understanding the diseases of the newborn that affect the hematologic system. Without this knowledge the nurse will miss many of the subtle signs and symptoms that indicate that a problem has arisen. This chapter discusses the hematologic and hemostatic systems, as well as the most common hematologic diseases of the newborn period.

OVERVIEW OF THE HEMATOLOGIC SYSTEM

Hematopoiesis

The hematopoietic system is characterized by the presence of pluripotent stem cells that differentiate into the three types of circulating blood cells: red blood cells (RBCs), white blood cells (WBCs), and thrombocytes (platelets). The formation, production, and maintenance of blood cells are referred to as hematopoiesis. Hematopoiesis is a continuous process that involves cell maturation and destruction concurrent with new cell production. Gestational age and postnatal age influence maturation and govern individual cell components, the level of activity, and the site of production.

The liver becomes the main site for hematopoiesis beginning at approximately 5 to 6 weeks gestation. The production peaks at 4 to 5 months of age, then slowly regresses, with the bone marrow predominating from 22 weeks gestation on. Also helping with hematopoiesis during the fetal period are extramedullary sites of the spleen, lymph nodes, thymus, and kidneys while the long bones are small (Yoder, 2011).

Red Blood Cells

Erythropoiesis, the production of RBCs, begins at approximately 3 to 4 weeks gestation. The RBCs are initially primitive megaloblasts, but when the liver becomes the primary site of hematopoiesis, a definitive line of RBCs is formed from the normoblasts, which progresses through several phases of refinement and accrue hemoglobin before reaching maturation. When the hemoglobin concentration of the normoblast reaches 34%, the nucleus is extruded and the cell becomes a reticulocyte. Approximately 1 to 2 days later, the reticulocyte becomes a mature RBC and is released into the bloodstream. The development of the RBC is identical in the bone marrow when it becomes the primary site of erythrocyte production.

The role of the RBC is to exchange oxygen and carbon dioxide between the lungs and tissues. Tissue oxygenation occurs by hemoglobin transport, whereas carbon dioxide removal is a reaction with carbonic anhydrase. RBCs also serve as a buffer to maintain acid–base balance.

The life span of fetal and newborn RBCs is much shorter than the adult RBC life span of 120 days. The term newborn's erythrocyte can last 60 to 70 days, that of a preterm infant, 35 to 50 days. One theoretic reason for this is the diminished deformability of the neonatal erythrocyte. Because of its larger size and cylindrical shape, the neonatal erythrocyte is more prone to destruction in the narrow sinusoids of the spleen (Obis, 2011).

The mean RBC count in the term newborn is in the range of 5.8 million per milliliter, with an elevated reticulocyte count of 3% to 7% during the first 24 to 48 hours of life. Mean RBC counts in the premature infant range from 4.6 million to 5.3 million per milliliter, with a greater number of circulating immature RBCs reflected in a higher reticulocyte count of 3% to 10% (Brugnara & Platt, 2009). In both groups of infants, the reticulocyte count falls abruptly to about 1% and the erythropoietin level drops to low, often undetectable, levels by the first week of life.

Hemoglobin

At 10 weeks gestation, hemoglobin synthesis changes from the embryonic to the fetal form (hemoglobin F). This event coincides with the transition of the site of erythropoiesis from the yolk sac to the fetal liver (Wilbur, Nienhuis, & Persons, 2011). The mechanism by which stem cells and progenitor cells perform this changeover remains unclear. Although low levels of a third form of hemoglobin, adult hemoglobin (hemoglobin A), are detectable at this time, hemoglobin F remains the predominant form during fetal development. At 30 weeks gestation, 90% to 100% of hemoglobin is the fetal form; the remainder is hemoglobin A. Between 30 and 32 weeks, the percentage of hemoglobin F starts to decline. At 40 weeks, 50% to 75% of RBCs contain fetal hemoglobin; at 6 months of age, 5% to 8%; and at 1 year of age, 1%.

Each type of hemoglobin has properties that make it valuable at the time of its synthesis. Each has a different affinity for oxygen that varies its uptake and release to the tissue (Figure 13.1). Fetal hemoglobin has a high affinity for oxygen, binding it more readily at the intervillous spaces in the placenta when the fetal partial pressure of oxygen (PO_2) averages between 25 and 30 mmHg. Adult hemoglobin has a decreased affinity for oxygen, which allows easier release of oxygen to the tissues when metabolic needs are high and the lungs are functional.

Erythropoietin

The single most important factor in regulating RBC production is tissue oxygenation. The main stimulus for RBC production at times of low oxygen is the hormone erythropoietin. This circulating glycoprotein hormone, the gene of which is located on the seventh chromosome, is an obligate growth factor that stimulates stem cells to become committed progenitors of the erythrocyte (Figure 13.2). In adults, the kidneys produce 90% to 95% of erythropoietin, but in the fetus the liver is considered the predominant site of production throughout most of gestation.

The major stimulus for erythropoietin release is diminished tissue oxygenation. In the absence of erythropoietin, hypoxia has no effect on the production of RBCs. However,

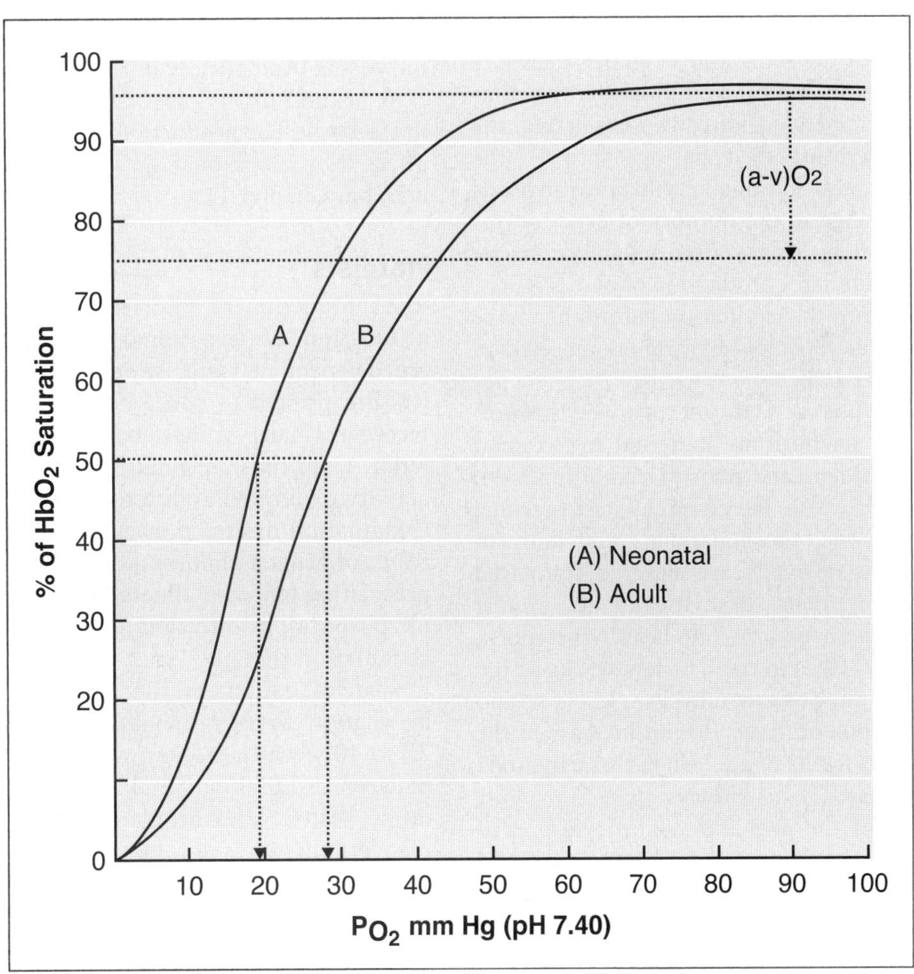

FIGURE 13.1 The affinity for oxygen (i.e., the ability of the hemoglobin molecule to bind and hold the oxygen molecule) is markedly different between fetal and adult hemoglobin. Fetal hemoglobin has a greater affinity for oxygen. It is able to bind to oxygen more readily at the intervillous spaces of the placenta, a property that is useful in the low partial pressure of oxygen (PO_2) environment of the fetus. Adult hemoglobin has a diminished affinity for oxygen, which allows easier release of oxygen to the tissue when metabolic needs are higher than those that arise in the fetus.

Adapted from Sacks and Delivoria-Papadopoulos (1984).

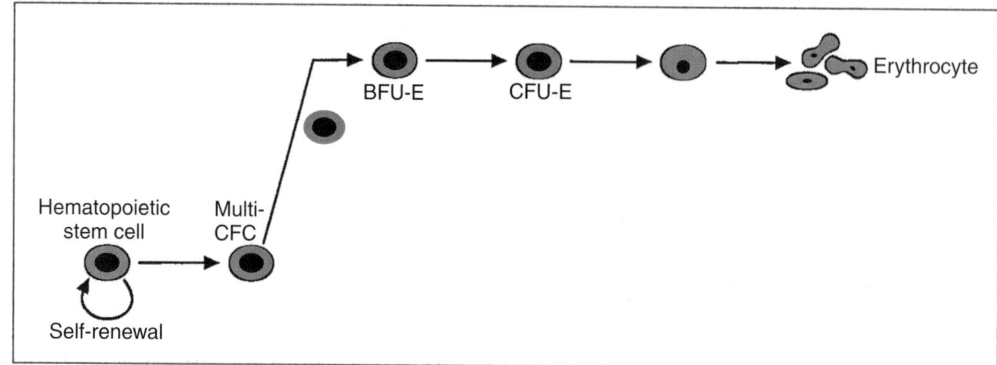

FIGURE 13.2 Hematopoietic stem cells stimulated to become erythrocytes initially develop into multipotent colony-forming cells (multi-CFC). A portion of the multi-CFC become erythroid progenitor cells, the early and late erythroid burst-forming units (BFU-E), which eventually differentiate into erythroid colony-forming units (CFU-E). These progenitor cells progress to form the normoblast, the erythrocyte precursor. Multiple divisions and alterations of the normoblast lead to the development of the reticulocyte. When the reticulocyte extrudes its nucleus, it normally moves out of the predominant production sites (i.e., the liver or bone marrow) and into the blood.
Modified from Luchtman-Jones and Wilson (2011).

if erythropoietin production is intact, hypoxia stimulates a rapid increase in erythropoietin levels, which remain elevated until hypoxia no longer exists. Although the liver is less responsive to hypoxia than the kidneys, production of erythropoietin in the fetus and newborn increases within minutes to hours after a precipitating event such as hypoxia. Erythropoietin acts by directly stimulating the RBC precursors, accelerating their passage through the various maturational stages. Although erythropoietin levels increase rapidly, no change in the number of erythrocytes is noted for approximately 5 days after a hypoxic stress. When erythropoietin stimulates production of excess RBCs, the RBCs are released into the circulation before they have reached maturity (i.e., as reticulocytes); this is reflected in an elevated reticulocyte count.

Factors besides hypoxia that increase erythropoietin production in the newborn are maternal hypoxemia, smallness for gestational age, and poor placental function. Erythropoietin levels are also increased by testosterone, estrogen, thyroid hormone, prostaglandins, and lipoproteins. Cord blood levels normally are elevated compared with adult values but drop dramatically to almost undetectable levels in the newborn. The healthy newborn, therefore, produces few RBCs in the first few weeks of life because the hypoxic stimuli of low fetal PO_2 levels are no longer present. Erythropoietin levels do not increase in the term infant until 8 to 10 weeks of age, when tissue hypoxia caused by anemia is sensed by the kidneys.

The characteristics of the neonatal erythrocyte predispose both preterm and term infants to problems associated with hemolysis and immature hepatic response to erythrocyte destruction, as well as to the effects of shortened erythrocyte life span (as is seen in physiologic neonatal anemia and anemia of the premature infant). In addition to maturational influences, preexisting maternal diseases and intrauterine abnormalities can impair RBC function and production, resulting in increased oxygen and nutritional requirements for the growing fetus (Obis, 2011).

White Blood Cells

The formation of the WBCs begins in the liver at approximately 5 to 7 weeks gestation and then in the lymph nodes at 12 weeks gestation, with the number of circulating WBCs increasing dramatically during the third trimester. The purpose of the WBC is to work against foreign proteins found in the body. The production and function of WBCs are also affected by gestational age; this subject is covered in more detail in Chapter 11.

Platelets

The production of platelets and clotting factors is also a function of gestational age. Although some factors are deficient at birth, several clotting factors and platelets are present in concentrations similar to adult levels. However, many of these components are functionally different from those of adults, possibly because of impaired activity or limited ability to respond to heightened needs. Coagulation dysfunction in the newborn may also be the result of genetic abnormalities (e.g., X-linked hemophilia), preexisting maternal illness (e.g., immune thrombocytopenic purpura), or infection (e.g., disseminated intravascular coagulation [DIC]).

Platelet counts in the newborn do not vary much in relation to gestational age. Counts are similar from 27 to 40 weeks gestation, with the range of normal falling between 215,000/mm^3 and 378,000/mm^3. At 32 weeks gestation, platelet levels are comparable to those of an adult, but platelet function is not. Platelet counts under 150,000/mm^3 are considered thrombocytopenic.

Blood Volume

Normal blood values found shortly after birth reflect a time of maximum change. Blood values at birth depend on (1) the timing of cord clamping, (2) the infant's gestational age, (3) the blood sampling site, and (4) the technique used to obtain adequate blood flow.

The timing of cord clamping and the positional differences between the infant and the placenta can significantly influence newborn blood volume. Complete emptying of placental vessels before clamping can increase blood volume by 61%; one quarter of the placental transfusion occurs within the first 15 seconds, and half of the transfusion is complete by 1 minute. Controversy remains on whether to clamp the cord immediately or to delay cord clamping. Recent studies have shown in both term and preterm infants that delayed cord clamping (up to 180 seconds for term and 30–45 seconds for preterm infants) led to higher hematocrits (Hct), a decreased need for transfusion and higher ferritin levels, lower incidence of iron deficiency, and lower incidence of neonatal anemia (Anderson, Hellstrom-Westas, Andersson, & Domellof, 2011; McDonald & Middleton, 2008; Oh et al., 2011).

The average blood volume is approximately 85 mL/kg of body weight in the term infant, though it can be as high as to 90 to 105 mL/kg in the preterm infant. The younger the infant's gestational age, the greater the blood volume will be per kilogram of body weight. The hemoglobin concentration and Hct are also functions of gestational age, especially in infants born before 32 weeks gestation. The average mean hemoglobin concentration at 26 to 30 weeks is 13.4 g/dL, with an average mean Hct of 41.5%. In the term infant, mean hemoglobin values range from 16.5 to 18.5 g/dL, with mean Hct values between 51% and 56% (Brugnara & Platt, 2009). Mean hemoglobin values in post mature infants are higher than in the term infant, possibly as a result of progressive placental dysfunction and of oxygen deficit, which stimulates the release of erythropoietin. Table 13.1 summarizes the differences in hematologic values as a function of increasing gestational and postnatal age.

It is important to consider the sampling site and the quality of blood flow when interpreting laboratory values. The hemoglobin levels of capillary blood are 10% to 20% higher than those of venous and arterial blood. This discrepancy can be minimized by warming the extremity before drawing blood to enhance peripheral perfusion, allowing better spontaneous blood flow. Discarding the first few drops obtained on a capillary draw also improves the accuracy of the sample. Sampling by the venous route also requires care; poor blood flow through small-bore needles increases the chance of hemolysis, which can lead to sampling errors. Greater accuracy can be obtained by using the largest possible bore needle and removing the needle from the syringe before placing the sample in the specimen container. Gestational age also affects the discrepancy between reported capillary and venous results: the younger the gestational age, the larger the discrepancy. The key to accuracy in hematology laboratory values lies in the use of a consistent sampling site.

Blood Group Type

The RBCs have antigens located on the surface of the cell membranes that can cause antigen-antibody reactions. Blood is classified by group and types based on the antigens that are found on the RBC. The four major blood types are A, B, O, and AB. The most common blood types in the population are O at 47% and A at 41% (Hall, 2011). Antibodies to the antigens of different blood types occur naturally in the plasma (Table 13.2). For example, type A blood has A antigens on the cell surface but has circulating anti-B antibodies in the plasma. Type B blood has just the opposite, B antigens on the cell surface and anti-A antibodies in the plasma. Type AB blood has A and B antigens on the cell

TABLE 13.1

AGE-SPECIFIC NORMAL BLOOD CELL VALUES IN FETAL SAMPLES (26–30 WEEKS GESTATION) AND NEONATAL SAMPLES (28–44 WEEKS GESTATION)

Age	Hb (gm/dL)[a]	HCT (%)[a]	MCV (fL)[a]	MCHC (g/dL RBC)[a]	Reticulocytes	WBCs (× 10^3/mL)[b]	Platelets (10^3/mL)[b]
26–30 weeks gestation[c]	13.4 (11)	41.5 (34.9)	118.2 (106.7)	37.9 (30.6)	—	4.4 (2.7)	254 (180–327)
28 weeks	14.5	45	120	31.0	(5–10)	—	275
32 weeks	15.0	47	118	32.0	(3–10)	—	290
Term[d] (cord)	16.5 (13.5)	51 (42)	108 (98)	33.0 (30.0)	(3–7)	18.1(9–30)[d]	290
1–3 days	18.5 (14.5)	56 (45)	108 (95)	33.0 (29.0)	(1.8–4.6)	18.9 (9.4–34)	192
2 weeks	16.6 (13.4)	53 (41)	105 (88)	31.4 (28.1)	—	11.4 (5–20)	252
1 month	13.9 (10.7)	44 (33)	101 (91)	31.8 (28.1)	(0.1–1.7)	10.8 (4–19.5)	—

Hb, Hemoglobin; Hct, hematocrit; MCV, mean corpuscular volume; MCHC, mean corpuscular hemoglobin concentration; WBCs, white blood cells.

[a] Data are mean (number in parenthesis is –2 standard deviations [SD]).

[b] Data are mean (number in parenthesis is –2 SD).

[c] In infants younger than 1 month, capillary Hb exceeds venous Hb: at 1 hour old, the difference is 3.6 g; at 5 days, 2.2 g; at 3 weeks, 1.1 g.

[d] Mean (95% confidence limits).

Modified from Ashan and Noether (2011).

TABLE 13.2

BLOOD GROUPS AND THEIR ANTIGENS AND ANTIBODIES

Blood Group Type	Antigens	Antibodies
Ox	None	Anti-A
A	A	Anti-B
B	B	Anti-A
AB	A and B	None

Modified from Hall (2011).

surface and neither antibody in the plasma, and type O blood has neither antigen on the cell surface and both anti-A nor anti-B antibodies in the plasma. Antigens usually are polypeptides and complex proteins; antibodies are immunoglobulins (mostly IgG and IgM).

The other type of antigen is Rh antigens. Chromosome 1 stores the genetic material governing Rh antigens, and in most individuals two genes, *CD240CE* and *CD240D*, determine the Rh blood group (Liley, 2009). There are three presumed Rh gene loci with the capability of producing five recognized antigens in the Rh complex: C, D, E, c, d, and e. Each individual has a paired set of these factors, having inherited a single set of C or c, D or d, and E or e from each parent. A predilection exists toward three particular combinations, two Rh positive (CDe and cDE) and one Rh negative (cde). Of these six factors, the two involved in Rh determination are D and d. The D antigen is most prevalent; its presence on the RBC indicates an Rh-positive cell, whereas its absence indicates an Rh-negative cell. Approximately 85% of Caucasians are Rh positive and 15% Rh negative. African Americans are approximately 95% Rh positive, and Africans are virtually 100% Rh positive (Hall, 2011). Because of single-set inheritance from each parent, the potential exists for three different combinations of paired antigens: one pair being both d (Rh negative, homozygous), another pair being both D (Rh positive, homozygous), and the third pair being a combination of d and D (Rh positive, heterozygous). The end product is the production or absence of Rh antigen positioned on the surface of the RBC. The Rh antigen can be detected as early as 38 days gestation on the fetal RBC and attains complete development during fetal life. This antigen is necessary for normal function of the RBC membrane, and, unlike A and B antigens, which can be found in other tissues, it is confined exclusively to the RBC. Antibodies never occur naturally in the Rh system; exposure to the antigen is necessary to produce antibodies.

Hemostatic System

The components involved in blood coagulation and fibrinolysis (dissolution of a formed clot) are produced in the liver, vascular wall, and tissue during early fetal life. Many of the clotting factors (procoagulants) and anticoagulants (inhibitors) can be identified during the 8th to 12th weeks of gestation. However, procoagulants, anticoagulants, and the substances responsible for dissolution of a clot, fibrinolytics, do not increase in number and function or reach adult levels simultaneously (Tables 13.3 through 13.5). Some components increase with increasing gestational age, whereas others achieve normal adult levels several weeks to months

TABLE 13.3

NORMAL COAGULATION TEST RESULTS AND BLOOD LEVELS OF COAGULATION FACTORS IN THE FETUS (19–27 WEEKS GESTATION) AND NEWBORN (28 WEEKS GESTATION TO TERM)

Test/Factor	19–27 Weeks Mean ± SD	28–31 Weeks Mean (Boundary)	30–36 Weeks, Day 1 Mean (Boundary)	30–36 Weeks, Day 5 Mean (Boundary)	Full Term, Day 1 Mean (Boundary)	Full Term, Day 5 Mean (Boundary)
Test						
Prothrombin time (PT) (seconds)	—	15.4 (14.6–16.9)	13 (10.6–16.2)	12.5 (10–15.3)	13 (10.1–15.9)	12.4 (10–15.3)
Activated partial thromboplastin time (AAPTT) (seconds)	—	108 (80–168)	53.6 (27.5–79.4)	50.5 (26.9–74.1)	42.9 (31.3–54.5)	42.6 (25.4–59.8)
Thrombin clotting time (TCT) (seconds)	—	—	24.8 (19.2–30.4)	24.1 (18.8–29.4)	23.5 (19–28.3)	23.1 (18–29.2)
Factor						
Fibrinogen (g/L)	1 ± 0.4	2.56 (1.6–5.5)	2.43 (1.5–3.73)	2.8 (1.6–4.18)	2.83 (1.67–3.99)	3.12 (1.62–4.62)
Factor II (units/mL)	0.12 ± 0.02	0.31 (0.19–0.54)	0.45 (0.2–0.77)	0.57 (0.29–0.85)	0.48 (0.26–0.7)	0.63 (0.33–0.93)

(*continued*)

TABLE 13.3

NORMAL COAGULATION TEST RESULTS AND BLOOD LEVELS OF COAGULATION FACTORS IN THE FETUS (19–27 WEEKS GESTATION) AND NEWBORN (28 WEEKS GESTATION TO TERM) (CONTINUED)

Test/Factor	19–27 Weeks Mean ± SD	28–31 Weeks Mean (Boundary)	30–36 Weeks, Day 1 Mean (Boundary)	30–36 Weeks, Day 5 Mean (Boundary)	Full Term, Day 1 Mean (Boundary)	Full Term, Day 5 Mean (Boundary)
Factor V (units/mL)	0.41 ± 0.1	0.65 (0.43–0.8)	0.88 (0.41–1.44)	1 (0.46–1.54)	0.72 (0.34–1.08)	0.95 (0.45–1.45)
Factor VII (units/mL)	0.28 ± 0.04	0.37 (0.24–0.76)	0.67 (0.21–1.13)	0.84 (0.3–1.38)	0.66 (0.28–1.04)	0.89 (0.35–1.43)
Factor VIII (units/mL)	0.39 ± 0.14	0.79 (0.37–1.26)	1.11 (0.5–2.13)	1.15 (0.53–2.05)	1 (0.5–1.78)	0.88 (0.5–1.54)
von Willebrand factor (vWF) (units/mL)	0.64 ± 0.13	1.41 (0.83–2.23)	1.36 (0.78–2.1)	1.33 (0.72–2.19)	1.53 (0.5–2.87)	1.4 (0.5–2.54)
Factor IX (units/mL)	0.1 ± 0.01	0.18 (0.17–0.2)	0.35 (0.19–0.65)	0.42 (0.14–0.74)	0.53 (0.15–0.91)	0.53 (0.15–0.91)
Factor X (units/mL)	0.21 ± 0.03	0.36 (0.25–0.64)	0.41 (0.11–0.71)	0.51 (0.19–0.83)	0.4 (0.12–0.68)	0.49 (0.19–0.79)
Factor XI (units/mL)	—	0.23 (0.11–0.33)	0.3 (0.08–0.52)	0.41 (0.13–0.69)	0.38 (0.1–0.66)	0.55 (0.23–0.87)
Factor XII (units/ml)	0.22 ± 0.03	0.25 (0.05–0.35)	0.38 (0.1–0.66)	0.39 (0.09–0.69)	0.53 (0.13–0.93)	0.47 (0.11–0.83)
Prekallikrein (PK) (units/mL)	—	0.26 (0.15–0.32)	0.33 (0.09–0.57)	0.45 (0.26–0.75)	0.37 (0.18–0.69)	0.48 (0.2–0.76)
High-molecular-weight kininogen	—	0.32 (0.19–0.52)	0.49 (0.09–0.89)	0.62 (0.24–1)	0.54 (0.06–1.02)	0.74 (0.16–1.32)
(HMWK) (units/mL)						
Factor XIIIa (units/mL)	—	—	0.7 (0.32–1.08)	1.01 (0.57–1.45)	0.79 (0.27–1.31)	0.94 (0.44–1.44)
Factor XIIIb (units/mL)	—	—	0.81 (0.35–1.27)	1.1 (0.68–1.58)	0.76 (0.3–1.22)	1.06 (0.32–1.8)
Plasminogen (units/mL)	—	—	1.7 (1.12–2.48)	1.91 (1.21–2.61)	1.95 0.35 (44)	2.17 ± 0.38 (60)

Modified from Andrew et al. (1990).

TABLE 13.4

NORMAL BLOOD LEVELS OF COAGULATION INHIBITORS IN NEWBORNS (30 WEEKS GESTATION TO TERM)

Coagulation Inhibitors	30–36 Weeks Gestation		Full Term	
	Day 1 Mean (Boundary)	Day 5 Mean (Boundary)	Day 1 Mean (Boundary)	Day 5 Mean (Boundary)
Antithrombin III (ATIII) (units/mL)	0.38 (0.14–0.62)	0.56 (0.3–0.82)	0.63 (0.39–0.87)	0.67 (0.41–0.93)
Alpha2-macroglobulin (α2-M) (units/mL)	1.1 (0.56–1.82)	1.25 (0.71–1.77)	1.39 (0.95–1.83)	1.48 (0.98–1.98)
C1 esterase inhibitor (C1E-NH) (units/mL)	0.65 (0.31–0.99)	0.83 (0.45–1.21)	0.72 (0.36–1.08)	0.90 (0.6–1.2)
Alpha1-antitrypsin (α1-AT) (units/mL)	0.9 (0.36–1.44)	0.94 (0.42–1.46)	0.93 (0.49–1.37)	0.89 (0.49–1.29)

(continued)

TABLE 13.4

NORMAL BLOOD LEVELS OF COAGULATION INHIBITORS IN NEWBORNS (30 WEEKS GESTATION TO TERM) (CONTINUED)

Coagulation Inhibitors	30–36 Weeks Gestation		Full Term	
	Day 1 Mean (Boundary)	Day 5 Mean (Boundary)	Day 1 Mean (Boundary)	Day 5 Mean (Boundary)
Heparin cofactor II (HCII) (units/mL)	0.32 (0.1–0.6)	0.34 (0.1–0.69)	0.43 (0.1–0.93)	0.48 (0.1–0.96)
Protein C (units/mL)	0.28 (0.12–0.44)	0.31 (0.11–0.51)	0.35 (0.17–0.53)	0.42 (0.2–0.64)
Protein S (units/mL)	0.26 (0.14–0.38)	0.37 (0.13–0.61)	0.36 (0.12–0.6)	0.5 (0.22–0.78)

Modified from Andrew et al. (1990).

TABLE 13.5

NORMAL BLOOD LEVELS OF FIBRINOLYTIC COMPONENTS IN PREMATURE AND TERM NEWBORNS

Fibrinolytic Component	Premature Infants		Full-Term Infants	
	Day 1 Mean (Boundary)	Day 5 Mean (Boundary)	Day 1 Mean (Boundary)	Day 5 Mean (Boundary)
Plasminogen (units/mL)	1.7 (1.12–2.48)	1.91 (1.21–2.61)	1.95 (1.25–2.65)	2.17 (1.41–2.93)
Tissue plasminogen activator (TPA) (ng/mL)	8.48 (3–16.7)	3.97 (2–6.93)	9.6 (5–18.9)	5.6 (4–10)
Alpha2-antiplasmin (α2-AP) (units/mL)	0.78 (0.4–1.16)	0.81 (0.49–1.13)	0.85 (0.55–1.15)	1 (0.7–1.3)
Plasminogen activator inhibitor (PAI) (units/mL)	5.4 (0–12.2)	2.5 (0–7.1)	6.4 (2–15.1)	2.3 (0–8.1)

Modified from Andrew et al. (1990).

before the fetus reaches term. Still other components do not achieve normal adult levels until several weeks to months after birth. Although the function of coagulation factors and anticoagulants in the fetus is not identical to that in an older child or adult, initial vascular response to injury by release of tissue thromboplastin is functional in the fetus as early as 8 weeks.

Hemostasis consists of a delicate and dynamic balance between factors that prevent exsanguination and those that keep the blood in a fluid form. The balanced interrelationship among four distinct components ensures orderly hemostasis and fibrinolysis when vascular integrity is destroyed or interrupted. The four constituents are vascular spasm, platelets and their activating substances, coagulation or plasma factors, and the fibrinolytic pathway.

INITIAL STEPS IN HEMOSTASIS

Vascular Spasm

Initial hemostasis in a ruptured blood vessel consists of vascular spasm, which is a consequence of multiple mediator interactions, nervous reflexes, and localized muscle spasm. Although nervous reflexes are a response to pain, most of the vascular spasm is due to muscle contraction in the vessel wall secondary to direct injury. This vascular response to injury is present in an 8-week fetus and at term is the equivalent of adult norms in regard to capillary fragility and bleeding time. This component is gestational age dependent, as is evident in the increased capillary fragility shown by the preterm infant.

Platelet Plug Formation

The second mechanism of hemostasis after vascular injury is the formation of the platelet plug. Platelets coming into contact with an injured vascular wall adhere to the wall and form a platelet plug. This hemostatic plug is the primary means of closing small vascular holes at the capillary and small-vessel level. The platelets' ability to adhere on contact to a denuded vascular wall requires a glycoprotein, von Willebrand factor (vWF), which is synthesized by vascular endothelial cells and megakaryocytes vWF complexes with Factor VIII (antihemophilic factor) and both circulate jointly.

Platelets also have the ability to aggregate (stick to other platelets), forming large clumps. Aggregation is made possible by the platelet's ability to modify its shape and to secrete many biochemical substances (platelet release reaction) that enhance cohesion. When platelets and associated glycoproteins are activated by excess release of these biochemical substances during times of stress, fibrinogen receptors appear on the surface of the platelet. These receptors enhance the platelets' ability to bind fibrinogen, which in turn cross-links the platelets, allowing them to aggregate. This provides a tight mesh of clot around an injured vessel that controls bleeding (Figure 13.3). After 32 weeks gestation, average platelet counts are comparable to those of term infants and adults, but the ability of platelets to aggregate is relatively diminished (Diacovo, 2011).

Coagulation

When bleeding cannot be controlled with merely a platelet plug, circulating plasma coagulation factors are triggered to form a network of fibrin that turns the existing plug into a hemostatic seal, which in turn completes hemostasis. Fibrin threads, necessary for clot formation, can develop within 15 to 20 seconds in the presence of normal coagulation factors. Within 3 to 6 minutes after vascular rupture, the entire opening is occluded by clot; within 30 to 60 minutes, the clot begins to retract, pulling the injured vascular portions together and further sealing the vascular end. This coagulation reaction involves several plasma proteins and three distinct phases. The first phase involves the formation of prothrombin activator, followed by the activation of prothrombin to thrombin (formation of thrombin), and then concludes with the conversion of soluble fibrinogen to fibrin (fibrin clot formation) (Hall, 2011).

■ Phase I: Formation of Prothrombin Activator. According to the earliest theories on coagulation (cascade theory), prothrombin activator can be generated by two separate pathways, the intrinsic and extrinsic pathways. The intrinsic pathway is triggered by trauma or damage that occurs inside the vessel or to the blood itself and the extrinsic pathway is triggered by the production of tissue thromboplastin that is generated by vessel wall damage. This bimodal pathway can be interrupted or negated by a deficiency in platelets or any of the plasma coagulation factors or by the presence of inhibitors (anticoagulants) in the plasma. Selective activation of one of these pathways depends on the site and severity of injury.

Activation of the intrinsic pathway is slower because it lacks the major stimulus of the extrinsic pathway, tissue thromboplastin generated by vessel wall damage. The intrinsic pathway relies on blood trauma or injury within the vessel to alter platelets and plasma proteins and to convert dormant factors (zymogens), naturally found in circulating blood, into active proteolytic enzymes (Figure 13.4). Each activated enzyme subsequently reacts with the succeeding factor, changing it into its activated form. The steps of intrinsic activation of coagulation are as follows:

1. An activator (blood trauma, injury within the vessel, or contact with collagen) activates Factor XII, converting it to Factor XIIa, while simultaneously damaging platelets, which causes a release of platelet phospholipids.

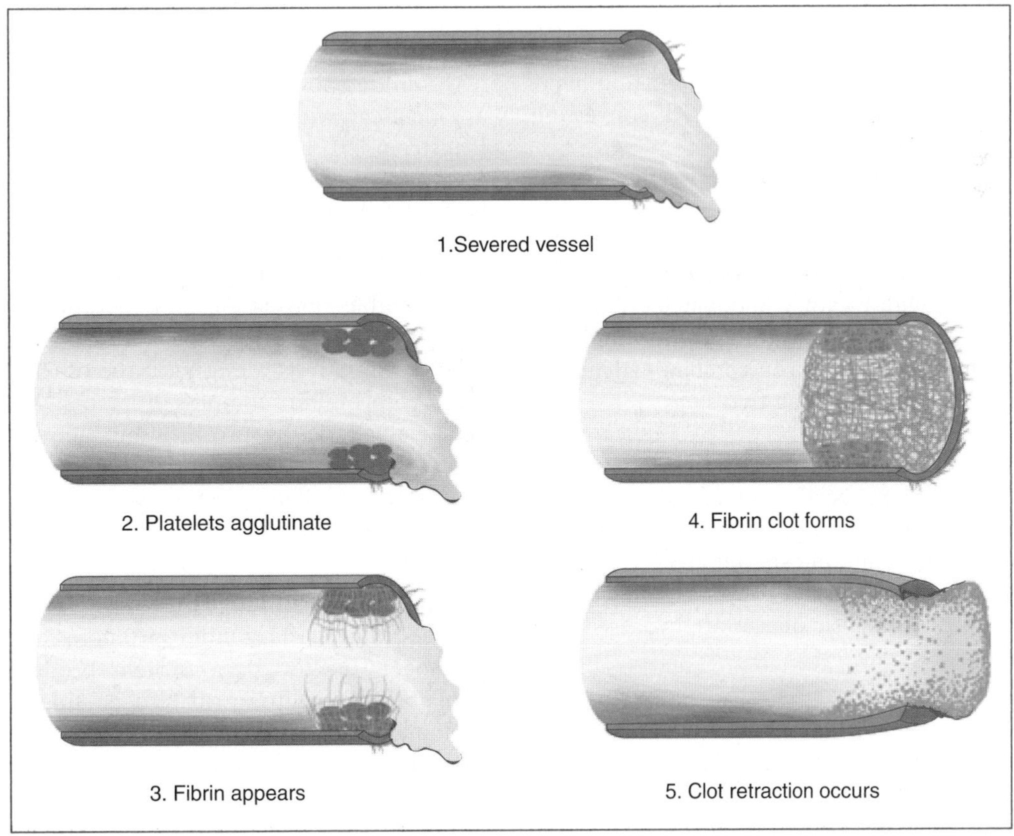

FIGURE 13.3 When vessel wall injury occurs, the initial clotting process begins with the formation of a platelet plug. Platelet activation stimulates fibrinogen receptors found on the surface of the platelets, which enhance their aggregation with other platelets and fibrinogen. The fibrin clot that forms retracts and occludes the damaged vascular wall.
Redrawn from Hall (2011) and Witt (1948).

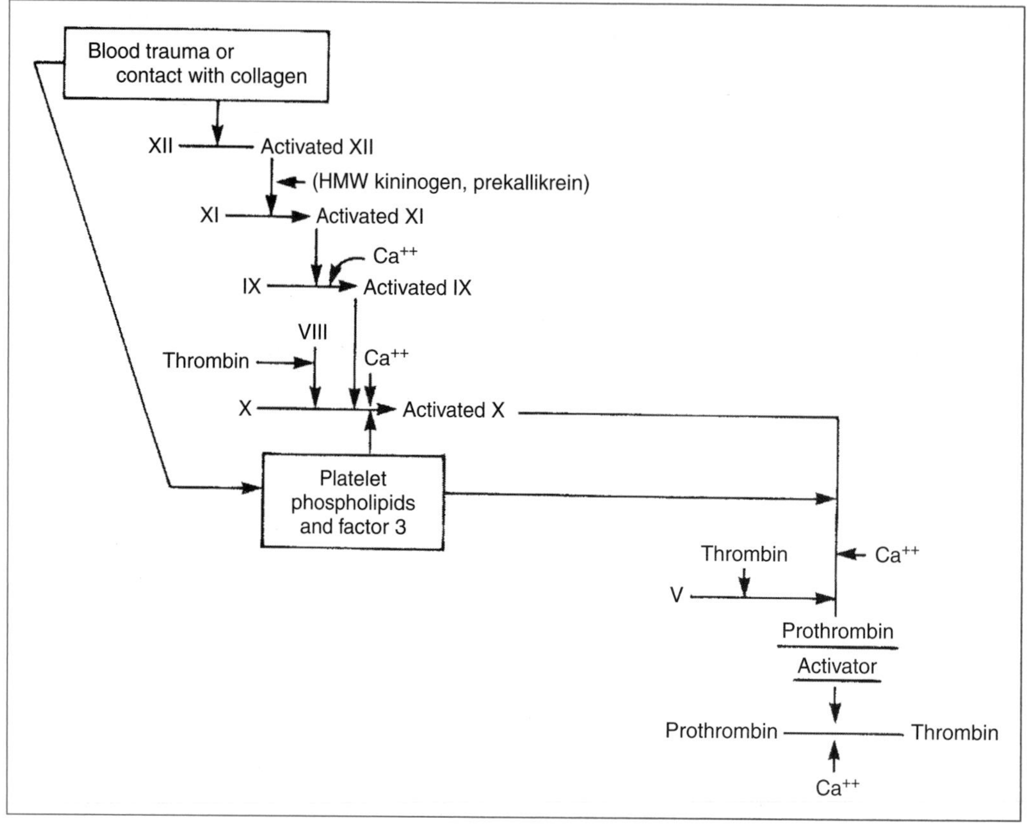

FIGURE 13.4 The intrinsic pathway for initiating the clotting cascade is activated by trauma to the blood, injury within the vessel, or contact with collagen. HMW, high molecular weight.
From Hall (2011).

2. Factor XIIa, in conjunction with prekallikrein and high-molar-weight kininogen, activates Factor XI, converting it to Factor XIa.
3. Factor XIa activates Factor IX, converting it to Factor IXa.
4. Factor IXa, platelet phospholipid, and Factor VIII combine to activate Factor X, converting it to Factor Xa.
5. Factor Xa combines with Factor V and platelet phospholipids to form prothrombin activator (prothrombinase), which releases thrombin from prothrombin. Calcium is required for this and the preceding two steps.

The extrinsic pathway can generate thrombin in a matter of seconds when injury occurs outside the vascular space (Figure 13.5). Tissue thromboplastin (tissue factor), composed of glycoproteins and phospholipids, is produced when tissue is injured. When plasma comes in contact with this substance, the initial intrinsic phases are bypassed and the following responses occur:

1. Tissue thromboplastin or tissue factor (Factor III) activates Factor VII to Factor VIIa. These two factors form a complex with glycoprotein in the presence of ionized calcium (tissue factor–Factor VIIa complex) that activates Factor X, converting it to Factor Xa.
2. In the presence of calcium, Factor Xa forms complexes with phospholipids and Factor V to form prothrombin activator.

From this point on, the intrinsic and extrinsic pathways are identical, with both proceeding to phase II (Monagie & Hagstrom, 2011).

■ **Phase II: Formation of Thrombin.** Prothrombin activator from either of the two pathways continues the clotting cascade by further influencing the breakdown of the unstable plasma protein prothrombin. Prothrombin (Factor II) is synthesized by the liver under the influence of vitamin K, along with the other factors that form the prothrombin complex (Factors VII, IX, and X). When acted on by prothrombin activator, prothrombin forms the potent coagulant thrombin. The newly formed thrombin stimulates completion of the third and final phase of coagulation.

■ Phase III: Fibrin Clot Formation

Procoagulants. Thrombin promotes the conversion of fibrinogen (Factor I), a protein produced by the liver, into fibrin by splitting off two peptides from the soluble fibrinogen molecule. This exposes two sites, to which other split fibrin molecules can cross-link, forming an insoluble fibrin chain. Fibrin stabilizing factor (Factor XIII) further strengthens the tight bond of this developing fibrin mesh. Fibrin stabilizing factor is naturally found in the plasma and is also secreted by entrapped platelets. The forming fibrin clot begins to contract and retract with the help of platelets

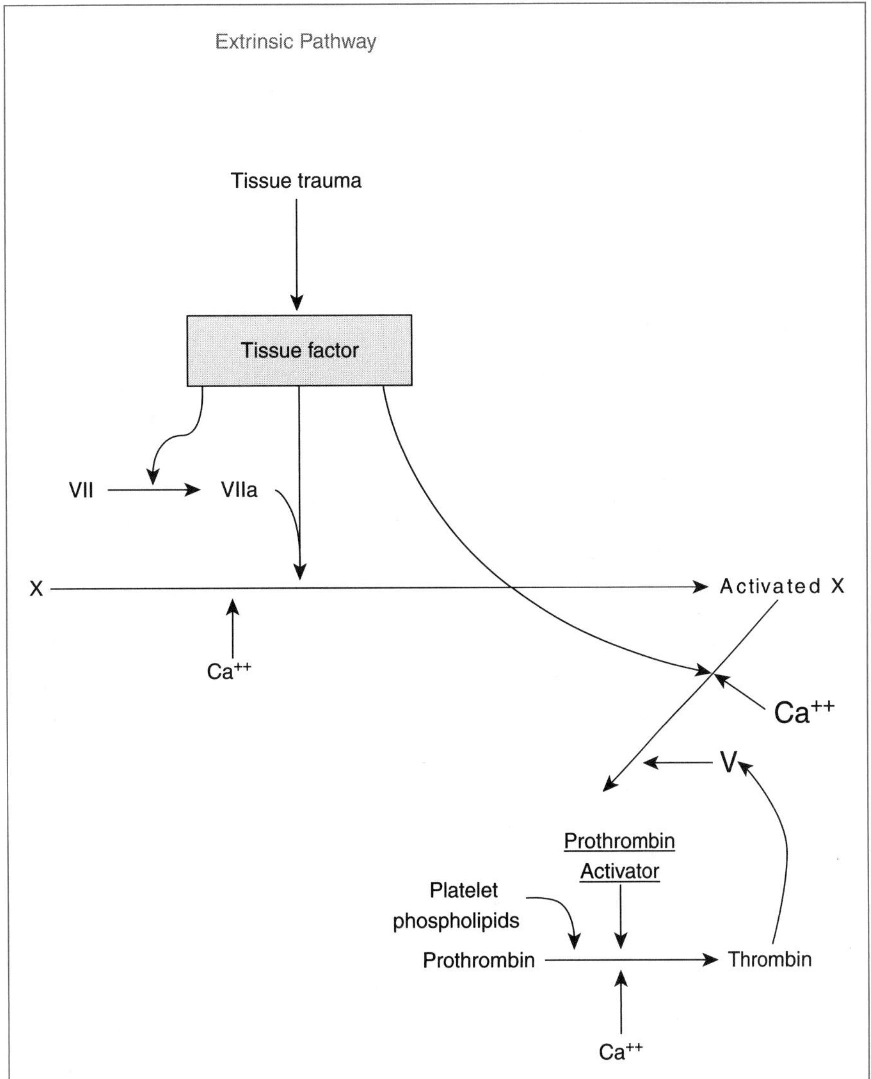

FIGURE 13.5 The extrinsic pathway for initiating the clotting cascade can generate thrombin rapidly as a result of thromboplastin release from injured tissue.
From Hall (2011).

that have actin-myosin action, the same action by which a muscle works. Extension of the clot into the surrounding circulating blood promotes further thrombosis. Thrombin from the clot has the ability to cleave prothrombin into more thrombin and enhances the production of prothrombin activator, thus acting as a potent biofeedback system for perpetuation of the clotting cascade.

Anticoagulants. Throughout the entire coagulation pathway, the action of the activated enzymes is modulated at each stage by multiple and specific inhibitors (anticoagulants). Consequently, coagulation is a process of balance between coagulation factors and naturally occurring inhibitors. Some of these anticoagulants are endothelial surface factors that prevent coagulation until the vessel's endothelial wall is damaged. One such factor is the smoothness of the wall, which prevents any adherence and subsequent activation; another is the monomolecular layer of protein covering the wall, which repels plasma clotting factors and platelets.

Two inhibitors, α1-antitrypsin and C1 esterase inhibitor, interfere with the coagulation factors involved in the initial activation of the intrinsic pathway, as does Factor Xa despite its role in cleaving prothrombin into thrombin. Factor Xa rapidly binds with a tissue factor pathway inhibitor (TFPI) found in the plasma. This complex, TFPI–Factor Xa, joins with the tissue factor–Factor VIIa complex to form a quaternary complex that inhibits further activation of Factor X by tissue factor.

Thrombin also acts as its own inhibitor by stimulating activation of protein C, which inactivates Factors V and VIII in the presence of another vitamin K–dependent inhibitor, protein S. A deficiency of these two proteins has been implicated in cases of neonatal thrombosis.

Other inhibitors of thrombin formation are (1) fibrin threads created during clot formation, which absorb thrombin, thus removing it from circulation and eliminating its potential for further coagulation; (2) thrombomodulin, found on the endothelial surfaces of the body and in the plasma complexes with thrombin, which eliminates thrombin's ability to cleave fibrinogen; (3) α2-macroglobulin, which inhibits proteases, including thrombin; (4) antithrombin III, which combines with thrombin, blocking the conversion of fibrinogen into fibrin; and (5) heparin cofactor II, which removes several activated procoagulants. Both antithrombin III and heparin are produced in the precapillary connective tissue of the lungs and liver (Monagie & Hagstrom, 2011).

Fibrinolysis. Once a clot develops, it can be invaded by fibroblasts that lay down connective tissue throughout the clot or it can be dissolved. The process of dissolution occurs by activation of naturally occurring factors that lyse the clot. Fibrinolysis is activated simultaneously with stimulation of the coagulation system, with powerful but inactivated anticoagulants built right into the clot (Figure 13.6). One of these anticoagulants, plasminogen, is manufactured by the liver, kidneys, and eosinophils. Under the influence of thrombin, activated Factor XII, tissue plasminogen activator (t-PA; located on the vascular endothelium), and urokinase plasminogen activator (u-PA; found in the urine), plasminogen is converted into plasmin, a proteolytic enzyme that breaks down fibrin into fibrin split products. Plasmin not only digests the fibrin chains but also deactivates fibrinogen; Factors V, VII, and XII; and prothrombin. Plasmin can be inactivated by its inhibitor, α2-antiplasmin; t-PA can be inactivated by its inhibitor, plasminogen activator inhibitor-1.

In summary, both term and preterm newborns have the ability to create a balance between transitory deficiencies in the amount and function of a variety of clotting factors, platelets, and anticoagulant factors. The homeostasis between clotting factors and anticoagulants places the newborn in a mildly hypercoagulable state at birth. Compared with older children and adults, therefore, the newborn has no greater tendency to bleed but does have several differences in regard to coagulation components and reserves, including (1) gestational age-dependent variations in the concentrations of coagulation factors, anticoagulants, and fibrinolytics; (2) a faster turnover rate of components; (3) a slower rate of synthesis of components; and (4) limited ability to supply necessary components during times of increased need (Monagie & Hagstrom, 2011).

ASSESSMENT OF HEMATOLOGIC FUNCTION

Because infants respond to a variety of problems in a similar manner, many clinical findings (e.g., hypoglycemia, hypocalcemia, hypothermia, apnea, bradycardia, cyanosis,

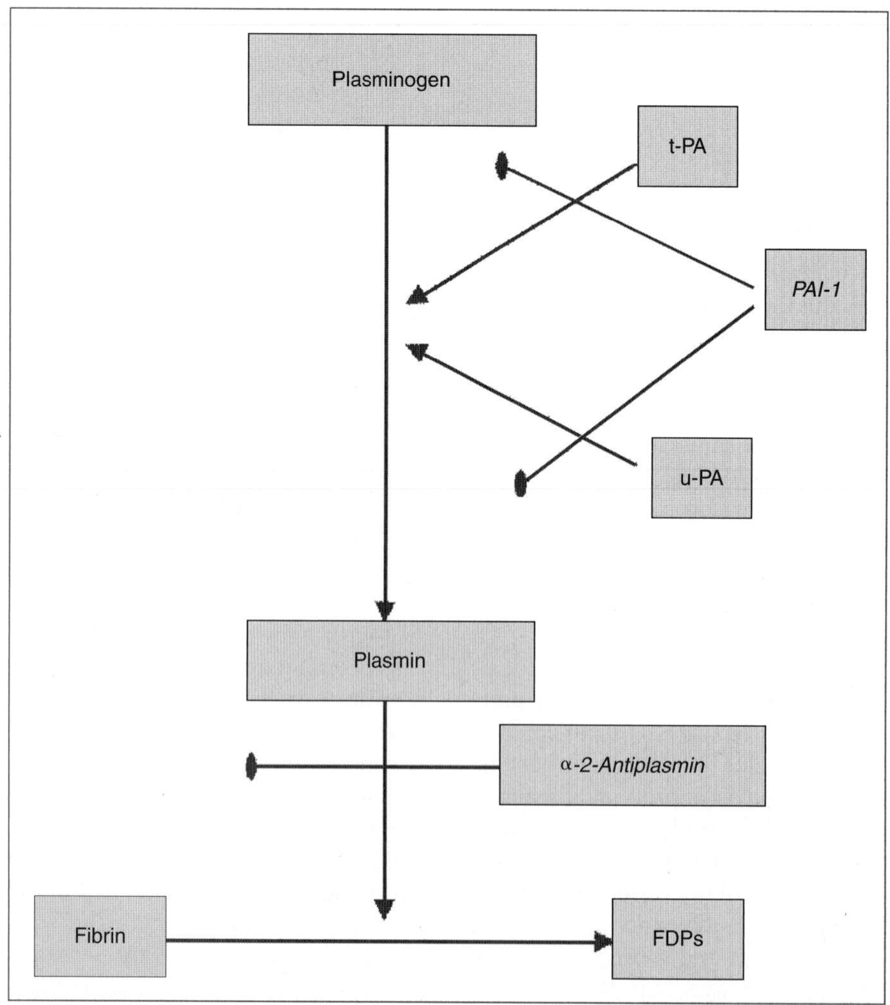

FIGURE 13.6 The components of the fibrinolytic system involved in the lysis of a fibrin clot. t-PA, tissue plasminogen activator; PAI-1, plasminogen activator inhibitor; u-PA, urokinase plasminogen activator; FDPs, fibrin degradation products.
Modified from Edstrom (2000).

lethargy, poor feeding) warrant at least a complete blood count (CBC) to determine if a hematologic reason exists for these symptoms. With active bleeding, platelet counts, clotting studies, fibrinogen levels, and measurements of products of fibrinolysis (e.g., d-dimer, fibrin split products, or fibrin degradation products) can shed light on the type of blood dyscrasia present and can direct the caregiver to the appropriate therapeutic response. These studies also provide a way to monitor and evaluate treatments. However, laboratory data are most helpful when they are used in conjunction with astute observation and physical assessment skills.

Several physical findings can help determine the well-being and homeostasis of the hematologic system (Box 13.1). Cutaneous abnormalities such as hematomas, abrasions, petechiae, and bleeding should alert the nurse to the possibility of a hematologic abnormality. Hepatosplenomegaly also can indicate abnormal breakdown of RBCs. Hepatosplenomegaly concurrent with hyperbilirubinemia and hemolysis can signal alloimmune problems (e.g., Rh and ABO incompatibilities) or acquired, congenital, or postnatal infection (e.g., cytomegalovirus infection, toxoplasmosis, herpes simplex infection, or hepatitis).

COMMON HEMATOLOGIC DISORDERS

Blood Group Incompatibilities

Blood group incompatibilities were first recognized in the 1940s with the discovery of the Rh grouping and the first test for detection of antibody-coated RBCs, devised by Coombs in 1946. Before the introduction of Rh immune globulin (i.e., RhIgG, RhIG, RhoGAM, Rhophylac) in 1964 and its release for general use in 1968, Rh incompatibility accounted for one third of all blood group incompatibilities. With the use of RhIgG, the frequency of Rh incompatibility has dropped significantly, and ABO has become the main blood group incompatibility, with sensitization occurring in 3% of all infants. Both incompatibilities involve maternal antibody response to fetal antigen, leading to RBC destruction by hemolysis. Rh antibody response is elicited on exposure to antigen and does not exist spontaneously, whereas anti-A and anti-B antibodies occur naturally. These entities also differ in the severity of the effect on the fetus and newborn and in the method of treatment.

> **BOX 13.1**
>
> **PHYSICAL FINDINGS HELPFUL IN EVALUATING THE INTEGRITY OF THE HEMATOLOGIC SYSTEM**
>
> Ecchymosis
> Hematomas
> Hepatosplenomegaly
> Jaundice
> Obvious blood loss—hemorrhage
> Pallor
> Petechiae
> Plethora

Other minor blood groupings (e.g., Kell, C, E, Duffy, and Kidd) may also be involved in incompatibilities that result in hyperbilirubinemia, but Rh and ABO incompatibilities are the most common, accounting for 98% of all cases. There are 400 known RBC antigens that can induce antibody production. Some of these antibodies are induced after transfusion therapy with incompatible blood; others occur in response to the transfer of incompatible fetal blood cells into the maternal circulation during pregnancy. The Rh system alone has 40 discrete antigens, but only 6 (C, D, E, c, d, and e) are important.

ABO Incompatibility

Antigens or agglutinogens present on the RBC surface of each blood type react with antibodies or agglutinins found in the plasma of opposing blood types. Of the 30 common antigens involved in antigen–antibody reactions, the ABO antigens are one of two groups most likely to be a problem, the other being the Rh group (Hall, 2011). As discussed earlier in this chapter, the four major blood types are A, B, O, and AB, with the antibodies to the antigens of different blood types occurring naturally in the plasma (Table 13.2).

With antigen and antibody in harmony, no RBC destruction occurs, but when a conflicting antibody is introduced into the circulation, RBC destruction may occur. RBCs have multiple binding sites to which opposing antibodies can attach. An antibody is capable of simultaneously attaching to several RBCs, thus creating a clump of cells. This clumping of cells, known as agglutination, can cause occlusion of small vessels and impair local circulation and tissue oxygenation. Fetal RBCs coated with antibodies attract phagocytes and macrophages that eventually destroy these agglutinated RBCs, usually through hemolysis by the reticuloendothelial cells in the spleen. Hemolysis can occur without preliminary agglutination, but it is a more delayed process because the body must first activate its complement system. High antibody titers (hemolysins) are required to stimulate this system, which causes the release of proteolytic enzymes that rupture the cell membrane.

In a transfusion reaction, when opposing blood types are mixed, the donor's RBCs are agglutinated, and the recipient's blood cells tend to be protected. The plasma portion of donor blood that contains antibodies becomes diluted by the recipient's blood volume, thus reducing donor antibody titers in the recipient's circulation. However, recipient antibody titers are adequate to destroy the donor RBCs by agglutination and hemolysis or by hemolysis alone. This is the situation in ABO incompatibility. In such cases, the maternal blood type usually is O, containing anti-A and anti-B antibodies in the serum, whereas the fetus or newborn is type A or B. Although incompatibility can occur between A and B types, it is not seen as frequently as AO or BO because of the globulin composition of the antibodies. In the O-type mother, the antibodies are usually IgG and can cross the placenta, whereas the antibodies of the type

A or B mother frequently are IgM, which are too large to cross the placenta.

When transplacental hemorrhage (TPH) occurs between an ABO-incompatible mother and fetus, fetal blood entering the maternal circulation undergoes agglutination and hemolysis by maternal antibodies. This rapid response prevents the development of antibodies to other antigens present on fetal RBCs, because a time lapse is required for activation of the immune system. Consequently, fetal RBCs that are Rh positive in addition to being type A or type B are destroyed by naturally occurring anti-A or anti-B antibodies before any maternal antibodies to Rh factor (anti-D) can be produced. This naturally occurring phenomenon is the basis for the use of RhIgG, in which extrinsic anti-D destroys fetal cells before the maternal immune system can be activated to produce antibodies.

Despite this destruction of fetal RBCs, maternal anti-A or anti-B antibodies of the IgG form can freely cross the placenta and adhere to RBCs in the fetal circulation. For this reason, ABO incompatibility can occur in the first pregnancy (40%–50% of total occurrences involve primigravidas) because TPH and inoculation of the mother with fetal blood are not necessary for the development of these naturally occurring antibodies. Since the A and B antigens on the fetal and neonatal RBCs are not well developed, only a small amount of maternal antibody actually attaches to the antigen. Other body tissues and secretions also have antigen sites to which some of the circulating antibodies can adhere, thereby decreasing the potential for RBC destruction. The resulting small amounts of IgG in the plasma do not stimulate activation of the complement system; therefore hemolysis is minimal. This lack of stimulation of the complement system and the above factors may explain why only 3% to 20% of infants of the 15% to 22% who are ABO incompatible with their mothers become symptomatic (Ozolek, Watchko, & Mimouni, 1994).

Erythrocyte antibodies are not usually present in the circulating blood until 2 to 8 months of postnatal age, which prevents maternal inoculation with fetal anti-A or anti-B antibodies. Antibody production then increases, reaching a maximum titer at 8 to 10 years of age (Hall, 2011). The newborn becomes inoculated with A and B antigens after birth through ingestion of food and the resulting bacterial colonization. This initiates production of anti-A or anti-B antibodies that circulate in the plasma, depending on the antigens present on the RBCs.

■ Clinical Manifestations. The chief symptom of ABO incompatibility is jaundice within the first 24 hours of life; 90% of all affected infants are female. Hemolysis and anemia are minimal, although signs of a mildly compensated hemolytic state are reflected in certain CBC values. The peripheral blood smear may show evidence of spherocytes, or RBCs lacking the normal central pallor and biconcave, disklike shape of the normal RBC. Because they are smaller than normal RBCs, spherocytes appear thicker. These physical characteristics result in abnormal fragility under osmotic stress. Spherocytes are not distensible or compressible because they lack the normal amount of loose cell membrane, making them more susceptible to destruction in the splenic sinusoids.

Additional laboratory findings include a positive direct Coombs test result in 3% to 32% of cases (Ozolek et al., 1994) and positive results on both direct and indirect Coombs tests in 80% of cases when micro techniques are used. The direct Coombs test is a measurement of the presence of antibody on the RBC surface; the indirect Coombs test is a measurement of antibody in the serum. ABO incompatibility can also be identified by the performance of an eluate test, which involves washing the RBCs of the newborn and testing the wash for anti-A or anti-B antibodies.

On physical examination, hepatosplenomegaly can be observed, a reflection of extramedullary erythropoiesis generated by the fetus in response to significant hemolysis. In an effort to compensate for increased cell destruction, the liver and spleen manufacture RBCs for a longer period than usually is seen in the fetus and newborn. Engorgement of the splenic sinusoids by hemolyzed RBCs contributes to splenomegaly.

■ Treatment. Since the antibodies involved in ABO incompatibility occur naturally, elimination of this type of incompatibility is virtually impossible. However, its effects on the fetus and newborn are much less dramatic and life threatening than those of Rh incompatibility; therefore amniocentesis and monitoring of amniotic fluid bilirubin levels, intrauterine transfusions, and early delivery usually are not necessary. Nevertheless, problems associated with postnatal bilirubin clearance do arise, and phototherapy and possible exchange transfusion become part of the repertoire of care. These two treatment methods are discussed in further detail later in the chapter.

Rh Incompatibility

Incompatibilities involving the Rh system are the second most common alloimmune problem, but the severity of complications far surpasses that of ABO incompatibility. Antibodies never occur naturally in the Rh system; exposure to the antigen is necessary to produce antibodies. Such exposure is thought to occur through maternal inoculation with fetal RBCs by TPH or through undetectable hemorrhage during labor, abortion, ectopic pregnancy, or amniocentesis.

Spontaneous TPH occurs in 50% to 75% of all pregnancies, with the greatest and most severe occurrence at the time of delivery. Fetal RBCs can be found in 6.7% of all pregnancies during the first trimester, 15% in the second trimester, and 28.9% in the third trimester (Porter, Peltier, & Branch, 2003). Spontaneous TPH allows fetal RBCs to pass into the maternal circulation, where antibodies develop in response to any foreign RBC antigen the mother does not possess. The risk of immunization depends on the ABO status of both mother and fetus and the size of the hemorrhage. On the basis of blood type, the risk for maternal Rh immunization in an ABO-compatible Rh-negative mother and Rh-positive fetus is 16%, whereas an ABO-incompatible pregnancy with an Rh-negative mother and Rh-positive fetus runs a 1.5% to 2% risk with each pregnancy. On the basis of the volume of TPH, if the hemorrhage is less than 0.1 mL RBCs, the overall risk for immunization is 3%; if the hemorrhage is greater than 5 mL, the risk increases to 50% to 65%.

The maternal Rh antibody is slow to develop and initially may consist exclusively of IgM, which cannot cross the placenta because of its molecular size. This is followed by the production of IgG, which can cross the placenta into the fetal circulation. The maximum concentration of the IgG form of antibody occurs within 2 to 4 months after termination of the first sensitizing pregnancy (Hall, 2011). If initial immunization occurs shortly before or at the time of delivery, the first Rh-positive infant born to such a mother may trigger the initial antibody response, but the infant will not be affected. However, subsequent exposure to RBCs of Rh-positive fetuses produces a rapid antibody response that consists mostly of IgG. This response results in antibody attachment to antigen sites on the fetal RBCs of these fetuses. The antibody coating of the RBCs forms the basis for a positive result on the direct Coombs test. The affected RBCs undergo agglutination, phagocytosis, and eventually extravascular hemolysis in the spleen. The by-products of hemolysis, especially bilirubin, pass through the placenta into the maternal circulation to be metabolized and conjugated by the maternal liver. The rate of destruction of fetal RBCs depends on the amount of anti-D antibodies on the cells, the effectiveness of anti-D antibodies in promoting phagocytosis, and the capability of the spleen's reticuloendothelial system to remove antibody-coated cells.

TABLE 13.6

CONTRAST BETWEEN Rh AND ABO INCOMPATIBILITY

	Rh Incompatibility	ABO Incompatibility
Rh-negative mom	Yes	No
First pregnancy affected	Rarely	Often
Cord bilirubin elevated	Yes	Sometimes
Early anemia prominent	Yes	No
Jaundice in first 24 hours	Yes	Yes
Hepatospleenomegaly	Yes	Sometimes
Nucleated RBC	Very common	Quite common
Spherocytes	No	Yes
Reticulocytosis	Yes	Yes
Maternal antibodies	Yes	Not always
Direct Coombs test	Positive	Positive or negative
Indirect Coombs test	Negative	Positive

Modified from Ohls (2001).

Erythroblastosis Fetalis

Hemolysis in the fetus caused by Rh incompatibility results in the disease known as erythroblastosis fetalis (EBF); the major consequences are anemia and hyperbilirubinemia. The name is derived from the presence of immature circulating RBCs (erythroblasts), which are forced into the circulation of affected fetuses to compensate for rapid destruction of fetal blood cells. The severity of the disease depends on the degree of hemolysis and the ability of the fetus's erythropoietic system to counteract the ensuing anemia. In an attempt to compensate for rapid destruction, the fetus continues to use extramedullary organs, such as the liver and spleen, which normally would have ceased RBC production after the seventh month of gestation.

■ **Clinical Manifestations.** The clinical manifestations of EBF are similar to those of ABO incompatibility but often are more intense (see Table 13.6). Jaundice results from an exaggerated rise in bilirubin, with the premature infant exhibiting an earlier rise and a more prolonged period of elevation. Hepatosplenomegaly may be found on physical examination, along with varying degrees of hydrops. Hydrops fetalis is a severe, total body edema often accompanied by ascites and pleural effusions. This is only seen in approximately 25% of infants affected. Although the pathogenesis is unclear, it is thought to be the result of congestive heart failure and intrauterine hypoxia from severe anemia, portal and umbilical venous hypertension caused by hepatic hematopoiesis, and low plasma colloid osmotic pressure induced by hypoalbuminemia. Low serum albumin levels are a consequence of altered hepatic synthesis, which may be due to local cellular necrosis and compromised intrahepatic circulation. All these factors can lead to portal and venous hypertension and edema. The severity of the anemia and hypoalbuminemia affects the degree of extravasation of fluid into the tissue.

Altered hepatic synthesis can impair production of vitamin K and vitamin K–dependent clotting factors, which can lead to hemorrhage in these infants. Petechiae and prolonged bleeding from cord and blood sampling sites may be initial signs of clotting abnormalities. Hypoglycemia that occurs secondary to hyperplasia of the pancreatic islet cells also is associated with EBF. Products of RBC hemolysis are thought to inactivate circulating insulin, promoting increased insulin release and subsequent pancreatic α-cell hyperplasia. Another theory suggests that potassium or amino acids released from hemolyzed cells may directly stimulate insulin production or indirectly produce this effect by increasing glucagon secretion. Approximately one third of surviving erythroblastotic infants have low blood glucose levels and elevated plasma insulin levels.

■ **Antenatal Therapy.** Adequate antenatal care is important in safeguarding the fetus that may be affected by EBF. Proper screening of any pregnant woman at her first prenatal visit is essential and should include blood type and Rh factor. If the mother is Rh negative, the father's blood type should also be ascertained. If the father is Rh positive, it is essential to determine Rh immunization of the mother by Coombs testing, specifically the indirect Coombs test. In addition to blood typing, a concise obstetrical history regarding any previous spontaneous or therapeutic abortions or delivery of an affected infant is important to ensure appropriate management of the current pregnancy. Women who are sensitized require more surveillance throughout the pregnancy than their unsensitized counterparts, and women who have previously given birth to affected infants require the greatest degree of care.

The unsensitized Rh-negative mothers can benefit from antenatal and postpartum administration of RhIgG. The Kleihauer–Betke test for fetal cells in the maternal circulation and the erythrocyte rosetting test that detects Rh-positive fetal cells may be useful screens for determining maternal candidates for RhIgG. Before the inception of RhIgG in 1964, when the first clinical trials were conducted, the frequency of Rh immunization was 7% to 8% in ABO-compatible pregnancies and 1% in ABO-incompatible pregnancies, with close to 50% of all perinatal deaths attributable to EBF. With the use of RhIgG after delivery, the incidence of Rh immunization was dramatically reduced to 1% to 1.8%. Because sensitization was known to occur without evidence of TPH at the time of delivery, the question was raised whether antenatal sensitization occurred in response to frequent, small, and undetectable hemorrhage before or during labor. For this reason, antenatal administration of RhIgG was initiated to eliminate such cases of alloimmunization. Antenatal administration has further reduced the incidence to as low as 0.1%. However, there will always be pregnancies in which RhIgG fails to suppress the formation of antibodies or in which administration is not feasible. Immunization is not effective if sensitization occurs before the initial antenatal screening or if the RhIgG dosage is inadequate to neutralize a massive TPH. For these reasons, it is estimated that the incidence cannot be reduced beyond 4 in 10,000 pregnancies even with the use of RhIgG.

The manner in which RhIgG works to prevent sensitization of the D antigen is not fully understood. Two known effects of the anti-D antibody is that it prevents antigen-induced B lymphocyte antibody production in the mother as well as it adheres to the D-antigen sites on the RBCs in the fetus that could cross the placenta and enter the maternal circulation, which then interferes with the immune response to the D antigen. Agglutination, hemolysis, and removal of these foreign RBCs occur before the maternal immune system can recognize the invasion and develop antibodies that would transplacentally cross into the fetus (Hall, 2011).

Several obstetrical conditions, which may require RhIgG prophylaxis because they can increase the risk of sensitization by increasing the chances of TPH, are

- Therapeutic or spontaneous abortion of any type; the incidence of TPH is higher with therapeutic abortion (3 in 30 women may be sensitized)
- Any procedure that could cause TPH such as an amniocentesis (which has a 10% chance of causing TPH), chorionic villus sampling, or percutaneous umbilical sampling
- Ectopic pregnancies or hydatidiform moles
- Abdominal trauma
- Antepartum bleeding, as with placental abruption or placenta previa

Failure to administer RhIgG after such occurrences may leave these women at risk for sensitization. The American Congress of Obstetricians and Gynecologists, formerly the American College of Obstetricians and Gynecologists (1999, reaffirmed, 2007) recommends a dose of 50 mcg for high-risk situations that arise before 13 weeks gestation and 300 mcg after 13 weeks gestation, with the 300-mcg dose repeated at 28 weeks gestation.

RhIgG has a half-life of 23 to 26 days and is effective for approximately 2 weeks after antigen exposure. It is essential to maintain an adequate level of Anti D throughout pregnancy to maintain protection, so if it is given prior to 28 weeks gestation, it is advised to repeat it every 12 weeks until delivery (Mintz, 2005).

The timing of the dose after delivery is important; administration within 72 hours of delivery is recommended. The dose after delivery allows a maximum estimated fetal transfusion of 30 mL of whole blood or 15 mL of packed RBCs, which leaves 1% of postpartum mothers without full coverage. If massive TPH is suspected, the dose of RhIgG may need to be increased to provide adequate amounts of anti-D antibodies. After administration of RhIgG, the Kleihauer–Betke test can be performed on the mother's blood to check for RBCs with fetal hemoglobin and to help determine the need for additional RhIgG.

By reducing the incidence of EBF, there was at one time a fear of having a reduced supply of RhIgG, as there would be a reduced number of available immunized donors. While there are still women who have had their children and ask to be sensitized to help others, the majority of donors now are male who have been DNA typed to the RBCs that are used to sensitize them. DNA typing prevents the donors from developing Anti-C, Kell, and other antibodies. A monoclonal antibody has been developed, but it did not have the same success rates as the polyclonal antibodies on the market.

Other methods of monitoring the status and treating the fetus with EBF include ultrasonography, flow Doppler studies, amniocentesis, cordocentesis, intrauterine transfusions, and pharmacologic agent administration.

■ **Treatment.** On delivery of an infant with EBF, assessment of the newborn's cardiorespiratory status is of utmost importance. Because of ascites, pleural effusions, and circulatory collapse, these infants often require stabilization of the airway by intubation and mechanical ventilation. If peritoneal or pleural fluid prevents adequate chest excursion, paracentesis may be required to remove fluid from the abdominal cavity, or thoracentesis may be needed to drain excess pleural fluid.

Delivery of an infant shortly after intraperitoneal transfusion may not allow adequate time for absorption of blood from the peritoneal cavity. The unabsorbed portion could lead to diminished lung expansion, resulting in respiratory failure or restricted mechanical ventilation. Such infants may require paracentesis for removal of blood from the peritoneal cavity.

After initiation of respiratory support, the infant should be assessed for adequacy of circulating blood volume. If the infant is severely hydropic, the inevitable anemia must be corrected with transfusions of packed RBCs, since an exchange transfusion may not be tolerated until the intravascular RBC volume is replenished. Transfusion is accomplished with O-negative or type-specific Rh-negative blood cross-matched against maternal blood. Initial use of a single-volume or partial exchange may offer a degree of cardiovascular stability before a double-volume exchange is attempted. Congestive heart failure, not present at the time of intravascular volume depletion, may become apparent as the infant is transfused. At times a severely affected infant may benefit from digitalization and diuretic therapy.

Prenatal damage to the liver can adversely affect the production of coagulation factors in such infants, making them prone to bleeding disorders. Hepatic damage can intensify any hyperbilirubinemia present, because the hepatic substances required for conjugation may also be impaired. Laboratory evaluation of the infant affected by EBF should consist of liver function studies, Hct determinations, and evaluation of coagulation status.

Nursing care of the infant affected by EBF involves scrupulous attention to the infant's cardiorespiratory status and vital signs. The infant needs to be positioned so as to reduce abdominal pressure on the diaphragm which will permit better chest expansion. Maintaining a normal PaO_2 and avoiding overventilation may prevent barotrauma to lungs already compromised by pleural effusions. The lungs may be hypoplastic if their growth has been sufficiently compromised by hydrops in utero, making ventilation difficult and predisposing the infant to extraventilatory air. Vital signs usually are assessed every hour until the infant's condition has stabilized. Hct and bilirubin levels should be checked frequently during the first few hours and days of life to maintain adequate circulating blood volumes and to prevent toxic levels of bilirubin by timely initiation of therapy. If the cord bilirubin levels are significantly elevated, exchange transfusion may be necessary shortly after birth. A newer therapy that has been proven to be safe and effective is the administration of intravenous immunoglobulin (IVIG) to the neonate with hemolytic disease that has a rapidly rising serum bilirubin level despite intense phototherapy (American Academy of Pediatrics [AAP], 2004, Smits-Wintjens, Walther, & Lopriore, 2008; Walsh & Malloy, 2009).

If bilirubin levels do not require immediate exchange, blood levels should be checked every 4 to 8 hours, depending on the initial cord blood levels and subsequent rate of rise. In Rh incompatibility, exchange is imminent if the rate of rise exceeds 1 mg/hr for the first 6 hours of life. The interval of blood sampling for bilirubin may be increased to 6 to 12 hours after the first 48 hours of life.

The major therapies used to control excessive unconjugated bilirubin levels are similar for all problems resulting in elevated unconjugated bilirubin levels. Phototherapy and exchange transfusion, the most frequently used therapies, are discussed later in the chapter.

Analysis of Laboratory Data. The following laboratory data can be helpful in the diagnosis and treatment of EBF:

- The mother's and infant's blood and Rh types
- Coombs reactivity: The infant's RBCs are coated with anti-D antibodies, resulting in a positive direct Coombs test result; on occasion, the heavy coating of neonatal RBCs with antibody can lead to a false Rh typing (Rh negative); if the direct Coombs test result is positive, the infant should be considered Rh positive.
- The infant's Hct, reticulocyte count, and RBC morphologic characteristics: The presence of immature cells or spherocytes helps distinguish Rh incompatibility from ABO incompatibility.
- Plasma bilirubin levels: The initial cord-blood bilirubin level and the rate of rise determine the appropriate timing of any exchange transfusion needed to control bilirubin levels. Cord bilirubin levels are closely associated with the severity of the disease and the mortality rate.

BILIRUBIN METABOLISM AND HYPERBILIRUBINEMIA

Bilirubin production begins as early as 12 weeks gestation. It is the primary degradation product of hemoglobin, although 20% to 30% is derived from nonerythroid sources such as tissue heme. Bilirubin is produced after completion of the natural life span of the RBC, but ineffective erythropoiesis or premature destruction of blood cells can increase its production. In RBC destruction, the aging or hemolyzed RBC membrane ruptures, releasing hemoglobin that is phagocytized by macrophages. The hemoglobin molecule then splits into a heme portion and a globin portion. Bilirubin is derived from the degradation of the heme ring in the heme portion that binds to heme oxygenase. The ferric heme breaks down to the ferrous form and then is cleaved to form carbon monoxide and biliverdin. Biliverdin is further reduced to form bilirubin, and carbon monoxide joins with heme to form carboxyhemoglobin.

The four forms of circulating bilirubin are (1) conjugated bilirubin (which is excretable through the kidneys and intestines), (2) conjugated covalently bound bilirubin (which is attached to serum albumin and not found in neonates younger than 2 weeks of age), (3) unconjugated bilirubin (which is reversibly bound to albumin), and (4) free bilirubin (which is unconjugated and unbound). The measurement of conjugated (direct) bilirubin identifies the amount of bilirubin that reacts directly with van den Bergh's reagent. The portion of bilirubin reversibly bound to albumin is lipid soluble. It does not react with van den Bergh's reagent until it is combined with alcohol, hence the term *unconjugated (indirect) bilirubin*. Free bilirubin is not attached to albumin and can easily cross the blood–brain barrier, causing the damage seen in kernicterus. Measurements of conjugated and unconjugated bilirubin are important in the evaluation of the hyperbilirubinemic infant and provide valuable information for the diagnosis and method of treatment (Smits-Wintjens, Walther, & Lopriore, 2008; Walsh & Malloy, 2009).

Although bilirubin is found in stool and amniotic fluid, the major route of elimination in the fetus is through the placenta. For this reason, bilirubin must be retained in the form that allows its passage into the maternal circulation. Consequently, the enzyme systems found in the fetus enhance the retention of bilirubin in the unconjugated form.

Persistence of some of these fetal mechanisms during the newborn period can contribute to jaundice. Plasma concentrations of bilirubin usually are low in the fetus, except in cases of severe hemolytic disease. All bilirubin in the cord blood of the fetus is the unconjugated variety, which is effectively metabolized, conjugated, and excreted by the maternal liver and gallbladder. The mean cord blood bilirubin concentration in an infant unaffected by hemolytic disease is 1.8 mg/dL, regardless of the infant's gestational age or weight.

In the newborn, the major routes of bilirubin excretion are through the intestine and the kidneys. As the production of bilirubin exceeds the newborn liver's capacity to conjugate and eliminate it, plasma levels begin to rise rapidly. Jaundice becomes noticeable when the serum concentration reaches three times the amount normally present in the serum. The conjunctivae become visibly jaundiced at serum levels exceeding 2.5 mg/dL. In the full-term infant, jaundice usually becomes apparent within 2 to 4 days after birth and lasts until the sixth day, reaching a peak concentration of 6 to 7 mg/dL. Although infants born at 37 weeks gestation or later are considered term, they are more likely to reach or exceed serum bilirubin levels of 13 mg/dL or higher than are infants born at 40 weeks gestation. The preterm infant has cord-blood bilirubin levels similar to those of the term infant, but peak levels are higher, jaundice lasts longer, and levels peak later, at 5 to 7 days. Among preterm infants, 63% reach levels of 10 to 19 mg/dL, and 22% reach levels above 15 mg/dL.

Although the neonatal liver's conjugating mechanisms are reduced during the first few days of life, the liver is able to metabolize and excrete two thirds to three quarters of the bilirubin circulating throughout the body. Initially, bilirubin is transported in the plasma, bound to albumin at two sites—a primary binding site that has a strong bond and a secondary site that has a weak bond. When available albumin binding sites are saturated, bilirubin circulates freely in the plasma. It is this portion of unconjugated bilirubin that can migrate into brain cells, causing damage known as kernicterus. The occurrence of kernicterus is related to the amount of diffusible, loosely bound bilirubin, and the availability of albumin binding sites (Smits-Wintjens, Walther, & Lopriore, 2008; Walsh & Malloy, 2009).

When bilirubin reaches the liver, it is transferred from plasma albumin, across the cell membrane of the liver, and into the liver cell. Two proteins, Y and Z, also called ligands, affect bilirubin transfer from plasma to liver. Here the bilirubin is either stored in the cell cytoplasm or removed from the ligands and conjugated in the hepatic endoplasmic reticulum. Conjugation is essential for the excretion of bilirubin into bile. Eighty percent of bilirubin is conjugated with glucuronic acid, becoming bilirubin glucuronide. Glucuronosyltransferase is the important hepatic enzyme required for the production of bilirubin glucuronide. Ninety-five percent of bilirubin glucuronide is excreted into bile and subsequently into the intestine.

Effective excretion of bilirubin from the intestine depends on the length of time needed for the passage of stool and on the presence of substances that break down conjugated bilirubin. The newborn may have diminished bowel motility and delayed meconium passage, which allow longer exposure of stool to bilirubin glucuronidase, the enzyme responsible for breaking down conjugated bilirubin. The action of this enzyme, in conjunction with the newborn's lack of the intestinal flora required to reduce bilirubin to urobilinogen, converts the conjugated form to the unconjugated form, which is then reabsorbed by the intestine (Smits-Wintjens, Walther, & Lopriore, 2008; Walsh & Malloy, 2009).

Kernicterus

Kernicterus, the chronic form of bilirubin encephalopathy, was rarely seen between the 1960s and the 1990s, but its incidence has risen since the mid-1990s with the advent of earlier home discharges. The exact incidence of kernicterus is unknown, but a voluntary Kernicterus Registry in the United States showed 125 babies enrolled in the registry between 1984 and 2002. Of the 125 babies in the registry, 97% had been discharged home prior to 72 hours of age (Johnson, Bhutani, & Brown, 2002). Other possible causes that could be involved with the reemergence of kernicterus besides early hospital discharge are: lack of understanding of the risks associated with increased bilirubin levels in healthy term and late-preterm infants, an increased incidence of breastfeeding, health care cost constraints, lack of monitoring of newborns' jaundice once discharged home and demonstration that bilirubin is an antioxidant (Bergeron & Gourley, 2009). The AAP recognizing this alarming trend, reissued its hyperbilirubinemia guidelines in 2004, stating that if infants are discharged home prior to 48 hours of age a follow-up visit should be done within 48 hours (AAP, 2004). Unfortunately, many health care professionals do not follow these guidelines.

Kernicterus occurs when the albumin binding sites are filled which allows for increased amounts of free bilirubin to pass into the central nervous system (CNS). Free bilirubin easily crosses the blood–brain barrier and is transferred into the brain cells, causing obvious yellow staining of the brain tissue (kernicterus) that is similar to the effect on the skin. The areas of the brain usually affected by the staining are the basal ganglia, hippocampus, dentate nucleus, substania nigra, cerebellum, and nuclei of the floor of the fourth ventricle (Bergeron & Gourley, 2009; Springer, 2010). Kernicterus is associated with varying degrees of neurologic damage, but a direct correlation cannot be drawn between serum bilirubin levels and the severity of involvement.

Many factors can influence the bilirubin binding capacity and increase the risk of kernicterus at lower bilirubin levels, including the following:

- The total amount of available serum albumin: Premature infants normally experience a relative hypoproteinemia and have fewer albumin binding sites available for free bilirubin.
- The presence of other substances competing for available binding sites: Certain drugs (e.g., sulfisoxazole, salicylates, sodium benzoate) compete with bilirubin

for binding sites or replace bilirubin loosely attached to binding sites.

- Acidosis and hypoxia: Increased production of hydrogen ions and implementation of anaerobic metabolism can impede bilirubin binding. Albumin's ability to bind bilirubin drops to half its potential at a serum pH of 7.1, with free fatty acids produced during anaerobic metabolism competing for albumin binding sites. The simultaneous presence of acidosis and hypoxia, which can open the blood–brain barrier, can expose a sick infant to kernicterus at much lower serum bilirubin levels. Evidence also suggests that tests evaluating bilirubin binding capacity, rather than serum bilirubin concentrations, are better correlated with the appearance of subsequent CNS abnormalities (Cashore, 2011; Rund-Hansen, 2011).

■ Clinical Manifestations. Kernicterus usually becomes evident during the first 5 days of life. Its signs include lethargy or irritability, hypotonia, paralysis of upward gaze, high-pitched cry, poor eating, opisthotonic posturing, and spasticity. It is also associated with deafness, cerebral palsy, and tooth enamel abnormalities. The overall risk for kernicterus is 50% if serum bilirubin levels are 30 mg/dL or higher and 10% if levels are between 20 and 25 mg/dL. Preventing elevated levels of free bilirubin is the primary means of eliminating kernicterus. Prevention may require phototherapy for slowly rising levels but almost certainly demands exchange transfusion if the rise is rapid and marked.

Nonimmune Causes of Hyperbilirubinemia

Elevated bilirubin levels within the first 24 hours of life or levels exceeding 12 mg/dL are not considered physiologic and deserve investigation. Many conditions other than blood group incompatibilities can cause jaundice in the newborn. Most of the commonly seen disorders result in elevated levels of unconjugated rather than conjugated bilirubin. These pathologic conditions can be classified as (1) those that cause increased breakdown of RBCs (e.g., sepsis, drug reactions, and extravascular blood); (2) those that interfere with bilirubin conjugation (e.g., breast milk jaundice, drug interactions, hypothyroidism, acidosis, and hypoxia); and (3) those that cause abnormal bilirubin excretion (e.g., hypoxia or asphyxia, bowel obstruction, ileus, and congestive heart failure). The single factor most implicated in hyperbilirubinemia is prematurity, with the severity of jaundice directly correlated to declining gestational age. The premature infant is thought to be subject to a combination of increased RBC breakdown secondary to reduced RBC life span and impaired bilirubin conjugation as a result of liver immaturity (Cashore, 2011).

Increased Red Blood Cell Breakdown

Several problems that arise in the perinatal period are associated with excessive and premature destruction of the RBCs by hemolysis. Neonatal bacterial and viral infections and intrauterine viral infections, especially those of the TORCH complex (toxoplasmosis, other agents, rubella, cytomegalovirus, and herpes simplex), have been implicated in the hemolytic destruction of RBCs. Certain medications, such as the synthetic analogues of vitamin K or large doses of natural vitamin K, also induce RBC destruction. Other conditions prevalent in the premature and term newborn can result in the extravasation of large amounts of blood (e.g., cephalhematoma and pulmonary or intracerebral hemorrhages). These extravascular collections of blood cells must undergo hemolysis to be reabsorbed by the body. Significant hemolysis, regardless of the cause, increases the bilirubin load on a metabolically immature neonatal liver. This increased load often results in hyperbilirubinemia in the newborn.

Interference With Bilirubin Conjugation

■ Breast Milk Jaundice. Breast milk jaundice affects approximately 2% to 4% of all breastfed babies and can be divided into two types, breastfeeding jaundice and breast milk jaundice, each with a different time of onset and a different underlying cause. In breastfeeding jaundice, the infant is affected within the first few days of life. The etiology of this condition is not fully understood, but is thought to be due to a combination of maternal and infant factors that lead to diminished fluid intake and dehydration. Predisposing maternal factors include limited maternal milk supply, engorgement, cracked nipples, poor feeding technique, and maternal illness or fatigue. Neonatal factors include poor suck, illness, lethargy that accompanies hyperbilirubinemia, and dehydration. Poor intake leads to poor stool output and increased enterohepatic resorption of bilirubin. The recommended treatment is phototherapy and alleviation of dehydration. Frequent breastfeedings with avoidance of supplementation, in addition to lactation counseling, are advised.

Breast milk jaundice is a separate entity that is attributed to a change in the chemical or physical composition of breast milk; it usually occurs after the first 4 to 7 days of life (Deshpande, 2012). Bilirubin levels can reach 12 to 20 mg/dL between 8 and 15 days and may remain elevated for as long as 2 months. The infant appears healthy, and no evidence of RBC hemolysis is seen. This jaundice is not well understood, but the following factors are believed to play a role: (1) Two substances found in breast milk, pregnanediol and nonesterified fatty acids, interfere with bilirubin conjugation or increase enterohepatic circulation, resulting in resorption of bilirubin from the intestine. They are thought to inhibit glucuronyl transferase, the enzyme necessary for bilirubin conjugation in the liver. However, the role of these two substances in the interference with glucuronyl transferase remains questionable. (2) An increase in enterohepatic bilirubin due to increase of β-gluconronidase activity in breast milk and the intestines of breastfed babies as well as the delayed establishment of enteric flora in breastfed babies. (3) A defect in UGT gene *UGT1A1*, which is responsible for conjugation and elimination of bilirubin. (4) Mutation of the solute carrier organic anion transporter protein SLCO1B1 which results in reduced hepatic uptake of unconjugated bilirubin. (5) Presence of inflammatory cytokines in human milk, in particular IL-1β and IL-6. Both of these are known to be cholestatic and reduce uptake, metabolism, and excretion of bilirubin. (6) High levels of epidermal growth factor (EGF) in breast milk and the serum have been found in neonates with breast milk jaundice. It is thought that the reduced GI motility and increased bilirubin absorption and uptake are the mechanisms responsible for the jaundice as well as (7) serum alpha-feto-protein levels are higher in these babies, but the significance of this is yet unknown (Deshpande, 2012).

When breastfeeding is discontinued, the bilirubin level falls within 24 to 48 hours, dropping to half its previous peak level by 48 hours. With resumption of breastfeeding, the bilirubin level starts to rise but at a much slower pace. Interruption of breastfeeding is not recommended; instead, continued and frequent breastfeeding is encouraged. However, the health care provider has the option to supplement nursing with formula or to interrupt breastfeeding and substitute formula, depending on the degree of bilirubin elevation. Supplementation of nursing with water or glucose water does not appear to have any effect on bilirubin levels in healthy term infants.

■ Drugs That Interfere With Bilirubin Conjugation Certain medications ingested by the mother and passed transplacentally to the fetus (e.g., salicylates, sulfa preparations) can interfere with the ability of albumin to bind bilirubin. Administration of these drugs to the newborn can produce the same effect. Other medications, such as sodium benzoate, a commonly used preservative, compete with bilirubin for albumin binding sites.

■ Hypothyroidism. Hypothyroidism is one of the more common metabolic disorders associated with hyperbilirubinemia. Of all infants with hypothyroidism, 20% have elevated bilirubin levels lasting 3 to 4 weeks, with normalization of levels requiring up to 4 months. The suspected mechanism for jaundice is theorized to be a delay in glucuronosyltransferase synthesis or impairment of hepatic proteins that bind bilirubin and remove it from the plasma. The plasma membrane of liver cells may also be altered, resulting in decreased bilirubin influx into the hepatic cells.

■ Acidosis and Hypoxia. As previously stated in the discussion of kernicterus, a drop in serum pH alters albumin's ability to bind bilirubin. The accompanying increase in the production of free fatty acids promotes competition between fatty acids and bilirubin for binding sites. In animal models, respiratory acidosis but not metabolic acidosis increases movement of bilirubin across the blood–brain barrier.

■ Abnormal Bilirubin Excretion. Any disease state resulting in abnormal bilirubin excretion can raise serum bilirubin levels significantly. This is seen in hepatic dysfunction secondary to such entities as hypoxia or asphyxia, bowel obstruction, ileus, and congestive heart failure. However, these conditions have a tendency to elevate both the conjugated and unconjugated bilirubin levels. The diminished bowel motility associated with these conditions lengthens the time during which beta-glucuronidase, which is naturally present in the gut, can act on conjugated bilirubin in the stool. This enzymatic reaction converts conjugated bilirubin into the unconjugated form, which is reabsorbed into the intravascular compartment through the enterohepatic circulation. Direct hepatocellular damage associated with cholestasis and bacterial and viral infections can further impair the liver's ability to metabolize bilirubin (Cashore, 2011).

Treatment of Hyperbilirubinemia

■ Phototherapy. Phototherapy reduces unconjugated bilirubin through photo-oxidation and photo-isomerization, which changes bilirubin into water-soluble and excretable forms. Photo-oxidation involves the oxidation of bilirubin pigment deposited in the skin and its conversion into colorless products that can be excreted into the urine. Of the total body bilirubin concentration, 15% can undergo photodegradation through oxidation. Photoisomerization involves the conversion of bilirubin polymers present in the skin into excretable isomers. When the natural form of bilirubin is exposed to blue light at certain wavelengths, it undergoes photoisomerization. This changes it from a tetrapyrrole, a lipid-soluble substance, into five water-soluble isomers. Four of these isomers are excreted into bile without undergoing conjugation. Two are unstable isomers that are incorporated into bile and must be promptly eliminated from the gastrointestinal tract as a component of stool or they revert back to their natural forms, resulting in resorption of bilirubin from the gut and recirculation into the plasma. Two other isomers remain relatively stable and account for most of the bilirubin found in bile. The fifth isomer, lumibilirubin, is a stable, water-soluble form of bilirubin that is eliminated through urine and bile (Bhutani and the Committee on Fetus and Newborn, 2011).

Phototherapy is also thought to enhance hepatic excretion of unconjugated bilirubin and to increase bowel transit time. When phototherapy is begun early, a 20% to 35% reduction in the serum bilirubin concentrations is noted by day 2 of life and a reduction of 41% to 55% by day 4. This reduction is more significant than the naturally occurring drop in the untreated infant.

Although no significant adverse effects are attributed to the use of phototherapy, it is not without associated side effects. Some of these problems include dermal rash, lethargy, abdominal distention, possible eye damage, dehydration caused by increased insensible water loss through the skin and digestive tract, thrombocytopenia, hypocalcemia, and secretory diarrhea possibly as a result of a temporary intestinal lactose deficiency. Another effect of phototherapy seen in infants with a significant direct bilirubin component is "bronze baby" syndrome. This syndrome is thought to be due to skin deposition or a photoproduct of bilirubin decomposition, possibly copper porphyrins, which cause bronzing of the skin and urine. Although no harmful effects can be attributed to the bronzing, it can last for several weeks to several months and is somewhat alarming to parents (Bhutani et al., 2011).

Phototherapy is not adequate therapy for a rapidly rising bilirubin level, but it is effective in treating moderate hyperbilirubinemia that has not reached or exceeded levels known to be associated with kernicterus and in reducing the need for exchange transfusions after the first 12 hours of life. Intensive phototherapy can produce a decline of 2 mg/dL of total serum bilirubin (TSB) within 4 to 6 hours (AAP, 2004; Bhutani et al., 2011). This is a reflection of the length of exposure necessary for phototherapy to exhibit its effectiveness. The AAP (2004) revised a set of guidelines for the initiation of phototherapy and exchange transfusion in the term, healthy newborn (Figure 13.7). Suggested bilirubin levels for initiation of therapy based on birth weight and gestational age, including very low birth weight, are found in Table 13.7. Recommended levels for the use of phototherapy or exchange transfusion must be adjusted downward for prematurity, acidosis, hypoxia, respiratory distress, asphyxia, and neurologic decompensation (Figure 13.8). Diminished bilirubin-binding capacity of albumin, decreased amounts of circulating albumin, and increased permeability of the CNS expose these infants to increased amounts of free bilirubin, which can easily cross the blood–brain barrier.

Although administration of IVIG to the mother has produced contradictory results, its administration to infants with Rh or ABO hemolytic disease can be beneficial. Administration of IVIG to a group of infants with Rh incompatibility was associated with a reduction in the rate of exchange transfusion to 12.5%, compared with 69% in the control group. Huizing, Roislien, and Hansen (2008) found that exchange transfusions in their neonatal intensive care unit (NICU) of 750 admissions per year dropped to 0 to 2 per year with the use of IVIG. It is hypothesized that IVIG may interfere with receptors in the reticuloendothelium that are required to induce hemolysis. The AAP 2004 Guidelines on Hyperbilirubinemia recommends 500 to 1,000 mg/kg intravenously over 2 hours for TSB rising despite intensive phototherapy or if the TSB is within 2 to 3 mg/dL of the exchange level (Hansen, 2012; Huizing, Roislien, & Hansen, 2008).

The administration of albumin to an infant undergoing phototherapy may reduce the amount of bilirubin available in the skin for photoisomerization. In an attempt to saturate the increased available albumin binding sites, free bilirubin is drawn into the vascular compartment from the skin, where phototherapy exerts its effect. For this reason, use of albumin in the infant undergoing phototherapy should be carefully weighed.

■ Collaborative Management. Infants who require phototherapy benefit most from blue light in the wavelength range at which photoisomerization occurs most efficiently: that is, 420 to 460 nm. In addition to the appropriate wavelength, effective illumination must be maintained. Spectroradiometric readings of 4 to 6 mcW/cm²/nm are considered to be in the effective therapeutic range. For optimum therapy, phototherapy units should be checked for adequacy of light levels by nursing or bioengineering staff. Prolonged exposure to phototherapy lights may cause retinal damage, which can be minimized with adequate eye protection.

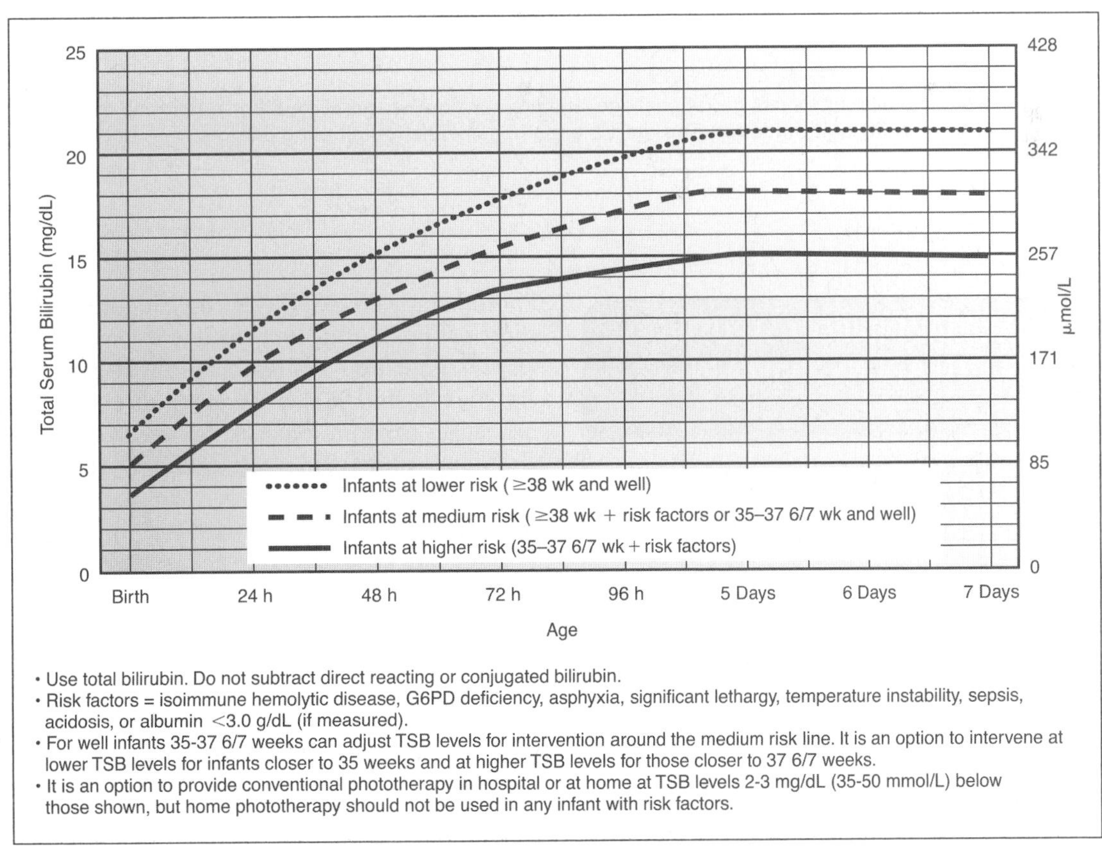

FIGURE 13.7 Guidelines for phototherapy in hospitalized infants of 35 or more weeks gestation.
From American Academy of Pediatrics, Subcommittee on Hyperbilirubinemia (2004). Copyright © 2004 American Academy of Pediatrics.

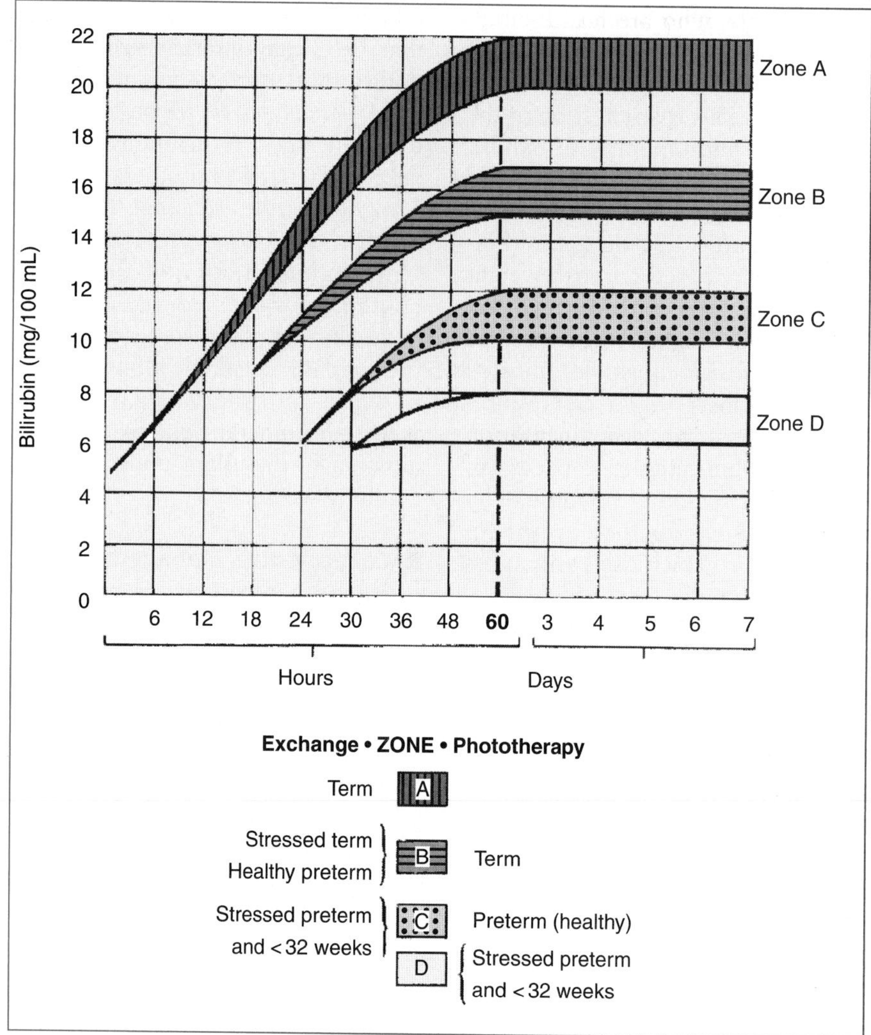

FIGURE 13.8 The rate of increase in bilirubin levels, gestational age, and the newborn's general condition determine the type of treatment for hyperbilirubinemia and the rapidity of its initiation. This chart is a useful guideline for initiating phototherapy or exchange transfusion in hyperbilirubinemic infants.
From Pernoll et al. (1986).

TABLE 13.7

SUGGESTED MAXIMAL INDIRECT SERUM BILIRUBIN CONCENTRATIONS (mg/dL) IN PRETERM INFANTS

Birth Weight (g)	Uncomplicated[a]	Complicated[a]
<1,000	12–13	10–12
1,000–1,250	12–14	10–12
1,251–1,499	14–16	12–14
1,500–1,999	16–20	15–17
2,000–2,500	20–22	18–20

[a] Complications include perinatal asphyxia, acidosis, hypoxia, hypothermia, hypoalbuminemia, meningitis, intraventricular hemorrhage, hemolysis, hypoglycemia, or signs of kernicterus. Phototherapy is usually started at 50% to 70% of the maximal indirect level. If values greatly exceed this level, if phototherapy is unsuccessful in reducing maximal bilirubin level, or if signs of kernicterus are evident, exchange transfusion is indicated.
From Ambalavanan and Carlo (2011).

Phototherapy units and eye protection should be removed for short periods throughout the day to provide the infant with visual stimulation and interaction with parents and caregivers. Nurses should also be aware that they may experience headaches from prolonged exposure to phototherapy lights.

Infants undergoing phototherapy require temperature stabilization appropriate for their size and overall condition. A larger infant who is basically well can be nursed in an open crib, but the sick term, premature, or low-birth-weight (LBW) infant requires temperature control through the use of open warmers or closed incubators. Adequate fluid intake and compensatory fluid adjustments for increased insensible water and stool loss may be required to prevent dehydration in these infants. While the infant is receiving phototherapy, bilirubin levels must be monitored frequently to assess the effectiveness of therapy and the need for exchange transfusion. Because phototherapy lights can alter blood bilirubin results, the lights should be turned off when drawing blood for serum bilirubin determinations.

Many hyperbilirubinemic infants, who are healthy and not in need of thermoregulation or exchange transfusion, can be cared for at home as long as the AAP guidelines are met. The parents of these infants must have access to home phototherapy equipment and a medical supply company to service the equipment, as well as the support of their medical caregiver. If the infant can remain normothermic in an open crib without clothing, home phototherapy may be considered a cost-effective alternative to hospitalization. The same precautions regarding protective eye covering and adequate fluid intake must be observed in these infants. Frequent determination of bilirubin levels is required to ensure adequate treatment, and blood may be drawn daily for this purpose at the physician's office, at the neighborhood hospital laboratory, or by a home health care worker.

■ Pharmacologic Agents. Phenobarbital is thought to accelerate bilirubin excretion by increasing its uptake and conjugation by the liver and by increasing its excretion by enhancing bile flow. However, no increased benefit is noted that cannot be achieved with phototherapy alone. No medications have been approved in the United States as therapy for inhibition of bilirubin synthesis, but clinical trials have shown that metalloporphyrins may be effective in controlling hyperbilirubinemia in the term and preterm infant. Metalloporphyrins are inhibitors of heme oxygenase, the enzyme involved in the degradation of heme to biliverdin, an intermediate in the synthesis of bilirubin. Tin-mesoporphyrin and tin-protoporphyrin are the two heme oxygenase inhibitors used in clinical trials as a prophylaxis and as treatment. Although these studies have shown beneficial effects, they are still not approved by the U.S. Food and Drug Administration.

■ Exchange Transfusion. Once done frequently in neonatal intensive care units, exchange transfusions are now rarely done and only to treat extreme hyperbilirubinemia or metabolic issues. An exchange transfusion may be necessary, if bilirubin levels start to approach those associated with kernicterus despite phototherapy, to protect the CNS status of the jaundiced infant. The object of this procedure is to remove bilirubin and the antibody-coated RBCs from the newborn's circulation. In addition, exchange transfusion removes some of the circulating maternal antibodies and Rh-positive fetal RBCs while potentially normalizing the Hct. After a single-volume exchange, 75% of the newborn's RBC mass is removed; a double-volume exchange removes 85% to 90% of the cells. However, bilirubin removal is much less effective; only 25% of the infant's total body bilirubin is removed during a double-volume exchange. This probably occurs because the major portion of bilirubin is in the extravascular compartment, an area not affected by the exchange of blood volume. Rebound in bilirubin levels occurs within 1 hour of the exchange, with posttransfusion levels rising as high as 55% of preexchange values.

Although EBF remains the primary condition requiring exchange transfusion, the procedure also can be used to reduce levels of circulating metabolic toxins or exogenous drugs and to reestablish a normal Hct without further volume overload in anemia-induced congestive heart failure. The mortality rate for exchange transfusions is approximately 3 in 1,000 procedures. This rate includes death during the procedure or within 6 hours after its completion but excludes hydropic, kernicteric, or moribund infants (AAP, 2004; Luchtman, and Wilson, 2011).

The following criteria are used to determine the need for and timing of exchange transfusions, particularly in infants with EBF (AAP, 2004):

- A cord blood bilirubin level over 4.5 mg/dL in term infants and 3.5 mg/dL in preterm infants
- A hemoglobin level under 8 g/dL and a bilirubin level over 6 mg/dL within 1 hour of delivery in a term infant
- A hemoglobin level under 11.5 g/dL and a bilirubin level over 3.5 mg/dL within 1 hour of delivery in a preterm infant
- An increase in bilirubin levels by 0.5 mg/dL/hr despite phototherapy
- A bilirubin level over 20 to 25 mg/dL in an uncompromised term infant, 18 mg/dL in the high-risk term newborn, and 10 to 18 mg/dL in the preterm infant, depending on gestational age and condition (Figure 13.9)
- A bilirubin level over 10 to 17 mg/dL in a stressed or very immature preterm infant, over 10 to 12 mg/dL if hypoxia and acidosis are present

Identical criteria are used to determine the need for repeated exchange transfusion. With more liberal use of phototherapy and appropriate fluid management, exchange transfusions are infrequently necessary (Luchtman & Wilson, 2011).

Side Effects of Exchange Transfusion

Exchange transfusion can have a marked effect on the cardiovascular status and the intravascular compartment, which is reflected in pressure changes, volume fluctuations, and biochemical balance. Significant morbidities such as apnea/bradycardia, anemia, air embolism, infection, cyanosis, necrotizing enterocolitis, vasospasm, thromboembolism and death can also occur as a result of an exchange transfusion.

■ Collaborative Management of the Infant Undergoing an Exchange Transfusion. In addition to the general nursing care required by a sick infant, specific stabilization procedures are necessary for a successful exchange transfusion.

ANEMIA

Pathophysiology

An infant is considered anemic if the hemoglobin or Hct value is more than two standard deviations below normal for his or her gestational age group (Baker, Greer, & Committee on Nutrition, 2010). During the neonatal period, several abnormalities can evoke states of both acute and chronic anemia in the newborn. These forms of anemia often precede and occur independently of the natural propensity for physiologic

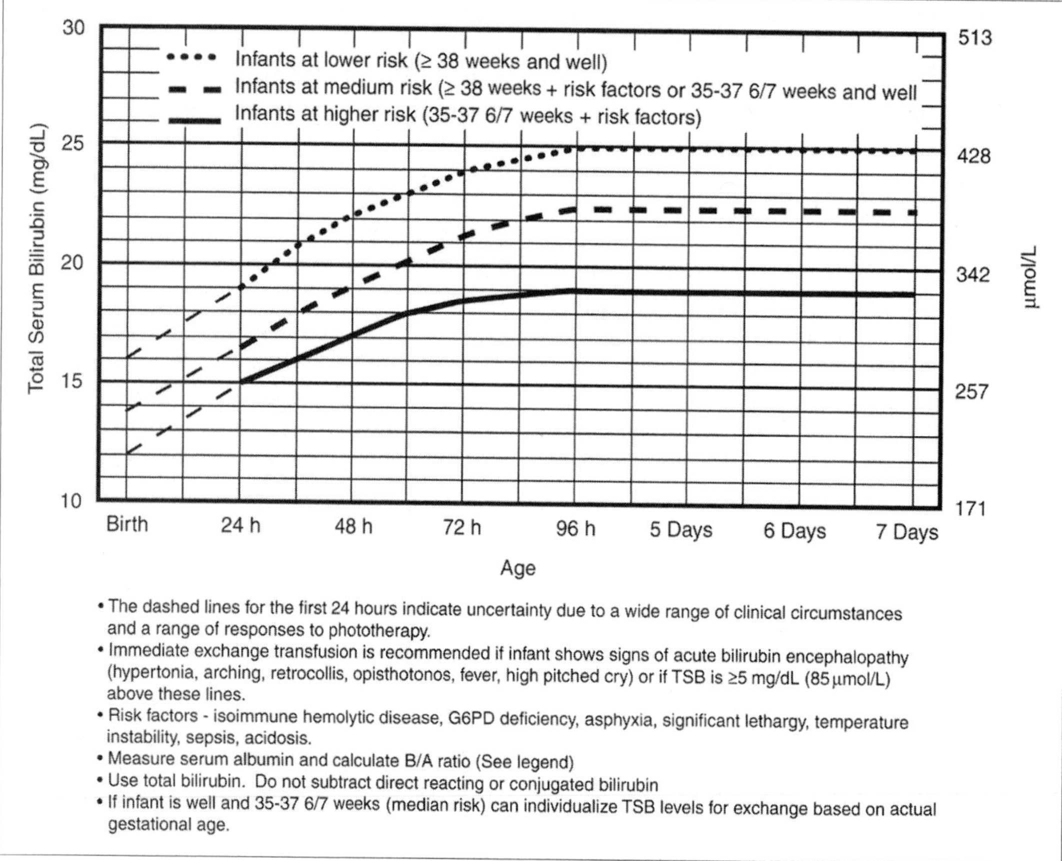

FIGURE 13.9 Guidelines for exchange transfusion in infants 35 or more weeks gestation.
From American Academy of Pediatrics, Subcommittee on Hyperbilirubinemia (2004). Copyright © 2004 American Academy of Pediatrics.

anemia that exists as a common entity among all infants, both term and preterm. The conditions that most commonly trigger these pathologic anemias are acute or chronic episodes of hemorrhage, acute or chronic RBC destruction and hemolysis, and blood sampling for laboratory analysis.

■ **Acute Anemia.** The physical presentation of acute anemia is more intense than that seen in the chronic form, because the causes of acute anemia are more emergent, life-threatening, and disruptive to the homeostasis of the infant (Box 13.2). The resulting cardiovascular collapse, followed closely by respiratory failure, can overwhelm the neonate with only marginal reserves. Immediate intervention and replacement of lost intravascular volume often are required to achieve stabilization. An infant experiencing an acute anemic episode (hemorrhage being the most common cause) has symptoms reflecting compromise of the cardiorespiratory system: shock, poor peripheral perfusion, poor respiratory effort or respiratory distress, tachycardia, pallor, lethargy, and hypotension. Before signs of acute anemia become apparent, the hemoglobin level must fall precipitously below 12 g/dL.

Acute blood loss results in a recognizable sequence of symptoms based on the volume loss:

- 7.5% to 15% volume loss: Little change is noted in heart rate and blood pressure, but stroke volume and subsequent cardiac output are reduced. Peripheral vasoconstriction occurs, resulting in diminished blood flow to the skeletal muscles, gut, and carcass.
- 20% to 25% volume loss: Hypotension and shock become apparent. Cardiac output is reduced, and peripheral vasoconstriction is present. Low tissue oxygen levels and acidosis become apparent.

■ **Chronic Anemia.** Prolonged, or chronic, anemia may not require rapid intravascular volume expansion, but it is by no means completely benign, as is seen with EBF or chronic twin-to-twin transfusion (Box 13.3). In both of these conditions, infants may require removal of intravascular volume and replacement with a volume of a higher Hct before stabilization is achieved. Because these infants have had considerable time to adjust to chronic blood loss or hemolysis, the changes in vital signs may reflect poor oxygen-carrying capacity rather than hypovolemia. On physical examination, pallor usually is accompanied by hepatosplenomegaly, a reflection of the body's attempt to compensate for blood loss through extramedullary hematopoiesis. The blood smear may also reflect the long-standing nature of the problem; RBCs appear hypochromic and small, and a greater number of immature RBCs are seen.

Common Causes of Pathologic Anemia in the Newborn

■ **Hemorrhage.** Hemorrhage is one of the most common causes of pathologic anemia in the newborn. There are many different types of hemorrhage, but they can be classified into four distinct categories, each of which will be discussed below.

BOX 13.2

CAUSES OF ACUTE ANEMIA IN THE NEWBORN

Obstetric Accidents, Malformations of the Placenta and Cord

Rupture of a normal umbilical cord

- Precipitous delivery
- Entanglement

Hematoma of the cord or placenta

Rupture of an abnormal umbilical cord

- Varices
- Aneurysm

Rupture of anomalous vessels

- Aberrant vessel
- Velamentous insertion
- Communicating vessels in multilobed placenta

Incision of placenta during cesarean section

Placenta previa

Abruptio placentae

Occult Hemorrhage Before Birth

Fetoplacental

- Tight nuchal cord

Cesarean section

Placental hematoma

Fetomaternal

- Traumatic amniocentesis
- After external cephalic version, manual removal of placenta, use of oxytocin
- Spontaneous
- Chorioangioma of the placenta
- Choriocarcinoma

Twin-to-twin

- Chronic
- Acute

Internal Hemorrhage

Intracranial

Giant cephalhematoma, subgaleal, caput succedaneum

Adrenal

Retroperitoneal

Ruptured liver, ruptured spleen

Pulmonary

Iatrogenic Blood Loss

Modified from Brugnara and Platt (2009).

BOX 13.3

CAUSES OF CHRONIC ANEMIA IN THE NEWBORN

Immunity Disorders

- Rh incompatibility
- ABO incompatibility
- Minor blood group incompatibility
- Maternal autoimmune hemolytic anemia
- Drug-induced hemolytic anemia

Infection

- Bacterial sepsis
- Viral infections

Congenital infections

- Syphilis
- Malaria
- Cytomegalovirus
- Rubella
- Toxoplasmosis
- Disseminated herpes
- Disseminated intravascular coagulation

Macroangiopathic and Microangiopathic Hemolytic Anemias

- Cavernous hemangioma
- Large-vessel thrombi
- Renal artery stenosis
- Severe coarctation of aorta

Iron Deficiency Anemia

Galactosemia

Hereditary Disorders of the Red Cell Membrane

- Hereditary spherocytosis
- Hereditary elliptocytosis
- Hereditary stomatocytosis
- Other rare membrane disorders

Pyknocytosis

Red Cell Enzyme Deficiencies

- Most commonly glucose-6-phosphate dehydrogenase deficiency, pyruvate kinase deficiency, 5′-nucleotidase deficiency, and glucose-6-phosphate isomerase deficiency

Alpha-Thalassemia Syndrome

Alpha-Chain Structural Abnormalities

Gamma-Thalassemia Syndromes

Gamma-Chain Structural Abnormalities

Modified from Brugnara and Platt (2009).

■ **Fetal–Maternal Transfusion Caused by Transplacental Hemorrhage.** This phenomenon occurs in approximately 50% to 75% of all pregnancies and can be an acute or chronic process. An estimated 5.6% of pregnancies involve a fetal-maternal transfusion in the range of 11 to 30 mL of blood; another 1% involve an exchange of more than 30 mL. Fetal–maternal transfusions can be verified by the presence of fetal cells in the maternal circulation, which can be detected with the erythrocyte rosette test and the Kleihauer–Betke acid elution test for fetal hemoglobin in maternal blood. The erythrocyte rosette test specifically detects fetal RBCs. The Kleihauer–Betke test consists of an acid wash of a maternal blood smear followed by staining. Fetal hemoglobin resists elution from intact RBCs in an acid solution. Intact cells containing fetal hemoglobin can be distinguished microscopically, when stained, from adult erythrocytes. The presence of stained erythrocytes suggests contamination of maternal blood by fetal blood. This test is useful in identifying fetal RBCs in the mother's blood as long as no underlying condition increases the amount of fetal hemoglobin in the mother's blood.

■ **Twin-to-Twin Transfusion.** This phenomenon, which can be both acute and chronic, occurs in 15% to 33% of all monochorionic (monozygotic) twins, in which the placentas tend to be fused. The anastomosis usually is between an artery of one placenta and the vein of the other, although vascular connections may be artery to artery or vein to vein. In the chronic form of twin-to-twin transfusion, the size difference between twins can be helpful in determining the donor and the recipient. When the weight difference exceeds 20%, the smaller twin is always the donor. When the weight difference is less than 20%, either twin may be the donor. In such cases, Hct values prove useful in determining the donor and the recipient. The donor twin is anemic, and the blood count reflects increased hematopoiesis, as evidenced by an elevated reticulocyte count and increased numbers of immature RBCs. The recipient develops polycythemia but can exhibit signs of congestive heart failure and pulmonary or systemic hypertension. Laboratory data usually show a difference of 5 g/dL between donor and recipient hemoglobin values. Stillbirths are common in twin-to-twin transfusion, and both twins are at risk.

■ **Obstetrical Accidents.** Many obstetrical problems, especially those that occur before labor and delivery, can result in chronic as well as acute blood loss. Long-standing problems, such as placenta previa or partial abruption, usually result in anemia. However, acute hemorrhage rather than anemia is the case in problems that occur at the time of delivery. Examples are severe abruption, severing of the placenta during cesarean section, or umbilical cord rupture as a result of sudden tension on a short or tangled cord. A tight nuchal cord can reduce blood volume in a newborn by approximately 20%. Holding a newly delivered infant above the placenta can also reduce the Hct and blood volume because of the gravitational drainage of blood from the newborn into the placenta.

■ **Internal Hemorrhage.** A drop in the Hct during the first 24 to 72 hours that is not associated with hyperbilirubinemia usually is attributed to internal hemorrhage. Bleeding can occur in various parts of the body secondary to birth trauma or preexisting anomalies. The areas of potential hemorrhage in the head include the subdural, subarachnoid, intraventricular, intracranial, and subgaleal spaces. Infants can lose an estimated 10% to 15% of their blood during an intraventricular or intracranial hemorrhage. In cases of traumatic delivery or vacuum extraction, extensive scalp bleeding can result in significant blood loss, which can be estimated by measuring the increase in the head circumference. Each centimeter of increase represents an estimated 38 mL of blood lost from the intravascular compartment. Hemorrhage into the liver, kidneys, spleen, or retroperitoneal space can also occur in association with traumatic and breech deliveries.

Hepatic rupture occurs in approximately 1.2% to 5.6% of stillbirths and neonatal deaths; half of the hemorrhages are subcapsular. Infants with this disorder tend to be stable for 24 to 48 hours and then suddenly deteriorate. This deterioration seems to coincide with rupture of the capsule and hemoperitoneum. Hepatic rupture carries a poor prognosis, but rapid surgery preceded by multiple transfusions can save the infant. Splenic rupture is associated with severe EBF and should be suspected at the time of exchange transfusion if the central venous pressure is low rather than elevated. Signs of splenic rupture include scrotal swelling and peritoneal effusion without free air. Adrenal hemorrhage is seen more often in the infant of a diabetic or prediabetic mother and is characterized by a flank mass with bluish discoloration of the overlying skin.

RED BLOOD CELL DESTRUCTION AND HEMOLYSIS

Maternal–Fetal Blood Group Incompatibilities

Isoimmunization, as in ABO and Rh incompatibility, accounts for most cases of neonatal hemolysis. A reduced RBC life span caused by hemolysis usually is associated with a rise in the bilirubin level, 1 g of hemoglobin yielding 35 mg of bilirubin. Infants who have received intrauterine transfusions or exchange transfusions for blood group incompatibilities are predisposed to a hyporegenerative anemia that develops within the first few months of life. The pathophysiology is considered to be bone marrow suppression, possibly as a result of the increased amount of hemoglobin A received during the blood transfusions.

■ **Acquired Defects of the Red Blood Cells.** This hemolytic problem is seen in bacterial sepsis and viral infections, especially of the TORCH variety. Drug-induced RBC destruction, caused by either maternal ingestion or direct administration of the drug to the newborn, is another common cause of hemolysis. An example of this would be the hemolysis that could occur with administration of iron supplements to an infant with vitamin E deficiency.

■ **Congenital Defects of the Red Blood Cells.** Defects resulting in destruction of the RBCs can involve the cell membrane, enzymatic system, or hemoglobin component, as in glucose-6-phosphate dehydrogenase deficiency, thalassemia, and hereditary spherocytosis. Although these conditions can cause hemolysis in the newborn period, they are rare diseases.

■ **Blood Sampling.** Blood loss that occurs secondary to sampling is one of the two most frequent causes of chronic anemia in infants, the other being physiologic anemia of the newborn and premature infant. In premature infants weekly phlebotomy losses in the first 2 weeks of life average 10% to 30% of their total blood volume, which is 10 to 25 mL/kg (Widness et al., 2005). Prudent blood sampling may eliminate unnecessary blood volume depletion and reduce the need for replacement transfusion therapy. Accurate recording of blood lost to sampling can prove beneficial in the assessment of a sick infant's circulatory status and volume needs. However, perfusion status and Hct values may be better determinants of the need for volume expansion or blood transfusions.

Differential Diagnosis

History. Acute and chronic anemia often can be distinguished from each other and from other problems by analyzing the family history for anemia or jaundice. The maternal history should be carefully examined for evidence of drug ingestion that may affect RBC life span or production, bleeding during the pregnancy or labor, or other incidents surrounding the delivery that may contribute to blood loss in the newborn.

Laboratory Findings. The type of anemia often can be identified on the basis of laboratory studies that evaluate RBC content and form.

- Hct and hemoglobin levels can define the type as well as the degree of anemia. Blood loss during acute hemorrhage is rapid, with little evidence of the compensatory hematopoiesis seen in chronic anemia. RBCs are of normal size and have a normal hemoglobin mass, and no significant increase is seen in the number of immature RBCs. Hemoglobin values initially may not reflect hemorrhage because the intravascular volume contracts and masks volume loss. It may take several hours for intravascular equilibration to occur before the hemoglobin accurately reflects the extent of the hemorrhage. The site of hemoglobin or Hct sampling is important for obtaining accurate information, because capillary sticks on an infant in shock reflect venous stasis. A more accurate sample at this time would be from an arterial or venous source.
- Reticulocyte counts are useful in differentiating chronic and acute forms of anemia. Increased numbers of immature RBCs reflect the degree of hematopoietic activity in response to anemia. Increased hematopoiesis requires a time lapse between the occurrence of anemia and stimulation of the hematopoietic centers.
- Peripheral blood smears are helpful in evaluating iron content and the size and shape of the RBC, which vary in different forms of anemia.
- Blood typing, Rh determination, and Coombs testing can help identify blood group incompatibilities as causes of anemia.

Treatment

Collaborative Management of the Infant With Acute Anemia. The following measures are used to stabilize the condition of an infant with acute anemia:

- Basic resuscitation of the infant experiencing precipitous blood loss often includes stabilization of the airway by means of intubation and ventilation.
- Rapid line placement for fluid replacement, volume expansion, and blood sampling may require use of the umbilical vein or artery. Central venous pressure measurements can be helpful in assessing the degree of volume loss and the amount of replacement needed.
- If acute volume expansion is required, normal saline is the volume expander of choice at 10 to 20 mL/kg. If time allows fresh frozen plasma or low-titer, type O-negative blood can be used at the dosing of normal saline until a type and cross-match replacement is available. In an emergency situation, blood taken from the fetal side of the placenta after it is delivered in a sterile manner can also be infused into the neonate. Failure to respond may indicate continuing internal hemorrhage.
- After the infant's condition has been stabilized, laboratory tests and a physical examination should be performed to determine the cause of the anemia and to rectify the problem.
- Examination of the placenta and maternal blood sample testing for fetal hemoglobin may prove useful in determining the cause of the blood loss.

As with all newborns, the principles of care (provision of warmth, monitoring of vital signs, ongoing assessment, and accurate determination of intake and output) are essential to the well-being of the infant who has suffered acute blood loss. After initial stabilization, nursing care must include modifications that either eliminate recurrence of precipitous events or prevent further blood loss. Providing safe care to such infants requires adequate knowledge of the principles and procedures involved in volume expansion and the use of blood products. A review of the use of blood products can be found at the conclusion of this chapter.

Collaborative Management of the Infant With Chronic Anemia. The major focus of therapy for the infant with chronic anemia is control or elimination of the cause of the anemia. Several forms of chronic anemia in term and preterm infants are linked to dietary deficiencies that can be eradicated by replacement therapy. Chronic forms of anemia requiring symptomatic therapy can also be treated with transfusion therapy and erythropoietin.

Dietary Supplementation. The three major dietary factors that affect RBC production are iron, folate, and vitamin E. Because all three increase in amount with increasing gestational age, premature birth predisposes the immature infant to anemia as a result of insufficient stores.

Without benefit of iron supplementation, the hematopoiesis necessary to maintain a normal hemoglobin level depletes the infant's iron reserves by the time birth weight is doubled. Various factors can further contribute to iron deficiency anemia, such as low birth weight, low initial hemoglobin levels, and blood loss through trauma, hemorrhage, or sampling. In the term infant, exhaustion of iron reserves normally occurs by 20 to 24 weeks postnatal age, but this happens much earlier in the preterm infant. Iron stores needed for hemoglobin production are present in insufficient quantities at birth in the premature infant, making supplementation necessary during the first 2 to 4 months to prevent iron deficiency anemia.

In any gestational age group, iron depletion first becomes evident in reduced serum ferritin levels (serum ferritin being a measure of accumulated iron stores) and in the disappearance of stainable iron from the bone marrow. A subsequent reduction in the mean corpuscular volume of the RBC is followed by a drop in the hemoglobin level. Although prophylactic iron supplementation does not prevent the initial fall in hemoglobin, the administration of 1 mg/kg for exclusively breastfed infants or breastfed infants that receive 50% of their nutrition through breast milk starting at 4 months of age and 2 mg/kg/d of supplemental iron should supply preterm infants starting at 1 month of age with adequate reserves; 2 to 4 mg/kg/d is recommended in iron-deficient infants or those receiving erythropoietin. Term infants on formula do not need supplementation as commercial formula has iron (Baker et al., 2010).

Folate is the generic description for folic acid and its related compounds. Folate is a component of the B-complex vitamins involved in the maturation of RBCs, particularly the synthesis of DNA, which controls nuclear maturation and division. Because bone marrow is one of the body's faster growing and proliferative tissues, folic acid deficiency diminishes its ability to produce RBCs, resulting in a megaloblastic anemia.

High amounts of folate are present at birth in both term and preterm infants, but these levels drop rapidly, especially in LBW infants. It is estimated that approximately 68% of infants weighing less than 1,700 g have subnormal levels of folate at 1 to 3 months of age. However, only a few infants actually develop anemia. Human milk and soy-based products contain an adequate amount of natural folate, but commonly used commercial products must be artificially enriched. Premature infant formulas are adequately enriched to satisfy a premature infant's folate needs provided that intake is sufficient. Because folate is absorbed in the duodenum and jejunum, any disease or medication that affects the absorptive surface of these areas can impair folate absorption (Brugnara & Platt, 2009).

Vitamin E, an antioxidant, is valuable in protecting the RBC membrane from destruction due to lipid peroxidation. Deficiency of this nutrient shortens the life span of the cell by exposing the unprotected, unsaturated membrane lipids to peroxidation and hemolysis. Infants are born in a state of relative vitamin E deficiency that is more intense in the smaller and more premature infants. Vitamin E is required in increasing amounts as the intake of polyunsaturated fatty acids increases. Deficiency becomes apparent in infants of birth weights less than 1,500 g at approximately 4 to 6 weeks of age, resulting in decreased hemoglobin levels ranging from 7 to 10 g/dL. The administration of iron supplementation in the presence of Vitamin E deficiency will intensify the hemolytic response. Signs and symptoms, as with many neonatal diseases, mimic those of other disease entities that occur in the neonatal period. One of the more obvious symptoms is edema of the feet, lower extremities, and scrotal area. The appearance of the RBC may vary, but abnormalities usually include fragmented or irregularly shaped cells, presence of spherocytes, and thrombocytopenia. Infant formulas are now enriched with adequate amounts of vitamin E, provided formula intake is sufficient.

■ Transfusion Therapy. In the past of all preterm infants admitted to a NICU, approximately 90% receive one transfusion in the first 6 weeks of life; 50% receive cumulative transfusions in excess of their total circulating RBC mass. Today, transfusions have declined as the result of the improved treatment and prevention of neonatal lung disease, the reduction of blood loss from gas and chemistry analysis and the use of transfusion guidelines (Brugnara & Platt, 2009). In determining which infants may need subsequent transfusions after the first 2 weeks of life, gestational age of less than 30 weeks is the best predictor, regardless of severity of illness, number of transfusions during the first week, complications, or Hct level at birth. Only 14% of infants of more than 30 weeks gestation require transfusions after 2 weeks of age.

Although a critically ill infant generally is maintained with an Hct above 40%, the benefits of transfusion therapy in the convalescent infant remain controversial. When the effects of transfusion therapy in the convalescent infant were studied, the elimination of symptoms attributed to anemia was not a consistent finding. In premature infants with an Hct below 30%, apnea, bradycardia, dyspnea, feeding difficulties, poor weight gain despite good calorie intake, lethargy, tachypnea, tachycardia, and increased cardiac output and oxygen consumption appear to be relieved by transfusion therapy in some studies. There appears to be no overall relationship between Hct values and physiologic symptoms such as apnea, bradycardia, or changes in heart and respiratory rates, nor does abatement of these symptoms follow transfusion therapy (Brugnara & Platt, 2009).

In light of the controversy surrounding transfusions, evidence of impaired tissue oxygenation remains the ultimate criterion for the use of blood products. Measurement of lactic acid levels may prove helpful in determining which infants may benefit from transfusion therapy. When the oxygen-carrying capacity of hemoglobin is insufficient for tissue needs, anaerobic metabolism occurs, leading to excess production of lactic acid. Monitoring of lactic acid levels and transfusing only those infants with elevated levels may aid in establishing more sound criteria for transfusion therapy.

Several methods of blood preparation and use have been evaluated to minimize donor exposure and reduce the potential for transmitted disease. Studies suggest that packed RBCs with a shelf life of more than 5 days, and up to 42 days, are safe for use in neonatal transfusions (Nunes dos Santos & Trindade, 2011). This finding, combined with use of a sterile connection device that allows multiple aseptic entries into a unit of blood, would permit use of a designated unit for each infant at risk for multiple transfusions, thereby significantly reducing donor exposure (Nunes dos Santos & Trindade, 2011). The desire to limit donor exposure must inevitably be balanced by the limited availability of banked blood. Multiple users on a blood unit may reduce wastage but may possibly expose an infant to multiple donors.

Blood administered to the newborn is often irradiated, which causes cell membrane disruption and potassium leakage from the cell. The decision by the U.S. Food and Drug Administration to change its recommendations for the maximum storage time of irradiated blood from 42 to 28 days affects the length of use of a designated unit. Although older blood appears to be safe to administer, it is not recommended for rapid transfusions, administration of large aliquots, exchange transfusions, or treatment of coagulopathies.

The establishment of transfusion criteria can effectively minimize donor exposure. These guidelines help determine which infants would benefit from transfusion on the basis of symptoms, Hct value, and severity of illness (Nunes dos Santos & Trindade, 2011).

■ Recombinant Human Erythropoietin Therapy

Cloning of the human erythropoietin (HuEPO) gene in 1985 resulted in the production of large amounts of HuEPO for use as an exogenous stimulant of erythroid progenitor cells in patients with anemia. HuEPO acts primarily on CFU-E, derivatives of the hematopoietic stem cells in the bone marrow and the precursors of the RBCs (Figure 13.10). Studies from the United States and England have shown the use of recombinant erythropoietin to be an effective replacement for transfusion therapy in raising the hemoglobin level in hyporegenerative anemia and end-stage renal disease. Further studies of preterm infants have demonstrated that HuEPO maintains the Hct level during the phase of normal anemia of the premature infant, with good proliferation of erythroid progenitor cells in response to HuEPO.

HuEPO had attained recognition as a standard of care for anemia of prematurity, because several clinical trials have established its effectiveness in reducing both the number of transfusions and the cumulative volume of transfused blood needed in treated patients (Messer, Haddad, Donato, & Matis, 1993; Maier, Obladen, & Wardrop, 1994; Meyer et al., 1994; Ohls, Hunter, & Christensen, 1993, 1995). Donato and associates (2000) noted increased reticulocytosis in infants started early on erythropoietin but failed to see a reduction in transfusion requirements in those infants. A Cochrane review of literature by Aher and Ohlsson (2010a) showed in comparing early versus late erythropoietin usage for preventing RBC transfusion for preterm and/or low-birth-weight infants that early erythropoietin(before 8 days of age) did not significantly reduce the use of one or more RBC transfusions or the number of transfusions per infant compared to late administration of erythropoietin. They did find a statistically significant increased risk of retinopathy of prematurity of any stage in those in the early treatment groups as well as for retinopathy greater than stage 3, which is concerning. Aher and Ohlsson also looked at late erythropoietin usage to prevent RBC transfusion in preterm and/or low-birth-weight infants. In this review they found that the administration of erythropoietin at 8 days or after did decrease the use of one or more RBC transfusions and the number of transfusions per infant. There was no decrease or increase in clinically important adverse outcomes with the late use of erythropoietin. They noted that donor exposure was not reduced as all infants had had a transfusion prior to the administration of the erythropoietin.

The use of erythropoietin in treating anemia of prematurity varies according to the physician and institution where the neonate is hospitalized. If used, the usual response in preterm infants given HuEPO is an increase in blood levels of erythropoietin and reticulocytes, as well as RBC volume, 2 to 3 weeks after initiation of therapy. The accepted dosage of erythropoietin is 500 to 1250 units/kg/wk divided into two to five doses. The commonly used dose is 250 units/kg/dose. The dose is given subcutaneously in rotating sites three times a week for 10 doses (Lexi Comp Online, 2012).

HuEPO has been evaluated for its effectiveness as an alternative to transfusion therapy for treatment of anemia in premature infants caused by (1) blood sampling, with administration beginning within the first 2 days of life (Maier et al., 1994; Ohls et al., 1995); (2) physiologic anemia of prematurity, with therapy starting at 1 to 4 weeks of age (Messer et al., 1993; Meyer et al., 1994; Shannon et al., 1995); and (3) anemia of bronchopulmonary dysplasia, with treatment starting at 3 months of age (Ohls et al., 1993).

Serum ferritin levels decline rapidly after initiation of HuEPO therapy in infants with normal pretreatment ferritin levels, despite prophylactic iron supplementation of 2 mg/kg/d. This predisposition to the development of iron

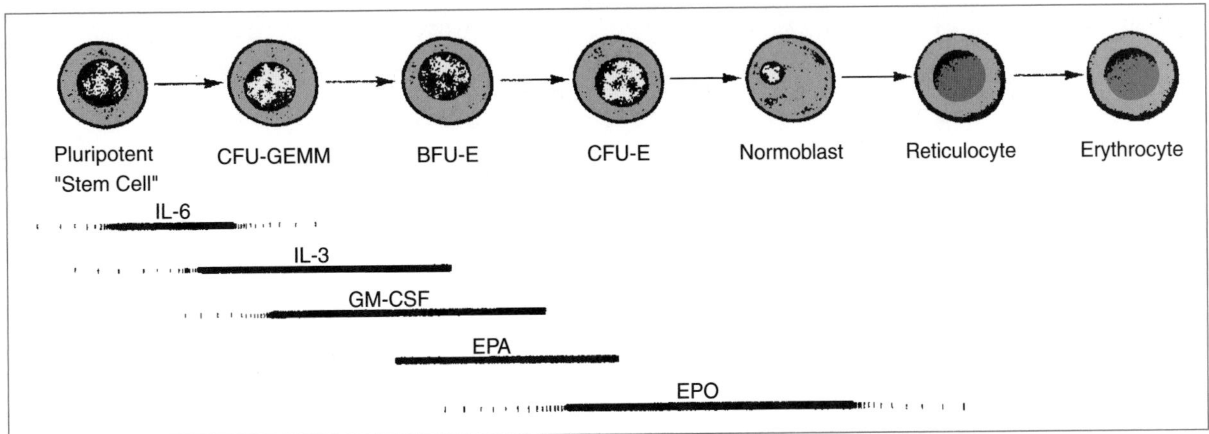

FIGURE 13.10 The principal action of human recombinant erythropoietin is on the derivatives of the hematopoietic stem cells in the bone marrow that have been designated erythrocyte colony-forming units (CFU-E), the precursors of the red blood cell (RBC). CFU-GEMM, colony-forming units—granulocytes, erythroid cells, macrophages, and megakaryocytes; BFU-E, erythrocyte burst-forming units; IL-6, interleukin-6; IL-3, interleukin-3; GM-CSF, granulocyte-macrophage colony-stimulating factor; EPA, erythroid potentiating activity; EPO, erythropoietin.
From Christensen (1989).

deficiency anemia underlines the need for increased iron supplementation in infants treated with HuEPO. Also documented as a side effect of HuEPO therapy are transient thrombocytosis shortly after the initiation of therapy and transient neutropenia. The transient neutropenia can last as long as 2 months after discontinuation of therapy. It has been postulated that this phenomenon is due to a stimulant effect of HuEPO on megakaryocyte progenitors and a negative effect on granulocyte-monocyte progenitor cells. Before HuEPO was proven effective in raising Hct levels, its use was projected to eliminate the need for one third of all transfusions in premature infants.

PHYSIOLOGIC ANEMIA OF THE NEWBORN AND ANEMIA OF THE PREMATURE INFANT

Shortly after birth, the physiologic regulator of RBC production, erythropoietin, falls to barely perceptible levels because the relative intrauterine hypoxia that stimulated its release in utero is no longer present. Erythropoietin levels remain low until another hypoxic stimulus occurs, one created by the normal drop in the hemoglobin level that marks physiologic anemia of the newborn. This drop in the hemoglobin level is due to decreased marrow production of RBCs secondary to diminished circulating erythropoietin levels, a shorter life span of the neonatal RBC with destruction of fetal hemoglobin, and hemodilution caused by growth.

The drop in hemoglobin that prompts the postnatal rise in erythropoietin directly correlates with the infant's gestational age and birth weight (Figure 13.11). The smaller and more immature infant reaches a lower nadir at an earlier postnatal age. The hemoglobin level in the term newborn reaches a nadir of 11.4 g/dL ± 0.9 in the first 2 to 3 months of life and plateaus at this level for approximately 2 more months before it gradually increases. Although there is no significant difference in cord blood hemoglobin levels between term infants and preterm infants born after 32 weeks gestation, the drop in hemoglobin occurs earlier in the preterm infant, is more precipitous, and reaches a lower nadir. Starting at 2 weeks of age, the preterm infant has a drop in hemoglobin of 1 g/dL/wk for the first several weeks; the nadir at 6 to 8 weeks of age is 2 to 3 g/dL lower than that of the term infant. An infant weighing 1,000 to 1,500 g at birth will have a mean hemoglobin nadir of 8 g/dL at 4 to 6 weeks of age.

Infants who have undergone exchange transfusion or multiple transfusions also have a greater fall in their hemoglobin level in the first 3 months of life. This phenomenon theoretically may be due to improved oxygen delivery to tissue associated with the replacement of fetal with adult hemoglobin. Adult hemoglobin has less affinity for oxygen because of the structural difference of the globin portion of the hemoglobin molecule. This, coupled with the increased amount of 2,3-disphosphoglycerate present in the blood, allows adult hemoglobin to release oxygen to the tissue more easily. Improved tissue oxygenation effectively lowers serum erythropoietin levels (Figure 13.12), resulting in decreased RBC production. Consequently, an infant undergoing intrauterine transfusion, exchange transfusion, or frequent postnatal transfusions has improved tissue oxygenation and a decreased erythropoietin level.

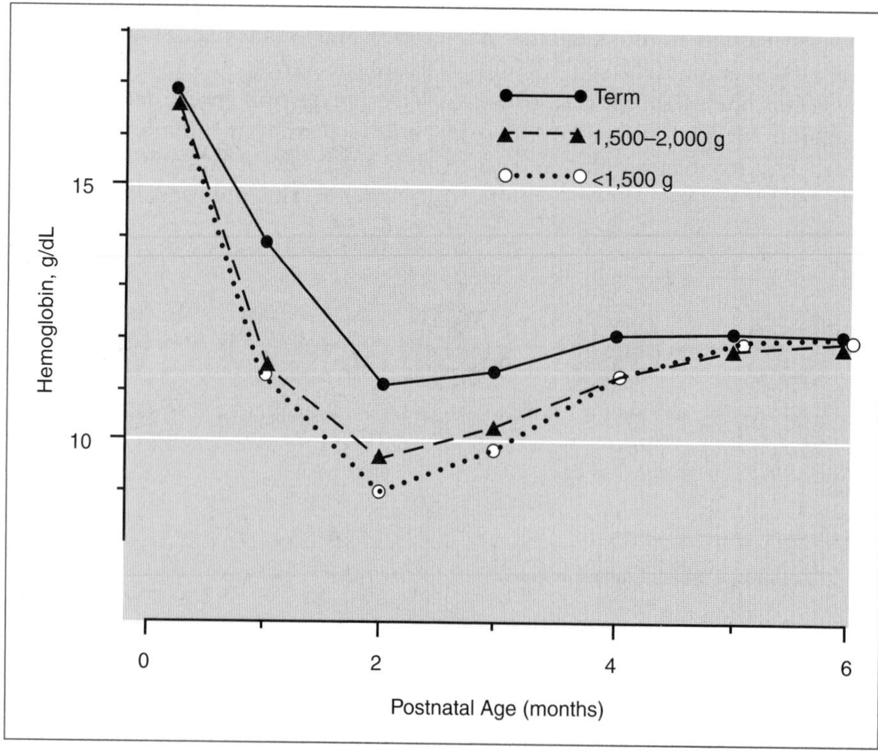

FIGURE 13.11 Gestational age and birth weight are directly correlated with the timing of the postnatal drop in hemoglobin and with the nadir of the drop. Shown here are the differences between term infants and two groups of preterm infants, one weighing 1,500 to 2,000 g and the other less than 1,500 g.
From Brown (1988).

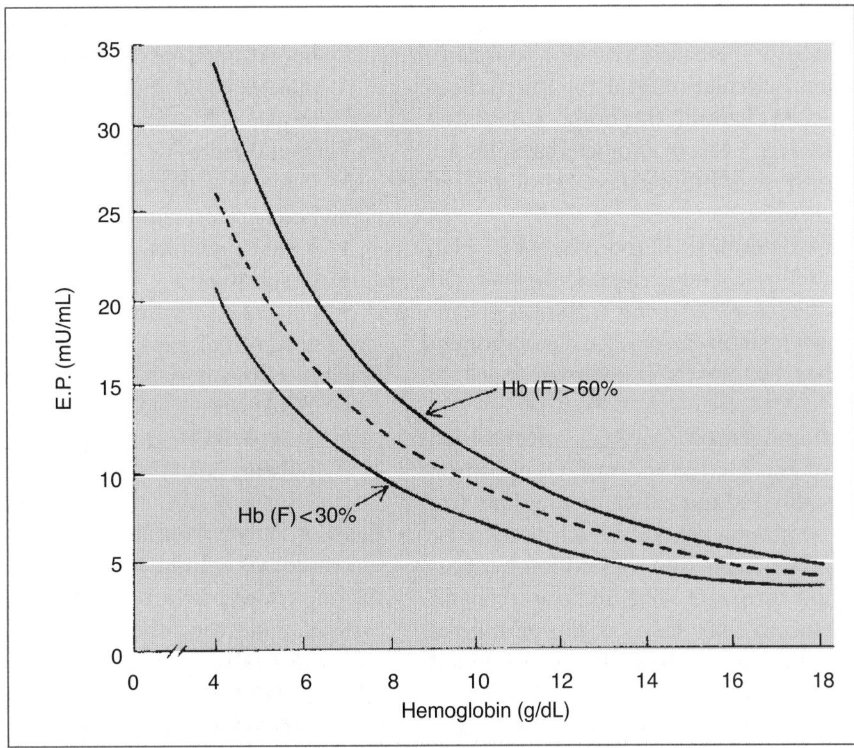

FIGURE 13.12 Because of the differences in oxygen affinity between adult and fetal hemoglobin, variations in the percentage of available fetal hemoglobin (hemoglobin F) affect erythropoietin levels. Improved oxygen uptake but decreased unloading at the tissue level is associated with hemoglobin F. Therefore the stimulus for erythropoietin production is diminished with lower concentrations of hemoglobin F (<30%). With higher concentrations (60%) of hemoglobin F, the stimulus response is an increase in erythropoietin production. At identical total hemoglobin levels, the stimulus for erythropoietin production is increased whenever the percentage of hemoglobin F exceeds the adult norm.
Adapted from Stockman et al. (1977). Copyright © 1977 Massachusetts Medical Society.

The switch in the predominant site of erythropoietin production during fetal life from the liver to the kidneys occurs concurrently with the change in hemoglobin to a more mature form. Hepatic production of erythropoietin in response to hypoxia is not as rapid as the kidneys' response, an adjustment that actually spares the fetus from polycythemia in utero. However, persistence of this hepatic pathway after premature birth may explain why the premature infant's Hct values reach a lower nadir that persists longer compared with the term infant. Although erythropoietin levels are reduced in the early newborn period, the erythroid progenitor cells in the bone marrow are exceedingly sensitive to erythropoietin and respond rapidly as blood levels increase. The normal erythropoietin level in infants beyond the newborn period is 10 to 20 units/mL.

Treatment

Physiologic anemia does not usually require any form of treatment. With good nutrition, the hemoglobin level in the term infant should start to rise by 3 months of age. With adequate nutrition and iron supplementation, the hemoglobin level in the preterm infant should start to increase by 5 months of age, eventually attaining hemoglobin values comparable to those of the term infant. It is the preterm infant with symptomatic anemia of prematurity who poses the question of transfusion versus HuEPO therapy, a question that has not yet been answered conclusively.

Polycythemia

■ **Pathophysiology.** Polycythemia, defined as a peripheral venous Hct over 65%, occurs in 4% to 5% of the total population of newborns, in 2% to 4% of term infants appropriate for gestational age, and in 10% to 15% of infants either small or large for gestational age. It has not been observed in infants of less than 34 weeks gestation. Although the fetus lives in a low-PO_2 environment that should induce a polycythemic response, it protects itself by keeping Hct levels below 60%. This may be a function of slower fetal hepatic response to hypoxia compared with rapid renal response after birth. The average Hct on the first day of life is approximately 50% in the term infant and the preterm infant of more than 32 weeks gestation and 45% in the preterm infant of less than 32 weeks gestation. During the first 4 to 12 hours of life, hemoglobin and Hct values tend to rise and then equilibrate, especially in infants receiving large placental transfusions.

The choice of sampling site can affect Hct values considerably, particularly during the early newborn period when peripheral circulation may be somewhat sluggish. Infants younger than 1 day of age either lack or have diminished cutaneous vasoregulatory mechanisms that reduce peripheral perfusion. Polycythemia further impairs peripheral circulation by increasing blood viscosity and reducing the flow rate. As blood viscosity increases, vascular resistance increases in the peripheral circulation and the microcirculation of the capillaries throughout the body. Compared with venous samples, the Hct levels of capillary samples are 5% to 15% higher, and those of umbilical vessel or arterial samples are 6% to 8% lower.

Three major factors determine blood viscosity: Hct, plasma viscosity (osmolality), and deformability of the RBCs. With Hct levels below 60% to 65%, blood viscosity increases in a linear fashion, but viscosity exponentially increases at higher Hct levels (Luchtman-Jones & Wilson, 2011).

Variations in the components of plasma affect blood viscosity independent of the Hct. Abnormal composition of plasma protein, electrolytes, and other metabolites can either decrease or increase plasma viscosity. Such an increase in the presence of a high Hct further increases blood viscosity and reduces the blood flow rate. The ability of cells to modify their shape to successfully traverse the peripheral vascular bed and microcirculation also affects the blood flow rate. The degree of deformability of the cell determines its ability to pass through small vascular spaces; the greater the deformability of the cell, the quicker its passage. Less deformable cells can increase blood viscosity by occluding small vessels, causing sludging in the microcirculation that can lead to thrombosis and tissue ischemia.

The two major types of polycythemia are (1) the active form, which is caused by the production of an excess number of RBCs in response to hypoxia and other poorly defined stimuli; and (2) the passive form, which is caused by RBC transfusion to an infant secondary to maternal–fetal transfusion, twin-to-twin transfusion, or delayed cord clamping (Luchtman-Jones & Wilson, 2011).

Active Polycythemia. Tissue hypoxia, regardless of the cause, elicits an increase in erythropoietin that stimulates RBC production. In the fetus, erythropoietin is produced initially by the liver and then by the kidneys, the adult production site. The kidneys' potential to release erythropoietin is active by 34 weeks gestation. At this time, a renal erythropoietic factor reacts with a substance in the plasma to produce erythropoietin, the RBC stimulating factor. Hypoxia of the tissues adjacent to the renal tubules, where erythropoietin is produced, is the potent stimulator of this factor's release.

Many factors can lead to tissue hypoxia associated with the active form of polycythemia. These factors include the following:

1. Maternal factors that result in reduced placental blood flow
   - Pregnancy-induced hypertension
   - Older maternal age
   - Maternal renal or heart disease
   - Severe maternal diabetes (Hct values of 64% or higher are found in 42% of infants of a diabetic mother and 30% of gestational infants of a diabetic mother)
   - Oligohydramnios
   - Maternal smoking (the mechanism is thought to be production of carbon monoxide that crosses the placenta and induces a state of tissue hypoxia in the fetus)
2. Placental factors
   - Placental infarction
   - Placenta previa
   - Viral infections, especially TORCH
   - Postmaturity
   - Placental dysfunction that results in a small-for-gestational-age (SGA) infant
3. Fetal syndromes
   - Trisomies 13, 18, and 21
   - Beckwith–Wiedemann syndrome (Luchtman-Jones & Wilson, 2011)

Passive Polycythemia. Passive polycythemia is a result of increased fetal blood volume caused by maternal–fetal transfusion; twin-to-twin transfusion, with one twin being polycythemic and the other anemic; or delayed cord clamping. A diagnosis of maternal–fetal transfusion can be considered when (1) the infant's blood is found to contain larger amounts than expected of adult hemoglobin, IgA, or IgM; (2) RBCs in the infant's blood have maternal blood group antigens, if the mother's and the infant's blood groups are different; or (3) XX cells are found in an XY infant. In twin-to-twin transfusion, morbidity and mortality are comparable in both groups of affected infants, with one twin being anemic and the other polycythemic. In the past it was believed that delayed cord clamping with the positioning of the baby below the level of the placenta was the most common cause of passive polycythemia. However, a systematic review and meta-analysis by Hutton and Hassen in 2007 of 15 trials with 1,912 neonates showed that late cord clamping up to 3 minutes, of those who were placed on their mothers abdomen or chest, did show more polycythemia versus the ones who had early cord clamping. None of the babies in the studies were symptomatic or required admission to a NICU. Hutton and Hassan (2007) identified one possible explanation for the increased polycythemia as the artificially low lab values based on babies who had immediate cord clamping at birth.

■ Clinical Manifestations. Symptoms of polycythemic hyperviscosity, which usually are evident within the first few days after birth, reflect compromise of various organ systems. The most commonly seen findings include the following:

1. Neurologic symptoms
   - Lethargy
   - Hypotonia
   - Tremulousness
   - Exaggerated startle
   - Poor suck
   - Vomiting
   - Seizures
   - Apnea
2. Cardiovascular symptoms
   - Plethora
   - Cardiomegaly

- Electrocardiographic changes (right and left atrial hypertrophy, right ventricular hypertrophy)

3. Respiratory symptoms
   - Respiratory distress
   - Central cyanosis
   - Pleural effusions
   - Pulmonary congestion and edema
4. Hematologic symptoms
   - Thrombocytopenia
   - Elevated reticulocyte level
   - Hepatosplenomegaly
5. Metabolic symptoms
   - Hypocalcemia
   - Hyperbilirubinemia
   - Hypoglycemia

Hypoglycemia found in conjunction with polycythemia can be a reflection of (1) increased glucose consumption by an overabundant number of RBCs; (2) increased cerebral extraction of glucose secondary to hypoxia; (3) a state of hyperinsulinemia caused by increased erythropoietin levels; or (4) decreased hepatic glucose production as a result of sluggish hepatic circulation. Hyperbilirubinemia associated with polycythemia is a reflection of increased by-products of RBC destruction.

The complications of polycythemia center around the increased resistance to blood flow related to hyperviscosity; blood flow to all organ systems is impaired by sluggish circulation. Pulmonary blood flow can be dramatically compromised, resulting in pulmonary hypertension, retained lung fluid, and respiratory distress syndrome. Taxation of the heart by an increased vascular load can lead to congestive heart failure and left to right shunting across the foramen ovale or ductus arteriosus. Sludging of blood in the microcirculation of the kidneys can lead to renal vein thrombosis and renal failure. Impairment of blood flow to the bowel can lead to necrotizing enterocolitis (Lessaris, 2012).

■ Treatment. Although most infants with polycythemia are asymptomatic or minimally symptomatic, the Hct level and the presence of symptoms, even if minimal, should form the basis of treatment. Because Hct levels of 65% can lead to neurologic abnormalities and levels of 75% or higher are always associated with neurologic changes, an infant with a venous Hct of 65% or higher should be considered for partial exchange transfusion.

Partial exchange results in dramatic improvement in symptomatic infants, relieving congestive failure and improving CNS function. It also corrects hypoglycemia, relieves respiratory distress and cyanosis, and improves renal function (Lessaris, 2012).

Partial exchange transfusion should be done as the venous Hct approaches 65% and as symptoms appear; normal saline is the replacement fluid of choice for the removed aliquot of blood. Plasmanate, 5% albumin, or fresh frozen plasma has been used in the past, but due to the advent of stricter precautions for prevention of viral transmission by blood products, use of these items would not seem advisable (Lessaris, 2012). The formula for calculating the partial replacement of blood volume is: [blood volume (patient's Hct − desired hct)]/patient's Hct. The blood volume is patient's weight × 90 mL/kg of blood.

■ Collaborative Management of the Infant With Polycythemia. The care of any newborn infant should include a screening Hct determination for polycythemia by 12 hours of age. This allows both detection of any infant with polycythemia and adequate observation before symptoms become apparent. Because the initial sample usually is obtained by heel stick or finger stick, detection of a high value should be followed by venipuncture confirmation. The infant should be kept adequately hydrated and closely monitored for hypoglycemia and hypocalcemia. A Hct value over 65% should prompt careful observation of the infant for any symptoms associated with hyperviscosity. If symptoms appear, the infant should undergo partial exchange transfusion. During the partial exchange, the same care should be provided as that given during a single-volume or double-volume exchange transfusion.

COMMON COAGULATION DISORDERS IN THE NEWBORN

Hemorrhagic Disease of the Newborn

The liver produces most of the clotting factors, including those of the prothrombin complex. Adequate function of this complex requires the specific action of vitamin K, which is continuously synthesized by bacteria in the bowel. Vitamin K is not directly involved in the synthesis of these factors but is required for the conversion of precursor proteins produced by the liver into active factors having coagulant capabilities. Vitamin K is especially necessary for conversion of prothrombin binding sites into forms that can bind calcium, which is required for the completion of many steps in the clotting cascade.

Vitamin K–dependent factors reach approximately 30% to 70% of adult levels in the cord blood of term infants but quickly drop to half that amount if the infant is not given vitamin K. Because these factors are gestational age dependent, the more premature the infant, the lower the levels at birth. The exaggerated drop after birth may be due to poor placental transfer of maternal vitamin K, immature liver function, and delayed synthesis of vitamin K by the bowel. Vitamin K–dependent factors slowly rise but do not reach normal adult levels until approximately 9 months of age. Administration of approximately 0.5 to 1.0 mg of vitamin K can prevent this decline and normalize the prothrombin time (AAP, 2007, 2009).

Hemorrhage during the early neonatal period that can be attributed to a deficiency of vitamin K–dependent factors is classified as hemorrhagic disease of the newborn, of which there are three identified forms. The early form, the least common type, is characterized by bleeding within the first 24 hours of life, usually associated with maternal anticonvulsant therapy. It is theorized that anticonvulsants may induce fetal hepatic enzymes involved in the degradation of already low levels of fetal vitamin K. Early neonatal bleeding cannot be prevented by postnatal administration of vitamin K. Daily antenatal administration of large doses of oral vitamin K (10 mg) to mothers receiving anticonvulsant therapy for at least 10 days before delivery was found to be beneficial to the newborn. Vitamin K crosses the placenta, elevating newborn levels of vitamin K for 10 days after birth, with the increase in levels correlating with the timing of the last prenatal dose.

The classic form of hemorrhagic disease usually occurs during the first 2 to 5 days of life and manifests as generalized and, occasionally, dramatic bleeding. The most common sites are the gastrointestinal tract, umbilicus, circumcision site, skin, and internal organs. The usual cause is inadequate intake of breast milk in an infant who has not received prophylactic vitamin K. Breast milk provides adequate vitamin K to prevent this disorder if it is taken in sufficient quantities.

The late form of hemorrhagic disease, which occurs after the first week of life, is more devastating than the early form because of the higher incidence of intracranial hemorrhage (the risk approaches 63%). Permanent neurologic sequelae are seen in 24% of affected infants, and the mortality rate can be as high as 14%. This form of hemorrhagic disease is associated with chronic disease states that interfere with fat absorption or the performance of intestinal flora. Both early and late hemorrhagic disease of the newborn is intensified in breastfed infants. Definitive diagnosis rests on a history of lack of vitamin K prophylaxis at birth and a prolonged prothrombin time that measures the prothrombin complex clotting factors (Factors II, VII, IX, and X). One test, the protein induced by vitamin K absence or antagonist-II (PIVKA-II) test, is useful in identifying proteins induced by vitamin K deficiency that appear in the plasma of vitamin K–deficient infants. These proteins consist of the inert and functionally defective precursors of prothrombin that are produced when vitamin K levels are deficient.

Several factors can predispose an infant to hemorrhagic disease of the newborn. Almost all these factors involve some form of hepatic dysfunction. The most obvious predisposing factor is failure of an infant to receive prophylactic vitamin K postnatally. Other risk factors include maternal ingestion of anticonvulsants and coumarin anticoagulants (which interfere with the action of the prothrombin complex factors), birth asphyxia, prolonged labor, and breastfeeding.

Human milk has lower vitamin K content than cow's milk. Infants receiving a commercial formula for 24 hours have prothrombin times similar to those of infants receiving vitamin K after birth. Infants with hepatic dysfunction or bowel malabsorption, although not found strictly in the early neonatal period, can develop vitamin K deficiency despite having received prophylaxis at birth. Such disorders as chronic diarrhea, biliary atresia, hepatitis, cystic fibrosis, and prolonged parenteral nutrition do not allow adequate vitamin K production and can result in low prothrombin complex factors. These infants benefit from weekly vitamin K supplementation (1 mg given intramuscularly), the dose recommended by the AAP (2007, 2009) for postnatal newborn prophylaxis. The suggested preparation for administration to the newborn is the natural aqueous solution of vitamin K rather than the synthetic preparation, which can cause hemolysis. Because of preterm infants' hepatic immaturity and inability to effectively synthesize clotting factors, these infants' response to vitamin K is not as predictable as that of term infants.

Controversy continues over whether intramuscular or oral prophylaxis should be used. At one time, intramuscular administration of vitamin K was linked to the occurrence of childhood cancers; however, this charge has not been substantiated by research. The use of one or two oral doses of vitamin K as an effective treatment is also disputed, and research is needed to determine its efficacy. Research continues in an effort to determine the appropriate timing and number of oral doses of vitamin K and to develop a better oral preparation. Alternative therapies are also being investigated, including antenatal maternal dosing to prevent antenatal intraventricular hemorrhage and postnatal maternal dosing as prophylaxis in the breastfed infant.

Active bleeding caused by hemorrhagic disease of the newborn may require blood replacement or the use of fresh frozen plasma for immediate clotting factor replacement.

Hemophilia

■ Pathophysiology. Hemophilia A and B are the most common inherited bleeding disorders. Classic hemophilia (hemophilia A) is the most frequently inherited coagulation abnormality, accounting for 90% of all genetically linked coagulopathies and 80% to 85% of all hemophilias, whereas hemophilia B (Christmas disease) occurs in 10% to 15%. Both diseases are passed from mother to son as an X-linked trait. Hemophilia A is caused by Factor VIII deficiency and hemophilia B is caused by a Factor IX deficiency. Both factors are essential in normal thrombin production. They are needed for the activation of pathway of Factor X, which converts prothrombin to thrombin. The absence of either factor severely impairs the body's ability to generate both thrombin and fibrin. A hemophiliac's problem is not that of bleeding more rapidly, but of abnormal clot formation. This results in hemorrhage with a potential for significant blood loss. When the clot does form it is often fragile, and rebleeding can occur if proper treatment does not occur.

The severity of the disease is dependent on the baseline level of Factor VIII or Factor IX. Levels of 1% to 2% are associated with severe disease, 2% to 5% with moderate disease, and over 5% with mild disease, a level at which active bleeding rarely occurs. In a retrospective study of hemophiliacs, approximately 44% of a group of severe hemophiliacs were symptomatic during the first week of life, whereas only 14% of a mildly affected group displayed any bleeding during the first 7 days of life (Schulman, 1962).

■ Diagnosis. Infants affected with hemophilia have a prolonged partial thromboplastin time and decreased factor, but the prothrombin time, thrombin time, and platelet count are relatively normal. The major symptom of hemophilia is bleeding, most often from the circumcision site, scalp, umbilicus, and brain. Not all severe hemophiliacs bleed after circumcision in the early newborn period. The reason for this is unknown, but it has been suggested that tissue thromboplastin release, caused by the circumcision clamp on the foreskin, may initiate the extrinsic pathway and clotting cascade, preventing excessive bleeding.

Prenatal diagnosis is possible through amniocentesis or chorionic villus biopsy. Diagnosis involves measurement of the ratio of factor antigen to coagulant antigen on blood samples of fetuses of more than 20 weeks gestation. If diagnosed with Factor VIII deficiency, the infant should also be evaluated for von Willebrand disease.

■ Treatment. The ultimate goal in the treatment of hemophilia is to raise the defective or deficient factor to a level that will prevent bleeding. In order to have replacement products be as free as possible of transfusion-transmissible diseases, it is recommended that recombinant products be used rather than plasma-derived products. Recombinant factor VIII concentrates are preferred for hemophilia A, whereas recombinant Factor IX is preferred for hemophilia B (Luchtman-Jones & Wilson, 2011; Zaiden, 2012).

Desmopressin (DDAVP, 1-desamino-8-d-arginine vasopressin) is now the treatment of choice for mild to moderate hemophilia A or von Willebrand disease. This medication is not effective in the treatment of hemophilia B. The effectiveness and applicability of this therapy in the newborn are still unknown, but currently it is not recommended if the infant is younger than 3 months of age (Lexi-Comp Online). Amicar and tranexamic acid, antifibrinolytic agents that are being used, show some benefit in the treatment of hemophilia (Luchtman-Jones & Wilson, 2011).

Von Willebrand Disease

Von Willebrand disease is a disorder of the vWF, which contributes to the adherence of platelets to the endothelium and serves as a carrier protein for Factor VIII. A deficiency in this factor leads to mucocutaneous and post-surgical bleeding or if it is absent or markedly reduced can lead to bleeding in joints and muscles similar to hemophilia A due to the reduction of Factor VIII. vWF levels are high at birth and in the neonatal period; thus the chance of any bleeding being from von Willebrand disease is low. Since vWF serves as a carrier for Factor VIII, those who do present with bleeding will have signs and symptoms consistent with factor VIII deficiency.

Infants with von Willebrand disease will present with similar symptoms as hemophilias with bleeding into the joints and intracranially. Lab tests to diagnose von Willebrand disease are a bleeding time, activated partial thromboplastin time, platelet function screen, blood type, factor VIII coagulant activity, vWF antigen, vWF activity, and multimetric analysis (Luchtman-Jones & Wilson, 2011). Treatment is similar as those for hemophilia.

Thrombocytopenia

The normal range of platelets is 150,000 to 450,000/mm^3; the average count in the newborn is approximately 250,000/mm^3. Platelet counts below 150,000/mm^3 are considered abnormal and should be subject to investigation for a possible pathologic process. Platelet function in the neonate reaches normal adult levels between the fifth and ninth postnatal days. Although 14% of all preterm infants and 4% of all term infants are thrombocytopenic, with platelet counts below 150,000/mm^3, not all of these infants are ill.

Thrombocytopenia is the most common bleeding disorder in the newborn, with 20% to 35% of all NICU admissions and 70% of infants born at less than 1,000 g having the diagnosis during their NICU stay (Sollman & Sola-Visner, 2012). Of the affected infants, 50% will have platelet counts <100,000/mm^3 and 20% will have platelet counts <50,000/mm^3 (Cantor, 2009). However, the pathogenesis of the thrombocytopenia can be determined in only 60% of these infants. Abnormalities of the platelet count are due to increased destruction or decreased production, and the underlying cause is mediated by maternal, placental, neonatal, or iatrogenic factors. In most thrombocytopenic newborns, platelet counts are low as a result of increased destruction rather than bone marrow depression. The overall mortality rate for infants with thrombocytopenia is 34%; 22% of these infants exhibit a bleeding diathesis. Infants with a platelet count below 20,000/mm^3 are at particularly high risk for bleeding.

■ Maternal Factors. Thrombocytopenia is the most common form of hemostatic problem present during pregnancy; 5% to 7% of healthy mothers have platelet counts below 150,000/mm^3. Some of the maternal factors associated with thrombocytopenia are maternal drug ingestion (e.g., chloramphenicol, hydralazine, tolbutamide, and thiazides), maternal eclampsia and hypertension, placental infarction, and immune-mediated maternal platelet antibodies.

■ Immune-Mediated Maternal Platelet Antibodies

Idiopathic Thrombocytopenia. With immune-mediated thrombocytopenia, in which maternal antibodies destroy platelets, 80% of cases are caused by the autoimmune form, or maternal idiopathic thrombocytopenic purpura (ITP), which strikes women during the second to third decade of life. ITP, now also referred to as autoimmune thrombocytopenia, is a preexisting condition in which maternal lymphocytes produce IgG antiplatelet antibodies (PAIgG) that attack maternal platelets, usually reducing the platelet count to below 150,000/mm^3. These antibodies are specifically directed at platelet antigen and bind to platelets, which are then phagocytized by cells carrying a specific receptor, the Fc receptor. The greatest number of cells with this receptor is found in the reticuloendothelial system of the spleen, which is also the major site of PAIgG production. ITP is often confused with HELLP syndrome, which, in addition to a low platelet count, involves hemolysis and elevated liver enzymes.

Because IgG can cross the placenta, fetal platelets can also be destroyed by the transplacental passage of platelet antibodies, resulting in thrombocytopenia in the fetus and newborn. The mortality rate is 1% to 10% in these affected infants, and the condition can persist postnatally for as long as 4 months.

Neonatal Alloimmune Thrombocytopenia. The remaining 20% of immune-mediated thrombocytopenia are caused by an alloimmune (isoimmune) reaction in which maternal antibodies are produced against foreign fetal platelets (paternally inherited), whereas maternal platelet levels remain normal. This reaction occurs when fetal platelets, which have an antigen not found on maternal platelets, pass into the maternal circulation. The resultant generation of maternal antibodies in response to the fetal platelets is similar to the mechanism behind Rh incompatibility. Unlike Rh incompatibility, alloimmune thrombocytopenia affects 335 to 50% of first pregnancies. The mother develops IgG antibodies that eventually cross into the fetal circulation, resulting in platelet destruction. The PlA1 alloantibodies are responsible for 50% to 80% of neonates with alloimmune thrombocytopenia. This phenomenon occurs in approximately 1 in 2,000 to 1 in 5,000 live births. The mortality rate of 10% to 15% in alloimmune thrombocytopenia is higher than that in ITP, because bleeding tends to be more severe. The incidence of intracranial hemorrhage in utero is reported to be as high as 10% to 15%, with most cases occurring between 30 and 35 weeks gestation. Treatment consists of transfusion of maternal platelets, exchange transfusion, and use of IVIG. Platelets usually normalize in the newborn by 4 weeks of age.

■ Antenatal Treatment. The cornerstone of antenatal treatment is maternal administration of corticosteroids and administration of IVIG to the newborn (Berkowitz et al., 2006). Steroids and IVIG work in similar fashion by (1) diminishing the production of antiplatelet antibodies, (2) interfering with antibody attachment to the surface of the platelets, and (3) reducing platelet destruction by interfering with phagocytic receptors in the reticuloendothelial system. Pacheo et al. (2012) developed an algorithm based on risk stratification for the administration of steroid and IVIG therapy. In the algorithm, the administration of steroids and IVIG is based on previous infants with thrombocytopenia with no intracranial bleeding (ICH) after 28 weeks gestation or before 28 weeks gestation. For mothers who had a no previous infant with an ICH, at 20 weeks gestation IVIG would be started at 1 g/kg/wk and prednisone 0.5 mg/kg/d or IVIG 2 mg/kg/wk. At 32 weeks IVIG would be given at 2 mg/kg/wk and prednisone at 0.5 mg/kg/d. Delivery of the baby by cesarean section at 37 to 38 weeks gestation after lung maturity tests documented. For mothers who have had a previous infant with thrombocytopenia with a ICH after 28 weeks gestation, they would receive 1 g/kg/wk of IVIG starting at 12 weeks gestation, increasing the dose to 2 g/kg/wk at 20 weeks or adding prednisone 0.5 mg/kg/d and at 28 weeks gestation give 2 mg/kg/wk of IVIG and prednisone 0.5 mg/kg/d with delivery by cesarean section at 35 to 36 weeks gestation after lung maturity tests documented. And for the mothers who had a previous infant with and ICH before 28 weeks gestation, she should receive IVIG 2 g/kg/wk at 12 weeks gestation, add prednisone at 0.5 mg/kg/d at 20 weeks gestation and deliver the baby at 35 to 36 weeks gestation by cesarean section after lung maturity tests are documented. For all three categories, vaginal deliveries are recommended only if percutaneous umbilical cord sampling at 32 weeks shows a platelet count of more than 100,000/mm^3 (Pacheo et al., 2012).

■ Postnatal Treatment. Postnatal treatment consists of platelet transfusion, exchange transfusion with blood less than 2 days old, steroid therapy (prednisone, 1 to 5 mg/kg/d), and IVIG. The major difference in therapy between ITP and alloimmune thrombocytopenia is the use of washed, irradiated, maternal platelets in infants with alloimmune thrombocytopenia.

Neonatal Factors

Neonatal factors associated with thrombocytopenia include asphyxia, an Apgar score of less than 7, DIC, exchange transfusion, infection, smallness for gestational age, necrotizing enterocolitis, hyperbilirubinemia and phototherapy, meconium aspiration, cold injury, polycythemia, pulmonary hypertension, and cardiopulmonary bypass procedure. Treatment of thrombocytopenia caused by neonatal factors consists initially of amelioration of the underlying problem, followed by symptomatic treatment with platelet transfusion. Transfusion therapy should be considered if platelet counts are in the range of 50,000/mm^3 to 100,000/mm^3 and active bleeding is present. Platelet transfusion should be considered when the level is below 50,000/mm^3 even if active bleeding is not present. Transfusion with 10 to 15 mL/kg of platelets will generally yield an increase of 50,000 uL to 100,000 u/L as long as there are no predisposing factors for continued platelet destruction (Luchtman-Jones & Wilson, 2011; Pacheo et al., 2012).

Disseminated Intravascular Coagulopathy

DIC is marked by a generalized deficiency of coagulation factors and platelets, which leave the infant predisposed to hemorrhage. Because this condition is triggered by a preexisting illness and does not occur independently, treatment consists of identification and resolution of the underlying problem. Releases of tissue factor and substantial injury to endothelial cells are the two major mechanisms that precipitate DIC (Hall, 2011). The factors most often associated with bleeding that occurs secondary to DIC are obstetrical complications, respiratory distress syndrome, hypoxia, hypotension, necrotizing enterocolitis, and sepsis. Occasionally thrombosis of large vessels can trap platelets and consume an amount of clotting factors sufficient to cause DIC. Mortality rates reach 60% to 80% in infants with DIC who experience severe bleeding (Luchtman-Jones & Wilson, 2011).

The hematologic picture of DIC (Table 13.8) reflects a depletion of platelets, prothrombin, fibrinogen, angiotensin III (AT III), protein C, and Factors V, VIII, and XIII. The prothrombin time and partial thromboplastin time are prolonged and are not corrected by the addition of fresh frozen plasma to the blood sample. The fibrinolytic system is also stimulated, as evidenced by the presence of degradation products of fibrinolysis (i.e., fibrin degradation products or fibrinolytic split products). A commonly used test, measurement of d-dimer, serves as an evaluation of the activation of the fibrinolytic system in that it measures degradation of cross-linked fibrin. However, the D-dimer test may not be very helpful in the newborn because the result commonly is positive in infants who do not have a consumptive coagulopathy (Luchtman-Jones & Wilson, 2011).

TABLE 13.8

LABORATORY FINDINGS IN DISSEMINATED INTRAVASCULAR COAGULATION

Laboratory Test	Results
Platelet count	Decreased
PT	Prolonged
PTT	Prolonged
Fibrinogen	Decreased
Factor V and VIII	Decreased
Factor VII and IX	Normal
AT III	Decreased
Protein C	Decreased
Heparin co-factor II	Decreased
Fibrin	Elevated
Fibrinogen degradation products	Elevated
D-dimer	Increased
Hematocrit	Decreased
Bleeding time	Prolonged
Red blood cell on smear	Fragmented

Information from Luchtman-Jones and Wilson (2011).

Successful treatment of DIC depends on alleviation of the underlying cause. Palliative treatment consists of replacement of deficient clotting factors with fresh frozen plasma and cryoprecipitate, platelet transfusions, and exchange transfusion. Heparin is used infrequently because it carries a higher risk of hemorrhage; it is used only when large-vessel thrombosis occurs (Luchtman-Jones & Wilson, 2011).

■ **Protein C and S Deficiency.** Protein C and S are two of several anticoagulant proteins and are inherited in an autosomal dominant pattern. Heterozygous deficiency causes increased incidence of thrombosis, but are rare in the neonatal period. Homozygous Protein C or S deficiency will present in the neonatal period and can occur in the first few hours to days of life. Patients affected by a protein C or S deficiency will present with purpura fuliminans, severe DIC, and life-threatening thrombosis. Diagnosis is done with laboratory tests that are consistent with DIC, and there is no measurable protein by assay. Treatment if done early can improve clinical outcomes. Treatment consists of the administration of fresh frozen plasma. A protein C concentrate is available in the United States for compassionate use only. Patients with this disease will need to be on lifelong warfarin therapy (Luchtman-Jones & Wilson, 2011).

Differential Diagnosis of Newborn Coagulopathies

Analysis of a number of factors often can aid in the identification of the specific coagulopathy affecting an infant. Careful evaluation of the following factors can pinpoint the correct diagnosis and influence the choice of therapy or intervention:

- A familial history of a bleeding disorder, such as hemophilia
- A maternal history of a bleeding disorder, as in autoimmune thrombocytopenia
- An obstetrical history that suggests a possible abnormality, as in maternal alloimmunization or hypofibrinogenemia
- An adverse neonatal history, such as with hypoxia or asphyxia
- Failure to administer prophylactic vitamin K at birth
- Physical manifestations of a bleeding disorder (e.g., obvious bleeding, the presence or absence of petechiae or ecchymosis) and the infant's overall condition
- Laboratory data that identify specific abnormalities, such as specific coagulation factor deficiencies, thrombocytopenia, and prolonged prothrombin time, partial thromboplastin time, and clotting times

Collaborative Management of a Coagulopathy

Care of an infant with a bleeding diathesis should be aimed at prevention of further injury or bleeding. Supportive care of fragile tissue and limiting the number of blood draws from sites other than central catheters are of great importance in the infant who lacks adequate clotting factors to control bleeding. Appropriate administration of platelets, clotting factors, or blood products requires the correct equipment, the correct method of administration, and conscientious monitoring of vital signs to ensure effective therapy without causing further harm to the infant. Wise decisions regarding replacement blood products are now important in light of the severe and potentially lethal sequelae of acquired infection. Adopting guidelines for transfusion therapy may safeguard infants and eliminate unnecessary exposure to blood products (see guideline at end of chapter). Monitoring of laboratory tests to determine continuing needs and the efficacy of therapy is important throughout the infant's course of therapy.

When blood or blood products are administered, the infant must be evaluated continuously for signs of fluid overload and untoward reaction. Although blood reactions are rare in the newborn, they tend to occur within the first 15 minutes of blood or blood product administration. Signs of such reactions include rashes, tachycardia, hypertension, hematuria, cyanosis, and hyperthermia. Throughout the acute course of illness, the Hct values and the state of perfusion, rather than the percentage of the infant's blood volume removed, should govern the decision on whether to transfuse. Symptoms of hypovolemia include metabolic acidosis, hypotension, poor perfusion, tachycardia, cyanosis, and shock (Luchtman-Jones & Wilson, 2011).

SUPPORT OF THE FAMILY OF THE INFANT WITH HEMATOLOGIC DISORDER

An ill neonate is a crisis for families as no one expects their baby to be born prematurely or ill. When a diagnosis of a hematologic disorder occurs, the physician should discuss with the parents the disease, cause, treatment and outcomes. Parents have a role in deciding the goals of the care to be delivered to their baby, but they cannot make an informed decision unless they have been presented complete and reliable information. Unfortunately, many times this type of information may not be available until after the acute phase of the disease.

During care of the infant with a hematologic disorder, health care professionals should keep the parents informed of what is occurring to their newborn and parents' wishes should be honored, if appropriate. More discussion of the care of the family is discussed in the chapters in Unit VI.

BLOOD COMPONENT REPLACEMENT THERAPY

Whole Blood

This product is not used for routine volume expansion because of the Hct dilution that occurs. It is used in surgical procedures that require large volumes of blood for replacement, for exchange transfusions, and for priming heart-lung oxygenators for extracorporeal membrane oxygenation (Fasano & Luban, 2010; Young, 2011).

Packed Red Blood Cells

Blood is "hard spun" to concentrate cells (Hct 70 to 90) and to allow the supernatant to be removed. Because of this form of preparation, less volume can be administered. Packed RBCs can be reconstituted with normal saline, 5% albumin, or fresh frozen plasma. Packed RBCs can be used in exchange transfusions or in the treatment of anemia in the acutely ill or symptomatic convalescent infant (Fasano & Luban, 2010; Young, 2011).

Washed Red Blood Cells

For additional protection, RBCs can be washed to remove as much of the plasma, nonviable RBCs, WBCs, and metabolic wastes as possible. To further eliminate the possibility of a graft-versus-host reaction, cells can be irradiated with 5,000 rad; this prevents T-lymphocyte proliferation and, when done in conjunction with washing, can remove up to 95% of T lymphocytes (Fasano & Luban, 2010; Young, 2011).

Frozen Deglycerolized Red Cells

Frozen storage of deglycerolized RBCs allows preservation of rare units of blood, but the cost of preparation increases considerably. In addition, this product tends to have a higher potassium content and hemoglobin concentration. Centrifuging it, removing the supernatant, and diluting it to the desired Hct tend to control these problems (Fasano & Luban, 2010; Young, 2011).

Fresh Frozen Plasma

A whole unit of fresh frozen plasma can be thawed, but once entered, it is good for only 6 hours. If, however, it is packaged in aliquots, such as a quad pack, before freezing and then thawed, the quad pack unit is good for 24 hours once it has thawed. Fresh frozen plasma provides a rich source of coagulation factors; 10 to 15 mL/kg, which contains 1 IU/mL of all clotting factors, raises the overall level of clotting factor activity by 20% to 30%. Fresh frozen plasma often can normalize prolonged prothrombin and partial thromboplastin times in the newborn who has a generalized deficiency in quantity and activity of available clotting factors (Fasano & Luban, 2010; Young, 2011).

Platelets

The number of platelets available for circulation after transfusion depends on the storage time. In transfusions using platelet bags less than 7 days old, the rise in platelet levels is comparable to the rise seen with the use of fresh platelets. Use of packs older than 7 days achieves only 70% of the rise seen with the use of fresh platelets. Platelets also can be concentrated by centrifuge if smaller volumes are required. An important caveat: Platelets require a special administration set for proper infusion (Fasano & Luban, 2010; Young, 2011).

Granulocytes

Granulocytes, which are used for infusion in septic infants with severe neutropenia, are prepared from fresh donor blood through the process of plasmapheresis. WBCs are removed from the unit of blood, but a large number of RBCs remain. For this reason, the donor unit must be typed and cross-matched to the infant for blood type and Rh compatibility. WBCs usually are irradiated to eliminate donor T cells in an effort to prevent graft-versus-host responses. The use of granulocyte transfusions remains controversial (Fasano & Luban, 2010; Young, 2011).

Cryoprecipitate

This form of plasma preparation is rich in Factors VIII and XIII and fibrinogen and is useful in the treatment of hemophilia. Because it is a single-donor collection, the risk for infection is lower than with pooled substances. Each unit of cryoprecipitate transfused raises fibrinogen levels by 200 mg/dL per 100 mL of the infant's blood volume (Fasano & Luban, 2010; Young, 2011).

Factor Concentrates

Factor concentrates are used as specific therapy for identified factor deficiencies. They are obtained from pooled plasma and expose the recipient to multiple donors, thereby increasing the potential for infection, especially with hepatitis B, CMV, and AIDS. Eighty percent of cases of hepatitis B-infected blood can be identified by the third-generation screening tests, and blood screening is also available for CMV. Because the risk for transmission of HIV is increased by pooled concentrates, it is now recommended that concentrates be treated with heat, solvent, steam, detergent, or ultraviolet light to kill any virus that may be present. Currently, it is unclear whether such treatment alters or inactivates the clotting activity of factor concentrates (Fasano & Luban, 2010; Young, 2011).

Protocols

■ Management of Jaundice in the Newborn Nursery

Nearly two thirds of the 4 million newborns born in the United States will develop clinical jaundice, but the majority will not develop any severe sequelae as a result of the hyperbilirubinemia (Kaplan, Wong, Sibley, & Stevenson, 2010). Knowing which neonate will or will not develop sequelae as a result of the hyperbilirubinimia is the challenge that health care professionals must face when caring for the newborn.

A major factor that makes a newborn more prone to developing more severe jaundice is prematurity. The more premature a baby is, the greater the risk. Several reasons for this is the premature infant liver has a delay in reaching maximum concentrations of uridine diphosphoglucouronate glucuronosyltransferase (UGT), the substance that helps with the breakdown of bilirubin. The premature baby may feed less than a term baby, which leads to fewer bowel movements, another essential component in eliminating bilirubin from the body (Kaplan et al., 2010).

As stated earlier in this chapter the sequelae related to hyperbilirubinemia is acute bilirubin encephalopathy (transient mild encephalopathy) and chronic bilirubin encephalopathy (kernicterus) (Kaplan et al., 2010). Kernicterus is a preventable disease if a newborn's jaundice is recognized and managed properly. The AAP in 1994 developed guidelines for health care professionals to manage hyperbilirubinemia in the newborn and revised them in 2004. A study by Burke et al. (2009) showed that since the implementation of the AAP 1994 guidelines the incidence of hospitalizations with a diagnosis of kernicterus in the United States has decreased, showing that proper adherence to the AAP guidelines helps to prevent long-term sequelae of hyperbilirubinemia.

Example of Transfusion Guidelines

- A central Hct should be obtained on admission, and no further Hct should be obtained unless specifically ordered.
- Transfusions generally should be considered only if acute blood loss of >10% associated with symptoms of decreased oxygen delivery occurs or if significant hemorrhage of >20% total blood volume occurs.
- In term and preterm infants, a transfusion should be considered if an immediate need for increased oxygen delivery to tissues is suspected clinically.
- Transfuse 20 mL/kg packed red cells unless the Hct is >29% (0.29). A volume of 20 mL/kg also could be used if significant phlebotomy losses are anticipated in smaller infants whose Hcts are >29% (0.29). The volume may be administered in two 10 mL/kg aliquots.
- For infants receiving erythropoietin, considerations of the above guidelines should be made regarding the rate of decrease in hemoglobin or Hct, the infant's reticulocyte count, the postnatal day of age, the need for supplemental oxygen, and the overall stability of the infant.
- Central measurements of hemoglobin or Hct are preferred; alternatively, heel stick measurements may be obtained after warming the heel adequately. An infant meeting the following criteria should not be transfused automatically, but a transfusion should or can be considered for the following:

1. A transfusion should be considered if acute blood loss of >10% associated with symptoms of decreased oxygen delivery occurs or if significant hemorrhage of >20% total blood volume occurs.
2. For infants requiring moderate or significant mechanical ventilation, defined as mean arterial pressure (MAP) >8 cm H_2O and FiO_2 >0.40 on a conventional ventilator or MAP >14 and FiO_2 >0.40 on high-frequency ventilator, transfusions can be considered if the Hct is <30% (0.30) (hemoglobin <10 g/dL [100 g/L]).
3. For infants requiring minimal mechanical ventilation, defined as MAP <8 cm H_2O and/or FiO_2 <0.40 on a conventional ventilator or MAP <14 and/or FiO_2 <0.40 on a high-frequency ventilator, transfusions can be considered if the Hct is <25% (0.25) (hemoglobin <8 g/dL [8 g/L]).
4. For infants receiving supplemental oxygen who do not require mechanical ventilation, transfusions can be considered if the Hct is <20% (0.20) (hemoglobin <7 g/dL [70 g/L]), and one or more of the following is present:
   - >24 hours of tachycardia (heart rate >180 beats/min) or tachypnea (respiratory rate >60 breaths/min)
   - A doubling of the oxygen requirement from the previous 48 hours
   - Lactate >2.5 mEq/L (2.5 mmol/L) or an acute metabolic acidosis (pH <7.20)
   - Weight gain <10 g/kg/d over the previous 4 days while receiving >120 kcal/kg/d
   - If the infant will undergo major surgery within 72 hours
5. For infants who have no symptoms, transfusions can be considered if the Hct is <18% (0.18) (hemoglobin <6 g/dL [60 g/L]) associated with an absolute reticulocyte count of <100_103/mcL (100_109/L) (<2%) (Ohls, 2012).

EVIDENCE-BASED PRACTICE BOX

Hyperbilirubinemia is the most common hematologic condition in the newborn period. If it is not treated properly, the levels of unconjugated bilirubin can rise and cross the blood–brain barrier causing kernicterus. Kernicterus is a devastating disease to an otherwise healthy neonate. Traditionally, hyperbilirubinemia has been treated with the use of phototherapy and if needed, an exchange transfusion. Emerging research in this area has focused on the use of immunoglobulins and metalloporphyrins to reduce the incidence and severity of hyperbilirubinemia and more importantly the resulting kernicterus.

A review of seven research studies by Alcock and Liley (2009) yielded only three that met the inclusion criteria of randomized or quasi-randomized controlled trials for the administration of IVIGs for isoimmune hemolytic disease. There were a total of 189 term and preterm infants in these three trials. IVIG was found to decrease significantly the need for exchange transfusion when compared to the control groups as well as decrease the mean number of exchange transfusions in the immunoglobulin treated group. Unfortunately, no long-term outcomes were reported of the infants in the studies. Due to the small number of studies and infants included in the studies, as well as no long-term outcomes being reported, the applicability of these studies is limited until further studies are done.

Another new treatment modality is the use of metalloporphyrins. Suresh, Martin, and Soll (2009) reviewed three small randomized control trial studies for a total of 170 preterm and term infants who received metalloporphyrins for unconjugated hyperbilirubinemia for any cause. They found that the infants who received metalloporphyrins appeared to have a lower maximum plasma bilirubin level, a lower frequency of severe hyperbilirubinemia, a decreased need for phototherapy, fewer bilirubin measurements, and a shorter hospital course than those who did not receive the metalloporphyrins. In both studies, neither group of infants needed an exchange transfusion. There was a small group of infants in both groups that did develop a photosensitivity rash, but the numbers are too small to rule out an increase in photosensitivity or other adverse reactions in the metalloporphyrin-treated infants. As in the immunoglobulin studies, neither of these studies reported on long outcomes of these infants, and the applicability of these studies is limited until larger studies is done.

Due to the limited studies on these two treatment modalities, the mainstay for treating hyperbilirubinemia in the neonate remains phototherapy and exchange transfusion, if needed.

CASE STUDY

■ Identification of Problem. A 4-day-old infant is admitted to the NICU with a history of jaundice and lethargy from his local pediatrician's office. A TSB test drawn at the pediatrician's office had a result of 38 mg%.

■ Assessment: History and Physical. The baby boy was born at 37 weeks gestation at 3.2 kg to a 28-year-old gravida 2 para 1 AB 1 mother of Asian descent. The pregnancy was complicated by a positive Group B bacterial streptococcal cultures, and the mother was treated with prophylactic antibiotics prior to delivery. The baby was born by vacuum-assisted vaginal delivery. The baby was vigorous at birth with Apgar scores of 8 and 9. The mother's blood type was O positive and the baby's blood type was A positive. The Coomb's test was positive. The breastfed infant had an unremarkable course at the delivery hospital but was noted to be jaundiced at 32 hours of age. A TSB was done with a result of 12.8%. He was discharged home at 46 hours of age.

On admission to the NICU, the infant was noted to be severely jaundiced but pink. His vital signs were within normal limits with an axillary temperature of 98.5° F, heart rate of 150 beats/min, respiratory rate of 55 breaths/min, and blood pressure of 60/36 mmHg with a mean of 48 mmHg. His weight on admission was noted to be 2.72 kg, a 15% loss. His examination was nonremarkable, except for his decreased response to stimuli, poor muscle tone, poor suck and a decreased Moro. His glucose screen was 50.

■ Differential Diagnosis. Many conditions are known to cause jaundice and lethargy in the newborn. The most common are hyperbilirubinemia, ABO incompatibility, G6PD, hypothyroidism, dehydration secondary to inadequate breastfeeding, sepsis, and kernicterus.

■ Diagnostic Tests. To determine the cause of the jaundice and lethargy, a CBC with differential, repeat TSB, electrolytes, calcium, glucose, liver function tests, and T4/TSH, G6PD screen, a hemoglobin electrophoresis, and blood culture all need to be ordered.

■ Working Diagnosis. The baby's repeat bilirubin was 40%; his CBC showed a WBC of 12.2/mm^3, with 35% segs, and 4% bands; his hemoglobin was 10.0 g%; his Hct was 28%, and his reticulocyte count was 3%. The G6PD screen was adequate. Electrolytes, liver function tests, calcium, and glucose were all within normal limits, and the free T4 was 1.1 ng/dL (NL: 0.9–2.1), but TSH was 25.76 mIU (NL: 1.7–9.1). The hemoglobin electrophoresis was "A, F". These test results suggest a working diagnosis of hyperbilirubinemia secondary to ABO incompatability and hypothyroidism.

■ Development of Management Plan. The main goal for an infant with a bilirubin of 40% is to reduce the bilirubin level as quickly as possible to prevent kernicterus. While the blood is being typed and cross-matched, the infant needs to be placed in a neutral thermal environment, made NPO, have a peripheral IV placed and IV fluids of D10.2NS with 20 KCL/L at 120 mL/kg/hr, and started on antibiotics. An attempt should be made to do a cutdown of the umbilical cord to place an umbilical vein and arterial catheter for the exchange transfusion. Double phototherapy lights need to be started immediately.

■ Implementation and Evaluation of Effectiveness A double volume exchange transfusion was done over 3 hours. The infant received calcium and glucose boluses during the transfusion for low calcium and glucose. Phototherapy lights were continued after the transfusion. His laboratory tests of TSB, electrolytes, CBC with differential, glucose, and calcium were repeated after the exchange transfusion was completed. His postprocedure TSB level was 23%.

During the exchange transfusion the baby became apneic, which required intubation and the need for ventilation for 1 day. He received antibiotics for 2 days as phototherapy for 4 days. He was started on Synthroid for his abnormal TSH.

On day of life 10, the TSB was 10 mg%. On examination, the infant was slightly hypertonic. A BAER was normal, but an MRI was consistent with kernicterus. He was discharged home with a referral made to the neonatal developmental clinic and early intervention to follow his developmental status.

ONLINE RESOURCES

Cochrane Library
http://www.cochranelibrary.com
Cochrane Reviews
http://www.cochrane.org/cochrane-reviews
Emedicine
http://www.emedicine.medscape.com
Kernicterus and Newborn Jaundice Online
http://www.kernicterus.org
MedlinePlus
http://www.nlm.nih.gov/medlineplus
National Blood Clot Alliance
http://www.stoptheclot.org
National Hemophilia Organization
http://www.hemophilia.org
Neonatology on the Web
http://www.neonatology.org
Pubmed
http://www.ncbi.nlm.nih.gov/pubmedhealth

REFERENCES

Aher, S. M., & Ohlsson, A. (2010a, January 20). Early vs late erythropoietin for preventing red blood cell transfusion in preterm and or low birth weight infants. *Cochrane Reviews.*

Aher, S. M., & Ohlsson, A. (2010b, April 14). Late erythropoietin for preventing red blood cell transfusion in preterm and or low birth weight infants. *Cochrane Reviews.*

Alcock, G. S., & Liley, H. (2009, January 21). Immunoglobulin infusion for isoimmune haemolytic jaundice in neonates. *Cochrane Reviews.* doi: 10.1002/14651858.CD003313

Ambalavanan, N., & Carlo, W. A. (2011). Kernicterus. In R. M. Kliegman, B. F. Stanton, St. J. W. Geme, N. F. Schor, & R. E. Behrman (Eds.), *Nelson textbook of pediatrics* (19th ed.). Philadelphia, PA: Elsevier.

American Congress of Obstetrics and Gynecology. (1999, May). Prevention of RhD alloimmunization. *ACOG Practice Bulletin, 4.* Reaffirmed 2007 Clinical management guidelines for obstetricians and gynecologists. *American College of Obstetrics and Gynecology.*

American Academy of Pediatric (AAP) & The American College of Obstetrics and Gynecology (ACOG). (2007). *Guidelines for perinatal care* (6th ed.). Elk Grove, IL: AAP.

American Academy of Pediatrics (AAP) & Committee on Fetus and Newborn. (2009). Controversies concerning vitamin K and the newborn. *Pediatrics, 112*(1), 191–192, Reaffirmed 2006, September 1 and 2009, August 1.

American Academy of Pediatrics, Provisional Committee for Quality Improvement, & Subcommittee on Hyperbilirubinemia. (2004). Management of hyperbilirubinemia in the newborn infant 35 or more weeks of gestation. *Pediatrics, 114,* 297–316.

Andersson, O., Hellström-Westas, L., Andersson, D., & Domellöf, M. (2011). Effect of delayed versus early umbilical cord clamping on neonatal outcomes and iron status at 4 months: A randomised controlled trial. *British Medical Journal, 343,* d7157. doi:10.1136/bmj.d7157

Andrew, M., et al. (1990). Development of the hemostatic system in the neonate and young infant. *American Journal of Pediatric Hematology/Oncology, 12,* 97–98.

Ashan, S., & Noether, J. (2011). *Harriet Lane handbook* (19th ed.). Philadelphia, PA: Elsevier.

Baker, R. D., Greer, F. A., & The Committee on Nutrition. (2010). Diagnosis and prevention of iron deficiency and iron deficiency anemia in infants and young children (0–3 years age). *Pediatrics, 126,* 1040–1050.

Bergeron, M. J., & Gourley, G. R. (2009). Disorders of bilirubin metabolism. In S. H. Orkin, D. G. Nathan, D. Ginsburg, A. T. Lock, D. E. Fisher., & S. E. Lux (Eds.), *Nathan and Oski's hematology in infancy and childhood* (7th ed.). Philadelphia, PA: Saunders/Elsevier.

Berkowitz, R. L., Kolb, E. A., McFarland, J. G., Wissert, M., Primani, A., & Lesser, M. (2006). Parallel randomized trials of risk-based therapy for fetal alloimmune thrombocytopenia. *Obstetrics Gynecology, 107,* 91–96.

Bhutani, V. K., & The Committee on Fetus and Newborn. (2011). Phototherapy to prevent severe neonatal hyperbilirubinemia in the newborn infant 35 or more weeks of gestation. *Pediatrics, 128,* e1046–e1052.

Brown, M. (1988). Physiologic anemia of infancy: Normal red cell values and physiology of neonatal erythropoiesis. In J. Stockman & C. Pochedly (Eds.), *Developmental and neonatal hematology.* New York, NY: Raven Press.

Brugnara, C., & Platt, O. S. (2009). The neonatal erythrocyte and its disorders. In S. H. Orkin, D. G. Nathan, D. Ginsburg, A. T. Lock, D. E. Fisher, & S. E. Lux (Eds.), *Nathan and Oski's hematology in infancy and childhood* (7th ed.). Philadelphia, PA: Saunders/Elsevier.

Burke, B. L., Robbins, J. M., Bird, T. M., Hobbs, C. A., Nesmith, C., & Tifford, J. M. (2009). Trends in hospitalizations for neonatal jaundice and kernicterus in the United States, 1988–2005. *Pediatrics, 123*(2), 524–532.

Cantor, A. B. (2008). Developmental hemostasis: Relevance to newborns and infants. In S. H. Orkin, D. G. Nathan, D. Ginsburg, A. T. Lock, D. E. Fisher, & S. E. Lux (Eds.), *Nathan and Oski's hematology in infancy and childhood* (7th ed.). Philadelphia, PA: Saunders/Elsevier.

Cashore, W. (2011). Neonatal bilirubin metabolism (pp. 1291–1295). In R. Polin, W. Fox, & S. Abman (Eds.), *Fetal and neonatal physiology*. Philadelphia, PA: Saunders.

Christensen, R. (1989). Recombinant erythropoietic growth factors as an alternative to erythrocyte transfusion for patients with anemia of prematurity. *Pediatrics, 83*, 793–796.

Deshpande, P. G. (2012). Breast milk jaundice. *eMedicine*. Retrieved from http://emedicine.medscape.com/article/973629

Diacovo, T. (2011). Platelet-vessel wall interactions (pp. 1547–1552). In R. Polin, W. Fox, & S. Abman (Eds.), *Fetal and neonatal physiology*. Philadelphia, PA: Saunders.

Donato, H., Vain, N., Rendo, P., Vivas, N., Prudent, L., Larquia, M., ... Gorenstein, A. (2000). Effect of early versus late administration of human recombinant erythropoietin on transfusion requirements in premature infants: Results of randomized, placebo controlled, multicenter trial. *Pediatrics, 105*, 1066–1072.

Edstrom, C., et al. (2000). Developmental aspects of blood hemostasis and disorders of coagulation and fibrinolysis in the neonatal period. In R. Christensen (Ed.), *Hematologic problems of the neonate*. Philadelphia, PA: Saunders.

Fasano, R., & Luban, N. (2010). Blood component therapy for the neonate. In R. Martin, A. Fanaroff, & M. Walsh (Eds.), *Neonatal-perinatal medicine. Diseases of the fetus and newborn* (9th ed., pp. 1360–1374). Boston, MA: Mosby.

Hall, J. E. (2011). *Guyton and hall textbook of medical physiology* (12th ed.). Philadelphia, PA: Saunders/Elsevier.

Hansen, T. W. R. (2012). Neonatal jaundice treatment and management. *eMedicine*. Retrieved from http://emedicine.medscape.com/article/974786

Huizing, K., Roislien, J., & Hansen, T. (2008). Intravenous immune globulin reduces the need for exchange transfusions in Rhesus and ABO incompatibility. *Acta Paediatrica, 97*(10), 1362–1365.

Hutton, E. K., & Hassan, E. S. (2007). Late vs early clamping of the umbilical cord in full term neonates: Systematic review and metaanalysis of controlled trials. *Journal of the American Medical Association, 297*(11), 1241–1252.

Johnson, L. H., Bhutani, V. K., & Brown, A. K. (2002). System-based approach to management of neonatal jaundice and prevention of kernicterus. *Journal of Pediatrics, 140*(4), 396–403.

Kaplan, M., Wong, R., Sibley, E., & Stevenson, D. (2010). Neonatal jaundice and liver disease. In R. Martin, A. Fanaroff, & M. Walsh (Eds.), *Neonatal-perinatal medicine. Diseases of the fetus and newborn* (9th ed., pp. 1443–1496). Boston, MA: Mosby.

Lessaris, K. J. (2012). Polycythemia in the newborn. *eMedicine*. Retrieved from http://emedicine.medscape.com/article/976319

Lexi-Comp Online. *Lexi-Drugs Online*. Hudson, OH: Lexi-Comp Inc.

Liley, H. G. (2009). Immune hemolytic disease in the newborn. In S. H. Orkin, D. G. Nathan, D. Ginsburg, A. T. Lock, D. E. Fisher, & S. E. Lux (Eds.), *Nathan and Oski's hematology in infancy and childhood* (7th ed.). Philadelphia, PA: Saunders/Elsevier.

Luchtman-Jones, L., & Wilson, D. B. (2011). The blood and hematopoietic system. In R. J. Martin, A. A. Fanaroff, & M. C. Walsh (Eds.), *Fanaroff and Martin's neonatal-perinatal medicine: Diseases of the fetus and infant* (9th ed.). St. Louis, MO: Elsevier/Mosby.

Maier, R. F., Obladen, M., & Wardrop, C. A. (1994). The effect of epoetin-beta (recombinant human erythropoietin) on the need for transfusion in very-low-birth-weight infants. *New England Journal of Medicine, 330*, 1173–1178.

McDonald, S. J., & Middleton, P. (2008, April 16). Effect of timing of umbilical cord clamping on term infants on maternal and neonatal outcome. *Cochrane Database Systemic Reviews*, (2).

Messer, J., Haddad, J., Donato, L., & Matis, J. (1993). Early treatment of premature infants with recombinant human erythropoietin. *Pediatrics, 92*, 519–523.

Meyer, M. P., Meyer, J. H., Commerford, A., Hann, F. M., Sive, A. A., Moller, G., ... Malan, A. F. (1994). Recombinant human erythropoietin in the treatment of anemia of prematurity: Results of a double-blind, placebo-controlled study. *Pediatrics, 93*, 918–923.

Mintz, P. D. (2005). Rh immune globin. In P. D. Mintz (Ed.), *Transfusion therapy: Clinical principles and practice* (2nd ed.). Bethesda, MD: AABB Press.

Monagie, P., & Hagstrom, J. (2011). Developmental hemostasis. In R. Polin, W. Fox, & S. Abman (Eds.), *Fetal and neonatal physiology* (pp. 1538–1546). Philadelphia, PA: Saunders.

Nunes dos Santos, A. M., & Trindade, C. E. P. (2011). Red blood cell transfusions in the neonate. *Neoreviews, 12*, e13. doi:10.1542/neo.12-1-e13

Obis, R. (2011). Developmental erythropoiesis. In R. Polin, W. Fox, & S. Abman (Eds.), *Fetal and neonatal physiology* (pp. 1495–1519). Philadelphia, PA: Saunders.

Oh, W., Fanaroff, A. A., Carlo, W. A., Donovan, E. F., McDonald, S. A., Poole, W. K., & Eunice Kennedy Shriver National Institute of Child Health and Human Development Neonatal Research Network. (2011, April). Effects of delayed cord clamping in very-low-birth-weight infants. *Journal of Perinatology* (Suppl. 1), *31*, S68–S71.

Ohls, R. (2001). Anemia in the newborn. In R. Polin, et al. (Eds.), *Workbook in practical neonatology* (3rd ed.). Philadelphia, PA: Saunders.

Ohls, R. (2012). Red blood cell transfusions in the newborn. In D. H. Mahoney & J. A. Garcia-Prats (Eds.), *UptoDate*. Waltham, MA: UptoDate.

Ohls, R. K., Hunter, D. D., & Christensen, R. D. (1993). A randomized, double-blind, placebo-controlled trial of recombinant erythropoietin in treatment of the anemia of bronchopulmonary dysplasia. *Journal of Pediatrics, 23*, 996–1000.

Ohls, R. K., Osborne, K. A., & Christensen, R. D. (1995). Efficacy and cost analysis of treating very-low-birth-weight infants with erythropoietin during their first 2 weeks of life: A randomized, placebo-controlled trial. *Journal of Pediatrics, 126*, 421–426.

Ozolek, J. A., Watchko, J. F., & Mimouni, F. B. (1994). Prevalence and lack of clinical significance of blood group incompatibility in mothers with blood type A or B. *Journal of Pediatrics, 125*, 87–91.

Pacheo, L. D., Berkowitz, R. L., Moise, K. J., Bussel, J. B., McFarland, J. G., & Saade, G. R. (2012). Fetal and neonatal alloimmune thrombocytopenia: A management algorithm based on risk stratification. *Obstetrics and Gynecology, 118*(5), 1157–1163.

Pernoll, M., et al. (1986). Neonatal hyperbilirubinemia and prevention of kernicterus. In M. Pernoll et al. (Ed.), *Diagnosis and management of the fetus and neonate at risk* (5 th ed.). St Louis, MO: Mosby.

Porter, T. F., Peltier, M., & Branch, D. W. (2003). Immunologic disorders in pregnancy. In J. R. Scott & D. N. Danforth (Eds.), *Danforth's obstetrics and gynecology* (9th ed.). Philadelphia, PA: Lippincott.

Rund-Hansen, T. (2011). Mechanisms of bilirubin-induced brain injury. In R. Polin, W. Fox, & S. Abman (Eds.), *Fetal and neonatal physiology* (pp. 1295–1306). Philadelphia, PA: Saunders.

Sacks, L., & Delivoria-Papadopoulos, M. (1984). Hemoglobin-oxygen interactions. *Seminars in Perinatology, 8*:168–183.

Schulman, I. (1962). Pediatric aspects of the mild hemophilias. *Medical Clinics of North America, 46*, 93–105.

Shannon, K. M., Keith, J. F., 3rd., Mentzer, W. C., Ehrenkranz, R. A., Brown, M. S., Widness, J. A., ... Davis, C. B. (1995). Recombinant human erythropoietin stimulates erythropoiesis and reduces erythrocyte transfusions in very-low-birth-weight preterm infants. *Pediatrics, 95*, 1–8.

Smits-Wintjens, V. E., Walther, F. J., & Lopriore, E. (2008). Rhesus haemolytic disease of the newborn: Postnatal management, associated morbidity and long-term outcome. *Seminars Fetal Neonatal Medicine, 13*, 265–271.

Sollman, H., & Sola-Visner, M. (2012). Clincal and research issues in neonatal anemia and thrombocytopenia. *Current Opinion in Pediatrics, 24*(1), 16–22.

Springer, S. C. (2010). Kernicterus. *eMedicine*. Retrieved from http://emedicine.medscape.com/article/975276

Stockman, J. et al. (1977). The anemia of infancy and the anemia of prematurity: Factors governing the erythropoietin response. *New England Journal of Medicine, 296*, 647.

Suresh, G., Martin, C. L., & Soll, R. (2009, January 21). Metalloporphyrins for treatment of unconjugated hyperbiliruinemia in neonates. *Cochrane Review*. doi: 10.1002/14651858.CD004207

Walsh, S., & Molloy, E. J. (2009). Is intravenous immunoglobulin superior to exchange transfusion in the management of hyperbilirubinemia in term neonates? *Archive Diseases in Childhood, 94*(9), 739–741.

Widness, J. A., Madan, A., Grindeanu, L. A., Zimmerman, M. B., Wong, D. K., & Stevenson, D. K. (2005). Reduction in red blood cell transfusions among preterm infants: Results of a randomized trial with an in-line blood gas and chemistry monitor. *Pediatrics, 115*(5), 1299–1306.

Wilburm, A., Nienhuis, A. W., & Persons, D. A. (2011). Transcriptional regulation of fetal to adult hemoglobin switching: New therapeutic opportunities. *Blood, 117*(15), 3945–3953.

Witt, S. (1948). *Hemostatic agents*. Springfield, IL: Charles C. Thomas Publishers, Ltd.

Yoder, M. (2011). Developmental biology of stem cells: From the embryo to the adult. In R. Polin, W. Fox, & S. Abman (Eds.), *Fetal and neonatal physiology* (pp. 1459–1468). Philadelphia, PA: Saunders.

Young, G. (2011). Hemostatic disorders of the newborn. In C. A. Gleason & S. Devasker (Eds.), *Avery's diseases of the newborn* (9th ed., pp. 1056–1079). Philadelphia, PA: Saunders.

Zaiden, R. A. (2012). Hemophilia A and B. *Emedicine*. Retrieved from http://emedicine.medscape.com/article/77934

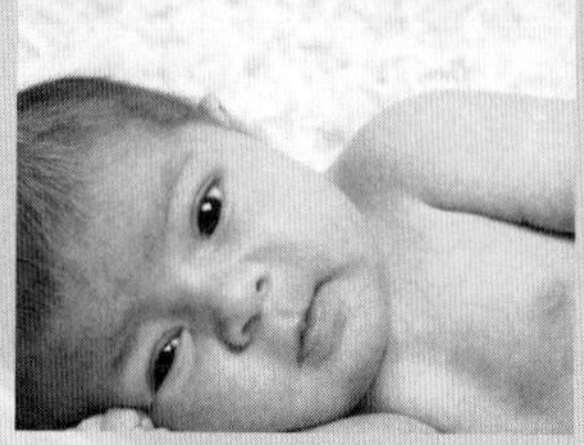

CHAPTER

14

Musculoskeletal System

■ Joyce M. Butler and Beth Mullins

Abnormalities of the neonatal musculoskeletal system range from a subtle brachydactyly to a fatalistic form of osteogenesis imperfecta (OI) congenita. Causes range from uterine malpositioning of the fetus to autosomal dominant disorders. Regardless of the clinical significance, an overt structural defect can become the focus of parental attention. Assessment of the musculoskeletal system—which can have multiple normal variants—and knowledge of pathogenesis, sequelae, treatment, and prognoses for deformities of this system are imperative to the clinician (Box 14.1). Delay in diagnosis and treatment may be implicated as a cause of a less than favorable outcome of the musculoskeletal deformity. Appropriate education of the family by the health care professional is often paramount to a beneficial outcome because many musculoskeletal disorders require compliance with long-term therapy.

BOX 14.1

COMMON MUSCULOSKELETAL CONDITIONS

Skeletal Dysplasias

- OI
- Achondroplasia
- Arthrogryposis
- Congenital hip dislocation

Limb Defects

- Clubfoot
- Syndactyly
- Polydactyly
- Amniotic band syndrome
- Birth trauma
- Torticollis

The following are common terms that are used when discussing the musculoskeletal system:

- Valgus refers to a deformity in which a body part is bent outward and away from the midline of the body; it is a part that is in abduction.
- Varus implies a body part positioned inward, toward the midline of the body; it is a part that is in adduction.
- Talipes refers to any one of various foot deformities.
- Reduction is restoration to a normal position.
- Avulsion is the tearing away of a part or segment.
- Plagiocephaly describes a misshapen skull/head.
- Subluxation describes an incomplete dislocation or a displaced joint.

Deformities of the musculoskeletal system create not only functional problems but, in some cases, visible defects as well. The type of dysfunction may greatly affect how the parent views the neonate and the infant's potential for positive growth and development.

This chapter describes musculoskeletal problems seen in the neonatal period. The collaborative management of these problems is discussed, as well as the long-term implications of the functional and aesthetic problems encountered with musculoskeletal dysfunction.

EMBRYOLOGY

The embryonic period is characterized by maximal organogenesis and lasts from the end of the first week until the eighth week of gestation. The embryo originates from three cell layers—termed the ectoderm, endoderm, and mesoderm. The embryonic mesoderm gives rise to the articular, muscular, and skeletal systems.

The articular system, or joints, can be classified into three types: fibrous, cartilaginous, and synovial. Fibrous joints are those in which two bones are separated only by dense fibrous connective tissue, as seen in cranial sutures. Cartilaginous joints (such as the symphysis pubis and between the intervertebral discs of the spine) have hyaline cartilage or fibrocartilage between the two bony surfaces. The elbow and knee are examples of synovial joints. In these joints, the adjoining bone ends are covered with a thin cartilaginous layer and joined by a ligament lined with a synovial membrane. This synovial membrane secretes a lubricant referred to as synovial fluid, a source of nutrition for the articular cartilage. The synovial joints are the most movable. The articular system begins to develop during the sixth week of gestation, with functional joints being present by the end of the eighth week.

Groups of myotubes, the primordia of skeletal or striated muscle, are apparent by the end of the eighth week of gestation. As the myotubes enlarge, the appearance of myofilaments is evident in interior regions. Growth of myofilaments leads to mature muscle fibers. Postnatal development of muscle fibers continues both in number and in size. Muscle development depends on proper innervation, evident at 8 to 10 weeks of gestation. Without this innervation, the muscles atrophy. The mother can detect intrauterine fetal movements at 16 weeks of gestation. The upper limbs develop more quickly than the lower limbs, and several days elapse between the development of the upper limbs and that of the lower limbs.

The skeleton develops by intramembranous bone formation and endochondral ossification. The vertebral column is initially of a cartilaginous form, with ossification beginning during the embryonic period and reaching completion in early adulthood. Ossification is evident in all long bones by 12 weeks gestation.

Rapid cell division during organogenesis renders an organ vulnerable to any disturbance that might result in aberrant development. Functional and minor morphologic abnormalities may occur any time during gestation. The skeletal system, because of rapid growth through puberty, has a prolonged period of sensitivity.

ASSESSMENT

Detailed observation is the key tool for assessing the neonatal musculoskeletal system. Visual inspection should begin in one body region—that is, cephalic or caudal—and progress along the body in an organized fashion. For the initial examination, place the infant in a quiet resting state to assess posture, positioning, and identification of any obvious anomalies. Active movement by the infant allows the clinician to view muscle tone and active ranges of motion. Manipulation is used to assess passive range of motion, including joint mobility. Radiologic studies as well as simple body measurements aid the health care provider in the identification of covert or hidden musculoskeletal deformities such as hip dysplasias and absence of bony structures to name a few.

Maternal history is reviewed for uterine anomalies that may compromise fetal movement and growth, such as the bifid uterus, which describes the division of the uterine cavity into two segments. Additional maternal and a family history that are important include previous family members, especially siblings, with musculoskeletal anomalies; presence of oligohydramnios; and fetal movement during gestation and the birthing process.

In developing a differential diagnosis, the clinician must be aware that a combination of deformities present in a neonate may be a small part of a larger syndrome. Conversely, congenital anomalies that present in combination may be a coincidental finding (Box 14.1).

TYPES OF MUSCULOSKELETAL DYSFUNCTION

Osteogenesis Imperfecta

Osteogenesis imperfecta (OI), sometimes called the "brittle bone disease," is a disorder caused by a genetic mutation affecting collagen, the major extracellular protein. The incidence of this disorder is about 1 per 20,000 births. Most patients with OI have a mutation on the *COL1A1* or *COL1A2* genes. Collagen is found in bone, sclera, ligaments, skin, and teeth. In this disorder, all of these tissues may be affected (Sillence & Danks, 1978).

The clinical presentation of OI varies greatly, depending on the particular type. There is also a wide range of severity and symptoms within each type. The classification system described by Sillence and Danks outlines four basic types of OI. Additional types described in the literature do not appear to have defects in the collagen genes.

Types of OI and Clinical Presentation

OI type I has an autosomal dominant inheritance pattern. In general, type I is the mildest type of OI, but the clinical appearance of affected individuals may range from mild to severe, even within the same family. A small number of patients with this type may present with fractures in the neonatal period. An increased rate of fractures may be seen as the child begins to walk. Persons with this type are generally of normal height and stature. Sclerae are blue, and the teeth are also affected. In adults with type I OI, hearing loss may occur (Bishop, 2010). Premature or accelerated bone loss following menopause is also seen.

OI type II is also referred to as the lethal perinatal type. This is an autosomal recessive disorder that generally results in death either in utero or in the perinatal/neonatal period. The likelihood of prenatal diagnosis is increased with type II, due to the multiple fractures and bowing of extremities seen in utero. Death can occur secondary to damage of vital organs (brain, liver, and lungs) that are not protected by the fragile bony structures. Severe respiratory distress is seen secondary to the narrow and shortened ribcage. Infants with type II OI are small for gestational age with shortened body and legs, with the head appearing large for body size. The extremities tend to be shortened and deformed with multiple fractures. X-rays demonstrate multiple fractures, both old and new. Ribs and smaller bones may also appear thin and difficult to discern on x-ray. The trauma of birth takes a further toll on the appearance of these infants and contributes to the maceration of the head and limbs.

OI type III is a severe form with an autosomal recessive inheritance pattern. This is the most severe type for those surviving the neonatal period. Multiple fractures of the long bones may occur both before and after birth. There is significant deformity of the bones over time, with scoliosis and hearing loss. Sclerae may be blue. Infants with type III may have normal height and weight at birth. This deteriorates over time, with very short stature seen in childhood/adulthood. The severe deformities of the spine and thorax seen in type III can restrict breathing, leading to significant respiratory complications in adulthood. The life expectancy may be shortened due to these problems (Marini, 2011).

OI type IV is similar to type I in that it is an autosomal dominant disorder with variable penetrance. OI type IV resembles type I in terms of presentation. Newborns rarely have identified fractures, but a number of fractures occur as the child begins to ambulate, with increased weight bearing. These infants also present with growth that is average for gestational age. The growth pattern can change as the child matures secondary to increased bowing of extremities and kyphoscoliosis, with a short stature compared to a normal height at maturity with the milder forms of type I. OI type IV can also progress to a more severe form, depending on the degree of kyphoscoliosis and vertebral compression fractures, often resembling type III. Unlike type III, life span in type IV is not affected.

As stated earlier, additional types of OI have been identified since the original classification system was developed. These are described as types V, VI, VII, VIII. These types do not have defects in the collagen genes. However, the clinical features and management are similar to the other types of OI.

Diagnosis

OI may be suspected prenatally if there is a positive family history. Fractures and other deformities of the skeleton may be seen on ultrasound prior to birth. After birth, the diagnostic process is based largely on physical exam findings of fractures and deformities of the extremities. A skin biopsy can provide a definitive diagnosis through examination of collagen (Steiner, Pepin, & Byers, 2005).

Collaborative Management

Neonates with OI should be handled very gently to avoid causing new fractures and to reduce the pain of existing injuries. During care, they should be lifted by using the hands to gently support the buttocks and head. These patients should never be lifted by pulling the extremities, or with hands under the armpits. With diaper changes, it is important to never lift the baby by the ankles, but to move the diaper by lifting the buttocks. When dressing these infants, the caregiver should gently bring the garments over the arms and legs, while avoiding pulling the extremities through the sleeves and legs of the garments. Simple garments with wide openings for extremities are best. At discharge, a special car bed that allows prone positioning may be required (Neonatal and Nursery Care, 2012).

Feeding ability may be compromised with these infants, due to respiratory compromise and difficulty with positioning and handling. Gentle rubbing should be used for burping to avoid rib fractures. If these infants require prolonged immobilization during healing of fractures, measures to protect the skin and facilitate frequent repositioning may be used, such as gel pads or foam wedges. Pain management is also an important part of the care plan when fractures are present. IV medications or oral sucrose may be used, as well as other nursing measures to improve comfort and positioning (McLean, 2004).

The long-term medical management of patients with OI is focused on avoiding fractures and correcting deformities of bones, while maintaining maximal mobility and physical function. Intravenous bisphosphonates have shown some benefit by improving bone volume, though this does not change the essential defect of collagen (Monti et al., 2010). Growth hormone has also been used with the milder types of OI.

SKELETAL DYSPLASIA

Skeletal dysplasia is a term used to identify a group of clinical disorders that involve abnormal endochondral ossification. It includes achondroplasia, hypochondroplasia, and thanatophoric dysplasia, all of which present with a short-limbed skeletal dysplasia at varying ages of development.

Achondroplasia

Although the word *achondroplasia* was once used to describe any form of dwarfism, it is not recognized as one distinct type of dwarfism having characteristic features. Achondroplasia has an autosomal dominant pattern of inheritance (Wilkin et al., 1998) and is the most common nonlethal skeletal dysplasia. Most cases occur by spontaneous mutation, so many of these children have parents of normal stature. A mutation of the gene encoding fibroblast growth factor receptor-3 (FGFR3) has been implicated in this disorder. The incidence of achondroplasia has varied in the past as a result of multiple forms of skeletal dysplasia diagnosed as achondroplasia. The current incidence is 1 in 10,000 to 30,000 live births. One risk factor for spontaneous mutation that involves achondroplasia appears to be advanced paternal age.

Achondroplastic infants can be identified at birth with a rhizomelic shortening of the extremities. In other words, when the arms are viewed, the upper arm (humerus bone) will appear more severely shortened when compared to the lower arm (radius and ulnar bones). The same holds for the lower extremities, where the thigh (femur) will appear more severely shortened than the lower leg (tibia and fibular bones). The infant who is affected with achondroplasia also presents with a disproportionately large head with frontal bossing and depressed nasal bridge. The hands are small with a trident configuration that describes the appearance of the fingers and an increased spacing between the long and ring fingers (Horton & Hecht, 2011).

Identification of mild hypotonia and limitation of elbow extension with laxity in most other joints is also noted in the achondroplastic child. These neuromuscular and skeletal anomalies—including the mild hypotonia, rhizomelia, joint laxity, and reduced elbow extension—can produce a delay in gross motor milestones but generally improve to normal over the first few years of life. Central intelligence is normal in most cases.

Hypochondroplasia

Hypochondroplasia is rarely noted at birth, as the length of the infant is often normal. The short stature becomes clinically apparent around 24 months of age. This condition is rarely diagnosed in the neonatal period but may present with macrocephaly. Hypochondroplastic children and adults experience some of the similar orthopedic complications as the achondroplastic individual. Some of these include joint and lower back pain.

Thanatophoric Dysplasia

Thanatophoric dysplasia is the third in this series of common skeletal dysplasias. The name of this disorder is derived from the Greek word "thanatos," meaning "death." It is a lethal defect and is often compared to OI, type II, in terms of its clinical scenario after birth. Death usually occurs within a few hours or days secondary to respiratory failure from severe pulmonary hypoplasia. The clinical presentation of thanatophoric dysplasia describes a fetal environment of reduced fetal movements and polyhydramnios. Hypotonia in the neonate with macrocephaly, often presenting as a cloverleaf-shaped skull, is believed to be secondary to early fusion of the coronal and lambdoidal sutures. The limbs are short and bowed with severe brachydactyly or short digits. The thorax is very narrow and short, reminding the clinician of the abnormal pulmonary development and severe pulmonary hypoplasia. The abdomen has a protuberant appearance (Figures 14.1 and 14.2). Almost all cases of thanatophoric dysplasia result from a new genetic mutation, with a low risk of recurrence in subsequent pregnancies. As with other skeletal dysplasias, there is a defect in *FGFR3*, the *FGFR3* gene (Miller, Blaser, Shannon, & Widjaja, 2009).

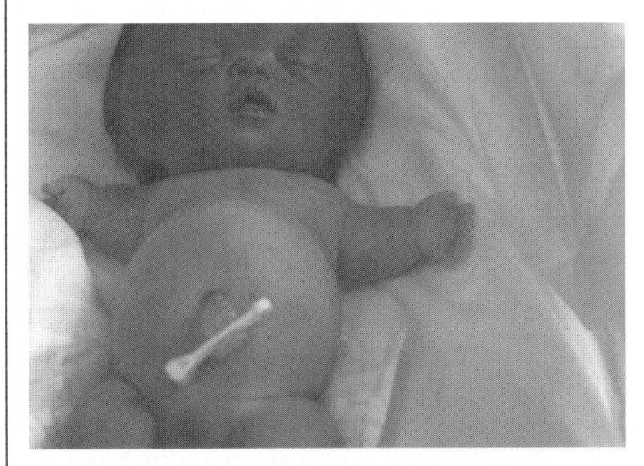

FIGURE 14.1 Thanatophoric dysplasia: narrow thorax and protuberant abdomen.

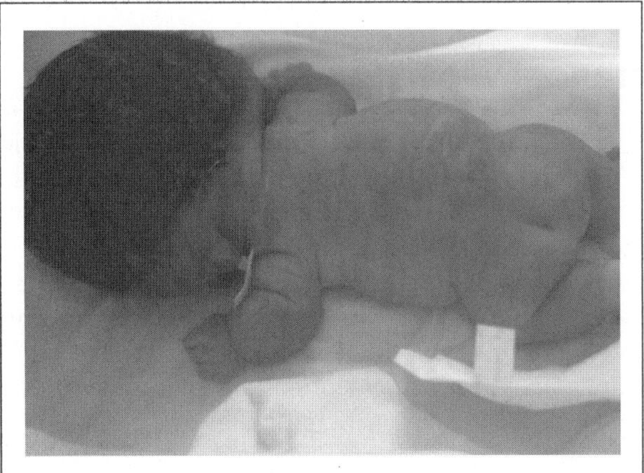

FIGURE 14.2 Thanatophoric dysplasia: shortened lower extremities.

Differential Diagnosis

The differential diagnosis of a neonate with dwarflike appearance includes achondroplasia, OI type II, thanatophoric dwarfism, asphyxiating thoracic dysplasia, lethal short limb-polydactyly syndromes, and achondrogenesis. In achondroplasia, the patients has markedly shortened limbs and often bowing of the lower limbs, but radiographic studies do not show evidence of multiple fractures and long-bone crumbling as seen in OI type II. Thanatophoric dwarfism and achondrogenesis, both typically fatal in the neonatal period, are characterized by an extremely narrow chest and marked defective ossification, respectively (Shirley & Ain, 2009). These disorders may be detected prenatally through ultrasound identification of the abnormal skeletal features.

Management

Management of skeletal dysplasias depends on the long-term outcome for the specific type of dysplasia. As noted in the previous section, some of the skeletal dysplasias are lethal during the newborn period. With nonlethal varieties, the complications are primarily neurologic and involve the spinal nerves. Anatomic configuration of the intraspinal canal results in pressure on the cord and spinal nerves. This pressure produces chronic backache and, in the most severe scenario, paraplegia. Referrals to physical and occupational therapists, along with long-term orthopedic follow-up, can reduce some of the complications. If these changes in the spinal column do occur, the child is at greatest risk for development of increased respiratory difficulties, mobility problems, self-concept and self-esteem concerns, physical pain, and central or peripheral nervous system neuropathies. Other common long-term complications include recurrent otitis media, hearing loss, dental overcrowding, and sleep apnea, which may present in childhood (Sisk, Heatley, Borowski, Leverson, & Pauli, 1999).

Limb-lengthening techniques are sometimes used in management of skeletal dysplasias. This has been done in an attempt to reduce the functional and psychosocial difficulties associated with very short stature. The process of limb-lengthening is very arduous and surgically complex, with lengthy rehabilitation periods. Often, the physical outcome does not match the desired result, so the benefit of these procedures remains uncertain (Wright & Irving, 2012).

Because children with achondroplasia have a different appearance than their peers, any exaggeration of the condition can add to a faulty self-concept. As the child grows, continual assessment by health care professionals and the parents concerning the personal image that the child is developing is prelude to a positive self-esteem. Positive support of parents during the neonatal period through comments about what the infant is doing and how the infant looks may provide a role model of positive behavior that the parents can emulate with the child.

ARTHROGRYPOSIS

Historically, the term *arthrogryposis* (curved, hooked joint) has been used not only to provide a description of a clinical appearance but also as a diagnosis for various conditions (Figure 14.3). The one common denominator for conditions termed arthrogryposis is the presence of multiple congenital joint contractures. More than 150 known conditions feature multiple congenital contractures as the dominant feature. Many of these conditions are syndromes unrelated to a chromosomal or genetic problem.

Pathogenesis

Arthrogryposis describes limitation of movement in multiple joints that is present at birth. Due to the variety of conditions that may be associated with this condition, the etiology is varied, but decreased fetal movement is the common factor in all cases. With decreased movement, extra connective tissue forms around the joints of the fetus and fixes them in position. This may be related to abnormal development of the muscles, tendons, and/or joints as listed in Table 14.1. In some cases, the fetus may be kept from normal movement due to restrictions within the uterus from multiple pregnancy or abnormalities of the uterine structure. Maternal diseases such as myasthenia gravis or myotonic dystrophy may be related to arthrogryposis, as well as the use of certain medications or infections in the mother. Intrauterine vascular compromise is another potential associated factor, with damage to developing muscles and nerves due to decreased blood flow (O'Flaherty, 2001). Finally, abnormalities of the central nervous system in the fetus may be a cause, such as spinal muscle atrophy (SMA) or cerebro-oculo-facial-skeletal syndrome (Table 14.1).

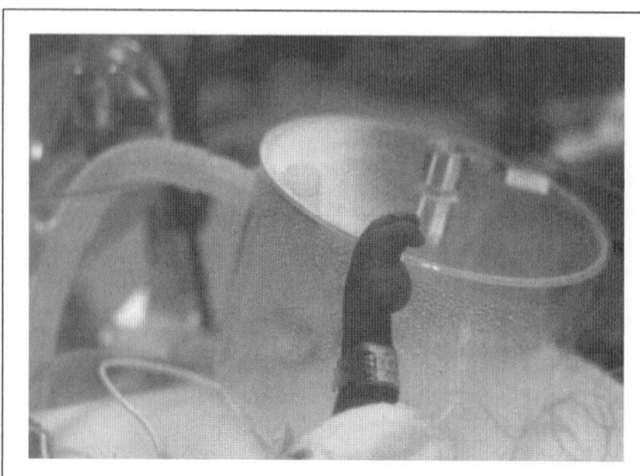

FIGURE 14.3 Distal fixed joints: arthrogryposis.

Clinical Manifestations

Arthrogryposis is characterized by limited movement of the affected joints. The distal joints are more frequently affected than proximal joints. Talipes equinovarus (clubfoot) is almost universal, and the wrists are typically flexed. The elbows and knees can be in a flexed or extended position. Dimpling may be noted at the elbows and knees. Shoulders are internally rotated. Normal skin creases overlying the joints are often absent, suggesting an onset of arthrogryposis in the early intrauterine period. Changes in facial features may also be seen, including micrognathia.

Diagnosis

A thorough evaluation is required to determine the cause of arthrogryposis. This process may begin prenatally. Decreased fetal movement and joint contractures are often seen on prenatal ultrasound. Polyhydramnios may be seen secondary to decreased fetal swallowing. Prenatal imaging may reveal other physical characteristics that lead to suspicion of certain syndromes. Amniocentesis may provide information leading to a genetic diagnosis. A detailed

TABLE 14.1

ETIOLOGY OF DECREASED FETAL MOVEMENT

Category	Examples
Myopathic	
Abnormal muscle function secondary to failure of muscle formation or degeneration	Congenital muscular dystrophy Absence of muscles
Neuropathic	
Abnormal nerve function or innervation that involves either CNS or peripheral nervous system	Drugs or toxins CNS malformations: decreased number of anterior horn cells
Abnormal connective tissue	Abnormal formation of bone, cartilage, tendons, or connective tissue
Mechanical Limitation	
Produces compression within the uterus	Twins Amniotic rupture Oligohydramnios Uterine myomas

family history is essential to detect evidence of an inherited disorder. Maternal pregnancy and labor/delivery history should be reviewed carefully. Physical examination of the infant with careful description of the affected joints is needed, as well as detailed evaluation of the muscle mass and tone and function of the nervous system. Radiographic and ultrasound evaluation is needed to determine the presence of other congenital anomalies, as this may help link the contractures to a specific syndrome. Detailed imaging of the brain and spinal cord is indicated. Muscle biopsy and nerve conduction tests may be recommended. Genetic testing is also required. If a specific genetic etiology or specific syndrome is detected, a more accurate assessment of long-term prognosis can be made.

Management

Excluding infants with severe central nervous system dysfunction, infants with multiple congenital contractures have a good prognosis. The goal of management is to achieve and maintain an acceptable range of motion in the affected joints. During the newborn period, it is often a challenge to hold and care for these infants due to the extended position of the extremities and the reduced ability to manipulate the contracted limbs. Physical therapy should be initiated early in the neonatal period, to begin strengthening muscles and improving range of motion. Splints are also used, specifically molded and shaped for each limb depending on severity of contractures and positioning (Figures 14.3 and 14.4). Physical therapy is a lifelong process, and parents can be taught techniques to use with the child. Family involvement is a key factor in the success of therapy for these infants. Creativity on the part of the health care professional, as well as on the part of the parents, complements efforts to manipulate the rather rigid infant during feedings, sleeping, holding, and daily care activities. Parents may need referrals to agencies providing respite care or assistance from volunteers to maintain daily care needs.

Prognosis

The long-term prognosis for multiple congenital contractures depends on the extent of involvement. Mortality rates are low for those without central nervous system (CNS) involvement (1%–7%). For those with CNS involvement, mortality rates rise to almost 50%. Ventilator dependence at birth is associated with a poor prognosis (Bianchi & Van Marter, 1994).

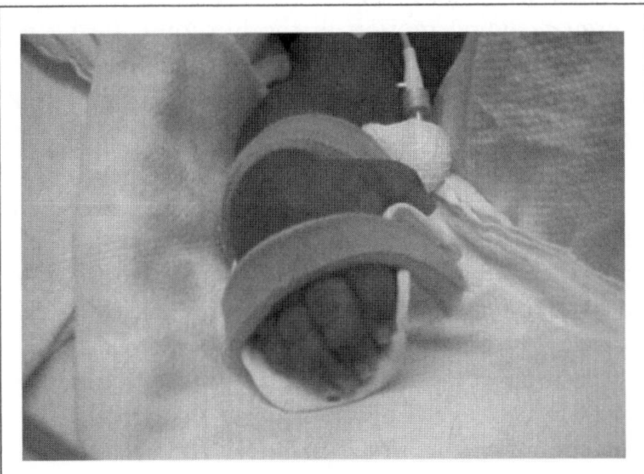

FIGURE 14.4 Hand splint with arthrogryposis.

DEVELOPMENTAL DYSPLASIA OF THE HIP

Developmental dysplasia of the hip (DDH) refers to any manifestation of hip instability, ranging from subluxation to complete dislocation. DDH remains a common problem despite almost universal neonatal screening. Although controversy surrounds the usefulness of clinical neonatal screening programs for the diagnosis of DDH, these programs have led to earlier diagnosis and treatment for many infants. Additional studies have noted improved diagnosis of hip dysplasia with the use of ultrasound. It is recognized that up to 88% of unstable hips will normalize without treatment. The use of early clinical exams and targeted ultrasounds for those infants with high-risk factors are the primary screening tools currently used. Those infants with high-risk factors include a family member with congenital/developmental hip dysplasia, infants with breech presentation and those with feet deformities (Shorter, Hong, & Osborn, 2011).

Incidence and Risk Factors

Reports of the incidence of DDH vary. The incidence of DDH in the United States is approximately 4 in 1,000 live births. Differences in DDH incidence rates across ethnic groups can be attributed to genetic, ethnic, and environmental influences. Other influential factors include the age of the infant at the time of examination, the expertise of the examiner, and the definition used by the examiner for the diagnosis of DDH.

Incidence of DDH is increased in first-born children. This increase may be due to the unstretched uterine and abdominal muscles, oligohydramnios, and the high association of fetal breech positioning in primigravidas. A definite preponderance toward DDH occurs in female children. The ratio of occurrence of DDH in girls to boys is 6 to 1. Females account for 80% of all cases of DDH. Factors that may contribute to this finding include the fact that twice as many females as males present in the breech position, and females appear to have heightened laxity in response to maternal relaxin hormones.

The breech position remains a major contributory factor to the development of DDH. Specific incidences of DDH in relationship to positioning are 0.7% for cephalic, 2% for footling, and 20% for single breech. The incidence of DDH for infants in the breech presentation is not altered by delivery methods. Breech-positioned infants delivered by cesarean section have the same predisposition to hip dislocation as those delivered vaginally. The left hip is involved three times more often than the right hip. Approximately 60% of DDH is on the left side, 20% on the right side, and 20% bilateral. This finding is attributed to the tendency of the fetus to lie with its left thigh against the maternal sacrum. This position forces the left hip into a posture of flexion and adduction. Thus the femoral head is covered more by the joint capsule than by the acetabulum.

For infants born with other musculoskeletal and congenital renal abnormalities, such as torticollis and Potter's association, the incidence of DDH is increased. Congenital renal abnormalities can result in fetal oliguria, thus subsequently producing oligohydramnios. Oligohydramnios can cause postural deformities because of the mechanical pressure on the fetus. Torticollis, arthrogryposis, and metatarsus adductus are thought to result from intrauterine compression, as does DDH.

After 40 weeks gestation, the femoral head in the normal infant is firmly seated in the acetabulum and remains positioned there by the surface tension of the synovial fluid. The hips of a normal infant are difficult to dislocate. Conversely, the infant with a dysplastic hip has a loosely fitting femoral head and acetabulum. Because of this pathophysiologic phenomenon, the femoral head can assume several abnormal positions in an infant with DDH. One such position is termed subluxation. Subluxation occurs when the femoral head can be moved to the edge of the acetabulum but not completely out of it. Another position is termed a dislocatable hip. A dislocatable hip exists when the femoral head can be displaced from the acetabulum by manipulation but returns to the acetabulum afterward. The femoral head can also be found in a completely dislocated position at birth. Dislocated hips may or may not be reduced by manipulation.

DDH is a dynamic disorder that may improve or deteriorate with or without treatment. Thus the joint may spontaneously dislocate and reduce (return to normal position) with normal neonatal movement. With time, this simple mechanism progresses in complexity secondary to adaptive changes. DDH can eventually progress either to permanent reduction, complete dislocation, or dysplasia (abnormal development). More than 60% of infants with hip instability stabilize within the first week of life, and 88% stabilize postnatally within the second month. Only 12% of infants with initial hip instability are considered to have DDH with potential for progression.

When complete dislocation occurs, pathologic changes occur to the femoral head, acetabulum, and ilium. This complete dislocation is due to the adaptive changes that occur in the adjacent tissue and bone. The long-term complication of dislocation, when adequate treatment has not occurred, is degenerative changes of both the femoral head and the acetabulum. Once adaptive changes occur, risk for progressive degeneration despite treatment increases. The subluxated hip, when not diagnosed in the neonatal period, is generally diagnosed at adolescence, when the strain of puberty and rapid growth spurts occur. With subluxation, the femoral head is laterally displaced and pushed upward into the joint; it is not completely out of the acetabulum. As the child grows and increased weight bearing occurs, the femoral head slides around and moves to the joint's edge. Degenerative changes result from this continual sliding. Sclerosis of the underlying bone, loss of cartilage, and formation of degenerative cysts are the most common degenerative changes (Cooperman & Thompson, 2002). Early arthritis is a common complication of those with DDH, often requiring surgical intervention for improved mobility (Stelzeneder et al., 2012).

Diagnosis and Clinical Manifestations

In the neonatal period, the Ortolani and Barlow maneuvers are useful in making the diagnosis of DDH. The Ortolani test is used to determine dislocation in the hip of a newborn, and the Barlow test is used to determine whether the hip is dislocatable (Barlow, 1962; Ortolani, 1976). In practice, both procedures are done in sequence. For examination, the infant is placed on a firm surface in the supine position.

The infant should be relaxed and quiet. Only one hip should be examined at a time. To perform the Ortolani test, the clinician stabilizes the infant's pelvis with one hand and with the other hand grasps the infant's thigh on the side to be tested. The examiner's middle finger is located over the greater trochanter (lateral aspect of the upper thigh), and the thumb is across the knee. The hip is flexed to 90° while bending the infant's knee. The infant's leg is then gently abducted with an anterior lift. In a positive Ortolani test, a "clunk" is heard with abduction. This clunk occurs as the dislocated femoral head slides over the posterior rim of the acetabulum and into the hip socket. Next, the hip is adducted, and, for the infant with DDH, a second clunk can be heard as the femoral head is displaced out of the acetabulum.

False-positive diagnoses of DDH have occurred when the examiner misinterprets a normal "click" (high-pitched sound) for a clunk. A click is not a sign of DDH. Clicks may be heard as a result of snapping of ligaments or tendons, and the majority are normal.

Barlow's test determines instability of the hip and identifies those hips that can be dislocated upon manipulation. Both hips and knees are flexed, with the hip to be tested in slight adduction. The examiner's middle finger remains positioned as for the Ortolani test, over the greater trochanter. However, the thumb is located over the medial aspect of the infant's lower thigh. Gentle pressure is exerted by the thumb posteriorly and laterally (down and out). For the infant with DDH, the femoral head can be felt to move out of the acetabulum with the typical clunk. The hip can then be reduced by the Ortolani maneuver or simply by releasing thumb pressure and abducting and flexing the hips.

When the femoral head is subluxated, the examiner may observe a sliding motion in the hip joint during physical examination. This sliding motion can be characteristic of an unstable hip joint. Most cases of unstable hips spontaneously resolve without treatment.

The American Academy of Pediatrics (AAP) committee on quality improvement has issued guidelines to assist in the diagnosis and management of the infant with DDH. All newborns should receive a screening exam. The Barlow and Ortolani maneuvers are not useful after 8 to 12 weeks of age. Ultrasonography is not recommended as a universal screening tool but is useful as a targeted screening tool. If the physical exam of the neonate is equivocal, a repeat exam should be performed at 2 weeks of age. Certain physical signs that would result in an equivocal hip exam for DDH would include a persistent soft click. If the Ortolani/

Barlow exam is positive with a hip clunk at 2 weeks of age, a referral to an orthopedic specialist is required. This is not an emergency but should be completed in a timely matter over the next few weeks. The infant presenting at 2 weeks with a persistent soft click should receive ultrasonography of the hip within the next 3 to 4 weeks or referral to an orthopedic specialist at this time. For the infant who exhibits a normal hip exam with resolution of the soft hip click, routine screening with well baby checks during the first year of life is the recommendation. It is important to note that, according to the AAP recommendations, a newborn who is discharged before 48 hours of age should receive repeat hip exam at 2 to 4 days after discharge.

If the family has a history of DDH, the incidence increases 9.4/1,000 in males and 44/1,000 in females. Because of this increased risk, even with a negative hip exam, an ultrasound at 6 weeks should be considered, or an x-ray of the hips at 4 months can be an alternative (Morey, 2001).

Collaborative Management

The goal of collaborative management is to achieve and maintain reduction of the unstable hip. The sooner treatment is implemented, the greater the chance for successful outcome. Various splinting devices are used to treat DDH in infants. Examples of splints include the Pavlik harness, von Rosen splint, Denis Browne hip adduction splint, and Frejka pillow splint. The most commonly used splint for neonates is the Pavlik harness.

The Pavlik harness allows for spontaneous hip and lower extremity movement while maintaining reduction of the hip joint. It can be worn comfortably during all aspects of normal newborn care, including diaper changes. The Pavlik harness can be adjusted for growth. It is indicated for use in newborns and infants up to 6 months of age. Use of the Pavlik harness is contraindicated for infants able to stand and for those infants in whom the hip joint is not reducible by manipulation. A major factor influencing the success of the Pavlik harness is parental compliance with the treatment. With this condition extensive parental education is imperative.

Parent and Family Education and Support

In addition to providing information regarding the pathology and treatment goals of DDH, the nurse should provide the parents with an opportunity to remove and reapply the harness while under supervision. Parental support groups can help parents adjust to the infant's temporary awkward condition. Parents should also be educated in the procedure used to reduce the dislocated hip because complete reduction must be achieved before the harness is applied.

Long-Term Consequences and Complications

As with most therapeutic treatments, the potential for iatrogenic complications exists. Complications observed following DDH treatment include avascular necrosis, redislocation, and acetabular dysplasia. Complications can result from either inadequate or overly aggressive treatment.

An additional complication that has been reported with the use of the Pavlik harness is the development of brachial plexus palsy (Mostert, Tulp, & Castelein, 2000). The tension of the shoulder harness appears related to this complication. The harness may be applied too tightly or may not be modified with the infant's growth, thus causing downward pressure on the brachial plexus nerves and subsequent neuropathy.

Such alternatives include closed reduction with traction or open reduction with casting. A hip spica cast is most often used with these infants. Care then includes observance for poor pedal pulses, decreased peripheral circulation, pain, skin excoriation or abrasions, and possible development of respiratory infections resulting from decreased mobility. An adjustment in car seats is required with the harness and any casting and parental education should be documented prior to discharge of the infant.

CLUBFOOT

The classic clubfoot, talipes equinovarus, refers to a dysmorphic-appearing foot with hindfoot equinus (heel is pulled upward as if walking on the toes), forefoot adduction (toes are pointed inward), and midfoot supination. The term *clubfoot* may also be used to describe milder talipes conditions, including talipes calcaneus and talipes varus.

Foot deformities are among the most common birth defects. Clubfoot has an incidence of 1 in 1,000 live births. Males are affected nearly twice as often as females, and, in infants with unilateral presentation, the majority appear on the right.

Pathology

The precise mechanism of development of clubfoot has not been irrefutably established. Some researchers allude to the theory of intrauterine malposition, whereas others, noting a higher incidence of clubfoot in families with a positive history of the disorder, ascribe it to a genetic cause.

A popular theory is that clubfoot is a multifactorial disorder involving a genetic predisposition coupled with environmental forces such as oligohydramnios, primiparity, macrosomia, and multiple fetuses.

Clinical Manifestations

Clubfoot deformities are apparent at birth. The skin overlying the lateral aspect of the foot may be taut, whereas the medial aspect may have increased skin folds. The affected foot may be smaller in size than a normal foot. In older children, the calf muscle may be noticeably decreased in size. Milder talipes conditions may be returned to the neutral position by manipulation.

Collaborative Management

Early diagnosis and treatment of clubfoot are essential. In the early newborn period, joints, muscles, and ligaments may be more compliant to corrective manipulation without surgical intervention. This may involve serial casting as frequently as 2- to 4-day intervals. As many as 50% of clubfoot deformities may require surgery. Difficulty with skin closure has been reported as a complication following correction of severe clubfoot. This is especially true if the affected foot has received prior surgery. Special shoe splints or braces may be used toward the end of any successful treatment.

Parental education includes implementation of routine newborn care for an infant wearing either splints or bilateral casts. Problems and solutions associated with clothing, sleeping, feeding, and bathing should be addressed. Compliance by parents in using splints may vary. Because consistent treatment is necessary for a favorable outcome, health care professionals must explore parental feelings and actions while providing anticipatory guidance.

SYNDACTYLY

Fusion, or webbing, between two digits is referred to as syndactyly. This condition is the most common anomaly of the hand, with an incidence of 1 in 2,250 live births. Males are affected slightly more than females. Half of the time, both hands are involved in a symmetric presentation. Syndactyly of the fingers may be accompanied by syndactyly of the toes.

Pathology

Although most occurrences of syndactyly appear to be through spontaneous mutation, familial predisposition has been reported, thus indicating an autosomal dominant pattern. Syndactyly may also be associated with a specific syndrome such as Apert syndrome.

There are four classifications of syndactyly. Complete syndactyly occurs when the fusion is from the base to the tip of the digit. Fusion that does not extend to the tip of the digit is termed incomplete. Simple syndactyly refers to digits connected by skin and soft tissue. Fused digits involving an osseous connection is considered complex. Abnormal nerve and vessel configurations may accompany complex syndactyly.

Treatment

The type and timing of treatment of syndactyly depend on its classification. Surgery is directed toward promoting normal function and appearance. Fingers of unequal length should be separated within 6 to 12 months of age to prevent curvature of the longer finger from deviating toward the shorter finger. If more than two adjacent digits are involved, surgery should be performed in stages to prevent vascular compromise of the middle digits.

Prognosis

Prognosis is favorable for normal function and appearance, except in cases of complex syndactyly involving not only bone but also vascular and nervous tissue. These cases may be associated with some postoperative loss of function.

Collaborative Management

Parents of infants with syndactyly are instructed in physical therapy, specifically in massage of the interconnecting skin. Massaging of the webbed area prior to surgery allows some stretching of the skin, which permits easier repair.

POLYDACTYLY

Polydactyly is any duplication of digits beyond the normal five. It is the second most common hand anomaly. Polydactyly is believed to be caused by duplication of a single embryonic bud. African Americans are affected 10 times more often than Caucasians. African Americans more often have postaxial polydactyly (duplication of the little finger), whereas preaxial polydactyly (duplication of the thumb) occurs primarily in Caucasians. In African Americans, postaxial polydactyly is typically an isolated incidence, whereas in Caucasians it is associated with syndromes and chromosomal anomalies. Central axial polydactyly is the duplication of the ring, long, or index finger. Central axial polydactyly is often associated with complex syndactyly. Polydactyly may be further classified into three types. Type I is merely a rudimentary soft tissue mass connected by a pedicle. Treatment of this type involves simple excision, which can be done prior to discharge from the nursery per the parents' request. To avoid any residual tag after excision, these babies are often referred to plastic surgery for a more complete removal. Type II is a partial duplication with involvement of the phalanges. Type III, a rare occurrence, involves complete duplication of the metacarpal and phalanges.

Collaborative Management

Treatment of polydactyly types II and III centers around functional capacity first and appearance second. The infant is observed for which duplication is dominant and most functional, and efforts are made to remove the least functional counterpart. If both duplicated digits appear to be equally functional, surgery should then be used to promote aesthetic appearance. Reparative surgery should be completed by 3 years of age.

AMNIOTIC BAND SYNDROME

Amniotic band syndrome (ABS; also referred to as amniotic rupture sequence or constriction band syndrome), is associated with asymmetric fetal deformities. Deformities that have been attributed to the ABS include congenital limb amputation, syndactyly, constriction bands, clubfoot, craniofacial defects such as cleft lip and palate, and visceral defects such as gastroschisis and omphalocele (Baraitser & Winter, 1996). Early fetal evaluation has linked ABS with skull and brain defects (Lee, Lee, Kim, Son, & Namgung, 2011).

Diagnosis

Many clinicians believe that amniotic bands must be present for the diagnosis of ABS to be made. However, others believe that the presence of fetal deformities in a nonanatomic pattern, without obvious bands, is sufficient to establish the diagnosis of the syndrome. Congenital deformations, such as the visceral and craniofacial types, in the absence of amniotic bands may go undiagnosed as ABS because they could represent a faulty midline developmental pattern during the first trimester of pregnancy instead of the production of amniotic bands that constricted or restricted growth. Therefore the true incidence of this syndrome may be much higher than it generally appears—not only because of the difficulty establishing a diagnosis but also because of the high mortality rate that exists during gestation.

ABS has been implicated in fetal deaths secondary to cord compression by the constricting bands. Strauss and colleagues provide a clinical report of fetal demise involving a normal karyotype male secondary to torsion and strangulation of the umbilical cord by an amniotic band. The only significant history in the gestation was an early second-trimester amniocentesis. It has been speculated that amniotic rupture may follow amniocentesis and fetal blood sampling. Strangulation furrows, limb reduction defects, and cleft lip or palate can be late sequelae of invasive prenatal procedures in animal models.

Pathophysiology

Etiologic factors in the ABS are unclear. Part of the difficulty is that some of the same deformities that occur with this syndrome can also occur for other reasons. Thus the exact cause of the deformities is not always clear, but the primary theory is the association with early amnion rupture and fetal entanglement of the resulting fibrous bands.

Two theories—endogenous and exogenous—explain the cause of ABS. The endogenous theory postulates that the deformities are caused by an innate derangement of the primary embryonic cell layers from which the tissues and organs develop. The presence of amniotic bands, according to the endogenous theory, is a late development with no clinical significance.

The exogenous—and seemingly more popular—theory contends that early amnionic rupture allows the fetus to move into close approximation to the chorion by entering the chorionic cavity. The ruptured amnion then forms fibrous strings or bands. These bands can adhere to the skin, thus altering normal morphogenesis (e.g., cleft lip or palate, omphalocele) or disrupt the vascular integrity, resulting in gastroschisis. Amniotic bands have been found encircling normally developed structures, thus resulting in congenital amputations, constriction rings with lymphedema distal to the ring, and facial clefts in nonanatomic distribution. Postural deformities such as clubfoot are believed to be caused by the fetus's close approximation to the chorion.

Figure 14.5 is an example of an amniotic band constriction ring noted on the arm of an infant with unilateral cleft lip and palate. Evidence of this constriction ring indicates that development of the lip and palate were at one time normal, but development was altered with the presence of amniotic bands.

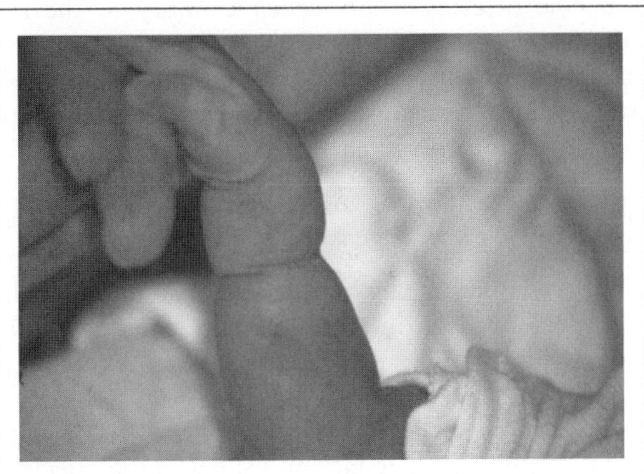

FIGURE 14.5 Constriction ring.

Collaborative Management

Notwithstanding the inherent problems associated with omphaloceles, gastroschisis, encephaloceles, clubfoot, syndactyly, and facial clefts, the clinician must be attuned to the unique complications of constricting bands. Constricting bands are usually associated with edema distal to the band. The resulting edema and vascular compromise contribute to complications such as skin breakdown, necrosis, thromboemboli formation that results from venostasis, and infection. Care should include frequent vascular checks to assess perfusion. Trauma and tissue breakdown are discouraged through positioning and skin care. Observation for localized areas of necrosis is stressed.

As with other aesthetically disappointing musculoskeletal disorders, the family requires emotional and psychological support as adjustment to and acceptance of the infant are allowed to occur. Parents may be fearful that an extremity will be lost because of necrotic tissue formation or infection. These fears may be justified, and the parents should be prepared for such a possibility. Complete surgical repair may not be possible during the infant's initial hospitalization, thus necessitating frequent hospitalizations during the early developing years. The delay in repair may necessitate that parents be taught to observe for vascular perfusion of an extremity, to recognize signs of infection, and to change dressings over open or healing areas. Preparation for discharge requires a multidisciplinary approach. The family may need surgical supplies, follow-up visitations by a home-visiting nurse, orthopedic or surgical consultations, pediatrician visits for general well-child care, and support of social or financial services to meet the long-term responsibilities of caring for their infants.

In addition, the nurse, working with the perinatal social worker, must attempt to provide opportunities for parent-infant bonding if the parents are to feel somewhat prepared for discharge. While the infant is still in the hospital, the parents must be encouraged to touch and talk to the infant and to participate in the infant's care. They must also be encouraged to verbalize their own feelings about their infant's condition. Every attempt should be made to attend to their fears, concerns, or misconceptions about the cause of their infant's problem. Only then will positive transition to home be possible.

BIRTH TRAUMA

Birth trauma encompasses both mechanical and asphyxial events occurring during delivery. This trauma may be due to pressure and distortion. Trauma can occur despite exemplary obstetrical care. Birth trauma occurs in approximately 2 to 7 in 1,000 live births. A positive association exists between birth trauma and macrosomia, prematurity, breech presentation, dystocia, and cephalopelvic disproportion.

Clinical Manifestations

Birth trauma includes abrasions, ecchymoses, erythema, cephalohematomas, caput succedaneum, fractures (especially of the clavicle), brachial plexus damage, and nerve palsies. Clavicular fractures are the most common fractures diagnosed as birth trauma. Clavicles are at an increased risk for fractures during shoulder dystocias in a vertex presentation or with arms extended during a breech delivery (Cooperman & Thompson, 2002).

Physical examination findings related to birth trauma may appear only as bruising, abrasions, and petechiae that overlie the affected part. Further diagnostic methods should be used when the infant exhibits pain on movement, limited motion, and abnormal passive positioning of an extremity or head movement.

Skull fractures may present as cephalohematomas. Skull fractures are most often linear and typically involve the parietal bones. Symptomatic evidence of a nondepressed skull fracture may resemble signs of increased intracranial pressure secondary to epidural hemorrhage. Clinical presentation may include changes in tone, hypertonicity or hypotonicity, arching of the back with the head in hyperextension, and respiratory compromise. Usually, no treatment is indicated for asymptomatic skull fractures. Depressed skull fractures, however, may require elevation of the depressed area.

A rare, but possible, fatal delivery complication is subgaleal hemorrhage. This may present as a cephalohematoma with small area of swelling on the scalp as early as 4 hours of age. This often progresses and unlike the cephalohematoma, crosses suture lines and involves the nape of the neck. The volume of blood loss may be high, causing hypovolemic shock.

Vertebral fractures are incurred in difficult breech deliveries in which longitudinal traction in combination with a twisting motion may occur. These features commonly involve the seventh cervical and first thoracic vertebrae. Treatment depends on the extent of resultant nerve damage but often requires traction.

The most common nerve injury attributed to birth trauma is brachial plexus damage and resulting nerve palsy. This injury involves damage to the network of nerve fibers in the neck and shoulders referred to as the brachial plexus. Involvement may occur in the upper portion (Erb-Duchenne palsy), lower portion (Klumpke's paralysis), or both portions (complete brachial plexus palsy).

Erb-Duchenne paralysis is the most common form. The affected arm is limp and in a position of elbow extension and internal rotation. The Moro reflex is diminished and the grasp reflex intact. Klumpke's paralysis involves paralysis of the hand and wrist. Complete brachial plexus paralysis results in paralysis of the entire arm.

Diagnosis

Diagnosis of birth trauma is based on physical assessment findings. These are usually fairly visible at birth or in the immediate postnatal period. Physical findings should be confirmed, when necessary, by radiologic evaluation to establish whether a fracture is present. For significant scalp swelling, evaluation of the skull by x-ray is prudent.

Collaborative Management

Treatment of birth trauma depends on the type and severity of the trauma. Often, supportive measures may be the only intervention required. For instance, brachial plexus injuries require immobilization in a neutral position using braces or splints. Passive range-of-motion exercises should be instituted at 7 to 10 days.

Clavicular fractures also respond to supportive management. Typically, the arm is held flexed, and the elbow is held against the chest. This position limits movement, thereby decreasing pain and possible trauma to the site. Callus formation stabilizes the fracture by 10 days of age. A hard, palpable knot can often be felt with this callus formation.

Parental Education and Support

Diagnosing a disorder resulting from birth trauma can evoke anxiety in a parent. Birth trauma may connote thoughts of violence. The manner in which such information is taken from and conveyed to the family is important. Nonjudgmental, supportive care by health professionals along with consistent primary care by one individual may diminish some anxiety and allow the parents to establish trust. The mother may especially feel that she is to blame for the neonatal problem. Calm reassurance about the nature of the trauma is important. It also helps to allay fears that something was done incorrectly during the delivery process if parents understand that many of these injuries cannot be avoided or anticipated. Parental education is prerequisite if the parents are to understand the need for continued, long-term treatment, which many of these infants require. Many birth trauma injuries require long-term follow-up care by orthopedists, neurologists, or physical and occupational specialists.

CONGENITAL MUSCULAR TORTICOLLIS

Congenital muscular torticollis, with an incidence of 0.4% of all live births, is another musculoskeletal deformity with unknown pathogenesis. It is known to be primarily a disorder of the sternocleidomastoid muscle.

Pathophysiology

Several theories exist as to the cause of congenital torticollis, including genetics, abnormal uterine positioning, neurogenic disorders, and ischemic injury to the sternocleidomastoid muscle. Whatever the cause, this pathologic disorder consists of a fibrous contraction of the sternocleidomastoid muscle. Typically, the ipsilateral trapezius muscle is atrophic.

Diagnosis

Congenital torticollis can present within the neonatal period. Presentation may include a 1- to 3-cm hard palpable mass in the neck on the affected side accompanied by an abnormal positioning of the head. Infants with congenital torticollis tilt the head to the affected side, and the chin is pointed upward in the opposite direction. Facial asymmetry may be a later sign. The face and skull on the affected side appear smaller.

In children with untreated congenital torticollis or in cases with torticollis unresponsive to therapy, the shoulder on the affected side is raised to compensate for the abnormal head positioning. This form of compensation may lead to cervical and lumbar scoliosis as well as chronic back pain.

Collaborative Management

Traditionally, physical therapy for congenital torticollis is instituted immediately. Because congenital torticollis may resolve naturally within the first year of life, surgery is typically delayed pending results of therapy.

Severe fibrosis of the sternocleidomastoid muscle is often reversible and will require surgery. In one study, 98% of those infants diagnosed with torticollis responded to physical therapy. Duration of therapy was dependent on severity of the muscular fibrosis (Lee et al., 2011).

Physical therapists and orthopedic surgeons should be consulted to assist in the management and subsequent follow-up of these infants. Family members should be taught home physical therapy, which should be performed at least twice daily. Parents should be counseled regarding the possibility of a neck brace to be postoperatively worn by the infant. It is usually the nurse's responsibility to coordinate consultations and to prepare the family with discharge instructions. In addition, the nurse must determine whether the family lives in an area accessible to follow-up care. If not, a referral to social services or financial counseling may be needed so the family can participate in follow-up.

CRANIOSYNOSTOSIS

The bones that constitute the skull are joined with fibrous joints. These joints are lined with a thin layer of fibrous tissue. Separation of these joints allows for remodeling of the skull at the time of delivery and for rapid growth of the head during the early developmental years. The skull consists of five main sutures: coronal, lambdoidal, squamosal, sagittal, and metopic. The signal for normal closure of these sutures remains unclear, but is believed to be secondary to multiple factors. The various sutures of the skull begin to close clinically in the first year of life, and the process continues into childhood. Complete ossification of these sutures is anticipated in the second or third decade of life. Figures 14.6 and 14.7 illustrate the newborn's cranial sutures.

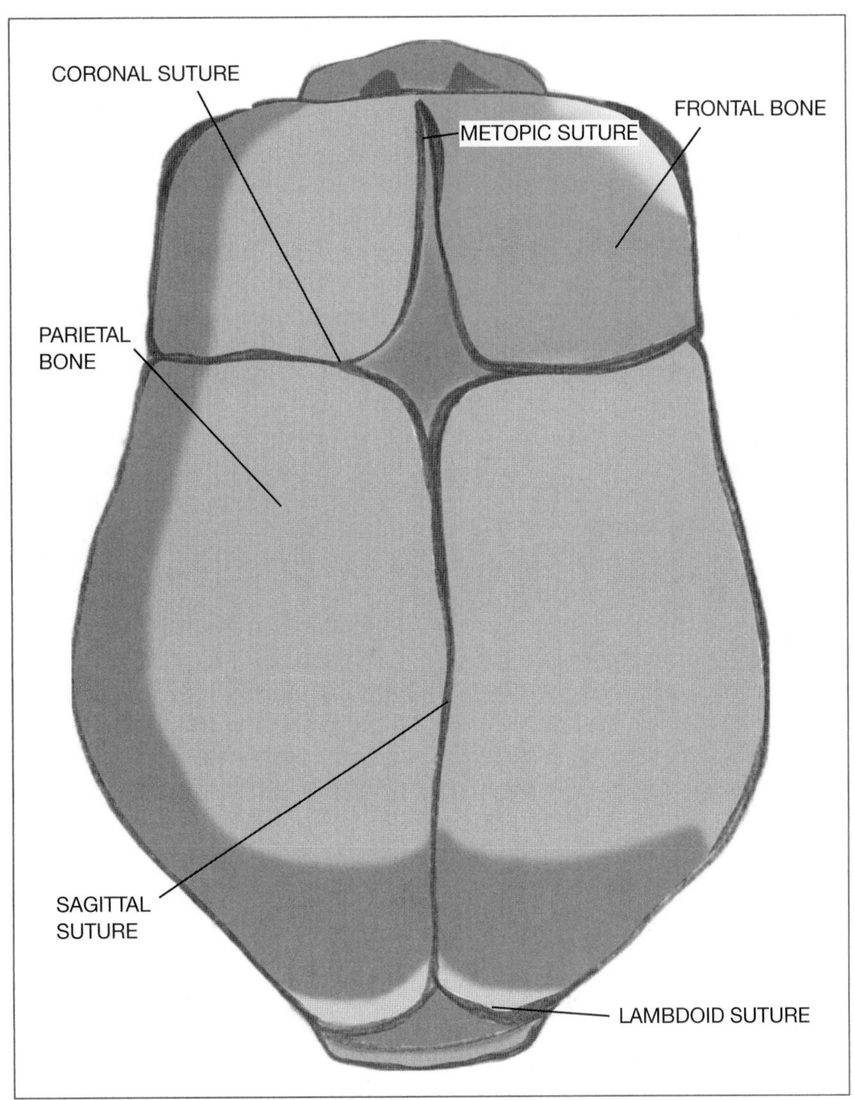

FIGURE 14.6 Cranial sutures.
Illustration by Wren (2012).

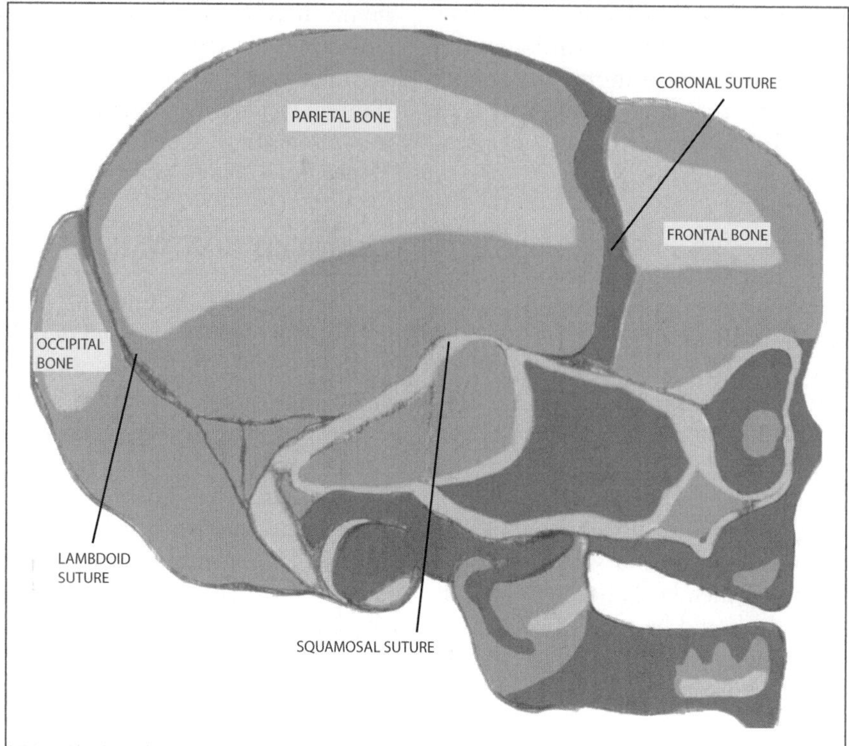

FIGURE 14.7 Cranial sutures.
Illustration by Wren (2012).

Premature closure of any suture in the skull results in a clinical condition called craniosynostosis. The early closure of a cranial suture typically starts at one point and progresses along the suture line. Premature closure may occur prenatally or postnatally. Only one suture may be prematurely fused, or multiple sutures may be involved. Simple craniosynostosis, which involves one suture, generally occurs as an isolated defect. Complex craniosynostosis describes the premature closure of two or more sutures. This is usually associated with a genetic syndrome, such as Apert syndrome or Crouzon syndrome.

Pathology and Clinical Characteristics

Clinical characteristics depend on which suture is affected. The closure of one suture does not allow growth in that area, but generally increases growth in the other areas of the skull. The sagittal suture is the most commonly affected suture. When this suture is involved, the head presents as dolichocephalic, with a long and narrow appearance of the skull and increased length from front to back. Bossing of the frontal and occipital regions is also seen. The coronal suture is the second most common suture involved in premature closure. Bilateral closure of the coronal suture leads to the clinical appearance of a skull that is wide from side to side, but short from front to back (also termed *brachycephaly*). Unilateral closure of a coronal suture results in plagiocephaly, or twisted skull, with prominence of the forehead on the unaffected side, as the skull grows in this direction. The forehead is flattened and the eyebrow is raised on the affected side. Bilateral lambdoidal craniosynostosis could be identified with a flattened occipital region, whereas unilateral lambdoidal craniosynostosis has a flattened area on one side of the occiput and appears asymmetrical when compared to the other side. Long-term supine positioning of the infant can also produce this appearance.

Positional asymmetric skull appearance, not related to abnormal suture closure, may be seen in those infants with a neuromuscular defect that will not allow the child to move its head from side to side spontaneously. Congenital torticollis can result in an asymmetrically flat occipital region as the infant tilts the head toward the affected side. Isolated metopic craniosynostosis will produce a deformity with a narrow, protruding forehead. Facial development of the skull is also affected, and orbital hypotelorism is also noted with this defect.

Diagnosis and Management

Diagnosis is preceded by suspicion of the abnormal physical appearance of the skull. There is persistent or progressive abnormal skull growth, often with the head circumference intact for age. Craniosynostosis is usually confirmed with a computed tomography (CT) scan of the skull, with three-dimensional CT required for more detailed preoperative examination. Surgery is required to correct this defect. This will take place in a specialized pediatric hospital with a multidisciplinary team of providers. The complexity of the procedure increases with the number of sutures involved and the cranial remodeling at the time of surgery. The type of repair is dependent on the suture(s) involved. Surgery generally takes place in early infancy (3–9 months of age). The goal is to achieve early correction of the synostosis and avoid extreme cranial deformities as the skull grows rapidly in the first year of life. In recent years, endoscopic procedures have shown good results in reducing the excessive blood loss and extended hospital stays that were previously associated with repair of craniosynostosis.

TAR SYNDROME: THROMBOCYTOPENIA-ABSENT RADIUS

TAR syndrome is characterized by the bilateral absence of radii and severe thrombocytopenia in the neonatal period. Hypoplasia or absence of the ulna may also be seen. The thumbs are always present in this syndrome (Scott & Montgomery, 2011). Congenital heart defects and renal anomalies also occur in a significant percentage of these patients. Skeletal anomalies of the lower limbs may also be present, although this is highly variable.

Pathology

The inheritance pattern is uncertain in this disorder, although a microdeletion on chromosome 1 is part of the genetic signature. The greatest pathology occurs in the neonatal period and correlates to the severity of thrombocytopenia, which can lead to intracranial and gastrointestinal hemorrhages (Sola, Del Vecchio, & Rimsza, 2000). The thrombocytopenia is quite significant in many patients, with counts as low as 10,000. Hematologic complications improve with age, hence the reduced mortality and morbidity associated with this syndrome after the first year of life. Platelet counts are generally normal by childhood.

A complication encountered as the child matures is the gross motor developmental delay experienced by the abnormal hands and arms. Most children who are affected with this syndrome might require some type of adaptive device but rarely perform well with prostheses, as they learn to compensate with their existing limbs. If no significant intracranial hemorrhage occurs in the neonatal period, intelligence is expected to be normal.

Management

The primary management in the newborn period centers on the platelet levels. Because of increased risk of bleeding, platelet transfusions may be required. In addition, handling and phlebotomy via heelsticks should be kept to a minimum to reduce bruising. Cow's milk allergy is seen in many patients with TAR syndrome. The introduction of cow's milk may lead to worsening of thrombocytopenia, and this factor should be considered in management (Toriello, 2011).

SUMMARY

Although the majority of musculoskeletal defects in the newborn are nonlethal and often not functional problems, they may become the focus of the parents' attention. This can be attributed to the perception that the infant does not meet their preconceived idea of the "perfect child." An understanding of the development of the musculoskeletal system and pathology for various defects can assist the clinician in teaching and supporting the family and infant. In addition, recognizing the subtle abnormalities can prompt the clinician to evaluate for additional, often subtle, associated defects that could have serious genetic implications.

When a clinician recounts a case involving a musculoskeletal defect, it is often one of the more rare, yet clinically impressive, defects such as thanatophoric dwarfism and OI. This chapter helps to identify the epidemiological and clinical aspects of the rare and the common defects in an effort to improve the understanding of the defect as well as to provide guidelines for management based on the pathology, complications, and prognosis of the defect.

CASE STUDY

■ **Identification of the Problem.** Female infant born at term gestation, noted on initial physical exam to have abnormalities of the upper extremities.

■ **Assessment: History and Physical Examination.** The infant was born by vaginal delivery at 37 weeks gestation to a 16-year-old Caucasian female, G1P0. The mother received late and limited prenatal care, with the pregnancy remaining unacknowledged until the third trimester secondary to young maternal age. Delivery was uncomplicated. The 1-minute Apgar score was 9, and the infant did not require resuscitation or other special care at delivery. The birth weight was 2,850 g. Infant was noted on general inspection to have abnormalities of the upper extremities.

Physical exam on admission to the transition nursery:

- GENERAL: pink, well-developed female infant; vital signs in the normal range; oxygen saturation was 98% on room air
- HEENT: normocephalic, anterior fontanelle open and flat, eyes normal, ears normally formed, nares patent, palate intact
- LUNGS: bilateral breath sounds clear and equal, good respiratory effort
- CV: RRR, soft murmur, good peripheral perfusion, femoral and pedal pulses palpable
- ABD: soft, active bowel sounds, no organomegaly or masses, three-vessel cord
- GU: normal term female features, patent anus

- NEURO: appropriate tone for gestational age, active and responsive
- NECK: full range of motion, no masses
- SPINE: intact
- EXTREMITIES: bilateral malformed upper extremities with thumbs present; lower extremities normal
- SKIN: pink, scattered petechiae over the trunk and face

■ Suspected Diagnosis. In this patient, the physical exam findings led to a strong suspicion of TAR syndrome. Immediate evaluation is indicated to assess platelet count, which can be very low with risk of hemorrhage. Cranial ultrasound should be done to rule out intracranial bleeding. Evaluation of the skeletal structure of the upper extremities is also needed. Echocardiogram should be performed to rule out cardiac defects, which are present in a large percentage of patients with this disorder.

■ Diagnostic Tests

1. Complete blood count with differential: WBC 12.7, hematocrit 39%, platelet count 28,000/mm^3
2. X-rays of upper extremities: bilateral absence of radii, with hypoplasia of the ulnae bilaterally; the humeri were present and normal bilaterally; x-rays of lower extremities revealed no abnormalities
3. Echocardiogram: patent ductus arteriosus, no significant structural abnormalities
4. Cranial ultrasound: no evidence of intracranial hemorrhage

■ Development of Management Plan

- Platelet transfusion
- Gentle handling of infant to avoid bruising and bleeding
- Close monitoring of the platelet count

■ Implementation of Management Plan. The infant was transferred to the neonatal intensive care unit to obtain a peripheral IV and to have the necessary studies completed. The platelet count was repeated 12 hours after the transfusion with a value of 49,000/mm^3. The infant received an additional transfusion of platelets with improvement to 72,000/mm^3. The infant remained hospitalized for an additional week while receiving ad lib breastfeedings. She remained stable. Repeat cranial ultrasound at 7 days of age was again normal.

The infant was discharged home at 10 days of age with platelet count 80,000/mm^3. She returned to the newborn outpatient clinic 3 days later with platelet count 43,000/mm^3. An additional platelet transfusion was given in the outpatient clinic with no complications. The platelet count on a follow-up visit the next day was 85,000/mm^3. The infant continued to receive periodic follow-up visits for complete blood count monitoring over the next 3 months. She required no further platelet transfusion.

■ Outcome. Infant was seen at 6 months of age in the newborn follow-up clinic with normal growth and development. Platelet count was normal.

EVIDENCE-BASED PRACTICE BOX

Osteogenesis imperfecta (OI), often called "brittle bone disease," is a condition caused by a genetic mutation affecting collagen. The complications of OI stem primarily from bone fractures. The treatment of these patients focuses chiefly on preventing fractures, therefore minimizing pain and improving long-term mobility and function. A number of research studies have investigated the use of bisphosphonates to reduce fracture rates in patients with OI. Biphosphonates act by decreasing the activity of osteoclasts, therefore reducing the rate of bone resorption. These drugs are used successfully in adults with osteoporosis to improve bone strength and density.

A recent review by Bishop (2010) examined the early use of intravenous pamidronate in neonates in the first year of life. The drug was given on a cyclical basis at varying intervals. A reduced rate of fractures was seen in these infants, as well as improved growth. No severe side effects were documented. There are concerns regarding the difficulty of maintaining reliable central venous access in a small infant. Also, the long-term effects of this therapy remain unknown. It should be noted that the drug does not change the process of abnormal collagen formation.

Growth hormone, which is known to stimulate bone growth and collagen synthesis, has also been examined as a potential treatment for OI. A review by Monti and colleagues (2010) examined the available information. Data from limited studies suggest that growth hormone can improve growth and exert a beneficial effect on muscle mass and strength, therefore improving capacity for exercise; no increased rate of fractures was noted. This increase in physical activity in OI patients may improve skeletal health and overall physical well-being. Growth hormone is considered a promising therapy in patients with moderate forms of OI. Patients with the more severe types of the disorder did not see a benefit.

Research in the arena of genetics is very promising. Investigators hope to identify more specific causative factors at the molecular level, as well as to explore the possibility of manipulating the disorder's genetic expression. Bone marrow transplant is also being examined as a potential treatment. Limited data suggest that bone marrow transplant can be used to introduce stem cells into the body that can produce normal bone. These modalities remain in early stages of development.

ONLINE RESOURCES

Evaluation and Care of the Normal Neonates
http://www.merckmanuals.com/professional/pediatrics/approach_to_the_care_of_normal_infants_and_children/evaluation_and_care_of_the_normal_neonate.html

Musculoskeletal Implications of Preterm Infant Positioning in the NICU
http://www.ncbi.nlm.nih.gov/pubmed/12083295

Musculoskeletal Sonography
http://www.monash.edu.au/pubs/handbooks/units/SON4024.html

REFERENCES

Baraitser, M., & Winter, R. M. (1996). *Color atlas of congenital malformation syndromes*. St Louis, MO: Mosby.

Barlow, T. G. (1962). Early diagnosis and treatment of congenital dislocation of the hip. *Journal of Bone and Joint Surgery, 44B*, 292–301.

Bianchi, D. W., & Van Marter, L. J. (1994). An approach to ventilator-dependent neonates with arthrogryposis. *Pediatrics, 94*(5), 682–686.

Bishop, N. (2010). Characterising and treating osteogenesis imperfecta. *Early Human Development, 86*, 743–746.

Cooperman, D. R., & Thompson, G. H. (2002). Neonatal orthopedics. In A. A. Fanaroff & R. J. Martin (Eds.), *Neonatal-perinatal medicine: Diseases of the fetus and infant* (7th ed.). St Louis, MO: Mosby.

Horton, W. A., & Hecht, J. T. (2011). Disorders involving transmembrane receptors. In R. M. Kliegman, B. F. Stanton, J. W. St Geme III, N. F. Schor, & R. E. Behrman (Eds.), *Nelson textbook of pediatrics* (19th ed.). Philadelphia, PA: Elsevier Saunders.

Lee, S. H., Lee, M., Kim, M., Son, G., & Namgung, K. (2011). Fetal MR imaging of constriction band syndrome involving the skull and brain. *Journal of Computer Assisted Tomography, 35*(6), 685–687.

Lee, Y. T., Yoon, K., Kim, Y. B., Chung, P. W., Hwang, J. H., Park, Y. S., . . . Han, B. H. (2011). Clinical features and outcome of physiotherapy in early presenting congenital muscular torticollis with severe fibrosis on ultrasonography. A prospective study. *Journal of Pediatric Surgery, 46*(8), 1526–1531.

Marini, J. C. (2011). Osteogenesis imperfecta. In R. M. Kliegman, B. F. Stanton, J. W. St Geme III, N. F. Schor, & R. E. Behrman (Eds.), *Nelson textbook of pediatrics* (19th ed.). Philadelphia, PA: Elsevier Saunders.

McLean, K. R. (2004). Osteogenesis imperfecta. *Neonatal Network, 23*(2), 7–14.

Miller, E., Blaser, S., Shannon, P., & Widjaja, E. (2009). Brain and bone abnormalities of thanatophoric dwarfism. *American Journal of Roentgenology, 192*(1), 48–51.

Monti, E., Mottes, M., Fraschini, P., Brunelli, P., Forlino, A., Venturi, G., . . . Antoniazzi, F. (2010). Current and emerging treatments for the management of osteogenesis imperfecta. *Therapeutics and Clinical Risk Management, 6*, 367–381.

Morey, S. S. (2001). The American Academy of Pediatrics: AAP develops guidelines for early detection of dislocated hips. *American Family Physician, 63*, 565–566.

Mostert, A. K., Tulp, N. J., & Castelein, R. M. (2000). Results of Pavlik harness treatment for neonatal hip dislocation to Graf's sonographic classification. *Journal of Pediatric Orthopedics, 20*, 306–310.

Neonatal and nursery care. (2012). *Osteogenesis imperfecta foundation*. Retrieved from http://www.oif.org/site/DocServer/Neonatal_and_Nursery_Care_pdf

O'Flaherty, P. (2001). Arthrogryposis multiplex congenita. *Neonatal Network, 20*(4), 13–20.

Ortolani, M. (1976). Congenital hip dysplasia in the light of early and very early diagnosis. *Clinical Orthopedics and Related Research, 119*, 6–10.

Scott, J. P., & Montgomery, R. R. (2011). Neonatal thrombocytopenia. In R. M. Kliegman, B. F. Stanton, J. W. St Geme III, N. F. Schor, & R. E. Behrman (Eds.), *Nelson textbook of pediatrics* (19th ed.). Philadelphia, PA: Elsevier Saunders.

Shirley, E. D., & Ain, M. C. (2009). Achondroplasia: Manifestations and treatment. *Journal of the American Academy of Orthopedic Surgeons, 17*(4), 231–241.

Shorter, D., Hong, T., & Osborn, D. A. (2011). Screening programmes for developmental dysplasia of the hip in newborn infants. *Cochrane Database of Systematic Reviews*, CD004595.

Sillence, D., & Danks, D. (1978). The differentiation of genetically distinct varieties of osteogenesis imperfecta in the newborn period. *Clinical Research, 26*, 178A.

Sisk, E. A., Heatley, D. G., Borowski, B. J., Leverson, G. E., & Pauli, R. M. (1999). Obstructive sleep apnea in children with achondroplasia: Surgical and anesthetic considerations. *Otolaryngology-Head and Neck Surgery, 120*, 248–254.

Sola, M. C., Del Vecchio, A., & Rimsza, L. M. (2000). Evaluation and treatment of thrombocytopenia in the neonatal intensive care unit. *Clinics in Perinatology, 27*(3), 655–679.

Steiner, R. D., Pepin, M. G., & Byers, P. H. (2005, January 28). *Osteogenesis imperfecta*. Gene Reviews. Retrieved from http://www.ncbi.nlm.nih.gov/books/NBK1295

Stelzeneder, D., Mamisch, T. C., Kress, I., Domayer, S. E., Werlen, S., Bixby, S. D., . . . Kim, Y. J. (2012). Patterns of joint damage seen on MRI in early hip osteoarthritis due to structural hip deformities. *Osteoarthritis and Cartilage, 20*(7), 661–669.

Toriello, H. V. (2011). Thrombocytopenia-absent radius syndrome. *Seminars in Thrombosis and Hemostasis, 37*(6), 707–712.

Wilkin, D. J., Szabo, J. K., Cameron, R., Henderson, S., Bellus, G. A., Mack, M. L., . . . Francomano, C. A. (1998). Mutations in fibroblast growth-factor receptor 3 in sporadic cases of achondroplasia occur exclusively on the paternally derived chromosome. *American Journal of Human Genetics, 63*, 711–716.

Wright, M. J., & Irving, M. D. (2012). Clinical management of achondroplasia. *Archives of Disease in Childhood, 97*(2), 129–134.

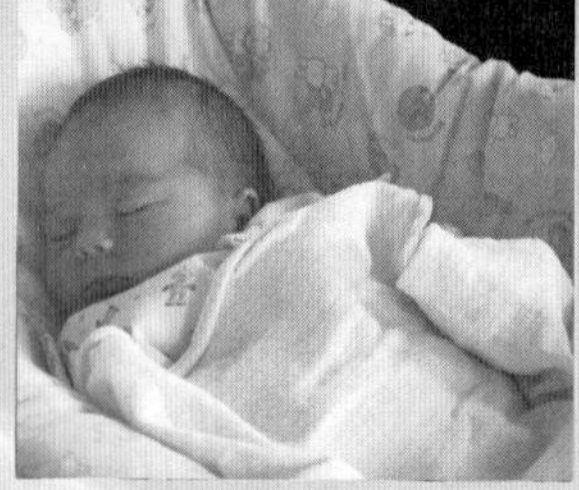

CHAPTER

15

Neurologic System

■ Georgia R. Ditzenberger and Susan Tucker Blackburn

The central nervous system (CNS) is one of the extraordinarily complex systems of the human body. Normal function of the CNS is critical to the function of every organ in the body and for the integration of organ systems that coordinate physiologic and neurobehavioral processes. Neurologic dysfunction during the neonatal period can arise from insults that occur before, during, or after birth. Such insults can affect the infant's ability to survive in the perinatal and neonatal periods and can have implications for later developmental and cognitive outcomes. Thus, alterations in neurologic function in the neonate have significant immediate and long-term consequences for the infant and family. Early recognition of infants at risk for neurologic dysfunction and prompt implementation of appropriate interventions are crucial for both the survival and reduction of long-term morbidity.

This chapter examines the structural and functional development of the CNS in the embryo, fetus, and neonate and the basis for common congenital and developmental anomalies. Neurologic assessment of the neonate and related diagnostic techniques are also presented, as are selected pathophysiologic problems that affect the central and peripheral nervous systems. The neurologic problems examined include neonatal seizures, intracranial hemorrhage, white-matter injuries (WMIs), hypoxic-ischemic encephalopathy (HIE), structural alterations, and birth injuries. Figure 15.1 shows the general structure of the newborn brain.

CNS DEVELOPMENT AND STRUCTURAL ABNORMALITIES

Many disorders of the neurologic system are related to defects in the development of the CNS. The development of the CNS can be divided into six stages: (1) neurulation, (2) prosencephalic development, (3) neuronal proliferation, (4) neuronal migration, (5) organization, and (6) myelinization. These stages overlap, and development progresses at different rates in various sections of the CNS. Embryologic development of the CNS begins shortly after fertilization, and maturation continues after birth until adulthood. The CNS therefore is one of the earliest systems to begin development and one of the last to reach maturity. The stages of CNS development are summarized in Table 15.1. CNS development is controlled by developmental genes in a complex cascade of signaling molecules, neurotropic growth factors, and vitamins (such as vitamin A and folic acid) mediating gene expression along the anterior-posterior axis of the embryo (Lew & Kothbauer, 2007; Rennie, 2005; Volpe, 2008).

Neurulation

Neurulation is the process by which the formation of the brain and spinal cord occurs as a result of inductive events within the dorsal aspect of the embryo (Table 15.1). The inductive events are separated into two stages: primary neurulation, the events related to the formation of the brain and spinal cord excluding the caudal segments of the lumbar region, and secondary neurulation, the events related to the caudal neural tube formation (Lew & Kothbauer, 2007; Volpe, 2008).

Primary neurulation occurs during the first 3 to 4 weeks of gestation and involves the formation of the primitive brain and spinal cord except the lower sacral and coccygeal segments. The CNS arises as a thickening of the ectoderm on the dorsal portion of the embryo at about 18 days gestation. The brain and spinal cord develop from this thickening, which is called the neural plate. The neural plate invaginates, forming the midline neural groove along the dorsal surface of the embryo. The parallel folds of tissue on either side of this groove are called the neural folds. The neural folds eventually form the forebrain, midbrain, hindbrain, and spinal cord. By the end of the third postconceptional week, the neural folds fuse to form the neural tube. The cranial portion of the lumen of the neural tube forms the ventricles; the caudal portion forms the central canal of the spinal cord. The tissues of the neural tube interact with surrounding mesoderm tissue (somites) to stimulate development of the bony structures, the skull and vertebrae, of the CNS (Creuzet, 2009; Moore, Persaud, & Torchia, 2012; Volpe, 2008).

In the fusion of the neural folds, some of the neuroectodermal cells on the upper margins are not incorporated into the neural tube. These cells form the neural crest, which lies

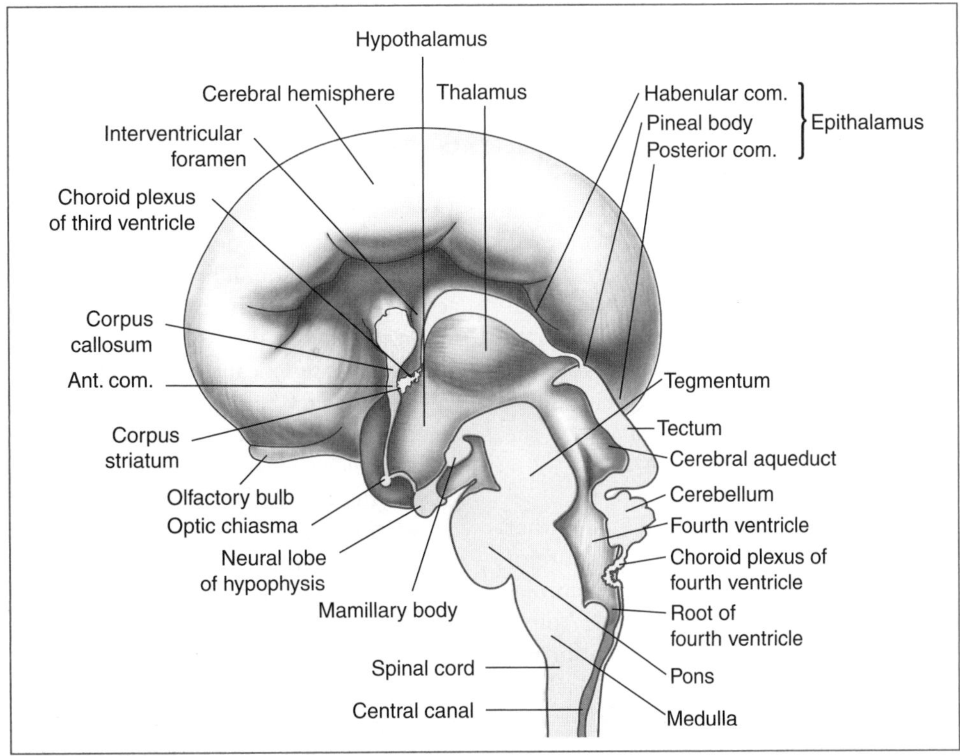

FIGURE 15.1 Cerebral anatomy.

TABLE 15.1

STAGES IN THE DEVELOPMENT OF THE CNS AND RELATED DEVELOPMENTAL DEFECTS

Stage	Peak Period of Occurrence	Developmental Defects
Neurulation	3–4 weeks gestation	Neural tube defects, anencephaly, encephalocele, spina bifida cystica (meningocele, myelomeningocele, myeloschisis), dermal sinus
Prosencephalic development	2–3 months gestation	Holoprosencephaly, holotelencephaly
Neuronal proliferation	3–4 months gestation	Microcephaly vera, macrencephaly, neurofibromatosis, other neurocutaneous disorders
Neuronal migration	3–5 months gestation	Hypoplasia or agenesis of the corpus callosum, schizencephaly, lissencephaly, pachygyria, polymicrogyria
Organization	6 months gestation–1 year of age	Alterations in brain development secondary to the effects of Down syndrome and trisomies 13, 14, and 15; behavioral alterations; mental retardation
Myelinization	8 months gestation–1 year of age	Brain hypoplasia, neurologic deficits

Compiled from Gressens and Huppi (2006); Volpe, et al. (2009); and Volpe (2008).

between the neural tube and the surface ectodermal layer. The neural crest tissue forms the peripheral nervous system, which includes the cranial, spinal, and autonomic system ganglia and nerves, Schwann cells, melanocyte (pigment) cells, meninges, and skeletal and muscular components of the head (Creuzet, 2009; Moore et al., 2012; Volpe, 2008).

Closure of the neural tube begins in the occipitocervical region at about 22 days gestation. The neural folds do not fuse simultaneously; fusion proceeds in cephalic and caudal directions from this site. For several days the neural tube is fused toward the central area but is open at both ends. The end areas are known as the rostral (anterior) and the caudal (posterior) neuropores. The cranial end of the neural tube closes at approximately 24 days gestation. Fusion of the cranial portion forms the forebrain. Failure of closure leads to anencephaly. The caudal neuropore, which is in the future lumbosacral area, closes in a rostrocaudal direction at approximately 26 days gestation (Lew & Kothbauer, 2007; Volpe, 2008). Once both neuropores are closed, the neural tube is a closed, fluid-filled system that has no further connection to the amniotic cavity unless a defect is present. Failure of the neuropores to close gives rise to neural tube defects (NTDs). Because differentiation of the surrounding mesodermal tissue (somites) into vertebrae, cranium, and dura depends on interaction with the neural tube, NTDs involve not only the neural elements but also the bony structures and meninges (Blackburn, 2013; Moore et al., 2012; Stoll, Dott, Alembik, & Roth, 2011; Volpe, 2008).

Secondary neurulation consists of two sequential phases: canalization and regressive differentiation. These phases form the spinal cord of the sacral and coccygeal segments. Canalization begins at 28 to 32 days gestation and continues through the seventh week of gestation and involves the development of the lower lumbar, sacral, and coccygeal areas from an undifferentiated cell mass at the caudal end of the neural tube. Vacuoles develop that gradually coalesce, enlarge, and contact the caudal end of the neural tube. The second phase, regressive differentiation, begins about the seventh week and continues until sometime after birth. Regressive differentiation is characterized by regression of much of the caudal cell mass, leaving behind the ventriculus terminalis, which is located in the conus medullaris, and the filum terminale (Blackburn, 2013; Volpe, 2008).

■ Disorders of Neurulation. Congenital anomalies that arise during the period of neurulation result from failure of neural tube closure, of which 80% occur at either the cranial or caudal end (Blackburn, 2013; Moore et al., 2012; Volpe, 2008). NTDs are one of the most common CNS malformations, occurring in 0.5 to 5 per 1,000 live births (Back & Plawner, 2012; Detrait et al., 2005; Kanekar, Kaneda, & Shively, 2011). Incidence varies with ethnicity, diet, geographical area, and socioeconomic status and is difficult to ascertain (Back & Plawner, 2013; Hockley & Salanki, 2009). NTDs usually are accompanied by alterations in vertebral, meningeal, vascular, and dermal structures and include craniorachischisis totalis, anencephaly, encephalocele, spina bifida occulta and cystica (meningocele, myelomeningocele, and myeloschisis), and Chiari type II malformations (Blackburn, 2013; Stoll et al., 2011; Volpe, 2008). The most common NTD presentations are myelomeningocele and anencephaly (Back & Plawner, 2012; Detrait et al., 2005).

NTDs arise from genetic, nutritional, and/or environmental influences (Blackburn, 2013; Detrait et al., 2005; Volpe, 2008). There is a familial incidence and an increased genetic susceptibility within immediate families. There is a three- to fivefold increase in the risk for NTD in subsequent offspring after one affected child; the risk increases to tenfold with two or more affected family members (Back & Plawner, 2012; Bassuk & Kibar, 2009). In addition, the risk of NTD is greater if the previously affected family member had a lesion at T11 or higher (Volpe, 2008). In the general population, increased risk of NTD is associated with maternal diabetes, maternal obesity, prior miscarriages, maternal folate deficiency, and maternal exposure to drugs such as valproic acid and folic acid antagonists such as trimethoprim and carbamazepine (Au, Ashley-Koch, & Northrup, 2010; Detrait, 2005; Hockley & Salanki, 2009; Jentink et al., 2010).

Folic acid supplementation at conception reduces the rate of NTDs (Blackburn, 2013; Breimer & Nilsson, 2012; Detrait et al., 2005; Mosley et al., 2009). Folate is a cofactor for enzymes needed in DNA and RNA synthesis and is important to a cell's ability to methylate proteins, lipids, and myelin and to the actions of other B vitamins. The American Academy of Pediatrics (AAP) recommends that women of childbearing age consume 0.4 mg of folate daily; for women who previously have had an infant with a NTD, the recommendation is 4 mg daily (American Academy of Pediatrics Committee on Genetics [AAP], 2007).

Antenatal screening for NTDs involves maternal serum alpha-fetoprotein screening (MSAFP), ultrasound examination, and/or measurement of the alpha-fetoprotein (AFP) level of the amniotic fluid. Analysis of MSAFP is performed between 15 and 20 weeks gestation, with the optimal time between 16 and 18 weeks gestation. AFP is a major fetal glycoprotein, similar to the albumin produced in the fetal liver from 6 weeks gestation; concentrations of AFP peak at 13 to 15 weeks gestation. Normally, the AFP concentration of the cerebrospinal fluid (CSF) is significantly higher than that of the amniotic fluid; therefore when CSF leaks into the amniotic fluid, as occurs with an open NTD, the AFP level of the amniotic fluid and maternal serum is elevated. Between 75% and 90% of open NTD and greater than or equal to 95% of anencephaly are detectable by increased MSAFP levels. MSAFP levels of greater than 2.0 to 2.5 multiples of the median for singleton pregnancies and 4.0 to 5.0 multiples of the median in pregnancies involving multiple fetuses are considered elevated and require further investigation for diagnosis. Some pregnancies may require an analysis of amniotic fluid for AFP and acetylcholinesterase levels to confirm the diagnosis, particularly if the MSAFP level is borderline high-normal (Cunniff & Hudgins, 2010; Driscoll, Gross, & Professional Practice Guidelines Committee, 2009). Elevated AFP levels, either serum or amniotic fluid, are often followed up with examination by fetal ultrasonography to determine if the elevated AFP levels are the result of open NTD or other causes, such as open abdominal wall defects (gastroschisis and omphalocele), congenital nephrosis, or fetal demise (Cameron & Moran, 2009; Chaoui & Nicolaides, 2010; Driscoll et al., 2009). Neither maternal serum nor amniotic AFP is useful for closed NTD, which comprise 10% of all NTD, since fetal CSF does not leak into the amniotic fluid or maternal blood. Closed NTDs can be detected with two-dimensional fetal ultrasonography. Three-dimensional ultrasonography is gaining accuracy with improved diagnostic views for fetal defects and may replace the use of serum and/or amniotic AFP as the primary method of diagnosis of NTDs (Cameron & Moran, 2009; Chaoui & Nicolaides, 2010; Hockley & Salanki, 2009; Pooh & Pooh, 2009).

Craniorachischisis totalis results from the total failure of neurulation, in which only the formation of the neural plate-like structure occurs without further development of the overlying tissue. Most spontaneously abort during the embryonic period, with very few progressing to fetal stage. As a result, the incidence is not known (Gressens & Huppi, 2006; Volpe, 2008).

Anencephaly. Anencephaly is caused by failure of the anterior neural tube to fuse in the cranial area. Since the advent of perinatal diagnosis and folic acid therapy, the incidence of anencephaly has declined to 0.2 per 1,000 live births. Because fusion of the anterior neural tube forms the forebrain, anencephalic infants have minimal development of brain tissue. The brain tissue that does develop is poorly differentiated and becomes necrotic with exposure to amniotic fluid; this results in a mass of vascular tissue with neuronal and glial elements and a choroid plexus marked by partial absence of the skull bones. Because anencephaly is caused by failure of the neural tube to close cranially, this defect occurs before 24 to 26 days gestation, around the period of closure of the rostral neuropore (Bassuk & Kibar, 2009; Blackburn, 2013; Volpe, 2008).

Anencephalic infants often have other anomalies. Three fourths are stillborn; live-borns die within the first postnatal month, generally by the end of the first week (Volpe, 2008). Management of infants with anencephaly is supportive, involving provision of warmth and comfort until the infant dies. Families require emotional support and assistance in coping with their grief over the birth of an infant with a defect and the death of their infant.

Encephalocele. Encephaloceles arise from failure of closure of a portion of the neural tube in the anterior region. The incidence of encephalocele is reported to be 0.8 to 5.6 per 10,000 live births (Rowland, Correa, Cragan, & Alverson, 2006; Wen, Ethen, Langlois, & Mitchell, 2007). Although this defect can occur in any region, approximately three fourths occur in the occipital region. The sac protrudes from the back of the head or the base of the neck. The next most common area is the frontal region, with involvement of the orbit, nose, and/or nasopharynx. Rarely do encephaloceles occur in the temporal or parietal areas (Gressens & Huppi, 2006; Volpe, 2008). Hydrocephalus, which may be present at birth or develop after surgical repair, occurs with 50% of occipital encephaloceles because of alterations in the posterior fossa (Gressens & Huppi, 2006). Encephalocele may occur in association with chromosomal abnormalities, such as trisomy 13, 18, and 21, Meckel–Gruber syndrome, or Walker–Warburg syndrome (Jones, 2006; Wen et al., 2007).

The protruding sac varies considerably in size; however, the size of the external sac does not correlate with the presence of neural elements. For example, a large occipital sac may contain minimal neural tissue, whereas a small sac may contain parts of the cerebellum or accessory lobes; some occipital lesions have no neural elements in the sac (Gressens, & Huppi, 2006; Volpe, 2008). Neural tissue generally displays normal gyration and white matter, and is connected to the brain by a slender neck-like structure (Gressens & Huppi, 2006). If the sac is leaking CSF at birth, immediate repair is necessary. If the defect is covered by skin, surgery may be delayed until a complete workup, including skull radiography, computed tomography (CT) or cranial ultrasonography, magnetic resonance imaging (MRI), and EEG can be performed. Surgical closure helps prevent infection and facilitates feeding and other care. A ventriculoperitoneal shunt is inserted if hydrocephalus is present. Other management includes prevention of infection and trauma and positioning to avoid pressure on the defect. Maintenance of normal body temperature is essential, especially in infants with CSF leakage, because these infants are at risk for thermoregulatory problems caused by evaporative losses. Postoperative management includes assessment of ventilation and perfusion, comfort measures, monitoring of neurologic and motor function, promotion of normothermia, prevention of infection, positioning to prevent pressure on the operative site, and monitoring of the site for CSF leakage. The mortality rate and later outcome are significantly better for infants with anterior defects than for those with posterior defects. The prognosis is poor if significant brain tissue is contained within the sac (Back & Plawner, 2012).

Families of infants with an encephalocele need initial and continuing support and counseling. Initial parental care involves assisting parents with the shock of the defect and its appearance and with their grief over having an infant with an anomaly, as well as helping the parents deal with the outcome implications of this defect. Nursing care also involves enhancing parent–infant interaction and involving the parents in the infant's care when they are ready. Teaching before discharge includes skin care, positioning, exercises, handling and feeding techniques, and activities to promote growth and development.

Spina Bifida. Spina bifida is a general term used to describe defects in closure of the caudal neural tube that are associated with malformations of the spinal cord and vertebrae. Spina bifida arises from defects in closure of the caudal neuropore (open defects) or during secondary neurulation (closed defects). Defects range from minor malformations of minimal clinical significance to major disorders that result in paraplegia or quadriplegia and loss of bladder and bowel control. The two major forms of spina bifida are spina bifida occulta and spina bifida cystic (Blackburn, 2013; Moore et al., 2012).

Spina bifida occulta is a vertebral defect at L5 or S1 that arises from failure of the vertebral arch to grow and fuse between 5 weeks gestation and the early fetal period. Frequently, only one vertebra is involved in the defect and the spinal cord and nerves are not involved, so there usually are no neurologic symptoms. The dermal layer is intact over the vertebral defect; occasionally the defect is indicated by a dimple or tuft of hair. Incidence is difficult to determine as most go unrecognized due to minimal/no physical problems arising from the presence of this defect. Spina bifida occulta is estimated to occur in 3% to 20% of the normal population and is most often discovered in radiographs of the lumbar and sacral regions (Moore et al., 2012). A few individuals have underlying abnormalities of the spinal cord or the nerve roots, or both, such as diastematomyelia or dermal sinus (dermoids). Diastematomyelia results from the division of the spinal cord or nerve roots in an anteroposterior direction by a bony spicule or cartilaginous band. A dermal sinus is a tract of squamous epithelium that connects to the dura mater and is found in the midline, usually in the lumbosacral area corresponding to the location of the caudal neuropore. A dermal sinus occasionally is recognized at birth, but more often it is diagnosed later, after repeated episodes of meningitis (Volpe, 2008). Spina bifida occulta occurs in the atlas of the cervical region in about 3% of the normal population. The defect is rare at other cervical levels but if present, is occasionally accompanied by other abnormalities of the cervical region (Moore et al., 2012).

Spina bifida cystica is a generic term for NTDs characterized by a cystic sac containing meninges or spinal cord elements, or both, along with vertebral defects. Epithelium or a thin membrane covers the sac. This defect occurs in approximately 1 in 1,000 live births, and, as with anencephaly, the incidence has declined in recent years (Moore et al., 2012). Spina bifida cystica can occur anywhere along the spinal column but is seen most often in the lumbar or lumbosacral area. The three main forms of spina bifida cystica are meningocele, myelomeningocele, and myeloschisis (Moore et al., 2012; Blackburn, 2013; Sandler, 2010; Volpe, 2008).

A meningocele involves a sac that contains meninges and CSF, but the spinal cord and nerve roots are in their normal position. Neurologic deficits are not typically associated with meningocele. Meningoceles account for about 5% of spina bifida cystica (Blackburn, 2013; Gressens & Huppi, 2006; Moore et al., 2012).

Myelomeningocele refers to a sac containing spinal cord or nerve roots, or both, in addition to meninges and CSF and accounts for 80% of spina bifida cystica. This defect occurs at 26 to 30 days gestation, around the time of closure of the caudal neuropore. During development, the nerve tissues become incorporated into the wall of the sac, impairing differentiation of nerve fibers. The spinal cord and/or nerve roots are displaced dorsally, and defects of the muscle and bony structures are present. These lesions are covered with skin or meninges or both and are usually located in the lumbosacral area. The level of the impairment of the spinal cord dictates the severity of the neurologic deficit as the nerve tissues below the sac are impaired. The sensory level generally tends to approximate the motor level but may be several segments lower because of differences in the pattern of innervation between sensory and motor fibers (Blackburn, 2013; Volpe, 2008). Approximately 80% to 90% of these malformations occur in the lumbar area, which is the final area of neural tube fusion (Blackburn, 2013; Moore et al., 2012; Volpe, 2008). If the sac is covered with meninges, there is a risk of rupture during delivery, along with leakage of CSF and the risk of infection and dehydration. Infants with this defect have altered tone and activity of the lower extremities and may assume a froglike posture. With bowel and bladder involvement, dribbling of urine and feces may be noted. Many infants also have an associated Chiari malformation type II with a noncommunicating form of hydrocephalus (Blackburn, 2013; Gressens & Huppi, 2006; Hockley & Salanki, 2009; Moore et al., 2012; Volpe, 2008).

Myeloschisis is a severe defect in which no cystic covering exists, leaving the spinal cord open and exposed. Myeloschisis is thought to arise from a local overgrowth of the neural plate, which prevents neural tube closure. This defect probably occurs between 18 and 23 days gestation. The spinal cord in affected patients is a flattened mass of neural tissue. Infants with myeloschisis have a poor prognosis. These infants have significant neurologic deficits and are at great risk for infection, and many die of sepsis in the neonatal period. This defect can involve the entire length of the spinal cord and can occur in association with anencephaly (Blackburn, 2013; Moore et al., 2012; Volpe, 2008).

Chiari Type II Malformation. Chiari type II malformation is a defect in neural tube closure involving several anomalies, including displacement of the medulla, fourth ventricle, and lower cerebellum into the cervical canal; bony defects of the occiput, foramen magnum, and cervical vertebrae; and obstruction of the foramen magnum, leading to hydrocephalus (Gressens & Huppi, 2006; Volpe, 2008). The resulting hydrocephalus is caused primarily by one, or both, of two defects—either a hindbrain malformation blocking normal flow of the spinal fluid from fourth ventricular outflow and/or through the posterior fossa, or there may be aqueductal stenosis causing disruption of normal spinal fluid flow. Chiari type II malformation occurs with nearly every case of myelomeningocele located at the thoracolumbar, lumbar, and lumbosacral levels (Hockley & Salanki, 2009; Volpe, 2008).

Immediate management for all NTDs includes stabilization and prevention of trauma to or infection of the sac, if present, and its contents. The infant is monitored for signs of infection, including signs of sepsis or meningitis and localized infection, including redness or discharge from the sac. Warmth and hydration are provided, and fluid and electrolyte status is monitored. These infants are at greater risk of hypothermia and dehydration because of the open lesion, which lacks the normal protective skin covering. Infants with NTDs may have evidence of hydrocephalus at birth. Ultrasonography, CT, or MRI can be used to determine the size of the ventricular system, to rule out Chiari type II malformation, and to monitor ventricular status and the development of hydrocephalus. Renal dysfunction may develop as a result of recurring urinary tract infections. Infants with NTDs may also have cardiac, intestinal, orthopedic, and other neurologic anomalies (Blackburn, 2013; Gressens & Huppi, 2006; Hockley & Salanki, 2009; Volpe, 2008).

The infant with NTD is positioned prone or on the side to reduce tension on the sac. A roll between the legs at hip level assists in maintaining abduction of the legs; a foot roll is used to maintain the feet in a neutral position. Change of position from prone to side lying or side to side, as well as range-of-motion exercises, helps prevent skin breakdown and contractures. If the infant must be temporarily placed in a supine position for a procedure, a donut roll can be used to prevent pressure on the sac. Postoperative positioning also involves use of the prone or side-lying position, maintenance of body alignment, prevention of hip abduction, and prevention of pressure on the operative site with holding. Lumbar/sacral defects must be kept free of fecal or urine contamination. Meticulous skin care, with attention to keeping the skin clean and dry and removing urine and stool, helps prevent skin breakdown and infection. The timing and characteristics of urination and stool excretion are observed to help determine the degree of deficit.

For many infants with NTDs, immediate closure and aggressive care constitute the appropriate management (Hockley & Salanki, 2009; Piatt, 2010; Volpe, 2008). Unless the defect is severe or is associated with multiple life-threatening anomalies, more than 90% of infants with myelomeningocele survive the neonatal period. If the defect goes untreated, 15% to 30% survive and are left with a handicapping condition. Immediate closure, therefore, is the treatment of choice for most infants (Piatt, 2010; Volpe, 2008). Immediate closure reduces the risk of infection and improves the prognosis by reducing further deterioration of the spinal cord and nerve tracts. Early closure also facilitates caregiving. A large defect may require several surgical procedures for complete closure. If the defect is completely covered by epithelium, surgery may be delayed for a short period so that function can be evaluated further. All infants with NTDs are evaluated and monitored for hydrocephalus. Urologic function and renal function also are assessed continually. All infants with involvement of the spinal cord or nerve roots, or both, require multidisciplinary follow-up and continuing care to deal with neurologic, urologic, orthopedic, and psychologic problems (Hockley & Salanki, 2009; Piatt, 2010).

Families of infants with NTDs need initial and continuing support and counseling. Initial parental care involves assisting parents with the shock of the defect and its appearance and with their grief over having an infant with an anomaly. Nursing care also involves enhancing parent–infant interaction and involving the parents in the infant's care when they are ready. Teaching before discharge includes skin care, positioning, exercises, handling and feeding techniques, and provision of activities to promote development. Many areas have spina bifida associations and parent-to-parent support programs to which parents can be referred for peer support.

In utero repair of NTDs, specifically myelomeningocele, performed before 26 weeks gestation has been reported with mixed results to reduce postnatal complications such as hindbrain herniation, hydrocephalus, and urologic dysfunction. Significant improvement in sensorimotor function has not been reported and an increase in obstetrical complications, such as preterm labor, oligohydramnios, premature rupture of the membranes, and surgical risks involved with two cesarean sections (one for fetal surgery and one for delivery) have been reported in several small studies (Adzick et al., 2011; Bebbington, Danzer, Johnson, & Adzick, 2011; Bruner, 2007; Danzer, Johnson, & Adzick, 2012; Hirose & Farmer, 2009; Hockley & Salanki, 2009; Volpe, 2008). In an effort to determine whether prenatal repair of myelomeningocele improved outcomes over postnatal surgical repair, a large, prospective randomized clinical trial, the Management of Myelomeningocele Study funded by National Institutes of Health (NIH), was done at three maternal-fetal surgery centers. The results showed that in utero repair of myelomeningocele reduced the need for postnatal shunting and improved motor outcomes at 30 months but is associated with maternal and fetal risks. Maternal risks included oligohydramnios, chorioamniotic separation, placental abruption, and spontaneous membrane rupture. An area of dehiscence or a very thin prenatal uterine surgical scar was present at the time of delivery in one third of the women who underwent in utero surgery. Fetal complications included premature delivery, with an average gestational age of 34.1 weeks, versus 37.1 weeks in postnatal surgical group, and nearly 13% delivered before 30 weeks gestation (vs. none in postnatal surgical group), and respiratory distress syndrome, which was likely primarily attributable to prematurity. No other significant fetal/neonatal complications were reported for the in utero surgical group. Postnatal shunt placement for hydrocephalus was significantly reduced for infants who underwent fetal repair, with 40% requiring shunts versus 82% of the postnatal repair group by a year of age. The prenatal surgical group also had a lower rate of moderate or severe hindbrain herniation (25%) than the postnatal surgical group (67%). There were no significant differences between the groups for epidermoid cysts. The prenatal surgical group required more procedures for delayed spinal cord tethering than did the postnatal surgical group. Infants in the prenatal surgical group (32%) had significantly improved function that was two or more levels better than expected according to the anatomical level than the postnatal surgical group (12%). The prenatal surgical group was also less likely to have worse than predicted levels of function (prenatal surgery 12% versus postnatal surgery 28%). Parent-reported self-care and mobility were also significantly better in the prenatal surgical group than the postnatal group. There were no differences in cognitive scores between groups (Adzick et al., 2011; Danzer et al., 2012). While the results of this multicenter randomized trial reflect promising support for prenatal surgical intervention for myelomeningocele repair, it is clear that fetal surgery is not the cure; timing and techniques of the actual surgery must be improved and made uniform; and the increased risk to maternal and fetal welfare and the availability of expert fetal surgical practitioners must be taken into consideration prior to generalized recommendations for fetal surgery (Danzer et al., 2012; Hockley & Salanki, 2009).

The prognosis associated with NTDs varies with the level and severity of the defect. Most infants with lesions lower than S1 will walk unaided; those with lesions higher than L2 generally will have some wheelchair dependency; bowel and bladder function are controlled at the level of S2 to S4 (Cohen & Walsh, 2006; Mitchell et al., 2004). However, these limitations are changing as a result of improved perinatal management and new technologies, and more children are ambulatory now than they were previously. Infants with a myelomeningocele involving a small lumbosacral lesion, without accompanying hydrocephalus or other anomalies, have some degree of neurologic deficit. These infants may be paraplegic but have a good prognosis for eventual independent function. The prognosis has also improved with the current early and aggressive treatment of infants without major cerebral lesions, hemorrhage, infection, high spinal cord lesions, or advanced hydrocephalus (Mitchell et al., 2004; Thompson, 2009; Volpe, 2008).

Prosencephalic Development

Prosencephalic development, or ventral induction, involves early development of the brain and ventricular system, which occurs during the second to third month of gestation (peaking at 5–6 weeks). The brain develops from the cranial end of the neural tube, beginning at the end of the fourth week. During this period, the three primary brain bulges (or vesicles) and cavities are formed, after fusion of the neural folds in the cranial area. Development of the face is associated with prosencephalic development of the CNS; consequently, alterations in brain development often result in facial malformations (Back & Plawner, 2012; Kanekar, Shively, & Kaneda, 2011; Volpe, 2008; Volpe, Campobasso, De Robertis, & Rembouskos, 2009).

The primary brain bulges are the forebrain (prosencephalon), the midbrain (mesencephalon), and the hindbrain (rhombencephalon). During the fifth week, the forebrain divides into two secondary vesicles, the telencephalon and the diencephalon, and the hindbrain divides into the metencephalon and the myelencephalon. The derivatives of each of these structures form the structures of the definitive brain. The third and fourth ventricles are formed from cavities within the rhombencephalon and diencephalon; the aqueduct of Sylvius links these two ventricles. The lateral ventricles arise from cavities in the cerebral hemispheres and are connected to the third ventricle by the foramen of Monro (see Figure 15.1). Early growth of the neural tube is most rapid in the forebrain region. To give these structures space to grow, the neural tube bends at several points, forming the mesencephalic (midbrain area), cervical (junction of the hindbrain and spinal cord), and pontine flexures (Back & Plawner, 2012; Hockley & Salanki, 2009; Volpe, 2008; Volpe et al., 2009).

■ Disorders of Prosencephalic Development. Malformations that occur during this period generally are thought to arise around the fifth to sixth weeks of gestation. Infants with these anomalies have a poor prognosis, and many are lost in early pregnancy or are stillborn. Malformations of the forebrain include holoprosencephaly and holotelencephaly. Holoprosencephaly is an abnormality in cleavage of the hemispheres that arises from genetic or possibly environmental alterations. Failure of horizontal, transverse, and sagittal cleavage of the prosencephalon disrupts formation of the telencephalon and the diencephalon and their derivatives. The resultant brain has a single monoventricular cerebral mass enclosed by a membrane; aplasia of the optic tract with absence of the olfactory tracts and bulbs, and agenesis of the corpus callosum, also is characteristic. Microcephaly, hydrocephaly, and facial anomalies also may be seen (Back & Plawner, 2012; Volpe, 2008; Volpe et al., 2009). With holotelencephaly, the parts of the brain that develop from the telencephalon form a single spheroid structure; the diencephalon and its derivatives are less affected. Congenital hydrocephalus can also arise during this period. At about 6 weeks gestation, three critical events occur that are related to the formation and circulation of CSF: (1) development of secretory epithelium in the choroid plexus, (2) perforation of the roof of the fourth ventricle, and (3) formation of the subarachnoid space. Alterations in the second and third events give rise to a communicating form of hydrocephalus (Volpe, 2008).

Neuronal Proliferation

The development of neurons and glial cells involves proliferation in the germinal matrix; migration (to their final destination) in the next stage of CNS development; differentiation of glial cells (during the period of organization) into specific cell types; alignment of neurons; and the development of interneuron and glial-neuron relationships. The peak period of neuronal proliferation lasts from 2 to 4 months gestation. During this stage, further development occurs in the subventricular and ventricular zones, where neurons and glial cells are derived from stem cells in the germinal matrix. Initial proliferation involves primarily neurons and radial glia, which are needed for neuron migration. Proliferation of other glia and their derivatives (astrocytes and oligodendrocytes) occurs intensively during the stage of organization, at 5 to 8 months gestation. During the most intense period of proliferation, before 32 to 34 weeks gestation, the periventricular area receives a large proportion of the cerebral blood flow. This area is vulnerable to hemorrhage in preterm infants (Blackburn, 2013; Volpe, 2008).

■ Disorders of Neuronal Proliferation. Disorders of proliferation arise from inadequate or excessive proliferation of neuronal derivatives, glial derivatives, or glial cell derivatives. Because mature neurons cannot divide, the eventual number of neurons is determined early in gestation. Insults may alter the neuronal-glial stem cells, which reduces the number of neurons or glial cells, or may alter cell growth, which results in smaller cells. The resulting disorders include micrencephaly, macrencephaly, and neurofibromatosis (Abuelo, 2007; Olney, 2007; Volpe, 2008). Micrencephaly may be due to a reduction in either the size or number of stem cells (Abuelo, 2007; Back & Plawner, 2012; Blackburn, 2013; Volpe, 2008). Micrencephaly vera is associated with a small brain caused by a decrease in the size of the proliferating units as a result of genetic or environmental factors and occurs at 2 to 4 months gestation. These infants often do not have marked neurologic deficits or seizures during the neonatal period, and in general the brain is well formed; however, the infants later manifest mental delays. Genetic factors associated with micrencephaly vera include autosomal recessive or dominant trait, X-linked recessive trait, or translocation. Micrencephaly vera is associated with environmental factors such as irradiation, metabolic alteration, maternal rubella, fetal alcohol syndrome, maternal cocaine use, and maternal phenylketonuria with elevated phenylalanine levels during pregnancy.

Micrencephaly caused by decreased number of stem cells is called radial microbrain and is familial, most likely autosomal recessive. Infants affected by this rare and more severe form of micrencephaly generally die within the first month of life (Back & Plawner, 2012; Blackburn, 2013; Pomeroy & Ullrich, 2004; Volpe, 2008).

Macrencephaly results in a large brain size because of excessive proliferation of neuronal elements or nonneuronal elements, or a combination of both. Macrencephaly is associated with genetic disorders including Beckwith–Wiedemann syndrome, Sturge–Weber syndrome, Weaver syndrome, and achondroplasia; chromosomal disorders such as Klinefelter and fragile X syndromes, and partial trisomy of chromosome 7; and neurocutaneous disorders, such as neurofibromatosis. Neurofibromatosis is an autosomal dominant genetic disorder involving excessive proliferation of nonneuronal elements in the CNS and mesodermal structures of the body, with cutaneous stigmata (Back & Plawner, 2012; Blackburn, 2013; Kanekar Kaneda, & Shively, 2011; Volpe, 2008). Neurofibromatosis often presents with alterations of skin pigmentation (café-au-lait macules), Lisch nodules of the iris, buphthalmos (enlarged eyeball), skin nodules and multiple benign neurofibromas. Infants with more than five café-au-lait macules larger than 5 mm in diameter at birth should be further evaluated for neurofibromatosis. Neurofibromatosis is associated with learning disabilities and, later in life, possible development of skeletal abnormalities, vascular disease, CNS tumors, or malignant peripheral nerve sheath tumors (Blackburn, 2013; Jett & Friedman, 2010; Isaacs, 2010; Volpe, 2008).

Neuronal Migration

The peak period for the neuronal migration stage is 3 to 5 months gestation. This stage is characterized by the movement of millions of cells from their point of origin in the subependymal germinal matrix of the periventricular region to their eventual loci in the cerebral cortex and cerebellum (see Figure 15.1). The process of neuronal migration is critical to the formation of the neocortex, gyri, and deep nuclear structures. Development of the gyri and sulci follows a predictable pattern that is linked to gestational age. At 21 to 25 weeks gestation, the central ventricles are large and the brain agyric; gyral development begins by the end of this period (Blackburn, 2013; Guerrini & Parrini, 2010; Kuijpers & Hoogenraad, 2011; Valiente & Marin, 2010; Volpe, 2008).

The mechanisms that guide neuronal migration are not completely understood, but they are mediated by signaling proteins, surface molecules, and receptors on both the neurons and the radial glia (Guerrini & Parrini, 2010; Valiente & Marin, 2010). Radial glia act as guides for migrating cells and then later transform into astrocytes (Guerrini & Parrini, 2010; Valiente & Marin, 2010; Volpe, 2008). The cerebral cortex has essentially achieved its full complement of neurons by 20 to 24 weeks gestation. Later, migration predominantly involves glial cells. The migration of the neurons to both the cortex and the cerebellum is assisted by the radial glia (Volpe, 2008).

■ Disorders of Neuronal Migration. Errors or exogenous insults before or after birth can alter migration of neurons and glial cells. Alterations in migration can result in hypoplasia or agenesis of the corpus callosum, agenesis of a part of the cerebral wall (schizencephaly), or gyral anomalies (pachygyria, lissencephaly, and polymicrogyria). The preterm infant may be especially vulnerable to gyral alterations. Rapid development of the gyri begins at 26 to 28 weeks gestation and continues through the third trimester into the postbirth period. Development of gyri results in a marked increase in cerebral surface area (Back & Plawner, 2012; Guerrini & Parrini, 2010; Mochida, 2009; Valiente & Marin, 2010; Volpe, 2008).

Organization

The peak period for organization is about the fifth month of gestation to a few years after birth. However, organizational processes continue throughout childhood, particularly in the cerebellum. Some processes, such as synaptogenesis, continue until death. Organizational processes allow the nervous system to act as an integrated whole. These processes include (1) establishment of subplate neurons, which serve as transient "way stations" by providing a place of synaptic contact for axons that ascend from the thalamus and other areas in which connecting cortical neurons are not yet in place; (2) attainment of the proper alignment, orientation, and layering of cortical neurons; (3) arborization or differentiation and branching of axons and dendrites; (4) differentiation of the glial cells; (5) development of synaptic connections ("wiring" of the brain); (6) balancing of excitatory and inhibitory synapses; and (7) cell death and selective elimination of neuronal processes (Blackburn, 2013; Volpe, 2008).

Subplate neurons are critical structures in the development of the neocortex, with maximal size and vulnerability reached by 26 to 30 weeks. Thus subplate neurons are vulnerable to perinatal injury. Subplate neurons are a site of initial synaptogenesis between areas within the cortex and are critical in guiding axons to their final loci and in establishing functional connections between different areas of the brain (Kling, 1989; Verklan, 2009; Volpe, Kinney, Jensen, & Rosenberg, 2011).

Glial cells serve as supportive structures with the CNS. The three forms of glia are (1) myelin-producing glia (oligodendrocytes in the CNS; Schwann cells in the peripheral nervous system); (2) guiding glia (radial glia for neuron migration during CNS development; Schwann cells for guiding peripheral nerves); and (3) "clean-up" glia (astroglia and microglia), which remove waste and dead tissue. Astroglia also provide support for neurons, assist in integration of information within the CNS, and are important in the structure and function of the blood–brain barrier. Microglia are capable of phagocytosis and function as brain macrophages and may be involved in developmental apoptosis (Blackburn, 2013; Kling, 1989; Vandertak, 2009; Verklan, 2009; Verney et al., 2011; Volpe, 2008; Volpe et al., 2011). When activated by inflammation or ischemia, as occurs with WMI, microglia can lead to further cellular injury. During the premyelinating period, oligodendrocytes are especially vulnerable to hypoxic-ischemic injury (see the later section in this chapter, WMI in Preterm Infants) (Deng, Pleasure, & Pleasure, 2008; Verklan, 2009; Verney, Monier, Fallet-Bianco, & Gressens, 2010; Volpe et al., 2011).

The process of cell death and selective elimination of neuronal processes is important in adjusting the size of individual neurons to their anticipated need. It is also an important component of brain plasticity in infants. In the developing brain, neuronal processes targeted for elimination can be saved if they are needed because of damage to other processes; by this means, functional ability is preserved. Excitatory neurotransmitters, such as glutamate, mediate neural development and organization by acting on N-methyl-D-aspartate (NMDA) receptors, and also likely, on GluR2-deficient alpha-amino-3-hyrdroxy-5-methyl-4-isoxazolenpropionic acid (AMPA) receptors and by opening voltage-dependent calcium channels (Volpe, 2008).

There is a striking increase in the cerebral cortical volume and gyral changes during this period of development and organization of cortical neurons, especially from around 28 to 40 weeks gestation in fetal growth. Recent advances in diffusion-based MRI, referred to as tractography, is proving to be useful in following changes in fiber tract development in premature infants (de Bruïne et al., 2011; Huang, 2010; Thompson et al., 2011; Volpe, 2008).

■ Disorders of Organization. Organization of the brain is susceptible to insults from errors of metabolism, abnormal chromosomes, and perinatal insults. Organizational processes are particularly vulnerable in the preterm infant being cared for in an intensive care unit during this period. Alterations in arborization and wiring of the brain can lead to hypersensitivity, poorly modulated behavior, and all-or-nothing responses. Alterations in organization are seen in infants with Down syndrome, who have abnormal development of the axons and dendrites and altered synaptic formation, fragile X syndrome (the most common cause of inherited mental retardation in males), Angelman syndrome (microdeletion on the long arm of maternal chromosome 15), infantile autism, Duchenne muscular dystrophy, mental retardation (with or without seizures), and Rett syndrome. Rett syndrome is one of the most common causes of mental retardation in females and is characterized by onset of decreasing head growth, loss of purposeful movement with the development of stereotypical, random hand movements, and autism (Volpe, 2008).

Myelinization

The myelinization stage involves development of myelin sheaths around nerve fibers in the nervous system. Oligodendrocytes, the nerve fibers of the CNS or Schwann cells, the nerve fibers of the peripheral nerves, form sheaths. The lipoprotein plasma membranes of these cells wrap themselves around the nerve fibers for several layers. Myelinization of fiber tracts tends to occur before maturation of functional ability (Blackburn, 2013; Moore et al., 2012; Volpe, 2008).

Myelinization begins early in pregnancy and continues to adulthood. Myelinization occurs between 8 months gestation and 2 years of age, with the peak period thought to be occurring within the first 8 postnatal months of life (Blackburn, 2013; Volpe, 2008). This process begins before birth in the peripheral areas, first in the peripheral motor nerves and then in the peripheral sensory nerves. Myelinization also begins before birth in the CNS, moving upward from the brainstem. In the CNS, myelinization occurs first in the sensory areas and then in the motor areas. Myelinization of ascending pathways in the spinal cord, brainstem, and thalamus is completed by about 30 weeks gestation, and myelinization from the thalamus to the cortex is completed by 37 weeks (Volpe, 2008). From birth to adulthood, myelinization proceeds within the cerebral hemispheres in conjunction with development of higher associative and sensory functions. Myelinization is important in most nerve tracts in the CNS because it insulates individual fibers to enhance specificity of connections, increases the number of alternative pathways, and markedly increases the speed of transmission (Blackburn, 2013; Beggs & Fitzgerald, 2007; Volpe, 2008). This has implications for neonatal pain management, particularly for preterm infants (Grunau & Tu, 2007; Blackburn, 2013).

■ **Disorders of Myelinization.** Myelinization is susceptible to damage from diverse exogenous influences, particularly malnutrition, which can lead to a range of neurologic deficits in which hypoplasia of the cerebral white matter occurs. Primary hypoplasia of the white matter with vacuolization of the myelin occurs in inadequate postnatal nutrition, congenital hypothyroidism, 18q-syndrome, and amino and organic acidopathies such as maple syrup urine disease, homocystinuria, and phenylketonuria. This defect in myelinization can lead to severe neurologic deficits in these infants (Volpe, 2008).

Neurologic Assessment

Assessment of neurologic function is an initial step in evaluating an infant's response to the transition to extrauterine life and the impact of perinatal events and pathophysiologic problems on the central and peripheral nervous systems. Assessment of neurologic function and identification of dysfunction encompass several components, including the history, physical examination, neurologic examination, laboratory tests, and other diagnostic techniques.

History

Risk factors noted in the maternal, obstetrical, and neonatal histories can be useful in identifying infants at risk for neurologic dysfunction and specific pathophysiologic factors. Specific risk factors for each problem discussed here are identified later in individual sections. General maternal or family historical factors that must be examined include a family history of NTDs; chromosomal or genetic abnormalities or other malformations; maternal substance abuse; chronic maternal health problems; maternal age, nutritional status, and exposure to teratogens; and the outcome of previous pregnancies (Heaberlin, 2009).

Obstetrical risk factors include prematurity, postmaturity, placental problems (e.g., abruptio placentae and placenta previa), use of analgesia or anesthesia, and maternal problems (e.g., infection, hypertension, and substance abuse). A large-for-gestational-age infant, prolonged or precipitate labor, forceps delivery, and abnormal presentation increase the risk of birth trauma and hemorrhage. Alterations in intrauterine growth and polyhydramnios may be present with an infant who has a CNS malformation. Fetal distress, hypoxia, ischemia, and low Apgar scores are associated with intracranial hemorrhage, and HIE (Blackburn, 2013; Bonifacio, Gonzalez, & Ferriero, 2012; Volpe, 2008).

Because neurologic dysfunction also can arise from postnatal problems, the infant's postnatal history is evaluated for status at birth, whether resuscitation was required, ischemic or hypoxic episodes, shock, hypoperfusion ± subsequent reperfusion, hemorrhage, infection, and metabolic or electrolyte aberrations. The infant's record is also reviewed for clinical signs, such as seizures or alterations in activity, tone, and state, which are associated with neurologic dysfunction (Bonifacio et al., 2012; Volpe, 2008).

Physical Examination

A comprehensive physical examination is an important component of the assessment of any infant at risk for or showing evidence of neurologic dysfunction. Infants are examined especially for evidence of infection and birth trauma, such as ecchymosis, edema, lacerations, and fractures. Temperature, blood pressure, color, and respiratory patterns also are assessed. The infant is examined for signs of vascular alterations, such as a port wine stain along trigeminal nerve branches, which may indicate Sturge–Weber syndrome. The characteristics of the infant's cry (e.g., robustness, presence in response to aversive stimuli, and pitch) may also be useful. Funduscopic examination may be performed to assess for chorioretinitis (associated with intrauterine viral infection), papilledema (seen with cerebral edema, although less reliably in neonates), and congenital anomalies (Amiel-Tison & Gosselin, 2009; Smith, 2012).

Specific parameters that are particularly important for the nurse to assess in infants with neurologic problems are (1) the head size, shape, and rate of growth; (2) the sutures and fontanelles; (3) whether major and minor anomalies are present; and (4) the vertebral column. Because CNS anomalies often are associated with other anomalies and syndromes, the infant also is examined for major anomalies of body systems and for isolated or clustered minor malformations, such as low-set or abnormally shaped ears, micrognathia, and hypertelorism of the eyes. The vertebral column is inspected and palpated for evidence of NTDs. Signs that may indicate an underlying defect include hair tufts, dimples, and fistulae (Amiel-Tison & Gosselin, 2009; Smith, 2012).

■ Head Size, Shape, and Rate of Growth. The monitoring and plotting of head circumference are basic components of health care for all infants, regardless of gestation or health status. The largest circumference is measured, which usually is the occipitofrontal circumference, about 1 cm above the eyes. The measurement is plotted on the appropriate growth grid for the infant's gender and gestation. The most accurate measurements are made with a metal or plastic tape marked in centimeters. Paper tapes tend to stretch and are less accurate but can be used for initial screening and for infants whose head size raises no concern. The occipitofrontal circumference generally ranges from 32.6 to 37.2 cm in term infants. Infants with caput succedaneum or overriding sutures may need to be re measured after 3 days to obtain a more accurate measurement (Amiel-Tison & Gosselin, 2009). The head usually grows 0.1 to 0.6 cm per week in infants 24 to 40 weeks gestation (Ditzenberger, 2010).

Serial measurements must be made to identify changes in the rate of growth as well as in size. Changes in the growth rate are important because an infant may have a significant increase or decrease in head growth but remain within the 10th to 90th percentiles on standard head growth grids. The occipitofrontal circumference should be measured several times over the first days after birth to obtain an accurate baseline after molding and edema from birth have resolved. Head circumference is measured weekly on preterm or ill infants. More frequent measurements may be made if the infant is at risk of developing progressive ventricular dilatation. Head shape can also reflect perinatal events and specific anomalies. The forces of labor and delivery may deform the head, but these changes are transient and disappear within a few days. Infants with craniosynostosis (premature closure of one or more sutures) and hydrocephalus have abnormal head configurations (Gomella, Cunningham, & Eyal, 2009).

■ Sutures and Fontanelles. The entire head is inspected and palpated, and each suture and fontanelle is assessed. The anterior fontanelle is assessed while the infant is in a quiet state and in a semiupright or sitting position. The fontanelle should be open, soft, and flat. Pulsation may be felt normally in a newborn but can be associated with elevated blood pressure. A sunken or depressed fontanelle is seen with dehydration, and a bulging fontanelle is noted with increased intracranial pressure (ICP). The anterior fontanelle usually is diamond shaped and may be small at birth if molding and overriding of the sutures are present; the size increases within a few days to the usual dimensions seen in term infants (i.e., 3–4 cm long by 1–3 cm wide). The anterior fontanelle closes at 8 to 16 months of age. The anterior fontanelle may bulge slightly with increased tension when the infant cries and may be slightly depressed when the infant is placed in an upright position. The posterior fontanelle closes any time from 8 months gestation to 2 months after birth. If open at birth, it is 1 to 3 cm wide and has a triangular shape. In rare cases, a "third fontanelle" may be palpated along the sagittal suture between the anterior and posterior fontanelles; this is not a true fontanelle but a defect in the parietal bone. It can be palpated in normal infants, but it is also seen in infants with Down syndrome or hypothyroidism (Heaberlin, 2009). A 4- to 5-mm separation (up to 1 cm) of all the sutures except the squamosal (temporoparietal) suture is normal in the newborn. The squamosal suture should not be separated more than 2 to 3 mm, especially in the term or near-term (late preterm) infant. Overriding of the bones and molding from delivery may modify this finding in the first few days after birth. Abnormal findings include persistence of suture separation over time, increased separation of the sutures, and separation of the squamosal suture by more than 2 to 3 mm. With increased ICP, separation of the sutures occurs in a specific order: sagittal, coronal, metopic, lambdoidal, and squamosal; therefore separation of the squamosal suture is the most clinically significant (Amiel-Tison & Gosselin, 2009). The cranial bones are inspected and palpated so that fractures, extradural hemorrhage, edema, and areas of uneven ossification of the cranial bones or craniotabes can be identified.

Neurologic Examination

The neurologic examination is useful for evaluating for the presence and determining the extent of neurologic dysfunction in the neonate, for monitoring recovery, and as a prognostic indicator. Factors such as gestational age, health status, the infant's state, medications, and timing of feedings must be considered in the interpretation of neurologic findings. Parameters examined in the assessment of neurologic status include level of consciousness, activity, tone, posture, reflexes, and evaluation of selected cranial nerves (Amiel-Tison & Gosselin, 2009; Heaberlin, 2009; Volpe, 2008). The optimum state of the infant during a neurologic examination is quiet and alert, after awakening naturally from a sleep state. It may be difficult to find such a perfect moment, and often the infant must be aroused from a sleep state or quieted from a state of heightened arousal. It is important to determine the state of the infant prior to a neurologic examination, since the infant's level of alertness has an effect on the interpretation of the infant's neurologic status (Amiel-Tison & Gosselin, 2009).

■ Observation of State: Level of Consciousness Neurologic insults frequently alter the infant's level of consciousness. The level of consciousness may range from normal states of consciousness for gestation to hyperexcitability, irritability, lethargy, hyperalertness, and stupor or coma. The three clinical levels of consciousness that best correlate with outcome are hyperalertness, lethargy, and stupor or coma. In the hyperalert state, the infant has an increased sensitivity to sensory stimulation, with wide-open eyes but with a diminished blink response and ability to fixate and follow (Amiel-Tison & Gosselin, 2009; Volpe, 2008). A lethargic infant responds to tactile and noxious stimuli, but the responses are delayed. A stuporous or obtunded infant's response is limited to noxious stimuli, and a comatose infant shows no response to tactile or noxious stimuli (Amiel-Tison & Gosselin, 2009; Volpe, 2008). Hyperexcitability and irritability can be assessed by noting an infant's response to caregiving actions and medical procedures, as well as the baby's state between caregiving intervals to assess the infant's ability to use self-consoling measures.

■ Posture, Tone, and Activity. Because normal tone requires integrated functioning of the entire nervous system, disturbances in either the central or peripheral nervous system may manifest in alterations in neonatal position, tone, and activity (Fenichel, 2007). The infant first is assessed while lying in a resting position. A frog-leg position while supine is seen in immature infants, after breech delivery, and in infants who have experienced severe asphyxia or who have major health problems or neuromuscular disorders (Amiel-Tison & Gosselin, 2009). The quality and symmetry of activity with spontaneous and elicited movement are assessed. Alterations in symmetry of the trunk, face, and extremities at rest or with spontaneous movement suggest congenital anomalies, birth injury, or neurologic insult. Tight fisting is an abnormal sign. A cortical thumb (inside thumb on closure of the hand) may be normal, but it is abnormal if persistent. Opisthotonos and decerebrate or decorticate posturing may also occur (Amiel-Tison & Gosselin, 2009; Fenichel, 2007; Heaberlin, 2009; Volpe, 2008).

Abnormal movements include seizure activity, jitteriness, and tremors, although the last two findings often are normal. Tremors and jitteriness must be differentiated from seizures. The characteristic movements seen with tremors in the neonate vary with the underlying disorder. Tremors associated with metabolic abnormalities usually are low-amplitude, high-frequency movements, whereas tremors associated with CNS complications usually are high-amplitude, low-frequency movements. Jitteriness is a common finding in infants because of the lack of myelinization of the pyramidal tracts. A major function of these tracts is to inhibit spinal reflexes. In the neonate, these unmyelinated tracts respond in a mass way to central arousal with peripheral hyperexcitability. Jitteriness is stimulus sensitive and is not marked by gaze or eye deviations. The predominant movement in jitteriness is tremulousness, rather than the clonic movement seen in seizures, which ceases with passive flexion. Spontaneous or elicited movement can set off tremors. Tremors can also be associated with metabolic abnormalities, asphyxia, or drug withdrawal (Volpe, 2008).

Resting, passive, and active tone is assessed. Resting tone is evaluated by observing the infant at rest in a supine position. Passive tone is evaluated by examining extensibility, which involves maneuvers used in the neuromuscular component of the assessment of gestational age. Assessment of active tone involves altering the infant's posture to obtain directed motor responses (Amiel-Tison & Gosselin, 2009).

Common maneuvers are righting reactions of the legs and trunk and examination of neck flexors and extensors. Righting reactions are elicited by holding the infant upright with the feet on a firm surface. The infant's ability to straighten the legs and trunk is assessed. Neck flexors and extensors are assessed using the pull-to-sit maneuver (Amiel-Tison & Gosselin, 2009; Fenichel, 2007). Infants with peripheral nerve injuries, neuromuscular disorders, alterations at the neuromuscular junction, and spinal cord injuries tend to be hypotonic and have muscle weakness. Infants with CNS disturbances secondary to asphyxia, intracranial hemorrhage, chromosomal disorders or other genetic defects, or metabolic disturbances tend to be hypotonic without muscle weakness (Amiel-Tison & Gosselin, 2009; Dastgir, Chan, & Darras, 2012; Fenichel, 2007). Hypertonia is seen less often than hypotonia in neonates with neurologic problems. Marked extensor hypertonia with arching of the back (opisthotonus) may be seen in association with severe hypoxic-ischemic injury, bacterial meningitis, or massive intraventricular hemorrhage (IVH) (Amiel-Tison & Gosselin, 2009; Heaberlin, 2009; Volpe, 2008).

■ Reflexes. In infants with neurologic dysfunction, primary and tendon reflexes may be diminished, absent, or accentuated. Primary reflexes are affected by gestational age, but all are present to some degree by 28 to 32 weeks gestation and include sucking, grasping, crossed extension, automatic walking (stepping), and the Moro reflex. These reflexes should be present, symmetric, and reproducible in the neonatal period and should gradually disappear during infancy (Amiel-Tison & Gosselin, 2009). The tendon reflexes assessed in the neonate are the biceps, knee, and ankle jerk. All should be present after about 33 weeks gestation, but are not very helpful beyond confirming symmetry in the neonatal period (Amiel-Tison & Gosselin, 2009).

■ Examination of Selected Cranial Nerves. Full cranial nerve assessment generally is not performed on the neonate. However, function of these nerves can be evaluated using several relatively simple maneuvers: fixation and following, pupillary responses, doll's eye response, hearing, vestibular response, and suck and swallow (Table 15.2) (Amiel-Tison & Gosselin, 2009; Fenichel, 2007; Heaberlin, 2009; Rennie, 2005).

■ Clinical Signs Associated With Neurologic Dysfunction Clinical manifestations of neurologic dysfunction can be specific or nonspecific. Five types of clinical signs are commonly seen in infants with neurologic problems: (1) CNS depression, (2) hyperirritability, (3) increased ICP, (4) seizures, and

TABLE 15.2

NURSING ASSESSMENT OF SELECTED CRANIAL NERVES IN THE NEWBORN

Nerve	Assessment	Implications
Optic (II)	Blink in response to light (consistent by 28 weeks gestation) Fixation on object placed approximately 19 cm in front of infant's face (consistent by 32 weeks gestation) Follows object with eyes and by turning head (consistent by 37 weeks gestation) Examination of external eye	Visual system intact to the level of the superior colliculi (does not indicate visual cortex function) Presence of vision
Oculomotor (III), trochlear (IV), and abducens (VI)	Funduscopic examination (ophthalmoscope set at 2–4 diopters) Pupillary reactivity (equal and responsive to light; appears by 28 weeks gestation and consistent by 32 weeks) Doll's eye maneuver (vestibular response; present by 25 weeks gestation): hold infant in an upright position at arm's length and rotate in both directions	Evaluation of abnormalities (e.g., cataracts, irregularities of size or shape, microphthalmos, or scleral hemangiomas) Normal newborn optic disc is pale or grayish-white; observe for abnormalities (e.g., retinal hemorrhage or lesion) Intact cranial nerve III; unequal or nonresponsive pupils in infants over 32 weeks gestation are associated with increased ICP or hemorrhage Stimulation of semicircular canals with impulses sent to the brainstem via nerves III, VI, and VII. Normal response is isotonic deviation of the eyes away from the direction of movement; lack of response is associated with brainstem dysfunction or excessive administration of sedatives such as phenobarbital; disconjugate eye movements and some nystagmoid movements occasionally are seen normally during the first 3 weeks
Trigeminal (V)	Elicit the corneal reflex (may not be reliable in newborn) or observe for a grimace on pinprick Elicit sucking and ability of infant to bite down on examiner's finger	Facial sensation (not usually done routinely but may be useful with an infant with facial paralysis) Masticatory power
Facial (VII)	Observe appearance and symmetry of face at rest and during spontaneous and elicited movement	Abnormalities associated with birth injury and cerebral insults
Acoustic (VIII)	Evaluate auditory function by noting response (blink or startle) to sudden loud noise (seen by 28 weeks gestation) or (in more mature infants) by cessation of movement and turning to sound while in a quiet, alert state	A gross assessment of auditory function; failure of the infant to respond while in a quiet, alert state in a quiet environment on repeated examinations indicates the need for examination of auditory function
Trigeminal (V), facial (VII), glossopharyngeal (IX), vagus (X), and hypoglossal (XII)	Evaluate sucking (V, VII, XII), swallowing (IX and X), and gag reflex (IX and X)	Impairment interferes with feeding and may indicate or be associated with cerebral insult

Compiled from Amiel-Tison and Gosselin (2009); Rennie (2005); and Volpe (2008).

(5) movement alterations. Seizures are discussed later. Signs and symptoms of CNS depression, hyperirritability, increased ICP, and movement alterations are listed in Table 15.3.

Diagnostic Techniques

Diagnostic techniques that may be used with infants suspected of neurologic problems include neurophysiologic studies, structural brain imaging and assessment of cerebral blood flow, and laboratory tests. Neurophysiologic studies used in the neurologic assessment of the newborn include brainstem auditory evoked responses, visual evoked responses, somatosensory evoked responses, and electroencephalogram (EEG) and amplitude-integrated EEG (aEEG) (Lehmann, 2009; Trollmann, Nüsken, & Wenzel, 2010). The brainstem auditory evoked response test is the reflection of the electrical events generated in the auditory pathways detected via small external sensors and indicates the response of the infant to auditory stimulus. This test is easily performed and is currently the most often used technique for routine hearing screening in newborn nurseries. Visual evoked and somatosensory evoked responses are part of a more extensive neurologic examination to aid in determining the extent of the disturbance in the vision and peripheral sensation (Lehmann, 2009; Trollmann, Nüsken, & Wenzel, 2010; Volpe, 2008). EEG and aEEG will be discussed in the section on neonatal seizures.

TABLE 15.3

CLINICAL MANIFESTATIONS OF CNS DYSFUNCTION

Alteration	Clinical Manifestations
CNS depression	Altered level of consciousness
	Weak, absent cry
	Weak, absent primary reflexes
	Poor feeding
	Decreased activity
	Decreased passive tone
	Decreased active tone
	Altered respirations
Hyperirritability	Sharp, excessive crying
	Hyperactivity
	Exaggerated passive tone
	Hypertonia
	Difficult to console
	Low sensory threshold
Increased ICP	Irritability
	Lethargy
	Increased head circumference
	Palpable sutures, especially squamous
	Bulging, tense fontanelle
	Increased extensor tone of neck
	Downward deviation of eyes
	Vomiting (late)
	Dilated head veins (late)
Seizures	See Table 15.5
Movement alterations	Jitteriness, tremors
	Decerebrate posturing
	Decorticate posturing
	Opisthotonos

Compiled from Amiel-Tison and Gosselin (2009); Heaberlin (2009); and Rennie (2005).

The three types of brain structural imaging most often used are ultrasonography, CT, and MRI. Head, or cranial, ultrasound examination is used most often to evaluate intracranial structures and is most frequently the imaging modality of choice to evaluate germinal and IVH in the premature infant, with an estimated 90% accuracy level (Ramenghi & Huppi, 2007). Ultrasonography is portable, safe, convenient, and readily available at the bedside, utilizing nonionizing radiation with minimal/no need for sedation. Cranial and sagittal images can be evaluated by means of the anterior fontanelle and periventricular leukomalacia (PVL) by means of the posterior fontanelle. Doppler sonography, which is done as part of a complete head ultrasound, can be used to evaluate cerebral blood flow. Head ultrasonography is not generally useful for evaluating the posterior fossa and interparenchymal and meningeal areas (Fenichel, 2007; Koufman, Zanelli, Cantey, & Sanchez, 2012; Lehmann, 2009; Ramenghi & Huppi, 2007; Volpe, 2008). CT uses ionizing radiation coupled with computerized image reconstruction to provide high-resolution images within a few minutes of scanning. A CT of the newborn brain provides information regarding calcifications and cranial bony abnormalities, most parenchymal disorders, hemorrhage or fluid in the subdural and subarachnoid spaces, and most posterior fossa lesions. The MRI, which uses nonionizing radiation, is useful for diagnosing many abnormalities, some of which may be missed by sonography or CT, such as partial agenesis of the corpus callosum, arteriovenous malformations, acute or chronic focal cerebral ischemic lesions (infarcts), venous thrombosis, PVL, hemorrhagic lesions, and virtually all lesions in the posterior fossa and spinal cord (Girard & Raybaud, 2011; Koufman et al., 2012; Volpe, 2008). Both CT and MRI require transportation and sedation, however, which may prove to be detrimental for the critically ill infant. Using these modalities often necessitates waiting until the infant has recovered from the initial critical condition to be performed (Volpe, 2008).

Laboratory tests are performed to assist in the diagnosis of specific neurologic disorders and to identify underlying causes. The CSF is examined for signs of hemorrhage (increased red blood cells, increased protein, decreased glucose, and xanthochromia) and to rule out infection (culture, turbidity of the fluid, and increased or decreased white cells, protein and/or glucose) (Gomella et al., 2009). Xanthochromia often is a late sign and may reflect an elevated protein level rather than the presence of blood. Other laboratory evaluations include complete blood count with differential (e.g., white and red blood cell counts, hemoglobin, hematocrit (Hct), neutrophils, bands, and platelet count), serum glucose and calcium levels, electrolyte levels, blood gases, and acid–base status. A sepsis workup or screening for toxoplasmosis, rubella, cytomegalovirus, herpes simplex, and syphilis is performed if intrauterine infection or neonatal sepsis and meningitis are suspected. A genetic workup and other metabolic studies are performed if errors of metabolism or other inherited disorders are thought to be present (duPlessis, 2008a; Lehmann, 2009; Volpe, 2008).

GENERAL MANAGEMENT

Management specific to each type of neurologic dysfunction is described in later sections. However, in the nursing care of infants with neurologic dysfunction, common nursing diagnoses and management techniques that must be considered with all infants and their families are listed below. Those marked with an asterisk (*) are discussed in other chapters.

1. Alteration in level of consciousness
    - Monitor infant's state, activity level, responsiveness, eye movements, head circumference, and vital signs; also monitor for seizure activity and signs of increased ICP
    - Position infant so as to promote skin integrity, prevent contractures, and reduce ICP (i.e., head in midline and slightly elevated)

- Monitor fluid and electrolyte status
- Maintain adequate ventilation and perfusion
- Implement comfort measures
- Maintain an appropriate thermal environment
- Reduce environmental stressors
- Promote neurobehavioral stability

2. Potential for injury related to trauma or infection
   - Use sterile technique
   - Position infant to prevent contamination of defects or operative sites
   - Monitor for signs of localized infection or neonatal sepsis
   - Handle infant gently
   - Position infant to reduce potential of trauma or contamination
3. Impairment of skin integrity
   - Position infant in alignment and change position regularly
   - Use foam, sheepskin, lambskin, or waterbeds
   - Massage skin gently to stimulate circulation
   - Use appropriate skin care measures
4. Alteration in comfort*
5. Impaired mobility
   - Position infant in alignment and change position regularly
   - Promote skin integrity
   - Use gentle range-of-motion exercises
6. Alteration in thermoregulation*
7. Alteration in nutrition*
8. Promote neurobehavioral organization and development*
9. Altered family processes*
10. Grieving (family)*

NEONATAL SEIZURES

Seizures are the most common neurologic sign during the neonatal period and are more common in the newborn stage than at any other time in childhood. The reported incidence of neonatal seizures is approximately 1.8 to 5 per 1,000 live term births and 30 to 130 per 1,000 live preterm births (Scher, 2012a; Rennie & Boylan, 2009). Neonatal seizures usually are acute, with a third occurring on the first day and another third on the second day of life, then disappearing within the first few weeks after birth. Perinatal hypoxia-ischemia accounts for 50% to 60% of all neonatal seizures (Scher, 2012a; Rennie & Boylan, 2009).

Seizures are not a disease in themselves but a sign of underlying disease processes that have resulted in an acute disturbance within the brain. There is increasing evidence suggesting these seizures exacerbate brain injury, which increases the necessity for prompt recognition, efficient observation and monitoring methods, and effective therapeutic interventions (Bassan et al., 2008; Glass & Wirrell, 2009; Jensen, 2009; Scher, 2012a; Shah, Boylan, & Rennie, 2012; Toet & Lemmers, 2009; Volpe, 2008). If left untreated, these disorders can lead to permanent damage of the CNS or other tissues. Disease processes associated with seizures in the neonate include primary CNS disorders, hypoxic-ischemic events, systemic diseases, and metabolic insults. Seizure activity may be an acute, recurrent, or chronic phenomenon. Recurrent or continuous seizures increase the risk of neurologic damage from the seizure activity itself (Rennie & Boylan, 2009; Scher, 2012a; Shah et al., 2012; Volpe, 2008).

Pathophysiology

Seizures are the result of excessive, synchronous electrical discharge or depolarization in the brain that produces stereotypic, repetitive behaviors. Depolarization and repolarization of the nerves are caused by the movement of sodium and potassium across the cell membrane. The inward migration of sodium ions (Na^+) results in depolarization; repolarization is produced by the outward migration of potassium ions (K^+). These processes require an energy-dependent pump and energy in the form of adenosine triphosphate (ATP). The specific mechanism that causes neonatal seizures is unknown but might be the result of one or more of these mechanisms: (1) disturbances in energy production and the Na^+-K^+ pump, (2) altered neuronal membrane permeability to sodium, and (3) imbalances in excitatory and inhibitory neurotransmitters (Rennie & Boylan, 2009; Scher, 2012a; Volpe, 2008). A disturbance in energy production, with changes in the movement of Na^+ and K^+ across the neuronal membrane, may lead to an imbalance between depolarization and repolarization. The movement of K^+ (repolarization) unbalances the movement of Na^+ (depolarization). Changes in energy production may result from hypoxemia, ischemia, and/or hypoglycemia. Alterations in the permeability of the neuronal membrane to sodium can occur with hypocalcemia. Calcium normally binds with proteins in the cell membrane to inhibit Na^+ movement. A decrease in the availability of calcium would increase inward movement of Na^+ and lead to depolarization. Hypomagnesemia also increases membrane permeability to Na^+, and alkalosis or hyponatremia also leads to seizures through this mechanism. Imbalances in neurotransmitters lead to a relative excess of excitatory neurotransmitter (glutamate or acetylcholine) over inhibitory neurotransmitter (gamma-aminobutyric acid [GABA]) and increases the rate of depolarization. This can occur as a result of an excess of excitatory substance (associated with hypoxemia, ischemia, and hypoglycemia) or a deficiency of inhibitory substance. Pyridoxine deficiency leads to an inhibitory neurotransmitter deficiency by depressing the activity of the enzyme responsible for synthesis of GABA. Elevated levels of excitatory inhibitors derived from ammonia are seen in infants who have liver dysfunction after severe hypoxic-ischemic events (Jensen, 2009; Rennie & Boylan, 2009; Scher, 2012a; Volpe, 2008).

Biochemical Effects of Seizures

Seizures result in increased energy expenditure, which leads to the following sequence of biochemical events: (1) breakdown of ATP to adenosine diphosphate with release of energy; (2) increased glycolysis, stimulated by adenosine diphosphate, with conversion of glycogen to glucose; (3) increased production of pyruvate, which is used by the mitochondria in ATP production; (4) increased oxygen and glucose consumption; (5) increased production of lactate from pyruvate, stimulated by increased adenosine diphosphate; and (6) lactate/H^+-stimulated local vasodilation, which increases local blood flow and substrate availability (Rennie & Boylan, 2009; Scher, 2012a; Volpe, 2008). The rise in blood pressure associated with seizures also increases cerebral blood flow and substrate availability. Seizures result in a marked decrease in brain glucose concentrations because the cells to replenish ATP supplies use much of the available glucose. Repetitive seizures in the neonate eventually alter brain lipid and protein metabolism and energy metabolism, resulting in a reduction in total brain DNA, RNA, protein, and cholesterol. In animal models these deficiencies lead to impairment of cellular proliferation, differentiation, and myelinization (Volpe, 2008). The effects in the human neonate are unclear but of concern. Brain damage caused by seizure activity could be the result of alterations in protein metabolism or the energy supply, or it could be the result of damage from asphyxia or edema (Scher, 2012a, 2012b; Volpe, 2008).

Seizures in Neonates Compared With Those in Older Children and Adults

Seizures are expressed differently in the neonate than in older individuals because of structural and functional differences in the neonatal brain (Blackburn, 2009a; Silverstein & Jensen, 2007; Volpe, 2008). The peak time for organizational processes in the brain is from the sixth month of gestation to 1 year after birth; therefore term and especially preterm infants have relatively immature brain organization. This lack of organization results in an inability to propagate and sustain generalized seizures. For example, the neonate's brain lacks the arborization and synaptic connections (wiring) necessary for a firing neuron to recruit adjacent neurons to fire synchronously. Inadequate organization also leads to a slower response to stimuli (Blackburn, 2009a, 2009b; Volpe, 2008). The lower rate of nerve conduction, limited myelinization, and smaller number of connections between neurons alter the threshold for neuron firing and ability to propagate seizures (Blackburn, 2009a, 2009b; Scher, 2012a, 2012b; Volpe, 2008).

The neonate has increased inhibitory synapses compared to excitatory synapses which may actually be a protective mechanism because it reduces the chance that a generalized seizure will be propagated in the cerebral cortex. As a result, cortical seizures are rare in neonates (Blackburn, 2009b; Volpe, 2008). The newborn has more excitatory (glutamate) than inhibitory neurotransmitters. In addition, GABA, the main inhibitory neurotransmitter in adults, is excitatory in the newborn. The glutamate level is increased (it is needed by the brain for neuronal development and organization); maturation of the inhibitory system is delayed; and the number of NMDA receptors that respond to glutamate is increased (Blackburn, 2009a, 2009b; Jensen, 2009; Rennie & Boylan, 2009). Seizure activity in these infants is more likely to be generated in areas of the brain that are more mature, such as the temporal lobe and subcortical structures, especially in the limbic area. The limbic area, located above the corpus callosum, is one of the oldest parts of the brain in terms of embryologic development. This area is involved with behaviors such as sucking, drooling, chewing, swallowing, oculomotor deviations, and apneic episodes, behaviors typical of those seen with subtle seizures in the neonate (Blackburn, 2009b; Volpe, 2008).

Assessment

Seizures are a clinical manifestation associated with various underlying pathologic processes (Table 15.4), including hypoxia, ischemia, hypoglycemia, hypocalcemia, intracranial hemorrhage, infection (meningitis, congenital viral infections, viral encephalopathy), congenital anomalies of the CNS, and other metabolic disturbances, such as alkalosis, hypomagnesemia, hypernatremia, and hyponatremia. Less common causes of seizures are drug withdrawal from opiates or barbiturates, genetic disorders of amino and organic acid metabolism, kernicterus, hyperviscosity, and local anesthetic intoxication (Rennie & Boylan, 2009; Scher, 2012a; Volpe, 2008).

Seizures can be difficult to recognize in neonates because the clinical manifestations often are subtle and can be associated with other disorders or can involve individual behaviors such as grimacing, startle, sucking, and twitching. Seizures also can occur with minimal or no outward signs. Recognition of seizures in the neonatal period requires careful, continuous assessment by the nurse of all infants at risk. Clinical manifestations may include abnormal movements or alterations in tone of the trunk or extremities; abnormal and repetitive facial, oral, tongue, or ocular movements such as blinking, lip smacking, or chewing motions; and increases in blood pressure and apneic events (Glass & Wirrell, 2009; Rennie & Boylan, 2009; Volpe, 2008). Specific examples of each of these are listed in Table 15.5.

Types of Seizures

Various classifications of neonatal seizures are used, some focusing primarily on clinical and behavioral manifestations, others on the presence or absence of electroencephalographic correlates (Rennie & Boylan, 2009; Scher, 2012a). There is increasing evidence supporting a combination of clinical categories with electrographical confirmation, especially with the recent advances in digital technology that makes it possible to archive and review huge amounts of data generated by bedside video-EEG monitoring (Rennie & Boylan, 2009; Scher, 2012a, 2012b; Tao & Mathur, 2010; Toet & DeVries, 2012). The addition of simultaneous, continuous video-EEG and aEEG (method of displaying one or two channels of compressed and filtered EEG readings) monitoring may refine diagnosis and management of newborns, with seizure activity categorized within traditional classifications. The aEEG monitoring technique is a relatively easy method of detection of seizure activity and is in use with increasing regularity and reliability for monitoring neurologic status of infants with hypoxic-ischemic encephalopathy (Barnes, 2007; Bonifacio, Glass, Peloquin, & Ferriero, 2011; Hellstrom-Westas & DeVries, 2007; Rennie & Boylan, 2009; Tao & Mathur, 2010; Toet & Lemmers, 2009; Toet & DeVries, 2012).

TABLE 15.4

MAJOR CAUSES OF NEONATAL SEIZURES

Cause and Frequency (% of Total)	Usual Age at Onset (Days)	Predominant Type of Seizure
Hypoxic-ischemic injury (50%–60%)	After 1 (often 6–18 hours after birth); 90% in first 72 hours	Subtle (all), generalized tonic, multifocal clonic
Intracranial hemorrhage (10%)		
IVH	1–4	Subtle progressing to tonic
SAH	2–3	Any type
SDH	1–2	May be focal
Hypocalcemia (15%)		
Early	1–3	Usually focal or multifocal
Late	4–7	Usually focal or multifocal
Hypoglycemia (10%)	1–2	Usually focal or multifocal
Infections (5%–10%)		
Bacterial meningitis	4–7	Any type; may be tonic
Viral encephalopathy	2–15	Any type
Congenital viral infection	3–7	Tonic, myoclonic
CNS malformations (<5%–10%)	2–10 (often not until several months of age)	Tonic, myoclonic
Drug withdrawal (rare)	3–34	Tonic or myoclonic
Local anesthetic intoxication[a] (uncommon)	Before 1 (1–6 hours after birth)	Tonic

[a] Caused by accidental injection of local anesthetic into the scalp during placement of paracervical, pudendal, or epidural blocks or during injection of local anesthetics at delivery.

Compiled from Rennie and Boylan (2009); Scher (2012a, 2012b); Volpe (2008); and duPlessis (2008).

Traditional clinical seizure classification identifies the following seizure types: subtle, tonic, clonic (multifocal or migratory, and focal), and myoclonic (Rennie & Boylan, 2009; Scher, 2012a; Volpe, 2008). Subtle seizures are the most common type of seizure seen in neonates, particularly among preterm infants. This type of seizure often is missed because the clinical manifestations may be difficult to recognize and distinguish from other events. The behaviors most commonly seen with subtle seizures are (1) tonic, horizontal deviations of the eyes with or without nystagmoid jerking; (2) repetitive blinking or fluttering of the eyelids; (3) drooling, sucking, or tongue thrusting; and (4) swimming or rowing movements of the arms with occasional bicycling movements of the legs. Apnea may occur but usually is the result of the underlying cause of the seizure in the preterm, rather than of the seizure, and rarely occurs as an isolated seizure event (Rennie & Boylan, 2009; Scher, 2012a, 2012b; Volpe, 2008).

The most common form of tonic seizure is the generalized tonic seizure, which usually involves tonic extension of all the extremities but sometimes is limited to a single extremity or is manifested by tonic flexion of all limbs. Generalized tonic seizures can be confused with decorticate or decerebrate posturing. Other signs may include eye deviations, apnea, and occasional clonic movements. This type of seizure is the one seen most frequently in preterm infants, especially those with IVH and hypoxic-ischemic insults. Generalized tonic seizures often are accompanied by apnea or decerebrate-type postures or both. Occasionally, focal tonic seizures may occur, which are characterized by sustained asymmetric posturing of the limbs, trunk, or neck. Focal tonic seizure activity may be difficult to differentiate from voluntary movement (Rennie & Boylan, 2009; Scher, 2012a; Volpe, 2008).

Clonic seizures may be multifocal or focal. Because multifocal or migratory clonic seizures involve the cortex, they are more characteristic of term infants but occasionally may be seen in older preterm infants. This type of seizure involves rhythmic, jerky clonic movements of one or more limbs that migrate to other parts of the body in a random fashion. Multifocal clonic seizures can be confused with jitteriness. These seizures are associated with diffuse hyperexcitability of the cortex, such as occurs with metabolic derangements (Volpe, 2008).

Focal clonic seizures also are seen more frequently in term than in preterm infants. This form of seizure is characterized by localized clonic jerking that usually is present in one limb or the face. Focal clonic seizures may be associated with focal traumatic CNS injuries, such as cerebral contusions and infarcts, or may be a response to a severe metabolic disturbance or asphyxia and occur in combination with other seizure types (Scher, 2012a).

Myoclonic seizures are uncommon in term infants and are rarely seen in preterm infants. These seizures are characterized by single or multiple sudden jerks with flexion of the upper (most common) or lower extremities and occasionally

TABLE 15.5

CLINICAL MANIFESTATIONS OF SEIZURES IN THE NEONATE

Type of Manifestation	Specific Alterations
Abnormal movement or alterations of tone in the trunk and extremities	Clonic (generalized or multifocal, migratory)
	Altering hemiclonic tonic (single extremity), extension of arms and legs ("decerebrate-like"), extension of legs and flexion of arms ("decorticate-like"), or generalized
	Myoclonic (isolated or general)
	Bicycling movements of legs
	Swimming or rowing arm movements
	Loss of tone with general flaccidity
Facial, oral, and tongue movements	Sucking
	Grimacing
	Twitching
	Chewing, swallowing, yawning
Ocular movements	Tonic horizontal eye deviation
	Staring, blinking
	Nystagmoid jerks
Respiratory manifestations	Apnea (usually preceded or accompanied by one or more subtle manifestations)
	Hyperpneic or stertorous breathing

Compiled from Jensen (2009); Scher (2012); Bassan, Bental, Shany, Berger, Froom, Levi, and Shiff (2008); and Heaberlin (2009).

the trunk and neck. Myoclonic seizures are most often seen with inborn errors of metabolism or other metabolic problems (Rennie & Boylan, 2009; Scher, 2012b; Volpe, 2008).

Management

Management of neonatal seizures has two goals: (1) to determine and treat the underlying cause of the seizures and (2) to protect the infant from injury during and after the seizure. Determining the cause involves assessment of the perinatal and neonatal history, a physical examination, laboratory evaluation, and other diagnostic studies. Previous events that may indicate the underlying cause include the delivery history, bleeding, birth trauma, hypoxic-ischemic events, exposure to infectious agents and other teratogens, maternal substance abuse, and postbirth illnesses.

The physical examination includes evaluation of the infant's general health and neurologic status. Routine laboratory studies include electrolyte levels; glucose, calcium, magnesium, and blood urea nitrogen (BUN) levels; Hct value; blood gases; and pH. A blood culture and lumbar puncture also are often performed. A lumbar puncture helps to rule out both infection and CNS bleeding. Other laboratory and diagnostic studies may include screening for congenital viral infections, amino acid screening (for inborn errors of metabolism), CT, ultrasonography, MRI, skull radiography, or EEG. The results of a continuous video-EEG can provide information for the prognosis, more so in a term than a preterm infant (Scher, 2012a).

Seizures must be recognized, seizure activity documented, and the infant protected and supported during and after the seizure. Observing and documenting seizure activity involves noting and recording (1) the time the seizure begins and ends; (2) the body parts involved (e.g., extremities, eyes, head); (3) a description of motor movement, eye deviations, and pupillary reactions; and (4) the infant's respiratory status, color, state, level of consciousness, and postictal status. During the seizure, the infant's airway must be maintained, vital signs monitored, and the infant assessed for adequacy of respiration and heart rate to maintain ventilation and perfusion. To protect the infant from injury during the seizure, the nurse should not force anything into the infant's mouth or try to restrain the infant's extremities. The nurse should try to turn the infant's head to the side, if possible. After the seizure, the infant's condition should be monitored, and supportive care should be provided so that ventilation, oxygenation, adequate fluids, glucose, and warmth are maintained. The nurse also should assess the infant for signs related to the events that can cause seizure activity in the neonate to help determine the cause of the seizure and prevent additional seizures (Scher, 2012a).

The overall goal of treatment of neonatal seizures is to prevent long-term brain damage through management of the underlying cause of the seizures and cessation of the clinical and electrical seizure activity (Scher, 2012b; Volpe, 2008). Treatment of the underlying cause of the seizure is a priority for preventing more seizures and neurologic damage. Continual monitoring of blood gases, acid–base status, serum glucose, and fluid and electrolyte status is important for any infant with seizures. Infants who have seizures, regardless of the cause, require intravenous administration of glucose because seizure activity depletes brain glucose and energy supplies (Scher, 2012b). Alterations in oxygenation and acid–base status can occur as a complication of the apnea associated with a seizure or the physiologic consequences of seizure activity. Fluid and electrolyte management should be appropriate to the underlying cause of the seizures. For example, fluids are restricted initially in infants with cerebral edema and perinatal hypoxic-ischemic injury (Scher, 2012b; Volpe, 2008). Management of intracranial hemorrhage and CNS anomalies is discussed later in this chapter. Management of other conditions, such as hypoxic-ischemic events, metabolic and electrolyte disorders, infections, and drug withdrawal, are discussed in detail in other chapters.

The issues of when to treat with anticonvulsant drugs, which drug or combination of drugs to use, and duration of treatment are controversial (Bassan et al., 2008; Gomella et al., 2009; Scher, 2012a; Silverstein & Jensen, 2007). Some clinicians favor early, aggressive therapy, whereas others do not because neonatal seizures often abate spontaneously

(Glass & Wirrell, 2009). Recurrent or prolonged seizures require treatment with anticonvulsants to reduce the risk of brain injury. Controversy over what medications to use to provide control of neonatal seizures persists due to the diversity of etiology, complexities of diagnosis, and the limited efficacy of the known anticonvulsants available in treating neonatal seizures (Silverstein & Jensen, 2007). In general, however, the current consensus is that the first-line anticonvulsant used for seizure control in the newborn continues to be phenobarbital; phenytoin (Dilantin) is second-line if seizures persist (Bassan et al., 2008; Fenichel, 2007; Glass & Wirrell, 2009; Scher, 2012a; Silverstein & Jensen, 2007). Other drugs used include fosphenytoin (recommended for IV use over phenytoin) and benzodiazepines such as lorazepam and midazolam (Rennie & Boylan, 2009; Scher, 2012a; Volpe, 2008). Phenobarbital, phenytoin, and fosphenytoin doses may be given incrementally to reach therapeutic blood levels, which then must be monitored carefully to maintain therapeutic effect and prevent toxicity. Refractory seizure may require alternative agents such as clonazepam, lidocaine, carbamazepine, diazepam, valproate, or primidone (Fenichel, 2007; Glass & Wirrell, 2009; Rennie & Boylan, 2009; Scher, 2012a; Volpe, 2008). Recently, newer drugs, such as levetiracetam (which may inhibit burst firing) and topiramate (which is broad-spectrum antiepileptic), are being recommended for rigorous clinical trials to determine efficacy, pharmacokinetics, and safety in newborns due to small case report successes (Glass & Wirrell, 2009; Scher, 2012a).

Length of treatment after seizure activity has been controlled and after the infant has recovered is undefined at this point. Often the duration of treatment is clinically determined by etiology of the seizures, the time taken and amount of medications required to control the seizure activity. It may range from length of hospitalization to 2 years post discharge, provided there is no further seizure activity or perceived neurologic indication for extending treatment (Glass & Wirrell, 2009; Scher, 2012a; Volpe, 2008).

Because anticonvulsants can be respiratory or myocardial, and CNS depressants can compete with bilirubin for albumin binding, the infant's cardiorespiratory status, color, and neurologic status are monitored in addition to drug effectiveness. Parent teaching includes helping the family to understand the cause and significance of the seizure or seizures and any diagnostic tests that are planned. Discharge teaching of parents includes recognition of seizure manifestations, care of the infant during and after a seizure, and administration of anticonvulsants (dosage and side effects) if administration of these drugs is to be continued after discharge.

Outcomes

The mortality rate for infants with seizures has declined in recent years, from approximately 40% before 1969 to less than 15%. Currently (Scher, 2012b; Silverstein & Jensen, 2007). Two thirds of infants with seizures, especially premature infants and/or those with repeated seizures, have adverse neurologic sequelae, from epilepsy (20%–25%) to motor deficits, mental retardation, and subtle deficits, such as learning disabilities or poor social adjustment in teen years. Benign seizures in otherwise healthy infants during the first week have a good prognosis (Scher, 2012b). Preterm infants tend to recover more rapidly from a seizure than do term infants; however, mortality and later morbidity are higher in preterm infants. The prognosis for infants who have seizures during the neonatal period is influenced by (1) the time of onset, (2) the cause of the seizure, (3) continuous video-EEG results, (4) responsivity to treatment, and (5) the frequency and duration of the seizures (Fenichel, 2007; Rennie & Boylan, 2009; Scher, 2012a; Volpe, 2008). Seizure onset less than 48 hours after birth has a poor prognosis, whereas onset after 4 days generally has a good prognosis. Clonic seizures have a better prognosis than the other types. The EEG results appear to be a better prognostic sign in term than in preterm infants (Scher, 2012a, 2012b; Silverstein & Jensen, 2007; Tao & Mathur, 2010; Toet & Lemmers, 2009; Volpe, 2008).

The poorest prognosis is seen with seizures associated with severe hypoxic-ischemic injury, grade III or grade IV IVH, herpes infection, some bacterial meningitis, and CNS malformations. The best prognosis is seen in infants with seizures secondary to late hypocalcemia, hyponatremia, and uncomplicated subarachnoid hemorrhage (SAH). Other causes have a mixed prognosis. Repeated or prolonged seizures can lead to brain injury by altering cerebral blood flow and delivery of oxygen and nutrients, by depleting brain glucose and energy stores, and by interfering with ventilation (Volpe, 2008).

HIE

HIE (hypoxic ischemic encephalopathy) is an injury to the brain caused by oxygen deficit resulting from either systemic hypoxemia (decreased oxygen in blood supply) or ischemia (diminished cerebral blood perfusion) or a combination of the two conditions. The hypoxemia and ischemia may occur simultaneously or sequentially, and it appears from recent evidence that ischemia is the more important of the two oxygen deprivation states in causing the brain injury. In addition, the subsequent reperfusion of the affected brain area has been shown to be the time at which the majority of the injury to the brain occurs. Glucose deprivation also plays a part in the severity of the brain injury (Greisen, 2009; Sorem, Smith, & Druzin, 2009; Volpe, 2008). HIE may occur secondary to prenatal, intrapartum, or postnatal insults in both preterm and term infants. The site of injury varies with maturational changes in the vascular anatomy and metabolic activity of the brain. In the preterm infant younger than 32 to 34 weeks gestation, hypoxic-ischemic damage usually is associated with germinal matrix hemorrhage/IVH. The incidence of severe forms of HIE has declined markedly as a result of advances in perinatal care. Most perinatal hypoxic-ischemic events are mild with minimal effects. The insult is significant enough to cause transient organ dysfunction in 4 to 6 per 1,000 live births and result in death or significant neurologic sequelae in 1 per 1,000 (Bonifacio et al., 2012; de Vries & Jongmans,

2010; Dickey, Long, & Hunt, 2011; Roland & Hill, 2007; Wachtel & Hendricks-Münoz, 2011).

Pathophysiology

After 33 to 34 weeks gestation, blood flow and brain metabolic activity become less prominent in the germinal matrix and periventricular area and shift to the cortical area. Hypoxia and ischemia in older preterm and term infants, therefore, are more likely to damage areas of the peripheral and dorsal cerebral cortex. Five types of lesions have been identified in infants with HIE: (1) selective neuronal necrosis; (2) status marmoratus of the neurons of the basal ganglia and thalamus, with loss of neurons in these areas; (3) parasagittal cerebral injury; (4) PVL (primarily in preterm infants); and (5) focal or multifocal ischemic brain necrosis (Hill, 2005; Volpe, 2008).

The primary lesion for the hypoxic injury is neuronal necrosis in the cortices of the cerebrum and cerebellum, with damage to the gray matter at the depths of the sulci. Neurons of the brainstem may also be injured. Areas of necrosis may extend into the white matter and into the gray matter of the basal ganglia. The primary ischemic injury occurs in the posterior portion of the parasagittal region secondary to watershed or border zone infarcts. The border zone is at the junctions of the anterior, middle, and posterior cerebral arteries and the superior and inferior cerebellar arteries. This area is farthest from the major cerebral vessels which are the source of the blood supply for the brain. Thus, with localized ischemia, such as occurs when the infant has systemic hypotension or hypoperfusion, this area receives the least amount of blood. With hypoxia and systemic hypotension, cerebral perfusion is maintained at first by cerebral vasodilation and redistribution of blood flow to the brain from other organs. If the hypoxia continues, cerebral blood flow is altered; energy is depleted; ischemia and edema develop; and neurophysiologic activity is disrupted. At the cellular level, neurologic injury is caused by energy depletion, accumulation of extracellular glutamate, and activation of glutamate NMDA receptors. This process occurs in two phases. The initial insult and effects of hypoxia lead to hyperpolarization with an influx of sodium, potassium, and water into the cell. This interferes with the cell's ability to produce an action potential, leading to failure of the sodium-potassium pump and cell edema. Calcium moves into the cell via voltage-dependent ion channels opened by the changes in the sodium-potassium pump. This reduces calcium currents and release of neurotransmitters. These events may be protective mechanisms to reduce neuronal excitability and conserve oxygen. However, reperfusion and reoxygenation may lead to buildup of free oxygen radicals and primary neuronal death. If the hypoxia and ischemia persist, NMDA receptors are activated, which further increases intracellular calcium (entering the cell via glutamate-controlled ion channels). More glutamate is released and accumulates to toxic levels. Nitric oxide (NO) is also released and accumulates. NO, which at normal levels promotes vasodilation and increased blood flow, reaches toxic levels, leading to production of excess free oxygen radicals and further activation of NMDA receptors. NO combines with superoxide free radicals to produce the toxic peroxynitrates, causing further cell damage. This late reperfusion phase (usually beginning 6–12 or more hours after the initial insult) is characterized by hyperexcitability and cytotoxic edema and damage caused by the release of free oxygen radicals and NO, inflammatory changes, and imbalances in inhibitory and excitatory neurotransmitters with secondary neuronal death due to necrosis or apoptosis (Dickey et al., 2011; Hill, 2005; Johnston, Fatemi, Wilson, & Northington, 2011; Sorem et al., 2009; Stola & Perlman, 2008; Volpe, 2008). After a hypoxic-ischemic insult, the entire cortex initially may be edematous, and further ischemic damage may occur as a result of compression of the cortex against the skull.

Assessment

Most term infants with HIE demonstrate a characteristic pattern of neurologic findings over the first 72 hours of life, including seizures, altered levels of consciousness, altered tone, altered activity, irregular respirations, apnea, poor or absent Moro reflex, abnormal cry, poor suck, and altered pupillary responses and eye movements. Clinical signs categorizing the severity of HIE have been classified in three stages first by Sarnat and Sarnat and is summarized in Table 15.6 (Sarnat & Sarnat, 1976). Stage 1, mild HIE, is characterized by mild depression or hyperalertness, irritability, and sympathetic nervous system excitation (tachycardia, dilated pupils). These infants have a good Moro reflex and deep tendon reflexes and generally are symptomatic for less than 24 hours or so. Infants in Stage 2, moderate HIE, demonstrate lethargy interspersed with brief arousal, decreased tone, altered primary reflexes, and increased parasympathetic tone (bradycardia, decreased pupil size and blood pressure) and may develop seizures. Infants in Stage 3, severe HIE, have varying levels of consciousness initially but then become stuporous or comatose. These infants have depressed deep tendon and Moro reflexes, as well as hypotonia, and most develop seizures. Seizures occur in up to 60% of infants with HIE, with a usual onset at 12 to 14 hours of age. The types of seizures most often seen are multifocal clonic seizures in term infants, although myoclonic clonic and subtle seizures may also be seen (Johnston et al., 2011; Roland & Hill, 2007; Volpe, 2008).

Management

Infants with HIE have multiorgan and multisystem problems that arise from the original hypoxic-ischemic insult (Sarkar, Barks, Bhagat, & Donn, 2009; Tagin, Woolcott, Vincer, Whyte, & Stinson, 2012; Zanelli, Buck, & Fairchild, 2012). As a result, management of these infants is complex and requires a coordinated team effort. Acute management of infants with HIE focuses on delivery room resuscitation and stabilization and management of the primary problem and related alterations in the cardiovascular, pulmonary, gastrointestinal, and renal systems. Prompt identification and treatment of seizures are needed to prevent further alterations in ICP and cerebral blood flow. Management of these infants in relation to neurologic problems focuses on elimination of the cause of the original hypoxia,

TABLE 15.6

STAGES OF HIE

	Stage 1: Mild	Stage 2: Moderate	Stage 3: Severe
Level of consciousness	Hyperalert	Lethargic; obtunded	Stuporous
Pupils	Dilated	Constricted	Variable; unequal
Heart rate	Tachycardic	Bradycardic	Variable
Muscle tone	Normal	Mildly hypotonic	Flaccid
Myoclonus	Present	Present	Absent
Sucking reflex	Weak	Weak; absent	Absent
Salivary secretions	Sparse	Profuse	Absent
Moro embrace reflex	Strong	Weak; incomplete	Absent
Seizures	None	Common; focal or multifocal	Uncommon
Duration of symptoms and recovery	< 24 hours	2–14 days	Hours to weeks

Compiled from Sarnat and Sarnat (1976); Chirinian and Mann (2011); Sarkar, Barks, Bhagat, and Donn (2009); Fenichel (2007); and Gomella, Cunningham, and Eyal (2009).

alleviation of tissue hypoxia, and promotion of adequate cerebral perfusion and brain oxygenation with maintenance of an adequate glucose supply (Kelen & Robertson, 2010; Stola & Perlman, 2008; Volpe, 2008; Wachtel & Hendricks-Münoz, 2011).

Interventions are directed toward establishing ventilation and adequate perfusion and preventing or minimizing hypotension, hypoxia, acidosis, rapid alterations in cerebral blood flow and systemic blood pressure, and severe apneic and bradycardic episodes. Hyperoxia is also avoided because this state can result in cerebral vasoconstriction and diminished perfusion. The infant's neurologic status is continually monitored and documented, as are oxygenation, temperature, and blood pressure (Stola & Perlman, 2008; Wachtel & Hendricks-Münoz, 2011). HIE must be differentiated from other neurologic dysfunctions caused by trauma, infection, or CNS anomalies. An extensive workup to define the type, extent, and location of the injury may include cranial ultrasonography, brainstem auditory evoked potentials, MRI, EEG, and measurements of cerebral blood flow, ICP, and the creatinine kinase level (Gunny & Lin, 2012; Tao & Mathur, 2010; Toet & DeVries, 2012; Toet & Lemmers, 2009; Stola & Perlman, 2008; Wachtel & Hendricks-Müoz, 2011; Walsh, Murray, & Boylan, 2011).

Other parameters that are monitored are the serum and urinary electrolyte levels and osmolality; BUN, serum creatinine, and glucose levels; and fluid and electrolyte balance. These infants are at risk for hypocalcemia secondary to release of excessive phosphorus from the breakdown of ATP that occurred to produce energy; the need for energy arises in response to the stress induced by perinatal hypoxic-ischemic injury. The excess phosphorus is also related to use of bicarbonate to correct acidosis induced by these events. After hypoxic-ischemic events, an infant is at risk for hypoglycemia as a result of depletion of stores from high energy; therefore, provision of adequate glucose for energy and interventions to reduce energy expenditure are important. Fluid status and intake and output are monitored to prevent fluid overload and to reduce localized increases in pressure; fluids are restricted, although the effectiveness of this intervention has not been evaluated with clinical trials. Fluid management is critical not only for treating the cerebral edema but also for managing the alterations in renal function and problems such as acute tubular necrosis that frequently accompany moderate to severe stages of HIE (Stola & Perlman, 2008; Wachtel & Hendricks-Münoz, 2011).

Induced mild hypothermia has been shown to provide neuroprotection and reduce the extent of tissue injury and is increasingly the treatment of choice for infants greater than or equal to 36 weeks gestation with moderate to severe HIE (Bonifacio et al., 2012; Hoehn et al., 2008; Laptook, 2012; Pfister & Soll, 2010; Rutherford et al., 2010; Stola & Perlman, 2008). Potential mechanisms for these effects with hypothermic therapy include inhibition of glutamate release, reduction of cerebral metabolism, and preservation of high-energy phosphates. Additional neuroprotective mechanisms include decreases of intracellular acidosis and lactic acid accumulation, preservation of endogenous antioxidants, reduction of NO production, decrease in protein kinase inhibition, improved protein synthesis, reduction of leukotriene production, minimiztion of blood–brain barrier disruption, reduced brain edema, and apoptosis inhibition (Hoehn et al., 2008; Pfister & Soll, 2010; Stola & Perlman, 2008). Techniques studied include either selective head cooling or whole-body cooling to attain mild systemic hypothermia of 32°C to 34°C core body temperature (Barks, 2008; Hoehn et al., 2008; Kelen & Robertson, 2010; Laptook, 2012; Stola & Perlman, 2008). Infants are assessed to determine whether hypothermia criteria are met before the cooling regimen is initiated. Current criteria used to determine if a newborn is a candidate for hypothermia are (1) term infants ≥36 weeks gestation without major congenital anomalies, IUGR (≤1,800 g) or known chromosomal anomaly; (2) admitted at less than or equal to 6 hours of age to neonatal intensive care unit (NICU); (3) assessed to be in Stage 2 moderate HIE, or Stage 3, severe HIE by neonatologist and/or pediatric neurologist (Gancia & Pomero, 2011; Hoehn et al., 2008). The cooling regimen continues for 72 hours and is begun as soon as possible after birth, by 5.5 to 6 hours postbirth and optimally before seizure activity is noted (Bonifacio et al., 2011; Bonifacio et al., 2012; Hoehn et al., 2008; Laptook, 2012; Stola & Perlman, 2008; Volpe, 2008). Within 6 hours of birth is a therapeutic window demonstrated in sheep between insult and further cell death for neuroprotective interventions; early hypothermia studies indicate that cooling may be less effective if started after onset of seizures or in infants with most severe EEG changes before therapy (Gancia & Pomero, 2011; Gluckman et al., 2005; Gunn et al., 2008; Volpe, 2008).

Hypothermia therapy has multisystem effects in addition to the effects resulting from HIE (Table 15.7) (Battin et al., 2009; Glass, 2010; Lista et al., 2011; Reynolds & Talmage, 2011; Selway, 2010; Vandertak, 2009; Verklan, 2009). The infants undergoing a cooling regimen, either selective head cooling or whole-body cooling, require optimal care and attention at the bedside; this intervention is only being done in tertiary NICU settings (Barks, 2008; Reynolds & Talmage, 2011; Selway, 2010; Zanelli, Buck, & Fairchild, 2011). Delays in transport are critical and should be avoided. Induced hypothermia is not recommended either prior to or during transport. Care should be taken that the infants not become hyperthermic with core temperatures greater than 37°C (Glass, 2010; Hoehn et al., 2008; Pfister & Soll, 2010).

Fluctuations in systemic blood pressure with increased ICP and altered cerebral hemodynamics can occur as a result of caregiving or environmental stress; therefore developmentally supportive care of these infants to reduce stress is essential. As the infant recovers, opportunities for sensory experiences are an important part of care. These experiences can be introduced slowly, as the infant can tolerate them without becoming stressed and overloaded. Physiologic and neurologic status is monitored and documented at regular intervals. The infant is observed for changes in level of consciousness, tone, and activity and for evidence of seizures. Seizures are recognized and treated promptly to prevent further injury. Positioning and skin care are important, especially for hypoactive, obtunded, or comatose infants. Physiologic and clinical effects and supportive measures for infants treated with hypothermia are summarized in Table 15.7.

Parents need initial and continuing support in dealing with their infant's critical illness; the lack of infant responsiveness if the infant is hypoactive, stuporous, or comatose; the possibility of death; and the implications for later neurologic deficits. Parent teaching focuses on promoting an understanding of the infant's health status and care and providing anticipatory guidance regarding changes in the infant's state, as well as the outcome (Long & Brandon, 2007; Selway, 2010). The parents need to be shown how to interact with and care for their infant in a developmentally appropriate manner, with the goal of promoting opportunities for interaction while minimizing stressful events. The nurse can model this type of care for the parents and provide anticipatory guidance in the ways the infant's needs and care will change as the baby matures. Parents can also be involved in devising and implementing a developmental plan of care for their infant (Gudsnuk & Champagne, 2011; Sullivan, Perry, Sloan, Kleinhaus, & Burtchen, 2011).

Outcomes

The prognosis, which varies with the extent and severity of the insult and the resulting brain injury, ranges from perinatal death to severe neurologic impairment to minimal or no sequelae. Specific sequelae may not be apparent for several months or longer. Some infants make a significant recovery, although the rate and degree of recovery vary. MRI or CT can be used to assess the location, degree, and extent of the injury (de Vries & Jongmans, 2010; Epelman, Daneman, Chauvin, & Hirsch, 2012; Gunn et al., 2008; Gunny & Lin, 2012; Lodygensky, Menache, & Huppi, 2012; Lori et al., 2011). Sequelae of HIE in term infants are related to the site of injury (e.g., the cortex) and include mental retardation, microcephaly, cortical blindness, hearing deficits, and epilepsy. Generally, infants with mild HIE do well. Infants with moderate HIE or severe HIE have a higher mortality rate and later cognitive and motor problems (de Vries & Jongmans, 2010; Gunn et al., 2008; Wyatt et al., 2007).

The advent of hypothermia therapy as a treatment modality appears to have improved the general outcome, especially for infants with Stage 2 moderate HIE. Most human studies report beneficial effects of hypothermia therapy in terms of improved survival and outcome with no significant adverse effects for infants with Stage 2 moderate HIE (Bonifacio et al., 2012; Gunn et al., 2008; Rutherford et al., 2010; Volpe, 2008). A recent meta-analysis comparing head cooling with total body cooling technique showed both to be effective treatments for moderate to severe HIE, resulting in reduction in the risk of death or major neurodevelopmental disability at 18 months, particularly for infants with moderate HIE (Tagin, Woolcott, Vincer, Whyte, & Stinson, 2012). Guillet et al. reported subtle cognitive and motor neurological disabilities at school age (7–8 years) follow-up of the CoolCap study (Guillet et al., 2012). The authors also reported support for long-term predictive value of a favorable outcome at 18 months of age.

GERMINAL MATRIX-INTRAVENTRICULAR HEMORRHAGE

Germinal matrix-intraventricular hemorrhage (GM-IVH, GMH/IVH, or, most commonly, IVH) is the most common type of intracranial hemorrhage seen in the neonatal period (Bassan, 2009; Blackburn, 2009; McCrea & Ment, 2008; Takenouchi & Perlman, 2012; Volpe, 2008). IVH is seen almost exclusively in preterm infants, particularly those weighing less than 1,500 g. Decreasing gestational age increases the risk and severity of IVH. Incidence of IVH in premature infants less than 1,500 g has remained fairly stable for the past decade at 15% to 25%; 10% to 15% suffer more severe IVH, particularly those < 1,000 g (Ballabh, 2010; Bassan, 2009; Inder & Volpe, 2011; McCrea & Ment, 2008; Perlman, 2011; Takenouchi & Perlman, 2012; Volpe, 2008). The major risk factors for IVH in the neonate are prematurity

TABLE 15.7

POTENTIAL PHYSIOLOGIC EFFECTS OF HYPOTHERMIA BY SYSTEMS WITH MEDICAL AND NURSING INTERVENTIONS

System	Potential Physiologic Effects	Medical and Nursing Interventions
Neurologic	Decreased cerebral blood flow	Observe for seizure activity
	Decreased cerebral metabolic rate	Monitor infant's state of arousal
	Amplitude and frequency	EEGs, continuous with video; aEEGs
Respiratory	Decreased respiratory drive	Monitor respiratory rate, effort; may need intubation, ventilation
	Increased pulmonary vascular resistance	Monitor systemic blood pressure,
	increased Co_2 and o_2 solubility	Monitor blood gases (preferably arterial)
	Decreased Co_2 production and 0_2 consumption	Adjust assisted ventilation as needed to prevent hypercarbia, hypoxia
	Increased pH by 0.0016 for every 1P C decrease in temperature	Monitor saturations with pulse oximetry to prevent hypoxia
	Decreased minute ventilation to preserve normal $PaCO_2$	
Cardiovascular	Decreased heart rate by 14–60 bpm	Monitor continuous cardiorespiratory monitoring
	Increased systemic vascular resistance	Monitor invasive arterial blood pressure
	Decreased cardiac output	Observe changes in perfusion status, urine output
	Decreased intravascular volume	Maintain blood pressure within parameters with vasopressors, boluses
	Potential for ECG changes: prolonged PR, QRS, QT	Monitor cardiac strips; obtain ECG as needed
Renal	Decreased renal perfusion and glomerular filtration rate	Monitor fluid intake, urine output
	Impaired salt and water reabsorption	Obtain electrolytes every 4–8 hours as needed
	Diuresis	
	Potential for hypokalemia with increased intracellular uptake	Maintain normal potassium level
	Potential for hyperkalemia during rewarming	
	Potential for decreased calcium, magnesium, phosphorus	
Gastrointestinal	Decreased intestinal blood flow	Provide parenteral nutrition
		Begin enteral nutrition cautiously after rewarming; monitor for intolerance
Hematologic	Decreased platelet count; thrombocytopenia	Monitor platelet count every 6–12 hours as indicated
	Increased activation and aggregation (clumping)	
	Increased PT, PTT	Monitor PT, PTT every 12–24 hours as indicated
Immunologic	Impaired neutrophil release and function	Monitor CBC with differential at least every 24 hours
	Decreased leukocyte chemotaxis	
	Decreased phagocytosis and killing	

Compiled from Zanelli, Buck, and Fairchild (2011); Toet and DeVries (2012); Chirinian and Mann (2011); Verklan (2009); Vandertak (2009); Wachtel and Hendricks-Muñoz (2011); Reynolds and Talmage (2011); Selway (2010); and Lista, Castoldi, Cavigioli, Bianchi, Fontana, and La Verde (2011).

and hypoxic events interrelated with the anatomic and physiologic processes that make the periventricular site particularly vulnerable. IVH occurs but is rare after 35 to 36 weeks gestation because of the involution of the subependymal germinal matrix and alterations in cerebral blood flow patterns that occur after this time. Any perinatal or neonatal event that results in hypoxia or alters cerebral blood flow or intravascular pressure increases the risk of IVH (Bassan, 2009; McCrea & Ment, 2008; Volpe, 2008).

IVH is classified by the location and severity of the hemorrhage. A grade I or slight hemorrhage is characterized by isolated germinal matrix hemorrhage; a grade II or small hemorrhage by IVH with normal ventricular size; and a grade III or moderate hemorrhage IVH with acute ventricular dilation. A grade IV or severe hemorrhage involves both intraventricular and brain parenchyma hemorrhage IVH (Bassan, 2009; McCrea & Ment, 2008; Volpe, 2008).

Pathophysiology

The neuropathophysiology of IVH involves a complex interaction of intravascular, vascular, and extravascular factors. In infants of less than 28 to 32 weeks gestation, the hemorrhage generally arises from the subependymal germinal matrix at the head of the caudate nucleus near the foramen of Monro. On those rare occasions when IVH occurs in term infants, bleeding usually arises from the choroid plexus rather than from the germinal matrix (Bassan, 2009; Volpe, 2008). The germinal matrix includes the tissue underlying the ependymal wall of the lateral ventricles. In many preterm infants, the hemorrhage begins as a microvascular event in the germinal matrix and is confined to the subependymal area. In the rest, the original hemorrhage ruptures into the lateral ventricles and then into the third and fourth ventricles. The blood eventually collects in the subarachnoid space of the posterior fossa, often extending into the basal cistern (see Figure 15.1) (Ballabh, 2010; Bonifacio et al., 2012; Perlman, 2011). Rupture of the hemorrhage from the germinal matrix into the ventricles may serve a protective function by decompressing the hemorrhagic area and reducing further tissue destruction. Progressive ventricular dilation may occur as the result of obstruction of CSF flow by an obliterative arachnoiditis or as the result of blood clots at the level of the aqueduct of Sylvius or the foramen of Monro. With severe hemorrhages, blood may also be found in the periventricular white matter. This usually is due not to extravasation of blood from the ventricles but to an associated insult in the white matter that increases the risk of adverse neuromotor outcome (Bassan, 2009).

The neuropathologic consequences of IVH include (1) destruction of the germinal matrix and its glial precursor cells, (2) infarction and necrosis of periventricular white matter, and (3) posthemorrhagic hydrocephalus (Bassan, 2009; Perlman, 2011; Volpe, 2008). As the IVH moves from the germinal matrix area into the surrounding white matter, periventricular hemorrhagic infarction associated with intraparenchymal echodensities develops. The appearance of this parenchymal lesion is associated with increased mortality and neurodevelopmental sequelae. Infants with IVH may also have PVL. However, PVL may be a consequence of hypoxic-ischemic injury and may not be a result of the IVH (Bassan, 2009; McCrea & Ment, 2008; Volpe, 2008).

■ **Intravascular Factors.** Intravascular hemodynamic factors play a prominent role in the pathogenesis of IVH. These factors include distribution of blood to the periventricular region, pressure-passive cerebral blood flow, and venous hemodynamics. The stages of CNS development characteristic of preterm infants born at less than 32 to 33 weeks gestation increase the risk of hemorrhage in the periventricular area (Bassan, 2009; McCrea & Ment, 2008; Volpe, 2008).

■ **Periventricular Blood Flow.** The subependymal germinal matrix is a transient structure that begins to thin after 14 weeks and has almost completely involuted by 36 weeks gestation (Levene & DeVries, 2009; Volpe, 2008). This is the site where neuroectodermal cells that serve as precursors for neurons (before about 24 weeks gestation) and glial cells develop. These cells subsequently migrate to their eventual locus in the cerebral cortex. Processes involved in the proliferation, differentiation, and migration of these cells result in an area that is highly vascularized and metabolically active. Before 32 weeks gestation, a significant portion of the total cerebral blood flow goes to the periventricular germinal matrix, primarily to support neuroblast and glioblast mitotic activity and migration. Any factor that increases cerebral blood flow can result in overperfusion of the periventricular region. After 32 to 34 weeks gestation, cell proliferation and migration decline. The germinal matrix becomes less prominent and receives a smaller proportion of the cerebral blood supply. At this point, the greater proportion of blood flow is to the rapidly differentiating cerebral cortex (Bassan, 2009; Blackburn, 2009b; Bonifacio et al., 2012; Levene & DeVries, 2009; Volpe, 2008).

■ **Cerebral Autoregulation.** The blood vessels of the brain normally are protected from marked alterations in flow by autoregulatory processes. If cerebral autoregulation is intact, the arterioles constrict or dilate to maintain a constant cerebral blood flow despite fluctuations in systemic blood pressure. Hypoxia and hypoxemia in the neonate alter cerebral autoregulation. This alteration can lead to a pressure-passive system in which cerebral blood flow varies directly with arterial pressure. Subsequent alterations in systemic blood pressure or cerebral blood flow, or both, are transmitted directly to the brain and, in particular, to the area receiving the greatest proportion of cerebral blood flow, that is, the fragile, thin-walled vessels of the germinal matrix. Thus rapid fluctuations in systemic blood pressure or cerebral blood flow (i.e., moving from increased to decreased flow and vice versa) also increase the risk of vessel rupture (Bonifacio et al., 2012; duPlessis, 2008b; Levene & DeVries, 2009; Perlman, 2011; Volpe, 2008). Altered hemodynamics with fluctuations in blood flow can occur with positive pressure ventilation, rapid volume expansion, hypercapnia, and possibly reduced Hct and blood glucose values. Increased systemic blood pressure and, potentially, cerebral blood flow also can occur with caregiving events, such as handling, suctioning, and chest physical therapy (duPlessis, 2008a; Perlman, 2011; Takenouchi & Perlman, 2012; Volpe, 2008).

■ Venous Hemodynamics. Increased venous pressure, arising from events such as myocardial failure or positive pressure ventilation, can also be transmitted directly to the capillaries of the germinal matrix. These events can impede cerebral venous return, leading to stasis and venous congestion, which then lead to increased venous pressure and vessel rupture. The point of vulnerability in the venous drainage system of the brain is at the level of the foramen of Monro and the caudate nucleus (the usual site of IVH). At this location there is a U-shaped turn in the venous drainage system where the confluence of the thalamostriate, terminal, and choroidal veins forms the internal cerebral vein, which empties into the great vein of Galen. This results in a sharp change in the direction of blood flow and predisposes to turbulent venous flow with stasis and thrombus formation and an area vulnerable to increased intravascular pressure (Volpe, 2008). In addition, the pliable skull of the preterm infant can easily be deformed, obstructing the major venous sinuses and increasing venous pressure.

■ Vascular Factors. The capillary bed of the germinal matrix is immature and has large, irregular, thin-walled vessels, a feature that increases its vulnerability to rupture. The capillary walls thicken with increasing gestational age. The fragility of these vessels is due partly to the lack of thickness and strength of the basement membrane and the lack of collagen and smooth muscle. With migration of the neuronal and glial cells and their derivatives, the germinal matrix undergoes involution. The immature capillary bed is remodeled into the definitive, mature capillary bed (Takenouchi & Perlman, 2012; Volpe, 2008). The epithelial cells of these capillaries are dependent on oxidative metabolism and thus are easily injured by hypoxic events. This characteristic increases the likelihood of leakage or rupture if transmural pressure increases. Because these vessels require an adequate supply of oxygen to maintain their functional integrity, decreased cerebral blood flow can lead to hypoxic-ischemic injury. These vessels are also susceptible to ischemia because they tend to lie in the vascular border zone, or "watershed" area. Both increased and decreased cerebral blood flow, therefore, can be involved in the pathogenesis of IVH (Ballabh, 2010; Levene & DeVries, 2009; Volpe, 2008).

■ Extravascular Factors. The capillary bed of the highly vascularized germinal matrix is embedded in gelatinous material deficient in supportive mesenchymal elements, thus providing poor support for the fragile blood vessels. In addition, excessive fibrinolytic activity occurs in the periventricular area. As a result, a small initial bleed may not clot off and be localized, but rather may continue to enlarge and rupture into the ventricles, or the cerebral parenchyma, or both (Ballabh, 2010; Volpe, 2008).

■ Genetic Factors. There have been recent indications that genetic factors could contribute to the predisposition of IVH occurring in some premature infants and not in others. This may explain why some stable premature infants can and do develop IVH, whereas some clinically hemodynamically unstable premature infants do not develop IVH. In addition, despite measures to provide stable management in the form of ventilatory and hemodynamic support, the incidence of IVH has not appreciably changed over the past decade. Genetic factors may potentiate alterations in intravascular coagulation, germinal matrix structure, the integrity of cerebral autoregulation, and inflammatory mechanisms, all of which could therefore predispose certain vulnerable premature infants to develop IVH (Bassan, 2009; McCrea & Ment, 2008).

Assessment

Perinatal events associated with fetal and neonatal hypoxia include maternal bleeding, fetal distress, perinatal hypoxic-ischemic injury, prolonged labor, maternal infection, preterm labor, and abnormal presentation. Neonatal hypoxic events, such as respiratory distress, apnea, and hypotension, further increase the risk of IVH (Hill, 2005; Inder & Volpe, 2011; Levene & DeVries, 2009; Volpe, 2008). Events associated with impairment of venous return, increased venous pressure, or both include assisted ventilation, high positive inspiratory pressure, prolonged duration of inspiration, continuous positive airway pressure (CPAP), and air leak. Venous pressure can also be increased by compression of the infant's skull during vaginal delivery, application of forceps, and use of constricting head bands. Rapid administration of hypertonic solutions (e.g., sodium bicarbonate and glucose), rapid volume expansion, hypernatremia, hypercarbia, caregiving interventions, and environmental stress can increase cerebral blood flow. Hypercarbia causes cerebral vasodilation, thus increasing blood flow. Hypertonic solutions given rapidly or in a large bolus alter osmotic gradients between the brain and the blood. Repeated or prolonged seizures raise the blood pressure and can lead to hypoxia (Hill, 2005; Inder & Volpe, 2011; Levene & DeVries, 2009; McCrea & Ment, 2008; Volpe, 2008).

The clinical manifestations of this disorder often are nonspecific and are not well correlated with later sonographic evidence of bleeding. Therefore a high index of suspicion, along with careful monitoring, is important for infants at risk. The diagnosis is generally made by cranial ultrasonography to determine the presence and severity of IVH and the progression of the hemorrhage, as well as to monitor later complications such as PVL, progressive ventricular dilation, and posthemorrhagic hydrocephalus (Inder & Volpe, 2011; Levene & DeVries, 2009; McCrea & Ment, 2008; Takenouchi & Perlman, 2012; Volpe, 2008).

More than 90% of infants with IVH bleed within the first 72 hours after birth; 50% of the bleeding occurs in the first 24 hours after birth (Ballabh, 2010; Bassan, 2009; Levene & DeVries, 2009; Volpe, 2008). Approximately 10% to 20% of infants observed serially with cranial ultrasonography after bleeding demonstrate progressive increases in the size of the hemorrhage over a 24- to 48-hour period (Levene & DeVries, 2009).

Late hemorrhages are seen after a few days or weeks in about 10% of infants, primarily in preterm infants with severe, prolonged respiratory problems. A new hemorrhage or an extension of a previous one may develop in these infants. IVH may also develop before birth in some infants (Hill, 2005; Volpe, 2008).

The signs and symptoms of IVH are often nonspecific and subtle. Clinical signs that correlate most closely with CT evidence of hemorrhage are (1) a full anterior fontanelle; (2) changes in activity level; and (3) decreased tone (Volpe, 2008). Other clinical signs associated with IVH are impaired visual tracking, increased tone of the lower limbs, hypotonia of the neck, and brisk tendon reflexes (Levene & DeVries, 2009).

Besides a declining Hct or failure of the Hct to increase after transfusion, laboratory evidence suggestive of IVH involves CSF findings indicative of hemorrhage: increased red blood cell levels, increased protein levels, decreased glucose levels, and xanthochromia (often a later finding and caused by increased protein). Extremely low CSF glucose levels, or hypoglycorrhachia, can be found several days to a week (usually 5–15 days) after the hemorrhage in some infants.

The patterns of clinical manifestations seen in individual infants vary widely and range from silent or subtle to catastrophic. At one end of the continuum are the 25% to 50% of infants with IVH who have only silent, subependymal bleeding with no or minimal clinical signs. The hemorrhage is discovered during routine ultrasonographic screening. Other clinical manifestations, if present, include alterations in level of consciousness or stupor, hypotonia, abnormal eye movements or positions, and altered mobility. These infants generally survive. Later developmental outcome varies, depending on the severity of the hemorrhage (Bassan, 2009; Takenouchi & Perlman, 2012; Volpe, 2008).

Catastrophic deterioration usually involves major hemorrhages that evolve rapidly over several minutes or hours. Clinical findings include stupor progressing to coma, respiratory distress progressing to apnea, generalized tonic seizures, decerebrate posturing, fixation of pupils to light, and flaccid quadriparesis. This clinical presentation is associated with a declining Hct value, bulging fontanelle, hypotension, bradycardia, temperature alterations, hypoglycemia, and syndrome of inappropriate antidiuretic hormone. Infants with catastrophic hemorrhages have a high mortality rate and, if they survive, a poor prognosis for later development (Bassan, 2009; Levene & DeVries, 2009; Volpe, 2008).

Management

Management of IVH involves prevention of hemorrhage in infants at risk, acute care of infants with current bleeding, pharmacologic therapies, and management of posthemorrhagic ventricular dilation. Routine ultrasonographic screening of infants at risk for IVH can identify infants with silent bleeding or bleeding associated with nonspecific, subtle symptoms. Prevention or risk reduction begins in the perinatal period, with the prevention of preterm birth, perinatal hypoxic-ischemic injury, and birth trauma. Administration of antenatal steroids is associated with a decreased incidence of IVH (Bassan, 2009; McCrea & Ment, 2008; Volpe, 2008).

Postbirth prevention and risk-reduction activities include resuscitation by a trained NICU team and interventions to prevent or reduce hypoxic or ischemic events; to prevent rapid changes in cerebral blood flow, fluctuations in systemic blood pressure, and hyperosmolarity; and to prevent or minimize fluctuations in ICP. By identifying these vulnerable infants, interventions can be instituted to prevent new bleeding or extensions of existing hemorrhage. Continual assessment of fetal and neonatal oxygenation and perfusion is important so that subtle alterations can be recognized and clinicians can intervene early to prevent cerebral hyperperfusion and stabilize cerebral blood flow and pressures. Prompt resuscitation at birth minimizes hypoxemia and hypercarbia, which can alter cerebral autoregulation. Hypertonic solutions and volume expanders are administered slowly, with careful monitoring of vital signs and color. Activities that can increase ICP or cause wide swings in arterial or venous pressure are avoided or minimized when possible, especially during the first 72 hours of life. Because seizures can alter cerebral blood flow and ICP, they must be recognized promptly and treated (Bassan, 2009; Levene & DeVries, 2009; McCrea & Ment, 2008; Takenouchi & Perlman, 2012; Volpe, 2008).

Acute treatment of infants with IVH involves providing physiologic support by maintaining oxygenation, perfusion, normothermia, and normoglycemia. Physical manipulations, handling, and environmental stressors are minimized to reduce the risk of hypoxia and of fluctuations in arterial blood pressure and cerebral blood flow. The infant's position is also important. The infant can be placed prone or side lying. The head is positioned in the midline or to the side, but without flexing the neck. The head of the bed can be elevated slightly. The Trendelenburg position is avoided. Vital signs, blood pressure, tone, activity, and level of consciousness are monitored frequently. The care of infants with progressive ventricular dilation is discussed in the section on hydrocephalus. Developmental interventions, such as containment or swaddling during aversive procedures such as endotracheal suctioning, may promote greater physiologic stability during these procedures and a more rapid return to baseline (Kling, 1989; Owens, 2005; Pitcher, Schneider, Drysdale, Ridding, & Owens, 2011). Specific interventions are listed in Table 15.8.

Pharmacologic therapies, including administration of phenobarbital, indomethacin, vitamin E, and fibrinolytic agents, have been tried prophylactically to reduce the incidence of hemorrhage, to prevent more severe bleeding and/or neurologic damage, or both. Research findings have been inconsistent for all of these therapies, and some infants have done poorly with these therapies (Bassan, 2009; Hill, 2005; McCrea & Ment, 2008).

Parent care involves recognition and discussion of parental concerns about their infant's immediate and long-term prognosis and teaching regarding IVH, its implications and management. The parents need to be shown how to interact with and care for the infant at risk for IVH in a developmentally appropriate manner, with the goal of promoting opportunities for interaction while minimizing stressful events. The nurse can model this type of care for parents

TABLE 15.8

NURSING CARE TO REDUCE THE RISK OF GERMINAL MATRIX HEMORRHAGE/IVH[a]

Intervention	Rationale
1. Position the infant with the head in the midline and the head of the bed slightly elevated.	ICP is lowest with the head in the midline and the head of the bed elevated 30°.
	Turning the head sharply to the side causes obstruction of the ipsilateral jugular vein and can increase ICP.
2. Avoid tight, encircling phototherapy masks.	Pressure on the occiput can increase ICP by impeding venous drainage.
3. Avoid rapid fluid infusions for volume expansion. (a) Know the normal blood pressure (BP) for the infant's weight and age. (b) If the infant is not hypovolemic, suggest dopamine therapy to maintain BP.	Rapid increases in intravascular volume can rupture the capillaries in the germinal matrix, and this risk may be even greater if there is a history of hypoxia and hypotension. Even modest, abrupt increases in BP may cause IVH.
4. If sodium bicarbonate ($NaHCO_3$) therapy is necessary to correct a documented metabolic acidosis, give a dilute solution slowly.	The role of $NaHCO_3$ is unclear, but rapid infusions may cause elevations in carbon dioxide, possibly dilating cerebral vessels and contributing to a pressure-passive cerebral circulation.
5. Monitor BP diligently. Inform physician if there is fluctuating pattern in the arterial pressure tracing.	The blood flow velocity in the anterior cerebral artery is reflected by the pattern of the simultaneously recorded arterial BP.
6. Monitor closely for signs of pneumothorax, including: (a) Increase in mean BP, especially increases in diastolic BP (early) (b) Tachycardia (early) (c) Hypotension and bradycardia (late) (d) Changes in breath sounds (e) Diminished arterial oxygen pressure (PaO_2) (f) Increased arterial carbon dioxide pressure ($PaCO_2$) (g) Shift in cardiac point of maximum impulse	Pneumothorax may precede IVH. The sum of hemodynamic changes caused by pneumothorax is flow under increased pressure in the germinal matrix capillaries. Changes in vital signs can be early indicators of pneumothorax.
7. Maintain temperature in neutral thermal range.	Hypothermia has been associated with IVH.
8. Suction only as needed.	Even brief suctioning episodes (20 sec) can increase cerebral blood flow velocity, BP, and ICP and reduce oxygenation.
9. Avoid interventions that cause crying. (a) Consider long-term methods of achieving venous access to avoid frequent venipuncture. (b) Critically evaluate all manipulations and handling. (c) Use analgesics for stressful procedures.	Crying can impede venous return, increase cerebral blood volume.
10. Maintain blood gas values within a normal range. (a) Use continuous noninvasive monitoring of oxygenation. (b) Adjust the fractional concentration of oxygen in inspired gas (FiO_2) as needed to maintain the transcutaneous oxygen pressure ($TcPO_2$) or pulse oximeter values within desired range. (c) Avoid interventions that cause hypoxia.	Hypoxia and excessive hypercapnia are associated with the development of IVH. These events increase cerebral blood flow and may impair the neonate's already limited ability to autoregulate the cerebral blood flow. Hypoxia can injure the germinal matrix capillary endothelium.

[a] Premature neonates are most vulnerable to IVH during the first 4 days of life; approximately 50% of hemorrhages occur in the first 24 hours. Attempts to minimize the risk of IVH should begin immediately after birth, even before the infant has reached the special care nursery (Kling, 1989).

Modified from Owens (2005); Kling (1989); and Pitcher, Schneider, Drysdale, Ridding, and Owens (2011).

and provide anticipatory guidance in ways in which the infant's needs and care will change as the baby matures. Parents can also be involved in devising and implementing a developmental plan of care for their infant to reduce environmental stressors.

Management of Progressive Ventricular Dilation

Because progressive posthemorrhagic ventricular dilation is seen in 25% to 35% of IVH, infants with a history of IVH are followed with serial cranial ultrasonography. Posthemorrhagic hydrocephalus develops after birth at varying times after the initial insult. Head size can increase without increases in ICP (normopressive hydrocephalus) because of the neonate's soft, malleable skull and open sutures and fontanelle. A tense fontanelle may be noted when the infant is placed in an upright position when the fontanelle is typically soft. Progressive ventricular dilation initially may cause compression and damage to the cortex without causing any change in head size and may be apparent only on ultrasound. Signs of increased ICP (e.g., bulging anterior fontanelle, setting-sun sign, dilated scalp veins, and widely separated sutures) tend to be later findings. In most infants, the ventricular dilation occurs slowly, without increased ICP. Ventricular growth spontaneously arrests in approximately half of these infants within about 30 days. The remaining infants continue to demonstrate ventricular dilation and increased ICP (Bassan, 2009; Hill, 2005; McCrea & Ment, 2008; Volpe, 2008).

The initial treatment for normopressive hydrocephalus is observation, because in many of these infants, ventricular growth arrests spontaneously without therapy (Whitelaw & Aquilina, 2009). Progressive ventricular dilation with increasing ICP is managed with a ventriculoperitoneal shunt or, if the infant is too ill or too small for surgery, with temporary ventricular drainage. A ventriculoperitoneal shunt is the shunt of choice in infants and children because this type is easy to insert, revise, and uncoil as the infant grows. One end of a radiopaque catheter is placed in the lateral ventricle, usually on the right side, and the other end is placed in the peritoneal cavity. The catheter contains a one-way valve that is palpable on the side of the head near the ear. The shunt may need multiple revisions during childhood for growth and for malfunctioning. Major complications of ventriculoperitoneal shunts are infection and obstruction. Too-rapid drainage of CSF immediately after insertion of the shunt can lead to herniation of the brain or subdural hematoma (Solanki & Hockley, 2009).

After surgery, these infants are positioned on the side opposite the shunt, with the head of the bed flat or slightly elevated to prevent rapid loss of CSF and decompression. The position can be rotated to supine every few hours to prevent skin breakdown. The skin should be kept clean and dry. Infants with a shunt are observed for signs of localized or systemic infection, ileus, and shunt obstruction. Obstruction of the shunt leads to accumulation of CSF, enlargement of the head, and signs of increased ICP. Infection of the shunt may appear as localized redness or drainage around the incision, temperature instability, altered activity, or poor feeding. Fluid status and intake and output are monitored, and the infant is observed for signs of dehydration from too-rapid loss of CSF. Signs of too-rapid decompression include a sunken fontanelle, agitation or restlessness, increased urine output, and electrolyte abnormalities (Solanki & Hockley, 2009).

Parent teaching before discharge includes care of the infant and shunt, especially positioning and skin care. Parents must be comfortable in handling and caring for their infant before discharge. They should know the signs of shunt malfunction, increased ICP, infection, and dehydration. Continuing follow-up care of the infant and parental support are important. Parents may be referred to parent groups for peer support.

Outcomes

The severity and extent of the hemorrhage and the presence of associated problems (e.g., respiratory distress syndrome, perinatal hypoxic-ischemic injury, and sepsis) influence mortality and morbidity. Infants with a history of IVH are also at risk for developing posthemorrhagic ventricular dilation, which may be normopressive or associated with increased ICP. Infants with small or mild hemorrhages survive and generally have a good outcome, with a low incidence of major neurologic sequelae and posthemorrhagic ventricular dilation. Infants with moderate hemorrhage have a 5% to 20% mortality rate, and ventricular dilation develops in 15% to 25% of survivors. Mortality in infants with severe hemorrhage averages 50%, with development of progressive ventricular dilation in 55% to 80%. Although infants with severe hemorrhages tend to have significant motor and cognitive deficits, some seem to escape significant long-term sequelae. The incidence of neurologic sequelae ranges from 15% in infants with moderate hemorrhage to 35% to 90% in infants with severe hemorrhages. Sequelae include cerebral palsy, developmental delay, sensory and attention problems, learning disorders, and hydrocephalus (Bassan, 2009; Hill, 2005; Inder & Volpe, 2011; Levene & DeVries, 2009; McCrea & Ment, 2008; Myers & Ment, 2009; Takenouchi & Perlman, 2012; Volpe, 2008).

WHITE-MATTER INJURIES (WMI) IN PRETERM INFANTS

WMI are the most common severe neurologic insult seen in preterm infants (Bonifacio et al., 2012; de Vries, Counsell, & Levene, 2009). White-matter hypoxic-ischemic injury involves both cystic and noncystic focal necrotic lesions as well as diffuse WMI with damage to the premyelinating oligodendrocytes, astrogliosis, and microglial infiltration (Deng et al., 2008; Vandertak, 2009; Verklan, 2009; Verney et al., 2010; Verney et al., 2012; Volpe et al., 2011). This injury is referred to as PVL. Leukomalacia refers to change in the brain's white matter reflective of softening. Focal cystic necrotic lesions are seen in 3% to 15% of surviving very-low-birth-weight infants, and the more common diffuse noncystic lesions associated with disturbances in myelinization seen in up to 50% of survivors (de Vries et al., 2009; Vandertak, 2009; Verney et al., 2010; Volpe et al., 2011). WMI is often accompanied by secondary alterations in the brain characterized by axonal and neuronal alteration that may include damage to the thalamus, basal ganglia, cerebral cortex, and cerebellum (Kling, 1989; Vandertak, 2009; Volpe et al., 2011). WMI often is associated with IVH, but it is a separate lesion that may also occur in the absence of IVH. PVL is a symmetric, nonhemorrhagic, usually bilateral lesion caused by ischemia from alterations in arterial circulation. Time of onset is variable (Bonifacio et al., 2012; de Vries et al., 2009; Inder & Volpe, 2011; Volpe et al., 2011).

Risk factors include any event during the prenatal, intrapartal, or postbirth periods that results in cerebral ischemia; this includes asphyxia, IVH, hypoxia, hypercarbia, hypotension, cardiac arrest, and infection (in which blood flow is diminished by the action of endotoxins). The major risk factors are IVH, asphyxia, and chorioamnionitis (de Vries et al., 2009).

Pathophysiology

PVL begins with ischemic necrosis of the white-matter dorsal and lateral to the external angles of the lateral ventricles, especially in the border zone area. The border zone is the area farthest from the original source of the cerebral blood supply and thus is most susceptible to ischemic damage from diminished cerebral blood flow. PVL often extends into the cortical white matter (Volpe, 2008). Pathologic changes begin with patchy areas of focal ischemic coagulation that may occur as early as 5 to 8 hours after the initial hypoxic-ischemic insult. This is followed within a few days by proliferation of macrophages and astrocytes, along with endothelial and glial infiltration. Later changes include thinning of the white matter and liquefaction in the central portion of the necrotic area, as well as cavitation, cystic changes, and decreased myelinization (Verklan, 2009; Verney et al., 2012; Volpe, 2008). Cerebral atrophy leads to expansion of the lateral ventricles and hydrocephalus.

The pathogenesis of WMI is due to the interaction of three maturation-dependent factors: (1) immature vascular supply to the white matter that reduces oxygen delivery to vulnerable areas of the brain; (2) impairments in cerebral autoregulation; and (3) vulnerabilities of the premyelinating oligodendrites to damage from reactive oxygen and nitrogen species (free radicals), glutamate, adenosine, and cytokines (de Vries et al., 2009; Volpe et al., 2011). Damage to the premyelin-producing oligodendrites leads to release of cytokines (indicating an inflammatory process), glutamate, and free radicals. Oligodendrocyte development and survival are impaired, leading to hypomyelination with subsequent motor, cognitive, and behavioral neurodevelopmental problems. Axonal damage and disruption also occur. Perinatal infection and an immune-mediated inflammatory response with release of proinflammatory cytokines are increasingly thought to play a prominent role in the pathogenesis of PVL (Deng et al., 2008; Vandertak, 2009; Verklan, 2009; Verney et al., 2012; Volpe et al., 2011).

Assessment

PVL is a compilation of prenatal or postnatal insults or both. Often, no clinical findings are specific to PVL during the first weeks of life unless the damage is severe. Cranial ultrasonography can identify infants at risk for or who have early signs of PVL, although a head ultra-sound (HUS) is not as sensitive in the diagnosis of PVL as it is with IVH. MRI can identify changes early and is especially useful with diffuse WMI (El-Dib, Massaro, Bulas, & Aly, 2010; Lodygensky et al., 2012). Infants at risk for WMI should undergo serial cranial ultrasonographic examinations and again at discharge and with later follow-up. There is evidence that serial MRI may be of benefit for ongoing follow-up, especially for infants with severe damage with the increased association of neuromotor abnormalities and developing ventricular enlargement (Lodygensky et al., 2012). As the infant matures, neurologic and motor deficits become apparent.

Management

Initial management focuses on treating the primary insult and its attendant complications and preventing further hypoxic-ischemic damage. This involves preventing or minimizing hypotension, hypoxia, acidosis, and severe apneic and bradycardic episodes. HUS and MRI are used serially to diagnose PVL and to follow its progression in infants at risk. Later management involves care related to residual problems, such as spastic diplegia and hydrocephalus. Nursing interventions focus on acute management of the primary problem and supportive care for the infant and parents. Nurses have a major role in identifying signs of hypoxia and ischemia and instituting interventions to prevent further ischemic damage. These interventions are similar to those described earlier and in Table 15.8. Environmental stressors may increase the risk for development of IVH and subsequent PVL or may cause associated developmental problems. Developmental and environmental interventions, therefore, are important aspects of nursing care.

Parents need initial and continuing support in dealing with their infant's illness and the risk of later neurologic problems. Parent teaching should focus on promoting an understanding of the infant's health status and care and providing anticipatory guidance and follow-up care. The parents can be shown how to interact with and care for their infant in a developmentally appropriate manner to foster parent–infant interaction and to promote infant organization and development. The nurse can model this type of care for the parents and can provide anticipatory guidance as the infant's needs and care change.

Outcomes

Infants with PVL may die in the neonatal period, usually from the original hypoxic, hemorrhagic, or infectious insult rather than from PVL per se. Infants with WMI are at higher risk for later developmental problems that affect motor, cognitive, and visual function (Inder & Volpe, 2011; Mwaniki, Atieno, Lawn, & Newton, 2012; Myers & Ment, 2009; Volpe, 2008). The most prominent sequela in survivors, especially those with multifocal cystic lesions around the lateral ventricles, is spastic diplegia with or without hydrocephalus. In infants with spastic diplegia, descending fibers from the motor cortex cross the affected area around the ventricles. Because the leg motor fibers are closest to the ventricles, spastic diplegia of the leg is the most common sequela. With extension of the damage, arm involvement with spastic quadriplegia may occur. Infants with diffuse WMI are more likely to develop visual, cognitive, and neurobehavioral impairments (Takenouchi & Perlman, 2012).

CEREBELLAR INJURY IN PRETERM INFANTS

The cerebellum is one of the later structures to mature, with critical developmental events occurring at the end of the second and beginning of the third trimester, accompanied by a rapid growth spurt from 24 weeks through the third trimester and birth (Limperopoulos et al., 2005; Chirinian & Mann, 2001; Glass, 2010). The cerebellum is important in regulation of cognition, motor function, emotion, and social behavior, and acts as a neural distribution node with interconnections with the thalamus and cortex (Bolduc & Limperopoulos, 2009; Owens, 2005; Volpe, 2008). Preterm infants, especially those who are very low birth weight, are at risk for cerebellar injury. These injuries may alter motor and language development and cognitive, socio-emotional, and behavioral function (Bolduc & Limperopoulos, 2009; Glass, 2010; Kling, 1989; Limperopoulos, 2009; Limperopoulos, 2010; Owens, 2005; Vandertak, 2009).

BIRTH INJURIES

Traumatic injury to the central or peripheral nervous system can occur during the perinatal or postnatal period. Most of these injuries happen during the intrapartum period and may occur with perinatal hypoxic-ischemic events. Perinatal events most frequently associated with birth injury include midforceps delivery, shoulder dystocia, low forceps delivery, birth weight exceeding 3,500 g, and second stage of labor lasting longer than 60 minutes. The incidence of injury has declined markedly in recent years as a result of improvement in obstetrical care and increased use of cesarean sections for abnormal presentations. However, birth injuries can also arise from trauma during a cesarean section or resuscitation. Injuries that occur before the intrapartum period usually are caused by compression or pressure injuries from an unusual fetal position. The risk of injury to the central or peripheral nervous system is greater with malpresentation (especially breech), prolonged or precipitate labor, prematurity, multiple gestation, shoulder dystocia, macrosomia, and instrumental delivery. The most prevalent types of injury to the nervous system are extracranial hemorrhage, intracranial hemorrhage, skull fractures, spinal cord injury, and peripheral nerve injury (Bonifacio et al., 2012).

Extracranial Hemorrhage

Caput succedaneum and cephalohematoma are the most common types of birth injury, as well as the most benign. Caput succedaneum is characterized by soft, pitting, superficial edema that is several millimeters thick and overlies the presenting part in a vertex delivery. This edematous area lies above the periosteum and thus crosses suture lines. The edema consists of serum or blood, or both. Infants with caput succedaneum may also have ecchymosis, petechiae, or purpura over the presenting part. Caput succedaneum occurs in infants after a spontaneous vertex delivery or after the use of a vacuum extractor. This type of extracranial hemorrhage requires no care other than parent teaching regarding its cause and significance. It resolves within a few days after birth with no sequelae. Cephalohematoma occurs in 1.5% to 2.5% of newborns (Bonifacio et al., 2012; Waller, Gopalani, & Benedetti, 2012). It involves subperiosteal bleeding, usually over the parietal bone but possibly over other cranial bones. Cephalohematoma usually is unilateral but can be bilateral. This type of hemorrhage is seen most often in males, after the use of forceps, after a prolonged, difficult delivery, and in infants born to primiparas. The characteristic finding is a firm, fluctuant mass that does not cross the suture lines. The mass often enlarges slightly by 2 to 3 days of age. Approximately 5% of infants with unilateral and 18% with bilateral cephalohematomas have a linear skull fracture underlying the mass (Fenichel, 2007; Waller et al., 2012). In rare cases an infant may have a subdural or SAH.

Caput succedaneum and cephalohematoma over the occipital bone must be differentiated from encephalocele. In contrast to extracranial hemorrhage, an encephalocele is characterized by pulsations, increased pressure (tenseness) with crying, and the appearance of a bony defect on radiographic studies (Fenichel, 2007; Heaberlin, 2009). Infants with a cephalohematoma generally have no symptoms. Management includes parent teaching and monitoring for the development of hyperbilirubinemia (Watchko, 2009). Occasionally an infant with a large cephalohematoma becomes anemic. These infants should also be monitored for symptoms of intracranial hemorrhage or skull fracture. Generally, cephalohematomas resolve between 2 weeks and 6 months of age, and most resolve by 8 weeks. Calcium deposits occasionally develop, and the swelling may remain for the first year.

■ Subgaleal Hemorrhage. Subgaleal or subaponeurotic hemorrhage is the most serious form of extracranial hemorrhage in newborns (Schierholz & Walker, 2010; Waller et al., 2012). Subgaleal hemorrhage occurs in 4 per 10,000 spontaneous vaginal deliveries and 59 per 10,000 vacuum-assisted deliveries. The incidence is also increased with precipitous deliveries, macrosomia, and severe dystocia, and with failed vacuum deliveries requiring forceps. Use of soft silastic cups (rather than the rigid hard cup) with vacuum extractors is associated with fewer scalp injuries, although the soft cups are more likely to fail (Waller et al., 2012). Mortality is 17% to 25%; however, if the infant survives the hemorrhage and does not develop HIE, the hemorrhage usually resolves in 2 to 3 weeks and outcomes are good (Fenichel, 2007; Volpe, 2008).

Traction or application of intense shearing forces to the scalp pull the aponeurosis from the vault and rupture large emissary veins. Blood collects in a large potential space between the galea aponeurotica and the periosteum of the skull through which the large emissary veins pass (Schierholz & Walker, 2010; Volpe, 2008). The area is called a potential space because it is not present until blood separates the galea aponeurotica from the periosteum of the skull. This space can quickly expand to accommodate 260 to 280 mL of blood. Total newborn blood volume is 80 to 100 mL/kg, so this volume may be more than the entire blood volume of some newborns (Fenichel, 2007; Schierholz & Walker, 2010; Volpe, 2008).

Subgaleal hemorrhage is a clinical emergency. These infants usually present at birth or within a few hours after birth (Bonifacio et al., 2012; Fenichel, 2007; Schierholz & Walker, 2010; Volpe, 2008). Clinical findings include a firm, ballotable head mass that crosses sutures and fontanelles (often extending from the orbital ridge, around the ears to the neck) and increases in size after birth. Each centimeter of enlargement is estimated to be equivalent to 40 mL of blood loss (Fenichel, 2007; Schierholz & Walker, 2010; Volpe, 2008). The mass mimics edema and shifts with head repositioning. Infants usually show signs of pain on manipulation of the scalp or head. Infants may present with a rapidly falling Hct, anemia, hypovolemia, pallor, hypotension, tachycardia, tachypnea, hypotonia, and other signs of shock (Bonifacio et al., 2012; Fenichel, 2007; Schierholz & Walker, 2010; Volpe, 2008). Management includes rapid recognition, cardiovascular and respiratory monitoring, administration of blood and volume expanders, and control of bleeding (Fenichel, 2007; Schierholz & Walker, 2010; Volpe, 2008).

Other Types of Intracranial Hemorrhage

In addition to IVH, several other clinically important types of intracranial bleeding can occur in the neonate, including primary SAH, subdural hemorrhage, and intracerebellar hemorrhage. These types of hemorrhage arise from trauma or hypoxia during the perinatal period.

■ **Primary SAH.** Primary SAH is the most prevalent form of intracranial hemorrhage in neonates and the least clinically significant for most infants. SAH occurs in both preterm and term infants but is more common in preterm infants. SAH may occur alone (primary SAH) or as a secondary event with other forms of intracranial hemorrhage. For example, with IVH, blood moves into the subarachnoid space via the fourth ventricle (Levene & DeVries, 2009; Volpe, 2008).

Pathophysiology. Primary SAH consists of bleeding into the subarachnoid space that is not secondary to subdural or intraventricular bleeding. In neonates, the source of the bleeding is venous blood; in older children and adults, SAH usually involves arterial blood. With primary SAH, blood leaks from the leptomeningeal plexus, bridging veins, or ruptured vessels in the subarachnoid space (Levene & DeVries, 2009). This type of hemorrhage is associated with trauma or asphyxia. Trauma that causes increased intravascular pressure and capillary rupture is the underlying causal event in most term infants with SAH. In preterm infants, SAH usually is the result of asphyxial events. Factors that place an infant at risk for SAH include birth trauma, prolonged labor, difficult delivery, fetal distress, and perinatal hypoxic-ischemic events (Levene & DeVries, 2009; Volpe, 2008).

Assessment. Three clinical presentations have been described for infants with SAH (Volpe, 2008). The most common is a preterm infant with a minor SAH. These infants are asymptomatic. The hemorrhage is discovered accidentally, for example, during a lumbar puncture as part of a sepsis workup. With the second type of clinical presentation, term or preterm infants may show isolated seizure activity at 2 to 3 days of age, or preterm infants occasionally may present with apnea. Between seizures, the infant appears and acts healthy ("well baby with seizures"). Infants in both of these groups survive and usually do well developmentally. The third type of clinical presentation involves infants with a massive SAH that has a rapid and fatal course. This presentation is rare and often is associated with both a severe asphyxial event and birth trauma. Blood in the CSF on lumbar puncture indicates the possibility of SAH, but true hemorrhage must be distinguished from a bloody tap. MRI and CT also can help confirm the diagnosis; ultrasonography is unreliable with SAH (Levene & DeVries, 2009; Volpe, 2008).

Management. Management of these infants begins with efforts to prevent or reduce the risk of trauma and hypoxia during the perinatal period, so as to reduce the risk of development of SAH. Infants with SAH are observed for seizures and other neurologic signs during the early neonatal period. Nursing care is primarily supportive and includes maintenance of oxygenation and perfusion and provision of warmth, fluids, and nutrients. Nursing management also involves helping the parents to understand the basis for and cause and prognosis of SAH, as well as the care of their infant.

Outcomes. Generally, infants with SAH survive, and asymptomatic infants do well. Up to half of symptomatic infants with severe, sustained traumatic or hypoxic injury with further damage to the CNS have neurologic sequelae (Hill, 2005; Levene & DeVries, 2009; Volpe, 2008). Hydrocephalus occasionally develops in infants with a history of SAH as a result of obstruction of CSF flow by adhesions. These infants should undergo repeat ultrasonographic examinations to monitor ventricular dilation.

■ **Subdural Hemorrhage.** Subdural hemorrhage (SDH) is the least common of the hemorrhages seen in newborns; however, recognition of this hemorrhage is important as immediate intervention for large SDH can be lifesaving (Volpe, 2008). The incidence of SDH has declined markedly as a result of improvements in obstetrical care. This decrease has been particularly notable in term infants (Hill, 2005; Levene & DeVries, 2009). Risk factors include precipitous, prolonged, or difficult delivery, use of midforceps or high forceps, prematurity, cephalopelvic disproportion, and macrosomia. SDH is seen more often in infants born to primiparas, possibly because of the more rigid birth canal. Infants with abnormal presentations (e.g., breech, foot, brow, or face) are also at higher risk for SDH (Hill, 2005; Volpe, 2008; Waller et al., 2012).

Pathophysiology. SDH in newborns is almost always caused by trauma during the perinatal period. Unilateral or bilateral bleeding occurs between the dura and the arachnoid. The bleeding occurs over the cerebral hemispheres or posterior fossa with or without lacerations of the tentorium or falx cerebri (see Figure 15.1). The cerebral hemispheres are the most common site for SDH. Bleeding usually occurs over the temporal convexity, with rupture of superficial cerebral veins or of "bridging" veins between the superomedial aspect of the cerebrum and the superior sagittal sinus. Because the superficial veins over the cerebrum are poorly developed in the preterm infant, this type of hemorrhage is seen less often in these infants. Bleeding over the posterior fossa involves bleeding below the tentorium and compression of the brainstem. Dural tears at the junction of the falx and tentorium near the attachment of the great vein of Galen are also associated with compression of the brainstem and midbrain (Fenichel, 2007; Levene & DeVries, 2009; Volpe, 2008).

Assessment. SDH must be distinguished from other types of intracranial hemorrhage and neurologic problems. This differentiation often can be accomplished by evaluating the infant's history and presentation and, if the infant is having seizure activity, by ruling out other causes of seizures. SDH over the cerebral hemispheres often is associated with SAH. SDH also occurs with extracranial hemorrhages, such as cephalohematoma and subgaleal, subconjunctival, and retinal hemorrhages; skull fractures; and brachial plexus or facial palsies. MRI or CT can assist in confirming the diagnosis; CT appears to be the imaging modality of choice (Fenichel, 2007, Hill, 2005; Levene & DeVries, 2009; Volpe, 2008).

Clinical signs of SDH relate to the site of the bleeding and the severity of the hemorrhage. Three patterns are seen in infants with bleeding over the cerebral hemispheres (Volpe, 2008). The first pattern is seen in most neonates with SDH; these infants have a minor hemorrhage and are asymptomatic or have signs such as irritability and hyperalertness. With the second pattern, primarily focal seizures develop during the first 2 to 3 days of life. Other neurologic signs that may be seen include hemiparesis; pupils that are unequal and respond sluggishly to light; full or tense fontanelle; bradycardia; and irregular respirations. The third pattern is seen in a few infants who have no or nonspecific signs in the neonatal period but in whom signs appear at 4 weeks to 6 months of age. These infants generally show increasing head size as a result of continued hematoma formation, poor feeding, failure to thrive, altered level of consciousness and, occasionally, seizures caused by the chronic subdural effusion. Infants with abnormal neurologic signs from birth often have had bleeding over the posterior fossa with tentorial lacerations. Signs include stupor or coma, eye deviation, asymmetric pupil size, altered pupillary response to light, tachypnea, bradycardia, and opisthotonos. As the clot enlarges, these infants rapidly deteriorate, with signs of shock appearing over minutes to hours. The infant becomes comatose and has fixed, dilated pupils and altered respirations and heart rate, which culminate in respiratory arrest. Infants with small tears in the posterior fossa may have no clinical manifestations for the first 3 to 4 days of life. During this time, the clot gradually enlarges until signs of increased ICP appear. As the brainstem becomes compressed, the infant's condition deteriorates, and oculomotor abnormalities, altered respiration, bradycardia, and seizures occur (Fenichel, 2007; Volpe, 2008).

Management. Infants with a history of perinatal trauma or other risk factors are observed for seizures and other neurologic signs. Care is primarily supportive and includes maintenance of oxygenation and perfusion and provision of warmth, fluids, and nutrients. Nursing management also involves helping the parents to understand the basis for and the cause and prognosis of this type of hemorrhage, as well as the care of their infant.

Symptomatic infants with bleeding over the temporal convexity and increased ICP may require surgical evacuation if the infant's condition cannot be stabilized neurologically. Massive posterior fossa hemorrhage requires craniotomy and surgical aspiration of the clot (Fenichel, 2007; Levene & DeVries, 2009). Infants at risk for SDH should be monitored carefully over the first 4 to 6 months after birth for late signs of bleeding and hematoma formation. Monitoring of these infants includes observation of head size, growth, feeding, activity, and level of consciousness, as well as monitoring for seizure activity.

Outcomes. The prognosis varies with the location and severity of the hemorrhage. Infants with bleeding over the cerebral hemispheres who are asymptomatic do well, as do most infants who have transient seizures in the neonatal period if no associated cerebral injury is present. Early diagnosis with CT or MRI has improved the outcome for infants with posterior fossa hemorrhage. Most infants with bleeding over the tentorium or falx cerebri die; severe hydrocephalus and neurologic sequelae usually develop in those that survive (Hill, 2005; Volpe, 2008).

■ Intracerebellar Hemorrhage. Intracerebellar hemorrhage is rare and is thought to be multifactorial with primary importance of birth trauma (breech or forceps delivery) and circulatory events. These hemorrhages occur in both term and preterm infants but are more common in preterm infants. Intracerebellar hemorrhage is seen during autopsy in infants with a history of perinatal hypoxic-ischemic events or severe respiratory distress syndrome (or both) and IVH (Bonifacio et al., 2011; Fenichel, 2007; Volpe, 2008).

Two presentations have been described. Many infants are critically ill from birth, with rapidly progressive apnea, a declining Hct value, and death within 24 to 36 hours. Other infants are less ill initially, and symptoms develop up to 2 to 3 weeks of age. Clinical manifestations include apnea, bradycardia, hoarse or high-pitched cry, eye deviations, opisthotonos, seizures, vomiting, hypotonia, and diminished or absent Moro reflex. Hydrocephalus often develops in these infants as early as the end of the first week after birth. The prognosis is poor in survivors, especially those born prematurely or with severe hemorrhage (Bonifacio et al., 2011; Fenichel, 2007; Levene & DeVries, 2009; Volpe, 2008).

■ Perinatal Stroke. Ischemic strokes are more common in the perinatal period than at any other time of life and are the leading cause of hemiplegic cerebral palsy, yet until recently have been poorly understood and oftentimes not diagnosed in the neonatal period. As a result, incidence is estimated to be from fairly rare (17–93 per 100,000 live births) to relatively common (1 in 2,300–5,000 live births) (Benders et al., 2009; Chabrier, Husson, Dinomais, Landrieu, & Nguyen, 2011; Cheong & Cowan, 2009; Kirton & deVeber, 2009; Mineyko & Kirton, 2011; Myers & Ment, 2012). Evidence suggests that preterm infants are just as likely, if not more likely than term infants, to experience perinatal ischemic stroke (Benders et al., 2009; Cheong & Cowan, 2009; Myers & Ment, 2012; Lynch, 2009).

Perinatal stroke was defined in 2006 by the National Institute of Child Health and Human Development and the National Institute of Neurological Disorders as the result of a focal disruption of cerebral blood flow secondary to an arterial or venous thrombosis or embolism occurring between 20 weeks gestation and 28 postnatal day of life (Kirton & deVeber, 2009; Mineyko & Kirton, 2011; Myers & Ment, 2012). Perinatal strokes are further classified as fetal or neonatal. Fetal stroke is defined as having occurred between 20 weeks gestation and the onset of labor or cesarean section and neonatal stroke as having occurred between the onset of labor and actual delivery.

Presumed perinatal ischemic strokes are those identified by neuroimaging in infants greater than 28 days of life as having had a focal infarction at some point between 20 weeks gestation and postnatal day 28 (Chabrier et al., 2011; Kirton & deVeber, 2009; Myers & Ment, 2012; Lynch, 2009).

Risk factors for perinatal stroke seem to be multifactorial and are still being identified to determine which factors are associated with a predilection for or direct causation of stroke. The risk factors that are being studied can be grouped into maternal, pregnancy/labor-related, and fetal or neonatal conditions (Myers & Ment, 2012; Lynch, 2009). Maternal risk factors include: thrombophilias (Factor V Leiden, Factor VIII, protein S deficiency, protein C deficiency, prothrombin mutation, and antiphospholipid antibodies), preexisting conditions such as thyroid disease, diabetes mellitus, or gestational diabetes or history of infertility. Pregnancy/labor-related risk factors implicated in perinatal stroke include significant maternal trauma, primiparity, placental abnormalities, oligohydramnios, decreased fetal movement, prolonged rupture of membranes, chorioamnionitis, prolonged second stage of labor, or assisted delivery (vacuum or forceps). Fetal or neonatal risk factors include fetal distress during labor, cord abnormalities (tight nuchal or body cord, true cord knot), thrombophilias (same as maternal), congenital cardiac defects, and corrective surgery (Cheong & Cowan, 2009; Kirton & deVeber, 2009; Mineyko & Kirton, 2011; Myers & Ment, 2012). In addition, there may be a gender effect on incidence of stroke, with male gender being a risk factor over female gender (Chabrier et al., 2011; Cheong & Cowan, 2009; Kirton & deVeber, 2009; Myers & Ment, 2012).

Clinical signs and symptoms of perinatal stroke are determined by the timing of the initial insult. Seizures occur in 85% to 92% of affected newborns and are often the earliest manifestation of a perinatal stroke in an otherwise healthy appearing newborn. Most seizures happen within the first 72 hours of life; approximately 50% of seizures are focal motor, 33% generalized motor, and 17% subtle (Myers & Ment; 2012). Physical examination may reveal a bulging and/or pulsatile fontanel, dilated head and neck veins, papilledema, asymmetrical movements or primitive reflexes, or seizure-like activity (Kirton & deVeber, 2009). Transient hemiparesis or generalized tone anomalies, such as hypotonia, are seen in the early newborn phase (Myers & Ment, 2012). Other symptoms of stroke are hypotonia and apnea, which are generic symptoms of any aberration in the newborn period, necessitating differential diagnosis from hypoxic, metabolic, and infectious disorders. Infants not diagnosed during the newborn stage are typically identified at a median of 6 months when asymmetry of reach and grasp is noted. Seizures occurring after 28 days of life and language delay have also been reported (Kirton & deVeber, 2009; Myers & Ment, 2012).

Diagnostic work-up includes thorough history, newborn assessment, laboratory tests, and cardiac and neurologic imaging. Echocardiogram and electrocardiogram may be indicated to assess for cardiac dysfunction or rhythm disorders. EEG and neuroimaging are definitely indicated to evaluate for perinatal stroke (Kirton & deVeber, 2009; Mineyko & Kirton, 2011; Myers & Ment, 2012). During the past decade, rapid advances in the use of good quality early cranial ultrasonography and MRI with diffusion-weighted sequences has facilitated improved and rapid diagnosis in the neonatal period, allowing for earlier identification and treatment and support of the affected newborn (Cheong & Cowan, 2009; Kirton & deVeber, 2009; Myers & Ment, 2012). Treatment of perinatal stroke is supportive and is directed at minimizing secondary brain injury and optimize outcome. Blood glucose, temperature, ventilation, oxygenation, and blood volume and pressure should be normalized. Hyperthermia and hyperthermic environment should be avoided. Seizures are documented and treated aggressively (Kirton & deVeber, 2009; Myers & Ment, 2012).

Outcome for infants with perinatal stroke varies with area of original insult. It is estimated that 20% to 70% of hemiplegic cerebral palsy are associated with perinatal stroke, with the spasticity more marked in the upper extremities. Intelligence is within normal parameters for two thirds of affected infants (Myers & Ment, 2012).

Skull Fracture

Two types of skull fractures, linear and depressed, are uncommon but can be seen in newborns (Bonifacio et al., 2011; Fenichel, 2007; Gomella et al., 2009). Skull fractures occur in utero, during labor, with forceps delivery, or during a prolonged, difficult labor with compression and battering of the fetal skull against the maternal ischial spines, sacral promontory, or symphysis pubis (Bonifacio et al., 2011). The fetal skull often is able to tolerate mechanical stressors relatively well, because it is flexible, malleable, poorly ossified, and less mineralized than the adult skull. Depressed fractures occur after forceps delivery but occasionally are seen after a vaginal or cesarean birth. Compression of the skull causes buckling of the inner table without a break in the continuity of the skull. Linear fractures usually occur over the frontal or parietal bones. These fractures often are associated with extracranial hemorrhage and may underlie a cephalohematoma and are usually asymptomatic. Skull radiographs are required for the diagnosis (Tekes, Pinto, & Huisman, 2011). Intracranial hemorrhage rarely complicates linear fractures.

A depressed skull fracture is a visible, palpable depression, or dent in the skull, usually over the parietal area. These fractures often are described as resembling a ping-pong ball because the depression does not involve any loss of bone continuity. Unless underlying cerebral contusion or hemorrhage is present, no other signs or symptoms are seen (Bonifacio et al., 2011; Tekes et al., 2011). The diagnosis is confirmed with skull radiographs or CT scans. CT is performed to identify cerebral contusions or hemorrhage (Tekes et al., 2011).

Nursing assessment includes monitoring infants identified with skull fractures for signs of neurologic dysfunction, intracranial hemorrhage, meningitis, and seizures, although these findings are rare. Parents usually are concerned about their infant's appearance (with a depressed fracture) and the possibility of brain damage. They need support and teaching. Infants with uncomplicated linear fractures require no special management. Follow-up monitoring usually is recommended so that a growing fracture and development of a leptomeningeal cyst can be ruled out (Fenichel, 2007). Infants with basal fractures are treated for shock and hemorrhage.

In some infants with a depressed fracture, the fracture elevates spontaneously within the first week. Most clinicians recommend manually elevating an uncomplicated depressed fracture that does not elevate spontaneously within a few days (Fenichel, 2007; Tekes et al., 2011). After this time, manual elevation is more difficult or impossible. Surgical intervention usually is necessary if manual elevation fails, if the fracture is more severe and bone fragments are in the cerebrum, if neurologic deficits exist, or if ICP is increased.

Linear fractures heal spontaneously with no sequelae unless underlying cerebral damage or a growing fracture is present. Basal fractures are associated with high mortality and poor developmental outcome. Infants with depressed fractures that are small or treated early (or both) have a good prognosis. Infants with large fractures, especially if treatment is delayed, have a greater risk of sequelae. Unless a depressed fracture has lacerated the dura (a rare occurrence), neurologic deficits in these infants usually are caused by cerebral injury from the original trauma or a hypoxic event, or both, rather than by the fracture (Bonifacio et al., 2011; Fenichel, 2007). Infants with skull fractures should undergo regular evaluation of growth and development during infancy and early childhood.

Spinal Cord Injury

Spinal cord injuries are uncommon and usually occur in the midcervical to lower cervical and upper thoracic areas. Injury can occur at any point along the cord. Spinal cord injuries are caused by excessive traction, rotation, and torsion of the vertebral column and neck. Injury usually does not result from compression, but rather from stretching of the spinal cord, which is less flexible than the bony vertebral column. Damage to the spinal cord ranges from complete transection to laceration, edema, hemorrhage, and hematoma formation. Hemorrhage into the lining of the arteries may result in thrombosis, infarction, and ischemic cord damage. Risk factors are breech delivery (major factor), dystocia, macrosomia, and cephalopelvic disproportion (Bonifacio et al., 2012; Fenichel, 2007; Madsen, Frim, & Hansen, 2005; Volpe, 2008).

Infants with partial spinal cord injury have subtle neurologic signs and variable degrees of spasticity. Infants with high cervical or brainstem injuries are stillborn or die shortly after birth from respiratory depression, shock, and hypothermia. Infants with midcervical or upper cervical injury may be stillborn, born with marked respiratory depression, or have respiratory depression, with the neurologic injury going unrecognized until flaccidity, immobility of the legs, urine retention, or all three are noted. If born alive, these infants usually die within the first week, after development of progressive central respiratory depression that often is complicated by pneumonia. Other findings in this group of infants include relaxation of the abdominal wall, absent sensation in the lower half of the body, absent deep tendon and spontaneous reflexes, brachial plexus injury, and constipation. This group also includes infants with injuries at the C8 to T1 level who usually survive and may have a transient paraplegic paralysis at birth. Infants with mild injury may recover most or all of their function. Infants with moderate to severe damage are paraplegic or quadriplegic and have permanent neurologic damage (Bonifacio et al., 2011; Fenichel, 2007; Volpe, 2008).

Initially, clinical manifestations are those of spinal cord shock, with hypotonia, weakness, flaccid extremities, sensory deficits, relaxed abdominal muscles, diaphragmatic breathing, Horner syndrome (ipsilateral ptosis, anhidrosis, and miosis), and a distended bladder. Infants with low cervical lesions have shallow, paradoxical respirations; these infants do not sweat. The skin over the affected area is dry and warm. Pinprick and deep tendon reflexes are absent. Areflexia may be noted over the upper and lower extremities in some infants. The degree of neurologic insult often cannot be accurately evaluated until the infant has recovered from the initial period of spinal shock and any edema or hemorrhage has been reabsorbed (Fenichel, 2007; Madsen et al., 2005; Volpe, 2008). After several weeks or months, a paraplegic autonomic hyperreflexia develops that is characterized by periodic mass reflex response. This results in tonic spasms of extremities, spontaneous micturition, and profuse sweating over the paralyzed area (Volpe, 2008).

Initial management focuses on stabilization, treatment of associated problems (e.g., asphyxia, hemorrhage, shock), and management of respiratory depression. Infants with midcervical to upper cervical or brainstem lesions require assisted ventilation. Parents are in shock initially and need time to grieve. They need continuing support and teaching regarding the care of the infant. Ongoing management of these infants and their families requires a multidisciplinary team that includes the disciplines of nursing, medicine, neurology, neurosurgery, physical therapy, orthopedics, urology, social work, and psychology. Ultrasonography, CT, or MRI may be performed to determine the level and the extent of injury (Fenichel, 2007; Volpe, 2008).

Skin integrity over the paralyzed area must be maintained to prevent pressure areas and skin breakdown. Thermoregulation may be a problem, because evaporative loss through the skin is reduced over the affected body parts in the initial period of the recovery process. The infant is positioned and repositioned regularly to promote normal alignment of body parts and prevent development of contractures and decubiti. The affected areas should be kept clean and dry and massaged with gentle, passive range-of-motion exercises. These infants need meticulous bowel and bladder care to prevent urinary tract infection and skin excoriation. Glycerin suppositories at regular intervals can help normalize bowel function. Infants are also monitored for signs of respiratory infection and pneumonia. Parental teaching before discharge focuses on normal baby care issues and concerns, as well as the special needs of a paralyzed infant.

The prognosis depends on the level and severity of the injury, but it generally is poor. Many infants with spinal cord injury are stillborn or die shortly after birth, particularly those with midcervical to high cervical or brainstem injuries. Those who survive have varying degrees of residual paralysis, respiratory problems, and bowel and bladder dysfunction, depending on the level of the injury. Most surviving infants have a spastic quadriplegia. Infants with involvement of the intercostal muscles and diaphragm often are ventilator dependent (Bonifacio et al., 2011; Fenichel, 2007; Madsen et al., 2005; Volpe, 2008).

Peripheral Nerve Injuries

Peripheral nerve injuries result from stretching, compression, twisting, hyperextension, or separation of nerve tissue (Bonifacio et al., 2012; Fenichel, 2007; Hill, 2005; Levene, 2009; Volpe, 2008). Injury can occur before, during, or after birth. Damage can range from swelling of the nerve to complete peripheral degeneration (with later total recovery) to complete division of all structures. The more common sites affected are the brachial plexus and the facial, phrenic, radial, median, and sciatic nerves. This type of injury is seen predominantly in term or large for gestational age (LGA) infants (Bonifacio et al., 2012; Hill, 2005; Volpe, 2008).

Injury to the radial nerve usually results from compression of the nerve caused by fracture of the humerus during a breech delivery or by intrauterine compression of the arm. The infant has wrist drop with a normal grasp reflex. Recovery usually occurs over the first few weeks to months. Median and sciatic nerve injuries are typically postnatal iatrogenic events. Median nerve injury can be a complication of brachial or radial arterial punctures. These infants have diminished pincer grasp and thumb strength and a flexed fourth finger. Recovery is variable. Sciatic nerve injuries are often permanent. They arise from trauma from a misplaced intramuscular injection or from ischemia from an injection of hypertonic solutions into the gluteal muscle. Infants with this type of injury have diminished abduction and distal joint movement. Hip adduction, rotation, and flexion are unaffected (Levene, 2009).

■ **Facial Nerve Palsy.** Facial nerve palsy has an incidence of 0.23% (Levene, 2009). Injury to the peripheral nerve is caused by trauma from oblique application of forceps, prolonged pressure on the nerve during labor from the maternal sacral promontory, or pressure from an abnormal fetal posture. Although some investigators have not found any differences in incidence between forceps and spontaneous vaginal deliveries, others have noted a correlation between the type of forceps and the incidence of injury. The facial nerve of the newborn is superficial after it emerges from the stylomastoid foramen. As a result, the nerve is vulnerable to compression injury at this site or as it traverses the ramus of the mandible. The temporofacial and cervicofacial nerve branches are most often involved. The injury is most common on the left. Because the prognosis is favorable, the injury appears to be caused by hemorrhage or edema into the nerve sheath rather than by disruption of the nerve fibers (Levene, 2009; Volpe, 2008).

Facial nerve paralysis must be distinguished from asymmetric crying facies and nuclear agenesis. Asymmetric crying facies results from absence of the depressor muscle of the angle of the mouth. These infants close their eyes normally when crying, but the mouth does not move down and out. They suck without dribbling. This disorder generally is benign. Nuclear agenesis (Möbius syndrome) is a more significant disorder characterized by congenital paralysis of the facial muscles (Levene, 2009; Terzis & Anesti, 2011; Volpe, 2008).

Clinical manifestations vary, depending on whether the injury is to the central nerve, the peripheral nerve, or the peripheral nerve branch. The complete peripheral nerve injury results in a unilateral inability to close the eye or open the mouth. The lower lip on the affected side does not depress during crying, nor does the forehead wrinkle. The affected side appears full and smooth, with obliteration of the nasolabial fold. These infants dribble milk while feeding. The infant may be unable to close the eye on the affected side. Central injury usually results in a spastic paralysis of the lower portion of the face contralateral to the side of CNS injury without involvement of the eyes or forehead. Peripheral nerve branch injury results in varying degrees of paralysis of the forehead, eye, or lower face, depending on the branch involved. The paralysis is apparent at birth or within 1 to 2 days after birth.

Almost all infants recover completely. Improvement usually is apparent by 1 to 4 weeks, and complete recovery occurs after several months in most infants. Infants with severe nerve regeneration have a longer recovery period and may occasionally require later cosmetic surgery (Levene, 2009; Terzis & Anesti, 2011).

Nursing management involves parent counseling and teaching and prevention of complications. The eye on the affected side is patched, and 1% methylcellulose eye drops are instilled every 3 to 4 hours to prevent corneal damage. Dribbling with sucking can be a transient problem. A neurosurgical consultation is recommended if no improvement is noted by 7 to 10 days or if further loss of function occurs. With partial degeneration, physical therapy, massage, or electrical stimulation may be used, although the efficacy of these therapies is controversial and not well documented. Electromyography, nerve excitability, or nerve conduction latency examinations may be performed to evaluate the extent of the damage (Gomella et al., 2009; Terzis & Anesti, 2011).

■ **Brachial Plexus Injury.** Brachial plexus palsy involves injury of the C5 to T1 nerve roots and is seen almost exclusively in term infants. The incidence ranges from 0.5% to 2% (Volpe, 2008). Injury to the brachial plexus results from excessive lateral flexion, rotation, or traction on the neck. The degree of injury varies, ranging from edema and hemorrhage of the nerve sheath to avulsion of the nerve root from the spinal cord. With mild-to-moderate injury the axons are shattered, but the nerve sheaths remain intact. This degree of intactness of the nerve sheaths promotes regeneration of the nerve by 3 to 4 months, with full recovery by 3 to 15 months in most infants (Alfonso, 2011; Doumouchtsis & Arulkumaran, 2009; Fenichel, 2007; Levene, 2009; Volpe, 2008). Severe injuries result in radicular rupture or intraspinal tearing of the nerve and division of the nerve into radicles. If radicular rupture occurs, the root loses contact with the spinal cord. These injuries do not recover spontaneously (Alfonso, 2011; Doumouchtsis & Arulkumaran, 2009; Levene, 2009).

Brachial plexus injuries usually are unilateral and on the left side. Fracture of the clavicle may occur in conjunction with this type of injury. Brachial plexus injury can be seen in uncomplicated deliveries and after cesarean birth, but is usually associated with vaginal delivery of LGA infants, shoulder dystocia, breech presentations, and prolonged labor or difficult delivery. Spontaneous injuries may occur from compression of the shoulder as it passes over the sacral prominence (Alfonso, 2011; Doumouchtsis & Arulkumaran, 2009; Levene, 2009).

Clinical manifestations vary with the location and severity of the injury. Signs of injury usually are apparent from birth but may be delayed for several days to a few weeks in some infants. The major types of injury are Erb (Erb-Duchenne) palsy, an injury of the upper plexus involving C5 to C7, and Klumpke palsy or lower plexus injury at C5 to T1 (Fenichel, 2007; Levene, 2009). With Erb palsy, the shoulder and upper arm are involved, and denervation of the deltoid, supraspinous, biceps, and brachioradialis muscles occurs. The arm lies passively at the infant's side, abducted and internally rotated, and the forearm is pronated. The wrist and fingers are flexed. This posture is referred to as the "waiter's tip" position. The Moro reflex is absent, and the biceps and radial reflexes are diminished or absent on the affected side; the grasp reflex is normal.

Klumpke palsy is seen primarily in breech infants whose arm has been hyperabducted and delivered with the head affecting the flexors of the wrist and hand. Cervical sympathetic fibers may also be affected; sweating and sensation are absent in the affected hand and arm. The infant holds the affected arm at the side of the thorax with the hand in a claw hand posture. The Moro and grasp reflexes are absent, and the triceps reflex is diminished or absent on the affected side; biceps and radial reflexes are present. If the T1 root is affected, the infant manifests Horner syndrome (Bonifacio, 2011; Levene, 2009).

Erb-Klumpke (total) palsy is characterized by entire arm and hand involvement as a result of injury to the nerve roots of the brachial plexus from C5 to T1. Complete paralysis of the upper and lower arm and hand, flaccidity, and accompanying sensory, trophic, and circulatory changes are noted. Deep tendon and Moro reflexes are absent. If the C4 roots are also affected, an associated phrenic nerve (diaphragmatic) paralysis occurs. Involvement of the T1 root leads to Horner syndrome in about one third of these infants (Levene, 2009).

Brachial plexus palsy can also be hereditary and is difficult to discern from traumatic injury. The genetic disorder is autosomal dominant inheritance (mapped to 17q25), which results in myelin abnormalities that should be considered for an infant with brachial plexus palsy following an uncomplicated delivery and a positive family history (Fenichel, 2007).

Initial management focuses on protecting the arm until localized edema and pain subside. MRI or CT is used to visualize the degree of injury. The affected arm should not be splinted or immobilized, as it has not proven beneficial to prevent contractures and further stretching of the plexus as had previously been thought. After edema subsides, at about 7 to 10 days, physical therapy gradually is instituted as the infant can tolerate it. Gentle passive range-of-motion exercises have been shown to minimize formation of contractures and to reduce permanent disability. These infants have continued physical therapy consisting of massage and exercise over the first months until total or partial recovery occurs (Fenichel, 2007; Volpe, 2008). Infants with a brachial plexus injury should be evaluated for associated problems, including fractures and respiratory difficulty secondary to phrenic nerve paralysis. If improvement is not noted within the first few months, electromyography and nerve conduction studies are performed to determine the extent of the damage, to follow recovery, and to determine whether surgical intervention is needed (Volpe, 2008). Infants with brachial plexus injuries often experience considerable pain during movement of the affected arm in the first few weeks after birth. Nursing management is directed at reducing passive and active movement of the arm and providing comfort measures to reduce pain. The paralyzed arm is supported in a position of relaxation. Parent teaching regarding positioning, prevention of contractures, and exercise is essential.

The prognosis depends on the level and severity of the injury. Approximately 65% to 95% of infants have full recovery with supportive care. Many recover by 3 to 4 months of age and more than 90% by 2 to 3 years. Erb palsy, the most common type of injury, has the best prognosis for full recovery. Infants with total paralysis are most likely to have residual paralysis. Residual functional deficits include alteration in abduction and external rotation of the shoulder; restricted movement of the elbow, forearm, and hand; and hand weakness. These functional impairments can lead to abnormal muscle development and arm growth (Fenichel, 2007; Levene, 2009).

■ Phrenic Nerve Palsy. Phrenic nerve palsy is caused by injury of the cervical nerve roots at C3 to C5. The injury results from tearing of the nerve sheath, which is accompanied by edema and hemorrhage. Phrenic nerve palsy may occur as an isolated event or in association with brachial nerve palsy. Risk factors, especially breech delivery, are similar to those for brachial plexus injury. Paralysis of the diaphragm is a result of damage to the phrenic nerve. The injury usually is unilateral and on the right side. Because the diaphragm is paralyzed, infants with phrenic nerve injury have respiratory difficulty. This phenomenon must be differentiated from CNS, cardiac, and pulmonary problems (Levene, 2009; Volpe, 2008).

Infants with mild to moderate phrenic nerve injury may have early respiratory difficulty, suggestive of hypoventilation that stabilizes or improves. The infant may have recurrent episodes of cyanosis and dyspnea. Respiratory efforts result in primarily thoracic movement with minimal or no abdominal excursions, opposite of the normal newborn breathing pattern. Infants with complete avulsion or bilateral injury have severe respiratory distress from birth, with tachypnea, apnea, and a weak cry (Fenichel, 2007; Volpe, 2008).

Management focuses on promoting ventilation and oxygenation. Infants are not enterally fed initially until respiratory status improves. Infants with severe distress require positive pressure ventilation or constant positive airway pressure for support until recovery occurs. Surgical plication of the diaphragm is performed if no improvement is noted or if the infant is still ventilator dependent at 4 to 6 weeks of age (Fenichel, 2007; Volpe, 2008).

The infant is positioned on the affected side. If the infant cannot be fed, adequate fluid and calories must be provided. Feeding is instituted gradually, most likely by gavage tube initially. When oral feeding is started, the infant is fed slowly and given ample opportunity for rest and monitoring of respiratory status. Because recovery takes several months, parents must be taught feeding, positioning, and comfort techniques. The developmental needs of infants requiring prolonged hospitalization must be met; sensory input and play activities appropriate to their maturity and health status must be provided. Most infants recover by 6 to 12 months of age. Other infants recover clinically but have residual abnormalities of diaphragmatic movement on radiography (Volpe, 2008).

SUMMARY

Infants with neurologic dysfunction present a significant challenge to the neonatal nurse. The nurse must respond to infants with life-threatening conditions, such as perinatal hypoxic-ischemic injury and intracranial hemorrhage; to those with transient problems, such as an isolated seizure; and to those with chronic problems, such as NTDs. Nurses must also deal with their own responses and those of the families of infants who may die during the neonatal or early infancy periods or whose short-term and long-term outcome may be altered by the extent of neurologic insult. To optimally care for these infants and their families, nurses must understand the basis for and the implications of specific types of neurologic dysfunction; they must recognize the clinical manifestations of these types of dysfunction; and they must respond appropriately in concert with other health care professionals.

The nursing care of infants who have or who are at risk for neurologic dysfunction involves assessment and monitoring of the infant's neurologic status and responses to the extrauterine environment, as well as of subtle signs that may indicate a change in status. Nursing management of the infant involves activities to address alteration in level of consciousness, potential for injury related to trauma or infection, impairment of skin integrity, alterations in comfort, impaired mobility, alterations in thermoregulation, alterations in nutrition and fluid and electrolyte status, and promotion of neurobehavioral organization and development. The nurse must also assess family coping, interactive processes, knowledge, and grieving to assist the family in coping with the birth of an ill infant and, for many families, with the uncertainty or certainty of long-term neurologic deficits in their infant.

CASE STUDY

■ Identification of the Problem. Term female infant vaginal delivery with vacuum assist; presented with apnea, no tone, requiring resuscitation intervention.

■ Assessment: History and Physical Examination. The term female infant was delivered vaginally to a 24-year-old G2 P1 woman following prolonged labor at term after an uncomplicated pregnancy. The vaginal delivery was assisted with a vacuum apparatus. Gestational age was term with a birth weight of 3.3 kg.

Upon delivery, the infant was limp, cyanotic/pale, and apneic. The infant was successfully resuscitated following Neonatal Resuscitation Program (NRP©) guidelines; required 2 minutes positive pressure ventilation by T-piece resuscitator to initiate effective ventilation when spontaneous respirations were noted; infant received 10 minutes of CPAP via the T-piece resuscitator; heart rate was greater than 100 beats per minute by 1 minute of age. Pulse oximetry was initiated by 1 minute of age, reading 44% oxygen saturations initially and gradually improved to 85% by 5 minutes of life; room air was used throughout resuscitation.

She remained pale with thready pulses and poor peripheral perfusion at 10 minutes of life; spontaneous respiratory rate 40 to 60 seconds with easy respiratory effort without CPAP; pulse oximetry saturations 88% to 94%; heart rate 160 seconds. The infant was brought to the NICU for ongoing care.

Apgar scores were 4^1, 6^5, 8^{10}

■ Physical Examination on Admission to the NICU

GENERAL: pale with thready pulses, poor peripheral perfusion; heart rate 180 beats/min. Respiratory rate 46, shallow; saturations 88% to 92% in room air

HEENT: increasingly boggy, enlarging scalp hematoma; eyes open, no blink; pupils reactive to light; positive red reflex and normal facies

RESP: lung fields bilaterally clear and equal to bases; gasping respiratory effort

CV: rate regular with no murmur noted. Poor peripheral perfusion, capillary blood refill time greater than 5 seconds, and thready pulses were noted

ABD: abdomen soft and nontender with no hepatosplenomegaly or masses palpable; three-vessel cord. The anus appeared patent

GENITOURINARY: normal female infant genitalia

NEURO: decreased responses, with eyes open and unblinking; extremities were well formed; muscle tone was markedly decreased

SKIN: pale with general cyanotic undertones, pronounced circumoral and acrocyanosis

EXTREMITIES: well formed; 10 digits per extremity; generalized cool and mottled Umbilical arterial and venous catheters were placed, and 10 mL/kg normal saline was given for volume expansion; dopamine was initiated because of low blood pressure and ongoing poor perfusion. Labs were drawn via the umbilical arterial catheter: arterial blood gas, complete blood count (CBC)/differential, and disseminated intravascular coagulation (DIC) panel, transfusion panel (type and cross for transfusion). The scalp hematoma was noted to be rapidly enlarging during this time. The infant was immediately intubated and was given an emergency blood transfusion of 15 mL/kg.

■ Differential Diagnoses

- Subgaleal hemorrhage
- Perinatal hypoxic-ischemic injury
- Shock
- DIC
- Intracranial hemorrhage
- Sepsis screen
- Congenital cardiac defects screen

■ Diagnostic Tests

Laboratory tests:

- CBC/differential: WBC 10.3, segmented cells 44; bands 1; Hct 21%, platelet count 168,000/mm^3
- Coagulation (DIC) panel: prothrombin time (PT) greater than 100 seconds, partial thromboplastin time (PTT) greater than 100 seconds, fibrinogen 54 mg/dL, and D-dimers 2 to 4 mg/mL
- Blood, tracheal, and surface cultures for bacterial and/or viral infections: all negative

Imaging tests:

- Head CT scan (performed within 4 hours of age): extensive blood within the extracranial soft tissues, mild IVH and SAH
- Transcranial Doppler and nuclear medicine flow scan (performed at 24 hours of age): no cerebral blood flow
- EEG (performed on day of life 3): absence of cortical activity

■ Working Diagnosis

Extensive subgaleal hemorrhage with hematoma

Based on clinical, laboratory, and imaging findings, data from history and physical assessment

■ Development of Management Plan

Continuous monitoring of arterial blood pressure, vital signs, and neurologic status, every 2 to 4 hours Hct, platelet count, PT/PTT, and fibrinogen

Maintenance fluid support; fluid boluses to support intravascular volume

Ensure adequate blood volume, clotting factors: colloids (fresh-frozen plasma with cryoprecipitate, whole blood, packed red blood cells, platelets) as needed to treat DIC, anemia

Respiratory support with mechanical ventilation as needed

Vasopressors to maintain adequate blood pressure and cerebral blood flow

Antibiotics until cultures negative for 72 hours

■ Implementation and Evaluation of Effectiveness

Implementation of management plan: (immediately after initial assessment in the NICU)

The infant was intubated within the first half hour of life

Multiple blood transfusions, fresh-frozen plasma with cryoprecipitate, whole blood and packed red blood cell transfusions, and normal saline boluses given to normalize the coagulation studies by 24 hours of age, with a total of 476 mL neonatal red blood cells, 8 units of cryoprecipitate, and 140 mL of fresh-frozen plasma.

Dopamine 10 mcg/kg/min initiated by 1 hour of life; weaned to 5 mcg/kg/min by 36 hours

■ Effectiveness of Management Plan

Respiratory status stable by 2 hours of life

Blood pressures were normalized by 2 hours of life

Metabolic acidosis and coagulation panel results were normalized within the first 24 hours of life

Severe brain involvement was suspected on day of life 2, with dismal results of the Doppler and flow scan and flat EEG results

■ Outcome. Brain death was determined on day of life 3. Life support was terminated on day of life 4. The autopsy was remarkable for an extensive subgaleal hematoma and moderate subarachnoid and subdural hemorrhage.

CASE STUDY

■ Identification of the Problem. A 6-day-old former term infant turned blue at home on day of life 4 and was admitted to the local hospital.

■ Assessment: History and Physical Examination

A 6-day-old former term neonate was delivered vaginally following an uncomplicated pregnancy with a birth weight of 2,990 g. Prenatal laboratory results were remarkable for positive Group B streptococcus (GBS) vaginal culture, for which the mother received prophylactic perinatal antibiotics. The infant did well after delivery, breastfed vigorously, and was discharged home with his mother on day 2 of life. At the time of admission, his weight was 2,950 g, occipito-frontal circumference was 33 cm, and length was 49.5 cm.

After initial admission to local hospital, the infant was screened for sepsis (normal CBC and differential, negative cultures for viral and bacterial sepsis). On day 2, at the local hospital, the infant had a seizure consisting of lip smacking, apnea, cyanosis, and bicycling of lower extremities; was given 10 mg/kg phenobarbital; and was taken to CT, which showed a right IVH. The infant was transferred to the NICU of the tertiary care hospital.

Physical Examination

GENERAL: vital signs within normal limits; somewhat sleepy and irritable with handling

HEENT: anterior fontanelle large and soft, with sutures split to just above eyebrows, lateral sutures proximate. Pupils equal and reactive to light; bilateral positive red reflex; sunset eyes when crying; nares patent bilaterally; palate and clavicles intact

LUNGS: clear and bilaterally equal; easy work of breathing with spontaneous respirations

CV: heart regular rhythm and rate, no murmur; peripheral pulses 2+ in all extremities, good peripheral perfusion; capillary blood refill time ~3 seconds

ABD: abdomen was soft and nontender; liver right costal margin; no hepatosplenomegaly or masses palpable; umbilical stump dry

GU: normal male genitalia; testes bilaterally descended; well-developed scrotum

NEURO: arched with handling, moved all extremities with increased tone; occasional tongue thrust; positive sunset eyes, positive gag reflex, positive blink response; no clonus

EXTREMITIES: well formed with good muscle mass, 10 digits/extremity

SKIN: pale pink; good turgor and healing areas from previous lab draws and intravenous access attempts. No petechiae or rashes were noted

SOCIAL: maternal history is significant, for a cousin died of "fits" at 3 months of age; other relatives suffered frequent bone fractures or sundown eye sign; father is reportedly short-statured with short-statured children

Differential Diagnoses

- Seizures of unknown etiology
- Rule out herpes simplex infection and other viral or bacterial meningitis
- Rule out brain structure abnormalities
- Rule out nonaccidental trauma (NAT)
- Rule out intracranial and intraventricular hemorrhage
- Hypoventilation of unknown etiology

Diagnostic Tests

Laboratory tests:

- CBC/differential: WBC 10.6, segmented cells 27, bands 0, Hct 60.2%, platelet count 254,000/mm^3
- Electrolytes: sodium 132, potassium 4.7, chloride 96, bicarbonate 29, calcium 11.9, ionized calcium 1.42, phosphorus 2.9, alkaline phosphorus less than 5, ammonia 45, lactate 2.2, BUN less than 1, and serum glutamic-oxaloacetic transaminase (SGOT) 33
- Blood and central spinal fluid bacterial and viral cultures: negative
- Urine drug screen: negative

Imaging tests:

- Serial EEGs: excessive background discontinuity and prominent high-amplitude spikes and polyspikes, but no seizures; repeat EEG (hospital day 7) significantly improved but still mildly abnormal due to focal moderate amplitude, midline vertex, and negative spikes without seizure activity
- MRI of the brain: hemorrhage located either in subependymal location or cavum velum interpositum not consistent with shear injury
- Head CT: placement of the hemorrhage in the right thalamic area with extension into the lateral ventricles and stable ventricle size

Consults: (pediatric specialists)

- NAT team: ophthalmic examination: normal without ocular hemorrhages; skeletal radiographic study no fractures; evidence of metaphyseal fraying in the lower extremities consistent with developing rickets
  Neurology, metabolic, and endocrine services

Working Diagnosis

- Six-day-old infant with seizures due to probable hypophosphatemia
- Laboratory results effectively ruled out sepsis, meningitis, electrolyte imbalances, and metabolic disease as etiologies for seizure activity
- The extremely low-alkaline phosphorus, low phosphorus, and high calcium and ionized calcium levels were indicators for endocrine disease
- EEG was moderately abnormal due to excessive background discontinuity and prominent high-amplitude spikes and polyspikes, but no seizures and improved by hospital day 7
- Imaging results ruled out NAT and other structural causes for the clinical presentation of seizure-like activity
- Skeletal radiographic study gave further support for endocrine disease due to the early radiographic indication for rickets
- NAT team concluded that the seizures were not caused by brain injury due to NAT
- Neurology service concluded that the etiology of the seizures was not structural or related to brain injury but most likely due to pyridoxine deficiency or some endocrine or metabolic syndrome
- Endocrinologists considered the seizures to be related to hypophosphatasia

Development of Management Plan

- Monitor the infant
- Provide respiratory, fluid, and nutritional support with a low-calcium formula
- Initiate vitamin D supplements to delay bone decalcification and rickets
- Provide teaching and support for the parents
- Arrange follow-up with the primary care provider and the pediatric neurology, orthopedic, and endocrinology services

■ Implementation and Evaluation of Effectiveness During the examination phase, pyridoxine was given for a seizure-like event on hospital day 2 that included bicycling, sneezing, clonic-tonic movements with paroxysmal respiratory pattern. Maintenance pyridoxine was given until hospital day 10, when it was determined the seizures were caused by hypophosphatemia. The infant was NPO with peripheral intravenous fluids until a special low-calcium formula could be delivered, and vitamin D supplements were started to delay bone decalcification and rickets. At time of discharge, the infant was taking good amounts of the formula by nipple and gaining weight slowly. His mother was learning what little there is to know about this rare congenital disease and learning to prevent fractures as much as possible. Follow-up care was arranged with primary pediatrician, neurology, orthopedics, and endocrinology.

■ Outcome. The prognosis for symptomatic congenital hypophosphatasia is poor, with death usually occurring within the first year of life. Parents initially denied being told about infant's condition at first follow-up visit with primary pediatrician; however was feeding infant correct, formula and following all discharge instructions.

CASE STUDY

■ Identification of the Problem. A term infant male was limp and not breathing after home-birth delivery.

■ Assessment: History and Physical Examination. The infant boy was born at 40 6/7 weeks by vaginal delivery to a 24-year-old, G1 P0 >1 woman at home with a certified nurse midwife present. Prenatal laboratory results and history were unremarkable with negative GBS status. The pregnancy was uncomplicated. Membranes were spontaneously ruptured with clear fluid approximately 11 hours prior to delivery, and no maternal fever was documented; the mother received antibiotics about 4 hours prior to delivery. Active pushing in second stage was 4 hours, followed by shoulder dystocia after the infant's head was delivered. The infant was limp and apneic after delivery. The certified nurse midwife performed mask-delivered positive pressure ventilation with room air with improvement in respiratory effort. Apgar scores were 1^1, 2^5, 4^{10}, 5^{15} per the nurse midwife report.

The infant was emergently brought to the NICU.

Admission weight: 3,765 g, head circumference: 37 cm, and length: 54 cm.

HEENT: Anterior fontanelle was soft, flat, sutures opposed, proximate with a right cephalohematoma; eyes equal and reactive to light with a positive red reflex; nares bilaterally patent; palate and clavicles intact

RESP: breath sounds coarse bilaterally, slightly decreased over the lower right lung field. Increased work of breathing with increased subcostal and substernal retractions, slight tracheal tug, and flared nares

CV: Mildly tachycardic, no murmur; peripheral pulses 1+ in all extremities; poor peripheral perfusion and capillary blood refill time of greater than 4 seconds. Low-borderline cuff blood pressure

ABD: Abdomen soft and nontender; no hepatosplenomegaly or masses palpable; three-vessel cord

NEURO: Responsive and alert on admission

EXTREMITIES: well formed; slightly decreased muscle tone

SKIN: pale pink and slightly mottled, with acrocyanosis and circumoral cyanosis

■ Development of Management Plan

- Nasal CPAP to support respiratory effort
- Peripheral intravenous fluids at 80 mL/kg/day maintenance
- Fluid bolus 10 mg/kg normal saline as needed
- Place umbilical arterial and venous catheters
- Chest radiograph confirmed right pneumothorax
- Needle aspiration was performed for small amount of air
- Chest radiographs as needed
- Monitor for abnormal activity showed pneumothorax resolved. Infant initially improved but on day 2 of life developed apnea, tonguing, lip smacking, and rhythmic extremity movement.

■ Differential Diagnoses

The differential diagnoses for an infant following a difficult delivery with positive pressure ventilation include:

- Respiratory distress versus transient tachypnea of the newborn
- Rule out pneumothorax
- Rule out hypoxic-ischemic encephalopathy
- Rule out intracranial hemorrhage
- Sepsis screen
- Shock
- Rule out seizures
- Congenital cardiac defects
- Metabolic and/or endocrine defects

■ Diagnostic Tests

Laboratory tests:

- CBC with differential: WBC 11.7, segmented cells 33, bands 2; Hct: 56; platelets: 156,000/mm^3
- Blood cultures for bacterial and viral growth: negative
- Electrolytes, lactic acid, and ammonia levels, amino acid assays and urine organic acids, and liver function tests: normal

Imaging tests:

- Chest radiography: small right pneumothorax
- Head CT: (24 hours of life) no evidence of hydrocephalus, ischemia, or intracranial hemorrhage
- Serial EEGs: (48 hours of life) moderate to severely abnormal EEG due to discontinuous low-amplitude background with asynchrony and frequent, subclinical, electrographic seizures from midline vertex and left central region. Second EEG: (72 hours) improvement from initial EEG with no electrographic seizures. There were positive sharp transient waves that were of concern for underlying structural abnormalities and can be consistent with anoxic and hypoxic events as reflected with clinical presentation. Third EEG: (5 days) abnormal due to predominately right temporal sharp waves and possibly two brief electrographic seizures.
- MRI: (11 days) abnormalities on T2 and diffusion weighted imaging (DWI) consistent with perinatal HIE

Consult:

- Pediatric neurology: seizures due to HIE

■ Working Diagnoses

- Seizures due to HIE
- Respiratory distress
- Pneumothorax

■ Development of Management Plan

The management plan included:

- Monitoring
- Respiratory support with mechanical ventilation as needed
- Fluid support; initiate feeds
- Sepsis screen
- Antibiotics
- Needle aspiration of small right pneumothorax
- Chest tube insertion if indicated
- Lactic acid and ammonia levels, amino acid assays and urine organic acids
- Expedite state newborn screen testing

■ Implementation and Evaluation of Effectiveness

Implementation of management plan: (immediately after initial assessment in the NICU)

- Antibiotics were given for 48 hours for the sepsis screen
- Right pneumothorax was reduced with needle aspiration and resolved without further intervention
- Seizure activity noted on day of life 2, confirmed with EEG, given phenobarbital 15 mg/kg, with resolution of the seizure
- Subsequently intubated at approximately 36 hours of life for a prolonged apnea event requiring positive pressure ventilation, given another 15 mg/kg phenobarbital loading dose and initial lorazepam (Ativan) dose to control seizures
- Metabolic etiology was ruled out with normal lactic acid and ammonia levels and normal amino acid assays and urine organic acids results
- State metabolic screening results were normal
- Neurologic examination deteriorated over the first 4 days, with the infant presenting with no gag, no corneal reflex, passive hypertonicity, active hypotonia, consistent and rhythmic hyperventilation, and periodic apnea, clonic-tonic movements of predominately the left extremities by the end of day 3 of life, and persisting through day 5 of life
- Maintenance phenobarbital was initiated on day 3 of life, and lorazepam was given periodically for seizure activity during days 4 to 5 of life. Seizures were no longer observed after day 5 of life; infant gradually improved clinically with improved passive and active tone, improved gag, and positive corneal reflex
- Extubated on day 6 of life to high-flow nasal cannula of 2 L/min flow of room air; weaned quickly to room air without nasal cannula flow
- Feeds of expressed mother's milk had been initiated per gavage tube on day 3 of life; infant was tolerating full volume by day 7 by gavage every 3 hours. Breastfeeding and nipple feeds were initiated on day 8, but infant needed most of his feeds by gavage at time of discharge on day 18. Follow-up care was arranged for neurology clinic and EEG 1 month after discharge.

■ Outcome. Infant was discharged with phenobarbital and gavage feeds; was breastfeeding well, gaining weight, and thriving at the neurology follow-up appointment at 1 month of life.

EVIDENCE-BASED PRACTICE BOX

HIE is the major cause of encephalopathy in newborns. HIE is an injury to the brain caused by oxygen deficit resulting from either systemic hypoxemia or ischemia or a combination of the two conditions. The hypoxemia and ischemia may occur simultaneously or sequentially, and it appears from recent evidence that ischemia is the more important of the two oxygen deprivation states in causing the brain injury. Subsequent reperfusion of the affected brain area has been shown to be the time at which the majority of the injury to the brain occurs. Glucose deprivation also plays a part in the severity of the brain injury. HIE causes transient organ dysfunction in 4 to 6 in 1,000 live births and results in death or significant neurologic deficits in 1 per 1,000 live births. Traditionally, the newborns affected by HIE have been treated by symptoms of the resultant multiorgan and multisystem effects. A recent development in proactive treatment with the use of controlled hypothermia has proven to be effective for newborns with moderate to severe HIE.

Induced mild hypothermia is increasingly the treatment of choice for infants ≥36 weeks gestation with moderate-to-severe HIE in addition to establishing ventilation and adequate perfusion and preventing or minimizing hypotension, hypoxia, and acidosis, rapid alterations in cerebral blood flow and systemic blood pressure, and severe apneic and bradycardic episodes in providing supportive care. Mild hypothermia is induced using either selective head cooling or whole-body cooling. A systematic review and meta-analysis of seven randomized controlled trials including 1,214 newborns done by Tagin et al. (2012), provided evidence that hypothermia with either total body cooling or selective head cooling improves survival and protects neurodevelopment in newborns with moderate-to-severe HIE. Simbruner, Mittal, Rohlmann, Muche, and neo.nEURO.network Trial Participants (2010) reported that in their randomized control trial involving 129 newborns with neurodevelopmental follow-up for 111 infants at 18 months, hypothermia treatment provided strong neuroprotective effect for infants with severe HIE. A multicenter international randomized controlled trial done by Jacobs et al. (2011) provides supporting evidence that whole-body hypothermia reduced the risk of death or major disability at 2 years of age.

Selective hypothermia, if begun within 6 hours of life, is carefully controlled within a tertiary level NICU environment and is continued for 72 hours while providing multisystemic and multiorgan support, appears to reduce mortality and improve morbidity for newborns with moderate-to-severe HIE.

References

Jacobs, S. E., Morley, C. J., Inder, T. E., Stewart, M. J., Smith, K. R., McNamara, P. J., . . . Infant Cooling Evaluation Collaboration. (2011). Whole-body hypothermia for term and near-term newborns with hypoxic-ischemic encephalopathy: A randomized controlled trial. *Archives of Pediatrics & Adolescent Medicine, 165*(8), 692–700. doi:10.1001/archpediatrics.2011.43

Simbruner, G., Mittal, R. A., Rohlmann, F., Muche, R., & neo.nEURO.network Trial Participants. (2010). Systemic hypothermia after neonatal encephalopathy: Outcomes of neo.nEURO.network RCT. *Pediatrics, 126*(4), e771–e778. doi:10.1542/peds.2009-2441

Tagin, M. A., Woolcott, C. G., Vincer, M. J., Whyte, R. K., & Stinson, D. A. (2012). Hypothermia for neonatal hypoxic ischemic encephalopathy: An updated systematic review and meta-analysis. *Archives of Pediatrics & Adolescent Medicine.* doi:10.1001/archpediatrics.2011.1772

ONLINE RESOURCES

Embryological development of the neurological system from the University of New South Wales Embryology including animations
http://php.med.unsw.edu.au/embryology/index.php?title=Neural_System_Development

Genetic conditions affecting neurologic system from the Dolan DNA Leaning Center at Cold Spring Harbor Laboratory
http://www.ygyh.org

Neuron migration: illustration of a neuron (a granule cell is a small neuron) migrating along a radial glia
http://www.youtube.com/watch?v=ZRF-gKZHINk

Newborn physical assessment findings
http://newborns.stanford.edu/RNMDEducation.html

Prenatal brain development is an animation is a nice summary of major stages in brain development from conception to term
http://www.youtube.com/watch?v=mMDPP-Wy3sI

Recommendations for folic acid supplementation in childbearing women to reduce the risk of neural tube defects
http://www.uspreventiveservicestaskforce.org/uspstf09/folicacid/folicsum.htm

Telling Stories: Understanding Real Life Genetics
http://www.tellingstories.nhs.uk

REFERENCES

Abuelo, D. (2007). Microcephaly syndromes. *Seminars in Pediatric Neurology, 14*, 118–127.

Adzick, N. S., Thom, E. A., Spong, C. Y., Brock, J. W., Burrows, P. K., Johnson, M. P., . . . Farmer, D. L. (2011). A randomized trial of prenatal versus postnatal repair of myelomeningocele. *New England Journal of Medicine, 364*, 993–1004.

Alfonso, D. T. (2011). Causes of neonatal brachial plexus palsy. *Bulletin of the NYU Hospital for Joint Diseases, 69*, 11–16.

American Academy of Pediatrics Committee on Genetics. (1999). Folic acid for the prevention of neural tube defects. *Pediatrics, 100*, 143–152, reaffirmed 2007.

Amiel-Tison, C., & Gosselin, J. (2009). Clinical assessment of the infant nervous system. In M. I. Levene & F. A. Chervenak (Eds.),

Fetal and neonatal neurology and neurosurgery (pp. 128–154). Edinburgh, Scotland: Churchill Livingstone/Elsevier.

Au, K. S., Ashley-Koch, A., & Northrup, H. (2010). Epidemiologic and genetic aspects of spina bifida and other neural tube defects. *Developmental Disabilities Research Reviews, 16*, 6–15.

Back, S., & Plawner, L. L. (2012). Congenital malformations of the central nervous system. In H. W. Taeusch, R. A. Ballard & C. A. Gleason (Eds.), *Avery's diseases of the newborn* (pp. 844–867). Philadelphia, PA: Elsevier/Saunders.

Ballabh, P. (2010). Intraventricular hemorrhage in premature infants: Mechanism of disease. *Pediatric Research, 67*, 1–8.

Barks, J. (2008). Technical aspects of starting a neonatal cooling program. *Clinics in Perinatology, 35*, 765–776.

Barnes, G. N. (2007). Electroencephalography and evoked response. In G. M. Fenichel (Ed.), *Neonatal neurology* (pp. 199–222). Philadelphia, PA: Churchill/Livingstone/Elsevier.

Bassan, H. (2009). Intracranial hemorrhage in the preterm infants: Understanding it, preventing it. *Clinics in Perinatology, 36*, 737–762.

Bassan, H., Bental, Y., Shany, E., Berger, I., Froom, P., Levi, L., & Shiff, Y. (2008). Neonatal seizures: Dilemmas in workup and management. *Pediatric Neurology, 38*, 415–421.

Bassuk, A. G., & Kibar, Z. (2009). Genetic basis of neural tube defects. *Seminars in Pediatric Neurology, 16*, 101–110.

Battin, M. R., Thoresen, M., Robinson, E., Polin, R. A., Edwards, A. D., Gunn, A. J., & Group obotCCT. (2009). Does head cooling with mild systemic hypothermia affect requirement for blood pressure support? *Pediatrics, 123*, 1031–1036.

Bebbington, M. W., Danzer, E., Johnson, M. P., & Adzick, N. S. (2011). Open fetal surgery for myelomeningocele. *Prenatal Diagnosis, 31*, 689–694.

Beggs, S., & Fitzgerald, M. (2007). Development of peripheral and spinal nociceptive systems. In K. Anand, B. Stevens & P. McGrath (Eds.), *Pain in neonates and infants* (pp. 11–24). New York, NY: Elsevier.

Benders, MJNL, Groenendaal, F., & De Vries, L. S. (2009). Preterm arterial ischemic stroke. *Seminars in Fetal and Neonatal Medicine, 14*, 272–277.

Blackburn, S. T. (2009a). Central nervous system vulnerabilities in preterm infants, part I. *Journal of Perinatal & Neonatal Nursing, 23*, 12–14.

Blackburn, S. T. (2009b). Central nervous system vulnerabilities in preterm infants, part II. *Journal of Perinatal & Neonatal Nursing, 23*, 108–110.

Blackburn, S. T. (2012). *Maternal, fetal and neonatal physiology: A clinical perspective*. St. Louis, MO: Saunders/Elsevier Science.

Bolduc, M.-E., & Limperopoulos, C. (2009). Neurodevelopmental outcomes in children with cerebellar malformations: A systematic review. *Developmental Medicine & Child Neurology, 51*, 256–267.

Bonifacio, S. L., Glass, H. C., Peloquin, S., & Ferriero, D. M. (2011). A new neurological focus in neonatal intensive care. *Nature Reviews. Neurology, 7*, 485–494.

Bonifacio, S. L., Gonzalez, F., & Ferriero, D. M. (2012). Central nervous system injury and neuroprotection. In C. A. Gleason & S. Devaskar (Eds.), *Avery's diseases of the newborn* (pp. 869–891). Philadelphia, PA: Saunders/Elsevier.

Breimer, L. H., & Nilsson, T. K. (2012). Has folate a role in the developing nervous system after birth and not just during embryogenesis and gestation? *Scandinavian Journal of Clinical & Laboratory Investigation*, 72(3), 185–91. 1–7, Early Online.

Bruner, J. P. (2007). Intrauterine surgery in myelomeningocele. *Seminars in Fetal and Neonatal Medicine, 12*, 471–476.

Cameron, M., & Moran, P. (2009). Prenatal screening and diagnosis of neural tube defects. *Prenatal Diagnosis, 29*, 402–411.

Chabrier, S., Husson, B., Dinomais, M., Landrieu, P., & Nguyen The Tich, S. (2011). New insights (and new interrogations) in perinatal arterial ischemic stroke. *Thrombosis Research, 127*, 13–22.

Chaoui, R., & Nicolaides, K. H. (2010). From nuchal translucency to intracranial translucency: Towards the early detection of spina bifida. *Ultrasound in Obstetrics and Gynecology, 35*, 133–138.

Cheong, J. L. Y., & Cowan, F. M. (2009). Neonatal arterial ischaemic stroke: Obstetric issues. *Seminars in Fetal and Neonatal Medicine, 14*, 267–271.

Chirinian, N., & Mann, N. (2011). Therapeutic hypothermia for management of neonatal asphyxia: What nurses need to know. *Critical Care Nurse, 31*(3); e1–12.

Cohen, A. R., & Walsh, M. C. (2006). Myelomeningocele. In R. J. Martin, A. A. Fanaroff & M. C. Walsh (Eds.), *Neonatal-perinatal medicine: Diseases of the fetus and newborn* (pp. 1014–1016). Philadelphia, PA: Mosby/Elsevier.

Creuzet, S. E. (2009). Neural crest contribution to forebrain development. *Seminars in Cell & Developmental Biology, 20*, 751–759.

Cunniff, C., & Hudgins, L. (2010). Prenatal genetic screening and diagnosis for pediatricians. *Current Opinion in Pediatrics, 22*, 809–811.

Danzer, E., Johnson, M. P., & Adzick, N. S. (2012). Fetal surgery for myelomeningocele: Progress and perspectives. *Developmental Medicine & Child Neurology, 54*, 8–14.

Dastgir, J., Chan, K., & Darras, B. (2012). Neonatal hypotonia and neuromuscular disorders. In J. M. Perlman (Ed.), *Neurology*. Philadelphia, PA: Saunders/Elsevier.

de Bruïne, F., van Wezel-Meijler, G., Leijser, L., van den Berg-Huysmans, A., van Steenis, A., van Buchem, M., & van der Grond, J. (2011). Tractography of developing white matter of the internal capsule and corpus callosum in very preterm infants. *European Radiology, 21*, 538–547.

Deng, W., Pleasure, J., & Pleasure, D. (2008). Progress in periventricular leukomalacia. *Archives of Neurology, 65*, 1291–1295.

Detrait, E. R., George, T. M., Etchevers, H. C., Gilbert, J. R., Vekemans, M., & Speer, M. C. (2005). Human neural tube defects: Developmental biology, epidemiology and genetics. *Neurotoxicology and Teratology, 27*, 515–524.

de Vries, L. S., Counsell, S. J., & Levene, M. (2009). Cerebral ischemic lesions. In M. Levene & F. A. Chervenak (Eds.), *Fetal and neonatal neurology and neurosurgery* (pp. 431–471). Edinburgh, Scotland: Churchill Livingstone/Elsevier.

de Vries, L. S., & Jongmans, M. J. (2010). Long-term outcome after neonatal hypoxic-ischaemic encephalopathy. *Archives of Disease in Childhood—Fetal and Neonatal Edition, 95*, F220–F224.

Dickey, E. J., Long, S. N., & Hunt, R. W. (2011). Hypoxic ischemic encephalopathy—what can we learn from humans? *Journal of Veterinary Internal Medicine, 25*, 1231–1240.

Ditzenberger, G. R. (2010). Nutritional management. In M. T. Verklan & M. Walden (Eds.), *Core curriculum for neonatal intensive care nursing* (pp. 182–207). St. Louis, MO: Saunders/Elsevier.

Doumouchtsis, S., & Arulkumaran, S. (2009). Are all brachial plexus injuries caused by shoulder dystocia? *Obstetrical and Gynecological Survey, 64*, 615–623.

Driscoll, D. A., Gross, S. J., & Professional Practice Guidelines Committee. (2009). Screening for fetal aneuploidy and neural tube defects. *Genetics in Medicine, 11*, 818–821.

duPlessis, A. J. (2008a). Cerebrovascular injury in premature infants: Current understanding and challenges for future prevention. *Clinics in Perinatology, 35*, 609–642.

duPlessis, A. J. (2008b). Neonatal seizures. In J. P. Cloherty, E. C. Eichenwald & A. R. Stark (Eds.), *Manual of neonatal care* (pp. 483–498). Philadelphia, PA: Woters Kluwer/Lippincott Williams & Wilkins.

El-Dib, M., Massaro, A. N., Bulas, D., & Aly, H. (2010). Neuroimaging and neurodeveolopmental outcome of premature infants. *American Journal of Perinatology, 27*, 803–818.

Epelman, M., Daneman, A., Chauvin, N., & Hirsch, W. (2012). Head ultrasound and MR imaging in the evaluation of neonatal encephalopathy: Competitive or complementary imaging studies? *Magnetic resonance imaging clinics of North America, 20*, 93–115.

Fenichel, G. M. (2007). *Neonatal neurology* (p. 231). Philadelphia, PA: Churchill/Livingstone/Elsevier.

Gancia, P., & Pomero, G. (2011). Brain cooling and eligible newborns: Should we extend the indications? *Journal of Maternal-Fetal and Neonatal Medicine, 24*, 53–55.

Girard, N., & Raybaud, C. (2011). Neonates with seizures: What to consider, how to image. *Magnetic Resonance Imaging Clinics of North America, 19*, 685–708.

Glass, H. C. (2010). Neurocritical care for neonates. *Neurocritical Care, 12*, 421–429.

Glass, H. C., & Wirrell, E. (2009). Controversies in neonatal seizure management. *Journal of Child Neurology, 24*, 591–599.

Gluckman, P. D., Wyatt, J. S., Azzopardi, D., Ballard, R., Edwards, A. D., Ferriero, D. M., . . . Gunn, A. J. (2005). Selective head cooling with mild systemic hypothermia after neonatal encephalopathy: Multicentre randomised trial. *The Lancet, 365*, 663–670.

Gomella, T. L., Cunningham, M. D., & Eyal, F. G. (2009). *Neonatology: Management, procedures, on-call problems, diseases, and drugs* (p. 894). New York, NY: McGraw-Hill/Lange.

Greisen, G. (2009). Cerebral blood flow and energy metabolism in the developing brain. In M. Levene & F. A. Chervenak (Eds.), *Fetal and neonatal neurology and neurosurgery* (pp. 171–191). Edinburgh, Scotland: Churchill Livingstone/ Elsevier.

Gressens, P., & Huppi, P. S. (2006). The central nervous system, part 1: Normal and abnormal brain development. In R. J. Martin, A. A. Fanaroff & M. C. Walsh (Eds.), *Neonatal and perinatal medicine: Diseases of the fetus and infant* (pp. 883–908). Philadelphia, PA: Mosby/Elsevier.

Grunau, R. E., & Tu, M. T. (2007). Long-term consequences of pain in human neonates. In K. Anand, B. Stevens, & P. J. McGrath (Eds.), *Pain in neonates and infants* (pp. 45–56). New York, NY: Elsevier.

Gudsnuk, K. M., & Champagne, F. A. (2011). Epigenetic effects of early developmental experiences. *Clinics in Perinatology, 38*, 703–718.

Guerrini, R., & Parrini, E. (2010). Neuronal migration disorders. *Neurobiology of Disease, 38*, 154–166.

Guillet, R., Edwards, A. D., Thoresen, M., Ferriero, D. M., Gluckman, P. D., Whitelaw, A., & Gunn, A. J. (2012). Seven- to eight-year follow-up of the CoolCap trial of head cooling for neonatal encephalopathy. *Pediatric Research, 71*, 205–209.

Gunn, A. J., Wyatt, J. S., Whitelaw, A., Barks, J., Azzopardi, D., Ballard, R., . . . Thoresen, M. (2008). Therapeutic hypothermia changes the prognostic value of clinical evaluation of neonatal encephalopathy. *The Journal of Pediatrics, 152*, 55–58.e1.

Gunny, R. S., & Lin, D. (2012). Imaging of perinatal stroke. *Magnetic resonance imaging clinics of North America, 20*, 1–33.

Heaberlin, P. D. (2009). Neurologic assessment. In E. P. Tappero & M. E. Honeyfield (Eds.), *Physical assessment of the newborn: A comprehensive approach to the art of physical examination* (pp. 159–184). Santa Rosa, CA: NICU Ink.

Hellstrom-Westas, L., & deVries, L. S. (2007). EEG and evoked potentials in the neonatal period. In M. I. Levene & F. A. Chervenak (Eds.), *Fetal and neonatal neurology and neurosurgery* (pp. 192–221). Edinburgh, Scotland: Churchill Livingstone/ Elsevier.

Hill, A. (2005). Neurological and neuromuscular disorders. In M. G. MacDonald, M. D. Mullett & M. M. Seshia (Eds.), *Avery's neonatology: Pathophysiology & management of the newborn* (pp. 1384–1409). Philadelphia, PA: Lippincott Williams & Wilkins.

Hirose, S., & Farmer, D. L. (2009). Fetal surgery for myelomeningocele. *Clinics in Perinatology, 36*, 431–438.

Hockley, A. D., & Salanki, G. A. (2009). Surgical management of neural tube defects. In M. I. Levene & F. A. Chervenak (Eds.), *Fetal and neonatal neurology and neurosurgery* (pp. 847–855). Edinburgh, Scotland: Churchill Livingstone/Elsevier.

Hoehn, T., Hansmann, G., Bührer, C., Simbruner, G., Gunn, A. J., Yager, J., . . . Thoresen, M. (2008). Therapeutic hypothermia in neonates. Review of current clinical data, ILCOR recommendations and suggestions for implementation in neonatal intensive care units. *Resuscitation, 78*, 7–12.

Huang, H. (2010). Structure of the fetal brain: What we are learning from diffusion tensor imaging. *The Neuroscientist, 16*, 634–649.

Inder, T. E., & Volpe, J. J. (2011). Intraventricular hemorrhage in the neonate. In R. A. Polin, W. W. Fox & S. H. Abman (Eds.), *Fetal and neonatal physiology* (pp. 1830–1847). Philadelphia, PA: Saunders/Elsevier.

Isaacs, H. (2010). Perinatal neurofibromatosis: Two case reports and review of the literature. *American Journal of Perinatology, 27*, 285–292.

Jensen, F. E. (2009). Neonatal seizures: An update on mechanisms and management. *Clinics in Perinatology, 36*, 1–20.

Jentink, J., Loane, M. A., Dolk, H., Barisic, I., Garne, E., Morris, J. K., & de Jong-van den Berg, L. T. W. (2010). Valproic acid monotherapy in pregnancy and major congenital malformations. *New England Journal of Medicine, 362*, 2185–2193.

Jett, K., & Friedman, J. M. (2010). Clinical and genetic aspects of neurofibromatosis. *Genetics in Medicine, 12*, 1–11.

Johnston, M. V., Fatemi, A., Wilson, M. A., & Northington, F. (2011). Treatment advances in neonatal neuroprotection and neurointensive care. *The Lancet Neurology, 10*, 372–382.

Jones, K. L. (2006). *Smith's recognizable patterns of human malformation*. Philadelphia, PA: Saunders/Elsevier.

Kanekar, S., Kaneda, H., & Shively, A. (2011). Malformations of dorsal induction. *Seminars in Ultrasound, CT, and MRI, 32*, 189–199.

Kanekar, S., Shively, A., & Kaneda, H. (2011). Malformations of ventral induction. *Seminars in Ultrasound, CT, and MRI, 32*, 200–210.

Kelen, D., & Robertson, N. J. (2010). Experimental treatments for hypoxic ischaemic encephalopathy. *Early Human Development, 86*, 369–377.

Kirton, A., & deVeber, G. (2009). Advances in perinatal ischemic stroke. *Pediatric Neurology, 40*, 205–214.

Kling, P. (1989). Nursing interventions to decrease the risk of periventricular-intraventricular hemorrhage. *Journal of Obstetric, Gynecologic, & Neonatal Nursing, 8*, 462–470.

Koufman, D., Zanelli, S., Cantey, J. B., & Sanchez, P. J. (2012). Neonatal meningitis: Current treatment options. In J. M. Perlman (Ed.), *Neurology* (pp. 181–202). Philadelphia, PA: Saunders/Elsevier.

Kuijpers, M., & Hoogenraad, C. C. (2011). Centrosomes, microtubules and neuronal development. *Molecular and Cellular Neuroscience, 48*, 349–358.

Laptook, A. R. (2012). The use of hypothermia to provide neuroprotection for neonatal hypoxic-ischemic brain injury. In J. Perlman (Ed.), *Neurology* (pp. 63–76). Philadelphia, PA: Saunders/Elsevier.

Lehmann, C. U. (2009). Studies for neurologic evaluation. In T. L. Gomella (Ed.), *Neonatology: Management, procedures, on-call problems, diseases, and drugs* (pp. 155–162). New York, NY: McGraw-Hill Companies/Lange.

Levene, M. (2009). Disorders of the spinal cord, cranial and peripheral nerves. In M. Levene & F. A. Chervenak (Eds.), *Fetal and neonatal neurology and neurosurgery* (pp. 778–791). Edinburgh, Scotland: Churchill Livingstone/Elsevier.

Levene, M., & deVries, L. S. (2009). Neonatal intracranial hemorrhage. In M. Levene & F. A. Chervenak (Eds.), *Fetal and neonatal neurology and neurosurgery* (pp. 395–430). Edinburgh, Scotland: Churchill Livingstone/Elsevier.

Lew, S. M., & Kothbauer, K. F. (2007). Tethered cord syndrome: An updated review. *Pediatric Neurosurgery, 43*, 236–248.

Limperopoulos, C. (2009). Autism spectrum disorders in survivors of extreme prematurity. *Clinics in Perinatology, 36*, 791–806.

Limperopoulos, C. (2010). Extreme prematurity, cerebellar injury, and autism. *Seminars in Pediatric Neurology, 17*, 25–29.

Limperopoulos, C., Soul, J. S., Gauvreau, K., Huppi, P. S., Warfield, S. K., Bassan, H., Robertson, R. L., Volpe, J. J., and duPlesis, A. J. (2005). Late gestation cerebellar growth is rapid and impeded by premature birth. *Pediatrics* 115(3), 688-695.

Lista, G., Castoldi, F., Cavigioli, F., Bianchi, S., Fontana, P., & La Verde, A. (2011). Ventilatory management of asphyxiated infant during hypothermia. *Journal of Maternal-Fetal and Neonatal Medicine, 24*, 67–68.

Lodygensky, G. A., Menache, C. C., & Huppi, P. S. (2012). Magnetic resonance imaging's role in the care of the infant at risk for brain injury. In J. M. Perlman (Ed.), *Neonatology* (pp. 285–324). Philadelphia, PA: Saunders/Elsevier.

Long, M., & Brandon, D. H. (2007). Induced hypothermia for neonates with hypoxic-ischemic encephalopathy. *Journal of Obstetric, Gynecologic, & Neonatal Nursing, 36*, 293–298.

Lori, S., Bertini, G., Molesti, E., Gualandi, D., Gabbanini, S., Bastianelli, M. E., . . . Dani, C. (2011). The prognostic role of evoked potentials in neonatal hypoxic-ischemic insult. *Journal of Maternal-Fetal and Neonatal Medicine, 24*, 69–71.

Lynch, J. K. (2009). Epidemiology and classification of perinatal stroke. *Seminars in Fetal and Neonatal Medicine, 14*, 245–249.

Madsen, J. R., Frim, D. M., & Hansen, A. R. (2005). Neurosurgery of the newborn. In M. G. McDonald, M. D. Mullett & M. M. Seshia (Eds.), *Avrey's neonatology: Pathophysiology and management of the newborn* (pp. 1410–1427). Philadelphia, PA: Lippincott Williams and Wilkins.

McCrea, H., & Ment, L. R. (2008). The diagnosis, management, and postnatal prevention of intraventricular hemorrhage in the preterm neonate. *Clinics in Perinatology, 35*, 777–792.

Mineyko, A., & Kirton, A. (2011). The black box of perinatal ischemic stroke pathogenesis. *Journal of Child Neurology, 26*, 1154–1162.

Mitchell, L. E., Adzick, N. S., Melchionne, J., Pasquariello, P. S., Sutton, L. N., & Whitehead, A. S. (2004). Spina bifida. *The Lancet, 364*, 1885–1895.

Mochida, G. H. (2009). Genetics and biology of microcephaly and lissencephaly. *Seminars in Pediatric Neurology, 16*, 120–126.

Moore, K. L., Persaud, T. V. N., & Torchia, M. (2012). *The developing human: Clinically oriented embryology*. Philadelphia, PA: Saunders/Elsevier.

Mosley, B. S., Cleves, M. A., Siega-Riz, A. M., Shaw, G. M., Canfield, M. A., Waller, D. K., . . . Study FTNBDP. (2009). Neural tube defects and maternal folate intake among pregnancies conceived after folic acid fortification in the United States. *American Journal of Epidemiology, 169*, 9–17.

Mwaniki, M. K., Atieno, M., Lawn, J. E., & Newton, C. R. (2012). Long-term neurodevelopmental outcomes after intrauterine and neonatal insults: A systematic review. *Lancet, 379*, 445–452.

Myers, E., & Ment, L. R. (2009). Long-term outcome of preterm infants and the role of neuroimaging. *Clinics in Perinatology, 36*, 773–790.

Myers, E., & Ment, L. R. (2012). Perinatal stroke. In J. Perlman (Ed.), *Neurology* (pp. 91–108). Philadelphia, PA: Saunders/Elsevier.

Olney, A. H. (2007). Macrocephaly syndromes. *Seminars in Pediatric Neurology, 14*, 128–135.

Owens, R. (2005). Intraventricular hemorrhage in the premature neonate. *Neonatal Network: The Journal of Neonatal Nursing, 24*, 55–71.

Perlman, J. (2011). Cerebral blood flow in premature infants: Regulation, measurement, and pathophysiology of intraventricular hemorrhage. In R. A. Polin, W. W. Fox & S. H. Abman (Eds.), *Fetal and neonatal physiology* (pp. 1820–1829). Philadelphia, PA: Saunders/Elsevier.

Pfister, R., & Soll, R. (2010). Hypothermia for the treatment of infants with hypoxic–ischemic encephalopathy. *Journal of Perinatology, 30*, S82–S87.

Piatt, J. H. (2010). Treatment of myelomeningocele: A review of outcomes and continuing neurosurgical considerations among adults. *Journal of Neurosurgery: Pediatrics, 6*, 515–525.

Pitcher, J. B., Schneider, L. A., Drysdale, J. L., Ridding, M. C., & Owens, J. A. (2011). Motor system development of the preterm and low birthweight infant. *Clinics in Perinatology, 38*, 605–625.

Pomeroy, S. L., & Ullrich, N. J. (2004). Development of the nervous system. In R. A. Polin, W. W. Fox & S. H. Abman (Eds.), *Fetal and neonatal physiology* (pp. 1675–1698). Philadelphia, PA: Saunders/Elsevier.

Pooh, R. K., & Pooh, K. (2009). Antenatal assessment of CNS anomalies, including neural tube defects. In M. I. Levene & F. A. Chervenak (Eds.), *Fetal and neonatal neurology and neurosurgery* (pp. 291–338). Edinburgh, Scotland: Churchill Livingstone/Elsevier.

Ramenghi, L. A., & Huppi, P. S. (2007). Imaging the neonatal brain. In M. I. Levene & F. A. Chervenak (Eds.), *Fetal and neonatal neurology and neurosurgery* (pp. 68–102). Edinburgh, Scotland: Churchill/Livingstone/Elsevier.

Rennie, J. M. (2005). Neurological problems of the neonate: Assessment of the neonatal neurological system. In J. M. Rennie (Ed.), *Roberton's textbook of neonatology* (pp. 1093–1105). Edinburgh, Scotland: Churchill Livingstone/Elsevier.

Rennie, J. M., & Boylan, G. B. (2009). Seizure disorders of the neonate. In M. I. Levene & F. A. Chervenak (Eds.), *Fetal and neonatal neurology and neurosurgery* (pp. 698–710). Edinburgh, Scotland: Churchill Livingstone/Elsevier.

Reynolds, R., & Talmage, S. (2011). "Caution! Contents should be cold": Developing a whole-body hypothermia program. *Neonatal Network: The Journal of Neonatal Nursing, 30*, 225–230.

Roland, E. H., & Hill, A. (2007). Neonatal hypoxic-ischemic and hemorrhagic cerebral injury. In G. M. Fenichel (Ed.), *Neonatal neurology* (pp. 69–90). Philadelphia, PA: Churchill Livingstone/Elsevier.

Rowland, C. A., Correa, A., Cragan, J. D., & Alverson, C. J. (2006). Are encephaloceles neural tube defects? *Pediatrics, 118*, 916–923.

Rutherford, M., Ramenghi, L. A., Edwards, A. D., Brocklehurst, P., Halliday, H., Levene, M., . . . Azzopardi, D. (2010). Assessment of brain tissue injury after moderate hypothermia in neonates with hypoxic–ischaemic encephalopathy: A nested substudy of a randomised controlled trial. *The Lancet Neurology, 9*, 39–45.

Sandler, A. D. (2010). Children with spina bifida: Key clinical issues. *Pediatric Clinics of North America, 57*, 879–892.

Sarkar, S., Barks, J., Bhagat, I., & Donn, S. (2009). Effects of therapeutic hypothermia on multiorgan dysfunction in asphyxiated newborns: Whole-body cooling versus selective head cooling. *Journal of Perinatology, 29*, 558–563.

Sarnat, H., & Sarnat, M. (1976). A clinical and electroencephalographic study. *Archives of Neurology, 33*, 696–795.

Scher, M. S. (2012a). Diagnosis and treatment of neonatal seizures. In J. M. Perlman (Ed.), *Neurology* (pp. 109–141). Philadelphia, PA: Saunders/Elsevier.

Scher, M. S. (2012b). Neonatal seizures. In C. A. Gleason & S. Devaskar (Eds.), *Avery's diseases of the newborn* (pp. 901–919). Philadelphia, PA: Saunders/Elsevier.

Schierholz, E., & Walker, S. R. (2010). Responding to traumatic birth: Subgaleal hemorrhage, assessment, and management during transport. *Advances in Neonatal Care, 10*, 311–315.

Selway, L. D. (2010). State of the science: Hypoxic-ischemic encephalopathy and hypothermic intervention for neonates. *Advances in Neonatal Care, 10*, 60–66.

Shah, D. K., Boylan, G. B., & Rennie, J. M. (2012). Monitoring of seizures in the newborn. *Archives of Disease in Childhood—Fetal and Neonatal Edition, 97*, F65–F69.

Silverstein, F. S., & Jensen, F. E. (2007). Neonatal seizures. *Annals of Neurology, 62*, 112–120.

Smith, J. B. (2012). Initial evaluation: History and physical examination of the newborn. In C. A. Gleason & S. Devaskar (Eds.), *Avery's Diseases of the newborn* (pp. 277–299). Philadelphia, PA: Saunders/Elsevier.

Solanki, G. A., & Hockley, A. D. (2009). Neurosurgical management of hydrocephalus. In M. Levene & F. A. Chervenak (Eds.), *Fetal and neonatal neurology and neurosurgery* (pp. 834–846). Edinburgh, Scotland: Churchill Livingstone/Elsevier.

Sorem, K., Smith, J. F., & Druzin, M. L. (2009). Antenatal prediction of asphyxia. In M. Levene & F. A. Chervenak (Eds.), *Fetal and neonatal neurology and neurosurgery* (pp. 491–505). Edinburgh, Scotland: Churchill Livingstone/Elsevier.

Stola, A., & Perlman, J. (2008). Post-resuscitation strategies to avoid ongoing injury following intrapartum hypoxia–ischemia. *Seminars in Fetal and Neonatal Medicine, 13*, 424–431.

Stoll, C., Dott, B., Alembik, Y., & Roth, M.-P. (2011). Associated malformations among infants with neural tube defects. *American Journal of Medical Genetics Part A, 155*, 565–568.

Sullivan, R., Perry, R., Sloan, A., Kleinhaus, K., & Burtchen, N. (2011). Infant bonding and attachment to the caregiver: Insights from basic and clinical science. *Clinics in Perinatology, 38*, 643–656.

Tagin, M. A., Woolcott, C. G., Vincer, M. J., Whyte, R. K., & Stinson, D. A. (2012). Hypothermia for neonatal hypoxic ischemic encephalopathy: An updated systematic review and meta-analysis. *Archives of Pediatrics & Adolescent Medicine*. 166(6), 558–66.

Takenouchi, T., & Perlman, J. M. (2012). Intraventricular hemorrhage and white matter injury in the preterm infant. In J. Perlman (Ed.), *Neurology* (pp. 27–46). Philadelphia, PA: Saunders/Elsevier.

Tao, J. D., & Mathur, A. M. (2010). Using amplitude-integrated EEG in neonatal intensive care. *Journal of Perinatology, 30*, S73–S81.

Tekes, A., Pinto, P. S., & Huisman, T. A. G. M. (2011). Birth-related injury to the head and cervical spine in neonates. *Magnetic resonance imaging clinics of North America, 19*, 777–790.

Terzis, J. K., & Anesti, K. (2011). Developmental facial paralysis: A review. *Journal of Plastic, Reconstructive & Aesthetic Surgery, 64*, 1318–1333.

Thompson, D. K., Inder, T. E., Faggian, N., Johnston, L., Warfield, S. K., Anderson, P. J., . . . Egan, G. F. (2011). Characterization of the corpus callosum in very preterm and full-term infants utilizing MRI. *NeuroImage, 55*, 479–490.

Thompson, D. N. P. (2009). Postnatal management and outcome for neural tube defects including spina bifida and encephalocoeles. *Prenatal Diagnosis, 29*, 412–419.

Toet, M. C., & DeVries, L. S. (2012). Amplitude-integrated EEG and its potential role in augmenting management within the NICU. In J. M. Perlman (Ed.), *Neurology* (pp. 263–284). Philadelphia, PA: Saunders/Elsevier.

Toet, M. C., & Lemmers, P. M. A. (2009). Brain monitoring in neonates. *Early Human Development, 85*, 77–84.

Trollmann, R., Nüsken, E., & Wenzel, D. (2010). Neonatal somatosensory evoked potentials: Maturational aspects and prognostic value. *Pediatric Neurology, 42*, 427–433.

Valiente, M., & Marín, O. (2010). Neuronal migration mechanisms in development and disease. *Current Opinion in Neurobiology, 20*, 68–78.

Vandertak, K. (2009). Cool competence. The nursing challenges of therapeutic hypothermia. *Journal of Neonatal Nursing, 15*, 200–203.

Verklan, M. T. (2009). The chilling details: Hypoxic-ischemic encephalopathy. *Journal of Perinatal & Neonatal Nursing, 23*, 59–68.

Verney, C., Monier, A., Fallet-Bianco, C., & Gressens, P. (2010). Early microglial colonization of the human forebrain and possible involvement in periventricular white-matter injury of preterm infants. *Journal of Anatomy, 217*, 436–448.

Verney, C., Pogledic, I., Biran, V., Adle-Baissette, H., Fallet-Bianco, C., & Gressens, P. (2012). Microglial reaction in axonal crossroads is a hallmark of noncystic periventricular white matter injury in very preterm infants. *Journal of Neuropathology and Experimental Neurology, 71*, 251–264.

Volpe, J. J. (2008). *Neurology of the newborn*. Philadelphia, PA: Elsevier Inc/Saunders.

Volpe, J. J., Kinney, H. C., Jensen, F. E., & Rosenberg, P. A. (2011). The developing oligodendrocyte: Key cellular target in brain injury in the premature infant. *International Journal of Developmental Neuroscience, 29*, 423–440.

Volpe, P., Campobasso, G., De Robertis, V., & Rembouskos, G. (2009). Disorders of prosencephalic development. *Prenatal Diagnosis, 29*, 340–354.

Wachtel, E. V., & Hendricks-Muñoz, K. D. (2011). Current management of the infant who presents with neonatal encephalopathy. *Current Problems in Pediatric and Adolescent Health Care, 41*, 132–153.

Waller, S. A., Gopalani, S., & Benedetti, T. (2012). Complicated deliveries: Overview. In C. A. Gleason & S. Devaskar (Eds.), *Avery's diseases of the newborn* (pp. 146–158). Philadelphia, PA: Saunders/Elsevier.

Walsh, B. H., Murray, D. M., & Boylan, G. B. (2011). The use of conventional EEG for the assessment of hypoxic ischaemic encephalopathy in the newborn: A review. *Clinical Neurophysiology, 122*, 1284–1294.

Watchko, J. F. (2009). Identification of neonates at risk for hazardous hyperbilirubinemia: Emerging clinical insights. *Pediatric Clinics of North America, 56*, 671–687.

Wen, S., Ethen, M., Langlois, P. H., & Mitchell, L. E. (2007). Prevalence of encephalocele in Texas, 1999–2002. *American Journal of Medical Genetics Part A, 143A*, 2150–2155.

Whitelaw, A., & Aquilina, K. (2009). Neonatal hydrocephalus-clinical assessment and non-surgical treatment. In M. Levene & F. A. Chervenak (Eds.), *Fetal and neonatal neurology and neurosurgery* (pp. 819–833). Edinburgh, Scotland: Churchill Livingstone/Elsevier.

Wyatt, J. S., Gluckman, P. D., Liu, P. Y., Azzopardi, D., Ballard, R., Edwards, A. D., . . . & Group FTCS. (2007). Determinants of outcomes after head cooling for neonatal encephalopathy. *Pediatrics, 119*, 912–921.

Zanelli, S., Buck, M., & Fairchild, K. (2011). Physiologic and pharmacologic considerations for hypothermia therapy in neonates. *Journal of Perinatology, 31*(6), 377–86.

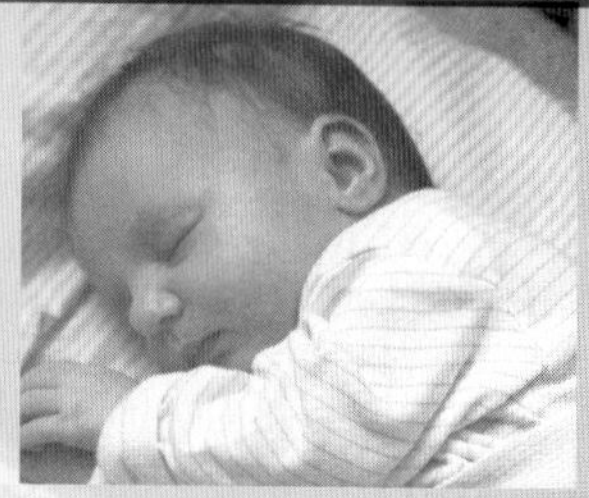

CHAPTER

16

Auditory System

■ Kathleen Haubrich

Hearing is a prerequisite to cognitive, social, and emotional development. Any impairment, either temporary or permanent, from birth to 18 months can have a profound effect on the auditory stimulation necessary for early language development (Kennedy et al., 2006). Auditory development, in particular development of speech, is dependent upon an exposure to a rich acoustic and linguistic environment. Hearing newborns are known to demonstrate a preference for listening to the sound of their mother voice, a skill that is developed via in utero exposure to the acoustic properties (DeCasper & Fifer, 1980; DeCasper, Lecanuent, Busnel, Granier-Deferre, & Maugeais, 1994).

Sensory deprivation affects the acquisition of communication skills, even though the hearing loss may be corrected. To prevent or minimize the detrimental effects on social, cognitive, and educational development, hearing impairment must be identified as early as possible (Kennedy et al., 2006). Permanent hearing loss is one of the most common congenital newborn disorders. Although, statistically, there is some variance in the data reported, incidence is currently about 1 to 6 per 1,000 newborn infants in a well-baby nursery and about 2 to 4 per 100 infants in the neonatal intensive care unit (Nelson, Bougatsos, & Nygren, 2008). Moderate to profound hearing impairment is reported in fewer than 2% of infants at risk, and approximately 1 in 1,000 infants are born deaf.

The importance of early identification of hearing impairment in the neonate has been well documented in the literature (Bachman, Johnston, & O'Malley, 1998; Fitzpatrick, Durieux-Smith, Eriks-Brophy, Olds, & Gaines, 2007; Kennedy et al., 2006; Nelson et al., 2008). A study of childhood language development and academic achievement reported that hearing impairment has a significant impact on the development of a child as evidenced by limited speech production skills (Sininger, Doyle, & Moore, 1999). Korver et al. (2010) looked at another aspect of childhood development, receptive and expressive language skills, and found that children with a hearing impairment demonstrated a significant delay in the development of these skills and slower academic achievement.

Historically, screening for hearing loss in infants and very young children was limited to observations of behavioral responses to sound such as the ringing of a bell outside of the view of a child. This method was fraught with difficulty and delay in early identification of hearing loss. During the past two decades, great strides have been made toward universal newborn hearing screening (UNHS) through early identification, development of reliable screening programs, consideration of adverse side effects, evaluation of availability and effectiveness, and evaluation of long-term outcomes for earlier diagnosis and interventions (Lim, Kim, & Chung, 2012; Patel & Feldman, 2011). Since the initial Joint Committee Position Statement on Infant Hearing (1994) through subsequent revisions (1999, 2007), the American Academy of Pediatrics (AAP) and the U.S. Preventative Task Force (USPSTF) (Nelson et al., 2008), having based recommendations on available evidence supported the practice of UNHS. UNHS has been widely accepted throughout developed regions of the world with research reports of screening modalities and program evaluation reported through scientific publications (De Capua et al., 2007; Korver et al., 2010; Langagne, Schmidt, Leveque, & Chays, 2008; Ohl, Dornier, Czajka, Chobaut, & Tavernier, 2009; Van Dommelen, Mohangoo, Verkerk, Van der Ploeg, & Van Straaten, 2010; Verhaert, Willems, Van Kerschaver, & Desloovere, 2008).

ANATOMY OF THE EAR

The ear is the anatomic unit involved in hearing and equilibrium. It consists of three parts: the external ear, the middle ear, and the inner ear. The external ear is composed of the auricle (pinna) and the external ear canal (Figure 16.1).

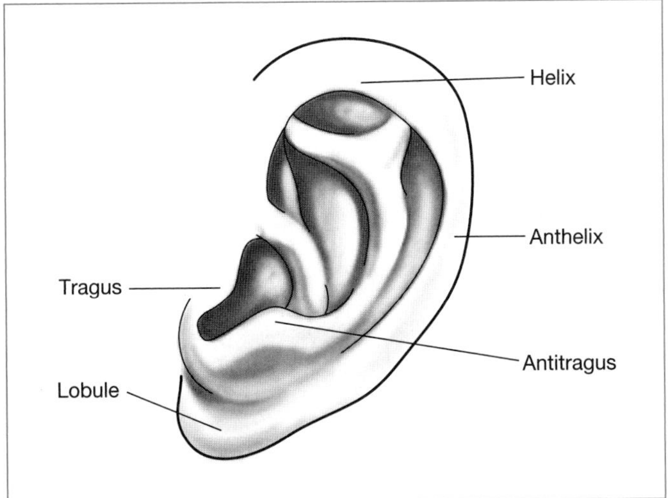

FIGURE 16.1 Anatomy of the external ear.

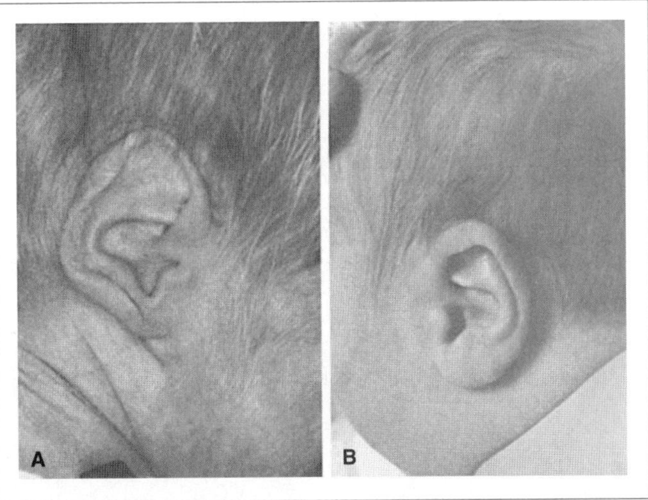

FIGURE 16.2 Premature (A) and full-term (B) ear. Adapted from Schreiner and Bradburn (1987).

A complex cartilage framework gives structure to the auricle. Because of this anatomic position, the auricle is susceptible to trauma from external forces. The external ear canal is curved posterosuperiorly and anteromedially. The canal is oval in shape, and the long axis is positioned superorinferiorly. Normally, the outer portion of the canal is cartilaginous, and the medial portion is bony. Before 34 weeks gestation, the pinna is a slightly formed, cartilage-free double thickness of skin. In the newborn, however, most of the canal is cartilaginous and collapsed (Moore & Linthicum, 2007). But as ear development ensues, the cartilage becomes firmer, making the outer two thirds of the canal more patent (Figure 16.2). Cerumen glands and tiny hairs are present in the outer portion of the cartilaginous canal. The medial two thirds of the canal lie immediately over a bony area and are referred to as the osseous region. The external auditory meatus assumes an irregular path from the concha to the tympanic membrane.

At the termination of the external canal is the eardrum, or tympanic membrane, which forms the boundary between the outer and the middle ear (Figure 16.3). The tympanic membrane has a complicated shape that loosely resembles a flat cone, and moves with changes in air pressure. Because the tympanic membrane is oval and translucent, the middle ear structure often can be visualized through it. The short and long processes of the malleus are attached to the fibrous layer of the tympanic membrane and are visible on the lateral surface. In the middle ear, the malleus, incus, and stapes occupy the region between the tympanic membrane and the oval window of the middle ear. During otoscopic examination, the long process of the incus often can be seen through the tympanic membrane. The middle ear cavity is an air-filled space connected by an air cell system posterior to the mastoid and by the Eustachian tube anterior to the nasopharynx. Neither of these is in a dependent position for drainage of fluids. Ciliated columnar cells cover the walls of the tympanic cavity and mastoid air cells. Secretory cells are distributed throughout the middle ear, with the greatest number in the Eustachian tube. The stapedius and the tensor muscles of the tympanic membrane attach in the middle ear to the malleus and the stapes by tendons. The chorda tympani nerve passes across the posterior surface. The medial wall of the middle ear cavity contains the oval and round windows. Between these two windows, the lower portion of the cochlea forms a prominence known as the promontorium tympani on the medial wall of the middle ear.

The inner ear consists of a bony labyrinth composed of three parts: the semicircular canals, the vestibule, and the cochlea. A dense, bony capsule in the petrous protein of the temporal bone surrounds these hollow spaces; this capsule contains perilymph and endolymph. Each of the semicircular canals has a dilated portion at the end, referred to as ampullae, which contain the crista ampullaris, a vestibular sense organ. In the vestibule, the utricle and saccules are formed; these structures contain sensory endings important for maintaining equilibrium.

The cochlea is a tubular structure with 2.5 turns; it closely resembles a snail shell, having a base and an apex. The cochlea is divided into the scala vestibuli, the scala media, and the scala tympani. The scala vestibuli begins at the oval window, and the scala tympani terminates at the round window. The basilar membrane side of the duct gives rise to the organ of Corti, the organ of hearing. The organ of Corti includes hair cells and supporting cells; attached to the hair cells is a gelatinous membrane called the tectorial membrane.

The membranous labyrinth of the inner ear is composed of connective tissue filled with endolymph that forms in the bony labyrinth. Hair cells of the cochlea and the vestibular labyrinth are attached by afferent nerve fibers to the neurons of the auditory system, the spiral ganglion, and the Scarpa ganglion in the temporal bone. Efferent nerve fibers from ganglia form the auditory and vestibular division of the eighth cranial nerve and exit the temporal bone on its posterior surface to enter the brainstem.

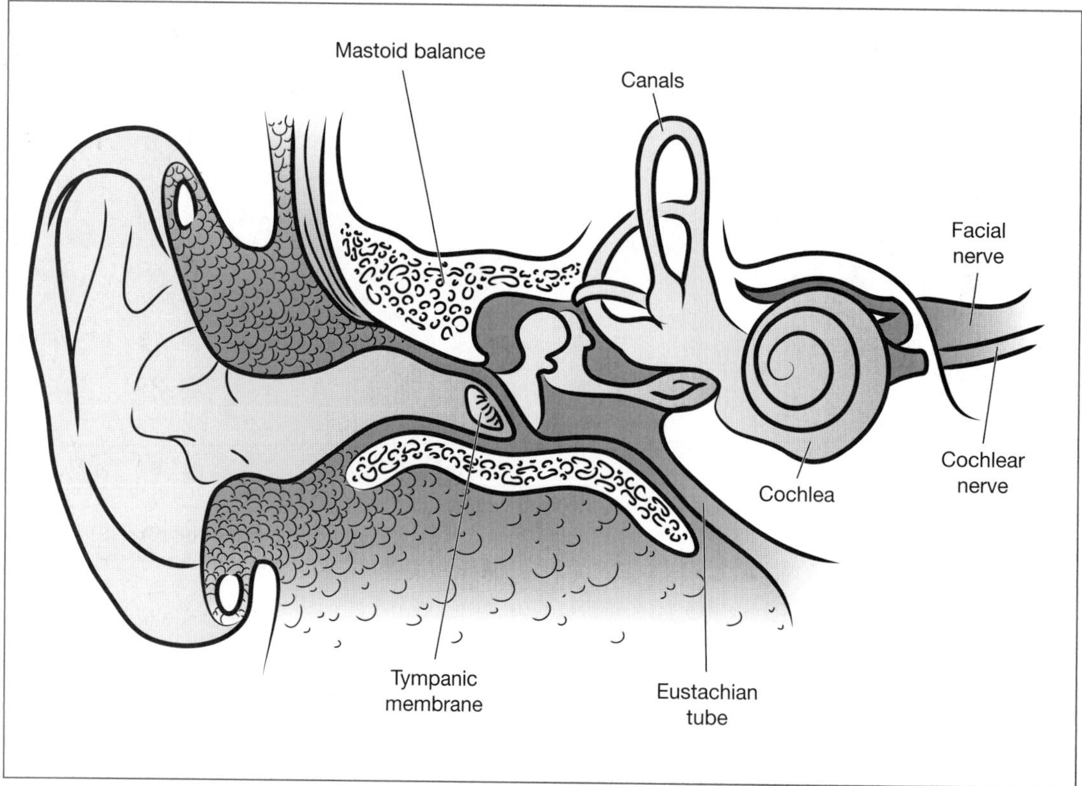

FIGURE 16.3 General framework of the outer, middle, and inner ear. Redrawn from Pappas (1985).

PHYSIOLOGY OF AUDIOLOGIC FUNCTION

External Ear

The external ear consists of the auricle (pinna) and the external auditory meatus (external canal). The primary function of the external ear is to funnel sound to the tympanic membrane. Absence of the auricle contributes to difficulty in sound localization.

Middle Ear

Advancing sound entering the auditory canal directly strikes the tympanic membrane. This membrane and the ossicles serve as transmitters from the outer ear to the inner ear. The malleus, which is continuous with the tympanic membrane and is connected with the incus and stapes, moves the ossicles. Ossicles transfer sound energy into the inner ear through the oval window, which holds the stapes by means of an angular ligament.

The middle ear is lined with respiratory mucosa composed of ciliated columnar epithelial cells, supporting cells, and secretory cells. Secretory cells secrete mucus that forms a complex mucous layer. The cilia of the middle ear interact with the mucus by transporting mastoid and middle ear secretions through the Eustachian tube to the nasopharynx, where they are swallowed. This mechanism is known as the mucociliary transport system. Glycoproteins in the mucus determine the viscosity and elasticity of the middle ear mucus. Mucus that is too thick or too thin impedes effective transport of bacteria and cellular debris from the mastoid and middle ear cleft: This transport has a protective effect against ear infections. In addition to serving as an exit for secretions into the nasopharynx, the Eustachian tube equalizes the pressure between the middle ear and the ambient atmosphere.

Inner Ear

Before this point in the hearing mechanism, all of the sound energy is contained in the air-filled spaces of the external and middle ear. From the stapes onward, the pathway for sound moves through fluid-filled spaces. When sound is transferred from the tympanic membrane to the inner ear, the stapes creates a fluid wave that is transmitted to the round window. This transmission creates fluid waves that travel from the basal aspect of the cochlea to the apex. As the fluid wave moves, it displaces the basilar membrane. Maximum movement of the basilar membrane occurs at the point specific to the frequency of sound entering the ear; that is, high-frequency sounds cause minimal disturbance at the basal end of the cochlea, and low-frequency sounds cause minimal disturbance at the apex.

Vibrations in the basilar membrane cause movement of the organ of Corti. This organ contains receptor hair cells that are on the basilar membrane. Vibrations of the hair on the hair cells cause either polarization or depolarization, depending on the direction of the bend. When sufficient depolarization occurs, action potentials are produced that are propagated along the auditory pathway to the auditory cortex. The cochlea provides input by coding information about loudness and frequency in the action potentials sent to the cortex, giving meaning to the sound. Hair cells of the spiral organ of Corti are stimulated as they touch the tectorial membrane. Hair cells act as transducers that convert mechanical energy into electrical impulses; this action occurs in the fibers of the spiral ganglion. Axons of these cells become the auditory nerve (vestibulocochlear nerve). Nerve fibers pass to the medulla, the pons, and the midbrain, and finally to the temporal lobes of the cortex, where the impulses are interpreted as sound.

The vestibular system is similar to the auditory system. Fluid moves within the vestibular labyrinth when the head moves. The semicircular canals respond to angular acceleration (rotation), and the utricle and saccule respond to linear acceleration (position). Movement of endolymph exerts force on the hairs of the sensory cells of the cristae and the maculae. Depolarization of the sensory cells produces action potentials, which are transmitted to the vestibular cortex. The vestibular apparatus functions in conjunction with proprioception and visual orientation to maintain balance.

HEARING IMPAIRMENT

The American Speech-Language-Hearing Association (ASHA) defines hearing impairment as "a loss of auditory sensitivity that can be measured at birth and for which intervention strategies are known and available." Hearing impairment represents a spectrum of hearing loss classified as mild, moderate, severe, or prolonged (Spivak, 1998).

Types of Hearing Impairment

The types of hearing impairment have been classified according to the location of the problem. Impairment may be one of three types: conductive, sensorineural, or a combination of these. Conductive losses arise from conditions that affect the outer and middle ear; sensorineural loss results from inner ear disorders; and combination losses result from disruptions in both areas of the ear.

Conductive hearing loss exists when dysfunction in the outer or middle ear disrupts the normal sequence of sound localization and vibration. Frequently, the external auditory meatus becomes occluded by cerumen (wax), which impedes the transmission of sound. Otitis media, an infection of the middle ear, is the most common cause of conductive hearing loss. In this instance, fluid accumulates in the middle ear, preventing the tympanic membrane and ossicular chain from vibrating normally (Boudewyns et al., 2011).

Congenital deformities of the outer ear also can inhibit the neonate's ability to hear. Because the function of the external ear is to funnel sound, variations in the structure and protrusion of the pinna may contribute to conductive hearing loss.

A missing or deformed pinna can result from a malformation of the auricular folds. Atresia of the auditory meatus or abnormal development of the ossicular chain may arise from defective development of the brachial chain (Jones, 2006).

Infants with conductive hearing loss have difficulty hearing low-frequency sounds (i.e., those in the 125- to 500-Hz range). Management of the neonate with conductive hearing loss is directed toward early observation, detection, and intervention to eliminate the source of infection, to remove the blockage, and to provide amplification, resulting in the restoration of normal hearing.

Sensorineural hearing impairment results from damage to the sensory nerve endings of the cochlea or dysfunction of the auditory nerve (eighth cranial nerve). A typical characteristic of inner ear dysfunction is the inability of the inner ear to interpret fluid changes in the cochlea. Sensorineural hearing loss may manifest as a congenital inner ear abnormality, resulting in congenital deafness. Other conditions that may cause sensorineural hearing loss are trauma to the inner ear, the effects of certain drugs, prolonged exposure to loud noise, infections, infectious conditions such as measles, and the effects of aging (Harlor & Bower, 2009).

IDENTIFICATION OF THE HEARING-IMPAIRED INFANT

Physical Examination

The physical examination of the infant should be performed in a quiet, warm, draft-free area appropriate for observation and inspection of auditory structures and function. Observing the infant's behavior before examining the ear yields baseline assessments. The alert, normal full-term newborn reacts by turning toward the sound of human speech or ring of a bell; this infant also startles to the stimulus of a loud noise. Observation of the preterm infant is deferred to a later time, prior to discharge when the behavioral response has matured. Observation of infant response alone provides only a crude estimate of neonatal hearing ability.

Inspection of the Ear

Inspection of the ear begins with the medial and lateral surfaces of the pinna and the surface of the scalp, face, and neck. Development of the pinna correlates with the infant's gestational age. At term, the pinna of the newborn is well shaped and has sufficient cartilage to maintain normal shape and resistance (Figure 16.2). Before 34 weeks gestation, the pinna is a slightly formed double thickness of cartilage. The relationship of the pinna to the other structures of the head and face is important in the initial assessment. With normal placement, the helix is located at the level of the outer canthus and the tragus is roughly level with the intraorbital rim. Low-set auricles frequently are associated with abnormalities of the urinary system. Unilateral conductive hearing loss may be present in children with normal-size pinnae and unilateral absence of the superior crus or in patients with a fused anthelix-helix; thickened, hypertrophied ear lobes; a "cup" ear; and a protruding pinna. The pinna may be abnormally small (microtia) or absent (anotia). Atresia (closure of the external auditory canal) may be observed. The condition is classified as mild, indicating a small ear canal; medium, indicating that a bony atretic plate has replaced the canal with ossicular malformation; or severe, indicating a small or absent ear canal and middle ear space.

Several combinations of atresia and microtia may be seen, therefore all children with these abnormalities should be suspected of having middle ear abnormalities. These infants may also have sensorineural hearing loss. Atresia often is observed with cranial, facial, mandibular, or acrofacial dysostoses. Abnormalities of the skeletal system or chromosomal aberration may also be accompanied by atresia. Aural atresia may be associated with facial, labial, or palatal clefts. Infants with atresia often have conductive hearing loss related to the inability of the ear canal to transmit sound.

Preauricular abnormalities, including pits or tags (Figure 16.4) and branchial fistulas, often are accompanied by external or middle ear malformations. These appendages may be present with an otherwise normal-appearing pinna. Preauricular tags or pits usually require only cosmetic surgery or excision if they are draining.

The pinna should be inspected for location and for its relationship to other facial structures. Normal attachment is to the side, level with the middle third of the face and fixed in position to the lateral aspect of the external auditory canal. The major convolutions of the pinna are the helix, anthelix, tragus, antitragus, and lobule. The lobule of the external ear has no cartilage. The angle of placement of the pinna is almost vertical, and if the angle is more than 10° off normal, it is considered abnormal. The superior helix is located at the outer canthus of the eye, and the tragus is roughly level with the infraorbital rim.

Low-set auricles frequently are associated with other abnormalities of the first and second branchial cleft and with abnormalities of the urinary system. Other abnormalities that may be noted are skin tags, sinuses, or pits, which often are associated with other auditory or renal malformations. The pinna often may be observed to have bruising from a forceps delivery. Depending on the degree of bruising, the discoloration should subside within the first week of life.

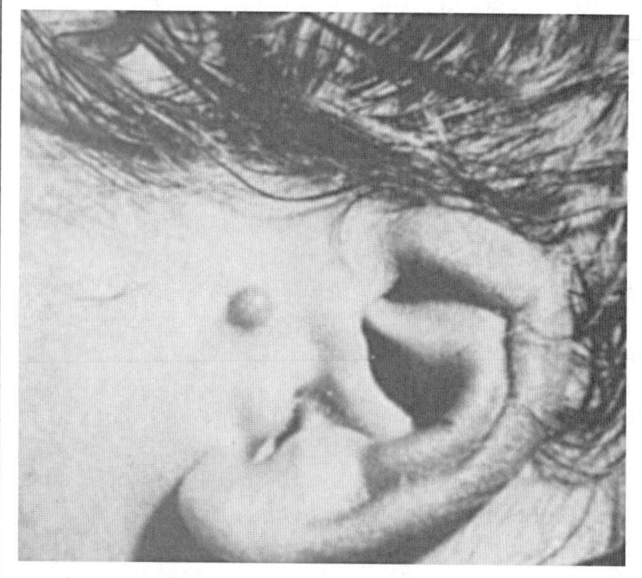

FIGURE 16.4 Preauricular tag.
Adapted from Schreiner and Bradburn (1987).

The external auditory meatus should then be observed for patency. Atresia or stenosis of the external meatus may be seen. This abnormality results in a conductive hearing loss because sound transmissions are blocked; the condition should be noted as part of the physical findings.

Inspection of the Middle Ear and Tympanic Membrane

The depths of the external meatus can be examined with a brightly illuminated pneumatic otoscope. Vernix caseosa frequently is encountered in the ear canal of the neonate. The otoscope is introduced into the ear canal by exerting gentle traction posterosuperiorly on the auricle. In the neonate, the tympanic membrane lies in a nearly horizontal plane. The tympanic membrane is visualized through the collapsed neonatal ear by gently dilating the ear canal with the speculum as the cartilaginous canal is traversed. The tympanic membrane should be examined for thickness, vascularity, and contour. All areas, including the area above the short process of the malleus (pars flaccida), should be visualized for completeness. Normally the tympanic membrane appears translucent. White shadows of the ossicles usually can be seen through the membrane. The mobility of the tympanic membrane can be assessed by applying intermittent pressure through a bulb or by blowing through a polyethylene tube connected to an otoscope.

Otitis media can occur in the first days of life and can be diagnosed by otoscopic examination. Otitis media often manifests as a poorly mobile, bulging, yellow, opacified tympanic membrane. Complications of otitis media are common. Otitis media with middle ear effusion may cause hearing loss, perforation of the tympanic membrane, and possibly intracranial complications, including meningitis, encephalitis, and brain abscess (Vartiainen, 2000). Middle ear effusion occurs in both outpatient and inpatient groups of neonates.

Inspection of the Head and Neck

The anatomy of the head and neck should be assessed for deficits as part of the screening process for all neonates. Ear anomalies associated with head and neck anomalies may occur as a result of a primary regional defect; secondary to a primary defect in an area contiguous to the temporal bone; as part of an inherited defect involving the skeletal system; or as part of a chromosomal disorder. Malformations of the head and neck may be relatively simple or complex. Any neonate with a defect, even a minor one, should be closely examined for hidden major malformations.

■ **Nose.** Examination of the nose should be directed toward identification of suspicious defects, such as unusual broadness with a flat base and a short length (saddle nose), small nostrils, and notched alae. Deformities of the nose often appear with other craniofacial abnormalities.

■ **Mouth.** Defects in the oral cavity are the most common defect associated with hearing impairment. A child with cleft lip or palate has a deficiency in the palate musculature that is primarily related to the inability of the tensor muscle of

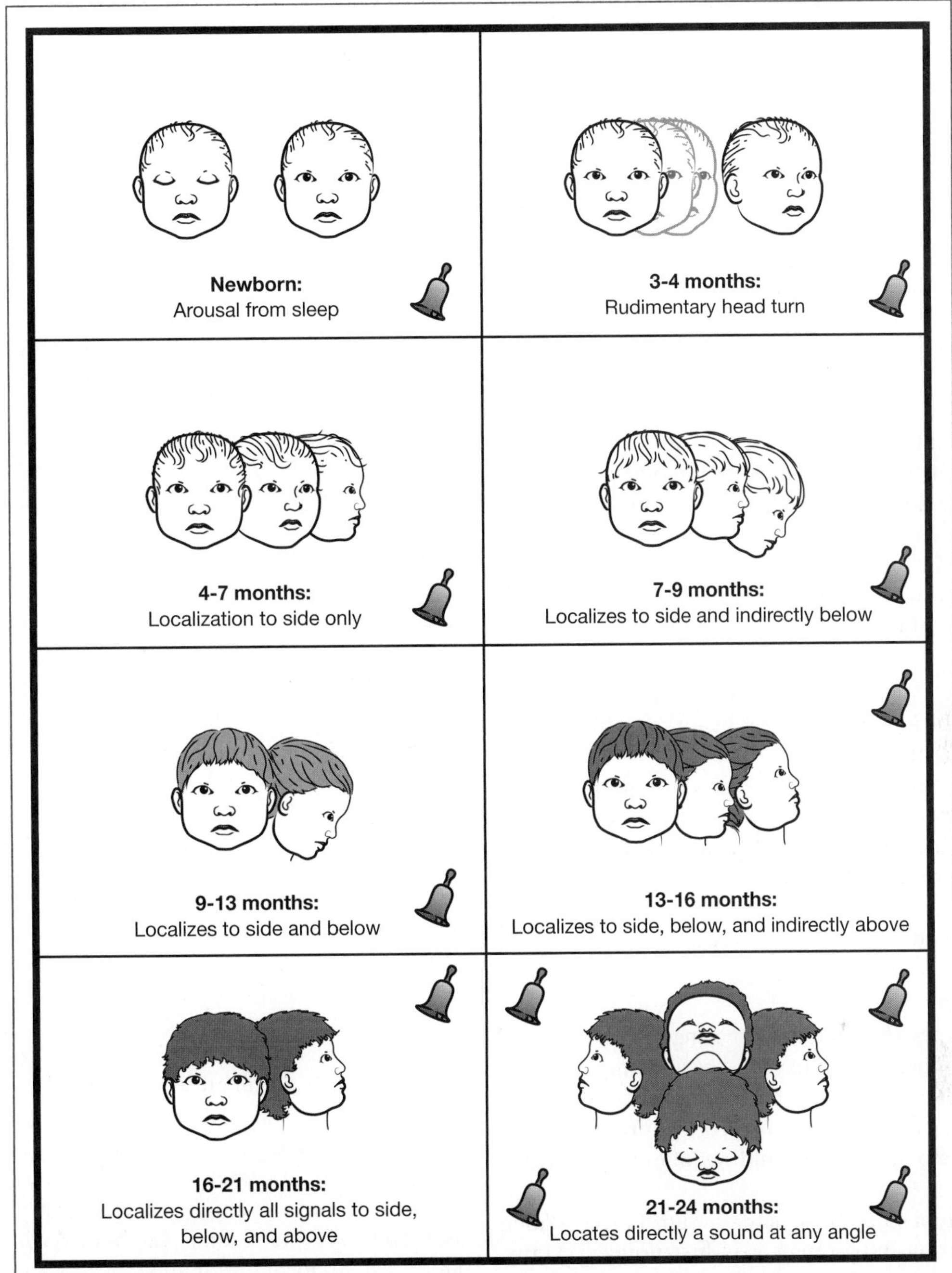
Newborn:
Arousal from sleep
3-4 months:
Rudimentary head turn
4-7 months:
Localization to side only
7-9 months:
Localizes to side and indirectly below
9-13 months:
Localizes to side and below
13-16 months:
Localizes to side, below, and indirectly above
16-21 months:
Localizes directly all signals to side, below, and above
21-24 months:
Locates directly a sound at any angle

FIGURE 16.5 Maturation of auditory response.
Redrawn from Northern and Downs (2002).

the velum palatinum to dilate the Eustachian tube actively during swallowing. Hearing problems may be observed in patients with cleft palate, depending on the patient's age on examination and the means of the exploration.

Cleft lip or palate leaves the child vulnerable to the effusion of fluid and, as a result, to varying degrees of hearing loss. The consequences of effusion raise the rate of otitis media, for which 50% to 90% incidences have been reported. The hearing loss associated with cleft lip or palate generally is conductive; however, sensorineural and combination losses have been reported. Infants younger than 12 months of age who had cleft palate that was surgically repaired often have a detectable degree of hearing loss. The degree of loss is directly related to the severity of the palatal defect.

■ **Eyes.** Deformities of the eyelids are the most common abnormality involving the eyes. A variation in eyelid configuration has been noted in which the upper eyelid forms an almost vertical curve at the level of the medial limit of the cornea and fuses with the lower eyelid. The distance of the two medial angles is increased. These findings typically are noted in Waardenburg syndrome, an autosomal dominant disorder that results in mild to severe sensorineural hearing loss in 50% of patients. The hearing loss may be unilateral or bilateral and progressive.

Epicanthal folds that are true vertical folds extending from the nasal fold into the upper eyelid are commonly noted in infants with Down syndrome, or trisomy 21. Other physical features seen in Down syndrome are low-set ears, small pinnae, and a narrow external ear canal. Infants with this syndrome tend to have recurrent otitis media and anomalies of the middle ear ossicles. The incidence of hearing loss is high, and the condition may be the sensorineural, conductive, or combination type.

■ **Hair.** An unusual hair texture or hairline should raise suspicion in the assessment for abnormalities associated with hearing loss. Twisted hair (pili torti) has been associated with sensorineural hearing loss. The hair may be twisted, dry, brittle, or easily broken. Aberrant scalp hair patterns may also be significant.

■ **Neck.** Defects of the neck that may be associated with hearing impairment are branchial cleft fistulas and mildly webbed or shortened neck. Not all infants with defects of the head or neck also have hearing impairments; many variations may be observed in the normal neonate population. The presence of such defects does increase the risk of hearing impairment, however, and should be followed up in the long-term interest of the child.

History

The importance of a comprehensive history for identifying the infant at risk cannot be overemphasized. The newborn carries a history extending back to the time of conception and is influenced by both perinatal events and parental genetic composition. Gathering of data on the infant's history is the first step in identifying infants at risk for hearing impairment. A thorough history of familial hearing loss, either presenting at birth or childhood through adolescence, is significant.

Family History

More than 50 types of hereditary hearing loss have been described. A significant number of hearing impairments may be classified as genetically based. Hereditary hearing loss must be identified on the basis of a thorough medical and family history, which should include the following components:

1. Determination of the cause and circumstances under which the hearing impairment was first noticed: Many different circumstances surrounding the onset of the hearing loss may cause it to be labeled as congenital or hereditary, or both. An example of hearing loss that is hereditary and not congenital is Alport syndrome, an autosomal dominant trait resulting in deafness that begins in preadolescence.
2. A complete family history: This should include a history of previous and current pregnancies.
3. An extended family history of data relating to hearing impairments of both immediate and extended family members.
4. A thorough physical examination: The head and neck region, particularly, should be examined for abnormalities.
5. Selective testing procedures for assessing possible causes of sensorineural hearing loss.

A questionnaire can be used to obtain information on familial hearing loss from the mother. Although the questions easily may be asked orally, the form provides a structure that can ensure consistency and is the preferred method of data gathering in most settings. The questionnaire should be given to all new mothers and should be completed prior to discharge. The questionnaire provides an excellent opportunity for educating the mother on normal speech and language development.

HEREDITARY HEARING LOSS

Autosomal Dominant Inheritance

Autosomal dominant inheritance accounts for 10% to 25% of cases of hereditary hearing impairment. The hearing loss may be unilateral or bilateral, and males and females are affected equally. Autosomal dominant hearing disorders vary in severity ("variable expressivity") and in progression of hearing loss. A typical example of an autosomal dominant hearing disorder occurs in Waardenburg syndrome, which is characterized by hypertelorism, a high nasal bridge, synophrys, and hypoplastic alae nasi. Pigmentation abnormalities include a white forelock, partial albinism, hypopigmentation of the fundi, blue irises, and premature graying. In this syndrome, severe to profound bilateral sensorineural hearing loss is present with integumentary system involvement. The histopathologic characteristics are absence of the organ of Corti and atrophy of the spiral ganglion.

Another example of an autosomal dominant hearing loss with incomplete penetrance and variable expression occurs in Treacher Collins syndrome. Major features of the syndrome include facial anomalies; small, displaced, or absent external ears; external auditory canal atresia; and poorly developed or malformed tympanic ossicles. Deafness generally is complete and conductive.

Klippel–Feil syndrome, if familial, is another example of autosomal dominance with variable expression. The characteristics of this syndrome are craniofacial disorders, fusion of some or all of the cervical vertebrae, cleft palate (occasionally), and severe sensorineural hearing loss. Crouzon disease is another disorder in which hearing loss is attributed to autosomal dominance with variable expression. An abnormally shaped head, a beaked nose, and marked bilateral exophthalmos caused by premature closure of the cranial sutures characterize this disease. Hearing loss may be conductive because of middle ear deformities or sensorineural abnormalities.

Autosomal Recessive Inheritance

Autosomal recessive inheritance accounts for about 40% of childhood deafness. An estimated one in eight individuals is a carrier for a recessive form of hearing impairment. The incidence of recessive inheritance is higher in marriages of recent common ancestry, such as siblings or cousins. This type of union increases the possibility that each parent will be the carrier of an identical defective gene that may express itself as an abnormal trait. Hearing loss in people with an autosomal recessive gene tends to be more severe than in those with autosomal dominant inheritance, because most cases of recessive hearing loss are associated with the Scheibe deformity of the cochlea. With Scheibe dysplasia, the entire organ of Corti is rudimentary; hair cells are missing, and the supporting cells are distorted or collapsed. The vestibular membrane usually is collapsed. Pendred syndrome, a condition marked by hearing loss and goiter detected in the first 2 years of life, is an example of an autosomal recessive disorder.

■ X-Linked Disorders. Approximately 3% of hereditary deafness is due to the X-linked mode of transmission (Northern & Downs, 2002). The mutant gene is on the X chromosome, and males transmit only Y chromosomes to their male offspring; therefore only males are affected. The female is the carrier and has the chance to transmit the gene to 50% of her sons, who manifest the disease, and 50% of her daughters, who carry the abnormality. The hearing loss characteristically is not present at birth but develops in infancy to varying degrees. X-linked hearing losses, with exceptions, are sensorineural, and some retention of hearing in all frequencies often occurs. Recessive, or X-linked, Duchenne muscular dystrophy is an example of this type of disorder. Characterized by muscle wasting, the severe infantile form of muscular dystrophy also is associated with mild to moderate sensorineural hearing loss.

■ Cytogenetic Disorders. Cytogenetic disorders are caused by structural changes in one or more of the chromosomes or by errors in the distribution of the chromosomes. Down syndrome, which is caused by an extra chromosome 21, is the most common chromosomal aberration syndrome, with an incidence of 1 in 600 to 800 births. Approximately 5% of cases of Down syndrome are due to translocation and fusion of part of chromosome 21 to chromosome 14. Children with trisomy 21 have a high incidence of hearing loss.

Characteristic otologic findings that have an impact on the hearing performance of these children during the early years are a high incidence of: (1) stenosis of the external auditory canal, (2) serous otitis media, and (3) a cholesteatoma-persistent growth of squamous epithelium from the ear canal into the middle ear or mastoid through a tear in the tympanic membrane. The narrowed segment is located at the junction of the cartilaginous and bony portions of the canal. With increasing age, the canal has been noted to assume a more typical appearance as the thickened tissue recedes.

The degree of hearing loss in these infants varies, but is rarely profound. On examination of the aperture, some of these children are found to have congenital ossicular malformations and destruction caused by inflammations arising from chronic infection.

Mental retardation is a clinical condition frequently seen with Down syndrome. The impact of the otologic handicap on the developmental potential of these children is uncertain. Because of the high incidence of hearing loss in this group, early and frequent monitoring is imperative. Collaborative research studies need be done to identify factors affecting the otologic problems of infants with Down syndrome and to devise early strategies to optimize these infants' potential (Park, Wilson, Stevens, Harward, & Hohler, 2012).

Differential Diagnosis

No differential diagnosis exists for deafness, although generally a differential diagnosis to determine the etiology of the hearing impairment is listed.

Diagnostic Test

- Laboratory testing is not of benefit in the diagnosis of deafness; however, if a genetic syndrome is suspected, biochemical evidence may be of benefit in determining the etiology.
- Connexin-26 is a genetic marker for deafness (Wang et al., 2011).
- Laboratory testing for perinatal infections such as cytomegalovirus (CMV), syphilis, and other TORCH infections may be indicated.
- For bilateral hearing loss, markers for general inflammatory disease, such as sedimentation rate, rheumatoid factor, or 68-kD protein a marker especially for autoimmune ear disease, may be evaluated.
- CT scanning and MRI imaging may be used to establish a malformation of the cochlea or cochlear nerve. MRI scanning may be used to identify an enlarged vestibula aqueduct, in the case of a sensitive ear in a child with a minor head trauma who presents with deteriorating hearing.

SCREENING METHODS FOR IDENTIFICATION OF HEARING LOSS

In the past 15 years, programs and procedures for screening newborns have been developed, modified, and improved. The goal of any screening program is to accomplish the task rapidly, accurately, and economically. Early hearing detection and intervention (EHDI) refers to the practice of screening every newborn for hearing loss prior to hospital discharge. All 50 states and the District of Columbia have EHDI laws or voluntary compliance programs that screen hearing. The EHDI program is responsible for creating, operating, and continuously improving a system. In addition, institutions are advised to use the risk factors associated with permanent congenital, delayed onset, and/or progressive hearing loss in children. Box 16.1 is a guide to identifying infants whose history indicates that degenerative disease or intrauterine infection may cause progressive, fluctuating, or late-onset hearing loss. In these cases it is recommended that the child have follow-up for 2 years in addition to initial screening.

The AAP Task Force on Newborn and Infant Hearing (2007) has endorsed universal screening of all newborns. In all cases, before discharge the parents should be informed about speech and hearing milestones and should be provided with information about community agencies available for long-term follow-up if needed (Figure 16.5).

Peripheral Measurements of Hearing Function

Assessment of hearing function in the neonate has focused on a two-tiered approach in which the evoked otoacoustic emissions (OAEs) test is used initially, and the automated auditory brainstem response (ABR) test is used as follow-up for infants who show hearing impairment on the initial screening. OAEs are low-intensity sounds that can be measured by placing a sensitive microphone in the ear canal. Hearing screening using OAEs is quick, inexpensive, and relatively accurate. Newborns delivered at home, or at birthing centers without hearing screening facilities need to have some referral mechanism for newborn hearing screening and follow-up mechanism.

If hearing impairment is detected on the OAE test, the ABR test can confirm the validity of that result. The ABR test records the electrical potentials that arise from the auditory nerve system. During this test, disk electrodes are attached to the vertex and mastoid areas, and repetitive sounds are presented to the ear in the form of clicks caused by a direct current pulse. The recorded response is a sequence of waves that represents the action potential of the auditory nerve. The wave latencies in infants at risk tend to show smaller and more prolonged responses. The absolute latency of the ABR waves depends on the intensity of the click stimulus. Reducing the click stimuli from 60 dB to 30 to 40 dB identifies thresholds of hearing. Absence of all waves indicates the presence of a peripheral lesion.

An abnormal ABR result may be defined as one that shows an absence of response at 40 dB or a wave V latency that exceeds the norm by two standard deviations. Wave V responses are used to determine abnormality because they are highly repeatable in infants and show little variability in normal-hearing subjects. The ABR test appears to be a sensitive method in that no false-negative results have been reported. Considering that any screening method should be quick, inexpensive, and easily administered and should allow easy interpretation of a large number of infants, the drawback to the ABR test is that it is more costly than the OAE test. Nevertheless, the ABR test can be justified as the initial neonatal hearing test, especially in preterm or high-risk infants. The Joint Committee on Infant Hearing (AAP, 1994, 1999, 2007) specifies that an audiologist should supervise the infant hearing screening program.

In some infants whose initial ABR test results are passing, but the infant meets risk criteria, continuing audiologic follow-up and management may be appropriate as designated by USPSTF for the following three years. Those infants include one with risk factors associated with possible progressive or fluctuating loss, such as a family history of progressive hearing loss, CMV infection, and persistent fetal circulation.

Infants who do not demonstrate a repeatable ABR wave V to the signal presented at 40 dB in at least one ear should have a comprehensive hearing evaluation at no later than 6 months of age. This follow-up includes a general physical examination, including examination of the head and neck; otoscopy; identification of relevant physical abnormalities; and laboratory tests for perinatal infections. A comprehensive audiologic evaluation may include additional evoked potential evaluation and acoustic immittance measurements. Although precise data on hearing sensitivity cannot be obtained until the infant can respond to operant conditioning test procedures at approximately 6 months of age, habilitation should not be delayed.

Infants can be fitted with hearing aids before 3 months of age. Attention to early identification, amplification, and education does not necessarily ensure speech and language acquisition but certainly facilitates it, even in the most profoundly hearing-impaired child.

BOX 16.1

RISK FACTORS ASSOCIATED WITH PERMANENT CONGENITAL, DELAYED ONSET, AND/OR PROGRESSIVE HEARING LOSS IN CHILDREN

1. Family history of permanent childhood hearing loss
2. Neonatal intensive care for 2 days or more or any of the following: extracorporeal membrane oxygenation-assisted ventilation, exposure to ototoxic medications (gentamicin and tobramycin) or loop diuretics (furosemide/Lasix), and hyperbilirubinemia requiring exchange transfusion
3. In utero exposure to infections such as CMV, herpes, rubella, syphilis, and toxoplasmosis
4. Craniofacial anomalies, including those that involve the pinna, ear canal, ear tags, ear pits, and temporal bone anomalies
5. Syndromes associated with hearing loss or progressive or late onset hearing loss, such as Waardenburg, Alport, Pendred, Ushers, and neurofibromatosis
6. Neurodegenerative disorders such as Hunter syndrome
7. Culture-positive postnatal infections associated with sensorineural hearing loss, including confirmed bacterial and viral meningitis
8. Head trauma
9. Chemotherapy
10. Recurrent or persistant otitis media
11. Concerned parent; child may have hearing loss

Adapted from U.S. Preventive Services Task Force (2008).

DEVELOPMENT OF A TREATMENT PLAN FOR THE HEARING-IMPAIRED NEONATE

Hearing screening of all infants should be completed before discharge or no later than 1 month of age. Those who do not pass the newborn screening should undergo audiologic and medical evaluation before 3 months of age for confirmatory testing. If confirmation of a diagnosis is made, then a treatment plan and habilitation can begin. Infants whose history indicates that they are at risk for late-onset hearing loss should be observed by periodic audiologic testing for 3 years.

For the infant with a confirmed hearing loss, efforts are directed at treatment. In accordance with Public Law 99, early intervention services are (1) evaluation and assessment and (2) development of an individualized family service plan. The full evaluation plan is to be completed within 45 days of referral. This plan may include various methods directed at treatment of serous otitis media, which is a major cause of temporary conductive hearing loss. For the infant with a permanent conductive hearing loss, amplification with a hearing aid may facilitate stimulation in the early critical period.

Infants can be fitted with a hearing aid device as soon as the impairment is diagnosed. In addition to amplification, the family should be taught total communication skills that will enhance interaction between the sender and the receiver. The basic premise is to use every means to communicate, such as gesturing, touching, and attending to stimuli.

The infant with severe to profound hearing impairment who is not at risk for recurrent otitis media and who does not get satisfactory results with a hearing aid is a candidate for cochlear implants (discussed below). For the hearing-impaired infant, multiple referral sources exist in which a multidisciplinary approach optimizes the infant's potential for growth and development.

Cochlear Implants

Cochlear implants are not new, but they increasingly are being used to treat infants with severe to profound sensorineural hearing loss. Cochlear implants are electronic devices that are surgically implanted in the inner ear and bypass the damaged part of the ear to deliver electrical signals to the hearing nerve. A cochlear implant system is composed of a microphone, an external sound processor, transmitter, internal cochlear receiver, and electrode array. The external sound processor captures sound with a microphone and converts the sound to digital information. The digital signal is sent to the internal receiver and converted to electrical signals, which stimulate tiny electrodes in the inner ear. The electrodes send the electrical signal to the hearing nerve. These signals are then interpreted by the brain as sound. Implants work only if some spiral ganglion cells are present to transmit the auditory signal. An issue for patients of any age with any type of cochlear implant is the comfortable level of sound. This sometimes is difficult to determine in infants, who cannot provide feedback as to what they are hearing.

Cochlear implants are Food and Drug Administration approved for adults and children as young as 12 months of age. Research has shown that earlier implantation is associated with better speech and language development (Svirsky, Teoh, & Neuburger, 2004). It is critical that infants with hearing loss be diagnosed and early intervention be initiated without delay. The later the child receives the implants, the more likely it is that speech and language development will be delayed.

Hearing screening is a task for a team of professionals that includes pediatricians, otolaryngologists, audiologists, neurologists, and nurse practitioners. Local public health agencies may provide services such as data collection and referral. Many large metropolitan medical centers have speech and hearing centers as part of a broad base of services ranging from diagnosis to rehabilitation.

Implementation and Evaluation

The overall goal of any treatment program for the hearing impaired is to optimize the infant's potential communication skills and abilities. To achieve this goal, a comprehensive evaluation, follow-up, and management system must be implemented.

Parental Support

Support for the parents of a hearing-impaired child is based on the foundation of trust and acceptance between the practitioner and the family. Notification of a hearing impairment is an extremely traumatic and deeply disturbing situation for the parents, one that often provokes denial. Often, identification of the problem is delayed because the parents cannot admit that something is wrong. Some practices in the diagnostic workup for hearing impairment seem to favor separation of the parents from the diagnostic process. OAE and ABR testing may foster denial because the findings are abstract, and parents need to have visible, tangible evidence of the impairment. The practitioner plays a major role in reiterating, interpreting, and reinforcing the information conveyed by the audiologist. Sensitivity to the parents' need to grieve the loss of the "perfect child" is important. Acceptance of the handicap can be aided by enlisting the parents as codiagnosticians. Asking the parents what they think the problem is and making them part of the decision-making process objectifies the diagnoses and aids future compliance with the habilitative regimen. Through encouraging dialogue with other parents with similar children's needs and coaching parents with question prompts, the facilitator simulates decision making (Coulter & Ellins, 2007). By listening to the parents' feelings of inadequacy and by indirect teaching, practitioners can help the parents acquire more fruitful coping strategies. Sices et al. (2009) investigated parents' and early intervention specialists' beliefs and experiences regarding discussing child development in primary care. Focus groups were used to collect data from mothers of young children with typical development as well as those who received early intervention and early intervention specialists. Themes from the data revealed that most mothers preferred a nonalarmist style of communication when developmental delays are suspected. Some mothers preferred a more direct approach, including the use of labels to help them understand. The importance of preparation to accept development delays emerged as a theme in all groups. Elements of preparedness included: information about expected developmental skills, suggestion for promoting skills, and a time frame for follow-up.

The mother–infant relationship is potentially damaged when the infant is hearing impaired. Reciprocal communication that normally occurs between the mother and the infant on an affective and a verbal level has been reported to be diminished with infants who are hearing impaired. The handicapped infant may miss intended signals from parents and may emit signals that are not understood. The parents must capture their infant's visual attention so that their efforts are effectively stimulating. An asynchrony may develop that can retard the infant's ability to acquire language even beyond the limits of the hearing loss itself. The family can be taught total communication skills (gesturing, touching, and attending) to support interaction with the infant.

EVIDENCE-BASED PRACTICE BOX

The multidisciplinary, multiservices approach should be instituted only when all components are available to the infant and the family (ASHA, 2007).

In addition to qualified professionals and services, other factors influence the management and habilitation of the hearing-impaired infant. These factors can facilitate or hamper entry into the system and compliance with the treatment regimen (Box 16.2).

Outcome measures of the treatment program include early identification and implementation of a comprehensive habilitation plan, in order to maximize communication potential and parental acceptance of the infant's disability. Bailey and coauthors (2004), in a nationally representative sample of families of children (average age of diagnosis 7.4 months of age) with or at risk for disability, reported very positive first experiences with early intervention. A small percentage experienced significant delays and wanted more involvement, and nearly 20% were unaware of the existence of a written plan for service. Pappas et al. (2008), in a study of belief in and practice of speech language pathologists in service planning and delivery for children with hearing impairment, revealed that stated beliefs don't always reflect practice: decision making was therapist centered rather than family centered. McCracken and coauthors (2008), in a qualitative study of parental reflections on very early audiologic management, concluded that to be most effective, the focus should be on the infant sooner, rather than on the child later. Inber and Dromi (2010) examined the actual versus desired family-centered practice in early intervention for children with hearing loss from the professional and parental viewpoint. Results revealed that parental involvement in the program was perceived positively, however, a wide range of programs need to be offered for parents.

References

ASHA (American Speech-Language-Hearing Association). (2007). Childhood apraxia of speech [Position Statement]. Available from www.asha.org/policy

Bailey, D. B., Hebbeler, K., Scarborough, A., Spiker, D., & Mallik, S. (2004). First experiences with early intervention: A national perspective. *Pediatrics, 113*(4), 887–896.

Ingber, S., Al-Yagon, M., & Dromi, E. (2010). Mothers' involvement in early intervention for children with hearing loss: The role of maternal characteristics and context-based perceptions. *Journal of Early Intervention, 32*, 351–369.

McCracken, S. G., & Marsh, J. C. 2008. Practitioner expertise in evidence-based practice decision making. *Research in Social Work Practice* (18), 301–310.

BOX 16.2

FACTORS INFLUENCING THE MANAGEMENT AND HABILITATION OF THE HEARING-IMPAIRED INFANT

Factors That Facilitate Management

- Preparation to accept information about development delays; a nonalarmist style of communication
- Information about expected developmental skills, suggestion for promoting skills, and a time frame for follow-up
- Parental involvement, offering a wide range of programs that are family-centered focused
- Expeditious arrangements for referral

Factors That Hamper Management

- Long waiting lists
- Poor communication between speech and hearing departments

ONLINE RESOURCES

ASHA
http://www.asha.org

National Center for Hearing Assessment and Management
http://www.infanthearing.org

National Institute on Deafness and other Communication Disorders

National Resource Center for Early Detection of Hearing Disorders in Infants (EHDI)
http://www.infanthearing.org

U.S. Preventative Services Task Force (USPSTF) Universal Screening for Hearing Loss in Newborns: Recommendation Statement
http:// www.ahrq.gov/clinc/uspstf/uspsnbhr.html
(Additional USPSTF recommendations regarding screening test for newborns can be assessed at **http://www.ahrq.gov/clinc/cps3dix.html#pediatric**)

Wise Ears
http://www.nih.gov/nidcd/health/wise

REFERENCES

American Academy of Pediatrics. (1994). Joint Committee on Infant Hearing 1994 Position Statement. *Pediatrics, 95*, 152–156.

American Academy of Pediatrics, Task Force on Newborn and Infant Hearing. (1999). Newborn and infant hearing loss: Detection and intervention. *Pediatrics, 103*(2), 527–530.

American Academy of Pediatrics, Joint Committee on Infant Hearing. (2007). Year 2007 position statement: Principles and guidelines for early hearing detection and intervention programs. *Pediatrics, 120*(4), 898–921.

Bachman, J. G., Johnston, L. D., & O'Malley, P. M. (1998). Explaining recent increases in students' marijuana use: Impacts of perceived risks and disapproval, 1976 through 1996. *American Journal of Public Health, 88*, 887–892.

Boudewyns, A., Declau, F., Van den Ende, J., Van Kerschaver, E., Dirckx, S., Hofkens-Van den Brandt, A., & Van de Heyning, P. (2011). Otitis media with effusion: An underestimated cause of hearing loss in infants. *Otology & Neurotology, 32*(5), 799–804.

Coulter, A., & Ellins, J. (2007). Effectiveness of strategies for informing, educating, and involving patients. *BMJ, 335*(7609), 24–27.

De Capua, B., Costantini, D., Martufi, C., Latini, G., Gentile, M., & De Felice, C. (2007). Universal neonatal hearing screening: The Siena (Italy) experience on 19,700 newborns. *Early Human Development, 83*(9), 601–606.

DeCasper, A. J., & Fifer, W. P. (1980). Of human bonding: Newborns prefer their mothers' voices. *Science, 208*(4448), 1174–1176.

DeCasper, A. J., Lecanuent, J., Busnel, M., Granier-Deferre, C., & Maugeais, R. (1994). Fetal reactions to recurrent maternal speech. *Infant Behavior and Development, 17*, 159–164.

Fitzpatrick, E., Durieux-Smith, A., Eriks-Brophy, A., Olds, J., & Gaines, R. (2007). The impact of newborn hearing screening on communication development. *Journal of Medical Screening, 14*(3), 123–131.

Harlor, A. D., Jr., & Bower, C. (2009). Hearing assessment in infants and children: Recommendations beyond neonatal screening. *Pediatrics, 124*(4), 1252–1263.

Jones, K. L. (2006). *Smith's recognizable patterns of human malformation* (6th ed.). Philadelphia, PA: Elsevier, Saunders.

Kennedy, C. R., McCann, D. C., Campbell, M. J., Law, C. M., Mullee, M., Petrou, S., . . . Stevenson, J. (2006). Language ability after early detection of permanent childhood hearing impairment. *The New England Journal of Medicine, 354*(20), 2131–2141.

Korver, A. M., Konings, S., Dekker, F. W., Beers, M., Wever, C. C., Frijns, J. H., & Oudesluys-Murphy, A. M. (2010). Newborn hearing screening vs later hearing screening and developmental outcomes in children with permanent childhood hearing impairment. *JAMA, 304*(15), 1701–1708.

Langagne, T., Schmidt, P., Leveque, M., & Chays, A. (2008). [Universal hearing screening in the Champagne-Ardenne regions: Results and consideration after 55,000 births from January 2004 to June 2007]. *Rev Laryngol Otol Rhinol (Bord), 129*(3), 153–158.

Lim, H. W., Kim, E. A., & Chung, J. W. (2012). Audiological follow-up results after newborn hearing screening program. *Clinical & Experimental Otorhinolaryngology, 5*(2), 57–61.

Moore, J. K., & Linthicum, F. H., Jr. (2007). The human auditory system: A timeline of development. *International Journal of Audiology, 46*(9), 460–478.

Nelson, H. D., Bougatsos, C., & Nygren, P. (2008). Universal newborn hearing screening: Systematic review to update the 2001 US preventive services task force recommendation. *Pediatrics, 122*(1), e266–e276.

Northern, J. L., & Downs, M. P. (2002). *Hearing in children* (5th ed.). Baltimore, MD: Lippincott Williams & Wilkins.

Ohl, C., Dornier, L., Czajka, C., Chobaut, J. C., & Tavernier, L. (2009). Newborn hearing screening on infants at risk. *International Journal of Pediatric Otorhinolaryngology, 73*(12), 1691–1695.

Pappas, D. (1985). *Diagnosis and treatment of hearing impairment in children*. San Diego, CA: College-Hill Press.

Pappas, N. W., McLeod, S., McAllister, L., & McKinnon, D. H. (2008). Parental involvement in speech intervention: A national survey. *Clinical Linguistics and Phonetics, 22*(4–5), 335–344.

Park, A. H., Wilson, M. A., Stevens, P. T., Harward, R., & Hohler, N. (2012). Identification of hearing loss in pediatric patients with Down syndrome. *Otolaryngology-Head and Neck Surgery, 146*(1), 135–140.

Patel, H., & Feldman, M. (2011). Universal newborn hearing screening. *Paediatrics & Child Health, 16*(5), 301–310.

Schreiner, R. L., & Bradburn, N. C. (1987). *Care of the newborn* (2nd ed.). New York, NY: Raven Press.

Sices, L., Egbert, L., & Mercer, M. B. (2009). Sugar-coaters and straight talkers: Communicating about developmental delays in primary care. *Pediatrics, 124*(4), e705–e713.

Sininger, Y. S., Doyle, K. J., & Moore, J. K. (1999). The case for early identification of hearing loss in children. Auditory system development, experimental auditory deprivation, and development of speech perception and hearing. *Pediatric Clinics of North America, 46*(1), 1–14.

Spivak, L. G. (Ed.). (1998). *Universal newborn hearing screening*. New York, NY: Thieme.

Svirsky, M. A., Teoh, S. W., & Neuburger, H. (2004). Development of language and speech perception in congenitally, profoundly deaf children as a function of age at cochlear implantation. *Audiol Neurootol, 9*(4), 224–233.

Task Force on Newborn and Infant Hearing. (1999). *Early identification of hearing impairment in infants and young children*. Elk Grove Village, IL: American Academy of Pediatrics.

U.S. Preventive Services Task Force. (2008). Universal screening for hearing loss in newborns. U.S. Preventive Services Task Force recommendation statement. *American Family Physician, 122*(1), 143–148.

Van Dommelen, P., Mohangoo, A. D., Verkerk, P. H., Van der Ploeg, C. P., & Van Straaten, H. L. (2010). Risk indicators for hearing loss in infants treated in different neonatal intensive care units. *Acta Paediatrica, 99*(3), 344–349.

Vartiainen, E. (2000). Otitis media with effusion in children with congenital or early-onset hearing impairment. *Journal of Otolaryngology, 29*(4), 221–223.

Verhaert, N., Willems, M., Van Kerschaver, E., & Desloovere, C. (2008). Impact of early hearing screening and treatment on language development and education level: Evaluation of 6 years of universal newborn hearing screening (ALGO) in Flanders, Belgium. *International Journal of Pediatric Otorhinolaryngology, 72*(5), 599–608.

Wang, Q. J., Zhao, Y. L., Rao, S. Q., Guo, Y. F., He, Y., Lan, L., . . . Shen, Y. (2011). Newborn hearing concurrent gene screening can improve care for hearing loss: A study on 14,913 Chinese newborns. *International Journal of Pediatric Otorhinolaryngology, 75*(4), 535–542.

CHAPTER

17

Ophthalmic System

■ Lori Baas Rubarth and Debra M. Parker

The eyes of the newborn infant begin to grow and develop early in gestation, making it susceptible to malformation, deformation, and disruption injuries. Neonatal visual problems can occur because of infection, congenital malformation, or oxygen and drug exposure. Visual disturbances in the newborn can range from minor refractory problems to complete blindness. In addition, other diseases and disorders can affect the eyes. Early detection and treatment of eye disorders are essential for the best possible outcome.

This chapter briefly outlines the embryologic development of the eye, reviews the methods of assessment of a newborn's eyes, describes specific ophthalmic disorders of the eye, and describes diseases that can affect the eyes, including prematurity. Collaborative management, family support, and appropriate nursing care are also discussed in this chapter.

EMBRYOLOGY

The newborn eye develops from a variety of embryonic tissues. The lens and part of the cornea develop from ectoderm. The pigmented epithelium and part of the retina develop from neuroectoderm. Part of the cornea, the ciliary and iris muscles, part of the choroid, and the sclera develop from neural crest cells. Part of the choroid and part of the cornea also develop from mesoderm (Figure 17.1).

Eye development actually has its beginnings during gastrulation and neurulation, with the formation of a single eye field in the neural plate (Schoenwolf, Bleyl, Brauer, & Francis-West, 2009). Many transcription factors early in development regulate and induce eye development. Without these transcription factors and other enzymes or proteins, anomalies can occur. The initial single eye field is stimulated to split into two separate optic primordia. Without this early splitting stimulation, holoprosencephaly (failure of brain to split into two hemispheres) and cyclopia (a single, midline eye) would occur (Schoenwolf et al., 2009).

Rudimentary eye formation is seen at the beginning of the fourth week of fetal life, or about 22 days after fertilization, with the indentation called the optic sulcus (Schoenwolf et al., 2009). Bilateral invaginations of the neural tube occur with formation of the optic vesicles. These two optic vesicles remain in contact with the developing brain. By about 32 to 34 days, the optic vesicles change shape to appear as a "goblet," with an additional invagination of ectoderm inward becoming the lens of the eye (Schoenwolf et al., 2009, p. 602). The fibers within the lens become transparent with the assistance of crystallins, which are soluble proteins within the eye. With the invagination of the optic cup, there are two layers formed that develop into the inner retina containing rods and cones and the outer melanin containing pigmented epithelium. These two layers of the retina do not ever fuse completely, but can separate, causing a retinal detachment. Both layers expand over the lens from the edges of the optic cup becoming the iris. The color of the iris is either light blue or gray at birth but becomes fully developed with increased pigment by about 6 months of age.

Cellular differentiation and development continue within the eye throughout fetal life. Macular differentiation occurs during the sixth month, and the fovea centralis, the area needed for sharp, high-acuity vision, does not mature until months into the postpartum period (Schoenwolf et al., 2009). Therefore, the term newborn's vision is present, but limited, during the first few days and weeks of life. Infants are most interested in high-contrast shapes that are about 8 to 12 inches from the eyes.

The eyelids develop as surface ectoderm folds over the cornea by about the sixth week of fetal life. Then the eyelids fuse together by the eighth week, but separate again sometime between the fifth and seventh months of fetal life. The lacrimal glands also form from ectoderm, but are still immature until about 6 weeks after birth (Schoenwolf et al., 2009). Tear production in newborns is limited until that time.

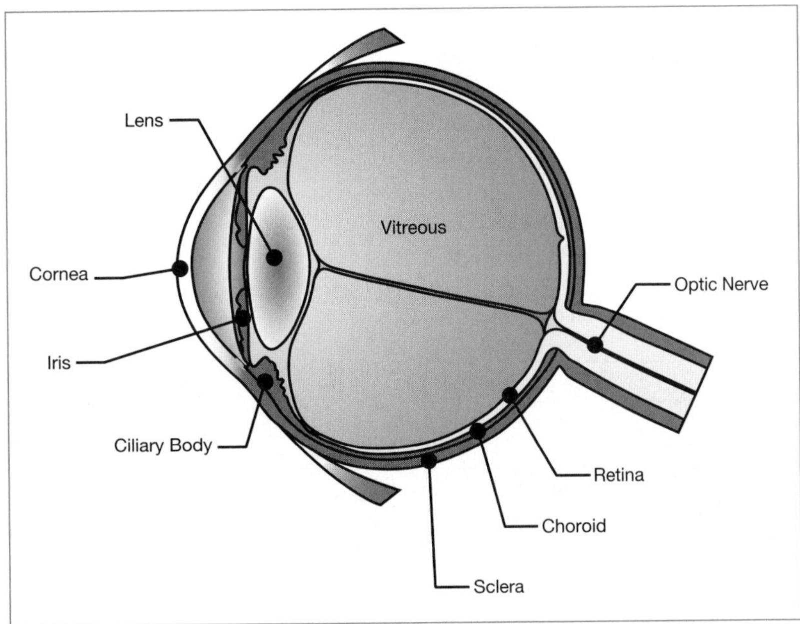

FIGURE 17.1 Anatomy of the eye.

ASSESSMENT

History

A thorough history is imperative to determine whether risk factors for eye problems are present. A complete family, medical, pregnancy, and psychosocial history, along with a maternal review of systems, should be obtained. The health care provider should ask questions related to the family history of vision problems (e.g., strabismus, glaucoma, and retinoblastoma) and refractive errors (e.g., myopia) and understand the terminology involved in assessment (Table 17.1). The maternal history should include questions about exposure to infectious diseases such as gonorrhea, chlamydia, rubella, and cytomegalovirus (CMV) infection, which are known to cause significant eye problems in newborns. The perinatal history should include questions about any difficulties that might have resulted in hypoxia or anoxia, conditions associated with adverse optical changes. Previous pregnancies that resulted in preterm births can provide important information about prior experience with retinopathy of prematurity (ROP).

Examination

Examining the eyes of a newborn can be a challenge. Care must be taken during the examination process to protect the newborn from injury and cold stress. The infant's state is also important for a successful examination. Newborns in the quiet, alert state are more responsive to visual stimuli.

Examination of the external features of the eye should occur first. Most of the important information about the eyes of the newborn can be obtained from inspection and observation. An examination with an ophthalmoscope is indicated to check for red reflex, but routine retinal examinations on all normal newborns are not indicated. A retinal exam or ophthalmology consult is indicated for the premature infant at risk for ROP or if physical examination findings suggest serious problems, such as cataracts or glaucoma.

It is easier to examine the newborn's eyes when they are spontaneously open. Dimming the lights, talking to the infant, and holding the baby upright may facilitate natural opening of the eyes. Newborn eyes should be assessed for their shape, symmetry, and size and for the presence of obvious features, such as eyebrows and eyelashes. The eyes should appear clear and without swelling or discharge. The eyelids should also be evaluated for redness, swelling, or evidence of colobomas and abnormal tumor masses. Inability to elevate the eyelids or ptosis (drooping) of one or both eyelids may lead to amblyopia or poor visual development. The presence of unusual folds and the slant of the eye should be noted.

The pupils should be checked for size, shape, symmetry, reaction to light, and accommodation. The color, clarity, and intensity of the red reflex should be checked and compared bilaterally. In African American infants, the red reflex may be pale orange or gray rather than red (Tappero & Honeyfield, 2009). An abnormal red reflex would be a white reflex (leukocoria), dark spots noted (possible cataracts), or a significant variation between the eyes. The onset of pupillary constriction in response to light is present by about 30 to 34 weeks gestation.

The cornea should be evaluated for clarity and size. A cloudy cornea may be caused by congenital glaucoma, errors of metabolism, or congenital corneal dystrophy. Leukocoria is the term for a whitish-appearing pupil or opaque cornea. This condition is almost always indicative of a serious eye problem. The differential diagnosis of leukocoria includes cataract, retinoblastoma, chorioretinal or optic nerve head coloboma, persistent hyperplastic primary vitreous, retinal detachment, ROP, persistent fetal vasculature, familial exudative vitreoretinopathy, toxocariasis,

TABLE 17.1

DEFINITIONS

Amblyopia	Known as "lazy eye" where one eye wanders from a straight line of vision
Aniridia	Much or all of the iris is missing
Anophthalmos	Complete absence of the ocular tissue within the orbit
Anti-Mongoloid slant	An inner canthus that is higher than the outer canthus
Blennorrhea	Excessive mucus discharge from the eye
Brushfield spots	Speckled iris; frequently associated with Down syndrome
Coloboma	Defect or opening that results from failure of part of the eye to close during embryogenesis; can occur in the iris or eyelids
Ectropion	A condition in which the eyelid is turned outward
Endophthalmitis	Inflammation of the internal eye tissues and fluid
Epicanthal fold	Skin that appears to overlap and partially obscure the inner canthus
Epiphora	Excessive tearing
Exophthalmos	An eye that appears to be bulging
Heterochromia	Pigmentation of the two irises is different
Inner canthus	The angle of the eyelid nearest the nose
Interpupillary distance	The distance between the centers of each pupil
Leukocoria	"White" reflex instead of red
Microphthalmia/ microphalmos	Small eyes
Mongoloid slant	An outer canthus that is higher than the inner canthus
Myopia	Near-sightedness
Nystagmus	The involuntary rhythmic or oscillating movements of the eyes
Outer canthus	The outer angle of the eyelid
Palpebral width	Width of the eyelid opening from inner canthus to outer canthus
Proptosis	Bulging of the eyes (exophthalmos)
Ptosis	Drooping of the upper eyelid
Strabismus	Cross-eyed; a condition where the eyes aim in different directions
Synophrys	An abnormal extension of the eyebrows so that they meet in the middle (midline)

uveitis, Peter's anomaly, and Coats' disease (Achim & Yen, 2012; de Alba Campomanes, Binenbaum, & Quinn, 2012). Trauma at birth can result in injury to the cornea, giving the cornea a hazy appearance. Preterm infants may also have a transient haziness of the cornea during the first week of life.

The iris is examined for coloboma and color. The iris eye color of dark-skinned Caucasian and African American infants is often darker due to earlier melanin deposition. As stated earlier, the deposition of color in most infants occurs by 6 months of age.

Heterochromia is a color variation, where the two eyes are different colors, or it can be that there are two colors within the same eye. Heterochromia can be a clue to the development of other disorders, including Sturge–Weber syndrome or Waardenburg syndrome, and would indicate the need for further follow-up (Rehman, 2008). The iris must be examined for coloboma resembling a keyhole with the pupil. The presence of coloboma may indicate a need to look for abnormalities in other systems. Infants with fetal alcohol syndrome can have colobomas, cataracts, and microphthalmos. The presence of these findings should alert the care provider to look for other features of the syndrome. The maternal history should also be reevaluated for alcohol use during the pregnancy.

Directly behind the iris is the lens. Cloudiness or opacity in the lens is by definition a cataract. An ophthalmologist should evaluate any cataract found in a newborn as soon as possible to determine if it is visually significant. Surgery should be performed to remove vision-threatening cataracts as soon as the infant is able to tolerate the procedure. Early surgery is critical to the prevention of amblyopia (lazy eye), which develops in these eyes when the condition is ignored for longer than a few months.

The sclera is examined for color and hemorrhage. The sclera of term infants should be white in color. A blue tint is indicative of possible osteogenesis imperfecta. Due to the thin sclera of preterm infants, the color can appear bluish. Subconjunctival hemorrhages are common following normal vaginal delivery and present no significant long-term complication for the term or preterm infant.

Attention should also be given to an eye motility examination. In the neonate, the position of the eyes varies greatly. Most infants display intermittent outward deviation (exotropia), which usually disappears within the first few months of life. Any constant inward (esotropia) or outward deviation should be evaluated for a possible nerve or muscle palsy. Intermittent nystagmus (rapid back and forth movements of the eye) is a common finding in the newborn. Persistent nystagmus is abnormal; patients with this disorder should be referred for further evaluation (Tappero & Honeyfield, 2009).

The infant's ability to see can be assessed immediately after birth. An infant who sees will look at and follow brightly colored objects. The examiner should hold the object steady about 7 to 9 inches from the infant's eye until the newborn fixates on it (the examiner notes the reflection of the object in the middle of the newborn's pupil). Newborns should be able to follow an object in either direction from a midline or central position. Care should be taken to eliminate distractions and to avoid talking because infants respond best to the presentation of one stimulus at a time.

Determining visual acuity in a newborn is difficult. Several methods can be used, including visual preference charts and visual evoked potentials. At term, newborn visual acuity ranges from 20/100 to 20/400, depending on the testing method used. This improves to 20/80 to 20/200 by 4 months of age, 20/40 to 20/80 by 12 months of age, and 20/20 by 2 years of age. According to one study looking at refractive errors at birth and gestational age, the authors state that all newborns are born with some degree of myopia (Varughese et al., 2005). They examined 1,200 newborns in the first week of life, who were born between 24 and 43 weeks gestation. The degree of myopia was inversely proportional to the gestational age, with the most significant myopia seen in very-low-birth-weight infants. Approximately 68% of the infants also had astigmatism.

Several important measurements should be obtained during an eye examination. The interpupillary distance and the width of the palpebral fissure should be determined; abnormal values may indicate an underlying syndrome, such as fetal alcohol syndrome. The interpupillary distance (the distance from midpupil to midpupil when the eyes are looking forward) determines whether the eyes are spaced appropriately. Abnormal findings are hypotelorism (eyes too close together) or hypertelorism (eyes too far apart). The width of the palpebral fissure is the distance from the medial canthus to the lateral canthus of each eye; this measurement determines the appropriateness of the opening for the eye (Table 17.2). The measurements obtained should be compared with published norms to determine if the value is normal or abnormal. Infants of diabetic mothers should be carefully examined for displaced inner canthi, lens opacity, microphthalmos, tear duct obstruction, and ocular lipoma.

Though not a routine procedure on normal newborns, a retinal exam can be done with an ophthalmoscope and pupil dilation if needed. About 34% of newborns will have retinal hemorrhages, most often in the posterior pole (Emerson, Pieramici, Stoessel, Berreen, & Gariano, 2001). The risk of retinal hemorrhage is greater with vacuum-assisted delivery and diminished with delivery by cesarean section. Most retinal hemorrhages from birth resolve within 2 weeks; however, resolution of retinal hemorrhages in the newborns of women who have had induced labor or forcep deliveries may take up to 8 weeks to resolve and would need to be part of a differential diagnosis with a shaken baby evaluation (Hughes, May, Talbot, & Parsons, 2006).

TABLE 17.2

EXTERNAL EYE DIMENSIONS (TERM NEWBORN)

Interpupillary distance	33–46 mm (average 39 mm)
Inner canthal distance	13–26 mm (average 20 mm)
Palpebral width (medial to lateral canthus)	17–22 mm (average 18 mm)
Pupil size	2–4 mm
Cornea	9–10 mm

Adapted from Jones (2006); Kaufman et al. (2010); and Scanlon, Nelson, Grylack, and Smith (1979).

Eye Drops

Great care must be taken in the selection of dilating drops for use in newborns. Systemic absorption of eye drops, although unavoidable to some extent, can cause severe reactions, especially in higher concentrations. Cardiovascular consequences, including arterial hypertension, a predisposing factor for intracranial hemorrhage, have been reported in premature infants (Jalali et al., 2003). Necrotizing enterocolitis (NEC), gastric distension, and feeding intolerance have also been reported in premature infants after eye examinations (Nair, Pai, daCosta, & Khusaiby, 2000; Sarici, Yurdakok, & Unal, 2001).

Excess medication that flows out of the eyelids is easily absorbed through the porous skin of the newborn and should be wiped off to prevent systemic absorption. Medication can also be absorbed from the nasolacrimal system; this can be minimized by applying pressure with a fingertip over the nasolacrimal duct for approximately 1 minute after instillation of the drops.

The mydriatics most often used are cyclopentolate, phenylephrine, and tropicamide. For maximum dilation and minimum risk of side effects, a combination of drugs routinely is used in most clinical settings. According to Chew, Ropilah, Shafie, and Mohamad (2005), the combination of cyclopentolate 0.2% and phenylephrine 1% produced better mydriasis with fewer systemic side effects in infants with dark irises. This randomized, double-blinded clinical trial compared cyclopentolate 1% and phenylephrine 2.5%, tropicamide 1% and phenylephrine 2.5%, and cyclopentolate 0.2% and phenylephrine 1% in preterm infants undergoing screening for ROP. Although all three regimens resulted in pupillary dilation, the higher dosed mydriatics were associated with significant increases in blood pressure and more feeding intolerance. In another prospective, randomized study, eight different regimens were studied in a population of full-term infants (Ogut et al., 1996). The drug associated with maximum side effects was phenylephrine 2.5%. The safest drug was tropicamide 1%, whereas cyclopentolate 0.5% in combination with tropicamide 0.5% and phenylephrine 2.5% produced the best mydriasis. According to Bolt, Benz, Koerner, and Bossi (1992), phenylephrine 2.5% with tropicamide 0.5% produced mydriasis in preterm infants without systemic adverse effects.

After the examination, the infant's eyes should be shielded from light until the pupils return to normal size. The eyes can be covered with occlusive eye shields, such as phototherapy shields, or a cover can be placed over the baby's incubator. Unshielded, dilated eyes are very sensitive to light. Excessive light entering a dilated pupil may cause intense pain. In premature infants or those with underlying health problems, the reaction to the pain may involve systemic responses, such as apnea, bradycardia, cyanosis, and agitation (Wood & Kaufman, 2009).

NEONATAL CONJUNCTIVITIS

Any conjunctivitis that occurs in the first 28 days of life is classified as neonatal conjunctivitis, according to the World Health Organization (WHO). Neonatal conjunctivitis can be classified as aseptic or septic. Aseptic conjunctivitis is often a chemical reaction to prophylactic medication administered shortly after birth to prevent gonorrheal disease of the newborn's eyes. The Centers for Disease Control's National Nosocomial Infections Surveillance (NNIS) program defines conjunctivitis as the isolation of culture positive pathogens from purulent discharge obtained from the conjunctiva or contiguous tissues such as eyelids or cornea, or redness and/or pain in the conjunctiva or eye and the presence of one of the following: purulent discharge, organisms and/or white blood cells present in the Gram stain of the exudate, positive antigen test, positive viral culture, positive single antibody titer, or the presence of multinucleated giant cells visible under microscopy (Horan & Gaynes, 2004). This definition is used for infections in neonatal intensive care units, although it has been shown to miss 38% of the cases of neonatal conjunctivitis in two large neonatal intensive care units (Haas, Larson, Ross, See, & Saiman, 2005).

Septic conjunctivitis in the newborn is an infection of the conjunctiva (the thin, translucent mucous membrane covering the cornea) caused by a variety of bacteria, viruses, and other organisms. The incidence of septic neonatal conjunctivitis in the United States is 1% to 2%. Chlamydial infection has replaced gonorrhea as the most common cause of septic eye infection in many countries (Rours et al., 2008). Septic neonatal conjunctivitis usually manifests with a discharge that develops shortly after birth. Because the origins of newborn conjunctivitis can vary, laboratory investigations are important in determining the exact cause. In some cases of conjunctivitis, rapid treatment is important to prevent vision loss.

The presentation of neonatal conjunctivitis varies with the cause of the inflammation or infection. Some findings, such as purulent eye discharge and erythema and edema of the eyelids and conjunctiva, are present in most cases. Transient tearing or watery discharge may be noticed early in the infection process.

Aseptic Neonatal Conjunctivitis

Most of the United States requires prophylaxis against neonatal gonorrheal conjunctivitis. According to the American Academy of Pediatrics (AAP), topical 1% silver nitrate solution, 0.5% erythromycin ointment, and 1% tetracycline ointment are equally effective (AAP, 2012). Although not available commercially in the United States as single-dose vials or tubes, 2.5% povidone-iodine solution is another safe treatment option (Richter et al., 2006). Erythromycin ophthalmic ointment (0.5%) is the *only* Centers for Disease Control and Prevention (CDC) recommended therapy for prophylaxis of ophthalmia neonatorum available in the United States (Mabry-Hernandez & Oliverio-Hoffman, 2010).

Silver nitrate was first used as a prophylactic agent against ophthalmia neonatorum caused by the bacteria *Neisseria gonorrhea* and other bacteria in 1881. One drop of 1% silver nitrate into the eyes of newborns prevented gonococcal infection, corneal scarring, and possible blindness. During the early 1900s, many state legislatures passed laws requiring physicians to treat all newborns with a silver nitrate solution. The problem that occurred in the majority of infants was that silver nitrate caused a chemical conjunctivitis with a purulent discharge, inflammation, and swelling of the eyes. The chemical conjunctivitis usually resolved within 24 to 48 hours after birth (Standler, 2006). Although penicillins were discovered in the late 1940s, silver nitrate continued to be used as the main prophylactic agent until the mid-1990s. Today, silver nitrate solutions have been replaced by erythromycin as the drug of choice for neonatal ocular prophylaxis in the United States as recommended by the AAP, since tetracycline 1% is no longer available in the United States (Mabry-Hernandez & Oliverio-Hoffman, 2010). WHO recommends either 1% silver nitrate solution or 1% tetracycline ointment, with additional treatment for infants born to mothers with gonorrhea (WHO, 2004). Silver nitrate was effective against *Neisseria gonorrhea* and most bacteria; however, it was not effective against Chlamydia organisms. For this reason, erythromycin ointment is now used for routine prophylaxis in newborn eyes after birth. Erythromycin and tetracycline ointments are both effective against a variety of microorganisms, including chlamydia and gonorrhea. These ointments rarely cause irritation to the newborn's eyes. Because erythromycin is only about 70% to 80% effective, a second dose may be needed.

Chlamydial Conjunctivitis (Inclusion Conjunctivitis)

Chlamydia trachomatis has been recognized as the most common cause of conjunctivitis in the newborn. The bacteria are transmitted from the infected mother to the infant at birth, and conjunctivitis usually appears 4 to 14 days later. The condition may be mild or moderate, and with proper treatment it resolves within 6 weeks. Clinical symptoms include swelling of one or both eyelids and mucopurulent discharge. Chronic infection can lead to more serious consequences, such as conjunctival scarring, adhesions of the eyelid, and deposits of connective tissue under the cornea.

The diagnosis is made from laboratory tests. The conjunctiva is scraped with a spatula, and a smear is made for Giemsa staining; classically this reveals a dark-staining cytoplasmic inclusion body. Cell cultures, direct fluorescent antibody (DFA) staining, enzyme immunoassay (EIA), nucleic acid amplification testing (NAAT), or polymerase chain reaction (PCR) methods should be done to confirm the diagnosis. The organisms of the chlamydia species are obligate intracellular organisms, so the specimens collected must be obtained from the conjunctival cells, not just the drainage (Chandran & Boykan, 2009). In one study in Iran, PCR had the highest sensitivity, 100% with 96% specificity, whereas Giemsa staining sensitivity was 58%, and cell cultures were only positive in 13% of the infants (Tabatabaei et al., 2012).

Topical eye treatment should consist of application of sulfacetamide drops or ointment for 3 weeks. Although the eye infection generally is not serious, a chlamydial pneumonitis develops in 3% to 18% of infected neonates (Kakar et al., 2010). Systemic therapy with oral erythromycin for 3 weeks often is necessary to eradicate the organism from the respiratory tract.

Gonorrheal Conjunctivitis

Routine prophylaxis of neonates has greatly reduced the incidence of gonorrheal conjunctivitis. Because of the potential for blindness from this infection, early detection and prompt treatment are critical. Gonorrheal conjunctivitis typically manifests as an acute, purulent, bilateral conjunctivitis with eyelid edema. If not treated appropriately and quickly, the infection may progress to corneal ulceration, endophthalmitis, and perforation of the globe (de Alba Campomanes et al., 2012). Gram stains and cultures should be performed routinely in all cases of neonatal conjunctivitis. The presence of *N. gonorrhea* confirms the diagnosis. Treatment consists of administration of intravenous or intramuscular antibiotics and application of topical ointment to the eye. Irrigation of the eye with sterile saline may be necessary to remove drainage.

Staphylococcal Conjunctivitis

Staphylococcal conjunctivitis is a bacterial infection usually acquired during vaginal delivery or by contact with an infected mother or nursery personnel. Symptoms normally appear 2 to 4 weeks after birth. In most cases the conjunctivitis is mild and produces a purulent discharge. It may progress to corneal ulceration, endophthalmitis, or generalized skin infection. The diagnosis is made with cultures and Gram stain. Because staphylococci can be found in the conjunctiva of healthy neonates, laboratory results should be interpreted cautiously. Treatment includes application of topical bacitracin or erythromycin ointment and cleansing of exudate from the eyelids.

Herpes Simplex Conjunctivitis

Herpes simplex infection at birth may be a feature of either localized or systemic disease. The neonate is usually infected during passage through the birth canal. The conjunctivitis manifests with eyelid swelling, conjunctival inflammation, corneal opacity, and epithelial dendrites. The dendrites can best be seen if the cornea is stained with a fluorescein dye and then examined under the blue light of a portable slit-lamp. The onset of the conjunctivitis usually is 2 to 14 days after birth. The disseminated form of the disease may also lead to cataracts, optic neuritis, apnea, respiratory distress, and death.

Diagnosis through laboratory findings is based on conjunctival epithelial scrapings for Giemsa staining and tissue cultures. The Giemsa stain should reveal multinucleated giant cells and intranuclear inclusion. Fluorescent antibody techniques are also helpful for making the diagnosis. This disease should always be kept in mind when the mother or father has a history of genital herpes. Treatment should be instituted with application of the topical antiviral trifluridine. Systemic treatment (intravenous) is necessary for infants whose conjunctivitis has spread to be a systemic infection.

Infectious Conjunctivitis Caused by Other Microorganisms

Case reports describing neonatal infectious conjunctivitis caused by unusual microorganisms have increased in the professional literature. Although most of the case reports describe infections in hospitalized premature infants, including preterm infants with meningitis, some reports concerned term infants who were readmitted with conjunctivitis caused by *Neisseria meningitides* (Dinakaran & Desai, 1999; Kurlenda, Pabich, & Grinholc, 2010; Lehman, 1999). All infants required local and systemic treatment. Because *Neisseria meningitidis* can cause a serious infection resulting in significant morbidity and mortality, it is important to differentiate this organism from other gram-negative diplococci, such as *Neisseria gonorrhea* (Lehman, 1999). Individuals exposed to *Neisseria meningitidis* are considered high-risk contacts and should be treated with chemoprophylaxis (Lehman, 1999).

There have been quite a few case reports of serious eye infections in preterm infants caused by *Pseudomonas aeruginosa*. Many were cases of endophthalmitis, which is an infection of the vitreous humor and the internal tissues of the eye, resulting from bacteria crossing the blood-ocular barrier (Figueiredo, Joao, Mateus, Varandas, & Ferraz, 2009; O'Keefe, Nolan, Lanigan, & Murphy, 2005; Wasserman, Sondhi, & Carr, 1999). On physical exam, the infants developed a purulent discharge from the eyes following a systemic infection. This is called endogenous (coming from internal sources) endophthalmitis. Exogenous (coming from the outside) endophthalmitis is caused by bacteria gaining access to the internal eye via trauma or perforation. Most neonatal cases of endophthalmitis are endogenous. According to a recent study, the incidence of neonatal endophthalmitis is decreasing in the United States, and most of the infants with endophthalmitis also have a systemic bacteremia or Candidemia and are very-low-birth-weight infants (Egan, 2011; Moshfeghi, Charalel, Hernandez-Boussard, Mortan, & Moshfeghi, 2011).

Premature infants in the neonatal intensive care units (NICU) frequently are colonized with a variety of *Candida* species. Despite the increased incidence of *Candida* sepsis in premature infants, ocular involvement usually is limited to a chorioretinitis that resolves with systemic antifungal therapy (Shah, McKey, Spirn, & Maguire, 2008). Several reports have been published describing severe candidal eye disease that required surgical intervention with lensectomy and vitrectomy (Drohan, Colby, Brindle, Sanislo, & Ariagno, 2002; Johnston & Cogen, 2000; Shah, Vander, & Eagle, 2000; Stern, Calvano, & Simon, 2001). These reports described the development of either cataracts or glaucoma in very-low-birth-weight infants born between 24 and 26 weeks with systemic *Candida* infections. So even with the decreasing rates of endophthalmitis, the very-low-birth-weight infants are at significant risk for these serious and often deadly complications.

The conjunctiva can also be the portal of entry of nosocomial pathogens or hospital-acquired conjunctivitis in the NICU. Organisms seen were coagulase-negative *Staphylococcus* as the most common (22%), *Klebsiella pneumonia* (7%–18%), *Escherichia coli* (5%–16%), methicillin-susceptible *Staphylococcus aureus* (4%–13%), and *enterococcus* species (1%–5%), with gram-positive cocci being most resistant (Borer et al., 2010). A case report from Italy describes the horizontal transmission of *Candida parapsilosis*, a pathogen normally associated with indwelling catheters (e.g., percutaneously inserted central lines), from the nursing staff to a preterm infant (Lupetti et al., 2002). The preterm infant developed candidemia. Molecular typing determined the organism was transferred from the hands of two nurses to the infant's conjunctiva, and then to the bloodstream.

Adenovirus type 8 was the cause of outbreaks of keratoconjunctivitis in NICUs in Europe and the Middle East (Chaberny, Schnitzler, Geiss, & Wendt, 2003; Ersoy et al., 2012; Percivalle et al., 2003). The virus was identified with PCR, and antibody technologies were used to document the presence of the virus in patients and nursery staff.

LACRIMAL DYSFUNCTION

Obstructed Nasolacrimal Duct

Blockage of the nasolacrimal duct occurs when the duct fails to canalize at the entrance to the nose, leaving a thin mucosal membrane. This blockage occurs in 5% to 6% of all newborns and is a common cause of chronic conjunctivitis in infants (de Alba Campomanes et al., 2012). After 1 month of age, the infant shows excessive tearing and mucus discharge in the inner canthal region. Pressure on the lacrimal sac area usually causes pus or mucus to exude from the puncta. Because the problem resolves spontaneously in most affected neonates by 6 months of age, conservative treatment involving lacrimal massage and application of topical antibiotics is recommended. Dacryocystitis can occur as a result of this temporary obstruction. Dacryocystitis is a secondary infection of the lacrimal sac. Obstruction that lasts beyond 6 to 12 months may require lacrimal probing. Nasolacrimal duct blockage must be differentiated from other causes of conjunctivitis, a foreign body on the eye, or corneal injury.

Mucocele

Mucoceles occur because of the one-way valve effect at the end of the nasolacrimal duct. Mucus accumulates or amniotic fluid is trapped in the nasolacrimal sac, and the infant develops a bluish mass in the inferomedial region of the eyelid. This swelling most often is confused with a hemangioma. If simple massage does not decompress the mucocele, probing of the nasolacrimal duct may be necessary.

ROP

ROP, a disease arising from proliferation of abnormal blood vessels in the newborn retina, was first reported by Terry in 1942. His description of a fibrous growth behind the lens and retinal detachment in premature infants gave birth to the name retrolental fibroplasia (RLF). The name was changed to ROP in 1984 by an international committee charged with providing a uniform classification system for the disease. The original classification system, International Classification of Retinopathy of Prematurity (ICROP), used a standard description of the location of retinopathy (using zones and clock hours), the severity of the disease (stage), the presence of special risk factors (plus disease), and the features of regression (International Committee for the Classification of ROP, 1984) (see Figure 17.2 for zone diagram).

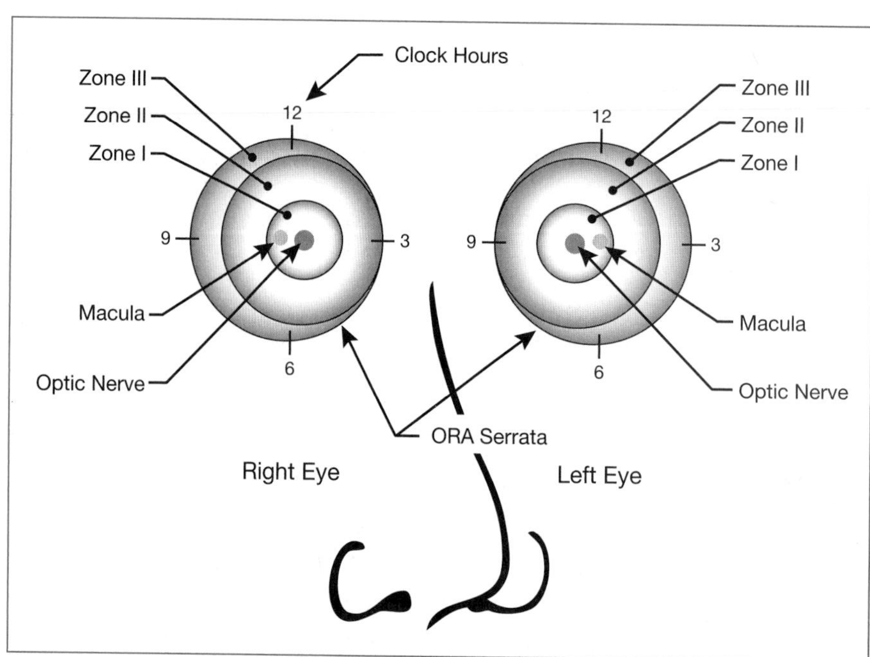

FIGURE 17.2 Diagram of zones of the eyes.

In 2005, the International Committee for the Classification of ROP published updates to the original ICROP. Three changes to the ICROP were introduced: (1) recognition of a more virulent form of ROP, aggressive posterior ROP (AP-ROP); (2) an intermediate grade of plus disease (pre plus) that occurs between normal posterior pole vessels and frank plus disease; and (3) a clinical tool for estimating the extent of zone I involvement.

AP-ROP is defined as a rapid, progressive form of ROP that quickly progresses to stage 5 ROP if left untreated. Characteristics of AP-ROP include posterior location and prominence of plus disease, usually in zone I, but may be in posterior zone II. Because of the aggressive nature of this disease, the diagnosis of AP-ROP is normally made during a single examination. The diagnosis of plus disease was modified from presence of vascular dilatation and tortuosity in four quadrants to two quadrants. The new recommendations also included adding the + symbol after the ROP stage number to designate the presence of plus disease (e.g., stage 3+). The new term of preplus disease was defined as vascular abnormalities of the posterior pole that are insufficient for the diagnosis of plus disease but that demonstrate more arterial tortuosity and more venous dilatation than normal.

The 1986 multicenter CRYO-ROP trial led to the definition of threshold and prethreshold ROP. Threshold disease was considered the minimum disease needed for treatment. The 2000 to 2002 multicenter ET-ROP trial results substituted type 1 and type 2 as the equivalent but newly defined intervention and pre intervention point. Type 1 is defined as zone 1, any stage ROP with plus disease; zone I, stage 3 ROP without plus disease; or zone II, stage 2 or 3 with plus disease. Type 2 ROP is defined as zone I, stage 1 or 2 ROP without plus disease; or zone II, stage 3 ROP without plus disease (Reynolds, 2010).

ROP was responsible for an epidemic of blindness in young children in the 1940s and early 1950s until the link to supplemental oxygen therapy was made in 1952. Subsequently, the practice of limiting oxygen administration in the care of premature infants led to the near disappearance of the disorder; however, cerebral palsy and death increased. Improvements in neonatal health care in the past 35 years have increased the survival of tinier and sicker infants. As technology helped these smaller infants survive, the rate of ROP rose. The younger the gestational age and the lower the birth weight the more strongly these correlate with the incidence of ROP (Drack, 2006). Results from the CRYO-ROP, LIGHT-ROP, and ET-ROP multicenter trials, revealed that ROP occurs in 65% to 70% of premature infants with birth weights of 1,250 g or less (ET-ROP, 2003, 2005; Reynolds et al., 2002; Reynolds, 2010) (see Table 17.3 for information on research studies relating to the risk factors, incidence, treatment, and severity of ROP).

Pathophysiology

ROP is a disease caused by an abnormal adaptation of normal maturational processes in the face of physiologic stress. The disease develops gradually and is divided into five stages of increasing clinical severity (Table 17.4). Some ophthalmologists will use the term stage 0 if the retina's vascularity is immature.

The key factor in the development of ROP, especially in premature infants, is the developing retinal blood vessels. The pathophysiology of ROP occurs in two phases. Phase I is delayed growth of the retinal vascularity following preterm birth. Phase II occurs when the hypoxia created during phase I stimulates the growth of new blood vessels (Smith, 2003). Retinal vascularization begins at the optic nerve at about 16 weeks gestation. Retinal vascular development proceeds slowly and reaches the retinal periphery (ora serrata retinae) during the ninth month of gestation (Vander, 1994). The incompletely vascularized retina has a peripheral avascular zone that varies with the degree of immaturity of the retina (Smith, 2003). The in utero growth of retinal blood vessels is stimulated by the release of vascular endothelial growth factor (VEGF) and insulin-like growth factor-1 (IGF-1). VEGF is found at the front line of the growing retinal blood vessels, whereas IGF-1 is maintained at a constant level in the retina microenvironment. VEGF is a cytokine regulated by the amount of oxygen (hypoxia). IGF-1 is a nonoxygen-regulated cytokine involved in the regulation of endothelial cell survival and proliferation (Smith, 2004).

Following preterm birth, the normal growth of the retina vascularity stops and some of the already developed vessels are lost. The retina, however, remains metabolically active and becomes hypoxic because of the lack of blood vessels. This hypoxia becomes a potent inducer of new vessel growth (neovascularization) by stimulating the expression of VEGF at 32 to 34 weeks postmenstrual age. As the new blood vessels proliferate, they tend to grow into the vitreous and cause bleeding and the formation of fibrous tissue (Smith, 2003).

Many preterm infants in the NICU receive supplemental oxygen to treat their respiratory distress. The hyperoxia caused by oxygen use suppresses VEGF and IGF-1, resulting in programmed cell death, or apoptosis, of vascular endothelial cells, which in turn causes hyperoxia-induced vaso-obliteration and scarring of the retinal vessels (Smith, 2004).

As the preterm infant matures, the growing retina triggers a release of VEGF; IGF-1 levels will also rise. This creates an environment for new vessel growth (neovascular proliferation) that leads to the progression of retinopathy (Smith, 2003). Milder degrees of ROP are often transient and regress once the abnormal stimuli are removed or corrected. Moderate retinopathy can lead to excessive fibrous tissue formation or scarring in the peripheral retina, which may lead to traction on the macula and reduced vision. In severe cases of ROP, fibrous tissue development may lead to retinal detachment and blindness. Severely affected neonates may also have leukocoria, glaucoma, or both.

Risk Factors

ROP is a multifactorial disease that occurs primarily in premature infants. Although many risk factors have been identified, prematurity and low birth weight remain the most important factors leading to the development of ROP (Allegaert, deCoen, Devilieger, & EpiBel Study Group, 2004; Chiang, Arons, Flynn, and Starren, 2004; Markestad et al.,

TABLE 17.3

ROP SCREENING GUIDELINES

Recommending Group	Infant Criteria	First Examination Date
American Academy of Pediatrics (AAP) American Academy of Ophthalmology (AAO) American Association of Pediatric Ophthalmology & Strabimus (AAPOS)	Birth weight < 1,500 g or gestational age ≤ 32 weeks Selected infants between 1,500 and 2,000 g with an unstable clinical course	GA at birth (weeks) / Age at initial exam (weeks) 22 / 9 23 / 8 24 / 7 25 / 6 26 / 5 27–32 / 4
Canadian Pediatric Society Canadian Association of Pediatric Ophthalmologists	Birth weight ≤ 1,250 g OR Gestational age ≤ 30 6/7 weeks	≤ 26 6/7 weeks at birth, age at initial exam should be at 31 weeks PMA ≥ 27 weeks at birth, infant should be 4 weeks chronologic age
Royal College of Ophthalmologists	Birth weight < 1,501 g or < 32 weeks at birth SHOULD be screened Birth weight < 1,251 g or < 31 weeks at birth MUST be screened	< 27 weeks at birth, initial exam should be at 30–31 weeks PMA 27–32 weeks at birth, initial exam should be at 4–5 weeks chronologic age > 32 weeks at birth, but with birth weight < 1,501 g, initial exam should be at 4–5 weeks chronologic age

From Section on Ophthalmology, American Academy of Pediatrics (AAP), American Academy of Ophthalmology (AAO), and American Association of Pediatric Ophthalmology and Strabimus (AAPOS) (2006).

TABLE 17.4

STAGES OF ROP WITH POSSIBLE OUTCOMES

Stage	Finding	Possible Outcome
1	Demarcation line at avascular retina	Complete resolution probable
2	Ridge with height and width	May resolve
3	Ridge with fibrosis extending into vitreous	May resolve; prevention of detachment needed if plus disease
4	Partial retinal detachment with or without fovea	Visual impairment
5	Complete retinal detachment	Visual impairment/Blindness

Adapted from Fleck and McIntosh (2009).

2005; Reynolds, 2010). According to Reynolds (2010), the incidence of ROP strongly correlates with birth weight and gestational age at birth. ROP is twice as common in infants born at less than 750 g than infants born between 1,000 and 1,250 g. Even more dramatic, these two groups have a seven-fold difference in the incidence of threshold ROP.

Other epidemiologic facts include a higher risk of ROP in White infants than Black infants, infants born at outlying hospitals that require transport to a Level III NICU, and infants of multiple births (Reynolds, 2010). Other risk factors are associated with the management of the extremely preterm infant; supplemental oxygen, fluctuating oxygen saturations, continuous positive pressure ventilation, intraventricular hemorrhage (IVH), acidosis, blood transfusions, maternal preeclampsia, and intrauterine growth restriction (Allegaert, de Coen, Devlieger, & the EpiBel Study Group, 2004; Anderson, Benitz, & Madan, 2004; Darlow et al., 2005; Reynolds, 2010; York, Landers, Kirby, Arbogast, & Penn, 2004).

According to Chow et al. (2003), the rate of severe, stage 3 and 4 ROP was reduced from 38% to 12% in infants with a birth weight less than 750 g by strictly maintaining oxygen saturations between 85% and 95% (and between 83%–93% on the smallest infants). The studies that keep oxygen saturations in the low 90% level can reduce the rate of severe ROP significantly (Drack, 2006). Recently, the BOOST II Collaborative Group (2013) published data showing a lower mortality rate in infants less than 28 weeks who were kept in lower oxygen (with saturations less than 90%) as compared to infants whose saturations remained higher than 90%. Their study shows that even though the rates of ROP can be lowered with lowered oxygen saturations, the higher risk of death in these tiny infants must also be considered. Therefore, many NICUs are now keeping oxygen saturation levels of the extremely premature infants in the low 90s.

Other factors such as breast milk feedings and the use of nitric oxide in the treatment of respiratory distress in preterm infants may provide some protection against the development of ROP. Hylander, Strobino, Pezzullo, and Dhanireddy (2001) found that preterm infants weighing less than 1,500 g at birth who received human milk feedings had a lower incidence of ROP when compared to preterm infants who were formula fed. The positive benefit of human milk feeding remained after adjusting for confounding variables such as birth weight, race, and duration of oxygen therapy. Mestan, Marks, Hecox, Huo, and Schreiber (2005) reported that treatment with nitric oxide improved the neurodevelopmental outcomes of preterm infants at 2 years of age. The incidence of severe ROP was 24% in the nitric oxide group and 46% in the placebo group of preterm infants.

Although most ROP occurs in premature infants, rare cases of the disease have been reported in full-term infants, stillborn infants, and infants who have not received supplemental oxygen. In several studies, variations in the Norrie disease gene, a gene responsible for an X-linked form of congenital retinal detachment or dysgenesis, were more common in infants with severe ROP than in those in whom the disease resolved on its own. Each individual carries genetic predispositions to certain disorders, but less understood are the genetic proclivities toward outside effects—trauma, hypoxia, and premature birth among them (Drack, 2006). Further research is needed to increase our understanding of the cause and the pathophysiology of this disease.

Treatment

Treatment of ROP can be divided into three categories: preventive, interdictive, and corrective. Until premature birth can be eradicated, the major focus of ROP treatment is early detection and appropriate follow-up of significant disease. Javitt, DeiCas, and Chiang (1993) estimated that properly timed screening and treatment for ROP is not only cost saving but may also save approximately 320 infants per year from a lifetime of blindness. Despite the international effort to standardize ROP and the efforts of the several multicenter, randomized clinical trials, no universally accepted guidelines exist for the screening of premature infants. Screening protocols vary from institution to institution, among different countries, and even with the level of development of the countries. Several widely used, published guidelines are summarized in Table 17.5 (American Academy of Pediatrics, 2006; Jefferies, 2010; Royal College of Ophthalmologists, 2008).

According to Roth et al. (2001), indirect ophthalmoscopy by an experienced ophthalmologist in the NICU has traditionally been considered the criterion standard method for detection of ROP. These examinations can be physiologically stressful for the infants, time consuming for the ophthalmologist, and costly for the medical system. A mydriatic agent (e.g., phenylephrine 2.5%, cyclopentolate 0.5%, or tropicamide 0.5%) is instilled topically for pupil dilation approximately 30 to 45 minutes prior to the exam. A topical anesthetic, such as 0.5% proparacaine HCl ophthalmic solution, should be instilled in each eye, to dull the corneal and conjunctival sensitivity and decrease the newborn's pain before the exam. A lid speculum and a sclera depressor, individually sterilized for each infant's examination, is used to visualize the peripheral retina and ora serrata, the anterior border of retinal vascularization, or retinopathy (Figure 17.3). Examinations are performed with the binocular indirect ophthalmoscope and 30-diopter lens, first evaluating the posterior pole and then the periphery with sclera depression. The presence or absence of ROP disease, its location and extent, and the presence or absence of plus disease are documented at the time of examination according to the international classification of ROP.

A wide-field digital camera (RetCam) is being used as an alternative to indirect ophthalmoscopy for screening infants for ROP. Retinal images taken by the camera can be stored, transmitted to an expert, reviewed, analyzed and sequentially compared over time and are useful for telemedicine purposes (Chawla et al., 2012). The same eye drops must be utilized to dilate the pupils and anesthetize the area. The eyelid speculum is also used, but the scleral depressor is not needed. A water-soluble gel is applied to serve as a barrier between the eye and the lens.

Timing for eye exams can be frustrating for not only the NICU staff, but also for the ophthalmologist. Often, the ophthalmologist may arrive to examine an infant when the infant is due to eat, or the infant has just completed his feed, or during the infant's scheduled "quiet time." Use of the RetCam allows examinations to be scheduled at the convenience of the NICU staff, are less traumatic to the infant, and provide for permanent documentation through the digital images (Roth et al., 2001) (Figure 17.4).

Oxygen monitoring has been the major emphasis in the prevention of ROP. Elaborate policies and practices for continuous monitoring of oxygenation have evolved over the years, including evasive methods (fiberoptic umbilical catheters) and noninvasive techniques (transcutaneous oxygen monitoring, and pulse oximetry). Despite these efforts, little data indicate a safe level of oxygenation in premature infants at risk for ROP (Saugstad, 2005). Early efforts at restricting oxygen delivery in the 1950s and 1960s traded visual problems for neurologic sequelae. Recent practice changes are aimed at minimizing oxygen exposure while preserving optimum functioning of vital organs. Further research is being done to determine appropriate strategies.

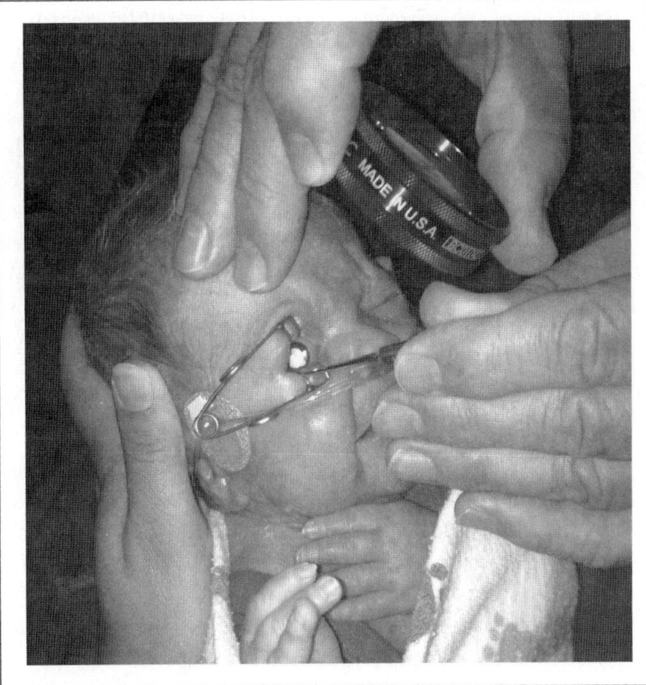

FIGURE 17.3 Photo of premature infant during eye exam undergoing indirect ophthalmoscopy using eyelid speculum and sclera depressor.

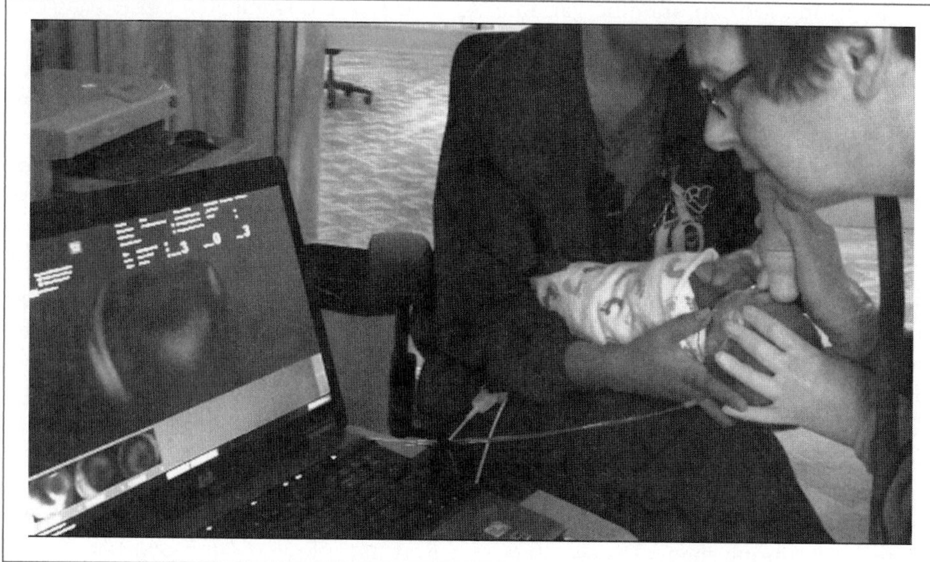

FIGURE 17.4 Photo of premature infant during retinal evaluation using the RetCam.

Environmental lighting in NICUs has been implicated as a contributing factor in the development of ROP. Although some clinical studies claimed to show this relationship, they had many limitations. A large multi-centered, randomized controlled trial (RCT) was completed and published in 1998, which showed that there was no statistically significant difference between the infants exposed to ambient lighting and those wearing light-reduction goggles during their first few weeks of life (Reynolds et al., 1998). Despite this evidence, many NICUs continue to institute reduced environmental lighting and shielding of incubators as part of a developmental approach to care.

The second strategy for treating ROP focuses on therapies aimed at minimizing or preventing blindness once the disease has developed. Interdictive therapies include cryotherapy, laser photocoagulation, and possibly treatment with bevacizumab.

Cryotherapy was developed in Japan in the 1970s. It gained popularity in the United States in the 1980s after the release of data from the Cryotherapy for ROP Study. Cryotherapy is a surgical procedure involving insertion of a probe cooled with liquid nitrogen on the medial aspect of the eye. Confluent spots on the avascular retina are ablated (destroyed by freezing), reducing the release of angiogenic factors that appear to induce retinal vasoproliferation.

Transpupillary laser photocoagulation delivered through an indirect ophthalmoscope has essentially replaced cryotherapy as the treatment of choice for ROP (Coats & Reddy, 2009). Argon and infrared diode lasers are used to ablate the avascular retina in a manner similar to that used in cryotherapy. Advantages of the laser photocoagulation therapy include the technical ease of performance and its usefulness in posterior ROP that was difficult to treat with cryotherapy, requires less eye manipulation. In addition, it is less traumatic for the patient, and there are fewer delayed consequences of myopia and retinal detachment. Using cost-utility analysis, health care economists have determined that laser ablation surgery for threshold ROP is cost effective (Brown & Brown, 2005; Brown, Brown, & Sharma, 2004).

Treatment can be performed in either the operating room or within the NICU. Sedation and either retrobulbar anesthesia or general anesthesia can be utilized, dependent on the preferences of the ophthalmologist and anesthesiologist, and the medical condition of the infant. Major potential complications of laser treatment include diminished peripheral vision, intraocular bleeding, cataract formation, myopia, and retinal detachment (Coats, 2009). A known side effect of laser ablation therapy is angle-closure glaucoma in infants with severe ROP (Trigler, Weaver, O'Neil, Barondes, & Freedman, 2005).

Results of multicenter clinical trials suggest that earlier treatment of ROP is more important than the type of treatment. The Early Treatment for ROP (ET-ROP) clinical trial found that unfavorable outcomes at the 9-month follow-up appointment were significantly reduced in the early treatment of eyes (ET-ROP Cooperative Group, 2003). Both cryotherapy and laser photocoagulation were used in the clinical trial, and the study group recommended retinal ablation therapy "for any eye with type 1 ROP" and serial examinations for those with type 2 ROP. In another study comparing early versus conventional treatment of prethreshold disease, no significant differences were noted in the prevalence of myopia (Davitt et al., 2005). Thus, it appears that early treatment of ROP is beneficial to the infant.

Recent research with bevacizumab has revealed a new treatment for ROP that is showing promising results. The U.S. Food and Drug Administration approved the use of bevacizumab for the treatment of metastatic colorectal cancer in 2004. The drug was shown to reduce the size and number of new vessels feeding the area of metastasis. Off-label use of bevacizumab for the treatment of neovascular ophthalmologic diseases began shortly thereafter (Bryant, 2011).

According to Mintz-Hittner, Kennedy, Chuang, and BEAT-ROP Cooperative Group (2011), bevacizumab is relatively inexpensive and is available for recommended use in infants with zone I posterior stage 3+ disease. Administration of the drug decreases the high levels of VEGF in the vitreous

TABLE 17.5

ROP STUDIES

First Author	Location	Years Included	Gestational Age of Subjects	Birth Weight of Subjects	Type of Study	Significant Findings
Good (Chair)	US ET-ROP	2000–2002		<1,250 g	Prospective	Incidence of ROP 68% with more zone I and prethreshold disease than in the CRYO-ROP study of 1986–1987. Incidence unchanged by race; however, more prethreshold disease seen in White infants
Markestad	Sweden	1999–2000	22–27 weeks	500–999 g	Prospective, observational	33% of 23 weeks preterm infants needed ROP treatment compared to 0% >25 weeks
Chiang	US	1996–2000	All newborns hospitalized for >28 days		Population-based cohort	ROP incidence by BW: <600 g—32% 600–799 g—38% 800–999 g—30% 1,000–1,199 g—17% 1,200–1,499 g—8% 1,500–1,999 g—4% 2,000–2,499 g—2%
Hussain	US	1989–1997	22–36 weeks	600–1,832 g	Retrospective	All ROP—21% ≥Stage 3—5% >32 weeks—0%
Gilbert	International NO-ROP Group	1996–2002	25.3–33.5 weeks	410–2,700 g	Observational	Mean GA/BW for severe ROP for: *Highly developed countries:* Canada 25.6/759 US 25.4/763 UK 25.3/737 *Moderately developed countries:* Argentina 30.2/1263 Brazil 27.7/952 Chile 26.8/903 Colombia 29.2/1,122 Cuba 30.7/1,285 Ecuador 33.5/1,259 Peru 29.1/1,051 *Poorly developed countries:* India 29.3/1,243 Vietnam 29.9/1,284
Lee	Canada	1996–1997	All admissions to Level 3 NICUs		Population-based cohort	Incidence of ROP: <1,500 g 43% >stage 3 11%
Larsson	Sweden	1988–1990 1998–2000		<1,500 g	Prospective comparison to 1988–1990 data in same geographic region	Total ROP stayed the same (36.4% 2000 vs. 40% 1990 Change in distribution noted: Incidence by GA: ≤26 weeks—23% vs. 14% 27–29 weeks—42% vs. 48% 30–32 weeks—32% vs. 30% ≥33 weeks—4% vs. 9% Incidence by BW: ≤750 g—9% vs. 5% 751–1,000 g—27% vs. 24% >1000 g—64% vs. 72%

(continued)

TABLE 17.5

ROP STUDIES (CONTINUED)

First Author	Location	Years Included	Gestational Age of Subjects	Birth Weight of Subjects	Type of Study	Significant Findings
Hameed	UK	1990–1994 1995–1999		≤1,250 g	Observational comparison in same geographic region	Survival—76% (1995–1999) Survival—62% (1990–1994) ≥Stage 3—12% (1995–1999) ≥Stage 3—4% (1990–1994)
O'Connor	US	1994–2000		≤1,250 g	Retrospective	Incidence of ROP increased from 2% to 5% Highest incidence and severity seen in BW <750 g
Fledelius	Denmark	1993–1997		<1,750 g	Retrospective	Incidence of ROP—10%
Mintz-Hittner	US Multicenter BEAT-ROP		<30 weeks	<1,500 g	Prospective, Randomized, Controlled	Increased efficacy of intravitreal bevacizumab as compared with conventional laser therapy for stage 3+ ROP when both zones I and II are considered
STOP-ROP	US Multicenter STOP-ROP	1994–1999			Prospective, Randomized, Controlled	Use of supplemental oxygen with pulse oximetry saturations of 96% to 99% did not cause additional progression of prethreshold ROP. But it also did not significantly reduce the number of infants requiring peripheral ablation surgery.
Reynolds	US Multicenter LIGHT-ROP	1995–1997	<31 weeks	<1,251 g	Prospective, Randomized, Controlled	A reduction in the ambient light exposure does not alter the incidence of ROP.
BOOST II	UK, Australia, New Zealand	2006–2010	<28 weeks	<1,100 grams	Prospective, Randomized Controlled	Targeting of oxygen saturation monitoring at levels less than 90% was associated with an increased death rate

gel; which are not reduced by conventional laser therapy. Development of peripheral retinal vessels continues after treatment with intravitreal bevacizumab, whereas conventional laser therapy leads to the permanent destruction of the peripheral retina. Compared to laser ablation surgery, where the infant requires intubation and where there is known peripheral field loss and possibly myopia, the use of bevacizumab is relatively benign; anesthesia is achieved through topical drops. The drug is administered intravitreously using a tiny needle. Ocular inflammation has been observed after seven or more injections of the drug.

The focus of corrective treatment is surgery for the repair of the detached retina. Scleral buckling, vitrectomy, or both, with or without lensectomy, are the techniques most often used. Scleral buckling involves the placement of a silicone or plastic band around the globe of the eye. The band is tightened which brings the sclera closer to the retina, facilitating retinal reattachment. This procedure is often performed in conjunction with laser therapy to salvage any remaining vision (Kaufman, Miller, & Gupta, 2010).

When retinal detachment progresses beyond the point of scleral buckling, the ophthalmologist must consider anatomic reattachment of the retina. Vitrectomy involves surgically opening the eye, removing the lens, and gently excising the proliferative scar tissue; this allows the retina to lie against the pigmented epithelium and, hopefully reattach. Despite the skill required for these procedures, most infants who undergo corrective therapy do not experience significant improvement in their vision. The best surgical reattachment rates (>50%) occurred when the surgery was performed on infants between 2 and 9 months of age. In addition, the level of visual function did not correlate with the degree of retinal reattachment. Poor visual outcomes have occurred regardless of the timeliness or delay in surgical reattachment (Ertzbischoff, 2004).

Outcome studies suggest that the incidence of long-term problems associated with ROP has been underestimated. Although studies on the natural history of ROP in the post-surfactant era consistently support an increased rate of mild ROP, which usually regresses, the consequences of severe ROP, especially stage 3 or greater, disease remain less than desirable. At 18 months of age, 34.5% of preterm infants with threshold ROP had complications consisting of strabismus, nystagmus, myopia, and late retinal detachment (O'Connor, Vohr, Tucker, & Cashore, 2003). Fifteen percent of the infants were legally blind.

Prematurity without ROP is also associated with poor visual outcomes. According to Cooke, Foulder-Hughes, Newsham, and Clarke (2004), preterm infants are three times more likely to wear glasses, three to four times more likely to have poor visual acuity or stereopsis (3D vision or depth perception), and 10 times more likely to have strabismus. Poor school performance in this population of preterm infants was also attributed to visual impairments. Because none of the infants with poor visual outcomes had IVH s or periventricular leukomalacia (PVL), poor school performance could not be explained by neurologic problems. Larsson, Rydberg, and Holmstrom (2005) showed that preterm infants have decreased distance and near vision acuities when compared to full-term infants.

Collaborative Care

Health professionals have to be concerned about care of the individual infant with ROP and the families of those infants. A nursery nurse may be caring for a convalescing infant who is being transported back to a community hospital, or an infant who is discharged prior to the first ROP screening examination. Attar, Gates, Iatrow, Lang, and Bratton (2005) found that infants transported back to a community hospital often missed their follow-up eye examinations when compared to those discharged directly from the regional perinatal-neonatal unit. The same authors found that infants discharged prior to their first ROP exam were more likely to miss follow-up eye care than those infants who had their first examination while in the NICU. It is imperative that there is clear, concise communication to the receiving hospital and to the parents about the importance of initial and follow-up eye examinations.

The development of ROP is concerning to parents of premature infants. Open communication between the neonatal health care team and the parents is crucial for helping the parents successfully cope with the stress of a hospitalized premature infant. At first, general information about the relationship of ROP and prematurity can be shared with the parents. After the initial eye examination has been performed, the information can be specific to their baby. The neonatal health care team must work closely with the ophthalmologist to provide a consistent message to the family. Parent teaching should focus on providing a basic understanding of ROP, the purpose of the screening examinations, and the importance of regular vision testing for their infant after discharge. Misconceptions about the disease and the use of oxygen need to be corrected.

Once ROP is diagnosed in an infant, parents may need more support than usual. Some parents may exhibit denial because they cannot see any physical evidence of a problem. Families of infants who need surgical intervention may feel greater stress from their concern for their infant's vision and may need the added communication with an ophthalmologist or retinal surgeon. NICU staff members can help parents cope by providing support during decision-making sessions with the eye specialists, by asking questions to clarify information, and by reinforcing information provided. It is also important to determine if parents are obtaining information from outside sources on the Internet. An analysis of 114 Internet sources on ROP found that 62.5% of the sites evaluated contained poor to fair information (Martins & Morse, 2005). Of the websites analyzed, 25% were academic, 20% were organizational, and 55% were commercial.

Information given to the parents about the prognosis of ROP in their infant must be included in any discharge planning. Parents need to understand that eye problems are more common in premature infants and may develop in infants with regressed ROP. Myopia (nearsightedness), strabismus (crossed eye), astigmatism, and amblyopia (lazy eye) are common sequelae. Glaucoma and late retinal detachment are common sequelae in infants with severe ROP.

Clearly, early detection and referral to programs for visual impairment are essential. Parents need to understand the importance of regular eye examinations by a pediatric ophthalmologist or by an ophthalmologist knowledgeable about ROP and its complications. Many families may benefit from referral to community resources, support groups, and special programs for children with visual problems.

Lastly, the nursing staff and unit managers have to maintain vigilance about infection control practices during eye examinations, laser ablation surgery, or intravitreal injections that occur within the NICU. Major risk factors for nosocomial infection are unwashed or poorly washed hands, and the sterility of instruments such as eyelid speculums and eye probes. In a study of NICU nurse managers representing 290 units, 72% reported that the unit provided that the instruments for eye examinations and 17% reported instruments were provided by the ophthalmologist (Hered, 2004). Nineteen percent of units reported that they reuse instruments. Eye infections occurring after ROP screening were acknowledged by 9% of the units. This study revealed that there is no consistency in practice regarding the cleaning and/or sterilization of ophthalmic instruments.

CONGENITAL DEFECTS

Aniridia

Aniridia is a severe ocular abnormality that manifests as a bilateral absence of the iris. Cataracts, corneal pannus, macular dysfunction, and glaucoma usually accompany the defect. Most of these infants have significantly diminished visual acuity, to a level of 20/200 or worse. About 25% of children with the noninherited form of aniridia eventually develop Wilms' tumor of the kidney with a deletion of the short arm of chromosome 11 (11p13) (Kaufman et al., 2010).

Persistent Hyperplastic Primary Vitreous

Persistent hyperplastic primary vitreous is a unilateral disorder that affects both genders equally. It results from persistence of the hyaloid vessels that connect the optic nerve and the posterior surface of the lens during fetal development. It should be considered in the differential diagnosis of leukocoria. The involved eye is usually small with an absent red reflex. Surgery may improve the integrity of the eye, and useful vision is sometimes restored.

Capillary Hemangioma of the Eyelid

Capillary hemangiomas of the eyelids are relatively common in newborns. They tend to appear on the eyelids and nape of the neck, and are sometimes referred to as salmon patches or stork bites. They usually disappear over time and require no treatment. The larger and deeper strawberry hemangiomas tends to enlarge, stabilize, and then regress by the time the child is between 5 and 10 years old. These hemangiomas are usually elevated and reddish purple at their peak size. There are also larger and deeper hemangiomas called cavernous hemangiomas that usually grow larger under the skin. No treatment is usually necessary, but treatment would depend on the location of the growth. Superficial tumors of the eyelid may cause cosmetic and visual problems. Parents often are concerned with hemangiomas on the face and want them removed, but no treatment is the best option to prevent scarring. Pressure on the globe from the tumor may result in significant astigmatism and subsequently amblyopia. These hemangiomas, may be treated with surgical removal, radiation, or steroid injections. Tumors that are exclusively cosmetic should be allowed to regress without intervention.

Another type of hemangioma is called the port-wine stain, because of its dark purple pigmentation and location on the face. It is also called nevus flammeus and is associated with Sturge–Weber syndrome. These birth marks are extensive and usually removed with laser therapy.

Ptosis

Ptosis is a drooping of one or both eyelids as a result of neurologic, muscular, or mechanical factors. If the ptosis is significant enough to cover the pupil, a dense amblyopia may result. If bilateral ptosis is present, the infant may have slowed motor development and delayed ambulation later in life. Congenital ptosis is usually caused by an abnormality in the development of the levator palpebrae muscle, but other causes can be third nerve palsy, Horner's syndrome, and plepharophimosis syndrome (de Alba Campomanes et al., 2012). A thorough family history should be obtained as well as ruling out birth trauma to the cervical ganglion. Direct trauma to the eyelid or a tumor in the eyelid may also cause ptosis. Surgical repair corrects this defect.

Congenital Glaucoma

Primary congenital glaucoma occurs rarely, but has been found to be an autosomal recessive eye disorder with its locus on the chromosome 2p21 (Stoilov, Akarsu, & Sarfarazi, 1997). Glaucoma is a disease in which the intraocular pressure is elevated to a level sufficient to damage the optic nerve. Because of the blinding potential of this disease, glaucoma must be detected early and treated properly. The affected neonate shows tearing, light sensitivity, eyelid spasm, and a large, cloudy cornea. The disease is slightly more common in males than in females. The diagnosis is often missed until the child is about 2 to 3 months of age. Conditions associated with glaucoma include trisomy 21, congenital rubella, Marfan syndrome, neurofibromatosis, oculodentodigital syndrome, Rieger's syndrome, Sturge–Weber syndrome, Rubinstein-Taybi syndrome, and Weill-Marchesani syndrome (Kaufman et al., 2010).

It is critical that congenital glaucoma be differentiated from other diseases that have similar symptoms. Nasolacrimal duct obstruction involves tearing but does not cause light sensitivity or a cloudy cornea. Difficult labor or forceps injury may damage the cornea and cause temporary clouding, but the intraocular pressure is not elevated, a hallmark feature of glaucoma. The large eyes of the infant with congenital glaucoma may appear beautiful to the parents, but health professionals should be alert to the possibility of this disease.

The abnormality in congenital glaucoma is a deformity of the filtering system that controls the level of intraocular pressure in the eye. Congenital glaucoma is treated surgically. The results usually are good, but parents must be educated about the need for continued monitoring of this condition throughout the child's life.

Congenital Cataracts

The causes of significant lens opacity in the newborn are numerous. Cataracts are an important cause of blindness because they may interfere with the process of visual development early in the infant's life. For this reason, visually significant cataracts must be detected and treated before they cause amblyopia; which may be unresponsive to the most persistent treatment.

Heredity is an important cause of congenital cataracts. A thorough family history is critical in determining the cause of the lens opacity. The inheritance pattern may be autosomal dominant, autosomal recessive, or sex linked. A maternal history of diabetes, x-ray exposure, or malnutrition may be an important factor in cataract formation. In premature infants, transient cataracts or insignificant opacities are commonly seen as a result of remnants of developmental tissues. ROP can also lead to cataracts in premature infants. Several inborn errors of metabolism cause cataracts, including galactosemia, Alport's syndrome, Fabry's disease, and Lowe syndrome. Intrauterine rubella infection is also associated with cataracts in the neonate.

Cataract surgery early in life is critical to the infant's visual rehabilitation. Useful vision is especially difficult to achieve in eyes with monocular cataracts. It is important for nurses to work closely with the infant's parents. The parents' persistence in handling contact lenses and in amblyopia therapy often determines the outcome for their child's vision.

Retinoblastoma

Retinoblastoma is the most common intraocular neoplasm in childhood. The tumor occurs in approximately 1 in 15,000 live births in the United States (Ray & Gombos, 2012). Most cases appear sporadically and occur in infants with no family history of the disease. An autosomal dominant pattern usually is responsible for the 5% to 10% of inherited retinoblastomas, most of which are bilateral. Autosomal dominant transmission occurs with an estimated 85% penetrance (Brantley & Harbour, 2001). A somatic mutation affecting the gene on chromosome 13q14 accounts for 80% of unilateral tumors (Ray & Gombos, 2012).

The most common presenting symptom is leukocoria. Most of the tumors are not detected in the neonatal period, except in infants with a positive family history. The tumor is highly malignant and may spread to the bone marrow, central nervous system (CNS), or other organs. Untreated patients rarely survive. The standard treatment for advanced cases of retinoblastoma is enucleation. Less severe cases are treated with radiation, laser photocoagulation, or cryotherapy. Children with this tumor require close follow-up for possible recurrence after treatment. Parents must be educated about the disease so that they are aware of the need for constant monitoring of their child.

CONGENITAL INFECTIONS

CMV Infection

Congenital CMV infection occurs in most infants with symptomatic disease and infrequently in asymptomatic infants. Ocular lesions include chorioretinitis, optic nerve atrophy, strabismus, cataract, macular scarring, and visual impairment. In a recent report from the Congenital CMV Longitudinal Study Group, 22% of the infants with symptomatic CMV disease had moderate to severe vision impairment, compared with 1% of the asymptomatic infants with CMV disease (Coats et al., 2000). The two common causes of severe visual impairment were optic atrophy and cortical visual impairment. Strabismus was also present in many of the symptomatic infants (Coats et al., 2000). Because of the risk for later development of strabismus and amblyopia, the authors recommend lifelong eye examinations for symptomatic infants (Coats et al., 2000).

Like many of the herpes family viruses, CMV can become active after periods of dormancy. Parents should be advised of this so that they can seek appropriate eye care if their child develops vision problems later in life.

Rubella

Congenital rubella is responsible for a wide variety of ocular complications, including pigmentary retinopathy, glaucoma, cataract, and microphthalmos. Although the clinical presentations range across a wide spectrum, newborns classically have hearing, eye, and cardiac defects.

Currently the incidence of congenital rubella syndrome is very low due to mandatory vaccination for rubella measles, but the incidence may increase as more parents withhold vaccinations in their children. Also, new information from long-term follow-up studies suggests that the prevalence of ocular problems is nearly twice the previously thought rate (78% instead of 43%). Several trends have also been noted, including an increase in cases of delayed disease and new associations of combination problems. Microphthalmia, cataracts, and glaucoma are more likely to occur in combination than independently. Pigmentary retinopathy produces a characteristic salt-and-pepper appearance and can result in sudden vision loss during adulthood. Poor visual acuity and diabetic retinopathy are also of concern in individuals with congenital rubella syndrome. The parents of an infant with congenital rubella need to understand that vision problems may occur at any time and that they must have their child screened regularly.

Herpes Simplex Virus

Herpes simplex virus causes a wide variety of eye disorders in newborns. Corey and Flynn (2000) reported a case of congenital herpes simplex infection that resulted in bilateral persistent fetal vasculature of the eye. Persistent fetal vasculature occurs when intraocular vessels fail to involute in utero. This involution is a normal part of eye development. Other eye conditions that can be seen with a herpes virus infection are conjunctivitis, chorioretinitis, and cataracts (de Alba Campomanes et al., 2012).

Varicella

Although rare, congenital infection caused by varicella, commonly known as chickenpox, produces eye anomalies in more than 50% of affected infants. These defects include microphthalmia, chorioretinitis, enophthalmia, cataract, optic nerve atrophy, nystagmus, and anisocoria (Choong, Patole, & Whitehall, 2000).

Toxoplasmosis

Toxoplasma gondii is a parasitic organism with an affinity for brain and eye tissue. As with many other congenital infections, ocular anomalies vary depending on fetal age at the time of infection. The most common clinical presentation is a focal necrotizing chorioretinitis. Other ocular manifestations include microphthalmia, traction retinal detachment, nystagmus, strabismus, cataracts, disruption of the retinal pigment epithelium, retinal dysplasia, and vitreitis (Berk, Oner, & Saatci, 2000; Roberts et al., 2001). Another study of congenital toxoplasmosis suggests that the inflammatory response mounted by the fetus and newborn contributes to irreversible retinal damage (Roberts et al., 2001).

Lymphocytic Choriomeningitis Virus

Another viral infection, lymphocytic choriomeningitis virus (LCV), can also cause ocular defects (Barton, Mets, & Beauchamp, 2002). Congenital LCV infection was first reported in the United States in 1993. LCV is a single-strand RNA virus found in rodents, including house mice and hamsters. Outbreaks of LCV infection associated with mice tend to occur in trailer parks, inner-city dwellings, and substandard housing. Laboratory mice and hamsters can also cause outbreaks among laboratory personnel. The virus is probably transmitted by airborne droplets and by food contaminated by rodent urine or feces. It also may be transmitted by the bite of an infected animal (Barton, Mets, & Beauchamp, 2002; Mets, Barton, Khan, & Ksiazek, 2000).

Neonates with congenital infection usually have microcephaly, hydrocephaly, and chorioretinitis. In one report, a 3-day-old boy who had microcephaly at birth was found to have chorioretinitis, conjunctivitis, congenital glaucoma, and a serious cardiac defect (single ventricle and pulmonary atresia). Further testing revealed positive antibody titers for LCV (Mets et al., 2000). Mets and colleagues concluded that "congenital LCV infection may be more common than previously appreciated" and that "serologic testing ... should be part of the standard workup for congenital chorioretinitis" (Mets et al., 2000). It also might be prudent to counsel women to avoid handling pet mice and hamsters during pregnancy.

OTHER DISORDERS THAT AFFECT THE EYES

Fetal Alcohol Syndrome

Ocular abnormalities are often overlooked in infants with fetal alcohol syndrome (FAS) because of the CNS damage, facial dysmorphia, and severe intrauterine growth restriction present in these infants. Abnormalities of the eyes common in infants with FAS include microphthalmos, coloboma, nystagmus, cataracts, glaucoma, microcornea, amblyopia, persistent hyperplastic primary vitreous, and refractive errors. Most affected infants have diminished visual acuity. One study found ocular evidence of FAS in previously undiagnosed children evaluated for developmental delay or hyperactivity disorders or both (Hug, Fitzgerald, & Cibis, 2000). This study suggests that FAS should be included in the differential diagnosis of infants undergoing eye examination for developmental delay or hyperactivity disorders.

Maternal Diabetes

Although maternal diabetes is recognized for its teratogenic effects, craniofacial anomalies are rarely reported. The presence of oculoauriculovertebral (OAV) complex in 14 infants of diabetic mothers who were insulin dependent or who were treated with oral hyperglycemic medications throughout their pregnancies has been reported (Ewart-Toland et al., 2000). Women with gestational diabetes were excluded from the study. The specific ocular anomalies noted in these infants were lens opacity, microphthalmia, optic nerve hypoplasia, laterally displaced inner canthi, tear duct obstruction, and ocular lipomas. Wang, Martinez-Frias, and Graham (2002) suggest that OAV occurs as a result of faulty neural crest cell migration in diabetic women with poor control during pregnancy.

PVL

PVL is a major cause of visual impairment in premature infants. Impairments found in infants with PVL included diminished visual acuity, eye movement disorders, and visual field restriction. Other eye problems included optic disc anomalies, nystagmus, strabismus, delayed visual maturation, and visual perceptual-cognitive problems (Jacobson & Dutton, 2000).

IVH

IVH without PVL is also associated with ocular morbidity (O'Keefe, Kafil-Hussain, Flitcroft, & Lanigan, 2001). Strabismus was present in 47% of infants with grade I and grade II IVH and in 42% of infants with grade III and grade IV IVH. Optical atrophy was present in 25% of infants with IVH. The incidence of ROP was also higher in this population of infants; no significant relationship to the grade of IVH was noted. Visual impairments were also common in infants with IVH, including smaller than average visual field, poor grating acuity, and poor recognition acuity (O'Keefe et al., 2001).

SUMMARY

Visual disturbances, although sometimes difficult to detect in newborns, can have a dramatic impact on a newborn's behavioral and psychosocial development. PVL has replaced ROP as the most common cause of serious eye disease in premature infants. Despite significant advances in the diagnosis, treatment, and follow-up of infants with very low birth weight and prematurity, visual morbidity continues to be a concern as smaller neonates survive neonatal intensive care.

Treatment of vision problems requires collaborative efforts among the neonatal health care team, the ophthalmologist, and the families of affected children. Clear, consistent communication between health care providers and parents, parental education, and good follow-up are important to the quality of care.

CASE STUDY

■ **Identification of the Problem.** Premature infants, especially those weighing less than 1,500 g, are at risk for complications from immature development of the eyes and the effects of supplemental oxygen on the developing eyes. As a result of the supportive therapies used in the neonatal intensive care unit, ROP can develop. This case study presents a patient born at 25 weeks of gestation who is presently 11 weeks of age or 36 weeks corrected gestational age. Due to his early birth, the infant has chronic lung disease (CLD), is on a mild diuretic, and continues to require a low amount of oxygen via nasal cannula. The plan is to discharge to home within 5 to 7 days.

■ Assessment: History and Physical Examination

Baby Boy TS was born on June 4, 2012 at 25 weeks gestation to a 23-year-old, gravida 1, para 0 mother whose pregnancy was complicated by preterm labor. She received prenatal care and delivered spontaneously by vaginal route following 2 days of unsuccessful tocolysis treatment and rupture of membranes approximately 15 hours prior to birth. Baby Boy TS was born with minimal respiratory effort, requiring intubation, bagging, and surfactant treatment in the delivery room, but was extubated to nasal continuous positive airway pressure (CPAP). By 4 hours of age, he required moderate ventilation and his condition deteriorated, requiring high-frequency oscillatory ventilation by 24 hours of age. He received a second dose of surfactant and remained on ventilation for approximately 3 weeks. He was weaned to nasal CPAP, to high-flow oxygen, and then to low-flow oxygen. He remains on 200 to 250 mL/min of oxygen via nasal cannula. He had umbilical lines placed after birth, PICC line for 12 days, started on NG feedings that were well-tolerated and advanced to full feedings. He has been nippling feeds with occasional apnea and bradycardia.

■ Physical Examination

- GENERAL: preterm, male infant
- HEENT: slight dolichocephaly, anterior fontanel soft and flat with widened sagittal sutures; eyes clear, no drainage

or redness; pupils reactive to light; positive red reflex OU; eyes and ears normoset with palate intact

- RESPIRATORY: lung fields clear and equal bilaterally; minimal respiratory effort; respiratory rate = 48 with saturations 89% to 93% on 200 ml/L nasal cannula oxygen
- CARDIOVASCULAR: regular rate and rhythm with no murmur; pulses strong, regular and equal in all extremities; good peripheral perfusion 2+/4+ and capillary blood refill time less than 3 seconds
- ABDOMEN: soft and nontender with no masses palpable and positive bowel sounds throughout; liver edge down 2 cm below right costal margin; no splenomegaly; patent anus
- GENITOURINARY: normal male genitalia with testes descended into scrotum bilaterally
- NEURO: awake and active; cries when distressed or disturbed; sleep pattern appropriate for near-term infant; normal tone and responsiveness for gestational age
- EXTREMITIES: moves all four extremities with normal range of motion; hips—no click; clavicles—no crepitus; good muscle tone of all extremities; ten digits per extremity
- SKIN: pink, warm, dry, and intact; no rashes or bruising noted; mucous membranes pink and moist

Premature infants are at risk for many complications due to their immaturity and treatments.

■ Premature Diagnoses

- Respiratory distress syndrome—can develop into CLD
- Hypoglycemia
- At risk for patent ductus arteriosus
- Possible sepsis/pneumonia
- At risk for IVH
- At risk for ROP
- Apnea of prematurity
- Anemia of prematurity

■ Rop Examinations

Dates	Age (weeks)	Gestational Age (weeks)	Results	Plan
July 16, 2012	6	31	Immature vascularity in both eyes (stage 0, zones 2–3 bilaterally)	Follow-up in 2 weeks
July 30, 2012	8	33	Stage 1–2, zone 2 with questionable plus disease	Follow-up in 1 week
August 6, 2012	9	34	Stage 2–3+, zone 2 on right; stage 2+, zone 2 on left	Referral for laser treatment
August 8, 2012	9 ½	34 ½	Stage 3+, zone 2 bilaterally	Laser photocoagulation was performed

According to the AAP, the first eye exam would be done at 6 weeks gestation.

■ Discharge Diagnoses

- Premature male infant
- CLD
- Apnea of prematurity
- ROP

EVIDENCE-BASED PRACTICE BOX

In evaluating infants with ROP, neonatal researchers have conducted studies to assess the effects of supplemental oxygen provided to preterm infants in the neonatal intensive care unit. There have been numerous studies on neonates with ROP or prevention of ROP (see Table 17.5). This table provides an in-depth look at studies between 1988 and 2010 on neonatal ROP prevention from around the world. The significant findings are listed within the table. On searching for meta-analyses of ROP studies, the Cochrane reviews (http://www.cochrane.org) has listed 20 literature summaries dealing with ROP in neonatal care. These summaries involve a variety of prevention methods, including uses of supplemental oxygen, early light reduction, retinal ablation therapy, and early versus late oxygen reduction.

On searching eye disorders, there are two literature summaries in neonatal care. There continue to be many studies on the prevention of eye disease and disorders, especially ROP. By searching Internet sites, nurses can find the newest evidence-based protocols for prevention of ROP and other eye disorders.

ONLINE RESOURCES

Family Practice Notebook—Newborn Eye Exam **http://www.fpnotebook.com/Nicu/Exam/NwbrnEyExm.htm**

University of Illinois Department of Ophthalmology and Visual Sciences EYE FACTS **http://www.uic.edu/com/eye/LearningAboutVision/EyeFacts/BabyEyes.shtml**

REFERENCES

Achim, C., & Yen, K. G. (2012). An infant with leukocoria. *Medscape ophthalmology—interactive case series*. Retrieved from http://www.medscape.com/viewarticle/759475

Allegaert, K., deCoen, K., Devilieger, H., & EpiBel Study Group. (2004). Threshold retinopathy at threshold of viability: The EpiBel study. *British Journal of Ophthalmology, 88*, 239–242.

American Academy of Pediatrics (AAP) Committee on Infectious Disease. (2012). *Red Book 2012, Section 5: Antimicrobial Prophylaxis, Prevention of Neonatal Ophthalmia* (pp. 880–881). Elk Grove Village, IL: AAP.

Anderson, C. G., Benitz, W. E., & Madan, A. (2004). Retinopathy of prematurity and pulse oximetry: A national survey of recent practices. *Journal of Perinatology, 24*, 164–168.

Attar, M. A., Gates, M. R., Iatrow, A. M., Lang, S. W., & Bratton, S. L. (2005). Barriers to screening infants for retinopathy of prematurity after discharge or transfer from a neonatal intensive care unit. *Journal of Perinatology, 25*(1), 36–40.

Barton, L. L., Mets, M. B., & Beauchamp, C. L. (2002). Lymphocytic choriomeningitis virus: Emerging fetal teratogen. *American Journal of Obstetrics and Gynecology, 187*(6), 1715–1716.

Berk, T. A., Oner, R. H., & Saatci, A. O. (2000). Underlying pathologies in secondary strabismus. *Strabismus, 8*(2), 69–75.

Bolt, B., Benz, B., Koerner, F., & Bossi, E. (1992). A mydriatic eye drop combination without systemic effects for premature infants: A prospective double-blind study. *Journal of Pediatric Ophthalmology and Strabismus, 29*(3), 157–162.

BOOST II Collaborative Groups—United Kingdom, Australia, & New Zealand (2013). Outcome saturations and outcomes in preterm infants. *New England Journal of Medicine, 368*, 1949–1950. doi: 10.1056/NEJMoa1302298

Borer, A., Livshiz-Rivenc, I., Golan, A., Saidel-Odes, L., Zmora, E., Raz, C., . . . Peled, N. (2010). Hospital-acquired conjunctivitis in a neonatal intensive care unit: Bacterial etiology and susceptibility patterns. *American Journal of Infection Control, 38*, 650–652.

Brantley, M. A., & Harbour, J. W. (2001). The molecular biology of retinoblastoma [Review]. *Ocular Immunology and Inflammation, 9*(1), 1–8.

Brown, M. M., & Brown, G. C. (2005). How to interpret a health care economic analysis. *Current Opinion in Ophthalmology, 16*(3), 191–194.

Brown, M. M., Brown, G. C., & Sharma, S. (2004). Value-based medicine and vitreoretinal diseases. *Current Opinion in Ophthalmology, 15*(3), 167–172.

Bryant, C. (2011). Research with bevacizumab offers hope in treatment of retinopathy of prematurity. *NANN Central, 27*(2), 4.

Chaberny, I. F., Schnitzler, P., Geiss, H. K., & Wendt, C. (2003). An outbreak of epidemic keratoconjunctivitis in a pediatric unit due to Adenovirus Type 8. *Infection Control and Hospital Epidemiology, 24*(7), 514–519.

Chandran, L., & Boykan, R. (2009). Chlamydial infections in children and adolescents. *Pediatrics in Review, 30*, 243–250. doi:10.1542/pir.30-7-243

Chawla, D., Agarwal, R., Deorari, A., Paul, V. K., Parijat, C., & Azad, R. V. (2012). Retinopathy of Prematurity. *Indian Journal of Pediatrics, 79*(4), 501–509.

Chew, C., Ropilah, A. R., Shafie, S. M., & Mohamad, Z. (2005). Comparison of mydriatic regimens used in screening for retinopathy of prematurity in preterm infants with dark irises. *Journal of Pediatric Ophthalmology and Strabismus, 42*(3), 166–173.

Chiang, M. F., Arons, R. R., Flynn, J. T., & Starren, J. B. (2004). Incidence of retinopathy of prematurity from 1996 to 2000: Analysis of a comprehensive New York State patient database. *Ophthalmology, 111*, 1317–1325.

Choong, C. S., Patole, S., & Whitehall, J. (2000). Congenital varicella syndrome in the absence of cutaneous lesions. *Journal of Paediatrics and Child Health, 36*(2), 184–185.

Chow, L.C., Wright, K.W., Sola, A., & the CSMC Oxygen Administration Study Group. (2003). Can changes in clinical practice decrease the incidence of severe retinopathy of prematurity in very low birth weight infants? *Pediatrics, 111* (2), 339-345. doi: 10.1542/peds.111.2.339

Coats, D. K., Demmler, G. J., Paysse, E. A., Du, L. T., Libby, C., & The Congenital CMV Longitudinal Study Group. (2000). Ophthalmologic findings in children with congenital cytomegalovirus infection. *Journal of American Association for Pediatric Ophthalmology and Strabismus, 4*(2), 110–116.

Coats, D. K., & Reddy, A. K. (2009). Retinopathy of prematurity. In M. E. Wilson, R. A. Saunders, & R. H. Trivedi (Eds), *Pediatric ophthalmology* (pp. 376–384). Berlin: Springer-Verlag.

Cooke, R.W. I., Foulder-Hughes, L., Newsham, D., & Clarke, D. (2004). Ophthalmic impairment at 7 years of age in children born very preterm. *Archives of Diseases in Childhood—Fetal-Neonatal Edition, 89*, F249-F253. doi: 10.1136/adc.2002.023374

Corey, R. P., & Flynn, J. T. (2000). Maternal intrauterine herpes simplex virus infection leading to persistent fetal vasculature. *Archives of Ophthalmology, 18*(6), 837–840.

Darlow, B. A., Hutchinson, J. L., Henderson-Smart, D. J., Donoghue, D. A., Simpson, J. M., Evans, N. J., & The Australian and New Zealand Neonatal Network. (2005). Prenatal risk factors for severe retinopathy of prematurity among very preterm infants of the Australian and New Zealand Neonatal Network. *Pediatrics, 115*(4), 990–996.

Davitt, B. V., Dobson, V., Good, W. V., Hardy, R. J., Quinn, G. E., Siatkowski, R. M., ... The Early Treatment for ROP Cooperative Group. (2005). Prevalence of myopia at 9 months in infants with high-risk prethreshold retinopathy of prematurity. *Ophthalmology, 112*, 1564–1568.

de Alba Campomanes, A. G., Binenbaum, G., & Quinn, G. E. (2012). Disorders of the eye. In C. A. Gleason & S. U. DeVaskar (Eds.), *Avery's diseases of the newborn* (9th ed.). Philadelphia, PA: Elsevier.

Dinakaran, S., & Desai, S. P. (1999). Central serous retinopathy associated with Weber-Christian disease. *European Journal of Ophthalmology, 9*(2), 139–141.

Drack, A. (2006). Retinopathy of prematurity. *Advances in Pediatrics, 53*, 211–226.

Drohan, L., Colby, C. E., Brindle, M. E., Sanislo, S., & Ariagno, R. L. (2002). Candida (Amphotericin-sensitive) lens abscess associated with decreasing arterial blood flow in a very low birth weight preterm infant. *Pediatrics, 110*, e65–e68. doi:10. 1542/peds.110.5.e65

Early Treatment for Retinopathy of Prematurity Cooperative Group (ET-ROP). (2003). Revised indications for the treatment of retinopathy of prematurity: Results of the early treatment for retinopathy of prematurity randomized trial. *Archives of Ophthalmology, 121*(12), 1684–1694.

Early Treatment for Retinopathy of Prematurity Cooperative Group (ET-ROP). (2005). The incidence and course of retinopathy of prematurity: Findings from the early treatment for retinopathy of prematurity study. *Pediatrics, 115*(1), 15–23. doi:10.1542/peds.2004-1413

Egan, D. J., Peters, J. R., & Peak, D. A. (2011). Endophthalmitis. *Medscape reference*. Retrieved from http://emedicine.medscape.com/article/799431-overview

Emerson, M. V., Pieramici, D. J., Stoessel, K. M., Berreen, J. P., & Gariano, R. F. (2001). Incidence and rate of disappearance of retinal hemorrhage in newborns. *Ophthalmology, 108*, 36–39.

Enzenauer, R. W., McCourt, E. A., Jatla, K. K., & Zhao, F. Neonatal Conjunctivitis. *Medscape reference*. Retrieved from http://emedicine.medscape.com/article/1192190-overview

Ersoy, Y., Otlu, B., Turkcuoglu, P., Yetkin, F., Aker, S., & Kuzucu, C. (2012). Outbreak of adenovirus serotype 8 conjunctivitis in preterm infants in a neonatal intensive care unit. *Journal of Hospital Infection, 80*, 144–149.

Ertzbischoff, L. M. (2004). A systematic review of anatomical and visual function outcomes in preterm infants after scleral buckle and vitrectomy for retinal detachment. *Advances in Neonatal Care, 4*(1), 10–19.

Ewart-Toland, A., Yankowitz, J., Winder, A., Imagire, R., Cox, V. A., Aylsworth, A. S., & Golabi, M. (2000). Oculoauriculovertebral abnormalities in children of diabetic mothers. *American Journal of Medical Genetics, 90*(4), 303–309.

Figueiredo, S., Joao, A., Mateus, M., Varandas, R., & Ferraz, L. (2009). Endogenous endophthalmitis caused by Pseudomonas aeruginosa in a preterm infant: A case report. *Cases Journal, 2*, 9304. Retrieved from http://www.casesjournal.com/content/2/1/9304

Fleck, B. W., & McIntosh, N. (2009). Retinopathy of prematurity: Recent developments. *NeoReviews, 10*(1), e20–e30. doi: 10.1542/neo.10-1-e20

Fledelius, H. C., Gote, H., Greisen, G., & Jensen, H. (2004). Surveillance for retinopathy of prematurity in a Copenhagen high-risk sample 1999–2001. Has progress reached a plateau? *Acta Ophthalmolologica Scandinavica, 82*, 32–37.

Gilbert, C., Fielder, A., Gordillo, L., Quinn, G., Semiglia, R., Visintin, P., . . . The International NO-ROP Group. (2005). Characteristics of infants with severe retinopathy of prematurity in countries with low, moderate, and high levels of development: Implications for screening programs. *Pediatrics, 115*(5), 518–525.

Haas, J., Larson, E., Ross, B., See, B., & Saiman, L. (2005). Epidemiology and diagnosis of hospital-acquired conjunctivitis among neonatal intensive care unit patients. *Pediatric Infectious Disease Journal, 24*(7), 586–589.

Hameed, B., Shyamanur, K., Kotecha, S., Manktelow, B. N., Woodruff, G., Graper, E. S., & Field, D. (2004). Trends in the incidence of severe retinopathy of prematurity in a geographically defined population over a 10-year period. *Pediatrics, 113*, 1653–1657.

Hered, R. W. (2004). Use of non-sterile instruments for examination for retinopathy of prematurity in the neonatal intensive care unit. *Journal of Pediatrics, 145*(3), 308–311.

Horan, T. C., & Gaynes, R. P. (2004). Surveillance of nosocomial infections. In C. G. Mayhall (Ed.), *Hospital epidemiology and infection control* (3rd ed., pp 1659–1702). Philadelphia, PA: Lippincott Williams & Wilkins.

Hug, T. E., Fitzgerald, K. M., & Cibis, G. W. (2000). Clinical and electroretinographic findings in fetal alcohol syndrome. *Journal of American Association for Pediatric Ophthalmology and Strabismus, 4*, 200–204.

Hughes, L. A., May, K., Talbot, J. F., & Parsons, M. A. (2006). Incidence, distribution, and duration of birth-related retinal hemorrhages: A prospective study. *Journal of American Association for Pediatric Ophthalmology and Strabismus, 10*, 102–106.

Hussain, N., Clive, J., & Bhandari, V. (1999). Current incidence of retinopathy of prematurity, 1989–1997. *Pediatrics, 104*(3), e26–e34.

Hylander, M. A., Strobino, D. M., Pessullo, J. C., & Dhanireddy, R. (2001). Association of human milk feedings with a reduction in retinopathy of prematurity among very low birth weight infants. *Journal of Perinatology, 21*(6), 356–362.

International Committee for the Classification of Retinopathy of Prematurity. (2005). The international classification of retinopathy of prematurity revisited. *Archives of Ophthalmology, 123*(7), 991–999.

International Committee on Retinopathy of Prematurity (ICROP). (1984). An international classification of retinopathy of prematurity. *Pediatrics, 74*(1), 127–133.

Jacobson, L. K., & Dutton, G. N. (2000). Periventricular leukomalacia: An important cause of visual and ocular motility dysfunction in children [review]. *Survey of Ophthalmology, 45*(1), 1–13.

Jalali, S., Anand, R., Kumar, H., Dogra, M. R., Azad, R., & Gopal, L. (2003). Programme planning and screening strategy in retinopathy of prematurity. *Indian Journal of Ophthalmology, 51*, 89–97.

Javitt, J., DeiCas, R., & Chiang, Y.-P. (1993). Cost-effectiveness of screening and cryotherapy for threshold retinopathy of prematurity. *Pediatrics, 91*, 859–866.

Jefferies, A. L. (2010). Retinopathy of prematurity: Recommendations for screening. *Paediatric Child Health, 15*(10), 667–674.

Johnston, W. T., & Cogen, M. S. (2000). Systemic candidiasis with cataract formation in a premature infant. *Journal of American Association for Pediatric Ophthalmology and Strabismus, 4*, 386–388.

Jones, K. L. (2006). *Chapter 6: Normal standards. Smith's recognizable patterns of human malformation* (6th ed., pp. 856–859), Philadelphia, PA: Elsevier-Saunders.

Kakar, S., Bhalla, P., Maria, A., Rana, M., Chawla, R., & Mathur, N. B. (2010). *Chlamydia trachomatis* causing neonatal conjunctivitis in a tertiary care center. *Indian Journal of Medical Microbiology, 28*, 45–47.

Kaufman, L. M., Miller, M. T., & Gupta, B. K. (2010). The Eye, Part 1: Examination and common problems. In R. J. Martin, A. A. Fanaroff & M. C. Walsh (Eds.), *Neonatal-perinatal medicine: Diseases of the fetus and infant* (9th ed.). Philadelphia, PA: Mosby.

Kurlenda, J., Pabich, A. K., & Grinholc, M. (2010). Neonatal intrauterine infection with *Neisseria meningitides* B. *Clinical Pediatrics, 49*(4), 388–390.

Larsson, E. K., Rydberg, A. C., & Holmstrom, G. E. (2005). A population-based study on the visual outcome in 10-year-old preterm and full-term children. *Archives of Ophthalmology, 123*, 825–832.

Lehman, S. S. (1999). An uncommon cause of ophthalmia neonatorum: *Neisseria meningitidis*. *Journal of American Association for Pediatric Ophthalmology and Strabismus, 3*(5), 316.

Lupetti, A., Tavanti, A., Davini, P., Ghelardi, E., Corsini, V., Merusi, I., . . . Senesi, S. (2002). Horizontal transmission of *Candida parapsilosis* candidemia in a neonatal intensive care unit. *Journal of Clinical Microbiology, 40*, 2363–2369. doi:10.1128/JCM.40.7.2363–2369.2002

Mabry-Hernandez, I., & Oliverio-Hoffman, R. (2010). *Ocular prophylaxis for gonococcal ophthalmia neonatorum: Evidence update for the U.S. Preventive Services Task Force reaffirmation recommendation statement*. Retrieved from http://www.uspreventiveservicestaskforce.org/uspstf10/gonoculproph/gonocup.htm#ref12

Markestad, T., Kaaresen, P. I., Ronnestad, A., Reigstad, H., Lossius, K., Medbo, S., . . . Irgens, L. M. (2005). Early death, morbidity, and need of treatment among extremely premature infants. *Pediatrics, 115*(5), 1289–1298. doi:10.1542/peds.2004-1482

Martins, E. N., & Morse, L. S. (2005). Evaluation of Internet websites about retinopathy of prematurity patient education. *British Journal of Ophthalmology, 89*(5), 565–568. doi:10.1136/bjo.2004.055111

Mestan, K. K., Marks, J. D., Hecox, K., Huo, D., & Schreiber, M. D. (2005). Neurodevelopmental outcomes of premature infants treated with inhaled nitric oxide. *New England Journal of Medicine, 353*, 23–32.

Mets, M. B., Barton, L. L., Khan, A. S., & Ksiazek, T. G. (2000). Lymphocytic choriomeningitis virus: An underdiagnosed cause of congenital chorioretinitis. *American Journal of Ophthalmology, 130*(2), 209–215.

Mintz-Hittner, H. A., Kennedy, K. A., Chuang, A. Z., & BEAT-ROP Coorperative Group. (2011). Efficacy of intravitreal bevacizumab for stage 3+ retinopathy of prematurity. *New England Journal of Medicine, 364*(7), 603–615.

Moshfeghi, A. A., Charalel, R. A., Hernandez-Boussard, T., Mortan, J. M., & Moshfeghi, D. M. (2011). Declining incidence of neonatal endophthalmitis in the United States. *American Journal of Ophthalmology, 151*(1), 59–65. doi:10.1016/j.ajo.2010.07.008

Nair, A. K., Pai, M. G., daCosta, D. E., & Al Khusaiby, S. M. (2000). Necrotising enterocolitis following ophthalmological examination in preterm neonates. *Indian Pediatrics, 37*, 417–421.

O'Connor, M. T., Vohr, B. R., Tucker, R., & Cashore, W. (2003). Is retinopathy of prematurity increasing among infants less than 1250 g birth weight? *Journal of Perinatology, 23*, 673–678.

Ogut, M. S., Bozkurt, N., Ozek, E., Birgen, H., Kazokoglu, H., & Ogut, M. (1996). Effects and side effects of mydriatic eyedrops in neonates. *European Journal of Ophthalmology, 6*(2):192–196.

O'Keefe, M., Kafil-Hussain, N., Flitcroft, I., & Lanigan, B. (2001). Ocular significance of intraventricular haemorrhage in premature infants. *British Journal of Ophthalmology, 85*, 357–359.

O'Keefe, M., Nolan, L., Lanigan, B., & Murphy, J. (2005). *Pseudomonas aeruginosa* endophthalmitis in a preterm infant. *Journal of the American Association for Pediatric Ophthalmology and Strabismus, 9*(3), 288–289.

Percivalle, E., Sarasini, A., Torsellini, M., Bruschi, L., Antoniazzi, E., Revello, M. G., & Gerna, G. (2003). A comparison of methods for detecting adenovirus type 8 keratoconjunctivitis during a nosocomial outbreak in a neonatal intensive care unit. *Journal of Clinical Virology, 28*, 257–264.

Ray, A., & Gombos, D. S. (2012). Retinoblastoma: An overview. *Indian Journal of Pediatrics, 79*, Online version. Retrieved from http://www.springerlink.com/content/a463357772274002/abstract/.doi:10.1007/s12098-012-0726-8

Rehman, H. U. (2008). Heterochromia. *Canadian Medical Association Journal, 179*(5), 447–448. doi:10.1503/cmaj.070497

Reynolds, J. D. (2010). Retinopathy of prematurity. *International Ophthalmology Clinics, 50*(4), 1–13.

Reynolds, J. D., Dobson, V., Quinn, G. E., Fielder, A. R., Plamer, E. A., Saunders, R. A., . . . CRYO-ROP & LIGHT-ROP Coorperative Groups. (2002). Evidenced-based screening criteria for retinopathy of prematurity, natural history data from the CRYO-ROP and LIGHT-ROP studies. *Archives of Ophthalmology, 120*, 1470–1476.

Reynolds, J. D., Hardy, R. J., Kennedy, K. A., Spencer, R., van Heuven, W. A., & Fielder, A. R. (1998). Light Reduction in Retinopathy of Prematurity (LIGHT-ROP) Cooperative Group. *New England Journal of Medicine, 338*, 1572–1576.

Richter, R., Below, H., Kadow, I., Kramer, A., Muller, C., & Fusch, C. (2006). Effect of topical 1.25% Povidone-Iodine eye drops used for prophylaxis of opthalmia neonatorum on renal iodine excretion and thyroid-stimulating hormone level. *The Journal of Pediatrics, 148*, 401–403.

Roberts, F., Mets, M. B., Ferguson, D. J., O'Grady, R., O'Grady, C., Thulliez, P., . . . McLeod, R. (2001). Histopathological features of ocular toxoplasmosis in the fetus and infant. *Archives of Ophthalmology, 119*, 51–58.

Roth, D. B., Morales, D., Feuer, W. J., Hess, D., Johnson, R. A., & Flynn, J. T. (2001). Screening for Retinopathy of Prematurity Employing the RetCam 120. *Archives of Ophthalmology, 119*, 268–272.

Rours, I. G., Hammerschlag, M. R., Ott, A., DeFaber, T. J., Verbruch, H. A., deGroot, R., & Verkooyen, R. P. (2008). *Chlamydia trachomatis* as a cause of neonatal conjunctivitis in Dutch infants. *Pediatrics, 121*(2), e321–e326.

Royal College of Ophthalmologists. (2008). *Guideline for the screening and treatment of retinopathy of prematurity*. Retrieved from http://www.rcophth.ac.uk/core/core_picker/download.asp?id=339

Sarici, S. U., Yurdakok, M., & Unal, S. (2001). Acute gastric dilatation complicating the use of mydriatics in a preterm newborn. *Pediatric Radiology, 31*, 581–583.

Saugstad, O. D. (2005). Oxygen for newborns: How much is too much? *Journal of Perinatology 25*(Suppl. 2), S45–S49.

Scanlon, J. W., Nelson, T., Grylack, L. J., & Smith, Y. F. (1979). *A system of newborn physical examination*. Baltimore, MD: University Park Press.

Schoenwolf, G. C., Bleyl, S. B., Brauer, P. R., & Francis-West, P. H. (2009). *Larsen's human embryology* (4th ed.). Philadelphia, PA: Churchill Livingstone, Elsevier.

Section on Ophthalmology, American Academy of Pediatrics (AAP), American Academy of Ophthalmology (AAO), & American Association of Pediatric Ophthalmology and Strabimus (AAPOS). (2006). Screening examination of premature infants for retinopathy of prematurity. *Pediatrics, 117*(2), 572–576. doi:10.1542/peds.2005-2749

Shah, C. P., McKey, J., Spirn, M. J., & Maguire, J. (2008). Ocular candidiasis: A review. *British Journal of Ophthalmology, 92*(4), 466–468.

Shah, G. K., Vander, J., & Eagle, R. C. (2000). Intralenticular *Candida* species abscess in a premature infant. *American Journal of Ophthalmology, 129*(3), 390–391.

Smith, L. E. (2003). Pathogenesis of retinopathy of prematurity. *Seminars in Neonatology, 8*, 469–473.

Smith, L. E. (2004). Pathogenesis of retinopathy of prematurity. *Growth Hormone & IGF Research, 14*(Suppl. A), S140–S144.

Standler, R. B. (2006). *Statutory law in the USA: Requiring silver nitrate in eyes of newborns*. Retrieved from http://www.rbs2.com/SilvNitr.pdf

Stern, J. H., Calvano, C., & Simon, J. W. (2001). Recurrent endogenous candida endophthalmitis in a premature infant. *American Association of Pediatric Ophthalmology and Strabismus, 5*(1), 50–51. doi:10.1067/mpa.2001.111136

Stoilov, I., Akarsu, A. N., & Sarfarazi, M. (1997). Identification of three different truncating mutations in cytochrome P4501B1 (CYP1B1) as the principal cause of primary congenital glaucoma (Buphthalmos) in families linked to the GLC3A locus on chromosome 2p21. *Human Molecular Genetics, 6*(4), 641–647.

STOP-ROP Multicenter Study Group (STOP-ROP). (2000). Supplemental therapeutic oxygen for prethreshold retinopathy of prematurity (STOP-ROP), A randomized, controlled trial. *Pediatrics, 105*(2), 295–310. doi:10.1542/peds.105.2.295

Tabatabaei, S. R., Afjeiee, S. A., Fallah, F., Zanjani, N. T., Shiva, F., Fard, A. T., . . . Kariimi, A. (2012). The use of polymerase chain reaction assay versus cell culture in detecting neonatal chlamydial conjunctivitis. *Archives of Iranian Medicine, 15*(3), 171–175.

Tappero, E. P., & Honeyfield, M. E. (2009). *Physical assessment of the newborn: A comprehensive approach to the art of physical examination* (4th ed.). Santa Rosa, CA: NICU Ink.

Trigler, L., Weaver, R. G., O'Neil, J. W., Barondes, M. J., & Freedman, S. F. (2005). Case series of angle-closure glaucoma after laser treatment for retinopathy of prematurity. *Journal of the American Association for Pediatric Ophthalmology and Strabismus, 9*, 17–21.

Vander, J. F. (1994). Retinopathy of prematurity: Diagnosis and management. *Journal of Ophthalmic Nursing and Technology, 13*(5), 207–212.

Varughese, S., Varghese, R. M., Gupta, N., Ojha, R., Sreenivas, V., & Puliyel, J. M. (2005). Refractive error at birth and its relation to gestational age. *Current Eye Research, 30*(6), 423–428. doi:10.1080/02713680590959295

Wang, R., Martinez-Frias, M. L., & Graham, J. M. (2002). Infants of diabetic mother are at increased risk for the oculo-auriculo-vertebral sequence: A case-based and case-control approach. *Journal of Pediatrics, 141*, 611–617.

Wasserman, B. N., Sondhi, N., & Carr, B. L. (1999). Pseudomonas-induced bilateral endophthalmitis with corneal perforation in a neonate. *Journal of the American Association for Pediatric Ophthalmology and Strabismus, 3*, 183–184.

Wood, M. G., & Kaufman, L. M. (2009). Apnea and bradycardia in two premature infants during routine outpatient retinopathy of prematurity screening. *Journal of the American Association for Pediatric Ophthalmology and Strabismus, 13*, 501–503.

World Health Organization (WHO). (2004). *ISDB WHO Single medicines review: Silver nitrate eye drops*. Retrieved from http://archives.who.int/eml/expcom/expcom14/silver_nitrate_eye_soln/1_ISDB_WHO_silver_nitrate.pdf

York, J. R., Landers, S., Kirby, R. S., Arbogast, P. G., & Penn, J. S. (2004). Arterial oxygen fluctuation and retinopathy of prematurity in very-low-birth-weight infants. *Journal of Perinatology, 24*, 82–87.

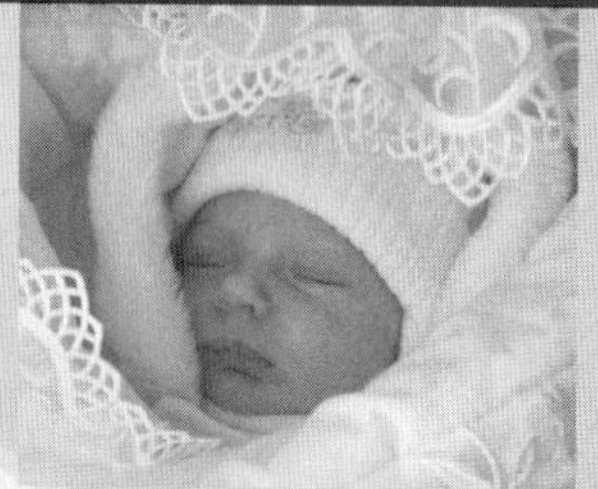

CHAPTER 18

Genitourinary System

■ Leslie A. Parker

Comprehensive nursing care of infants with renal or genital disorders requires a thorough understanding of normal anatomy and physiology. Development of renal and genital systems arises from shared structures; therefore abnormalities in one system may indicate abnormal development in the other. Because nurses provide hands-on care to infants in both the newborn nursery and neonatal intensive care unit (NICU), they are often the first to recognize abnormalities in the renal and genital systems. To readily identify such disorders and participate in their collaborative management, nurses need a clear understanding of the normal anatomy and physiology of the genital and renal systems and the pathologic processes that may be present in the neonatal patient.

The kidneys function to maintain fluid, electrolyte, and acid–base balance as well as to rid the body of nitrogenous and other waste products. Perinatal depression, medical management for common neonatal conditions, and dehydration are only a few of the many factors placing the newborn at risk for renal compromise. Timely, accurate nursing assessment and intervention is of utmost priority to ensure optimal outcome for both the infants and their family.

This chapter outlines embryologic development and anatomy, physiology, and assessment of the genitourinary system. It also describes various abnormalities and disease processes commonly identified in the neonatal period, including pathophysiology, risk factors, clinical manifestations, diagnosis, collaborative management, and prognosis.

EMBRYOLOGIC DEVELOPMENT OF THE UROGENITAL SYSTEM

During the first weeks of gestation, the mesoderm is divided into three segments: the lateral, intermediate, and paraxial. The intermediate mesoderm separates from the paraxial mesoderm and migrates ventrally as the nephrogenic cords located on either side of the primitive aorta. Cells on the dorsal end of the nephrogenic cords join to form the urogenital ridges from which components of both the urinary and genital structures are developed.

The Urinary System

The urinary system consists of the kidneys, ureters, urinary bladder, and the urethra (Figure 18.1). Development of the primary excretory organ begins around the fourth week of gestation with the production of fetal urine by week 10. At approximately 36 weeks, renal anatomic development is completed. Functional maturity increases after birth and continues until approximately 2 years of age.

Development of the kidneys occurs with the progressive formation of three nephric structures within the nephrogenic cord: the pronephros, the mesonephros, and the metanephros. The pronephros or primitive kidney develops during the first month of gestation, and then gradually degenerates, thus contributing the duct system for the next developmental stage. The pronephros has no excretory function.

The second excretory organ to develop is the mesonephros. The mesonephric development begins at the caudal end of the pronephros during the fourth to sixth week of gestation. The mesonephros contains thin-walled glomeruli and tubules that are functional. Ultra-urine is produced by these mesonephric nephrons at 8 to 10 weeks. Mesonephric nephrons that are located more cranially along the nephrogenic cord begin to degenerate as those located more caudally are still developing. During this time, approximately the fourth week, the gonadal blastema begins to form in the genital ridge located on the medial aspect of each mesonephros, thus creating a urogenital ridge between the developing kidney and the genitals. As the mesonephric structure begins to degenerate in a caudal direction, it leaves a duct system for the following stage. In addition, the mesonephric duct eventually matures into the epididymis, vas deferens, and ejaculatory duct in the male or the vestigial Garner in the female. Thus failure of the mesonephric duct to develop may result in anomalies in both the urinary and genital systems.

The third and final stage of kidney development, beginning in the fifth week of gestation, is the formation of

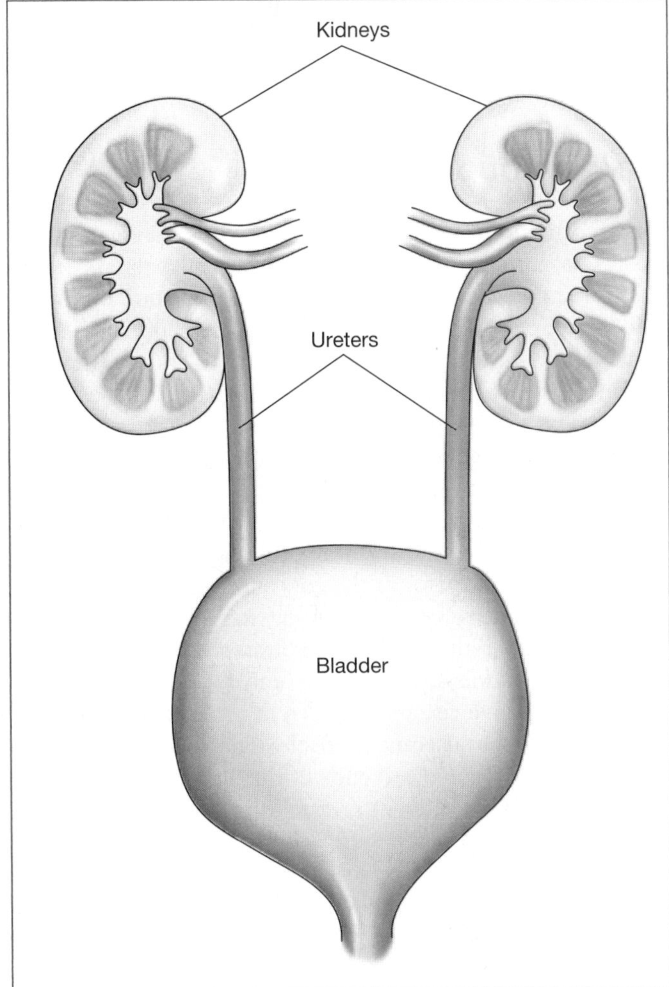

FIGURE 18.1 The renal system.
From Guyton and Hall (1997).

the metanephros or definitive kidney. The metanephros develops from the induction of the metanephrogenic blastema (metanephric mesoderm) by the ureteric bud. The ureteric bud, also called the metanephric diverticulum, is an outgrowth of the mesonephric duct, and the metanephrogenic blastema originates from the lower segment of the nephrogenic cord. As this stage progresses, the stalk of ureteric bud becomes the ureter. The development of the renal pelvis, major and minor calices, and finally the collecting tubes occurs through the continued elongating and branching of the cranial end of the ureteric bud. At the ends of the collecting tubules, the cells of the metanephric blastema clump and stimulate the formation of the glomerulus, proximal tubule, loop of Henle, and distal tubule, which eventually empties into the collecting duct, thereby forming a nephron (Moore & Persaud, 2011).

To complete the formation of the urinary system, a bladder and urethra are produced. The epithelium of the bladder and most of the urethra derive from the embryologic hindgut. The expanded terminal end of the hindgut is the cloaca. The allantois, an outgrowth of the yolk sac, is attached to the ventral side of the cloaca. The urorectal septum creates a compartmentalized cloaca that consists of the anorectal canal and the urogenital sinus. With the exception of the bladder trigone—the area between the urethra and ureters—the bladder arises from this urogenital sinus. The primitive structures regress, fibrose, or become a part of the newly formed structures. The point of origin of ureteric bud marks the point of insertion for the ureters. The ureters, formerly the metanephric ducts, then open bilaterally into the urinary bladder as the developing bladder reabsorbs the distal portions of the mesonephric ducts into its dorsal wall (trigone).

The allantois narrows into a fibrous band called the urachus that runs from the apex of the bladder to the umbilicus. Abnormalities of the urachus occur when it either remains patent or forms an urachal sinus. A patent urachus may occur in association with another anomalous condition and may allow development of a functional kidney by alleviating the effects of urinary obstruction. An urachal sinus is usually an isolated anomaly and causes leakage of urine from the umbilical stump.

Urethral development in the male and female begins in the same manner. The urogenital sinus is visible at 6 weeks and consists of a narrow portion near the bladder, the pelvic urethra, and an expanded portion near the urogenital membrane (cloacal membrane), called the phallic urethra. Through several processes and stages, the phallic end of the urogenital sinus eventually becomes the bulbar and the penile urethra, and the pelvic urethra develops into the permanent urethra and vagina. Differentiation of the urethra in the male and female fetus can be detected by 12 to 14 weeks gestation.

Initially, the kidneys are located within the pelvic region. They make a gradual ascent into their final location in the flank position or lumbothoracic area. Normal renal ascent is achieved as the result of caudal growth of the fetal spine, lengthening of the ureter, molding of the renal parenchyma, and fixation of the kidney to the retroperitoneum (Moore & Persaud, 2011). Failure of normal ascent of the kidneys results in abnormalities such as horseshoe kidneys or pelvic kidneys. Blood supply to the ascending kidneys changes from lower arteries that gradually regress to arteries that arise from the aorta.

In utero, the placenta functions as the excretory organ for the fetus. Functional kidneys are therefore not necessary for fetal homeostasis. Consequently, pathological problems such as aplastic, hypoplastic, and otherwise nonfunctioning kidneys may not be detected until the neonatal period. Fetal urination, swallowing, and breathing impact amniotic fluid volume. Excretion of fetal urine contributes significantly to amniotic fluid volume, especially during the third trimester. A reduction in fetal urine excretion results in oligohydramnios. Failure of the fetus to swallow amniotic fluid because of gastrointestinal obstruction or central nervous system anomaly results in overaccumulation of amniotic fluid or polyhydramnios. Abnormalities in amniotic fluid volume can therefore signal pathology in various fetal organ systems (Mehler, 2011).

A balance between genetic influences, cellular mediators, and the interaction of various molecular mechanisms is necessary for the initiation and development of the kidney.

Depending on the timing of development, insult or failure of the primitive structures to grow or to branch appropriately may result in a variety of uropathies, including dysplasia and renal agenesis.

PHYSIOLOGY OF KIDNEY FUNCTION

Kidney structure includes the cortex, the major and minor calices, and the renal pelvis (Figure 18.2). The kidney is divided into two sections, the outer renal cortex and the inner medulla. The kidney functions to regulate fluid and electrolyte balance and arterial blood pressure, as well as excrete toxic and waste substances. These regulatory mechanisms are all intimately tied to formation of urine that involves three basic processes; ultrafiltration of plasma by the glomerulus, reabsorption of water and solutes from the ultrafiltrate, and secretion of certain solutes into the tubular fluid (Koeppen & Stanton, 2006).

The nephron is the functional unit of the kidney and is the site of urine formation. It consists of a glomerulus (Bowman's capsule and glomerular capillaries) and a renal tubule that has three sections: a proximal convoluted tubule, the loop of Henle, and a distal convoluted tubule (Figure 18.3). After urine is produced by the nephron, it drains into the minor and major calyces. From there it drains into a single large cavity called the renal pelvis, then out through the ureter, and into the bladder.

Nephron formation (nephrogenesis) begins during the second month of gestation and is anatomically complete by approximately 35 weeks. Although anatomic formation may be complete, functional immaturity of the nephrons continues throughout infancy. At the completion of nephrogenesis, each kidney contains approximately 1 million nephrons. Nephrogenesis begins deep within the renal cortex near the medulla in the juxtamedullary region and continues outwardly (Koeppen & Stanton, 2006). The juxtamedullary nephrons differ from the superficial cortical nephrons in that their glomeruli are larger, the loop of Henle is longer, and the efferent arteriole forms a more complex vascular system. The less mature superficial cortical nephrons make up the majority of nephrons, while the more mature juxtamedullary nephrons account for a very small percentage of the total number. Altered renal function in the premature infant may therefore be caused by both anatomic and physiologic immaturity.

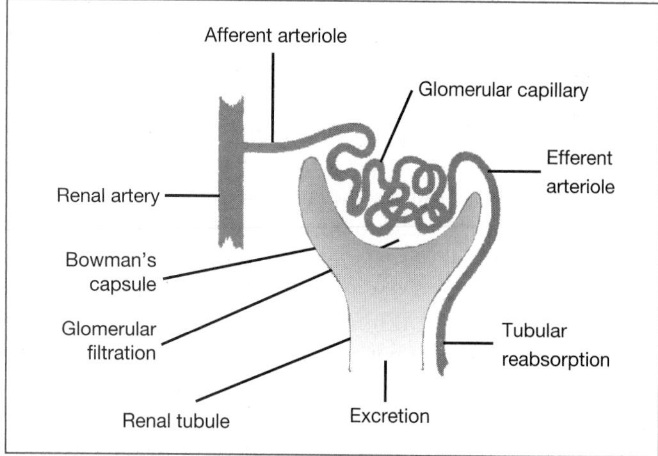

FIGURE 18.2 Glomerular apparatus.
From Guyton and Hall (1997).

RENAL BLOOD FLOW

Urine formation begins with blood flow. The pressure-driven process of ultrafiltration depends on optimal arterial pressure and is regulated by the dilatation and constriction of afferent and efferent arterioles (Koeppen & Stanton, 2006). Adequate renal blood flow is therefore essential to kidney function. During the first 12 hours of life, 4% to 6% of the cardiac output goes to the kidney, which increases to 8% to 10% over the next few days. This is compared to the 25% of cardiac output that reaches the adult kidney. Renal blood flow not only provides oxygen and nutrients to the kidneys but also affects the rate of solute and water reabsorption by the proximal tubule, participates in the concentration and dilution of the urine, and delivers substrates for excretion in the urine.

The left and right renal arteries arise from the aorta. After entering the kidneys, they divide and branch several times to eventually give rise to the afferent arterioles. Each nephron receives one afferent arteriole that divides and forms the glomerulus. The distal ends of the glomerular capillaries merge to form the efferent arterioles that carry blood away from the glomerulus. The efferent arterioles divide to form the peritubular capillaries, which surround the tubular parts of the nephron in the renal cortex. Other vessels called the vasa recta also arise from the efferent arterioles to surround the tubular parts of the nephron in the renal medulla. The peritubular capillaries empty into the venous system and eventually leave the kidneys in the form of the renal vein. The fetus and infant have a decreased renal blood flow due to increased renal vascular resistance and decreased mean arterial pressure. Renal vascular resistance is elevated in the fetus because fetal renal function is required only for production of amniotic fluid (Blackburn, 2012). Renal blood flow increases with both advancing gestational and chronologic age.

GLOMERULAR FILTRATION RATE

As blood flows into the kidney via the renal artery, it is directed into the afferent arteriole and carried into the glomerulus. The glomerulus consists of the glomerular capillaries and Bowman's capsule. Plasma driven through the glomerular capillaries is filtered through the filtration barrier, and the protein-free plasma, or ultrafiltrate, is forced into the Bowman's capsule or leaves via the efferent arteriole and enters into the renal vein. To produce ultrafiltrate, the glomerulus functions as a filtering site. Glomerular capillaries are lined with epithelial cells called podocytes forming one of the layers of Bowman's capsule (see Figure 18.3). The endothelial cells of the glomerular capillaries are covered by a basement membrane also surrounded by podocytes. The basement membrane, podocytes, and the endothelial cells of the glomerular capillaries form the filtration barrier. The epithelial cells of this filtration barrier express negatively charged glycoproteins and contain many small openings called fenestrations.

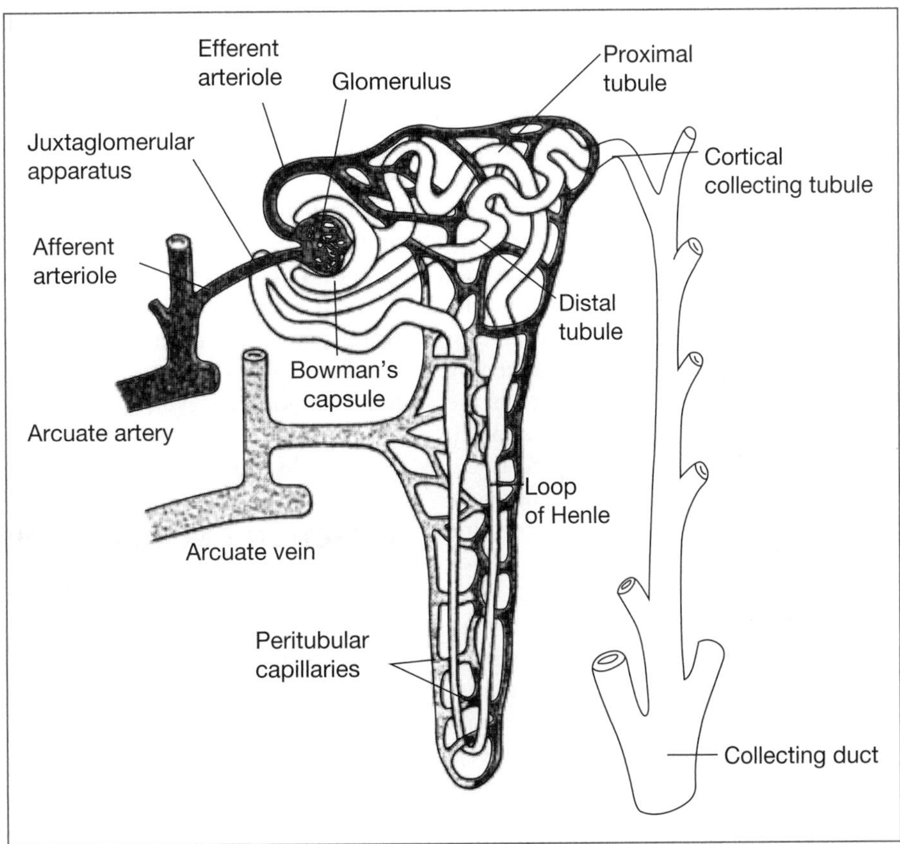

FIGURE 18.3 The nephron.
From Guyton and Hall (1997).

The size of the fenestrations inhibits passage of large proteins such as blood cells and platelets but is highly permeable to the passage of water, small solutes, urea, and glucose. In addition, positively charged large proteins are repelled by the cationic cell membrane (Koeppen & Stanton, 2006).

The glomerular filtration rate (GFR) is the rate at which fluid is filtered through the glomerulus. Because it is equal to the sum of all filtration rates of all nephrons in both kidneys, the GFR reflects kidney function and a decrease in GFR signifies renal disease. Oncotic and hydrostatic pressures (Starling forces) drive the ultrafiltration process. Oncotic pressure is osmotic pressure generated by large proteins or colloids. Hydrostatic pressure is pressure exerted by fluids in equilibrium and depends on arterial pressure and vascular resistance (Koeppen & Stanton, 2006). Oncotic pressure in Bowman's space is very near zero because ultrafiltrate is nearly protein-free. Filtration at this level is therefore driven by hydrostatic pressure across the glomerular capillaries. Hydrostatic pressure within Bowman's space and glomerular oncotic pressure oppose glomerular hydrostatic pressure in the capillaries. The GFR is proportional to the sum of hydrostatic and oncotic pressures existing along the renal capillaries multiplied by the ultrafiltration coefficient. The difference between the permeability of the glomerular capillary and the glomerular surface area available for filtration is the ultrafiltration coefficient (Koeppen & Stanton, 2006). GFR is therefore affected by changes in arterial blood pressure, vascular resistance, concentration of plasma proteins, and glomerular capillary permeability. Alteration in the permeability of the glomerular capillaries may result from inherent damage to the capillary, thus altering the pore size or changing the electrical charge within the membrane. GFR may also be negatively affected by urinary system obstruction.

Fetal GFR is relatively low due to increased renal vascular resistance and decreased renal blood flow and then rapidly increases during the first few hours following birth. GFR increases with both advancing gestational and chronologic age due to increased number and growth of the nephrons and reaches full-term levels by 32 to 35 weeks gestation (Blackburn, 2012). In the preterm infant functional maturation is determined by conceptional age, not by postnatal age (Solhaug, Bolger, & Jose, 2004). When corrected for body surface area, GFR is 10 mL/min/1.73 m^2 at 28 weeks gestation and rises to 30 mL/min/1.73 m^2 at term. GFR does not rise due to an increase in the number of nephrons, but rather it is believed to reflect a decrease in vascular resistance and an increase in glomerular surface area (Riccabona, 2004). Even in term infants, GFR is low compared to an older infant or child. This low GFR is adequate in normal circumstances, but in conditions such as sepsis, hypoxia, or the administration of nephrotoxic medications, the GFR may not meet the physiologic needs of the infant. Medications administered prenatally can also have detrimental effects on fetal GFR and subsequent neonatal renal function. Examples of these drugs include prostaglandin inhibitors (indomethacin), nonsteroidal anti-inflammatories, diuretics and antibiotics especially aminoglycosidesangiotensin-converting enzyme inhibitors (Gubhaju, Suterland, Hons, & Black, 2011).

Assessment of GFR is important in evaluating renal function. One method of assessing GFR is measurement of the renal clearance of a substance. Renal clearance represents a volume of plasma completely cleared of a substance by the kidneys over a specified period of time (Koeppen & Stanton, 2006). Various substances are used as markers for measuring GFR. Marker substances must have the following characteristics: (1) freely filter across the glomerulus into Bowman's space; (2) not be reabsorbed or secreted by the nephron; (3) not be metabolized or produced by the kidney; and (4) not alter GFR (Koeppen & Stanton, 2006). Para-aminohippurate (PAH) is a substance not produced by the body, is secreted by the proximal tubules, and meets the marker criteria. PAH, which is nearly completely cleared, moves through the renal tubules so that it is effectively cleared via plasma movement within the kidney. Therefore measurement of the renal clearance of PAH can determine the effective renal plasma flow, which is a direct way of determining renal function. Since PAH is not produced by the body, it must be administered by infusion. Insulin may also be used as a tag substance for testing the intactness of the kidney's filtering system and GFR and is also administered via infusion (Koeppen & Stanton, 2006).

Creatinine, a by-product of muscle metabolism, also meets the marker criteria. Measurement of serum creatinine levels are clinically the most useful method of estimating renal function in neonates. Because creatinine readily crosses the placenta, levels obtained during the first week reflect maternal levels (Boer, de Rijke, Hop, Cransberg, & Dorresteijn, 2010). After birth, the GFR in term infants increases as renal blood flow increases and vascular resistance decreases. This increase in function generally occurs over the first week of life and results in a drop in creatinine levels to nearly 0.4 mg/dL, depending on clinical status and gestational age. Glomerular filtration rate does not increase as drastically until completion of nephrogenesis. Therefore premature infants do not demonstrate the same decline in serum creatinine levels as infants born after 36 weeks gestation (Subramanian, Agarwal, Deorari, Paul, & Bagga, 2011). Small increases in serum creatinine levels may indicate a significant decrease in GFR. Monitoring trends in serial creatinine levels may therefore render a more accurate evaluation of renal function.

Regulation of renal blood flow and consequently GFR is achieved by hormonal and sympathetic nervous system (SNS) influences. The renal vessels, including the afferent and efferent arterioles, are highly innervated by sympathetic nerve fibers. Mild stimulation of the SNS does not cause a change in renal vascular tone. However, under severe physiologic stress such as that caused by significant fluid loss, activation of the renal sympathetic nerve fibers causes vasoconstriction of the renal arteries, which in turn decreases GFR.

Hormonal control is exerted mainly via activation of the renin-angiotensin-aldosterone system (RAS). The RAS plays a significant role in blood pressure regulation and sodium homeostasis and is found in the fetus, beginning at about 3 months gestation. Renin is an enzyme found in high levels in the plasma and is produced and stored in specialized cells of the juxtaglomerular apparatus. Newborns have a significantly higher renin level than adults due to the neonate's altered GFR, increased vascular resistance, and decreased renal blood flow.

When renal blood flow is diminished due to decreased arterial pressure, the vessel walls of the afferent arterioles are less stretched and the release of renin is stimulated. Release of renin causes production of angiotensin I from angiotensin, which is then converted by angiotensin-converting enzyme to angiotensin II. Angiotensin II stimulates secretion of aldosterone by the adrenal cortex. Aldosterone in turn triggers increased reabsorption of sodium and water, thereby increasing extracellular fluid volume and renal perfusion (Figure 18.4). The ultimate goal of the renin-angiotensin cycle is to maintain an adequate systemic blood flow to supply the body's vital organs (Tortora & Grabowski, 2011).

SECRETION AND REABSORPTION

The kidneys control fluid and electrolyte balance by reabsorption and secretion of sodium and water. The four segments of the nephron, the proximal tubule, loop of

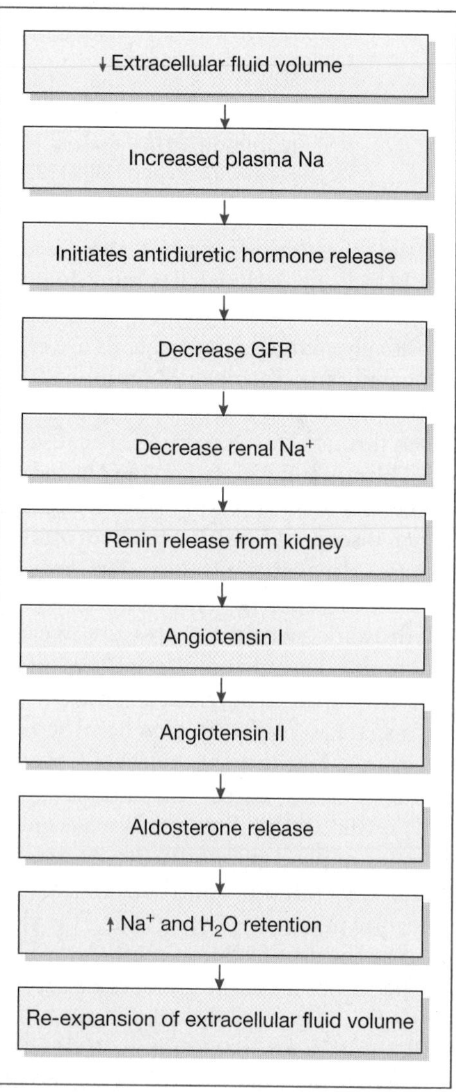

FIGURE 18.4 The renin-angiotensin-aldosterone regulation of extracellular fluid.

Henle, distal tubule, and the collecting duct, determine the composition and volume of urine.

Because nephron formation begins in the medullary area, the thin ascending portion of the nephron controlling reabsorption is not fully formed in the neonate. By birth, nephron formation has extended from the medullary to the juxtamedullary area. The descending portion of the tubular system, which controls urine secretion, is therefore more fully developed than the ascending segment at birth. Thus a newborns ability to concentrate urine is decreased because although urine secretion occurs readily, reabsorption is limited. Infants are therefore more likely to lose sodium, glucose, and other solutes in their urine. This process is further altered in preterm infants resulting in possibly significant fluid and electrolyte disturbances.

Tubular reabsorption, secretion, and excretion are closely tied together and function in maintenance of internal homeostasis and regulation of fluids and electrolytes. Tubular reabsorption is the process whereby substances from the tubular lumen move into the capillary system through simple diffusion and active transport. Many of the body's nutrients, electrolytes, and 99% of the filtered water are reabsorbed, thus achieving a balance for continued growth and normal physiologic function. Simple diffusion involves movement of substances down a gradient, from an area of higher to an area of lower concentration. Active transport requires energy derived directly from adenosine triphosphate because the net movement of substances is against a gradient. Molecular structures may link together to piggyback, or carry one another, across the membrane. Sodium first undergoes simple diffusion across the tubular membrane and then is transported via active transport by the sodium pump into the interstitial fluid. Because sodium filtration depends on GFR, a higher GFR increases sodium reabsorption into the vascular space. If the extracellular fluid volume increases, sodium reabsorption is decreased.

Water follows sodium ions across the membrane and into the capillary bed. This type of transport of a second substance is called secondary active transport. Simple facilitated diffusion is similar to active transport in that a carrier substance is used, but the net movement is not against a gradient. Glucose is a substance that secondary active transport carries along with sodium across the membrane. Glucose is reabsorbed by the proximal tubules, thus appearing in the urine only when the renal threshold or the maximal tubular transport capacity has been exceeded or when the permeability of the filtering capillaries has been altered. Amino acids, water-soluble vitamins, albumin, and lactate are also transported in this fashion.

Tubular secretion moves substances such as potassium and hydrogen from the epithelial lining of the tubules' capillaries into the interstitial fluid and finally into the tubular lumen. Tubular excretion is the process whereby substances enter the filtrate that will eventually exit the body as urine. Ions such as potassium, which are secreted in the distal tubule (a portion is also reabsorbed in the proximal tubule), find their way into the urine when the body has no need for higher concentration levels. The movement of hydrogen ions influences the excretion of potassium; therefore metabolic acidosis and alkalosis affect the potassium level. Hormones and drugs, especially diuretics, can also affect the movement of potassium with aldactone causing potassium secretion and the thiazides resulting in potassium excretion. Other filtrates present in the urine include urea, creatinine, and other ions not needed by the body.

ASSESSMENT OF THE GENITOURINARY SYSTEM

History

A thorough family history is imperative for all infants suspected of having a urogenital abnormality. Many urogenital problems have an inheritance pattern suggesting a genetic predisposition. The history should focus on family members who have had a renal transplant or have undergone dialysis, those with a history of renal failure, and those with cystic kidney disease or anomalies of the GU system. A review of family history should also include fetal or neonatal deaths and the presence of individuals with external genitalia abnormalities such as hypospadias, ambiguous genitalia, or undescended testicles. The prenatal history should be reviewed for antepartal factors associated with renal abnormalities, including oligohydramnios, an abnormal prenatal ultrasound or perinatal depression.

The neonatal history should include the following questions:

1. Has the infant urinated, and if so how long following delivery? Normal voiding occurs within the first 24 hours of life. Care should be taken to note whether the infant voided in the delivery room.
2. Has the infant undergone any significant hypoxic episodes that may result in decreased renal blood flow?
3. Is the fluid intake sufficient relative to the infant's clinical status, gestational age, and immediate environment (radiant warmer or humidified isolette)? A radiant warmer can increase insensible water losses, thereby increasing fluid requirements.
4. Is the infant under treatment for jaundice? (Phototherapy increases insensible water losses.)
5. Is the infant experiencing any bleeding or increased gastrointestinal losses from nasogastric suctioning, vomiting, diarrhea, or increased ostomy output?
6. What is the specific gravity of urine? (Normal range is 1.003 to 1.015.)
7. What is the infant's gestational and chronological age?
8. Has the infant received any nephrotoxic medications?
9. What is the infant's blood pressure? (Hypotension can indicate volume depletion, whereas hypertension may be associated with an underlying renal abnormality.)

PHYSICAL ASSESSMENT

Physical examination should include inspection, palpation, and percussion. Auscultation is generally not useful in assessment of the renal system.

Inspection

Observation of the abdominal region is essential in infants suspected of having renal abnormalities. One should note the presence of abdominal distention including whether the distention is localized to one side or is generalized. Any abdominal asymmetry is considered an abnormal finding. The presence of bladder distention should also be noted. While mild abdominal protuberance in the neonate may be normal due to the relative weakness of the abdominal musculature compared to infants who are several months older, an absence of muscle tone is characteristic of prune-belly syndrome. The umbilicus should be assessed for hernias and/or drainage. If possible, the urinary stream should be assessed. A continuous, straight stream is considered normal.

The genital and perineal area should be carefully inspected. Peritoneal tissue leading to the anal opening should be intact and smooth in appearance. Any abnormal openings, depressions, or swellings should be noted. The anus is normally located midline and can be tested for patency by gentle insertion of a gloved, well-lubricated small finger. Gentle stroking of the anal tissue and observation for anal sphincter constriction tests the anal wink indicating adequate muscle tone.

Male infants require inspection of the skin covering the scrotum for color, and the presence of rugae, edema, or ecchymosis. If the infant is full-term, the scrotal sac should be full, and rugae should be present. The premature male infant exhibits a generally flaccid, smooth scrotal sac. The scrotum is generally darkly pigmented, without bluish discoloration that could denote disruption of circulation to the area, indicating the possible presence of a testicular torsion. An enlarged or edematous scrotum may accompany a hydrocele (a trapping of fluid in the tunica vaginalis), or may result from pressure during the birth process, especially during a breech delivery. If a hydrocele is suspected, transillumination of the scrotum with a good light source, such as a transilluminator or a flashlight, helps determine the presence of fluid. When transilluminated, fluid will allow light to pass through what appears as a highly lightened area.

Penile size, resting position, and position of the urinary meatus should also be assessed. An abnormally large or small penis may indicate a genital abnormality. A micropenis is suspected when the penis measures less than 2 to 2.5 cm in length and can be associated with renal, genital, and chromosomal abnormalities. Priapism, or a constantly erect penis, is also an abnormal finding. The urinary meatus should be located midline on the ventral portion of the glans penis. Dorsal or ventral placement of the meatus can occur anywhere along the shaft of the penis and is considered abnormal. A urinary meatus located on the dorsum of the penis is known as an epispadias and a hypospadias if the opening is displaced along the ventral penile surface. A hypospadias can be associated with a downward curvation, bowing, or chordee of the penis. The foreskin of the uncircumcised male may be gently retracted for accurate observation of meatal location and then returned to its unretracted state to avoid swelling and possible decreased penile circulation.

Female infants require inspection of the labia, clitoris, urinary meatus, and external vaginal orifice. The labia minora in the term infant should be well formed and the labia majora should be present and extend beyond the labia minora. As gestational age decreases, the labia majoria is smaller and in premature infants, the labia minora may be larger than the labia majora. The labia may be darkly pigmented and is of no clinical significance. Because the labia may not be fully developed in premature infants, the clitoris in infants born preterm may appear prominent but if of normal size is considered normal. The urinary meatus should be patent and anterior to the vaginal orifice. The vagina should be inspected for patency, and any vaginal secretions should be noted. A white, milky vaginal secretion in the first few days of life, followed by pseudomenses or slight vaginal bleeding, is a normal finding. A hymenal tag may be present, usually disappearing within the first few weeks, and is considered a normal finding.

In both male and females, bruising and swelling of the genitalia may occur following a breech delivery. Ecchymosis and sometimes hematomas may also occur after traumatic delivery. These birth-related findings are transient and can be expected to resolve within several days. The inguinal areas should be assessed for the presence of an inguinal hernia. The genital and peritoneal regions must be observed to ensure there is a clear differentiation of the sexes. If not, ambiguous genitalia must be considered (see Chapter 10).

Palpitation

This portion of the physical examination may be stressful to the infant and thus is best left until last. Place the infant in the supine position with the knees and hips flexed and provide a means of nonnutritive sucking for the infant. This position generally places the infant at ease and facilitates relaxation of the abdominal muscles. The abdomen is then gently palpated with a gradual downward movement, anteriorly to posteriorly. To palpate the kidneys, place the fingers of one hand along the flank while the thumb palpates the abdomen. This allows the examiner to trap the kidney's pole between the fingers and the thumb (ballottement). Deep palpitation is required to manually assess the kidneys and is therefore reserved only for infants suspected of having a genitourinary or renal abnormality. The kidneys are only reliably palpated in the first 1 to 2 days of life (Hernandez & Glass, 2005).

In males, palpate the scrotal sac for each testis and cord. If the testis is absent, palpate along the canal to assess location. The scrotal sac may be palpated by gentle pressing of the tissue between two fingers, one on the anterior surface and the other on the posterior surface. Gentle movement of the fingers upward over the scrotum until the testes are detected bilaterally indicates whether one or both testes are descended and their location in relationship to the internal ring in the inguinal canal. Until 28 weeks gestation, the testes are abdominal organs and between 28 and 30 weeks, they begin to descend into the inguinal canal. The cremasteric reflex, recoil of the testes toward the inguinal canal, may be elicited by gentle stroking of the upper thigh or scrotal sac.

Percussion

If bladder distention is palpated or observed, percussion should be performed. This technique is useful in determining whether the area is fluid filled or a solid mass. If the bladder is filled with fluid, percussion will invoke a somewhat tympanic sound, while a dull sound will be noted if the mass is solid. Percussion may also be used over the entire abdominal region. Examination of the abdomen and gastrointestinal system is discussed in depth in Chapter 8.

Related Findings

All infants should be inspected for general characteristics suggesting renal abnormalities. Potter's facies (flattened, beak-like nose; wide-set eyes; micrognathia; disproportionately large ears; short neck) accompanied by abnormal positioning of the hands and feet and pulmonary hypoplasia are associated with oligohydramnios and may indicate the presence of a renal disorder. Since genetic syndromes commonly have associated renal abnormalities, one should assess for characteristics consistent with the presence of a genetic abnormalities. A single umbilical artery is present in 0.3% of newborns (Gornall, Kurinczuk, & Konje, 2003). Historically, the presence of a single umbilical artery was thought to be strongly associated with renal abnormalities, and therefore a renal ultrasound was recommended. Recent evidence has suggested the association is not as strong as previously thought, and an ultrasound may only be indicated in infants with other symptoms of renal disease (de Boom et al., 2010; Deshpande, Jog, Watson, & Gornal, 2009). The ears should be assessed for abnormalities since preauricular tags have been associated with urinary tract abnormalities (Srinivasan & Arora, 2005). Meningomyelocele and other neural tube defects may cause decreased or absent bladder innervation resulting in a neurogenic bladder and bladder distention. If untreated, the associated urinary stasis may result in a urinary tract infection (UTI). Syndromes associated with renal and genital problems are listed in Table 18.1.

Urine Collection

Urine collection is a relatively simple procedure in the neonate and several adhesive-backed collection bags are currently available. When placing urine collection bags, care should be taken to not include the rectum or scrotum within the opening of the bag. The penis should not be left in urine because infection and skin irritation may occur. To avoid skin irritation when using adhesive-backed collection bags, care should be taken to maintain skin integrity. Alternative collection systems can be used if accurate measurement of urine output is not needed. Cotton balls can be placed inside diapers to catch a small specimen for dipstick analysis or for measurement of specific gravity. Many institutions now use super-absorbency disposable diapers, which can potentially alter the result of urine tests. Nursing research is needed to evaluate the accuracy of specific laboratory tests when using these newer products.

When sterile urine specimens are required for culture, a suprapubic bladder tap or urethral catheterization must be performed. Performance of a suprapubic tap requires minimal equipment and time. The lower abdomen is prepared with an antimicrobial solution and allowed to dry. If the infant has voided within the previous hour, the attempt

TABLE 18.1

SYNDROMES ASSOCIATED WITH THE DEVELOPMENT OF UROGENITAL DISORDERS

Syndromes	Renal Component	Genital Component
Potter's association	Renal agenesis	Absence of vas deferens, seminal vesicle, upper vagina, uterus
Meckel's syndrome	Polycystic kidneys	Ambiguous genitalia Hypoplastic phallus Cryptorchidism
Trisomy 21	Cystic kidneys and other renal anomalies	Hypoplastic penis and scrotum Cryptorchidism
Trisomy 18	Dysplastic renal system	Hypoplastic clitoris and labia minora Cryptorchidism
Turner's syndrome	Horseshoe kidney	Infantile genitalia Duplications of the collecting system
Prune-belly syndrome Urinary tract dysplasia	Bladder and ureter dilation	Patent urachus Cryptorchidism
Errors of metabolism	Renal tubular dysfunction	Galactosemia Tyrosinemia Glycogen storage (Gierke's) disease
Adrenogenital syndrome	Masculinization of the female clitoral hypertrophy	Incomplete masculinization of the male Hypospadias Hypoplastic penis Cryptorchidism

should be delayed until the infant's bladder is full. If severe dehydration, abdominal congenital anomalies, inguinal hernias or distention are present, a suprapubic tap may be contraindicated. Nonpharmacological and/or pharmacological pain relief should be provided. The procedure is usually performed with a 3-mL syringe and a 23- to 25-gauge straight needle. The needle is placed midline, 1 to 1.5cm above the symphysis pubis, and is inserted perpendicularly or at a slight angle, pointing toward the head. Entry into the bladder is determined when resistance decreases as the needle is inserted. A slight traction on the plunger facilitates aspiration of urine into the syringe. If no urine is obtained on the first attempt, a second attempt should be delayed until sufficient urine buildup has occurred. At the completion of the procedure, pressure should be applied over the puncture site until all evidence of bleeding has ceased.

Suprapubic aspiration can result in complications, including uterine and bowel perforation, trauma to other portions of the renal system, and infection. The procedure is not recommended for neonates with clotting disorders or disseminated intravascular coagulation. Urethral catheterization may also be performed to obtain sterile urine specimens. After prepping the area with an antimicrobial solution, a 3.5 French or 5 French feeding tube or urinary catheter is coated with lubricant and inserted into the urethra until urine returns. Discarding the initial 1 to 2 mL of urine obtained will increase the accuracy of the culture results (Peniakov, Antonelli, Naor, & Miron, 2004). Because bagged specimens have a significant risk of contamination, they are not recommended for Gram stain or culture.

Urinalysis

One of the first steps in a urogenital workup is a urinalysis. Variables normally assessed in a urinalysis include color, pH, specific gravity, white blood cells, blood, and protein. Urinalysis includes gross assessment as well as dipstick and microscopic evaluation. The urine is most often straw-colored, but this may be altered by the type and amount of solutes. Dipstick testing of urine can provide a wide range of information. This test requires that one to two drops of urine be placed on the dipstick, or the stick may be dipped into a specimen of urine. The results are generally obtained within 30 seconds to 1 minute; however, the exact timing required is based on the manufacturer's suggested procedure and can be found in either the instruction manual or on the dipstick bottle itself. In addition to pH, specific gravity, protein, and blood, the dipstick test may also assess the presence of leukocytes, nitrites, glucose, bilirubin, and ketones in the urine. The presence of leukocytes and nitrites can be indicative of a UTI (Cataldi, Italian Society of Neonatology Neonatal Nephrology Study Group, Zaffanello, Gnarra, & Fanos, 2010).

Renal regulation of acid–base balance has previously been discussed. Urinary pH values range from 4.5 to 8 and reflect the kidney's attempt to maintain acid–base balance. The newborn initially excretes alkalotic urine with a pH of approximately 6. Urine pH values in the newborn should be evaluated in relation to the serum bicarbonate values. Production of alkaline urine with documented metabolic acidosis may indicate renal pathology.

Specific gravity indicates the kidney's ability to concentrate and dilute urine, and normal levels typically range from 1.001 to 1.015. Since infants have a decreased ability to concentrate urine, specific gravity measurement in the newborn can be misleading. High specific gravities can be an indication of either dehydration or high solute excretion. Excretion of glucose and protein in the urine may artificially increase the specific gravity in the newborn. Urine osmolality or the number of solute particles dissolved in a given volume of solution is a more accurate measure.

Urine Chemistries

Urine chemistries can be helpful in determining fluid and electrolyte balance when evaluated in comparison to serum electrolyte levels. Sodium excretion is very high in the fetus

TABLE 18.2

DIFFERENCES IN RENAL FUNCTION BETWEEN FULL-TERM AND PRETERM INFANTS

Preterm	Full Term
Creatinine clearance	11 ± 5 46 ± 15
1 week after birth	(GA 25–[mL/min/1.73 m2] 28 weeks) 15 ± 6 (GA 29–34 weeks)
Plasma creatinine	1.4 ± 0.8 0.5 ± 0.1
1 week after birth (mg/dL)	(GA 25–28 weeks)
Maximum urine osmolality(mOsm/kg H2O)	400–700 600–900
Proteinuria (mg/m2/d)	88–377 68–309
Plasma bicarbonate (mEq/L)	19.5 ± 2.9 21.0 ± 1.8
Mean fractional excretion of sodium (%)	4 (GA < 30 weeks) < 2

GA, gestational age.
Adapted from Springate et al. (1987).

and premature infant but tends to decrease with increasing gestational age. While the term infant conserves renal sodium and renal sodium loss is small, sodium loss in the premature infant can be very high, necessitating correction in intravascular fluids or feedings. The increased sodium loss in premature infants is related to an impaired reabsorption of sodium in the renal tubules as well as unresponsiveness to aldosterone.

Potassium is freely filtered by the glomerulus, but urinary potassium levels are low because the majority of filtered potassium is reabsorbed by the proximal tubule and to a lesser extent, the loop of Henle. Urinary potassium levels reflect the amount secreted by the collecting tubule. As a result, increased potassium load can significantly increase serum potassium levels. Hyperkalemia can be a life-threatening situation and is defined as a potassium level greater than 6 mEq/L. Infants who are extremely low birth weight (less than 1,000 g) are at high risk of hyperkalemia due to a reduced GFR, acidosis, and an immature tubular response to aldosterone.

Blood Urea Nitrogen and Creatinine

Evaluation of blood urea nitrogen (BUN) and creatinine levels is essential when assessing renal function. Creatinine is a breakdown product of creatinine phosphate in muscles. It is freely filtered by the glomerulus, and creatinine levels are the most common indicator of GFR (Boer et al., 2010). Creatinine levels at birth are relatively high and reflect maternal levels, gestational age, and the infant's GFR (Gubhaju et al., 2011). The level may temporarily increase on day 1 but then begins to decrease over the first few weeks of life (Boer et al., 2010). The more immature the infant, the higher the initial creatinine level and the longer it takes to reach normal levels. Serial levels are necessary to accurately evaluate renal function. Although these indices are not absolute indicators of long-term renal dysfunction, they can be used to identify and treat acute problems. During the first few days of life, BUN levels should not be greater than 20 mg/dL. Elevated BUN levels can result from significant dehydration, ingestion of high protein loads, as well as renal dysfunction. Table 18.2 provides a summary of blood and urine chemistries in both term and preterm infants.

Urine Culture

Urine culture in the newborn is used to assess for UTI. UTIs are common in the infant and can occur in association with urinary tract deformities, due to sepsis, or when organisms have been introduced via invasive procedures. Urine cultures should be obtained by either in-and-out catheterization or suprapubic tap to maintain the sterility of the specimen.

RADIOLOGIC EVALUATION

Radiologic examination includes a variety of tests available for determining anatomic and physiologic function.

Renal Ultrasonography

One of the safest and most useful tests to evaluate for the presence of renal anomalies is ultrasonography. Ultrasound is readily available, is noninvasive and inexpensive, and can detect most structural renal abnormalities. The two-dimensional mode and Doppler imaging are the usual techniques. The two-dimensional mode may be used to illustrate kidney structure, and Doppler imaging provides information relative to blood flow in the renal arteries and veins. Ultrasonography is useful in identifying renal obstruction, hydronephrosis, the presence of renal calculi, and in some cases, advanced parenchymal disease.

Prenatal Ultrasound

Currently, the majority of pregnant women undergo prenatal ultrasounds between 16 and 20 weeks gestation. Seventy percent of renal and UTIs are now diagnosed during prenatal ultrasound (Bhide, Sairam, Farrugia, Boddy, & Thilaganathan, 2005). Prenatal ultrasound is proficient in providing information regarding amniotic fluid volume, degree of urinary tract obstruction, as well as the presence of hydronephrosis. The presence of abnormally sized kidneys, renal cysts, hydronephrosis, abnormal bladder size, and oligohydramnios suggests significant renal or urinary tract abnormality. Amniotic fluid is predominately produced by the kidneys, and anhydramnios or severe oligohydramnios may be indicative of severe kidney disease (Morris, Malin, Khan, & Kilby, 2010). Normal amniotic fluid levels are critical for normal lung development, and severe oligohydramnios can result in pulmonary hypoplasia.

Prenatal diagnosis of renal abnormalities provides an opportunity for family counselling and if necessary allows the family time to make treatment decisions including elective termination if the anomaly is incompatible with life. It also allows maternal transfer prior to a tertiary care center so that the infant can be provided optimal care in the delivery room and immediately following delivery. Because of prenatal diagnosis, treatment of neonatal renal disease may be initiated prior to the onset of symptoms, potentially improving long-term prognosis. Prenatal diagnosis of renal abnormalities can cause significant family stress, and families require honest, accurate information. To become a source of this information, nurses require an understanding of the disease process and treatment options for renal abnormalities (Hubert & Palmer, 2007).

Prenatal ultrasound also provides an opportunity for in utero treatment of certain disorders. Placement of a vesicoamniotic shunt (a shunt placed in the bladder to drain urine into the amniotic fluid) can be used to increase amniotic fluid volume and reduce the complications of oligohydramnios (Chandler & Gauderer, 2004) (Figure 18.5). The goals of in utero shunting include restoration of adequate amniotic volume for lung development and preservation of renal function by relieving obstruction (Morris et al., 2010). Unfortunately, this procedure generally results in minimal improvement in outcome (Becker & Baum, 2006). Complications of vesicoamniotic shunt placement include dislodgement, premature labor, urinary ascites, and chorioamnionitis (Morris et al., 2010).

Voiding Cystourethrogram (VCUG)

During a VCUG, a urinary catheter is placed into the bladder, contrast material is instilled, and fluoroscopy is then

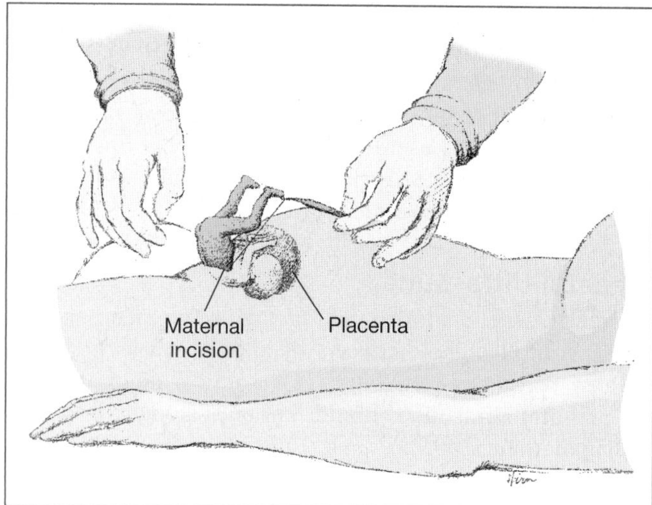

FIGURE 18.5 Fetal surgery to prevent hydronephrosis.

used to monitor bladder filling and voiding mechanisms and to assess for the presence of vesicoureteric reflux (Darge, 2010). VCUGs are primarily used to assess for the presence of vesicoureteric reflux (Darge, 2010) but can also assess bladder and urethral function and anatomy (Riccabona, 2002).

Renal Scintigraphy With Dimercaptosuccinic Acid (DMSA) Scan

This test is considered the gold standard for assessment of renal parenchyma and is usually performed to evaluate renal function and assess for renal damage. It involves IV administration of an actively labeled substance (radioisotope) radioactive isotope. The most commonly used radioisotope is technetium-99m mercaptoacetyltriglycine (99mTC-MAG-3). The radioactive isotope is taken up by the renal parenchyma to identify regions of decreased update representing inflammation or renal scarring. It can also be used to visualize kidney mass as well as ureter and bladder outline. In the premature infant, contrast material should only be used when absolutely necessary since the hyperosmolarity of the solution can lead to further renal compromise.

Diuretic Renography

A diuretic renography is another radionuclide test that is most often used to differentiate between obstructive and nonobstructive uropathies and to assess renal function. A radioisotope injection is administered, followed 15 to 30 minutes later by a diuretic injection. The diuretic facilitates the movement of the radioisotope through the renal system, and a gamma computer tracks the isotope's movement. If urinary obstruction is present, the isotope's progress is slowed or impeded and is shown as retention of the radioactive substance. If dilation exists along the renal system, urine is retained at the uteropelvic junction until overflow occurs with diuretic action. Stretching of the muscle fibers at this point causes strong contractions, release of urine, and rapid movement of the isotope with a sharp, immediate decline in isotope concentration. In a normal kidney, the isotope takes about 25 minutes to clear the system.

Computed Tomography (CT) and Magnetic Resonance Imaging (MRI)

CT and MRI provide high-resolution cross-sectional imaging. There is little advantage to the use of these modalities over other renal imaging techniques, and their use is limited to situations where other tests are inconclusive.

MANAGEMENT

Fluid, Electrolytes, and Nutrition

When renal failure is suspected, serum electrolytes, phosphorus, and calcium levels should be monitored as frequently as clinically indicated to prevent derangement. Fluids should be carefully managed relative to the clinical presentation and response to therapy.

Abnormalities in fluid status, including both dehydration and overhydration, are common and must be carefully monitored. Nursing management involves the ongoing assessment and reporting of signs and symptoms consistent with abnormities in hydration. Daily or twice-daily weights may be required for determination of excessive fluid retention or loss. Accurate intake and output must be measured, and urine-specific gravity should be frequently monitored. The presence of edema due to fluid overload can be assessed by observing for the presence of periorbital edema and edema of the hands, feet, labia, and scrotum. Pitting should be determined by gentle depression of a fingertip into the suspected edematous site.

Hyponatremia is common and is usually related to fluid overload and increased antidiuretic hormone (ADH) production (Karlowicz & Adelman, 2005). A sodium level less than 120 mEq/L can result in seizures and must be treated with sodium replacement therapy. Careful monitoring of fluid status and restricting fluid intake to insensible water loss plus urinary output is imperative to prevent hyponatremia in infants with severe oliguria.

Due to oliguria or anuria, hyperkalemia is also a potential complication of renal failure and maintenance of appropriate potassium levels is imperative. If hyperkalemia is associated with ECG changes, it may result in a medical emergency; careful cardiac monitoring is essential to detect any abnormal rhythms or patterns resulting from alterations in potassium levels. Potassium should not be added to parenteral fluids until an appropriate urine output has been established. The goals of hyperkalemia management are to decrease myocardial excitability, enhance cellular potassium uptake, and facilitate potassium excretion. Administration of intravenous calcium gluconate aids in decreasing myocardial excitability. Cellular uptake of potassium can often be achieved through combined administration of glucose and insulin as well as administration of sodium bicarbonate (1 mEq/kg). These measures are only temporary solutions to the problem since they do not remove the excess potassium from the body. Exchange transfusions and administration of Kayexelate can facilitate potassium excretion.

The administration of a cation-exchange resin such as Kayexelate binds the serum potassium and actively removes it from the body. Each gram per kilogram administered will decrease the potassium level by 1 mEq/L (Karlowicz & Adelman, 2005). Since the mechanism of action is exchange of a sodium ion for a potassium ion, hypernatremia, fluid overload, and congestive heart failure are potential side effects of Kayexelate (Karlowicz & Adelman, 2005). Administration of Kayexelate is not an immediate solution for hyperkalemia since it takes several hours to take effect. If the hyperkalemia is severe or if conventional therapies are unsuccessful, dialysis may be necessary.

Because of decreased excretion, hyperphosphatemia may also occur with renal disease, causing severe hypocalcemia and even tetany. Aluminum hydroxide is a treatment option by binding phosphorus in the intestines, but dialysis is often indicated for treatment of severe hyperphosphatemia. A low-phosphorus formula such as Similac PM 60/40 (Ross Laboratories, Columbus, OH) or spinal muscle atrophy (SMA) (Wyeth, Madison, NJ) may be indicated in infants receiving enteral nutrition.

Hypocalcemia is common and, if symptomatic, can be treated with calcium supplements. Close nursing observation is necessary during intravenous administration since rapid administration can precipitate cardiac arrest. Vitamin D supplementation is a useful adjunct for correction of calcium levels through facilitation of intestinal calcium absorption during enteral feedings. Metabolic acidosis often occurs in conjunction with renal disease due to decreased secretion and increased production of hydrogen ions. Sodium bicarbonate is indicated if the pH falls to less than 7.2.

Growth and nutrition may be compromised due to the necessary fluid and protein restriction necessitating meticulous attention to nutrition and fluid status. A positive nutritional status positively affects both the short- and long-term outcome of infants with renal disorders. If fluid restriction is necessary, attempts should be made to increase the total caloric consumption without increasing the overall fluid volume. The overall goal of nutritional therapy is to preserve a positive nitrogen balance while avoiding increases in nitrogenous waste products and increased BUN levels. Protein intake should be determined by overall caloric intake and BUN levels, and recommendations usually include 1 to 2 gm/kg/d (Drukker & Guignard, 2002).

Skin Management

Impaired skin integrity is common, especially in the presence of severe edema. The infant's position should be changed every 2 hours to decrease the effects of dependent edema and to improve circulation. The skin around any operative site should be inspected with every dressing change for signs of irritation or infection and should be kept clean and dry to prevent skin breakdown and infection.

Respiratory Management

Due to oligohydramnios, respiratory compromise is common in infants with alterations in urinary elimination. During fetal life, insufficient amniotic fluid is linked to decreased development of the respiratory tree (see discussion on Potter's syndrome). Varying degrees of lung hypoplasia may exist, resulting in potentially significant respiratory distress.

Before extensive therapy is initiated for the treatment of renal anomalies, careful evaluation of respiratory status should be performed (see Chapter 6). Measures to improve renal function may not be considered if respiratory capacity is insufficient to support life.

General Preoperative Management

If surgical intervention is indicated, preoperative care is directed toward achieving and maintaining fluid and electrolyte balance and ensuring hemodynamic stability. Ongoing assessment for signs of a UTI including poor feeding, temperature instability, cyanosis, and other subtle signs of infection is necessary. Surgery should be delayed until the infant is free from any possible infection including UTIs (Riccabona, 2004).

General Postoperative Management

Postoperatively, nursing management is again focused on careful assessment and monitoring of the fluid and electrolyte status as well as the hemodynamic system. Vital signs including blood pressure, pulse, and respiration should be monitored every 2 to 4 hours after the initial post-op period. Accurate measurement of fluid intake and output is critical. Dressings should be inspected for bloody drainage or secretions. Initially, a small amount of bleeding at the site is common, but prolonged or heavy bleeding should be reported to the medical team. Depending on the overall clinical status of the infant, feedings can usually be resumed once bowel sounds can be auscultated and the nasogastric tube has been removed.

If renal function is at risk due to a blockage at the level of the ureter, surgical placement of a nephrostomy tube may be indicated. Generally, nephrostomy tubes are considered only for severe bilateral obstruction with renal failure or if there is evidence of renal insufficiently in a severely obstructed unilateral kidney (Riccabona, 2004). Because the renal system is highly vascularized, the chance for bleeding and infection is increased. After insertion of a nephrostomy tube, pink-tinged urine or even urine with visible bloody streaks is common. Because they are located within the renal pelvis, these tubes should not be irrigated. The tubes should be connected to a closed drainage system to maintain sterility, and a clean dressing surrounding the tube should be used to maintain the position and protect the underlying skin. Upon removal, leakage of urine at the site for up to 48 hours is considered normal.

Parental Support

Parental response to a critically ill infant will vary and must be addressed individually. Consenting to a major surgical procedure on their infant so early in life may be very difficult. The parents must be given accurate information regarding their infant's prognosis and should be encouraged to express their concerns. Use of an interdisciplinary team is essential. Collaboration among the neonatologist, pediatric urologist, nurse, clergy, and social worker will help the parents adjust to this frightening situation. If the infant's clinical status is terminal, early identification and involvement of their support network, including family, friends, and clergy, can assist the parents in coping with the reality that their child may not survive. In order for the family's needs to be met, the bedside nurse must anticipate their needs and respond appropriately (Wright, 2008).

The general principles of collaborative management have been outlined. The remainder of the chapter addresses the most common GU neonatal problems.

URINARY TRACT INFECTIONS

Pathophysiology

UTIs are common in infants and are defined as infection of the kidney and/or bladder. Infection occurring in the kidney is called pyelonephritis, while infection of the bladder is cystitis. The presence of a UTI results in acute morbidity in the neonatal population and if not properly treated can result in long-term sequelae, including decreased renal function, renal scarring, and hypertension (Cataldi, Mussap, & Fanos, 2006).

Risk Factors

The incidence of UTIs is 0.1% to 2% in all newborns and 20% in preterm and high risk infants. UTIs are more common in male infants potentially due to an increased risk of UTI in uncircumcised males (Shaikh, Morone, Bost, & Farrell, 2008). Traditionally, it was thought that UTIs were strongly associated with the presence of vesicoureteral reflux, but recent evidence has refuted this assumption (Yamazaki, Shiroyanagi, Matsuno, & Nishi, 2009). The presence of a neurogenic bladder may also increase the incidence of UTIs. Neurogenic bladders are associated with neural tube defects, including meningomyelocele, and occurs when the bladder lacks innervation and therefore fails to completely empty.

Clinical Manifestations

During the first 1 to 2 months of life, clinical manifestations of UTIs are often nonspecific and subtle and include temperature instability, poor feeding, cyanosis, abdominal distention, poor weight gain, hepatomegaly, jaundice, and fever (Biyikli, Alpay, Ozek, Akman, & Bilgen, 2004; Catalde et al., 2010). A urine dipstick is often positive for protein, blood, nitrites, or leukocytes. The presence of a UTI may also be discovered during a general sepsis evaluation.

Diagnosis

Initial examination of the infant suspected of having a UTI should include a thorough family and perinatal history. Any positive familial history of pyelonephritis or nephritis as well as maternal infections should be noted. Neonatal procedures including suprapubic bladder taps and bladder catheterization should be noted along with the dates these procedures were performed in order to estimate the incubation time for possible infection. Infants with signs of a UTI may have nonspecific inflammatory markers, including an elevated or decreased white blood cell count, a left-shift on complete band count, and an elevated c-reactive protein (CRP). A urinalysis or dipstick positive for either leukocytes or nitrites should be considered evidence of a UTI until urine culture results are obtained. The presence of protein and blood in the urine suggests a UTI but is not conclusive.

A urine Gram stain and culture should be obtained using either suprapubic aspiration or sterile bladder catheterization. Bagged urine specimens should never be used for culture purposes due to the high likelihood of perineal contamination (American Academy of Pediatrics [AAP], 2011). False-positive culture results obtained from bagged specimens can lead to misdiagnosis and inappropriate treatment. Any bacteria obtained from a suprapubic aspiration must be considered diagnostic, whereas urine obtained via catheterization can have up to 10^5 CFUs (colony-forming units) before a UTI is diagnosed. Because of the strong possibility of systemic infection, a blood culture should also be obtained. All Gram stains and cultures should be obtained prior to the initiation of antibiotic therapy, allowing appropriate diagnosis and identification of pathogens (AAP, 2011).

Prognosis

With prompt diagnosis and treatment, the prognosis is generally excellent for isolated UTIs. If left untreated, the potential for serious complications, including severe damage to the renal system exists, including renal scarring, decreased renal function, and hypertension (Biyikli et al., 2004; Wald, 2004). The prognosis of UTIs associated with renal abnormalities is dependent on the severity and type of underlying abnormality.

Collaborative Management

Prompt treatment is imperative to prevent complications, including renal scarring, which can lead to hypertension or permanent kidney failure. Empiric broad-spectrum IV antibiotic therapy should be initiated following completion of the diagnostic workup and continued for 7 to 14 days IV (AAP, 2011). Following identification of the infective organism on culture and specification of sensitivities, antibiotic coverage may be adjusted. A repeat urine culture should be obtained 48 to 72 hours following initiation of treatment. The majority of UTIs are caused by *Escherichia coli*; however, *Klebsiella, Pseudomonas, Proteus, Enterococcus, Staphylococcus*, and *Candida* are becoming more common as causative agents in the NICU (Nese et al., 2004). UTIs commonly occur in conjunction with systemic sepsis, and it may be difficult to determine whether the UTI is a result of the sepsis or is the underlying cause of the sepsis.

Historically, infants diagnosed with a UTI underwent a VCUG to assess for vesicourethral reflux (VUR) because of a believed strong association between VUR and UTIs. Evidence now exists that the risk of recurrent UTI is not significantly affected by VUR, and the AAP currently recommends that a VCUG not be performed following the first UTI unless the renal ultrasound indicates abnormalities, including hydronephrosis, renal scarring, severe VUR, or obstructive uropathy (AAP, 2011; Ismaili et al., 2011). A VCUG is also indicated if the infant is affected by future UTIs. A renal ultrasound is recommended following all UTIs. It is a safe and easy procedure that may provide important information regarding an underlying renal abnormality (AAP, 2011). Controversy exists concerning the necessity of prescribing prophylactic antibiotic therapy to all infants until the presence of reflux has been eliminated. It has been recently shown that prophylactic antibiotics do not fully prevent UTIs or scarring associated with reflux, and the incidence of UTI does not increase without antibiotics (Hayashi & Kojima, 2010).

Nursing Management

Nurses play a key role in monitoring infants in the NICU for symptoms of sepsis and UTI. When such signs present or if an infant has abnormalities including positive leukocytes, nitrites, blood or protein in the urine, these should be reported to the medical team for further diagnostic workup. If the infant requires a VCUG, it is important to realize the procedure is uncomfortable to the infant and stressful to the family. Nonpharmacologic interventions, including sucrose nipples, swaddling, and nonnutritive sucking, should be used to soothe the infant. Pharmacologic pain interventions are rarely needed but should be administered if the infant has elevated pain scores. If an infant has had a UTI, discharge teaching must include instructions regarding symptoms of a UTI, and parents should be instructed to seek medical care immediately if symptoms occur (AAP, 2011).

CIRCUMCISION

Circumcision is defined as removal of the prepuce from the glans of the penis (Ahmed & Ellsworth, 2012). Although the function of the prepuce is not entirely understood, it is probably involved in protection of the glans (Lukong, 2011). Circumcision is one of the most commonly performed procedures in the United States, with approximately 1.1 million neonates undergoing this procedure yearly (Lukong, 2011). There are currently three commonly utilized methods of circumcision, including the Gomco clamp, the Plastibell device, and the Mogen clamp. The method utilized is generally dependent upon individual preference and familiarity.

Circumcision dates back to medieval times and is presently performed for generally cultural and religious indications. The practice of circumcision has been a source of extreme controversy over the past several decades, and this controversy has increased dramatically during the last several years. Until 1989, the AAP recommended against routine circumcision based on lack of medical indication for the procedure (AAP, 1971, 1975, 1983). In 1989, a multidisciplinary Task Force on Circumcision established by the AAP summarized the pros and cons of circumcision but did not make specific recommendation regarding the necessity of routine circumcision (AAP, 1989). In 1999 this same task force again summarized the existing scientific evidence stating that although potential benefits to circumcision existed, there was insufficient data to recommend routine circumcision. They recommended that parents be provided with accurate and unbiased information and allowed to make the decision whether to circumcise their child (AAP, 1999). The World Health Organization takes a more proactive stance, stating that circumcision should be considered an effective intervention of HIV prevention in areas with heterosexual HIV epidemics and a low rate of male circumcision (WHO, 2012).

Complications associated with not performing neonatal circumcision include infection of the prepuce (prosthitis), glans (balanitis) or both (balanoprosthitis), and obstruction of the urethra (phimosis) (Tobian & Gray, 2011). An increased rate of UTI in uncircumcised males has also been reported with an increase from 2.3% to 20.7% in the first year of life (Shaikh et al., 2008). This increased risk is thought to be due to the higher periurethral colonization of bacteria in uncircumcised males that can be introduced into the urethral opening.

There has been an increased interest in the potential long-term benefits of circumcision. Three large randomized clinical trial conducted in sub-Saharan Africa reported a 60% increased rate of HIV in noncircumcised males and suggested there was strong evidence to support the protective effects of circumcision (Avert et al., 2005; Bailey et al., 2007; Gray et al., 2007). Circumcision is associated with a 28% reduction in risk of herpes simplex virus (Gray et al., 2010) as well as a decreased rate of human papillovirus (Tobian et al., 2009). It can be argued that the HIV rate in heterosexual men in the United States is much lower than in sub-Saharan Africa and therefore the protective effects are not as impressive. Sanson et al. in 2010 presented a model of the potential effect of neonatal circumcision on the risk of HIV in men born in the United States. They found a life time reduction for acquiring HIV of 16%, which they argue would significantly lower the expected cost of HIV. Circumcision has also been associated in a meta-analysis with a substantially reduced risk of penile cancer probably due to a decrease in the incidence of phimosis (Larke, Thomas, dos Santos Silva, & Weiss, 2011). However in 2009, the American Cancer Society stated that due to the low risk of penile cancer among uncircumcised males in the United States, circumcision should not be recommended only to prevent penile cancer (American Cancer Society, 2009).

Complications of circumcision are rare occurring in 0.2% to 3% of cases (Weiss, Larke, Halperin, & Schenker, 2010). Most complications are minor and include bleeding, pain, inadequate skin removal, and mild infection. Bleeding is by far the most common complication occurring in 1% of infants undergoing circumcision (Krill, Palmer, & Palmer, 2011). A hematologic workup is warranted in patients who have persistent or significant bleeding associated with the procedure. More serious complications including amputation of the glans, glandular necrosis, and meatal stenosis are rare (Krill et al., 2011). Complications occur most often when the wrong-sized equipment is used or when the clinician performing the procedure is inexperienced or untrained (Weiss et al., 2010). While the complication rate of circumcision is higher in older individuals, there is concern that the parents are providing consent for what is considered by most to be a nonessential procedure and perhaps the procedure should be delayed until the child reaches adolescence and can make an independent and informed decision.

It is well known that performing circumcision without analgesia produces significant pain and physiologic stress, underscoring the necessity of appropriate procedural analgesia; the use of analgesic is recommended by the AAP. The use of a dorsal penile nerve block, a ring block, and eutectic mixture of local anesthetics (EMLA) have all been shown to decrease the pain associated with circumcision, with the dorsal penile nerve block being found most effective in pain control (Brady-Fryer, Wiebe, & Lander, 2004, 2011). Effective adjuncts to nerve blocks include nonnutritive sucking, sucrose nipples, and padded chairs; these therapies should be provided in addition to more invasive pain relief.

Nursing Management

Nursing care following circumcision includes assessment for symptoms of bleeding every 30 minutes for at least 2 hours. Assessment and documentation of the first void following circumcision are also necessary to evaluate for urinary obstruction related to penile injury or edema. Petroleum gauze should be applied to the circumcision site and should be changed frequently to protect the site and prevent bleeding. Parent education prior to discharge is necessary and should include care of the site as well as potential complications requiring medical care. Parents should be told that normal bathing is safe and be provided instructions regarding the petroleum-based dressing. Parents should also be advised to seek medical care if the child presents with pain, fever, lethargy, separation of the edges of the skin, unusual swelling or bleeding, and difficulty with urination.

ACUTE RENAL FAILURE

Pathophysiology

Acute renal failure (ARF) is associated with a significant increase in both the mortality and morbidity of infants in the NICU. ARF occurs when the GFR abruptly decreases or completely ceases, leading to impairment in fluid and electrolyte regulation and acid–base homeostasis (Andreoli, 2004; Barletta & Bunchman, 2004). ARF can be either oligoanuric or nonoliguric. Oligoanuric renal failure is suspected when urinary output falls below 1 mL/kg/hr and serum creatinine levels rise to greater than 1.5 mg/dL. Nonoliguric renal failure occurs in 30% of cases and has an elevated creatinine level, but urine output is either normal or elevated. Other indicators of ARF include a serum creatinine level that rises by 0.3 mg/dL/d or fails to fall below the maternal levels within 5 to 7 days of life (Subramanian et al., 2011).

ARF can be classified as prerenal, intrinsic, or postrenal. Prerenal failure is by far the most common, accounting for 75% to 80% of cases and is due to inadequate perfusion to a normal kidney (Agras et al., 2004). Decreased perfusion may be caused by increased fluid losses from hemorrhage, increased insensible water loss, third spacing or by decreased renal blood flow due to congestive heart failure, hypotension, or hypoxia (Andreoli, 2004). Persistent hypoxia may lead to shunting of blood away from the kidneys toward the more critical organs of the body, causing renal hypoperfusion. Failure to adequately recognize and treat prerenal failure can result in permanent kidney damage.

Intrinsic renal failure results from damage to the renal parenchyma and can occur due to progression of either prerenal or postrenal failure, infection, renal vein thrombosis (RVT), or nephrotoxicity from medications such as aminoglycosides, indomethacin, and amphotericin B (Patzer, 2008). Acute tubular necrosis (ATN) is the most common cause of intrinsic renal failure and is a renal tubular cellular injury due to severe hypoxia, dehydration, sepsis, or blood loss (Patzer, 2008). Other causes of intrinsic renal failure include structural abnormalities of the kidney, including renal dysplasia and polycystic or multicystic kidney disease (MKD).

Postrenal failure is caused by obstruction of the urinary tract with resultant disruption in antegrade urine flow (Basu, Devarajan, Wong, & Wheeler, 2011). Obstruction can be caused by posturethral valves, ureteropelvic and ureterovesical junction obstruction, prune-belly syndrome, and neurogenic bladder. Back flow of urine into the kidney pelvis can result in hydronephrosis and subsequent damage to the renal parenchyma.

Risk Factors

Acute kidney injury is common in the neonatal population and is estimated to occur in close to 24% of neonates admitted to the NICU (Drukker & Guignard, 2002). This estimate may not accurately reflect the true incidence since cases of nonoliguric renal failure are often not included in the analysis (Drukker & Guignard, 2002). Any condition that interferes with normal kidney function can cause acute kidney injury (Table 18.3). Asphyxia is one of the most common causes of ARF with 30% to 56% of affected infants presenting with ARF (Agras et al., 2004). Severity of the asphyxia is correlated with both the incidence and severity of the ARF. ARF is common in very-low-birth-weight infants with the most premature infants being the most susceptible to injury (Koralkar et al., 2011).

Clinical Manifestations

Acute kidney injury should be suspected in all critically ill infants in the NICU, especially those with underlying risk factors for ARF. The cardinal symptoms of ARF include a urine output less than 1 mL/kg/hr and an elevated creatinine level. However, one must not rely on the presence of oliguria to signify ARF since those with nonoliguric renal failure may either have a normal or high urine output. The infant may also appear edematous due to fluid overload resulting from a decreased urinary output and be hypertensive from fluid overload or an increased secretion of renin and aldosterone from the damaged kidney. Physical examination may reveal a flank mass, abnormal genitalia, or the presence of other associated congenital anomalies.

Serum electrolytes will show an elevated BUN and creatinine level and possibly hyperphosphatemia, hyponatremia,

TABLE 18.3

MAJOR CAUSES OF ACUTE RENAL FAILURE IN THE NEWBORN

Prerenal Failure	Intrinsic Renal Failure	Postrenal Failure
Systemic hypovolemia	Acute tubular necrosis	Congenital malformations
Fetal/neonatal hemorrhage	Congenital malformations	Imperforate anus
Septic shock	Bilateral agenesis	Urethral stricture
Necrotizing enterocolitis	Renal dysplasia	
Polycystic kidney disease	Posterior urethral valves	
Dehydration		Urethral diverticulum
Renal hypoperfusion	Glomerular immaturity	Primary vesicoureteral reflux
Perinatal asphyxia	Infection Congenital syphilis	
Congestive heart failure	Toxoplasmosis	Ureterocele Megacystis megaureter
Cardiac surgery	Pyelonephritis	
Respiratory distress syndrome	Renal vascular Renal artery thrombosis	Eagle-Barrett syndrome (prune-belly syndrome)
Pharmacologic	Renal venous thrombosis	
Tolazoline	Disseminated intravascular coagulation	Ureteropelvic junction obstruction
Captopril		
Indomethacin		Extrinsic compression
	Nephrotoxins	
	Aminoglycosides	Sacrococcygeal teratoma
	Indomethacin	
	Amphotericin B	Hematocolpos
	Contrast media	Intrinsic obstruction
	Intrarenal obstruction	
		Renal calculi
	Uric acid nephropathy	Fangus balls
		Neurogenic bladder
	Myoglobinuria	
	Hemoglobinuria	

Modified from Vogt (2006).

acidosis, and hypocalcemia. Hematuria and proteinuria on urine dipstick and urinalysis are also common signs of intrinsic renal failure (Leung & Wong, 2010). A urine-to-plasma osmolality ratio of 1 to 1 or less is also indicative of renal failure. Renal compromise can be detected in utero through evaluation of fetal urine samples. The maximum fetal urine electrolyte levels considered within normal limits are sodium, 100 mEq/L; chloride, 90 mEq/L; and osmolality, 210 mOsm/kg. When these levels are increased, renal failure is suspected.

Diagnosis

ARF is often a manifestation of other underlying disease processes, and diagnosis is aimed at both determining the presence of ARF and identifying the causative element. Specific diagnostic testing is determined by the suspected contributing process. Table 18.4 provides a list of diagnostic indices for neonatal ARF.

A careful prenatal, perinatal, and postnatal history is necessary when evaluating an infant with symptoms of renal failure. A family history and prenatal history including prenatal ultrasound results and amniotic fluid measurements should be evaluated. Information should be collected regarding a history of perinatal depression, conditions associated with decreased renal blood flow, and administration of nephrotoxic medications.

To differentiate between prerenal and intrinsic renal failure, a fluid challenge of 10 to 20 mg/kg of an intravenous

TABLE 18.4

DIAGNOSTIC INDICES IN NEONATAL ACUTE RENAL FAILURE

	Prerenal Oliguria Without Renal Failure	Prerenal and Intrinsic Renal Failure
Serum Findings		
Na	Normal or elevated	Low normal or elevated
K	Normal or elevated	Normal or elevated
BUN	Normal or elevated	Elevated
Creatinine	Normal or elevated	Elevated
Ca	Normal	Low
P	Normal	Normal or elevated
Urine Findings		
RBC, protein, casts, and tubular cell casts	Usually absent	Present
Specific gravity	Increased	Low
Urine volume	Low	Low in 60%–80% (1 mL/kg/hr), normal or high in 40% (>2.4 mL/kg/hr)
Urine osmolarity	Increased	Decreased
(mOsm/kg water)	>300–400	<300
Urine Na (mEq/L)	<30 mEq/L (preterm infant) <20 mEq/L	>30 mEq/L
Creatinine clearance	Normal or decreased	Decreased
U/P creatinine	>20:1	<10:1
U/P urea	>20:1	<10:1
U/P osmolarity	<1.5:1	>1.5:1
FENa%	<1% (term infant) <3% (preterm infant)	>2% (term infant) >3% (preterm infant)
RFI	<3%	>3%

BUN, blood urea nitrogen; RFI, renal failure index; U/P, urine/plasma ratio.
Modified from John and Yeh (1985). Reprinted with permission.

isotonic solution may be administered (Subramanian et al., 2011). A urine output of at least 1 mL/kg/hr within 2 hours of the fluid infusion strongly suggests a prerenal cause for the renal failure. The use of a diuretic following the fluid challenge may be necessary if urine output does not immediately increase. A fractional excretion of sodium (FeNa) and a renal failure index may be calculated to further differentiate between prerenal and intrinsic renal failure. A FeNa greater than 3% and a renal failure index greater than 3 suggest a prerenal etiology. Unfortunately, both of these indices are only accurate after 48 hours following delivery, suggesting a need for alternative mechanisms for acute kidney injury within the first 48 hours of life (Durkan & Alexander, 2011). Certain biomarkers, including urinary beta 2-microglobulin (B2M) and N-acetyl-beta-D-glucosaminidase (NAG), may be more specific urinary markers for renal tubular damage (Willis, Summers, Minutillo, & Hewitt, 1997).

Postrenal failure originating in the lower urinary system can be diagnosed by a positive urinary output following placement of a urinary catheter. A renal ultrasound is indicated to evaluate the etiology of both intrinsic and postrenal failure. Other diagnostic testing is indicated by individual clinical manifestations and suspected underlying etiology of the renal failure.

Prognosis

The prognosis of ARF is related to both the severity of the underlying disease and the ability to treat the underlying problem. The presence of ARF is an independent risk factor for infant mortality and is associated with both short- and long-term complications (Barrantes, Tian, Vazquez, Amoateng-Adjepong, & Manthous, 2008). At least 40% of infants diagnosed with ARF experience residual renal dysfunction and/or hypertension.

Collaborative Management

Early recognition and treatment of ARF may prevent further renal failure and improve outcome. The overall treatment goal is to prevent the long-term complications of ARF. ARF is treated symptomatically until a definitive cause is determined to guide more specific treatment. Prerenal failure is treated by increasing renal perfusion through administration of increased intravascular fluids and possibly administration of low-dose dopamine.

In infants with intrinsic renal failure, fluid administration is limited to replacement of insensible water losses, other fluid losses, and urine output. Accurate calculation of fluid intake, electrolytes, and urine output is vital to prevent fluid overload and subsequent hypertension, edema, and hyponatremia. Hyponatremia can occur because of fluid overload due to oliguria and increased renal sodium losses in infants with nonoliguric renal failure (Subramanian et al., 2011). If the infant is symptomatic or the serum sodium level is less than 120 mEq/L, correction with 3% hypertonic 5 mL/kg over 4 to 5 hours is warranted (Subramanian et al., 2011). Hyponatremia unresponsive to treatment may require dialysis.

Since excess phosphorus is excreted by the kidney, hyperphosphatemia can occur with renal failure. Treatment includes phosphorus restriction and administration of oral calcium carbonate, which binds phosphate and prevents absorption (Haycock, 2003). Hypocalcemia is also common and may require additional calcium supplementation.

Potassium is excreted by the kidney, and infants with intrinsic renal failure are at significant risk of hyperkalemia. Hyperkalemia can be a life-threatening situation because of the possibility of cardiac rhythm abnormalities. Therefore the intake of potassium should be eliminated or extremely limited and monitored carefully. Fresh blood should be used for transfusions since older blood is more likely to contain hemolyzed cells, with a resultant elevation in potassium. Treatment of hyperkalemia includes administration of sodium bicarbonate and a combination of insulin and dextrose to drive potassium from the intracellular space into the extracellular space, thereby reducing the serum level of potassium. Administration of IV calcium can be used to protect the heart against arrhythmias but does not reduce the serum potassium level. Kayexelate can be administered rectally to increase elimination of potassium through the intestinal tract. Kayexelate may be ineffective in infants less than 29 weeks gestation and may be contraindicated due to a possible increased risk of necrotizing enterocolitis (Karlowicz & Adelman, 2005). Uncontrolled hyperkalemia is the most common reason that dialysis is necessary.

Since the kidneys function to excrete excess hydrogen from the body, metabolic acidosis is common in infants with intrinsic renal failure. Treatment with either additional sodium acetate in IV solution or administration of sodium bicarbonate orally or parenterally may be necessary. Sodium bicarbonate should be administered with caution due to its hypertonic nature and its association with an increased incidence of intraventricular hemorrhage in premature infants.

Due to decreased production and release of erythropoietin from the affected kidney, anemia is a potential complication of renal failure. Careful monitoring of the hematocrit is essential, and treatment with Epogen or packed red blood cell transfusion may be necessary.

Hypertension secondary to fluid overload or increased renin secretion from the damaged kidney is common and may require treatment with sodium and fluid restriction. Antihypertensive agents such as hydralazine, nicardipine, and nitroprusside may be required if the hypertension is severe and/or uncontrollable (Karlowicz & Adelman, 2005).

Because many medications are eliminated through the kidney, certain drugs including aminoglycosides, penicillins, cephalosporins, theophylline, indomethacin, tolazoline, amphotericin, and magnesium should be used with caution and levels carefully monitored.

Adequate nutrition is critically important in order to prevent catabolism and malnutrition but is challenging due to the necessary protein and fluid restriction. Because of their decreased sodium potassium and phosphorous loads, infants receiving enteral nutrition may benefit from feedings of breast milk, Similac PM 60/40 (Ross Laboratories, Columbus, OH), or SMA (Wyeth, Madison, NJ). Infants with intrinsic renal failure are unable to excrete the by-products of protein breakdown, and BUN and ammonia levels may become significantly elevated. Protein administration is thereby generally limited to 1 to 2 g/kg/d.

If the infant's condition continues to deteriorate and high BUN and creatinine levels coupled with increasing ammonia levels are present, dialysis may be necessary. Dialysis is a process that removes solutes by diffusion from across a semipermeable membrane (Goldstein, 2011). Dialysis is generally indicated when maximal medical therapy has failed, and specific recommendations include hyperkalemia, severe hyponatremia, acidosis, hypocalcemia, hyperphosphatemia, volume overload, and malnutrition (Karlowicz & Adelman, 2005; Subramanian et al., 2011). Although survival of infants requiring dialysis has increased over the last several decades, it remains a challenge in the neonatal patient (Wedekin, Jochen, Ehrich, & Pape, 2010).

Currently, two types of dialysis are used in neonatal patients: peritoneal dialysis and hemofiltration. Peritoneal dialysis is simple, less invasive, is associated with improved hemodynamic tolerance and is currently the most common type of dialysis performed in the neonatal population (Bonilla-Feliz, 2009). During peritoneal dialysis, hyperosmolar dialysate is infused into the peritoneal cavity through a surgically placed Silastic Tenckhoff catheter, and following dialysis, the fluid is drained from the cavity. Depending on the need for solute and fluid removal, cycle time, dwell time, volume, and the osmolar concentration of the fluid can be adjusted.

Hemofiltration is used when peritoneal dialysis is contraindicated, such as in infants with NEC or those that have undergone abdominal surgery (Subramanian et al., 2011). Hemofiltration is a continuous filtration process and includes continuous arteriovenous and continuous venovenous hemofiltration. Continuous arteriovenous hemofiltration (CAVM) involves cannulation of both an artery and a vein. Blood is removed via the artery driven across a filter and replaced via the vein. Continuous venovenous hemofiltration involves either cannulation of two veins or placement of a double-lumen venous line, and a pump is used to draw blood into the filtration circuit.

Nursing Management

Accurate calculation of fluid intake and output is vital to prevent fluid overload and its associated hypertension, hyponatremia, and edema. Frequent monitoring of electrolytes is essential to assess for abnormalities, including hyponatremia, which if severe can result in seizures and hyperkalemia, which may produce life-threatening cardiac arrhythmias. Bedside EKG monitors need careful monitoring for cardiac arrthymias in infants with intrinsic renal failure at risk for hyperkalemia. Changes in vital signs, activity level, or color should be frequently assessed to ensure subtle changes, indicating anemia may be promptly detected. Infants with renal failure are prone to infection due to multiple invasive procedures and their extended hospitalization. They should therefore be monitored for signs of infection, and any abnormality reported to ensure timely diagnosis and treatment.

Nursing care responsibilities for infants on dialysis include monitoring the equipment, monitoring the cycles if performed manually, performing clotting studies, and administration of heparin and other drugs via the dialysis apparatus. Catheter care includes maintenance of aseptic technique, prevention of hemorrhage and clotting, and observation of the insertion site for signs of infection or dislodgment. The infant should be observed for signs and symptoms of chemical imbalances during the entire dialysis procedure. Accurate measurement of fluid intake and output and electrolyte levels is critical. Fluid shifts affecting blood pressure and electrolyte balance can occur rapidly, causing cardiac arrhythmias, muscle spasms, seizures, and shock.

POTTER'S SYNDROME

Pathophysiology

Potter's syndrome occurs in approximately 1 in 10,000 births with an increased incidence in males. Defects associated with this syndrome can be due to bilateral renal agenesis resulting when the ureteric bud fails to divide and develop culminating in complete absence of the kidney. The etiology can also include completely dysfunctional kidneys due to autosomal recessive polycystic kidney disease (ARPKD), dysplastic kidneys, renal hypoplasia, and obstructive uropathies. The developing fetus continuously swallows amniotic fluid, which is absorbed by the gastrointestinal system and is then secreted into the amniotic cavity by the kidney. When there is little to no urinary output, severe oligohydramnios occurs, resulting in the deformities seen in Potter's syndrome (Potter, 1965). The presence of an adequate amount of amniotic fluid is also necessary for normal pulmonary development. In the presence of severe oligohydramnios, normal pulmonary development fails to occur, resulting in the development of hypoplastic lungs.

Diagnosis

Infants are often born premature, small for gestational age, and in the breech position. Many affected fetuses are stillborn. The effect of severe oligohydramnios on the face includes low-set, malformed ears and micrognathia, "senile" appearance, wrinkled skin, parrot-beak nose, and widely-set eyes with epicanthal folds. Depending on the degree of oligohydramnios, variable degrees of respiratory distress due to pulmonary hypoplasia are present. Contractures of the limbs due to intrauterine compression are often present (Potter, 1965).

Potter's syndrome is readily identifiable on direct observation because of its characteristic features. Prenatal history includes severe oligohydramnios and bilateral renal agenesis or other renal disorders. Regardless of prenatal ultrasound results, an abdominal ultrasound following birth is indicated to confirm the diagnosis.

Collaborative Management

Potter's syndrome is almost universally fatal due to pulmonary hypoplasia and subsequent respiratory failure. Because of the irreversible pulmonary hypoplasia, treatment does not include renal transplantation or long-term dialysis.

Assisting the family to cope during and after the death of their infant is the primary aspect of nursing care of infants with Potter's syndrome. The nurse should encourage parents to visit and hold their infant. Support from pastoral services or social work is imperative during this difficult time.

UNILATERAL RENAL APLASIA

Pathophysiology

When one of the ureteric buds fails to form in utero, unilateral renal aplasia, or absence of the kidney occurs. The incidence of unilateral renal aplasia may be as high as 1 in 500 births and is often associated with other structural defects, such as VACTLRL association (vertebral anomalies, tracheoesophageal atresia, esophageal atresia, renal agenesis, renal dysplasia, and limb defects), caudal regression syndrome as well as chromosomal abnormalities (Durson et al., 2005). This condition may often go undetected in the newborn period and may be an incidental finding later in life.

Clinical Manifestations

If the unaffected kidney is normal, infants with unilateral renal aplasia are often asymptomatic. Unfortunately, the contralateral kidney is often abnormal and findings of VUR, ureteropelvic junction (UPJ) obstruction, renal dysplasia, and ureterocele are common. When the contralateral kidney is abnormal, symptoms are directly associated with the type of renal abnormality. If function of the remaining kidney is significantly decreased, the infant may exhibit signs of renal failure. Diagnosis centers on confirmation of the presence of a single kidney and investigation of the contralateral kidney for abnormalities. This is best accomplished by renal ultrasonography with future testing being determined by results of the ultrasound.

Collaborative Management

If kidney function is not compromised, no nursing care beyond normal newborn care is usually necessary. Information regarding the nursing care and treatment of the specific disorders affecting the contralateral kidney is contained in the appropriate section. The prognosis for infants diagnosed with unilateral renal atresia is excellent if the contralateral kidney is normal. If the remaining kidney is abnormal, the prognosis is depending on the specific disease process.

CYSTIC KIDNEY DISEASE

Cystic disease of the kidney occurs when normal kidney tissue is replaced with nonfunctioning cysts. These cysts may occur unilaterally or bilaterally, and the amount of cystic formation within each kidney determines severity of the disease. Severely affected kidneys often have an associated ureteral agenesis. Cystic disease includes polycystic kidney disease and MKD.

POLYCYSTIC KIDNEY DISEASE

Pathophysiology

Polycystic kidney disease is a bilateral process involving micro- or macroscopic cysts distributed throughout the renal parenchyma (Thomas, 2002). There are two types of polycystic kidney disease: autosomal dominant polycystic kidney disease (ADPKD) and autosomal recessive polycystic kidney disease (ARPKD). ADPKD rarely presents in the neonatal period, with symptoms presenting in the fourth to fifth decade of life. In contrast, ARPKD presents in the neonatal period with enlarged kidneys and replacement of the kidney parenchyma with nonfunctional cysts. The pelvis, calyces, and ureter are all normal (Figure 18.6) (Avni & Hall, 2010). Liver involvement, including hepatic fibrosis, is nearly universal, but symptoms rarely occur in the neonatal period.

Risk Factors

The incidence of ARPKD is 1 in 20,000. The majority present as a sporadic anomaly but an association with other syndromes has been reported. The genetic cause of ARPKD is mutations in the *PKHD1* gene located on chromosome 6p21 (Bergmann et al., 2005).

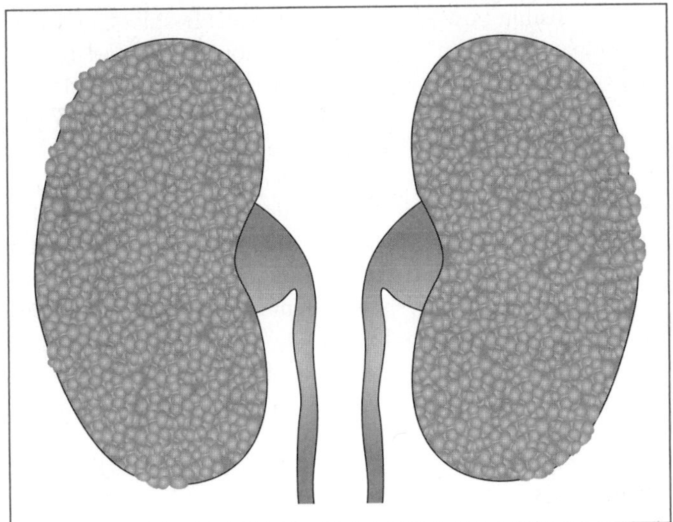

FIGURE 18.6 Autosomal recessive polycystic kidney disease. From Thomas (2002).

Clinical Manifestations

Symptoms include bilateral abdominal masses and hypertension. Respiratory distress may also be present due to pressure from the enlarged kidneys on the diaphragm or from pulmonary hypoplasia due to oligohydramnios (Srinath & Shneider, 2012).

Diagnosis

ARPKD may be diagnosed on prenatal ultrasound showing enlarged kidneys with increased echodensity. Postnatal diagnosis is through ultrasound findings of small cysts in the collecting ducts. After discussion with the family, a positive family history for ARPKD is often discovered.

Prognosis

Six to thirty percent of affected infants will die in the neonatal period usually as a result of respiratory failure from pulmonary hypoplasia. In those who survive the neonatal period, 70% to 87% are alive at 1 year and 70% to 88% are alive at 5 years (Capisonda et al., 2003). An additional 50% of infants will eventually advance to end-stage renal disease, requiring dialysis and renal transplantation. Hepatic complications are common and include portal hypertension and biliary disease (Shneider & Magid, 2005).

Collaborative Management

Treatment of ARPKD is mainly supportive and includes treatment of renal failure, ventilatory support if significant respiratory distress is present, and treatment for hypertension. Hypertension associated with ARPKD may be difficult to control, requiring treatment with fluid restriction and antihypertensive medications (Thomas, 2002). Nephrectomy may be indicated if severe respiratory distress occurs due to pressure on the diaphragm and/or lungs from the enlarged kidney (Mesrobian, Balcom, & Durkee, 2004).

MKD

Pathophysiology

MKD is characterized by a collection of different-sized noncommunicating cysts with a complete lack of renal function occurring due to early obstruction of the ureter leading to kidney maldevelopment (Chiappinelli, Savanelli, Farina, & Settimi, 2011). MKD is generally a unilateral disease; however, if both kidneys are affected, the prognosis is grim due to respiratory failure from pulmonary hypoplasia.

Risk Factors

MKD has an incidence of 1 in 4,300 (Narchi, 2005).

Clinical Manifestations and Diagnosis

The majority (86%) of cases are diagnosed via antenatal ultrasound (Mansoor et al., 2011). If not diagnosed prenatally, most infants present with a palpable flank mass.

Postnatal diagnosis is through renal ultrasound indicating multiple noncommunicating renal cysts with no normal renal parenchyma or renal pelvis (Avni & Hall, 2010). A radionuclide renal scan will indicate a complete lack of renal function of the affected kidney (Kuwertz-Broeking et al., 2004). Vesico-ureteral reflux and UPJ obstruction frequently occurs in the contralateral kidney, requiring careful evaluation either via ultrasound and possibly VCUG (Mansoor et al., 2011). The contralateral kidney is also at risk for decreased function both in the neonatal period and childhood.

Collaborate Management

Historically, management included nephrectomy of the affected kidney to confirm diagnosis and prevent hypertension and renal malignancy. It is now known that spontaneous involution of the multicystic kidney generally occurs and only a minimal risk of either hypertension or malignancy exists (Chiappinelli et al., 2011). Spontaneous involution of the multicystic kidney occurs at a mean age of 29.5 +/–18 months and conservative treatment is now recommended (Mansoor et al., 2011). Follow-up care includes clinical and ultrasound assessment every 6 months for the first 2 years and yearly afterward until complete involution of the kidney (Chiappinelli et al., 2011). Proponents of prophylactic nephrectomy argue that frequent follow-up is burdensome to the family and child and more cost is incurred than with early removal of the kidney (Cambio, Evans, & Kurzrock, 2008). Since long-term dysfunction in the remaining kidney is common, careful long-term evaluation for kidney function is warranted.

PRUNE-BELLY SYNDROME (EAGLE-BARRETT SYNDROME)

Pathophysiology

Prune-belly syndrome consists of a triad of anomalies, including lack of appropriate abdominal musculature, undescended testicles, and urinary tract malformations (Figure 18.7). Associated urinary abnormalities include an enlarged, poorly functioning bladder, vesicoureteral reflux, and urethral obstruction. The ureters may be tortuous and severely dilated, and the kidneys may be dysplastic due to urinary tract obstruction with reflux of urine into the kidneys. Other associated abnormalities include orthopedic, cardiovascuar, and respiratory anomalies as well as imperforate anus and patent urachus (Hassett, Smith, & Holland, 2012).

Two theories currently exist concerning the etiology of prune-belly syndrome. The first suggests that in utero urethral obstruction results in backup of urine into the bladder leading to severe bladder dilation. This extreme dilation places pressure on the abdominal muscles with subsequent abnormal abdominal wall muscle development (Leeners, Sauer, Schefels, Cotarelo, & Funk, 2000). The second and most prevalent theory is that a generalized mesodermal abnormality occurs during the 4th to 10th weeks of fetal development. During this time the bladder is taking shape and is being separated from the allantois, and formation of the abdominal wall is occurring. The abnormal mesodermal development leads to the triad of defects seen with prune-belly syndrome (Strand, 2004).

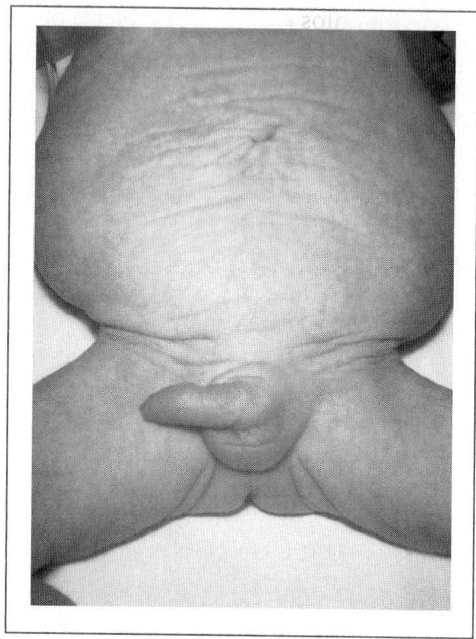

FIGURE 18.7 Prune-belly syndrome.
From Clark (2000).

Risk Factors

Prune-belly syndrome predominantly affects males and only rarely occurs in females. It is 20 times more common in males and has an incidence of approximately 3.76 cases per 100,000 live births (Routh, Huang, Retik, & Nelson, 2010).

Clinical Manifestations

If the abdominal muscles are severely weakened, the abdominal region may appear wrinkled, much like a prune's surface. Due to the lack of abdominal musculature, there may be visible bowel loops and observable spleen and liver (Woods & Brandon, 2007). The abdomen will feel flaccid, and there will be a lack muscle tone. A large distended bladder and large kidneys will be present on palpitation (Woods & Brandon, 2007). Although the spleen is rarely palpable in neonates, one can often feel the spleen in infants with prune-belly syndrome due to lack of abdominal muscle tone. The liver may also be easily palpable, with more than 1 to 3 cm of liver appreciated even if no hepatomegaly is present. Bilateral cryptochorism is universally present in males (Strand, 2004). Infants with pulmonary hypoplasia due to oligohydramnios may present with varying degrees of respiratory distress and those with cardiac anomalies may have symptoms of cardiac disease.

Diagnosis

A diagnosis of prune-belly syndrome can be made as early as 13 weeks on prenatal ultrasound (Papantoniou et al.,

2010). Oligohydramnios may be present if fetal renal function is compromised. The presence of a distended bladder, dilated ureters, large kidneys, and an abnormal abdominal wall on prenatal ultrasound is highly suggestive of prune-belly syndrome. Following birth, the diagnosis of prune-belly syndrome is generally obvious upon initial examination. A postnatal ultrasound will indicate bladder and urethra distension, hydroureter, and hydronephrosis (Strand, 2004). Determination of renal function is necessary and an electrolyte panel including creatinine and BUN levels should be obtained. Urinary output and fluid status must be meticulously monitored. Following stabilization, a VCUG is generally indicated to assess for VUR, and a radionuclide renal scan may be scheduled to determine the degree of renal function.

Woodard classified patients with prune-belly syndrome into three groups. The first group accounts for 20% of cases and presents with severe renal dysplasia, pulmonary hypoplasia and has a mortality rate of nearly 100%. Group two accounts for 40% of patients and presents with significant urinary tract abnormalities but adequate renal function. Future renal compromise may occur due to renal obstruction or infection. The last group, accounting for 40% of patients, presents with mild urinary tract abnormalities and normal kidney function (Woodard, 1978).

Prognosis

The prognosis of prune-belly syndrome is directly related to the severity of any underlying renal dysfunction, whether there is pulmonary hypoplasia, and the presence of other associated anomalies. The mortality rate is 10% to 20%, and another 25% to 30% will develop chronic renal dysfunction, potentially requiring ultimate dialysis and transplant (Routh el al., 2010).

Collaborative Management

This triadic anomaly generally results in severe urinary tract complications. The bladder is usually extremely distended and has a large postvoid residual often requiring bladder decompression for prevention of stasis and resultant reflux of urine into the kidney. Bladder decompression generally requires bladder catheterization and an urethrotomy may be required if urethral obstruction is present. If urinary stasis results in UTIs, a vesicostomy may be indicated (Strand, 2004; Woods & Brandon, 2007). Other urinary tract correction is dependent on the type and severity of the underlying abnormalities.

The main goal of therapy is preservation of existing kidney function. Urinary stasis, reflux, and infection can potentially lead to progressive deterioration in renal function. Careful monitoring and prompt diagnosis and treatment are necessary to preserve existing renal function. In infants with decreased renal function, careful attention to fluid and electrolyte balance, removal of wastes, and adequate nutrition for growth and development is required. Prophylactic antibiotics are recommended if VUR is present.

The prenatal placement of a vesicoamniotic shunt may be considered in the presence of oligohydramnios, a large distended bladder, and severe hydronephrosis when there is evidence of functioning kidneys. This procedure has been successful in decreasing the degree of oligohydramnios and its associated complications and improving subsequent renal function (Leeners et al., 2000).

Muscle tone has been shown to improve with time, but abdominoplasty may be performed to improve the appearance of the abdomen and has been shown to increase self-esteem and improve abdominal strength (Denes, Arap, Giron, Silva, & Arap, 2004). The resultant improvement in abdominal strength may also decrease constipation associated with an inability to perform the necessary Valsalva maneuver required for intestinal evacuation. Strengthening the abdominal muscles may also decrease the number of respiratory infections occurring due to lack of abdominal support and an inability to produce an effective cough as well as improve the child's posture.

Undescended testes are present in all males affected with prune-belly syndrome, and orchiopexy is generally recommended prior to 6 months of age to avoid potential future testicular cancer; however, it is often delayed for 1 year to allow repair in conjunction with urinary tract reconstruction (Strand, 2004). Some recommend a nonoperative approach unless significant renal compromise is present, while others feel early urinary reconstruction to eliminate urinary stasis, correct reflux, and improve bladder drainage is necessary. Evidence suggests concurrent early urinary reconstruction and bilateral orchiopexy; and abdominoplasty is associated with improved results (Denes et al., 2004).

Nursing Management

If bladder distention and urinary retention continue when the infant is ready for discharge, parents should be taught to empty the infant's bladder by intermittent catheterization. Parents must also be educated regarding the signs and symptoms of a UTI such as increased irritability with urination, temperature instability, increase or decrease in urine output, and cloudy or foul-smelling urine. They must understand the importance of early detection and intervention to prevent long-term renal compromise. If a vesicostomy or other urinary diversion procedure has been performed, parents will need specific discharge instructions regarding care of the device.

Consideration of parental feelings concerning the physical appearance of their infant is mandatory. Because American culture places significant value on an individual's appearance, it may be difficult for parents to accept the loss of their "perfect" dream infant. Significant parental support from social and pastoral services may be necessary. To increase parent–infant interaction, nurses should attempt to include the family as much as possible in the daily care of their infant. Infants diagnosed with prune-belly syndrome often require frequent hospitalizations, and parents need to be prepared for this possibility.

EXSTROPHY OF THE BLADDER

Pathophysiology

Exstrophy of the bladder is a rare but severe congenital defect where the anterior abdominal wall fails to close at the point of the bladder. During the first 4 weeks of gestation, the abdominal wall begins to fuse. Exstrophy results when the mesenchymal cells fail to migrate over the abdomen, and a thin membrane forms over the abdominal contents. This membrane later ruptures and leaves the bladder exposed. Exstrophy of the bladder is the most common condition in a spectrum of anomalies ranging from simple epispadias to classic bladder exstrophy (Ebert, Reutter, Ludwig, & Rosch, 2009).

Risk Factors

The incidence of this defect is 1 in 10,000 live births, with males being affected more often than females (Huether, 2004). There are no known risk factors or causative agents.

Clinical Manifestations

In classic bladder exstrophy, the bladder region appears open or uncovered and the posterior wall of the bladder is exposed. The implantation of the ureters may be visible as urine continues to pass from the orifices. Bilateral inguinal hernias are commonly present (Ebert et al., 2009). A concomitant defect exists in the genitalia, and males present with epispadias with a short, flat, and angulated penis. In the female, the labia do not meet in the midline, and a divided clitoris exists. Exstrophy of the bladder is generally not associated with other anomalies, and the kidneys are generally normal. Prolapse of the rectum may also be evident prior to surgical correction. Failure of the pubic bones to meet anteriorly causes the hips to rotate outward (Kiddoo, Carr, Dulczak, & Canning, 2004). Cloacal exstrophy is the most severe expression in this spectrum of anomalies and presents with all the features of classic bladder exstrophy along with an omphalocele, imperforate anus, spinal defects, and UPJ obstruction (Ebert et al., 2009). Neural tube defects and spinal dysraphisms are also commonly present.

Diagnosis

Prenatal ultrasound may suggest the presence of bladder exstrophy, but definitive diagnosis does not occur until after birth when the defect is obvious on visual inspection (Figure 18.8).

Prognosis

Prognosis is generally favorable with most children leading nearly normal lives (Hammouda & Dotb, 2004). Long-term complications include incontinence as well as sexual and fertility problems.

Collaborative Management

Treatment goals for infants with exstrophy of the bladder include successful bladder and abdominal wall closure, urinary continence, preservation of the upper urinary tract, and normal-appearing genitalia. Prior to or immediately following delivery, the infant should be transported to a tertiary care facility experienced with care of the infant with this defect. Because bladder exstrophy exposes the urinary tract to the environment, careful attention to prevention of infection is essential both before and after surgical correction. Broad-spectrum antibiotic therapy is initiated prior to surgery and continued for at least 7 days. Because wound dehiscence is often caused by infection, strict observation of aseptic technique and aggressive management of infection is mandatory.

Two types of repair are currently performed for correction of bladder exstrophy. In the 3-stage repair, the bladder is closed within 48 to 72 hours following birth. Epispadias repair is delayed until the infant is 6 to 9 months of age, and bladder neck reconstruction is performed around 3.5 to 5 years of age (Kiddoo et al., 2004). The 2-staged repair combines the last two stages and the single stage where the complete repair occurs at around 6 weeks of age (Hammouda & Dotb, 2004; Kiddoo et al., 2004). A suprapubic catheter and bilateral ureteral stents may be placed during surgery to allow drainage of urine while the bladder heals. The infant may be immobilized for several weeks following surgery with traction to facilitate wound healing. Vesicoureteral reflux is common and may require an anti-reflux procedure (Purves, 2011).

Nursing Management

Immediately following birth, the exposed bladder should be covered with plastic wrap or a similar material to protect it from injury until closure is complete (Ebert et al., 2009). The area should also be protected by avoiding petrolatum or gauze due to the possibility of becoming dry and adhering to the tissue, using a tie instead of a clamp for umbilical care, changing dressings as needed to prevent skin irritation, and using humidified incubators to prevent excess drying. Diapers should be kept folded well below the defect

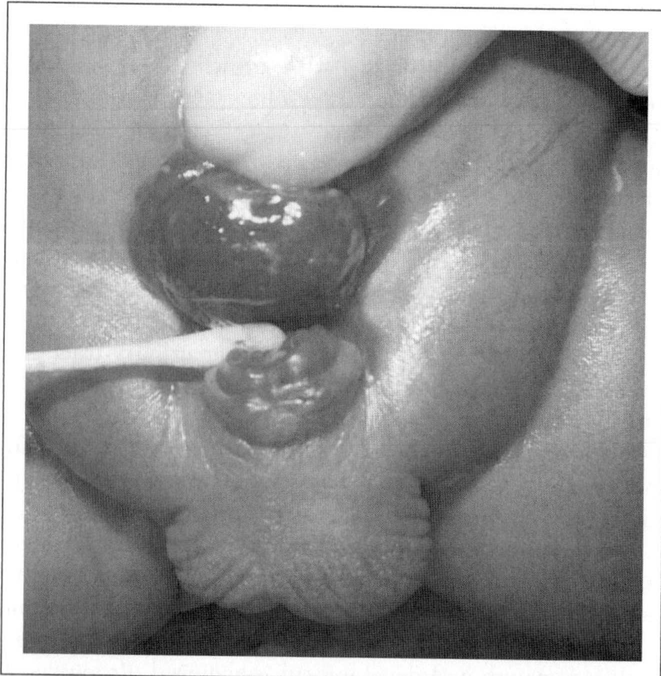

FIGURE 18.8 Exstrophy of the bladder.
From Clark (2000).

to not only protect the area from irritation but to prevent wound infection.

RVT

Pathophysiology

RVT is a rare occurrence in the neonate that can potentially result in renal failure, renal atrophy, and hypertension (Kraft, Brandon, & Navarro, 2011). The thrombus may be unilateral or bilateral and often extends into the inferior venocava (IVC) (Messinger, Sheaffer, & Mrozeck, 2006).

Risk Factors

RVT occurs in approximately 0.5 of 1,000 admissions to the NICU. Although the presence of an umbilical catheter is a risk factor, the majority of RVTs are noncatheter related and the exact etiology is often unknown (Kraft et al., 2011). Up to 80% of affected infants have one or more risk factors including male gender, hyperviscosity and polycythemia, perinatal asphyxia, maternal diabetes, prematurity, dehydration, and infection (Kraft et al., 2011; Lau et al., 2007). Most risk factors are thought to be related to an associated decreased kidney perfusion leading to vasoconstriction and a subsequent decreased venous blood flow and thrombosis. Neonates are at a greater risk for RVT than older children due to a low renal perfusion pressure, decreased levels of natural anticoagulants, and lower levels of fibrinolytic components (Elsaify, 2009).

Up to 50% affected with RVT have inherited prothrombotic risk factors, including hypercoagulation disorders such as protein C deficiency, homocystinuria, and Factor V Leiden (Lau et al., 2007; Marks et al., 2005).

Clinical Manifestations

The mean age of onset is 3 days with 7.3% of RVTs presenting in utero, 67% within the first 3 days following delivery and 26% later than 3 days of life (Kraft et al., 2011; Lau et al., 2007). RVT often occurs in critically ill infants and may be incidentally discovered when the infant is imaged for other reasons. The classic triad of symptoms include a palpable flank mass, hematuria, and thrombocytopenia, however only 13% to 22% of infants actually present with all three symptoms (Winyard et al., 2006). However, the majority of infants present with at least one of the three symptoms. Other clinical manifestations include symptoms of decreased renal function including decreased urinary output, elevated creatinine, and anemia (Anochie & Eke, 2004; Brandao, Simpson & Lau, 2011; Marks et al., 2005).

Diagnosis

Diagnosis is through Doppler ultrasound showing an enlarged kidney, provides information regarding renal blood flow, and may reveal the presence of a thrombosis located in the renal vein (Kraft et al., 2011). A radionuclide renal scan may be performed to assess renal function of the affected kidney. Since RVTs may not present with the typical triad of symptoms (flank mass, hematuria, and thrombocytopenia), a high degree of suspicion is necessary to increase the likelihood of prompt diagnosis and appropriate treatment (Brandao et al., 2011).

Prognosis

Prognosis is dependent on the extent of the thrombus and whether the lesion is unilateral or bilateral. While the mortality rate is relatively low (5%) and often related to the underlying critical nature of the infant rather than the RVT, the risk of both acute and chronic complications is significant. Acute complications include adrenal hemorrhage, thromboemboli, and pulmonary embolism. Hypertension, renal atrophy, and chronic renal failure, including end-stage renal disease are long-term complications (Kraft et al., 2011; Lau et al., 2007; Marks et al., 2005). Hypertension (HTN) occurs in 19% to 22% of survivors and may require nephrectomy if severe (Marks et al., 2005). Chronic renal insufficiency occurs in up to 71% of affected infants with 3% of infants ultimately experiencing end-stage renal failure (Lau et al., 2007).

Collaborative Management

Treatment is dependent on the severity of the RVT, whether it is unilateral or bilateral, and the presence of impaired renal function (Brandao et al., 2011). Currently no specific guidelines exist for RVT treatment, and therapy varies between institutions and individual clinicians. Therapy may include supportive care, degradation of the clot with urokinase, streptokinase, or tissue plasminogen activator, or anticoagulation with low-molecular-weight heparin. If signs of renal failure occur, careful monitoring of fluid and electrolyte status is necessary as well as treatment of any hypertension. In cases of severe renal failure, dialysis may be required (Kraft et al., 2011). Due to the association of RVT with anticoagulant deficiencies, the infant will require a diagnostic workup for these disorders. All infants will require long-term monitoring for hypertension, HTN, renal atrophy, and chronic renal insufficiency.

Nursing Management

Nurses are a critical element in successful evaluation and treatment of RVT. They are often the first clinicians to recognize the presence of risk factors and clinical manifestations, and it is therefore necessary for nurses to have a strong knowledge base concerning RVTs. Careful monitoring for hypertension is necessary as well as following dipstick urine analysis for hematuria and proteinuria. Strict monitoring of input and output as well as electrolyte status is also necessary. The use of thrombolytic agents or heparin requires careful monitoring of coagulation status, and extreme caution is warranted when using these agents in very-low-birth-weight infants due to the risk of intraventricular hemorrhage (Weinschenk, Pelidis, & Fiascone, 2001).

HYDRONEPHROSIS

Pathophysiology

Hydronephrosis is the accumulation of urine within the renal pelvis and calices to the point of overdistention. If left untreated, this buildup of fluid can cause irreversible kidney damage. Hydronephrosis can be caused by obstruction of urine flow at the junction of the ureteropelvis, the ureterovesical valve, or the urethrovesical valve. Nonobstructive abnormalities such as VUR and prune-belly syndrome can also cause hydronephrosis. Secondary etiologies include obstruction such as kidney stones or tumors (Yang, Hou, Niu, & Wang, 2010). The severity of hydronephrosis is classified from grade I to grade V depending on the diameter of the renal pelvis.

Clinical Manifestations

Hydronephrosis is usually detected during a prenatal ultrasound. If the hydronephrosis is severe and bilateral, the presence of oligohydramnios may also be appreciated. If diagnosis is delayed until after birth, hydronephrosis often presents as a large, smooth, solid, palpable abdominal mass in the region of the kidney. Since the presence of an abdominal mass can signify many disease processes, including cystic kidney disease, urogenital tumors, and RVT, determination of the mass's etiology is essential.

Depending on the amount of functioning kidney, infants with hydronephrosis may have a decreased or normal urine output. When only one kidney is involved, urine output may be normal because a single kidney is sufficient for adequate removal of water and waste. Severe bilateral hydronephrosis may present with signs and symptoms of kidney failure, including a low or nonexistent urine output as well as a high creatinine and BUN level. Infants born with bilateral severe hydronephrosis may also exhibit features consistent with Potter's syndrome, including pulmonary hypoplasia due to the presence of oligohydramnios. Since UTIs are often associated with hydronephrosis, infants may present with signs of an UTI including fever, subtle signs of sepsis, hematuria, proteinuria, and the presence of white blood cells on urinalysis.

Diagnosis

Since the almost universal use of prenatal ultrasound, hydronephrosis is most commonly diagnosed on prenatal ultrasound. It can be detected as early as 12 weeks gestation as and is indicated by the presence of a dilated renal pelvis (Maayan-Metzger et al., 2011). Hydronephrosis is the most common renal abnormality detected prenatally and is present in 2.3% of all pregnancies (Sairam, Al-Habib, Sasson, & Thilaganathan, 2001).

The first diagnostic study indicated in infants suspected of having hydronephrosis or who have hydronephrosis on prenatal ultrasound is a renal ultrasound. In clinically stable infants, ultrasound should be delayed until the infant is 24 to 72 hours of age since the newly born infant's relative dehydration may mask the presence of hydronephrosis (Riccabona, 2004). Controversy exists regarding the benefit of early ultrasounds. While these early ultrasounds provide information regarding the extent of the hydronephrosis and the need for additional diagnostic studies, treatment is rarely indicated prior to 3 months of age. Based on this information, some advocate delay of the initial ultrasound. A VCUG is recommended to assess for the presence of reflux if the hydronephrosis is severe (Maayan-Metzger et al., 2011). Although administration of prophylactic antibiotics for prevention of UTI is somewhat controversial, most clinicians will prescribe until the presence of reflux has been excluded.

Prognosis

Prognosis depends on the underlying causative factor, the severity, and the presence of any permanent renal damage. Outcome ranges from complete resolution to end-stage renal disease requiring dialysis and renal transplant. Most cases of hydronephrosis occur without significant obstruction and can be managed conservatively without surgery (Tekgul et al., 2009). Complications of hydronephrosis include hypertension, UTI, and progressive renal damage. Hydronephrosis secondary to VUR generally spontaneously resolves (Penido et al., 2006). Antenatally diagnosed hydronephrosis can indicate obstruction or other serious abnormalities but can also represent a transient developmental change that may spontaneously resolve prior to birth (Yang et al., 2010).

Collaborative Management

Preservation of renal function is the main goal of treatment and treatment is dependent upon severity of the hydronephrosis. Mild to moderate hydronephrosis is usually managed conservatively with close ultrasound monitoring. A VCUG is generally indicated to evaluate for vesicorenal reflux. Although severe hydronephrosis is initially managed with conservative treatment, some cases will ultimately require pyeloplasty due to deteriorating renal function. When reflux is present, prophylactic antibiotics are usually prescribed for UTI prophylasix.

When severe hydronephrosis is prenatally diagnosed, vesicoamniotic shunting (placement of a catheter into the bladder to drain urine) may be performed to reduce oligohydramnios and its associated complications as well as to sustain kidney function (Chandler & Gauderer, 2004). After birth, definitive surgery is necessary to correct the obstructive defect or to provide a diversion for urine flow.

Nursing Management

Careful assessment is imperative in infants diagnosed with hydronephrosis. Vital signs, including blood pressure, must be monitored at least every 4 hours and more frequently if unstable. Monitoring blood pressure is especially important since hypertension is a common complication in infants with severe hydronephrosis. Fluid and electrolyte status including serum creatinine and BUN must also be carefully monitored. Fluid intake and output should be recorded at least every 2 to 4 hours.

OBSTRUCTIVE UROPATHY

Pathophysiology

When obstruction occurs in the urinary tract, changes referred to as obstructive uropathy can occur. Obstruction to urinary flow can cause reflux of urine into the kidney, with resultant hydronephrosis and irreversible kidney damage (Becker & Baum, 2006). Urinary obstruction can be unilateral or bilateral and can occur at the ureterovesical junction, the UPJ, or due to posturethral valves (Chevalier, 2004) (Figure 18.9). The most common cause of urinary obstruction is UPJ obstruction. UPJ obstruction occurs due to obstruction of urinary flow from the pelvis of the kidney into the ureter and is caused by stenosis of the ureter and/or its associated valves or by an insertion anomaly of the ureter. Ureterovesical junction obstruction is caused by obstruction of flow from the ureter into the bladder.

Risk Factors

UPJ obstruction is the most common cause of obstructive uropathy, with an incidence of 1 in 2,000, and is increased in males (Woodward & Frank, 2002). Ureterovesical junction obstruction also occurs more often in males (Becker & Baum, 2006). Information concerning posturethral valves may be found in the section below.

Clinical Manifestations

Signs of urinary tract obstruction include symptoms of a UTI, or if significant hydronephrosis is present an abdominal mass may be appreciated. Severe, bilateral obstruction can also be associated with symptoms of renal failure.

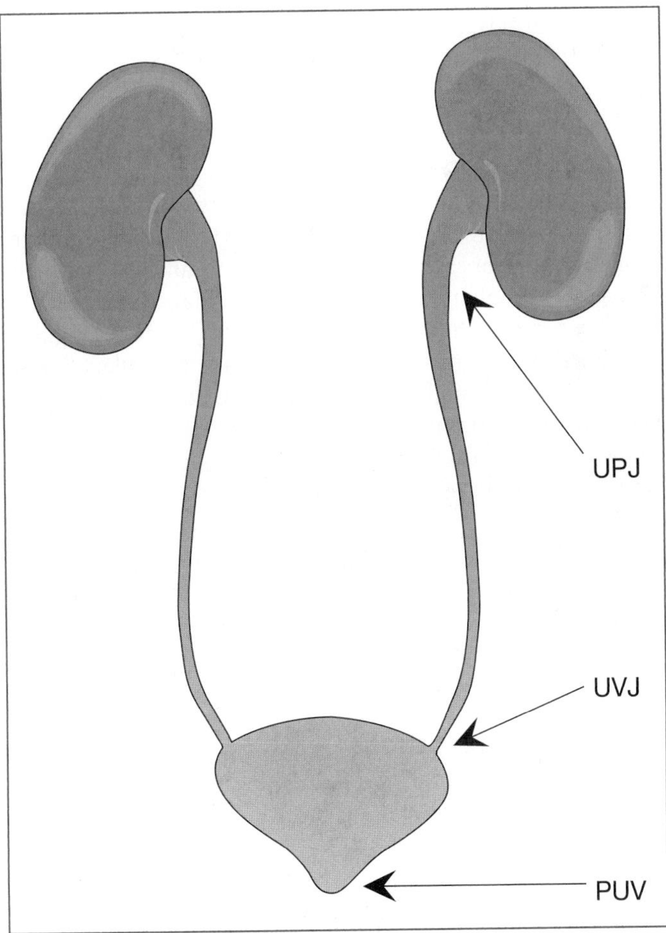

FIGURE 18.9 Location of most common sites of congenital urinary tract obstruction. UPJ, ureteropelvic junction; UVJ, ureterovesical junction; PUV, posterior urethral valves.
From Chevalier (2004).

Diagnosis

Urinary tract obstruction can be diagnosed on prenatal ultrasound as early as 16 to 17 weeks gestation with evidence of hydronephrosis (Becker & Baum, 2006). Ultrasound findings range from mild hydronephrosis to extreme obstruction with oligohydramnios.

Postnatal diagnosis is via renal ultrasound followed by a VCUG to assess for reflux. A radionuclide renal scan is also recommended to assess renal function.

Prognosis

Obstructive uropathy can result in chronic renal failure and is a common cause of pediatric kidney transplantations.

Collaborative Management

Treatment depends on the severity of the obstruction and on whether the obstruction is unilateral or bilateral. If mild, conservative management is appropriate with frequent renal assessment. Prophylactic antibiotics may be indicated to prevent UTIs and the possibility of associated renal damage.

If the obstruction is severe, surgical intervention may be indicated to relieve the obstruction. Insertion of a urinary diversion such as a pyelostomy tube inserted into the renal pelvis may be indicated if the infant is too clinically unstable to tolerate surgery. If the obstruction is severe, significant diuresis may follow urinary diversion; meticulous monitoring of fluid and electrolytes and replacement of losses are critical to avoid dehydration. Long-term follow-up is essential for the early detection of chronic renal problems (Holmdahl & Sillen, 2005; Ylinen, Ala-Houhala, & Wikström, 2004).

Prenatal treatment, including insertion of a vesicoamniotic shunt, may be indicated if severe obstruction is present to increase the amniotic fluid volume and decrease the potential for renal failure. Complications of this procedure include shunt displacement and clogging of the shunt.

POSTERIOR URETHRAL VALVES

Pathophysiology

Posterior urethral valves (PUV) are the most common cause of urinary tract obstruction and cause severe obstruction uropathy, often resulting in end-stage renal failure (Eckoldt, Healing, Woderich, & Wolke, 2004; Youssif et al., 2009). PUV occurs when urine is obstructed at the level of the bladder outlet due to the presence of enlarged valves. Severity ranges from mild obstruction to severe disease, with obstructive uropathy and massive hydronephrosis (Krishnan, de Souza, Konijeti, & Baskin, 2006). Urinary obstruction can increase pressure in the bladder and upper urinary tract, resulting in abnormal bladder function and renal injury (Hodges, Patel, McLorie, & Atala, 2009).

Risk Factors

Posturethral valves is a rare disease occurring exclusively in males with an incidence of 1 in 3,000 to 1 in 8,000 live births (Yohannes & Hanna, 2002). The specific etiology is unknown. Other associated urinary tract anomalies including veiscourethral reflux are common (Kibar, Ashley, Roth, Frimberger, & Kropp, 2011).

Clinical Manifestations

Neonatal symptoms of PUV include a palpable bladder, anuria or oliguria, a weak urinary stream, urosepsis, and urinary ascites (Kibar et al., 2011; Nasir, Ameh, Abdur-Rahman, Adeniran, & Abraham, 2011). If severe oligohydramnios is present prenatally, respiratory symptoms due to pulmonary hypoplasia may be present (Nasir et al., 2011).

Diagnosis

Posturethral valves are often diagnosed on prenatal ultrasound with the presence of bilateral hydronephrosis, a distended bladder, a dilated posterior urethra, and a thickened bladder wall (Casella, Tomaszewski, & Ost, 2012). Following delivery, an ultrasound is required to evaluate the presence and degree of hydronephrosis, the presence of bladder wall thickening, and the general health of the kidneys. However, the gold-standard for diagnosis is through a VCUG showing a dilated posterior urethra, a trabeculated bladder, vesicouretral reflux, and sometimes visualization of the enlarged valve leaflets (Hodges et al., 2009). Renal scintigraphy for evaluation of renal function is usually deferred for approximately 4 weeks following birth to allow maturation of developing kidneys (Nasir et al., 2011).

Prognosis

The diagnosis of PUVs is associated with significant long-term morbidity, which is dependent on the amount of renal damage caused by the PUVs (Youssif et al., 2009). Over 50% of infants diagnosed with PUV will progress to end-stage renal disease in 10 years often requiring dialysis and/or renal transplantation (Kibar et al., 2011). Bladder dysfunction in childhood is common, including bladder overactivity resulting in urgency, urge incontinence, and nocturnal enuresis. The bladder can also become overdistended and overcompliant, causing ineffective bladder emptying and possibly requiring intermittent catheterization. Urethral strictures are also a possible complication occurring later in childhood (Caione & Nappo, 2011).

Collaborative Management

The initial treatment of posturethral valves is immediate urinary diversion with either bladder catheterization or suprapubic diversion to relieve the obstruction and reduce the pressure on the urinary tract to maintain normal bladder and kidney function (Hodges et al., 2009; Youssif et al., 2009). Due to the increased risk of long-term complications, suprapubic diversion is only performed if bladder catherization is impossible or if early correction of the defect is impossible because of the infant's small size or if the urethra is too small, precluding insertion of the endoscope for valve ablation. The infant may also require stabilization, including administration of IV fluids, correction of electrolyte or acid/base abnormalities, and antibiotics to prevent infection. Mechanical ventilation may be required if pulmonary hypoplasia is present. Definitive treatment of PUV is transurethral endoscopic ablation (rupture) of the enlarged valves (Youssif et al., 2009). Prophylactic antibiotics are required to prevent UTIs and subsequent renal injury, and long-term follow-up is essential to monitor bladder and renal function.

Unfortunately, prenatal treatment is difficult to perform and has not been shown to improve the mortality or morbidity of infants with PUV. In cases of oligohydramnios associated pulmonary hypoplasia, some clinicians favor prenatal treatment with urinary diversion to increase the amniotic fluid level (Youssif et al., 2009). In the future, prenatal valve ablation may be possible, thereby avoiding the renal and urinary tract damage that often occurs early in gestation prior to diagnosis of the defect (Hodges et al., 2009).

Nursing Management

Immediately following delivery, the bladder should be catheterized under sterile conditions using a small 5- or 6-gauge feeding tube to allow passage through the constricted urethra. The use of balloon catheters is contraindicated due to the possibility of bladder spams. Parents should be educated regarding the necessity of close postdischarge follow-up to ensure early detection of chronic renal disease and bladder dysfunction (Holmdahl & Sillen, 2005).

HYDROCELE

Pathophysiology

A hydrocele, the collection of fluid in the scrotal sac, is a common occurrence in the neonate. The fluid originates from the peritoneal cavity, which communicates with the scrotum through a patent processus vaginalis. The only difference between the presence of a hydrocele and an inguinal hernia is the size of the process vaginalis (Madden, 2007). If the process vaginalis is small, only fluid can move into the scrotum, resulting in a hydrocele. Larger passageways may allow escape of a bowel segment into the scrotum, resulting in an inguinal hernia.

Risk Factors

The risk of a patent processus vaginalis is elevated with increased abdominal pressure secondary to a ventriculoperitoneal shunt or high ventilatory pressures and prematurity (Madden, 2007).

Clinical Manifestations

Clinical manifestations include the presence of painless scrotal swelling that is readily transilluminated.

Diagnosis

The most critical aspect of diagnosis is differentiating whether scrotal swelling is due to the presence of a hydrocele or the more serious diagnosis of either an inguinal hernia or testicular torsion. Upon palpitation, inguinal hernias are generally reducible whereas hydroceles are not. When transilluminated, the hydrocele will show a fluid-filled scrotum, while an inguinal hernia will appear as a solid mass. If the examiner encounters loops of intestine near the vas deferens or the ductus deferens within the scrotal sac, an inguinal hernia is present. Ultrasound may also assist in differentiation (Clark, 2010).

Collaborative Management

Treatment for hydroceles is rarely indicated; the majority will spontaneously resolve within 1 to 2 years due to closure of the processus vaginalis (Lau, Lee, & Caty, 2007; Madden, 2007). Indications for surgical correction generally include failure to resolve within the first year of life, although some surgeons will wait 2 years if there are no complications. Surgery entails drainage of fluid from the scrotal sac and closure of the processus vaginalis (Clarke, 2010). Until resolution of the hydrocele, the infant should be closely monitored for signs of intestinal herniation. If an inguinal hernia is suspected, surgical intervention is indicated.

Nursing Management

Parents should be taught the signs of intestinal herniation and incarceration and the need for prompt medical attention if symptoms occur. These signs include the presence of a lump in the groin (this lump is especially noticeable when the infant is crying) and increased irritability. Careful attention must be paid to skin care of the edematous scrotum to avoid irritation and breakdown.

INGUINAL HERNIA

Pathophysiology

An inguinal hernia occurs when the intestines descend into either the inguinal canal or the scrotum through an open processus vaginalis (Clark, 2010) (Figure 18.10). During fetal life, as the testes descend into the scrotum, they bring a small part of the peritoneum that is the processus vaginalis (Madden, 2007). When the processus vaginalis is open, fluid or intestines can pass through the opening, resulting in either a hydrocele or an inguinal hernia. The presence of a hydrocele or inguinal hernia is dependent on the size of the opening. The processus vaginalis becomes obliterated between 38 and 48 weeks gestational age.

Risk Factors

Due to the presence of an open processus vaginalis during fetal life, the incidence of inguinal hernias is inversely related to gestational age and birth weight. The incidence is also nine times more prevalent in male infants. Sixty percent of inguinal hernias occur in the right and 15% are bilateral (Lau et al., 2007). Additional risk factors include cystic fibrosis, congenital hip dysplasia, the presence of a ventriculoperitoneal shunt, and abdominal wall defects.

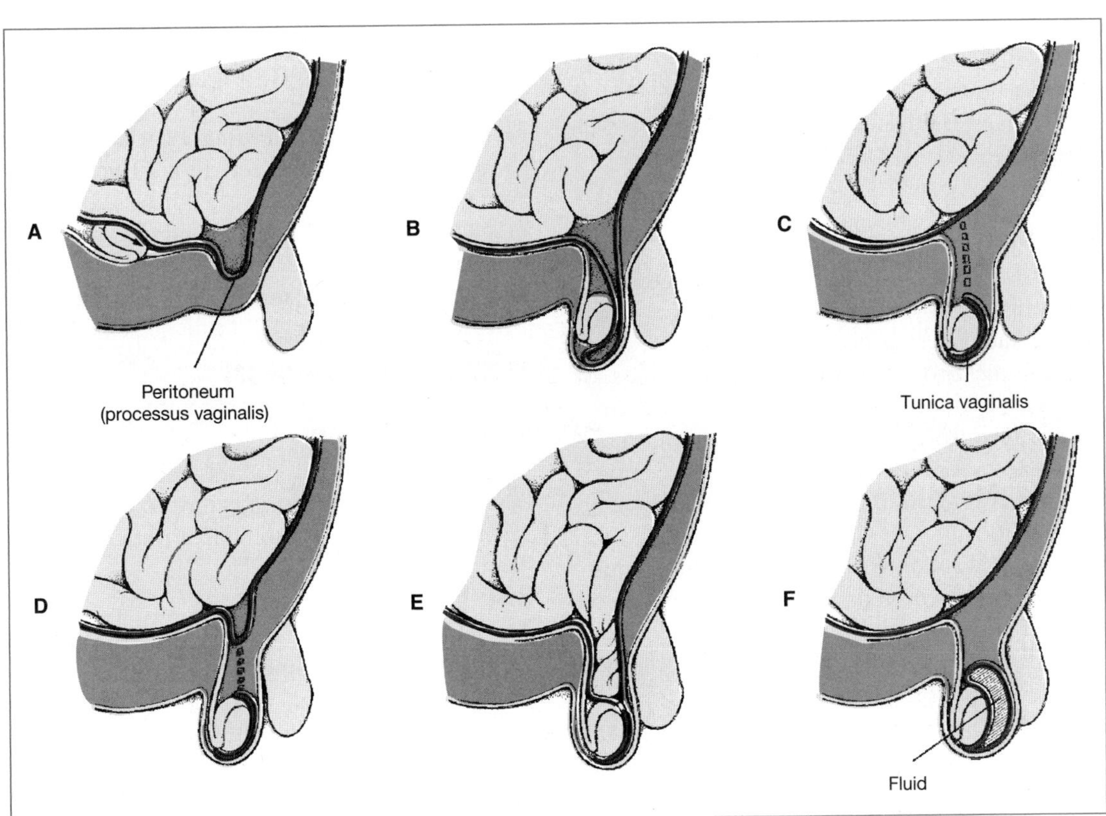

FIGURE 18.10 Development of inguinal hernias. (A and B) Prenatal migration of processus vaginalis. (C) Normal. (D) Partially obliterated processus vaginalis. (E) Hernia. (F) Hydrocele.
From Hockenberry (2003).

Prognosis

The most severe complication of inguinal hernia is an incarcerated hernia with subsequent intestinal necrosis. The highest risk of incarceration occurs in early infancy, and the risk of incarceration in premature infants is up to 31% (Misra, 2001). When inguinal hernias are surgically repaired prior to incarceration, complications are rare. The incidence of reoccurrence after surgical repair is 1% to 2% (Madden, 2007).

Clinical Manifestations

The most common clinical manifestation of an inguinal hernia is the presence of an inguinal bulge or mass as the omentum of the small intestine slides through the open processus vaginalis (Clark, 2010). Crying or increased abdominal pressure often causes the inguinal hernia to appear more prominent. When a hernia is reducible, the intestine can be gently manipulated back into the abdomen cavity.

Diagnosis

The most important component of diagnosis is determining whether the mass is an inguinal hernia or other scrotal mass, including a hydrocele or testicular torsion. If the scrotum can be transilluminated, the mass may be either a hydrocele or an inguinal hernia (Benjamin, 2002). Testicular torsion should be suspected if the scrotum contains a hard, solid mass. This is a surgical emergency and must be immediately reported to the surgical team (Benjamin, 2002). If it is not possible to distinguish between an inguinal hernia and a hydrocele, a rectal examination while palpating the scrotum simultaneously may reveal whether an intestinal loop is present in the scrotal sac rather than a fluid-filled hydrocele. The use of ultrasound may also prove beneficial in differentiating between the two processes.

Collaborative Management

Inguinal hernias should be reduced daily and as needed by applying gentle pressure to assess for incarceration of the hernia. An incarcerated hernia occurs when the intestines are caught within the processus vaginalis. Symptoms of incarcerated hernias include inability to reduce, vomiting, a firm tense mass, inconsolable crying, and abdominal distention. When incarceration occurs, circulation is compromised and intestinal necrosis is possible, necessitating an immediate surgical consult.

If the inguinal hernia is nonreducible, advanced attempts at reduction are often attempted. After the infant is well sedated and placed in the Trendelenburg position, ice packs are placed on the hernia to reduce intestinal edema. If gentle reduction is successful, surgery may be delayed for 24 to 48 hours. Surgery for incarcerated hernias includes reduction of the hernia and if necrotic bowel is present resection of the affected intestine (Lau et al., 2007).

Because of the high risk of incarceration, it is generally recommended that surgical repair of inguinal hernias occur as soon as possible. Surgery may be delayed in premature infants due to the technical difficulty of operating and an increased risk of complications including testicular atrophy and recurrent hernia. Exact timing of surgical intervention in the premature infant is controversial; however, the majority of surgeons will correct the defect prior to discharge from the hospital. Surgery may be performed either through an open procedure or more recently by laparoscopic surgery. Surgical correction involves separation of the hernia sac from surrounding structures (Clark, 2010). The contralateral side may be explored to detect a patent process or a nonclinically evident hernia (Lau et al., 2007). Whether or not to explore the contralateral side is controversial. The goal of this exploration is to avoid future inguinal hernias, thereby reducing the risk of a second surgery and possible incarceration. However, it also increases the risk of infection, pain, and the cost of surgery (Lau et al., 2007). The risk of complications associated with surgical correction of inguinal hernias is generally low; however, premature infants are at high risk for postoperative apnea and should be monitored for at least 24 hours following surgery. Apnea following surgery may be decreased with the use of spinal anesthesia.

Nursing Management

Reduction of all inguinal hernias should take place daily, and an inability to reduce the hernia should immediately be reported to the medical and surgical team. The postoperative course is similar following open procedures or laparotomy and includes observation for apnea and adherence to aseptic technique with regard to suture line maintenance. The infant should be placed in a side-lying or supine position with the head turned to the side to prevent disruption of the suture line. Operative dressings should be observed for any drainage and bleeding, kept dry, and underlying skin should be regularly inspected for irritation and breakdown. Pain should be assessed every 4 hours, and appropriate pain management should be provided when indicated. Since discharge is often 24 hours after surgery, the parents need to be instructed on proper surgical site and dressing care.

TESTICULAR TORSION

Pathophysiology

Torsion of the testicle occurs when the testis and coverings twist inside the scrotum, compromising blood flow, frequently resulting in a nonviable testicle.

Risk Factors

The incidence of testicular torsion is 6.1 per 100,000 (John, Kooner, Matthew, Almed, & Kenny, 2008). Although it is most often unilateral, bilateral torsion can unfortunately occur, resulting in complete lack of testicular development (Callewaert & Kerrebroeck, 2010). Risk factors include vaginal delivery, prolonged labor, gestational diabetes, and macrosomia, and it appears that fetal stress and mechanical factors may be contributing factors (Arena et al., 2006; Kaye et al., 2008).

Prognosis

An 8.96% salvage rate for testicular torsion in the neonatal population has been reported. This may increase to 21.7% if surgery is emergent. Unfortunately, salvage of antenatally occurring torsion is extremely rare (Nandl & Murphy, 2011).

Clinical Manifestations

Testicular torsion presents with unilateral acute pain and scrotal swelling. The scrotum is firm to the touch, tender, and often discolored. The abdomen may be significantly discolored and be either plethoric or cyanotic. The clinical presentation of testicular torsion is similar to other scrotal abnormalities such as hydrocele, inguinal hernia, and trauma; however, it can often be distinguished due to the presence of scrotal discoloration and an inability to be transilluminated. Information related to testicular blood flow can be obtained via the use of color Doppler ultrasound (van der Sluijis, den Hollander, Lequin, Nijman, & Robben, 2004). Because of the emergent need for surgical intervention, the diagnosis of testicular torsion must be considered in all infants presenting with scrotal swelling.

Collaborative Management

Treatment of acute testicular torsion is immediate surgery to untwist the testicle and restore blood supply. Timing of the intervention is critical, and a delay in surgical intervention of 4 to 6 hours following initiation of symptoms offers little to no chance of testicular survival. If the torsion occurs antenatally, the chance for testicular survival is nearly nonexistent and surgical intervention may be futile. The most important determinant in the decision to perform surgery is the appearance of the scrotum in the delivery room. If the scrotum appears normal initially and then becomes acutely painful, swollen, and discolored, immediate surgery is indicated in an attempt to salvage the testicle. If the scrotum appears blue, hard, and painless immediately after birth, the torsion occurred prenatally and the testicle has already become necrotic.

Controversy exists regarding the treatment of antenatally occurring testicular torsion. Some advocate conservative treatment with regular ultrasound examination to monitor for testicular atrophy (van der Sluijis et al., 2004). Others suggest contralateral orchiopexy is necessary to prevent the possibility of torsion and subsequent necrosis of both testes (Fuhrer et al., 2005; Yerkes et al., 2005).

Nursing Management

The focus of nursing care is on keeping the infant as comfortable and quiet as possible. The abdominal girth should be measured every 4 hours to assess for distention. The infant should be positioned supine with head turned to the side or in a side-lying position to avoid excessive pressure on the abdominal and scrotal areas.

If surgery is required, nursing care is centered on stability of the vital signs and prevention of infection. The suture line is generally small but still requires aseptic technique. The site should be assessed for edema, drainage, or discoloration.

NEPHROBLASTOMA (WILMS' TUMOR)

Pathophysiology

Wilms' tumor (nephroblastoma) is a well-encapsulated heterogeneous malignant tumor of the kidney. It is thought to be due to persistent nephrogenic embryologic cells that fail to develop appropriately. Wilms' tumor is associated with other anomalies, including aniridia (lack of development or absence of the iris), GU tract anomalies, and Beckwith-Wiedemann syndrome (Powis, 2010).

Risk Factors

The incidence of Wilms' tumor in neonates is 0.2%, and this incidence increases in the young infant and child. Wilms' tumor is generally a sporadic condition, but 1% of those affected have a family history of the disease (Powis, 2010).

Clinical Manifestations

The typical presentation of Wilms' tumor is a unilateral smooth, solid abdominal or flank mass that does not cross the midline in an otherwise well-appearing infant (Powis, 2010). Microscopic hematuria may be present, and hypertension may occur if associated renal artery stenosis or increased renin secretion is present (Hartman & MacLennan, 2005; Leclair et al., 2005).

Diagnosis

Fifteen percent of infants with Wilms' tumor are diagnosed on prenatal ultrasound (Issac, 2008). Other fetal indicators of Wilms' tumor include an increased risk of fetal distress, hydrops, and prematurity (Leclair et al., 2005). Postnatally, the initial diagnostic procedure is an abdominal ultrasound to determine the origin of the abdominal mass (Powis, 2010). This is generally followed by either CT or MRI to make a definitive diagnosis and to determine cancer stage (Powis, 2010). Biopsies are usually unnecessary in infants under 6 months of age.

Prognosis

Prognosis is related to the stage of disease and size of the tumor. Children younger than 2 years of age generally have a very favorable prognosis since the cancer is most often at a lower stage (van den Heuvel-Ebrink et al., 2008).

Collaborative Management

Because of the possibility that the encapsulated tumor may rupture and seed other areas of the body, repeated abdominal examinations should be avoided. Treatment of unilateral Wilms' tumor generally includes only nephroureteroctomy in the neonate. If the tumor is bilateral, if shrinkage is necessary prior to removal, or if metastasis has occurred, chemotherapy may be required (Powis, 2010). The diagnosis of cancer in a young infant can be devastating to the family. Clear, easy-to-understand information related to treatment and prognosis is required to assist parents to have realistic expectations related to their infant's diagnosis.

SUMMARY

The infant presenting with a genitourinary abnormality presents unique challenges to the neonatal care team. Although aberrations in the genital system are not life threatening, their appearance can be traumatic for the parents. Urinary tract pathology, on the other hand, can result in emergent life-threatening events at any age. Renal abnormality and diseases manifesting in the neonatal period can have lifelong consequences. The neonatal nurse must be able to accurately assess and respond to alterations in renal function. Astute nursing care of the infant and parents is paramount to optimal management and outcome. The neonatal nurse is in the position to be the first member of the health care team to detect minor changes in neonatal physiologic functions that may signify onset of significant compromise. To do this, the neonatal nurse must have knowledge of normal and abnormal renal and urinary tract physiology and pathophysiology. Parental support is another aspect of nursing care that is of major importance when caring for the infant with GU conditions. Timely assessment of parental coping mechanisms, alterations in parent–infant attachment, and evaluation of the parents' response to teaching provide vital information that will ultimately affect the infant's overall well-being.

CASE STUDY

■ **Identification of the Problem.** Infant with an average urinary output of 0.4ml/kg/hr for the last 24 hours.

■ **Assessment: History and Physical Examination.** The child is a 3-day-old, 900-g, 28-weeks gestational age infant born to a 28-year-old gravida 1, para 0 mother. Blood type is A+ and all serologies including Venereal Disease Research Laboratory (VDRL), HbsAg, GC, and HIV are negative. The mother received good prenatal care during this pregnancy. No smoking or drug or alcohol use reported. Delivery was via cesarean section due to placental abruption at 28 weeks gestation. No antibiotics or prenatal steroids were administered prior to delivery. Infant required intubation at delivery because of apnea and low heart rate. Apgar scores were 4 at 1 minute and 8 at 5 minutes. Infant was transferred to the Level 3 NICU. His problems included the following:

- Fluid, electrolytes, and nutrition: he is currently on minimal enteral feedings of 1 mL every 12 hours and tolerating these well; his total fluid volume is 120 mL/kg/d of total parenteral nutrition
- Respiratory: received two doses of artificial surfactant for a chest radiograph consistent with hyaline membrane disease; he remains intubated on moderate ventilatory settings
- Cardiovascular: infant has had several episodes of hypotension that have resolved spontaneously without treatment; heart rate is 175; current blood pressure has a mean arterial pressure of 28
- Infectious disease; receiving ampicillin and gentamicin for suspected sepsis; no culture-proven sepsis
- Hematologic: hematocrit is 35%; under phototherapy for hyperbilirubinemia
- Neurologic: a cranial ultrasound has been ordered for 1 week of life
- Social: Parents are married; this is their first child; they are appropriately concerned and have been updated at the bedside daily

■ **Physical Assessment**

- GENERAL: no obvious anomalies noted
- HEENT: anterior fontanelle soft and flat; eyes clear without drainage, red reflex present; pupils equally reactive to light; nares patent bilaterally; no clefts or abnormalities of mouth noted; ear canals patent bilaterally
- CHEST AND LUNGS: heart rate regular without murmur; pulses equal in all four extremities; quiet precordium; capillary refill time is 2 seconds; lungs equal with fine crackles bilaterally
- ABDOMEN: soft and nondistended; positive bowel sounds auscultated in all four quadrants; no masses felt; umbilical cord normal; liver felt 2 cm below right intercostal margin.
- GU: normal female infant; genitalia appropriate for gestational age
- SKELETAL: moves all extremities well; no obvious anomalies noted
- NEUROLOGIC: all reflexes present; tone appropriate for gestational age

■ **Differential Diagnoses.** The differential diagnosis of oliguria in this infant includes:

- Prerenal failure associated with decreased renal blood due to low systemic blood pressure or inadequate fluid intake
- Intrinsic renal failure due to the administration of nephrotoxic medications (gentamicin) or ATN due to perinatal depression related to the placental abruption as evidenced by the low Apgar scores
- Postrenal obstruction due to a neurogenic bladder related to fentanyl administration

■ **Diagnostic Tests.** Palpate the abdomen for the presence of a distended bladder and perform an in-and-out catheterization.

- Electrolytes: sodium 148, potassium 3.5; creatinine 0.4; BUN 10
- Weight is 780 g
- Gentamicin trough is 0.4mg/L
- Urine-specific gravity is 1,020, no protein, blood, or WBCs are present in the urine

The next step should be administration of 10 to 20 mL/kg of normal saline via IV. Use of a diuretic after the fluid challenge may be necessary if urine output does not increase immediately after the fluid challenge.

■ Working Diagnosis. The bladder is not distended. No urine is obtained via in-and-out catheterization, thus ruling out postrenal failure.

Physical assessment is impressive for lack of abdominal masses that would possibly indicate an enlarged kidney and associated intrinsic renal failure. Tachycardia is present, possibly indicating mild dehydration. A borderline mean arterial pressure may indicate decreased intravascular volume or decreased systemic blood flow.

Infant has lost 120 g over the past 3 days.

Gentamicin level is normal and does not support the presence of intrinsic renal failure.

The sodium level and specific gravity are elevated, which are both consistent with prerenal failure.

The creatinine and BUN are normal. If elevated, they would support a diagnosis of intrinsic renal failure.

There is no blood or protein in the urine. The presence of these substances would also support a diagnosis of intrinsic renal failure.

The administration of a fluid challenge produced a urine output of over 1 mL/kg/hr, thus indicating a diagnosis of prerenal failure.

No other workup such as a renal ultrasound would be indicated at this time.

■ Development of Management Plan. Ensure administration of an adequate fluid volume by increasing fluid volume appropriately to ensure a urine output over 1 mL/kg/hr. Compensate for fluid losses due to insensible water losses including losses from phototherapy.

Low-dose dopamine may increase renal blood flow.

Ensure appropriate renal blood flow by increasing mean arterial pressure. If increase in fluid volume does not increase blood pressure sufficiently, inotropes such as higher dose dopamine or dobutamine may be administered.

■ Implementation and Evaluation of Effectiveness Monitor skin turgor and fontanelles for signs of dehydration.

- Monitor serum electrolytes closely to ensure normalization of sodium levels
- Monitor vital signs every 3 to 4 hours to ensure normalization of blood pressure and heart rate
- Carefully monitor intake and output to ensure that infant is receiving adequate volume to result in a urine output of over 1 mL/kg/hr
- Daily or twice daily weights
- Monitor specific gravity to ensure resolution to a normal range

EVIDENCE-BASED PRACTICE BOX

UTIs are common in infants and are defined as infection of the kidney and/or bladder. They are estimated to occur in 0.1% to 2% of all newborns and in 20% of preterm and critically ill infants. UTIs can increase morbidity and if not properly treated can result in decreased renal function, renal scarring, and hypertension (Cataldi et al., 2006). Treatment of UTIs consists of antibiotic therapy, and traditionally due to concerns of vesicoureteral reflux (VUR), a VCUG and prophylactic antibiotic therapy were recommended in all infants diagnosed with a UTI. Unfortunately a VCUG is not a benign procedure and is associated with both infant pain and family stress.

Evidence now exists that the risk of recurrent UTI is not significantly affected by VUR, and the AAP currently recommends that a VCUG not be performed following the first UTI unless the renal ultrasound indicates abnormalities including hydronephrosis, renal scarring, severe VUR, or obstructive uropathy (AAP, 2011; Ismaille et al., 2011). A meta-analysis of six studies including data on 1,091 infants indicated no benefit in providing prophylactic antibiotics to prevent future UTIs in infants with grade I-IV VUR, and there was insufficient data regarding use in infants with Grade V VUR (AAP, 2011). Furthermore, it is estimated that only 1% of infants diagnosed with a UTI has Grade V VUR (AAP, 2011). Therefore the use of a VCUG or prophylactic antibiotic therapy is not recommended following an initial UTI (AAP, 2011). If an infant is diagnosed with subsequent UTIs, a VCUG is required at that time (AAP, 2011).

ONLINE RESOURCES

American Academy of Pediatrics Guidelines for Circumcision
http://www.pediatrics.aappublications.org/content/103/3/686.full

American Academy of Pediatrics Guidelines for Treatment of Urinary Tract Infections
http://www.pediatrics.aappublications.org/content/128/3/595.abstract?ijkey=36070040942fafabc8fed8e6a2680afbd0dd06c3&keytype2=tf_ipsecsha

American Urological Association Foundation
http://www.auanet.org

International Pediatric Endosurgery Group Guidelines for Inguinal Hernias and Hydroceles
http://www.ipeg.org/education/guidelines/hernia.html

The National Kidney Foundation
http://www.kidney.org

U.S. Department of Health and Human Services

National Kidney and Urologic Diseases Information Clearinghouse (NKUDIC). A service of the National Institute of Diabetes and

Digestive and Kidney Diseases (NIDDK), National Institutes of Health (NIH)
http://www.kidney.niddk.nih.gov/kudiseases/a-z.aspx

REFERENCES

Agras, P. L., Tarcan, A., Baskin, E., Cengiz, N., Gürakan, B., & Saatci, U. (2004). Acute renal failure in the neonatal period. *Renal Failure, 26*, 305–309.

Almed, A., & Ellsworth, P. (2012). To circ or not: A reappraisal. *Urologic Nursing, 32*(1), 10–18.

American Academy of Pediatrics: Committee on the Fetus and Newborn (1971). *Standards and recommendations for hospital care of newborn infants*. Evanston, IL: Author.

American Academy of Pediatrics: Committee on the Fetus and Newborn (1975). Reports of the Ad Hoc Task Force on Circumcision. *Pediatrics, 56*, 610–611.

American Academy of Pediatrics: Committee on the Fetus and Newborn (1983). *Guidelines for perinatal care*. Elk Grove Village, IL: Author.

American Academy of Pediatrics. (1989). Report of the Task Force on Circumcision. *Pediatrics, 84*, 388–391.

American Academy of Pediatrics. (1999). Report of the Task Force on Circumcision. Circumcision policy statement. *Pediatrics, 103*, 686–693.

American Academy of Pediatrics. (2011). Urinary tract infection: Clinical practice guidelines for the diagnosis and management of the initial UTI in febrile infants and children, 2 to 24 months. *Pediatrics, 128*(3), 595–610.

American Cancer Society. (2009). *Can penile cancer be prevented?* Retrieved from www.cancer.org/cancer/penilcancer/detailedguide/penile-cancer-prevention

Andreoli, S. P. (2004). Acute renal failure in the newborn. *Seminars in Perinatology, 28*, 112–123.

Anochie, I. C., & Eke, F. (2004). Renal vein thrombosis in the neonate: A case report and review of the literature. *Journal of the National Medical Association, 96*(12), 1648–1652.

Arena, F., Nicòtina, P. A., Romeo, C., Zimbaro, G., Arena, S., Zuccarello, B., & Romeo, G. (2006). Prenatal testicular torsion: Ultrasonographic features, management and histopathological findings. *International Journal of Urology, 13*(2), 135–141.

Avert, B., Taljaard, D., Lagarde, E., Sobngwi-Tambekou, J., Sitta, R., & Puren, A. (2005). Randomized controlled intervention trial of male circumcision for reduction HIV infection risk: The ANRS 1265 Trial. *PLoS Med, 2*, e298.

Avni, F. E., & Hall, M. (2010). Renal cystic disease in children: New concepts. *Pediatric Radiology, 40*, 939–946.

Bailey, R. C., Moses, S., Parker, C. B., Agot, K., Maclean, I., Krieger, J. N., . . . Ndinya-Achola, J. O. (2007). Male circumcision for HIV prevention in young men in Kisumu, Kenya: A randomized controlled trial. *Lancet, 369*, 643–656.

Barletta, G. M., & Bunchman, T. E. (2004). Acute renal failure in children and infants. *Current Opinions in Critical Care, 10*, 499–504.

Barrantes, F., Tian, J., Vazquez, R., Amoateng-Adjepong, Y., & Manthous, C. A. (2008). Acute kidney injury criteria predict outcomes of critically ill patients. *Critical Care Medicine, 36*, 1397–1403.

Basu, R. K., Devarajan, P., Wong, H., & Wheeler, D. S. (2011). An update and review of acute kidney injury in pediatrics. *Pediatric Critical Care, 12*(3), 339–347.

Becker, A. & Baum, M. (2006). Obstructive uropathy. *Early Human Development, 82*, 15–22.

Benjamin, K. (2002). Scrotal and inguinal masses in the newborn period. *Advances in Neonatal Care, 2*, 140–148.

Bergmann, C., Senderek, J., Windelen, E., Küpper, F., Middeldorf, I., Schneider, F., . . . Arbeitsgemeinschaft für Pädiatrische Nephrologie. (2005). Clinical consequences of PKHD1 mutations in 164 patients with autosomal recessive polycystic disease (ARPKD). *Kidney International, 67*, 829–848.

Bhide, A., Sairam, S., Farrugia, M. K., Boddy, S. A., & Thilaganathan, B. (2005). The sensitivity of antenatal ultrasound for predicting renal tract surgery in early childhood. *Ultrasound Obstetrics and Gynecology, 25*, 489–492.

Biyikli, N. K., Alpay, H., Ozek, E., Akman, I., & Bilgen, H. (2004). Neonatal urinary tract infections: Analysis of the patients and recurrences. *Pediatrics International, 46*, 21–25.

Blackburn, S. T. (2012). *Maternal, fetal and neonatal physiology: A clinical perspective*. Philadelphia, PA: Saunders.

Boer, D. P., de Rijke, Y. B., Hop, W. C., Cransberg, K., & Dorresteijn, E. M. (2010). Reference values for serum creatinine in children younger than 1 year of age. *Pediatric Nephrology, 25*, 2107–2113.

Bonilla-Feliz, M. (2009). Peritoneal dialysis in the pediatric intensive care unit setting. *Peritoneal Dialysis International, 29*(Suppl. 2), S183–S185.

Brady-Fryer, B. Wiebe, N., & Lander, J. A. (2004). Pain relief for neonatal circumcision. *Cochrane Database of Systematic Reviews* Oct *18*(4):CD004217.

Brady-Fryer, B., Wiebe, N., & Lander, J. A. (2011). Pain relief for neonatal circumcision. *Cochrane Database of Systematic Reviews, 18*(4), CD004217.

Brandao, L. R., Simpson, E. A., & Lau, K. K. (2011). Neonatal renal vein thrombosis. *Seminars in Fetal and Neonatal Medicine, 16*, 323–328.

Caione, P., & Nappo, S. G. (2011). Posterior urethral valves: Long-term outcome. *Pediatric Surgery International, 27*, 1027–1035.

Callewaert, P. R., & Van Kerrebroech, P. (2010). New insights into testicular torsion. *European Journal of Pediatrics, 169*, 705–712.

Cambio, A. J., Evans, C. P., & Kurzrock, E. A. (2008). Non-surgical management of multicystic dysplastic kidney. *British Journal of Urology International, 3*, 48–52.

Capisonda, R., Phan, V., Traubuci, J., Daneman, A., Balfe, J. W., & Guay-Woodford, L. M. (2003). Autosomal recessive polycystic kidney disease: Outcomes from a single-center experience. *Pediatric Nephrology, 18*, 19–26.

Casella, D. P., Tomaszewski, J. J., & Ost, M. C. (2012). Posterior urethral valves: Renal failure and prenatal treatment. *International Journal of Nephrology, 2012*, 351067.

Cataldi, L., Italian Society of Neonatology Neonatal Nephrology Study Group, Zaffanello, M., Gnarra, M., & Fanos, V. (2010). Urinary tract infection in the newborn and the infant: State of the art. *The Journal of Maternal-Fetal and Neonatal Medicine, 23*(Suppl. 3), 90–93.

Cataldi, L., Mussap, M., & Fanos, V. (2006). Urinary tract infections in infants and children. *Journal of Chemotherapy, 18*, 5–84.

Chandler, J. C., & Gauderer, M. W. (2004). The neonate with an abdominal mass. *Pediatric Clinics of North America, 51*, 979–997.

Chevalier, R. L. (2004). Perinatal obstructive nephropathy. *Seminars in Perinatology, 28*, 124–131.

Chiappinelli, A., Savanelli, A., Farina, A., & Settimi, A. (2011). Multicystic dysplastic kidney: Our experience in non-surgical management. *Pediatric Surgery International, 27*, 757–779.

Clark, D. A. (2000). *Atlas of neonatology*. Philadelphia, PA: Saunders.

Clark, S. (2010). Pediatric inguinal hernia and hydrocele: An evidence-based review in the era of minimal access surgery. *Journal of Laparoendoscopic and Advanced Surgical Techniques, 20*(3), 305–309.

Darge, K. (2010). Voiding urosonography with U.S. contrast agent for the diagnosis of veiscoureteric reflux in children: An update. *Pediatric Radiology, 40*, 956–962.

de Boom, M. L., Kist-van Holthe, J. E., Sramek, A., Lardenoye, S. W., Walther, F. J., & Lopriore, E. (2010). Is screening for renal anomalies warranted in neonates with isolated umbilical artery? *Neonatology, 97*, 225–227.

Denes, F. T., Arap, M. A., Giron, A. M., Silva, F. A., & Arap, S. (2004). Comprehensive surgical treatment of prune belly syndrome: 17 years' experience with 32 patients. *Urology, 64*, 790–794.

Deshpande, S. A., Jog, S., Watson, H., & Gornall, A. (2009). Do babies with isolated single umbilical artery need routine postnatal renal ultrasound? *Archives of Disease of Childhood Fetal and Neonatal Edition, 94*, F265–F267.

Drukker, A., & Guignard, J. P. (2002). Renal aspects of the term and preterm infant: A selective update. *Current Opinions in Pediatrics, 14*, 175–182.

Durkan, A. M., & Alexander, R. T. (2011). Acute kidney injury post neonatal asphyxia. *The Journal of Pediatrics, 158*(Suppl. 2), e29–e33.

Durson, H., Bayazit, A. K., Büyükçelik, M., Soran, M., Noyan, A., & Anarat, A. (2005). Associated anomalies in children with congenital solitary functioning kidney. *Pediatric Surgery International, 21*, 456–459.

Ebert, A. K., Reutter, H., Ludwig, M., & Rosch, W. H. (2009). The extrophy-epidspadias complex. *Orphanet Journal of Rare Diseases*. Retrieved from http:/www.ojrd.com/content/4/1/23

Eckoldt, F., Healing, F., Woderich, R., Wolke, S. (2004). Posterior urethral valves: Prenatal diagnostic signs and outcome. *Urology International, 73*, 296.

Elsaify, W. M. (2009). Neonatal renal vein thrombosis: Grey-scale and Doppler Ultrasonic features. *Abdominal Imaging, 34*, 413–418.

Fuhrer, S., May, M., Koch, A., Marusch, F., Gunia, S., Erler, T., & Gastinger, I. (2005). Intrauterine torsion of a testicular teratoma: A case report. *Journal of Perinatology, 25*, 220–222.

Goldstein, S. L. (2011). Continuous renal replacement therapy: Mechanism of clearance, fluid removal, indications and outcomes. *Current Opinions in Pediatrics, 23*, 181–185.

Gornall, A. S., Kurinczuk, J. J., & Konje, J. C. (2003). Antenatal detection of a single umbilical artery: Does it matter? *Prenatal Diagnosis, 23*, 117–123.

Gray, R. H., Kigozi, G., Serwadda, D., Makumbi, F., Watya, S., Nalugoda, F., . . . Wawer, M. J. (2007). Male circumcision for HIV prevention in men in Rakai, Uganda: A randomized trial. *Lancet, 369*, 657–666.

Gray, R. H., Serwadda, D., Kong, X., Makumbi, F., Kigozi, G., Gravitt, P. E., . . . Wawer, M. J. (2010). Male circumcision decreases acquisition and increases clearance of high-risk human papilloma virus in HIV-negative men: A randomized trial in Rakai, Uganda. *Journal of Infectious Diseases, 201*(10), 1455–1462.

Gubhaju, L., Suterland, M. R., Hons, B., & Black, M. J. (2011). Preterm birth and the kidney: Implications for long-term renal health. *Reproductive Sciences, 18*(4), 322–333.

Guyton, A. C., & Hall, J. E. (1997). *Human physiology and mechanisms of disease* (6th ed.). Philadelphia, PA: Saunders.

Hammouda, H. M., & Dotb, H. (2004). Complete primary repair of bladder exstrophy: Initial experience with 33 cases. *Journal of Urology, 172*, 1441–1444.

Hartman, D. J., & MacLennan, G. T. (2005). Wilms' tumor. *Journal of Urology, 173*, 2147.

Hassett, S., Smith, G. H., & Holland, A. J. (2012). Prune belly syndrome. *Pediatric Surgery International, 28*(3), 219–228.

Hayashi, Y., & Kojima, Y. (2010). Is antibiotic prophylaxis effective in preventing urinary tract infections in patients with vesicoureteral reflux? *Expert Review of Antibiotic and Infective Therapy, 8*, 51–58.

Haycock, G. B. (2003). Management of acute and chronic renal failure in the newborn. *Seminars in Neonatology, 8*, 325–334.

Hernandez, J. A., & Glass, S. M. (2004). Physical assessment of the newborn. In P. J. Thureen et al. (Eds.), *Assessment and care of the well newborn*. St Louis, MO: Saunders.

Hockenberry, M. J. (2003). *Wong's nursing care of infants and children* (7th ed., p. 478). St Louis, MO: Mosby.

Hodges, S. J., Patel, B., McLorie, G., & Atala, A. (2009). Posterior urethral valves. *The Scientific World Journal, 9*, 1119–1126.

Holmdahl, G., & Sillen, U. (2005). Boys with posterior urethral valves: Outcome concerning renal function, bladder function and paternity at ages 31–44 years. *Journal of Urology, 174*, 1031–1034.

Hubert, K. C., & Palmer, J. S. (2007). Current diagnosis and management of fetal genitourinary abnormalities. *Urologic Clinics of North America, 34*, 89–101.

Huether, S. E. (2004). Alterations of renal and urinary tract function in children. In K. L. McCance & S. E. Huether (Eds.), *Pathophysiology: The basis for disease in adults and children*. St Louis, MO: Mosby.

Ismaili, K., Lolin, K., Damry, N., Alexander, M., Lepage, P., & Hall, M. (2011). Febrile urinary tract infections in 0- to 3-month-old infants: Prospective follow-up study. *Journal of Pediatrics, 158*, 91–94.

Issac, H. (2008). Fetal and neonatal renal tumors. *Journal of Pediatric Surgery, 43*, 1587–1595.

John, C. M., Kooner, G., Matthew, D. E., Almed, S., & Kenny, S. E. (2008). Neonatal testicular torsion—a lost cause? *Acta Paediatrics, 97*, 502–504.

John, E. G., & Yeh, T. F. (1985). Renal failure. In T. F. Yeh TF (Ed.), *Drug therapy in the neonate and small infant*. Chicago, IL: Year Book Medical Publishers.

Karlowicz, M. G., & Adelman, R. D. (2005). Acute renal failure. In A. R. Spitzer (Ed.), *Intensive care of the fetus and neonate*. Philadelphia, PA: Mosby.

Kaye, J. D., Levitt, S. B., Friedman, S. C., Franco, I., Gitlin, J., & Palmer, L. S. (2008). Neonatal torsion: A 14-year experience and proposed algorithm for management. *Journal of Urology, 179*(6), 2377–2383.

Kibar, Y., Ashley, R. A., Roth, C. C., Frimberger, D., & Kropp, B. P. (2011). Timing of posterior urethral valve diagnosis and its impact on clinical outcome. *Journal of Pediatric Urology, 7*, 538–542.

Kiddoo, D. A., Carr, M. C., Dulczak, S., & Canning, D. A. (2004). Initial management of complex urological disorders: Bladder exstrophy. *Urologic Clinics of North America, 31*, 417–426.

Koeppen, B., & Stanton, B. (2006). *Renal physiology*. St Louis, MO: Mosby.

Koralkar, R. (2011). Acute kidney injury reduces survival in very low birth weight infants. *Pediatric Research, 69*(4), 354–358.

Kraft, J. K., Brandio, R., & Navarro, O. M. (2011). Sonography of renal venous thrombosis in neonates and infants: Can we predict outcome? *Pediatric Radiology, 41*, 299–307.

Krill, A. J., Palmer, L. S., & Palmer, J. S. (2011). Complications of circumcision. *The Scientific World Journal, 11*, 2458–2468.

Krishnan, A., de Souza, A., Konijeti, R., & Baskin, L. S. (2006). The anatomy and embryology of posterior urethral valves. *Journal of Urology, 175*, 1214.

Kuwertz-Broeking, E., Brinkmann, O. A., Von Lengerke, H. J., Sciuk, J., Fruend, S., Bulla, M., . . . Hertle, L. (2004). Unilateral multicystic dysplastic kidney: Experience in children. *British Journal of Urology International, 93*, 388–392.

Larke, N. L., Thomas, S. L., dos Santos Silva, I., & Weiss, H. A. (2011). Male circumcision and penile cancer: A systematic review and meta-analysis. *Cancer Causes Control, 22*(8), 1097–1110.

Lau, K. K., Stoffman, J. M., Williams, S., McCusker, P., Brandao, L., Patel, S., . . . Canadian Pediatric Thrombosis and Hemostasis Network. (2007). Neonatal renal vein thrombosis: Review of the English-language literature between 1992 and 2006. *Pediatrics, 120*, e1278–e1284.

Lau, S., Lee, Y., & Caty, M. (2007). Current management of hernias and hydroceles. *Seminars in Pediatric Surgery, 16*, 50–57.

Leclair, M. D., El-Ghoneimi, A., Audry, G., Ravasse, P., Moscovici, J., Heloury, Y., & French Pediatric Urology Study Group. (2005). The outcome of prenatally diagnosed renal tumors. *Journal of Urology, 173*, 186–189.

Leeners, B., Sauer, I., Schefels, J., Cotarelo, C. L., & Funk, A. (2000). Prune-belly syndrome: Therapeutic options including in utero placement of a vesicoamniotic shunt. *Journal of Clinical Ultrasound, 28*, 500–507.

Leung, A. K. C., & Wong, A. H. C. (2010). Proteinuria in children. *American Academy of Family Physicians, 82*(6), 645–651.

Lukong, C. S. (2011). Circumcision: Controversies and prospects. *Journal of Surgical Technique and Case Report, 3*(2), 65–66.

Maayan-Metzger, A., Lotan, D., Jacobson, J. M., Raviv-Zilka, L., Ben-Shlush, A., Kuint, J., & Mor, Y. (2011). The yield of early postnatal ultrasound scan in neonates with documented antenatal hydronephrosis. *American Journal of Perinatology, 28*(8), 613–617.

Madden, N. (2007). Testis, hydrocele and varicocele. *Essentials in Paediatric Urology, 1691*, 130.

Mansoor, O., Chandar, J., Rodriguez, M. M., Abitbol, C. L., Seeherunvong, W., Freundlich, M., & Zilleruelo, G. (2011). Long-term risk of chronic kidney disease in unilateral mulitidysplastic kidney. *Pediatric Nephrology, 26*, 595–603.

Marks, S. D., Massicotte, M. P., Steele, B. T., Matsell, D. G., Filler, G., Shah, P. S . . . Shah, V. S. (2005). Neonatal renal venous thrombosis: Clinical outcomes and prevalence of prothrombotic disorders. *Journal of Pediatrics, 146*, 811–816.

Mehler, K., Beck, B. B., Kaul, I., Rahimi, G., Hopper, B., & Kribs, A. (2011). Respiratory and general outcome in neonates with oligohycramnios – a single-centre experience. *Nephrology Dialysis and Transplant, 26*, 3514–3522.

Mesrobian, H. G., Balcom, A. H., & Durkee, C. T. (2004). Urologic problems of the neonate. *Pediatric Clinics of North America, 51*, 1051–1062.

Messinger, Y., Sheaffer, J. W., & Mrozek, J. (2006). Renal outcome of neonatal renal venous thrombosis: Review of 28 patients and effectiveness of fibrinolytics and heparin in 10 patients. *Pediatrics. 118*, e478–e484.

Misra, D. (2001). Inguinal hernias in premature babies: Wait or operate? *Acta Paediatrics, 90*, 370–371.

Moore, K. L., & Persaud, T. V. N. (2011). *The developing human: Clinically oriented embryology*. Philadelphia, PA: Elsevier.

Morris, R. K., Malin, G. L., Khan, K. S., & Kilby, M. D. (2010). Systematic review of the effectiveness of antenatal intervention for the treatment of congenital lower urinary tract obstruction. *International Journal of Obstetrics and Gynecology, 17*, 382–390.

Nandl, R., & Murphy, F. L. (2011). Neonatal testicular torsion: A systematic literature review. *Pediatric Surgery International, 27*, 1037–1040.

Narchi, H. (2005). Risk of hypertension with multicystic kidney disease: A systematic review. *Archives of Diseases in Childhood, 90*, 921–924.

Nasir, A. A., Ameh, E. A., Abdur-Rahman, L. O., Adeniran, J. O., & Abraham, M. K. (2011). Posterior urethral valves. *World Journal of Pediatrics, 7*(3), 205–216.

Papantoniou, N., Papoutsis, D., Daskalakis, G., Chatzipapas, I., Sindos, M., Papaspyrou, I., . . . Antsaklis, A. (2010). Prenatal diagnosis of prune-belly syndrome at 13 weeks of gestation: Case report and review of literature. *The Journal of Maternal-Fetal and Neonatal Medicine, 23*(10), 1263–1267.

Patzer, L. (2008). Nephrotoxity as a cause of acute kidney injury in children. *Pediatric Nephrology, 23*(12), 2159–2173.

Peniakov, M., Antonelli, J., Naor, O., & Miron, D. (2004). Reduction in contamination of urine samples obtained by in-out catheterization by culturing the later urine stream. *Pediatric Emergency Care, 20*, 1–3.

Penido Silva, J. M., Oliveira, E. A., Diniz, J. S., Bouzada, M. C., Vergara, R. M., & Souza, B. C. (2006). Clinical course of prenatally detected primary vesicoureteral reflux. *Pediatric Nephrology, 21*, 86–91.

Potter, E. L. (1965). Bilateral absence of ureters and kidneys: A report of 50 cases. *Obstetrics & Gynecology, 25*, 3–12.

Powis, M. (2010). Neonatal renal tumours. *Early Human Development, 86*, 607–612.

Purves, J. T. (2011). Modern approaches in primary exstrophy closure. *Seminars in Pediatric Surgery, 20*, 79–84.

Riccabona, M. (2002). Cystography in infants and children: A critical appraisal of the many forms with special regards to voiding cystourethrography. *European Radiology, 12*, 2910–2918.

Riccabona, M. (2004). Assessment and management of newborn hydronephrosis. *World Journal of Urology, 22*, 73–78.

Routh, J. C., Huang, L., Retik, A. B., & Nelson, C. P. (2010). Contemporary epidemiology and characterization of newborn males with prune belly syndrome. *Urology, 76*, 44–48.

Sairam, S., Al-Habib, A., Sasson, S., & Thilaganathan, B. (2001). Natural history of fetal hydronephrosis diagnosed on mid-trimester ultrasound. *Ultrasound in Obstetrics and Gynecology, 17*, 191–196.

Sanson, S. L., Prabhu, V. S., Hutchinson, A. B., An, Q., Hall, H. I., Shrestha, R. K., . . . Taylor, A. W. (2010). Cost-effectiveness of newborn circumcision in reducing lifetime HIV risk among U.S. males. *PLoS, 5*(1), e8723, 1–8.

Shaikh, N., Morone, N. E., Bost, J. E., & Farrell, M. H. (2008). Prevalence of urinary tract infection in childhood: A meta-analysis. *Pediatric Infectious Disease Journal, 27*, 302–308.

Shneider, B. L., & Magid, M. S. (2005). Liver disease in autosomal recessive polycystic kidney disease. *Pediatric Transplantation, 9*, 634–639.

Solhaug, M. J., Bolger, P. M., & Jose, P. A. (2004). The developing kidney and environmental toxins. *Pediatrics, 113*, 1084–1091.

Springate, J. E. et al. (1987). Assessment of renal function in newborn infants. *Pediatrics in Review*, 9(2):56.

Srinath, A., & Shneider, B. L. (2012). Congenital hepatic fibrosis and autosomal recessive polycystic kidney disease. *Journal of Pediatric and Gastroenteral Nutrition, 54*(5), 580–587.

Srinivasan, R., & Arora, R. S. (2005). Do well infants born with an isolated single umbilical artery need investigation? *Archives of Disease in Childhood, 90*, 100–101.

Strand, W. R. (2004). Initial management of complex pediatric disorders: Prune-belly syndrome, posterior urethral valves. *Urologic Clinics of North America, 31*, 399–415.

Subramanian, S., Agarwal, R., Deorari, A. K., Paul, V. K., & Bagga, A. (2011). Acute renal failure in neonates. *Indian Journal of Pediatrics, 73*, 385–391.

Tekgul, S., et al. (2009). Dilatation of the upper urinary tract. EAU Guidelines of paediatric urology. Retrieved from http://www.uroweb.org/fileadmin/tx_eauguidelines/2009/Full/Paediatric_Urology.pdf

Thomas, D. F. M. (2002). Cystic renal disease. In D. F. M. Thomas, et al. (Eds.), *Essentials of paediatric urology*. London, UK: Martin Dunitz.

Tobian, A. A., & Gray, R. H. (2011). The Medical benefits of male circumcision. *Journal of the American Medical Association, 306*, 1479–1480.

Tobian, A. A., Serwadda, D., Quinn, T. C., Kigozi, G., Gravitt, P. E., Laeyendecker, O., . . . Gray, R. H. (2009). Male circumcision for the prevention of HSV-2 and HPV infections and syphilis. *New England Journal of Medicine, 360*, 1298–1309.

Tortora, G. J., & Grabowski, S. R. (2011). *Principles of anatomy and physiology*. New York, NY: Wiley.

Van den Heuvel-Ebrink, M. M., Grundy, P., Graf, N., Pritchard-Jones, K., Bergeron, C., Patte, C., . . . de Kraker, J. (2008). Characteristics and survival of 750 children diagnosed with a renal tumor in the first seven months of life: A collaborative study by the SHOP/GPOH/SFOP, NWTSG, and UKCCSG Wilms tumor study groups. *Pediatric Blood Cancer, 50*, 1130–1134.

van der Sluijis, J. W., den Hollander, J. C., Lequin, M. H., Nijman, R. M., & Robben, S. G. (2004). Prenatal testicular torsion: Diagnosis and natural course: An ultrasonographic study. *European Radiology, 14*, 250–255.

Vogt, B. A., et al. (2006). The kidney and urinary tract. In A. A. Fanaroff et al. (Eds.), *Neonatal-perinatal medicine: Diseases of the fetus and infant* (8th ed.). Philadelphia, PA: Mosby.

Wald, E. (2004). Urinary tract infections in infants and children: A comprehensive overview. *Current Opinion in Pediatrics, 16*, 85–88.

Wedekin, M., Ehrich, J. H. H., Offner, G., & Pape, L. (2010). Renal replacement therapy in infants with chronic renal failure in the first year of life. *Clinical Journal of American Society of Nephrology, 5*, 18–23.

Weinschenk, N., Pelidis, M., & Fiascone, J. (2001). Combination thrombolytic and anticoagulant therapy for bilateral renal vein thrombosis in a premature infant. *American Journal of Perinatology, 18*, 293–297.

Weiss, H. A., Larke, N., Halperin, D., & Schenker, I. (2010). Complications of circumcision in male neonates, infants and children: A systematic review. *BioMed Central Urology, 10*, 2.

Willis, F., Summers, J., Minutillo, C., & Hewitt, I. (1997). Indices of renal tubular function in perinatal asphyxia. *Archives of Diseases in Childhood Fetal and Neonatal Edition, 77*, F57–F60.

Winyard, P. J., Bharucha, T., De Bruyn, R., Dillon, M. J., van't Hoff, W., Trompeter, R. S., . . . Rees, L. (2006). Perinatal renal vein thrombosis: Presenting renal length predicts outcome. *Archives of Diseases in Children Fetal and Neonatal Edition, 91*, F273–F278.

Woodard, J. R. (1978). The prune belly syndrome. *Urology Clinics of North America, 5*, 75–93.

Woods, A. G., & Brandon, D. H. (2007). Prune belly syndrome. *Advances in Neonatal Care, 7*(3), 132–143.

Woodward, M., & Frank, D. (2002). Postnatal management of antenatal hydronephrosis. *British Journal of Urology International, 89*, 149–156.

World Health Organization. (2012). *Male circumcision for HIV prevention*. Retrieved from www.who.int/hiv/topics/malecircumcision/en/

Wright, J. A. (2008). Prenatal and postnatal diagnosis of infant disability: Breaking the news to mothers. *Journal of Perinatal Education, 17*(3), 27–32.

Yamazaki, Y., Shiroyanagi, Y., Matsuno, D., & Nishi, M. (2009). Predicting early recurrent urinary tract infection in pre-toilet trained children with vesicoureteral reflux. *Journal of Urology, 182*(Suppl. 4), 1699–1702.

Yang, Y., Hou, Y., Niu, Z. B., & Want, C. L. (2010). Long-term follow-up and management of prenatally detected, isolated hydronephrosis. *Journal of Pediatric Surgery, 45*, 1701–1706.

Yerkes, E. B., Robertson, F. M., Jordan, G., Martin, K., Cain, M. P., & Rink, R. C. (2005). Management of perinatal torsion: Today, tomorrow or never? *Journal of Urology, 174*, 1579–1582.

Ylinen, E., Ala-Houhala, M., & Wikström, S. (2004). Prognostic factors of posterior urethral valves and the role of antenatal detection. *Pediatric Nephrology, 19*, 874–879.

Yohannes, P., & Hanna, M. (2002). Current trends in the management of posterior urethral valves in the pediatric population. *Urology, 60*, 947.

Youssif, M., Dawood, W., Shabaan, S., Mokhless, I., & Hanno, A. (2009). Early valve ablation can decrease the incidence of bladder dysfunction in boys with posterior urethral valves. *The Journal of Urology, 182*, 1765–1768.

UNIT IV: SPECIAL CONSIDERATIONS

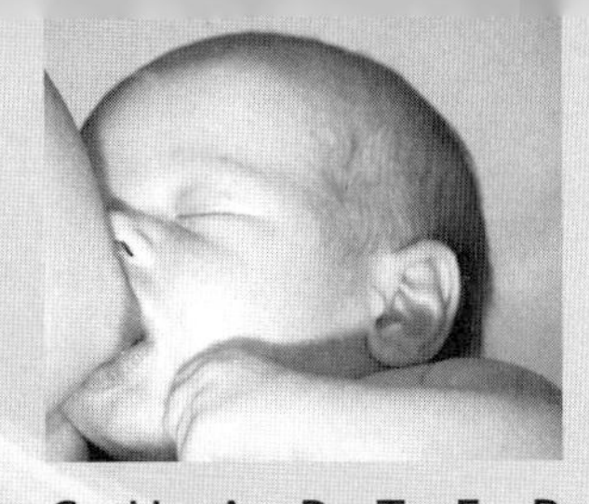

CHAPTER

19

Fluids, Electrolytes, Vitamins, and Minerals

■ Sergio DeMarini and Linda L. Rath

Water and electrolytes are vital components of the body at any age. The laws that regulate fluid and electrolyte balance in the newborn are the same as those that control this process in children and adults. However, the newborn's body water distribution is both quantitatively and qualitatively different. Furthermore, rapid changes occur at the time of birth, and sick newborns pose additional challenges. Consequently, water and electrolyte homeostasis is of vital importance and special care is required to maintain an appropriate balance, especially in very-low-birth-weight (VLBW) infants.

In this discussion, the recommendations of the American Academy of Pediatrics (AAP) have been followed whenever possible. In all other instances the conclusions drawn are based on current medical evidence in the field.

WATER AND ELECTROLYTES

Water

■ Physiology. Water is the main component of the human body. It is distributed both inside and outside the cells: Therefore a practical simplification is to classify total body water (TBW) as intracellular water (ICW) and extracellular water (ECW). ICW is the total amount of water in all the body's cells. ECW is the total amount of water outside the cells; it comprises the water in the interstitial space and in the intravascular space (plasma).

The distribution of TBW between intracellular and extracellular spaces depends on the water's relative content of solutes (electrolytes, proteins), that is, on its relative osmolality. The total number of solute particles in solution determines the osmolality of a solution. Osmolality values are expressed in osmoles or milliosmoles per kilogram of water (Osm/kg or mOsm/kg). Because cell membranes are completely permeable to water but not to most solutes, water shifts from one compartment to the other until equilibrium is established between the osmolalities on both sides of the membrane. The osmolality of intracellular and extracellular spaces, therefore, is equal, although the composition of ICW is different from that of ECW; sodium (Na) is the main extracellular ion, whereas potassium (K) is the main intracellular ion. The size of a compartment depends on the number of osmoles in it, which in turn determines the water content.

In each compartment, a main solute acts to keep water in the compartment:

- The volume of the intracellular compartment is maintained mainly by potassium salts and is regulated by the Na-K cellular pump.
- The volume of the extracellular compartment is maintained mainly by sodium salts and is regulated by the kidneys.
- In the extracellular space, the volume of the intravascular compartment is maintained mainly by the colloidal osmotic pressure of plasma proteins.

Changes in Water Distribution

TBW declines with growth (Figure 19.1). It constitutes more than 90% of the total body weight in the first trimester of gestation, about 80% at 32 weeks gestation, about 78% at 40 weeks gestation, and approximately 60% to 65% at the end of the first year of life. The ratio of ECW to ICW also changes with growth. ECW declines from approximately 60% of body weight in the second trimester to about 45% at term. Correspondingly, ICW increases from about 25% of body weight in the second trimester to approximately 33% at term.

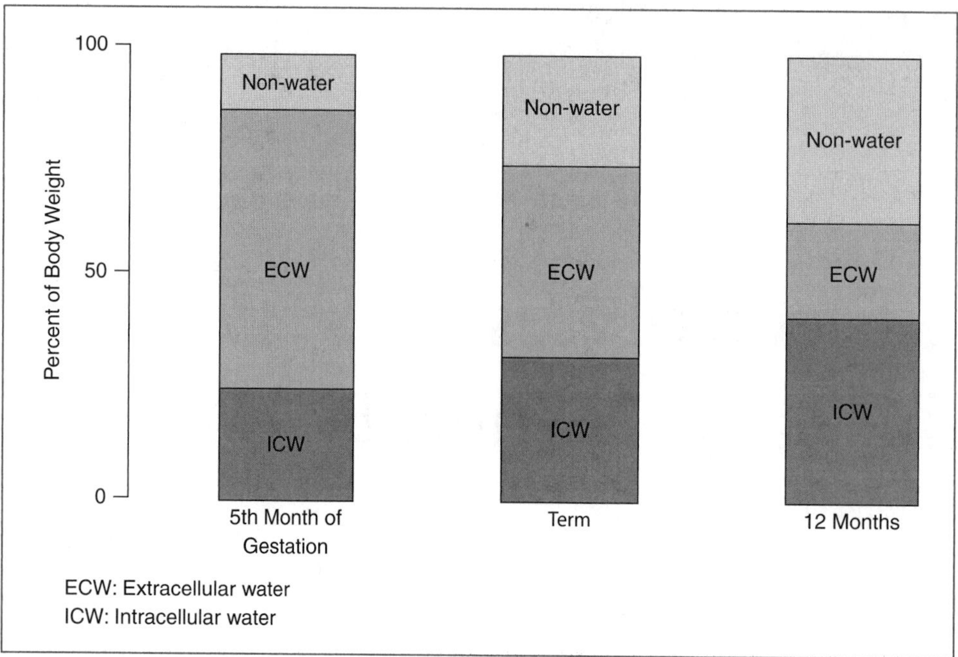

FIGURE 19.1 Changes in body water distribution.

At birth an acute expansion of ECW is superimposed on the gradual changes that took place during fetal life. This is due to (a) placental transfusion, (b) reabsorption of lung fluid, and (c) shift of water and electrolytes from the intracellular to the extracellular space (Baumgart & Costarino, 2000). The newborn at birth, therefore, is in a state of excess extracellular fluid, a condition that is particularly prominent in preterm infants (TBW and ECW are greater at lower gestational ages). Because the excess ECW is lost through diuresis, some weight loss (5%–10% in term infants) usually occurs as a consequence of these physiologic changes in body water distribution. Postnatal loss and regaining of weight reflect changes in the interstitial water component of ECW, whereas plasma volume remains essentially unchanged. In preterm infants, the postnatal weight loss is greater (usually 10%–20%) and occurs more frequently in the smallest infants. As long as the intravascular volume is adequate and serum electrolytes are normal, it appears inappropriate to replace all fluid losses during the first days of life. Administration of large amounts of fluids increases the risk of symptomatic patent ductus arteriosus (PDA) and bronchopulmonary dysplasia (BPD).

Water Balance and Body Metabolism

The human body loses a variable amount of water and electrolytes daily. To maintain body fluid balance, fluid losses must be replaced periodically. Maintenance fluid requirements are calculated to replace water and electrolytes normally lost through urine, stool, skin, and the respiratory tract. Water turnover is part of cellular metabolism and usually is related precisely to the basal metabolic rate. The basal metabolic rate is the amount of energy the body must produce to maintain homeostasis at rest and in a thermally neutral environment. Carbohydrates, lipids, and proteins are the substances used to produce energy. Waste products are heat, nitrogen, carbon dioxide, and water. To excrete waste products, the body normally loses water through the kidneys (to eliminate nitrogen), the skin (to eliminate excess heat), and the respiratory tract (to eliminate carbon dioxide). Therefore a high body energy expenditure means a large amount of waste products and, consequently, large water losses.

The cells generate some water as a byproduct of cell metabolism (i.e., water of oxidation). This amount of water, which must be subtracted from fluid requirements, is approximately equal to water losses in stools; therefore the latter can be omitted from the usual calculations of required water intake.

Water Requirements

Maintaining the overall body water and salt composition requires replacement of renal water and electrolyte losses and insensible water losses (IWLs) from the respiratory tract and skin evaporation. An approximate estimate of maintenance fluids is: 100 mL of water is needed for each 100 kcal of energy expended.

Although this relationship between metabolic rate and water loss holds true in full-term infants, it is not valid in preterm infants. Immature renal function, very high IWLs as a result of skin immaturity and a higher body surface area to body mass ratio, and neonatal illnesses significantly affect fluid balance (Baumgart & Costarino, 2000). Although values for fluid requirements are available (Table 19.1), they provide only an approximate guideline for the individual infant.

Fluid requirements may be determined more accurately if factors that influence IWL are taken into account (Table 19.2). For example, radiant warmers and phototherapy increase IWL, whereas use of a plastic blanket under a radiant warmer or adequate humidification in an incubator reduces IWL.

TABLE 19.1

APPROXIMATE WATER REQUIREMENTS OF NEWBORNS IN THE FIRST WEEK OF LIFE[a]

	Birth Weight			
Time Period	**Under 1,000 g**	**1,000–1,500 g**	**1,501–2,000 g**	**Full Term**
First 48 hours	80–140	60–100	60–80	40–60
End of first week	150–200	140–160	110–150	100–150

[a]Amounts are given as mL/kg/d.

TABLE 19.2

FACTORS AFFECTING WATER LOSS IN NEONATES

Increases Water Loss	**Reduces Water Loss**
Water Loss From the Skin	
Low gestational age	High humidity in incubator
Forced convection in	Double-walled incubator
Radiant warmer	Plastic heat shield
Hyperthermia	Plastic blanket
Activity	Semipermeable skin patches
Phototherapy	
Water Loss From the Respiratory Tract	
Tachypnea	Continuous distending pressure with humidified gas
Inadequate humidification	Artificial ventilation with humidification
Renal Water Loss	
Diuretics	Renal failure
Osmotic diuresis (hyperglycemia, mannitol)	Inappropriate secretion of antidiuretic hormone
Congenital adrenal hyperplasia	Congestive heart failure

Postnatal Adaptation

Fluid management is easier if one remembers a few simple principles: (1) to separate water from sodium requirements; (2) to keep maintenance fluids separate from fluids given to correct electrolyte abnormalities; (3) to recognize the pattern of neonatal diuresis. Monitoring a newborn's urine output (UOP) can help to individualize fluid requirements. According to Lorenz, Kleinman, Ahmed, and Markarian (1995), most preterm infants show a definite postnatal pattern of diuresis, which has three phases: the prediuretic phase, the diuretic phase, and the homeostatic phase (Table 19.3). The *prediuretic phase* occurs in the first 48 to 72 hours of life. In this phase, the glomerular filtration rate, UOP, and sodium and potassium excretion are all very low. Water is lost mainly by IWL. Because only water is lost through the skin, the appropriate steps in calculating fluid intake during this phase are the following:

- Intake is limited to IWLs
- No sodium, chloride, or potassium is given
- The standard intravenous (IV) solution should provide glucose at a rate of 4 to 6 mg/kg/min (with increasing amounts of amino acids)

As only skin water losses occur during this phase, preterm infants appear to be predisposed to hypernatremia. Early sodium supplementation offers no advantage and increases the risk of hypernatremia.

The *diuretic phase* usually begins on day 2 to 5 of life. UOP and sodium and potassium excretion all increase abruptly. This phase seems to be triggered by atrial natriuretic peptide (ANP), which is released by myocardial cells in response to atrial stretching. The proposed mechanism in falling pulmonary vascular resistance leads to increased venous return to the left atrium and to release of ANP. ANP in turn causes increased natriuresis (Modi, 2003). In this phase, fluid intake is adjusted as follows:

- Water intake is increased to maintain a normal serum sodium concentration and to obtain a total weight loss

TABLE 19.3

PATTERN OF POSTNATAL DIURESIS IN PRETERM INFANTS DURING THE FIRST WEEK OF LIFE

	Phases of Postnatal Diuresis		
Factors	**Prediuretic**	**Diuretic**	**Homeostatic**
Age	First 2 days	2–5 days	After 2–5 days
Diuresis	Very low	Sudden increase	Varies with intake
Urine	Very low	Sudden increase	Varies with intake
	Interventions		
Water	Fluid restriction	Allow physiologic weight loss	Provide calories for growth
Sodium	None	Provide enough to maintain normal serum sodium level	Provide growth allowance

Adapted from Lorenz et al. (1995).

of about 10% in term newborns and between 10% and 20% in preterm infants.

- Sodium (to keep the serum sodium level normal) and potassium (when the serum potassium level declines) should be added to the IV solution.

In the *homeostatic phase*, which follows the diuretic phase, diuresis stabilizes. The goal of fluid and electrolyte intake in this phase is to allow an adequate caloric intake and growth, without causing fluid overload.

Appropriate administration of fluid is important, because both excessive fluid restriction and fluid overload lead to clinical consequences. Excessive fluid restriction may lead to dehydration, hyperosmolality, hypoglycemia, and hyperbilirubinemia. In preterm infants, high volumes of parenteral fluids have been associated with a higher incidence of PDA, BPD, and necrotizing enterocolitis. It is important to realize that the occurrence of BPD has been correlated with fluid volume administered during the first 4 days of life. Maintaining the fluid and electrolyte balance, therefore, is extremely important in preterm infants. Close monitoring of clinical hydration, body weight, UOP, and the serum sodium concentration should allow the best possible decisions on fluid administration.

■ **Sodium.** Sodium is the main extracellular ion, constituting, with its salts, more than 90% of the total amount of solutes in the extracellular space. Sodium is absorbed in both the small intestine and the colon; the largest amount is absorbed in the jejunum. Sodium absorption involves several mechanisms:

- Passive absorption, after glucose absorption, secondary to the flow of water
- Active absorption, stimulated by glucose and amino acids
- Active absorption, uncoupled with glucose, involving the Na-K pump
- Active absorption in exchange with hydrogen ions

The overall process is very efficient. Adults normally absorb 98% of ingested sodium.

The kidneys excrete sodium, which is filtered by glomeruli and reabsorbed throughout the tubules and the collecting ducts. Most of the sodium is absorbed with chloride (Cl), but small amounts are absorbed in exchange with potassium ions (K^+) or hydrogen ions (H^+). Under normal circumstances, 96% to 99% of filtered sodium is reabsorbed. The main factors involved in the regulation of sodium resorption are the oncotic and hydrostatic pressures in the peritubular capillaries and the action of aldosterone, which increases the absorption of sodium in exchange with K^+ or H^+. Although antidiuretic hormone does not affect the excretion of sodium directly, it can influence the serum sodium concentration indirectly because it regulates the excretion or resorption of free water.

The sodium concentration in human milk is 12 to 20 mEq/L (12–20 mmol/L). The current recommendation for standard formulas is 20–60 mg/100 kcal (6–17 mEq/419 kJ) (AAP, 2009). The recommendation for growing preterm infants is 3 to 5 mEq/kg/d (Tsang, Lucas, Uauy, & Zlotkin, 2005). Because of their high urinary loss of sodium, VLBW infants (those weighing less than 1,500 g) may temporarily require up to 8 mEq/kg/d by the end of the first week of life. Thereafter, urinary losses in these infants are gradually reduced. The normal serum sodium concentration ranges from 130 to 150 mEq/L. Disorders of sodium balance are listed in Box 19.1.

■ **Hyponatremia.** Hyponatremia (a serum sodium level below 130 mEq/L) is caused by retention of water relative to sodium. When the serum sodium concentration and, therefore, serum osmolality decline, water moves into cells. The increased water content in the brain causes the signs and symptoms of hyponatremia. Vomiting, lethargy, and apnea may occur with various degrees of hyponatremia, but seizures and coma usually are not seen unless the serum sodium concentration falls below 115 mEq/L. Neonatal hyponatremia usually is classified as early or late, depending on the timing of the occurrence.

■ **Early Hyponatremia.** Early hyponatremia, which often occurs in the first 2 days of life, is caused by extrinsic

BOX 19.1
DISORDERS OF SODIUM BALANCE

Hyponatremia

- *Early*
  Perinatal asphyxia
  RDS
  Diuretics
  Nebulization associated with nasal CPAP
  Hypotonic fluid administered to mother during labor
- *Late*
  VLBW infant fed human milk or standard formula
  With overhydration: CHF, renal failure
  With dehydration: adrenal insufficiency, vomiting, diarrhea, peritonitis

Hypernatremia

- *With Dehydration*
  Vomiting, diarrhea with inadequate fluid replacement
  Osmotic diuresis (hyperglycemia, mannitol)
  Radiant warmers
  "Hyperosmolar state" in infants weighing less than 800 g
- *With Overhydration*
  Excessive administration of sodium bicarbonate ($NaHCO_3$)
  Errors in administration of sodium chloride (NaCl)

perinatal factors. It is not influenced by parenteral administration of additional sodium and water.

Early hyponatremia most often is caused by perinatal asphyxia. The mechanism is diminished excretion of free water, which is caused by increased secretion of antidiuretic hormone (syndrome of inappropriate secretion of antidiuretic hormone, or SIADH) and impairment of renal function by hypoxia. Severe respiratory distress syndrome (RDS) also predisposes newborns to hyponatremia, probably for the same reasons.

Early hyponatremia can be iatrogenic in origin. Possible causes include administration of large volumes of hypotonic fluid to the mother during labor; nebulization with nasal continuous positive airway pressure (CPAP), resulting in water overload and use of diuretics with excessive free water replacement. Infants with early hyponatremia usually are in a state of excess water, and fluid restriction is the appropriate treatment.

■ **Late Hyponatremia.** The most common form of late hyponatremia typically is seen after the first week of life in growing VLBW infants fed either human milk or standard formulas. These infants have a negative sodium balance in the first weeks of life because of a combination of factors, including an inadequate sodium intake and temporary unresponsiveness of the renal tubules to aldosterone (Baumgart & Costarino, 2000; Thureen & Hay, 2006). VLBW infants initially may require amounts such as 8 mEq/kg/d or higher to obtain a positive sodium balance. Usually, the lower is the gestational age, the higher is the sodium intake needed. Spontaneous improvement in sodium balance within weeks is the rule.

At any time, neonatal hyponatremia may occur in association with overhydration (dilutional hyponatremia) or dehydration (true hyponatremia).

Hyponatremia with overhydration may occur in newborns with congestive heart failure (CHF) (congenital heart disease, PDA), renal failure, or SIADH. Because total body sodium is increased but TBW is even more increased, administration of sodium would only cause additional expansion of the extracellular space, which can aggravate the infant's condition. Fluid restriction is the treatment.

Either renal or extrarenal sodium and water losses can cause hyponatremia with dehydration. Renal losses usually result from adrenal insufficiency (salt-losing type of congenital adrenal hyperplasia, adrenal hemorrhage), although infants with a urinary tract obstruction occasionally may have similar electrolyte disorders. Extrarenal losses may result from disorders such as vomiting, diarrhea, and peritonitis. Treatment is directed both at the underlying disorder and at volume replacement with sodium chloride (NaCl)–containing solutions. The amount of sodium needed to correct a low serum sodium level can be calculated according to the standard formula:

$$\text{Na to be given (mEq / mmol)} = 0.6 \times \text{Weight (kg)} \times \text{(Desired serum} - \text{Na actual serum Na)}$$

The correction usually is made over several hours, and the target is a serum sodium concentration of about 135 mEq/L. However, this general rule has two important exceptions:

- If shock is present or impending, normal saline should be given IV and rapidly at 10 to 20 mL/kg over 20 to 30 minutes; this treatment is repeated until arterial blood pressure is normal.
- With symptomatic hyponatremia, which almost always occurs only when the serum sodium level is below 115 mEq/L, hypertonic saline should be infused. However, because either an abrupt or a large increase in osmolality carries the risk of intracranial hemorrhage and CHF, the aim of the initial correction in this case should be a lower than normal serum sodium concentration, such as 120 to 125 mEq/L. Even if hyponatremia is asymptomatic, hypertonic saline is used if serum sodium is below 120 mEq/L to prevent symptoms.

Hyponatremia in preterm infants has been associated with adverse neurological outcome at 2 years of age.

Additionally, the risk appears to increase in proportion to the magnitude of the variation of serum sodium during the NICU stay (Baraton et al., 2009).

Postoperative hyponatremia can be a problem at any age. Although there are no randomized trials in newborns, it should be remembered that, in children, the risk of postoperative hyponatremia can be decreased significantly using isotonic solutions as opposed to hypotonic solution (Choong et al., 2011).

■ Hypernatremia. Hypernatremia (a serum sodium level over 150 mEq/L) is an increase in the serum sodium concentration. It may be accompanied by dehydration or, in rare cases, by overhydration. Hypernatremia with dehydration is caused by an insufficient water intake, by increased renal or extrarenal water losses, or by a combination of these two factors. Hypernatremia with overhydration usually is iatrogenic in origin.

When hypernatremia and, therefore, hyperosmolality develop, water moves out of the cells into the extracellular space to achieve an osmotic equilibrium between intracellular and extracellular fluid. This attempt to equilibrate intracellular and extracellular fluids results in volume depletion of the intracellular space. Brain cells can protect themselves, maintaining their intracellular volume by generating new solutes, called idiogenic osmoles. Idiogenic osmoles are substances (amino acids, polyols, trimethylamines) synthesized by the brain as a protective response to serum hyperosmolality. Idiogenic osmoles are neither produced nor catabolized rapidly, therefore this mechanism is effective within certain limits and only if hyperosmolality does not develop too rapidly. Similarly, correction of hypernatremia with hypotonic solutions should not be performed rapidly, because idiogenic osmoles cannot be metabolized quickly and cerebral edema can occur as a result of movement of water into brain cells.

In VLBW infants, sodium restriction during the first 3 to 5 days of life (i.e., no sodium other than with transfusions) may prevent hypernatremia and reduce the need for parenteral fluid.

Hypernatremia With Dehydration. Hypernatremia with dehydration results from water losses for which fluid replacement is inadequate. Water loss may occur from the gastrointestinal tract (vomiting, diarrhea). Inadequate replacement of fluids may include failure to provide the appropriate water intake, especially when this shortcoming is compounded by administration of high-solute fluids. Renal water loss may occur when an increased amount of solute, such as glucose or mannitol, must be excreted (osmotic diuresis). Significant IWL through the skin occurs when infants are placed under radiant warmers and the magnitude of these losses is inversely related to gestational age.

Hypernatremia with dehydration must be corrected slowly, because cerebral edema can easily develop. Intravascular *volume* should be restored *quickly* with isotonic fluids, but *water deficits* should be corrected *slowly* and with great caution by administration of hypotonic fluids.

As a general rule, serum sodium should *not* increase by more than 0.5 mEq/kg/hr. A hyperosmolar state can occur in the first days of life in infants of less than 26 weeks gestation who weigh less than 800 g. These infants' immature skin and large surface allow massive evaporative losses of free water, which results in significant dehydration (weight loss of 20% or more in the first 48 hours) accompanied by hypernatremia, hyperkalemia, and hyperglycemia, without oliguria (Baumgart & Costarino, 2000). Once this hyperosmolar state is fully established, correction involves the risk of volume overload. The suggested strategy for preventing this syndrome is as follows:

- IWL through the skin is reduced by using an incubator with a high relative humidity (instead of an overhead warmer), with or without a plastic shield or Saran wrap blanket or semipermeable membranes (such as Tegaderm).
- The infant's weight, UOP, serum sodium level, and glucose concentration are monitored frequently.
- Sodium is restricted, and the smallest volume of fluids is given that allows the serum sodium concentration to be maintained within normal limits (the initial rate is 80 to 100 mL/kg/d with subsequent increases, usually without exceeding 150 mL/kg/d).

Hypernatremia With Overhydration. Hypernatremia with overhydration is almost always iatrogenic in origin. It may occur after administration of sodium bicarbonate during cardiopulmonary resuscitation or for acidosis or RDS, or it may arise from errors in the administration of NaCl with fluids. Because administration of sodium increases serum osmolality, it results in a shift of water into the intravascular space. An acute expansion of plasma volume may result in intracranial bleeding and heart failure with pulmonary edema. Treatment of hypernatremia with overhydration involves restricting sodium intake and providing diuretic therapy.

■ Potassium. Potassium is the main intracellular cation. Its concentration in cells is maintained by the membrane sodium-potassium adenosine triphosphatase (Na^+, K^+-ATPase) pump. Because potassium is involved in the regulation of cell membrane potential, variations in the serum potassium concentration have important effects. Although every cell is susceptible to fluctuations in the serum potassium concentration, the effects on myocardial cells are the most prominent and severe.

Dietary potassium is mainly absorbed in the small intestine by passive absorption, and it is actively secreted in the colon. The kidneys excrete potassium. Probably all filtered potassium is reabsorbed in the proximal tubule. Potassium is then secreted by the distal tubules in exchange with sodium in a process regulated by aldosterone. The amount of potassium secreted normally is proportional to intake, so that balance is maintained. Stable, growing preterm infants have a potassium retention rate similar to the fetus (about 1.0–1.5 mEq/kg/d).

The potassium requirement for both preterm and full-term infants is 2 to 3 mEq/kg/d. The current recommendation for standard infant formulas is 80 to 200 mg/100 kcal (14–34 mEq/419 kJ) (AAP, 2009). The recommendation for growing preterm infants is 1.5 to 2.7 mEq/419 kJ (Tsang et al., 2005).

The normal serum concentrations are 3.5 to 5 mEq/L. Disorders of potassium balance are listed in Box 19.2.

■ Hypokalemia. Hypokalemia (a serum potassium level below 3.5 mEq/L) can be caused by inadequate intake, gastrointestinal losses (diarrhea, vomiting, continuous aspiration, and removal of gastrointestinal contents), and renal losses (diuretics, steroid therapy, renal tubular acidosis, Bartter syndrome).

The consequences of hypokalemia are related to the effects on muscle cells. Although abdominal distention and diminished bowel motility may occur, the cardiac effects are of much greater concern, and an electrocardiogram (EKG) may be a better measure of serious toxicity than the serum potassium concentration. EKG changes include a depressed ST segment, a flattened T wave, and a higher U wave. A prolonged P-R interval, a widening QRS complex, and various arrhythmias may follow, particularly in newborns treated with digoxin.

Treatment involves potassium replacement. Potassium chloride should be given very slowly (< 0.3 mEq/kg/hr), and the serum potassium concentration or EKG, or both, should be checked frequently. Rapid IV administration of potassium may cause fatal arrhythmias.

■ Hyperkalemia. Hyperkalemia (usually defined as a serum potassium level over 6.5 mEq/L) can be caused by an excessive intake of potassium, impaired excretion (renal failure, salt-losing congenital adrenal hyperplasia), or increased movement of potassium from intracellular to extracellular space (catabolic states, acidosis of any origin). Spurious hyperkalemia that is caused by venipuncture (injury to red blood cells) must be ruled out. Hyperkalemia occurs in approximately 50% of infants whose birth weight is less than 1,000 g, and it is especially common in infants with low UOP in the first hours of life. The proposed mechanism is an increased potassium flow from the intracellular to the extracellular compartment, caused by a decline in the activity of Na^+, K^+-ATPase. Increased catabolism does not seem to play a significant role. Cardiac toxicity is the main issue and is better reflected by EKG changes than by the serum potassium concentration. The typical EKG sequence is peaked T waves, disappearance of P waves, and a widening QRS complex, which fuses with the T wave to form a sine wave. Ventricular fibrillation may follow.

Treatment is directed at the underlying disorder, but several temporary measures can be taken, including administration of the following:

- 10% calcium gluconate (1 mL/kg, IV), to antagonize the effect of hyperkalemia on the myocardium
- Sodium bicarbonate (1–2 mEq/kg, IV), to raise the blood pH and consequently increase potassium influx into cells
- Salbutamol, by aerosol, to try to increase cellular uptake of potassium
- Infusion of glucose and insulin, at a ratio of 4 g of glucose to 1 unit of insulin, to increase cellular uptake of potassium
- Furosemide (1 mg/kg, IV), to increase renal excretion
- A potassium-binding resin, Kayexalate (1 g/kg, by rectum or by mouth), to increase intestinal excretion

All these measures are temporary. If the serum potassium concentration continues to rise and exceeds 8 mEq/L, peritoneal dialysis or exchange blood transfusions, using a mixture of washed red blood cells (RBCs) and fresh-frozen plasma (to avoid a high blood potassium level), should be instituted.

BOX 19.2

DISORDERS OF POTASSIUM BALANCE

Hypokalemia

Inadequate intake

Gastrointestinal losses: vomiting, diarrhea, continuous gastric aspiration

Renal losses: diuretics, steroids, renal tubular acidosis

Hyperkalemia

Excessive intake

Impaired excretion: renal failure, congenital adrenal hyperplasia

Movement of potassium out of cells: catabolic states, acidosis

■ Chloride. Chloride is the main inorganic anion in the extracellular fluid, and together with sodium, it is essential for maintenance of plasma volume. Chloride is administered as NaCl in the diet. Intestinal absorption is passive in the jejunum and occurs secondary to sodium absorption. In the ileum and colon, chloride is actively absorbed in exchange with bicarbonate. Normally only minimal amounts of chloride are lost in the feces. Chloride is excreted by the kidneys: like sodium, it is filtered by the glomeruli and reabsorbed throughout the tubules and collecting ducts. Normally 99% of the filtered chloride is reabsorbed.

Chloride resorption is inversely related to bicarbonate resorption. The serum concentrations of chloride and bicarbonate are also inversely correlated, which keeps the total anion concentration (Cl^- and HCO_3^-) constant. For this reason, although chloride has no buffer effect, it plays an important part in acid–base regulation. When chloride is retained in the body, the serum bicarbonate level declines and metabolic acidosis follows. When chloride is lost from the body, the serum bicarbonate level rises and metabolic alkalosis ensues.

The current chloride recommendation for infant formulas is 55 to 150 mg/100 kcal (10–28 mEq/419 kJ) (AAP, 2009). The recommendation for growing preterm infants is 2.3 to 6.4 mEq/419 kJ (Tsang et al., 2005). Normal serum Cl concentrations are 90 to 112 mEq/L in full-term infants and 100 to 115 mEq/L in preterm infants. Disorders of chloride balance are listed in Box 19.3.

■ Hypochloremia. Hypochloremia (a serum Cl level below 90 mEq/L) may be caused by diminished intake or by increased loss of chloride (gastrointestinal or renal). Clinical manifestations include metabolic alkalosis, hypokalemia, and, in the case of a chronic disturbance, failure to thrive.

Insufficient intake has occurred with some old soy formulas that had a very low chloride content. The diagnosis of insufficient chloride intake is based on the dietary history and on the absence of urinary chloride, which indicates a normal ability to retain chloride to compensate for the low intake. Prolonged vomiting (pyloric stenosis) or continuous aspiration and removal of gastric contents (e.g., necrotizing enterocolitis, abdominal surgery) can increase gastrointestinal losses of chloride as hydrochloric acid (HCl).

Congenital chloridorrhea is a rare disorder of severe diarrhea, beginning at birth, caused by impairment of the active Cl transport system in the ileum and colon. Analysis of feces shows an acid pH and a greatly increased Cl concentration. Diarrhea is caused by the osmotic effect of excess chloride, and hypokalemia ensues as a secondary consequence of diarrhea. Treatment involves a diet low in NaCl and potassium supplementation. The most common cause of increased renal loss of chloride is diuretic therapy. Frequent indications for this treatment in infancy are CHF and BPD.

Chronic administration of furosemide, which often is part of the treatment for BPD, may cause chloride deficiency with secondary metabolic alkalosis. Alkalosis, in turn, causes hypo-ventilation and an increase in the arterial carbon dioxide pressure ($PaCO_2$). This clinical picture can simulate pulmonary edema, but in this case the treatment should not be additional diuretic therapy (as in pulmonary edema), but rather correction of the hypochloremia.

Metabolic alkalosis with hypochloremia and hypokalemia caused by increased renal loss of chloride is the characteristic feature of Bartter syndrome, in which the underlying mechanism is a defect in tubular resorption of chloride. Elevated urinary Cl and prostaglandin concentrations are diagnostic. Replacement with NaCl and potassium chloride (KCl) or treatment with indomethacin (a prostaglandin antagonist), or both, is usually effective.

■ Hyperchloremia. Hyperchloremia (a serum Cl level over 115 mEq/L) usually is associated with metabolic acidosis and can be caused either by bicarbonate depletion or by an excessive chloride intake. Diarrhea is the most common cause of hyperchloremic metabolic acidosis, because in the intestine chloride is absorbed with sodium, and bicarbonate is excreted with potassium. Increased loss of bicarbonate occurs with renal tubular acidosis. Usually only the proximal type is diagnosed in the neonatal period, and it occurs mainly in male infants. The renal threshold for bicarbonate drops below normal, and the acidity of the urine is not diminished in this condition. The result is a hyperchloremic metabolic acidosis. The condition is self-limited, and the diagnosis is based on the demonstration that the renal bicarbonate threshold is lower than normal. When the serum bicarbonate concentration is lower than the normal threshold, bicarbonate is retained and acid urine is produced.

Hyperchloremia may follow excessive administration of NaCl. Overtreatment with NaCl may be absolute, as in accidental errors in administration, or relative, as in renal failure. In the latter case, excretion is impaired and can be exceeded by an otherwise "normal" intake; NaCl administration, therefore, must be reduced accordingly. Finally, apparent hyperchloremia, together with increased serum concentrations of other electrolytes, can occur with dehydration when there is a water deficit in relation to solute.

BOX 19.3

DISORDERS OF CHLORIDE BALANCE

Hypochloremia

Decreased intake: some soy formulas

Increased gastrointestinal losses: vomiting (pyloric stenosis), continuous gastric aspiration, congenital chloridorrhea

Increased renal losses: diuretics, Bartter syndrome

Hyperchloremia

Increased bicarbonate losses: renal tubular acidosis

Excessive administration of NaCl: absolute or relative (renal failure)

Hypertonic dehydration (apparent hyperchloremia)

■ Calcium and Phosphorus. Calcium (Ca) is the most abundant mineral in the human body. It is an essential component of the skeleton and plays an important role in muscle contraction, neural transmission, and blood coagulation. Phosphorus (P) is essential for bone mineralization, erythrocyte function, cell metabolism, and generation and storage of energy.

The calcium content of human milk is about 39 mg/100 kcal (0.97 mmol/419 kJ), and the phosphorus content is about 19 mg/100 kcal (0.61 mmol/419 kJ). The current recommendations for standard formulas are 60 mg/100 kcal (1.5 mmol/419 kJ) for calcium and 30 mg/100 kcal (0.97 mmol/419 kJ) for phosphorus (AAP, 2009). The recommendations for growing preterm infants are 1.9 to 5.0 mmol/419 k for calcium and 1.5 to 4.1 mmol/419 kJ for phosphorus (Tsang et al., 2005). With parenteral nutrition, a calcium intake of 60 to 80 mg/kg/d (1.5–2.0 mmol/kg/d) and a phosphorus intake of 45 to 60 mg/kg/d (1.5–1.9 mmol/kg/d) is recommended (Tsang et al., 2005).

To avoid precipitation in the parenteral solution, the calcium concentration should be maintained between 500 and 600 mg/L (12.5–15 mmol/L), and the phosphorus concentration should be maintained between 390 and 470 mg/L (12.5–15 mmol/L).

■ **Calcium.** Calcium transport in the intestine occurs by both passive and active processes. Active intestinal transport involves carriers called calcium-binding proteins. Vitamin D in its active form, 1,25-dihydroxyvitamin D, is essential for the active process. Parathyroid hormone (PTH) is involved only through stimulation of production of 1,25-dihydroxyvitamin D. Vitamin D deficiency and almost any form of intestinal malabsorption can impair calcium transport. Corticosteroids diminish calcium absorption by inhibiting its transfer in the intestinal mucosa. Anticonvulsants can directly inhibit intestinal transfer of calcium (phenytoin) or can interfere with vitamin D metabolism (phenobarbital and phenytoin).

The serum calcium concentration is maintained within narrow limits by the action of PTH, 1,25-dihydroxyvitamin D, and calcitonin. PTH and 1,25-dihydroxyvitamin D increase the serum calcium level, and calcitonin reduces it. PTH secretion is determined by the serum ionized calcium concentration via the calcium-sensing receptors of the parathyroid cells.

The kidneys excrete calcium, and filtered calcium is reabsorbed in most segments of the tubules. PTH increases tubular resorption of calcium, whereas calcitonin is thought to increase calcium excretion. Disorders of calcium balance are listed in Box 19.4.

BOX 19.4
DISORDERS OF CALCIUM BALANCE

Hypocalcemia

- *Early*
  - Preterm infant
  - Infant of insulin-dependent diabetic mother
  - Perinatal asphyxia
- *Late*
  - Cow milk–based formula
  - Hypomagnesemia
  - Hypoparathyroidism
  - Maternal vitamin D deficiency
  - Osteopetrosis

Hypercalcemia

Excessive administration of calcium or vitamin D (or both)
Subcutaneous fat necrosis
Williams syndrome
Idiopathic hypercalcemia
Hyperparathyroidism
Hypophosphatasia
Bartter syndrome
Congenital carbohydrate malabsorptions
Familial hypocalciuric hypercalcemia

■ **Hypocalcemia.** Neonatal hypocalcemia is defined as an ionized serum calcium concentration below 4.4 mg/dL (1.1 mmol/L) in full-term infants. For preterm infants, for whom insufficient normative data on ionized calcium are available, a total serum calcium concentration below 7 mg/dL (1.75 mmol/L) continues to be a reasonable definition. Hypocalcemia conventionally is divided into early hypocalcemia, which occurs in the first 2 days of life, and late hypocalcemia, which occurs after the first 2 days, usually at about 1 week of age. Neonatal hypocalcemia may be asymptomatic or can cause symptoms such as irritability, tremors, poor feeding, muscle twitching, and seizures.

Early hypocalcemia is relatively common and sometimes is caused by perinatal factors. Approximately 30% of pre-term infants (those <37 weeks gestation), 35% of birth-asphyxiated infants, 17% to 32% of infants of insulin-dependent diabetic mothers, and up to 90% of VLBW infants (those weighing <1,500 g) develop hypocalcemia in the first days of life. Several factors appear to be involved, including abrupt termination of maternal calcium supply, temporary functional hypoparathyroidism (in infants of diabetic mothers), an increased calcitonin concentration (in asphyxiated and preterm infants), and, possibly, 1,25-dihydroxyvitamin D resistance (in VLBW infants).

Late hypocalcemia typically occurs by the end of the first week of life and is caused by a relative increase in the dietary phosphate load. Maternal vitamin D deficiency may be a predisposing factor. Phototherapy appears to be a cofactor associated with neonatal hypocalcemia, especially in preterm infants. The mechanism is incompletely understood.

In rare cases, late hypocalcemia can occur as a consequence of subclinical maternal hyperparathyroidism: Maternal hypercalcemia leads to fetal hypercalcemia, which suppresses the fetal parathyroid glands. After birth, when the maternal source of calcium is no longer available, the suppressed parathyroid glands are unable to maintain a normal serum calcium concentration. Because the maternal hyperparathyroidism often is asymptomatic, neonatal hypocalcemia may provide the initial clue to the maternal disease. Another uncommon but serious condition that can cause symptomatic hypocalcemia is severe hypomagnesemia (see the section on Magnesium later in the chapter).

Several factors complicate the choice of treatment for neonatal hypocalcemia: (1) it may coexist with other perinatal complications, such as asphyxia and hypoglycemia, which can cause similar clinical signs; (2) it may be associated with seizures without being the cause of the seizures; and (3) in most cases, the condition is asymptomatic and self-limited.

If the hypocalcemia is asymptomatic, 10% calcium gluconate (9.4 mg of elemental calcium per milliliter) may be given orally (PO) at a rate of 75 mg/kg/d divided into six equal doses. If hypocalcemia is symptomatic (e.g., seizures), 10% calcium gluconate must be given IV at a rate of 2 mL/kg over 10 minutes; the heart rate should be closely monitored and the infusion stopped immediately at the first sign of bradycardia.

■ **Hypercalcemia.** Hypercalcemic disorders (a serum calcium level over 11 mg/dL [2.75 mmol/L]), such as subcutaneous fat necrosis, Williams syndrome, congenital hyperparathyroidism, hyperthyroidism, neonatal Bartter's syndrome, osteopetrosis, and familial hypocalciuric hypercalcemia, are all exceedingly rare among newborns. Hypercalcemia usually is of iatrogenic origin and results from excessive administration of calcium or vitamin D, or by insufficient phosphorus intake. Consequently, before embarking on elaborate differential diagnosis and expensive tests, one should carefully review the actual Ca, P, and vitamin D intakes.

Clinical signs, which are nonspecific, include constipation, polyuria, and bradycardia. Nephrocalcinosis and nephrolithiasis caused by hypercalcemia can be aggravated by dehydration and administration of furosemide.

Treatment of hypercalcemia is as follows:

- Calcium and vitamin D supplementation is suspended, and dietary intake of calcium and vitamin D is restricted (human milk or vitamin D–free formula is given).
- Urinary excretion of calcium is promoted by fluid administration (about twice the maintenance requirement).
- In the case of vitamin D excess, glucocorticoids are given to reduce intestinal absorption and bone resorption of calcium.
- With failure of other interventions, pamidronate can be given, although experience with biphosphonates in newborns is limited. Pamidronate is generally given at a dose of 1 mg/kg, as a single 4-hour infusion. In case an additional dose is needed, it should not be given prior to 6 to 7 days, as serum calcium nadir usually occurs by day 6.

■ **Phosphorus.** Phosphorus is absorbed mainly in the jejunum by both active and passive diffusion. Absorption depends mainly on the absolute amount of phosphorus in the diet, the relative concentrations of calcium and phosphorus (an excessive amount of either can diminish absorption of the other), and whether substances are present that bind to phosphorus and make it unavailable for absorption (e.g., phytates in soy-based formulas).

The kidneys excrete phosphorus; normally about 10% to 15% of the filtered phosphorus is excreted. PTH directly influences phosphorus excretion through its phosphaturic effect. Disorders of phosphorus balance are listed in Box 19.5.

BOX 19.5

DISORDERS OF PHOSPHORUS BALANCE

Hypophosphatemia

Rickets/osteopenia of prematurity

Inadequate parenteral phosphorus administration

Malabsorption

Familial hypophosphatemias: vitamin D-resistant rickets, X-linked hypophosphatemia, Fanconi syndrome

Hyperphosphatemia

Impaired excretion of phosphorus: renal failure

Hypoparathyroidism

Excessive parenteral or enteral administration of phosphorus

■ **Hypophosphatemia.** Hypophosphatemia (a serum phosphorus level below 4 mg/dL [1.29 mmol/L]) is a common feature in preterm infants with rickets of prematurity, which is caused by insufficient intake of calcium and phosphorus. Rickets of prematurity is common in VLBW infants fed regular formulas, especially human milk with a low phosphorus content. Preterm formulas provide a higher concentration of calcium and phosphorus and can produce bone mineralization similar to intrauterine bone mineralization. In very rare cases, hypophosphatemia is caused by neonatal hyperparathyroidism.

In infancy, hypophosphatemia can be caused by diseases of vitamin D metabolism (vitamin D–dependent rickets) or by disorders of renal phosphorus transport (hypophosphatemic rickets).

Severe hypophosphatemia (a serum phosphorus level below 1 mg/dL [0.32 mmol/L]) is uncommon and may occur only in newborns receiving parenteral alimentation with an inadequate amount of phosphorus. Respiratory failure and decreased myocardial performance have been described as possible consequences of severe hypophosphatemia.

■ **Hyperphosphatemia.** Neonatal hyperphosphatemia (a serum phosphorus level over 7 mg/dL [2.26 mmol/L]) can be caused by ingestion of milk formulas containing high amounts of phosphorus, by excessive parenteral administration of phosphorus, by impaired phosphorus excretion (renal failure), or by defects in hormonal regulation (hypoparathyroidism). Severe hyperphosphatemia may cause metastatic calcifications and hypocalcemia. Management includes alimentation with human milk or with a low-phosphorus formula, and calcium supplementation to increase binding to phosphorus and its fecal excretion. Reducing the parenteral phosphorus intake usually resolves parenteral hyperphosphatemia. In renal failure, 1,25-dihydroxyvitamin D, which exerts its effects independent of functioning renal tissue, can be given to counteract hypocalcemia secondary to hyperphosphatemia.

Supplementation with 1,25-dihydroxyvitamin D and calcium may be used to treat hypoparathyroidism that arises from maternal hyperparathyroidism (transient secondary hypoparathyroidism) or from permanent primary hypoparathyroidism (sporadic or hereditary).

■ **Magnesium.** Magnesium (Mg) is distributed primarily in the skeleton and the intracellular space. It is involved in energy production, cell membrane function, mitochondrial function, and protein synthesis.

Magnesium is absorbed by passive diffusion throughout the small intestine. Absorption is related to intake, and approximately 50% to 70% of dietary magnesium is absorbed. The kidneys primarily regulate the serum magnesium concentration; under normal circumstances, less than 5% of the filtered magnesium is excreted. PTH increases the serum magnesium concentration, possibly through mobilization from bone. An acute decline in the serum magnesium concentration increases secretion of PTH, but chronic magnesium deficiency reduces PTH secretion and therefore may cause hypocalcemia.

The magnesium content of human milk is about 5 mg/100 kcal (0.21 mmol/419 kJ). The recommendation for standard formulas is 6 mg/100 kcal (0.25 mmol/419 kJ) (AAP, 2009). The recommendation for growing preterm infants is 0.3 to 0.6 mmol/419 kJ (Tsang et al., 2005).

In parenteral nutrition, an intake of 4.3 to 7.2 mg/kg/d (0.2–0.3 mmol/kg/d) is recommended. The magnesium concentration in the parenteral solution should be maintained between 36 and 48 mg/L (1.5–2 mmol/L) to avoid precipitation. Disorders of magnesium balance are listed in Box 19.6.

■ **Hypomagnesemia.** Theoretically, magnesium transfer from mother to fetus might be impaired with placental malfunction, and placental insufficiency appears to predispose the infant to neonatal hypomagnesemia (a serum magnesium level below 1.6 mg/dL [0.66 mmol/L]). In infants of diabetic mothers, hypomagnesemia appears to be a consequence of maternal magnesium depletion. Any severe malabsorption syndrome can cause magnesium deficiency, and an isolated defect in intestinal absorption of magnesium has been described.

Hypomagnesemia in the neonatal period usually is transient (except in malabsorption cases) and asymptomatic, but it can cause hyperexcitability and, occasionally, severe intractable hypocalcemic seizures that are unresponsive to calcium infusion and anticonvulsants. The mechanism of the resultant hypocalcemia is diminished secretion of PTH caused by magnesium depletion. The treatment is 0.2 ml/kg of 50% magnesium sulfate ($MgSO_4$) given intramuscularly (IM) or IV. This dose can be repeated, with monitoring of the serum magnesium concentration every 12 hours, until normomagnesemia is achieved.

BOX 19.6
DISORDERS OF MAGNESIUM BALANCE

Hypomagnesemia

Infant of diabetic mother

Infant small for gestational age

Malabsorption syndromes

Isolated intestinal magnesium malabsorption

Hypermagnesemia

Maternal treatment with $MgSO_4$ (e.g., for tocolysis, preeclampsia)

Excessive magnesium administration with parenteral nutrition

■ **Hypermagnesemia.** Neonatal hypermagnesemia (a serum magnesium level over 2.8 mg/dL [1.15 mmol/L]) is an iatrogenic event caused either by parenteral nutrition or, more commonly, by maternal treatment with $MgSO_4$ for tocolysis or preeclampsia. Other causes are administration of magnesium-containing antacid for treatment of stress ulcers and treatment of persistent pulmonary hypertension of the newborn with $MgSO_4$. Reported clinical signs of hypermagnesemia include hyporeflexia, lethargy, and respiratory depression. Neonatal serum magnesium concentrations rarely rise to potentially dangerous levels and gradually return to normal after several days. Hypermagnesemia does not cause hypocalcemia in the neonatal period and appears to be associated only with hypotonia. Usually no treatment is necessary. In severe cases, exchange blood transfusion has been used to lower the elevated serum concentrations.

WATER-SOLUBLE VITAMINS

Thiamine (Vitamin B_1)

Thiamine is a necessary coenzyme in carbohydrate and amino acid metabolism. Intestinal absorption is both active and passive; transport is active at physiologic concentrations and passive at pharmacologic concentrations. Thiamine is absorbed throughout the small intestine, but mainly in the duodenum. The kidneys excrete thiamine, and urinary excretion varies according to dietary intake.

The thiamine content of human milk is about 210 mcg/L. For standard formulas, the AAP (2009) recommends a minimum content of 40 mcg/100 kcal (0.12 μmol/419 kJ). The recommendation for growing preterm infants is 0.5 to 0.7 μmol/kg/d (Tsang, 2005). Both breast milk and formulas provide adequate amounts of thiamine. The recommended parenteral intake for stable preterm infants is 0.6 to 1.0 μmol/kg/d.

■ **Deficiency.** Thiamine deficiency results in beriberi, but it is never seen in the neonatal period. Infantile beriberi occurs only in breastfed infants of thiamine-deficient mothers. The clinical signs, which become apparent after 1 to 4 months, include aphonia, cardiac signs (dyspnea and cyanosis), and neurologic signs (bulging fontanelle and seizures). Thiamine deficiency can be determined from reduced activity of the erythrocyte enzyme transketolase or by measuring the whole blood thiamine concentration.

■ **Toxicity.** Thiamine toxicity has not been reported with oral administration and is very rare in parenteral administration. Very large IV doses of thiamine have caused anaphylaxis and respiratory depression in adults.

Riboflavin (Vitamin B_2)

As part of the coenzymes flavin adenine dinucleotide (FAD) and flavin mononucleotide (FMN), riboflavin is involved in electron transport and is essential to glucose, amino acid, and lipid metabolism. Riboflavin is absorbed in the proximal part of the small intestine, and amounts in excess of needs are excreted unchanged in the urine. The average riboflavin content of human milk is approximately 350 mcg/L (Tsang et al., 2005). The AAP (2009) recommends a concentration of 60 mcg/100 kcal (0.16 μmol/419 kJ) for standard formulas and 200 to 300 mcg/100 kcal (0.53–0.80 μmol/419 kJ) for stable preterm infants. Riboflavin is degraded by light (both sunlight and phototherapy), but is resistant to pasteurization.

■ **Deficiency.** Riboflavin deficiency results in epithelial abnormalities (stomatitis, cheilosis, glossitis, seborrheic dermatitis), normocytic anemia, and vascularization of the cornea. Riboflavin intake may not be sufficient in preterm infants fed human milk, especially if the infant undergoes phototherapy and if human milk is given by continuous drip and therefore remains exposed to light. The significance of this deficiency is unclear, as clinical riboflavin deficiency caused by phototherapy has never been reported, but supplementation may be reasonable.

■ **Toxicity.** There are no toxic effects of riboflavin. However, grossly abnormal parenteral intakes have been associated with obstructive uropathy in a preterm infant.

Vitamin B_6

Vitamin B_6 is the generic term used to describe three substances: pyridoxine, pyridoxal, and pyridoxamine. The metabolic functions of these vitamins include synthesis of neurotransmitters, heme, and prostaglandins and interconversion of amino acids. Absorption occurs in the proximal small intestine by passive diffusion, and phosphorylation takes place in the liver. Vitamin B_6 needs are related to protein intake, the mean vitamin/protein ratio being 15 mcg/g.

The vitamin B_6 content of human milk ranges from 130 to 310 mcg/L, depending on maternal intake of the vitamin (Tsang et al., 2005). The AAP (2009) recommends a concentration of 60 mcg/100 kcal (0.29 μmol/419 kJ) for standard formulas and 125 to 175 mcg/100 kcal (0.61–0.85 μmol/419 kJ) for preterm infants. Vitamin B_6 is inactivated by light. Pyridoxal and pyridoxamine are heat labile, whereas pyridoxine is heat stable and is used for milk fortification.

■ **Deficiency.** Vitamin B_6 deficiency can develop with any severe malabsorption and with dietary deprivation (human milk low in vitamin B_6, improperly sterilized milk, goat milk). Clinical signs include hypochromic microcytic anemia, failure to thrive, irritability, and seizures. Isoniazid binds to and inactivates vitamin B_6; therefore infants receiving this drug may need vitamin B_6 supplementation. Neonatal pyridoxine-dependent seizures are caused by a congenital abnormality of vitamin B_6 metabolism, and pharmacologic doses of vitamin B_6 are needed.

■ **Toxicity.** There are no reports of vitamin B_6 toxicity in newborns. However, seizures and sensory neuropathy have been reported in adults taking large doses of pyridoxine.

Cyanocobalamin (Vitamin B_{12})

Vitamin B_{12} is essential to (a) synthesis of DNA nucleotides, (b) carbohydrate and lipid metabolism, and (c) myelin formation. Vitamin B_{12} is also necessary in cell folate metabolism. It can be synthesized only by microorganisms and is absent in plants, thus causing deficiency in strict vegetarians. Absorption of vitamin B_{12} takes place in the distal third of the ileum and requires the presence of intrinsic factor, a glycoprotein secreted by the stomach. The vitamin is transported in plasma by a specific protein (transcobalamin II). Vitamin B_{12} is stored in the liver, and preterm infants have much lower stores than term newborns.

The average cobalamin concentration in mature human milk is about 0.7 mcg/L (0.51 nmol/L). The AAP (2009) recommends a cobalamin content of 0.15 mcg/100 kcal (0.11 nmol/419 kJ) in standard formulas and 0.25 mcg/100 kcal (0.18 nmol/419 kJ) for preterm ones. The current recommended intake for growing preterm infants is 0.3 mcg/kg/d (0.22 nmol/kg/d) (Tsang et al., 2005).

■ **Deficiency.** Vitamin B_{12} deficiency causes hematologic changes (megaloblastic anemia, thrombocytopenia, leukopenia with hypersegmentation of neutrophils) and neurologic changes (hypotonia due to demyelination of the spinal cord and mental retardation). Neurologic manifestations may precede anemia. Because liver stores at birth are very large and usually sufficient for most of the first year of life, vitamin B_{12} deficiency rarely develops in early infancy.

Since body stores significantly exceed needs, nutritional deficiency occurs exclusively in infants fed breast milk from unsupplemented strictly vegetarian (vegan) mothers. Deficiency in such infants has been described at as early as 4 months of age: Signs include developmental delay and anemia. Both vegan mothers and their infants have high urinary concentrations of methylmalonic acid, as a biochemical marker. Vitamin B_{12} deficiency can develop in infants with short bowel syndrome if the terminal ileum (the site of absorption) is resected. The onset of vitamin B_{12} deficiency from intrinsic factor deficiency occurs at about 6 months of age. Congenital transcobalamin II deficiency is a rare but important cause of vitamin B_{12} deficiency; signs can occur after only 6 weeks of life, and mental retardation is invariably present. Because both folic acid and vitamin B_{12} deficiency can cause megaloblastic anemia and because folic acid can interfere with vitamin B_{12} metabolism, the differential diagnosis becomes important. A large folate intake may mask the hematologic signs of vitamin B_{12} deficiency and can aggravate the neurologic damage.

■ **Toxicity.** Toxicity from vitamin B_{12} has not been reported.

Folic Acid

Folic acid is essential to the synthesis of nucleic acids and to the metabolism of some amino acids. It is found in plants and synthesized by bacteria. Maximum absorption of folic acid takes place in the proximal jejunum. Absorption is active with physiologic doses of folic acid and mainly passive with pharmacologic doses. Folic acid is stored in the liver in small amounts, but its half-life is prolonged by enterohepatic recirculation. Folic acid can be synthesized by intestinal bacteria.

The average folate concentration in mature human milk is approximately 85 mcg/L (191 nmol/L), although heat treatment reduces the concentration in milk. The current recommendation for standard formulas is 4 mcg/100 kcal (9 nmol/419 kJ), as this intake is associated with normal blood cell morphology (AAP, 2009). For preterm infants, the current recommended intake is 25 to 50 mcg/kg/d (56–113 nmol/kg/d) (Tsang et al., 2005).

■ **Deficiency.** Signs of deficiency include hypersegmentation of neutrophils, megaloblastic anemia, poor growth, irritability, and hypotonia. Neurologic disorders, such as seizures and mental retardation, are seen only with the congenital, isolated defect of folic acid absorption. Folic acid deficiency may be associated with prematurity (rapid growth and diminished hepatic stores), hemolytic disease of the newborn (increased erythropoiesis), anticonvulsant therapy (interference with absorption), prolonged antibiotic therapy (diminished production from intestinal bacterial flora), and any malabsorption syndrome.

■ **Toxicity.** There are no reports on toxic effects of folic acid in infancy. However, at least theoretically, very large doses of folic acid may reduce the serum concentration of phenytoin. In preterm infants, folic acid may diminish zinc absorption.

Ascorbic Acid (Vitamin C)

Vitamin C is required for collagen synthesis, for normal function of osteoblasts and fibroblasts, for metabolism of some amino acids, and for synthesis of neurotransmitters. It also acts as an antioxidant. Ascorbic acid is actively absorbed in the small intestine, and a feedback mechanism apparently regulates absorption of the vitamin. Very large doses of vitamin C appear to diminish the efficiency of intestinal absorption and to leave affected individuals prone to rebound deficiency once intake declines. Vitamin C is excreted by the kidneys either unchanged or as oxalic acid.

The vitamin C concentration in human milk is about 50 mg/L (284 μmol/L). The AAP (2009) recommends a concentration of 8 mg/100 kcal (45 μmol/419 kJ) for standard formulas. The recommendations for stable preterm infants are 18 to 24 mg/kg/d (102–136 μmol/kg/d) (Tsang et al., 2005). Heat treatment (e.g., pasteurization) significantly reduces vitamin C content in milk.

■ **Deficiency.** Vitamin C deficiency is very rare but can occur in infants fed pasteurized, unsupplemented cow milk or vitamin C–deficient breast milk. Vitamin C deficiency is associated with transient tyrosinemia and neonatal scurvy.

Transient tyrosinemia arises from a partial enzymatic deficiency that causes an elevation in the serum concentration of the amino acid tyrosine. The tyrosine concentration declines with administration of vitamin C. Transient tyrosinemia is common, occurring in as many as 10% of full-term infants and 30% of preterm infants during the first week of life. The amount of dietary tyrosine also plays a role, because a high-protein intake and casein-predominant formulas can increase the serum tyrosine concentration. With the current whey-based formula, this does not appear to be a significant problem. Additionally, since these transiently elevated concentrations are so common, it seems unlikely that they could be regarded as abnormal.

Neonatal scurvy is very rare. It is characterized by hemorrhages in the skin, subperiosteal spaces, and costochondral cartilage; by anemia resulting from diminished iron absorption; and by failure to thrive. Rebound scurvy, or scurvy that develops after abrupt discontinuation of a large vitamin C intake, has been reported in infants of mothers who took large amounts of vitamin C during their pregnancy (Schanler, 1997).

■ **Toxicity.** Large doses of vitamin C may diminish vitamin B_{12} absorption, increase iron absorption, and increase the incidence of nephrolithiasis in congenital disorders such as oxalosis and cystinuria.

Niacin

Niacin includes nicotinic acid and its amide, nicotinamide. As components of the coenzymes nicotinamide adenine dinucleotide (NAD) and nicotinamide adenine dinucleotide phosphate (NADP), niacin is involved in mitochondrial electron transport, lipid synthesis, and glycolysis.

Niacin can also derive from the amino acid tryptophan: Consequently, dietary intake of both niacin and tryptophan is evaluated to calculate niacin requirements. For this reason, it is customary to use niacin equivalents (1 mg of niacin = 1 niacin equivalent = 60 mg of tryptophan).

The average concentration of niacin in human milk is 0.8 niacin equivalents/100 kcal, which also is the recommended concentration for standard formulas (AAP, 2009). The recommendation for growing preterm infants is 3.6 to 4.8 mg/kg/d (30–40 μmol/kg/d) (Tsang et al., 2005). Heating and storage do not significantly affect the niacin content in milk.

■ **Deficiency.** Pellagra (rough skin) is the consequence of niacin deficiency. In adults, signs include dermatitis and inflammation of the mucous membranes, diarrhea, and dementia.

■ **Toxicity.** Toxicity is related to the proportion of nicotinic acid and may manifest in adults as cutaneous vasodilation, arrhythmias, and increases in intestinal motility and gastric acid secretion.

FAT-SOLUBLE VITAMINS

Vitamin A

Vitamin A exists in many isomeric forms; the basic and most active component is all-trans retinol. Vitamin A can be administered in different forms (retinol itself, palmitate esters of retinol, provitamins) and in different units (micrograms, international units [IU]). Vitamin A activity usually is defined as the equivalent weight of retinol (retinol equivalent [RE]). One RE is equal to 1 mcg or 3.33 IU of retinol and to 6 mcg or 10 IU of the provitamin beta carotene. Dietary retinol is absorbed in the proximal intestine, and under normal circumstances, about 50% is absorbed. Retinol is incorporated into chylomicrons and transported to the liver, where it is stored as retinyl esters, mainly in the stellate cells. From the liver, retinol is released into the circulation according to needs. It is transported in plasma, bound to retinol-binding protein, and delivered to tissues. Although liver stores are the main body reserve, vitamin A is stored also in eyes and lungs. Retinol facilitates the visual process in the rod cells of the retina and plays a role in regulating and differentiating epithelial cells. Retinol appears to be necessary for normal lung growth.

With parenteral nutrition, a considerable amount of retinol is lost during delivery, due to both photodegradation and adherence to tubing. Loss during infusion may be minimized by adding vitamin A to IV lipids. The average vitamin A concentration in mature human milk is approximately 600 to 2,000 IU/L. The AAP (2009) recommends a concentration of 250 to 750 IU (75–225 RE/100 kcal) for standard formulas. The recommendation for growing preterm infants is 700 to 1,500 IU/kg/d (Tsang et al., 2005). Higher intakes (2,000–3,000 IU/kg/d) may be needed in infants with chronic lung disease (Greer, 2005).

■ **Deficiency.** The classic signs of vitamin A deficiency (night blindness, dryness of the cornea progressing to ulceration, perifollicular dermatitis) are of no value in the neonatal period. In clinical practice, a serum retinol concentration below 10 mcg/dL (0.35 μmol/L) is accepted as indicative of unequivocal vitamin A deficiency. In preterm infants, deficiency is commonly defined by a serum retinol concentration below 20 mcg/dL (0.7 μmol/L).

Vitamin A deficiency may occur with any form of fat malabsorption (diminished absorption), in preterm infants (low hepatic stores and diminish intake), in infants given parenteral nutrition (adherence of retinol to plastic tubing), and in infants with BPD. In infants with BPD, vitamin A deficiency may not be absolute but relative, possibly owing to an increased requirement for vitamin A. Based on this hypothesis, several trials have been conducted to prevent BPD with large parenteral doses of vitamin A. The results have been analyzed in a review (Darlow & Graham, 2011). At dosages of 2,000 to 5,000 IU given IM three times a week, there was no overall difference in oxygen use at one month of age. Vitamin A supplementation was associated with a significant but small reduction in oxygen use at 36 weeks postconceptional age from 62% to 55% (RR: 0.85). There was no difference in length of stay. As BPD is typically a multifactorial disease and shows marked variations among units, there is no uniform consensus on such therapy.

■ **Toxicity.** Vitamin A toxicity occurs from significant overdosage. The clinical signs are those of increased intracranial pressure: bulging anterior fontanelle, vomiting, and other neurologic symptoms. Doses of up to 8,500 IU/kg/d have been given to preterm infants without recognizable side effects (Mactier & Weaver, 2005).

Vitamin D

Vitamin D is essential for normal metabolism of calcium and phosphorus. Through the effects of its active form, 1,25-dihydroxyvitamin D, it is necessary for PTH action in mobilizing calcium and phosphorus from bone; for intestinal absorption of calcium and phosphorus; and, indirectly, for bone formation.

Vitamin D can be obtained through the diet or can be synthesized by the skin after exposure to sunlight. Regardless of its origin, vitamin D is transported to the liver, where it is converted into 25-hydroxyvitamin D (25-OHD), and subsequently to the kidneys, where it is converted into the final, active metabolite, 1,25-dihydroxyvitamin D. 25-OHD is the major circulating vitamin D metabolite, and it is regarded as an indicator of vitamin D status. It is transferred from mother to fetus, and maternal vitamin D deficiency may be a predisposing factor for late neonatal hypocalcemia.

The serum concentration of 1,25-dihydroxyvitamin D appears to be tightly regulated. The synthesis of 1,25-dihydroxyvitamin D is facilitated by PTH, hypocalcemia, and hypophosphatemia. Placental transfer of 1,25-dihydroxyvitamin D has been demonstrated only after pharmacologic maternal doses. It is not clear if maternal-fetal transfer occurs, at least in significant amounts, under normal circumstances.

The current recommendation is a daily intake of 400 IU for both full-term and preterm infants during the first year of life (Abrams, 2011). Reliance on sunlight exposure is not recommended.

■ **Deficiency.** Vitamin D deficiency results in bone demineralization or rickets. Clinical signs are craniotabes, frontal bossing, widened ribs with enlargement of the costochondral junctions, and muscle weakness.

Laboratory findings include a low serum 25-OHD concentration (<20 ng/mL or 50 nmol/L), as a result of diminished intake); an increased serum PTH level, stimulated by a transiently low blood calcium level (to maintain a normal serum calcium level); normal or increased 1,25-dihydroxyvitamin D level (as a result of PTH stimulation); and restored serum calcium and low serum phosphorus concentrations (as a result of the effects of PTH).

Rickets can be caused by inadequate vitamin D intake, by inadequate exposure to sunlight, and by any form of fat malabsorption. Rickets or osteopenia of prematurity, a common disorder in VLBW infants, is caused neither by dietary vitamin D deficiency nor by abnormality of vitamin D metabolism, but by insufficient intake of calcium and phosphorus.

■ **Toxicity.** Excessive doses of vitamin D can cause hypercalcemia, restlessness, polyuria, and failure to thrive. Calcinosis occurs mainly in the kidneys but may also occur in the cardiovascular system, lungs, and intestine.

Vitamin E

Vitamin E is made up of several compounds, named tocopherols, which are important biologic antioxidants; among these, alpha-tocopherol is believed to be most active. Vitamin E acts as a free radical scavenger and protects the polyunsaturated fatty acid of biologic membranes from peroxidation.

Oral administration of either alpha-tocopherol or alpha-tocopherol acetate results in satisfactory absorption. However, fixed oral daily doses of vitamin E can produce variable serum concentrations. Moreover, absorption may be diminished in sick infants. Tocopherols are absorbed in the jejunum and transported by either chylomicrons or low-density lipoproteins to body tissues. The serum tocopherol concentration may not reflect the tissue concentration, because tocopherol is carried by plasma lipoproteins, which are diminished in the newborn. Vitamin E is stored mainly in adipose tissue and in the liver.

Vitamin E is excreted mainly in feces. Biliary excretion is small, and urine excretion is almost negligible. The half-life of tocopherol is approximately 2 days. Because excretion is minimal, vitamin E is cleared from serum by tissue uptake or metabolic degradation, or both.

The average vitamin E concentration in mature human milk is about 2 to 3 IU/L. The recommendation of the AAP (2009) for standard formulas is based on both caloric intake and dietary content of polyunsaturated fatty acids: 0.7 IU of vitamin E/100 kcal or at least 0.71 IU of vitamin E per gram of linoleic acid. During the first 2 to 3 weeks of life of enterally fed preterm infants, intake usually is too low to achieve vitamin E sufficiency; therefore the vitamin should be supplemented at a dosage of 6 to 12 IU/kg/d (Tsang et al., 2005).

Pharmacologic doses of vitamin E have shown no benefit for physiologic anemia of prematurity or BPD, and the effects on retinopathy of prematurity (ROP) and on intraventricular hemorrhage (IVH) remain controversial. Vitamin E supplementation is associated with an increased risk of neonatal sepsis (Brion, Bell, & Raghuveer, 2003). Doses exceeding 25 IU/kg/d may result in tissue concentrations greater than those needed for maximum antioxidant effect.

■ **Deficiency.** Vitamin E deficiency can occur in infants with severe forms of fat malabsorption: neurologic and myopathic abnormalities develop over several years.

■ **Toxicity.** Very large doses of vitamin E can cause calcification at injection sites, creatinuria, inhibition of wound healing, and fibrinolysis. An increased incidence of necrotizing enterocolitis has been associated with high oral doses of a hyperosmolar preparation. In the past, an IV preparation, tocopherol acetate in polysorbate, has been associated with a fatal syndrome consisting of renal failure, thrombocytopenia, hepatomegaly, cholestasis, and ascites.

Vitamin K

Two forms of vitamin K are naturally available: vitamin K_1, or phylloquinone, which is synthesized by plants, and vitamin K_2, or menaquinone, which is synthesized by bacteria.

Vitamin K is required for the synthesis of coagulation factors II, VII, IX, and X and for conversion of inactive precursors into active clotting factors. Other vitamin K-dependent proteins include plasma protein C and S, osteocalcin, and renal Gla protein. Dietary vitamin K is absorbed in the small intestine and transported with chylomicrons through the lymphatic system. Intestinal bacteria synthesize vitamin K, and this form probably is absorbed in the colon. In adults, about 50% of the total amount of vitamin K in the body comes from intestinal bacteria. The intestine is sterile at birth, and no significant synthesis of vitamin K by the intestinal flora occurs in the first few days of life. The usual intestinal bacteria of breastfed infants do not appear to synthesize vitamin K. The vitamin is stored in the liver, but storage capacity appears to be limited. Excretion occurs mainly with bile in the feces; urinary excretion is quantitatively less important.

The concentration of phylloquinone in human milk is about 2.1 mcg/mL (4.6 μmol/L); it is about 4.9 mcg/mL (10.9 μmol/L) in cow milk and 55 to 58 mcg/mL (122–129 μmol/L) in formulas. Dietary intake of vitamin K, therefore, depends on both the quality and quantity of ingested milk. A deficiency state is seen almost exclusively in breastfed infants who do not receive vitamin K.

The following recommendations have been made for vitamin K supplementation:

- *At birth:* 0.5 to 1.0 mg (1.1–2.2 μmol) given IM in all infants greater than 1,000 g; below 1,000 g, 0.3 mg/kg (0.66 μmol/kg) appear adequate
- *Infants receiving total parenteral nutrition (TPN):* daily supplementation at a dosage of 10 mcg/kg (22 nmol/kg)
- *Standard formulas:* a minimum concentration of 4 mcg/100 kcal (9 nmol/419 kJ) (AAP, 2009)
- *Preterm infants:* an intake of 6.66 to 8.33 mcg/100 kcal (15–18.5 nmol/419 kJ)

■ **Deficiency.** Vitamin K deficiency may result in vitamin K deficiency bleeding (VKDB). Bleeding usually occurs from the umbilical stump or after minor procedures (e.g., circumcision, blood sampling), but serious events such as gastrointestinal and cerebral hemorrhages are also possible.

Three clinical forms of VKDB, early, classic, and late, have been recognized.

- The *early type* has been reported, on the first day of life, in infants born to mothers receiving anticonvulsant therapy (phenytoin, phenobarbital). These infants should be given vitamin K IM immediately after birth. This form of the disease may be prevented by antepartum maternal vitamin K supplementation.

- The *classic type* occurs between 2 and 10 days of life in breastfed infants who were not given vitamin K at birth. This form can be prevented by both IM and oral vitamin K supplementation.
- The *late type*, the most common form of the disease, occurs at 2 to 12 weeks of age, in breastfed infants with inadequate or no prophylaxis and in infants with fat malabsorption. This type is frequently complicated by intracranial bleeding, and it has a high mortality rate.

According to the AAP, vitamin K should be given to all newborns as a single intramuscular dose of 0.5 to 1 mg (AAP, 2003). Such a prophylaxis prevents the late form of VKDB, with the rare exception of severe malabsorption syndromes (Von Kries, 1999). Multiple oral doses (1 mg per week), during the first 12 weeks of life, may be as effective as a single dose given IM (Hansen, Minousis, & Ebbesen, 2003).

■ **Toxicity.** There is no evidence of vitamin K toxicity, except for RBC hemolysis and hyperbilirubinemia after administration of large doses of the synthetic vitamin K_3 (menadione).

TRACE MINERALS

Zinc

Zinc, as a cofactor, is necessary for the synthesis of nucleic acids and for the metabolism of proteins, lipids, and carbohydrates; it therefore is essential to normal growth and development.

Zinc accumulation in the fetus mainly occurs during the third trimester. Consequently, preterm infants have lower body stores than full-term infants. However, stores are limited in both full-term and preterm infants, and dietary intake is essential for maintaining optimum zinc status in the newborn. Zinc is absorbed in the duodenum and proximal jejunum. Although cases of zinc deficiency in breastfed infants have been reported, zinc absorption is greater from human milk than from formulas. Excretion occurs mainly through feces; urinary excretion is far less important.

The zinc concentration in human milk ranges from 60 to 22 μmol/L (Thureen & Hay, 2006) and declines over time. Healthy preterm infants given 23 μmol/kg/d show a retention rate similar to the intrauterine accretion rate (Wastney, Angelus, Barnes, & Subramanian, 1999).

The recommended concentration of zinc for standard formulas is 500 mcg/100 kcal (7.5 μmol/419 kJ) (AAP, 2009). The current recommendation for enteral feedings in growing preterm infants is 1,000 to 3,000 mcg/kg/d (15.3–45.9 μmol/kg/d) (Tsang et al., 2005). With parenteral nutrition, a zinc intake of 400 mcg/kg/d (6.1 μmol/kg/d) is recommended for stable preterm infants.

■ **Deficiency.** Zinc deficiency can arise from inadequate intake, diminished absorption (preterm infant), or increased loss (malabsorption syndromes, ostomies). A serum zinc concentration below 40 mcg/dL (6.1 μmol/L) is generally accepted as an indication of deficiency. However, in mild, subclinical zinc deficiency, serum zinc concentration can be in the low normal range.

Dietary zinc deficiency has been reported only in breastfed preterm infants, owing to the large variations in the zinc concentration of human milk. Signs of deficiency include reduced growth velocity, acro-orificial rash, hypoproteinemia, and generalized edema. In preterm infants, postnatal zinc supplementation seems to have a positive effect on linear growth (Diaz-Gomez et al., 2003). Acrodermatitis enteropathica is an autosomal recessive disease that involves a defect in the intestinal absorption of zinc. The disease is characterized by a dermatitis that affects the extremities and perioral/perigenital areas; diarrhea; and failure to thrive, which progresses to thymic atrophy and immunodeficiency.

■ **Toxicity.** Zinc toxicity has not been reported in newborns. Overdosage may result in copper deficiency and an increase in the serum cholesterol concentration.

Copper

Copper is necessary for normal functioning of oxidative enzymes (e.g., cytochrome oxydase) and for synthesis of collagen, melanin, and catecholamines. Both full-term and preterm infants are born with significant liver stores. Active absorption takes place mainly in the duodenum. Copper absorption appears to be greater with human milk than with formulas. In plasma, approximately two thirds of copper is bound to ceruloplasmin. In newborns, limited ceruloplasmin synthesis results in low plasma ceruloplasmin and, consequently, a low-serum copper concentration. Neither the serum copper level nor the ceruloplasmin concentration is an adequate index of copper status in the first weeks of life. Preterm infants show lower copper and ceruloplasmin levels than term infants for many months. Copper excretion occurs almost exclusively through the bile.

Despite wide variation in copper content, human milk appears adequate for both full-term and preterm infants. The recommended copper concentration for standard formulas is 60 mcg/100 kcal (0.93 μmol/419 kJ) (AAP, 2009). The recommendation for stable, growing preterm infants is 120 to 150 mcg/kg/d (1.9–2.4 μmol/kg/d). With parenteral nutrition, a copper intake of 20 mcg/kg/d (0.31 μmol/kg/d) is recommended for stable preterm infants (Tsang et al., 2005)

■ **Deficiency.** Copper deficiency can result from inadequate intake (cow milk, TPN) or increased loss (malabsorption syndromes, ostomies).

Clinical signs of copper deficiency include pallor (as a result of anemia and hypopigmentation), hypotonia, psychomotor retardation, hypochromic anemia unresponsive to iron therapy, neutropenia, osteoporosis, pseudoscurvy, and failure to thrive (Atkinson & Zlotkin, 1997; Hoyle, Schwartz, & Auringer, 1999). Signs are usually identified after the first month of life.

■ **Toxicity.** Copper toxicity has not been reported in newborns. However, IV administration of normal amounts to infants with cholestasis results in liver damage, because excess copper cannot be excreted.

NURSING MANAGEMENT

Obtaining vascular access in a sick newborn has become as routine a part of the admission procedure as obtaining vital signs and weighing the patient. Nurses are responsible for providing peripheral or central vascular access and ensuring safe delivery of IV fluids. They also must be able to recognize the signs and symptoms of disorders in hydration and prevent complications that may be associated with fluid and electrolyte administration.

Assessment and Evaluation in Fluid and Electrolyte Therapy

The estimation of a patient's fluid and nutritional needs depends on the infant's age and weight and the disease process involved. The fluid and electrolyte needs of a 4-kg infant with perinatal asphyxia and seizures are different from those of a 32-week, 1,750-g infant with RDS or a 23-week, 460-g infant with multiple complex needs. These infants represent varying points on the continuum of fetal growth and development. Each represents a different disease process, and each also requires careful management of fluid and electrolytes to maintain homeostasis.

Fluid needs can be calculated using body weight, body surface area, or caloric expenditure (Behrman, Kleigman, & Jenson, 2004). Caloric expenditure is an easy method in which the infant's caloric needs are calculated, and fluid and electrolyte requirements are related to it. To begin these calculations, it must be remembered that 1 kcal is the amount of heat needed to raise 1 L of water 1°C. Caloric expenditures up to 10 kg = 100 cal/kg/24 hr. For example, a 1,700-g infant would expend 170 calories in 24 hours, whereas a 460-g infant would expend 46 calories in 24 hours. This can be expressed as Energy intake = Energy stored + Energy expended + Energy excreted (Ambalavanan, 2012).

Caloric expenditures can be modified by an increase or decrease in body temperature and by specific disease states. Caloric expenditure can be used to determine water needs, because for every 100 calories metabolized, 100 mL of fluid is needed (Behrman et al., 2004). Water needs are determined by calculating IWL from the skin and pulmonary system and actual losses from the urine, stool, and sweat (Table 19.4).

IWL can be affected by a variety of factors, including skin integrity and the degree of that integrity. An example of this is the newborn infant with a large gastroschisis. This midline abdominal wall defect predisposes the infant to large IWLs because of the exposed abdominal organs and absent omentum or peritoneum. Another example is a 23-week, 400-g infant with the typical "translucent" skin that has not yet formed a protective keratin layer; this condition predisposes the infant to dehydration secondary to large IWL through the skin. Environmental factors also affect IWL; these factors include the presence or absence of humidity and increased or decreased ambient temperature. The use of radiant warmers has long been understood to affect an infant's fluid status by increasing insensible losses in a relatively open, unprotected environment. Phototherapy has similar effects, with the additional problem of thermoregulation. Increases in the metabolic rate, body temperature, and activity all must be included in the calculation of fluid needs.

TABLE 19.4

FLUID INTAKE AND OUTPUT IN NEONATES

	Range (mL/100 cal/24 hr)	Average[a] (mL/100 cal/24 hr)
	Output	
Insensible Water Losses		
Pulmonary	10–20	15
Skin	25–35	30
Urine	50–70	60
Stool	5–10	7
Sweat	0–20	0
	Intake	
All fluids consumed		112
Water of oxidation		−12

[a]Average maintenance requirement is 100 mL/100 cal/d.

Fluids usually are calculated on a daily basis, taking into consideration past losses, projected losses, and maintenance requirements. However, depending on the disease process, fluids may need to be calculated more often, even as often as every 4 hours, to keep up with losses and to make appropriate adjustments in fluid therapy. A general estimate of fluid requirements can be calculated on the basis of the guidelines presented in Table 19.1. Again, these are just guidelines; requirements differ according to gestational age and disease process. The fluid requirement for a premature, low-birth-weight infant may be as high as 150 to 200 mL/kg/d in some cases during the first 24 hours of life; on the other hand, for a full-term, asphyxiated infant, fluids may be restricted to no more than 40 to 50 ml/kg/d for the first 72 hours of life.

Electrolyte requirements usually are calculated on the basis of 100 calories metabolized:

- Sodium: 2 to 3 mEq/100 cal/24 hr (2–3 mEq/kg/d)
- Potassium: 1 to 2 mEq/100 cal/24 hr (1–2 mEq/kg/d)

Standard IV solutions containing a predetermined amount of sodium are routinely used in neonatal intensive care units (e.g., 5% dextrose in 0.45% NaCl) with potassium chloride and other electrolytes or minerals added as indicated (Table 19.5).

Caloric requirements cannot be met solely by the IV solutions commonly used in NICUs (i.e., 5% or 10% dextrose). These solutions are relatively low in calories, as there are only 4 calories per gram of glucose

TABLE 19.5

ELECTROLYTE COMPONENTS OF INTRAVENOUS FLUIDS

Solution	mEq Na/1000 ml	mEq Na/100 ml
D_5W ½ NS (dextrose 5%, ½ strength, normal saline)	77	7.7
D_5W ¼ NS	38.5	

Na, sodium.

(carbohydrate). The number of calories in IV solutions is calculated on a percent solution and based on grams per 100 mL. Therefore 5% dextrose in water (D_5W) contains 5 g of dextrose per 100 mL of fluid, 10% dextrose in water ($D_{10}W$) contains 10 g/100 ml, and so on. To carry this calculation further, D_5W and $D_{10}W$ IV solutions contain 20 and 40 calories, respectively (D_5W = 5 g/100 mL at 4 cal/g = 20 cal).

The dextrose concentration used also depends on the infant's gestational age and renal function. The premature kidneys, unable to concentrate urine and conserve electrolytes and glucose, may alter glucose excretion, "spilling sugar" into the urine. An essential test of the infant's response to IV glucose therapy can easily be done at the bedside with a urine dipstick and a few drops of urine. This test can detect glucose, protein, ketones, and blood in the urine and can determine the pH level, an important indicator of acid–base balance.

Determination of the specific gravity is another essential bedside test that requires only a few drops of urine. The specific gravity, which normally is between 1.008 and 1.012, is an early indicator of hydration status. The urine dipstick and specific gravity tests should be performed at least every shift while the infant is receiving IV fluids and more often as the infant's condition warrants.

Fluid intake and output should be strictly monitored to ensure adequate hydration. Giving too much or too little fluid affects UOP, as do disease processes such as acute renal failure and drug administration (e.g., indomethacin or aminoglycoside antibiotics). UOP is monitored and calculated hourly over a 24-hour period. It should be no less than 1 mL/kg/hr/d. For example, for a 2-kg infant:

$$\text{UOP} = 240 \text{ mL/24 hr} = 10 \text{ mL/2 kg} = 5 \text{ mL/kg/hr}$$

This is an adequate UOP for an infant of this weight and gestation.

For infants requiring long-term IV therapy, TPN is used to improve nutritional status, and it may be started within the first 24 to 72 hours of life. TPN spares protein, increases calories and, when used in conjunction with intralipid (an IV fat emulsion preparation), further maximizes caloric intake. If the TPN solution is infused through a peripheral vein, the glucose concentration is limited to no more than 12.5% because of the risks of tissue irritation and sloughing with infiltration; however, if the solution is infused through central lines, a higher glucose concentration may be used. With this route, in addition to the increased glucose concentration (which increases calories), higher concentrations of protein, fat, and other essential minerals and trace elements may be infused.

Caloric supplementation with TPN is as follows:

- Glucose: (4 cal/g): 2.5 to 12.5 g/100 cc (e.g., 2.5%–12.5% solutions)
- Protein (4 cal/g): 1 to 3 g/kg/d; 4 to 12 cal/kg/d
- Fat (9 cal/g): Up to 4 g/kg/d; (20% emulsion, 2 cal/mL)

The nurse is responsible for monitoring hourly fluid intake and should always double-check fluid orders to ensure that the ordered rate and solution are appropriate for that infant.

Weight is an important indicator of overall fluid status. Infants are usually weighed daily; extremely-low-birth-weight (ELBW) infants and infants with excessive fluid losses and needs may be weighed more often (i.e., every 12 hours or even every 6 hours), with fluid needs recalculated on the basis of weight changes. It is important to weigh infants carefully, because inaccuracies that show extreme weight fluctuations can have a detrimental impact on therapy. For example, an inaccurate weight measurement showing an increase of 100 g in a 12-hour period for an infant with severe RDS may result in giving that infant an unnecessary dose of furosemide. The infant should be weighed nude, with as much extraneous equipment removed as possible (e.g., ECG leads, probes), at the same time each day, and on the same scale. In-bed scales that give constant weight readouts simplify the weighing process and cause the infant minimal stress. It is common practice to use birth weight to calculate daily fluid needs during the first week of life, as the infant may lose up to 20% of birth weight during this time. After the infant has regained birth weight, the daily weights are used to calculate daily fluid needs.

The physical examination can reveal changes in the infant's fluid status and should be used in conjunction with laboratory data to plan interventions in fluid and electrolyte therapy. A general assessment for hydration status includes the infant's color, skin turgor, activity, mucous membranes, fontanelles, vital signs, and UOP, as follows:

- *Color:* Pink and well perfused, rather than pale and mottled (indicates dehydration)
- *Skin turgor:* Good turgor, rather than "tenting" (indicates dehydration) or edematous and shiny (indicates fluid overload)
- *Activity:* Active with good tone, rather than lethargic and hypotonic (indicates dehydration or overhydration)
- *Mucous membranes:* Pink and moist, rather than dry and gray (indicates dehydration)

- *Fontanelles:* Soft and flat, rather than depressed (indicates dehydration) or tense and full (may indicate overhydration)
- *Vital signs:* Heart rate, rhythm, blood pressure and temperature within normal range for gestational age
- *UOP:* Normal (e.g., ~1 cc/kg/hr), rather than excessive (indicates overhydration), diminished, or absent (indicating dehydration)

SUMMARY

The care of infants with alterations in fluid and electrolyte balance presents a management challenge for both physicians and nurses. A thorough understanding of the underlying pathophysiology and the rationale for therapy enables the health care team to provide more informed care for these infants and to anticipate and prevent problems.

CASE STUDY

■ **Identification of the Problem.** Preterm female infant developed necrotizing enterocolitis, resulting in a small bowel resection. Nutritional management presents daily challenges.

■ **Assessment: History and Physical Examination** Former 30-week, 1,250-g, AGA Caucasian female infant born by an uncomplicated vaginal delivery to a 32-year-old G_3/P_2 mother, with Apgars of $6^1/8^5$. Hospital course included a short course of respiratory distress requiring a maximum of 60% oxygen per oxyhood and a low-placed UAC for 36 hours. On DOL #8, the infant developed abdominal tenderness and distention, with guaiac-positive stools. Continued deterioration resulted in a small bowel resection 12 hours later, which left a 60-cm section of intact ileum, an intact ileocecal valve, intact colon, and placement of an ileostomy and jejunostomy. A central venous line (i.e., Broviac) was placed during surgery. Nutritional support continues with TPN (10% Dextrose, 2 g amino acids, 1.5 g fat), Intralipids through the central line, and slowly increasing enteral feeds for a total fluid load of 160 cc/kg/d and 120 cal/kg/d. Enteral nutrition is by Nutramigen 10 cc/kg/d via continuous infusion.

- PE on DOL #36: weight 1,550 gm, V.S. WNL
- GENERAL: quiet, alert, and slightly pale in room air
- HEENT: normocephalic, AF soft and flat, normal facies, pupils reactive to light, positive red reflex bilaterally, responsive to voice, nares patent, thyroid not palpable
- RESP: bilateral breath sounds equal and clear
- CV: regular rate and rhythm without murmur; pulses = +1; brisk capillary refill
- ABD: soft, round, and nontender with two stomas intact and pink; no H-Smegaly or palpable masses + bowel sounds
- GU: normal female genitalia
- NEURO-M/S: actively responsive to voice and touch, good muscle tone, and movement in all extremities
- SKIN: intact without redness or rashes; slight tenting of abdominal skin; broviac site intact

■ **Differential Diagnoses**

- Failure to thrive
- Malabsorption syndrome
- Hypothyroidism

■ **Diagnostic Tests**

- CBC
- Metabolic panel
- "Growth panel" including zinc
- Thyroid panel

■ **Working Diagnosis**

- ~35 weeks postconceptual age AGA WF infant
- S/P small bowel resection with ileostomy and jejonostomy
- Poor weight gain 2° malabsorption
- Nutritional deficiencies

■ **Development of Management Plan**

- TPN/intralipids must provide adequate carbohydrate, protein and fat calories, vitamins, and micronutrients for growth. This infant needs to have more calories from carbohydrates, protein and fats.
  - Dextrose should provide ~12 to 14 mg/kg/min (monitor serum and urine glucose for tolerance)
  - Provide proteins as amino acids (e.g., taurine, tyrosine, cysteine, and carnitine) to ~4 g/kg/d as tolerated
  - Daily pediatric multivitamins should include vitamin K, and trace elements of copper, zinc, chromium, manganese, and selenium
  - May need an additional 10 mcg/mL of zinc, as excessive losses may occur through ostomy output/diarrhea
- Increase enteral nutrition by 10 to 20 cc/kg/d (with concomitant decrease in TPN/IL volume to maintain 180–200 cc/kg/d) by continuous infusion as tolerated (e.g., monitor stool output).
- Close monitoring of intake and output for toleration of increased intestinal load, with special attention to stool output as enteral feedings increase in volume.
- Weekly growth parameters (e.g., weight, length, and head circumference) and growth labs must be monitored to insure adequate growth.
- If abnormal thyroid panel, initiate thyroid pharmacotherapy as indicated.

■ Implementation and Evaluation of Effectiveness This infant is not showing adequate growth at this point in her recovery and needs to have meticulous nutritional management.

- Increase TPN/IL sequentially over the next several days as tolerated to provide a maximum of 200 cc/kg/d; dextrose 14 mg/kg/min; proteins 4 g/kg/d; fats 3 g/kg/d
- Increase enteral feedings by 10 to 20 cc/kg/d as tolerated to maximum of 200 cc/kg/d with concomitant decrease in TPN/IL
- Daily weights, weekly measurement of length and head circumference
- Weekly CBC with diff/platelets, electrolytes, renal panel, metabolic profile/liver function tests

■ Effectiveness of Management Plan

- Improved growth and nutritional status
- Normal lab results with improved nutritional status

■ OUTCOME. Improved nutritional status improved growth. Infant was discharged at 46 weeks postconceptual age after successful reanastomosis, on full enteral feeds.

EVIDENCE-BASED PRACTICE BOX

Virtually all VLBW infants need IV fluid infusions for a variable length of time, depending on the degree of prematurity and on the number and severity of neonatal complications. The optimal amount of fluids is difficult to define. A low-fluid volume is associated with dehydration, hypernatremia, and jaundice, whereas a high-fluid volume has been related to increased rates of PDA and chronic lung disease.

A review of the available evidence has been published in 2010 by Bell and Acarregui. The aim of the review was to investigate the effect of different water intakes (liberal vs. restricted) on neonatal morbidities in preterm infants. Five studies were included in the analysis.

The water intake in the "Restricted Fluids" group ranged from 50 mL/kg/d to 122 mL/kg/d. Intake in the "Liberal Fluids" group ranged from 80 mL/kg/d to 169 mL/kg/d. Studies included in the review investigated the rates of the following neonatal complications in the two groups: weight loss, PDA, IVH, BPD and necrotizing enterocolitis.

The analysis results favored fluid restriction over liberal water intake. The risk of PDA was lower with restricted fluid intake: RR was 0.52 and number needed to treat was 7. The risk of necrotizing enterocolitis, a devastating disease, was also lower with restricted fluids: RR was 0.43 and number needed to treat was 20. The risk of BPD and IVH did not differ between the two fluid regimens.

In conclusion, the risk of two potentially serious neonatal complications can be significantly decreased by a very simple intervention.

Reference

Bell, E. F., & Acarregui, M. J. (2010). Restricted versus liberal water intake for preventing morbidity and mortality in preterm infants. *Cochrane Database of Systematic Reviews*, 1, *CD000503*. doi:10.1002/14651858.CD000503.pub2

ONLINE RESOURCES

Gaining and growing: Assuring nutritional care of preterm infants **http://www.depts.washington.edu/growing/Assess/SBS.htm**

Growth charts: Fenton growth curve **http://www.members.shaw.ca/growthchart**

National Center for Education in Maternal and Child Health **http://www.ncemch.org**

Olsen growth curve **http://www.nursing.upenn.edu/media/infantgrowthcurves/Documents/Olsen-NewIUGrowthCurves_2010permission.pdf**

Pediatric short bowel syndrome **http://www.emedicine.medscape.com/article/931855-overview**

Short bowel syndrome: National Digestive Diseases Information Clearinghouse (NDDIC) **http://www.digestive.niddk.nih.gov/ddiseases/pubs/shortbowel**

World Health Organization (WHO) Growth Curve **http://www.cdc.gov/growthcharts/who_charts.htm**

REFERENCES

Abrams, S. A. (2011). Dietary guidelines for calcium and vitamin D: A new era. *Pediatrics, 127*, 566–568.

Ambalavanan, N. (2012). Fluid, electrolyte, and nutrition management of the newborn. Retrieved April 23, 2012, from http://www.emedicine.com

American Academy of Pediatrics, Committee on Nutrition. (2009). *Pediatric nutrition handbook*. Elk Grove Village, IL: American Academy of Pediatrics.

American Academy of Pediatrics, Committee on Fetus and Newborn. (2003). Controversies concerning vitamin K and the newborn. *Pediatrics, 112*, 191–192.

Atkinson, S. A., & Zlotkin, S. H. (1997). Recognizing deficiencies and excesses of zinc, copper, and other trace elements. In R. C. Tsang & B. L. Nichols (Eds.), *Nutrition during infancy*. Cincinnati, OH: Digital Educational Publishing.

Baraton, L., Ancel, P. Y., Flamant, C., Orsonneau, C., Darmaun, D., & Rozé, J. C. (2009). Impact of changes in serum sodium level on 2-year neurologic outcome in very preterm infants. *Pediatrics*, *124*, e655–e661.

Baumgart, S., & Costarino, A. T. (2000). Water and electrolyte metabolism in the micropremie. *Clinics in Perinatology*, *27*, 131–146.

Behrman, R. E., Kleigman, R., & Jenson, H. B. (2004). *Nelson textbook of pediatrics* (17th ed.). Philadelphia, PA: WB Saunders.

Brion, L. P., Bell, E. F., & Raghuveer, T. S. (2003). Vitamin E supplementation for prevention of morbidity and mortality in preterm infants. *Cochrane Database Systematic Review, 3, CD003665*.

Choong, K., Arora, S., Cheng, J., Farrokhyar, F., Reddy, D., Thabane, L., & Walton, J. M. (2011). Hypotonic versus isotonic maintenance fluids after surgery for children: A randomized controlled trial. *Pediatrics*, *128*, 857–866.

Darlow, B. A., & Graham, P. J. (2011). Vitamin A supplementation for preventing morbidity and mortality in very low birth weight infants (Cochrane Review). In *The Cochrane Library* (Issue 2). Oxford. *Cochrane Database of Systematic Reviews 2002, 4. Art. No.: CD000501.* doi:10.1002/14651858.CD000501

Diaz-Gomez, N. M., Domenech, E., Barroso, F., Castells, S., Cortabarria, C., & Jiménez, A. (2003). The effect of zinc supplementation on linear growth, body composition, and growth factors in preterm infants. *Pediatrics*, *111*, 1002–1009.

Greer, F. R. (2005). Vitamin A, E and K. In R. C. Tsang, R. Uauy, B. Koletzko & S. H. Zlotkin (Eds.), *Nutritional needs of the Preterm Infant: Scientific basis and practical guidelines*. Cincinnati, OH: Digital Educational Publishing.

Hansen, K. N., Minousis, M., Ebbesen, F. (2003). Weekly oral vitamin K prophylaxis in Denmark. *Acta Paediatrica*, *92*, 802–805.

Hoyle, G.S., Schwartz, R. P., & Auringer, S. T. (1999). Pseudoscurvy caused by copper deficiency. *Journal of pediatrics*, *134*, 379.

Lorenz, J. M., Kleinman, L. I., Ahmed, G., & Markarian, K. (1995). Phases of fluid and electrolyte homeostasis in the extremely low birth weight infant. *Pediatrics*, *196*, 484–489.

Mactier, H., & Weaver, L.T. (2005). Vitamin A and preterm infants: What we know, what we don't know and what we need to know. *Archives of Diseases of Childhood (Fetal and Neonatal Edition)*, *90*, F103–F108.

Modi, N. (2003). Clinical implications of postnatal alterations in body water distribution. *Seminars in Neonatology, 8*, 301–306.

Schanler, R. J. (1997). Who needs water-soluble vitamins? In R. C. Tsang & B. L. Nichols (Eds.), *Nutrition during infancy*. Cincinnati, OH: Digital Educational Publishing.

Thureen, P. J., & Hay, W. W. (2006). *Neonatal Nutrition and Metabolism*. Cambridge, UK: Cambridge University Press.

Tsang, R.C., Lucas, A., Uauy, R., & Zlotkin, S. (2005). *Nutritional needs of the preterm infant: Scientific basis and practical guidelines*. Cincinnati, OH: Digital Educational Publishing.

Von Kries, R. (1999). Oral versus intramuscular phytomenadione: Safety and efficacy compared. *Drug Safety, 21*, 1–6.

Wastney, M. E., Angelus, P. A., Barnes, R. M., & Subramanian, K. N. (1999). Zinc absorption, distribution, excretion, and retention by healthy preterm infants. *Pediatric Research*, *45*, 191–196.

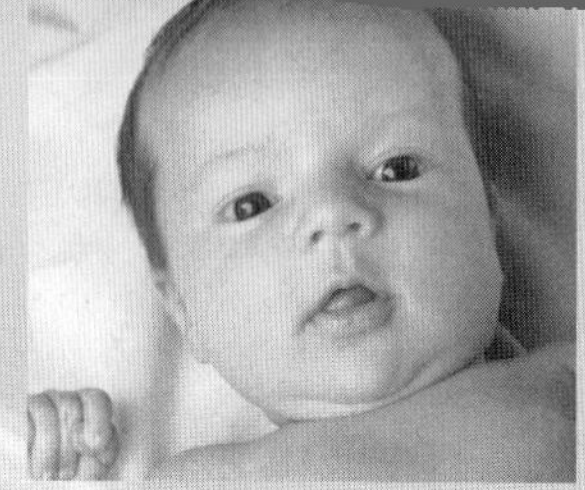

CHAPTER 20

Nutrition Management of Premature Infants

■ Diane M. Anderson

Meeting the nutritional needs of premature and sick infants is essential to their survival (Heird, Driscoll, Schullinger, Grebin, & Winters, 1972). Under conditions of total starvation, these infants have reserves for only 4.5 days, and daily provision of intravenous glucose will prolong survival only about 7 days. Therefore, the mandate is to meet the basic nutrient requirements of these infants and to understand their metabolic limitations to avoid physiologic stress and morbidity related to the delivery of enteral and parenteral nutrition (PN). Nutrition management of the premature infant continues shortly after birth with intravenous fluids, PN, and/or enteral feedings depending on the infant's gestational age and clinical condition. The goal is for the premature infant to grow at the same rate and composition of the fetus of the same gestational age without imposing undue metabolic stress (American Academy of Pediatrics Committee on Nutrition, 2009a). The goal for the premature infant differs from that of the healthy term infant that is breastfeeding. The premature infant has increased nutrient demands and will require fortification of human milk to meet nutrient needs. Due to illness and immaturity, PN and gavage feedings will be needed. Premature infants are at nutrition risks for many reasons including: early birth, which limits nutrient stores such as calcium, iron, and fat; rapid growth, which increases nutrient demand; illness, which may alter nutrient need, nutrient tolerance, and feeding modality; immature gastrointestinal tract, which presents as decreased gut motility, decreased digestive abilities, and decreased tolerance of feedings; and cold stress increasing energy demand.

After birth, infants lose weight due to fluid losses and low nutrient intakes. Once birth weight is regained, the premature infant will gain weight at the intrauterine rate of 15 g/kg/d and parallel their birth weight curve. By discharge, many infants will have a weight less than the 10th percentile for their postmenstrual age and be classified as extrauterine growth restriction (EUGR) (Ehrenkranz, 2010). Improved nutrition during week 1 of life has been associated with better weights at discharge and improved developmental outcomes at 18 months corrected age (Stephens et al., 2009; Valentine et al., 2009). Nutrition and a neonate's nutritional status impact the growth patterns—both immediate and long term. Evidence is mounting to support the need for good nutrition for the premature or sick neonate if short- and long-term complications are to be minimized.

This chapter will start with a brief review of the metabolism of nutrients, minerals, and vitamins in the neonate. It will then discuss the developmental and physiologic issues that are unique to the premature and sick infant. A discussion of neonatal nutrition with special emphasis on the premature infant describes the challenges of providing appropriate nutrients. The various nutrition routes are included.

NUTRIENTS

Protein

Protein must be broken down into amino acids to be absorbed. Protein digestion and absorption take place in the stomach, small intestinal lumen, and the intestinal cell, the enterocyte (Neu & Mshvildadze, 2011). Protein digestion begins in the stomach by the gastric acid, hydrochloric acid, and the enzyme, pepsin. Protein digestion continues in the intestinal lumen by the presence of pancreatic enzymes. Protein is now in the form of peptides (group of amino acids). In the enterocyte, the peptides are further broken down to amino acids. The amino acids are then absorbed into the blood. The intestine of the infant is immature, and intact proteins can cross into the bloodstream and perhaps induce an allergic reaction to milk protein. The openness of the intestine wall to intact protein is greater with infants born at less than 33 weeks gestation, but closure does occur a few days after birth (Neu & Mshvildadze, 2011). In the fetus, gastric acid production has been found from 13 to 28 weeks gestation, and gastric levels are lower in premature infants than levels seen with term infants.

Gastric enzymes appear at 16 weeks gestation and pancreatic enzymes by 24 weeks gestation. Protein digestion and absorption does not appear impaired with premature infants (Neu & Mshvildadze, 2011).

Fat

Food fat is mainly present as triglycerides which are three fatty acids attached to the carbohydrate, glycerol. Fat is digested in a two-step process in the intestine. The first step is to make the triglyceride water soluble with the mixing of bile salts from the liver. The second step breaks the triglyceride into two fatty acids and a monoglyceride by the pancreatic lipases, lingual lipase, gastric lipase, intestinal lipase, or milk bile acid stimulated lipase present in human milk. The monoglyceride and free fatty acids can be directly absorbed into the enterocyte or enter by transporter protein for fatty acids (Neu & Mshvildadze, 2011). Once in the enterocyte, triglycerides are made and are grouped with cholesterol, lipoproteins, and other lipids to form chylomicrons. The chylomicrons circulate by the lymphatic system into the blood system and then into cells throughout the body. Fat digestion and absorption are limited in infants due to decreased levels of bile salts and lipase levels. Bile acids levels are low due to decreased syntheses and decreased intestinal reabsorption. Fetal lipase levels are detected at 21 weeks gestation, but do not reach adult concentrations until 6 month of age in the term infant. Premature infants have lower lipase levels at birth than term infants. Fat is 40% to 50% of the dietary calories from human milk or infant formula, so it is a major component of intake by infants for their growth.

Medium chain triglyceride (MCT) oil has been added to premature infant formulas. MCT oils do not require bile salts or pancreatic lipases to be digested and are absorbed directly into the bloodstream by the infant. The addition of MCT does not help the premature infant absorb more fat, but may be helpful for infants with major absorption problems such as infants with short gut syndrome.

Carbohydrate

Carbohydrate must be in its simple form or as monosaccharides to be absorbed. Lactose is the major carbohydrate in human milk and is composed of the monosaccharides glucose and galactose. Starch consists of glucose polymers, and sucrose contains glucose and fructose. Digestion of carbohydrate begins in the mouth with salivary amylase to break it down to smaller-size carbohydrates or oligosaccharides. The digestion continues with pancreatic amylase enzymes in the stomach and intestine. The final digestion occurs on the brush border of the enterocyte with the enzymes lactase, maltase, and sucrase used to break down lactose, starch, and sucrose. The monosaccharides are carried into the enterocyte by a transport protein and into the blood by a different transport protein. Premature infants have decreased levels of the enzymes, lactase, maltase, and sucrase, but after birth with lactose containing human milk, the lactase enzymes are increased by 2 weeks of age (Neu & Mshvildadze, 2011). Formulas for premature infants contain a blend of lactose and glucose polymers that are well tolerated. Infants who have intestinal damage following necrotizing enterocolitis (NEC) or have developed short gut syndrome may not tolerate lactose and will need a formula continuing glucose polymers.

Summary

The absorption of the three major nutrients is relatively inefficient in the preterm as well as the term infant. Diets such as human milk or premature infant formulas are well tolerated. For nurses, a basic understanding of these mechanisms of absorption is essential so that the rationale for various dietary adjustments can be understood.

VITAMINS, MACROMINERALS, AND TRACE MINERALS

Infants received most of their fat-soluble vitamin stores during the last trimester of pregnancy. Premature infants will have lower vitamin A, D, E, and K stores than the term infant. Premature infants do not absorb fat soluble vitamins well because of their poor ability to digest and absorb fat (Greer, 2006). Premature infants have decreased bile salts and pancreatic lipase concentrations, both of which are needed for fat and fat-soluble vitamins to be absorbed. Premature infants have increased vitamin needs due to limited vitamin stores, increased demand for growth, and limited absorptive capabilities.

Water-soluble vitamins—B-complex and vitamin C—are less likely to create deficiency states owing to their relative availability and method of absorption in infants. Information on water-soluble vitamin needs are limited for the premature infant, and there is much to be learned (Greer, 2006).

The absorption of sodium, potassium, chloride, and bicarbonate across the intestinal mucosa in the infant appears to differ from that in the adult. Under normal circumstances, this difference appears to be of no consequence. In unusual circumstances, such as when hypertonic feedings are used or diarrhea occurs, the increased intestinal permeability leads to large intestinal losses of these electrolytes as well as water. This causes the infant to develop dehydration and electrolyte imbalance more rapidly than later in life. Basic requirements also vary in the infant because renal absorption and excretion of these minerals are not well regulated owing to organ immaturity, which is accentuated in the premature infant.

Calcium absorption occurs through a carrier-mediated mechanism and passive diffusion. The carrier-mediated mechanism is dependent on a vitamin D metabolite. Passive diffusion occurs across the intestinal mucosa against a concentration gradient. If bulk water flow through the intestinal tract occurs, as with diarrhea, calcium losses will be exaggerated.

Zinc that has been ingested is absorbed in the proximal small bowel. Absorption varies based on the bioavailability of the source and the presence of other minerals in the diet such as iron and copper, which are known to interfere with absorption.

GASTROINTESTINAL FUNCTION OF THE PREMATURE INFANT

Research on the developing fetus has determined that much of the gastrointestinal tract begins to function early in fetal life. Anatomically, the fore- and hindgut are present as early as 4 weeks gestation, with the intestinal villi appearing at 8 weeks. It is clear, however, that even in the full-term infant, the gastrointestinal tract is inefficient in its ability to propel, absorb, and utilize nutrients and maintain homeostasis during stress.

Developmentally, the issues of the premature infant begin with the inability to suck, swallow, and breathe in a coordinated fashion. This problem places a heavy burden on the caregiver to provide adequate nutrient intake via all artificial methods. Suck, swallow, and breath coordination matures around 32 to 34 weeks gestation. There are many reasons why this coordination can be delayed. For example, it is common to observe late coordination in infants who have cardiorespiratory disease and who are physiologically unstable. Another large group of infants who cannot regulate their own intake are those who remain on assisted ventilation. The sequence of the infant suck, swallow, and breathe pattern has been described as mature when the suck/swallow/respiration has a 1:1:1 to 2:2:2 pattern (Amaizu, Shulman, Schanler, & Lau, 2008). This sequence not only presumes maturity of the infant but also depends on physiologic stability. Nonnutritive sucking has obvious differences from nutritive sucking that make it only one of several indicators of feeding readiness.

The second physiologic issue of the premature is the absence or weakness of the gag and cough reflexes. This challenge increases the risks to premature infants when gastric enteral feedings are used. The risk of aspiration must be considered when the stomach is used for feeding. The assessment for presence of the gag reflex is easy to do by direct observation while passing a feeding tube. It is nearly impossible to assess the adequacy of the gag reflex in the prevention of aspiration if vomiting or reflex occurs. The risk of aspiration should be considered in all premature infants when started on enteral feeding. In addition, if the infant actually vomits owing to this challenge, chronic loss of nutrients becomes problematic. Reflux has frequently been linked as a cause of apnea. New research suggests that often they occur together, but it is the apnea that leads to the gastric reflux (Miller & Martin, 2011). During an apnea episode, the respiratory neural output is decreased and is accompanied by relaxation of the lower esophageal tone and results in gastroesophageal reflux. On rare occasions, reflux can result in apnea.

The third challenge is the relative relaxation of the lower esophageal sphincter. The purpose of this sphincter is to allow food to pass into the stomach. Inappropriate relaxation may lead to reflux of food back into the esophagus (Field & Hellemeir, 2011). Inadequate sphincter function adds an additional risk factor for all premature infants when orally fed.

Delayed gastric emptying is the fourth physiologic challenge in premature infants. Gastric emptying appears to be relatively delayed in all infants. This process is delayed in disease states, and nurses find that milk feedings do not predictably empty in preterm infants or sick term infants. This challenge may be the single limiting factor when the preterm infant is placed on enteral feeds in that little can be done toward feeding progression until stomach emptying occurs. If the stomach emptying remains a limiting factor, it can be bypassed with transpyloric feedings.

Intestinal motility is the fifth major challenge in the premature infant. Although this challenge is obvious to most clinicians the point of improvement seems to be around 32 weeks gestation. If there are central nervous system abnormalities, then motility can be adversely affected. If intestinal motility is the limiting factor in the progression of enteral feedings, it should be identified as such before multiple formula changes are made. It is always essential to identify the specific challenge as the causative factor when addressing a plan for the delivery of enteral nutrients.

Incompetence of the ileocecal valve, the sixth challenge, is not plainly assessed by the clinician. This valve acts as a barrier between small and large bowel contents, thus separating bacterial flora as well as regulating the time for the small bowel to absorb nutrients before its contents are delivered to the colon for water absorption. When reflux through this valve occurs, the small bowel is colonized with bacteria. With the presence of undigested nutrients in the small bowel and bacteria proliferation, hydrogen gas is produced. This mechanism is part of one sequence of events hypothesized to lead to NEC.

The seventh and last challenge is the premature infant's impaired rectosphincteric reflex, which creates a delay in stool evacuation, sometimes to the point of a functional obstruction. Although the first stool in a premature infant is slightly delayed when compared to the term infant, failure to pass meconium by 72 hours of life should alert the health professional to a potential problem.

Summary

The premature infant has many developmental and mechanical challenges that make the use of the gastrointestinal tract difficult or impossible. The tract matures with postnatal age and physiologic stability and needs to be reassessed regularly. Feeding assessment needs to be monitored to make changes in feedings as indicated.

PARENTERAL NUTRITION (PN)

Indications

PN describes a form of providing nutrients—food and fluid—by an intravenous route other than orally. PN is indicated for very-low-birth-weight (VLBW) infants to supplement the advancement of enteral feedings; infants with congenital abdominal or cardiac anomalies that preclude enteral nutrition; and infants that develop the gastrointestinal illnesses, NEC, short bowel syndrome, or intractable diarrhea requiring bowel rest or limitation of feedings. PN may begin the first day of life to provide hydration, glucose homeostasis, positive nitrogen balance, and normal blood calcium levels. Nutrient concentrations will be advanced as tolerated.

Infants are started on PN the first day of life when slow feeding advancement is anticipated. Starter PN may be used that contain a set concentration of glucose, protein, and perhaps calcium. The starter PN is available 24/7 and can be infused shortly after birth to infants to promote hydration, glucose homeostasis, and nitrogen balance. Early initiation of PN for the VLBW infant improves nitrogen balance, glucose tolerance, and growth (Poindexter,

Langer, Dusick, & Ehrenkranz, 2006; Thureen, Melara, Fennessey, & Hay, 2003; Valentine et al., 2009). Electrolytes are not indicated on day 1 of age. Vitamins may not be added to the standard starter PN solutions, for they decrease the shelf life. PN can then be advanced as described below. In Tables 20.1 and 20.2 the guidelines for PN are given. Table 20.3 provides parenteral calculations.

Energy

Energy intakes of 30 to 50 kcal/kg are adequate for nitrogen balance the first days of life (Denne & Poindexter, 2007). Energy intakes of 90 to 100 kcal/kg are the goal for growth with PN. For enteral feedings, 105 to 130 kcal/kg/d will meet the needs of most premature infants (American Academy of Pediatrics Committee on Nutrition, 2009a).

Glucose

Glucose homeostasis is an issue for premature infants, and blood levels should be monitored as parenteral glucose loads are advanced to ensure tolerance. Premature infants are at risk for hyperglycemia for many reasons including: if an excessive glucose load is provided, gluconeogenesis continues in the presence of elevated blood glucose levels, insulin production is decreased, insulin resistance exists, stress, or the development of sepsis (Schanler & Anderson, 2008).

Neonates usually produce glucose at the rate of 3 to 5 mg/kg/min for the term infant and up to 8 to 9 mg/kg/min in the extremely-low-birth-weight infant (Kalhan & Devaskar, 2011). Glucose tolerance is impaired in the VLBW infant, and starting glucose at less than 6 mg/kg/min is recommended (American Academy of Pediatrics Committee on Nutrition, 2009a). Often 4.5 to 6 mg/kg/min is provided to the premature infant and advanced slowly to a goal of 11 to 12 mg/kg/min to meet energy needs for growth (American Academy of Pediatrics Committee on Nutrition, 2009a). Glucose can be advanced by 1 to 2 mg/kg/min (Schanler & Anderson, 2008). The addition of parenteral protein enhances insulin release and the tolerance of the glucose load (Thureen et al., 2003). By monitoring blood glucose loads, slowly advancing glucose loads, and providing parenteral protein, the need for additional insulin may be avoided. Insulin will decrease hyperglycemia, but it does increase the incidence of hypoglycemia (Alsweiler,

TABLE 20.1

GROWING PREMATURE INFANTS—PARENTERAL GUIDELINES: ENERGY, PROTEIN, MINERALS

Nutrient	Unit (kg/d, Except as Noted)
Energy, kcal	90–100
Glucose, mg/kg/min	11–12
Carbohydrate, g	16–17
Protein, g	2.7–3.5, up to 4
Fat, g	3
Calcium, mg	60–80
Phosphorus, mg	39–67
Magnesium, mg	4.3–7.2
Sodium, mEq	2–4
Potassium, mEq	1.5–2
Chloride, mEq	2–4
Zinc, mcg	400
Copper, mcg	20
Selenium, mcg	2
Chromium, mcg	0.2
Manganese, mcg	1

Data from American Academy of Pediatrics Committee on Nutrition (2009a).

TABLE 20.2

PEDIATRIC MULTIVITAMIN BY DOSAGE FOR INFANTS

Vitamin	2 mL/kg Infant < 2.5 kg	5 mL/d Infants ≥ 2.5 kg
Vitamin A, IU	920	2,300
Vitamin E, IU	2.8	7
Vitamin K, mcg	80	200
Vitamin D, IU	160	400
Vitamin C, mg	32	80
Thiamin, mg	0.48	1.2
Riboflavin, mg	0.56	1.4
Niacin, mg	6.8	17
Vitamin B_6, mg	0.4	1
Folate, mcg	56	140
Vitamin B_{12}, mcg	0.4	1
Biotin, mcg	8	20
Pantothenic acid, mg	2	5

Data from American Academy of Pediatrics Committee on Nutrition (2009a).

TABLE 20.3

CALCULATIONS FOR PN

Nutrient	Calculations
Dextrose	3.4 kcal/g
Protein	4 kcal/g
20% lipid	10 kcal/g (which is 9 fat kcal and 1 glycerol kcal) or 2 kcal/mL (1 fat gram/5 mL)
Glucose infusion rate (GIR) mg/kg/min	[(mL/kg/d) × (grams glucose/100 mL) × (1,000 mg/g)]/1,440 min/d i.e., Infant receiving 130 mL/kg/d of 12.5% Dextrose [(130 mL/kg/d) × (12.5 g Dextrose/100 mL) × (1,000 mg/g)]/1,440 GIR = 11.3 mg/kg/min

Harding, & Bloomfield, 2012). Increased weight gain and increased head circumference growth with decreased linear growth has been reported, which may reflect greater adipose deposition (Alsweiler et al., 2012). Serum glucose levels above 150 mg/dL is the definition of hyperglycemia for premature infants (Poindexter & Denne, 2011). Decreasing the glucose load is the first step in preventing increases in blood glucose levels. Insulin use is reserved for infants with persistent blood glucose levels over 200 mg/dL (Poindexter & Denne, 2011). The precise blood glucose level used to indicate insulin therapy has not been defined. Tight blood glucose control is not recommended for premature infants because of the increased incidence of hypoglycemia and mortality (Alsweiler et al., 2012; Beardsall et al., 2008).

Premature infants are at risk for hypoglycemia due to poor glycogen stores, impaired gluconeogenesis, increased glucose need with acute illness (sepsis, respiratory distress), maternal therapy with beta-blockers, and hyperinsulinemia commonly seen with infants of diabetic mothers (Wilker, 2012). Hypoglycemia will occur when inadequate glucose is provided, glucose is not delivered due to intravenous line infiltration, PN has been rapidly discontinued, or insulin has been administered.

Protein

Protein may be started at 1.5 to 3 g/kg/d and results in normal plasma amino acid levels, increased nitrogen balance, and increased protein anabolism (American Academy of Pediatrics Committee on Nutrition, 2009a; Denne & Poindexter, 2007; Thureen et al., 2003). Early protein intake of 3g/kg/d is associated with better gain in weight, length, and head circumference at 36 weeks postmenstrual age, and decreased incidence of head circumference less than the 10th percentile at 22 months corrected age (Poindexter et al., 2006).

Protein is advanced to 3.5 to 4 g/kg/d. During the first week of life, blood urea nitrogen (BUN) does not consistently correlate to parenteral protein intake and should not be used to limit protein intake unless renal dysfunction is demonstrated by decreased urine output and elevated serum creatinine (Blanco, Falck, Green, Cornell, & Gong, 2008; Radmacher, Lewis, & Adamkin, 2009; Ridout, Melara, Rottinghaus, & Thureen, 2005). BUN level can reflect hydration status, excessive protein intake, inadequate protein or energy intake, illness, renal function, and hepatic synthesis (Radmacher et al., 2009).

Parenteral protein is provided as amino acids, and the use of the pediatric solutions is recommended. Three pediatric solutions are available in the United States and they are: Aminosyn-PF (Abbott), Premasol (Baxter), and TrophAmine (B. Braun) (Poindexter & Denne, 2011). These solutions provide a blend of amino acids to produce blood amino acid levels similar to those found with breastfed, term infants, or cord blood levels found with premature infants (Poindexter & Denne, 2011). The premature infant's ability to synthesize cysteine, tyrosine, and arginine is limited, so they should be provided in the early diet. Cysteine is not stable in solutions so it is added as cysteine hydrochloride acid. The addition of cystine improves nitrogen balance and increases the acidity of the solution, which allows greater amounts of calcium and phosphorous to be added (Soghier & Brion, 2010).

Lipids

Intravenous lipids are given to provide essential fatty acids and kilocalories. One half to 1 g of lipids will meet the essential fatty acid requirement of linoleic acid (Poindexter & Denne, 2011). Not providing lipids in the first week of life can result in biochemical fatty acid deficiency for premature infants with limited fat stores. Intravenous lipids may be started at 1 to 2 g/kg on day 1 of life and advanced to 3 g/kg/d (American Academy of Pediatrics Committee on Nutrition, 2009a). Infants who have decreased serum levels of lipoprotein lipase or suffer from metabolic stress may not clear lipids well. Infants most at risk include those who are small for gestation age, suffer from intrauterine growth restriction, are early gestational age, or have sepsis, liver disease, or have received steroids (American Academy of Pediatrics Committee on Nutrition, 2009a; Shulman & Phillips, 2003). To promote clearance of the triglycerides in lipids, the lipids should be provided over 24 hours, and 20% emulsions should be given (Poindexter & Denne, 2011; Schanler & Anderson, 2008). The phospholipid emulsifier decreases the clearance of fatty acids, and the concentration of emulsifier is the same in the 10% and 20% emulsions. By using 20% emulsion, less volume and less phospholipid will be given per gram of lipid at (5 versus 10 mL) (American Academy of Pediatrics Committee on Nutrition, 2009a). Serum triglycerides may be monitored, but acceptable levels have not been determined (Neu, 2009). A level less than 200 mg/dL has been suggested (American Academy of Pediatrics Committee on Nutrition, 2009a).

In the United States soy bean and safflower oil emulsions are available. These fat sources provide omega six fatty acids, linoleic acid, and arachidonic acid. A fish oil emulsion (Omegaven) from Europe is available for compassion use in the United States. These fish oils contain omega three fatty acids, docosahexaenoic acid (DHA), and eicosapentaenoic acid. The omega three fatty acids may be anti-inflammatory and have aided in the treatment of PN-associated cholestasis (Gura, 2010).

Carnitine

Carnitine facilitates the transport of long-chain fatty acids into the mitochondrial for oxidation. Premature infants have limited carnitine stores and a decreased ability to synthesize carnitine (Hay, 2008). Human milk and infant formula provide sources of carnitine, while parenteral solutions do not contain carnitine unless added. A dosage of 10 to 20 mg/kg/d may be provided for infants receiving PN for greater than 2 weeks (Schanler & Anderson, 2008).

Fluid and Electrolytes

Premature infants have high and variable fluid needs based on birth weight, gestational age, clinical condition, and the environment in which the infant is nursed (Dell, 2011). Constant monitoring and assessment are indicated to promote normal hydration status. Monitoring includes body weight, fluid intake, urine output, stool output and other fluid losses, serum electrolytes, and BUN (Bhatia, 2006). A weight loss up to 15% is common in the first week of life (Dell, 2011).

Sodium is not added in the first few days of life to allow for the diuresis of the extracellular fluid, but intravenous saline infusions or flushes may be indicated. These sources of sodium must be accounted for when prescribing PN sodium. The usual sodium requirement is 2 to 4 mEq/kg/d. Potassium is not needed the first day of life, but is added as renal function is established and serum potassium levels become normal. A potassium intake of 2 to 3 mEq/kg/d will usually meet the needs of the infants (Poindexter & Denne, 2011). Chloride may be provided with sodium and potassium. Acetate is indicated when acidosis occurs (Poindexter & Denne, 2011). All serum electrolytes require monitoring to ensure normal serum levels.

Calcium, Phosphorus, and Magnesium

Calcium, phosphorus, and magnesium are needed for metabolic management and bone mineralization. Calcium and phosphorus should be provided at a 1 to 1.3/1 molar ratio of calcium to phosphorus to promote normal blood levels and bone mineralization (Carlson, 2009). Calcium and phosphorus need to be provided together instead of in alternate day administrations to avoid urinary mineral wasting or abnormal blood calcium and phosphorus levels (Carlson, 2009).

Vitamins

Pediatric multivitamin injections are available but are not designed for the premature infant (American Academy of Pediatrics Committee on Nutrition, 2009a). The dosage schedule is based on the infant's weight and is shown in Table 20.2. At these intakes, adequate amounts of vitamins E and K are provided, low amounts of vitamins A and D are given, and many B vitamins are greater than recommendations (American Academy of Pediatrics Committee on Nutrition, 2009a). Parenteral vitamins are not available as single vitamins.

Trace Minerals

Trace mineral guidelines are shown in Table 20.1. Trace minerals are available as multimineral packets or as separate minerals. Extra zinc is indicated for infants with intestinal losses (Schanler & Anderson, 2008; Shulman, 1989). When cholestasis is present, copper and manganese intakes are decreased due to elimination of these trace minerals in the bile. Selenium and chromium intakes are limited with impaired renal function (American Academy of Pediatrics Committee on Nutrition, 2009a).

ENTERAL NUTRITION

Premature infants have increased nutrient needs to support fetal growth. Table 20.4 provides enteral nutrient guidelines. Enteral feedings are always the goal for the nourishment of premature infants. The infant should be evaluated daily for starting feeds, feeds advancement, milk fortification, or vitamin and mineral supplements.

Human Milk

The milk of choice for all infants is human milk, and pasteurized donor human milk is recommended as a supplement to the infant's own mother's milk for all premature infants (Eidelman, Schanler, & American Academy of Pediatrics Section on Breastfeeding, 2012). The human milk diet for the premature infant results in a decreased incidence of mortality, sepsis, and NEC, improved neurodevelopment, and a quicker time to full enteral feedings (Meinzen-Derr et al., 2009; Schanler, Shulman, & Lau, 1999; Sisk, Lovelady, Dillard, Gruber, & O 'Shea, 2007; Sullivan et al., 2010; Vohr et al., 2007).

Pasteurized donor milk needs to be obtained from one of the donor human milk banks or commercial banks to ensure safety of the product. Donors are screened for infections, medications, drugs, or high-risk activities, by history and blood tests. Mothers who would like to donate milk should be referred to one of the banks for proper screening. The Human Milk Banking Association of North America (http://www.hmbana.org) is a volunteer association that nonprofit Human Milk Banks may be a member of and whose members are required to meet the standards for human milk banking guidelines, set by the association guidelines (American Academy of Pediatrics Committee on Nutrition, 2009a).

Fortification by a multinutrient fortifier is indicated for VLBW infants to meet their increased nutrient demands. Bovine milk fortifiers are available as powder packets or liquid vials. These fortifiers contain carbohydrate, fat, protein, vitamins, and minerals. Iron supplements will be needed if a low-iron fortifier is used. The bovine fortifiers have been added at 100 mL/kg of human milk intake (Berseth, 2004). Donor human milk fortifiers contain human milk with concentrated protein and additives of calcium, phosphorus, and zinc. Multivitamins and iron supplements are needed with this fortifier. Donor human milk fortifiers have been added at 40 or 100 mL/kg of human milk intake (Sullivan et al., 2010). Table 20.5 compares human milks with the fortifiers fed at a standard volume of 150 mL/kg and at the usual milk kilocalorie concentrations.

The donor milk fortifier is available as 24, 26, 28, and 30 kcal/oz supplements. The 26 kcal fortification is often used to provide more protein and energy to support growth. The 28 and 30 kcal/oz supplements are helpful with infants who are fluid restricted.

Infant Formulas

Premature infant formulas are more nutrient dense than standard infant formulas and contain nutrients in a more easily digested form. Table 20.5 shows a selected nutrient comparison. Premature infant formulas come as 20, 24, and 30 kcal/oz milks. The 20 and 24 kcal/oz milks will meet the needs of most premature infants. The 30 kcal/oz milk is indicated for infants who are fluid restricted. The 30 kcal/oz milk can be mixed with 24 kcal/oz milk at different proportions to make milks greater than 24 kcal/oz. The 24 kcal/oz premature formulas are available as regular and high protein. See Table 20.6 for comparison of formulas fed at a standard volume of 150 mL/kg.

Postdischarge milks are designed for the premature infant at discharge. The nutrient composition is in between the composition of standard and premature infant formulas. Studies on these formulas have been on infants less than 1,800 g birth weight (Carver et al., 2001; Koo & Hockman, 2006; Lucas et al., 2001). Studies have shown both improved growth and poorer growth for premature infants

TABLE 20.4

ENTERAL NUTRIENT GUIDELINES FOR GROWING PREMATURE INFANTS (UNIT/KG/D)

Nutrient	Amount	Nutrient	Amount
Energy, kcal	105–130	Selenium, mcg	1.3–4.5
Protein, g	3.5–4	Iodine, mcg	10–60
Carbohydrate, g	10–14	Vitamin A, IU	700–1,500
Fat, g	5–7	Vitamin D, IU	150–400[a]
Calcium, mg	100–220	Vitamin E, IU	6–12
Phosphorus, mg	60–140	Vitamin K, mcg	8–10
Magnesium, mg	7.9–15	Vitamin C, mg	18–24
Sodium, mEq	3–5	Thiamin, mcg	180–240
Potassium, mEq	2–3	Riboflavin, mcg	250–360
Chloride, mEq	3–7	Niacin, mg	3.6–4.8
Iron, mg	2–4	Vitamin B_6, mcg	150–210
Zinc, mcg	1,000–3,000	Folate, mcg	25–50
Copper, mcg	120–150	Vitamin B_{12}, mcg	0.3
Chromium, mcg	0.1–2.25	Biotin, mcg	3.6–6
Manganese, mcg	0.7–7.75	Pantothenic acid, mg	1.2–1.7

[a] Vitamin D intake is per day.

Data from American Academy of Pediatrics Committee on Nutrition (2009a) and Tsang, Uauy, Koletzko, and Zlotkin (2005).

fed postdischarge formula as compared to the term formulas. This lack of agreement has made the recommendation for formula usage unclear (American Academy of Pediatrics Committee on Nutrition, 2009a). There have been reports of better growth for infants fed these formulas for 6 to 9 months (Carver et al., 2001; Lucas et al., 2001). A recommendation has been made that the infant's weight for length be consistent at the 25th percentile to discontinue the discharge milks (American Academy of Pediatrics Committee on Nutrition, 2009b). Premature infants will require additional vitamin D with the postdischarge formulas to achieve 400 IU of vitamin D per day to meet the Dietary Reference Intakes for Term Infants (Institute of Medicine [IOM], 2010). Infants will receive 2 mg/kg/d of iron on these formulas at normal volume intake. The iron guideline is 2 to 4 mg/kg/d (Baker, Greer, & American Academy of Pediatrics Committee on Nutrition, 2010). Additional iron may be provided if needed.

Soy infant formulas are not recommended for premature infants, because the phytates bind phosphorus leading to decreased absorption of calcium and phosphorus and the development of osteopenia (Bhatia, Greer, & the American Academy of Pediatrics Committee on Nutrition, 2008). Decreased soy protein absorption and utilization has been reported (American Academy of Pediatrics Committee on Nutrition, 2009a).

TABLE 20.5

SELECTIVE NUTRIENT COMPARISON OF HUMAN MILK WITH FORTIFICATION—150 ML/KG*

Nutrient	AAP 2009 (per kg)	Human Milk (20 kcal/oz)	Human Milk + Bovine Milk Fortifier (24 kcal/oz)	Human Milk + Donor Milk Fortifier (24 kcal/oz)
Energy, kcal	105–130	101	120	120
Protein, g	3.5–4	1.4	2.9–3.9	2.9
Calcium, mg	100–220	35	173–204	182
Iron, mg	2–4	0.1	0.7–2.3	0.3
Zinc, mg	1–3	0.3	1.5–1.8	1.4
Vitamin D, IU	150–400/d	1.5	177–237	41

*Representing usual volume intakes and milk concentrations without vitamin and mineral supplementation.

Data from American Academy of Pediatrics Committee on Nutrition (2009c); Abbott Nutrition; Mead Johnson Nutrition; Gerber Good Start Formulas for Premature Infants (2012, April 30); and Prolact + H²MF™Nutrient Values and Prolacta Bioscience MKT-0164 Rev-1.2009.

TABLE 20.6

SELECTIVE NUTRIENT COMPARISON OF INFANT FORMULAS—150 ML/KG*

Nutrient	AAP 2009 (per kg)	Standard (Term) (20 kcal/oz)	Premature (24 kcal/oz)	Postdischarge (22 kcal/oz)
Energy, kcal	105–130	101	120	120
Protein, g	3.5–4	2.1	3.6–4.2	3.2
Calcium, mg	100–220	68–80	197–219	117–135
Iron, mg	2–4	1.5–1.8	2.1–2.3	2–2.1
Zinc, mg	1–3	0.8–1.1	1.5–1.8	1.4
Vitamin D, IU	150–400/d	60–62	183–293	78–80

*Representing usual volume intakes and milk concentrations without vitamin and mineral supplementation.

Data taken from Abbott Nutrition; Mead Johnson Nutrition; and Gerber Good Start Formulas for Premature Infants (2012, April 30).

Specialized infant formulas including the protein hydrolysates and free amino acid formulas are used for infants who have malabsorption problems such as short gut who do not tolerate human milk. Vitamin or mineral supplementation may be needed with these formulas, as they are not designed to meet the needs of the premature infant.

Feeding Management

Enteral feedings should be considered for all infants. Trophic feedings that are small feedings to feed the gut and do not serve as a major nutrition source are frequently used for infants who are VLBW or clinically stressed. Studies have ranged from 1 to 25 mL/kg/d, and human milk is the milk of choice (American Academy of Pediatrics Committee on Nutrition, 2009a). Reported benefits of early small feedings include decreased incidence of indirect hyperbilirubinemia, cholestatic jaundice, and metabolic bone disease, increased concentrations of gastric hormones, full feedings achieved more quickly, maturation of intestinal motility patterns mature faster, increased lactase activity, and reduced intestinal permeability (Berseth, 1992; Dunn, Hulman, Meetze et al., 1992; Shulman et al., 1998a, 1998b; Weiner & Kliegman, 1988). By meta-analysis, the incidence of NEC was not increased with trophic feedings (Bombell & McGuire, 2009). There is no standard time for the length of trophic feedings as the studies have used different lengths of time for trophic feeding, different days of life to initiate feedings, and different milks. Trophic feedings can be initiated with the umbilical catheters in place (Davey, Wagner, Cox, & Kendig, 1994).

Nutritive feedings are often advanced by 10 to 20 mL/kg/d for VLBW infants. One report compared 15 versus 35 mL/kg of premature 20 kcal/oz formula (Rayyis, Ambalavanan, Wright, & Carlo, 1999). No difference was reported in the incidence of NEC, and the group fed the higher volume significantly achieved full feedings earlier, regaining birth weight sooner.

Several investigations report that the implementation of a standardized feeding guideline in the neonatal intensive care unit (NICU) is associated with a decrease in the incidence of NEC (McCallie et al., 2011; Patole & de Klerk, 2005).

Feeding Method

The feeding method for the infant will depend on the infant's gestational age, weight, clinical condition, and the experience of the nursery nursing staff (American Academy of Pediatrics Committee on Nutrition, 2009a). The premature infant does not coordinate sucking, swallowing, and breathing until 32 to 34 weeks gestation. Nasogastric and orogastric feedings are used for infants too young or ill to breast or bottle feed (American Academy of Pediatrics Committee on Nutrition, 2009a). Transpyloric feedings are used for infants with persistent gastric residuals or emesis without intestinal pathology present, but research is lacking to support this method for routine feeding of premature infants (Hay, 2008; Schanler & Anderson, 2008). Continuous milk infusion is needed for infants fed via transpyloric feedings, as the intestine has limited compliance (Schanler & Anderson, 2008). Gastrostomy feedings are indicated for infants with congenital anomalies or neurological impairment (Sapsford, 2009; Schanler & Anderson, 2008).

Continuous and bolus feedings are used with gastric feedings, and there have been numerous studies suggesting that each method is best (Hay, 2008). One concern with continuous infusion is the reported loss of fat and calcium (Rogers, Hicks, Hamzo, Veit, & Abrams, 2010).

Feeding Assessment

Feeding assessment is indicated for premature infants because they do not tolerate feedings well and are at risk for illness. Consensus is lacking on the criteria to evaluate feeding tolerance (Schanler & Anderson, 2008). Clinical assessment may include physical exam of the abdomen, the presence or absence of bowel sounds and their quality, gastric residuals, emesis, and changes in stool (Schanler & Anderson, 2008). Gastric residuals may be due to immature intestinal motor activity, feeding intolerance, NEC, or intestinal obstruction (Anderson, 2012). Residuals are frequently noted before feedings are initiated and during trophic feedings. These residuals may be ignored if no other signs of feeding tolerance or illness are present. Residuals at 50% or greater of a bolus feeding or 1.5 times an hourly rate for continuous feedings had been suggested to evaluate the infant for intolerance/illness (Schanler et al., 1999). A residual volume of 2 to 3 mL/kg per feed has also been used (Anderson, 2012). Recently, Shulman, Ou, and Smith (2011) reported that the premature infant's gastric residuals do not correlate with the obtaining of full gavage feedings. The bilious residual may be due to the feeding tube moving into the intestine, bile reflux into the stomach, or intestinal obstruction (Schanler & Anderson, 2008).

The tonicity of the abdomen should be evaluated. An increase in tonicity will occur with air swallowing, feeding intolerance, infrequent stooling, or NEC. Visual loop of bowel may indicate illness. A work-up for obstruction, NEC, and sepsis may be indicated, especially if other signs of illness are present, such as an increased number of apneas and bradycardias, an increased number of desaturation events, or the presence of lethargy (Schanler & Anderson, 2008).

Blood in the residual or stool is a worry and needs to be evaluated. Etiologies include a sign of illness, feeding-tube irritation of the intestine, anal fissure, or blood swallowed during delivery (Anderson, 2012).

GROWTH AND GROWTH CHARTS

Daily weights, weekly lengths, and weekly head circumferences should be obtained, and weekly measures should be plotted on intrauterine growth curves. The intrauterine charts are developed from the birth weight, birth length, and birth head circumferences from a large group of infants (Fenton & Kim, 2013; Olsen, Groveman, Lawson, Clark, & Zemel, 2010). Premature infants can be plotted against these charts to assess how their growth compares to the goal of fetal growth (American Academy of Pediatrics Committee on Nutrition, 2009a). The Fenton chart is a fetal-infant chart that goes from 22 weeks gestation to 50 weeks postmenstrual age (Fenton & Kim, 2013). The fetal portion is based on infants from Germany, the United States, Italy, Australia, Scotland, and Canada and the 40 to 50 weeks is taken from the World Health Organization (WHO) growth charts. The Fenton chart is electronically available from the website (http://ucalgary.ca/fenton) (Figures 20.1a and 20.1b).

The Olsen chart is based on a large, racially diverse sample from the United States and goes from 23 to 41 weeks gestation (Olsen et al., 2010). The gender-based charts include weight, length, and head circumference. These charts may be downloaded for individual patient use at the following: http://www.nursing.upenn.edu/media/infantgrowthcurves/Documents/Olsen-NewIUGrowthCurves_2010permission.pdf.

Once the premature infant reaches 40 weeks postmenstrual age, the WHO growth charts can be used to assess catch-up growth (Grummer-Strawn, Reinold, & Krebs, 2010). These charts are based on the growth of infants who were predominately breastfed for the first year of life and represent ideal growth. The WHO growth charts can be downloaded from www.cdc.gov/growthcharts/who_charts.htm.

The first week of life premature infants can lose up to 15% of their birth weight, which is the loss of extracellular fluid (Dell, 2011). Goals for weekly rate of gain are given in Table 20.7. Since weights are obtained daily, a weekly rate can be calculated daily. Closely monitoring growth is important to ensure the best growth for these high-risk infants and their future development. Extremely-low-birth-weight infants have demonstrated improved neurological outcomes and growth at 18 to 22 months of corrected age when their growth rates in the nursery were greater than 18 g/kg/d for weight or 0.9 cm/wk for head circumference (Ehrenkranz et al, 2006). When poor growth occurs, assessment of the etiology should be explored. Poor growth may be related to medical conditions or nutrition management. Medical issues that may contribute to poor growth include acidosis, hyponatremia, increased work of breathing, cold stress, anemia, infections, and the use of steroids (Anderson, 2012). These conditions require treatment before nutrition can be fully utilized. Issues related to nutrition are given in Box 20.1.

TABLE 20.7

GROWTH GOALS

Weight gain	15–20 g/kg/d for infants < 2 kg 20–30 g/d for infants > 2 kg
Length gain	0.7–1 cm/wk
Head circumference	0.7–1 cm/wk

Data from Anderson (2012).

BOX 20.1

CONSIDERATIONS FOR POOR GROWTH—NUTRITION FACTORS

Feeding intolerance—abnormal stools, excessive residuals, or emesis

Full nutrition just achieved that meets nutrient guidelines

Nutrition not optimized

- Parenteral nutrient concentrations not adequate
- Incorrect amount of fortifier not added to human milk
- Incorrect calculations

Human milk

- Continuous infusions will lead to fat losses
- Use of foremilk that is low in fat and kilocalories

Ordered diet not received

- Infant not able to consume adequate milk and is not supplemented with gavage feedings
- Feedings held for tests
- Volume of feedings ordered per kg has not kept up with weight gain

Nutrition solution not prepared correctly, or incorrect milk feeding provided

- Intravenous fluid administration has been held to provide medication or blood
- Ostomy output is excessive so parenteral fluids will need to be increased and enteral feedings decreased to meet infant's nutrition needs

Data from Anderson (2012).

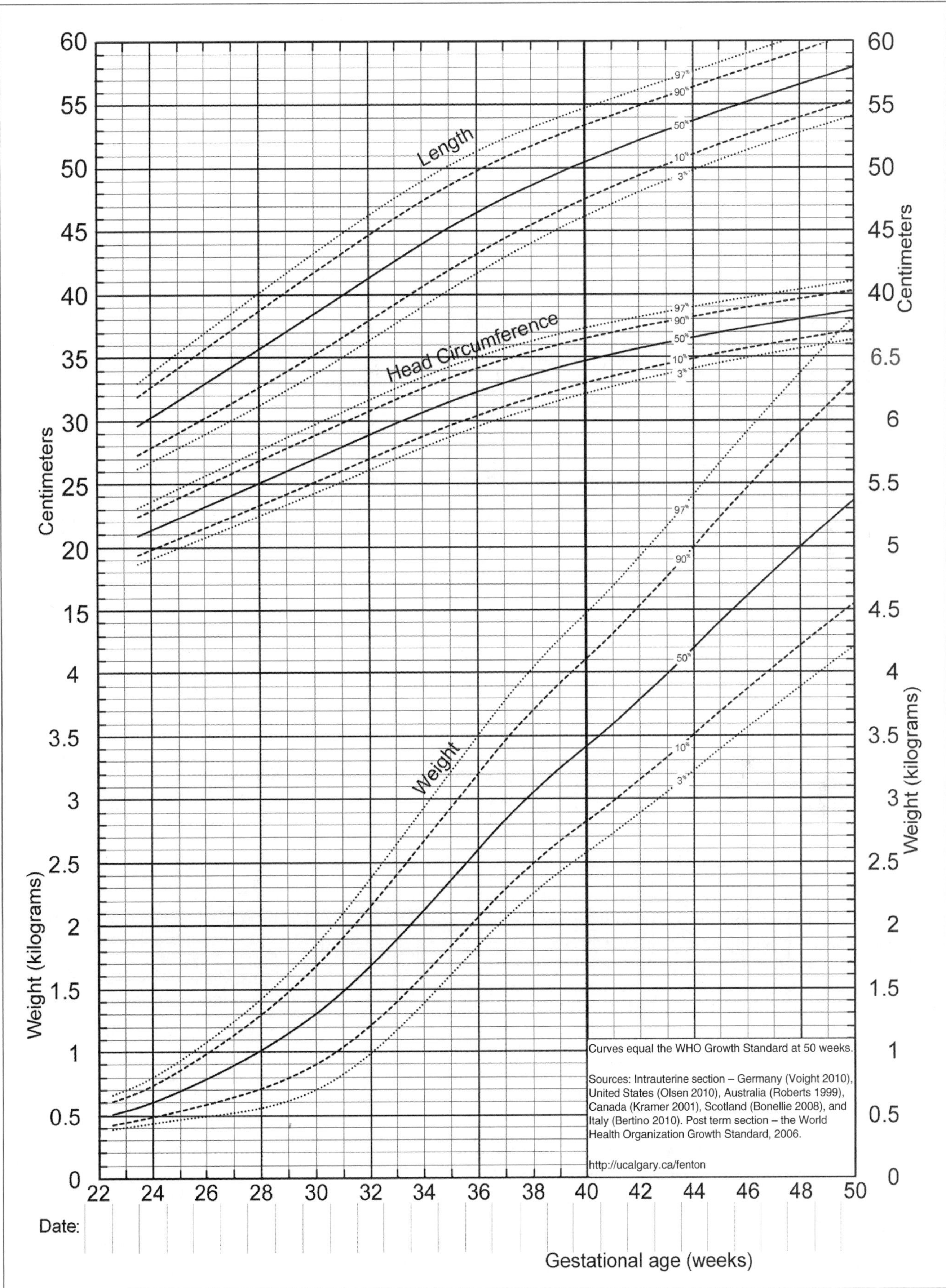

FIGURE 20.1a Fenton preterm growth chart for girls.

Chart may be downloaded from http://ucalgary.ca/fenton

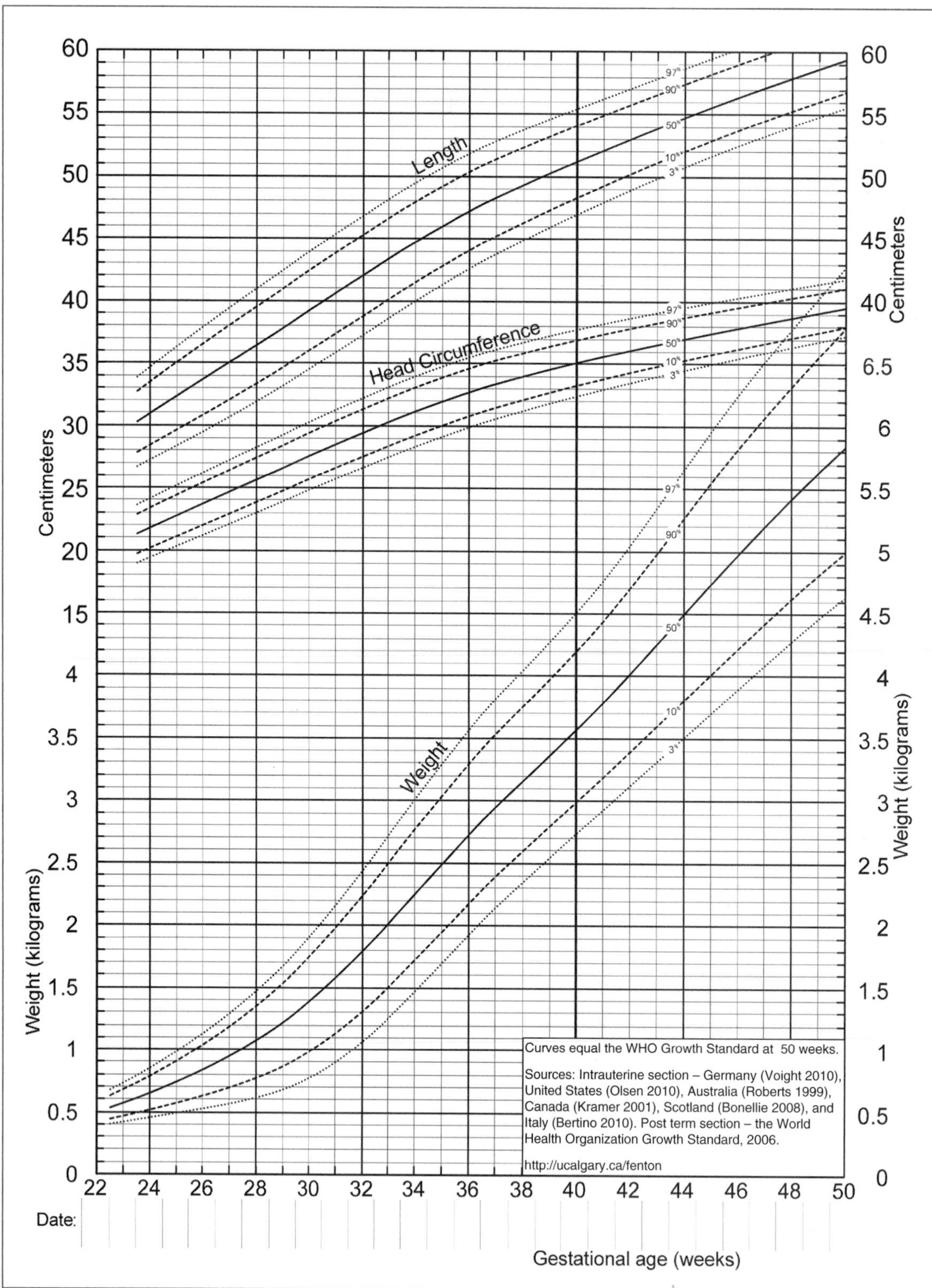

FIGURE 20.1b Fenton preterm growth chart for boys.
Chart may be downloaded from http://ucalgary.ca/fenton

Biochemical Indices

Serum electrolytes, glucose, BUN, and creatinine will be monitored daily or more frequently if abnormal the first week of life. Once stable, these serum values will be obtained once to twice a week for the infant receiving PN or receiving diuretics or for the infant who has an abnormal value (Anderson, 2012). While on PN, serum conjugated bilirubin and serum alanine aminotransferase (ALT, serum glutamic-pyruvic transaminase) will be drawn weekly starting at 2 weeks of PN therapy to detect liver disease associated with PN. Serum phosphorus and alkaline phosphatase activity levels are drawn on infants at risk for osteopenia, which includes VLBW infants and infants with a prolonged course of PN or milk intake of a formula not designed for premature infants. If alkaline phosphatase activity levels reach 800 IL/L, a radiograph of the wrist/knees (rickets survey) can be used to document osteopenia of prematurity (Mitchell et al., 2009). Hematocrit and hemoglobin levels are obtained as needed (Schanler & Anderson, 2008).

POSTDISCHARGE NUTRITION

Prior to discharge, the infant's nutritional status should be assessed for present growth status, feeding volume allowed and infant's actual volume intake, presence of any abnormal serum levels that require treatment, and the mother's desire to breastfeed. Depending on the infant's history regarding osteopenia, ability to nurse, and fluid allowance, the infant's feeding recommendation will be individualized. The infant should be placed on the discharge diet prior to discharge to assess growth and feeding tolerance to the plan. Parents need to demonstrate their ability to feed their infant, administer supplements, and prepare special milks if indicated.

The breastfed infant will need multivitamins and iron to provide vitamin D at 400 IU/d and iron at 2 to 4 mg/kg/d (American Academy of Pediatrics Committee on Nutrition, 2009a; IOM, 2010). Infants may require formula supplementation to meet needs for growth, and 2 to 3 feeds per day may be provided to increase nutrient intake. By using bottle feedings of formula instead of formula powder added to expressed human milk, the mother can actually breastfeed her infant and possibly avoid bacterial contamination of powder infant formulas. Nutrient intake can be greater with the use of two to three bottles of formula than making all the human milk 22 kcal/oz with formula powder. Mothers should be referred to lactation consultation for postdischarge.

In a recent study, discharged premature infants were for 12 weeks fed their mothers' milk, which was fortified with bovine human milk fortifier for half of their feedings, and the other half of feedings were breastfed or expressed milk (O'Connor et al., 2008). This group of infants was compared to a group of premature infants fed their mothers' milk supplemented with iron and vitamins. At 12 weeks postdischarge, the bovine human milk fortified group was longer and had greater head circumferences. At 1 year corrected age, the infants who received the bovine-fortified milk were longer, had greater head circumferences, and had greater weights (Aimone et al., 2009). No differences were noted in development at 18 months corrected age (Aimone et al., 2009).

The postdischarge formula may be used for infants who are not breastfed. Vitamin D supplementation of 200 IU/d in addition to the vitamin D in the formula should meet the infant's needs. Iron supplements may be provided if indicated (Baker et al., 2010).

Infants should be referred to the Special Supplemental Nutrition Program for Women, Infant and Children (WIC) and to the early children intervention programs. A medical home should provide the necessary assessment and management of the infant's nutrition needs related to growth and normal development.

SUMMARY

This chapter has reviewed the basic physiology of digestion and the importance of adequate neonatal nutrition for positive growth and development. Different routes of feeding as well as different formulas and breast milk feeding have been discussed. Neonatal nutrition is a challenge but sets the course for a lifetime of health.

CASE STUDY

■ Identification of the Problem. Premature infant not gaining weight

■ Assessment: History and Physical Examination. The premature female infant was delivered by spontaneous vaginal delivery following one course of antenatal steroids to a 30-year-old G2 P1 woman. The infant required oxygen at birth and was weaned to room air by 12 hours of age. Sepsis work-up was completed for preterm delivery, and results were negative. Her Apgar scores were 6^1, 8^5. She was placed into a humidified incubator. She developed hyperbilirubinemia and was treated with phototherapy from day of age 2 to 5.

She was born at 28 weeks gestation with a birth weight of 900 g, length of 37 cm, and head circumference of 26.5 cm. She is classified as appropriate for gestational age, for her birth weight is between the 10th and 50th percentile. Her length and head circumference are between the 10th and 50th percentile. She is now 21 days of age and 31 weeks postmenstrual age. She regained birth weight by 2 weeks of age and now weighs 950 g, which is below the 10th percentile. Her rate of weight gain this past week was 8 g/kg/d. Her length is 38 cm, and her head circumference is 27 cm.

She was started on PN day 1 of age at 80 mL/kg/d providing 45 kcal/kg, GIR of 5.2 mg/kg/min of glucose, 2.4 g protein/kg, and 1 g of lipid per kg. Mom's milk was started day 2 of age at 20 mL/kg/d and provided for 3 days as trophic feedings before advancing milk by 20 mL/kg/d to a volume of 150 mL/kg/d. PN was advanced to meet guidelines and was discontinued when 120 mL/kg of human milk feedings were achieved on day 9 of age. Today's diet order is human milk fortified with bovine human milk fortifier to 24 kcal/oz at 150 mL/kg/d by a continuous infusion of 5.5 mL/hr by a nasogastric tube. Diet should provide 120 kcal/kg and 3.9 g protein/kg/d.

Physical examination is normal.

■ Differential Diagnoses

- Infant needs formula supplement
- Infant not receiving diet as ordered
- Infant has increased requirements
- Diet order incorrect
- Infant just achieved appropriate diet
- Infant has abnormal labs
- Infant has a low temperature
- Infant is not tolerating feedings

- Documented weight incorrect
- Inadequate intake

Diagnostic Tests

- Check incubator temperature management: baby was on manual control mode at 35°C
- Recheck diet orders: at 5.5 mL/hr the infant is only receiving 140 mL/kg/d; order placed in the computer was for 22 kcal/oz milk instead of 24 kcal/oz; infant actually receiving 102 kcal/kg and 2.5 g protein/kg/d
- Review infant's flow sheet for output: no emesis, no stool for 2 days, abdomen soft
- Review vitals: yesterday the baby's skin temperature was 35°C
- Review labs: labs from 3 days ago; serum sodium 140 mEq/dL, potassium 5 mEq/dL, chloride 108 mEq/dL, BUN 12 mg/dL, hemoglobin 11 g/dL, and hematocrit 33%
- Review daily weight: slow, steady increase of 10 g/d; no large increases or decreases; weight is probably accurate

Working Diagnosis

- Infant cold stressed
- Inadequate nutrition intake

Development of Management Plan

- Change incubator temperature management to servo control mode at 37°C
- Change feeding order to 6 mL/hr to provide 150 mL/kg
- Order 24 kcal/oz human milk with bovine human milk fortifier

Implementation and Evaluation of Effectiveness

- Feeding order changed today
- Daily weights followed closely for the next 3 to 5 days to ensure good weight gain, weight gain since change in diet is 13 g/kg/d
- Change to bolus feedings to increase nutrient delivery; weight gain is now 15 g/kg/d; length and head circumferences have increase 1 cm each this past week
- Once infant demonstrated good weight gain, incubator temperature management changed back to manual control mode

Outcome. Growth can occur when infant's temperature is maintained. Human milk fortified with bovine human milk fortifier to 24 kcal/oz at 150 mL/kg given as a bolus meets infant's nutritional needs. Infant's growth is appropriate on human milk fortified to 24 kcal/oz diet at 150 mL/kg.

EVIDENCE-BASED PRACTICE BOX

Cysteine is an amino acid that is a precursor for taurine and glutathione, or cysteine may go directly into protein formation (Soghier & Brion, 2010). Cysteine may be semi-essential for the premature infant due to the infant's limited ability to synthesize cysteine from methionine (Poindexter & Denne, 2011). Cystathionase, the enzyme responsible for cysteine syntheses, has been reported at low concentrations in the livers of premature infants, but yet the extrahepatic tissue may contain adequate amounts of this enzyme. Not all studies with premature infants report limited ability to synthesize cysteine (Poindexter & Denne, 2011). Early studies did not show a positive nitrogen balance with the addition of cysteine, which may have been related to the low level of energy provided and the lack of tyrosine in some amino acid solutions (Soghier & Brion, 2010).

A recent meta-analysis compared six studies that were randomized control trials or quasi-randomized trials (Soghier & Brion, 2010). Five studies added cysteine to cysteine-free PN and compared nitrogen balance to those infants not receiving cysteine. The sixth study added N-acetyl-cysteine (cysteine precursor) to a parenteral solution containing a little cysteine. Four of the five studies with the addition of cysteine reported a positive nitrogen balance, which was significant by meta-analysis. The N-acetyl-cysteine additive did not improve nitrogen balance. Growth was only examined by two studies that reported no gains in growth. No studies reported mortality or morbidity information. Four trials examined serum cysteine levels that were significantly elevated as compared to infants not receiving cysteine. More research is needed to explore the effects of parenteral cysteine on infant growth to include changes in weight, length, head circumference, body composition, and bone mineralization (Soghier & Brion, 2010). The addition of cysteine hydrochloride increases the acidity of the parenteral solutions and permits more calcium and phosphorus to be added without precipitation of the minerals occurring (Poindexter & Denne, 2011; Schanler & Anderson, 2008; Soghier & Brion, 2010). The addition of the cysteine hydrochloride may result in metabolic acidosis in the infant, and acetate may be added to the parenteral solution to correct or prevent the acidosis.

ONLINE RESOURCES

American Academy of Pediatrics
http://www.aap.org

Fenton Growth Curve
http://www.ucalvary.ca/fenton

Human Milk Banking Association of North America
http://www.hmbana.org

National Center for Education in Maternal and Child Health
http://www.ncemch.org

Olsen Growth Curve
http://www.nursing.upenn.edu/media/infantgrowthcurves/Documents/Olsen-NewIUGrowthCurves_2010permission.pdf

World Health Organization (WHO) Growth Curve
http://www.cdc.gov/growthcharts/who_charts.htm

REFERENCES

Abbott Nutrition. Our products. (2012). Retrieved from www.abbottnutrition.com/our-products/our-products.aspx

Aimone, A., Rovet, J., Ward, W., Jefferies, A., Campbell, D. M., Asztalos, E., . . . O'Connor, D. L. (2009). Growth and body composition of human milk-fed premature infants provided with extra energy and nutrients early after hospital discharge: 1-year follow-up. *Journal of Pediatric Gastroenterology and Nutrition, 49*, 456–466.

Alsweiler, J. M., Harding, J. E., & Bloomfield, F. H. (2012). Tight glycemic control with insulin in hyperglycemic preterm babies: A randomized controlled trial. *Pediatrics, 129*, 639–647. doi:10.1542/peds.2011–2470

Amaizu, N., Shulman, R. J., Schanler, R. J., & Lau, C. (2008). Maturation of oral feeding skills in preterm infants. *Acta Paediatrica, 97*, 61–67.

American Academy of Pediatrics Committee on Nutrition. (2009a). Nutritional needs of preterm infants. In R. E. Kleinman (Ed.), *Pediatric nutrition handbook* (6th ed., pp. 79–112). Elk Grove Village, IL: Author.

American Academy of Pediatrics Committee on Nutrition. (2009b). Failure to thrive. In R. E. Kleinman (Ed.), *Pediatric nutrition handbook* (6th ed., pp. 601–636). Elk Grove Village, IL: Author.

American Academy of Pediatrics Committee on Nutrition. (2009c). In. R. E. Kleinman (Ed.), *Pediatric nutrition handbook*. (6th ed., pp. 1199–1200). Elk Grove Village, IL: Author [Appendix C. Table C-1 Representative values for constituents of human milk].

Anderson, D. M. (2012). Nutrition for premature infants. In P. Q. Samour & K. King (Eds.), *Pediatric nutrition* (4th ed., pp. 53–69). Sunbury, MA: Jones & Bartlett Learning.

Baker, R. D., Greer, F. R., & American Academy of Pediatrics Committee on Nutrition. (2010). Diagnosis and prevention of iron deficiency and iron-deficiency anemia in infants and young children (0-3 years of age). *Pediatrics, 126*, 1040–1050. doi:10.1542/peds.2010-2576

Beardsall, K., Vanhaesebrouck, S., Ogilvy-Stuart, A. L., Vanhol, C., Palmer, C. R., van Weissenbruch, M., . . . Dunger, D. B. (2008). Early insulin therapy in very-low-birth-weight infants. *New England Journal of Medicine, 359*, 1873–1884.

Berseth, C. L. (1992). Effect of early feeding on maturation of the preterm infant's small intestine. *Journal of Pediatrics, 120*, 947–953.

Berseth, C. L. (2004). Growth, efficacy, and safety of feeding an iron-fortified human milk fortifier. *Pediatrics, 114*, e699–e706. doi:10.1542/peds.2004-0911

Bhatia, J. (2006). Fluid and electrolyte management in the very low birth weight neonate. *Journal of Perinatology, 26*, S19–S21. doi:10.1038/sj.jp.7211466

Bhatia, J., Greer, F., & American Academy of Pediatrics Committee on Nutrition. (2008). Use of soy protein-based formulas in infant feeding. *Pediatrics, 121*, 1062–1068. doi:10.1542/peds.2008-0564

Blanco, C. L., Falck, A., Green, B. K., Cornell, J. E., & Gong, A. K. (2008). Metabolic responses to early and high protein supplementation in a randomized trial evaluating the prevention of hyperkalemia in extremely low birth weight infants. *Journal of Pediatrics, 153*, 535–540. doi:1016/j.peds.2008.04.059

Bombell, S., & McGuire, W. (2009). Early trophic feeding for very low birth weight infants. *Cochrane Database of Systematic Reviews (1), CD000504*. doi:10.1002/14651858.CD00054.pub3

Carlson, S. J. (2009). Parenteral nutrition. In S. Groh-Wargo, M. Thompson & J. H. Cox (Eds.), *ADA pocket guide to neonatal nutrition* (pp. 29–63). Chicago, IL: American Dietetic Association.

Carver, J. D., Wu, P. Y. K., Hall, R. T., Ziegler E. E., Sosa, R., Jacobs, J., . . . Lloyd, B. (2001). Growth of preterm infants fed nutrient-enriched or term formula after hospital discharge. *Pediatrics, 107*, 683–689.

Davey, A. M., Wagner, C. L., Cox, C., & Kendig, J.W. (1994). Feeding premature infants while low umbilical artery catheters are in place: A prospective, randomized trial. *Journal of Pediatrics, 124*, 795–799.

Dell, K. R. (2011). Fluid, electrolytes, and acid–base homeostasis. In R. J. Martin, A. A. Fanaroff, & M. C. Walsh (Eds.), *Neonatal-perinatal medicine: Diseases of the fetus and infant* (9th ed., vol. 1., pp. 669–684). St. Louis, MO: Elsevier.

Denne, S. C., & Poindexter, B. B. (2007). Evidence supporting early nutritional support with parenteral amino acid infusion. *Seminars in Perinatology, 31*, 56–60. doi:10.1053/j.semperi.2007.02.225

Dunn, L., Hulman, S., Weiner, J., & Kliegman, R. (1988). Beneficial effects of early hypocaloric enteral feeding on neonatal gastrointestinal function: Preliminary report of a randomized trial. *Journal of Pediatrics, 112*, 622–629.

Ehrenkranz, R. A. (2010). Early nutritional support and outcomes in ELBW infants. *Early Human Development, 86*, S21–S25. doi:10.1016/j.earlhumdev.2010.01.014

Ehrenkranz, R. A., Dusick, A. M., Vohr, B. R., Wright, L. L., Wrage, L. A., & Poole, W. K. (2006). Growth in the neonatal intensive care unit influences neurodevelopmental and growth outcomes of extremely low birth weight infants. *Pediatrics, 117*, 1253–1261. doi:0.1542/peds.2005-1368

Eidelman, A. I., Schanler, R. J., & American Academy of Pediatrics Section on Breastfeeding. (2012). Breastfeeding and the use of human milk. *Pediatrics, 129*, e827–e841. doi:10.1542/peds.2011-3552

Fenton, T. R., & Kim, J.H. (2013). A systematic review and meta-analysis to revise the Fenton growth chart for preterm infants. *BMC Pediatrics,* 13, 59. Retrieved http://www.biomedcentral.com/1471-2431/13/59

Field, D. G., & Hillemeir, A. C. (2011). Fetal and neonatal intestinal motility. In R. A. Polin, W. W. Fox, & S. H. Abman (Eds.), *Fetal and neonatal physiology* (4th ed., pp. 1226–1229)G5, Philadelphia, PA: Elsevier.

Gerber Good Start Formulas for Premature Infants. (2012, April 30). Gerber Handout PIFNRCO412 (2012 Nestle).

Greer, F. R. (2006). Vitamins. In P. J. Thureen & W. W. Hays (Eds.), *Neonatal nutrition and metabolism* (2nd ed., pp. 161–184). New York, NY: Cambridge University Press.

Grummer-Strawn, L. M., Reinold, C., & Krebs, N. F. (2010). Use of World Health Organization and CDC growth charts for children aged 0-59 months in the U.S. *Morbidity and Mortality Weekly Report, 59*(RR-9), 1–15. www.cdc.gov/mmwr

Gura, K. M. (2010). Potential benefits of parenteral fish oil lipid emulsions in parenteral nutrition-associated liver disease. *ICAN: Infant, Child, & Adolescent Nutrition, 2*, 251–257. doi:10.1177/1941406410376239

Hay, W. W. (2008). Strategies for feeding the preterm infant. *Neonatology, 94*, 245–254. doi:10.1159/000151643

Heird, W. C., Driscoll, J. M., Schullinger, J. N., Grebin, B., & Winters, R. W. (1972). Intravenous alimentation in pediatric patients. *Journal of Pediatrics, 80*, 351–372.

Institute of Medicine. (2010, November). *Dietary reference intakes for calcium and vitamin D*. Report Brief. Retrieved from www.iom.edu/vitamind

Kalhan, S. C., & Devaskar, S. U. (2011). Disorders of carbohydrate metabolism. In R. J. Martin, A. A. Fanaroff, & M. C. Walsh (Eds.), *Neonatal-perinatal medicine: Diseases of the fetus and infant* (9th ed., Vol. 2., pp. 1497–1523). St. Louis, MO: Elsevier.

Koo, W. W. K., & Hockman, E. M. (2006). Posthospital discharge feeding for preterm infants: Effects of standard compared with enriched milk formula on growth, bone mass, and body composition. *American Journal of Clinical Nutrition, 84*, 1357–1364.

Lucas, A., Fewtrell, M. S., Morley, R., Singhal, A., Abbott, R. A., Isaacs, E., . . . Clements, H. (2001). Randomized trial of nutrient-enriched formula versus standard formula for postdischarge preterm infants. *Pediatrics, 108*, 703–711. doi:10.1542/peds.108.3.703

McCallie, K. R., Lee, H. C., Mayer, O., Cohen, R. S., Hintz, S. R., & Rhine, W. D. (2011). Improved outcomes with a standardized feeding protocol for very low birth weight infants. *Journal of Perinatology, 31*, S61–S67.

Mead Johnson Nutrition. (2012). Professional center, product information. Retrieved from www.meadjohnson.com/professional/productinformation

Meetze, W. H., Valentine, C., McGuigan, J. E., Conlon, M., Sacks, N., & Neu, J. (1992). Gastrointestinal priming prior to full enteral nutrition in very low birth weight infants. *Journal of Pediatric Gastroenterology and Nutrition, 15*, 163–170.

Meinzen-Derr, J., Poindexter, B., Wrage, L., Morrow, A., Stoll, B., & Donovan, E. F. (2009). Role of human milk in extremely low birth weight infants' risk of necrotizing enterocolitis or death. *Journal of Perinatology, 29*, 57–62. doi:10.1038/jp.2008.117

Miller, M. J., & Martin, R. J. (2011). Pathophysiology of apnea of prematurity. In R. A. Polin, W. W. Fox, & S. H. Abman (Eds.), *Fetal and neonatal physiology* (4th ed., pp. 998–1011). Philadelphia, PA: Elsevier.

Mitchell, S. M., Rogers, S. P., Hicks, P. D., Hawthorne, K. M., Parker, B. R., & Abrams, S. A. (2009). High frequencies of elevated alkaline phosphatase activity and rickets exist in extremely low birth weight infants despite current nutritional support. *BMC Pediatrics, 9*, 47. doi:10.1186/1471-2431-9-47

Neu, J. (2009). Is it time to stop starving premature infants? *Journal of Perinatology, 29*, 399–400. doi:10.1038/jp.2009.46

Neu, J., & Mshvildadze, M. (2011). Digestive-absorption functions in fetuses. infants, and children. In R. A. Polin, W. W. Fox, & S. H. Abman (Eds.), *Fetal and neonatal physiology* (4th ed., pp. 1240–1249). Philadelphia, PA: Elsevier.

O'Connor, D. L., Khan, S., Weishuhn, K., Vaughan, J., Jefferies, A., Campbell, D. M., . . . Whyte, H. (2008). Growth and nutrient intakes of human milk-fed preterm infants provided with extra energy and nutrients after hospital discharge. *Pediatrics, 121*, 766–776. doi:10.1542/peds.2007-0054

Olsen, I. E., Grovemean, S. A., Lawson, L., Clark, R. H., & Zemel, B. S. (2010). New intrauterine growth curves based on United States data. *Pediatrics, 125*, e214–e224. doi:10.1542/peds.2009-0913

Patole, S. K., & de Klerk, N. (2005). Impact of standardised feeding regimens on incidence of neonatal necrotising enterocolitis: A systematic review and meta-analysis of observational studies. *Archives of Disease in Childhood. Fetal and Neonatal Edition, 90*(2), F147–F151.

Poindexter, B., & Denne, S. (2011). Nutrition and metabolism in the high-risk neonate. In R. J. Martin, A. A. Fanaroff, & M. C. Walsh (Eds.), *Neonatal-perinatal medicine: Diseases of the fetus and infant* (9th ed., Vol. 1., pp. 643–668). St. Louis, MO: Elsevier.

Poindexter, B., Langer, J. C., Dusick, A. M., & Ehrenkranz, R. A. (2006). Early provision of parenteral amino acids in extremely low birth weight infants: Relation to growth and neurodevelopmental outcome. *Journal of Pediatrics, 148*, 300–305.

Radmacher, P. G., Lewis, S. L., & Adamkin, D. H. (2009). Early amino acids and the metabolic response of ELBW infants (≤1000 g) in three time periods. *Journal of Perinatology, 29*, 433–437. doi:10.1038/jp.2009.36

Rayyis, S. F., Ambalavanan, N., Wright, L., & Carlo, W. A. (1999). Randomized trial of "slow" versus "fast" feed advancements on the incidence of necrotizing enterocolitis in very low birth weight infants. *Journal of Pediatrics, 134*, 293–297.

Ridout, E., Mclara, D., Rottinghaus, S., & Thureen, P. J. (2005). Blood urea nitrogen concentration as a marker of amino-acid intolerance in neonates with birth weight less than 1250 g. *Journal of Perinatology, 25*, 130–133. doi:10.1038/sj.jp.72111215

Rogers, S. P., Hicks, P. D., Hamzo, M., Veit, L. E., & Abrams, S. A. (2010). Continuous feedings of fortified human milk lead to nutrient losses of fat, calcium and phosphorous. *Nutrients, 2*, 230–240. doi:10.3390/nu2030240

Sapsford, A. (2009). Enteral nutrition. In S. Groh-Wargo, M. Thompson, & J. H. Cox (Eds.), *ADA pocket guide to neonatal nutrition* (pp. 64–103). Chicago, IL: American Dietetic Association.

Schanler, R. J., & Anderson, D. M. (2008). Nutrition support of the low birth weight infant. In C. Duggan, J. B. Watkins & W. A. Walker (Eds.), *Nutrition in pediatrics* (4th ed., pp. 377–394). Hamilton, ON: BC Decker, Inc.

Schanler, R. J., Shulman, R. J., & Lau, C. (1999). Feeding strategies for premature infants: Beneficial outcomes of feeding fortified human milk versus preterm formula. *Pediatrics, 103*, 1150–1157.

Shulman, R. J. (1989). Zinc and copper balance studies in infants receiving total parenteral nutrition. *American Journal of Clinical Nutrition, 49*, 879–883.

Shulman, R. J., Ou, C. N., & Smith, E. O. (2011). Evaluation of potential factors predicting attainment of full gavage feedings in preterm infants. *Neonatology, 99*, 38–44. doi:10.1159/000302020

Shulman, R. J., & Phillips, S. (2003). Parenteral nutrition in infants and children. *Journal of Pediatric Gastroenterology and Nutrition, 36*, 587–607.

Shulman, R. J., Schanler, R. J., Lau, C., Heitkemper, M., Ou, C-N., & Smith, E. O. (1998a). Early feeding, feeding tolerance, and lactase activity in preterm infants. *Journal of Pediatrics, 133*, 645–649.

Shulman, R. J., Schanler, R. J., Lau, C., Heitkemper, M., Ou, C-N., & Smith, E.O. (1998b). Early feeding, antenatal glucocorticoids, and human milk decrease intestinal permeability in preterm infants. *Pediatric Research, 44*, 519–523. doi:10.1203/00006450-199810000-00009

Sisk, P. M., Lovelady, C. A., Dillard, R. G., Gruber, K. J., & O'Shea, T. M. (2007). Early human milk feeding is associated with a lower risk of necrotizing enterocolitis in very low birth weight infant. *Journal of Perinatology, 27*, 428–433. doi:10.1038/sj.jp.7211758

Soghier, L. M., & Brion, L. P. (2010). Cysteine, cystine or N-acetylcysteine supplementation in parenterally fed neonates. *Cochrane Database of Systematic Reviews, (4), CD004869.* doi:10.1002/14651858.CD004869.pub2

Stephens, B. E., Walden, R. V., Gargus, R. A., Tucker, R., McKinley, L., Mance, M., . . . Vohr, B. R. (2009). First-week protein and energy intakes are associated with 18-month developmental outcomes in extremely low birth weight infants. *Pediatrics, 123*, 1337–1343. doi:10.1542/peds.2008-0211

Sullivan, S., Schanler, R. J., Kim, J. H., Patel, A. L., Trawoger, R., Kiechi-Kohlendorfer, U., . . . Lucas, A. (2010). An exclusively human milk-based diet is associated with a lower rate of necrotizing enterocolitis than a diet of human milk and bovine milk-based products. *Journal of Pediatrics, 156*, 562–567.

Thureen, P. J., Melara, D., Fennessey, P. V., & Hay, W. W. (2003). Effect of low *versus* high intravenous amino acid intake on very low birth weight infants in the early neonatal period. *Pediatric Research, 53*, 24–32. doi:10.1203/01.PDR.0000042441.34920.77

Tsang, R.C., Uauy, R., Koletzko, B., Zlotkin, S.H. (eds.). (2005). *Nutrition of the preterm infant: Scientific basis and practical guidelines*. (pp. 417–418). Cincinnati, OH: Digital Educational Publishing.

Valentine, C. J., Fernandez, S., Rogers, L. K., Gulati, P., Hayes, J., Lore, P., . . . Welty, S. E. (2009). Early amino-acid administration improves preterm infant weight. *Journal of Perinatology, 29*, 428–432. doi:10.1038/jp.2009.51

Vohr, B. R., Poindexter, B. B., Dusick A. M., McKinley, L. T., Higgins, R. D., Langer, J. C., & Poole, W. K. (2007). Persistent beneficial effects of breast milk ingested in the neonatal intensive care unit on outcomes of extremely low birth weight infants at 30 months of age. *Pediatrics, 120*, e953–e959. doi:10.1542/peds.2006-3227

Wilker, R. E. (2012). Hypoglycemia and hyperglycemia. In J. P. Cloherty, E. C. Eichenwald, A. R. Hansen, & A. R. Stark. *Manual of neonatal care* (7th ed., pp. 284–296). Philadelphia, PA: Wolters Kluwer/Lippincott Williams & Wilkins.

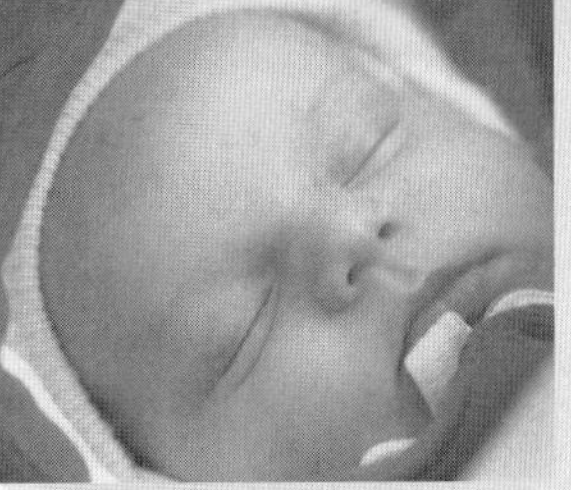

CHAPTER

21

Neonatal and Infant Pharmacology

■ Beth Shields

Neonatal and infant pharmacology requires an understanding of the impact of immature organ systems on pharmacologic drug response. Research in pharmacology has lagged behind the enhanced survival rates for sick newborn infants of all birth-weight subgroups. Optimal understanding of infant pharmacology is of vital importance, as the average number of drugs administered to premature infants weighing less than 1,000 g ranges from 15 to 20. Few well-controlled trials or road maps outline the use of medications in this high-risk patient population (Clark, Bloom, Spitzer, & Gerstmann, 2006; Raj, 2005). This chapter reviews the basic principles of neonatal and infant drug therapy. Discussion of the nursing implications is included.

DRUG THERAPY: EVIDENCE-BASED MEDICINE

The individualization of drug therapy in premature and term infants is essential because of rapid and variable maturation of all physiologic and pharmacologic processes. The phrase *therapeutic orphans*, coined more than 25 years ago, stresses the relative lack of drug safety and efficacy information in the pediatric population (Shirkey, 1968). Thirty years later, published literature on the use of medications in the pediatric population remains sparse. Conducting well-controlled trials is difficult, and therapeutic regimens are often supported by case reports, small studies, or past experiences of a particular clinician (Bell, 2010; Committee on Drugs, 2010; Golec, 2009). Advances in clinical medicine, study design, sampling techniques, and analytical techniques are accelerating the move to the concept of therapeutic orphans in a more historical perspective (Reed, 2011).

PEDIATRIC LABELING

The Food and Drug Administration (FDA) approved the initial labeling of a medication. Since the early 1970s, over 75% of medications were approved with no pediatric indications. However, once a drug is FDA approved, it may be prescribed by a licensed provider for any indication deemed appropriate. Most infants in the neonatal intensive care unit (NICU) are prescribed at least one medication that is used off-label, that is the use of a medication in any age group for a condition which is not included in the medical labeling (Bell, 2010; Kumar et al., 2008). Over the past several years, legislation has been passed to encourage the collection of safety, pharmacogenomic, pharmacokinetic, and pharmacodynamic data to aid in pediatric-specific labeling for medications. The Best Pharmaceuticals for Children Act and the Pediatric Research Equity Act are important pieces of legislation with an emphasis on therapeutic areas and specific pediatric subpopulations. The strongest incentive of these acts is a 6-month patent exclusivity awarded to a product if pediatric labeling is obtained (Bell, 2010; Clark et al., 2006). A list of drugs with a current exclusivity provision is outlined in the Pediatric Exclusivity Provision Best Pharmaceuticals Act for Children Priority List of Needs in Pediatric Pharmacotherapeutics, 2011, http://www.accessdata.fda.gov.

PEDIATRIC DOSING METHODS

Infants are not small adults and, as such, cannot simply be given a portion of an adult dose. Drug dosages must be prescribed for each infant on an individual basis. Their unique pharmacotherapeutic requirements predispose this population to errors in individual dosage calculations. Guidelines have been developed in an attempt to prevent dosing errors in this diverse patient population (Sentinel Event Alert, 2008; Stavroudis et al., 2010) Several dosing methods have been used to calculate the optimal drug dose for both preterm and full-term infants. Pediatric dosage handbooks employ dosing methods based on age, body weight, and body surface area (BSA) as well as pharmacokinetic dosing (Reed, 2011; Taketomo, Hodding, & Kraus, 2011;

Young & Mangum, 2011). Each method provides only an estimate, and dosages must constantly be reevaluated and adjusted according to clinical efficacy and toxicity. To calculate a drug dosage based on age or body weight, it is important to understand the meaning of terms commonly used in the pediatric population (Table 21.1). Because of ease of calculation, dosing based on weight (mg/kg/dose or mg/kg/d) is the most common method. Weight-based dosing is expressed as a dosage range versus an absolute dose. Dosing based on BSA (body surface area) (mg/m^2/dose) requires both a weight and height to accurately assess an infant's BSA. Lack of appropriate pediatric dosing information makes this method impractical with the exception of steroids and chemotherapeutic agents. Pharmacokinetic dosing is discussed in detail in the following sections.

ADVERSE DRUG EFFECTS

Like the elderly, infants are prone to adverse drug effects (ADEs). An ADE is an injury (both preventable and not preventable) that results from the use of a drug (Clark et al., 2006; Leonard, 2010; Woods, Thomas, Holl, Altman, & Brennan, 2005). Unique drug delivery factors, including individual dosage calculations, preparation of small doses from concentrated commercial solutions, multiple commercial concentrations, and slow IV rates, make neonates more prone to ADEs. Neonates are particularly predisposed to ADEs because of immature metabolic and excretion pathways as well as potential drug exposures during pregnancy, delivery, and lactation. In some instances, medications used for years have recently come into question. For example, acetaminophen with codeine products, commonly prescribed for pain in the postpartum period, have recently been shown to have the potential for central nervous system (CNS) depression and apnea in a cohort of breastfed infants. Such adverse effects may be related to unique metabolic pathways in some mothers (Madadi et al., 2009).

Several classic neonatal ADEs have occurred because of lack of knowledge or forethought regarding developmental differences between neonates and older infants and children. Examples of such ADEs include chloramphenicol-associated gray baby syndrome, neonatal gasping syndrome, and numerous case reports of ADEs caused by absorption of drugs through the skin of newborn infants (Robertson, 2003a, 2003b). The enhanced survival of extremely premature infants must raise awareness concerning the increased risk of serious short- and long-term adverse effects of neonatal drug therapy. Recent data support an increased incidence of neurodevelopmental delay and cerebral palsy in infants treated with high dose systemic dexamethasone in an attempt to decrease the incidence of bronchopulmonary dysplasia (Committee on Fetus and Newborn & American Academy of Pediatrics, 2010; Leonard, 2010).

MEDICATION ERRORS

Medication errors in the neonatal population are an iatrogenic cause of ADEs. Such errors have been noted at a rate three to eight times that published in the adult patient population. Medication errors can occur at any stage of the medication use process. Errors are particularly high risk in the neonatal population due to the need for multiple dosing calculations, immature renal, hepatic and immune pathways, and extended length of stays. Prevention strategies include

TABLE 21.1

PEDIATRIC DRUG DOSING: AGE/WEIGHT TERMINOLOGY

Term	Definition
Gestational age (GA)	By dates: number of weeks from the onset of mother's last menstrual period until birth
	By examination: assessment of gestation (time from conception until birth) by a physical and neuromuscular examination
Low birth weight (LBW)	Birth weight of less than 2,500 g
Very low birth weight (VLBW)	Birth weight of less than 1,500 g
Small for gestational age (SGA)	Birth weight less than 10th percentile for GA
Appropriate for gestational age	Birth weight between age (AGA) 10th and 90th percentile for GA
Large for gestational age (LGA)	Birth weight greater than 90th percentile for GA
Postnatal age (PNA)	Chronologic age (in days) after birth
Postconceptional age (PCA)	GA at birth plus PNA
Preterm infant	Less than 37 completed weeks GA at birth
Full-term infant	38–42 weeks GA at birth
Neonate	0–28 days PNA
Infant	1 month–1 year of age
Child	1–12 years of age

Adapted from Committee on Fetus and Newborn, American Academy of Pediatrics (2004).

collaborative efforts of a multidisciplinary health care team, use of computerized physician order entry systems, barcode medication administration, and standardization of doses and medication concentrations (Leonard, 2010; Poole & Carleton, 2008; Sauberan, Dean, Fiedelak, & Abraham, 2009; Sentinel Event Alert, 2008; Simpson & Grant, 2004). The use of standard concentrations is suggested by both the Institute for Safe Medication Practices (ISMP) and the Vermont Oxford Network (VON) for the neonatal patient population http://www.ISMP.org/tools (ISMP Medication Safety Alert, 2007).

In recent years, several overdoses of heparin have gained a great deal of press in the neonatal literature. Heparin is on the Institute for Safe Medication Practices high alert list and can cause considerable patient harm. In addition to the issues outlined above, stocking of look-alike products with 100- or 1,000-fold strength differences has contributed to these errors (Arimura, Poole, Jeng, Rhine, & Sharek, 2008; Leonard, 2010; Monagle, Studdert, & Newall, 2011; Sowan, Vaidya, Soeken, & Hilmas, 2010). Changes in packaging have resulted from the medication errors with heparin in particular. Many institutions now use checklists for medications, requiring two people to review the orders and what is to be administered before the medication is actually given. Medication Administration Records and physician order entry systems now have built-in checks and balances for drug incompatibilities and wrong dosages. A required system override is necessary in order to dispense a drug that is not considered within a safe range. That being said, many institutions have not used these electronic systems yet and systems are only as good as the information that is placed in them.

DEVELOPMENTAL PHARMACOKINETICS

Pharmacokinetics is the study of a drug concentration versus time and encompasses the absorption, distribution, metabolism, and elimination (ADME) of a drug and its metabolites in the body. Developmental pharmacokinetics—or the change in the ADME of drugs with organ maturation—is a well-known phenomenon (Figure 21.1).

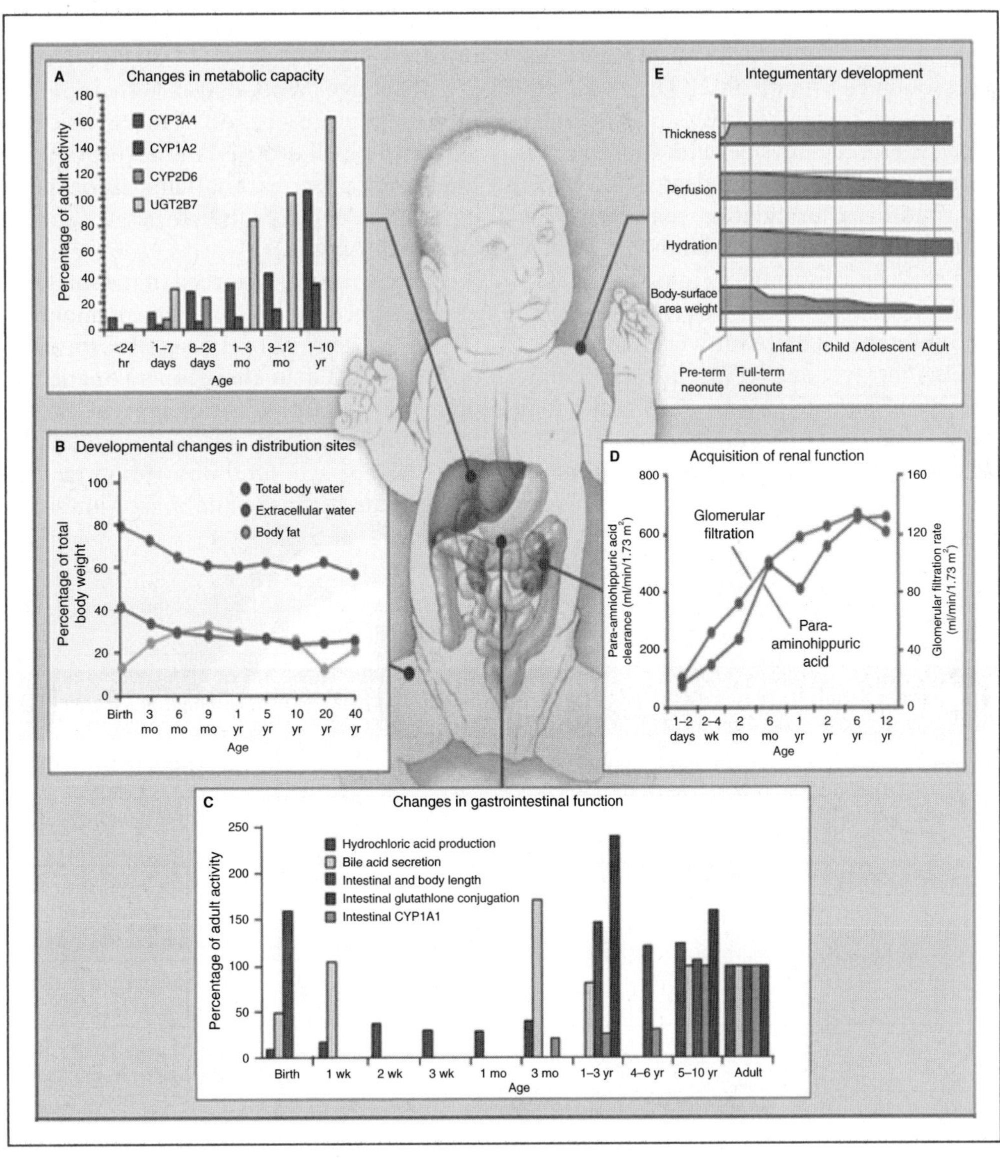

FIGURE 21.1 Age-dependent changes in both the structure and function of the gastrointestinal tract.
Adapted from Kearns (2003).

To fully comprehend the ADME of drugs, pharmacokinetic terminology must be applied. Standard pharmacokinetic terminology is used when describing the ADME of medications (Table 21.2). In addition to the pharmacokinetics of a drug, the pharmacodynamics of a particular medication is also important. Pharmacodynamics is the relationship between the pharmacokinetics of a drug and its therapeutic or toxic effects in a specific patient. Pediatric drug-dosing regimens are influenced by both the effect of the body on a drug (pharmacokinetics) and the effect of a drug on the body (pharmacodynamics). Recent data support age-dependent differences in the interaction of a drug and its receptors, ultimately resulting in an altered pharmacodynamic response (Kearns et al., 2003).

Absorption

Absorption refers to the translocation of a drug from the site of administration into the systemic circulation. With the exception of the intravenous route, all other routes of administration require a drug to cross membranes in order to reach the systemic circulation and exert its pharmacologic effects. Bioavailability is the pharmacokinetic term that has been used to describe the extent to which a drug enters the systemic circulation (Soldin & Soldin, 2002). Drugs administered via the intravenous route are 100% bioavailable. Drug absorption depends on the physiochemical properties of the drug—including molecular weight, degree of ionization, lipid solubility, and drug formulation characteristics. In addition, patient-dependent factors, many of which are age-related, affect drug absorption (Johnson, 2011; Kearns et al., 2003).

Medications are administered to infants via many routes including oral (PO), intravenous (IV), intramuscular (IM), intraosseous (IO), percutaneous, intranasal, and rectal administration. Parenteral administration (IV) of drugs is important when a rapid response is desired or clinical status precludes oral absorption. Muscle tone, muscle mass, and regional blood flow to the area influence absorption of medications from an IM injection. Neonates, particularly premature neonates, may have significantly decreased muscle mass, as muscle mass is directly proportional to an infant's gestational age (GA) (Kearns et al., 2003). The IM injection of a medication may result in a delay in peak serum concentrations due to poor or erratic absorption. Medications commonly administered to neonates via the IM route include vitamin K, ampicillin, and gentamicin.

Absorption from the gastrointestinal tract depends on factors including gastric acidity, gastric emptying time, bacterial colonization of the gastrointestinal tract, intestinal transit time and permeability, and biliary and pancreatic function (Johnson, 2011; Kearns et al., 2003). The maturation of gastric pH differs in preterm versus term infants and seems to correlate with postnatal age rather than postconceptional age. The gastric pH at birth approaches 6 to 8 because of the presence of residual amniotic fluid, falls to approximately 1.5 to 3 several hours after birth, and then slowly increases over the next 10 days in term infants. The lack of gastric acid output early in postnatal life is called relative achlorhydria. Gastric pH will reach adult values by 2 years of age (Woo, 2004). Gastric pH affects drug ionization and drug absorption. A more basic environment (higher gastric pH) will decrease the absorption of acidic drugs (i.e., phenytoin, phenobarbital) and favor the oral absorption of more basic or acid-labile drugs (i.e., ampicillin, penicillin, and erythromycin).

Most drugs are absorbed in the small intestine. Therefore gastric emptying time will play an important role in both the rate and extent of oral drug absorption. Gastric emptying time is delayed in the neonatal patient, especially in the premature infant. Gastric emptying may be prolonged up to 6 to 8 hours and may not attain adult values until 6 to 8 months of age. Oral absorption may also be delayed in the neonate because of decreased intestinal transit time and

TABLE 21.2

PHARMACOKINETIC TERMINOLOGY

Pharmacokinetic Term	Abbreviation	Definition
Bioavailability	F	The extent to which a drug enters the systemic circulation
Volume of distribution	Vd	The relation between the distribution amount of drug in the body and the measured plasma concentration
Clearance	Cl	The ability of eliminating organs to remove a drug from the blood or plasma
Elimination half-life	$t^{1/2s}$	The time required for half the amount of drug present in the blood to disappear
Steady-state concentration	Cpss	A concentration at which the rate of drug administration is equal to the rate of drug elimination

Adapted from Soldin and Soldin (2002).

activity of pancreatic enzymes as well as low concentrations of intraluminal bile acids (Kearns et al., 2003; Woo, 2004).

Percutaneous absorption or absorption through the skin depends on skin integrity, blood flow to the skin, thickness of the epidermal layer (i.e., stratum corneum), skin hydration, and the ratio of surface area per kilogram of body weight (BSA to weight ratio). Percutaneous absorption may be increased substantially in newborn infants because of an underdeveloped stratum corneum, smaller amounts of subcutaneous fat, and increased skin hydration. Maturation of premature skin is related to postnatal age, and the attainment of an epidermal layer similar to that of a full-term neonate occurs within 3 weeks of postnatal life.

The greater the BSA-to-weight ratio, the greater the absorption of a drug is on a per-kilogram basis with topical medications. The ratio of a newborn's skin to BSA is approximately three times that of an adult. Systemic toxicity has been described in neonates after the administration of topical iodine, hexachlorophene, salicylic acid, epinephrine, and corticosteroids (Woo, 2004). The rectal mucosa may serve as a site of drug absorption in neonates who are unable to take medications by mouth, and in whom rapid IV access cannot be achieved. Rectal absorption is dependent on regional blood flow, retention of the drug in the rectum, and chemical properties of the drug. The rectal route of administration results in less efficient absorption when compared to the oral route, and in many instances higher mg/kg doses may be required. Medications commonly administered via the rectal route in infants include acetaminophen, diazepam, chloral hydrate, and sodium polystyrene sulfonate.

Distribution

Once a medication has reached the bloodstream, it will distribute among various organs, fluids, and tissues. The distribution of drugs within the body is influenced by many factors, including total body water, total body fat, plasma and tissue binding, membrane permeability, and the infant's hemodynamic status. The pharmacokinetic term used to describe the relation between the amount of drug in the body and the measured plasma concentration is the apparent volume of distribution (Vd) (Johnson, 2011).

Total body water can be divided into intracellular and extracellular spaces. At birth, a full-term neonate is approximately 80% water, with 45% as extracellular and 35% as intracellular fluid. By 1 year of age a child is approximately 60% water, with 20% extracellular and 40% intracellular fluid (Kearns et al., 2003) (Figure 21.1). Body fat is approximately 1% of the total body composition of a premature infant at 29 weeks GA, increases to approximately 15% at term, and is 25% of total body composition between 1 and 2 years of age. Water-soluble medications have a much higher volume of distribution in neonates than in adults; therefore, neonatal dosing is higher on a per-kilogram basis (i.e., gentamicin, vancomycin). Fat-soluble medications have a much smaller distribution volume in a neonate than in an adult. Neonatal dosing of medications that are fat-soluble is lower on a per-kilogram basis (Kearns et al., 2003; Woo, 2004).

Several physiologic variables can produce both quantitative and qualitative differences in plasma and tissue binding of drugs. In general, neonatal plasma protein binding of drugs is decreased in comparison to adults. The decrease in plasma protein binding in neonates is a result of several factors, including the decreased formation of plasma proteins by the immature neonatal liver. Albumin is the major drug-binding protein in plasma and binds primarily to acidic drugs (i.e., phenobarbital, phenytoin). A lower plasma pH may decrease protein binding of acidic drugs, and the presence of endogenous substances may compete for protein-binding sites. Endogenous substances in the neonate include free fatty acids and bilirubin, as well as transplacentally acquired interfering substances such as hormones and pharmacologic agents. Reduction in protein binding of drugs leads to an increase in the unbound or active component of the drug (Kearns et al., 2003).

Metabolism

Drug metabolism is influenced by genetic factors (pharmacogenomics), age, and the activity of drug-metabolizing enzymes. Most drugs are fat soluble and require biotransformation into more water-soluble substances before elimination from the body. This process of biotransformation occurs mainly in the liver, and produces active as well as inactive metabolites.

The two main types of drug metabolism are phase I (nonsynthetic) and phase II (synthetic) reactions. Phase I reactions include oxidation, reduction, methylation, hydrolysis, and hydroxylation. The cytochrome P450 mixed-function oxidase system is responsible for most phase I reactions. Phase II reactions include conjugation with glycine, glucuronic acid, and sulfate. Phase I reactions appear to mature more rapidly, meeting or exceeding adult capacity by 6 months of age.

Phase II reactions reach adult levels in children by 3 to 4 years of age. Maturation of these enzymatic pathways will affect neonatal metabolism of medications and thereby affect the clinical response to medications (Figure 21.1). Examples of drug toxicity in neonates with immature metabolic pathways include the gray-baby syndrome, caused by decreased capacity to glucuronidate chloramphenicol, as well as neonatal gasping syndrome, which results from the decreased capacity of infants to glycinate benzyl alcohol. Benzyl alcohol is a preservative found in multi-dose medications and flush solutions (Robertson, 2003a).

Neonates may use different pathways to metabolize drugs than older infants and children use. These pathways may result in a modified pharmacologic response to medications. For example, neonates are not able to metabolize morphine adequately to its 6-glucuronide metabolite, a metabolite that is 20 times more active than morphine as an analgesic. Theophylline, a drug used for the treatment of apnea of prematurity, presents another example of altered metabolic pathways. Theophylline is oxidized to inactive components in adults but is N-methylated to caffeine, a pharmacologically active agent in the neonate.

Maturation of hepatic enzymes may also be influenced by prenatal or postnatal exposure to enzyme-inducing (i.e., phenobarbital, phenytoin, rifampin) or enzyme-inhibiting (i.e., cimetidine, erythromycin) agents. One drug may alter the metabolism of another medication, thereby increasing or decreasing effectiveness, creating toxicity, or producing subtherapeutic levels. Drug activity may also be interfered with by concurrent disease states. Interferences such as these are referred to as drug–disease state interactions (Kearns, 2003).

Elimination

Systemic clearance (Cl) is the ability of the eliminating organs (kidney, liver, lung, skin) to remove a drug from the blood or plasma. Drugs and their metabolites are primarily eliminated by the kidneys. The principal renal mechanisms responsible for drug excretion include glomerular filtration, tubular secretion, and tubular reabsorption, all of which are immature at birth. Overall renal function increases with age, although as with hepatic metabolism, the maturation rate of individual physiologic functions varies (Figure 21.1). Glomerular filtration matures several months before tubular secretion; tubular reabsorption is the last to mature. The glomerular filtration is directly proportional to GA after 34 weeks gestation. The increase in glomerular filtration after birth depends on postconceptional age and is influenced by increased cardiac output, decreased peripheral vascular resistance, increased mean arterial pressure, and increased surface area for filtration. The clinical importance of increases in glomerular filtration becomes apparent when one examines drugs excreted primarily by filtration such as gentamicin and vancomycin. Tubular reabsorption and secretion are also decreased in the neonate. Ampicillin, a drug commonly used in the neonatal population, undergoes tubular secretion (Woo, 2004).

The elimination half-life ($t^{1/2}$) of a drug refers to the time it takes for half the amount of drug in the blood to be eliminated. The volume of distribution and clearance of a medication are determinants of a drug's half-life. Half-life is an important factor in determining the appropriate interval between drug doses. Drugs with a long half-life are given at less frequent dosing intervals, whereas those with shorter half-lives may need to be given via a continuous infusion (Johnson, 2011).

With constant drug dosing, the elimination half-life will determine the time to reach the so-called steady-state serum concentration. Steady state refers to the time at which the rate of drug administration equals the rate of drug elimination. When drug concentrations are monitored in clinical practice, steady-state concentrations should be obtained. Steady-state concentrations are reached in approximately five half-lives. This factor explains the rationale for administering a loading dose for medications with long half-lives. A loading dose is a single dose of a medication that is used to rapidly attain a serum concentration and therefore the desired clinical effect. A loading dose produces a higher circulating concentration earlier in the therapeutic course as opposed to waiting five half-lives. In neonates, loading doses are commonly administered for caffeine, phenobarbital, phenytoin, digoxin, and levetiracetam (Johnson, 2011).

THERAPEUTIC DRUG MONITORING

Therapeutic drug monitoring (TDM) is the use of serum drug concentrations and pharmacokinetic and pharmacodynamic principles to regulate drug dosages. TDM is of particular importance in the neonatal population, which may under- or overrespond to the usual dosing regimens. Additional unique considerations in the neonate include the precise delivery of very small doses and volumes of medications, the availability of blood for measurement of drug concentrations, interference of endogenous substances with drug assays, frequent changes in neonatal pharmacokinetic parameters, and the extrapolation of therapeutic serum concentrations from adult data to the neonatal population (Gal, 2009; Johnson, 2011; Touw, Westerman, & Sprij, 2009).

TDM is used for drugs in which a correlation between the measured plasma concentration and drug efficacy or toxicity exists. Drugs with narrow therapeutic indexes are ideal candidates for TDM. A drug exhibits a narrow therapeutic index if the plasma concentration required for therapeutic effects is relatively close to the concentration known to produce toxicity. Drugs for which TDM is used in the neonatal population include caffeine, phenobarbital, phenytoin, levetiracetam, gentamicin, tobramycin, amikacin, vancomycin, and digoxin. TDM allows the clinician to aim for a therapeutic range, which is usually safe and effective, with minimal drug toxicity.

With the exception of drugs administered via a continuous infusion, drug concentrations in the plasma are not static. The time of blood sampling relative to the time of drug administration is of utmost importance. For some medications both trough and peak concentrations are monitored, whereas with other medications it is routine to monitor trough concentrations. Obtaining levels once a patient achieves steady-state concentrations provides the most accurate information with regard to drug efficacy or toxicity. Patients with altered organ function or rapidly changing clinical status may require closer monitoring of serum concentrations than do other patients.

Certain medications such as phenytoin are highly plasma protein-bound. For these medications, two types of assays are available, including total and free serum concentrations. Free levels indicate the amount of free, unbound drug that is available to exert its effects on target tissues. When free phenytoin serum assays are not available, caution must be used in the interpretation of total serum concentrations. Levels may be falsely interpreted as low when the actual amount of active drug is adequate or toxic (Soldin et al., 2003).

FETAL AND INFANT EXPOSURE TO MATERNAL MEDICATIONS

Fetal Exposure

Virtually any medication or substance given to the mother, either intentionally or inadvertently, can cross the placental membrane. The amount of drug that passes into the fetal circulation depends on several factors—including the molecular weight, protein binding, lipid solubility, and ionization of the drug; maternal drug serum concentrations; and integrity of the placental barrier. Physiologic changes during pregnancy can affect absorption, distribution, metabolism, and excretion of medications in the mother. Pregnancy results in many pharmacokinetic changes in the mother, including a greater volume of distribution, additional fat stores, and lower protein binding. Fetal exposure to a medication may lead to deleterious effects on the exposed fetus or may result in minimal or no adverse outcomes.

In recent years, the FDA has worked to collect and include more comprehensive information on drug labels regarding the drug's effects during pregnancy, including revisions to the product labeling. The Pregnancy and Lactation Labeling Rule continues to be under discussion (Pregnancy and lactation labeling, FDA, 2011). Labeling a drug as a teratogen indicates the potential of a medication to produce congenital malformations in an infant. A medication may not be a teratogen but may produce other untoward effects on the infant, such as respiratory depression or sedation, which has been seen with maternal narcotic administration just prior to delivery. Drug companies have been required since 1983 to assign each medication a pregnancy risk category (Table 21.3) (Demler, 2011; St Onge & Motycka, 2004). In recent years, there has been the suggestion to eliminate the current pregnancy categories A, B, C, D, and X due to their limited ability to convey risk and benefits of therapy during pregnancy. A new manner of categorizing pregnancy risk labeling has been proposed (Box 21.1).

Lactation Exposure

An often-overlooked source of exposure to medications is transfer from the maternal circulation into breast milk. The safety and potential risks to the nursing infant must be considered during maternal drug use. Maternal drug use includes over-the-counter drugs, prescription drugs, illicit drugs, and herbal products. The pH and size of a drug molecule, protein-binding properties, lipid and water solubility, and diffusion rate will all influence the quantity of drug that passes from maternal serum into breast milk. Additional considerations include the time the medication is taken in relation to the period of nursing, the dose and frequency of a medication, the pharmacokinetics of the drug, the length of nursing, and the amount of milk ingested. Published literature outlines guidelines regarding the transfer of drugs and chemicals into human milk. Only a small number of medications, including radiopharmaceuticals and chemotherapeutic medications, are considered contraindicated in the breastfeeding infant (American Academy of Pediatrics, 2005). In addition, websites are available that provide the most recent information on newer drugs and breastfeeding (Hale, 2011).

TABLE 21.3

CURRENT PREGNANCY RISK CATEGORIES

Category	Description
A	Adequate, well-controlled studies in pregnant women have not shown an increased risk of fetal abnormalities.
B	Animal studies have revealed no evidence of harm to the fetus; however, there are no adequate and well-controlled studies in pregnant women. Or, animal studies have shown an adverse effect, but adequate and well-controlled studies in pregnant women have failed to demonstrate a risk to the fetus.
C	Animal studies have shown an adverse effect, or no animal studies have been conducted, and there are no adequate and well-controlled studies in pregnant women.
D	Adequate, well-controlled, or observational studies in pregnant women have demonstrated a risk to the fetus. However, the benefits of therapy may outweigh the potential risk.
X	Adequate, well-controlled, or observational studies in animals or pregnant women have demonstrated positive evidence of fetal abnormalities. The use of the product is contraindicated in women who are or may become pregnant.

Adapted from Demler (2011).

BOX 21.1

PROPOSED PREGNANCY RISK CATEGORIES

Category Description

Fetal Risk Summary

This summary would begin with a risk conclusion statement that characterizes the likelihood that the drug increases the risk of four types of developmental abnormalities: structural anomalies, fetal and infant mortality, impaired physiologic function, and alternations to growth. The standardized statement would include whether it was based on animal or human data. For example: "Human data do not indicate that Drug X increases the overall risk of structural anomalies." More than one risk conclusion may be needed to characterize the likelihood of risk for different developmental abnormalities, doses, durations of exposure, or gestational ages at exposure.

For human data, the risk conclusion must also be followed by a paragraph describing the most important data about the effects of the drug on the fetus, such as the specific developmental abnormality (e.g., neural tube defects); the incidence, seriousness, reversibility, and correct ability of the abnormality; and the effect on the risk of dose, duration of exposure, and gestational timing of exposure.

Clinical Considerations

This component would address three main topics that are important when counseling with, and prescribing for, women who are pregnant, lactating, or of childbearing age: inadvertent drug exposure to the fetus during early pregnancy, prescribing decisions for pregnant women, and drug effects during labor or delivery.

Data

This section would have a more detailed discussion of available data, with human data appearing before animal data.

Adapted from Demler (2011).

MEDICATION ADMINISTRATION

Once an appropriate drug dosage is established, the optimal route and method of drug administration are also of utmost importance. Many commercially available dosage forms are not suitable for use in the pediatric patient population. Developmental considerations with regard to medication administration must also be considered.

Oral Administration

Many drugs prescribed for infants and children are not available in oral dosage forms that can be easily administered to small infants and children. Oral medications are administered to an infant via a nipple, dropper, syringe, or feeding tube. The preferred dosage form for infants is an alcohol-free, sugar-free, dye-free, and low-osmolality liquid preparation. However, orally administered medications may only be commercially available as tablets or capsules or as concentrated oral solutions or suspensions. High-osmolality substances administered to the neonate have been associated with many adverse effects, including the development of necrotizing enterocolitis and decreased intestinal transit time.

Preparation and delivery of small therapeutic doses from concentrated commercial oral solutions may be difficult. Alteration (dilution or compounding) of an adult dosage form raises issues regarding compatibility, stability, and the risk for medication errors. Commonly prescribed oral medications that are not commercially available in an appropriate liquid formulation include hydrocortisone, captopril, enalapril, and spironolactone. Oral medications may also contain silent or inactive ingredients that supply the "delivery system" of the drug or serve to flavor, sweeten, and preserve the drug. Such inert ingredients may be harmless in adults but may, when administered frequently to neonates, result in toxicity (Mennella & Beauchamp, 2008; Robertson, 2003b).

Intravenous Administration

The most effective means of rapid drug delivery in a critically ill neonate is IV administration. As with oral medications, small doses and delivery volumes complicate the delivery of IV medications. Furthermore, IV medication delivery is often delayed, prolonged, or incomplete in the neonatal patient. A distal drug delivery site, and slow infusion rates delay intravenous drug delivery. A major impact of delayed drug delivery is the potential for subtherapeutic plasma concentrations or even clinical failure with some medications. This is particularly important for medications that may require TDM (El-Chaar, 2003). In addition, touch contamination, wrong delivery route or method in the extremely vulnerable premature infants makes the use of closed IV systems of utmost importance. Central-line bundle initiatives have been instituted in many institutions in an effort to reduce central-line-associated bloodstream infections (CLABSI) (Douma, 2010).

Several techniques are currently used to administer parenteral medications in the neonatal population and include IV push, intramuscular, and use of smart infusion pumps. The infusion device, IV tubing, a container holding the medication (i.e., syringe, IV bag), dead space at injection ports, and IV in-line filters will affect drug delivery. Patient-specific factors such as body position and vascular occlusion may also affect IV drug delivery (Harding, 2011; Larsen, Parker, Cash, O'Connell, & Grant, 2005).

Administration of medications using the IV push method allows rapid drug delivery but is not appropriate for many medications. Drug delivery with a smart IV infusion pump and microbore tubing is the preferred method of IV drug administration in the neonatal population. A syringe pump allows absolute control over the rate of drug delivery with minimal IV fluid volume, at a rate that is independent of the primary IV rate. Microbore tubing allows the use of minimal volumes of flush solution. In addition to intermittent medications, continuous infusion medications such as pressors and inotropes may be administered via a syringe pump. Recently, "smart pump" technology has become available. Smart pumps incorporate computer technology, allowing the use of drug libraries, standard drug concentrations, and sophisticated checks, including soft- and hard-dosing limits. A potential disadvantage of syringe pumps, in particular the smart pumps, is the capital expense required to purchase the pump (Harding, 2011; Larsen et al., 2005).

Many of the problems that plague commercially available oral medications can also be found in commercial IV medications. IV medications may be available in concentrations that prohibit accurate measurement and administration of small neonatal doses. In selection of parenteral medications, not only drug concentration but also preservatives and other ingredients in the parenteral preparation are factors. Benzyl alcohol is a common preservative added to parenteral drug products. Severe toxicity has been reported in neonates after the use of flush solutions that contain benzyl alcohol. Whenever possible; preservative-free parenteral products should be used in the neonatal population for the first 2 months of life.

The osmolality of a drug solution is an important delivery factor. Tissue irritation or pain at the injection site can occur when a drug solution with an osmolality significantly different from that of the serum (275–295 mOsm/kg) is administered intravenously. As a point of reference, the osmolarity of dextrose 10% in water, an IV solution used commonly in the newborn infant, is 505 mOsm/kg. Infiltration of a hypotonic or hypertonic solution can cause trauma and necrosis of the injection site (Association of Women's Health, Obstetric and Neonatal Nurses [AWHONN], 2007; Ramasethu, 2004).

Premature infants typically have fluid restrictions as well as limited intravenous access, and the question of IV drug compatibilities often comes into play. Drug compatibility involves the question of both physical (visual) and chemical (nonvisual) compatibilities. IV drug compatibility is not clear-cut. This is true because of the influence of alterations in drug concentration, order of drug infusion, pH, and temperature. For these reasons, reference books and articles may provide conflicting information with regard to drug compatibilities. Two drugs are physically incompatible when turbidity, cloudiness, or a precipitate is formed after two or more drugs are mixed together. A physical incompatibility results when calcium gluconate and sodium bicarbonate–containing or phosphorus-containing solutions are mixed in the same IV solution or IV tubing. Chemical incompatibility implies a loss of potency or formation of a toxic byproduct when two or more substances are mixed. Epinephrine and sodium bicarbonate are chemically incompatible when co-infused (Taketomo et al., 2011; Trissel, 2010; Young & Mangum, 2011).

Extravasation and infiltration are used interchangeably in the literature; both terms reflect a leakage of IV fluid or medication out of a vein and into surrounding tissues (Ramasethu, 2004; Thigpen, 2007). Extravasation in neonates with circulatory compromise can lead to significant morbidity, functional impairment, or cosmetic defects. Many medications (i.e., potassium, calcium, parenteral nutrition, and dopamine) that are incorporated into the drug regimens of patients in the NICU are capable of causing tissue damage if extravasation occurs. The use of small or superficial venous access sites in areas that are difficult to immobilize should be avoided for administration of these agents unless absolutely necessary. Particularly tenuous sites include areas surrounding tendons, nerves, or arteries or near the face and forehead (AWHONN, 2007). The degree of cellular injury is often directly related to the physiochemical characteristics of the infusant—including osmolarity, pH, molecular weight, volume and location, and mechanical compression due to trapped fluid in tissues.

The treatment of extravasation injuries that result from infiltration of medications and IV solutions is controversial. Many infiltrates resolve spontaneously following the removal of the IV catheter. Treatment involves the use of specific antidotes and may be based on the staging of the infiltrate. Three possible antidotes—hyaluronidase, phentolamine, and topical nitroglycerin paste—have been studied most extensively in the neonatal population. The mechanism by which IV fluids and medications cause tissue necrosis varies, and optimal treatment choices vary with each extravasated agent (AWHONN, 2007; Ramasethu, 2004; Taketomo et al., 2011; Thigpen, 2007) (Table 21.4).

Intraosseous Administration

Intraosseous placement, medication administration directly into the marrow of a bone, may be a viable

TABLE 21.4

EXTRAVASATION TREATMENT

Extravasated Drug/Fluid	Treatment
Parenteral nutrition	Topical nitroglycerin, hyaluronidase
Calcium	Topical nitroglycerin, hyaluronidase
Dopamine	Phentolamine, topical nitroglycerin
Dobutamine	Phentolamine
Epinephrine	Phentolamine

Adapted from Ramasethu (2004).

alternative for parenteral drug delivery in neonates. This route of administration may be considered when IV access cannot be readily obtained. Use of intraosseous access is widely accepted in the pediatric population during resuscitation efforts. A recent study examined the use of intraosseous medication administration as opposed to umbilical venous cannulation (UVC) in a simulated neonatal resuscitation in the delivery room. Intraosseous access was faster and was not perceived as more technically difficult in this simulated trial. Intraosseous medication administration may be a viable alternative to UVC placement in certain neonatal resuscitations (Rajani, Chitkara, Oehlert, & Halamek, 2011).

Intranasal Administration

Intranasal delivery allows use of the highly vascularized nasal mucosa and olfactory tissue to facilitate the rapid transport of specific medications into the bloodstream and brain. The onset of intransal administration approaches that of parenteral medication delivery. In addition to the ease of administration, the fact that no needlestick is involved makes this an attractive medication delivery modality. Key factors to the intransal administration of medications include the use of both nares to increase available surface area for drug absorption and the use of concentrated medications (Wolfe & Braude, 2010).

Aerosol Administration

The use of aerosolized medications in the neonatal setting has increased with the resurgence of bronchopulmonary dysplasia, and the increased prevalence of pulmonary hypertension. The rationale for aerosol medication delivery includes direct delivery to the target organ (lungs) with decreased systemic adverse drug effects. A classic example of a medication with a myriad of systemic side effects is furosemide. Side effects including electrolyte imbalances, metabolic alkalosis, hearing loss, and nephrocalcinosis may be mitigated with the use of aerosolized furosemide, although the efficacy is still debatable (Sahni & Phelps, 2011).

Overall, the therapeutic efficacy of aerosolized medications is dependent on the delivery of an adequate dose of medication to the target sites within the lung. The primary factors that influence lung deposition include particle size, mode of assisted ventilation, inhaler device and placement, and age of the infant. The available methods to aerosolize medications in the neonate include nebulization either intermittently or continuously or a metered-dose inhaler (MDI) with a spacing device. Studies have revealed conflicting results with regard to the optimal method and efficacy of aerosol drug delivery in the neonate, including systems for mechanically ventilated infants. Those infants on oscillatory ventilation present further unique medication delivery challenges (Mazela & Polin, 2011).

Medication Administration in Extracorporeal Membrane Oxygenation

Extracorporeal membrane oxygenation (ECMO) is a highly technical and invasive technique used to treat cardiorespiratory failure when conventional means and technologies fail. ECMO is used for a variety of indications in the neonatal population, including those with persistent pulmonary hypertension, meconium aspiration, sepsis, respiratory distress syndrome, pneumonia, congenital diaphragmatic hernia, and in postoperative congenital heart disease patients. Patients who undergo ECMO receive on average more than 10 different medications, including antibiotics, sedatives, analgesics, inotropes, diuretics, antiepileptics, and medications that are used to maintain the ECMO circuit. Varying pharmacokinetics may be observed, depending on the actual site of injection. There is substantial variability between individual circuits. In general, larger volumes of distribution and decreased drug clearance are observed.

Medications may be administered to ECMO patients either into the ECMO circuit before or after the filter or directly into the patient. Distribution and delivery of medication are more consistent when drugs are injected after the filter. Administration into this site places the patient at risk for development of air emboli, and administration of medications should be done with great caution. Medications injected directly into the reservoir or before the filter usually result in a prolonged time of actual drug delivery to the patient and incomplete drug administration. A large part of the ECMO circuit consists of disposable polyvinyl chloride or silicone tubing of varying length, oxygenators, and centrifugal pumps. The amounts of tubing and other components contribute to a large surface area with the potential for drug binding, particularly for highly lipophilic medications. Therefore increased doses may be required initially when these medications are used or when the circuit is changed or primed with blood or crystalloid during ECMO therapy (Mehta, Halwick, Dodson, Thompson, & Arnold, 2007; Wildschut, Allegaert, Ahsman, Mathot, & Tibboel, 2010).

Interpretation of pharmacokinetic parameters in this type of patient is often difficult because of the influences of the site of injection, flow rate of the ECMO circuit, and clinical status and organ function of the patient. Gentamicin and vancomycin are two antibiotics that are commonly administered to infants on ECMO. Pharmacokinetics for these agents vary, not only with the ECMO circuit but also with the clinical status of the infant—including altered renal function in a sick infant. In addition, pharmacokinetics was found to vary with the infant's GA, postnatal age, and weight. Peak effect for these patients is often delayed, thus resulting in false interpretation of serum peak levels for aminoglycoside antibiotics (Mehta et al., 2007; Wildschut et al., 2010).

MEDICATION SHORTAGES

In 2011, the White House focused legislation to curb drug shortages of life-sustaining or supporting medications. Such medications are those whose discontinuation could have life-threatening consequences, including medications used to treat specific neonatal conditions. The focus of drug shortages also targets those drug companies that voluntarily choose to discontinue a medication which then may lead to a national drug shortage. Companies are to notify the FDA 6 months in advance of their intent to discontinue production of such a medication. The neonatal population has seen the impact of such national shortages over the past several years. Parenteral electrolytes including sodium, potassium, and calcium salts have led to restricted use of such agents based on availability. In addition, restrictions in parenteral nutrition solutions of essential trace elements and multivitamins may have long-term consequences for the growth and development of infants. Some institutions find themselves with a shortage of parenteral vitamin K, an agent used routinely to prevent hemorrhagic disease of the newborn (Traynor, 2011; Ventola, 2011).

SUMMARY

The individualization of drug therapy is critical in the neonatal population. The neonatal population presents a unique challenge with regard to both medication dosing and administration. Drug dosing on an mg/kg basis is the most common method because of the ease of calculation. A lack of large, well-controlled trials in this unique patient population results in drug dosing based on extrapolation from the adult literature or anecdotal experience. Furthermore, developmental pharmacokinetics—or the change in ADME of drugs—creates a population whose drug dosing is constantly changing. Once an appropriate dosing regimen is determined, the optimal drug administration technique is equally important to avoid iatrogenic adverse medication events.

CASE STUDY

■ Identification of the Problem. Term male infant born vaginally at 39 weeks GA (3.87 kg) to a mother with no prenatal care and with maternal fever.

■ Assessment: History and Physical Examination. The term male infant was delivered vaginally to a 21-year-old G2 P1 woman who reported to the emergency department with complaints of abdominal pain. There was maternal fever and suspicion of chorioamnionitis. The mother reports daily marijuana use and no prenatal care as she did not know she was pregnant. Due to the precipitous nature of the delivery in the emergency department, the mother did not receive any antibiotics prior to delivery. Upon delivery, the infant was intubated and suctioned for meconium aspiration, with no meconium noted below the cords. The infant was then placed on continuous positive airway pressure (CPAP) +6, with pulse oximetry saturations at 88%. The infant was brought to the NICU for ongoing care. Apgar scores were 3^1, 7^5, 9^{10}.

■ Physical Examination on Admission to the NICU

- GENERAL: active and reactive for age, heart rate 172 beats/min, respiratory rate 47
- HEENT: normocephalic, anterior fontanelle is open, soft and flat; lids open, eyes clear with no drainage, ears normally set, nares patent, oropharynx clear without cleft, moist mucus membranes
- CHEST: mild to moderate retractions, equal air entry and breath sounds
- CARDIAC: rate regular and rhythm, normal S1 and S2, femoral pulses equal, brisk capillary refill
- ABDOMEN: soft, nontender, nondistended, no hepatosplenomegaly or masses palpable; three-vessel cord; the anus appeared patent
- GENITOURINARY: normal male infant genitalia
- NEUROLOGIC: active and responsive, normal tone and reflexes for GA
- EXTREMITIES: well formed; 10 digits per extremity; good perfusion

The infant was admitted to NICU for closer observation for meconium aspiration, maternal hepatitis B status unknown, sepsis, and a chest x-ray was obtained. A peripheral IV was started to begin D10W at 60 mL/kg/d and to begin antimicrobial therapy.

■ Differential Diagnoses

- Neonatal sepsis
  - Maternal fever prior to delivery
  - Mother did not receive antibiotic therapy prior to delivery
  - Mother negative for Group B beta hemolytic streptococcus (GBBS), positive urine culture
- Pneumomediastinum
  - Initial chest x-ray findings consistent with pneumomediastinum
- Transient tachypnea of the newborn
- Maternal hepatitis B status unknown
- Intrauterine drug exposure—marijuana daily in mother during pregnancy

■ Diagnostic Tests

- Maternal tests: hepatitis B surface antigen
- Follow placental pathology
- Maternal urine culture—at delivery positive for *E. coli*

■ Laboratory Tests

Maternal:

- Hepatitis B surface antigen—negative
- Placental pathology—fetal membranes with early acute chorioamnionitis and pigment-laden macrophages consistent with meconium

Infant:

- Complete blood count (CBC)/differential: WBC 17.3, neutrophils 78; bands 16, I: T 0.36, platelet count 110,000/mm^3
- LP: WBC 26 (neutrophils 1, lymphocytes 11, monocytes 88), glucose 133, protein 109, RBC 0
- CRP: 24.2 (birth labs), 56 (@ 24 hours of life)
- Blood culture—no growth @ 24 hours
- Urine culture—no growth @ 24 hours
- CSF culture—no growth @ 24 hours

■ Working Diagnosis

- Pneumomediastinum—resolving per subsequent chest x-ray (infant weaned from CPAP to room air within 24 hours), respiratory distress resolved
- Presumed neonatal sepsis—maternal chorioamnionitis, maternal urine culture at delivery positive for pansensitive *E. coli*

■ Development of Management Plan. Initiate antimicrobials in infant and monitor urine output, antimicrobial levels, and cultures:

- Ampicillin 100 mg/kg/dose IV q12 h (× 7 days)
- Gentamicin 4 mg/kg/dose IV q24 h (× 7 days)
- Monitor infant blood, urine, CSF cultures all negative at 72 hours
  - Appropriate neonatal antibiotics empiric (maternal *E. coli* from urine pansensitive, including sensitivity to ampicillin) for 7 days of treatment (watch neonatal cultures for any positive growth)
  - Repeat infant CBC to monitor for resolution of initial bandemia
  - Monitor antimicrobial drug levels as appropriate, urine output
  - Monitor infant temperature
- Maintenance fluid support until able to tolerate oral feedings
- Respiratory support as needed, CX-ray resolution of pneumomediastinum
  - Respiratory support as needed

■ Implementation and Evaluation of Effectiveness

Implementation of management plan:

- The infant was off all respiratory support within 24 hours of birth, CX-ray with resolution of pneumomediastinum
- Maternal hepatitis B status unknown (hepatitis B vaccine administered on day of birth)
- Neonatal sepsis
  - All infant cultures remain negative @ 72 hours and final readings
  - CRP 10.2 after 72 hours of antimicrobial therapy
  - Ampicillin and gentamicin completed 7 days of therapy
  - Gentamicin levels around third dose, gentamicin trough 0.9 mcg/mL (30 minutes predose), gentamicin peak 6.7 mcg/mL (30 minutes post end infusion), urine output 4 to 6 mL/kg/hr, SCr 0.37 to 0.67
  - Infant normothermic
  - Infant CBC resolved (repeat CBC at 72 hours WBC 9.4 [43 S, 45L, 6M])

■ Outcome. Infant respiratory distress resolved and 7 days of antimicrobial treatment completed. Infant sent home with mother on full formula feeds with follow-up appointment with pediatrician in 3 days. Newborn screen sent and in progress. Social worker met with mother regarding marijuana use, strong social support and follow-up on discharge.

EVIDENCE-BASED PRACTICE BOX

Retinopathy of prematurity (ROP) involves abnormal blood vessel development in the retina of the eye and affects approximately 50% of infants with a birth weight of less than 1,250 g. ROP develops in two phases. The first phase occurs at birth to approximately 32 weeks postconceptual age and is marked by vessel loss and incomplete vascularization of the retinal and peripheral avascular zones. The second phase of ROP occurs at 32 to 34 weeks postconceptual age and is characterized by vascular proliferation of the premature retina and increased levels of vascular endothelial growth factor (VEGF). New vessel formation leads to scar tissue, which can result in retinal detachment. ROP is a major cause of blindness in infants and children.

For the past 20 years, treatment for ROP has ranged from cryotherapy (freezing of vessels) in the 1980s and laser ablation therapy in the 1990s. Both of these therapies are nonspecific and can lead to decreased visual acuity as the infant grows and matures.

A recent advance has expanded the available treatment option of ROP to include antivascular endothelial growth factor (anti-VEGF) agents such as bevacizumab (Avastin). VEGF is a key regulator in new blood vessel formation, which is referred to as angiogenesis. Anti-VEGF agents such as bevacizumab have been used in the adult treatment of age-related macular degeneration. Extrapolation of adult therapies to infants and children can often lead to novel and efficacious therapies.

Several small studies in neonates to date suggest the efficacy of bevacizumab in certain stages of ROP. In the largest study to date, the BEAT-ROP trial (Mintz-Hittner et al., 2011), the efficacy of intravitreal bevacizumab in zone I and zone II stage 3+ ROP was studied. The BEAT-ROP trial demonstrated that infants with zone I stage 3+ ROP showed a significant decrease in the recurrence of revascularization, which is associated with ROP. Furthermore, the time to recurrence when it did occur was prolonged with bevacizumab therapy compared to traditional laser therapy. Pharmacokinetics of intravitreal bevacizumab in the neonate remains unknown. More data is needed to determine the long-term structural and systemic outcomes using this therapy.

Reference

Mintz-Hittner, H. A., Kennedy, K. A., Chuang, A. Z., & BEAT-ROP Cooperative Group. (2011). Efficacy of intravitreal bevacizumab for stage 3+ retinopathy of prematurity. *New England Journal of Medicine, 364*(7), 603–615.

ONLINE RESOURCES

Neonatal and Pediatric Patient Safety
http://www.youtube.com/watch?v=qmAvfiO_A4k
Neonatal Pharmacology Principles (a charge)
http://www.nccwebsite.org/Self-Assessment/WB1223Neonatal PharmacologyPrinciples2.aspx

REFERENCES

American Academy of Pediatrics Section on Breastfeeding Policy Statement. (2005). Breastfeeding and the use of human milk. *Pediatrics, 115*, 496–506.

Arimura, J., Poole, R. L., Jeng, M., Rhine, W., & Sharek, P. (2008). Neonatal heparin overdose—a multidisciplinary team approach to medication error prevention. *Journal of Pediatric Pharmacology and Therapeutics, 13*(2), 96–98.

Association of Women's Health, Obstetric and Neonatal Nurses. (2007). *Neonatal skin care: Evidence-based clinical practice guideline* (2nd ed., pp. 53–58). Washington, DC: Johnson and Johnson Consumer Company, Inc.

Bell, G. (2010). Off-label medication use in the NICU. *Neonatal Network, 29*(4), 253–255.

Clark, R., Bloom, B. T., Spitzer, A. R., & Gerstmann, D. R. (2006). Reported medication use in the neonatal intensive care unit: Data from a large national data set. *Pediatrics, 117*(6), 1979–1987.

Committee on Drugs. (2010). Clinical report- guidelines for the ethical conduct of studies to evaluate drugs in pediatric populations. *Pediatrics, 125*, 850–860.

Committee on Fetus and Newborn, & American Academy of Pediatrics (AAP). (2010). Postnatal corticosteroids to prevent or treat bronchopulmonary dysplasia. *Pediatrics, 126*(4), 800–808.

Committee on Fetus and Newborn, American Academy of Pediatrics (AAP) (2004). Age terminology during the perinatal period. *Pediatrics, 114*(5), 1326–1364.

Demler, T. L. (2011). Labeling guidelines for antipsychotics during pregnancy. *U.S. Pharmacist, 36*(11), 39–44.

Douma, C. (2010). Navigating a neonatal intensive care unit clinical practice change. *Journal of Pediatric Nursing, 25*, 221–223.

El-Chaar, G. (2003). Pharmaceutical care in premature infants. *US Pharmacist, 25*, HS13–HS31.

Gal, P. (2009). Optimum use of therapeutic drug monitoring and pharmacokinetics-pharmacodynamics in the NICU. *Journal of Pediatric Pharmacology and Therapeutics, 14*(2), 66–74.

Golec, L. (2009). The art of inconsistency: Evidence based practice my way. *Journal of Perinatology, 29*, 600–602.

Hale, R. (2011). Breastfeeding and medication forum. Retrieved from Dr Hale's pharmacology website: http://ibreastfeeding.com

Harding, A. (2011). Use of intravenous smart pumps for patient safety. *Journal of Emergency Nursing, 37*(1), 71–72.

Johnson, P. J. (2011). Neonatal pharmacology—pharmacokinetics. *Neonatal Network, 30*(1), 54–61.

Kearns, G. L., Abdel-Rahman, S. M., Alander, S. W., Blowey, D. L., Leeder, J. S., & Kauffman, R. E. (2003). Developmental pharmacology—drug disposition, action, and therapy in infants and children. *New England Journal of Medicine, 349*(12), 1157–1167.

Kumar, P., Walker, J. K., Hurt, K. M., Bennett, K. M., Grosshans, N., & Fotis, M. A. (2008). Medication use in the neonatal intensive care unit: Current patterns of off-label use of parenteral medications. *Journal of Pediatrics, 152*(3), 412–415.

Larsen, G. Y., Parker, H. B., Cash, J., O'Connell, M., & Grant, M. C. (2005). Standard drug concentrations and smart pump technology reduce continuous-medication-infusion errors in pediatric patients. *Pediatrics, 116*(1), 21–25.

Leonard, M. S. (2010). Patient safety and quality improvement: Medical errors and adverse events. *Pediatrics in Review, 31*(4), 151–158.

Madadi, P., Moretti, M., Djokanovic, N., Bozzo, P., Nulman, I., Ito, S., & Koren, G. (2009). Guidelines for maternal codeine use during breastfeeding. *Canadian Family Physician, 55*(11), 1077–1078.

Mazela, J., & Polin, R. (2011). Aerosol delivery to ventilated newborn infants: Historical challenges and new directions. *European Journal of Pediatrics, 170*(4), 433–444.

Mehta, N. M., Halwick, D. R., Dodson, B. L., Thompson, J. E., & Arnold, J. H. (2007). Potential drug sequestration during extracorporeal membrane oxygenation: Results from an ex vivo experiment. *Intensive Care Medicine, 33*, 1018–1024.

Mennella, J. A., & Beauchamp, G. K. (2008). Optimizing oral medications for children. *Clinical Therapeutics, 30*(11), 2120–2132.

Monagle, P., Studdert, D. M., & Newall, F. (2011, June 17). Infant deaths due to heparin overdose: Time for a concerted action on prevention. *Journal of Pediatrics and Child Health, 48*(5): 380–381.

Poole, R. L., & Carleton, B. C. (2008). Medication errors: Neonates, infants and children are the most vulnerable. *Journal of Pediatric Pharmacology and Therapeutics, 13*(2), 65–67.

Pregnancy and lactation labeling, FDA. (Updated 2011, February 11). Retrieved from www.fda.gov/Drugs/DevelopmentApproval/ProcessDevelopmentResources/Labeling/ucm93307.htm

Raj, T. N. (2005). Research in neonatology for the 21st century: Executive summary of the National Institute of Child Health and Human Development—American Academy of Pediatrics Workshop. Part I: Academic issues. *Pediatrics, 115*(2), 465–474.

Rajani, A., Chitkara, R., Oehlert, J., & Halamek, L. P. (2011). Comparison of umbilical venous and intraosseous access during simulated neonatal resuscitation. *Pediatrics, 128*(4), e954–e958.

Ramasethu, J. (2004). Pharmacology review: Prevention and management of extravasation injuries in neonates. *Neoreviews, 5*, 491–497.

Reed, M. D. (2011). Reversing the myths obstructing the determination of optimal age- and disease-based drug dosing in pediatrics. *Journal of Pediatric Pharmacology and Therapeutics, 16*(1), 4–13.

Robertson, A. F. (2003a). Reflections on errors in neonatology II. The heroic years, 1950 to 1970. *Journal of Perinatology, 23*(2), 54–161.

Robertson, A. F. (2003b). Reflections on errors in neonatology III. The experienced years, 1970 to 2000. *Journal of Perinatology, 23*(3), 240–249.

Sahni, J., & Phelps, S. (2011). Nebulized furosemide in the treatment of bronchopulmonary dysplasia in preterm infants. *Journal of Pediatric Pharmacology and Therapeutics, 16*, 14–22.

Sauberan, J. B., Dean, L. M., Fiedelak, J., & Abraham, J. A. (2009). Origins and solutions for neonatal medication-dispensing errors. *American Journal of Health System Pharmacy, 66*, e31–e38.

Sentinel event alert: Preventing pediatric medication errors. (2008, April 11). (39) Retrieved from www.jointcommission.org

Shirkey, H. (1968). Therapeutic orphans. *Journal of Pediatrics, 72*, 119.

Simpson, J. H., & Grant, J. (2004). Reducing medication errors in the neonatal intensive care unit. *Archives of Disease in Childhood Fetal and Neonatal Edition, 89*, F480–F482.

Soldin, O. P., & Soldin, S. J. (2002). Review: Therapeutic drug monitoring in pediatrics. *Therapeutic Drug Monitoring, 24*(1), 1–8.

Sowan, A. K., Vaidya, V. U., Soeken, K. L., & Hilmas, E. (2010). Computerized orders with standardized concentrations decrease dispensing errors of continuous infusion medications for pediatrics. *Journal of Pediatric Pharmacology and Therapeutics, 15*(3), 189–202.

St. Onge, E. L., & Motycka, C. A. (2004, June). Risks associated with medication use in pregnancy. *Drug Topics*, 84–91.

Stavroudis, T. A., Shore, A. D., Murlock, L., Hicks, R. W., Bundy, D., & Miller, M. R. (2010). Neonatal Intensive Care Unit medication errors: Identifying a risk profile for medication errors in the neonatal intensive care unit. *Journal of Perinatology, 30*, 459–468.

Summary of proposed rule on pregnancy and lactation labeling. FDA. (2009, November 12). Retrieved from www.fda.gov/Drugs//DevelopmentApproval Process/DevelopmentResources/Labeling/ucm933310.htm

Taketomo, C. K., Hodding, J. H., & Kraus, D. M. (2011). *Pediatric dosage handbook* (18th ed.). Hudson, OH: Lexi-Comp.

Thigpen, J. L. (2007). Peripheral intravenous extravasation: Nursing procedure for initial treatment. *Neonatal Network, 26*(6), 379–384.

Touw, D., Westerman, E., & Sprij, A. J. (2009). Therapeutic drug monitoring of aminoglycosides in neonates. *Clinical Pharmacokinetics, 48*(2), 71–88.

Traynor, K. (2011, December 1). White House addresses drug shortages. *American Society of Health System Pharmacists*, 21–22. Pharmacy News.

Trissel, L. A. (2010). Drug stability and compatibility issues in drug delivery. In L. A. Trissel (Ed.), *Handbook of injectable drugs* (16th ed.). Bethesda, MD: American Society of Health-System Pharmacists.

Ventola, C. L. (2011). The drug shortage crisis in the United States: Causes, impact, and management strategies. *Pharmacy and Therapeutics, 36*(11), 740–758.

Wildschut, E. D., Allegaert, A. K., Ahsman, M. J., Mathot, R. A., & Tibboel, D. (2010). Determinants of drug absorption in different ECMO circuits. *Intensive Care Medicine, 36*(12), 2109–2116.

Wolfe, T. R., & Braude, D. A. (2010). Intranasal medication delivery for children: A brief review and update. *Pediatrics, 126*(3), 532–537.

Woo, T. M. (2004). Pediatric pharmacology update: Essential concepts for prescribing. *Advance Nursing Practice, 12*(6), 22–27.

Woods, T. E., Thomas, E., Holl, J., Altman, S., & Brennan, T. (2005). Adverse events and preventable adverse events in children. *Pediatrics, 115*(1), 155–160.

Young, T. E., & Mangum, B. (2011). *Neofax* (24th ed.). New York, NY: Thomson Reuters.

CHAPTER 22

Emerging Technologies in Neonatal Care: Health Care Simulation for Neonatal Care

■ Jennifer Arnold

WHAT IS HEALTH CARE SIMULATION?

Over the past 6 years, the number of medical institutions opening health care simulation programs has increased exponentially (Arnold, LeMaster, Todd, & Wallin, 2012). The advent of advanced, high-fidelity simulation technology over the last 10 to 15 years has made this possible. Health care simulation is defined by David Gaba as, "a technique—not a technology—to replace or amplify real patient experiences with guided experiences, artificially contrived, that evoke or replicate substantial aspects of the real world in a fully interactive manner" (2004). Health care simulation involves four important components: (1) the scenario: the story where a participant is immersed in a realistic clinical situation (2) the simulator: a tool used to create a realistic physical space, equipment, and/or patient such as a mannequin, (3) the experience: suspension of disbelief and "near life" experience during the scenario by the participants, and (4) the debrief: reflective discussion where the learning occurs (see Figure 22.1).

Simulation in health care is an ever-evolving educational methodology that began over 20 years ago in the field of anesthesiology (Gaba, 1992; Rosen, 2008). It has taken a long time for the medical field to embrace simulation, likely due to the limitations of realistic simulators, but also due to the resistance in traditional medical education to try new methods of education, when tried and true methods such as lectures and bedside teaching have seemingly worked. However, simulation offers benefits that cannot be achieved in traditional lecture or bedside teaching with the mantra of *see one, do one, teach one* educational activities. It is based on adult learning principles, making it a very effective tool for educating health care providers (see Table 22.1) (Arnold, 2011). Adult learners, which include providers in neonatal care, are independent, self-directed, and motivated to learn when what they are learning applies to their professional roles (Murphy & Halamek, 2005). Adult learners also respond well to receiving immediate feedback on their performance and being able to apply their newly acquired knowledge right away. Additionally, simulation can provide education on demand with the opportunity to repeat high-risk situations until all participants manage a situation properly. Simulation bridges the gap between education and the acquisition of high-stakes, low-frequency skills in clinical practice that are essential for acquisition and maintenance of skills in high-risk patient care fields such as neonatal intensive care (Galloway, 2009).

Most importantly, simulation is an educational opportunity where it is safe to make mistakes—there is no risk

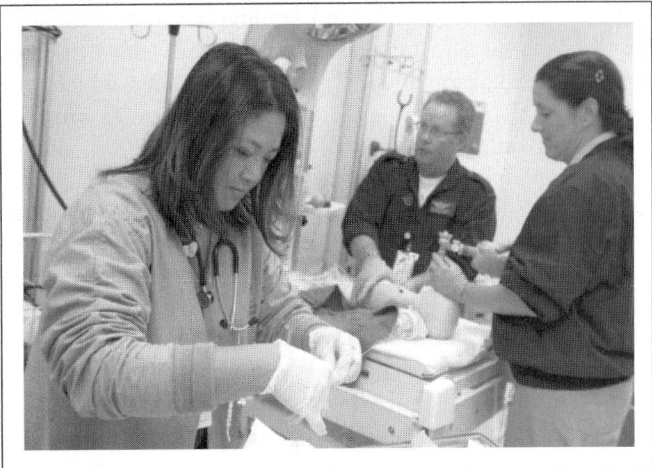

FIGURE 22.1 Near life experience in simulation.

TABLE 22.1

HOW ADULT LEARNING PRINCIPLES CORRELATE WITH HEALTH CARE SIMULATION

Adult Learning Principle	Simulation Curriculum Correlate
Adults prefer to apply what they learn soon after learning it	Simulation provides immediate, hands-on practice
Adults prefer learning concepts and principles	Preparation and presentation of key concepts prior to simulation allows for conceptual learning
Adults learn better at their own pace	Simulation provides repetitive and deliberate practice educational opportunities
Adults like to help set their own learning objectives	Learner-focused debriefings after simulation allow for reflection on personal objectives
Adults like to receive immediate feedback	Debriefing, enhanced with video review, of simulation scenarios is real time, immediate, and learner focused

Adapted from Arnold (2011).

to patients. In fact, the goal of high-fidelity simulation encounters is often for participants to make mistakes. Every mistake made in a simulation is a mistake that could then be prevented in the real world. Previously, other high-risk industries such as aviation and nuclear power have utilized simulation to improve safety and minimize risk.

Simulation-based research in health care continues to show that use of simulation-based learning methodologies enhances performance in both real-life clinical situations and simulated resuscitations (Andreatta, Saxton, Thompson, & Annich, 2011). In addition, use of debriefings after real or simulated resuscitations have been found to result in improved learning, knowledge, and skills (Rudolph, Taylor, & Foldy, 2001).

History of Health Care Simulation

Simulation, although a relatively new technique in health care education, is not new to many other high-risk industries. Military, aviation, and nuclear power have used simulation since they began to practice and prepare for rare and/or dangerous situations and highly strategic missions. Simulation in health care has learned many lessons from all these industries, but especially from the aviation industry. In the early years of aviation, simulation pilots practiced the technical skills of taking off, flying, and landing a plane as early as the first planes and gliders. From the early days of gliding, it was usual for "pilots" to sit in the glider, which was exposed to a strong facing wind, and "feel" how to keep the wings horizontal with their controls (Moore, 2008). Flight simulation has now moved forward to highly advanced and realistic technology cockpit simulators that allow pilots to practice flight crises they hope they will never encounter in their careers. However, despite very realistic and advanced flight simulation training in which all pilots participated, up until the 1980s the aviation industry was concerned about the frequency of major flight crises. So big was the problem that NASA launched an all-out study of jet transport accidents and incidents between 1968 and 1976 and found that the leading causes of these accidents were not deficiencies in the pilot's knowledge or skill, but more likely failures in teamwork, communication, and leadership (Cooper, White, & Lauber, 1980). With this information, aviation developed a new form of training, coined Crew Resource Management, which focused on training the whole aircraft team on human factors such as effective communication, flat hierarchy, teamwork, workload distribution, and situational awareness (Helmreich & Sexton, 2003; Helmreich, Wilhelm, Klinect, & Merritt, 2001). As a result of the initiation of Crew Resource Management in aviation in the 1980s, it is much safer to fly our blue skies.

Health care simulation has evolved from the lessons learned in aviation simulation. Although health care simulation began as early as the 1960s with the development of the first low-fidelity mannequin-based simulator, Resusci Anne® by Laerdal, as a field, simulation in health care has had a rapid surge in activity, technological advances, and research over the past 10 years. Resusci Anne, a low-fidelity or low-tech mannequin was developed and introduced in 1960 by Norwegian toy maker Asmund S. Laerdal (Laerdal Medical Company, 2012). He teamed up with two physicians, anesthesiologist Peter Safar, MD, and emergency medicine physician James Elam, MD, who developed mouth-to-mouth breathing (the airway component of cardiopulmonary resuscitation [CPR]), as a life-saving procedure. Together, they developed a life-sized doll to train medical and nonmedical personnel in CPR. Resusci Anne was modeled after a young girl whose body was pulled from the River Seine in Paris at the turn of the 19th century. Her death was a popular story in Europe at the time. It was assumed she had committed suicide over unrequited love, by jumping in the river, as there were no other visible causes of death. Because her identity could not be established, a death mask was made as was customary at the time. Moved by her story, Asmund S. Laerdal adopted her mask for the face of his new resuscitation-training mannequin.

Health care simulation has come a long way since Resusci Anne. We now have everything from virtual reality and haptic simulators to whole-body mannequins that are so realistic and interactive that health care providers forget a mannequin-based patient is not real. Whole-body, highly technical mannequins, are often referred to as high-fidelity mannequin-based simulators. These mannequins are so sophisticated that they have pulses and breathe, have heart and lung sounds, turn blue when cyanotic, talk or cry, sweat or bleed, and some move (Figure 22.2 and Figure 22.3). In neonatal simulation, there are four high-fidelity, whole-body mannequins now available (Table 22.2). Each has slightly different features, making the choice of the best simulator based on the needs of the specific simulation scenario one is trying to create.

What makes these mannequins so useful in health care is their ability to interact with providers. When a health care team administers a drug or intervention, the mannequin's

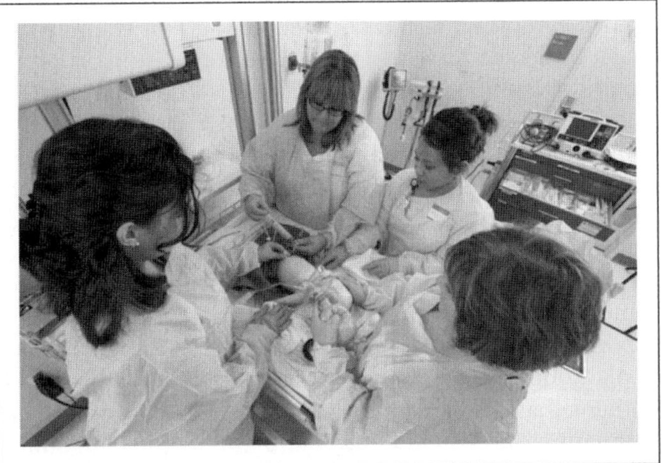

FIGURE 22.2 High-fidelity mannequin-based simulators. Courtesy of Texas Children's Hospital.

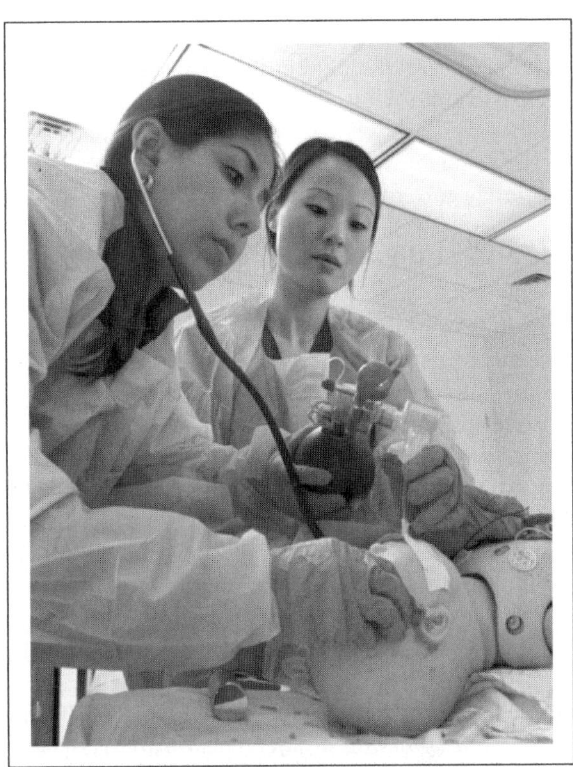

FIGURE 22.3 Sophisticated mannequin in neonatal simulation. Courtesy of Texas Children's Hospital.

TABLE 22.2

EXAMPLES OF HIGH-FIDELITY NEONATAL MANNEQUIN-BASED SIMULATORS

Features	SimNewB (Laerdal Medical)	Newborn Hal (Gaumard Scientific)	Premie Hal (Gaumard Scientific)	PEDI Blue Neonatal Simulator (Nasco)
Airway/Breathing	Realistic airway, normal and abnormal breath sounds, bilateral and unilateral chest rise, CO_2 exhalation	Realistic airway, normal and abnormal breath sounds, bilateral and unilateral chest rise	Realistic airway, normal and abnormal breath sounds, bilateral and unilateral chest rise	Realistic airway, bilateral chest rise
Cyanosis	Central, pulse oximetry	Central, pulse oximetry	Central, pulse oximetry	Peripheral and central
Circulation/EKG	Normal and abnormal heart sounds, central and peripheral pulses, EKG monitoring	Normal and abnormal heart sounds, central and peripheral pulses, EKG monitoring	Normal and abnormal heart sounds, central and peripheral pulses, EKG monitoring	None
Movement	All extremities: limp, tone, motion, seizure	Upper extremities: limp, tone, motion, seizure	None	None
Vocal Sounds	Cry, grunt, stridor, cough, hiccup	Cry, grunt, stridor	Cry, grunt, stridor	None
Access Procedures	Patent umbilical vein and arteries with blood flashback, bilateral intraosseous access	Patent umbilical vein with blood flashback, peripheral IV, bilateral intraosseous access	Patent umbilical vein with blood flashback, peripheral IV, bilateral intraosseous	Patent umbilical vein
Airway Procedures	BVM, intubation, LMA, needle thoracentesis	BVM, intubation, LMA	BVM, intubation, LMA	BVM, intubation
Control	Wireless handheld or tethered laptop	Wireless tablet PC	Wireless tablet PC	Tethered computer panel
Cost	$$$	$$$	$$$	$
Other	Interchangeable pupils, blood pressure	Gastric distention, bowel sounds, blood pressure	Premature newborn at 28 weeks	

BVM, bag-mask ventilation; LMA, laryngeal mask airway.

vital signs can change appropriately. Now a health care team is able to take care of a patient in a realistic environment in real time without the interruptions of a teacher telling them the vitals or asking what they might do in that situation. Now, the team must actively do all the things needed to appropriately care for their patient in a safe environment.

Simulation and Patient Safety

Simulation is an increasingly recognized tool to improve patient safety in health care. It provides an effective method to meet the needs of adult learners while improving patient safety and outcomes through a safe environment in which to improve and maintain skill proficiency.

Medical error accounts for approximately $24 billion in health care costs annually in the United States and 98,000 lives lost annually. It is the fifth leading cause of death in the United States. Both the Institute of Medicine (IOM) and The Joint Commission (TJC) have reported that medical errors result from deficiencies in teamwork, leadership, and communication rather than technical or cognitive deficiencies, similar to that of the aviation industry (JCAHO, 1998; Kohn, Corrigan, & Molla, 2000). In 1999, the IOM's *To Err Is Human: Building a Safer Healthcare System* found the leading cause of mistakes in medicine (70%) were due to human errors such as deficiencies in communication and leadership, not a lack of medical knowledge or skill on the part of the practitioner (Laerdal Medical Company, 2012). Similarly in 2004 and 2007, TJC during extensive review of sentinel events, found deficiencies in teamwork, communication and safety culture as the leading cause of error in these events. TJC has recommended that all health care institutions implement simulation-based training to improve teamwork and communication. Just as the aviation industry developed crew resource management to address deficiencies in teamwork, leadership, and communication, health care has developed Crisis Resource Management (CRM) training to address these deficiencies in health care. CRM in health care simulation was first described by David Gaba, MD, an anesthesiologist and father of modern health care simulation (Rall & Gaba, 2005). He reported 15 important CRM skills, such as role clarity, effective communication, personnel support, adequate use of all resources, and situational awareness, that all effective health care teams should embody to deliver safe care during high-risk clinical situations. Because simulation-based training focuses more on behavioral and teamwork skills than on individual technical skills, it provides the perfect opportunity for multidisciplinary teams to train together and practice these skills. Up until now, health care professionals have trained in silos: nurses in nursing school, physicians in medical school. But, when a patient crashes, health care providers are expected to work as a well-oiled team to successfully resuscitate a patient, even though they may have never had an opportunity to practice working together. In today's complex health care system, health care needs pit crews not cowboys. No longer are autonomy, knowledge and experience, and self-sufficiency enough to provide safe and effective health care. Now, more than ever, health care providers need to work as a team within a system to provide safe and effective care. High-fidelity simulation provides the only opportunity for health care teams to practice these important skills in a time-pressured, realistic, and safe environment.

There is a growing body of evidence that not only technical skills, but also behavioral skills are improved with simulation-based training, ultimately improving patient care outcomes and decreasing medical errors (Andreatta et al., 2006, 2011; Barsuk, Cohen, Feinglass, McGaghie, & Wayne, 2009). In obstetrics and gynecology, researchers have shown that team-based simulation training can result in decreased need for massive transfusion protocols in postpartum hemorrhage situations (Lockhart, Allen, Gunatilake, Hobbs, & Taekman, 2012). Additionally, units conducting simulation-based training on management of shoulder dystocia have shown improved neonatal Apgar scores, decreased incidence of brachial plexus injuries in newborns, and decreased incidence of neonatal hypoxic-ischemic encephalopathy (Draycott et al., 2008). Simulation-based team training has shown improved collaboration between obstetrics and neonatology (Zabari et al., 2006). In our field of neonatology, simulation-based training has shown increased success rates in neonatal intubations after simulation training (Arnold et al., 2008), but there is a need for additional research to show the impact of simulation-based training in neonatal patient outcomes.

Simulation in Neonatal Care

Simulation provides an opportunity to practice high-risk patient care situations so that providers are more competent in their abilities to manage these situations. Because neonatal intensive care involves unexpected high-risk clinical situations, simulation is a tool to improve patient care and patient outcomes.

Simulation-based training in neonatal care had its beginning in the Neonatal Resuscitation Program (NRP) (Halamek et al., 2000; Murphy & Halamek, 2005). With studies showing that cognitive and technical skills achieved are typically only retained for only 6 to 12 months, the goal of implementation of a simulation-based training curriculum was to improve learning and skills of health care providers caring for newborns requiring resuscitation at the time of delivery (Kaczorowski et al., 1998). It is not only recommended by national and international organizations including the International Liaison Committee on Resuscitation who oversee implementation of the NRP, but in its sixth edition, simulation-based training is now required (Perlman et al., 2010). Up until now, the NRP has focused on lectures accompanied by skill stations utilizing low-tech mannequins and did not use a formal debriefing process to give feedback, thereby only addressing knowledge and technical skills (Halamek, 2008). The incorporation of simulation-based methodology will now address the complex behavioral skills, such as effective teamwork and communication, that are essential in the resuscitation of the newborn. NRP instructors will now be required to have the knowledge and skills needed to conduct simulation-based training: how to design simulation scenarios and debrief using reflective questions. Although the NRP has been a leader in embracing simulation since early on, it is only the beginning for the many potential uses and benefits in neonatal care.

There is a growing body of evidence that not only technical skills, but also behavioral skills are improved with simulation-based training, ultimately improving patient care outcomes and decreasing medical errors (Andreatta et al., 2006, 2011; Barsuk et al., 2009; Draycott et al., 2008; Zabari et al., 2006). In the care of newborns, simulation-based training has been shown to improve provider success rates at endotracheal intubation, decreased incidence of hypoxic-ischemic encephalopathy, and improvement in APGAR scores (Arnold et al., 2008; Draycott et al., 2008).

Implementation of Simulation in Neonatal Care

The first step in the development of simulation-based neonatal activity is to determine the purpose of that activity. Five major categories in simulation can be used to help describe the purpose of simulation activity: (1) education, (2) competency and assessment, (3) research and development, (4) quality and patient safety, and (5) advocacy. Although simulation is an educational tool, it can be utilized for very different purposes beyond education. As a neonatal care provider is exploring developing simulation training opportunities, it is vital to determine the purpose of the initiative in order to develop a useful and successful simulation initiative.

■ Simulation for Educational Purposes. Using simulations to provide training to meet the educational demands of neonatal health care providers is the first category and most common use of simulation. Simulation-based education and training is primarily focused on delivering new knowledge/skills and/or providing practice and instruction to improve the learners' performance in a simulated event. It is important that all simulation-based educational activities are based on sound educational principles. (Please see the next section on simulation scenario design for key steps in this process.)

■ Simulation for Competency and Assessment. The goal of using simulation for assessment of skills and competency is growing. There is a need for development of validated simulation scenarios and assessment tools using validated and reliable measurement principles. Simulation has been shown to be helpful in demonstrating and evaluating competency in nursing training programs, advanced cardiac life support, advanced and emergency airway management, pediatric code resuscitation, CRM skills, laparoscopic surgical skills, and even bronchoscopy (Anderson, Murphy, Boyle, Yaeger, & Halamek, 2006; Calhoun, Rider, Meyer, Lamiani, & Truog, 2009; Konge, Arendrup, von Buchwald, & Ringsted, 2011; Lucisano & Talbot, 2012; Lutrell, Lenburg, Scherubel, Jacob, & Koch, 1999; Vaillancourt et al., 2011; Wayne et al., 2007).

In anesthesia and surgical fields, simulation is an accepted means for maintenance of certification for physicians. Currently, other certifying bodies already utilize simulation in their certification processes such as the Medical Council of Canada, General Medical Council (UK), National Board of Osteopathic Medical Examiners, and the United States Medical Licensing Examination (JCAHO, 2010). The discipline within neonatology that is most advanced in adoption of simulation to assess competency and skills are neonatal nurses and advanced practitioners or neonatal nurse practitioners (NNPs) (Cates & Wilson, 2011). Certification for NNPs and NICU nurses is provided by the National Certification Corporation (NCC). Although the NCC currently does not require simulation for recertification, research is currently ongoing to evaluate this as an official option for certification (National Council of State Boards of Nursing, 2012).

■ Simulation Research and Development. There is a need to foster and develop research and quality improvement studies to advance the science of health care simulation (Issenberg, McGaghie, Petrusa, Lee Gordon, & Scalese, 2005). If possible, all simulation-based activities should have measurable and publishable outcomes. Needed areas of research include, but are not limited to:

1. Identification of which debriefing techniques and adjuncts best enhance learning
2. Identification of the optimal simulation educational approach based on the level of learner, skill of the faculty, and specific learning objectives
3. Development of "best practices" for simulation training in health care
4. Procedural or technical skills simulation research:
    a. Number of times needed for practice of a skill before competence is achieved
    b. Duration of time before procedural skills deteriorate
    c. Training in technical skills in simulation extrapolate to improve performance in skill on patients
    d. Validation of task trainers, virtual reality, and computer-based simulators
    e. Simulation training to decrease time from novice to expert
5. Use of simulation methodology as an assessment tool of technical and behavioral skills in health care providers
    a. Determination of the number and content of simulations required to assure an acceptable level of reliability
    b. Development and validation of reproducible scenarios with reliable and valid assessment tools for evaluating professional competence for the purpose of promotion, certification, or licensure
6. Development of reliable reproducible simulation-based scenarios for use across multiple institutions
7. Effects of fatigue on health care performance: team behaviors, decision making, communications skills, and error rates

■ Simulation for Quality and Patient Safety. Ultimately, all health care simulation activities have the potential to improve quality and patient safety. The best way to achieve this is to align simulation-based activities with national, local, and institutional patient safety and quality goals and needs. By using qualitative research design and measurement, changes in patient care outcomes can be tracked and reported. Examples of this type of simulation include but are not limited to:

1. In-situ simulation to identify potential latent threats to patient safety in the clinical setting
2. Evaluation and testing of new hospital environments, technologies, equipment, or processes before being utilized in real patient care
3. Re-creation of near misses and serious safety events to help identify causes and prevent future events

■ Advocacy in Simulation. Using simulation as a tool for advocacy for patient care is broad. It involves supporting the larger community with simulation-based activities. This can include:

1. Promoting simulation at a national or local level through media and public relations opportunities so that laypersons understand and might support health care simulation
2. Lobbying for health care legislature to support funding for health care simulation
3. Providing simulation-based education to laypersons, such as parents, so that they are better prepared to care for medical emergencies and crises at home or out of hospital

SCENARIO DEVELOPMENT

Just as in other more traditional curricular development models, simulation scenario design must be standardized and evidence-based. It is important to realize that development of simulation educational events should be based on learning objectives and not on the features of mannequins or technology. Effective simulation scenario is essentially one where the learning objectives are achieved. Second, by incorporating real-life cases into scenarios, it not only improves the credibility of the cases for learners, but learners are also able to manage clinical problems and situations as they would in real-world practice. A series of steps are required to develop an effective and evidence-based scenario. For example, if one wanted to develop a scenario for educational purposes with the goal of training a health care team in how to manage a neonatal code, the process might look like this:

Step 1: Identification of the Purpose of the Scenario

Typically, when designing a scenario, it is recommended that the first step be to identify the purpose of the simulation: education, training, competency/assessment, research, or to address a patient safety goal. Once you know the goal of the simulation session, it is easy to write learning objectives and determine a clinical case that can be created to meet the desired goal. In this case the goal would be educational in nature.

Step 2: Identification of the Learning Objectives

The learning objectives should be determined based on the goal of the scenario. It is helpful to categorize learning objectives by their type: cognitive, technical, and behavioral. Although many simulation scenarios provide an opportunity to address many learning objectives, it is helpful to narrow the scope of the scenario to three or four at most so that the learners are able to synthesize these objectives.

Step 3: Identification of the Learners/Participants

It is important to identify who will be the participants. Will it be a single or multidisciplinary team? How many learners per group? For this scenario, a learner group might consist of two neonatal nurses, one neonatal physician, one NNP, and one neonatal respiratory therapist. In general, the number of learners per simulation should reflect the appropriate number and type of providers for the clinical case.

Step 4: Identification of a Clinical Case to Create in Order to Achieve the Desired Learning Objectives

A patient clinical scenario should be developed that will allow the learning objectives to be met. The clinical situation must be realistic and appropriate to the level of the learners. For example, one might not want to choose management of congenital diaphragmatic hernia for a group of new nurses or residents, but rather maybe a case of neonatal shock would be better aligned with their level of expertise. In this example case, one might choose a case of Group B strep septic shock to address the needed learning objectives.

Step 5: Completion of a Scenario Design Template

Many simulation programs have developed and tailored their own simulation scenario design templates. Certain important pieces of information must be known ahead of time in order to conduct an effective simulation. Most simulation education instructors utilize a scenario design template or script that identifies all the necessary equipment and technology needed, the learners, the roles of instructors, the room setup, the expected scenario flow (a script like a play or movie), the appropriate mannequin physiologic states based on actions of the learners, and the expected actions of the learners during a simulation. It is also very important to base the scenario and debriefing on the most recent evidence so that the educational experience is evidence-based.

Step 6: Development of Debriefing Script Based on Learning Objectives

Although many topics discussed during the debriefing after a simulation scenario will be based on the performance and actions of the participants, it is important to keep the debriefing focused on the learning objectives. Time during a debriefing is limited, and although many teachable points will be raised during a simulation scenario, it is important to prioritize the discussion to the planned learning objectives. Therefore it is often helpful to plan ahead with a few open-ended questions that will address the learning objectives. Some educators develop very detailed scripted debriefing questions to address these topics.

Step 7: Practice and Rehearsal of the Scenario

Every time a simulation scenario is run, the participants will likely act and perform differently. Therefore it is very important to practice a scenario so that the scenario developers can ensure that the appropriate cues are available and that the learning objectives are achieved. When conducting a dress rehearsal, one often identifies missing medical equipment or auditory and visual cues that may be missing in order for the learners to be able to share the same mental model of the case as you intended.

Step 8: Implementation and Evaluation of the Simulation Scenario

As with any educational intervention it is important to continuously reevaluate the effectiveness of the intervention. Getting feedback from learners and instructors is important so that simulation scenarios can be continuously refined and improved.

SUMMARY

Simulation is a highly effective and innovative educational tool. It can be used for many purposes in health care education, quality improvement, and patient safety. Although simulation can be a resource-intensive endeavor, when utilized appropriately it can greatly improve health care provider performance and patient care outcomes. Simulation provides a mechanism for bringing the health care team together—students or practicing professionals to learn and practice the art of working together in a safe environment. This is another way that patient safety and quality will be improved through simulated interprofessional experiences.

CASE STUDY

A sample of a simulation scenario in neonatal resuscitation.

■ Learning Objectives of the Scenario. By the end of the simulation session, learners should be able to:

- Cognitive
  1. Recognize the signs and symptoms of meconium aspiration syndrome in a neonate
  2. Develop a differential diagnosis of respiratory distress in a neonate
  3. Identify appropriate initial resuscitation and management steps in a newborn with meconium aspiration

- Technical
  1. Provide appropriate airway management skills for the neonate with meconium aspiration:
     a. Supplemental oxygen
     b. Tracheal intubation
     c. Positive pressure ventilation
     d. Surfactant replacement
     e. Inhaled nitrous oxide
  2. Obtain umbilical venous and arterial access
  3. Provide intravenous fluid resuscitation and dextrose as indicated

- Behavioral
  1. Utilize appropriate teamwork and communication skills during a neonatal resuscitation including:
     a. Identification of a team leader and other team roles
     b. Appropriate utilization of resources
     c. Effective communication, including closed-loop communication

■ Background for Learners of the Problem. This is a case of a newborn born with meconium aspiration syndrome who is to be managed by the NICU team post-initial resuscitation.

Assessment: History and Physical Examination

■ History

- Baby girl is a 3,800-g estimated 38-week female born to a 16-year-old G1P1 with good prenatal care
- Maternal prenatal labs: mother: O+/– HIV—RPR pending HbsAg-, UDS: positive for marijuana
- Mother presented to L&D with loss of fluid approximately 24 hours prior to presentation, at 10 cm and +5 station
- Infant was born via precipitous spontaneous vaginal delivery with thick, foul smelling meconium and fetal decels
- Mother developed fever to 102 at presentation
- At delivery no spontaneous respirations noted, infant taken to warmer and suctioned below cords ×2 with return of thick meconium and started on bag-mask ventilation for 30 seconds with spontaneous respirations noted
- Heart rate was greater than 100 throughout resuscitation
- Peripheral IV placed at L&D and started on 40% oxygen via facemask with continuous positive airway pressure (CPAP) for desaturation and increased work of breathing
- Patient brought to NICU immediately without further intervention for initiation of respiratory support and prolonged rupture of membranes with chorioamnionitis; Apgars were 6^1, 8^5

■ Physical Examination Upon Presentation to NICU

- GENERAL: pale with thready pulses, poor peripheral perfusion
- VITAL SIGNS: baseline vital signs
- Temp 98.3 HR 180 RR 78 BP 45/38 O_2 85% on 40% FiO_2 on FM with CPAP 8
- HEENT: AFOF, small caput, ears normal, palate intact, eyes open, pupils reactive to light; positive red reflex and normal facies
- RESP: lung fields bilaterally with course crackles and severe intracostal, subcostal, and substernal retractions noted; gasping respiratory effort on CPAP
- CV: rate regular with small II/VI systolic ejection murmur noted; poor peripheral perfusion, capillary blood refill time greater than 5 seconds, and thready pulses
- ABD: abdomen soft and nontender with no hepatosplenomegaly or masses; three-vessel cord; anus patent
- GENITOURINARY: normal female infant genitalia
- NEURO: decreased responses and tone
- EXTREMITIES: normal
- SKIN: pale with poor perfusion and mildly cyanotic; pronounced circumoral and acrocyanosis; no rashes or lesions

■ Differential Diagnoses

- Meconium aspiration syndrome
- Perinatal hypoxic-ischemic injury
- Shock
- DIC
- Sepsis
- Congenital cardiac defect

■ Diagnostic Tests

Laboratory tests:

- CBC/differential: WBC 20.3, segmented cells 44; bands 30; hematocrit (Hct) 48%, platelet count 168,000/mm^3
- Glucose: 68
- Baby blood type and Coombs: baby: O+/–

Imaging tests:

- Chest x-ray: bilaterally hazy with patchy areas of consolidation and atelectasis, hyperinflated to 10 ribs bilaterally, cardiac silhouette within normal limits

■ Simulation Scenario Setup and Logistics

Room Configuration (Setup). NICU inpatient room, infant warmer with neonatal high-fidelity mannequin on bed, covered up, no monitors on. Scenario starts with arrival of baby on CPAP from the labor and delivery room with transport team with portable warmer/isolette. Labor and delivery neonatal resuscitation team calls NICU when leaving L&D with brief handoff of patient to allow NICU team time to set up.

■ Equipment Needed

- High-fidelity neonatal mannequin with thick green moulage
- CPAP
- Ventilator (conventional and oscillator)
- Central-line access kit (umbilical)
- Neonatal crash cart
- Neonatal "fake" medications
- Airway supplies, including bag-mask and intubation equipment

■ Mannequins/Task Trainers/Confederates Needed

- High-fidelity neonatal mannequin: mannequin on admitting bed with a diaper and a hat only and some dark green thick moulage; peripheral intravenous (PIV) in place, CPAP on mannequin
- Low-fidelity neonatal mannequin: mannequin with hat and diaper on in transport isolette, attached to CPAP and FiO_2 at 40%, PIV in place
- Neonatal resuscitation team (confederate roles)
- Neonatal resuscitation team shows up with transport warmer/isolette with low-fidelity neonatal mannequin inside to start the scenario with a handoff to NICU admitting team.

■ Simulation Scenario Flow (Flow Chart)

Expected Scenario Flow. Neonatal Resuscitation Team (confederate team) arrives to bedside with transport warmer/ isolette (low-fidelity mannequin), and report is given to NICU admitting team (learner team), transport team relays important information and background of neonate's course and history in the delivery room. After handoff to the admitting NICU team, the high-fidelity mannequin should be exposed (blanket removed) and team should provide care to their new patient. The neonate should be placed on monitors. All appropriate providers should be in the room (nurses, physicians, respiratory therapists). Team should manage their patient until stabilized or 20 minutes of time has elapsed.

■ Expected Interventions of the Participants. Patient should be placed on monitors and vital signs assessed. Respiratory distress should be addressed first with noninvasive, then invasive ventilatory techniques. Recognition of possible meconium aspiration and sepsis should occur. Infant should be intubated and surfactant ordered. A chest x-ray should be obtained. Central access should be obtained, with appropriate labs sent and antibiotics ordered. Hypotension should be recognized and treated first with fluid resuscitation, then consider pressors. Failure of conventional ventilation should be recognized, and team should consider iNO and oscillator. Scenario ends when following are achieved:

- Intubation
- Central-line access
- Fluid resuscitation
- Ordering and/or administration of: surfactant, antibiotics, maintenance IVF, iNO, and ionotropes

Mannequin Operation: Scenario Flow Based on Participants Interventions and Time

■ Debriefing. At the completion of the scenario, the instructor should lead a facilitative, reflective discussion of the learner's performance during the simulation. Concepts of a safe and confidential learning environment should be reinforced. The debriefing should focus on the learning objectives and issues that arose during the simulation such as things done well or not as well as desired by the team, questions the learners have based on the scenario, or other items of interest to the learners or the instructor. If possible, the debriefing should use video-review of the scenario during the discussion. A typical debriefing lasts two to three times the duration of the simulation.

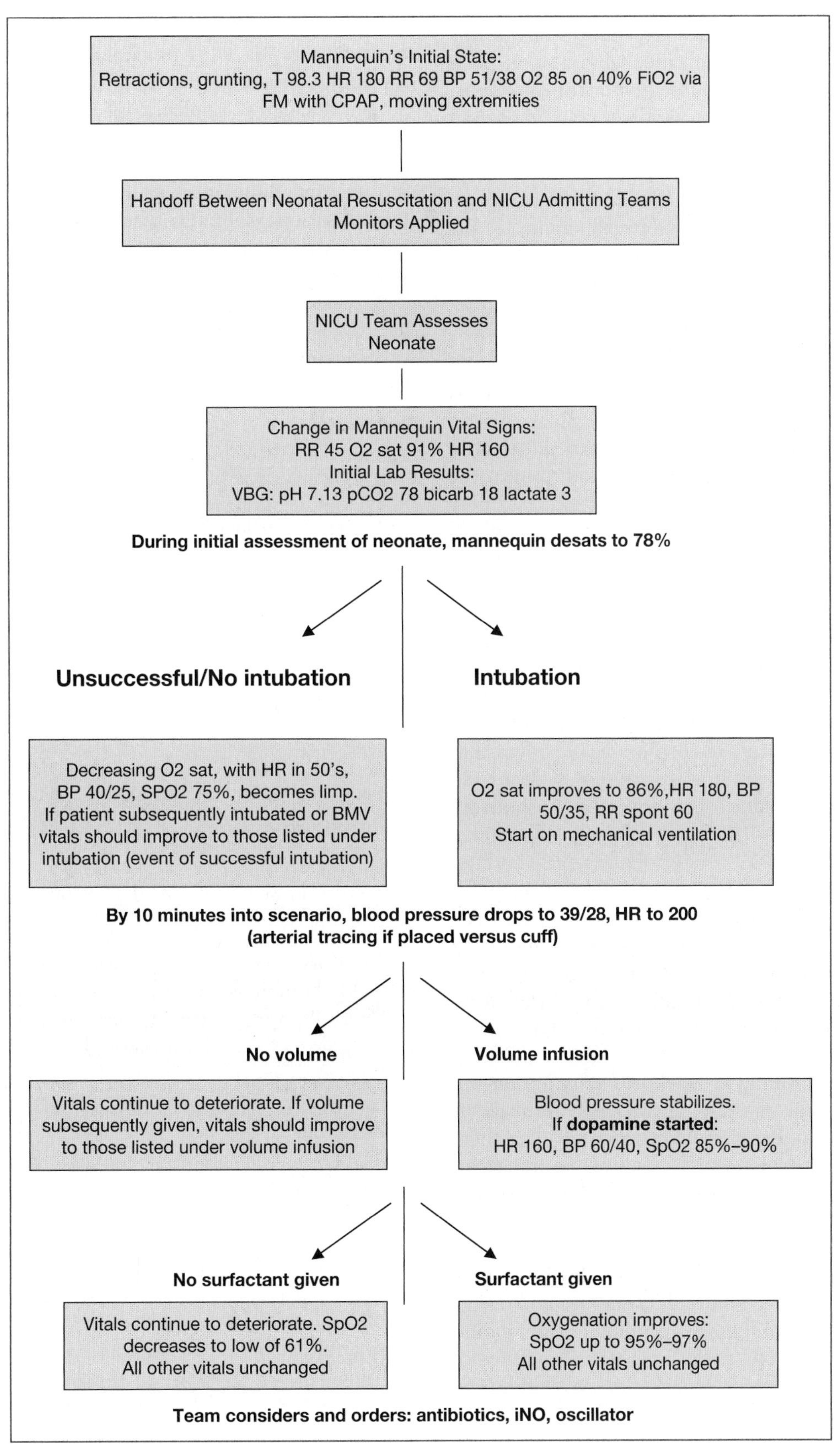

EVIDENCE-BASED PRACTICE BOX

Health care simulation is defined by David Gaba as "a technique—not a technology—to replace or amplify real patient experiences with guided experiences, artificially contrived, that evoke or replicate substantial aspects of the real world in a fully interactive manner" (Gaba, 2004). Health care simulation involves four important components: (1) the scenario: the story where a participant is immersed in a realistic clinical situation, (2) the simulator: a tool used to create a realistic physical space, equipment, and/or patient such as a mannequin, (3) the experience: suspension of disbelief and "near life" experience during the scenario by the participants, and (4) the debrief: reflective discussion where the learning occurs.

Simulation is an educational opportunity where it is safe to make mistakes—there is no risk to patients. In fact, the goal of high-fidelity simulation encounters is often for participants to make mistakes. Simulation is an increasingly recognized tool to improve patient safety in health care. It provides an effective method to meet the needs of adult learners, while improving patient safety and outcomes through a safe environment in which to improve and maintain skill proficiency. There is a growing body of evidence that clinician performance and patient care outcomes are improved with simulation-based training, ultimately improving patient care outcomes and decreasing medical errors (Andreatta, Saxton, Thompson, & Annich, 2011; Andreatta et al., 2006; Barsuk, Cohen, Feinglass, McGaghie, & Wayne, 2009). In obstetrics and gynecology, researchers have shown that team-based simulation training can result in decreased need for massive transfusion protocols in postpartum hemorrhage situations (Lockhart, Allen, Gunatilake, Hobbs, & Taekman, 2012). Additionally, units conducting simulation-based training on management of shoulder dystocia have shown improved neonatal APGAR scores, decreased incidence of brachial plexus injuries in newborns, and decreased incidence of neonatal hypoxic-ischemic encephalopathy (Draycott, 2008). Simulation-based team training has shown improved collaboration between obstetrics and neonatology (Zabari, 2006). Simulation-based training in newborn resuscitation has shown increased success rates in neonatal intubations after simulation training (Arnold et al., 2008), but there is a need for additional research to show the impact of simulation-based training in neonatal patient outcomes.

When developing and implementing simulation-based education, just as in other more traditional curricular development models, simulation scenario design must be standardized and evidence-based. It is important to realize that development of simulation educational events should be based on learning objectives and not the features of mannequins or technology. An effective simulation scenario is essentially one in which the learning objectives are achieved. A series of steps are required to develop an effective and evidence-based scenario. It is important that all simulation instructors receive formal training in how to implement and debrief simulation scenarios. Debriefing is a challenge, and most literature supports the need for educators to be trained in effective debriefing principles. Debriefing requires learner self-reflection and facilitative feedback in a psychologically safe environment (Rudolph, Simon, Dufresne, & Raemer, 2006; Rudolph, Simon, Raemer, & Eppich, 2008). An educator must take time to develop an evidence-based scenario and practice before implementation to ensure that learning objectives are achieved. Simulation is a highly effective and innovative educational tool. It can be used for many purposes in health care education, quality improvement, and patient safety. Although simulation can be a resource-intensive endeavor, when utilized appropriately it can greatly improve health care provider performance and patient care outcomes.

References

Andreatta, P. B., Woodrum, D. T., Birkmeyer, J. D., Yellamanchilli, R. K., Gerard, M., Doherty, G. M., . . . Minter, R. (2006). Laparoscopic skills are improved with LapMentor training: Results of a randomized, double-blinded study. *Annals of Surgery, 243*(6), 854–860.

Andreatta, P., Saxton, E., Thompson, M., & Annich, G. (2011). Simulation-based mock codes significantly correlate with improved pediatric patient cardiopulmonary arrest survival rates. *Pediatric Critical Care Medicine, 12*(1), 33–38.

Arnold, J., Hamilton, F., Kloesz, J., Clark, R., Kanter, S., Lowmaster, B., . . . Kochanek, P. (2008). *Effect of a high fidelity simulation curriculum on pediatric resident competency in neonatal airway management skills*. Pediatric Academic Societies Meeting, Honolulu, HI.

Barsuk, J. H., Cohen, E. R., Feinglass, J., McGaghie, W. C., & Wayne, D. B. (2009). Use of simulation-based education to reduce catheter-related bloodstream infections. *Archives of Internal Medicine, 169*(15), 1420–1423.

Draycott, T. J., Crofts, J. F., Ash, J. P., Wilson, L. V., Yard, E., Sibanda, T., & Whitelaw, A. (2008). Improving neonatal outcome through practical shoulder dystocia training. *Obstetrics and Gynecology, 112*(1), 14–20.

Gaba, D. (2004). *Crisis management in anesthesiology* (2nd ed.). Philadelphia, PA: Churchill Livingstone.

Lockhart, E., Allen, T., Gunatilake, R., Hobbs, G., & Taekman, J. (2012). *Use of human simulation for the development of a multidisciplinary obstetric massive transfusion protocol*. International Meeting for Simulation in Healthcare, San Diego, CA.

Rudolph, J. W., Simon, R., Raemer, D. B., & Eppich, W. (2008). Debriefing as formative assessment: Closing performance gaps in medical attention. *Academic Emergency Medicine, 15*, 1110Y–1116Y.

Rudolph, J. W., Simon, R., Dufresne, R. L., & Raemer, D. B. (2006). There's no such thing as a 'nonjudgmental' debriefing: A theory and method for debriefing with good judgment. *Simulation in Healthcare, 1*, 49Y–55Y.

Zabari, M., Suresh, G., Tomlinson, M., Lavin, J. P., Jr., Larison, K., Halamek, L., & Schriefer, J. A. (2006). Implementation and case-study results of potentially better practices for collaboration between obstetrics and neonatology to achieve improved perinatal outcomes. *Pediatrics, 118*(Suppl. 2), S153–S158.

ONLINE RESOURCES

A New Vision for Pediatric and Perinatal Education–Center for Advanced Pediatric & Perinatal Education
http://cape.lpch.org
Clinical Simulation in Nursing
http://www.nursingsimulation.org
Clinical Simulation to Improve Critical Thinking in the Neonatal Intensive Care
http://www.youtube.com/watch?v=Mf-RLRrc4XI
Deliberate practice using simulation improves neonatal resuscitation performance
http://www.ncbi.nlm.nih.gov/pubmed/21937960
Enhancing Patient Safety in Nursing Education through Patient Simulation
http://www.ahrq.gov/qual/nurseshdbk/docs/DurhamC_EPSNE.pdf
Neonatal Resuscitation
http://www.youtube.com/watch?v=TWaZBcjmxu8
Neonatal Simulation Center-Stony Brook Medicine
http://www.stonybrookmedicalcenter.org/pediatrics/neonatal_simulation
NOELLE® S550 Maternal and Neonatal Simulation System
http://www.stonybrookmedicalcenter.org/pediatrics/neonatal_simulation
SimNewB®
http://www.laerdal.com/us/doc/88/SimNewB

REFERENCES

Anderson, J. M., Murphy, A. A., Boyle, B. B., Yaeger, K. A., & Halamek, L. P. (2006). Simulating extracorporeal membrane oxygenation (ECMO) emergencies, Part II: Qualitative and quantitative assessment and validation. *Simulation in Healthcare, 1*, 228–232.

Andreatta, P., Saxton, E., Thompson, M., & Annich, G. (2011). Simulation-based mock codes significantly correlate with improved pediatric patient cardiopulmonary arrest survival rates. *Pediatric Critical Care Medicine, 12*(1), 33–38.

Andreatta, P. B., Woodrum, D. T., Birkmeyer, J. D., Yellamanchilli, R. K., Gerard, M., Doherty, G. M., . . . Minter, R. (2006). Laparoscopic skills are improved with LapMentor training: Results of a randomized, double-blinded study. *Annals of Surgery, 243*(6), 854–860.

Arnold, D., LeMaster, T., Todd, F., & Wallin, K. (2012). *Hospital-based simulation programs: Sharing operational models, practices, and strategies.* Abstract presentation at The International Meeting for Simulation in Healthcare, San Diego, CA.

Arnold, J. (2011). The neonatal resuscitation program comes of age. *Journal of Pediatrics, 159*(3), 357–358, el.

Arnold, J., Hamilton, F., Kloesz, J., Clark, R., Kanter, S., Lowmaster, B., . . . Kochanek, P. (2008). *Effect of a high fidelity simulation curriculum on pediatric resident competency in neonatal airway management skills.* Pediatric Academic Societies Meeting, Honolulu, HI.

Barsuk, J. H., Cohen, E. R., Feinglass, J., McGaghie, W. C., & Wayne, D. B. (2009). Use of simulation-based education to reduce catheter-related bloodstream infections. *Archives of Internal Medicine, 169*(15), 1420–1423.

Calhoun, A. W., Rider, E. A. M. S. W., Meyer, E. C., Lamiani, G. E., & Truog, R. D. (2009). Assessment of communication skills and self-appraisal in the simulated environment: Feasibility of multirater feedback with gap analysis. *Simulation in Healthcare, 4*, 22–29.

Cates, L. A., & Wilson, D. (2011). Acquisition and maintenance of competencies through simulation for neonatal nurse practitioners. *Advances in Neonatal Care, 11*(5), 1–7.

Cooper, G. E., White, M. D., & Lauber, J. K. (Eds.). (1980). *Resource management on the flightdeck: Proceedings of a NASA/Industry workshop (NASA CP –2120).* Moffett Field, CA: NASA-Ames Research Center.

Draycott, T. J., Crofts, J. F., Ash, J. P., Wilson, L. V., Yard, E., Sibanda, T., & Whitelaw, A. (2008). Improving neonatal outcome through practical shoulder dystocia training. *Obstetrics and Gynecology, 112*(1), 14–20.

Gaba, D. (2004). *Crisis management in anesthesiology* (2nd ed.). New York, NY: Churchill Livingstone.

Gaba, D. M. (1992). Improving anesthesiologist's performance by New York, NY: simulating reality. *Anesthesiology, 76*, 491–494.

Galloway, S. J. (2009). Simulation techniques to bridge the gap between healthcare professionals. *Online Journal of Issues in Nursing, 14*(2) manuscript 3.

Halamek, L. P. (2008). Educational perspectives: The genesis, adaptation, and evolution of the neonatal resuscitation program. *NeoReviews, 9*(4), 142–149.

Halamek, L. P., Kaegi, D. M., Gaba, D. M., Sowb, Y. A., Smith, B. C., Smith, B. E., & Howard, S. K. (2000). Time for a new paradigm in pediatric medical education: Teaching neonatal resuscitation in a simulated delivery room environment. *Pediatrics, 106* (4), e45–e53.

Helmreich, R. L., & Sexton, B. J. (2003). Analyzing cockpit communication: The links between language, performance, and workload. The University of Texas at Austin, Department of Psychology.

Helmreich, R. L., Wilhelm, J. A., Klinect, J. R., & Merritt, A. C. (2001). *Culture, error and crew resource management.* The University of Texas at Austin, Department of Psychology.

Issenberg, S. B., McGaghie, W. C., Petrusa, E. R., Lee Gordon, D., & Scalese, R. J. (2005). Features and uses of high-fidelity medical simulations that lead to effective learning: A BEME systematic review. *Medical Teacher, 27*, 10–28.

Joint Commission on Accreditation of Healthcare Organizations. (1998). *Sentinel events: Evaluating cause and planning improvement.* Oakbrook Terrace, IL: Joint Commission on Accreditation of Healthcare Organization.

Kaczorowski, J., Levitt, C., Hammond, M., Outerbridge, E., Grad, R., Rothman, A., & Graves, L. (1998). Retention of neonatal resuscitation skills and knowledge: A randomized controlled trial. *Family Medicine, 30*, 705–711.

Kohn, L. T., Corrigan, J. M., & Molla, S. D. (2000). *To err is human: Building a safer health system* (1st ed.). Washington, DC: National Academy Press.

Konge, L., Arendrup, H., von Buchwald, C., & Ringsted, C. (2011). Using performance in multiple simulated scenarios to assess bronchoscopy skills. *Respiration, 81*(6), 483–490.

Laerdal Medical Company. (2012). "The Girl from the River Seine". Retrieved from http://www.laerdal.com/us/doc/367/History

Lockhart, E., Allen, T., Gunatilake, R., Hobbs, G., & Taekman, J. (2012). *Use of human simulation for the development of a multidisciplinary obstetric massive transfusion protocol.* International Meeting for Simulation in Healthcare, San Diego, CA.

Lucisano, K. E., & Talbot, L. A. (2012). Simulation training for advanced airway management for anesthesia and other healthcare providers: A systematic review. *AANA Journal, 8*(1), 25–31.

Lutrell, M., Lenburg, C., Scherubel, J., Jacob, S., & Koch, R. (1999). Competency outcomes for learning and performance assessment: Redesigning a BSN curriculum. *Nursing and Health Care Perspectives, 20*, 134–141.

Moore, K. (2008). "A brief history of aircraft flight simulation," aircraft flight simulator. Kevin Moore, Retrieved from http://homepage.ntlworld.com/bleep/SimHist1.html

Murphy, A. A., & Halamek, L. P. (2005). Simulation-based training in neonatal resuscitation. *NeoReviews, 8*, e489–e492.

National Council of State Boards of Nursing. (2012). NCSBN national simulation study. Retrieved from https://www.ncsbn.org/2094.htm

Perlman, J. M., Wyllie, J., Kattwinkel, J., Atkins, D. L., Chameides, L., Goldsmith, J. P., . . . Neonatal Resuscitation Chapter Collaborators. (2010). The International Liaison Committee on Resuscitation (ILCOR) consensus on science with treatment recommendations for pediatric and neonatal patients: Neonatal resuscitation. *Pediatrics, 126*, e1319–e1344.

Rall, M., & Gaba, D. (2005). Human performance and patient safety. In R. Miller (Ed.), *Miller's anesthesia* (pp. 3021–3072). Philadelphia, PA: Elsevier Churchill Livingstone.

Rosen, K. R. (2008). History of medical simulation. *Journal of Critical Care, 23*, 157–166.

Rudolph, J. W., Taylor, S. S., & Foldy, E. G. (2001). Collaborative off-line reflection: A way to develop skill in action science and action inquiry. In P. Reason & H. Bradbury (Eds.), *Handbook of action research* (pp. 405–412). Thousand Oaks, CA: Sage.

The Joint Commission. (2010). Joint Commission Standard Frequently Asked Questions. Retrieved from http://www.jointcommission.org/search/default.aspx?Keywords=hospital%20accreditation%20standards

Vaillancourt, M., Ghaderi, I., Kaneva, P., Vassiliou, M., Kolozsvari, N., George, I., . . . Feldman, L. S. (2011). GOALS—incisional hernia: A valid assessment of simulation laparoscopic hernia repairs. *Surgical Innovations, 18*(1), 48–54.

Wayne, D. B., Didwania, A., Feinglass, J., Fudala, M. J., Barsuk, J. H., & McGaghie, W. C. (2007). Simulation-based education improves quality of care during cardiac arrest team responses at an academic teaching hospital: A case-control study. *Chest, 133*(1), 56–61. Retrieved from http://chestjournal.chestpubs.org/content/133/1/56.long

Zabari, M., Suresh, G., Tomlinson, M., Lavin, J. P., Jr., Larison, K., Halamek, L., & Schriefer, J. A. (2006). Implementation and case-study results of potentially better practices for collaboration between obstetrics and neonatology to achieve improved perinatal outcomes. *Pediatrics, 118*(Suppl. 2), S153–S158.

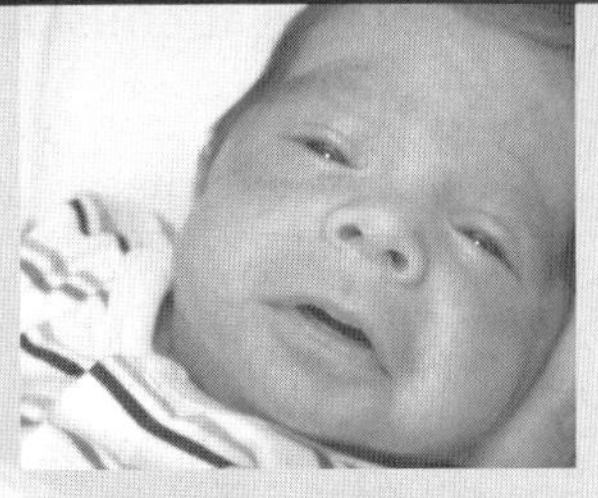

CHAPTER 23

Pain in the Newborn and Infant

■ Marlene Walden

Despite advances in neonatal pain assessment and management, nonpharmacologic and pharmacologic analgesic therapies continue to be underutilized to manage both acute and procedural pain (Carbajal et al., 2008; Simons, van Dijk, Anand, et al., 2003). Untreated acute, recurrent, or chronic pain related to disease or medical care may have significant and lifelong physiologic and psychologic consequences. As with all other medical conditions, the first step in the treatment process is the accurate diagnosis of the problem. Thus pain assessment provides the foundation for all pain treatment. This chapter reviews the developmental neurophysiology of pain, discusses methods to assess pain in infants, highlights factors that influence the pain experience, and discusses evidence-based strategies for managing infant pain.

DEFINING PAIN IN INFANTS

Pain is defined by the International Association for the Study of Pain (IASP) as "an unpleasant sensory and emotional experience associated with actual or potential tissue damage or described in terms of such damage"(Merskey, 1979). The IASP definition also states that pain is always subjective and is learned through experiences related to injury in early life. This definition is problematic when considering infants who are incapable of self-report and who may not have had previous experience with injury. Anand and Craig (1996) proposed that pain perception is an inherent quality of life that appears early in development to serve as a signaling system for tissue damage. This signaling includes behavioral and physiologic responses, which are valid indicators of pain that can be inferred by others. Broadening the definition of pain to include behavioral and physiologic indicators, in addition to self-report, can benefit preverbal, nonverbal, or cognitively impaired individuals who are experiencing pain by providing objective pain assessment.

Risk factors for pain along with a high index of suspicion should be used in determining whether an infant is in pain and is in need of appropriate pain-relieving treatment. The primary tenet is that pain in the newborn should be presumed in all situations usually considered to cause pain in adults and children, even in the absence of behavioral or physiologic signs (Agency for Health Care Policy and Research, 1992; National Association of Neonatal Nurses, 2012).

DEVELOPMENTAL NEUROPHYSIOLOGY OF PAIN

The basic mechanisms of pain perception in infants and children are similar to those of adults and include (1) transduction and transmission and (2) perception and modulation. However, because of neurophysiologic and cognitive immaturity, some differences exist. A brief review is presented here and emphasizes the developmental and maturational changes that occur during infancy and childhood (Fitzgerald & Howard, 2003).

Peripheral Transduction and Transmission

Noxious mechanical, thermal, or chemical stimuli excite primary afferent fibers that transmit information about the potentially injurious stimuli from the periphery to the dorsal horn of the spinal cord. A-delta (large, myelinated, and fast-conducting) and C (small, unmyelinated, and slow-conducting) fibers are primarily responsible for pain impulse transmission (nociception). However, these signals can be amplified or attenuated by activation of surrounding neurons in the periphery and spinal cord. For example, tissue injury causes the release of inflammatory mediators (e.g., potassium, bradykinin, prostaglandins, cytokines, nerve growth factors, catecholamines, and substance P) that sensitize A-delta and C fibers and recruit other neurons (silent nociceptors) and result in hyperalgesia. Stimulation of A-beta fibers that signal nonpainful touch and pressure can compete with the transmission of nociception in the dorsal horn of the spinal cord, thus reducing the intensity of the perceived pain.

Central Mechanisms and Modulation

Neurotransmitters in the spinal cord either amplify (e.g., substance P, calcitonin gene-related peptide, neurokinin A) or attenuate (e.g., endogenous opioids, norepinephrine, serotonin, GABA [gamma-aminobutyric acid], glycine) pain information from the periphery. Central sensitization occurs when excitatory amino acids act on NMDA (*N-Methyl-D-aspartate*) receptors to induce prolonged depolarization and windup.

Nociceptive sensory input reaches the thalamus through second-order neurons in the spinothalamic, spinoreticular, and spinomesencephalic tracts and is then widely distributed throughout the brain. The perception, emotional interpretation, and cognitive meaning of nociceptive stimuli occur within a distributive neuromatrix; no one "pain center" exists. The sensory-discriminative, affective-motivational, and evaluative dimensions of pain perception are mediated by past experience and the context of the painful event. For example, nociceptive stimuli activate areas of the limbic system thought to control emotion, particularly anxiety. Thus differences in physiologic, biochemical, and psychologic factors influence the perception of pain, making it an individual phenomenon.

Descending modulation occurs when efferent projections from supraspinal areas such as the periaqueductal gray, raphe nucleus, and locus coeruleus release inhibitory neurotransmitters. The major neurotransmitters that mediate descending inhibition are norepinephrine, serotonin, endogenous opioids, GABA, and acetylcholine.

Neurodevelopment of Pain Perception

Infants, even prematurely born infants, have the neurologic capacity to perceive pain at birth (Fitzgerald & Howard, 2003; Simons & Tibboel, 2006). The peripheral and central structures necessary for nociception are present and functional early in gestation (between the first and second trimesters). Functional maturation of the fetal cerebral cortex has been demonstrated by (1) electroencephalogram (EEG) patterns and cortical evoked potentials; (2) measurement of cerebral glucose use that shows maximal metabolic rates in sensory areas of the brain; and (3) well-defined periods of sleep and wakefulness that are regulated by cortical functioning from 28 weeks of gestation. The newborn infant possesses a well-developed hypothalamic-pituitary-adrenal axis and can mount a fight-or-flight response with the release of catecholamines and cortisol.

Research suggests that some differences in nociceptive processes between infants and adults exist. For example, pain impulse transmission in neonates occurs primarily along nonmyelinated C fibers rather than myelinated A-delta fibers. Less precision also occurs in pain signal transmission in the spinal cord, and descending inhibitory neurotransmitters are lacking (Fitzgerald & Howard, 2003). Thus young infants may perceive pain more intensely than older children or adults because their descending control mechanisms are immature and thus limit their ability to modulate the experience.

Long-Term Consequences of Pain

Although pain can serve as a warning of injury, the effects of pain are generally deleterious. Pain evokes negative physiologic, metabolic, and behavioral responses in infants. These responses include autonomic instability, pulmonary dysfunction, and hormonal stress (Goldschneider & Anand, 2003). Pain and stress contribute to an increased allostatic load of preterm neonates in the neonatal intensive care unit (NICU). *Allostatic load* is the resulting wear and tear on the body from repeatedly adapting to adverse situations (Grunau, Holsti, & Peters, 2006). Painful procedures may result in heightened pain sensitivity to routine handling as well as delayed recovery from noxious and routine caregiving procedures.

Learning about pain occurs with the first pain experience and may have effects on subsequent pain perception and responses. Memory of pain in infants is evident from differences in responses to painful vaccination in infants who had undergone unanesthetized circumcision in comparison to infants who were uncircumcised or who received analgesia during circumcision (Taddio, Goldbach, Ipp, Stevens, & Koren, 1995; Taddio, Katz, Ilersich, & Koren, 1997).

Research has suggested that pain syndromes may be related to early pain experiences. Grunau and colleagues reported that former extremely-low-birth-weight (ELBW) infants at 18 months were judged by their parents to be less sensitive to pain and have higher somatization (pain of unknown cause) compared with parents of full-term infants (Grunau, Whitfield, & Petrie, 1994). More recent research, however, has failed to demonstrate differences in somatization of former ELBW infants at age 9 years (Whitfield, Grunau, & Holsti, 1997) or at ages 17 to 19 years (Grunau et al., 2004). Further research is needed to learn about pain and its effects in infancy and beyond.

CLINICAL ASSESSMENT OF PAIN

Presently, no easily administered, widely accepted, uniform technique exists for assessing pain in infants (Duhn & Medves, 2004). A multidimensional pain assessment tool that includes measurements for both physiologic and behavioral indicators of pain is preferable given the multifaceted nature of pain (National Association of Neonatal Nurses, 2012; Walden, 2001). Selection of an appropriate clinical pain assessment method should be based first on the developmental age of the infant, and second on the type of pain experienced (e.g., for procedural pain or postoperative pain). Published validity and reliability should be considered when choosing a pain assessment tool.

Multidimensional Pain Tools

The most commonly used published multidimensional infant-specific pain assessment tools with psychometric data are listed in Table 23.1. The Premature Infant Pain Profile (PIPP) was originally developed to measure procedural pain (Stevens, Johnston, Petryshen, & Taddio, 1996), but recently has also been used in newborns to assess postoperative pain (El Sayed, Taddio, Fallah, De Silva, & Moore, 2007; McNair, Ballantyne, Dionne, Stephens, & Stevens, 2004). The PIPP has been tested in neonates ranging in ages from extremely preterm up to 40 weeks postconceptional age. The PIPP incorporates two contextual factors that may account for the infant's less robust pain responses that may result from their immaturity or behavioral state. By scoring infants who are younger or those who are asleep higher on the PIPP, the adjusted scores do not penalize infants who are known to be less capable of mounting a robust response to noxious stimuli. The PIPP contains two physiologic indicators (i.e., heart rate and oxygen saturation) and three facial indicators (i.e., brow bulge, eye squeeze, and nasolabial furrow). While total scores vary between 18 and 21 depending on the infant's gestational age, scores between 7 and 12 usually signify mild to moderate pain requiring nonpharmacologic pain relief measures and scores greater than 12 indicate moderate to severe pain requiring pharmacologic pain intervention in addition to comfort measures.

The CRIES was originally developed to assess postoperative pain in infants between 32 and 36 weeks gestational age (Krechel & Bildner, 1995), but recent studies have also documented its clinical utility in assessing procedural pain in preterm and term neonates (Ahn, 2006; Belda, Pallas, De la Cruz, & Tejada, 2004; Herrington, Olomu, & Geller, 2004). The CRIES is an acronym for the five parameters it measures: **C**rying, **R**equires oxygen to maintain saturation greater than 95%, **I**ncreased vital signs, **E**xpression, and **S**leepless. Total scores for the CRIES range from 0 to 10, with scores less than 4 indicative of mild pain requiring nonpharmacologic pain relief measures and scores greater than or equal to 5 consistent with moderate to severe pain requiring pharmacologic intervention in conjunction with comfort measures.

The Neonatal Infant Pain Scale (NIPS) was originally developed to assess procedural pain in preterm and term newborns (Lawrence et al., 1993), but recent literature also validates its utility with postoperative pain (Rouss, Gerber, Albisetti, Hug, & Bernet, 2007; Suraseranivongse et al., 2006). The NIPS examines five behavioral parameters (i.e., facial expression, crying, arms, legs, and state of arousal) and one physiologic parameter (i.e., breathing pattern). Total score ranges from 0 to 7. While the researchers of the NIPS do not provide guidelines for pain interventions based on total score, all pain instruments in neonates are based on the premise of increasing pain intensity. Therefore

TABLE 23.1

MOST COMMONLY USED MULTIDIMENSIONAL PAIN ASSESSMENT TOOLS IN NEWBORNS

Pain Instrument	Population	Indicators	Forms of Validity	Reliability Data
Premature infant pain profile (PIPP) (Stevens et al., 1996; Stevens, Johnston, Taddio, Gibbins, & Yamada, 2010)	Preterm and term neonates	Gestational age Behavioral state Heart rate Oxygen saturation Brow bulge Eye squeeze Nasolabial furrow	Face Content Construct	Inter- and intrarater reliability greater than 0.93
CRIES: Neonatal Postoperative Pain Assessment Score (Bildner & Krechel, 1996)	Neonates from 32–60 weeks	**C**rying **R**equires oxygen to maintain saturation 95% **I**ncreased blood pressure and heart rate **E**xpression **S**leep state	Face Content Discriminant Concurrent (r = 0.49–0.73)	Interrater reliability greater than 0.72
Neonatal Infant Pain Scale (NIPS) (Lawrence et al., 1993)	Preterm and term neonates	Facial expression Cry Breathing patterns Arm Movement Leg movement State of arousal	Face Construct Concurrent validity (r = 0.53–0.84)	Interrater reliability greater than 0.92
Neonatal Pain Agitation and Sedation Scale (N-PASS) (Hummel et al., 2008)	Preterm and term neonates	Crying/irritability Behavior/state Facial expression Extremities/tone Vital signs	Concurrent Discriminate	Interrater reliability greater than 0.90

in tools without scoring guidelines for pain management, when pain scores reach the midrange of the total possible points for that tool (i.e., approximately 4 or greater with the NIPS), the clinician may infer that the infant is experiencing moderate to severe pain and pharmacologic intervention for that pain is warranted.

The Neonatal Pain Agitation and Sedation Scale (N-PASS), developed by Hummel, Puchalski, Creech, and Weiss (2008), is a five-item scale that measures both pain/agitation and sedation in preterm and term neonates with prolonged pain postoperatively and during mechanical ventilation. The N-PASS examines four behavioral items (crying/irritability, behavior state, facial expression, extremities/tone) and one physiologic indicator (vital signs). Total pain scores range from 0 to –10, while sedation scores range from 0 to 10. Like the PIPP, the N-PASS includes gestational age as a contextual modifier of pain, thus adjusting the pain score to account for the preterm's limited ability to mount a robust pain response due to immaturity.

Factors That Influence Pain

Pain is unique among neurologic functions because of the degree of plasticity in pain neurophysiology. Although structural and functional maturity is reached at an early age, anatomic and functional changes occur throughout life and are related to the effects of each pain experience. This plasticity means that the perception and meaning of pain are unique to each individual and are not determined by maturation alone but are influenced by many individual and contextual factors. Currently available methods to assess pain in infants do not adequately or quantitatively incorporate all aspects of the context of pain that influence the pain experience. Thus the clinician must remain cognizant of the ways in which perception of pain may be positively or negatively influenced by these factors and subjectively incorporate them into the assessment of pain. These factors do not influence pain in isolation but are listed separately for clarity.

■ Behavioral State. The behavioral state of the infant, ranging from deep sleep to awake and crying, acts as a moderator of behavioral pain responses. The behavioral state of the infant immediately before the painful stimulus affects the robustness of the response. Infants in awake states demonstrate more robust reactions to pain than infants in sleep states. Infants in a drowsy or deep sleep state will show less vigorous facial expression in response to heelstick than infants who are alert or aroused before the heelstick (Grunau & Craig, 1987; Mathai, Naresh, & Sahu, 2011; Stevens, Johnston, & Horton, 1994).

■ Gestational Age. Gestational age affects infant pain responses, with younger infants displaying fewer and less vigorous behavioral responses to pain (Gibbins & Stevens, 2003; Stevens et al., 1994, 1996, 1999). In addition, preterm neonates may demonstrate unique behaviors in response to noxious stimuli. Several researchers have used the Newborn Individualized Developmental Care and Assessment Program (NIDCAP, Children's Hospital, Boston, MA) to examine responses of preterm neonates to a heelstick procedure and found that preterm neonates may uniquely respond to acute pain by increased flexion and extension of arms and legs, finger splay, fisting, frowning, and hand on face behaviors (Holsti, Grunau, Oberlander, & Whitfield, 2004).

■ Previous Pain Experience. Previous pain experience of preterm neonates may lead to alterations in pain signal processing. Infants who were subjected to more frequent painful procedures in the NICU had decreased behavioral and increased cardiovascular responses compared to infants who experienced less pain, even after controlling for gestational age–related differences in pain expression (Johnston & Stevens, 1996; Stevens et al., 1999).

■ Caregiver Handling. Term and healthy preterm newborns who were handled or immobilized before heelstick exhibited greater physiologic and behavioral reactivity, thus indicating that previous stress may result in greater instability in response to pain (Porter, Wolf, & Miller, 1998).

MANAGEMENT OF NEONATAL PAIN

The goals of pain management in infants are (1) to minimize the intensity, duration, and physiologic cost of the pain experience; (2) to maximize the infant's ability to cope with and recover from the painful experience; and (3) to maintain a balance between pain relief and adverse effects of analgesics (Carbajal, Gall, & Annequin, 2004). Depending on duration and severity, pain may be successfully managed with nonpharmacologic comfort measures and/or pharmacologic therapies.

Prevention of Pain

Painful procedures in the NICU are unavoidable; therefore it is vital that caregivers assist infants to cope with and recover from necessary but painful clinical procedures. Recent research suggests that greater neonatal procedural pain is associated with reduced white matter and impaired early brain development in very preterm infants (Brummelte et al., 2012). Therefore, strategies to prevent pain should be employed whenever possible, including grouping blood draws to minimize the number of venipunctures per day, establishing central vessel access when appropriate to minimize vein and artery punctures, and limiting adhesive tape and gentle removal of tape to minimize epidermal stripping.

Nonpharmacologic Comfort Management

Nonpharmacologic strategies are hypothesized to directly reduce pain by (1) blocking nociceptive transduction or transmission; (2) activating descending inhibitory pathways; or (3) activating attention or arousal systems that modulate pain. Nonpharmacologic strategies such as hand or blanket swaddling, nonnutritive sucking (NNS), oral sucrose, and skin-to-skin contact may help minimize neonatal pain and stress while maximizing the infant's own regulatory and coping abilities.

■ Swaddling or Facilitated Tucking. Containment strategies to limit excessive, immature motor responses have been demonstrated to be effective in minimizing pain responses in preterm neonates. Swaddling is thought to reduce pain by providing gentle stimulation across the proprioceptive, thermal, and tactile sensory systems. Several studies have been conducted in the preterm population using either hand or blanket swaddling. A hand-swaddling technique known as "facilitated tucking" (holding the infant's extremities flexed and contained close to the trunk) has been shown to attenuate pain responses in preterm neonates by decreasing heart rates, increasing oxygen saturations, decreasing crying time and sleep disruption times, and reducing pain scores during heelstick procedures and endotracheal suctioning (Cignacco et al., 2012; Obeidat, Kahalaf, Callister, & Froelicher, 2009).

■ NNS. NNS is the provision of a pacifier into the mouth to promote sucking without the provision of breast milk or formula for nutrition. NNS is thought to produce analgesia through stimulation of orotactile and mechanoreceptors when a pacifier is introduced into the infant's mouth. NNS is hypothesized to modulate transmission or processing of nociception through mediation by the endogenous nonopioid system (Blass, Fitzgerald, & Kehoe, 1987).

NNS has been shown to reduce pain responses in both term and preterm neonates (Pillai Riddell et al., 2011) during immunizations (Liaw et al., 2011) and heelstick procedures (Liaw et al., 2010). A study by Stevens and colleagues found that pain relief was greater in infants who received both NNS and sucrose (Stevens et al., 1999). A study by Campos (1989) reported a rebound in distress occurred when the NNS pacifier was removed from the infants' mouths. Therefore, the efficacy of NNS is immediate but appears to terminate almost immediately on cessation of sucking (Campos, 1989).

■ Sucrose. Sucrose with and without NNS has been the most widely studied nonpharmacologic intervention for infant pain management. Sucrose is a disaccharide comprised of fructose and glucose. A systematic review of 44 randomized control trials of full-term and preterm infants (N = 3,496) found that sucrose is safe and effective for reducing procedural pain in term and preterm neonates, particularly heelstick and venipuncture procedures (Stevens, Yamada, & Ohlsson, 2010). Doses of 24% sucrose or greater are most effective, although some additional benefit has been reported with doses of up to 50%. A pain-reduction response is noted with dose volumes ranging from 0.05 mL to 2 mL of a 24% solution administered approximately 2 minutes before the painful stimulus (Stevens, Yamada, et al., 2010). This 2-minute time interval appears to coincide with endogenous opioid release triggered by the sweet taste of sucrose (Blass, 1994). The effect of sucrose appears to last approximately 4 minutes; therefore, repeated doses may be necessary if procedures are prolonged (Stevens, Yamada, et al., 2010). The use of sucrose in combination with other behavioral interventions such as NNS, skin-to-skin holding, and containment may enhance the analgesic effect of sucrose.

Although relatively few contraindications to the provision of swaddling and NNS for management of pain in neonates exist, the absolute safety of sucrose has not been determined. Rare instances of choking and decreased oxygen saturation, all resolving spontaneously, have been reported (Gibbins et al., 2002). Although a study by Willis and colleagues reported an association between sucrose and necrotizing enterocolitis (NEC), more recent research found no significant differences in incidence rates for NEC between infants who received repeated doses of sucrose over 28 days of life compared to control groups (Stevens et al., 2005; Willis, Chabot, Radde, & Chance, 1977). Sucrose should be used with caution in extremely preterm neonates, critically ill newborns, neonates with unstable blood glucose levels, and infants at risk for NEC. Furthermore, sufficient evidence of the safety of repeated doses of sucrose in neonates to recommend its widespread use for repeated painful procedures is lacking (Stevens, Yamada, et al., 2010). Johnston and colleagues reported that preterm infants less than 31 weeks postmenstrual age who received repeated doses of sucrose for painful procedures showed poorer neurodevelopmental scores at 36 and 40 weeks (Johnston et al., 2002). However, a more recent study failed to demonstrate significant differences on neurobiological risk status outcomes between preterm infants who received sucrose plus pacifier, water plus pacifier or the standard care group (Stevens et al., 2005).

■ Skin-to-Skin Contact (Kangaroo Care). Skin-to-skin contact, or kangaroo care, has been demonstrated to significantly reduce pain responses in term newborns and preterm neonates greater than 28 weeks gestational age during heelstick procedures (Johnston et al., 2003, 2008). The 2008 study by Johnston and colleagues also showed that preterm neonates between 28 and 32 weeks gestational age demonstrated a shorter time to recovery as compared with control neonates who were swaddled and lying prone in an incubator during the heelstick procedure.

Pharmacologic Management

Pharmacologic agents are often required to alleviate moderate to severe procedural, postoperative, or disease-related pain in neonates. Systemic analgesia, topical anesthetics, nonopioid analgesia, and adjunctive medications are reviewed. The most commonly used drugs for analgesia in neonates are listed in Table 23.2.

■ Opioids. Opioid analgesics are considered the gold standard for pain relief. Opioids are often the preferred choice to manage moderate to severe pain in neonates. Morphine

TABLE 23.2

COMMONLY USED DRUGS FOR ANALGESIA IN NEONATES

Drugs	Routes	Dose	Administration Notes
Opioid Analgesics			
Morphine	Intermittent intravenous (IV), intramuscular, subcutaneous Continuous infusion Oral/parenteral ratio	0.05–0.2 mg/kg 0.01–0.02 mg/kg/hr	Give over at least 5 minutes Repeat as required (usually every 4 hours) Give loading dose of 0.1–0.15 mg/kg over 1 hour Oral dose is 3 to 5 times IV dose; for treatment of opioid dependence, begin at most recent IV morphine dose equivalent and taper 10%–20% per day as tolerated
Fentanyl	Intermittent intravenous (IV) Continuous infusion	0.5–4 mcg/kg 1–5 mcg/kg/hr	Repeat as required (usually every 2–4 hours) Tolerance may develop rapidly after constant infusion Adjust weaning schedule based on withdrawal symptoms
Nonsteroidal Anti-inflammatory			
Acetaminophen	PO Rectal	12–15 mg/kg 12–18 mg/kg	Give loading dose of 20–25 mg/kg Give loading dose of 30 mg/kg Maintenance intervals: Term infants: give every 6 hours. Preterm infants older than or equal to 32 weeks postconceptual age (PCA): give every 8 hours Preterm infants younger than 32 weeks PCA: give every 12 hours
Local/regional Anesthetics/Analgesia			
Eutectic mixture of local anesthetics (EMLA)	Topical	1–2 g	Apply and wrap with occlusive dressing; allow to remain intact for 60–90 minutes; remove and clean prior to procedure to avoid systemic absorption; monitor for methemoglobinemia
Local/regional Anesthetics/Analgesia			
Liposomal lidocaine cream (LMX 4%)	Topical	1 g	Use only on normal, intact skin; prepare the area by washing with mild soap and water; DO NOT use alcohol; apply a small amount of cream and gently massage into the skin, then apply the remainder of the dose in a 1/4-inch thick layer and cover with an occlusive dressing at least 30 minutes prior to the procedure; remove cream and cleanse area before beginning procedure
Amethocaine Gel (4%)[a]	Topical	0.5 g	Cover with occlusive dressing; do not spread or rub in; remove gel and dressing after 30 to 45 minutes; do not leave on for longer than 60 minutes; should not be used in premature infants or those younger than 1 month of age
Lidocaine 1%[b]	Subcutaneous	0.2–0.5 mL	Epinephrine should never be added to the lidocaine because of its vasoconstrictive properties and the risk of ischemia and necrosis; Infiltrate area using 25 G needle approximately 3 to 8 minutes prior to procedure

[a] O'Brien, Taddio, Lyszkiewicz, and Koren (2005); Orion Laboratories. Product Information Sheet.
[b] Pinheiro, Furdon, and Ochoa (1993); Regen and Whitehill (2012).

Adapted from Young and Manguml (2010).

and fentanyl are the most commonly used opioids in the NICU, although other drugs may also be used for pain control in the neonatal population. Opioids have (1) potent analgesic effects; (2) ability to produce sedation but no amnesic or hypnotic effects; (3) few hemodynamic side effects; and (4) availability of antagonist drugs such as naloxone to reverse adverse side effects (Walter-Nicolet, Annequin, Biran, Mitanchez, & Tourniaire, 2010). The most common adverse effects include respiratory depression, bronchospasm, reduced gastrointestinal motility, urinary retention, and pruritus.

Morphine. Morphine is the gold standard for opioid analgesia in critically ill and postoperative neonates. Morphine has a slower onset of analgesia due to lower lipid solubility, especially in preterm neonates. The onset of action is 5 minutes, and the peak effect occurs at 15 minutes (Walter-Nicolet et al., 2010).

Morphine has few effects on the neonatal cardiovascular system in the well-hydrated neonate. Hypotension, bradycardia, and flushing are part of the histamine response to morphine and can be decreased by slow intravenous bolus administration (over 10–20 minutes) and optimizing intravascular fluid volume (Anand, 2007). Although relatively uncommon, the effects of histamine release may also cause bronchospasm in infants with chronic lung disease (Anand, 2007). Decreased intestinal motility and abdominal distention may also occur causing a delay in the establishment of enteral feeding in the preterm neonate (Anand, 2007). Tolerance of enteral feeds may be improved by priming the gut with small volumes of milk.

Compared with fentanyl, morphine is less likely to cause dependence or withdrawal. Close monitoring and individual titration of the amount and frequency of doses for all neonates receiving morphine therapy is essential (Anand, 2007).

The effect of morphine therapy on neurologic outcomes of preterm neonates is unclear. Although two large randomized controlled trials (NEOPAIN [Neurologic Outcomes and Pre-emptive Analgesia in Neonates] and the EPIPAGE [Etude Epidemiologique sur lest Petits Ages Gestationalles]) suggest that morphine therapy does not have an adverse effect on the neurologic outcomes (Anand et al., 2004; Roze et al., 2008), a subsequent study evaluating neurobehavioral outcomes at 36 weeks of neonates enrolled in the NEOPAIN trial suggested that morphine analgesia may result in subtle neurobehavioral differences in preterm neonates (Rao et al., 2007).

The effectiveness of morphine for acute pain caused by invasive procedures remains unclear. Several studies support the effectiveness of morphine analgesia for acute pain (Anand et al., 1999; Taddio et al., 2006), while other studies have found no significant analgesic efficacy (Carbajal et al., 2005; Franck et al., 2000; Saarenmaa, Huttunen, Leppaluoto, Meretoja, & Fellman, 1999; Simons, van Dijk, van Lingen, et al., 2003).

Fentanyl. Randomized clinical trials in neonates have found that fentanyl is approximately 13 to 20 times more potent than morphine (Saarenmaa et al., 1999). Fentanyl is probably the most widely used analgesic in neonates and offers two distinct advantages over morphine (Anand, 2007). First, fentanyl causes less histamine release than morphine and may be more appropriate for neonates with hypovolemia or hemodynamic instability, congenital heart disease, or chronic lung disease (Walter-Nicolet et al., 2010). Second, fentanyl blunts increases in pulmonary vascular resistance. This finding makes it potentially useful in managing pain in neonates with persistent pulmonary hypertension (Walter-Nicolet et al., 2010).

Fentanyl has a more rapid onset (3 minutes) and shorter duration of action (30 minutes) compared with morphine and must be administered as a continuous infusion or as an intravenous bolus every 1 to 2 hours. Accumulation of fentanyl in fatty tissues with extended use may prolong its sedative and respiratory depressant effects and may be responsible for the rebound increase in plasma levels observed following discontinuation of therapy in neonates (Anand, 2007).

Tolerance may develop rapidly with fentanyl, especially with continuous infusions compared to bolus dosing. In addition, dependence and withdrawal are more significant with fentanyl as compared to morphine (Franck, Vilardi, Durand, & Powers, 1998).

Rarely, fentanyl can significantly reduce chest wall compliance (stiff chest syndrome). This naloxone-reversible side effect can be prevented by slow infusion (as opposed to rapid bolus administration) or concomitant use of muscle relaxants.

Prevention of Opioid Withdrawal Symptoms. Neonates who require opioid therapy for an extended period of time may develop physical dependence and withdrawal. Rapid weaning of opioids may lead to withdrawal symptoms such as irritability, crying, increased respiratory rate, jitteriness, hypertonicity, vomiting, diarrhea, sweating, skin abrasions, seizures, yawning, stuffy nose, sneezing, and hiccups. The goals of clinical management of opioid withdrawal are (1) to reduce withdrawal symptoms to promote regular sleep cycles and (2) to reduce agitation caused by care interventions (Anand et al., 2010). The prevalence of opioid withdrawal is greater in infants after continuous infusions of fentanyl than continuous infusions of morphine (Franck et al., 1998). Dominguez and colleagues reported a 53% incidence in opioid withdrawal in neonates who received a minimum of 24 hours of fentanyl by continuous infusion. In this study, the most significant risk factors for opioid withdrawal were higher total dose and longer infusion duration. In all neonates with withdrawal, onset of withdrawal symptoms occurred within 24 hours of discontinuation of the fentanyl infusion (Dominguez, Lomako, Katz, & Kelly, 2003).

Data are insufficient to determine the optimal weaning rate of opioids to prevent withdrawal symptoms in neonates on opioid therapy (Hudak et al., 2012). Ducharme and colleagues reported that adverse withdrawal symptoms in children who received continuous infusions of opioids and/or benzodiazepines could be prevented when the daily rate of weaning did not exceed 20% for children who received opioids/benzodiazepines for 1 to 3 days; 13% to 20% for 4 to 7 days; 8% to 13% for 8 to 14 days; 8% for 15 to 21 days; and 2% to 4% for more than 21 days, respectively (Ducharme, Carnevale, Clermont, & Shea, 2005). Abstinence scoring methods commonly used in the care of the infant with prenatal drug exposure must be employed in assessing the infant during withdrawal from prolonged opioid use. The Modified Finnegan's Neonatal Abstinence Scoring Tool (Hudak et al., 2012) is the most commonly used tool for assessment of neonatal abstinence syndrome in the United States (Sarkar & Donn, 2006).

Methadone. Methadone is a synthetic opioid that produces prolonged analgesia and has good oral bioavailability, thus making it an attractive option to manage neonatal abstinence syndrome (Hudak et al., 2012). When an infant is being weaned from opioid therapy to a longer-acting oral medication such as methadone, the starting dose of methadone should be calculated to provide a dose equivalent to the dose of opioid the neonate is receiving (Hudak et al., 2012). Further weaning should then be accomplished based on frequent reassessment to ensure that the patient is free of pain and withdrawal symptoms. Studies are needed to further establish the pharmacokinetics and dosing requirements of methadone in neonates.

■ Topical Application of Local Anesthetics. Topical anesthetics are useful for the management of procedure-related pain in neonates. While EMLA cream ([eutectic mixture of local anesthetics], lidocaine, and prilocaine; Astra Pharmaceuticals, London) has the best evidence for use in neonates, tetracaine 4% gel (Ametop; Smith & Nephew, London) and liposomal lidocaine cream (LMX 4%; Ferndale Laboratories, Michigan) have also been used in neonates.

EMLA Cream. EMLA cream (eutectic mixture of local anesthetics, lidocaine, and prilocaine; Astra Pharmaceuticals, London) is approved for use in infants at birth with a gestational age of 37 weeks or greater for a variety of clinical procedures. EMLA produces topical anesthesia when applied as a cream to the surface of intact skin and then covered with an occlusive dressing. The primary concern with the use of EMLA is methemoglobinemia caused by prilocaine toxicity. Neonates, particularly preterm neonates, are at increased risk because of a thinner stratum corneum and less active NADH-dependent (*NADH* dehydrogenase) methemoglobin reductase enzymes that result in higher plasma levels (Sethna & Koh, 2000). Neonates who have anemia, sepsis, hypoxemia, or metabolic acidosis and who are receiving other methemoglobin-inducing drugs such as acetaminophen, phenytoin, phenobarbital, or nitroprusside may also be at increased risk for development of systemic toxicity (Sethna & Koh, 2000). Although it is not routinely recommended for use in preterm neonates, one study found that a single dose of 0.5 g EMLA cream applied for 60 minutes to the intact skin of preterm infants older than 30 weeks gestation did not result in significant increases in blood methemoglobin concentrations (Taddio, Shennan, Stevens, Leeder, & Koren, 1995). In addition to the risk of methemoglobinemia, local skin reactions have been noted with EMLA cream and have included blanching, redness, and transient purpuric lesions (Sethna & Koh, 2000). Policies and procedures regarding application of EMLA cream should be established to maximize pain relief while minimizing the potential side effects.

Three primary factors determine the effectiveness of EMLA cream: dose, size of application area, and duration of exposure (Sethna & Koh, 2000). The depth of penetration of EMLA is approximately 2 to 3 mm (Walter-Nicolet et al., 2010). The recommended dose in neonates is 1 to 2 g applied to the procedure site 60 to 90 minutes before the procedure and covered with an occlusive dressing (*NEOFAX*, 2011). Multiple studies document the efficacy of EMLA in reducing pain associated with venipunctures and circumcisions (Anand et al., 2005). EMLA has also been documented to be effective in managing pain associated with lumbar puncture (Kaur, Gupta, & Kumar, 2003). EMLA has not been shown, however, to be effective in managing pain associated with the heelstick procedures (Anand et al., 2005).

Tetracaine 4% Gel. Tetracaine 4% gel (Ametop; Smith & Nephew, London) has also been investigated in neonates for management of procedural pain. Tetracaine 4% gel produces anesthesia within 30 to 45 minutes of application and has duration of action between 4 and 6 hours (O'Brien, Taddio, Lyszkiewicz, & Koren, 2005). A meta-analysis of six randomized controlled trials comparing tetracaine with EMLA found tetracaine significantly reduced pain associated with intravenous cannulation compared to EMLA. However, tetracaine is ineffective in reducing the pain of heelprick and peripherally inserted central catheters in neonates (Lander, Weltman, & So, 2006). The most commonly reported local skin reaction is transient local erythema.

LMX 4%. Another topical local anesthetic currently used in pediatrics for management of procedural pain is liposomal lidocaine cream (LMX 4%; Ferndale Laboratories, Michigan). Several studies have evaluated the efficacy of LMX and EMLA and found a 30-minute application of LMX to be as effective as a 60-minute application of EMLA for producing topical anesthesia for peripheral intravenous access in older children (Eichenfield, Funk, Fallon-Friedlander, & Cunningham, 2002; Kleiber, Sorenson, Whiteside, Gronstal, & Tannous, 2002; Koh et al., 2004). Similar results were found in a recent study in neonates that found LMX to be equally effective as EMLA in reducing the pain of circumcision in term newborns (Lehr et al., 2005). LMX may offer an improved risk-benefit profile compared to EMLA, considering the faster onset of action and no risk of methemoglobinemia. Further studies in neonates are needed to establish the safety and efficacy of LMX for management of procedural pain in neonates.

■ Nonopioid Analgesics

Acetaminophen. Acetaminophen is a nonopioid analgesic for short-term management of mild to moderate pain in neonates, but is ineffective for acute procedure-related pain. Acetaminophen has been commonly administered in neonates as an oral or rectal preparation. A recent study reports the safety of intravenous administration of acetaminophen in neonates (Zuppa et al., 2011). When acetaminophen is administered concurrently with opioid analgesia, the effect is additive and allows a reduction in dosages of both drugs, resulting in fewer adverse side effects (Menon, Anand, & McIntosh, 1998).

Little information is available on the pharmacokinetics of acetaminophen administration in neonates, especially administration by the rectal route. Peak concentrations of analgesic effect are reached approximately 60 minutes after an oral dose (*NEOFAX*, 2011). Elimination half-life is approximately 3 hours in term neonates, but can be as long as 11 hours in more preterm neonates requiring longer dosing intervals with decreasing gestational ages (*NEOFAX*, 2011). Acetaminophen is metabolized almost entirely by hepatic conjugation, and elimination may be prolonged in neonates with liver dysfunction.

At therapeutic doses, acetaminophen is well tolerated and has a low toxicity. Because acetaminophen does not inhibit prostaglandin synthesis in tissues other than the brain, common side effects of nonsteroidal anti-inflammatory drugs—such as inhibition of platelet function, renal insufficiency, and gastrointestinal irritation—do not occur (Anand, Menon, Narsinghani, & NcIntosh, 2000). The primary concern of acetaminophen is liver damage, but this should not be a concern in neonates if standard doses are used (*NEOFAX*, 2011). The use of acetaminophen in the first year of life seems to be associated with an increased risk of asthma, rhinoconjunctivitis, and eczema at age 6 to 7 years of age (Beasley et al., 2008). Further studies are needed to confirm these long-term adverse effects. Routine prophylactic use of acetaminophen at the time of vaccination is not recommended due to a potential reduction in antibody response (Prymula et al., 2009).

■ Use of Adjunctive Drugs. In the NICU, the use of sedatives, alone or in combination with analgesics, is controversial. Although sedatives suppress the behavioral expression of pain, they have no analgesic effects and can even increase pain. Sedatives should only be used when pain has been ruled out. When administered with opioids, sedatives may allow more optimal weaning of opioids in critically ill, ventilator-dependent neonates who have developed tolerance from prolonged opioid therapy. No research has been done to determine the safety or efficacy of combining sedatives and analgesics for the treatment of pain in infants. The most commonly administered sedatives in the NICU are benzodiazepines and chloral hydrate.

■ Benzodiazepines

Midazolam. Midazolam is a short-acting benzodiazepine that is frequently used as a hypnosedative in neonates. Recent concern about the safety of midazolam in neonates has been reported because of the large number of adverse neurologic effects associated with midazolam in term and preterm neonates. Severe hypotension, seizures, respiratory depression, and respiratory arrest have been reported in neonates following continuous infusions or rapid bolus administration (*NEOFAX*, 2011). Due to uncertainty about its safety, a Cochrane review concluded that data are insufficient to promote the use of intravenous midazolam infusions for sedation in neonates (Ng, Taddio, & Ohlsson, 2012).

Diazepam. Diazepam is not recommended for administration in neonates because of its very prolonged half-life (20–50 hours), its long-acting metabolites, and concern about the benzyl alcohol content. The dose of benzyl alcohol preservative in diazepam is, however, below the dose known to cause fatal toxicity in premature neonates (100–400 mg/kg/d). Diazepam displaces bilirubin from albumin-binding sites, thereby increasing the neonate's risk of kernicterus (Anand et al., 2000).

Chloral Hydrate. Chloral hydrate has been used in single doses to sedate neonates during pulmonary function, radiographic, and other diagnostic testing for which the patient must lie still. The onset of action is 10 to 15 minutes (*NEOFAX*, 2011). Adverse effects include bradycardia, gastric irritation, and paradoxical excitement (*NEOFAX*, 2011). Although clinically effective, concern has been raised about the potential carcinogenic effects of chloral hydrate administered to mice (*NEOFAX*, 2011). The extremely long half-life of chloral hydrate increases the risk of toxicity with repeated administration. Alternative sedatives (i.e., benzodiazepines) should be used when possible.

MANAGEMENT OF SPECIFIC PAIN TYPES

Pain management techniques may vary based on pain type and clinical situation. This section reviews special issues related to procedural pain, postoperative pain, preemptive analgesia for mechanical ventilation, and pain management at end of life (EOL).

Procedural Pain

It has been estimated that newborn infants, particularly those born preterm, are routinely subjected to an average of 61 invasive procedures performed from admission to discharge, with some of the youngest or sickest infants experiencing more than 450 painful procedures during their hospital stays (Barker & Rutter, 1995). Many of the procedures commonly performed in the neonate cause moderate to severe pain, with average pain scores of 5 on a 10-point scale (Simons et al., 2003). Substantial numbers of failed attempts at procedures dramatically increase the number of painful procedures that neonates are subjected to. Simons and colleagues found that the percentages of failed procedures for insertion of central venous catheters, insertion of peripheral arterial catheters, and intravenous cannula insertion were 45.6%, 37.5%, and 30.9%, respectively (Simons et al., 2003). These frequent, invasive, and noxious procedures occur randomly in the NICU, and many times are not routinely managed with either pharmacologic or nonpharmacologic interventions (Carbajal et al., 2008; Johnston, Barrington, Taddio, Carbajal, & Filion, 2011). Anand and the International

Evidence-Based Group for Neonatal Pain (2001) provide guidelines for preventing and treating neonatal procedural pain. Strategies for the management of procedures commonly performed in the NICU are summarized in Table 23.3 (Anand, 2001).

Local anesthesia may not be sufficient for procedures that affect deeper tissue, such as chest tube insertion or surgical cut down of vessels. Central analgesia is then required to prevent pain. For the nonventilated patient, in whom concern for the respiratory depressant effects of opioids exists, one-half the standard dose may be administered. The infant's respiratory status and responsiveness to pain stimuli can then be assessed before further drug administration. For the infant who is receiving opioid analgesics on a regular basis, a controlled infusion of a bolus dose may be required to provide adequate analgesia during an invasive procedure.

Postoperative Pain

Adequate analgesia is important during the immediate postoperative period for the optimal recovery of the patient. Unrelieved pain can interfere with ventilation and delay weaning. In general, it is thought that the use of low-dose continuous infusions of opioid analgesics provides more

TABLE 23.3

SUGGESTED MANAGEMENT OF PAINFUL PROCEDURES COMMONLY PERFORMED IN THE NICU

Pain Intensity	Procedure	Gentle Technique	NNS +/– Sucrose	Containment	Skin-to-Skin Holding	Topical Anesthetic	Opioids	Other/Notes
Mild	Tape removal	√	√	√	√			
↑	Endotracheal Suctioning	√	√	√	√			
	Oro/nasogastric tube insertion	√	√	√	√			
	Umbilical catheterization	√	√	√				
	Intramuscular injection	√	√	√	√	√		
	Venipuncture/arterial puncture	√	√	√	√	√		
Pain Intensity	Heel lance	√	√	√	√			Use spring-loaded lancet Consider venipuncture for term and older preterm infants
	Eye examination	√	√	√		√	√	Retinal surgery should be considered major surgery, and opioids should be provided
	Percutaneous/arterial venous line placement	√	√	√		√	√	
	Endotracheal intubation	√		√			√	Use combination of atropine, morphine/fentanyl, and nondepolarizing muscle relaxant
↓	Chest tube insertion	√		√		√	√	Consider subcutaneous infiltration of lidocaine
Severe	Circumcision	√	√	√		√		Dorsal penile nerve block or other regional block

Adapted from Anand (2001).

constant, effective pain relief with less medication than repeated, intermittent scheduled doses of opioids (Simons & Anand, 2006).

Preemptive Analgesia for Mechanical Ventilation

Opioids are frequently used to sedate, promote respiratory synchrony, produce physiologic stability, and relieve pain or discomfort in ventilated neonates. However, a systematic review and meta-analysis of 13 studies on 1,505 infants concluded that there is insufficient evidence available to recommend the routine use of opioids in mechanically ventilated neonates (Bellu, de Waal, & Zanini, 2010). These recommendations were attributed to failure to decrease pain scores during invasive procedures as well as the lack of overall benefits of morphine therapy on reduction of adverse outcomes such as death, intraventricular hemorrhage, and periventricular leukomalacia.

Pain Management at EOL

Pain management at EOL primarily centers on the provision of opioids to minimize pain and nonpharmacologic therapies to enhance the infant's comfort level (Walden, 2001). Pain assessment is extremely difficult in neonates at end of life. Therefore caregivers must often consider risk factors for pain and rely on physiologic measures such as increases in heart rate and decreases in oxygen saturation to make pain management decisions.

Continuous infusions of opioid therapy such as morphine and fentanyl are often required to manage pain at EOL and should be titrated to desired clinical response (analgesia). Opioid doses well beyond those described for standard analgesia are often required for infants who are in severe pain or who have developed tolerance (decreasing pain relief with the same dosage over time) after the prolonged use of opioids (Partridge & Wall, 1997). Physiologic comfort measures may palliate pain and distressing symptoms in infants at EOL and include reduction of noxious stimuli, organization of caregiving, and positioning and containment strategies (Walden, Sudia-Robinson, & Carrier, 2001).

PARENTS

Nurses who care for the infant in pain must care for the infant's family as well. Parents have many concerns and fears about their infants' pain and about the drugs used in the treatment of pain (Franck, Allen, Cox, & Winter, 2005; Gale, Franck, Kools, & Lynch, 2004). Parents may fear the effects of pain on their children's development. They may also fear that their infant may become "addicted" to the analgesics (Franck, Greenberg, & Stevens, 2000).

Parents should be educated on their infant's pain cues. A source of parental stress often occurs when there is a mismatch between parent and staff perceptions of the infant's pain (Gale et al., 2004). It is important to provide parents with consistent information about pain assessment and management. Debriefing with parents following a pain experience is a strategy that can be used to minimize disagreements between parents and nurses regarding pain intensity in the infant and may increase the potential for meaningful collaboration in improving the infant's pain care in the NICU.

Parents should be encouraged to participate in providing nonpharmacologic comfort measures to their infants during minor painful procedures. Several studies have shown that facilitated tucking by parents is an effective and safe pain management method during painful procedures in the NICU (Axelin, Lehtonen, Pelander, & Salantera, 2010; Axelin, Salantera, Kirjavainen, & Lehtonen, 2009; Axelin, Salantera, & Lehtonen, 2006). Increasing parental participation in providing comfort measures to their infant during painful procedures may help to moderate parental stress and optimize the parent–infant relationship (Miles & Holditch-Davis, 1997).

NEONATAL NURSE'S ROLE AND RESPONSIBILITIES

Provision of comfort and relief of pain are two primary goals of nursing care. To accomplish these goals, neonatal nurses must (1) prevent pain when possible; (2) assess pain in their neonatal patients who cannot verbalize their subjective experience of pain; (3) provide relief or reduction of pain through implementation of nonpharmacologic and/or pharmacologic measures; and (4) assist the infant in coping when pain cannot be prevented.

The effective management of infant pain requires nurses to collaborate with each other, with physicians, and with the infant's parents. Nurses must effectively communicate assessments and recommendations in an objective, concise manner and advocate for pain relief strategies with responsible health care team members. Neonatal nurses must remain informed about professional standards and clinical guidelines related to pain assessment and management in neonates. The nurse should also participate in ongoing pain education and review of new research and scientific developments.

SUMMARY

Pain in neonates is often assessed and managed inadequately in a large proportion of neonates in the NICU. It is clear, however, that caring for infants in pain requires attention not only to the immediate effects but also to the long-term developmental consequences of pain and pain treatment. Through ongoing research, objective assessment, effective collaboration, and systematic application of treatment plans, nurses will achieve greater comfort for individual patients and add to the body of knowledge in this rapidly evolving field.

CASE STUDY

■ Identification of the Problem. Term female infant with pain related to probable epidermolysis bullosa (EB) and extensive blistering of lower extremities

■ Assessment: History and Physical Examination. The term, 3,600-g female was born via vaginal delivery to a 19-year-old, unmarried, Hispanic, G2 P2, mother with minimal prenatal care. Maternal labs were unremarkable, including negative history for herpes. Maternal history positive for previous infant with confirmed EB. At birth, the infant was noted to have a vigorous respiratory effort at birth with Apgars 9 and 9 at 1 and 5 minutes of life, respectively. Significant bullous skin lesions were noted on the right lower leg and left ankle. She was transferred to the NICU for care.

Once in the NICU, she was placed in a dual radiant warmer/incubator bed and placed on continuous cardiorespiratory monitoring. An umbilical venous line was placed. Blood was sent for complete blood count (CBC) with differential and blood culture. Intravenous fluids were started along with small feedings of expressed breast milk or formula.

Physical examination on admission to the NICU was:

- VITAL SIGNS: heart rate 172; respiratory rate 38; temperature 97.6 axillary; blood pressure 68/47 MAP 54
- GENERAL: term-appearing infant with signs of pain and distress with handling
- HEENT: anterior fontanelle soft, flat, and large; sutures approximated; normocephalic; red reflex deferred; Nares patent; mucous membranes moist and pink
- RESP: bilateral lung sounds clear and equal; respirations unlabored and of normal rate; no retractions, grunting, or nasal flaring
- CV: regular rate and rhythm. S1 and S2 present without murmur; strong and equal brachial and femoral pulses; capillary fill time less than 3 seconds
- ABD: soft and slightly rounded; normal bowel sounds; no hepatosplenomegaly
- GENITOURINARY: female genitalia appropriate for gestation; anus patent and appropriately positioned
- NEURO: Normal tone and activity; good grasp, suck, moro. irritable with crying and facial grimacing
- SKIN: pink and warm; significant skin lesions on the right lower leg and left ankle
- EXTREMITIES: normotonic; full range of motion of all extremities; spine straight, midline without deformity

■ Diagnoses

- Term infant with probable EB
- Pain related to skin lesions

■ Diagnostic Tests

- CBC: WBC 13.2; Hgb 17; Hct 47.5; Plt 60; Segs 67; y Lymphs 15; Monos 4; Eos 0; Bands 12
- Glucose 93
- Chromosome panel: pending
- Will need skin biopsy and other tests as determined by consultations with Genetics and Dermatology for final diagnosis

■ Development of Management Plan for Pain

1. Use CRIES to assess for pain with vital signs and before, during, and after procedures or dressing changes.
2. Strategies for prevention of pain: Vital signs per monitor. Reduced frequency of BPs to every day to reduce friction to the skin. If nasogastric tube is needed for feedings, secure with nonadhesive methods such as TubiFast or silicone tape for fragile skin.
3. Dysphagia may occur secondary to pain, oral blistering, and scarring. Use a Haberman or Lamb's nipple to reduce oral friction with nippling. Consult with pharmacy regarding oral topical anesthetic to be administered before nippling.
4. Protect skin by using dressings on bony prominences, egg-crate mattresses, sheepskins, moist healing environment, avoiding tape, and avoiding trauma. Petrolatum-based emollients covered with antibiotic ointments and nonstick dressings (e.g., Mepitel dressings). Wrapping gauze, cotton mesh, or Coban around the dressing can protect and reduce friction.
5. Remove dressings carefully using gentle technique. Consider removing during bathing.
6. Reduce frequency of NICU interventions such as temperature taking, blood pressures, weighing, and so on.
7. Use mittens for the baby's hands and feet.
8. Administer fentanyl pro re nata (PRN) for CRIES scores 5 or above. Consider weaning to an oral opioid when intravenous access is no longer needed.
9. Administer fentanyl prior to dressing changes and procedures anticipated to be moderate to severe in intensity.
10. Consult Dermatology and Wound Care for further recommendations to maintain skin integrity and manage open wounds.
11. Educate parents on how to provide protective, prophylactic, and therapeutic care for their infant with EB.

EVIDENCE-BASED PRACTICE BOX

Reducing Pain Associated With Screening for Retinopathy of Prematurity

Infants born less than 1,500 g or less than 32 weeks are routinely subjected to necessary ophthalmological screening for retinopathy of prematurity (ROP). Screening examinations are a significant source of pain and discomfort and are associated with physiological instability in preterm neonates. Dempsey and colleagues published a Cochrane systematic review to determine the effect of instillation of topical anesthetic eye drops on pain responses of preterm neonates undergoing ROP screening (Dempsey & McCreery, 2011). Only two randomized crossover studies were identified for inclusion in the analyses. The authors concluded that the administration of proparacaine eye drops at least 30 seconds prior to the examination was associated with a reduction in pain scores, but was not effective in eliminating pain. The authors recommended that future studies should address the role of both nonpharmacological and pharmacological interventions, including different local anesthetic agents, NNS, sucrose, and swaddling to reduce pain associated with this common procedure.

Reference

Dempsey, E., & McCreery, K. (2011). Local anaesthetic eye drops for prevention of pain in preterm infants undergoing screening for retinopathy of prematurity [Meta-analysis review]. *Cochrane Database of Systematic Reviews* (9), CD007645. doi:10.1002/14651858.CD007645.pub2

REFERENCES

Agency for Health Care Policy and Research. (1992). *Acute pain management in infants, children, and adolescents: Operative and medical procedures: Quick reference guide for clinicians*. Rockville, MD: Department of Health and Human Services.

Ahn, Y. (2006). The relationship between behavioral states and pain responses to various NICU procedures in premature infants [Research Support, Non-U.S. Gov't]. *Journal of Tropical Pediatrics, 52*(3), 201–205. doi:10.1093/tropej/fmi099

Anand, K. J. (2001). Consensus statement for the prevention and management of pain in the newborn. *Archives of Pediatrics & Adolescent Medicine, 155*(2), 173–180. doi:poa00293 [pii]

Anand, K. J. (2007). Pharmacological approaches to the management of pain in the neonatal intensive care unit [Research Support, N.I.H., Extramural Review]. *Journal of Perinatology, 27*(Suppl. 1), S4–S11. doi:10.1038/sj.jp.7211712

Anand, K. J., Barton, B. A., McIntosh, N., Lagercrantz, H., Pelausa, E., Young, T. E., & Vasa, R. (1999). Analgesia and sedation in preterm neonates who require ventilatory support: Results from the NOPAIN trial. Neonatal outcome and prolonged analgesia in neonates. *Archives of Pediatrics & Adolescent Medicine, 153*(4), 331–338.

Anand, K. J., & Craig, K. D. (1996). New perspectives on the definition of pain [Editorial review]. *Pain, 67*(1), 3–6; discussion 209–211.

Anand, K. J., Hall, R. W., Desai, N., Shephard, B., Bergqvist, L. L., Young, T. E., & Group, N. T. I. (2004). Effects of morphine analgesia in ventilated preterm neonates: Primary outcomes from the NEOPAIN randomised trial [Clinical Trial Multicenter Study Randomized Controlled Trial Research Support, Non-U.S. Gov't Research Support, U.S. Gov't, P.H.S.]. *Lancet, 363*(9422), 1673–1682. doi:10.1016/S0140-6736(04)16251-X

Anand, K. J., Johnston, C. C., Oberlander, T. F., Taddio, A., Lehr, V. T., & Walco, G. A. (2005). Analgesia and local anesthesia during invasive procedures in the neonate [Research Support, N.I.H., Extramural Research Support, U.S. Gov't, Non-P.H.S. Research Support, U.S. Gov't, P.H.S. Review]. *Clinical Therapeutics, 27*(6), 844–876. doi:10.1016/j.clinthera.2005.06.018

Anand, K. J., Willson, D. F., Berger, J., Harrison, R., Meert, K. L., Zimmerman, J., . . . Human Development Collaborative Pediatric Critical Care Research Network. (2010). Tolerance and withdrawal from prolonged opioid use in critically ill children [Research Support, N.I.H., Extramural Review]. *Pediatrics, 125*(5), e1208–e1225. doi:10.1542/peds.2009-0489

Anand, K. J. S., Menon, G., Narsinghani, U., & NcIntosh, N. (2000). Systemic analgesic therapy. In K. J. S. Anand, B. J. Stevens, & P. J. McGrath (Eds.), *Pain in neonates* (2nd ed.). Amsterdam: Elsevier.

Axelin, A., Lehtonen, L., Pelander, T., & Salantera, S. (2010). Mothers' different styles of involvement in preterm infant pain care [Research Support, Non-U.S. Gov't]. *Journal of Obstetric, Gynecologic, and Neonatal Nursing, 39*(4), 415–424. doi:10.1111/j.1552-6909.2010.01150.x

Axelin, A., Salantera, S., Kirjavainen, J., & Lehtonen, L. (2009). Oral glucose and parental holding preferable to opioid in pain management in preterm infants [Randomized Controlled Trial Research Support, Non-U.S. Gov't]. *Clinical Journal of Pain, 25*(2), 138–145. doi:10.1097/AJP.0b013e318181ad81

Axelin, A., Salantera, S., & Lehtonen, L. (2006). Facilitated tucking by parents in pain management of preterm infants—a randomized crossover trial [Randomized Controlled Trial Research Support, Non-U.S. Gov't]. *Early Human Development, 82*(4), 241–247. doi:10.1016/j.earlhumdev.2005.09.012

Barker, D. P., & Rutter, N. (1995). Exposure to invasive procedures in neonatal intensive care unit admissions. *Archives of Disease in Childhood. Fetal and Neonatal Edition, 72*(1), F47–F48.

Beasley, R., Clayton, T., Crane, J., von Mutius, E., Lai, C. K., Montefort, S., . . . Group, I. P. T. S. (2008). Association between paracetamol use in infancy and childhood, and risk of asthma, rhinoconjunctivitis, and eczema in children aged 6-7 years: Analysis from Phase Three of the ISAAC programme [Research Support, Non-U.S. Gov't]. *Lancet, 372*(9643), 1039–1048. doi:10.1016/S0140-6736(08)61445-2

Belda, S., Pallas, C. R., De la Cruz, J., & Tejada, P. (2004). Screening for retinopathy of prematurity: Is it painful? *Biology of the Neonate, 86*(3), 195–200. doi:10.1159/000079542

Bellu, R., de Waal, K., & Zanini, R. (2010). Opioids for neonates receiving mechanical ventilation: A systematic review and meta-analysis [Meta-analysis review]. *Archives of Disease in Childhood. Fetal and Neonatal Edition, 95*(4), F241–F251. doi:10.1136/adc.2008.150318

Bildner, J., & Krechel, S. W. (1996). Increasing staff nurse awareness of postoperative pain management in the NICU. *Neonatal Network, 15*(1), 11–16.

Blass, E., Fitzgerald, E., & Kehoe, P. (1987). Interactions between sucrose, pain and isolation distress [Research Support, U.S. Gov't, P.H.S.]. *Pharmacology, Biochemistry and Behavior, 26*(3), 483–489.

Blass, E. M. (1994). Behavioral and physiological consequences of suckling in rat and human newborns [Review]. *Acta Paediatrica Supplement, 397*, 71–76.

Brummelte, S., Grunau, R. E., Chau, V., Poskitt, K. J., Brant, R., Vinall, J., . . . Miller, S. P. (2012). Procedural pain and brain development in premature newborns [Comparative Study Research Support, Non-U.S. Gov't]. *Annals of Neurology, 71*(3), 385–396. doi:10.1002/ana.22267

Campos, R. G. (1989). Soothing pain-elicited distress in infants with swaddling and pacifiers [Research Support, U.S. Gov't, P.H.S.]. *Child Development, 60*(4), 781–792.

Carbajal, R., Gall, O., & Annequin, D. (2004). Pain management in neonates [Review]. *Expert Review of Neurotherapeutics, 4*(3), 491–505. doi:10.1586/14737175.4.3.491

Carbajal, R., Lenclen, R., Jugie, M., Paupe, A., Barton, B. A., & Anand, K. J. (2005). Morphine does not provide adequate analgesia for acute procedural pain among preterm neonates [Clinical Trial Comparative Study Multicenter Study Randomized Controlled Trial Research Support, N.I.H., Extramural Research Support, Non-U.S. Gov't Research Support, U.S. Gov't, P.H.S.]. *Pediatrics, 115*(6), 1494–1500. doi:10.1542/peds.2004-1425

Carbajal, R., Rousset, A., Danan, C., Coquery, S., Nolent, P., Ducrocq, S., . . . Breart, G. (2008). Epidemiology and treatment of painful procedures in neonates in intensive care units. *JAMA, 300*(1), 60–70. doi:300/1/60 [pii] 10.1001/jama.300.1.60

Cignacco, E. L., Sellam, G., Stoffel, L., Gerull, R., Nelle, M., Anand, K. J., & Engberg, S. (2012). Oral sucrose and "facilitated tucking" for repeated pain relief in preterms: A randomized controlled trial. *Pediatrics, 129*(2), 299–308. doi:peds.2011-1879 [pii] 10.1542/peds.2011-1879

Dominguez, K. D., Lomako, D. M., Katz, R. W., & Kelly, H. W. (2003). Opioid withdrawal in critically ill neonates [Clinical Trial Research Support, U.S. Gov't, P.H.S.]. *Annals of Pharmacotherapy, 37*(4), 473–477.

Ducharme, C., Carnevale, F. A., Clermont, M. S., & Shea, S. (2005). A prospective study of adverse reactions to the weaning of opioids and benzodiazepines among critically ill children [Evaluation studies]. *Intensive & Critical Care Nursing, 21*(3), 179–186. doi:10.1016/j.iccn.2004.09.003

Duhn, L. J., & Medves, J. M. (2004). A systematic integrative review of infant pain assessment tools. *Advances in Neonatal Care, 4*(3), 126–140. doi:S1536090304001316 [pii]

Eichenfield, L. F., Funk, A., Fallon-Friedlander, S., & Cunningham, B. B. (2002). A clinical study to evaluate the efficacy of ELA-Max (4% liposomal lidocaine) as compared with eutectic mixture of local anesthetics cream for pain reduction of venipuncture in children [Clinical Trial Comparative Study Randomized Controlled Trial Research Support, Non-U.S. Gov't]. *Pediatrics, 109*(6), 1093–1099.

El Sayed, M. F., Taddio, A., Fallah, S., De Silva, N., & Moore, A. M. (2007). Safety profile of morphine following surgery in neonates. *Journal of Perinatology, 27*(7), 444–447. doi:10.1038/sj.jp.7211764

Fitzgerald, M., & Howard, R. F. (2003). The neurobiologic basis of pediatric pain. In N. L. Schechter, C. B. Berde, & M. Yaster (Eds.), *Pain in infants, children, and adolescents* (2nd ed.). Philadelphia, PA: Lippincott Williams & Wilkins.

Franck, L. S., Allen, A., Cox, S., & Winter, I. (2005). Parents' views about infant pain in neonatal intensive care. *Clinical Journal of Pain, 21*(2), 133–139. doi:00002508-200503000-00004 [pii]

Franck, L. S., Boyce, W. T., Gregory, G. A., Jemerin, J., Levine, J., & Miaskowski, C. (2000). Plasma norepinephrine levels, vagal tone index, and flexor reflex threshold in premature neonates receiving intravenous morphine during the postoperative period: A pilot study [Research Support, Non-U.S. Gov't Research Support, U.S. Gov't, P.H.S.]. *Clinical Journal of Pain, 16*(2), 95–104.

Franck, L. S., Greenberg, C. S., & Stevens, B. (2000). Pain assessment in infants and children. *Pediatric Clinics of North America, 47*(3), 487–512.

Franck, L. S., Vilardi, J., Durand, D., & Powers, R. (1998). Opioid withdrawal in neonates after continuous infusions of morphine or fentanyl during extracorporeal membrane oxygenation [Comparative study]. *American Journal of Critical Care, 7*(5), 364–369.

Gale, G., Franck, L. S., Kools, S., & Lynch, M. (2004). Parents' perceptions of their infant's pain experience in the NICU. *International Journal of Nursing Studies, 41*(1), 51–58. doi:S0020748903000968 [pii]

Gibbins, S., & Stevens, B. (2003). The influence of gestational age on the efficacy and short-term safety of sucrose for procedural pain relief [Clinical Trial Randomized Controlled Trial Research Support, Non-U.S. Gov't]. *Advances in Neonatal Care, 3*(5), 241–249.

Gibbins, S., Stevens, B., Hodnett, E., Pinelli, J., Ohlsson, A., & Darlington, G. (2002). Efficacy and safety of sucrose for procedural pain relief in preterm and term neonates [Clinical trial randomized controlled trial]. *Nursing Research, 51*(6), 375–382.

Goldschneider, K. R., & Anand, K. S. (2003). Long-term consequences of pain in neonates. In N. L. Schechter, C. B. Berde, & M. Yaster (Eds.), *Pain in infants, children, and adolescents* (2nd ed.). Philadelphia, PA: Lippincott Williams & Wilkins.

Grunau, R. E., Holsti, L., & Peters, J. W. (2006). Long-term consequences of pain in human neonates [Research Support, N.I.H., Extramural Research Support, Non-U.S. Gov't Review]. *Seminars in Fetal & Neonatal Medicine, 11*(4), 268–275. doi:10.1016/j.siny.2006.02.007

Grunau, R. E., Whitfield, M. F., & Fay, T. B. (2004). Psychosocial and academic characteristics of extremely low birth weight (< or =800 g) adolescents who are free of major impairment compared with term-born control subjects [Research support, Non-U.S. Gov't]. *Pediatrics, 114*(6), e725–e732. doi:10.1542/peds.2004-0932

Grunau, R. V., & Craig, K. D. (1987). Pain expression in neonates: Facial action and cry [Research Support, Non-U.S. Gov't]. *Pain, 28*(3), 395–410.

Grunau, R. V., Whitfield, M. F., & Petrie, J. H. (1994). Pain sensitivity and temperament in extremely low-birth-weight premature toddlers and preterm and full-term controls. *Pain, 58*(3), 341–346.

Herrington, C. J., Olomu, I. N., & Geller, S. M. (2004). Salivary cortisol as indicators of pain in preterm infants: A pilot study [Research Support, Non-U.S. Gov't Validation Studies]. *Clinical Nursing Research, 13*(1), 53–68. doi:10.1177/1054773803259665

Holsti, L., Grunau, R. E., Oberlander, T. F., & Whitfield, M. F. (2004). Specific Newborn Individualized Developmental Care and Assessment Program movements are associated with acute pain in preterm infants in the neonatal intensive care unit [Research Support, Non-U.S. Gov't Research Support, U.S. Gov't, P.H.S.]. *Pediatrics, 114*(1), 65–72.

Hudak, M. L., Tan, R. C., Committee on, Drugs and the Committee on Fetus and Newborn, & American Academy of Pediatrics. (2012). Neonatal drug withdrawal [Practice guideline]. *Pediatrics, 129*(2), e540–e560. doi:10.1542/peds.2011-3212

Hummel, P., Puchalski, M., Creech, S. D., & Weiss, M. G. (2008). Clinical reliability and validity of the N-PASS: Neonatal pain, agitation and sedation scale with prolonged pain [Research Support, Non-U.S. Gov't Validation Studies]. *Journal of Perinatol, 28*(1), 55–60. doi:10.1038/sj.jp.7211861

Johnston, C., Barrington, K. J., Taddio, A., Carbajal, R., & Filion, F. (2011). Pain in Canadian NICUs: Have we improved over the past 12 years? [Research Support, Non-U.S. Gov't]. *Clinical Journal of Pain, 27*(3), 225–232. doi:10.1097/AJP.0b013e3181fe14cf

Johnston, C. C., Filion, F., Campbell-Yeo, M., Goulet, C., Bell, L., McNaughton, K., . . . Walker, C. D. (2008). Kangaroo mother care diminishes pain from heel lance in very preterm neonates: A crossover trial. *BMC Pediatrics, 8*, 13. doi:1471-2431-8-13 [pii] 10.1186/1471-2431-8-13

Johnston, C. C., Filion, F., Snider, L., Majnemer, A., Limperopoulos, C., Walker, C. D., & Boyer, K. (2002). Routine sucrose analgesia during the first week of life in neonates younger than 31 weeks' postconceptional age [Clinical Trial Multicenter Study Randomized Controlled Trial Research Support, Non-U.S. Gov't]. *Pediatrics, 110*(3), 523–528.

Johnston, C. C., Stevens, B., Pinelli, J., Gibbins, S., Filion, F., Jack, A., . . . Veilleux, A. (2003). Kangaroo care is effective in diminishing pain response in preterm neonates. *Archives of Pediatrics & Adolescent Medicine, 157*(11), 1084–1088. doi:10.1001/archpedi.157.11.1084 157/11/1084 [pii]

Johnston, C. C., & Stevens, B. J. (1996). Experience in a neonatal intensive care unit affects pain response. *Pediatrics, 98*(5), 925–930.

Kaur, G., Gupta, P., & Kumar, A. (2003). A randomized trial of eutectic mixture of local anesthetics during lumbar puncture in newborns [Clinical Trial Randomized Controlled Trial]. *Archives of Pediatrics & Adolescent Medicine, 157*(11), 1065–1070. doi:10.1001/archpedi.157.11.1065

Kleiber, C., Sorenson, M., Whiteside, K., Gronstal, B. A., & Tannous, R. (2002). Topical anesthetics for intravenous insertion in children: A randomized equivalency study [Clinical Trial Comparative Study Randomized Controlled Trial Research Support, U.S. Gov't, P.H.S.]. *Pediatrics, 110*(4), 758–761.

Koh, J. L., Harrison, D., Myers, R., Dembinski, R., Turner, H., & McGraw, T. (2004). A randomized, double-blind comparison study of EMLA and ELA-Max for topical anesthesia in children undergoing intravenous insertion [Clinical Trial Comparative Study Randomized Controlled Trial]. *Paediatric Anaesthesia, 14*(12), 977–982. doi:10.1111/j.1460-9592.2004.01381.x

Krechel, S. W., & Bildner, J. (1995). CRIES: A new neonatal postoperative pain measurement score. Initial testing of validity and reliability. *Paediatric Anaesthesia, 5*(1), 53–61.

Lander, J. A., Weltman, B. J., & So, S. S. (2006). EMLA and amethocaine for reduction of children's pain associated with needle insertion. *Cochrane Database of Systematic Reviews, 19*(3), *CD004236*. doi:10.1002/14651858.CD004236.pub2

Lawrence, J., Alcock, D., McGrath, P., Kay, J., MacMurray, S. B., & Dulberg, C. (1993). The development of a tool to assess neonatal pain. *Neonatal Network, 12*(6), 59–66.

Lehr, V. T., Cepeda, E., Frattarelli, D. A., Thomas, R., LaMothe, J., & Aranda, J. V. (2005). Lidocaine 4% cream compared with lidocaine 2.5% and prilocaine 2.5% or dorsal penile block for circumcision [Comparative Study Randomized Controlled Trial Research Support, Non-U.S. Gov't]. *American Journal of Perinatology, 22*(5), 231–237. doi:10.1055/s-2005-871655

Liaw, J. J., Yang, L., Ti, Y., Blackburn, S. T., Chang, Y. C., & Sun, L. W. (2010). Non-nutritive sucking relieves pain for preterm infants during heel stick procedures in Taiwan [Research Support, Non-U.S. Gov't]. *Journal of Clinical Nursing, 19*(19–20), 2741–2751. doi:10.1111/j.1365-2702.2010.03300.x

Liaw, J. J., Zeng, W. P., Yang, L., Yuh, Y. S., Yin, T., & Yang, M. H. (2011). Nonnutritive sucking and oral sucrose relieve neonatal pain during intramuscular injection of hepatitis vaccine [Comparative Study Randomized Controlled Trial]. *Journal of Pain and Symptom Management, 42*(6), 918–930. doi:10.1016/j.jpainsymman.2011.02.016

Local AnGel 4%. (2005). Orion Laboratories. Product Information Sheet.

Mathai, S. S., Naresh, A., & Sahu, S. (2011). Behavioral response to pain in drowsy and sleeping neonates: A randomized control study [Randomized controlled trial]. *Indian Pediatrics, 48*(5), 390–392.

McNair, C., Ballantyne, M., Dionne, K., Stephens, D., & Stevens, B. (2004). Postoperative pain assessment in the neonatal intensive care unit [Clinical Trial Comparative Study Randomized Controlled Trial Research Support, Non-U.S. Gov't Validation Studies]. *Archives of Disease in Childhood. Fetal and Neonatal Edition, 89*(6), F537–F541. doi:10.1136/adc.2003.032961

Menon, G., Anand, K. J., & McIntosh, N. (1998). Practical approach to analgesia and sedation in the neonatal intensive care unit [Review]. *Seminars in Perinatology, 22*(5), 417–424.

Merskey, H. (1979). Pain terms: A list with definitions and notes on usage. Recommended by the IASP Subcommittee on Taxonomy. *Pain, 6*(3), 249.

Miles, M. S., & Holditch-Davis, D. (1997). Parenting the prematurely born child: Pathways of influence [Research Support, U.S. Gov't, P.H.S. Review]. *Seminars in Perinatology, 21*(3), 254–266.

National Association of Neonatal Nurses. (2012). *Newborn pain assessment and management: Guideline for practice*. Des Plaines, IL: Author.

NEOFAX. (2011). (24th ed.). Montvale, NJ: Thomson Reuters.

Ng, E., Taddio, A., & Ohlsson, A. (2012). Intravenous midazolam infusion for sedation of infants in the neonatal intensive care unit. *Cochrane Database of Systematic Reviews*, June 13;6:CD002052. doi: 10.1002/14651858.CD002052.pub2

Obeidat, H., Kahalaf, I., Callister, L. C., & Froelicher, E. S. (2009). Use of facilitated tucking for nonpharmacological pain management in preterm infants: A systematic review [Review]. *Journal of Perinatal & Neonatal Nursing, 23*(4), 372–377. doi:10.1097/JPN.0b013e3181bdcf77

O'Brien, L., Taddio, A., Lyszkiewicz, D. A., & Koren, G. (2005). A critical review of the topical local anesthetic amethocaine (Ametop) for pediatric pain. *Paediatric Drugs, 7*(1), 41–54.

Partridge, J. C., & Wall, S. N. (1997). Analgesia for dying infants whose life support is withdrawn or withheld [Research Support, U.S. Gov't, P.H.S.]. *Pediatrics, 99*(1), 76–79.

Pillai Riddell, R., Racine, N., Turcotte, K., Uman, L., Horton, R., Din Osmun, L., & Lisi, D. (2011). Nonpharmacological management of procedural pain in infants and young children: An abridged Cochrane review [Research Support, Non-U.S. Gov't Review]. *Pain Research & Management, 16*(5), 321–330.

Pinheiro, J. M., Furdon, S., & Ochoa, L. F. (1993). Role of local anesthesia during lumbar puncture in neonates. *Pediatrics, 91*(2), 379–382.

Porter, F. L., Wolf, C. M., & Miller, J. P. (1998). The effect of handling and immobilization on the response to acute pain in newborn infants [Clinical Trial Randomized Controlled Trial Research Support, U.S. Gov't, P.H.S.]. *Pediatrics, 102*(6), 1383–1389.

Prymula, R., Siegrist, C. A., Chlibek, R., Zemlickova, H., Vackova, M., Smetana, J., . . . Schuerman, L. (2009). Effect of prophylactic paracetamol administration at time of vaccination on febrile reactions and antibody responses in children: Two open-label, randomised controlled trials [Clinical Trial, Phase III Multicenter Study Randomized Controlled Trial Research

Support, Non-U.S. Gov't]. *Lancet, 374*(9698), 1339–1350. doi:10.1016/S0140-6736(09)61208-3

Rao, R., Sampers, J. S., Kronsberg, S. S., Brown, J. V., Desai, N. S., & Anand, K. J. (2007). Neurobehavior of preterm infants at 36 weeks postconception as a function of morphine analgesia [Randomized Controlled Trial Research Support, N.I.H., Extramural Research Support, Non-U.S. Gov't]. *American Journal of Perinatology, 24*(9), 511–517. doi:10.1055/s-2007-986675

Regen, R., & Whitehill, J. (2012). Drug considerations in circumcision. *U.S. Pharmacist, 27*(3), HS-2-5.

Rouss, K., Gerber, A., Albisetti, M., Hug, M., & Bernet, V. (2007). Long-term subcutaneous morphine administration after surgery in newborns. *Journal of Perinatal Medicine, 35*(1), 79–81. doi:10.1515/JPM.2007.013

Roze, J. C., Denizot, S., Carbajal, R., Ancel, P. Y., Kaminski, M., Arnaud, C., . . . Breart, G. (2008). Prolonged sedation and/or analgesia and 5-year neurodevelopment outcome in very preterm infants: Results from the EPIPAGE cohort [Comparative study]. *Archives of Pediatrics & Adolescent Medicine, 162*(8), 728–733. doi:10.1001/archpedi.162.8.728

Saarenmaa, E., Huttunen, P., Leppaluoto, J., Meretoja, O., & Fellman, V. (1999). Advantages of fentanyl over morphine in analgesia for ventilated newborn infants after birth: A randomized trial [Clinical Trial Comparative Study Randomized Controlled Trial]. *Journal of Pediatrics, 134*(2), 144–150.

Sarkar, S., & Donn, S. M. (2006). Management of neonatal abstinence syndrome in neonatal intensive care units: A national survey. *Journal of Perinatology, 26*(1), 15–17. doi:10.1038/sj.jp.7211427

Sethna, N. F., & Koh, J. L. (2000). Regional anesthesia and analgesia. In K. J. S. Anand, B. J. Stevens, & P. J. McGrath (Eds.), *Pain in neonates* (2nd ed.). Amsterdam: Elsevier.

Simons, S. H., & Anand, K. J. (2006). Pain control: Opioid dosing, population kinetics and side-effects. *Seminars in Fetal & Neonatal Medicine, 11*(4), 260–267. doi:S1744-165X(06)00028-X [pii] 10.1016/j.siny.2006.02.008

Simons, S. H., & Tibboel, D. (2006). Pain perception development and maturation [Review]. *Seminars in Fetal & Neonatal Medicine, 11*(4), 227–231. doi:10.1016/j.siny.2006.02.010

Simons, S. H., van Dijk, M., Anand, K. S., Roofthooft, D., van Lingen, R. A., & Tibboel, D. (2003). Do we still hurt newborn babies? A prospective study of procedural pain and analgesia in neonates. *Archives of Pediatrics & Adolescent Medicine, 157*(11), 1058–1064. doi:10.1001/archpedi.157.11.1058 157/11/1058 [pii]

Simons, S. H., van Dijk, M., van Lingen, R. A., Roofthooft, D., Duivenvoorden, H. J., Jongeneel, N., & Tibboel, D. (2003). Routine morphine infusion in preterm newborns who received ventilatory support: A randomized controlled trial. *JAMA, 290*(18), 2419–2427. doi:10.1001/jama.290.18.2419 290/18/2419 [pii]

Stevens, B., Johnston, C., Franck, L., Petryshen, P., Jack, A., & Foster, G. (1999). The efficacy of developmentally sensitive interventions and sucrose for relieving procedural pain in very low birth weight neonates [Clinical Trial Comparative Study Multicenter Study Randomized Controlled Trial Research Support, Non-U.S. Gov't Research Support, U.S. Gov't, P.H.S.]. *Nursing Research, 48*(1), 35–43.

Stevens, B., Johnston, C., Petryshen, P., & Taddio, A. (1996). Premature Infant Pain Profile: Development and initial validation [Clinical Trial Research Support, Non-U.S. Gov't]. *Clinical Journal Pain, 12*(1), 13–22.

Stevens, B., Johnston, C., Taddio, A., Gibbins, S., & Yamada, J. (2010). The premature infant pain profile: Evaluation 13 years after development [Research Support, Non-U.S. Gov't Review]. *Clinical Journal Pain, 26*(9), 813–830. doi:10.1097/AJP.0b013e3181ed1070

Stevens, B., Yamada, J., Beyene, J., Gibbins, S., Petryshen, P., Stinson, J., & Narciso, J. (2005). Consistent management of repeated procedural pain with sucrose in preterm neonates: Is it effective and safe for repeated use over time? *Clinical Journal Pain, 21*(6), 543–548. doi: 00002508-200511000-00011 [pii]

Stevens, B., Yamada, J., & Ohlsson, A. (2010). Sucrose for analgesia in newborn infants undergoing painful procedures [Meta-analysis review]. *Cochrane Database Systematic Reviews, (1), CD001069.* doi:10.1002/14651858.CD001069.pub3

Stevens, B. J., Johnston, C. C., & Horton, L. (1994). Factors that influence the behavioral pain responses of premature infants [Clinical Trial Research Support, Non-U.S. Gov't]. *Pain, 59*(1), 101–109.

Suraseranivongse, S., Kaosaard, R., Intakong, P., Pornsiriprasert, S., Karnchana, Y., Kaopinpruck, J., & Sangjeen, K. (2006). A comparison of postoperative pain scales in neonates [Comparative Study Research Support, Non-U.S. Gov't Validation Studies] *British Journal of Anaesthesia, 97*(4), 540–544. doi: 10.1093/bja/ael184

Taddio, A., Goldbach, M., Ipp, M., Stevens, B., & Koren, G. (1995). Effect of neonatal circumcision on pain responses during vaccination in boys [Research Support, Non-U.S. Gov't]. *Lancet, 345*(8945), 291–292.

Taddio, A., Katz, J., Ilersich, A. L., & Koren, G. (1997). Effect of neonatal circumcision on pain response during subsequent routine vaccination [Clinical Trial Randomized Controlled Trial Research Support, Non-U.S. Gov't]. *Lancet, 349*(9052), 599–603. doi: 10.1016/S0140-6736(96)10316-0

Taddio, A., Lee, C., Yip, A., Parvez, B., McNamara, P. J., & Shah, V. (2006). Intravenous morphine and topical tetracaine for treatment of pain in [corrected] neonates undergoing central line placement [Randomized Controlled Trial Research Support, Non-U.S. Gov't]. *JAMA, 295*(7), 793–800. doi: 10.1001/jama.295.7.793

Taddio, A., Shennan, A. T., Stevens, B., Leeder, J. S., & Koren, G. (1995). Safety of lidocaine-prilocaine cream in the treatment of preterm neonates. *Journal of Pediatrics, 127*(6), 1002–1005.

Walden, M. (2001). *Pain assessment and management: Guideline for practice.* Glenview, IL: National Association of Neonatal Nurses.

Walden, M., Penticuff, J. H., Stevens, B., Lotas, M. J., Kozinetz, C. A., Clark, A., & Avant, K. C. (2001). Maturational changes in physiologic and behavioral responses of preterm neonates to pain. *Advances in Neonatal Care, 1*(2), 94.

Walden, M., Sudia-Robinson, T., & Carrier, C. (2001). Comfort care for infants in the neonatal intensive care unit at end of life. *Newborn and Infant Nursing Reviews, 1*, 97–105.

Walter-Nicolet, E., Annequin, D., Biran, V., Mitanchez, D., & Tourniaire, B. (2010). Pain management in newborns: From prevention to treatment [Review]. *Paediatric Drugs, 12*(6), 353–365. doi:10.2165/11318900-000000000-00000

Whitfield, M. F., Grunau, R. V., & Holsti, L. (1997). Extremely premature (< or = 800 g) schoolchildren: Multiple areas of hidden disability. *Archives of Disease in Childhood. Fetal and Neonatal Edition, 77*(2), F85–F90.

Willis, D. M., Chabot, J., Radde, I. C., & Chance, G. W. (1977). Unsuspected hyperosmolality of oral solutions contributing to necrotizing enterocolitis in very-low-birth-weight infants. *Pediatrics, 60*(4), 535–538.

Young, T. E., & Manguml, B. (2010). *NeoFax* (23rd ed.). Montvale, NJ: Thomson Reuters and Lexicomp online 2012.

Zuppa, A. F., Hammer, G. B., Barrett, J. S., Kenney, B. F., Kassir, N., Mouksassi, S., & Royal, M. A. (2011). Safety and population pharmacokinetic analysis of intravenous acetaminophen in neonates, infants, children, and adolescents with pain or fever. *The Journal of Pediatric Pharmacology and Therapeutics, 16*(4), 246–261. doi:10.5863/1551-6776-16.4.246

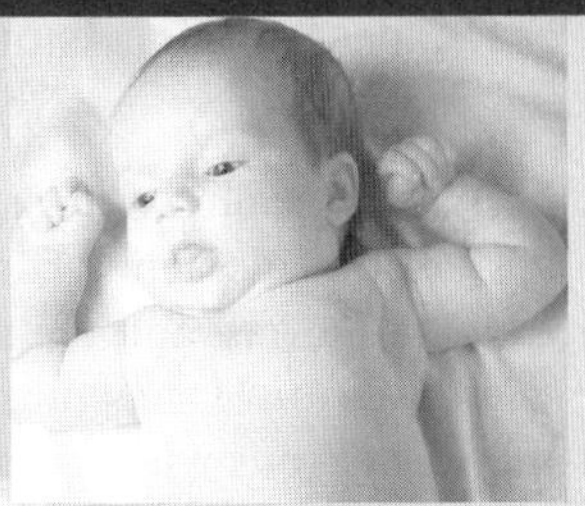

CHAPTER 24

Fetal Therapy

■ Jody A. Farrell

The fetus became a patient over three decades ago, and in the ensuing years, up to the present, this patient status has gained both wide acceptance and sophistication, while in utero treatment itself has improved significantly in strategy and technique. To a large extent, ultrasonography has unveiled that mystery, altered attitudes about the developing fetus, and has become the medium to document fetal growth and development unfolding in the womb. In addition, and perhaps more importantly, major advances in fetal imaging and diagnostic techniques have dramatically improved our ability to identify, comprehend, and, ironically by providing a means of following the natural history of the untreated disease, eventually manage many prenatally diagnosed malformations. Early diagnosis and close fetal monitoring have been key to determining which clinical features affect the outcome, as well as directing management approaches to improve the prognosis and outcome. For a number of these fetal defects, selection criteria for in utero intervention have been defined, and the anesthetic, tocolytic, and surgical techniques for hysterotomy and fetal surgery have been developed and refined (Harrison, 1996). As a result of these advances, the fetus has claimed a role as a patient in its own right.

What has become unequivocally clear with increasing experience is that, in fetal therapy, the patient is an inseparable, often complicated, dyad of mother and fetus. Fetal intervention is really maternal–fetal intervention. Thus, it became obvious early on that the profound challenge particular to fetal surgery was (and remains) that of weighing the benefits of an intervention against the potential risks to the mother, her health, her family, and her ability to have other children (Jelin & Lee, 2009). A multidisciplinary approach to the diagnosis and treatment of fetal diseases has distinguished advances in this specialized field of medicine. For nurses, fetal therapy presents complex challenges. Nurses contribute their counseling, teaching, organizational skills, and expertise to the treatment team, patients, and families. They also often provide significant insight and balance on the ethical considerations that arise in this evolving field.

Written from a nursing perspective for the nursing community, this chapter intends to: (1) provide a historical perspective of fetal treatment, including fetal surgery; (2) describe some key events of this multifaceted, complex area of medicine; (3) describe in detail the components and dynamics of collaborative team management of fetal therapy patients; and (4) outline emerging, future trends in this rapidly changing field.

HISTORICAL OVERVIEW

Designing a strategy for treating erythroblastosis fetalis, a life-threatening fetal and neonatal complication, prompted the first attempt at amelioration of a fetal condition. Sir William Liley made medical history in 1963 when he became the first doctor to give a fetus a blood transfusion before birth. Specifically, while working as a senior research fellow at an army hospital, he performed an in utero, fluoroscopy-guided exchange transfusion of red blood cells into the abdomen of a 32-week fetus to temporarily mitigate the effects of severe hemolytic disease, hydrops fetalis, caused by Rh sensitization-induced anemia (Liley, 1963). The significance of his achievement was not so much a major advance in the management of a serious fetal disease, but a first real demonstration that the fetus is accessible to skilled diagnosis and treatment. From a medical viewpoint, he opened the door for future fetal therapies; from a medical ethics point of view his work suggested the fetus has entitlement to be regarded as a patient.

Advances and improvements in imaging technology have been the hallmarks of the evolving field of fetal treatment. In the 1950s and 1960s, the use of ultrasonography as a diagnostic and imaging tool gave rise to farther-reaching implications in health care, and Ian Donald specifically is credited with developing its application in obstetrics.

Ultrasonography now can be reliably used to determine gestational age, fetal growth patterns and well-being, amniotic fluid levels, and the position of the placenta. It also can detect certain congenital anomalies (especially structural malformations when imaging is performed before 24 weeks gestation), and it is this capability that particularly links ultrasonography to fetal diagnosis and treatment.

Ultrasonography has also proved to be an essential adjunct to other prenatal diagnostic procedures such as amniocentesis, chorionic villus sampling, and percutaneous umbilical blood sampling (Laifer & Kuller, 1996). These techniques, coupled with ultrasonography, laid the groundwork for the new frontier of fetal treatment. Over the past decade, diagnostic advances have continued. The use of magnetic resonance imaging (MRI) has further defined anatomic abnormalities. Microarray-based comparative genomic hybridization (array CGH) is a type of cytogenetic testing. This technology evaluates important areas of our chromosomes to see if there are extra or missing DNA segments that could cause birth defects, mental retardation, or other medical or learning problems (Southard, Edelmann, & Gelb, 2012). Once abnormal fetal conditions could be detected early, many had the potential to become candidates for prenatal treatment. No longer were management options limited to termination of the pregnancy or postnatal treatment. Table 24.1 lists the fetal conditions that often prove amenable to medical or surgical treatment in utero.

In 1981 Michael Harrison and a multidisciplinary team at the University of California at San Francisco (UCSF) became the first group to clinically attempt correction of urinary tract obstruction in utero. Harrison and his coinvestigators hypothesized that if the outlet obstruction could be corrected before birth, then the devastating sequelae of fatal pulmonary hypoplasia or renal failure could be averted. The hypothesis was extensively tested in the fetal sheep model, and the surgical and anesthesia techniques were worked out. This experimental work paved the way for the first attempt at a closed surgical procedure in a human fetus with urinary obstruction.

Specifically, in the first human case in 1981, a catheter needle was passed through the maternal abdominal

TABLE 24.1

FETAL CONDITIONS AMENABLE TO IN UTERO TREATMENT

Condition	Intervention
Fetal Therapy: Medical Treatment	
Rh sensitization (anemia)	Red cell transfusion (into umbilical vessel or intraperitoneal)
Pulmonary immaturity	Betamethasone (transplacental)
Vitamin B_{12} deficiency	Vitamin B_{12} (transplacental)
Carboxylase deficiency	Biotin (transplacental)
Supraventricular tachycardia (SVT)	Digoxin, flecainide, or similar drug (transplacental)
Heart block	Betamimetics (transplacental)
Hypothyroidism	Thyroxine (transplacental)
Adrenal hyperplasia	Steroids
Intrauterine growth restriction (IUGR)	Protein calories (transamniotic)
SCID syndrome	Stem cell transplantation into umbilical vessel
Congenital cystic adenomatoid malformation (CCAM or CPAM)	Maternal steroid administration
Fetal Therapy: Surgical Treatment	
Urinary tract obstructions	Closed procedure (i.e., percutaneous catheter placement or fetal bladder cystoscopy)
TRAP	Closed procedure (interruption of blood flow to the abnormal fetus by ablating blood vessels)
Twin-to-twin transfusion syndrome	Closed procedure (laser ablation of intertwin vascular connections)
Diaphragmatic hernia	Closed procedure (i.e., temporary tracheal occlusion with a balloon)
MMC	Open procedure (i.e., open repair of spinal defect)
SCT	Closed procedure (i.e., interruption of blood flow to the tumor by ablating/sclerosing vessels) or open procedure (i.e., resection of tumor)
Pleural effusion	Closed procedure (i.e., placement of catheter for decompression)
Aortic stenosis (hypoplastic left heart syndrome)	Closed procedure (i.e., balloon valvuloplasty)
CHAOS	Closed procedure (i.e., bronchoscopy and passage of wire to relieve obstruction)

wall into the fetal bladder. An indwelling bladder catheter was then secured to drain fluid from the bladder into the amniotic sac; this catheter remained in place until birth. The procedure proved successful. Although the cause of the obstruction was not corrected until the neonatal period, the deleterious effects of the obstruction were averted while the fetus continued to grow and develop. The promising results of the intervention expanded the possibilities of fetal and neonatal medicine. Other physicians began to consider using this type of surgery for other anomalies.

About the same time, an international group of physicians, surgeons, and scientists met for an informal exchange of experiences and discussion that resulted in the formation of what is now called the International Fetal Medicine and Surgery Society (Manning, 1986). One of the organization's first tasks was to create an international registry to track the number, type, and outcome of fetal surgical attempts.

FETUS AS PATIENT: MATERNAL–FETAL RISKS AND BENEFITS

Although prenatal treatment of the fetus presents a formidable yet exciting challenge, fetal surgery is predicated on a profound responsibility to the mother to ensure her safety, because she, along with her unborn child, is a patient. The risk-benefit ratio of antenatal intervention favors the fetus with a lethal malformation, because without intervention, the mortality rate is almost uniformly 100%; with intervention, survival is possible. Justifying potential risks is most difficult for the mother, whose physical health usually is not jeopardized by her fetus's condition. Before clinical application of fetal surgery could be considered, it had to be proven that any intervention through the mother would not imperil her safety or affect her future fertility (Farrell et al., 1999; Wilson et al., 2004). As a result, fetal surgical procedures were tested first in the most rigorous animal model with an anatomy and physiology most closely resembling that of human pregnancy—the nonhuman primate.

In consideration of preserving the mother's reproductive capability, the ability to deliver subsequent pregnancies was evaluated in a number of studies (Farrell et al., 1999; Longaker et al., 1991; Wilson et al., 2004). Complications were reported as high as 35% of pregnancies of women who had undergone maternal–fetal surgery (Wilson et al., 2004). The anticipated risk of certain adverse outcomes led to several recommendations, including longer interpregnancy intervals and cesarean section for all future pregnancies following open fetal surgery. In the informed consent period, the woman must be counseled on the potential risks affecting the present pregnancy as well as future ones (Wilson et al., 2004).

ETHICAL CONSIDERATIONS

Fetal therapy presents new, often complex ethical dilemmas, rife with challenging questions and controversy, as the nature of this therapy involves operating on the fetus, located within the mother (Caniano, 2004). Balance is required, given that while the outcomes of fetal surgery have improved over the years, neonatal management of anomalies has also advanced (Evans, Harrison, Flake, & Johnson, 2002). Treatment of a fetus with a congenital anomaly confers no direct physical benefit to the mother and subjects her to risk. Maternal risk is primarily related to the high incidence of preterm labor and its corresponding morbidity, but as with any operation, fetal surgery also carries a risk of infection, bleeding, and damage to adjacent structures. Accordingly, the guiding principle for fetal surgery since its inception has been that all fetal interventions must be highly beneficial to the fetus while at the same time being safe for the mother. Fetal surgical procedures should only be considered if the in utero anomaly has been shown to have severe irreversible consequences and the procedure is safe and beneficial.

Ethical issues must be addressed carefully in the informed consent process. It is essential that the decision to proceed with the maternal–fetal intervention be based on informed, autonomous, and voluntary consent (Lyerly, Gates, Cefalo, & Sugarman, 2001). The informed consent process itself can be broken into three discrete elements: (1) disclosure from the medical team to the patient of adequate information concerning the patient's condition and its management; (2) the patient's understanding of that information; (3) a voluntary patient decision to authorize or refuse the proposed procedure (Chervenak, McCullough, Skupski, & Chasen, 2003).

EVOLUTION OF FETAL SURGICAL TECHNIQUES

The timing of open fetal surgery depends on the malformation and its pathophysiologic course. Difficulty determining an accurate diagnosis and the fragility of fetal tissue are limiting factors for performing procedures before 18 weeks gestation (Kiatano, 1999). After 30 weeks gestation, manipulation of the uterus is associated with a higher risk of premature rupture of the membranes (PROM) and preterm labor; thus, delivery of the fetus and treatment of the malformation with standard postnatal care becomes a more reasonable approach (Kiatano, 1999).

Open Fetal Surgery

In open fetal surgery, a general anesthetic is administered to the mother (and transferred to the fetus through the placenta), and a low abdominal transverse (Pfannenstiel) incision is made to open the maternal abdomen and visualize the uterus. Intraoperative ultrasound is then used to identify the position of the fetus and the location of the placenta. Depending on the placenta's location, an anterior or posterior hysterotomy is performed with a specially developed, absorbable uterine stapling device that provides hemostasis and seals the membranes to the myometrium. The fetus is given a narcotic and paralytic agent intramuscularly, and the appropriate fetal part(s) is exposed.

Throughout the procedure, warm lactated Ringer's solution is continuously infused around the fetus and open uterus to maintain fetal body temperature. Fetal monitoring during the surgery is done with a sterile pulse oximeter which records the fetal electrocardiogram. After the defect has been repaired, the fetus is returned to the womb, and amniotic fluid is restored with warm saline containing an antibiotic, such as nafcillin. The uterine incision is closed with two layers of absorbable suture.

Minimally Invasive Fetal Surgery

Although fetoscopic techniques for direct visualization of the fetus are not new, recent modifications of postnatal endoscopic techniques and the development of new fetoscopic instruments have resulted in minimal access fetal surgery. Minimally invasive fetal surgery techniques have been adapted from laparoscopic surgery and early fetoscopy. "Fetendo" is the name applied to fetoscopic intervention involving surgical manipulation of the fetus with very small instruments guided by direct fetoscopic view on a television monitor (Sydorak, Nijagal, & Albanese, 1991). As these techniques evolved and were refined, it was also discovered that the best method of visualizing the fetus in real time was to use both endoscopic (through the telescope) and sonographic (cross-sectional imaging of the fetus) techniques on separate screens. The combination of using two visual images to guide manipulation has proven to be quite powerful in solving a number of fetal problems. Fetendo intervention can be done either percutaneously or, in some circumstances, may require a maternal mini-laparotomy.

The mother is given spinal anesthesia. The surgeon performs the intervention using 1- to 5-mm trocars and scopes through the uterine wall. A continuous irrigation system introduced through the hysteroscope maintains a constant intrauterine fluid level, continuously washes the operative field, and exchanges out cloudy amniotic fluid to optimize visibility and keeps the fetus warm. The trocars are removed once the procedure is completed, and the port sites are closed. An overnight hospital stay may be needed. This less invasive approach avoids the maternal morbidity, primarily bleeding and preterm labor, associated with a large abdominal incision and hysterotomy, and allows vaginal delivery for this and all subsequent pregnancies.

"Fetal image-guided surgery for intervention or therapy" (FIGS-IT) describes the method of manipulating the fetus without either an incision in the uterus or an endoscopic view inside the uterus. The manipulation is done entirely under real-time view provided by the sonogram. This is the same sonogram as is used for diagnostic purposes, but in this case it is used to guide instruments such as in radiofrequency ablation for twin reversed arterial perfusion (TRAP). FIGS-IT, the least invasive fetal technique, results in the least amount of preterm labor, maternal discomfort, and hospitalization postprocedure. Disappointingly, however, neither fetendo nor FIGS-IT has completely eliminated the problem of preterm labor, and so monitoring and tocolytics may be necessary.

ANESTHESIA

All fetal interventional approaches, whether percutaneous or open, require anesthesia. The anesthesiologist evaluates a complex situation in which two patients are being anesthetized simultaneously. Because the particular hazards of anesthesia during pregnancy are related to physiologic changes in the mother and possible adverse effects on the fetus, anesthetizing a pregnant woman during major surgery requires specially trained anesthesiologists who can provide low-level anesthesia and pain management for the maternal–fetal unit while ensuring the mother's safety and minimal side effects for both patients (Collins, 1994).

In developing anesthetic techniques for fetal surgery, researchers had to consider the physiologic differences between healthy pregnant women and healthy nonpregnant women. Specifically, pregnancy causes the following:

- Decreased peripheral vascular resistance (cardiac output increases with no increase in blood pressure, resulting in a decrease in peripheral vascular resistance)
- Decreased functional residual capacity and an increase in alveolar ventilation (which speeds up induction with inhalation anesthetics)
- Increased oxygen consumption (decreased functional residual capacity combined with increased oxygen consumption predisposes pregnant women to hypoxia)
- Hypotension as a result of aortocaval compression (lying supine, a pregnant woman in the second and third trimesters experiences reduced blood flow back to the heart because of aortocaval compression by the gravid uterus)

Direct compression of the great vessels by the gravid uterus reduces uterine blood flow. Therefore the operating table is tilted laterally for all procedures to prevent uterine hypoperfusion. Finally, the anesthesiologist and the surgeons must maintain a continuous exchange of information throughout the procedure about the status of mother and fetus to ensure both patients' well-being.

As the pregnant uterus grows, the stomach is displaced cephalad and horizontally, which changes the angle of the gastroesophageal junction and predisposes the mother to passive regurgitation. This, along with an increase in gastric acid production, makes her more susceptible to regurgitation and aspiration when anesthetized. To reduce the acidity of the gastric juice, oral antacids are administered before general anesthesia is induced.

Pregnant women are also more sensitive to inhaled anesthetics because the endorphin level is elevated, and they therefore are more susceptible to overdosing. Regional anesthetics also require special attention. The increase in femoral venous and intra-abdominal pressure enlarges the epidural veins, which decreases the epidural space; thus less anesthetic is needed.

Fetal oxygenation depends on the maternal arterial oxygen content. If the mother's partial pressure of arterial oxygen, partial pressure of arterial carbon dioxide, and uterine blood flow are maintained within normal limits, fetal asphyxia does not occur. Although elevated maternal oxygen tension (which commonly occurs during anesthesia) is safe for the fetus, maternal hyperventilation can also cause fetal hypoxia and acidosis. Other causes of fetal asphyxia are maternal hypotension, which causes a decrease in uterine blood flow, as well as uterine vasoconstriction caused by anxiety, insufficient anesthesia, or vasoactive drugs.

When the mother is anesthetized for fetal surgery, the fetus also receives the anesthetic by means of placental transfer. Operating on an unanesthetized fetus results in stimulation of the autonomic nervous system and increases in hormonal activity and motor activity; for these reasons, general anesthesia is used for all open procedures to provide both maternal and fetal anesthesia.

Anesthesia of the mother and her baby is established with halogenated agents that also provide profound uterine relaxation. In the operating room, the mother is placed in left lateral decubitus position to prevent compression of the inferior vena cava by the gravid uterus. Maternal monitoring is accomplished with standard techniques, including pulse oximetry, large-bore intravenous catheters, measurement of urine output, and an electrocardiogram. In open fetal surgery procedures, insertion of an epidural catheter enhances postoperative pain control.

FETAL MALFORMATIONS AMENABLE TO SURGICAL CORRECTION

Prenatal diagnosis has defined a "hidden" mortality rate for some lesions (e.g., congenital diaphragmatic hernia [CDH], bilateral hydronephrosis, sacrococcygeal teratoma [SCT], and congenital cystic adenomatoid malformation [CCAM] of the lung). That is, these lesions, when first evaluated and treated postnatally, demonstrated a favorable selection bias. As a result, mortality rates were skewed, inaccurate, and seemingly lower because the most severely affected fetuses often died in utero or immediately after birth. These deaths, often unaccounted for, represent the hidden, often increased mortality for some anomalies. Although most prenatally diagnosed malformations are best managed by appropriate medical and surgical therapy after maternal transport and/or planned delivery at a tertiary care center, an expanding number of simple anatomic abnormalities with predictable, lethal consequences have been corrected before birth. The development of minimum access fetal surgery techniques, along with improvements in the treatment and prevention of preterm labor, have enabled the transition from treating only life-threatening defects to treating those that are not life-threatening but substantially morbid, such as myelomeningocele (MMC).

Obstructive Uropathy

Obstructive uropathy occurs in 1 per 1,000 live births. Unilateral urinary obstruction (e.g., ureteropelvic junction obstruction) has a favorable prognosis and usually does not require fetal intervention. However, fetuses with bilateral obstruction, principally male fetuses with posterior urethral valves, are potential candidates for prenatal intervention based on the degree and duration of the obstruction. Whereas newborns with partial bilateral obstruction may have only mild and reversible hydronephrosis, term infants with a high-grade obstruction may already have advanced hydronephrosis and renal dysplasia, both of which impact survival.

The outcome for patients with urinary tract obstruction depends primarily on whether oligohydramnios develops. Oligohydramnios, a condition characterized by too little amniotic fluid, is the result of decreased fetal urine production and can possibly lead to fatal pulmonary hypoplasia (Potter sequence). Prenatal ultrasound examination is reliable for detecting fetal hydronephrosis and for determining the level of the urinary obstruction. When sonography demonstrates bilateral hydronephrosis, the initial assessment for fetal renal function is determining the amount of amniotic fluid volume, because most of the amniotic fluid in middle and late pregnancy is the product of fetal urination. Normal amniotic fluid volume implies production and excretion of urine by at least one functioning kidney. Presence of bilateral hydronephrosis along with diminished amniotic fluid volume on serial ultrasound examinations with bilateral hydronephrosis usually indicates deteriorating renal function.

Renal function then can be assessed in two ways: appearance of the renal tissue on ultrasound examination and by laboratory analysis of urine obtained by bladder aspiration. The presence of cortical cysts or increased echogenicity is highly predictive of renal dysplasia; however, the absence of these findings does not preclude it. Direct sampling of the fetal urine provides critical information about fetal renal function. Normal fetal urinary chemistry levels are: sodium below 100 mEq/dL, chloride below 90 mEq/dL, osmolarity below 200 mOsm/L, and beta$_2$–microglobulin below 4 mg/dL. Higher levels of these components indicate the inability of the fetal kidney to reabsorb these molecules, and predict poor postnatal renal function. Three bladder aspirations must be performed with at least a 24-hour interval separating each succeeding procedure. The first aspiration empties stagnant bladder urine, and the second empties stagnant urine in the collecting system; therefore, the third specimen is most reflective of current kidney function.

The crucial question in the treatment of fetuses with hydronephrosis is how to select those with dilated urinary tracts that have a problem so severe that renal and pulmonary function may be compromised at birth, yet still have sufficient renal function to profit from prenatal intervention. Candidates for prenatal intervention must: (1) have or develop oligohydramnios; (2) have normal renal function (demonstrated by urine electrolyte and protein values); (3) be less than 30 weeks gestation; and (4) have no additional anomalies.

The strategy of prenatal intervention is to bypass or directly treat the obstruction. If the urinary tract is adequately drained, restoration of amniotic fluid enhances fetal lung growth and prevents further deterioration of renal function. Methods of urinary tract decompression include percutaneous placement of a vesicoamniotic shunt, fetoscopic vesicostomy, open vesicostomy, and fetoscopic fulguration of posterior urethral valves (Quintero et al., 1995).

Currently, the most widely used method of treating bladder outlet obstruction is percutaneous insertion of a double-J vesicoamniotic shunt. The actual surgical procedure varies, depending on the fetal renal disorder or the surgical team's preference. Posterior urethral valve obstruction may be treated by percutaneous placement of a shunt (catheter) from the fetal bladder to the amniotic sac (closed procedure). This shunt uses a Harrison French double-reversed pigtail catheter (Figure 24.1). The catheter or stent is shaped like a pigtail and has openings at either end. The diameters of the two ends are dissimilar—a safety feature in case the catheter

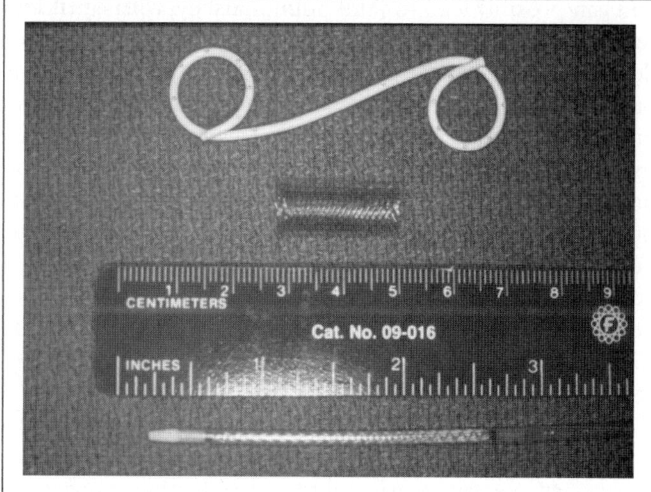

FIGURE 24.1 Harrison French double-reversed pigtail catheter.

becomes dislodged. The larger end is located in the amniotic cavity, so that the catheter would be more likely to move back into this cavity rather than into the fetal bladder.

A polyethylene catheter sometimes is used because it is more rigid and therefore less likely to bend or kink. The catheter is introduced through the maternal abdomen and uterus into the fetal abdomen and bladder by means of a needle and trocar guidance system, much as angiocatheters are used for intravenous therapy. When the catheter is in place, one end is in the renal pelvis and the other end is in the amniotic sac, providing a means to increase the amount of amniotic fluid in the latter. Once the guidance system is withdrawn, the tubing is left in place. More than one insertion attempt may be necessary for successful placement, as there is a 45% incidence rate of shunt complications, which include catheter migration or malfunction, and abdominal wall disruption (Johnson, 2001). Also during the neonatal period, the fetus must undergo corrective surgery to repair the bladder and abdominal wall and relieve the urethral obstruction.

Advances in the development of smaller instrumentation, fetoscopes, allow relief of the obstruction rather than mere diversion of the urine past the blockage. Fetoscopy with direct fetal cystoscopy may be useful in obstructive uropathy, both diagnostically and therapeutically. It has been used to assess lower urinary tract obstruction etiology, to successfully ablate posterior urethral valves, and to place a transurethral stent. These procedures are technically difficult, and the experience is limited; however, this technique avoids the complications of open surgery and may have improved outcomes over vesicoamniotic shunts (Holmes, Harrison, & Baskin, 2001). It should be emphasized that fetal intervention for obstructive uropathy should only be performed in patients who still have residual renal function with oligohydramnios, as stated in the criteria previously cited in this section.

To prevent long-term renal and pulmonary problems, treatment must be undertaken early. Fetal surgery for posterior urethral valve obstruction has been performed as early as 18 weeks gestation and as late as 26 weeks, but the ultimate goal remains the same—to prevent irreversible renal damage and pulmonary hypoplasia.

Congenital Diaphragmatic Hernia

Occurring in about 1 in 3,000 live births, CDH is a simple anatomic defect in which abdominal viscera herniate into the hemithorax, most often through a posterolateral defect in the diaphragm. Despite advances in prenatal care, maternal transport, neonatal resuscitation, and the availability of extracorporeal membrane oxygenation (ECMO), the devastating physiologic consequences of pulmonary hypoplasia and hypertension are associated with a high neonatal mortality rate and long-term morbidity (Harrison, Evans, Adzick, & Holzgreve, 2001). In fetal sheep, compression of the lungs during the last trimester, either with an intrathoracic balloon or by creation of a diaphragmatic hernia, resulted in fatal pulmonary hypoplasia. Removal of the compression allowed pulmonary growth and development to progress and increased the chances of survival.

Prenatal diagnosis of CDH is established when herniation of abdominal contents (e.g., loops of bowel, the stomach, or the left lobe of the liver) into the fetal thorax is seen on ultrasound evaluation. The function of certain fetal organs, such as the heart and kidneys, can be assessed in utero, but the fetal lungs do not exchange gas and therefore cannot be assessed directly. Several sonographically detectable predictors of the severity of CDH are used routinely. The two most important parameters are the lung to head ratio (LHR) (Lipshutz et al., 1997) and the position of the left lobe of the liver (Albanese et al., 1998). LHR is the calculated volume of the contralateral lung (the ipsilateral lung cannot be identified with CDH) indexed to head circumference to adjust for gestational age. Fetuses with an LHR of more than 1.0 have a favorable prognosis with tertiary postnatal care and therefore are not candidates for fetal intervention. In addition, fetuses with the liver in the normal abdominal position also tend to do well, and the survival rate is over 90% (Albanese et al., 1998). Determination of liver position is technically challenging and requires color Doppler ultrasonography to visualize the position of the branches of the left portal vein. Together, these prognostic indicators allow careful selection of severely affected fetuses that may benefit from fetal intervention.

The history and evolution of fetal diagnosis and therapy for CDH is perhaps the best illustration of both the success and disappointment of fetal surgery, as well as the innovation and refinement that occurs frequently and rapidly in the field. Open fetal surgery, in which a hysterotomy was performed and the diaphragm was repaired directly, presented many technical problems. Specifically, reduction of a herniated lobe of the liver during repair resulted in kinking of the intra-abdominal umbilical vein, cutting off blood flow from the placenta and led to fetal demise. Data from a 1994 National Institutes of Health (NIH)-sponsored single-center trial at the UCSF showed that repair of the diaphragm for fetuses without liver herniation was successful, but that the survival rate did not improve over that for standard postnatal care (Harrison et al., 1997). For the more severe form of CDH (i.e., liver herniation), a redirection in thinking about how to treat was necessary as complete repair was not technically feasible. Serendipity of nature provided a new paradigm for treating these severely affected fetuses. It had long been noted that fetuses with congenital high airway obstruction syndrome (CHAOS) caused by laryngeal or tracheal atresia have large, hyperextended lungs as a result of overdistention from lung fluid (Fetal Care Center of Cincinnati, 2005). While in the uterus the fetal lungs constantly produce fluid. As a result of this airway blockage, the lung fluid cannot escape out of the fetal mouth and the fetus's lungs become distended with fluid. Observation of the physiologic effects of CHAOS led investigators to apply these same principles of fluid dynamics to a new approach in fetal intervention for CDH. The strategy of in utero temporary tracheal occlusion (TO) is based on the premise that creating a temporary obstruction in the fetal trachea will interfere with the normal egress of lung fluid, expand and promote growth of the lungs, and therefore improve lung function. Occlusion was first accomplished with open fetal surgery to place a trachea plug and was later accomplished with the use of external tracheal clips. Both procedures were huge operations for the mother requiring a hysterotomy and resulted in preterm labor and early delivery. As smaller instrumentation evolved the procedure was accomplished using fetoscopic techniques, and this strategy of temporarily occluding the fetal trachea with a balloon to accelerate fetal lung growth was tested (Harrison et al., 1996, 1998) (Figure 24.2). The preliminary data showed this technique to have great promise and, in 1999, formed the basis for a second NIH-sponsored clinical trial of innovative fetal CDH treatment. In this randomized controlled trial (RCT), the fetal TO at 26 weeks gestation was compared with standard postnatal care for fetuses with a LHR less than 1.4 and liver herniation. The technique for removing the tracheal balloon is called the "ex utero intrapartum treatment" (EXIT) procedure (Crombleholme, Sylvester, Flake, & Adzick, 2000; DeCou, Jones, Jacobs, & Touloukian, 1998; Mychaliska et al., 1997). After the hysterotomy is performed, the fetal

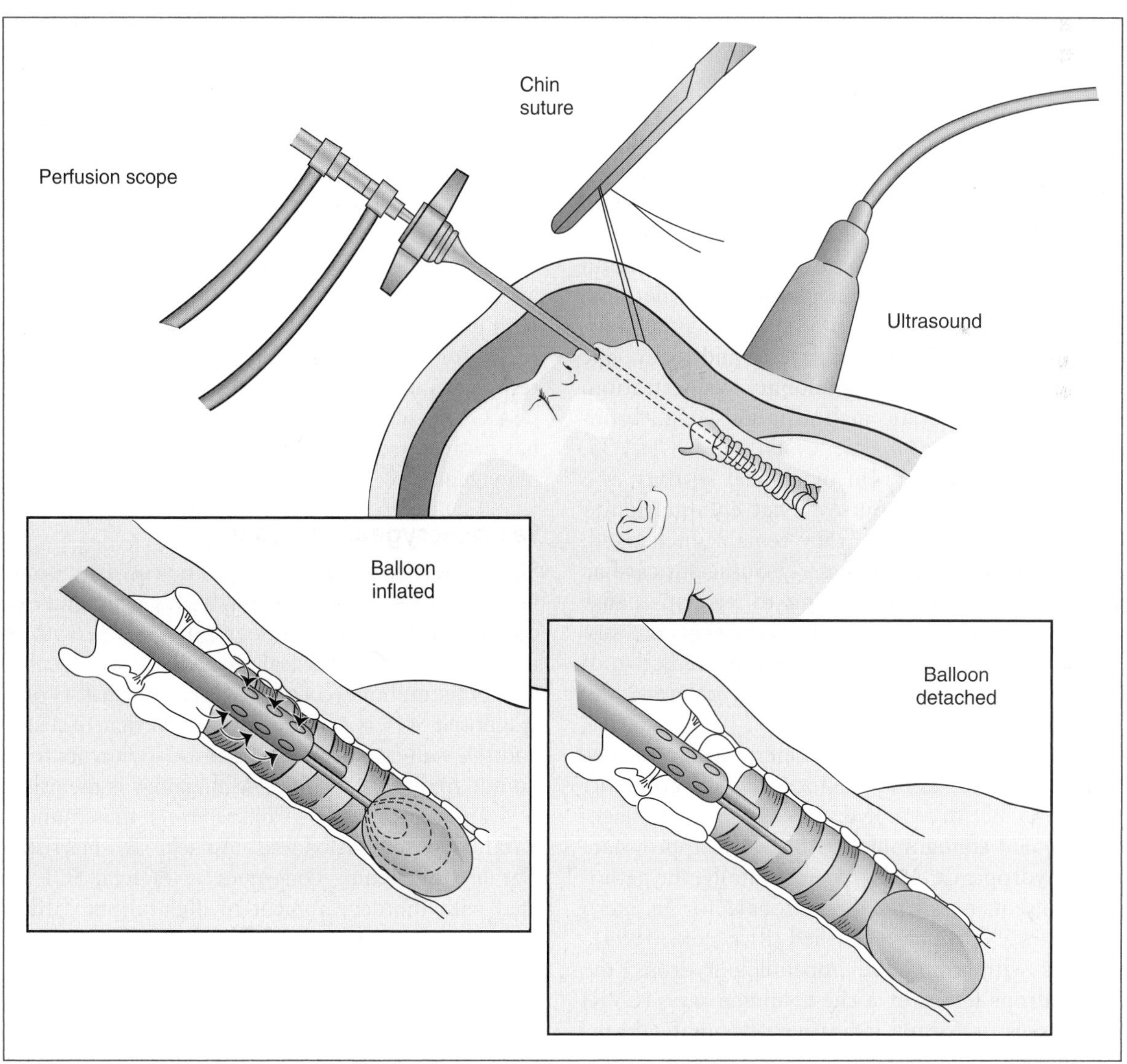

FIGURE 24.2 Fetal tracheal occlusion with balloon.

head and shoulders are delivered, but the cord is not clamped and the fetus remains on placental support. During the period, the pediatric surgeon inserts a bronchoscope, pops the balloon, and removes it with suction. The neonate is intubated; surfactant is administered; and mechanical hand ventilation is begun. Once the oxygen saturation increases, the cord is cut and the infant is delivered. The primary outcome variable was survival at 90 days. As with the previous trial, there was no demonstrable difference in the early mortality between the fetal surgery and standard postnatal care groups. What was surprising was an unexpectedly high survival rate shown in the standard care group (77%) that resulted in closing enrollment early (Harrison, 2003).

Evolution of technique continued and the European (EuroFetus Group) experiences with reversible balloon TO showed promise (Deprest et al., 2005). Advances in techniques and surgeon expertise now permit reversal of the TO (removal of the balloon) between 32 and 34 weeks gestation by minimally invasive techniques. Removing the balloon prior to birth has a twofold advantage: The mother can deliver vaginally, and unobstructing the trachea allows normal development of surfactant-producing type II pneumocytes. The subject population is women carrying fetuses with CDH, liver up, and an LHR less than 1.0, as their survival based on these prognostic factors is less than 60%. Clinical trials in both the United States and Europe continue to study this patient population with temporary TO.

Congenital Cystic Adenomatoid Malformation

CCAM of the lung is the most common type of fetal thoracic mass that can be detected by prenatal ultrasound examination as early as 16 weeks gestation, while most cases are diagnosed before 22 weeks. CCAM is a hamartoma of the lung that usually is unilateral and lobar. The differential diagnoses include pulmonary sequestration, CDH, other congenital cystic malformations (e.g., bronchogenic, enteric, or neurogenic cysts), and CHAOS. CCAMs have a broad spectrum of clinical severity and usually follow one of three courses: They enlarge significantly, leading to fetal hydrops; they remain unchanged; or they shrink and disappear prenatally. Sufficient cardiac and great vessel compression leading to hydrops cause fetal demise in 100% of pregnancies. However, the size and degree of mediastinal shift alone is not predictive of hydrops, which occurs in only the minority of prenatally diagnosed CCAMs.

Prenatal management of CCAMs is determined by the size and classification of the lesion, macrocystic or microcystic, as well as the presence of fetal hydrops. Expectant management with frequent sonographic evaluation is appropriate for small, nonhydropic CCAMs. Experimentally, the pathophysiologic consequences and the rationale for in utero treatment of CCAM have been clarified (Rice et al., 1994).

In the fetus with a CCAM, impending hydrops, the presence of hydrops fetalis or a chest volume ratio (CVR) greater than 1.6 is uniformly indicative of poor fetal outcome without prenatal intervention. A macrocystic form of CCAM is amenable to cyst decompression by needle aspiration or thoracoamniotic shunt placement, should they enlarge enough to cause the development of hydrops. Survival rates in hydropic fetuses with macrocystic lesions range from 50% to 69% (Cavoretto, Molina, Poggi, Davenport, & Nicolaides, 2008). Fetuses with microcystic CCAM are not amenable for thoracocentesis and cyst aspiration or thoracoamniotic shunting. Open fetal surgery with lobectomy in the presence of fetal hydrops has had a reported survival rate of 52% and mean gestational age at delivery of 31.3 weeks (Adzick, 2003; Crombleholme et al., 2002; Grethel et al., 2007). Unfortunately, morbidity and mortality remain high with open fetal surgical intervention.

In instances in which fetal surgery may not be an option, the use of maternal steroids had been reported to arrest the growth of fetal CCAMs. Although the mechanism of steroids' effect on CCAM is unknown, it is thought that the steroids stimulate the maturation of immature pulmonary cells of the microcystic CCAM (Curran et al., 2010). Initial experience of prenatal corticosteroid administration for CCAM was reported in 2003 (Tsao et al., 2003). In a cohort of three hydropic patients with large microcystic CCAMs, clinicians observed resolution of hydrops and survival through the neonatal period after maternal steroid administration. Two other institutions subsequently reported their experience with the use of prenatal steroids for fetal lung masses. Peranteau et al. (2007) reported 100% survival in a cohort of 11 fetuses with high-risk CCAM lesions (10/11 microcystic). They observed decreased lesion growth rates in 8/11 fetuses and resolution of hydrops in 4/5 fetuses. Most recently, Morris, Lim, Livingston, Polzin, and Crombleholme (2009) administered prenatal steroids for both macrocystic and microcystic lesions. For patients with microcystic lesions, there was 75% survival (6/8) and resolution of hydrops in 66% (4/6). Given these significant results, standard of care in the treatment of large microcystic CCAMs (chest volume ratio, CVR > 1.6) and/or hydrops has evolved from open fetal surgery techniques to medical management with the administration of maternal steroids.

Sacrococcygeal Teratoma

SCT is the most common tumor in newborns, occurring in 1 in 35,000 to 40,000 live births. SCT, a neural tube defect that can be detected by ultrasonography, is the growth of a tumor in the sacral and coccygeal areas of the spinal cord or at the base of the tailbone (coccyx). The natural history of prenatally diagnosed SCT is very different from that of neonatal SCT, and the well-established prognostic indicators for the latter do not apply for fetal SCT. Malignancy is the primary cause of death in neonatal SCT but is rare in these tumors in utero (Graf, Housely, Albanese, Adzick, & Harrison, 1998). The life-threatening consequences of fetal SCT are associated with the development of high-output cardiac failure, which results from a "vascular steal" phenomenon through the solid, highly vascular tumors.

Only 10% of fetal SCTs cause hydrops; if left untreated, the mortality rate is 100%. SCT also may lead to a potentially devastating maternal complication called maternal mirror (Ballantine) syndrome, in which the mother experiences progressive symptoms suggestive of preeclampsia, including hypertension, peripheral edema, proteinuria, and pulmonary edema, because of the release of endothelial cell toxins from the edematous placenta. This syndrome is reversed not by removing the SCT prenatally, but only by delivering the fetus and the placenta.

Prenatal sonographic diagnosis of SCT is based on detection of a characteristic sacral and/or obstetric sonography during midgestation; most SCTs can be diagnosed in utero. Fetal SCTs can be cystic, solid, or mixed in appearance (Westerburg et al., 2000); differential diagnoses include MMC and obstructive uropathy. Color flow Doppler ultrasonographic examination of large vascular tumors may show markedly increased distal aortic blood flow and shunting of blood away from the placenta to the tumor, a condition that almost uniformly leads to hydrops and makes the fetus a possible candidate for surgical intervention. Of the reported cases undergoing open fetal surgical resection of an SCT, there are few long-term survivors to date (Adzick, Crombleholme, Morgan, & Quinn, 1997; Graf, Albanese, Jennings, Farrell, & Harrison, 2000).

Fetal surgery for SCT involves tumor resection. Briefly, a maternal hysterotomy is performed, and the fetal buttocks and lower spine are exposed. If the lesion is small, a stapling device is used to apply pressure to the highly vascular tissue, gradually cutting off the blood supply to the tumor; this technique minimizes fetal blood loss. If the tumor is too large to be safely handled by stapling, umbilical tape can be pulled tightly over the tumor mass, binding it and cutting off the blood supply. The surgeon then can remove or resect the tumor with little risk of bleeding. Because these tumors sometimes recur or are not removed completely, further surgery may be required during the neonatal period.

Research efforts were redirected toward developing a minimally invasive approach to treatment in which, rather than debulking the mass, the tumor's blood supply is interrupted by coagulating the major feeding blood vessels (Westerburg et al., 1998). This approach can be accomplished percutaneously using radio frequency ablation (RFA). Most recently, Sago et al. reported a case of a fetus with large, solid, highly vascularized SCT diagnosed at 24 weeks gestation, with polyhydramnios and cardiac and placental enlargement. RFA was performed at 30 weeks gestation by percutaneously inserting the probe into the middle of the fetal tumor under ultrasonographic guidance. The blood supply to the tumor was successfully reduced with stabilization of high-output cardiac failure of the fetus. This case demonstrated that it is possible to use RFA to reduce the blood supply to the fetal SCT for prolongation of pregnancy (Sago et al., 2011).

Congenital High Airway Obstructive Syndrome

CHAOS usually is caused by laryngeal or tracheal atresia and in rare cases by isolated tracheal stenosis, mucosal web, or extrinsic compression by a large cervical mass (e.g., teratoma or lymphangioma) (Paek et al., 2001). Regardless of the etiology, fetal upper airway obstruction prevents egress of the fluid produced in the lungs, which normally travels from the airways into the amniotic space. This fluid usually is produced under a pressure that favors movement out through the fetal mouth, partly aided by fetal breathing movements. Sonographic findings of CHAOS include a bilaterally flattened or everted diaphragm; large, overdistended (i.e., fluid filled), echogenic lungs that compress the mediastinum; dilated large airways distal to the obstruction; and fetal ascites or hydrops (or both) resulting from compression of the heart and great vessel or vessels (Hedrick et al., 1994). If hydrops does not develop in utero, a fetus with CHAOS may be treated with the EXIT procedure, which maintains the baby on placental support until an airway is established via orotracheal intubation or tracheostomy (Mychaliska et al., 1997). However, if fetal hydrops develops, depending on the gestational age, early delivery or prenatal bronchoscopy as an attempt to relieve the obstruction is an option for treatment. Use of the EXIT procedure in CHAOS cases can offer an improved prognosis and the potential for excellent long-term outcome of these fetuses that otherwise would not survive. However, management of the airway, particularly with regard to long-term reconstruction in children with CHAOS, remains challenging (Shimabukuro et al., 2007).

Complications of Twin Pregnancies

Twin-to-twin transfusion syndrome (TTTS) is the most common complication in monochorionic-diamniotic twin pregnancies, occurring in 5% to 35% of these pregnancies. Although associated anomalies are rare, TTTS does carry a high risk of miscarriage, brain damage, perinatal death, and significant morbidity in survivors.

In TTTS, unequal sharing of the monochorionic placenta usually can be visualized sonographically: insertion of the smaller (or donor) twin's placental cord often is marginal or velamentous, whereas the larger (or recipient) twin's cord inserts into the placenta centrally. Vascular connections on the placental surface exist between the twins, and if these are unbalanced, a net shunting of blood occurs as a result of arteriovenous anastomoses, which can be detected by Doppler ultrasonography.

Ultrasonography commonly demonstrates severe oligohydramnios or anhydramnios in the sac of the donor twin (also known as the "stuck twin"). The differential diagnoses for a "stuck twin" include uteroplacental dysfunction, discordant aneuploidy, structural urinary tract malformations, or congenital infections. The recipient twin, on the other hand, develops polyhydramnios, pulmonary hypertension, and cardiomyopathy caused by chronic blood volume overload. The vessels in question are unpaired with flow from the donor fetus to the recipient fetus. Doppler studies demonstrate the characteristic pulsatile arterial blood flow on the donor's side, whereas the vessel shows a continuous venous flow on the recipient's side.

Once the diagnosis of TTTS is established, the severity of the condition may be assessed using the Quintero Staging System (Table 24.2). Not only does this staging system mirror the progression of disease, but it has also been shown to be important in establishing the prognosis (Quintero et al., 1999).

Untreated, TTTS that presents before 28 weeks gestation is associated with a poor survival rate and approximately 90% perinatal mortality rate, prompting a variety of treatment approaches. For example, studies have shown improved outcomes in patients treated with laser therapy compared to the traditional method of serial amnioreductions (Quintero et al., 2003; Senat et al., 2004; Yamamoto & Ville, 2006). In the European randomized trial, the study was interrupted prematurely because statistical improvement in pregnancy outcome in the laser therapy group was achieved at the time of an interval analysis (Senat et al., 2004).

Currently, the most effective treatment for Stages II, III, and IV TTTS is considered to be fetoscopic placental laser ablation of the intertwin vessels (Figure 24.3). The surgical procedure varies—some surgeons coagulate all vessels seen crossing the intertwin septum on the placental surface (Hecher, 1999), while others coagulate only the unpaired intertwin communicating vessels (De Lia, Kuhlmann, Harstad, & Cruikshank, 1995; Feldstein et al., 2000).

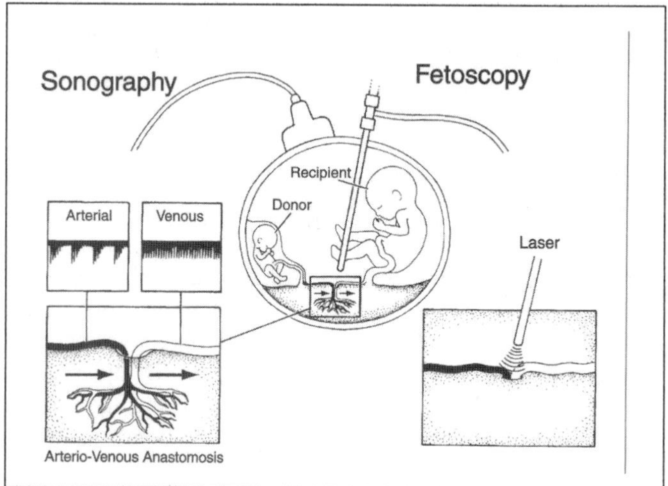

FIGURE 24.3 Fetoscopic placental laser ablation of the intertwin vessels.

Myelomeningocele

Open neural tube defects are a group of congenital abnormalities that arise by day 28 postconception when some portion of the neural tube fails to close. These defects are the most common and most severe of the congenital abnormalities affecting the central nervous system. Approximately 2,000 fetuses annually are affected with some sort of open neural tube defect in the United States, about half of which are open spina bifida. Health care costs are estimated by the Centers for Disease Control at $200 million per year (Centers for Disease Control and Prevention [CDC], 1989). Open spina bifida can occur either as a flat defect without a fluid filled sac covering (myeloschisis), with a membranous covering (meningocele), or membranous covering with extrusion of the spinal cord into the fluid filled sac (MMC).

Myelomeningocele, or spina bifida, is a midline defect that results in exposure of the contents of the spinal column. The defect usually is located in the lumbosacral portion of the vertebrae. Routine maternal serum alpha-fetoprotein (MSAFP) screening identifies more than 80% of pregnancies affected with MMC. When MSAFP values are outside the normal range, direct sonographic visualization of the fetal spine can be performed by 16 weeks gestation to confirm the presence of an MMC and other possible associated findings, including frontal bone scalloping (lemon sign), abnormality of the cerebellum (banana sign), Chiari II malformation (hindbrain herniation), hydrocephaly, microcephaly, and encephalocele. The Chiari II malformation (hindbrain herniation) and hydrocephalus in most cases are a result of altered cerebral spinal fluid dynamics. Damage to the exposed spinal cord can result in lifelong lower extremity neurological dysfunction, bowel and bladder incontinence, and skeletal deformities. This defect carries enormous personal, familial, and societal costs. The child is subjected to multiple hospitalizations, operations, and disability.

The clinical observation that, in fetuses with MMC, lower extremity function present early in the pregnancy was progressively lost in later gestation provided the rationale for considering prenatal intervention. It had been thought that the abnormally developed spinal cord did not allow the bones of the spinal column to form correctly, but now it is known that the opposite is true: The primary defect is in the bony aspect of the spinal column, which then exposes the normal spinal cord to trauma from amniotic fluid exposure and uterine wall friction. Creation and repair of the defect in animals showed that intrauterine repair of MMC may preserve peripheral neurologic function (Hutchins, 1996; Meuli et al., 1995a, b). Experimental studies also indicated that the Chiari II malformation, which is nearly always associated with MMC, may be prevented or reversed by prenatal repair (Paek et al., 2000).

The only options available to parents once a diagnosis was made prenatally were expectant management with delivery and postnatal therapy for the child, or pregnancy termination. By 1997, the first human fetal surgery cases of MMC repair were being performed at Children's

TABLE 24.2

QUINTERO STAGING SYSTEM

Stage I	The fetal bladder of the donor twin remains visible sonographically.
Stage II	The bladder of the donor twin is collapsed and not visible by ultrasound.
Stage III	Critically abnormal fetal Doppler studies noted. This may include absent or reversed end-diastolic velocity in the umbilical artery, absent or reverse flow in the ductus venosus, or pulsatile flow in the umbilical vein.
Stage IV	Fetal hydrops present
Stage V	Demise of either twin

Hospital of Philadelphia (CHOP), Vanderbilt University Medical Center (VUMC), and the UCSF (Adzick, Sutton, Crombleholme, & Flake, 1998). Clinical experience showed that open fetal surgery may improve neurologic function and more dramatically resolve the hindbrain herniation associated with MMC (Adzick et al., 1998; Bruner et al., 1999; Bruner, Richards, Tulipan, & Arney, 1999; Sutton et al., 1999; Tulipan, Hernanz-Schulman, & Bruner, 1998).

By 1999, both the CHOP and VUMC groups reported that results of their initial clinical experience with fetal repair suggested a decrease in hindbrain herniation, promising results regarding the decreased need for ventricular shunting and better than predicted lower extremity function (Bruner et al., 1999; Sutton et al., 1999). These promising results led to a cooperative agreement to answer the question correctly in a randomized controlled clinical trial of safety and efficacy—the NIH-sponsored Management of Myelomeningocele Study (MOMS). Although children with MMC suffer significant morbidity, this was the first fetal intervention offered in a nonlethal birth defect.

Trial enrollment and randomization began in 2002. The two primary endpoints were improvement of outcome, as measured by death or the need for ventricular decompressing shunting by 1 year of age; and improvement in neurologic function at 30 months corrected age as measured by a combined rank score of the Bayley Scales of Infant Development mental development index and the difference between the functional motor level versus anatomic lesion level. By December 2010, the MOMS' Data and Safety Monitoring Board (DSMB) recommended stopping recruitment for reasons of efficacy of prenatal surgery, not for safety concerns. Study endpoints were found to be statistically significantly different between the surgery groups. In short, the prenatal surgery group was not only found to have a decreased need for a ventriculoperitoneal shunt, but also had greater likelihood of walking (Adzick et al., 2011). The DSMB also recommended further follow-up of the children until school-aged to observe whether the results were sustained. That separate long-term follow-up study will be completed in 2016.

Amniotic Band Syndrome

The incidence of amniotic band syndrome is 1 in 12,000 to 15,000 live births. Early rupture of the amnion results in mesodermic bands that emanate from the chorionic side of the amnion and insert onto the fetal body. These bands may lead to amputations, constrictions, and postural deformities that occur secondary to immobilization. Crombleholme and colleagues produced amniotic band syndrome in fetal sheep so as to study the effects of fetoscopic release on morphometric outcome (Crombleholme et al., 1995).

It has been shown that the earlier the band occurs, the more severe is the resulting lesion (Strauss, Hasbargen, Paek, Bauerfeind, & Hepp, 2000). For example, amniotic rupture in the first weeks of pregnancy may result in craniofacial and visceral defects; with rupture during the second trimester, fetal morbidity ranges from formation of syndactyly to limb amputation. Umbilical cord constriction at any time in gestation may result in fetal death. For more severe forms, fetoscopic lysis of the bands may be useful (Quintero, Morales, Phillips, Kalter, & Angel, 1997). Development of smaller scopes has provided fetal access for cases of release of bands around a limb. Lysis of bands around extremities is now possible through minimally invasive procedures (Assaf, Llanes, & Chmait, 2012).

Hypoplastic Left Heart Syndrome

Prenatally diagnosed critical aortic valve stenosis leads to ventricular overload, chronic myocardial wall ischemia, and eventually hypoplastic left heart syndrome. Postnatal therapy involves staged surgical repairs, but mortality is up to 25% after the first operation and survivors face a lifetime of cardiac and neurologic dysfunction. In utero repair offers a promising alternative. Given a substantial body of knowledge regarding the fetal physiology and natural history of these lesions in utero and the success of balloon aortic and pulmonary valvuloplasty in preventing or reversing new onset ventricular dysfunction postnatally in infants, there is a theoretic rationale for intervention to relieve valvar stenosis or enlarge the atrial septal opening in fetal life. The theory has now been tested by numerous fetal cardiac intervention programs throughout the world. Percutaneous and open fetal aortic valvuloplasty have successfully relieved left ventricular obstruction and minimized left heart damage (Tworetzky et al., 2004).

MULTIDISCIPLINARY COLLABORATIVE APPROACH TO FETAL THERAPY

The fetus with an anomaly requires the attention of team specialists working together with the mother and fetus. Members of the team include a perinatologist, neonatologist, pediatric surgeon, urologist, neurosurgeon, sonologist, anesthesiologist, operating room and perinatal nurse specialists, physiologist, technicians, social worker, and nurse coordinator who can serve as a liaison for the family (Table 24.3).

In many instances, time is of the essence with fetal surgery cases; the legal window on the option of pregnancy termination may be closing, and delays can lead to substantial fetal morbidity and even mortality. For maximum possible benefit, fetal surgery candidates should be identified and referred before 23 weeks gestation. Early referral allows the fetal surgery team adequate time to consider the clinical situation carefully and to perform appropriately timed interventions. Box 24.1 outlines the multidisciplinary approach to specific interventions developed by the fetal surgery team at the University of California at San Francisco Benioff Children's Hospital.

Considerations for Collaborative Care Planning

When fetal surgery is chosen, the clinical case may be broken down into six phases: diagnosis, information and decision making, perioperative and postoperative care, home care and follow-up, delivery, and neonatal period.

TABLE 24.3

MILESTONES IN FETAL THERAPY

Therapy	Location	Year
Rh disease—IUT	New Zealand	1961
Hysterotomy for fetal vascular access and IUT	Puerto Rico	1964
Respiratory distress syndrome of prematurity—prenatal steroids	London	1972
Fetoscopy—diagnostic	Yale	1974
Experimental pathophysiology (sheep model)	UCSF	1980
Hysterotomy and maternal safety (monkey model)	UCSF	1981
Uropathy—vesicoamniotic shunt	UCSF	1982
Hydrocephalus—ventriculo-amniotic shunt	Denver	1982
Uropathy—open fetal surgery	UCSF	1983
International Fetal Medicine and Surgery Society (IFMSS) founded	Santa Barbara	1982
CCAM—resection	UCSF	1984
Intravascular transfusion	London	1985
CDH—open repair	UCSF	1989
Anomalous twin—cord ligation	London	1990
CDH—NIH trial; open repair	UCSF	1990
Aortic valvuloplasty	London	1991
SCT—resection	UCSF	1992
Laser ablation of placental vessels	Milwaukee; London	1995
EXIT procedure for airway obstruction	UCSF	1995
Uropathy—fetal bladder cystoscopy	Detroit	1995
Fetoscopic surgery (Fetendo)	UCSF	1996
XSCID—in utero stem cell transplant	Detroit	1996
Eurofetus founded	Leuven	1997
CDH—Fetendo clip → balloon	UCSF	1997
MMC—open repair	Vanderbilt	1997
Amniotic band—fetoscopic lysis	Tampa	1997
CDH—NIH trial: Fetendo balloon	UCSF	1998
TRAP—radiofrequency ablation	UCSF	1998
TRAP—cord electrocautery	Leuven	1999
Resection of pericardial teratoma	UCSF	2000
CCAM—prenatal steroid therapy	UCSF	2001
Resection of cervical teratoma	UCSF	2001
CDH—fetoscopic tracheal occlusion (FETO) trial	Leuven; London; Barcelona	2002
MMC—NIH trial: open repair	UCSF; CHOP; Vanderbilt	2002
Osteogenesis imperfecta—in utero stem cell transplant	Stockholm	2003
TTTS—amnioreduction vs. laser	Poissy; Eurofetus	2004
Hypoplastic left heart syndrome—balloon septotomy; valve dilation	Boston	2004
Hypoplastic left heart syndrome—laser atrial septotomy	Tampa	2005
North American Fetal Therapy Network (NAFTNet) founded	United States and Canada	2005
Amniotic collagen plug	Leuven	2007
CCAM—sclerotherapy	Venezuela; Tampa	2007

(*continued*)

TABLE 24.3

MILESTONES IN FETAL THERAPY (CONTINUED)

TRAP—radiofrequency ablation	NAFNET	2009
MMC—enrollment completion of the MOMS trial	UCSF, CHOP, Vanderbilt	2010

CCAM, congenital cystic adenomatoid malformation; CDH, congenital diaphragmatic hernia; IUT, intrauterine transfusion; MMC, myelomeningocele; MOMS, Management of Myelomeningocele Study; NIH, National Institutes of Health; SCT, sacrococcygeal teratoma; TRAP, twin reversed arterial perfusion; TTTS, twin-to-twin transfusion syndrome; UCSF, University of California, San Francisco, XSCID, in utero stem cell transplant.

■ **Diagnosis.** The diagnostic phase generally covers the period from referral to the fetal treatment center through the evaluation process. For the families, this typically is a waiting period, first for an appointment and then for the results. For many families this is the most difficult time, and the nurse should provide appropriate information about the process and suggest resources (e.g., social services, support groups, counseling) to help cushion the family against the challenges inherent in this situation. Technology has promoted better communication (e-mail) and patient education (Internet websites). The nurse must recognize that the family is enduring the loss of a normal pregnancy and experiencing the anxiety of an uncertain future. Also, during this phase the family's concerns often center on the diagnosis and cause of the fetal problem and their possible role in the cause. Families need explicit reassurance.

■ **Information and Decision Making.** Once the differential diagnoses are established, the family is presented with treatment options. These may include termination of the pregnancy (if still early enough in gestation), surgical intervention, or waiting to term for standard postnatal care. Whether invasive therapy should be offered and recommended or offered but not recommended is posed at this point. Such therapy should be offered and recommended only if two criteria are met: (1) the therapy is judged to have a high likelihood of being life-saving or of preventing serious, irreversible disease, injury, or disability for the fetus and the child to come; and (2) the therapy has a low risk of mortality

BOX 24.1

SAMPLE CARE MAP FOR WOMEN UNDERGOING OPEN FETAL SURGERY (CLINICAL PATHWAY)

The following care plan is used at the Fetal Treatment Center at the University of California, San Francisco.

1. *Informed consent and counseling*: Members of the team are included (perinatologist, fetal treatment center nurse coordinator, pediatric surgeon, operating room nurse specialist, sonographer, obstetric anesthesiologist, perinatal nurse specialist, perinatal social worker)
2. *Admission*: The evening before procedure
3. *Preoperative assessment*: Assessment includes baseline cervical examination (digital and by sonogram), baseline maternal vitals and oxygen saturation levels, electronic fetal heart rate, and uterine activity strip
4. *Tocolysis*: Patients receive tocolysis as follows:
   - *Indomethacin*: 50 mg by rectum (pr) given on call to operating room, then every 6 hours for at least 24 to 48 hours after procedure (decreasing dosage to 25 mg)
   - *Magnesium sulfate*: 6 g bolus at uterine closure, then 2 g/hr (titrated based on uterine contractions) given intravenously, initiated intraoperatively and continued until uterine activity has been controlled for 24 to 48 hours
   - *Nifedipine* (oral): If used, it begins when the magnesium sulfate is discontinued and given every 4 to 6 hours until delivery
5. *Coping and supportive care*: Nurse specialists and the perinatal social workers provide continuity for issues of coping
6. *Pain management*: Patients undergo general anesthesia for open fetal surgery procedures and have an epidural catheter placed postoperatively for pain management via epidurally administered narcotics and *-caine* anesthetics
7. *Medications*: Postoperatively, patients receive intravenous × 2 doses
8. *Monitoring*: Patients receive one-to-one care for 24 hours; electronic uterine-fetal monitoring is continuous
9. *Fluid management*: Strict measurement of intake and output is necessary to prevent or limit pulmonary edema; weighing the patient daily and continuous pulse oximetry help detect pulmonary edema early; adventitious lung sounds are a late sign.
10. *Oxygen therapy*: Oxygen is provided via nasal cannula to keep the arterial oxygen saturation above 95%; incentive spirometer is performed every 3 to 4 hours while awake; lungs are assessed every 6 hours
11. *Activity*: Complete bed rest is required until uterine activity is controlled; thigh-high TEDs (thrombo-embolic deterrents) and Venodyne boots with a sequential compression device are used while the patient is on complete bed rest to reduce the risk of emboli
12. *Hospitalization*: Discharge after 4 to 5 days when preterm labor is controlled on oral tocolytics and amniotic fluid level normal
13. *Follow-up*: The patient should return weekly for sonographic evaluation and examination by a perinatologist; biweekly NST and AFI should begin at 26 weeks

From information provided by the Fetal Treatment Center, University of California, San Francisco.

and a low or manageable risk of disease, injury, or disability to the fetus. Although risk to the mother is expected to be low or manageable, any surgical procedure carries some risk of morbidity and mortality, and this should be stated explicitly in the counseling and informed consent processes.

The decision-making phase often is when the family's worst fears are confirmed. As the grief reaction begins, the family's emotions and feelings may become more intense. They also must face the religious, moral, and ethical implications, as well as financial and practical considerations. The informed consent process must seek to minimize family and societal pressures. The individual obtaining the consent should make sure that the woman is alone and that some of the outside pressure is removed (Lyerly et al., 2001).

Before deciding what is best, the family meets with all members of the team. Team members provide detailed information about preoperative, intraoperative, and perioperative care, answer questions, and address concerns. The family also meets privately with the perinatal social worker, who makes a psychosocial assessment and evaluates the family's ability to cope. This evaluation includes assessment of the parental partnership, available support systems, coping strategies used in previous crises, prior experience of loss, current stress factors, unemployment or financial constraints, and other health problems. Collectively, this information assists in the team's assessment of how well the family will cope and what resources may be helpful.

■ **Perioperative and Postoperative Care.** If fetal intervention is chosen, nurses help prepare the family for the procedure and provide extensive preoperative teaching. It may also be an appropriate time to suggest and discuss coping strategies, in case fetal loss occurs at any time during the perioperative period.

■ **Postoperative Management.** Direct physical examination in the postoperative stage, daily fetal sonography and echocardiography provide insight and information about fetal status. During this 3- to 5-day period, too, epidural analgesics, spinal anesthesia, IV pain medication, or patient-controlled analgesia (PCA) are given to the mother to ease maternal stress and aid tocolysis. Nurses provide support, encouragement, and education at this critical time, when the mother and family face uncertainty about their fetus's survival and the possibility of uncontrollable preterm labor. Additional attention to the mother is important, because she must endure the effects of medications that may disrupt her mental status, comfort, and ability to sleep. She also may feel intimidated by the equipment used in postoperative care. The nurse should help promote flexible visiting hours, personalization of the room or bedside, and physical contact with significant others (Howell & Dunphy, 1999).

■ **Preterm Labor.** Preterm labor is the Achilles heel of open fetal surgery. Currently the tocolytic regimen begins with administration of indomethacin to the mother before surgery and over the next several days. Of the available tocolytics, indomethacin was chosen because of its ability to inhibit the synthesis of prostaglandins released during uterine manipulation. In contrast to their value in spontaneous labor, magnesium sulfate and nifedipine have been relatively ineffective and offer little advantage in the treatment of preterm labor induced by hysterotomy. Outpatient tocolysis usually consists of oral nifedipine. If membranes rupture or labor cannot be controlled, cesarean delivery is performed, usually before 36 weeks gestation (Harrison et al., 2001).

The mother may be concerned that something she does or fails to do will lead to preterm labor, PROM, or other harm to the fetus. Discharge planning includes thorough patient education on signs/symptoms of preterm labor.

■ **Home Care and Follow-Up.** The discharge to home can be a particularly anxious time. The mother often is restricted to modified bed rest and tocolytic therapy, and she may fear that something she does or fails to do will harm the fetus. For this reason, the patient and a family member or friend are encouraged and sometimes required to stay near the medical center so that they can return once or twice a week for fetal evaluation (i.e., nonstress test [NST] and amniotic fluid index [AFI]) and sonographic evaluation and assessment for signs of preterm labor. In some instances plans may be made for patients to stay at a nearby facility, such as a Ronald McDonald House (Harrison et al., 2001). If membranes rupture or shred (i.e., chorioamniotic separation) or if preterm labor cannot be controlled, the mother can be rehospitalized, kept on bed rest, and continuously monitored.

Extended separation from family and friends during this follow-up phase may be a significant emotional strain on the patient, and time away from work may be a financial hardship. The nurse coordinator should remain in daily contact with the family to maintain a sense of their emotional well-being and should suggest or provide whatever resources are appropriate to help ease the burden.

■ **Delivery.** Delivery of the infant is unpredictable and may take place any time after fetal surgery but most often occurs 4 to 12 weeks after the procedure, depending on a number of factors. During this phase, the parents' major concerns focus on the infant's chances of survival, and interestingly, but not surprisingly, on the infant's physical appearance at birth as a result of having undergone a surgical procedure. The parents should have the opportunity to see and touch the infant as soon as possible after birth, regardless of the outcome. If the infant does not survive, one of the nurse specialists should encourage the parents to hold, look at, and take pictures with their infant, because these actions help them accept the outcome and experience closure. If the infant survives, it is equally important for parents to see and touch the baby as soon as possible, to provide reassurance. If the physical conditions of both mother and infant make this contact difficult or impossible, a member of the treatment team should take pictures that can be given to the family immediately.

■ **Neonatal Period.** The final phase, the neonatal period, requires the team to work closely with the family's long-term health care providers to ensure appropriate management once the family leaves the fetal treatment center. Even if the infant does not survive, the nurse coordinator should maintain contact so that autopsy results and genetic counseling can be provided. One of the nurse specialists may want to initiate discussion of the various stages of the grief process with the parents. This is also an appropriate time to discuss the reactions of friends and family.

For the family whose infant has survived, the realization that the baby may require further surgery surfaces during this period, or the family may learn that the infant may not live long despite the fetal surgery. Even when the infant is doing well and has minimal risk of further illness, the family may not readily accept the information given. The family may require significant psychosocial support after the discharge to ensure a successful transition to home. This support can be provided through telephone contact, home visits, and clinic visits soon after discharge to assess the family's adjustment. Referrals to support groups, psychologists, or professionals of other disciplines should be made immediately if the family appears to be having trouble coping.

As can clearly be seen, the fetus with an anomaly requires the attention of a team of specialists (Harrison et al., 2001). Not only are there ethical issues that require the balancing of risks and benefits, but there are two patients, the mother and the fetus (Spitzer, 1996). Fetal surgery requires a collective approach to caregiving. The multidisciplinary team at a fetal treatment center requires meaningful collaboration involving the pediatric surgeon, perinatal obstetrician, sonographer, anesthesiologist, operating room and obstetrical nurses, geneticist, social worker, ethicist, and nurse coordinator (Taeusch & Ballard, 1998). Various defects require more subspecialties. Despite the multiple talents in the group, the role of the nurse in the team must not be discounted. Nursing represents a source of continuity in maternal–child care sessions; nurses provide care through all stages of fetal surgery and can be critical advocates for maternal and fetal surgery patients (Collins, 1994).

Fetal Therapy: New Horizons

Treatments for genetic problems are now being attempted through fetal therapy. For example, in conditions involving errors of metabolism the mother receives medication, vitamins, or the substance the fetus lacks, to be passed through the placenta to the fetus (see Chapters 1 and 38). Other therapeutic strategies have been aimed at correcting blood incompatibility problems. Fetuses with inherited diseases such as severe combined immunodeficiency (SCID), hemophilia, enzyme deficiencies, and sickle cell anemia, may benefit from gene therapy or stem cell transplantation. Most promising is that transplantation of allogeneic stem cells into the early gestational fetus, a treatment termed in utero hematopoietic cell transplantation (IUHCTx), could potentially overcome the limitations of bone marrow transplants, including graft rejection and the chronic immunosuppression required to prevent rejection. More exciting are recent findings by Nijagal et al. that there is a marked improvement in IUHCTx engraftment if the mother lacks T cells but not B cells, indicating that maternal T cells are the main barrier to engraftment. Furthermore, when the graft was matched to the mother, there was no difference in engraftment between syngeneic and allogeneic fetal recipients. Therefore, clinical success of IUHCTx may be improved by transplanting the fetus with cells matched to the mother (Nijagal et al., 2011).

Also key to the future of potential therapies is the discovery that the immune system of fetuses, and to some degree newborns, is designed specifically to tolerate foreign bodies to prevent it from attacking its own developing cells or its mothers. Essentially this is the opposite response of the adult immune system, which aggressively attacks threats such as tumors, viruses, bacteria, and fungi that cause infection. This discovery not only challenges the long-held assumption that fetuses and newborn babies have weak, immature immune systems that need time to build up to full strength after birth, but could also have profound effects on how to study and treat a wide variety of human ailments, from HIV and sickle cell disease, to childhood allergies. Prior to this work, it was generally believed that fetal immune cells were immature and nonfunctional. Instead researchers have found that the cells in the fetus are functional, and in fact have a robust, albeit nonaggressive, immune response against things that are foreign. When the fetal immune system senses an unfamiliar cell in the body, it releases a type of cell, known as a regulatory T cell that encourages tolerance. This is necessary for at least two reasons: first, because a fetus is developing rapidly, it could easily see its own cells as a threat, and second, maternal cells easily pass through the placenta, and an adult immune system might attack those healthy and necessary cells if it detected a threat.

Researchers hope to use fetal immune tolerance to prenatally treat and maybe even cure diseases before birth. One example is sickle cell disease, which can be cured with stem cell transplants that encourage the body to produce new, healthy blood cells. But transplant rejection has been a major obstacle. Doctors have tried to transplant stem cells into fetuses, to cure the disease before babies are born, but the cells have almost always been rejected, most likely because the mother's immune system is fighting them off. If the stem cells are a match to the mother, or better yet, if the mother's own cells could be transplanted, the infant could be born almost cured of the disease.

Stem cell therapy may also be a particularly promising solution to reverse spinal injury in MMC because of the immunotolerance unique to the developing fetus. Based on the exciting early clinical promise from the MOMS trial, researchers have assembled a multidisciplinary team that integrates extensive clinical and laboratory experience and expertise in the respective fields of pediatric and fetal surgery, neuroanatomy and neurobiology, spinal cord injury, bioengineering and nanotechnology. Preliminary research suggests that applying placental neural crest stem cells locally to the spinal cord during in utero MMC repair will allow for regeneration, restoration, and recovery of distal spinal cord function. In addition, the use of autologous neural crest stem cells derived from the fetus's own placenta at the time of diagnosis may circumvent the need for subsequent immunosuppression. These cells can be isolated and expanded in the period between diagnosis and repair in humans, and can be delivered via seeding onto biodegradable nanofibrous scaffolds that are surgically implanted at the time of in utero repair. The use of nanofibrous scaffolds as a delivery mechanism for stems cells is well established. These biomaterials play a new and promising role in the field of regenerative medicine because they can guide organized neo-tissue formation by providing a surface with the porosity to foster cellular attachment, migration, proliferation, and differentiation (Kurpinski & Patel, 2011; Zhu et al., 2011).

For many fetuses with severe disease, fetal surgery offers the best and sometimes only therapy. The efficacy of fetal intervention is still greatly limited by high rates of preterm labor and preterm birth, but as more is learned about the underlying mechanisms of preterm labor and strategies are developed to combat it, efficacy will increase and applications of fetal surgery will likely grow. In the near term, minimally invasive techniques will continue to improve and replace open techniques. More distantly, in utero gene therapy for metabolic deficiencies and tissue engineering for organ and tissue deficits promises to be the next frontier of fetal therapy.

Future of Fetal Surgery: Team Responsibilities

Increasingly sophisticated techniques for prenatal diagnosis and increasingly innovative, sometimes controversial treatment strategies have revolutionized the field of fetal medicine. The fetus has come a long way from its enigmatic identity as the biblical "seed" and the mystical "homunculus," to a unique individual with medical and surgical problems that can be diagnosed and treated. The relatively young but eventful history of fetal surgical intervention offers new hope for the fetus with an isolated congenital malformation. The great promise of fetal therapy is that, for some diseases, the earliest possible intervention (i.e., before birth) produces the best possible outcome (i.e., the best quality of life for the resources expended). However, the potential for cost-effective, preventive fetal therapy can be subverted by misguided clinical applications, such as performing a complex in utero procedure that "half saves" an otherwise doomed fetus for a life of intensive (and financially and emotionally expensive) care. Enthusiasm for fetal intervention must be tempered by reverence for the interests of the mother and her family, by careful study of the disease in experimental fetal animals and untreated human fetuses, and by a willingness to abandon therapy that does not prove both efficacious and cost-effective in properly controlled trials.

Recognizing the importance of safeguarding the interests of both the pregnant woman and the fetus, the American College of Obstetricians and Gynecologists (ACOG) and the American Academy of Pediatrics (AAP) made specific recommendations regarding maternal–fetal intervention and fetal care centers (ACOG/AAP, 2011):

1. Fetal intervention cannot be performed without informed consent.
2. Prospective parents should be informed of what is standard of care/evidence-based therapies versus innovative or experimental procedures. Research must be performed under the auspices of an IRB.
3. Informed consent should include risks/benefits, as well as the full range of pregnancy options.
4. Women considering fetal intervention should have access to a subject advocate who does not have ties to the experimental protocol.
5. Support services should be made available to families.
6. Maternal–fetal medicine centers should consist of a multidisciplinary team, and the organization should have institutional governance.
7. Cooperation between fetal care centers should be encouraged as a means to standardize clinical practice, further research efforts, and obtain outcomes data.

Short- and long-term clinical outcomes follow-up for this population is imperative and the responsibility of the clinical teams. While follow-up for the families focuses on general care needs of the child, it must also acknowledge and address the trauma and life-altering effects the fetal treatment itself has had on the family after birth and in the discharge period. This type of specialized care currently is delivered in only a few experienced neonatal intensive care units (NICUs), but it is likely to become more widespread as technology and knowledge of genetics expand. Nursing will have a significant role in providing expert input and shaping the future care of these patients.

Fetal Surgery or Fetal Care Units within specialty children's hospitals or centers now exist in many parts of the country. They are equipped for immediate care for a fetus/neonate that requires specialized services. Some examples of these units are the Fetal Care Center at Boston Children's Hospital, the Fetal Care Center of Cincinnati-Children's Hospital, Fetal Surgery at CHOP, and the Colorado Fetal Care Center-Children's Hospital of Colorado. The growth units demonstrate the increased usage of fetal surgery and the commitment to comprehensive maternal, fetal, and neonatal care.

SUMMARY

The primary goal of this chapter has been to describe fetal treatment and, in particular, fetal surgery. As this field rapidly evolves, expands, and broadens the options for treatment, more neonatal health care professionals will be approached by both colleagues and patients with questions on fetal intervention, including surgery. In this redefined clinical milieu, neonatal nurses must have a basic understanding of this area of medicine, including its associated technology and perhaps even the new ethical considerations it poses. This chapter recognizes the critical, complex, and often difficult role nurse specialists fulfill in fetal treatment, acting as both patient advocate and fetal treatment team representative. The responsibilities are complex, and the nurse specialist who fulfills them must be able to weigh, balance, interpret, and act on a variety of issues from a multifaceted, informed perspective. This chapter, then, is an acknowledgment of the talent, intellect, skill, and compassion that nursing professionals bring to the field of fetal treatment.

CASE STUDY

■ Identification of the Problem. A 31-year-old gravida 3 para 1, currently at 23 to 2/7 weeks, whose singleton gestation is complicated by a fetal MMC. The patient's amniocentesis results revealed a normal karyotype (46XX).

■ Assessment: History and Physical Examination

- Past medical history: unremarkable
- Surgical history: none
- Obstetric history: full-term NSVD 2 years ago (healthy male), followed by early first trimester SAB (spontaneous abortion)
- Meds: prenatal vitamins, Claritin, 1,600 mcg folic acid
- Allergies: NKDA (no known drug allergies)
- Social history: works as an accountant; her husband (present at today's visit) is employed as a police officer
- Family history: the patient's cousin may have had spina bifida, but the patient is unsure and at present has not been able to obtain records

■ Review of Systems

- GENERAL REVIEW OF SYSTEMS: negative
- CONSTITUTIONAL: she is oriented to person, place, and time; vital signs are normal; she appears well developed and well nourished
- HEAD: normocephalic and atraumatic
- EYES: conjunctivae and extra-ocular movement are normal; pupils are equal, round, and reactive to light
- NECK: normal range of motion; neck supple
- CARDIOVASCULAR: normal rate, regular rhythm, normal heart sounds, and intact distal pulses
- PULMONARY/CHEST: effort normal and breath sounds normal
- ABDOMINAL: soft; bowel sounds are normal
- GENITOURINARY: uterus gravid
- MUSCULOSKELETAL: normal range of motion
- NEUROLOGICAL: she is alert and oriented to person, place, and time, she has normal reflexes
- SKIN: skin is warm and dry
- PSYCHIATRIC: she has a normal mood and affect; her behavior is normal; judgment and thought content normal

■ Diagnostic Tests

1. Fetal echo: Structurally and functionally normal.
2. Obstetric ultrasound: Appropriately grown fetus with normal amniotic fluid volume. A severe Chiari II malformation is noted; there is ventriculomegaly measuring 17 mm on each side; the level of the defect is felt to be at L1 to L2, and there is also the finding of syringomyelia (syrinx). There is concern of no visible normal spinal cord below the level of the syrinx (just neural elements). The placenta is anterior, and the cervical length appears normal.
3. MRI: Small posterior fossa, and downward descent of the cerebellar tonsils down to the level of C4, and a lumbar MMC, consistent with Chiari II malformation. Abnormal T2 hyperintensity is noted in the spinal canal in the lower cervical region extending to the lower thoracic cord, concerning for syrinx.
4. Laboratory tests: B+, Rh positive, antibody screen negative; Hct = 42.3, Hgb = 13.5, rubella immune, VDRL negative, HBsAg negative, chlamydia and gonorrhea negative

■ Working Diagnosis. Pregnancy complicated with fetus with MMC

■ Development of Management Plan

Counseling. Discussed maternal and paternal history, the diagnostic findings, and the potential management options. Reviewed the MOMS trial that studied prenatal versus postnatal repair of MMC (Adzick et al., 2011). Reviewed the benefits of prenatal MMC repair seen in that trial, particularly the 40% reduction in need for shunting (primary outcome). Discussed the secondary outcomes of a potential decrease in ambulatory deficits, such as the need for a brace, or other motor functions such as bladder and bowel control. Patients who underwent prenatal repair appeared to have a benefit equivalent to a two level improvement in location of the lesion (e.g., deficits associated with a L2 lesion would potentially be closer to those normally seen with an L4 lesion). Discussed the risks of prenatal surgery, most significant of which are preterm birth and maternal risks such as those associated with a uterine hysterotomy.

Regarding Preterm Birth. Based on the MOMS trial results, there was an 80% incidence of preterm birth in patients who had the prenatal fetal surgery repair, compared with a 15% preterm birth in the nonsurgery or postnatal group. While this amounts to a fivefold higher risk of delivering preterm, if the patient elects prenatal surgery versus postnatal surgery, it is important to examine this more specifically by severity of the gestational age at the time of such a preterm birth. The greatest increased risk is in delivery under 30 weeks gestation because in patients who elected to have a postnatal repair, there were no births under this gestational age, whereas 12.8% of patients who had the prenatal repair delivered at less than 30 weeks. Overall, statistically 45% of patients who undergo prenatal surgery deliver at less than 34 weeks, whereas only 5% of patients who have a postnatal repair deliver at less than 34 weeks.

Risk involving the hysterotomy is potentially high and necessitates close surveillance. Of the 76 patients analyzed in the first publication of the MOMS trial who had prenatal surgery, 35.5% had thinning or dehiscence of their hysterotomy scar. For this reason it is imperative that patients who undergo prenatal surgical repair receive very close monitoring for contractions and are evaluated immediately if they complain of discomfort.

Other maternal risks include leakage of amniotic fluid through the hysterotomy site, which would lead to oligohydramnios and the potential need for long-term hospitalization for the remainder (or significant portions) of the pregnancy. For some patients, leakage of amniotic fluid is painful and inflammatory and leads to significant discomfort during the remainder of the pregnancy. Less common risks include other general operative risks such as bleeding, the need for blood transfusion, anesthetic complications, infection, blood clots, and complications resulting from any of the medications necessary to stabilize the patient postoperatively.

■ Pregnancy Management Options. Three management options:

The patient can elect to undergo a pregnancy termination. Legally this can be performed up to 24 weeks gestation.

The patient can elect to have standard postnatal repair. It is recommended that she undergo elective cesarean delivery at 39 weeks gestation in the same center prepared to offer postnatal MMC repair. Pregnancy recommendations are monthly growth scans antenatally as well as weekly NST beginning at 32 weeks.

The patient can elect to undergo prenatal repair. This would be scheduled prior to 26 weeks gestation. If the patient is over 24 weeks gestation at the time of surgery, there is the option of antenatal corticosteroids if she would choose to undergo an emergent cesarean delivery in the event of fetal distress. The patient understands that regardless of fetal status, she would have to have a cesarean delivery for this pregnancy (even in the event of an IUFD), as the fresh scar cannot undergo labor. For the prenatal surgery she would need both regional anesthesia (epidural) and general anesthesia. In the immediate postoperative period, the patient would be on IV magnesium and indomethacin. Once she no longer needed magnesium, the patient would begin oral nifedipine, which would continue until delivery. The usual postoperative course ranges between 4 and 5 days of inpatient hospitalization, followed by 2 to 3 weeks of local outpatient follow-up. If the patient has an uncomplicated outpatient postoperative course, she may be cleared to return home under the direct management of a perinatologist. Written guidelines for pregnancy management would be provided. Most importantly, as noted above, the patient should not be allowed to tolerate significant contractions or labor. She would need to be retocolyzed in the event of preterm labor, and delivered by cesarean section if labor was unstoppable. PPROM (preterm premature rupture of membranes), in the absence of contractions, can be managed as per usual protocol. Barring any other complications, the patient would have to undergo cesarean delivery by 37 weeks.

Regarding future pregnancies: There is no increased risk of infertility. There is also no option of vaginal birth after cesarean section, and all future pregnancies should be managed similar to having had a prior *classical scar* and should be delivered by early cesarean section. After a pregnancy involving a prenatal MMC repair, the uterus has a double scar (prenatal surgical hysterotomy plus delivery hysterotomy), which increases her risk in future pregnancies. It is advised that the patient adhere to a minimum interpregnancy interval of 16 months, and that, due to the double scar, future pregnancies be delivered at 36 weeks by repeat cesarean.

■ Outcome. Patient elected prenatal repair of fetal MMC. Surgery was performed the following week.

EVIDENCE-BASED PRACTICE BOX

Based on its most recent statistics, the CDC reports that birth defects affect 1 in 33 babies and are the leading cause of infant mortality in the United States, more so than low birth weight and prematurity, SIDS (sudden infant death syndrome), and maternal complications. Affected babies who survive are at increased risk for developing lifelong physical and cognitive challenges. Lifelong costs associated with birth defects, for example, and annual hospital stays, are a significant stressor on families and the health care system alike. Fortunately, advances in fetal diagnosis allow clinicians to both accurately identify most complex anomalies prenatally and, more often, stratify the severity of the birth defect. In many instances, because diagnosis can be made in the second trimester, clinicians can provide families information that enables them to make more informed decisions about the pregnancy and the delivery plan and to plan and prepare for the future.

Over the past four decades, fetal intervention for congenital anomalies has evolved from a mere concept to a full-fledged medical specialty. The strategy of fetal intervention is to ameliorate or reverse some of the progressive physiologic organ damage that occurs from a particular defect. Operative techniques used in fetal surgery, such as open hysterotomy, fetal endoscopy, and image-guided percutaneous procedures, were developed and tested extensively in animal models first, before clinical application. These advances in surgical techniques paralleled and complemented those in fetal imaging, prenatal diagnosis, and maternal tocolysis. In a relatively short time, fetal intervention has become an important option for the treatment of fetuses who would otherwise not survive gestation or who would endure significant morbidity and mortality after birth.

The evolution of fetal surgery from research hypothesis to medical specialty was not without many trials and tribulations. The fetal therapy community quickly learned that justification for in utero intervention based

(*continued*)

on anecdotal experience and retrospective studies of registry data was insufficient. Prospective controlled trials to determine the safety and efficacy of fetal interventions were necessary. As a result, in the mid-1980s, UCSF conducted the first NIH-sponsored trial examining open fetal surgical repair for CDH (Harrison et al., 1997). Upon completion of the trial, data suggested that fetal surgery for CDH, though physiologically sound and technically feasible, did not improve survival over standard postnatal treatment.

Three trends have dominated the field of fetal surgery. First, an emphasis has been placed on prospective RCTs instead of retrospective clinical trials to determine efficacy and effectiveness. The evolution of the interventions themselves represents a strategic shift from anatomic repair of a congenital anomaly to physiologic manipulation of the developmental consequences (e.g., from open in utero repair of the diaphragmatic defect in CDH to temporary TO to promote lung growth). Finally, innovation in techniques represents a movement toward developing minimally invasive procedures. These overarching themes emphasize the objective of a multidisciplinary team of obstetricians, surgeons, perinatologists, nurses, anesthesiologists, and sonologists: to promote maternal safety while improving outcomes for patients with fetal anomalies.

Many fetal treatment centers around the world have and are conducting clinical trials for fetal intervention. These centers have formed a cooperative and collaborative global community committed to reporting outcomes from fetal intervention, whether good or poor. These collaborations have already resulted in the successful completion of multicenter RCTs for TTTS and MMC. It is the dedication of these multidisciplinary teams that has helped establish fetal surgery as a medical specialty.

Prenatal screening, genetic testing, and improved imaging capabilities provide families more information earlier in their pregnancy. Potential parents are often not prepared for a poor prenatal diagnosis. Understandably, they react with fear and grief. All involved subspecialties have a very important, defined role. Clinicians have both the privilege and an ethical obligation to deliver services to families by educating parents about all their options, supporting them through the decision-making process, providing appropriate informed consent, and delivering competent and compassionate care. Providing care and support to the family faced with this news is of concern to all nurses who participate in their care. Nurses can be key planners/coordinators in the multidisciplinary team and have great potential to facilitate a healing environment for families facing the unexpected.

ONLINE RESOURCES

Advanced Fetal Care Center (AFCC) Boston Children's Hospital
http://www.childrenshospital.org/clinicalservices/Site2021/mainpageS2021P0.html

Colorado Fetal Care Center at the Colorado Institute for Maternal and Fetal Health
http://www.childrenscolorado.org/conditions/services/surgery/FetalSurgery/colorado-fetal-care-center.aspx

Fetal Care Center of Cincinnati
http://www.cincinnatichildrens.org/service/f/fetal-care/services/surgical/default

Fetal Surgery: The Children's Hospital of Philadelphia
http://www.chop.edu/service/fetal-diagnosis-and-treatment/about-our-services/fetal-surgery.html

Fetal Surgery-Garbose Family Story-Special Delivery Unit-Children's Hospital of Philadelphia
http://www.youtube.com/watch?v=UyVdhoNpFUA

Maternal Fetal Medicine Children's Hospital of Michigan
http://www.childrensdmc.org/?id=678&sid=1

University of California, San Francisco Fetal Treatment Center
http://fetus.ucsfmedicalcenter.org

REFERENCES

Adzick, N. S. (2003). Management of fetal lung lesions. *Clinics in Perinatology*, *30*(3), 481–492.

Adzick, N. S., Crombleholme, T. M., Morgan, M. A., & Quinn, T. M. (1997). A rapidly growing fetal teratoma. *Lancet*, *349*(9051), 538.

Adzick, N. S., Sutton, L. N., Crombleholme, T. M., & Flake, A. W. (1998). Successful fetal surgery for spina bifida. *Lancet*, *352*(9051), 1675–1676.

Adzick, N. S., Thom, E. A., Spong, C. Y., Brock, J. W., III, Burrows, P. K., Johnson, M. P., . . . MOMS Investigators. (2011). A randomized trial of prenatal versus postnatal repair of myelomeningocele. *New England Journal of Medicine*, *364*(11), 993–1004.

Albanese, C. T., Lopoo, J., Goldstein, R. B., Filly, R. A., Feldstein, V. A., Calen, P. W., . . . Harrison, M. R. (1998). Fetal liver position and perinatal outcome for congenital diaphragmatic hernia. *Prenatal Diagnosis*, *18*, 1138–1142.

American College of Obstetricians and Gynecologists, Committee on Ethics & American Academy of Pediatrics, Committee on Bioethics. (2011). Maternal–fetal intervention and fetal care centers. *Pediatrics*, *128*(2), 473–478.

Assaf, R., Llanes, A., & Chmait, R. (2012). In utero release of constriction amniotic bands via blunt dissection. *Fetal and Pediatric Pathology*, *31*(1), 25–29.

Bruner, J. P., Richards, W. O., Tulipan, N. B., & Arney, T. L. (1999). Endoscopic coverage of fetal myelomeningocele in utero. *American Journal of Obstetrics and Gynecology*, *180*, 153–158.

Bruner, J. P., Tulipan, N., Paschall, R. L., Boehm, F. H., Walsh, W. F., Silva, S. R., . . . Reed, G. W. (1999). Fetal surgery for myelomeningocele and the incidence of shunt-dependent hydrocephalus. *Journal of the American Medical Association*, *282*, 1819–1825.

Caniano, D. A. (2004). Ethical issues in the management of neonatal surgical anomalies. *Seminars in Perinatology*, 28, 240–245.

Cavoretto, P., Molina, F., Poggi, S., Davenport, M., & Nicolaides, K. H. (2008). Prenatal diagnosis and outcome of echogenic fetal lung lesions. *Ultrasound in Obstetrics and Gynecology*, *32*(6), 769–783.

Centers for Disease Control and Prevention. (1989). Current trends economic burden of spina bifida—United States, 1980–1990. *Morbidity and Mortality Weekly Report*, *38*(15), 264–267.

Chervenak, F. A., McCullough, L. B., Skupski, D., & Chasen, S. T. (2003). Ethical issues in the management of pregnancies complicated by fetal anomalies. *Obstetrical and Gynecological Survey*, *58*, 473–483.

Collins, J. E. (1994). Fetal surgery: Changing the outcome before birth. *Journal of Obstetric, Gynecologic, and Neonatal Nursing*, *23*, 166–169.

Crombleholme, T. M., Coleman, B., Hedrick, H., Liechty, K., Howell, L., Flake, A. W., . . . Adzick, N. S. (2002). Cystic adenomatoid malformation volume ratio predicts outcome in prenatally diagnosed cystic adenomatoid malformation of the lung. *Journal of Pediatric Surgery*, *37*(3), 331–338.

Crombleholme, T. M., Dirkes, K., Whitney, T. M., Alman, B., Garmel, S., & Connelly, R. J. (1995). Amniotic band syndrome in fetal lambs. I. Fetoscopic release and morphometric outcome. *Journal of Pediatric Surgery*, *30*, 974–978.

Crombleholme, T. M., Sylvester, K., Flake, A. W., & Adzick, N. S. (2000). Salvage of a fetus with congenital high airway obstruction syndrome by ex utero intrapartum treatment (EXIT) procedure. *Fetal Diagnosis and Therapy*, *15*, 280–282.

Curran, P., Jelin, E. B., Rand, L., Hirose, S., Feldstein, V. A., Goldstein, R. B., & Lee, H. (2010). Prenatal steroids for microcystic congenital cystic adenomatoid malformations. *Journal of Pediatric Surgery, 45*(1), 145–150.

DeCou, J. M., Jones, D. C., Jacobs, H. D., & Touloukian, R. J. (1998). Successful ex utero intrapartum treatment (EXIT) procedure for congenital high airway obstruction syndrome (CHAOS) owing to laryngeal atresia. *Journal of Pediatric Surgery*, *33*, 1563–1565.

De Lia, J. E., Kuhlmann, R. S., Harstad, T. W., & Cruikshank, D. P. (1995). Fetoscopic laser ablation of placental vessels in severe previable twin-twin transfusion syndrome. *American Journal of Obstetrics and Gynecology*, *172*, 1202–1208.

Deprest, J., Jani, J., Gratacos, E., Vandecruys, H., Naulaers, G., Delgado, J., . . . FETO Task Group. (2005). Fetal intervention for congenital diaphragmatic hernia: The European experience. *Seminars in Perinatology*, *29*(2), 94–103.

Evans, M. I., Harrison, M. R., Flake, A. W., & Johnson, M. P. (2002). Fetal therapy. *Best Practice and Research Clinical Obstetrics and Gynaecology*, *16*, 671–683.

Farrell, J. A., Albanese, C. T., Jennings, R. W., Kilpatrick, S. J., Bratton, B. J., & Harrison, M. R. (1999). Maternal fertility is not affected by fetal surgery. *Fetal Diagnosis and Therapy*, *14*, 190–192.

Feldstein, V. A., Machin, G. A., Albanese, C. T., Sandberg, P., Farrell, J. A., Farmer, D. L., & Harrison, M. R. (2000). Twin-twin transfusion syndrome: The "SELECT" procedure. *Fetal Diagnosis and Therapy*, *15*(5), 257–261.

Fetal Care Center of Cincinnati. (2005). Congenital High Airway Obstruction Syndrome/CHAOS. Retrieved from http://www.cincinnatichildrens.org/service/f/fetal-care/conditions/chaos/default

Graf, J. L., Albanese, C. T., Jennings, R. W., Farrell, J. A., & Harrison, M. R. (2000). Successful fetal sacrococcygeal teratoma resection in a hydropic fetus. *Journal of Pediatric Surgery*, *35*, 1489–1491.

Graf, J. L., Housely, H. T., Albanese, C. T., Adzick, N. S., & Harrison, M. R. (1998). A surprising histological evolution of preterm sacrococcygeal teratoma. *Journal of Pediatric Surgery*, *33*, 177–179.

Grethel, E. J., Wagner, A. J., Clifton, M. S., Cortes, R. A., Farmer, D. L., Harrison, M. R., . . . Lee, H. (2007). Fetal intervention for mass lesions and hydrops improves outcome: A 15-year experience. *Journal of Pediatric Surgery*, *42*, 117–123.

Harrison, M. R. (1996). Fetal surgery. *American Journal of Obstetrics and Gynecology*, *174*, 1255–1264.

Harrison, M. R. (2003). Fetal surgery: Trials, tribulations, and turf. *Journal of Pediatric Surgery*, *38*, 275–282.

Harrison, M, R., Adzick, N. S., Bullard, K. M., Farrell, J. A., Howell, L. J., Rosen, M. A., . . . Filly, R. A. (1997). Correction of congenital diaphragmatic hernia in utero. VII. A prospective trial. *Journal of Pediatric Surgery*, *32*, 1637–1642.

Harrison, M. R., Adzick, N. S., Flake, A. W., VanderWall, K. J., Bealer, J. F., Howell, L. J., . . . Goldberg, J. D. (1996). Correction of congenital diaphragmatic hernia in utero. VIII. Response of the hyperplastic lung to tracheal occlusion. *Journal of Pediatric Surgery*, *31*, 1339–1348.

Harrison, M. R., Evans, M., Adzick, N. S., & Holzgreve, W. (Eds.). (2001). *The unborn patient: The art and science of fetal therapy* (3rd ed.). Philadelphia, PA: Saunders.

Harrison, M. R., Mychaliska, G. B., Albanese, C. T., Jennings, R. W., Farrell, J. A., Hawgood, S., . . . Filly, R. A. (1998). Correction of congenital diaphragmatic hernia in utero. IX. Fetuses with poor prognosis (liver herniation and low LHR) can be saved by fetoscopic temporary tracheal occlusion. *Journal of Pediatric Surgery*, *33*, 1017–1022.

Hecher, K. (1999). Endoscopic laser surgery versus serial amniocentesis in the treatment of severe twin-twin transfusion syndrome. *American Journal of Obstetrics and Gynecology*, *180*, 717–724.

Hedrick, M. H., Ferro, M. M., Filly, R. A., Flake, A. W., Harrison, M. R., & Adzick, N. S. (1994). Congenital high airway obstruction syndrome (CHAOS): A potential for perinatal intervention. *Journal of Pediatric Surgery*, *29*, 271–274.

Holmes, N., Harrison, M. R., & Baskin, L. S. (2001). Fetal surgery for posterior urethral valves: Long-term postnatal outcomes. *Pediatrics*, *108*, 1–7.

Howell, L. J., & Dunphy, P. M. (1999). Fetal surgery: Exploring the challenges in nursing care. *Journal of Obstetric, Gynecologic, and Neonatal Nursing*, *28*, 427–432.

Hutchins, G. M. (1996). Acquired spinal cord injury in human fetuses with myelomeningocele. *Pediatric Pathology and Laboratory Medicine*, *16*, 701–702.

Jelin, E., & Lee, H. (2009). Tracheal occlusion for fetal congenital diaphragmatic hernia: The U.S. experience. *Clinics in Perinatology*, *36*, 349–361.

Johnson, M. P. (2001). Fetal obstructive uropathy. In M. R. Harrison, M. I. Evans, N. S. Adzick, & W. Holzgreve, (Eds.), *The unborn patient: The art and science of fetal therapy* (3rd ed., pp. 259–285). Philadelphia, PA: Saunders.

Kiatano, Y. (1999). Open fetal surgery for life-threatening fetal malformations. *Seminars in Perinatology*, *23*, 448–461.

Kurpinski, K., & Patel, S. (2011). Dura mater regeneration with a novel synthetic, bilayered nanofibrous dural substitute: An experimental study. *Nanomedicine*, *6*(2), 325–337.

Laifer, S. A., & Kuller, J. A. (1996). Percutaneous umbilical blood sampling. In J. A. Kuller, N. Chescheir, & R. C. Cefalo (Eds.), *Prenatal diagnosis and reproductive genetics*. St Louis, MO: Mosby.

Liley, A. W. (1963). Intrauterine transfusion of foetus in haemolytic disease. *British Medical Journal*, *5365*, 1107–1109.

Lipshutz, G. S., Albanese, C. T., Feldstein, V. A., Jennings, R. W., Housley, H. T., Beech, R., . . . Harrison, M. R. (1997). Prospective analysis of lung to head ratio predicts survival for patients with prenatally diagnosed congenital diaphragmatic hernia. *Journal of Pediatric Surgery*, *32*, 1634–1636.

Longaker, M. T., Golbus, M. S., Filly, R. A., Rosen, M. A., Chang, S. W., & Harrison, M. R. (1991). Maternal outcome after open fetal surgery. A review of the first 17 human cases. *Journal of the American Medical Association*, *265*, 737–741.

Lyerly, A. D., Gates, E. A., Cefalo, R. C., & Sugarman, J. (2001). Toward the ethical evaluation and use of maternal–fetal surgery. *The American College of Obstetricians and Gynecologists*, *98*, 689–697.

Manning, F. A. (1986). International Fetal Surgery Registry: 1985 update. *Clinical Obstetrics and Gynecology*, *29*, 551–557.

Meuli, M., Meuli-Simmen, C., Hutchins, G. M., Yingling, C. D., Hoffman, K. M., Harrison, M. R., & Adzick, N. S. (1995a). In utero surgery rescues neurologic function at birth in sheep with spina bifida. *Journal of Pediatric Surgery*, *30*, 342–347.

Meuli, M., Meuli-Simmen, C., Yingling, C. D., Hutchins, G. M., Hoffman, K. M., Harrison, M. R., & Adzick, N. S. (1995b). Creation of myelomeningocele in utero: A model of functional damage from spinal cord exposure in fetal sheep. *Journal of Pediatric Surgery*, *30*, 1028–1032.

Morris, L. M., Lim, F. Y., Livingston, J. C., Polzin, W. J., & Crombleholme, T. M. (2009). High-risk fetal congenital pulmonary airway malformations have a variable response to steroids. *Journal of Pediatric Surgery*, *44*, 60–65.

Mychaliska, G. B., Bealer, J. F., Graf, J. L., Rosen, M. A., Adzick, N. S., & Harrison, M. R. (1997). Operating on placental support: The ex utero intrapartum treatment (EXIT) procedure. *Journal of Pediatric Surgery*, *32*, 227–231.

Nijagal, A., Wegorzewska, M., Jarvis, E., Le, T., Tang, Q., & MacKenzie, T. C. (2011). Maternal T cells limit engraftment after in utero hematopoietic cell transplantation in mice. *Journal of Clinical Investigation*, *121*(2), 582–592.

Paek, B. W., Callen, P. W., Kitterman, J., Feldstein, V. A., Farrell, J., Harrison, M. R., & Albanese, C. T. (2001). CHAOS controlled: Successful fetal intervention for complete high airway obstruction syndrome. *Fetal Diagnosis and Therapy*, *17*(5), 272–276.

Paek, B. W., Farmer, D. L., Wilkinson, C. C., Albanese, C. T., Peacock, W., Harrison, M. R., & Jennings, R. W. (2000). Hindbrain herniation develops in surgically created myelomeningocele but is absent after repair in fetal lambs. *American Journal of Obstetrics and Gynecology*, *183*, 1119–1123.

Peranteau, W. H., Wilson, R. D., Liechty, K. W., Johnson, M. P., Bebbington, M. W., Hedrick, H. L., . . . Adzick, N. S. (2007). Effect of maternal betamethasone administration on prenatal congenital cystic adenomatoid malformation growth and fetal survival. *Fetal Diagnosis and Therapy, 22*, 365–371.

Quintero, R. A., Dickinson, J. E., Morales, W. J., Bornick, P. W., Bermúdez, C., Cincotta, R., . . . Allen, M. H. (2003). Stage-based treatment of twin-twin transfusion syndrome. *American Journal of Obstetrics and Gynecology*, *188*(5), 1333–1340.

Quintero, R. A., Johnson, M. P., Romero, R., Smith, C., Arias, F., Guevara-Zuloaga, F., . . . Evans, M. I. (1995). In utero percutaneous cystoscopy in the management of fetal lower obstructive uropathy. *Lancet*, *346*, 537–540.

Quintero, R. A., Morales, W. J., Allen, M. H., Bornick, P. W., Johnson, P. K., & Kruger, M. (1999). Staging of twin-twin transfusion syndrome. *Journal of Perinatology*, *19*(8 Pt 1), 550–555.

Quintero, R. A., Morales, W. J., Phillips, J., Kalter, C. S., & Angel, J. L. (1997). In utero lysis of amniotic bands. *Ultrasound in Obstetrics and Gynecology*, *10*, 316–320.

Rice, H. E., Estes, J. M., Hedrick, M. H., Bealer, J. F., Harrison, M. R., & Adzick, N. S. (1994). Congenital cystic adenomatoid malformation: A sheep model of fetal hydrops. *Journal of Pediatric Surgery*, *29*, 692–696.

Sago, H., Hayashi, S., Tanaka, H., Miyazaki, O., Nosaka, S., Matsuoka, K., . . . Honna, T. (2011). P22.01: Radiofrequency ablation of fetal sacrococcygeal teratoma. *Ultrasound in Obstetrics and Gynecology*, *38*, 241.

Senat, M. V., Deprest, J., Boulvain, M., Paupe, A., Winer, N., & Ville, Y. (2004). Endoscopic laser surgery versus serial amnioreduction for severe twin-twin perfusion syndrome. *New England Journal of Medicine*, *351*, 136–144.

Shimabukuro, F., Sakumoto, K., Masamoto, H., Asato, Y., Yoshida, T., Shinhama, A., . . . Aoki, Y. (2007). A case of congenital high airway obstruction syndrome managed by ex utero intrapartum treatment: Case report and review of the literature. *American Journal of Perinatology*, *24*(3), 197–201.

Southard, A. E., Edelmann, L. J., & Gelb, B. D. (2012). Role of copy number variants in structural birth defects. *Pediatrics*, *129*(4), 755–763.

Spitzer, A. R. (1996). *Intensive care of the fetus and neonate*. St Louis, MO: Mosby.

Strauss, A., Hasbargen, U., Paek, B., Bauerfeind, I., & Hepp, H. (2000). Intrauterine fetal demise caused by amniotic band syndrome after standard amniocentesis. *Fetal Diagnosis and Therapy*, *15*, 4–7.

Sutton, L. N., Adzick, N. S., Bilaniuk, L. T., Johnson, M. P., Crombleholme, T. M., & Flake, A. W. (1999). Improvement in hindbrain herniation demonstrated by serial fetal magnetic resonance imaging following fetal surgery for myelomeningocele. *Journal of the American Medical Association*, *282*, 1826–1831.

Sydorak, R. M., Nijagal, A., & Albanese, C. T. (1991). Endoscopic techniques in fetal surgery. *Yonsei Medical Journal*, *42*(6), 695–710.

Taeusch, H. W., & Ballard, R. A. (Eds.). (1998). *Avery's diseases of the newborn* (7th ed.). Philadelphia, PA: Saunders.

Tsao, K., Hawgood, S., Vu, L., Hirose, S., Sydorak, R., Albanese, C. T., . . . Lee, H. (2003). Resolution of hydrops fetalis in congenital cystic adenomatoid malformation after prenatal steroid therapy. *Journal of Pediatric Surgery*, *38*, 508–510.

Tulipan, N., Hernanz-Schulman, M., & Bruner, J. P. (1998). Reduced hindbrain herniation after intrauterine myelomeningocele repair: A report of four cases. *Pediatric Neurosurgery*, *29*, 274–278.

Tworetzky, W., Wilkins-Haug, L., Jennings, R. W., van der Velde, M. E., Marshall, A. C., Marx, G. R., . . . Perry, S. B. (2004). Balloon dilation of severe aortic stenosis in the fetus: Potential for prevention of hypoplastic left heart syndrome: Candidate selection, technique, and results of successful intervention. *Circulation*, *110*, 2125–2131.

Westerburg, B. W., Chiba, T., Gantert, W., Albanese, C. T., Harrison, M. R., & Jennings, R. W. (1998). Radio frequency ablation of the liver in the fetal sheep: A model for treatment of sacrococcygeal teratoma in the fetus. *Surgery Forum*, *49*, 461–463.

Westerburg, B., Feldstein, V. A., Sandberg, P. L., Lopoo, J. B., Harrison, M. R., & Albanese, C. T. (2000). Sonographic prognostic factors in fetuses with sacrococcygeal teratoma. *Journal of Pediatric Surgery*, *35*, 322–326.

Wilson, R. D., Johnson, M. P., Flake, A. W., Crombleholme, T. M., Hedrick, H. L., Wilson, J., & Adzick, N. S. (2004). Reproductive outcomes after pregnancy complicated by maternal–fetal surgery. *American Journal of Obstetrics and Gynecology*, *191*, 1430–1436.

Yamamoto, M., & Ville, Y. (2006). Recent finding on laser treatment of twin-to-twin transfusion syndrome. *Current Opinion in Obstetrics and Gynecology*, *18*, 87–92.

Zhu, Y., Wang, A., Patel, S., Kurpinski, K., Diao, E., Bao, X., . . . Li, S. (2011). Engineering bi-layer nanofibrous conduits for peripheral nerve regeneration. *Tissue Engineering Part C Methods*, *17*(7), 705–715.

Surgical Considerations in the Newborn and Infant

CHAPTER 25

■ Kaye Spence

Caring for an infant with a surgical condition is an exciting challenge that requires knowledge of pathophysiology and current neonatal care practices, training to recognize and respond to complications, and an ability to extend supportive care to the family. Optimum outcome is achieved through the skills of a multidisciplinary team that includes neonatal nurses, neonatologists, pediatric surgeons, radiologists, anesthesiologists, respiratory therapists, and parents. The members of this team must work together, guided by the knowledge that all of principles of neonatal care, as well as additional considerations related to surgical care, apply in each case. This chapter outlines the special considerations of the newborn and infant who undergo surgical procedures in the neonatal intensive care unit (NICU).

ANTENATAL CONSIDERATIONS

Neonatal surgery has been inextricably linked to the field of obstetrics with neonatologists and surgeons, along with fetal medicine specialists and obstetricians working together to characterize the development and well-being of fetuses with congenital malformations (Cass, 2011). Many congenital surgical defects are diagnosed in utero through routine prenatal screening, providing time for education and emotional support for the family. Women are transferred to a high-risk birth unit with skilled fetal–maternal specialists with access to a neonatal surgeon. If possible, a tour of the NICU should be arranged before delivery. It is recommended that the parents meet with members of the surgical and neonatal teams to discuss the findings and probable prognosis for their infant. Information given to the family should include the natural history of the abnormality, timing of surgery, anticipated surgical outcomes, possible long-term sequelae, and any other possible problems that may be involved with the neonate's course (Lakhoo, 2012). There have been many changes over the past decades in the care and management of newborn infants requiring surgery. Important areas of advancement have been in newborn intensive care and postoperative care. Another area of advancement has been in antenatal diagnosis and the early referral to NICUs for information and education regarding the expected course of treatment and the outcomes of surgical care for newborn infants. For more information on fetal surgery please see Chapter 24.

TRANSPORTATION OF INFANTS FOR SURGERY

Babies requiring surgery should be born in an appropriate tertiary perinatal center, adjacent to pediatric surgical facilities, in accordance with best practice. Pregnancies complicated by birth defects have variable rates of antenatal diagnosis and may require surgical repair in the newborn period. The success of antenatal transfer was found to be generally consistent with the sensitivity of antenatal diagnosis (Algert et al., 2008) and with regionalization; health care of women outside specific urban areas was not disadvantaged. For some specific conditions, such as congenital heart disease, transferring the mother for delivery to a high-risk center is preferred (Calisti et al., 2012) so that an expedited transfer from the birth unit to the NICU can occur in a matter of minutes. Advantages of antenatal referral of babies with congenital anomalies requiring surgery include:

1. Improved neonatal outcomes
2. The opportunity for parents to discuss the following issues with experienced staff:
    - Options for birth
    - Anticipated care of the baby
    - Likely neonatal outcomes
3. The reassurance of access to the best available obstetric and neonatal care
4. Women may also experience a reduction in stress and anxiety as an emergency transfer of the baby resulting in separation of mother and baby is avoided

Eighty percent of neonates with an antenatal diagnosis of a congenital anomaly require admission to a NICU and major surgery (NSW Department of Health, 2005). Emergency transport services retrieve neonates to tertiary referral centers for intensive care, diagnostic workup, or surgery. If birth occurs at an appropriate tertiary perinatal center, the potential for an emergency neonatal retrieval to a pediatric facility is avoided.

It is desirable for each maternity unit to have a policy on antenatal referral of mothers with babies known to have a congenital abnormality, likely one that would require surgery. The policy should emphasize antenatal consultation with the appropriate fetal, surgical, and other consultants (e.g., genetics, cardiac) in the preferred facility. It should note that the decision to make an antenatal maternal referral should take into account patient and clinician preferences. The policy should include options and processes for antenatal referral for more detailed fetal assessment and a plan for the optimal place of delivery. This referral will usually occur mid-pregnancy. If surgery or other critical therapy is likely to be required soon after birth, this plan should include delivery at a perinatal center with direct access to appropriate pediatric surgical services.

SURGICAL NEONATAL INTENSIVE CARE UNITS

Criteria for neonatal surgical units have been established in several countries to ensure that acceptable standards are met for infants who require surgery during the neonatal period. There are identified requirements for surgical services that provide operations and general anesthesia for newborn infants. These requirements relate to adequate training for the consultant surgeon and anesthetist with sufficient case loads to maintain skills (Royal College of Surgeons, 2007). In addition, adequately trained and experienced staff to care for the infant postoperatively need to be available in dedicated newborn surgical units.

There are arguments for and against large regional specialist pediatric centers being established for neonatal surgery. Benefits of regionalization include pooling of expertise, appropriate consultants, support services, and staff training. Disadvantages include children and their families having to travel long distances for care and the loss of expertise at a local level. However, the availability of a neonatal emergency transport service can provide expertise and support for transferring neonates to regional neonatal surgical intensive care centers (Ratnaval, 2009).

There are trends in some countries to ensure that surgical neonatal intensive care units (SNICUs) are located in children's hospitals with a co-located perinatal center (NSW Department of Health, 2005). This practice enables the women to deliver with a high-risk obstetric team as well as having a specialist pediatric/neonatal surgical team present to attend to the infant's well-being.

Staffing

The majority of the nursing staff in SNICUs require skills and competence in neonatal intensive care as well the specific management of neonatal surgical patients. Recommendations for staffing ratios vary; however, most infants will require dedicated nursing staff in the immediate postoperative period. During this period many infants will be unstable, and vigilant observation and assessment are required to avert postoperative complications. In addition, the families require additional support and explanation of many of the unique procedures seen in infants who have undergone surgery. A dedicated in-service program that includes a multidimensional approach to various conditions, altered pathophysiology, care paths, techniques, and procedures as well as counseling skills is recommended (Standards for PIC, 2010) A wide range of subspecialists, including cardiologists, gastroenterologists, endocrinologists, geneticists, infectious disease specialists, respiratory specialists, and anesthetists, are involved in the SNICU; this requires a coordinated effort of team meetings and communication. Nurses are in key positions to coordinate the information and develop care plans to ensure continuity when multiple specialist teams are involved. The combined skills of the pediatric surgeon, pediatric anesthetist, neonatologist, and neonatal nurse together with the resources available in a regional pediatric center will continue to contribute to the improvements in survival and quality of life of infants requiring neonatal surgery. However, there does need to be continuing debate on the surgical advances for infants with congenital malformations. Issues such as long-term outcomes and future quality of life need to be considered by the team together with the families. Other issues such as resources and cost effectiveness of the treatments need to be part of the community debate for future health care programs and according to present evidence, neonatal surgery yields good value for money and contributes to equity in health (Poley et al., 2008).

Family

Families will seek out information about their infant's prenatally diagnosed condition (Usui, Kamiyama, Tani, Kanagawa, & Fukuzawa, 2011) and require open and honest communication from the health care team regarding prognosis, treatment options, and outcomes. Decisions on the management and treatment of the infant require a team approach that includes parents, nurses, obstetricians, pediatric surgeons, neonatologists, nurse practitioners, and radiologists. Supportive services should be provided to the family as indicated to reduce some of the stressors of having their newborn infant undergo surgery (Diffin, Spence, Johnston, & Badawi, 2012).

Parents want comprehensive information, especially during the waiting periods. Parental coping may be greatly enhanced by timely updates from the operating room while the parents are waiting for their infant in surgery. It is also important for the surgeon to speak with the parents immediately after surgery to discuss findings and the infant's condition. Once the infant is back from the operating room, the parents should be encouraged to visit in a timely manner to reduce anticipatory stress. The nurse should discuss the infant's current condition, the equipment used, and anticipatory care in the short term.

In the postoperative period, parents need to be able to negotiate their parental role with the staff members caring for their infant and should be supported in their attempts to advocate for their infant. Parents should also be encouraged to participate in their child's care to the extent that it is comfortable for them. This participation means that parents must be provided with adequate information and guidance regarding their role to enable them to cope and use informal support structures to help allay their anxiety (McFadyen et al., 2012).

CLASSIFICATION OF NEONATAL SURGERY

Neonatal surgery is defined as surgery performed on infants who

- are less than 28 days old
- weigh less than 2,500 g regardless of age
- require care in a NICU regardless of age or weight

Approximately 0.6% of newborn infants undergo surgery in the first 4 weeks of life (Badawi et al., 2003). Some of the most common types of surgical procedures performed are gastrointestinal, cardiovascular, hernia, genitourinary, and neurosurgical.

Neonatal surgery can be classified into three groups for ease of management. Group 1 includes those infants with a life-threatening condition for whom a surgical operation is necessary within the first day of life, such as congenital diaphragmatic hernia, gastroschisis, or esophageal atresia with fistula and critical congenital cardiac malformations. In group 2 are those infants with an obvious abnormality but for whom a surgical operation may be deferred for days or months, such as exomphalos minor or cleft lip. Group 3 includes infants who have an obvious abnormality whose management may consist of interventions after due consideration, such as myelomeningocele.

PREANESTHETIC EVALUATION

Anesthetizing a preterm or critically ill neonate requires constant vigilance, rapid recognition of events and trends, and swift intervention. The anesthetic considerations in the preterm neonate are based on the physiological immaturity of the various body systems, the associated congenital disorders, and possible poor tolerance of anesthetic drugs and considerations regarding use of high concentrations of oxygen. The preoperative assessment should include consultation with the parents including the description of a likely deterioration in pulmonary function necessitating postoperative respiratory support. A complete examination should be undertaken, with special attention to the appearance of the upper airway and the possibility of difficult intubation (Taneja, Srivastava, & Saxena, 2012). Preterm and ex-premature infants can have dramatic responses with wide variability to narcotics and inhaled anesthetics.

Preoperative investigations include hemoglobin, hematocrit, and platelets, and the coagulation profile should be within acceptable limits. Serum electrolyte, glucose levels, arterial blood gas, and chest x-ray will aid in the intraoperative management and stabilization (Taneja et al., 2012). A blood cross-match must be available so that a transfusion can be given if the blood loss exceeds 10% of blood volume during the surgery.

PREPARATION FOR SURGERY

From the time of delivery, the goal is to reduce the likelihood of morbidity and mortality by continually assessing the infant and the responses to treatments instituted. Preparation for surgery starts with discussions with the family and gaining informed consent. The consent process is the responsibility of the surgical team; however, it is good practice for the nurse to be present when these discussions take place. If the parents are from a non-English-speaking background, then an interpreter needs to be present. Often nurses are asked to clarify issues that were discussed, and nurses are in a unique position to communicate misunderstandings back to the surgical team.

Many of the neonatal surgical procedures are performed on emergency operative lists; therefore the preparation needs to be coordinated and the many teams involved aware of the infant's condition prior to surgery. The anesthetist holds a key role in this coordination with multiple subspecialists, and the nurse is pivotal in ensuring the documentation is complete and the family informed and available. Each institution needs to have a clear and comprehensive system of evaluating infants during the preoperative period (Ferrari, 2004) to ensure effective use of operating time and to avoid undue delays and stress on the infant and family. An understanding of neonatal physiology is necessary to enable the team to provide appropriate care in three areas of homeostasis—temperature regulation, fluid and electrolyte balance, and acid–base balance (Taneja et al., 2012). In addition, specific practices for preparation for transfer to the operating room are described in this chapter. Each area is discussed in relation to the preparation of the infant for surgery.

Temperature Control

Heat loss can occur during transfer to the imaging department and the operating room due to the infant's high ratio of surface area to body weight. It remains important to maintain the core body temperature close to 37°C to minimize oxygen consumption. In the operating room, a low ambient temperature increases heat loss by both convection and radiation. It is ideal that the operating room be warmed to 28°C to 30°C for neonatal patients. The infant may be transferred on an open-care bed with a radiant warmer; some surgeons will operate on these beds to minimize the stress of heat loss. The infant undergoing surgical procedures where the organs are exposed is at particular risk of heat loss.

Prevention of hypothermia in the surgical neonate is imperative in the preoperative period. Maintaining a neutral thermal environment is a constant challenge. In a neutral thermal environment, metabolic activity is minimal because body temperature is kept stable. Oxygen consumption is reduced, and acidosis is prevented. Any prolonged deviations from the neutral thermal environment further stress the infant's already limited thermoregulatory abilities. Strategies such as wrapping the infant's head and limbs in cotton webbing can be useful in reducing some of the inevitable heat loss.

Heat loss occurs through evaporation, conduction, convection, and radiation. Evaporative heat loss occurs with exposure of the intestinal contents of a ruptured omphalocele or gastroschisis. In the case of an encephalocele or a myelomeningocele, the unprotected spinal cord may allow heat loss. The exposed bladder mucosa in exstrophy of the bladder also contributes to heat loss. This type of heat loss can be prevented by applying warm dressings to the defects and then covering these areas with plastic wrap.

Conductive heat loss occurs with direct skin contact with a cold surface, such as cold or wet linens, an operating table, radiographic plates, or an unwarmed bed. To prevent this type of heat loss, linens should be prewarmed as the bed or incubator is warmed. Operating or radiography tables can be warmed with heat lamps before and during procedures. Linens that become wet should be replaced with dry, warmed linens; radiographic plates and scales should be covered with warmed linens before the infant is placed on them.

Heat loss by convection occurs when air blows over the infant. Use of warmed oxygen in head hoods (boxes) and ventilators can reduce this type of heat loss. Also, it is essential that the incubator door not be open for prolonged periods. Insertion of nasogastric tubes, placement of intravenous lines, radiographic studies, physical examinations, and phlebotomy procedures should be performed through the incubator portholes to reduce heat loss. An additional heat source may be placed over the incubator when the door must be open.

Heat loss by radiation is the most difficult to control. This type of heat loss occurs during transportation of the neonate in cold hallways or in the cold operating room. To prevent this cold stress, the infant should be covered with warmed linens or wrapped during transport. Operating rooms should be prewarmed to well above the "comfortable" temperature. Nursing care that focuses on the thermoregulatory process of the neonate is vital to the prevention of complications related to poor temperature control. It is also beneficial to use warmed solutions for suctioning and dressing changes. Frequent monitoring of the infant's temperature is extremely important. Consistency in the method of measuring temperature and appropriate documentation are also essential.

Fluid and Electrolyte Balance

Adequate fluid volume is required to ensure the perfusion of all organ systems. An inadequate vascular volume interferes with the oxygen supply to peripheral tissues, resulting in cellular damage and acidosis. Precision in fluid management is essential; there is little margin for error. Particular care needs to be taken to ensure excessive volumes are not delivered with additional drugs used during the anesthesia. All fluid losses must be measured accurately to ensure adequate replacement. Estimation of insensible fluid losses is essential, including those caused by humidification through ventilation and radiant heating. Unexpected fluid losses and inadequate fluid replacement delay preoperative stabilization of the neonate's condition.

Infants with an esophageal atresia may have continuous losses of saliva suctioned from the esophageal pouch that needs to be considered in the fluid balance. The large exposed intestinal area seen with a ruptured omphalocele or gastroschisis results in large volumes of fluid losses. Replacement of these losses may involve up to twice the normal maintenance fluids of a neonate. If a membranous sac protects an omphalocele, the fluid requirement is less.

Gastrointestinal obstructions cause fluid losses from vomiting, aspiration, and the suctioning required for gastric decompression. Infants with open neural tube defects also have increased fluid losses. A leaking myelomeningocele requires increased fluid administration to keep up with the loss of cerebrospinal fluid.

Peritonitis, such as occurs with intestinal perforations in necrotizing enterocolitis, midgut volvulus, or ruptured meconium ileus, causes third-spacing of fluid (capillary leak syndrome) or fluid shifts into the bowel, necessitating increased fluid replacement. Third-spacing of fluids, or capillary leak syndrome, is the result of trauma to the gastrointestinal system. The capillary membrane's permeability is changed. This phenomenon may be due to natural fibronectin, a glycoprotein secreted by epithelial cells in the pulmonary and gastrointestinal trees. It is secreted in response to stimulation of the immune system to heal a wound. Fibronectin alters capillary permeability, shifting fluid and resulting in a "leaky capillary" and the third-spacing of fluid. The body's compensatory response to any gastrointestinal trauma, then, can result in a movement of fluid across this "leaky" membrane. Fluid moves out of the vascular compartment and into the tissues, and the infant develops generalized edema. Abdominal swelling exerts pressure on the thoracic cavity, increasing the work of breathing. Gas exchange and ventilation are compromised as a result of (1) the pressure; (2) the decreased circulation; (3) the increased workload of the heart, which delivers oxygen to the tissues; and (4) the increasing loss of the buffer system through the mechanisms of diminished kidney perfusion and gastric losses.

The numerous conditions that affect the surgical neonate may result in imbalances of serum electrolytes, especially sodium and potassium. Fluid losses and inadequate intake result in hypokalemia and hyponatremia.

Hyperkalemia occurs with acidosis, excessive potassium intake, and renal failure. Renal failure may result from genitourinary obstructions or from sepsis and poor perfusion, as is seen with necrotizing enterocolitis with perforation or peritonitis.

The causes of hypernatremia are generally iatrogenic. An excessive intake of sodium occurs with the administration of hypertonic solutions, intravenous flushes with normal saline or heparinized normal saline, or sodium bicarbonate for treatment of acidosis. Return to a fluid and electrolyte balance is needed to improve the neonate's ability to tolerate any necessary operative procedure and to reduce the likelihood of complications.

Maintenance of Glucose Levels

Fluctuation in the glucose level is a major indication of stress and infection. Preoperative hyperglycemia can result from sepsis or excessive intravenous administration of glucose. Hypoglycemia may result from a multitude of problems. For example, reduced glycogen stores are seen in premature infants and in infants with intrauterine growth restriction. Excessive insulin production occurs in the infant of a diabetic mother and with sudden or prolonged cessation of glucose infusions, as may occur with difficult or delayed insertion of intravenous lines. Abnormalities in glucose metabolism are evident with sepsis, shock, and asphyxia, as well as with various central nervous system (CNS) abnormalities. Glucose infusions must be carefully titrated to provide adequate hydration while the serum glucose is slowly restored to an acceptable concentration, avoiding extremes in the serum glucose level.

Acid–Base Balance

A variety of factors can alter the acid–base balance in the surgical neonate. Major conditions that can result in acidosis include inadequate respiratory support and fluid or electrolyte imbalances. The effects of sepsis and tissue necrosis are also significant causes of acidosis. Acidosis in the surgical neonate can be the respiratory, metabolic, or mixed type.

Respiratory acidosis could occur with decreased ventilation, resulting in an increased partial pressure of carbon dioxide (PCO_2) and a decreased pH. An overproduction of acids may occur with any condition that causes a decrease in oxygenation or perfusion. Impaired kidney function, such as that which occurs in acute renal failure or renal tubular necrosis, reduces elimination of hydrogen ions, contributing to the development of metabolic acidosis. Bicarbonate losses are increased with severe diarrhea, intestinal fistulas, vomiting, and gastric drainage, resulting in metabolic acidosis.

Poor tissue perfusion causes acidosis, as is seen with multiple gastrointestinal anomalies that are accompanied by large fluid losses. These anomalies include tracheoesophageal fistula with esophageal atresia, ruptured omphalocele and gastroschisis, bowel obstruction, and necrotizing enterocolitis. Adequately replenishing fluid or blood volume usually corrects this metabolic acidosis. When necrosis or perforation occurs, however, the acidosis may not be correctable until the necrotic bowel has been removed and any resulting sepsis treated.

Drugs

The role of prophylactic antibiotics for neonatal surgery remains controversial. However, with suspected gastrointestinal obstruction, antibiotics may be needed to treat peritonitis or enterocolitis. The progression of necrotizing enterocolitis may be slowed with vigorous antibiotic therapy. Treatment of omphalocele and gastroschisis may include antibiotics to protect the exposed gastrointestinal contents and to help prevent ischemic injury to the abdominal contents. If pneumonia accompanies an esophageal atresia with tracheoesophageal fistula, aggressive antibiotic therapy should be instituted to clear the pneumonia and promote optimum surgical repair of the defect. The infant with a myelomeningocele requires antibiotic treatment to prevent meningitis.

Inotropic agents may be necessary to improve cardiac function and thus improve organ perfusion impaired by sepsis and stress. The most frequently used agents are dobutamine and dopamine. Dobutamine hydrochloride achieves organ perfusion by increasing cardiac output. Dopamine hydrochloride, used in low to moderate doses, causes vasodilation with resultant improvement in cardiac, renal, gastrointestinal, and cerebral blood flow. Use of dopamine hydrochloride at high doses, however, causes vasoconstriction of renal and gastrointestinal vessels. This vasoconstriction could worsen the condition of a renal system affected by obstruction or poor flow status, as well as the gastrointestinal system already compromised by necrotizing enterocolitis, omphalocele, gastroschisis, or obstruction. Doses of dobutamine hydrochloride and dopamine hydrochloride, therefore, must be carefully calculated and continually titrated to achieve the desired effect. Furthermore, these medications are incompatible with many other drugs. For example, alkaline solutions (e.g., sodium bicarbonate, ampicillin, gentamicin, and furosemide) can inactivate dobutamine and dopamine. These inotropic agents are also irritating to vessels, and close monitoring of intravenous sites for infiltration is essential.

A buffering agent may be required to treat the acidosis that may accompany a diaphragmatic hernia, necrotizing enterocolitis, omphalocele, gastroschisis, or obstruction with resulting ischemic injury. Adequate ventilation and tissue perfusion must be established and maintained before medication is used to treat acidotic conditions.

Monitoring

Infants will require preoperative monitoring that continues during the operation into the postoperative period. At a minimum, cardiorespiratory monitoring is essential. The electrodes and leads should be placed with consideration of the operative area; this will enable the monitoring leads to be used during the surgery without the necessity of tissue damage from removal and re-siting. A pulse oximeter on an upper limb will enable the oxygen saturation levels to be monitored. The nurse needs to be mindful that some monitoring, such as transcutaneous oxygen, may be ineffective because of changes in skin perfusion during the procedure. The placement of a temperature probe can assist the anesthetist in monitoring the temperature during surgery. Amplitude electroencephalogram (aEEG) monitoring is recommended for neonates prior to surgery to aid in the postoperative course and as a way of determining cerebral insults that are possible during the anesthesia and surgery (Clancy, 2008).

Intravascular Lines

Ideally, a central venous catheter (CVC) will be required postoperatively for multiple drug infusions and parental nutrition (PN). It may be opportune for the CVC to be inserted during the operative procedure; this may be negotiated with the surgeon and anesthetist.

In addition, a peripheral arterial cannula will be required for the continuing measurement of the acid–base balance during the operation and in the postoperative period. It is best if this is inserted before the infant is transferred to the operating room. Precautions should be taken to ensure that all connections are Luer-Lok to avoid accidental disconnection when covered with surgical drapes. Caution needs to be taken if multiple drug infusions are required; incompatibilities and priority for access can be a challenge for complex conditions.

Nurse's Role

Adequate and thorough preparation of the infant can minimize stress during the process and help reduce the preparation and time of the surgery. Being prepared and anticipating the time and call for surgery can ensure that the infant is adequately prepared for transfer and surgery. If the nurse accompanies the infant to the operating room, continued monitoring and a smooth handover should occur. In some institutions, the neonatal nurse can remain in the operating room assisting the infant and helping with the monitoring of the oxygenation and temperature. This is, however, a contentious issue for some institutions and operating room staff.

The prospective site of the surgery needs to be prepared through the use of an antiseptic wash prior to the transfer for surgery. In the case of a stoma formation, the stoma therapist will indicate on the infant's abdomen the preferred location for the stoma. This type of preparation can make the postoperative care easier and avoid undue stress for the infant from a leaking stoma bag due to poor location. The surgeon makes a mark to indicate the side (right or left) for the operation to avoid a potential mistake during the operation.

Preoperative Checklist

A checklist may be helpful in ensuring that all the relevant information is available.

- Record infant's weight and gestational age
- Determine that preoperative condition is stable and optimal
- Identify associated conditions such as heart or lung disease, renal abnormalities
- Review preoperative investigations
- Ensure that venous access has been established
- Ensure that consent has been obtained
- Ensure blood has been cross-matched and available
- Reassure the parents

DURING SURGERY

Anesthesia

The developing brain in neonates is susceptible to the possible neurotoxic effects of general anesthesia (Sanders & Davidson, 2009). Other considerations that may contribute to neurodevelopmental outcomes include managing fluid, respiratory, cardiovascular, glucose and pain responses to surgery (Davidson, McCann, Morton & Myles, 2008). The timing of anesthesia needs to be considered and weighed in relation to the need for surgery and possible harmful effects, as the evidence in humans is yet to be determined.

The intraoperative period places the infant at risk of fluctuations in vital signs as well as stress. Many neonates will arrive at the operating room already intubated and ventilated. The endotracheal tube needs to be secure to ensure that accidental extubation does not occur. This is the responsibility of the anesthetist, who may elect to re-intubate prior to the surgery.

The choice of anesthetic agent will depend on the type of operation, the defect, and the infant's status. Muscle relaxants are commonly used together with controlled ventilation and humidified gases for neonates. Inhalation anesthetic agents are commonly administered in 100% oxygen during the anesthesia, and the use of opioids can limit episodes of hypoxic pulmonary vasoconstriction (Golianu & Hammer, 2005). How infants are positioned during surgery can predispose them to hypoxia. For example, when positioned in the lateral decubitus position for thoracic surgery, infants are at significant risk of hypoxia due to their increased consumption of oxygen (Golianu & Hammer, 2005). This type of information is useful when nurses are challenged to care for recovering infants in the postoperative period.

Anesthetic agents can cause respiratory depression, as can narcotic and sedative medications. The neonate has a limited capacity to tolerate prolonged anesthesia. Residual effects of anesthesia can delay recovery from the surgical procedure, as seen by the infant's diminished respiratory effort and apnea. For these reasons it remains unwise to extubate the infant in the immediate postoperative period. At least 24 hours of postoperative ventilation enables more control of the infant's condition and stability as well as enabling adequate postoperative pain management.

Stress Response

Early studies have shown that inadequate analgesia during surgery is associated with a large stress response that results in suboptimal postoperative recovery (Anand, Hansen, & Hickey, 1990). Despite this knowledge, neonates undergoing surgery continue to demonstrate a stress response and different approaches to anesthesia and analgesia are being considered (Wolf, 2012). Surgical stress occurs as a result of an insult to the specific organ(s), tissue damage and nociceptive stimulation presenting as an endocrine and metabolic response. The magnitude of the response is high in neonates due to the immature control of hormone secretion.

The effects of the response manifest as hyperglycemia, lactic academia, tachycardia, hypertension, and hypothermia. These changes continue into the postoperative period for several hours and can obscure other clinical signs.

Thermoregulation

Concerns regarding temperature regulation continue during the intraoperative period. Although achieving a normal core temperature in the infant before surgery is always helpful, it is not always possible. Body temperature should be monitored throughout the procedure using either a skin or a rectal probe. A radiant warmer should be used during line placement, preparation, draping, and induction of anesthesia. A warming blanket under the infant can also be used to achieve constant temperature control. In addition, the room temperature should be increased to help compensate for the neonate's inability to stabilize temperature. Another mechanism for improving temperature control is humidification and warming of anesthetic gases. Slightly warming blood products, irrigation fluids, and intravenous fluids also assists in temperature maintenance. Surgical drapes should be replaced, if possible, when they become wet.

Another challenge in temperature maintenance is encountered during transport of the neonate to and from the operating room. To ensure temperature stability, the infant should be covered with warmed linen during transport. During the operative procedure, the transfer bed should be warmed to allow for some warmth during transport postoperatively.

Fluid and Electrolyte Balance

The goal of intraoperative fluid management is to replace the fasting fluid deficit, maintenance and third-space fluid losses, and blood loss to maintain homeostasis. Constant monitoring of fluid balance should continue throughout the surgical procedure. During the operative procedure, the fluid choice reflects the most dominant fluid loss. Early treatment of hypovolemia is essential. Intravenous fluid administration rates must be monitored to prevent fluid boluses, which could compromise fluid and electrolyte balance. Fluid loss from the surgical defect and blood loss during the operative procedure must be monitored and replaced. The metabolic response to surgery may also alter the infant's fluid and electrolyte balance. Hyperglycemia is a common response to surgical stress. Cold stress adds to this metabolic response and consequent fluid needs.

Monitoring

The trends of the infant's vital signs of heart rate, oxygenation, and gases are useful indicators for the anesthetist. Continuous monitoring during the operative phase can be useful in reviewing the infant's course during the surgery.

POSTOPERATIVE CARE

Oxygenation and Ventilation

Respiratory care in the postoperative period can present a great challenge to the caregiver. Intubation, anesthetic gases, and the stress of the procedure can traumatize the infant's respiratory tract. Depression of respiratory drive may be seen as a residual effect of anesthesia, and airway clearance may be difficult to maintain. These alterations in respiratory mechanics may lead to respiratory insufficiency and the need for prolonged mechanical support. Although specific respiratory needs may vary depending on the surgical procedure, a conservative approach to respiratory care is essential to maintain optimum oxygenation. Different ventilation modalities, such as high-frequency oscillation (HFO) have been found to be useful when commenced early in reducing the duration of ventilation required postoperatively (Bojan, Gioanni, Mauriat, & Pouard, 2012). An aggressive plan of weaning may cause recurring acidosis, hypoxia, or damage to the surgical repair. Following cardiac surgery, infants' slow weaning may be associated with low cardiac output and respiratory compromise.

Postoperative care of neonates includes maintaining ventilation and ensuring adequate analgesia. Small, premature, or low-birth-weight infants have lung function that is already compromised. The stress of severe infection and the surgical procedure itself, as well as the prematurity of the lungs, may necessitate prolonged ventilation with a slow weaning process. However the majority of infants who undergo surgery for a congenital malformation have relatively normal lungs, and the ventilation can be quickly weaned while maintaining close observation on their work of breathing.

Pain Management

The assessment of the infant for postoperative pain is an important component of nursing care. Opioids remain the choice for pain management following major neonatal surgery. Morphine, in particular, has proved effective and has widespread use despite its well-recognized limitation of a prolonged duration of action in neonates. Fentanyl is being used more often during neonatal surgery and for postoperative pain management and the greater hemodynamic stability needs to be balanced against recognized disadvantages such as the early onset of tolerance (De Lima & Carmo, 2010).

Nurses need to have a good knowledge base for the physiologic responses, pharmacokinetics, and behavioral responses of the infant in pain. The use of a validated pain assessment tool and the reliability of the use of the tool between clinicians are important if postoperative pain is to be adequately managed (Spence, Gillies, Harrison, Johnston, & Nagy, 2005). Most infants will have a narcotic infusion in the immediate postoperative period. The use of narcotics is encouraged; however, the assessment of their effect is important. There remains a lack of information on the effectiveness of pain management strategies and outcomes of infants managed for pain with narcotics. The neonate's behavioral response and developmental capabilities are important components of the nurse's assessment. Research into the impact of the caregiving environment has revealed significant physiologic and behavioral responses to obviously painful and stressful procedures (Browne, 2011).

Fluid and Electrolyte Balance

A goal of postoperative care is to provide fluid and electrolyte balance without overhydration. Hypovolemia is a major cause of hypotension and must be resolved quickly to ensure adequate perfusion to all organ systems and to combat acidosis. However, extreme care must be taken in administering fluids because neonates are susceptible to third-spacing and edema. Neonates are also very easily overloaded with excessive fluids.

Vital signs should be monitored frequently, as changes in heart rate or blood pressure could indicate shock or undetected fluid loss for which the body is trying to compensate. Assessment of temperature continues to be an important factor and must be considered when evaluating fluid needs. The serum electrolyte and glucose levels are evaluated immediately postoperatively and then intermittently until the infant's condition is stable. The frequency of laboratory evaluation is individualized to the neonate's condition. Sodium losses may continue through wound drainage as well as through gastric decompression. Thus reevaluation of intravenous fluids, both maintenance and replacement, is required to achieve and maintain electrolyte balance. Glucose metabolism may be altered as a response to surgery. Serum glucose levels should be monitored regularly after surgery.

Replacement fluid therapy is designed to make up for abnormal fluid and electrolyte losses during therapy to reduce vomiting and for losses incurred through diarrhea, nasogastric tube drainage, stoma output, wound drainage, pleural fluid, and fistula losses. Because the constituents of these losses frequently are quite different from the composition of maintenance fluids, it may be hazardous to simply increase the volume of maintenance fluids in an attempt to compensate for these losses. In some cases, it is preferable to actually measure and analyze the electrolyte content of these losses and replace them milliequivalent for milliequivalent and milliliter for milliliter. Samples may be sent to the laboratory as needed for exact determination of the electrolyte content of these various body fluids.

Overzealous attempts to correct glucose or electrolyte problems can produce a rebound effect. The neonate may change from being hyperglycemic to being hypoglycemic without intervention over a period of minutes or hours. The neonate moves from a catabolic to an anabolic state fairly rapidly compared with an older child or adult. These phases may occur over a few days or weeks in the infant. Therefore it is best to obtain baseline serum electrolyte and glucose levels. These values should be obtained every 2 to 4 hours, depending on how extreme the levels are. When intervention is needed, the sodium, potassium, or other electrolyte should be increased or decreased slowly and in small increments. These incremental changes should be followed by repeated measurement of serum levels, which must be closely monitored.

Nutrition

The nutritional needs of infants with altered function of the gastrointestinal tract present unique problems. Enteral feeds may be unable to be commenced, and nutrition is supplied with PN. The use of PN with increased protein is associated with beneficial outcomes, such as improved wound healing and shorter time to hospital discharge (Reynolds, Bass, & Thureen, 2008). Neonates who undergo a stress response from abdominal surgery are able to achieve a positive protein balance with adequate support. When used, PN needs to be limited with the establishment of enteral feeds to avoid complications of PN-associated liver disease.

Feeding is usually initiated as soon as possible after surgery. This is largely controlled by the type of surgery performed and the responsiveness of the individual infant. Small trophic feeds of breast milk given every 3 to 4 hours can assist in the earlier feeding of many neonates who have undergone surgery. Infants who have undergone surgery on the gastrointestinal tract may take several days or indeed weeks before full enteral feeds are tolerated. A small stomach size with altered emptying ability, as is sometimes seen with a diaphragmatic hernia, gastroschisis, omphalocele, and bowel resection, may present paramount problems in providing proper nutrition when feedings are started. Use of continuous feedings may help with these problems. Feed tolerance is monitored with aspirations every 4 hours, the larger volumes being returned to avoid electrolyte imbalance occurring. The routine administration of excess calories may not be warranted in critically ill surgical neonates as they do not have an increase in their resting energy expenditure. The energy is redirected from what is normally used for growth to fuel the stress response. Diligent nursing care with attention to the infant's thermal environment and supportive positioning and handling can support the infant until the infant returns to normal homeostasis following surgery.

It is imperative that the mother understands that breast milk is the first choice and that she is involved in decisions regarding feeding. When her infant returns from the surgery, her presence and an open dialogue can facilitate her ability to express and store her milk in readiness for breastfeeding as soon as possible.

Wound Care

The neonate's susceptibility to infection following surgery is due to immune suppression as a result of the trauma of surgery. This is due to changes in the neuroendocrine balance, inflammatory mediators and both cellular and humoral components of the immune systems (Wolf, 2012). To prevent infection, nurses must provide careful handwashing and attention to wound care. Wound infections can occur during or after the surgical procedure, are related to the duration of the procedure, and can become a complicating factor (Allpress, Rosenthal, Goodrich, Lupinetti, & Zerr, 2004; Duque-Estrada, Duarte, Rodrigues, & Raphael, 2003). Infection occurs more often after "contaminated" surgeries, such as an intestinal perforation, compared with "clean" surgeries, such as ductal ligation. These wound infections may require treatment with antibiotics.

Nursing assessment of the site must be continual because these observations may provide the first indication of poor healing or wound infection. The neonatal or surgical team (or both) should be made aware of any changes. If any suspicion of infection exists, blood cultures should be taken before treatment is started with broad-spectrum antibiotics that target anaerobes, aerobes, and gram-positive and gram-negative organisms. Consideration should be given to pain relief during potentially painful removal of surgical and wound dressings. The use of oral sucrose for pain relief is recommended if given 2 minutes prior to the procedure. The small volume given is not contraindicated when the infant is ordered nothing by gastrointestinal tract. New approaches to surgical incisions are being considered to give a more cosmetic effect for later in life. Comparison of different types of incisions has found no difference in terms of their postoperative outcome (Suri & Langer, 2011).

OUTCOMES

Outcomes of neonatal surgery can be considered both short and long term. Short term focuses on issues such as recovery and establishment of feeds to enable discharge home.

Long-term consequences of neonatal surgery have been identified in several studies. Peters et al. (2005) concluded that prior tissue damage can contribute to long-term neurobiologic differences. Sternberg, Scorr, Smith, Ridgway, and Stout (2005) reported that early exposure to noxious or stressful stimuli such as surgery may induce long-lasting pain behavior changes into adulthood.

Research has shown that infants who underwent complex surgery in the newborn period to correct life-threatening birth defects performed significantly below population norms on a standardized test of infant development and at risk of abnormal development (Laing, Walker, Ungerer, Badawi, & Spence, 2011). This finding is concerning. Laing et al. (2011) recommend that all infants undergoing major newborn surgery be routinely enrolled in systematic multidisciplinary developmental follow-up. This recommendation is supported by other specialist groups (Liddell, Walker, & Davis, 2011) who recommend long-term follow-up for all survivors of congenital diaphragmatic hernia surgery. This long-term follow-up care is critical to identify and proactively manage comorbidities.

Neurodevelopmental outcomes in school-age children were found to be reduced in children who underwent an arterial-switch operation; however, there was no cognitive dysfunction (Hovels-Gurich et al., 2002). The deleterious effects of severe preoperative acidosis and hypoxia, and postoperative hemodynamic instability contribute to the risk of developmental impairment (Hovels-Gurich et al., 2002). Infant temperament following surgery for complex congenital heart disease was found to be a significant source of stress for the parents (Torowicz, Irving, Hanlon, Sumpter, & Medoff-Cooper, 2010), and predischarge guidance for the families is recommended. These outcomes need to be considered when following infants who have undergone neonatal surgery. It appears that the experience of surgery, neonatal intensive care, and hospitalization can be deleterious for sick infants and their families. Care needs to be taken to ensure that the stressors encountered are kept to a minimum, and nurses are in key positions to provide a quality focus to the care of these infants and families.

Socioeconomic and psychosocial factors are also important contributors to variability in longer-term outcomes for infants and families and indicate a link between parent factors and child developmental outcomes following newborn surgery for birth defects (Laing et al., 2011). Further research is needed to identify how best to incorporate nursing practices that enable caregivers to simultaneously meet the medical and developmental needs of vulnerable infants and promote positive parent–child interactions in a surgical neonatal context. Evaluating the appropriateness of such care practices may require a multimodal approach and may also be developmentally directed, family-centered, and humane care judged by common sense (Laing, Spence, McMahon, Ungerer, & Badawi, 2012).

Data on many specific congenital malformations requiring neonatal surgery are now being collected through specific registries, both national and international. These registries enable a more population-based measurement of outcomes and provide an opportunity for earlier and newer treatments to be considered.

SUMMARY

This chapter highlights the special considerations for the neonate and family undergoing surgery. The role of care coordination, and fluid, electrolyte, and nutrition management are essential elements of this care.

CASE STUDY

A 34-week-old infant was transferred to a regional referral center 5 hours after delivery due to increasing respiratory distress.

The transport team reported an inability to successfully intubate and aerate the infant.

Once in the unit, intubations were attempted again, and no bilateral breath sounds could be heard.

An ENT consult with a pediatric surgeon was done and an x-ray ordered.

The ENT specialist stated that after failed attempts to intubate by an experienced neonatologist, anesthesiologist, and ENT that the infant had to be trached.

The infant was placed in an open warmer; chest x-ray results were pending, and chest tube setup was in place.

It was determined that this procedure/surgery should be done in the NICU rather than move the infant to an OR suite.

The team of anesthesiologists, neonatologists, the ENT/pediatric surgeon, and nurses were prepared to begin the surgery.

- The x-ray results arrived
- The infant had no trachea
- Only lung buds were present despite the gestational age
- Nothing further could be done

This case presents the need for a team approach and also resulted in ethical issues regarding the transport decision separating the family from the baby. The family was referred to and seen by the palliative care team, and follow-up care was provided.

CASE STUDY

Laing et al. (2012) present an excellent case study on how difficult it is to conduct prospective research regarding developmental care when the infant has undergone surgery. This case can be found at http://www.earlyhumandevelopment.com/article/S0378-3782%2811%2900254-4/abstract.

EVIDENCE-BASED PRACTICE BOX

Esophageal atresia has been a long-standing complex neonatal problem. This condition has lifelong implications. Its treatment often requires multiple surgeries. At Boston Children's Hospital, Dr. John Foker developed a technique to treat long-gap esophageal atresia and tracheoesophageal fistula by stimulating the growth of both the upper and lower segments of the esophagus. This is accomplished through placing sutures on each end of the esophagus and then gradually tightening these sutures over the course of days to weeks. The treatment program and protocol is referred to as the Esophageal Atresia Treatment (EAT) Program. It has been the basis of multiple research studies, including new work using magnets to stretch the esophagus (Kunisaki & Foker, 2012; Oehlerking et al., 2011). For more information, see http://www.childrenshospital.org/clinicalservices/Site2807/mainpageS2807P16.html.

References

Kunisaki, S. M., & Foker, J. E. (2012). Surgical advances in the fetus and neonate: Esophageal atresia. *Clinics in Perinatology, 39*(2), 349–361.

Laing, S., Spence, K., McMahon, C., Ungerer, J., & Badawi, N. (2012). Challenges in conducting prospective research of developmentally directed care in surgical neonates: A case study. *Early Human Development*. Retrieved from http://www.earlyhumandevelopment.com/article/S0378-3782%2811%2900254-4/abstract

Oehlerking, A. L., Meredith, J. D., Nadeau, P. M., Smith, I. C., Gomez, T., Trimble, Z. A., ... Trumper, D. L. (2011). A hydraulically controlled nonoperative magnetic treatment for long-gap esophageal atresia. In *Proceedings of the 2011 Design of Medical Devices Conference DMD2011*. Minneapolis, MN, April 12–14, 2011.

ONLINE RESOURCES

Common Neonatal Surgical Conditions
http://www.ucsfbenioffchildrens.org/pdf/manuals/54_SurgicalConditions.pdf

Fetal and Neonatal Endoscopic Surgery
http://www.youtube.com/watch?v=vHaOKCn0kt8

Journal of Neonatal Surgery
http://www.jneonatalsurg.com

Neonatal Surgery
http://www.youtube.com/watch?v=_US087zMXCo

Neonatal Surgery: All Children's Hospital, Johns Hopkins Medicine
http://www.allkids.org/body.cfm?id=993

Truncus Arteriosus Repair: Premature Newborn
http://www.youtube.com/watch?v=qIyAvgEw8aA

REFERENCES

Algert, C. S., Bowen, J. R., Hadfield, R., Olive, E. C., Morris, J. M., & Roberts, C. L. (2008). Birth at hospitals with co-located paediatric units for infants with correctable birth defects. *Australian and New Zealand Journal of Obstetrics and Gynaecology, 48*, 273–279.

Allpress, A. L., Rosenthal, G. L., Goodrich, K. M., Lupinetti, F. M., & Zerr, D. M. (2004). Risk factors for surgical site infections after pediatric cardiovascular surgery. *Pediatric Infectious Disease Journal, 23*(3), 231–234.

Anand, K. J. S., Hansen, D. D., & Hickey, P. R. (1990). Hormonal-metabolic stress responses on neonates undergoing cardiac surgery. *Anesthesiology, 73*, 661–670.

Badawi, N., Adelson, P., Roberts, C., Spence, K., Laing, S., & Cass, D. (2003). Neonatal surgery in New South Wales, what is performed where? *Journal of Pediatric Surgery, 38*(7), 1025–1031.

Bojan, M., Gioanni, S., Mauriat, P., & Pouard, P. (2012). High-frequency oscillatory ventilation and short-term outcome in neonates and infants undergoing cardiac surgery. *Neonatal Intensive Care, 25*(2), 31–37.

Browne, J. V. (2011). Developmental care for high-risk newborns: Emerging science, clinical application, and continuity from Newborn Intensive Care Unit to community. *Clinical Perinatology, 38*, 719–729.

Calisti, A., Oriolo, L., Giannino, G., Spagnoi, L., Molle, P., Buffone, E., & Donadio, C. (2012, March 12). Delivery in a tertiary center with co-located surgical facilities makes the difference among neonates with prenatally diagnosed major abnormalities. *Journal of Maternal Fetal Neonatal Medicine*. [Epub ahead of print]

Cass, D. L. (2011). Impact of prenatal diagnosis and therapy on neonatal surgery. *Seminars in Fetal and Neonatal Medicine, 16*(3), 130–138.

Clancy, R. R. (2008). Neuroprotection in Infant heart surgery. *Clinics of Perinatology, 35*, 809–821.

Davidson, A., McCann, M., Morton, N., & Myles, P. (2008). Anesthesia and outcomes after neonatal surgery. *Anesthesiology, 109*, 941–944.

De Lima, J., & Carmo, K. B. (2010). Practical pain management in the neonate. *Best Practice & Research Clinical Anaesthesiology, 24*, 291–307.

Diffin, J., Spence, K., Johnston, L., & Badawi, N. (2012). Predictors of psychological distress in mothers and fathers of neonates admitted to the neonatal intensive care unit for surgical correction of a congenital anomaly. *Journal of Paediatrics and Child Health, 48*(Suppl. 1), 8–81.

Duque-Estrada, E. O., Duarte, M. R., Rodrigues, D. M., & Raphael, M. D. (2003). Wound infections in pediatric surgery: A study of 575 patients in a university hospital. *Pediatric Surgery International, 19*(6), 436–438.

Ferrari, L. (2004). Preoperative evaluation of pediatric surgical patients with multisystem considerations. *Anesthesia Analog, 99*, 1058–1069.

Golianu, B., & Hammer, G. B. (2005). Pediatric thoracic anesthesia. *Current Opinion in Anaesthesiology, 18*, 5–11.

Hovels-Gurich, H. H., Seghaye, M. C., Schnitker, R., Wiesner, M., Huber, W., Minkenberg, R., ... Von Bernuth, G. (2002). Long-term neurodevelopmental outcomes in school-aged children after neonatal arterial switch operation. *Journal of Thoracic Cardiovascular Surgery, 124*, 448–458.

Laing, S., Spence, K., McMahon, C., Ungerer, J., & Badawi, N. (2012). Challenges in conducting prospective research of developmentally directed care in surgical neonates: A case study. *Early Human Development, 88*(3), 171–178.

Laing, S., Walker, K., Ungerer, J., Badawi, N., & Spence, K. (2011). Early development of children with major birth defects requiring newborn surgery. *Journal of Paediatrics and Child Health, 47*(3), 140–147.

Lakhoo, K. (2012). Fetal counseling for surgical conditions. *Early Human Development, 88*, 9–13.

Liddell, M., Walker, G., & Davis, C. (2011). Modern management of congenital diaphragmatic hernia. *Infant, 7*(3), 92–97.

Mcfadyen, B. (2011). Exploring the impact of family care-giving following neonatal surgery: Caring for infants with surgically correctable congenital anomalies of the abdomen and airways. *Journal of Paediatrics and Child Health, 47*(Suppl. 1), 60–116.

Mcfadyen, B., Harms, L., Johnston, L., Anderson, P., Badawi, N., Evans, C., Hunt, R., Jordan, B., & Spence, K. (2011). Exploring the impact of family care-giving following neonatal surgery: Caring for infants with surgically correctable congenital anomalies of the abdomen and airways. *Journal of Paediatrics and Child Health, 47*(Suppl. 1), 60–116.

New South Wales Department of Health. (2005). *Antenatalmaternal referral/transfer: Known congenital anomalies likely to require surgery*. Retrieved from http://www.health.nsw.gov.au/policies/PD/2005/PD2005_158.html

The Paediatric Intensive Care Society London. (2010, June). *Appendices to standards for the care of critically ill children* (4th ed.). Retrieved from http://www.ukpics.org.uk/documents/PICS%20Appx%204th%20Edn%20V2%2020100707.pdf

Peters, J. W. B., Schouw, R., Anand, K. J. S., Dijk, M. V., Duivenvoorden, H. J., & Tibboel, D. (2005). Does neonatal surgery lead to increased pain sensitivity in later childhood? *Pain, 114*(3), 444–454.

Poley, M. J., Brouwer, W., Busschbach, J., Hazebroek, F., Tibboel, D., Rutten, F., & Molenaar, J. (2008). Cost-effectiveness of neonatal surgery: First greeted with scepticism, now increasingly accepted. *Pediatric Surgery International, 24*(2), 119–127.

Ratnaval, N. (2009). Safety and governance issues for neonatal transport services. *Early Human Development, 85*(8), 483–486.

Reynolds, R. M., Bass, K. D., & Thureen, P. J. (2008). Achieving positive protein balance in the immediate postoperative period in neonates undergoing abdominal surgery. *Journal of Pediatrics, 152*, 63–67.

Royal College of Surgeons of England. (2007). *Children's surgery: A first class service: Report of the paediatric forum of the RCSENG*. London: Professional Standards and Regulation.

Sanders, R., & Davidson, A. (2009). Anesthetic-induced neurotoxicity of the neonate: Time for clinical guidelines? *Pediatric Anesthesia, 19*, 1141–1146.

Spence, K., Gillies, D., Harrison, D., Johnston, L., & Nagy, S. (2005). A clinically reliable pain assessment tool for use in neonates. *Journal of Obstetric, Gynecologic, and Neonatal Nursing, 34*(1), 80–86.

Sternberg, W. F., Scorr, L., Smith, L. D., Ridgway, C. G., & Stout, M. (2005). Long-term effects of neonatal surgery on adulthood pain behaviour. *Pain, 113*(3), 347–353.

Suri, M., & Langer, J. C. (2011). A comparison of circumumbilical and transverse abdominal incisions for neonatal abdominal surgery. *Journal of Pediatric Surgery, 46*, 1076–1080.

Taneja, B., Srivastava, V., & Saxena, K. N. (2012). Physiological and anaesthetic considerations for the preterm neonate undergoing surgery. *Journal of Neonatal Surgery, 1*, 14.

Torowicz, D., Irving, S. Y., Hanlon, A. L., Sumpter, D. F., & Medoff-Cooper, B. (2010). Infant temperament and parent stress in 3 month old infants following surgery for congenital heart disease. *Journal of Developmental and Behavioral Pediatrics, 31*(3), 202–208.

Usui, N., Kamiyama, M., Tani, G., Kanagawa, T., & Fukuzawa, M. (2011). Use of the medical information on the Internet by pregnant patients with a prenatal diagnosis of neonatal disease requiring surgery. *Pediatric Surgery International, 27*(12), 1289–1293.

Wolf, A. (2012). Effects of regional analgesia on stress responses to pediatric surgery. *Pediatric Anesthesia, 22*, 19–24.

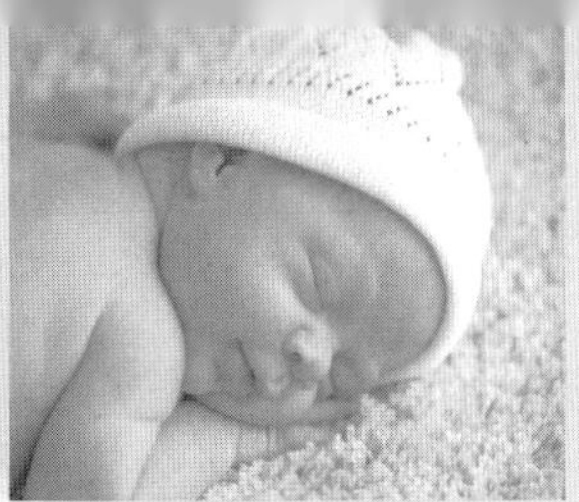

CHAPTER

26

Emerging Infections

■ Kathryn R. McLean

Emerging infections are those infectious agents whose incidence has increased within the past two decades or have the potential to increase in the near future. It includes those organisms that develop resistance to antimicrobials, new mutations, seldom-occurring pathogens recognized through new detection methods, zoonotic pathogens that have crossed over from an animal population, and reemergence of organisms that had been controlled in the past but are making a comeback (Greenfield & Bronze, 2010; Stramer et al., 2009). Scientists estimate that more than three new human pathogen species have been discovered each year since 1980 (Morgan, Kirkbride, Hewitt, Said, & Walsh, 2009). While not all of these pathogens have entered the neonatal intensive care unit (NICU), they all have the potential. Examples of each type will be given, but the majority of this chapter will focus on the development of resistance and methods to combat resistant organisms.

As we discuss these pathogens, it becomes evident that this is very much a global problem. Methicillin-resistant *Staphylococcus aureus* (MRSA) has been reported in NICUs in North and South America, Europe, and Asia (Chuang et al., 2004; Huang, Lien, Su, Chou, & Lin, 2011; Lepelletier et al., 2009; Nambiar, Herwaldt, & Singh, 2003; Regev-Yochay et al., 2005; Sakamoto, Yamada, Suzuki, Sugiura, & Tokuda, 2010; Seybold et al., 2008; Silva et al., 2009). Air travel allows transmission between hosts on different continents in a matter of hours. It is possible to travel between most countries in less time than the incubation period for many infectious diseases (Castillo-Salgado, 2010). The expanding human population and loss of animal habitats bring closer proximity to wildlife, reservoirs of zoonotic pathogens that can emerge in humans (Brouqui, 2009; Wendelboe, Grafe, & Carabin, 2010). Climate changes can allow range expansion of arthropods and rodents, vectors of viruses such as the hantavirus and tickborne protozoa such as *Babesia microti* (Gould, 2009).

It is important for the NICU team to understand how resistance develops and what steps can be taken to minimize the development of resistant organisms. Knowledge of chromosomal genetics and antimicrobial pharmacodynamics assists in this understanding. Infection control and antimicrobial stewardship are key elements to reduce the impact of resistance.

ANTIMICROBIAL RESISTANCE

Microorganisms demonstrate remarkable adaptability in response to antimicrobials. Penicillin was first used to treat human infections in 1941. Penicillin-resistant *Staphylococcus aureus* presented in 1944 and became widespread by the 1950s (Freeman, 1997; Rice, 2006; Tenover, 2006). Today 95% of *S. aureus* is resistant to penicillin due to penicillinase production (Andrews, 2003). Resistant strains of bacteria develop as new antimicrobials are introduced. The mechanisms of resistance vary with the antimicrobial actions of each antibiotic. Not only do the mechanisms vary, but the organisms have developed ingenious methods of transferring this resistance, making even existing susceptible organisms capable of developing resistance.

Natural or intrinsic resistance refers to the innate characteristics of an organism that interferes with the action of an antibiotic. Gram-negative bacteria wall structure, which includes an outer cell wall in addition to the peptidoglycan membrane layer and an intermediate space, can limit the uptake of a drug. This is an example of natural resistance. Acquired resistance occurs when a formerly susceptible organism becomes resistant (Andrews, 2003; Freeman, 1997; McManus, 1997; Mulvey & Simor, 2009). MRSA is an organism with acquired resistance.

Beta-lactam antibiotics (such as the penicillins, cephalosporins, and carbapenems) inhibit bacterial cell wall synthesis, specifically with the synthesis of the peptidoglycan layer (Andrews, 2003; Tenover, 2006). Interference requires the antibiotic bind to the cell wall at a target site called the penicillin-binding protein (PBP). Certain organisms have acquired genes encoding enzymes called beta-lactamases, which hydrolyze the amide bond of the beta-lactam ring and deactivate the antibiotic. Other organisms have evolved altered PBP structure, prohibiting the binding of the antibiotic (Andrews, 2003; Freeman, 1997; Mulvey & Simor,

2009; Shea & Jacobi, 2009). Bacteria may have genes encoding one or both of these methods.

Certain antibiotics must enter the microorganism in order to attach to a ribosome. They interfere with protein synthesis. Aminoglycosides, macrolides, and chloramphenicol are examples of these antibiotics. Passage through gram-negative bacteria walls often occurs through "porin" channels. Some bacteria have evolved the ability to close these porin (down regulation), blocking the entrance into the microorganism. Other bacteria have evolved efflux pumps with the ability to push the antibiotic out of the cell (Freeman, 1997; Shea & Jacobi, 2009; Tenover, 2006). The *mef* gene confers macrolide-specific efflux in resistant organisms (Andrews, 2003).

Other characteristics of microorganisms may influence the development of resistance. Certain bacteria develop biofilms. The microorganisms associate with and adhere to submerged surfaces (such as indwelling catheters). They become enclosed with a matrix, extracellular polymers composed primarily of polysaccharides, binding the cells to the submerged surface and to each other. This matrix prevents or impedes the diffusion of antimicrobials to the bacteria and protects the microorganisms from host defenses. In addition, oxygen and nutrient diffusion is impaired, decreasing the growth of the organisms themselves. Antibiotics that act on growth can be impaired (Donlan, 2000).

GENETIC MECHANISMS OF RESISTANCE

Natural or intrinsic resistance is stable and conferred by genes encoded in the chromosomal DNA. It is shared by all members of the genus. Acquired resistance involves a change in genetic material, either by mutation or by exchange of genetic material. Bacteria have multiple methods to exchange genetic material. Genetic material, including genes encoding for resistance, may exist outside of the chromosome on plasmids. Exchange of genetic material between bacteria occurs through conjugation, transduction, and transformation (Healy & Zervos, 1995; Johnson, 2012; McManus, 1997; Mulvey & Simor, 2009).

Conjugation involves the transfer of plasmids through elongated proteinaceous structures called sex pili, extending from the donor to recipient. Both donor and recipient have a copy of the plasmid. Transfer can be interspecies, even between gram-negative and gram-positive organisms (McManus, 1997; Tenover, 2006; Vrtis, 2008).

Transduction involves exchange of genetic material facilitated by viruses called bacteriophages. The genes may be of plasmid or chromosome origin. Transduction is a relatively rare event (McManus, 1997; Tenover, 2006; Vrtis, 2008).

Transformation involves acquisition of genetic material from the environment. When cell lysis occurs, DNA is released. The DNA binds to the cell surface of another bacterium. The bound DNA is taken up through the cell membrane and incorporated into its chromosome or a plasmid within the bacteria (McManus, 1997; Tenover, 2006; Vrtis, 2008).

Transposition enhances the spread of resistance. Genes may be flanked by insertion sequences at either end, creating a transposon. These transposons can "jump" to different locations on the chromosome or plasmids. A gene that was formerly on a chromosome or nontransferable plasmid can jump to a plasmid that can be exchanged between bacteria. This is the mechanism by which characteristics intrinsic to only one species can be transferred to a different species (Healy & Zervos, 1995; Johnson, 2012; McManus, 1997).

In some cases, the gene that confers resistance requires exposure to the antibiotic before the gene is activated. Bacteria with inducible resistance may initially test susceptible to an antimicrobial. With exposure to the antimicrobial the gene is activated and begins to produce enzymes such as beta-lactamases, inactivating the antimicrobial (McManus, 1997). The patient's condition worsens as the protected bacteria proliferate. The provider draws a second culture, and susceptibility shows the organism is now resistant to the original antibiotic.

PHARMACODYNAMICS AND RESISTANCE

Activity is measured based on minimal inhibitory concentrations (MICs) expressed in mcg/mL. The MIC is the lowest concentration of an antimicrobial agent that results in inhibition of bacterial growth. Antimicrobials are classified as either time-dependent or concentration-dependent. Time-dependent antimicrobials rely on serum concentrations that remain above the MIC for 60% to 70% of the treatment duration. These include beta-lactams and macrolides. Concentration-dependent antimicrobials rely on plasma concentrations within an area under the curve formed by plotting the plasma concentration of the drug versus time. Concentration-dependent antimicrobials include aminoglycosides, quinolones, and azilides (Andrews, 2003). Peak and trough drug levels are monitored for concentration-dependent medications. Peak/MIC ratio is used to describe optimal bactericidal effect based on higher peak concentration and increased dosing (Shea & Jacobi, 2009).

The MIC susceptibility breakpoints for antibiotic agents have been established and published by the Clinical and Laboratory Standards Institute (CLSI). Ranges exist for mildly resistant and highly resistant organisms (Shea & Jacobi, 2009). Culture and susceptibility reports interpret an isolate's activity based on these standards.

SELECTIVE ANTIBIOTIC PRESSURE

Selective antibiotic pressure is the trend for dominant antimicrobial species to evolve in response to the antibiotics chosen for treatment. Exposure to antibiotics creates an environment that inhibits or kills susceptible organisms but leaves resistant organisms alive and reproducing. Over time, resistant organisms may become the dominant species, colonizing the host. Within individual hospitals and the community, the specific antimicrobial selection can influence the development and predominance of resistant strains (Doyle, Buising, Thursky, Worth, & Richards, 2011; Mulvey & Simor, 2009). Indiscriminate over-the-counter use of antibiotics in China may have contributed to third-generation cephalosporin resistance in that country (Huang, Zhuang, & Du, 2007). Antimicrobials have also been used as a livestock growth promoter. Researchers found vancomycin–resistant enterococci (VRE) in the gut flora of poultry and swine (DeLisle & Perl, 2003; Shuford & Patel, 2005). Consumption of livestock colonized by antimicrobial-resistant organisms promotes the spread of these organisms to humans (Collignon, Powers, Chiller, Aidara-Kane, & Aarestrup, 2009). The impact of selective antibiotic pressure is a guiding principle for antimicrobial stewardship.

MRSA

Neonates are exposed to and their skin subsequently colonized with *S. aureus* shortly after birth. Colonization can also occur in the nasopharynx and gastrointestinal tract. Eighty percent of infants are colonized by day 10 of life (Bizzarro & Gallagher, 2007; Zingg, Posfay-Barbe, & Pittet, 2008). Of concern is the increasing prevalence of *S. aureus*, which is resistant to third-generation cephalosporins and semisynthetic penicillins such as methicillin. Premature and other compromised infants spend this early time period in NICUs where the selective pressure favors microorganisms with resistance. Outbreaks of MRSA infections were initially reported in the 1970s (Bizzarro & Gallagher, 2007). MRSA was first reported in a NICU in 1981 (Carey & Long, 2010; Gregory, Eichenwald, & Puopolo, 2009; Lessa et al., 2009; Sakamoto et al., 2010). MRSA outbreaks have now been reported in the United States, Brazil, Japan, Korea, Europe, India, and throughout the world (Gregory et al., 2009; Huang et al., 2011; Jain, Agarwal, & Bansal, 2004; Kamath, Mallaya, & Shenoy, 2010; Lepelletier et al., 2009; Nambiar et al., 2003; Park, Seo, Lim, Woo, & Youn, 2007; Saiman et al., 2003; Seybold et al., 2008; Silva et al., 2009; Zingg et al., 2008). MRSA colonization rates vary by geographic location and institution, ranging from 1.3% to 50% (Bizzarro & Gallagher, 2007; Carey, Della-Latta, et al., 2010; Carey, Duchon, Della-Latta, & Saiman, 2010; Gregory et al., 2009; Huang, Chou, Su, Lien, & Lin, 2006; Jain et al., 2004; Murillo, Cohen, & Kreiswirth, 2010; Sarda et al., 2009; Seybold et al., 2008; Song et al., 2010). Infection rates following colonization range from 14.7% to 81% (Bizzarro & Gallagher, 2007; Carey, Duchon et al., 2010; Gregory et al., 2009; Sarda et al., 2009; Silva et al., 2009; Song et al., 2010). From 1995 to 2004, the Centers for Disease Control and Prevention (CDC), National Nosocomial Infection Surveillance System (NNIS), reported that 23% of isolates causing infections in NICUs were methicillin-resistant (Lessa et al., 2009). The incidence of MRSA infection in U.S. NICUs increased 300% from 1995 to 2004 (Lessa et al., 2009; Milstone, Song, Coffin, & Elward, 2010). Certain areas of the world such as Taiwan have such a high percentage (95%) that MRSA is considered endemic (Huang et al., 2011).

Methicillin resistance is associated with specific genes: staphylococcal chromosome cassette (SCC) and *mecA*. The SCC gene complex and *mecA* gene confer resistance through changing the target site structure, creating (PBP)2A, which has a low affinity for beta-lactam antibiotics (Bizzarro & Gallagher, 2007; Carey & Long, 2010; Doyle et al., 2011).

MRSA infections are classified as either health care associated (HA-MRSA) or community acquired (CA-MRSA). Originally, HA-MRSA was the type more commonly seen in the NICU. Song et al. (2010) reported 67% with HA-MRSA compared with 33% with CA-MRSA in their unit. CA-MRSA is gaining in prevalence (Bizzarro & Gallagher, 2007; Carey, Della-Latta et al., 2010; Gregory et al., 2009). Pulse-field gel electrophoresis (PFGE) and polymerase chain reaction (PCR) allow identification of specific clones through molecular typing. Certain strains are associated with HA-MRSA. These strains differ in the type of SCC *mec* types: SCC *mecA* I-III. HA-MRSA strains include USA 100, USA 200, USA 500 to 800, and Rhine-Hessen (Healy, Hulten, Palazzi, Campbell, & Baker, 2004; Heinrich et al., 2011; Ramos et al., 2011; Seybold et al., 2008). Other strains are associated with CA-MRSA. These demonstrate SCC *mecA* IV-V. These include USA300 (majority), MW2, and USA400, USA 1000, USA 1100 (Carey, Della-Latta et al., 2010; Carey, Duchon et al., 2010; Carey, Saiman, & Polin, 2008; Healy et al., 2004; Seybold et al., 2008). The two types of MRSA infections differ in their resistance to antibiotics with HA-MRSA more resistant than CA-MRSA. CA-MRSA is usually susceptible to more non-beta-lactam antibiotics such as trimethoprim-sulfamethoxazole, clindamycin, and quinolone agents (Carey et al., 2008; Gregory et al., 2009; Ramos et al., 2011; Yee-Guardino et al., 2008). CA-MRSA may present with higher virulence. Certain strains produce Panton-Valentine leukocidin (PVL) and enterotoxins. PVL in particular has been implicated in the production of cytotoxins that attack the cell membrane, causing necrosis and cell lysis. CA-MRSA can present with severe necrotizing pneumonia and furunculosis (Carey & Long, 2010; Carey et al., 2008; Rice, 2006; Yee-Guardino et al., 2008).

Routes of transmission are primarily horizontal, with transfer from a colonized parent or health care worker, or from a colonized patient through contaminated hands or equipment (Maraqa et al., 2011; Zingg et al., 2008). The anterior nares are a major site of MRSA colonization (Huang et al., 2006; Maraqa et al., 2011; Singh et al., 2003). Other sites of colonization include the umbilicus, groin, axillae, hands, ears, gastrointestinal tract, and sinuses (Heinrich et al., 2011; Huang et al., 2006; Maraqa et al., 2011; Singh et al., 2003). Although some disagreement exists, the majority of practitioners consider screening of nares or nasopharynx sufficient to identify carriers (Maraqa et al., 2011; Lepelletier et al., 2009; Saiman et al., 2003; Singh et al., 2003). Detection is accomplished by either PCR or culture (Enomoto, Morioka, Morisawa, Yokoyama, & Matsuo, 2009; Francis et al., 2010). PCR has a turnaround time of hours as opposed to the 2 days required for culture (Francis et al., 2010). Francis et al. (2010) demonstrated that PCR had a sensitivity of 100% and specificity of 98%, recommending follow-up of positive results by culture. The necessity to culture all health care workers is controversial and usually confined to outbreaks (Grant, Charns, Rawot, & Benedetti, 2008). Transmission from health care workers is well documented (Burton, Edwards, Horan, Jernigan, & Fridkin, 2009; Gomez-Gonzalez, Alba, Otero, Sanz, & Chaves, 2007; Heinrich et al., 2011; Kim et al., 2007; Regev-Yochay et al., 2005; Seybold et al., 2008; Takei, Yokoyama, Katano, Tsukiji, & Ezaki, 2010). Transmission of MRSA from mother to infant has also been documented (Eckhardt, Halvosa, Ray, & Blumberg, 2003; Mongkolrattanothai, Mankin, Cranston, & Gray, 2010). Hospitals report a CA-MRSA vaginal colonization rate of 0.4% to 10.4% in pregnant women (Carey & Long, 2010; Carey et al., 2008), indicating a potential for transmission at birth. A positive culture obtained shortly after birth occurred in 1.7% of infants in a German hospital and 1.9% in a New Jersey hospital, suggesting such a transmission (Murillo et al., 2010; Seybold et al., 2008). Cases of transmission of CA-MRSA from contaminated breast milk (Behari, Englund, Alcasid, Garcia-Houchins, & Weber, 2004) and from father to infant (Al-Tawfiq, 2006) have also been reported.

MRSA infections may present as bloodstream infections (positive blood culture), surgical site infections, cellulitis, pustulosis, pneumonia, or osteomyelitis. Meningitis, urinary tract infections, and endocarditis are relatively rare (Carey & Long., 2010; Carey et al., 2008; Chuang et al., 2004; Gregory et al., 2009; Silva et al., 2009). The NNIS survey of MRSA infections from 149 nurseries from 1995 to 2004 classified 31% as bloodstream infections, 18% pneumonia, 17% conjunctivitis, 14% skin and soft tissue, 4% surgical, and 10% other (Lessa et al., 2009). Skin infection outbreaks have been reported in multiple otherwise normal full-term nurseries (Carey & Long, 2010). As with any infection, death is a possible outcome (Chuang et al., 2004). Symptoms remain the same as for any neonatal infection. The majority of risk factors also coincide with neonatal sepsis: extreme prematurity and low birth weight, indwelling central lines, prolonged hospitalization, endotracheal intubation, and previous exposure to antibiotics (Babazono et al., 2008; Burton et al., 2009; Couto, Pedrosa, Tofani, & Pedroso, 2006; Gerber et al., 2006; Khoury, Jones, Grimm, Dunne, & Fraser, 2005; Lessa et al., 2009; Maraqa et al., 2011; Nambiar et al., 2003; Seybold et al., 2008; Zingg et al., 2008). The NNIS reports rates of 5.4 infections per 1,000 catheter days for infants 1,001 to 1,500 g and 9.1 per 1,000 catheter days for infants weighing less than 1,000 g (Perlman, Saiman, & Larson, 2007). Colonization with MRSA frequently precedes infection (Gregory et al., 2009; Maraqa et al., 2011; Milstone, Budd et al., 2010). Maraqa et al. (2011) reported a relative risk (RR) of 37.75 as compared with noncolonized.

The gold standard of treatment remains vancomycin. Standard dosing is 15 mg/kg every 18 hours for neonates less than or equal to 29 weeks postconceptual age (PCA). Dosing interval decreases with increasing PCA: every 12 hours for infants with PCA between 30 and 36 weeks, and every 8 hours after 38 weeks. Peak concentrations reach 30 to 40 mcg, while trough levels should be between 5 and 10 mcg/mL. Some experts recommend trough levels of 15 to 20 mcg/mL when treating MRSA (Young & Magnum, 2010, pp. 96–97). The practitioner adjusts dosing to maintain levels. Duration of treatment depends on the type of infection, with most bacteremia requiring a 7 to 10 day course, while osteomyelitis may require 6 to 8 weeks for treatment (Carey & Long, 2010; Carey et al., 2008). Infectious disease specialists may be consulted for guidance. In the event an infant is allergic to vancomycin or resistance develops, linezolid is an option. The standard dose is 10 mg/kg every 12 hours for infants with a postnatal age (PNA) less than 8 days and every 8 hours for infants with PNA of 8 days or older (Carey & Long, 2010; Young & Magnum, pp. 58–59). For fulminant cases, gentamycin or rifampin may be added for synergy or better blood–brain barrier penetration. The monoclonal antibody tefibazumab has not proven effective (Carey & Long, 2010).

In addition to antibiotic coverage, additional measures are indicated to assure optimal outcomes. These measures include removal of indwelling catheters, drainage of any abscess, and documentation of sterilization of the bloodstream with follow-up blood cultures. The NICU team monitors the infant for any signs of osteomyelitis (Carey & Long, 2010).

Attempts to decolonize infants and care workers have achieved varied results. Intranasal mupirocin for five days is one measure. Multiple courses of mupirocen may be required (Carey, Della-Latta et al., 2010; Heinrich et al., 2011; Kim et al., 2007; Lepelletier et al., 2009; Nambiar et al., 2003). While chlorhexidine baths are often used in older patients (Doyle et al., 2011), concern over neurotoxicity limits its use in the neonatal population (Carey & Long, 2010). Units that use hexachlorophene baths often limit its use to infants with a birth weight of 1,500 g or higher (Saiman, 2006) or greater than 36 weeks gestation (Milstone, Budd et al., 2010). The baths may have more of a role in decolonization of the health care worker. Despite attempts to decolonize, many infants remain colonized at time of discharge (Francis et al., 2010; Kim et al., 2007; Lepelletier et al., 2009; Regev-Yochay et al., 2005). Contact isolation is usually maintained until a minimum of two consecutive cultures are obtained (Francis et al., 2010).

MRSA outbreaks can be particularly stubborn and require strict adherence to infection control methods and additional surveillance and isolation. In 2006 the Chicago Department of Public Health issued a consensus statement on control of MRSA in NICUs. These measures include strict adherence to hand hygiene, with the availability of waterless, alcohol-based hand-hygiene products at bedside. Hospital infection control professionals should provide education and direct observation to insure adherence. Nasopharyngeal surveillance cultures should be done on admission and then weekly. All positive cultures require contact precautions with gowns and gloves for all care, masks for suctioning. For nursing assignments, admissions can be cohorted in one group until cultures are available, infants with positive cultures in another group, and infants with negative cultures in a third group. Mupirocin may be used to decolonize MRSA-positive infants and health care workers. Culture of health care workers and the environment may be indicated. Molecular analysis such as PFGE should be performed to analyze the relationship between strains and to identify potential reservoirs and areas of infection control breakdown (Gerber et al., 2006). Extreme outbreaks with high persistence may require closure of the unit to new admissions until the organism is eradicated (Nambiar et al., 2003). Restriction of transfer of colonized patients prevents further contamination of outlying hospitals. Song et al. (2010) documented a stepwise approach using many of the Chicago consensus recommendations which took over 4 years to eradicate a MRSA outbreak in their nursery. In a Taiwan NICU where MRSA is endemic, it took 7 years (Huang et al., 2011).

The financial burden of MRSA can be tremendous. Gregory et al. (2009) reported screening costs alone during a 7-year period were $1.5 million at their hospital. It is estimated that each dollar spent on active surveillance can reduce health care cost by $10 through prevention of major outbreaks (Singh et al., 2003). Infections are associated with prolonged length of stay. Researchers estimate excess cost for neonatal patients attributed to methicillin-resistance to be $9,275 to $27,000 per patient. Some of this extra cost may be attributed to the delay in appropriate treatment while awaiting susceptibility results (Carey et al., 2008).

EXTENDED SPECTRUM BETA-LACTAMASE–PRODUCING ORGANISMS

Extended spectrum beta-lactamase (ESBL)–producing organisms were first discovered in 1983 in Germany (Huang et al., 2007). Gram-negative microorganisms which produce ESBLs include *Escherichia coli, Enterobacter cloacae, Klebsiella pneumoniae, Klebsiella oxytoca, Pseudomonas; Salmonella enterica,* and *Serratia marcescens* (Blaschke et al., 2009; Chiu, Huang, Lien, Chou, & Lin, 2005; Crivaro et al., 2007; Pessoa-Silva et al., 2002; Pessoa-Silva et al., 2003; Singh et al., 2002). Colonization rates of ESBL-producing organisms range from 5% to 53.8%, varying by geographic location and individual institutions (Murki, Jonnala, Mohammed, & Reddy, 2010; Ofek-Shlomai et al., 2011; Shakil, Ali, Akram, Ali, & Khan, 2010; Singh et al., 2002; Pessoa-Silva et al., 2003). Outbreaks have been reported worldwide (Abdel-Hady, Hawas, El-Daker, & El-Kady, 2008; Bagattini et al., 2006; Conte et al., 2005; Gundes et al., 2005; Huang et al., 2007; Iregbu & Anwaal, 2007; Kristóf et al., 2007; Lopez-Cerero et al., 2008; Mesa et al., 2006; Otman, Cavassin, Perugini, & Vidotto, 2002). Jain, Roy, Gupta, Kumar, and Agarwal (2003) reported ESBL in 86.6% of *Klebsiella* species, 73.4% of *Enterobacter* species, and 63.6% of *Escherichia coli* strains causing infections in their nursery in India. The NNIS reported similar rates of ESBL resistance: 81.8% of *Klebsiella* species, 73.1% of *E. coli*, and 60% *Enterobacter* species (Kamath et al., 2010). ESBL resistance has spread to *Neisseria gonorrhoeae* (Tapsall, 2009).

As previously described, beta-lactamase enzymes deactivate beta-lactam antibiotics through hydrolyzing the amide bond of the beta-lactam ring (Abdel-Hady et al., 2008; Andrews, 2003; Freeman, 1997; Huang et al., 2007; Mulvey & Simor, 2009; Shea & Jacobi, 2009). These enzymes extend resistance beyond penicillin to the extended-spectrum cephalosporins (ceftazidime, cefotaxime, ceftriaxone, etc.) and aztreonam (Abdel-Hady et al., 2008). Beta-lactamase enzymes make two of the four most common empirically prescribed antibiotics ineffective: ampicillin and cephalosporins. Inadequate empirical treatment is associated with higher mortality (Abdel-Hady et al., 2008; Grohskopf et al., 2005; Maragakis, 2010; Shea & Jacobi, 2009).

Most ESBLs are encoded on genes located on plasmids, promoting the transfer of resistance between bacteria of the same and other species (Crivaro et al., 2007; Healy & Zervos, 1995; Linkin, Fishman, Patel, Merrill, & Lautenbach, 2004). Identified genes associated with ESBL include SHV, TEM, CTX-M, and OXA (Abdel-Hady et al., 2008; Blaschke et al., 2009; Kristóf et al., 2007). As of 2002, 67 TEM-derived and 15 SHV-derived genes were identified (Jain et al., 2003). Crivaro et al. (2007) demonstrated the same plasmid in both *S. marcesans* and *K. pneumoniae* during investigation of ESBL in their NICU, indicating probable conjugal transfer of the plasmid between the two species. Other gram-negative bacilli may have chromosomal mutations that produce the gene AmpC, causing over production of beta-lactamase enzymes and making them resistant to even the beta-lactamase–beta-lactamase–inhibitor combination drugs (Kanj & Kanafani, 2011; Mulvey & Simor, 2009).

Horizontal transfer from contaminated patients through health care workers has been documented through PFGE analysis (Abdel-Hady et al., 2008; Boszczowski et al., 2005; Otman et al., 2002). Artificial fingernails on health care workers have been implicated in adult outbreaks (Boszczowski et al., 2005). Measures to control outbreaks are similar to those previously described for MRSA: strict hand hygiene, contact isolation, and cohorting of patients. Clinical improvement and sterilization of the bloodstream by antibiotics does not necessarily protect the gastrointestinal tract from colonization (Gundes et al., 2005). Screening for colonization is by stool or rectal culture (Singh et al., 2002).

Risk factors for infection with ESBL-producing organisms include lower gestational age, low birth weight, and longer length of stay. Previous exposure to third-generation cephalosporins has been implicated in all studies. Mixed results were found for endotracheal intubation duration (Jain et al., 2003; Kristóf et al., 2007; Linkin et al., 2004; Ofek-Shlomai et al., 2011; Pessoa-Silva et al., 2003; Shakil et al., 2010; Zingg et al., 2008). In contrast with MRSA, only one of the studies found the presence of a central line to be a risk factor (Pessoa-Silva et al., 2003). Colonization frequently precedes infection (Crivaro et al., 2007). Infections with ESBL-producing bacteria are associated with increased costs, prolonged length of stay, and higher mortality rates (Abdel-Hady et al., 2008; Gundes et al., 2005; Iregbu & Anwaal, 2007; Jain et al., 2003; Scheans, 2010).

Treatment is guided by susceptibility to antibiotics. Many of the ESBL-producing organisms are less susceptible to beta-lactam–beta-lactamase–inhibitor combinations due to higher production of ESBLs (Huang et al., 2007).

Carbapenems are often first-line agents used to treat ESBL-producing organisms (Kanj & Kanafani, 2011). The usual dose of meropenem is 20 mg/kg intravenous (IV). It is given every 12 hours if the infant is less than 32 weeks GA and less than or equal to 14 days PNA. Meropenem is also given every 12 hours in infants greater than 32 weeks but less than 8 days. Beyond those PNAs, the frequency is changed to every 8 hours. Imipenem dosing is 20 to 25 mg/kg per dose every 12 hours (Young & Magnum, 2010, pp. 60–61, 54–55). Synergy with gentamycin allows the beta-lactam antibiotic to be therapeutic in some cases of low resistance (Arias, Contreras, & Murray, 2010).

VANCOMYCIN-RESISTANT ENTEROCOCCUS

Vancomycin-resistant enterococcus (VRE) was first reported in 1986 in Europe (DeLisle & Perl, 2003). By 1995 VRE strains accounted for 10% of enterococci causing infections in the United States (Freeman, 1997). It had increased to 28.5% by 2004 (Bizzarro & Gallagher, 2007). VRE strains have been found in *Enterococcus faecium* and *Enterococcus faecilis* (Rice, 2006).

Enterococci have intrinsic resistance to many antimicrobials. Enterococci have long been resistant to beta-lactam antibiotics as they produce low-affinity PBP-5, interfering with the binding of the antibiotic to the cell wall. They can also bypass the block of folic acid synthesis by extracting folinic acid derivatives directly from their environment, interfering with trimethoprim-sulfamethoxazole. Aminoglycosides have difficulty crossing the cell wall unless paired with beta-lactams for synergy. Enterococci also produce enzymes that modify the ribosomes, decreasing the binding and bactericidal activity. Macrolides cannot stop protein synthesis because of a modified ribosomal target (DeLisle & Perl, 2003; Healy & Zervos, 1995; Tenover, 2006). Concern develops when acquired resistance occurs to one of the few antibiotics previously successful: vancomycin.

Vancomycin resistance is attributed to five gene clusters *vanA* to *vanE*, with *vanA* and *vanB* most significant. These clusters are associated with transposons that can move from chromosome to plasmids and transfer readily between bacteria. Glycopeptides normally interfere with cell wall synthesis by binding to the D-alaninyl-D-alanine terminus of a pentapeptide cell wall precursor. Resistance is conferred by substituting D-ala-D-lactate depsipeptide instead of the D-alaninyl-D-alanine, interfering with vancomycin binding and allowing cell wall synthesis to continue (DeLisle & Perl, 2003; Mulvey & Simor, 2009).

Transmission of VRE is horizontal, with transfer from colonized patients. VRE generally colonizes the gastrointestinal tract. Screening involves stool, rectal, or perirectal cultures. Patient-to-patient transfer can occur through contamination of health care workers' hands. The hospital environment provides many potential fomites, with survival of VRE up to 7 days on countertops (DeLisle & Perl, 2003; Healy & Zervos, 1995; Mulvey & Simor, 2009). Known cases require contact isolation until three stools obtained 1 week apart remain negative (DeLisle & Perl, 2003). Risk factors for infection include prior antimicrobial therapy with vancomycin or broad-spectrum cephalosporins (Louie, 2011; Mulvey & Simor, 2009).

Treatment of VRE is challenging and often involves a combination of agents. Microbial susceptibilities should guide treatment. Bacteriostatic agents such as chloramphenicol may need to be used (Bizzarro & Gallagher, 2007; DeLisle & Perl, 2003). Limited data suggest linezolid may be effective in some neonates (Bizzarro & Gallagher, 2007). Linezolid is an oxazolidinone antibiotic that interferes with ribosomal protein synthesis (Arias et al., 2010). Multiple blood cultures are recommended to confirm sterilization of the bloodstream (DeLisle & Perl, 2003). VRE is associated with higher mortality (Bizzarro & Gallagher, 2007). Methods to control outbreaks are similar to those described for MRSA: strict hand hygiene, screening, isolation, cohorting of patients and nurses, and environmental decontamination (DeLisle & Perl, 2003).

MULTIDRUG-RESISTANT ORGANISMS

Multidrug-resistant organisms (MDROs) are gram-negative bacteria that are resistant to more than two classes of antimicrobials. These organisms are typically resistant to penicillins, cephalosporins, fluoroquinolones, and aminoglycosides. Some have developed resistance to carbapenams, making treatment options difficult (Mulvey & Simor, 2009). MDROs include some strains of *Pseudomonas aeruginosa, Acinetobacter baumannii, E. coli, E. cloacae, K. pneumonia, K. oxytoca*, and *S. marcescens* (Mammina et al., 2007; Mulvey & Simor, 2009; Shea & Jacobi, 2009). These organisms often have multiple mechanisms for resistance. Energy-dependent efflux pumps located on the cytoplasmic membrane are encoded on the MexB gene. Regulation of outer membrane porin is encoded on the OprM gene. A protein that joins these genes is designated MexA. These combine to form the gene complexes MexAB-OprM, MexXY-OprM, MexCD-OprJ, and MexEF-OprN (Tenover, 2006). Efflux systems work against multiple classes of antimicrobials by lowering the concentration within the cell to a subtherapeutic level. Many already produce beta-lactamases, causing resistance to penicillins and cephalosporins (Freeman, 1997; Mammina et al., 2007). Recently, a carbapenum-resistant gene, VIM11, has been identified (Mammina et al., 2007). Carbapenemase production occurs in some species of *E. coli* and *K. pneumonia* (Kanj & Kanafani, 2011).

The usual reservoir of MDROs is the gastrointestinal tract. Screening is via stool culture. The proportion of colonized MDROs varies by geographic location and individual NICUs, ranging from 12% to 55.2% in nurseries with surveillance systems geared to detect these organisms. Breast milk proved protective in one study. Transfer is horizontal from patient to patient via contaminated health care worker hands or the environment. Identified risk factors for infection include early gestational age, low birth weight, and longer duration of NICU stay (Mammina et al., 2007).

MDROs have caused conjunctivitis, pneumonia, bloodstream infections, and death (Scheans, 2010). Treatment of MDROs should be guided by susceptibilities and may involve a combination of antimicrobials that are normally considered bacteriostatic instead of bacteriocidal. Clinicians may be forced to use antimicrobials that have few studies of the pharmacodynamics in neonates. Partnership between neonatologists, clinical pharmacists, and infectious disease specialists may present the best management. Outbreaks are managed through a combination of effective hand hygiene, isolation, cohorting of patients and nurses, and environmental decontamination (Maragakis, 2010; Zingg et al., 2008).

BABESIA

Babesia is an example of a pathogen with an animal vector that has been recognized by new detection methods as causing human infection (Stramer et al., 2009). Like Lyme disease, it is tickborne and found primarily in certain geographic locations. *Babesia microti*, the most common species, is an intraerythrocytic protozoa, which is detected by finding characteristic ring forms within the blood cell on blood smears (Aderinboye & Syed, 2010; Cable & Leiby, 2003; Dobroszycki et al., 1999; Fox et al., 2006; Herwaldt et al., 2011; Raju, Salazar, Leopold, & Krause, 2007; Snow, 2009). It can also be detected by PCR or serologic immunofluorescent antibody testing (Aderinboye & Syed, 2010; Cable & Leiby, 2003; Fox et al., 2006; Graham, Stockley, & Goldman, 2011).

Most cases of human babesiosis are associated with deer tick bites. Babesiosis is most common in five Northeastern states: Connecticut, Massachusetts, Rhode Island, New York, and New Jersey. It has also been found in two Midwestern states, Minnesota and Wisconsin. Other areas of the country such as the Pacific Northwest (Washington and California) are associated with a different species, *B. duncani* (Herwaldt et al., 2011). In contrast, the majority of neonatal infections are the result of blood transfusions from asymptomatic donors (Dobroszycki et al., 1999; Fox et al., 2006; Herwaldt et al., 2011). The first documented neonatal case occurred in 1982 (Dobroszycki et al., 1999; Raju et al., 2007). As of October 2011 there have been 18 neonatal cases (Herwaldt et al., 2011). Transfusions of blood from a single donor were implicated in a cluster of babesiosis in four neonates (Dobroszycki et al., 1999). There have been two reported congenital infections transmitted from a mother with babesiosis (Aderinboye & Syed, 2010; Fox et al., 2006). There are two reported cases of infants acquiring the infection postdischarge, with ticks removed from their bodies 2 weeks prior to the development of symptoms (Fox et al., 2006).

Babesiosis in neonates presents with jaundice, hepatosplenomegaly, hemolytic anemia, occasional thrombocytopenia, and occasional conjugated hyperbilirubinemia (Aderinboye & Syed, 2010; Dobroszycki et al., 1999; Fox et al., 2006). Unlike adult cases, fever is only reported in some cases (Aderinboye & Syed, 2010; Dobroszycki et al., 1999). Treatment includes the combination of clindamycin and quinine or the combination of azithromycin and atovaquone. Response is usually rapid with reduction or clearing of parasites within a few days. Treatment is continued for 7 to 14 days (Aderinboye & Syed, 2010; Dobroszycki et al., 1999; Fox et al., 2006; Raju et al., 2007). Packed red blood cell transfusions may be required for anemia. In severe cases an exchange transfusion may prove beneficial (Aderinboye & Syed, 2010; Fox et al., 2006). Cardiac monitoring will identify any arrhythmias, a potential adverse reaction associated with quinine (Raju et al., 2007). Hearing screening should follow treatment with quinine, as hearing loss and tinnitus are potential adverse reactions reported in adults (Krause et al., 2000; Snow, 2009).

No FDA-approved *Babesia* assay test is available to evaluate the blood supply used for transfusions (Cable & Leiby, 2003; Herwaldt et al., 2011). Current screening of donors for babesiosis is by questionnaire only, with only known cases excluded, and a question about exposure to tick bites not routinely included (Cable & Leiby, 2003; Dobroszycki et al., 1999; Germain & Goldman, 2002). Although supported in concept by the FDA's Blood Products Advisory Committee, regional screening of blood donors has not been instituted (Herwaldt et al., 2011). Asymptomatic donors with babesiosis remain undetected. The true extent of neonatal babesia exposure may be higher with asymptomatic infants undiagnosed. Until the blood supply is routinely screened, transfusion blood products for infants may be screened for babesiosis similar to our screening for cytomegalovirus (Cable & Leiby, 2003).

INFLUENZA A (H1N1)

H1N1 is an example of a viral illness that crossed from an animal population (swine) to the human population. In April 2009 the CDC identified two children with H1N1 influenza A, popularly known as "swine flu." The virus spread rapidly throughout the United States and worldwide, becoming pandemic by June of that year (Mosby, Rasmussen, & Jamieson, 2011; Pierce, Kurinczuk, Spark, Brocklehurst, & Knight, 2011). Pregnant women were at increased risk for serious illness requiring hospitalization or resulting in death (Mosby et al., 2011). In mothers, symptoms presented as fever 100.0°F or higher, cough, sore throat, and respiratory illness (Jamieson, Rasmussen, Uyeki, & Weinbaum, 2011; Varner et al., 2011). Varner et al. (2011) reported a maternal mortality rate of 1.1% related to respiratory failure. Premature delivery occurred in up to 30% of the H1N1-associated pregnancies (Mosby et al., 2011). Many of the premature births were for maternal indications due to the severity of her illness. In a series of 12 papers, 13 stillbirths and 8 neonatal deaths were documented. Most of the neonatal complications and deaths were related to premature births (Mosby et al., 2011). In the United Kingdom perinatal mortality was higher in infants born to women with H1N1 than in those born to uninfected women: 39 per 1,000 births versus 7 per 1,000 births (Pierce et al., 2011). Transfer of the virus to infants remained low, perhaps in response to strict isolation precautions. Among 45 neonates with documented testing, only six had positive tests (Mosby et al., 2011). Pierce et al. (2011) reported an increased prevalence of congenital anomalies in infants born to mothers with H1N1 when compared with the national rate in the United Kingdom: 32 per 1,000 births versus 17 per

1,000 births. Maternal fever and hyperthermia are thought to be the initiating mechanism behind the cleft lip and palate, cardiovascular, and neural tube defects seen in these infants (Mendez-Figueroa, Raker, & Anderson, 2011).

Mothers who smoked, were obese, or had chronic hypertension were at higher risk of developing severe illness (Mosby et al., 2011; Varner et al., 2011). Neuraminidase inhibitors administered within 48 hours of symptom onset significantly decreased the risk of severe disease, and up to 3 to 4 days conferred some benefit (Mosby et al., 2011). Oseltamivir was the neuraminidase inhibitor recommended by the CDC when a pregnant woman presented with influenza symptoms. No reports of potential negative neonatal outcomes occurred when pregnant women received any of the neuraminidase inhibitors (Rasmussen et al., 2011).

Seasonal influenza vaccination for pregnant woman has been recommended for all pregnant women since 2004 (Jamieson et al., 2011; Shah, Turcotte, & Meng, 2008). Coverage levels remain low: 32% for the year 2009. The H1N1 vaccination rate for 2009 was 46% (Jamieson, et al., 2011; Walker et al., 2011). Influenza vaccination of pregnant women provides transplacental transfer of antibodies to the fetus. Studies have shown a reduction by up to 63% in the rate of laboratory-confirmed influenza in infants less than 6 months old (Poehling et al., 2011; Rasmussen et al., 2011). Infants are ineligible for influenza immunizations until they reach 6 months of life; therefore, the only protection they receive is from their mothers and through "herd immunity" where their caretakers are immunized. In light of their susceptibility it is important for health care workers in NICUs and obstetric wards to also become immunized (Johnson & Talbot, 2011).

Isolation precautions were strenuous during the initial months of the 2009 H1N1 pandemic, often involving removal of the asymptomatic infant from the symptomatic mother (Gupta & Pursley, 2011; Rasmussen et al., 2011). Further evidence allowed more contact between mother and infant: by midpoint of the season, the CDC recommended separation limited to only until 48 hours of antiviral therapy received, fever resolved for 24 hours, and mother able to control her cough and respiratory secretions (Rasmussen et al., 2011). The Massachusetts Department of Public Health and 2010 CDC recommendations eliminated this separation, recommending that mothers be allowed to have infants in their room as long as they adhered to gown and mask with careful hand hygiene (Gupta & Pursley, 2011). Current recommendations include placing the mother on "droplet precaution" isolation in a separate room. These precautions are maintained until 7 days after onset of influenza symptoms or until 24 hours after fever and respiratory symptoms have resolved. Symptomatic parents and staff are restricted from nurseries. Infants are considered exposed, not infected, and receive droplet and standard precautions. Infants should be placed in isolettes with a minimum of 3 feet separating it from other isolettes or the mother's bed (Gupta & Pursley, 2011; Rasmussen et al., 2011). Parents and visitors require education on hand hygiene, "cough etiquette," and use of masks and other protective devices. Cough etiquette involves precautions for patients with a fever and cough: reporting symptoms to health care providers, wearing masks in public areas, covering their mouth when coughing, and using hand disinfection (Brouqui, 2009). If the mother plans on breastfeeding, a breast pump should be provided during any temporary separation.

HUMAN IMMUNODEFICIENCY VIRUS

Although human immunodeficiency virus (HIV) no longer meets the definition of an emerging infection in the NICU, the scope of the pandemic merits its continued surveillance by the CDC and discussion in this chapter. HIV is an evolving disease, with research providing new insights and improved management. The virus mutates and is at risk of developing antiretroviral resistance.

Acquired immunodeficiency syndrome (AIDS), the most severe expression of an HIV infection, was first recognized in 1981 among homosexual men in the United States. When a report in 1982 described an infant with noncongenital acquired immunodeficiency, epidemiologists failed to see a connection to the disease. Reports of AIDS shared by heterosexual men and women in Africa surfaced in 1983, prompting reexamination of the neonatal case and recognition of the disease in the neonatal population (Beckerman, 2005). The AIDS pandemic became the worst epidemic of the 20th century, killing more than 35 million people to date (Joint United Nations Programme on HIV/AIDS [UNAIDS], 2011; Quinn, 2012). The epidemic peaked in 1997. The annual new HIV infection rate fell 21% between 1997 and 2010, primarily through education and improved prevention of maternal–child transmission. In 2010, 390,000 children were diagnosed with HIV, over 30% fewer than at the peak of 560,000 in 2002 (Joint United Nations Programme on HIV/AIDS [UNAIDS], 2011). The majority of children acquired HIV during their infancy as a result of maternal–child transmission in utero, intrapartum, or from breastfeeding (Committee on Infectious Diseases, American Academy of Pediatrics, 2009; Panel on Treatment of HIV-infected Pregnant Women and Prevention of Perinatal Transmission, 2011). Despite advances in HIV maternal–child prophylaxis, 100 to 200 infants per year were infected in the United States (Centers for Disease Control and Prevention, 2007). The UNAIDS (2011) reported only 48% of pregnant HIV-infected women in developing countries such as in sub-Saharan Africa received effective regimens to prevent HIV transmission, placing many infants at risk. In contrast, 95% of pregnant women in New York received screening for HIV, infected women received antiretroviral treatment, and the transmission rate was only 2.1% (Birkhead et al., 2010). UNAIDS (2011) identified 22 countries still at high risk for maternal–child transmission, including countries in sub-Saharan Africa, the Caribbean, and India.

HIV is an RNA-containing retrovirus (Baley & Toltzis, 2006). Molecular studies suggest that HIV evolved from the simian immunodeficiency virus (SIV), making it originally a zoonotic pathogen (Quinn, 2012). The virus infects host cells by attaching to CD4+ receptor sites on T-helper cells (primary), B-lymphocytes, monocytes, macrophages, and glial cells of the brain (Bell, 2004). The virus binds to a cell at two receptor sites and then penetrates the cell. Viral RNA empties into the cell. Single strands of viral RNA are converted into double-stranded DNA by the reverse transcriptase enzyme (reverse transcription). Viral DNA combines with the cell's own DNA through the actions of the integrase enzyme (integration). During cell division, the viral DNA is copied and long chains of proteins are made (transcription). Sets of viral protein combine, forming the immature virus (assembly). The immature virus buds, pushing out of the cell while taking some of the host cell membrane (budding). This bud breaks free of the infected cell. Protease enzymes cut the protein chains in the viral particle into individual proteins. These proteins combine to make a working virus (maturation) (Beckerman, 2005).

HIV infections occur in three phases. During the primary infection a high viral load occurs. The host responds by mounting an antiviral immune response, resulting in anti-HIV antibodies and cytotoxic T cells. During the primary infection, CD4 cell death is countered by new CD4 production. In response to the immune response, viral load falls to a set point and the infection enters the latent phase. During the latent phase, the CD4 cell count continues to fall gradually. The virus continues to replicate. The infection will progress to AIDS without antiretroviral therapy (ART). AIDS presents with high viral load, low CD4 counts, and immunodeficiency. Immunodeficiency results from direct killing of the infected cells by the virus or host, apoptosis, abnormal cytokine production by infected cells, disruption of the architecture of lymphoid tissues, and disruption of hematopoiesis and lymphoid differentiation (Beckerman, 2005). Infants and children demonstrate a more rapid progress secondary to the low number of natural killer and T cells and the decreased function of those cells. In addition, the natural progress of growth in these children promotes high cell replication and high viral loads (Baley & Toltzis, 2006).

Maternal–child transmission rate of HIV infection was 25% to 30% if the mother did not receive ART. Significant progress in the fight against HIV transmission occurred in 1994 with the Pediatric AIDS Clinical Trials Group 076 (PACTG 076) study demonstrating that the administration of zidovudine to the pregnant woman and her infant reduced the transmission rate to 8.3% (Connor et al., 1994; Jamieson et al., 2007; Kriebs, 2006; Panel on Treatment of HIV-infected Pregnant Women and Prevention of Perinatal Transmission, 2011). Multiple studies showed even more significant reduction when combination antiretroviral prophylaxis was given to mothers antenatally. Triple combinations resulted in better results than dual combinations. Studies reported rate of transmission as low as 1.8% (ANRS 1201/1202 DITRAME PLUS Study Group, 2005; Haeri et al., 2009; Jamieson et al., 2007; Panel on Treatment of HIV-infected Pregnant Women and Prevention of Perinatal Transmission, 2011; The TEmAA ANRS 12109 Study Group, 2010; Warszawski et al., 2008). Subsequent clinical trials focused on determining the effectiveness of shorter, less expensive prophylactic regimens that could be easily implemented in developing countries (Bhoopat et al., 2005; Chi et al., 2005; Jamieson et al., 2007; The Kesho Bora Study Group, 2010). The CDC published a comprehensive review of the studies related to ART to reduce maternal–child transmission under "Lessons from Clinical Trials of Antiretroviral Interventions to Reduce Perinatal Transmission of HIV." This review can be retrieved at aidsinfo.nih.gov/contentfiles/IVguidelines/perinatalgl.pdf (Panel on Treatment of HIV-infected Pregnant Women and Prevention of Perinatal Transmission, 2011).

The current CDC recommendations for management of HIV-infected pregnant women and HIV-exposed infants are outlined in "Recommendations for Use of Antiretroviral Drugs in Pregnant HIV-1-Infected Women for Maternal Health and Interventions to reduce Perinatal HIV Transmission in the United States" (Panel on Treatment of HIV-infected Pregnant Women and Prevention of Perinatal Transmission, 2011). This guideline, updated last in September 2011, can be retrieved at aidsinfo.nih.gov/contentfiles/IVguidelines/perinatalgl.pdf. It reflects the most current research and infectious disease expertise. The guideline stresses the importance of early identification of HIV-infected women, implementation of a highly active ART (HAART) regimen as soon as it is safe for mother and fetus, continued monitoring of maternal HIV status (viral load and CD4 count), and neonatal ART for the first 6 weeks of life (Panel on Treatment of HIV-infected Pregnant Women and Prevention of Perinatal Transmission, 2011). HIV screening programs, which are "opt-out," screen more women than programs that are "opt-in." "Opt-in" programs require formal counseling and signed consent prior to the screening. "Opt-out" screening just require that the mother be informed of the test and has the right of refusal (Jamieson et al., 2007; Kriebs, 2006; Panel on Treatment of HIV-infected Pregnant Women and Prevention of Perinatal Transmission, 2011). Unscreened women should be tested during labor. While early HAART provides the most protection, even intrapartum prophylaxis can reduce the transmission of HIV to the neonate. The goal of HAART is to decrease the maternal viral load in blood and genital secretions. Intrapartum management includes zidovudine intravenous infusion during labor. Scalp electrode fetal monitoring, vacuum devices, and forceps are to be avoided. Elective cesarean sections are reserved for mothers with viral loads of more than 1,000 copies/mL (Jamieson et al., 2007; Kriebs, 2006; Panel on Treatment of HIV-infected Pregnant Women and Prevention of Perinatal Transmission, 2011). ART for the HIV-exposed infant begins shortly after birth and continues for 6 weeks (Panel on Treatment of HIV-infected Pregnant Women and Prevention of Perinatal Transmission, 2011).

Most triple HAART regimens include two nucleoside reverse transcriptase inhibitors (NRTIs) and one other drug, either a nonnucleoside reverse transcriptase inhibitor (NNRTI) or a protease inhibitor (PI). NRTIs act as fake nucleoside analogues, disrupting the formation of viral DNA (Riordan & Bugembe, 2009). Typical NRTIs include zidovudine, lamivudine, abacavir, didanosine, tenofovir disoproxil fumarate (TDF), and emtricitabine. The NRTIs stavudine and didanosine should not be used together as lactic acidosis, sometimes fatal, can occur in pregnant women receiving the combination. Stavudine should also be discontinued during intravenous zidovudine administration intrapartum, as it inactivates the zidovudine. Most NRTIs have minimal adverse effects on the fetus. TDF is associated with decreased fetal growth and increased bone porosity in monkeys (using double the usual dose in humans) and bone demineralization with chronic use in humans. At least one of the NRTIs should demonstrate high placental transfer (Panel on Treatment of HIV-infected Pregnant Women and Prevention of Perinatal Transmission, 2011; Riordan & Bugembe, 2009). NNRTIs bind directly to the reverse transcriptase enzyme, preventing it from copying the viral RNA (Riordan & Bugembe, 2009). NNRTIs include nevirapine and efavirenz. Efavirenz should not be used in the first trimester, as there is a known association with neural tube defects and facial clefts. Nevirapine is associated with hepatic toxicity in pregnant women with a CD4 count greater than 250/cubic mm (Panel on Treatment of HIV-infected Pregnant Women and Prevention of Perinatal Transmission, 2011; Riordan & Bugembe, 2009). PIs bind competitively with the protease enzyme, blocking viral maturation and resulting in immature and ineffective viral particles (Riordan & Bugembe, 2009). PIs include ritonavir-boosted lopinavir, ritonavir-boosted atazanavir, ritonavir, and saquinavir. These agents are associated with increased incidence of glucose intolerance and gestational diabetes in pregnant women receiving PIs (El Beitune et al., 2005). Saquinavir can cause prolonged PR or QT intervals—a baseline EKG is recommended. Indinavir may increase indirect bilirubin levels. Other drugs are available, but insufficient data exist to determine the safety of use in pregnancy. Other than efavirenz, ART is associated with few congenital anomalies. The most common anomaly is hypospadias in male infants (Watts et al., 2007). Some studies show a higher incidence of premature births with HAART (Hernandez et al., 2012; Panel on Treatment of HIV-infected Pregnant Women and Prevention of Perinatal Transmission, 2011; Townsend, Cortina-Borja, Pecham, & Tookey, 2007). Evidence is mixed as to the effect of HAART on growth, both intrauterine and postnatally (Briand et al., 2009; European Collaborative Study, 2005; Hernandez et al., 2012). Choice of drugs for the triple combination reflects previous regimens used to treat women diagnosed prior to their pregnancy, safety to the fetus depending on which trimester therapy is initiated, and presence of resistance (Panel on Treatment of HIV-infected Pregnant Women and Prevention of Perinatal Transmission, 2011).

The high number of HIV-1 particles produced daily provides many opportunities for mutations, including the genetic material coding for resistance. Antiretroviral drug resistance presents as persistent high viral loads despite ART. In the presence of a viral load in excess of 500 to 1,000 copies/mL, drug resistance testing should precede initiation of ART. Repeat viral load monitoring allows detection of ineffective therapy, resistance testing, and substitution of another effective drug. Development of resistance is associated with suboptimal adherence, such as occurs with maternal nausea and vomiting during the first trimester, and regimens that include short-term use of nevirapine (Jamieson et al., 2007; Panel on Treatment of HIV-infected Pregnant Women and Prevention of Perinatal Transmission, 2011).

ART in the HIV-exposed neonate is initiated within 6 to 12 hours after birth. Zidovudine prophylaxis is given for 6 weeks (Panel on Treatment of HIV-infected Pregnant Women and Prevention of Perinatal Transmission, 2011). The usual dosing in infants greater than or equal to 35 weeks is 2 mg/kg/dose given orally every 6 hours. The CDC currently recommends modifying that dosing to 4 mg/kg every 12 hours based on the results of many international studies. Twice daily administration is easier for parents. Premature infants between 30 and 34 weeks gestation receive a dose of 2 mg/kg given orally every 12 hours during the first 2 weeks of life, then every 8 hours from 3 to 6 weeks of life. Premature infants less than 30 weeks gestation receive 2 mg/kg/dose orally every 12 hours for the first 4 weeks of life, then every 8 hours for weeks 5 and 6. If an infant cannot tolerate oral feedings, zidovudine is given intravenously at a dose of 1.5 mg/kg (Panel on Treatment of HIV-infected Pregnant Women and Prevention of Perinatal Transmission, 2011; Young & Magnum, 2010, pp. 98–99). In the United Kingdom and other European countries, the regimen may be limited to 4 weeks duration if the mother received a triple HAART regimen during her pregnancy (Ferguson, Goode, Walsh, Gavin, & Butler, 2011). Some infants who are at higher risk warrant a two-drug regimen. Maternal–infant transmission is more likely to occur in cases where mothers had a high viral load at time of delivery, mothers did not receive antenatal prophylaxis or only received intrapartum prophylaxis, or there was an infection with drug-resistant viruses (Panel on Treatment of HIV-infected Pregnant Women and Prevention of Perinatal Transmission, 2011; Warszawski et al., 2008). Infants who are at higher risk should receive three doses of nevirapine during the first week of life in addition to the zidovudine course. The first dose is given within 48 hours of birth, the second 48 hours after the first, and the third dose 96 hours after the second. Nevirapine is not recommended for premature infants as their renal and hepatic function is immature, making them at increased risk of overdosing and toxicity (Mirochnick et al., 2008; Panel on Treatment of HIV-infected Pregnant Women and Prevention of Perinatal Transmission, 2011).

Breastfeeding is contraindicated in infants of mothers with HIV infection. In sub-Saharan Africa approximately 40% of HIV infections occur during the postnatal period due to breastmilk transmission (John-Stewart, 2012). Nurses and medical providers counsel HIV-infected women in the United States and other resource-rich countries not to breastfeed. Substitution of formula for breastfeeding is not an option in some developing countries. The lack of a safe water supply for formula preparation and loss of immunity offered by breastfeeding place infants who do not breastfeed at higher risk of death due to diarrhea, malnutrition, and other illnesses. Daily prophylaxis with nevirapine reduces transmission if breastfeeding is necessary (John-Stewart, 2012; Panel on Treatment of HIV-infected Pregnant Women and Prevention of Perinatal Transmission, 2011). Most studies limited prophylaxis to as short a duration as 6 weeks, but breastfeeding continued after the prophylaxis periods. While transmission was reduced during the initial study, long-term outcomes showed increased rate of seroconversion at 6 or more months. These findings suggest that prophylaxis should continue during the entire breastfeeding period or breastfeeding time be limited. All studies showed less transmission when breastfeeding was paired with prophylaxis than when a mix of formula and breastfeeding was paired with prophylaxis (Chung et al., 2005; John-Stewart, 2012; Kesho Bora Study Group, 2010).

HIV-infected mothers need counseling to avoid sharing food they have chewed with their infants. There are three case reports from the United States of possible transmission from premastication of infant food by infected caregivers. The caregivers had bleeding gums or sores in their mouth in two of the three cases (Committee on Infectious Diseases, American Academy of Pediatrics, 2009). Soft infant food should be prepared by mashing, use of blender or food processor, or commercially.

Infants require close monitoring for detection of infection or adverse reactions to ART. Recommended blood work after birth includes HIV-1 plasma viral load and a CBC with differential. Maternal HIV antibodies cross the placenta and will be detected in all HIV-exposed infants up to 18 months (Committee on Infectious Diseases, American Academy of Pediatrics, 2009; Panel on Treatment of HIV-infected Pregnant Women and Prevention of Perinatal Transmission, 2011). Most infants are HIV negative at birth, but can become seropositive within a few weeks (Baley & Toltzis, 2006). Virologic testing occurs within the first 14 to 21 days, at 1 to 2 months, and at 4 to 6 months. Two positive HIV DNA PCR or RNA viral assays are diagnostic. Newly diagnosed infants require viral resistance testing prior to starting combination ART. Definite exclusion of HIV follows obtaining negative HIV tests at 1 to 2 months and 4 to 6 months. Negative HIV status is often confirmed by a HIV antibody test at 12 to 18 months. Infants exposed to ART can develop mild and reversible anemia and/or neutropenia—monitor CBC as needed (Baley & Toltzis, 2006; Committee on Infectious Diseases, American Academy of Pediatrics, 2009; Feiterna-Sperling et al., 2007; Tighe, Rimsza, Christensen, Lew, & Sola, 2005). More severe cases of thrombocytopenia and anemia are associated with actual infections or HAART (Myers, Torrente, Hinthorn, & Clark, 2005; Tighe et al., 2005). Macrocytic anemia occurs in 1.1% of pediatric patients receiving zidovudine and 4% of pediatric patients receiving the combination of zidovudine and lamivudine (Myers et al., 2005). The long-term effects of in utero exposure to ART are unknown. If a child develops organ system abnormalities of unknown etiology, particularly of the heart or nervous system, mitochondrial dysfunction should be suspected. Clinical deterioration would prompt obtaining a serum lactate. Children require follow-up into adulthood to monitor for cancer (Committee on Infectious Diseases, American Academy of Pediatrics, 2009; Panel on Treatment of HIV-infected Pregnant Women and Prevention of Perinatal Transmission, 2011).

HIV positive infants are asymptomatic at birth but can become symptomatic within the first few years. The infant can present with unexplained fevers, recurrent bacterial infections such as otitis or pneumonias, persistent candidiasis (mucocutaneous and/or dermal), chronic diarrhea, or failure to thrive. Hepatosplenomegaly and lymphadenopathy can develop (Baley & Toltzis, 2006; Beckerman, 2005; Committee on Infectious Diseases, American Academy of Pediatrics, 2009). Lymphoid interstitial pneumonitis, one potential complication, presents with a chronic oxygen dependence (Baley & Toltzis, 2006). Infants are at risk for opportunistic infections by organisms that normally have a low pathogenicity. *Pneumocystis jirovecil* pneumonia (PCP), formerly known as *Pneumocystis carinii* pneumonia, is the most common opportunistic infection. It occurs most often during the first year of life, peaking at 3 to 6 months (Stokowski, 2009). In order to prevent this type of pneumonia, HIV-exposed infants receive prophylaxis with trimethoprim-sulfamethosazole (TMP-SMX). TMP-SMX is initiated after zidovudine prophylaxis is completed, beginning at 4 to 6 weeks (Panel on Treatment of HIV-infected Pregnant Women and Prevention of Perinatal Transmission, 2011). One fifth of HIV-infected infants present with neurologic or developmental issues by 2 years of life. Malignancies, such as Kaposi's sarcoma, are rare in infancy (Beckerman, 2005). A poor prognosis for survival is found in untreated infants, infants who present initially with high viral loads (greater than 100,000 copies/mL) and markedly decreased CD4 T-lymphocyte counts, and infants who develop severe manifestations of HIV infection (PCP, neurologic disease, or wasting)(Committee on Infectious Diseases, American Academy of Pediatrics, 2009). Survival and prognosis is dependent on adherence to a life-long therapy.

Prognosis and survival rates dramatically improved with the introduction of early HAART regimens. Before the introduction of HAART, approximately 20% of infants in Europe died or developed severe manifestations by their first year of life and 50% died by age 10 (Riordan & Bugembe, 2009). A study in the United Kingdom showed an 80% reduction of hospitalization rates, 50% reduction in clinical progression to AIDS, and fivefold decrease in mortality (Riordan & Bugembe, 2009). Recent studies in the United States and Europe indicated more than 95% of infected children survive at 16 years of life (Committee on Infectious Diseases, American Academy of Pediatrics, 2009).

Co-morbidities are more common in HIV-infected neonates. Case reports of HIV-associated tuberculosis, cytomegalovirus (CMV), malaria, and hepatitis C exist (Adhikari, Pillay, & Pillay, 1997; Khamduang et al., 2011; Mofenson, 2009; Slyker et al., 2009). Co-infection with malaria increases maternal HIV RNA levels, placing the infant at greater risk for maternal–child transmission of HIV (Mofenson, 2009). Maternal transmission of CMV and hepatitis C is increased in HIV-infected infants (Khamduang et al., 2011; Slyker et al., 2009). One high-risk group is made up of those women who have multiple sex partners or are prostitutes. These women are also at risk for sexually transmitted diseases such as gonorrhea or chlamydia. Another high-risk activity is intravenous drug use. Women who use intravenous drugs are also at increased risk for hepatitis B (Bell, 2004). Clinicians need to be aware of the possibility of additional congenital infections in HIV-exposed neonates.

MEASLES

Measles is an example of a disease that is re-emerging. Prevention is managed through a series of two vaccinations: the first at 12 to 15 months and the second at 5 to 6 years. Parents may elect to decline immunization, and their child may be protected by herd immunity. A paper from Italy documents seven cases of measles in infants: four were less than 3 months, and three were less than 12 months. Four of the mothers had no immunization and contracted measles themselves, while the other cases involved siblings with the disease (Bozzola et al., 2011).

COMBATING EMERGING INFECTIONS

The war against emerging infections begins with infection control. Many of the infection control methods such as isolation, cohorting patients, and surveillance are described in the section on MRSA. The goal of infection control is to reduce and control reservoirs. Hand hygiene remains an important action to protect our patients (Carey et al., 2008; Higgins, Baker, & Raju, 2010). The use of alcohol-based gel disinfectants at the bedside improves compliance (Carey et al., 2008; Saiman, 2006; Sakamoto et al., 2010).

Care bundles are a group of evidence-based actions which when implemented together have been successful in reducing infections. Central Line-Associated Blood Stream Infections (CLABSI) and Ventilator-Associated Pneumonia (VAP) are examples of care bundles (Doyle et al., 2011; Toth, Chambers, & Davis, 2010). A typical CLABSI bundle includes hand hygiene, use of full-barrier precautions during line insertion, effective skin antisepsis at the insertion site, minimizing catheter entry and disinfecting hub with alcohol when entry is required, use of closed medication systems, daily fluid and tubing changes using sterile technique, infection surveillance, and removal of catheter when appropriate (Doyle et al., 2011; Garland et al., 2008; Saiman, 2006). Removal of unnecessary catheters in particular is important as duration of catheter is a risk of CLABSI. Sengupta and colleagues reported incidence of CLABSI increased by 14% per day during the first 18 days, decreased by 20% during day 19 through 35, then increased by 33% per day after 35 days (Sengupta, Lehmann, Diener-West, Perl, & Milstone, 2010). VAP bundles have not been widely implemented in the neonatal population. A VAP bundle in the NICU might include hand hygiene, the use of in-line suction devices, limitation of saline administration, and surveillance.

Neonatal care providers continuously seek strategies to reduce the likelihood of colonization by antibiotic-resistant organisms. The use of probiotics is one strategy under investigation. The theory behind probiotics is viable nonpathogen bacteria, such as *Lactobacillus acidophilus* or *Bificobacterium infantis*, fed enterally compete with potential pathogen-producing antibiotic-resistant organisms. Results of studies are mixed, with optimal dosing, organism type, and effectiveness to be established (Saiman, 2006). The use of breast milk is protective, with decreased incidence of necrotizing enterocolitis and other infections documented. Breast milk contains 23 to 130 different oligosaccharides, a substance utilized by bifidobacteria. Lactoferrin in breast milk has anti-inflammatory, antimicrobial, and immunomodulatory properties (Higgins et al., 2010).

One strategy to reduce infections is the development of vaccines. This strategy effectively reduced the incidence of *Haemophilus influenza* serotype b (HIB) disease by 99% after it was introduced in 1990. Less than 1 case per 100,000 children under 5 years of age contracts this disease after the introduction of the immunization program (Centers for Disease Control and Prevention, 2008). Vaccine development is a goal in the fight against HIV. Infants remain at risk worldwide from perinatal transfer and through breastfeeding. A vaccine would be a lower cost alternative to detection and treatment of the disease. Current research involves nonhuman primate models and some studies in Africa with a population of neonates with known exposure (Cunningham & McFarland, 2008; Marthas & Miller, 2007). Research is in early stages, with safety and efficacy yet to be established.

The symptoms of sepsis are nonspecific in neonates, resulting in empiric treatment prior to obtaining a negative blood culture. Improved detection methods may help distinguish those episodes that are most likely sepsis-related from those that are related to other causes. Adjunctive tests such as C-reactive protein, procalcitonin, or interleukin-8 may help to distinguish cases of sepsis (Higgins et al., 2010; Patel et al., 2009; Zingg et al., 2011). Early detection also allows streamlining of antibiotics to those most likely to treat the microorganism. PCR tests are under investigation for some microorganisms such as Group B *Streptococcus*, *Escherichia coli*, *Candida albicans*, and MRSA (Enomoto, et al., 2009; Francis et al., 2010).

ANTIMICROBIAL STEWARDSHIP

Antimicrobial stewardship is the cornerstone in the battle against antimicrobial resistance. It is defined as "the optimal selection, dose, and duration of an antimicrobial that results in the best clinical outcome for the treatment or prevention of infection, with minimal toxicity to the patient, and minimal impact on subsequent resistance" (Lipsett, 2008; Louie, 2011). The goal of such a program is to preserve the effectiveness of prescribed antimicrobials by reducing resistance. Additional benefits include a reduction in costs, fewer antibiotic-related adverse events, and shorter hospital length of stay (Di Pentima & Chan, 2010; Louie, 2011; Newland & Hersh, 2010). Core strategies of antimicrobial stewardship include monitoring antimicrobial prescription and infectious agents, providing practitioners with feedback on this monitoring, and restricted use of certain antimicrobials to protect their effectiveness. Additional strategies include education, development of guidelines and policies, use of tools such as computerized order entry or automatic stop orders, dose optimization, cycling of antibiotics, and deescalation of therapy (Newland & Hersh, 2010). Programs can be highly structured with formulary restriction and preauthorization, formal committees including an infectious disease specialist and pharmacist, and computerized order templates (Lipsett, 2008; Louie, 2011). Medical providers prefer programs that offer guidance over those that restrict prescriptive privileges (Patel, Rosen, Zaoutis, Prasad, & Saiman, 2010).

Principles of appropriate antimicrobial usage include prescribing only when clinically indicated, basing empiric antimicrobial selection on local flora and antimicrobial resistance patterns, adjusting antimicrobials according to susceptibilities obtained and within as narrow of coverage as to be effective, assuring dose and timing provide therapeutic levels for the required duration, and stopping the drugs as soon as appropriate (Hart, 2011). It is estimated that antibiotic use is unnecessary or inappropriate in 50% of treatment episodes (Fishman, 2006). Patients and families can pressure practitioners to prescribe antimicrobials when they are not needed. Past practice in pediatrics included prescribing antibiotics for respiratory illnesses that were most likely viral and not affected by the antibiotics (Hart, 2011). This resulted in microorganisms exposed to many antimicrobials in their environment, contributing to the selective pressure favoring resistant organisms. Infectious disease committees for hospitals, state departments of health, and various surveillance systems tabulate statistics on infectious agents and their antimicrobial resistance patterns. This information can guide choice of empiric antibiotics. While early-onset infections are initially treated with ampicillin and gentamycin, late onset infections empiric choice reflect broad-spectrum coverage of those microorganisms most likely to cause infection. In the past, this empiric choice often involved a cephalosporin, contributing to the selective pressure for ESBL-producing microorganisms. Once culture and sensitivity results are obtained antimicrobial coverage should be adjusted to monotherapy with a narrower activity if possible (Fishman, 2006). Infection with multiple microorganisms may require multiple antibiotics (Vrtis, 2008). Failure to adjust to an appropriate antimicrobial can contribute to increased morbidity and mortality (Apisarnthanarak, Holzmann-Pazgal, Hamvas, Olsen, & Fraser, 2004). Monitoring of drug levels and compliance with recommended dose and frequency based on gestational and postconceptual age promotes maintenance of levels above the MIC. Subtherapeutic levels will target susceptible microorganisms while allowing resistant agents to proliferate. Suspected infections are generally screened by blood culture and covered by empiric antibiotics. Practitioners should stop antibiotics if cultures fail to turn positive in 48 hours, limiting unnecessary environmental exposure. Duration of antimicrobial coverage is governed by the type of infection and proof of sterilization of the infected site. Any protracted exposure beyond that necessary to treat the infection contributes to the selective pressure for resistance.

In an era of rising resistance and limited development of new classes of antimicrobials, it is essential to protect the effectiveness of the current antimicrobials. Restricted use of certain antimicrobials is a strategy to reduce resistance. Vancomycin is the drug most commonly restricted as it is associated with the development of VRE (Chiu et al., 2011; Louie, 2011; Mulvey & Simor, 2009). A vancomycin restriction policy at a Delaware children's hospital reduced the incidence of VRE (Di Pentima & Chan, 2010). Chiu et al. (2011) showed no increase in morbidity or mortality when vancomycin use was restricted to specific indications and no longer used for general empiric therapy. Its effectiveness in treating infections caused by ESBL-producing microorganisms is another reason to protect it. Other antimicrobials that may be restricted include carbapenums, linezolid, and fourth-generation cephalosporins. The substitution of beta-lactam-beta-lactamase inhibitors for cephalosporins resulted in decreased prevalence of ESBL-producing pathogens in a nursery in Korea (Lee et al., 2007). Restriction of cephalosporins in a nursery in India led to a 22% reduction in ESBL-producing gram-negative bacteria (Murki et al., 2010). Restrictions may come in the form of guidelines, preauthorization, or post-prescription review (Louie, 2011). Antibiotic cycling is another strategy. This cycling is a scheduled rotation of two or more antibiotic classes with similar range of activity over a specific time period, eventually returning to the original antibiotic class. Time periods vary from 1 to 4 months. The theory behind cycling is to reduce the selective pressure by limiting the exposure time to a particular antibiotic class. Evidence has not supported this strategy (Fishman, 2006; Lipsett, 2008).

Optimizing antimicrobial therapy involves tailoring dosing and method of antimicrobial administration to take advantage of the drug's pharmacodynamics. In the neonatal field this is an area of evolution with limited studies available. Potential alternate dosing regimens include continuous infusion or prolonged intermittent infusion. These alternate dosing methods can be effective for time-dependent antimicrobials, increasing the total time above the MIC (Shea & Jacobi, 2009). Inhaled antibiotic administration offers the potential for local action with minimal systemic adverse effects. Intermittent aerosolized administration of antibiotics has been used in older patients with *P. aeruginosa* pneumonia, particularly with patients with cystic fibrosis (Kanj & Kanafani, 2011). Antimicrobial stewardship promotes appropriate antimicrobial prescription through recommendations on antibiotic choice to narrow the therapy and eliminate redundancy, monitoring effectiveness, and providing reminders when antibiotics should be stopped (Hersh, Beekmann, Polgreen, Zaoutis, & Newland, 2009).

SUMMARY

Sepsis and the steps to reduce it are a part of the NICU life. When acuity increases and the census rises, it is easy to forget compliance with those mechanisms that protect our patients. Hand hygiene, isolation precautions, and surveillance are a necessary burden. Antimicrobial stewardship offers many benefits, including reduction of antimicrobial resistance. We may not be able to eliminate resistant organisms, but we can limit their spread and slow their development.

Thirty years ago, the emerging infectious disease was HIV, an evolved zoonotic pathogen. Today's emerging diseases focus on antimicrobial-resistant microorganisms. Tomorrow's emerging pathogens will be equally challenging. The development of new diagnostic tests and antimicrobial agents remains important and will involve research within and outside of the NICU.

CASE STUDY

■ **Identification of the Problem.** Baby W is a 1,060 g 27-week gestation female infant who presented with pustules on the right foot and right index finger on DOL 20.

■ **Assessment: History and Physical Examination** The mother presented in premature labor 3 days before delivery. Her membranes were intact, GBS status negative, and no other risk factors for sepsis were present. She received tocolytics, a betamethasone course, and magnesium sulfate. Labor progressed, membranes were ruptured artificially in the operating room (OR), and the infant was delivered by cesarean section due to breech presentation.

The infant was intubated in the OR for ineffective respiratory effort. Apgar scores were 4 at 1 minute and 6 at 5 minutes. The infant received assisted ventilation and two doses of Survanta, had umbilical lines placed, cultures and CBC with differential were drawn, and was placed on ampicillin and gentamycin. Baby W weaned on ventilator settings and was extubated to CPAP +8 on DOL 2. Caffeine was started for infrequent apnea. Cultures remained negative, and antibiotics were discontinued at 48 hours. On DOL 4 the infant weaned to high-flow nasal cannula 4 L/min. On DOL 10 the infant developed increased frequency of apnea/bradycardia/desaturation episodes and was placed back on CPAP. A systolic, grade II/VI murmur was noted, and an echocardiogram showed a patent ductus arteriosus (PDA). Treatment for the PDA consisted of a course of indomethacin—follow-up echocardiogram showed a miniscule, hemodynamic-insignificant PDA. The infant received parenteral nutrition from admission. Enteral feedings were initiated by DOL 4, advanced to full feedings by DOL 14, and then the infant was made NPO during treatment of the PDA. Reinitiation of feedings was hindered by feeding intolerance manifested by abdominal distention and nonbilious aspirants. Parenteral nutrition was resumed via a peripheral IV.

On DOL 20 the infant was on CPAP +8 FIO2 0.25. There were no episodes of apnea/bradycardia/desaturation. The vital signs were: respiratory rate 36 to 58, heart rate 158 to 180, mean blood pressure 41 to 54, temperature 36.7 to 37.6. Baby W had mild intercostal retractions, bilateral breath sounds clear and equal, a grade I/VI systolic murmur, peripheral and femoral pulses 2+ equal, a softly distended abdomen with good bowel sounds, good tone, and soft and flat fontanelles. Pustules were noted on the right foot and right index finger.

■ **Differential Diagnosis**

- Skin infection, organism unknown (possible organisms include staphylococcus, streptococcus, listeria, pseudomonas, candida, herpes)
- Erythema toxicum or other transient skin lesions

■ **Diagnostic Tests**

- Blood, urine, lesion, and CSF cultures
- CBC with differential
- Lumbar puncture for CSF culture, glucose, protein, cell count, and HSV

■ **Working Diagnosis.** A skin infection, potentially contagious and transmittable, was the most concerning potential diagnosis. The CBC showed an elevated white count of 26, with a differential of 40% neutrophils, 19% bands, and 21% lymphocytes. The immature-to-mature neutrophil ratio was 0.32, suggestive of sepsis. The infant also had a platelet count of 46 and a hematocrit of 33.

■ **Development of Management Plan.** The infant was placed on contact isolation. After cultures were drawn, empiric antibiotic treatment consisted of oxacillin and gentamycin. A repeat CBC showed platelets of 46 and a hematocrit of 29, prompting transfusions of both platelets and packed red blood cells. A serum chemistry was ordered and found to be normal. Infectious disease was consulted.

■ **Implementation and Evaluation of Effectiveness** Gram-positive cocci were seen in less than 24 hours, with positive identification of MRSA from both the pustules and blood. Sensitivities showed the organism resistant to both oxacillin and penicillin, but sensitive to vancomycin and gentamycin. Antibiotic coverage was switched from oxacillin to vancomycin, with gentamycin continued until other species could be ruled out. Vancomycin and gentamycin levels were monitored. Repeat blood cultures obtained on DOL 22 and 26 continued to be positive despite antibiotics, prompting a search for alternative infection sites. Cultures from a second lumbar puncture remained negative. An echocardiogram ruled out vegetation. Ultrasounds of the neck vessels and abdomen/kidneys ruled out septic emboli. Radiographic exam of the long bones ruled out osteomyelitis. On DOL 27 an MRI detected a brain abscess. The infant never demonstrated any seizure activity or focal deficits. Rifampin was added to the antibiotic coverage for improved CNS penetration, gentamycin was discontinued, and antibiotic coverage continued for 8 weeks (2 weeks beyond repeat MRI-documented absence of the brain abscess). Vancomycin dosing frequency was adjusted to maintain levels of 20 to 25 for troughs and peak level of 30 to 35. The medical team monitored weekly vancomycin levels, CBC with differential, chemistry profiles (including electrolytes, BUN, Creatinine, glucose), and liver function tests. Repeat blood cultures on day of life 28 and 31 were negative. The infant weaned to high flow nasal cannula on DOL 36. Placement of a percutaneous central line was postponed until negative cultures were obtained. Repeat skeletal films on DOL 48 showed a lucency on the right proximal femur indicative of osteomyelitis. The repeat MRI on DOL 48 showed the abscess reduced in size but still present. The infant required no additional length of antibiotic treatment due to concurrent treatment for the undrained brain abscess.

Baby W will require monitoring for hearing loss and motor skill/intelligence deficits. Her hearing will be screened prior to discharge. She will receive close neurodevelopmental follow-up through the hospital's follow-up clinic and referral to early intervention. The length of the right leg in comparison to the left leg will be closely monitored due to concerns for impaired growth secondary to the osteomyelitis.

Of note, the infant had routine surveillance MRSA cultures from both nares done on DOL 4, 32, and 36: all were negative. A second infant had a positive surveillance MRSA culture obtained 17 days after Baby W's infection. Molecular typing showed the second infant had the same strain as Baby W. The two infants shared nurses for multiple days.

EVIDENCE-BASED PRACTICE BOX

The evidence supporting antiretroviral prophylaxis to prevent mother-to-child transmission of HIV is extensive. For a complete summary of the major studies on this topic refer to Table 3 at http://www.aidsinfo.nih.gov/contentfiles/lVguidelines/perinatalgl.pdf. The majority of studies cited are randomized control with sufficient sample size. These studies include four comparing zidovudine to placebo, two comparing other antiretrovirals to zidovudine, 15 comparing various HAART regimens with zidovudine, and three comparing effectiveness of various HAART regimens with another regimen. Observational studies include two cohort studies looking at infants whose mothers received antenatal/intrapartum antiretrovirals versus those who received just postbirth ART. Each individual recommendation within the text of the guideline *Recommendations for Use of Antiretroviral Drugs in Pregnant HIV-1-Infected Women for Maternal Health and Interventions to Reduce Perinatal HIV Transmission in the United States* (*updated September 14, 2011*) is rated as to the strength and quality of the evidence. Recommendations are rated A (strong evidence), B (moderate evidence), or C (optional based on existing evidence). The quality of evidence is rated I, II, or III. The highest quality, I, has one or more randomized trials with clinical outcomes and/or validated laboratory endpoints supporting the evidence. Quality II is supported by one or more well-designed, nonrandomized or observational cohort studies with long-term clinical evidence. Quality III evidence is supported by expert opinion (Panel on Treatment of HIV-infected Pregnant Women and Prevention of Perinatal Transmission, 2011). The guideline is 207 pages in length and will not be published in this textbook. A discussion of the findings of these studies is contained within the text of this chapter.

ONLINE RESOURCES

Emerging Infections Program-Centers for Disease Control and Prevention
http://www.cdc.gov/ncezid/dpei/eip/index.html

Emerging Viral Infections in Neonatal Intensive Care Unit
http://www.ncbi.nlm.nih.gov/pubmed/21877999

H1N1 Influenza Vaccination During Pregnancy and Fetal and Neonatal Outcomes.
http://www.ncbi.nlm.nih.gov/pubmed/22515877

Rapid Whole-Genome Sequencing for Investigation Neonatal MRSA Outbreak
http://www.nejm.org/doi/full/10.1056/NEJMoa1109910

Worldwide Database of Health Care-Associated Outbreaks
http://www.outbreak-database.com

REFERENCES

Abdel-Hady, H., Hawas, S., El-Daker, M., & El-Kady, R. (2008). Extended-spectrum β-lactamase producing *Klebsiella pneumoniae* in neonatal intensive care unit. *Journal of Perinatology, 28*, 685–690.

Aderinboye, O., & Syed, S. S. (2010). Congenital babesiosis in a four-week-old female infant. *The Pediatric Infectious Disease Journal, 29*(2), 188.

Adhikari, M., Pillay, T., & Pillay, D. G. (1997). Tuberculosis in the newborn: An emerging disease. *The Pediatric Infectious Disease Journal, 16*(12), 1108–1112.

Al-Tawfiq, J. A. (2006). Father-to-infant transmission of community-acquired methicillin-resistant *Staphylococcus aureus* in a neonatal intensive care unit. *Infection Control and Hospital Epidemiology, 27*(6), 636–637.

Andrews, T. M. (2003). Current concepts in antibiotic resistance. *Current Opinion in Otolaryngology & Head and Neck Surgery, 11*, 409–415.

ANRS 1201/1202 DITRAME PLUS Study Group. (2005). Field efficacy of zidovudine, lamivudine and single-dose nevirapine to prevent peripartum HIV transmission. *AIDS, 19*(3), 309–318.

Apisarnthanarak, A., Holzmann-Pazgal, G., Hamvas, A., Olsen, M. A., & Fraser, V. J. (2004). Antimicrobial use and the influence of inadequate empiric antimicrobial therapy on the outcomes of nosocomial bloodstream infections in a neonatal intensive care unit. *Infection Control and Hospital Epidemiology, 25*(9), 735–741.

Arias, C. A., Contreras, G. A., & Murray, B. E. (2010). Management of multidrug-resistant enterococcal infections. *Clinical Microbiology and Infectious Diseases, 16*, 555–562.

Babazono, A., Kitajima, H., Nishimaki, S., Nakamura, T., Shiga, S., Hayakawa, M., . . . Doi, H. (2008). Risk factors for nosocomial infection in the neonatal intensive care unit by the Japanese Nosocomial Infection Surveillance (JANIS). *Acta Medica Okayama, 62*(4), 261–268.

Bagattini, M., Crivaro, V., Di Popolo, A., Gentile, F., Scarcella, A., Triassi, M., . . . Zarrilli, R. (2006). Molecular epidemiology of extended-spectrum beta-lactamase (ESBL)-producing *Klebsiella pneumoniae* in the neonatal intensive care unit of a university hospital in Italy. *Journal of Antimicrobial Chemotherapy, 57*(5), 979–982.

Baley, J. E., & Toltzis, P. (2006). Perinatal viral infections. In R. J. Martin, A. A. Fanaroff, & M. C. Walsh (Eds.), *Neonatal-perinatal medicine: Diseases of the fetus & infant* (8th ed., pp. 855–861). Philadelphia, PA: Mosby-Elsevier.

Beckerman, K. P. (2005). Identification, evaluation, and care of the human immunodeficiency virus-exposed neonate. In H. W. Taeusch, R. A. Ballard, & C. A. Gleason (Eds.), *Avery's diseases of the newborn* (8th ed., pp. 475–493). Philadelphia, PA: Elsevier Saunders.

Behari, P., Englund, J., Alcasid, G., Garcia-Houchins, S., & Weber, S. G. (2004). Transmission of methicillin-resistant *Staphylococcus aureus* to preterm infants through breast milk. *Infection Control and Hospital Epidemiology, 25*(9), 778–780.

Bell, S. G. (2004). Neonatal viral and fungal infections. In D. Fraser Askin (Ed.), *Infection in the neonate* (pp. 83–127). Santa Rosa, CA: NICU INK.

Bhoopat, L., Khunamornpong, S., Lerdsrimongkol, P., Sirivatanapa, P., Sethavanich, S., Limtrakul, A., . . . Bhoopat, T. (2005). Effectiveness of short-term and long-term zidovudine prophylaxis on detection of HIV-1 subtype E in human placenta and vertical transmission. *Journal of Acquired Immune Deficiency Syndromes, 40*(5), 545–550.

Birkhead, G. S., Pulver, W. P., Warren, B. L., Hackel, S., Rodriguez, D., & Smith, L. (2010). Acquiring human immunodeficiency virus during pregnancy and mother-to-child transmission in New York: 2002–2006. *Obstetrics & Gynecology, 115*(6), 1247–1255.

Bizzarro, M. J., & Gallagher, P. G. (2007). Antibiotic-resistant organisms in the neonatal intensive care unit. *Seminars in Perinatology, 31*, 26–32.

Blaschke, A. J., Korgenski, E. K., Daly, J. D., LaFleur, B., Pavia, A. T., & Byington, C. L. (2009). Extended-spectrum β-lactamase-producing pathogens in a children's hospital: A 5-year experience. *American Journal of Infection Control, 37*(6), 435–441.

Boszczowski, I., Nicoletti, C., Puccini, D. M. T., Pinheiro, M., Soares, R. E., Van Der Heijden, I. M., . . . Levin, A. S. (2005). Outbreak of extended spectrum β-lactamase-producing *Klebsiella pneumoniae* infection in a neonatal intensive care unit related to onychomycosis in a health care worker. *The Pediatric Infectious Disease Journal, 24*(7), 648–650.

Bozzola, E., Quondamcarlo, A., Krzysztofiak, A., Lancella, L., Romano, M., & Tozzi, A. (2011). Re-emergence of measles in young infants. *The Pediatric Infectious Disease Journal, 30*(3), 271.

Briand, N., Mandelbrot, L., Le Chenadec, J., Tubiana, R., Teglas, J.-P., Faye, A., . . . ANRS French Perinatal Cohort. (2009). No relation between in-utero exposure to HAART and intrauterine growth retardation. *AIDS, 23*(10), 1235–1243.

Brouqui, P. (2009). Facing highly infectious diseases: New trends and current concepts. *Clinical Microbiology and Infectious Diseases, 15*, 700–705.

Burton, D. C., Edwards, J. R., Horan, T. C., Jernigan, J. A., & Fridkin, S. K. 2009. Methicillin-resistant *Staphylococcus aureus* central line-associated bloodstream infections in US intensive care units, 1997–2007. *JAMA: The Journal of the American Medical Association, 301*(7), 727–736.

Cable, R. G., & Leiby, D. A. (2003). Risk and prevention of transfusion-transmitted babesiosis and other tick-borne diseases. *Current Opinion in Hematology, 10*(6), 405–411.

Carey, A. J., Della-Latta, P., Huard, R., Wu, F., Graham, P. L., Carp, D., & Saiman, L. (2010). Changes in the molecular epidemiological characteristics of methicillin-resistant *Staphylococcus aureus* in a neonatal intensive care unit. *Infection Control and Hospital Epidemiology, 31*(6), 613–619.

Carey, A. J., Duchon, J., Della-Latta, P., & Saiman, L. (2010). The epidemiology of methicillin-susceptible and methicillin-resistant *Staphylococcus aureus* in a neonatal intensive care unit, 2000–2007. *Journal of Perinatology, 30*(2), 135–139.

Carey, A. J., & Long, S. S. (2010). *Staphylococcus aureus*: A continuously evolving and formidable pathogen in the neonatal intensive care unit. *Clinics in Perinatology, 37*(3). Retrieved February 3, 2012, from OVID.

Carey, A. J., Saiman, L., & Polin, R. A. (2008). Hospital-acquired infections in the NICU: Epidemiology for the new millennium. *Clinics in Perinatology, 35*(1). Retrieved February 3, 2012, from OVID.

Castillo-Salgado, C. (2010). Trends and directions of global public health surveillance. *Epidemiologic Reviews, 32*, 93–109.

Centers for Disease Control and Prevention (CDC). (2008). *Haemophilus influenza* serotype b (HIB). Retrieved from www.cdc.gov/ncidod/dbmd/disease info/haeminfluerob_t.htm

Centers for Disease Control and Prevention (CDC). (2007). Mother-to-child (perinatal) HIV transmission and prevention. Retrieved from www.cdc.gov/hiv/topics/perinatal/resources/factsheets/pdf/perinatal.pdf

Chi, B. H., Wang, L., Read, J. S., Sheriff, M., Fiscus, S., Brown, E. R., . . . Goldenberg, R. (2005). Timing of maternal and neonatal dosing of nevirapine and the risk of mother-to-child transmission of HIV-1: HIVNET 024. *AIDS, 19*(16), 1857–1864.

Chiu, C.-H., Michelow, I. C., Cronin, J., Ringer, S. A., Ferris, T. G., & Puopolo, K. M. (2011). Effectiveness of a guideline to reduce vancomycin use in the neonatal intensive care unit. *The Pediatric Infectious Disease Journal, 30*(4), 273–278.

Chiu, S., Huang, Y.-C., Lien, R.-I., Chou, Y.-H., & Lin, T.-Y. (2005). Clinical features of nosocomial infections by extended-spectrum β-lactamase-producing *Enterobacteriaceae* in neonatal intensive care units. *Acta Paediatrica, 94*, 1644–1649.

Chuang, Y.-Y., Huang, Y.-C., Lee, C.-Y., Lin, T.-Y., Lien, R., & Chou, Y.-H. (2004). Methicillin-resistant *Staphylococcus aureus* bacteraemia in neonatal intensive care units: An analysis of 90 episodes. *Acta Paediatrica, 93*, 786–790.

Chung, M. H., Kiarie, J. N., Richardson, B. A., Lehman, D. A., Overbaugh, J., & John-Stewart, G. C. (2005). Breast milk HIV-1 suppression and decreased transmission: A randomized trial comparing HIVNET 012 nevirapine versus short-course zidovudine. *AIDS, 19*(13), 1415–1422.

Collignon, P., Powers, J. H., Chiller, T. M., Aidara-Kane, A., & Aarestrup, F. M. (2009). World Health Organization ranking of antimicrobials according to their importance in human medicine: A critical step for developing risk management strategies for the use of antimicrobials in food production animals. *Clinical Infectious Diseases, 49*(1), 132–141.

Committee on Infectious Diseases, American Academy of Pediatrics. (2009). *Red Book: 2009 Report of the Committee on Infectious Diseases* (28th ed., pp. 380–400). Elkgrove Village, IL: American Academy of Pediatrics.

Connor, E. M., Sperling, R. S., Gelber, R., Kiselev, P., Scott, G., O'Sullivan, M. J., . . . Balsley, J. (1994). Reduction of maternal-infant transmission of human immunodeficiency virus type 1 with zidovudine treatment: Pediatric AIDS clinical trials group protocol 076 study group. *New England Journal of Medicine, 331*, 1173–1180.

Conte, M. P., Venditti, M., Chiarini, F., D'Ettore, G., Zamboni, I., Scoarughi, G. L., . . . Orsi, G. B. (2005). Extended spectrum beta-lactamase–producing *Klebsiella pneumoniae* outbreaks during a third generation cephalosporin restriction policy. *Journal of Chemotherapy, 17*(1), 66–73.

Couto, R. C., Pedrosa, T. M. G., Tofani, Cde P., & Pedroso, E. R. P. (2006). Risk factors for nosocomial infection in a neonatal intensive care unit. *Infection Control and Hospital Epidemiology, 27*(6), 571–575.

Crivaro, V., Bagattini, M., Salza, M. F., Raimondi, F., Rossano, F., Triassi, M., & Zarrilli, R. (2007). Risk factors for extended-spectrum β-lactamase-producing *Serratia marcescens* and

Klebsiella pneumoniae acquisition in a neonatal intensive care unit. *Journal of Hospital Infection, 67*, 135–141.

Cunningham, C. K., & McFarland, E. (2008). Vaccines for prevention of mother-to-child transmission of HIV. *Current Opinion in HIV and AIDS, 3*(2), 151–154.

DeLisle, S., & Perl, T. M. (2003). Vancomycin-resistant enterococci: A road map on how to prevent the emergence and transmission of antimicrobial resistance. *CHEST, 123*, 504S–518S.

Di Pentima, M. C., & Chan, S. (2010). Impact of antimicrobial stewardship program on vancomycin use in a pediatric teaching hospital. *The Pediatric Infectious Disease Journal, 29*(8), 707–711.

Dobroszycki, J., Herwaldt, B. L., Boctor, F., Miller, J. R., Linden, J., Eberhard, M. L., . . . Wittner, M. (1999). A cluster of transfusion-associated babesiosis cases traced to a single asymptomatic donor. *JAMA: The Journal* of *the American Medical Association, 281*(10), 927–930.

Donlan, R. M. (2000). Role of biofilms in antimicrobial resistance. *ASAIO Journal, 46*, S47–S52.

Doyle, J. S., Buising, K. L., Thursky, K. A., Worth, L. J., & Richards, M. J. (2011). Epidemiology of infections acquired in intensive care units. *Seminars in Respiratory and Critical Care Medicine, 32*, 115–138.

Eckhardt, C., Halvosa, J. S., Ray, S. M., & Blumberg, H. M. (2003). Transmission of methicillin-resistant *Staphylococcus aureus* in the neonatal intensive care unit from a patient with community-acquired disease. *Infection Control and Hospital Epidemiology, 24*(6), 460–461.

El Beitune, P., Duarte, G., Foss, M. C., Montenegro, R. M., Quintana, S. M., Figueiró-Filho, E. A., & Nogueira, A. A. (2005). Effect of maternal use of antiretroviral agents on serum insulin levels of the newborn. *Diabetes Care, 28*(4), 856–859.

Enomoto, M., Morioka, I., Morisawa, T., Yokoyama, N., & Matsuo, M. (2009). A novel tool for detecting neonatal infections using multiplex polymerase chain reaction. *Neonatology, 96*(2), 102–108.

European Collaborative Study. (2005). Does exposure to antiretroviral therapy affect growth in the first 18 months of life in uninfected children born to HIV-infected women? *JAIDS Journal of Acquired Immune Deficiency Syndromes, 40*(3), 364–370.

Feiterna-Sperling, C., Weizsaecker, K., Bührer, C., Casteleyn, S., Loui, A., Schmitz, T., . . . Obladen, M. (2007). Hematologic effects of maternal antiretroviral therapy and transmission prophylaxis in HIV-1-exposed uninfected newborn infants. *JAIDS Journal of Acquired Immune Deficiency Syndromes, 45*(1), 43–51.

Ferguson, W., Goode, M., Walsh, A., Gavin, P., & Butler, K. (2011). Evaluation of 4 weeks' neonatal antiretroviral prophylaxis as a component of a prevention of mother-to-child transmission program in a resource-rich setting. *The Pediatric Infectious Disease Journal, 30*(5), 408–412.

Fishman, N. (2006). Antimicrobial stewardship. *American Journal of Infection Control, 34*, S55–S63.

Fox, L. M., Wingerter, S., Ahmed, A., Arnold, A., Chou, J., Rhein, L., & Levy, O. (2006). Neonatal babesiosis: Case report and review of the literature. *The Pediatric Infectious Disease Journal, 25*(2), 169–173.

Francis, S. T., Rawal, S., Roberts, H., Riley, P., Planche, T., & Kennea, N. L. (2010). Detection of methicillin-resistant *Staphylococcus aureus* (MRSA) colonization in newborn infants using real-time polymerase chain reaction (PCR). *Acta Paediatrica, 99*, 1691–1694.

Freeman, C. D. (1997). Antimicrobial resistance: Implications for the clinician. *Critical Care Nursing Quarterly, 20*(3), 21–35.

Garland, J. S., Alex, C. P., Sevallius, J. M., Murphy, D. M., Good, M. J., Volberding, A. M., . . . Maki, D. G. (2008). Cohort study of the pathogenesis and molecular epidemiology of catheter-related bloodstream infection in neonates with peripherally inserted central venous catheters. *Infection Control and Hospital Epidemiology, 29*(3), 243–249.

Gerber, S. I., Jones, R. C., Scott, M. V., Price, J. S., Dworkin, M. S., Filipell, M. B., . . . Noskin, G. A. (2006). Management of outbreaks of methicillin-resistant *Staphylococcus aureus* infection in the neonatal intensive care unit: A consensus statement. *Infection Control and Hospital Epidemiology, 27*(2), 139–145.

Germain, M., & Goldman, M. (2002). Blood donor selection and screening: Strategies to reduce recipient risk. *American Journal of Therapeutics, 9*(5), 406–410.

Gomez-Gonzalez, C., Alba, C., Otero, J. R., Sanz, F., & Chaves, F. (2007). Long persistence of methicillin-susceptible strains of *Staphylococcus aureus* causing sepsis in a neonatal intensive care unit. *Journal of Clinical Microbiology, 45*(7), 2301–2304.

Gould, E. (2009). Emerging viruses and the significance of climate change. *Clinics in Microbiology and Infections, 15*(6), 503.

Graham, J., Stockley, K., & Goldman, R. D. (2011). Tick-borne Illnesses: A CME update. *Pediatric Emergency Care, 27*(2), 141–147.

Grant, P. S., Charns, L. G., Rawot, B. W., & Benedetti, S. G. (2008). Consideration to culture health care workers related to increased methicillin-resistant *Staphylococcus aureus* activity in a neonatal intensive care unit. *American Journal Infection Control, 36*(9), 638–643.

Greenfield, R. A., & Bronze, M. S. (2010). Emerging pathogens and knowledge in infectious diseases. *The American Journal of the Medical Sciences, 340*(3), 177–180.

Gregory, M. L., Eichenwald, E. C., & Puopolo, K. M. (2009). Seven-year experience with a surveillance program to reduce methicillin-resistant *Staphylococcus aureus* colonization in a neonatal intensive care unit. *Pediatrics, 123*, e790–e796. Retrieved October 21, 2011 from OVID.

Grohskopf, L. A., Huskins, W. C., Sinkowitz-Cochran, R. L., Levine, G. L., Goldmann, D. A., Jarvis, W. R., & Pediatric Prevention Network. 2005. Use of antimicrobial agents in United States neonatal and pediatric intensive care patients. *The Pediatric Infectious Disease Journal, 24*(9), 766–773.

Gundes, S., Arisoy, A. E., Kolayli, F., Karaali, E., Turker, G., Sanic, A., . . . Vahaboglu, H. (2005). An outbreak of SHV-5 producing *Klebsiella pneumoniae* in a neonatal intensive care unit; meropenem failed to avoid fecal colonization. *The New Microbiologica, 28*(3), 231–236.

Gupta, M., & Pursley, D. M. (2011, June). A survey of infection control practices for influenza in mother and newborn units in US Hospitals. *American Journal of Obstetrics & Gynecology*, S77–S83. Retrieved October 21, 2011, from OVID.

Haeri, S., Shauer, M., Dale, M., Leslie, J., Baker, A. M., Saddlemire, S., & Boggess, K. (2009). Obstetric and newborn infant outcomes in human immunodeficiency virus-infected women who receive highly active antiretroviral therapy. *American Journal of Obstetrics and Gynecology, 201*(3), 315e1–315e5. Retrieved April 6, 2012, from OVID.

Hart, A. M. (2011, November). Antibiotic stewardship to preserve benefits. *The Clinical Advisor, 14*(11), 45–55.

Healy, C. M., Hulten, K. G., Palazzi, D. L., Campbell, J. R., & Baker, C. J. (2004). Emergence of new strains of methicillin-resistant *Staphylococcus aureus* in a neonatal intensive care unit. *Clinical Infectious Diseases, 39*(10), 1460–1466.

Healy, S. P., & Zervos, M. J. (1995). Mechanisms of resistance of enterococci to antimicrobial agents. *Reviews in Medical Microbiology, 6*(1), 70–76.

Heinrich, N., Mueller, A., Bartmann, P., Simon, A., Bierbaum, G., & Engelhart, S. (2011). Successful management of an MRSA outbreak in a neonatal intensive care unit. *European Journal of Clinical Microbiology & Infectious Diseases, 30*(7), 909–913.

Hernàndez, S., Morén, C., López, M., Coll, O., Cardellach, F., Gratacós, E., . . . Garrabou, G. (2012). Perinatal outcomes, mitochondrial toxicity and apoptosis in HIV-treated pregnant women and in-utero-exposed newborn. *AIDS, 26*(4), 419–428.

Hersh, A. L., Beekmann, S. E., Polgreen, P. M., Zaoutis, T. E., & Newland, J. G. (2009). Antimicrobial stewardship programs in pediatrics. *Infection Control and Hospital Epidemiology, 30*(12), 1211–1217.

Herwaldt, B. L., Linden, J. V., Bosserman, E., Young, C., Olkowska, D., & Wilson, M. (2011). Transfusion-associated babesiosis in the United States: A description of cases. *Annals of Internal Medicine, 155*(8), 509–519.

Higgins, R. D., Baker, C. J., & Raju, T. N. K. (2010). Executive summary of the workshop on infection in the high risk neonate. *Journal of Perinatology, 30*(6), 379–383.

Huang, Y.-C., Chou, Y.-H., Su, L.-H., Lien, R.-I., & Lin, T.-Y. (2006). Methicillin-resistant *Staphylococcus aureus* colonization and its association with infection among infants hospitalized in neonatal intensive care units. *Pediatrics, 118*(2), 469–474.

Huang, Y. C., Lien, R. I., Su, L. H., Chou, Y. H., & Lin, T. Y. (2011). Successful control of methicillin-resistant *Staphylococcus aureus* in endemic neonatal intensive care units—a 7-year campaign. *PLoS One*, e23001, Retrieved October 21, 2011 from OVID.

Huang, Y., Zhuang, S., & Du, M. (2007). Risk factors of nosocomial infection with extended-spectrum beta-lactamase-producing bacteria in a neonatal intensive care unit in China. *Infection, 35*(5), 339–345.

Iregbu, K. C., & Anwaal, U. (2007). Extended-spectrum beta-lactamase-producing *Klebsiella pneumoniae* septicaemia outbreak in the neonatal intensive care unit of a tertiary hospital in Nigeria. *African Journal of Medicine and Medical Sciences, 36*(3), 225–228.

Jain, A., Agarwal, J., & Bansal, S. (2004). Prevalence of methicillin-resistant, coagulase-negative staphylococci in neonatal intensive care units: Findings from a tertiary care hospital in India. *Journal of Medical Microbiology, 53*, 941–944.

Jain, A., Roy, I., Gupta, M. K., Kumar, M., & Agarwal, S. K. (2003). Prevalence of extended-spectrum β-lactamase-producing gram-negative bacteria in septicaemic neonates in a tertiary care hospital. *Journal of Medical Microbiology, 52*(5), 421–425.

Jamieson, D. J., Clark, J., Kourtis, A. P., Taylor, A. W., Lampe, M. A., Fowler, M. G., . . . Mofenson, L. M. (2007). Recommendations for human immunodeficiency virus screening, prophylaxis, and treatment for pregnant women in the United States. *American Journal of Obstetrics and Gynecology, 197*(3), S26–S32.

Jamieson, D. J., Rasmussen, S. A., Uyeki, T. M., & Weinbaum, C. (2011, June). Pandemic influenza and pregnancy revisited: Lessons learned from 2009 pandemic influenza A (H1N1). *American Journal of Obstetrics & Gynecology, 204*(Suppl. 6), S1–S3.

Johnson, J. G., & Talbot, T. R. (2011). New approaches for influenza vaccination of healthcare workers. *Current Opinion in Infectious Diseases, 24*(4), 363–369.

Johnson, P. J. (2012). Antibiotic resistance in the NICU. *Neonatal Network, 31*(2), 109–114.

John-Stewart, G. (2012). Prevention of HIV transmission through breastfeeding in resource-limited settings. Retrieved April 6, 2012, from *UpToDate*.

Joint United Nations Programme on HIV/AIDS. (2011). UNAIDS world AIDS day report. Retrieved April 6, 2012, from www.unaids.org/en/media/unaids/contentassets/documents/unaidspublication/2011/JC2216_ worldAIDSday_report_2011_en.pdf

Kamath, S., Mallaya, S., & Shenoy, S. (2010). Nosocomial infections in neonatal intensive care units: Profile, risk factor assessment and antibiogram. *Indian Journal of Pediatrics, 77*(1), 37–39.

Kanj, S. S., & Kanafani, Z. A. (2011). Current concepts in antimicrobial therapy against resistant gram-negative organisms: Extended-spectrum β-Lactamase-producing enterobacteriaceae, carbapenem-resistant enterobacteriaceae, and multidrug-resistant *Pseudomonas aeruginosa. Mayo Clinic Proceedings, 86*(3), 250–259.

The Kesho Bora Study Group. (2010). Eighteen-month follow-up of HIV-1-infected mothers and their children enrolled in the Kesho Bora study observational cohorts. *Journal of Acquired Immune Deficiency Syndromes, 54*(5), 533–541.

Khamduang, W., Jourdain, G., Sirirungsi, W., Layangool, P., Kanjanavanit, S., Krittigamas, P., . . . Program for HIV Prevention and Treatment (PHPT) Study Group. (2011). The interrelated transmission of HIV-1 and cytomegalovirus during gestation and delivery in the offspring of HIV-infected mothers. *JAIDS Journal of Acquired Immune Deficiency Syndromes, 58*(2), 188–192.

Khoury, J., Jones, M., Grimm, A., Dunne, W. M., & Fraser, V. (2005). Eradication of methicillin-resistant *Staphylococcus aureus* from a neonatal intensive care unit by active surveillance and aggressive infection control measures. *Infection Control and Hospital Epidemiology, 26*(7), 616–621.

Kim, Y. H., Chang, S. S., Kim, Y. S., Kim, E. A.-R., Yun, S. C., Kim, K. S., & Pi, S. Y. (2007). Clinical outcomes in methicillin-resistant *Staphylococcus aureus*-colonized neonates in the neonatal intensive care unit. *Neonatology, 91*, 241–247.

Krause, P. J., Lepore, T., Sikand, V. K., Gadbaw, J., Jr., Burke, G., Telford, S. R., 3rd, . . . Spielman, A. (2000). Atovaquone and azithromycin for the treatment of babesiosis. *New England Journal of Medicine, 343*, 1454–1458.

Kriebs, J. M. (2006). Changing the paradigm: HIV in pregnancy. *The Journal of Perinatal & Neonatal Nursing, 20*(1), 71–73.

Kristóf, K., Szabo, D., March, J. W., Cser, V., Janik, L., Rozgonyi, F., . . . Paterson, D. L. (2007). Extended-spectrum beta-lactamase-producing *Klebsiella* spp. in a neonatal intensive care unit: Risk factors for the infection and the dynamics of the molecular epidemiology. *European Journal of Clinical Microbiology and Infectious Disease, 26*, 563–570.

Lee, J., Pai, H., Kim, Y. K., Kim, N. H., Eun, B. W., Kang, H. J., . . . Ahn, H. S. (2007). Control of extended-spectrum β-lactamase-producing *Escherichia coli* and *Klebsiella pneumoniae* in a children's hospital by changing antimicrobial agent usage policy. *Journal of Antimicrobial Chemotherapy, 60*(3), 629–637.

Lepelletier, D., Corvec, S., Caillon, J., Reynaud, A., Rozé, J.-C., & Gras-Leguen, C. (2009). Eradication of methicillin-resistant *staphylococcus aureus* in a neonatal intensive care unit: Which measures for which success? *American Journal of Infection Control, 37*(3), 195–200.

Lessa, F. C., Edwards, J. R., Fridkin, S. K., Tenover, F. C., Horan, T. C., & Gorwitz, R. J. (2009). Trends in incidence of late-onset methicillin-resistant *Staphylococcus aureus* infection in neonatal intensive care units: Data from the National Nosocomial Infections Surveillance System, 1995–2004. *The Pediatric Infectious Disease Journal, 28*(7), 577–581.

Linkin, D. R., Fishman, N. O., Patel, J. B., Merrill, J. D., & Lautenbach, E. (2004). Risk factors for extended-spectrum beta-lactamase-producing *Enterobacteriaceae* in a neonatal intensive care unit. *Infection Control and Hospital Epidemiology, 25*(9), 781–783.

Lipsett, P. A. (2008). Antimicrobial stewardship in the ICU. *Contemporary Critical Care, 6*(5), 1–12.

Lopez-Cerero, L., De Cueto, M., Saenz, C., Navarro, D., Velasco, C., Rodriguez-Bano, J., & Pascual, A. (2008). Neonatal sepsis caused by a CTX-M-32-producing *Escherichia coli* isolate. *Journal of Medical Microbiology, 57*(10), 1303–1305.

Louie, T. (2011). Antimicrobial stewardship: A review. *Infectious Diseases in Clinical Practice, 19*(6), 382–387. Retrieved October 21, 2011 from OVID.

Mammina, C., Di Carlo, P., Cipolla, D., Giuffrè, M., Cassucio, A., Di Gaetano, V., . . . Corsello, G. (2007). Surveillance of multidrug-resistant gram-negative bacilli in a neonatal intensive care unit: Prominent role of cross transmission. *American Journal of Infection Control, 35*(4), 222–230.

Maragakis, L. L. (2010). Recognition and prevention of multidrug-resistant gram-negative bacteria in the intensive care unit. *Critical Care Medicine, 38S*, S345–S351.

Maraqa, N. F., Aigbivbalu, L., Masnia-Iusan, C., Wludyka, P., Shareef, Z., Bailey, C., & Rathore, M. H. (2011). Prevalence of and risk factors for methicillin-resistant *Staphylococcus aureus* colonization and infection among infants at a level III neonatal intensive care unit. *American Journal of Infection Control, 39*(1), 35–41.

Marthas, M., & Miller, C. J. (2007). Developing a neonatal HIV vaccine: Insights from macaque models of pediatric HIV/AIDS. *Current Opinion in HIV and AIDS, 2*(5), 367–374.

McManus, M. C. (1997). Mechanisms of bacterial resistance to antimicrobial agents. *American Journal of Health-System Pharmacy, 54*(12), 1420–1433.

Mendez-Figueroa, H., Raker, C., & Anderson, B. L. (2011, June). Neonatal characteristics and outcomes of pregnancies complicated by influenza infection during the 2009 pandemic. *American Journal of Obstetrics & Gynecology, 204*(Suppl. 6), S58–S63.

Mesa, R. J., Blanc, V., Blanch, A. R., Cortes, P., Gonzalez, J. J., Lavilla, S., . . . Navarro, F. (2006). Extended-spectrum β-lactamase (ESBL)-producing *Enterobacteriaceae* in different environments (humans, food, animal farms and sewage). *Journal of Antimicrobial Chemotherapy, 58*(1), 211–215.

Milstone, A. M., Budd, A., Shepard, J.W., Ross, T., Aucott, S., Carroll, K. C., & Perl, T. M. (2010). Role of decolonization in a comprehensive strategy to reduce methicillin-resistant *Staphylococcus aureus* infections in the neonatal intensive care unit: An observational cohort. *Infection Control and Hospital Epidemiology, 31*(5), 558–560.

Milstone, A. M., Song, X., Coffin, S., & Elward, A. (2010). Identification and eradication of methicillin-resistant *Staphylococcus aureus* colonization in the neonatal intensive care unit: Results of a national survey. *Infection Control and Hospital Epidemiology, 31*(7), 766–768.

Mirochnick, M., Nielsen-Saines, K., Henrique, J., Pinto, J., Jiménez, E., Velosa, V. G., . . . NICHD/HPTN 040/PACTG 1043 Protocol Team. (2008). Nevirapine concentrations in newborns receiving an extended prophylactic regimen. *Journal of Acquired Immune Deficiency Syndromes, 47*(3), 334–337.

Mofenson, L. M. (2009). Non-antiretroviral interventions to reduce perinatal HIV transmission in the developing world. Retrieved April 6, 2012, from *UpToDate*.

Mongkolrattanothai, K., Mankin, P., Cranston, J. B., & Gray, B. M. (2010). Molecular surveillance of *Staphylococcus aureus* colonization in a neonatal intensive care unit. *American Journal of Infection Control, 38*(8), 660–663.

Morgan, D., Kirkbride, H., Hewitt, K., Said, B., & Walsh, A. L. (2009). Assessing the risk from emerging infections. *Epidemiology & Infections, 137*, 1521–1530.

Mosby, L. G., Rasmussen, S. A., & Jamieson, D. J. (2011, July). 2009 pandemic influenza A (H1N1) in pregnancy: A systemic review of the literature. *American Journal of Obstetrics & Gynecology, 205*(1), 10–18.

Mulvey, M. R., & Simor, A. E. (2009). Antimicrobial resistance in hospitals: How concerned should we be? *CMAJ, 180*(4), 408–415.

Murillo, J. L., Cohen, M., & Kreiswirth, B. (2010). Results of nasal screening for methicillin-resistant *Staphylococcus aureus* during a neonatal intensive care unit outbreak. *American Journal of Perinatology, 27*, 79–82.

Murki, S., Jonnala, S., Mohammed, F., & Reddy, A. (2010). Restriction of cephalosporins and control of extended spectrum β-lactamase producing gram negative bacteria in a neonatal intensive care unit. *Indian Pediatrics, 47*, 785–788.

Myers, S. A., Torrente, S., Hinthorn, D., & Clark, P. L. (2005). Life-threatening maternal and fetal macrocytic anemia from antiretroviral therapy. *Obstetrics & Gynecology, 106*(5), 1189–1191.

Nambiar, S., Herwaldt, L. A., & Singh, N. (2003). Outbreak of invasive disease caused by methicillin-resistant *Staphylococcus aureus* in neonates and prevalence in the neonatal intensive care unit. *Pediatric Critical Care Medicine, 4*(2), 220–226.

Newland, J. G., & Hersh, A. L. (2010). Purpose and design of antimicrobial stewardship programs in pediatrics. *The Pediatric Infectious Disease Journal, 29*(9), 862–863.

Ofek-Shlomai, N., Benenson, S., Ergaz, Z., Peleg, O., Braunstein, R., & Bar-Oz, B. (2011). Gastrointestinal colonization with ESBL-producing *Klebsiella* in preterm babies—is vancomycin to blame? *European Journal of Clinical Microbiology & Infectious Diseases*, Retrieved August 4, 2011 from OVID.

Otman, J., Cavassin, E. D., Perugini, M. E., & Vidotto, M. C. (2002). An outbreak of extended-spectrum β-lactamase-producing *Klebsiella* species in a neonatal intensive care unit in Brazil. *Infection Control and Hospital Epidemiology, 23*(1), 8–9.

Panel on Treatment of HIV-infected Pregnant Women and Prevention of Perinatal Transmission. (2011, September 14). Recommendations for use of antiretroviral drugs in pregnant HIV-1-infected women for maternal health and interventions to reduce perinatal HIV transmission in the United States. pp. 1–207. Retrieved April 6, 2012, from http://aidsinfo.nih.gov/contentfiles/PerinatalGL.pdf.

Park, C.-H., Seo, J.-H., Lim, J.-Y., Woo, H.-O., & Youn, H. S. (2007). Changing trend of neonatal infection: Experience at a newly established regional medical center in Korea. *Pediatrics International, 49*, 24–30.

Patel, S. J., Oshodi, A., Prasad, P., Delamora, P., Larson, E., Zaoutis, T., & Saiman, L. (2009). Antibiotic use in neonatal intensive care units and adherence with centers for disease control and prevention 12 step campaign to prevent antimicrobial resistance. *The Pediatric Infectious Disease Journal, 28*(12), 1047–1051.

Patel, S. J., Rosen, E., Zaoutis, T., Prasad, P., & Saiman, L. (2010). Neonatologists' perceptions of antimicrobial resistance and stewardship in neonatal intensive care units. *Infection Control and Hospital Epidemiology, 31*(12), 1298–1299.

Perlman, S. E., Saiman, L., & Larson, E. L. (2007). Risk factors for late-onset health care-associated bloodstream infections in patients in neonatal intensive care units. *American Journal of Infection Control, 35*(3), 177–182.

Pessoa-Silva, C. L., Meurer Moreira, B., Camara Almeida, V., Flannery, B., Almeida Lins, M. C., Mello Sampaio, J. L., . . . Gerberding, J. L. (2003). Extended-spectrum β-lactamase-producing *Klebsiella pneumoniae* in a neonatal intensive care unit: Risk factors for infection and colonization. *Journal of Hospital Infection, 53*, 198–206.

Pessoa-Silva, C. L., Toscan, C. M., Meurer Moreira, B., Santos, A. L., Frota, A. C. C., Solari, C. A., . . . Jarvis, W. R. (2002). Infection due to extended-spectrum β-lactamase-producing *Salmonella enterica* subsp. *enterica* serotype infantis in a neonatal unit. *Journal of Pediatrics, 141*(3), 381–387.

Pierce, M., Kurinczuk, J. J., Spark, P., Brocklehurst, P., & Knight, M. (2011). Perinatal outcomes after maternal 2009/H1N1 infection: National cohort study. *BMJ, 342*, d3214, Retrieved October 21, 2011, from OVID.

Poehling, K. A., Szilagyi, P. G., Staat, M. A., Snively, B. M., Payne, D. C., Bridges, C. B., . . . New Vaccine Surveillance Network. (2011, June). Impact of maternal immunization on influenza hospitalization in infants. *American Journal of Obstetrics & Gynecology, 204*(Suppl. 6), S141–S148.

Quinn, T. C. (2012). The global human immunodeficiency virus pandemic. Retrieved April 6, 2012, from *UpToDate*.

Raju, M., Salazar, J. C., Leopold, H., & Krause, P. J. (2007). Atovaquone and azithromycin treatment for babesiosis in an infant. *The Pediatric Infectious Disease Journal, 26*(2), 181–183.

Ramos, E. R., Retzel, R., Jiang, Y., Hachem, R. Y., Chaftari, A. M., Chemaly, R. F., . . . Raad, I. I. (2011). Clinical effectiveness and risk of emerging resistance associated with prolonged use of antibiotic-impregnated catheters: More than 0.5 million catheter days and 7 years of clinical experience. *Critical Care Medicine, 39*(2), 245–251.

Rasmussen, S. A., Kissin, D. M., Yeung, L. F., MacFarlane, K., Chu, S. Y., Turcios-Ruiz, R. M., . . . Pandemic Influenza and Pregnancy Working Group. (2011, June). Preparing for influenza after 2009 H1N1: Special considerations for pregnant women and newborns. *American Journal of Obstetrics & Gynecology*, S13–S20. Retrieved October 21, 2011, from OVID.

Regev-Yochay, G., Rubinstein, E., Barzilai, A., Carmelli, Y., Kuint, J., Etienne, J., . . . Keller, N. (2005). Methicillin-resistant *Staphylococcus aureus* in neonatal intensive care unit. *Emerging Infectious Diseases, 11*(3), 453–456.

Rice, L. B. (2006). Antimicrobial resistance in gram-positive bacteria. *American Journal of Infection Control, 34*, S11–S19.

Riordan, A., & Bugembe, T. (2009). Update on antiretroviral therapy. *Archives of Disease in Childhood, 94*(1), 70–74.

Saiman, L. (2006). Strategies for prevention of nosocomial sepsis in the neonatal intensive care unit. *Current Opinion in Pediatrics, 18*, 101–106.

Saiman, L., Cronquist, A., Wu, F., Zhou, J., Rubenstein, D., Eisner, W., . . . Della-Latta, P. (2003). An outbreak of methicillin-resistant *Staphylococcus aureus* in a neonatal intensive care unit. *Infection Control and Hospital Epidemiology, 24*(5), 317–321.

Sakamoto, F., Yamada, H., Suzuki, C., Sugiura, H., & Tokuda, Y. (2010). Increased use of alcohol-based hand sanitizers and successful eradication of methicillin-resistant *Staphylococcus aureus* from a neonatal intensive care unit: A multivariate time series analysis. *American Journal of Infection Control, 38*(7), 529–534.

Sarda, V., Molloy, A., Kadkol, S., Janda, W. M., Hershow, R., & McGuinn, M. (2009). Active surveillance for methicillin-resistant *Staphylococcus aureus* in the neonatal intensive care unit. *Infection Control and Hospital Epidemiology, 30*(9), 854–860.

Scheans, P. (2010). Is your nursery full of MDROs? *Neonatal Network, 29*(6), 392–395.

Sengupta, A., Lehmann, C., Diener-West, M., Perl, T. M., & Milstone, A. M. (2010). Catheter duration and risk of CLA-BSI in neonates with PICCs. *Pediatrics, 125*(4), 648–653.

Seybold, U., Halvosa, J. S., White, N., Voris, V., Ray, S. M., & Blumberg, H. M. (2008). Emergence of and risk factors for methicillin-resistant *Staphylococcus aureus* of community origin in intensive care nurseries. *Pediatrics, 122*(5), 1039–1046.

Shah, S. I., Turcotte, F., & Meng, H. D. (2008). Influenza vaccination rates of expectant parents with neonatal intensive care admission. *The Journal of Maternal-Fetal and Neonatal Medicine, 21*(10), 752–757.

Shakil, S., Ali, S. Z., Akram, M., Ali, S. M., & Khan, A. U. (2010). Risk factors for extended-spectrum β-lactamase producing *Escherichia coli* and *Klebsiella pneumoniae* acquisition in a neonatal intensive care unit. *Journal of Tropical Pediatrics, 56*(2), 90–96.

Shea, K., & Jacobi, J. (2009). Maximizing the effectiveness of antibiotics: Challenges associated with multidrug gram-negative resistance and limited resources. *Contemporary Critical Care, 7*(4), 1–10.

Shuford, J. A., & Patel, R. (2005). Antimicrobial growth promoter use in livestock—implications for human health. *Reviews in Medical Microbiology, 16*, 17–24.

Silva, H. de A., Pereira, E. M., Schuenck, R. P., Pinto, R. C. M., Abdallah, V. O. S., Santos, K. R. N., & Gontijo-Filho, P. P. (2009). Molecular surveillance of methicillin-susceptible *Staphylococcus aureus* at a neonatal intensive care unit in Brazil. *American Journal Infection Control, 37*, 574–579.

Singh, K., Gavin, P. J., Vescio, T., Thomson, R. B., Deddish, R. B., Fisher, A., . . . Peterson, L. R. (2003). Microbiologic surveillance using nasal cultures alone is sufficient for detection of methicillin-resistant *Staphylococcus aureus* isolates in neonates. *Journal of Clinical Microbiology, 41*(6), 2755–2757.

Singh, N., Patel, K. M., Léger M.-M., Short, B., Sprague, B. M., Kalu, N., & Campos, J. M. (2002). Risk of resistant infections with *Enterobacteriaceae* in hospitalized neonates. *The Pediatric Infectious Disease Journal, 21*(11), 1029–1033.

Slyker, J. A., Lohman-Payne, B. L., Rowland-Jones, S. L., Otieno, P., Maleche-Obimbo, E., Richardson, B., . . . John-Stewart, G. C. (2009). The detection of cytomegalovirus DNA in maternal plasma is associated with mortality in HIV-1-infected women and their infants. *AIDS, 23*(1), 117–124.

Snow, M. (2009). Babesiosis: Another tick-borne disease. *Nursing, 39*(6), 55.

Song, X., Cheung, S., Klontz, K., Short, B., Campos, J., & Singh, N. (2010). A stepwise approach to control an outbreak and ongoing transmission of methicillin-resistant *Staphylococcus aureus* in a neonatal intensive care unit. *American Journal of Infection Control, 38*(8), 607–611.

Stokowski, L. A. (2009). Neonatal HIV Infection. *Advances in Neonatal Care, 9*(2), 50–51.

Stramer, S. L., Hollinger, F. B., Katz, L. M., Kleinman, S., Metzel, P. S., Gregory, K. R., & Dodd, R. Y. (2009). Emerging infectious disease agents and their potential threat to transfusion safety. *Transfusion, 49*, 1S–29S.

Takei, Y., Yokoyama, K., Katano, H., Tsukiji, M., & Ezaki, T. (2010). Molecular epidemiological analysis of methicillin-resistant staphylococci in a neonatal intensive care unit. *Biocontrol Science, 15*(4), 129–138.

Tapsall, J. W. (2009). *Neisseria gonorrhoeae* and emerging resistance to extended spectrum cephalosporins. *Current Opinions in Infectious Diseases, 22*, 87–91.

The TEmAA ANRS 12109 Study Group. (2010). Maternal and neonatal tenofovir and emtricitabine to prevent vertical transmission of HIV-1: Tolerance and resistance. *AIDS, 24*(16), 2481–2488.

Tenover, F. C. (2006). Mechanisms of antimicrobial resistance in bacteria. *American Journal of Infection Control, 34*, S3–S10.

Tighe, P., Rimsza, L. M., Christensen, R. D., Lew, J., & Sola, M. C. (2005). Severe thrombocytopenia in a neonate with congenital HIV infection. *The Journal of Pediatrics, 146*(3), 408–413.

Toth, N. R., Chambers, R. M., & Davis, S. L. (2010). Implementation of a care bundle for antimicrobial stewardship. *American Journal of Health-System Pharmacists, 67*, 746–749.

Townsend, C. L., Cortina-Borja, M., Peckham, C. S., & Tookey, P. A. (2007). Antiretroviral therapy and premature delivery in diagnosed HIV-infected women in the United Kingdom and Ireland. *AIDS, 21*(8), 1019–1026.

Varner, M. W., Rice, M. M., Anderson, B., Tolosa, J. E., Sheffield, J., Spong, C. Y., . . . Eunice Kennedy Shriver National Institute of Child Health and Human Development (NICHD) Maternal-Fetal Medicine Units Network (MFMU). (2011). Influenza-like illness in hospitalized pregnant and postpartum women during the 2009–2010 H1N1 pandemic. *Obstetrics and Gynecology, 118*(3), 593–600.

Vrtis, M. C. (2008). Is your patient taking the right antimicrobial? *AJN, 108*(6), 49–55.

Walker, D. K., Ball, S., Black, R., Izrael, D., Ding, H., Euler, G. L., . . . Centers for Disease Control and Prevention (CDC). (2011). Influenza vaccination coverage among pregnant women—United States, 2010–11 influenza season. *Morbidity and Mortality Weekly Report, 60*, 1078–1082.

Warszawski, J., Tubiana, R., Le Chenadec, J., Blanche, S., Teglas, J.-P., Dolifus, C., . . . ANRS French Perinatal Cohort.

(2008). Mother-to-child HIV transmission despite antiretroviral therapy in the ANRS french perinatal cohort. *AIDS, 22*(2), 289–299.

Watts, D. H., Li, D., Handelsman, E., Tilson, H., Paul, M., Foca, M., . . . Thompson, B. (2007). Assessment of birth defects according to maternal therapy among infants in the women and infants transmission study. *Journal of Acquired Immune Deficiency Syndromes, 44*(3), 299–305.

Wendelboe, A. M., Grafe, C., & Carabin, H. (2010). The benefits of transmission dynamics models in understanding emerging infectious diseases. *The American Journal of the Medical Sciences, 340*(3), 181–186.

Yee-Guardino, S., Kumar, D., Abughali, N., Tuohy, M., Hall, G. S., & Kumar, M. L. (2008). Recognition and treatment of neonatal community-acquired MRSA pneumonia and bacteremia. *Pediatric Pulmonology, 43*, 203–205.

Young, T. E., & Mangum, B. (2010). *Neofax 2010* (pp. 58–61, 96–99). Montvale, NJ: Thomson Reuters.

Zingg, W., Pfister, R., Posfay-Barbe, K. M., Huttner, B., Touveneau, S., & Pittet, D. (2011). Secular trends in antibiotic use among neonates: 2001–2008. *The Pediatric Infectious Disease Journal, 30*(5), 365–370.

Zingg, W., Posfay-Barbe, K. M., & Pittet, D. (2008). Healthcare-associated infections in neonates. *Current Opinion in Infectious Diseases, 21*, 228–234.

UNIT V: VULNERABLE POPULATIONS

CHAPTER 27

Newborn or Infant Transplant Patient

■ Linda MacKenna Ikuta and Kathleen P. Juco

Transplantation is not a common procedure in the neonatal period. The ability to perform various transplants on very small patients has risen as technology has improved to facilitate such surgery. Solid organ transplants such as liver, kidney, and heart are the most usual procedures. The use of stem cells is an exciting prospect for treating many limiting and sometimes fatal, congenital diseases, but this therapy is surrounded by controversy regarding the ethics of its use. Stem cell research is giving rise to regenerative medicine. Researchers are examining the stem cells in relationship to, for example, fetal liver development in order to determine how these cells regenerate under the right circumstances (Koike & Taniguchi, 2012). The ethics of transplantation in general is muddled and is even more complicated when a child's life is at stake. Some people do not believe it is always in the infant's best interest to do these procedures. This chapter addresses the most common types of transplants, procurement of organs and cells, and general procedures.

LIVER TRANSPLANTATION IN INFANTS AND CHILDREN

Liver transplantation has become a viable solution for some destructive liver diseases. In infants and small children, especially those weighing less than 15 pounds, a liver from a larger donor can be "trimmed" to fit the small recipient, which has reduced the wait for an ideal matching donor. The technique is applied in living-related liver transplants when a segment of liver from a relative is removed and transplanted into the recipient. The use of reduced-size organs from related donors has decreased mortality to as little as 4% in some transplant centers. Increase in survival and reduced hospitalization stays has led to a greater number of transplants being done for infants and children. Another measure done to reduce wait times for transplant candidates is registration of in utero transplant candidates (Organ Procurement and Transplantation Network [OPTN], 2012) ABO-incompatible liver transplant in infants. According to the OPTN and Scientific Registry of Transplant Recipients (SRTR) Annual Data Report 2010, children, like adults, are placed on a list of those persons awaiting transplants; the median number of months waiting for a liver-alone transplant for all blood types in pediatric recipients was 2.6 in 2009. Pretransplant mortality declined for patients wait-listed for a liver-alone transplant, from 14.4 deaths per 100 wait-list years in 1998 to 8.2 in 2008. Patients on the waiting list aged younger than 6 years have the highest death rate, but this improved from 23.2 deaths per 100 wait-list years in 1998 to 14.9 in 2008. The number of deceased donor liver transplants has remained steady, while the number of living donor transplants decreased from a peak of 120 in 2000 to 51 in 2009. The rate of pediatric liver transplants has increased since 2002 to the current rate of 83.1 transplants per 100 patient-years on the waiting list. Patient-year is "synonymous with life-years and refers to the total number of years lived by a group of people" (OPTN, 2012).

Patients aged 1 to 5 years are the most common transplant recipients. Whites accounted for more than half of recipients. The most common etiology of liver disease was cholestatic disease. Among children and adolescents who underwent transplant in 2007 to 2009, 58% were on the waiting list for 60 days or less. Fifteen percent of patients were status 1A at transplant, and 29% had a model for end-stage liver disease (MELD) and pediatric end-stage liver disease (PELD) score of 30 or higher. The MELD and PELD are numerical scales that are currently used for liver allocation. The MELD and PELD scores are based on a patient's risk of dying while waiting for a liver transplant and are based on objective and verifiable medical data. United Network for

Organ Sharing (UNOS, 2005) uses the PELD for patients who are younger than 12 years old. The PELD score is calculated using:

- Albumin (g/dL)
- Bilirubin (mg/dL)
- International normalized ratio (INR)
- Growth failure (based on gender, height, and weight ratio)
- Age at listing

Sixty-four percent of patients received a whole liver. Among living donor liver transplants, 72% were from related donors in 2009. Only a small number of transplants were from donation after cardiac death donors (OPTN/SRTR, 2012).

Etiology

In neonates, acute liver failure (ALF) is a rare but often fatal condition. Infants and younger children do not display the main symptom of ALF, hepatic encephalopathy, as do adults and older children, adding to the difficulty of diagnosis. Causes of ALF include congenital malformations, metabolic liver disease, hepatotoxins, idiopathic liver failure, malignant and benign neoplasms of the liver, infections, ischemic injury, congenital vascular or heart anomalies, and drugs.

Recognition of liver disease in a newborn is difficult because abnormal biochemical findings, such as hyperbilirubinemia and coagulopathy, may be due to various physiologic and pathophysiologic processes:

- Hepatic encephalopathy is difficult to identify in any infant and almost impossible to distinguish from other metabolic encephalopathies in an ill neonate, especially if the infant requires ventilation support.
- Neonatal liver failure is generally labeled as "acute," consistent with the adult definition of duration of less than 8 weeks. However, some infants clearly have liver failure from end-stage liver disease, with cirrhosis due to liver damage that occurred during gestation (Jackson & Roberts, 2001). Other causes of liver failure include biliary atresia.

Biliary Atresia

The hallmark of biliary atresia is a progressive inflammatory process beginning shortly after birth. Extrahepatic biliary atresia is the most common form. Biliary atresia occurs in 1 in 15,000 live births. The cause of the disease is unknown, but about 10% of the cases have other associated congenital defects of heart, blood vessels, intestine, and/or spleen involvement. The Kasai procedure or Roux-en-Y hepatoportojejunostomy is the treatment for biliary atresia. Of newborns younger than 3 months of age undergoing this procedure, 80% will have reestablishment of bile flow. The remaining 20% of infants will not be helped by the procedure. A liver transplant is the only other treatment option (Esquivel, 2005).

Errors of Metabolism

Inherited errors of metabolism contribute greatly to liver failure and must be diagnosed promptly in the neonatal period. Galactosemia, hereditary fructose intolerance, and tyrosinemia are the most common metabolic diseases. Newborn screening by tandem mass spectrometry identifies metabolic diseases in many states. Newborn screening leads to early identification and treatment. Neonatal hemochromatosis, an associated metabolic disease with acute liver disease is the most common cause of liver failure in infancy, linked with massive intrahepatic and extrahepatic iron deposition, sparing the reticuloendothelial system (Dhawan & Mieli-Vergani, 2005). Despite chelation therapy, many severely affected infants will require transplantation.

CONTRAINDICATIONS FOR LIVER TRANSPLANTATION

There are many contraindications or reasons why transplantation should not be performed: (1) positive test for acquired immunodeficiency syndrome (AIDS) or human immunodeficiency virus (HIV); (2) cancer outside the liver; (3) infection outside the liver; (4) technical infeasibility; and (5) other medical problems such as heart disease, lung failure, or epilepsy that would interfere with the success of the transplant (Esquivel, 2005).

TRANSPLANT SELECTION

The advent of partial liver transplant and the use of living liver donors have eased transplant selection by making more organs available for transplantation. Not all patients can receive a transplant. A liver function test based on the hepatic conversion of lidocaine to monoethylglycinexylidide (MEGX) can give prognostic information. This test has been used because of its rapid turnaround for real-time assessment of hepatic function in transplantation. The MEGX test provides information that can improve the decision-making process with respect to the selection of transplant candidates. Patients with a MEGX 15- or 30-minute test value less than 10 mcg/L have a particularly poor 1-year survival rate. Serial monitoring of liver graft recipients with the MEGX test after transplantation may alert the clinician to a major change in liver function; if used with other tests, such as serum hyaluronic acid concentrations, it may become more discriminatory. In critically ill patients, it has been found that an initially rapid decrease in MEGX test values is associated with an enhanced risk for the development of multiple organ dysfunction syndromes and a poor outcome. Further, this decrease appears to be associated with an enhanced systemic inflammatory response (Oellerich & Armstrong, 2001).

For purposes of Status 1A/1B definition and classification, candidates listed at younger than 18 years of age who remain on or have returned to the waiting list upon or after reaching age 18 may be considered Status 1A/1B and shall qualify for other pediatric classifications under the following criteria. There are five allowable diagnostic groups: (1) fulminant liver failure; (2) primary nonfunction; (3) hepatic artery thrombosis; (4) acute decompensated Wilson's disease; and (5) chronic liver disease. Candidates meeting criteria (1), (2), (3), or (4) may be listed as a Status 1A; those meeting criteria (5) may be listed as a Status 1B (OPTN, 2012).

NUTRITIONAL SUPPORT

Optimal nutrition is best achieved through the enteral route. Effective enteral administration is not always possible with patients with liver failure because of impaired absorption; total parenteral nutrition (TPN) may be needed to support hepatocellular function and improve altered metabolism and absorption. A thorough assessment of nutritional status can be difficult because of metabolic disturbances. The balanced dietary approach moderated to replenishment of substrates and calories as needed helps prevent complications. Protein is required for cellular structure and function. Proteins therefore impact organ function.

PRETRANSPLANT MANAGEMENT

Management of infants and children before the transplant is paramount for success. Prior to transplantation, an effort is made to optimize the patient's physical status, including correcting electrolyte imbalances, maximizing nutrition, decreasing ascites and edema, improving diuresis, and giving blood transfusions if indicated.

During the pretransplant evaluation, the recipient's immunizations are updated. Since the recipient's response to vaccinations may be suboptimal, it is recommended that vaccination should be given as soon as possible (Kline, 2009).

Recommended vaccinations include:

1. Inactivated polio virus
2. Tetanus-diphtheria toxoid
3. Influenza (yearly)
4. Pneumococcal
5. Varicella (if nonimmune)
6. Hepatitis B
7. Hepatitis A (if nonimmune)
8. Haemophilus influenza type B (pediatric candidates)
9. Measles-mumps-rubella (pediatric candidates)
10. Meningococcal vaccine (particularly for patients entering college and patients within the next 1–2 years) (Hockenberry-Eaton, 1998, p. 137)

PREPARING THE PATIENT FOR THE OR

Most transplant recipients are admitted in the intensive care unit (ICU), although in some cases patients are at home waiting or in a nearby center. If the patient is in the hospital, lab and transfusion orders are completed and antibiotics ordered for the OR. Patients are NPO in preparation for the surgery. The nurse will make sure that consent, history, and physical documentation of the patient are current. Importantly, a preoperative bath is given, and the intended surgical area is wiped with chlorhexidine gluconate prior to transport to the operating room to decrease infection risk.

For outpatients, the transplant coordinator contacts the family when a donor organ becomes available. The patient is then brought to the hospital and upon admission preoperative laboratory tests are obtained.

TYPES OF LIVER TRANSPLANTS

The typical liver transplant procedure takes approximately 8 to 12 hours; however, the timing is dependent upon the complexity of the case as well as organizational efficiency and other factors. Over 50% of infant transplants are done with reduced-size livers from older donors, again requiring time to retrofit the liver from adult to child. Once the donor liver arrives in the operating room, it is prepared at the back table; simultaneously, hepatectomy of the native liver is performed by a second surgical team. In some instances, the donor liver can be viewed and prepped prior to skin incision of the transplant recipient.

The transplant operation is accomplished in three phases: the removal of the native liver, the anhepatic phase during which the new organ is implanted, and the reperfusion phase. A bilateral subcostal incision is made to visualize major structures. This procedure is also known as the "Mercedes" incision. For status post-Kasai patients, an extension of the old incision is done. The abdomen is then retracted to provide a clear view of abdominal structures. The vena cava, portal vein, and hepatic artery are cross-clamped prior to hepatectomy. Anatomical anomalies such as preduodenal portal vein, retroperitoneal continuation of the inferior vena cava, left-sided vena cava, and situs inversus abdominus are usually seen in patients with biliary atresia. This phase of the surgery is the most hazardous in the transplant procedure, requiring close monitoring of anesthesia, precaution, and vigilance by the surgical team. The anhepatic phase of implantation of the new organ starts as soon as the diseased liver is dissected or removed from the abdominal cavity.

The orthotopic approach requires replacing the recipient liver with the donor liver. After the donor liver is removed, preserved, and packed for transport, it must be transplanted into the recipient within 12 to 18 hours. The surgery begins by removing the diseased liver from the four main blood vessels and other structures that hold it in place in the abdomen. After the recipient's liver is removed, the new healthy donor liver is then connected and blood flow is restored. The final connection is made to the bile duct, a small tube that carries bile made in the liver to the intestines.

Vascular anastomoses are performed in the following manner:

1. Suprahepatic inferior vena cava
2. Infrahepatic inferior vena cava
3. Hepatic artery

4. Bile duct reconstruction is performed with end-to-side Roux-en-Y limb
5. Duct-to-duct biliary reconstruction is often performed in children with an adequate biliary tree (recipients diagnosed with metabolic disorders or FHF [fulminant hepatic failure])

Reperfusion Phase

Reperfusion of the graft occurs after the portal vein anastomsis. During this time, various metabolic changes may occur. Calcium requirements may decrease or stop, the serum bicarbonate level rises, and potassium may fall. Additionally, the partial thromboplastin time may go up, and massive fluid shifts can result in intestinal edema, third-spacing edema-capillary leak syndrome, and renal compromise.

HETEROTOPIC LIVER TRANSPLANTATION

In heterotopic liver transplantation, the recipient's liver is left in place and a donor liver is sewn into an ectopic site (UNOS, 2005). The advantage of this type of transplant is that the patient retains the original liver with the donor liver helping. It is not as common as other types of liver transplantation in recent years because surgical procedures have improved.

REDUCED-SIZE LIVER TRANSPLANTATION

In reduced-sized liver transplantation, allografts of donor liver are divided into eight segments, each supplied by a different set of blood vessels. Two of these segments have been enough to save a patient in liver failure, especially if the patient is a child. It is therefore possible to transplant one liver into at least two patients. Liver tissue grows to accommodate its job so long as there is initially enough of the organ to use. Patients have survived with only 15% to 20% of their original liver, provided that the 15% to 20% were healthy (Carter et al., 2006).

LIVING DONOR TRANSPLANTATION

Living donor liver transplantation (LDLT) is a procedure in which a healthy, living person donates a portion of his or her liver to another person. The feasibility of LDLT was first demonstrated in the United States in 1989. The recipient was a child, who received a segment of his mother's liver. In the pediatric experience, survival of the recipient child and function of the transplanted liver (graft) at 1 year is about 90%. The transplanted liver grows to almost full size within 6 to 8 weeks and begins to function fully.

AUXILIARY LIVER TRANSPLANTATION

There are three levels of cells in the hepatic lineage that respond to injury: the mature hepatocyte, the ductular "bipolar" progenitor cell, and a putative periductular stem cell. Hepatocytes are numerous and respond rapidly to liver cell loss by one or two cell cycles. The liver ductular "bipolar" (a cell with two processes) progenitor cells are less numerous, may proliferate for more cycles than hepatocytes, and are generally considered "bipolar"; that is, they can give rise to biliary cells or hepatocytes. Periductular stem cells, though rare in the liver, can proliferate for a long time. Extrahepatic (bone marrow) origin of the periductular stem cells is supported by recent data showing that hepatocytes may express genetic markers of donor hematopoietic cells after bone marrow transplantation.

These different regenerative cells with variations in potential for proliferation and differentiation may provide different sources of cells for liver transplantation: hepatocytes for treatment of acute liver damage, liver progenitor cell lines for liver-directed gene therapy, and bone marrow-derived cells for chronic long-term liver replacement. A limiting factor in the success of liver cell transplantation is the condition of the hepatic microenvironment in which the cells must proliferate and set up housekeeping. In animal models portal vein pressure affected portal vein flow related to the amount of liver cells given (Meyburg & Hoffman, 2010). Few liver stem cell transplantations have taken place. Cases of mold and other infections have been associated with liver stem cell transplantations. Further evaluation is warranted before such transplantation is accepted as a therapy in end-stage liver disease.

PORTAL HYPERTENSION

Portal hypertension is abnormally high blood pressure in the portal vein, the primary vein that brings blood from the intestine to the liver. When this vein clots or when the liver develops scar tissue from disease and compresses the vein, the blood pressure in the vein goes up and portal hypertension develops. In most patients portal hypertension develops regardless of primary disease process with progressive cirrhosis.

The liver normally filters blood from the abdominal organs. Portal hypertension can prohibit the liver from doing its job by causing the growth of collateral circulation that connects blood flow from the intestine to the general circulation, bypassing the liver. When this occurs, substances that are normally removed by the liver pass into general circulation. If not treated, portal hypertension can be progressive and cause serious complications.

Pharmacologic management with medications such as vasopressin and octreotide has been used for acute portal hypertension. Complications of portal hypertension can include esophageal varices complicated by hemorrhage and hypersplenism. Treatment with endoscopic sclerotherapy has emerged as an effective treatment for bleeding esophageal varices. Sclerotherapy is the ideal, safe, and effective treatment for bleeding esophageal varices; it prevented bleeding in 88.1% of patients after variceal eradication (Zargar et al., 2004). Splenectomy is used for older children when hypersplenism and splenic sequestration of blood components are noted (leukopenia, thrombocytopenia, or anemia). In neonates and small children, splenectomy is rarely done, as fatal sepsis is a major complication; functional disorders, such as ascites and thrombocytopenia, should be treated with a more conservative approach.

INFECTION

The immune system of infants and children is compromised due to the immaturity and inexperience of the immune system. End-stage liver disease decreases further their ability to fight off infections, making them especially vulnerable to infections commonly seen during childhood such as colds, flu, and other childhood diseases (e.g., meningitis, otitis media, and pneumonia). Nosocomial exposure in the hospital from invasive procedures (liver biopsy, intravenous lines) and handling by the health care team further jeopardize the patient for infections. Standard precautions must be followed. According to the indications from the Centers for Disease Control and Prevention (CDC), infection can be decreased by as much as half with attention to handwashing, draping for procedures, rubbing IV hubs with alcohol before using them by at least 30 seconds, use of disinfectant before invasive events, and discontinuance of lines on a timely basis. Antibiotics are used when indicated by culture and sensitivity.

Vaccinations should be given to infants and children on a routine, scheduled basis when possible. Other immunizations advised before transplantation include hepatitis B, hepatitis A, and influenza for older children.

Respiratory syncytial virus (RSV) is the most common cause of bronchiolitis and pneumonia among infants and children younger than 1 year of age. RSV is highly infectious, and almost all babies get it before the age of 2. Palivizumab (Synagis; MedImmune, Gaithersburg, MD) is given for neonates at risk for RSV before transplant on a monthly basis per American Academy of Pediatrics (AAP) Red Book Pickering (2009).

POSTTRANSPLANT MANAGEMENT

In the operating room, two to three Jackson-Pratt (JP) drains are inserted. A t-tube for duct-to-duct reconstruction or a biliary catheter for Roux-en-Y is used.

Posttransplant management would include care given to any postoperative patient in addition to close monitoring for liver function or complications. Blood gases, laboratory reports, fluid balance, urinary output (1–2 mL/kg at least), and intravenous access are as usual watched closely. Drainage from the liver transplant is closely observed. Dark, black, bloody discharge can mean that the circulation to the transplant is not working, and the liver may be dead.

Prophylactic antibiotics are given before, during, and after surgery. Antifungal and antiherpes virus prophylaxis is also given.

Immunosuppressive Management

Immunosuppressive management usually starts with prednisone in infants and children. The calcineurin inhibitors cyclosporine and tacrolimus are also used; they have distinct advantages and drawbacks. It is important to tailor their use to the patient's tolerance. In some patients, the need to ameliorate the adverse effects of tacrolimus may necessitate a switch to cyclosporine-based therapy and vice versa. Some centers use azathioprine as part of an initial cyclosporine immunotherapy program. It is usually discontinued early in the posttransplant period.

Rejection is treated with steroid pulses, steroid recycling, or the monoclonal anti-T-cell antibody muromonab-CD3 (Orthoclone OKT3). Daily monitoring of immunosuppressive medications is necessary for proper dose adjustment in infants and children. Rescue therapy with a cyclosporine microemulsion–based (Neoral, Novartis Pharmaceuticals Corporation, East Hanover, NJ) regimen for transplant patients intolerant of tacrolimus has been evaluated to assess the best method of switching and determining the initial and maintenance doses in children. Transplant centers are evaluating this therapy at present (OPTN, 2012).

Drugs used for immunosuppression have been implicated in causing numerous long-term side effects, including nephrotoxicity, glucose intolerance, and hyperlipidemia. Calcineurin inhibitors are known to cause nephrotoxicity, which is of concern in pediatric liver transplant recipients. Almost all patients will require antihypertensive therapy. Posttransplant malignancies are among the most important complications in organ transplantation.

POSTOPERATIVE COMPLICATIONS

Most complications after liver transplantation are heralded by an increase in hepatocellular enzymes, often associated with malaise, fever, leukocytosis, and jaundice. The clinical picture defines hepatic allograft dysfunction, but it does not separate allograft rejection from other allograft complications such as primary nonfunction, bile duct abnormalities, hepatic artery thrombosis, or allograft infection. The use of real-time and Doppler ultrasonography to assess hepatic vasculature and the use of computed tomography (CT) and magnetic resonance imaging (MRI) are often necessary. Allograft biopsy is definitive when the cause of the graft abnormality is rejection; it can strongly support the diagnosis of viral infection or cholangitis when the characteristic histologic markers and microscopic appearance are seen. Definitive diagnosis of the cause of the allograft dysfunction should precede immunologic manipulation (OPTN, 2012).

POSTTRANSPLANT MANAGEMENT OF COMPLICATIONS

Most patients are taken to the pediatric ICU, intubated, and monitored for:

1. Hypothermia: common in infants due to prolonged exposure of the abdominal viscera during surgery; careful monitoring of patient's body temperature needed to prevent dysrhythmias, clotting abnormalities, and impaired renal function and delayed wound healing
2. Hemorrhage: increased blood in JP drains, increased abdominal girth, oozing from suture line, and change in cardiovascular status; will require blood products such as fresh frozen plasma, platelets, and cryoprecipitate

3. Fluid and electrolyte imbalance: decreased urine output less than 1 mL/kg/hr may indicate early graft dysfunction or nephrotoxicity; electrolytes monitoring every 6 hours
4. Neurologic status: encephalopathy/hepatic coma may indicate bad liver; "getting the shakes"—may indicate elevated levels of Prograf
5. GI status: watch for abdominal distention, rigid or painful abdomen, and stool color and consistency
6. Hepatic artery thrombosis: most common postoperative complication; watch for sudden spike in temperature, abdominal pain with increased LFTs, change in mental status, and biliary leaks
7. Portal vein thrombosis: presents with variceal bleeding or a slowly enlarging liver or spleen and low platelet count
8. Biliary leaks: leading cause of morbidity and mortality in children; a change in the color of fluid in the JP drains noted in the immediate postoperative period; will need surgical intervention
9. Rejection: early signs include low-grade fever, increased liver enzymes and bilirubin, pain over graft, irritability, and ascites

HEART TRANSPLANT

With advances in surgical techniques, younger and smaller patients are having heart transplants. The availability of organs is limited for small children. Many centers try to wait till the child is larger to accommodate a larger heart. Developmental studies have shown that young infants and children are at risk for growth failure, developmental delays, and serious neurologic sequelae.

Bridge to Transplant

Heart failure due to congenital defects and organ deterioration affects the entire body. Many patients waiting for a heart transplant are so debilitated that they may not be able to tolerate the surgery. To assist the body and improve the patients' physical status, several modalities are used to help the patient gain strength while awaiting transplant—hence a "bridge-to-transplant." Devices commonly used for bridge-to-transplant are the left ventricular assist device (LVAD), extracorporeal membrane oxygenation (ECMO) and, on a limited basis, the Berlin Heart.

Left Ventricular Assist Device

The LVAD is an implantable mechanical device to pump blood through the body. It takes over the work of the failing heart. Bridge-to-transplant facilities that have an aggressive approach to implantable LVAD placement may substantially improve the survival rate of patients with postcardiotomy heart failure (Garbade, Bittner, Barten, & Mohr, 2011).

Extracorporeal Membrane Oxygenation

ECMO currently comes in two varieties: venoarterial (VA) and venovenous (VV). VA ECMO takes deoxygenated blood from a central vein or the right atrium, pumps it past the oxygenator, and then returns the oxygenated blood, under pressure, to the arterial side of the circulation (typically, to the aorta). This form of ECMO partially supports the cardiac output as the flow through the ECMO circuit is in addition to the normal cardiac output.

VV ECMO takes blood from a large vein and returns oxygenated blood back to a large vein. VV ECMO does not support the circulation. VA ECMO helps support the cardiac output and delivers higher levels of oxygenation support than does VV ECMO. VA ECMO carries a higher risk of systemic emboli than does VV. The normalization of left heart filling pressures alleviates pulmonary edema and improves the child's physical status.

Berlin Heart

The Berlin Heart (Berlin Company, Berlin, Germany) has been used for infants and small children who can utilize neither LVAD nor ECMO. Named after the company in Berlin, Germany, that manufactures it, the Berlin Heart is a ventricular-assist device that works by helping the right ventricle of the heart pump blood to the lungs and the left ventricle to pump blood to the rest of the body. The bulk of the Berlin Heart is located outside of the body, with only the pumps connected to the heart emerging from the body. The device is run by a laptop computer. The Berlin Heart comes in various sizes for a range of patients and is the only mechanical heart small enough to be used in very young children.

PHYSIOLOGY OF THE TRANSPLANTED HEART

The physiology of the transplanted heart is distinctive. Both the recipient and donor atria are present but function separately, resulting in decreased atrial input. The transplanted heart does not experience angina because of denervation. Low cardiac output can result, as the transplanted heart has no innervation pacing the heartbeat.

Postoperative Management

Care of the heart transplant patient is similar to any other cardiac surgery. Good perfusion with adequate gas exchange and hemodynamic stability are goals after transplantation. Normal perfusion is evidenced by normalized blood gases, adequate urinary output, and adequate blood pressure.

A major complication from surgery is hemorrhage. This can be due to anticoagulation therapy secondary to end-stage heart disease, reoperation (prior cardiac surgery), and cardiopulmonary bypass during surgery, or clotting related to hepatic congestion secondary to severe right heart failure. The donor heart is smaller than the diseased heart it replaced. This results in the pericardial space acting as a reservoir for blood, resulting in cardiac tamponade. Frequent milking of the chest tubes helps decrease the blood volume in the pericardial space and maintains the patency of the chest tubes.

RENAL TRANSPLANTATION IN INFANTS AND CHILDREN

Renal transplantation in infants and children has been the most successful of all types of transplants. Recent advances in the techniques of dialysis and the management of end-stage renal disease (ESRD) in neonates have allowed many patients with complex urologic or hereditary abnormalities to reach the age and size at which transplantation is possible. These advances have permitted the implementation of renal transplantation, along with dialysis, as a complementary treatment in the care of infants with irreversible renal dysfunction.

Etiology

Acute renal failure in infants is most often the consequence of hemodynamic instability, hypoxia, or malperfusion, resulting in acute tubular necrosis. Most of these infants either recover sufficient function for normal long-term survival or die of multisystem failure. Chronic renal failure is uncommon in infants. Congenital nephrosis, dysplasia-hypoplasia, and other anatomic abnormalities associated with complex urogenital malformations are the common causes of ESRD in infants.

In children younger than 5 years of age who have glomerulonephritis, 46% have a congenital cause for ESRD. Lupus nephritis and recurrent pyelonephritis, which are more common in older patients, are uncommon causes of ESRD in the infant. Hereditary causes of renal failure are important to identify in planning the appropriate overall treatment strategy; evaluation of other family members and provision of genetic counseling, when needed, must also be considered. Appropriate identification of the cause of the ESRD also allows assessment of the potential for recurrence within a transplant allograft and consideration of living related-donor transplantation.

Pretransplant Management

Pretransplant tests are done to evaluate the patient's physical status and also to identify potential problems. The tests help determine whether transplantation is truly the best option and will increase the likelihood of success. Transplant feasibility consists of histocompatibility laboratory tests of tissue typing, panel reactive antibody, cross-match testing, and blood typing.

Dialysis

Dialysis is indicated in infants as in older children if complications of medical management of ESRD occur, namely, hyperkalemia, volume overload, acidosis, intractable hypertension, or uremic symptoms, such as vomiting. Dialysis can be accomplished by hemodialysis or peritoneal dialysis. Dialysis centers can take older children until a transplant is available. In neonates and small children, peritoneal dialysis is frequently utilized because (1) it avoids the multiple transfusions associated with hemodialysis; (2) it allows smoother gradual correction of electrolyte abnormalities, preventing cerebral disequilibrium syndrome in small infants; and (3) it is easier to perform. For long-term peritoneal dialysis, parents are taught how to care for the infant. This allows the parent to take the child home and be a family. The infant is given time to grow and normalize as much as possible. Glucose and electrolytes can be enhanced via peritoneal dialysis to enhance nutrition.

Nutritional Support

Nutritional support is a primary concern for the renal patient. Growth retardation is a major problem. The cause of this growth disturbance is multifactorial and includes both protein and calorie insufficiency, renal osteodystrophy, aluminum toxicity, acidosis, impaired somatomedin activity, and insulin resistance. A registered dietitian will need to constantly monitor the nutritional needs of the infant and child. The most intense period of growth occurs during the first 2 years of life. Head circumference is the key to monitoring growth, as it follows overall body development.

INTESTINAL TRANSPLANT

Data compiled by the international Intestinal Transplant Registry show that 55 intestinal transplant programs have performed 601 transplants, of which 402 were in children since 1985. Although not many infants and children have had intestinal transplants, the numbers are growing.

Intestinal Transplant Considerations

Patients with poor intestinal function who cannot be maintained on TPN via intravenous routes are potential candidates for transplantation. In some patients, most of the bowel has been surgically removed to treat the disease, or it became diseased. This produces short-gut syndrome, the most common cause of intestinal failure. For some infants and children, the entire intestine is present, but is unable to absorb adequate fluids and nutrients.

Transplantation is a potentially life-saving option for patients with intestinal failure who cannot tolerate TPN. The preferred type of transplant is isolated bowel transplants because the patient survival rate is better. Combined intestinal–liver transplants or cluster transplants are options for patients who have developed liver failure on TPN or for patients who have large, local tumors that can only be removed by removing several organs.

Diseases leading to intestinal transplantation include:

- Short-gut syndrome caused by volvulus, gastroschisis, trauma, necrotizing enterocolitis, ischemia, and Crohn's disease
- Poor absorption caused by microvillus inclusion, secretory diarrhea, and autoimmune enteritis
- Poor motility caused by pseudoobstruction, aganglionosis (Hirschsprung's disease), and visceral neuropathy
- Tumor or cancer such as desmoid tumor, familial polyposis (Gardner's disease)
- Congenital intestinal atresia
- Poor intestinal absorption
- Autoimmune disorders
- Brush-border element assembly problems
- Microvillus inclusion disease
- Severe disorders of motility resulting from intestinal pseudoobstruction (congenital or acquired)
- Desmoid tumors
- Serious complications of TPN therapy

- Thrombosis (blockage due to a blood clot) of two or more major central veins (subclavian, jugular, and femoral)
- Repeated episodes of line sepsis or line infections
- The decision to proceed with intestinal transplantation is made only after careful evaluation determines that the surgery is the child's most promising treatment option

Donor Options

Most intestinal grafts come from cadaver donors—people who have been declared dead in a hospital while attached to a ventilator (artificial breathing machine). Consent is given by the next of kin for organ removal and transplant. Occasionally, a portion of the bowel is taken from a living donor—a relative such as a parent or sibling.

Intestinal Transplant Evaluation

Small intestine transplant evaluation is similar to liver transplant evaluation. It is important that the child have a good history of central-line placement, IV access, upper gastrointestinal studies, number of gastrointestinal resections, and length of bowel to ensure that transplantation is the best medical option.

Studies done for evaluation include:

- Blood tests
- Chemistry panel
- Liver panel
- Hematology group
- Coagulation studies
- Blood typing and antibody screen
- Infectious diseases: hepatitis B, hepatitis C, HIV, cytomegalovirus, Epstein–Barr virus
- Imaging studies and other tests
- Ultrasound of the liver in combined intestinal–liver transplants
- CT scan
- MRI to map abdominal vasculature
- Endoscopy (EGD)
- Mobility studies
- Colonoscopy
- Liver biopsy for combined liver–intestinal patients to determine whether TPN damage is reversible
- Psychosocial and developmental evaluations
- Social worker
- Child development expert evaluation

If the child is a candidate for intestinal transplantation, his or her name is added to the transplant waiting list for an isolated intestinal transplant or for a combined liver and intestinal transplant, based on the severity of organ damage and dysfunction. Transplant waiting lists are maintained by the United Network of Organ Sharing (OPTN, 2012).

Postoperative Management

After the procedure, patients are placed on immunosuppressive drugs to prevent rejection of the transplanted organ. The doctors perform biopsies (take tissue samples of the intestine) at various intervals to check for signs of rejection. Rejection may be managed by adding immunosuppressive drugs or increasing dosages. Patients who have received intestinal transplants remain on immunosuppressive drugs indefinitely. Since patients on immunosuppressive drugs are vulnerable to infections by bacteria and viruses, they are monitored for signs and symptoms of infection. Particular attention is paid to wound care issues and fluid management. The multidisciplinary team performs a nutritional assessment to determine the child's caloric needs.

Intestinal Transplantation Survival

Improved antirejection drugs, refined surgical procedures, and a greater understanding of immunology have contributed to successful intestinal transplants. Short-term survival is now comparable to lung transplantation results. Most of the patients in the international Intestinal Transplant Registry have been followed for a brief time; it will take several years to obtain reliable data on long-term results (Intestinal Transplant Registry, 2005).

Until a few years ago, cyclosporine was used most often to prevent organ rejection. Tacrolimus (Prograf, Astellas Pharma US, Deerfield, IL) has been given to most intestinal transplant patients over the past 4 years. As of June 1995, 49% of all intestinal patients had died, usually from sepsis (42%) or multiple organ system failure (30%). Four patients (5%) died of rejection. Of the surviving patients, 78% had stopped TPN and had resumed a normal, oral diet.

To become the standard treatment for intestinal failure, transplantation must offer better survival, better quality of life, and lower costs than TPN. Considerable progress has been made toward these goals, but further refinements are needed before bowel transplantation becomes a routine surgical procedure.

Despite improved immunosuppression, the intestine offers more rejection than other organs.

Rejection of the intestine is also difficult to diagnose since there are no biochemical (blood) tests to indicate rejection. To prevent intestinal rejection, patients require higher doses of immunosuppression than with other types of transplantation. Now, because of new, more specific antirejection medications, the success of intestinal transplant has improved dramatically (Intestinal Transplant Registry, 2005).

ORGAN PROCUREMENT

Organ procurement is facilitated by the UNOS, a nonprofit, scientific and educational organization that administers the nation's only OPTN and was established by the U.S. Congress in 1984. Functions of OPTN include the following:

- Collects and manages data about every transplant event occurring in the United States
- Facilitates organ matching and placement process using UNOS-developed data technology and the UNOS Organ Center
- Brings together medical professionals, transplant recipients, and donor families to develop organ transplantation policy

UNOS was awarded the initial OPTN contract on September 30, 1986. UNOS is the only organization to ever manage the OPTN and has continued to administer the contract for more than 16 years and four successive contract renewals (OPTN, 2012).

Waiting List

The OPTN maintains the only national patient waiting list and features the most comprehensive data available in any single field of medicine (OPTN). UNetSM is the web-based electronic utility used by the contractor to conduct the business of OPTN. UNetSM comprises the Match System, all software, applications, and security architecture needed for the collection, modification, validation, reporting, management, and redundancy of data associated with the tasks and activities of the OPTN. The Organ Procurement Organization, having identified a potential organ donor, assumes responsibility for donor management and organ allocation. The Match System is the computerized algorithm used to prioritize candidates waiting for organs. It eliminates potential recipients whose size or ABO type is incompatible with that of a donor and then ranks those remaining potential recipients according to the ranking system (OPTN, 2012).

The waiting list is the computerized list of candidates waiting to be matched with specific donor organs in hopes of receiving transplants. Candidates are registered on the waiting list by member transplant centers. The candidate's transplant program is responsible for ensuring the accuracy of candidate ABO blood group system data on the waiting list. Each transplant program implements and operates procedures for online verification of a candidate's ABO data on the waiting list against the source documents by an individual. The transplant program maintains records documenting separate verification of the source documents against the entered ABO data. Upon entry of the candidate's waitlist data, the candidate will be added to the waitlist but will not be listed as an active candidate until separate verification of the candidate's ABO data has taken place (OPTN policy).

All transplant candidate interactions will be required to be completed through UNetSM by transplant programs. The Organ Center will facilitate candidate listings and modifications in the event of computer and/or Internet failure. When the Organ Center facilitates a candidate's listing or modification due to computer and/or Internet failure, the transplant center will be required to submit a statement explaining the event.

Each transplant candidate must be ABO typed on two separate occasions prior to listing. Two separate occasions is defined as two samples, taken at different times, sent to the same or different labs. Transplant candidates are listed on UNetSM with the candidate's actual blood type (OPTN, 2012).

PEDIATRIC CRITICAL PATHWAY

After brain death has been declared and consent granted for organ donation, pediatric specialists and organ procurement professionals should work together to care for the organ donor and family members. The UNOS (2005) (Figure 27.1) describes optimal care for the pediatric organ donor and maps the process to improve the outcome for successful organ transplantation.

STEM CELL TRANSPLANTATION

In recent years, human umbilical cord blood (CB) has become a source of hematopoietic progenitor cells. These stem cells are used to treat a variety of diseases such as malignancies, hemoglobinopathies, immunodeficiencies, and inborn errors of metabolism. Umbilical CB was used until recently to assess infants' health status. Otherwise, CB was discarded with all the other biologic tissues of birth: placenta, amniotic fluid, birth sac, and umbilical cord. These biologic tissues have been shown to be useful medically for other purposes. For example, it was found that a specific lung lipid isolated from amniotic fluid could ascertain the lung maturity of the fetus in the last trimester of pregnancy: the lecithin/sphingomyelin ratio.

Physiology

Umbilical CB is extremely rich in stem cells. Stem cells differ from other kinds of cells in the body. Regardless of their source, they have three general properties:

1. They are capable of dividing and renewing themselves for long periods
2. The cells are unspecialized
3. They give rise to specialized cells

There is controversy within the embryologist community regarding where stem cells and progenitor cells originate: in the yolk sac or aorta-gonad-mesonephros/intraembryonic splanchnopleura region. Stem cells move through the fetal liver and then the fetal circulation, where the numbers are high at birth (Ikuta, 2008).

In October 1988, the first CB transfusion was performed for a patient with Fanconi anemia: A sibling donor contributed the HLA-matched cells. Since this case several diseases have been successfully treated with stem cells. In a number of genetic, hematologic, and oncologic disorders, infusion of CB can be a potentially lifesaving procedure. Allogenic (related or unrelated) or autologous (self) bone marrow is the usual source of hematopoietic progenitor cells. One child in 2,700 might eventually benefit from an autologous stem cell transplant (Ikuta, 2008). Bone marrow is not always readily available. Umbilical CB can be a viable alternative for certain conditions (Table 27.1).

Collection of Cord Blood

CB can be collected from the placenta in situ during the third stage of labor or immediately after delivery of the placenta. About 50% to 70% of donated units are ineligible for storage, mainly because of low volume. Each unit should contain more than 40 mL of CB for a child weighing up to 30 kg. Maximal storage time is unknown, but under stable conditions the cells are likely to remain viable for decades.

Collaborative Practice	Phase I Identification and Referral	Phase II Preliminary Evaluation	Phase III Family Discussion and Consent	Phase IV Comprehensive Evaluation and Donor Management	Phase V Withdrawal of Support/ Pronouncement of Death/Organ Recovery
The following health care professionals may be involved in the Donation After Cardiac Death (DCD) donation process: Check all that apply: O Physician (MD) O Critical Care RN O Nurse Supervisor O Medical Examiner/ Coroner O Respiratory Therapy (RT) O Laboratory O Pharmacy O Radiology O Anesthesiology O OR/Surgery Staff O Clergy O Social Worker O Organ Procurement Coordinator (OPC) O Organ Procurement Organization (OPO)	Prior to withdrawing life support, contact local OPO for any patient who fulfills the following criteria: O Devastating neurologic injury and/or other organ failure requiring mechanical ventilatory or circulatory support O Family and/or care giving team initiate conversation about withdrawal of support Following referral, additional evaluation is done collaboratively to determine if death is likely to occur within 1 hour (or within a specified timeframe as determined by care giving team and OPO) following withdrawal of support Patient conditions might include the following: O **Ventilator dependent for respiratory insufficiency:** apneic or severe hypopneic; tachypnea ≥ 30 breaths/ min after DC ventilator O **Dependent on**	Physician O Supportive of withdrawal of care and has communicated grave prognosis to family O Review DCD procedure with OPC O Will be involved in withdrawal/ pronouncement O Will designate a person to be involved with withdrawal and/or pronouncement Family O Has received grave prognosis O Understands prognosis O In conjunction with care giving team, decide to withdraw support Patient O Age ______ O Weight ______ O Height ______ O ABO ______ O Medical Hx ______ O Surgical Hx ______ O Social Hx ______ O Death likely < 1 hour following withdrawal (determined collaboratively by	O Support services offered to family O OPC/hospital staff approach family about donation options O Legal next-of-kin (NOK) fully informed of donation options and recovery procedures O Legal NOK grants consent for DCD following withdrawal of support O Family offered opportunity to be present during withdrawal of support O OPC obtains _____ Witnessed consent from legal NOK for DCD _____ Signed consent Time ______ Date ______ _____ Detailed med/soc history Notification of donation O Hospital supervisor O ME/coroner notified _____ ME/coroner and releases for donation _____ ME/coroner has restrictions	O MD, in collaboration with OPO, implements management guidelines O Establish location and time of withdrawal of support O Review plan for withdrawal to include: – Pronouncing MD (should be in attendance for duration of withdrawal of support, determination of death, and may not be a member of the transplant team) – Comfort care – Extubation and discontinuation of ventilator support – Establish plan for continued supportive care if pt survives > 1 hour or predetermined time interval after withdrawal of support O Notify OR/Anesthesia _____ Review patient's clinical course, withdrawal plan, and potential organ recovery	O Withdrawal occurs in _____ OR _____ ICU _____ Other ______ O Family present for withdrawal of support _____ Yes _____ No O OR/room prepared and equipment set up O Transplant team in the OR (not in attendance during withdrawal) O Care giving team present O Administration of preapproved medication (e.g., heparin/Regitine) O **Withdrawal of support according to hospital/MD practice guidelines** **Time** ______ **Date** ______ O **Vital signs are monitored and recorded every minute (see attached sheet)** O **Pt pronounced dead and appropriate documentation completed**

FIGURE 27.1 Critical pathway for donation after cardiac death.
Adapted from UNOS (2005).

	mechanical circulatory support: LVAD; RVAD; V-A ECMO; pacemaker with unassisted rhythm < 30 beats/min O **Severe disruption in oxygenation:** PEEP ≥ 10 and SaO_2 ≤ 92%; FiO_2 ≥0.50 and SaO_2 ≤ 92%; V-V ECMO requirement O **Dependent upon pharmacologic circulatory assist:** norephinephrine, epinephrine, or phenylephrine ≥ 0.2 mcg/kg/min; dopamine ≥ 15 mcg/kg/min O **IABP and inotropic support:** IABP 1:1 and dobutamine or dopamine ≥ 10 mcg/kg/min and CI ≤ 2.2 L/min/M^2; IABP 1:1 and CI ≤ 1.5 L/min/M^2	evaluating injury, level of support, respiratory drive assessment)	*Stop pathway if –* O *Family, ME/coroner denies consent* O *Patient determined to be unsuitable candidate for DCD* O *Patient progresses to brain death during evaluation — refer to brain dead pathway*	procedures _____ Schedule OR time O Notify recovery teams O Prepare patient for transport to prearranged area for withdrawal of support O Patient transported to prearranged area O Note: Should the clinical situation require premortum femoral cannulation, the following should be reviewed: – Family consent or understanding – MD inserting cannula – Time and location of cannula insertion – If death does not occur, determine if cannula should be removed	**Time** _________ **Date** _________ **MD** _________ O **Transplant team initiates surgical recovery** at prescribed time following pronouncement of death O Allocation of organs per OPTN/UNOS policy O ***If cardiac death not established within 1 hour or predetermined time interval after withdrawal of support – Stop pathway Patient moved to predetermined area for continuation of supportive care*** O *Postmortem care administered*
Labs/Diagnostics		O ABO O Electrolytes O LFTs O PT/PTT O CBC with Diff O Beta HCG (female pts) O ABG		Repeat full panel of labs additionally: O Serology testing O Infectious disease profile O Blood cultures X2 O UA and urine culture O Sputum culture O Tissue typing	
Respiratory	O Maintain ventilator support O Pulmonary toilet PRN	→ O Respiratory drive assessment RR _________ VT _________ VE _________ NIF _________	→ O ABGs as requested O Notify RT of location and time of withdrawal of support	→ O Transport with mechanical ventilation using lowest FiO_2 possible while maintaining the SaO_2 > 90%	→

FIGURE 27.1 Critical pathway for donation after cardiac death. *(continued)*
Adapted from UNOS (2005).

		Minutes off ventilator ___ ○ Hemodynamics while off ventilator → HR ______ BP ______ SaO_2 ______			
Treatments/Ongoing Care	Maintain standard nursing care to include: → ○ Vital signs q 1 hour ○ I and O q 1 hour				○ Postmortem care at conclusion of case
Medications				○ Provide medications as directed by MD in consult OPC	○ Heparin and other medications prior to withdrawal of support
Optimal Outcomes	The potential DCD donor is identified, and a referral is made to the OPO	The donor is evaluated and found to be a suitable candidate for donation	The family is offered the option of donation, and their decision is supported	Optimal organ function is maintained, withdrawal of support plan is established, and personnel are prepared for potential organ recovery	Death occurs within 1 hour of withdrawal of support and all suitable organs and tissues are recovered for transplant

FIGURE 27.1 Critical pathway for donation after cardiac death.

Adapted from UNOS (2005).

TABLE 27.1

CONDITIONS FOR WHICH UMBILICAL CORD BLOOD CAN BE A VIABLE ALTERNATIVE

Disease	Indication	Blood Cell Transplantation
Leukemia, lymphomas	Engraftment of healthy cells	Effective
Bone and soft tissue sarcomas, Wilms' tumor, brain tumors	Very rarely indicated	Effectiveness unproven
Hematologic diseases	The new donor cells will produce normal white cells, red cells, and platelets	Effective
Immunodeficiency diseases	Engraftment of healthy allogenic cells	Effective
Hemoglobinopathies	The new donor cells will produce normal white cells, red cells, and platelets	Effective
Metabolic storage disorders	Donor cell will eventually produce the deficient enzyme	Controversial; may be effective in select patients
Genetic conditions	Cells from umbilical cord blood can be isolated, transduced, and engrafted to produce mature hematopoietic and lymphoid cells for at least several years	Effective in select diseases

Adapted from Baggott and Fochtman (2002) and Hockenberry-Eaton (1998).

CB is collected according to directions for the particular bank. In general, the samples are obtained from normal full-term deliveries under orders from the health care provider (physician, midwife, or nurse practitioner). Once labor has been established, the nurse will label the tubes, place them in a plastic zip-closure bag, and return them to the kit's Styrofoam box per instructions. The Styrofoam box will then be labeled with time, date, name, and initials of collector. The tops of the heparin vials are cleansed with alcohol, and 5 mL is drawn. The heparin is injected into labeled 60-mL syringes.

After the infant's birth, CB is collected within 10 minutes. CB is drawn from the umbilical vein with as much blood as possible. The syringes are inverted back and forth for 1 to 2 minutes to mix the blood and heparin well. The syringes are capped and put into the provided plastic bag. Then they are packaged into the Styrofoam box with provided absorbent pad. Blood should remain at room temperature to ensure viability of stem cells. CB is not refrigerated. It is usually the families' responsibility to ship the blood in a timely manner to the CB bank (Ikuta, 2008).

Cord Blood Banks

Private banks such as the Cord Blood Registry in San Bruno, California, offer collection kits to families. Private banks are accredited by the American Association of Blood Banks. Typical fees range from $1,000 to $1,500 for registration and collection. Storage fees are typically approximately $100 a year, but there are no additional fees for retrieving the cells for use. The costs are borne by the families.

Public cord banks accept collections only from affiliated hospitals. Units stored in them are available for any patient in need who is medically eligible for transplantation therapy. In the unlikely event that the donor or a member of his family develops an indication for a stem cell transplant, the stored cells could be traced and used. Public blood cord banks charge no fees for donation, but may charge $15,000 or more if the blood is actually used. The number of public banks is limited (Ikuta, 2008).

The AAP recommends that institutions or organizations (private or public) involved in CB banking should consider the following recommendations:

- Recruitment practices should be developed with an awareness of the possible emotional vulnerability of pregnant women and their families and friends. Efforts should be made to minimize the effect of this vulnerability on recruitment decisions.
- Accurate information about the potential benefits and limitations of allogenic and autologous CB banking and transplantation should be provided.
- A policy should be developed regarding disclosing to the parents any abnormal findings in the harvested blood.
- Specific permission for maintaining demographic medical information should be obtained and the potential risks of breaches of confidentiality disclosed.
- Written permission should be obtained during prenatal care and before the onset of labor. The practice of collecting blood first and obtaining permission afterward is considered unethical and should be discouraged.
- Consultation with the institutional review board or hospital ethics committee about recruitment strategies and the wording of consent forms is recommended.
- CB collection should not be done in complicated deliveries, and the CB stem collection program should

not alter routine practice for the timing of umbilical cord clamping.

- Because of the investigational status of CB banking and the high risk for its potential abuse, the regulatory agencies (e.g., U.S. Food and Drug Administration, Federal Trade Commission, state equivalent of these federal agencies) are encouraged to have an active role in providing oversight for the safety and welfare of the population (AAP, 1999; Ikuta, 2008).

Cord Blood Transfusion in Neonate

Families must be prepared for CB transfusion. Social services must conduct a psychosocial evaluation of the family for emotional stability, compliance to regimen, and financial support. The patient is evaluated for infections and physical functioning. If CB is given for malignancies, then chemotherapy and high-dose radiation is given to prepare the patient for CB transfusion.

There are two types of cord stem cell transfusions: frozen and fresh. Each type of transfusion is discussed in regard to considerations, side effects, and nursing care needed for the neonate. Frozen stem cells are used in autologous (collected from the patient) CB transplants. A preservative, dimethyl sulfoxide (DMSO), is added to the cells just prior to cryopreservation. It acts to coat the cells and prevent their lysis during the process of freezing and thawing. DMSO is infused to the patient with the transfusion of the cells. The garlic-like odor of DMSO is very distinctive and unpleasant. DMSO is excreted primarily through the respiratory system. DMSO is smelled and tasted as soon as it is infused, which can result in the baby having nausea and vomiting. Other side effects commonly seen are bradycardia and shortness of breath. Volume overload can occur as each bag of cells contains 50 to 100 mL.

Hypertension may require medication with antihypertensives and diuretics. Giving the transfusion over a 2- to 4-hours time period and in two different sessions may help lessen side effects. A significant reaction to DSMO may occur even without volume overload. The transfusion is thawed to break the ice crystals, so it is advised to keep the infant's environment as thermally neutral as possible with the use of a radiant warmer, isolette, or warm blankets. Monitor the temperature frequently. Stem cells should not be warmed as they may be damaged. After the transfusion, red urine may be seen as some of the cells will be excreted in the urine. Red urine will diminish over time. Hydration should be provided following infusion.

Fresh stem cells are given for allogenic transplants (related or unrelated) transplants within 48 hours of collection. Side effects may include hemolytic transfusion reactions, volume overload, pulmonary microemboli, and infection (as the transfusion is neither irradiated nor filtered) (Ikuta, 2008).

Assess the family's understanding of CB transfusion prior to the procedure and provide information and or education. For either transfusion type, careful monitoring of intake and output, oxygenation saturation, heart and respiratory rates, and blood pressures is warranted. Vital signs are taken before, during, and after the infusion. Interventions are based on the type of transfusion used (Table 27.2).

Umbilical CB transfusions offer hope to families of infants with various diseases requiring hematopoietic progenitor cells. It is not a common procedure as yet. In neonatal units affiliated with CB banks, studies of benefits versus ineffectiveness are occurring. It is still an uncommon

TABLE 27.2

POSSIBLE COMPLICATION SEQUENCE FOR CORD BLOOD TRANSFUSION

Immediate	Delayed (First Month)	Late Effects (After First Month)
Nausea/Vomiting	Bone marrow suppression	Immunosuppression
Diarrhea	Mucositis	Chronic graft-versus-host disease
Red urine	Hemorrhagic cystitis	Cataracts
Parotitis	Anorexia	Endocrine dysfunction
Hypertension	Capillary leak syndrome	Pulmonary restrictive disease
Volume overload	Venoocclusive disease	Genetic disease recurrence
Apnea/Bradycardia	Graft failure	Secondary malignancies
Tachypnea	Graft-versus-host disease	Bacterial infections
Respiratory distress	Acute renal failure	Cytomegalovirus infection
	Bacterial infection	Varicella zoster infection
	Viral infections (herpes simplex, cytomegalovirus)	Latent virus infections
	Fungal infection	*Pneumocystis carinii* pneumonia

Adapted from Baggott and Fochtman (2002) and Hockenberry-Eaton (1998).

procedure that can have far-reaching consequences. Thorough education of the family is required to deal with potential complications associated with stem cell infusion. Neonatal nurses need to be aware of the immediate, delayed, and late effects to give prompt intervention and treatment as needed.

Advantages and disadvantages of cord blood transfusion:

Advantages	Disadvantages
1. Easily obtained from cord at delivery of child. Not a good source of progenitor cells.	1. Can only be obtained at delivery if it is matched perfectly. Procedure for obtaining cord blood must be followed exactly. At times, not enough is collected or cannot be collected due to difficult delivery.
2. Can use unmatched cord blood from donors.	2. Need adequate volume of cord blood.
3. Decreased graft-versus-host disease with use of cord blood.	3. Slower engraftment of cells and delayed rebuilding of immune system, depending on hospital criteria for discharge, could mean greater length of stay.
4. Infection risk from blood-borne viruses lessened.	4. At risk longer from infection due to delayed rebuilding of immune system.

SUMMARY

In the past decade, transplantation has become more common but is more the exception than the rule. Transplants with solid organs were the mainstay but stem cell transplants are beginning to be explored. Transplants are a tertiary treatment. It is the last, best option for many patients. The next few years will likely see changes in indications for transplant, with earlier treatments and procedures.

The rise in the current number of transplant candidates, deaths of patients on the waitlist, and the shortage of donor organs have fueled the search for alternative measures in transplantation. One alternative is extracorporeal bioartificial livers containing functioning viable hepatocytes, which could provide temporary support for patients with fulminant hepatic failure or awaiting liver transplantation. Another solution is deemed possible in hepatocyte transplantation. Laboratory studies and experiences in small numbers of human subjects have demonstrated its efficacy. Unfortunately, cell transplantation therapy is also limited by the severe shortage of donor cells as well as low transplant efficiency.

The ultimate aim of cell transplantation, tissue engineering, and stem cells is to regenerate tissues and organs. With the development of whole-organ decellularized methods, the equation of organ shortage may dramatically change in the near future.

CASE STUDY

■ **Identification of Problem.** Late preterm twin female infants born vaginally; presented with lethargy, poor feeding, and weight loss at 3 days of age.

■ **Assessment: History and Physical Examination**
Twin female late preterm infants were delivered vaginally to a 28-year-old G2 P2 woman after an uncomplicated pregnancy. Infants were 36 weeks postmenstrual age with twin A's birth weight of 2.8 kg and twin B's birth weight of 2.7 kg. Twin A had Apgars of 9^1 9^5 and twin B had Apgars of 8^1 9^5. Admission to the NICU. Both infants had a gross normal physical exam upon admission. As late preterm infants, they had temperature instability requiring warming in isolettes. They are poor nipplers who require gavage feeds.

■ **Second Day of Life.** Newborn screens were sent on the second day of life. Screens are sent overnight for spectronomy.

■ **Differential Diagnosis**

1. Late preterm twins
2. Hypothermia
3. Feeding difficulties

■ **Diagnostic Tests.** Newborn screens

■ **Working Diagnosis.** Late preterm twins

■ **Third Day of Life.** These twins were born in a state that has expanded newborn screens. Expanded newborn screening results by spectronomy revealed a rare genetic disorder of methylmalonic acidemia (MMA). In most states these twins would have died before a diagnosis of MMA would have been made.

■ **Outcome.** The twins are late preterm infants whose appropriate acting masked their metabolic disorder. Both twins were diagnosed with MMA because of expanded newborn screening, which saved their lives. They were put on a low-protein diet and medications until they were big enough for a liver transplant. Liver transplants were done at 15 months of age. Transplants were done early in life to ward against the toxic effects to brain, kidney, and other organs. They remain on low-protein diets and medications. By having liver transplants, their chances at a long life have been improved greatly.

EVIDENCE-BASED PRACTICE BOX

Expanded Newborn Screening

Universal newborn screening is the practice of screening every newborn for genetic testing. Through early identification and treatment, newborn screening improves care. Primary intervention provides an opportunity for reduction in infant morbidity and mortality.

Expanded newborn screening using tandem mass spectrometry (MS/MS) can detect many genetic diseases. Every year approximately 4 million infants are screened. Of these screened infants 12,500 are diagnosed with one of the 29 core conditions of the uniform screening panel (Howell et al., 2012). Hearing loss, primary congenital hypothyroidism, cystic fibrosis, sickle cell disease, and medium-chain acyl-CoA dehydrogenase deficiency are the most common genetic entities detected in the United States. A group of experts assembled by the American College of Medical Genetics under the sponsorship of the Human Resources and Services Administration were assembled in 2006. These experts standardized tests of the expanded newborn screening for the United States. The new expanded-screening panel is composed of 29 core conditions. Within the panel are 20 inborn errors of metabolism, 3 hemoglobinopathies, and 6 other conditions (Howell et al., 2012).

Many of the diseases of the expanded newborn screen in the past were not diagnosed until after the child was very ill or died. Diagnosing disease early from the newborn screen can result in treatment before mortality or morbidity occurs. In the case of the twin infants with MMA, they had liver transplants to prevent the devastating effects of the disease. Therrell, Buechner, Lloyd-Puryear, van Dyck, & Mann (2008) noted that several studies provide data for the cost effectiveness of testing. Each infant with detectable disease leads to primary intervention, which leads to cost savings.

False-positive tests have been explored regarding parental stress and anxiety. It was hypothesized that the false-positive tests would cause undue emotional distress in parents and families. Several studies have addressed the false-positive tests and emotional distress of parents/families and concluded that benefits outweighed the distress (Sun, Lam, & Wong, 2012).

The expanded newborn screen has limitations of enough experts trained to care for neonates affected by complex rare conditions, laboratory capabilities, and possible false-positive results. Long-term follow-up of test results could answer these limitations. While the expanded newborn screen has helped many infants to be diagnosed and cared for earlier, there is still the question of which ones. Consumers need to be educated and be empowered to make informed decisions regarding the tests.

ONLINE RESOURCES

American Society of Transplantation (AST, 2012)
http://www.a-s-t.org/about/pediatric-community-practice-executive-committee

Organ Procurement and Transplantation Network (OPTN, 2012)
http://optn.transplant.hrsa.gov/members/committees.asp

The International Society for Heart & Lung Transplantation (ISHLT, 2012)
http://www.ishlt.org/about

United Network for Organ Sharing (UNOS, 2012)
http://www.unos.org

World Health Organization (2012). Organ Transplantation
http://www.who.int/transplantation/organ/en/index.html

REFERENCES

American Academy of Pediatrics. (1999). Cord blood banking for potential future transplantation (RE9860). *Pediatrics*, *104*, 116–118.

Baggott, C., & Fochtman, D. (2002). *Nursing care of children and adolescents with cancer*. Philadelphia, PA: Saunders.

Carter, B. A., et al. (2006). History of pediatric liver transplantation. Retrieved from http://www.emedicine.com/ped/topic2840.htm

Dhawan, A., & Mieli-Vergani, G. (2005). Acute liver failure in neonates. *Early Human Development*, *81*(12), 1005–1010.

Esquivel, C. (2005). *Liver transplantation in children*. Stanford University Medical School. Retrieved from http://med.stanford.edu/shs/txp/livertxp/HTML/selection.pediatric.html

Garbade, J., Bittner, H. B., Barten, M. J., & Mohr, F. (2011). Current trends in implantable left ventricular assist devices. *Cardiology Research and Practice*, Article ID 290561, 1–9.

Hockenberry-Eaton, M. J. (Ed.). (1998). *Essentials of pediatric oncology nursing: A core curriculum*. Glenview, IL: Association of Pediatric Oncology Nurses.

Howell, R., Terry, S., Tait, V. F., Olney, R., Hinton, C. F., Grosse, S., & Glidewell, J. (2012). CDC grand rounds: Newborn screening and improved outcomes. *MMWR: Morbidity & Mortality Weekly Report*, *61*(21), 390–393.

Ikuta, L. M. (2008). Human umbilical cord blood transplantation: What nurses need to know. *AACN Advanced Critical Care*, *19*(3), 264–267.

Intestinal Transplant Registry. (2005). The intestinal transplant registry. Retrieved from http://www.intestinaltransplant.org

Jackson, R., & Roberts, E. (2001). Identification of neonatal liver failure and perinatal hemochromatosis in Canada. *Paediatrics & Child Health*, *6*(5), 229–231.

Kline, N. E. (Ed.). (2009). *Essentials of pediatric hematology/oncology nursing: A core curriculum* (3rd ed.). Glenview, IL: Associate of Pediatric Oncology Nurses.

Koike, H., & Taniguchi, H. (2012). Characteristics of hepatic stem/progenitor cells in the fetal and adult liver. *Journal of Hepatobiliary Pancreatic Science*, *19*(6), 587–593. Epub.

Meyburg, J., & Hoffmann, G. F. (2010). Liver, liver cell and stem cell transplantation for the treatment of urea cycle defects. *Molecular Genetics and Metabolism*, *100*, 577–583.

Oellerich, M., & Armstrong, V. W. (2001). The MEGX Test: A tool for the real-time assessment of hepatic function. *Therapeutic Drug Monitoring*, *23*(2), 81–92.

Organ Procurement and Transplantation Network. (OPTN). (2012). Retrieved from http://optn.transplant.hrsa.gov

Organ Procurement and Transplantation Network (OPTN) and Scientific Registry of Transplant Recipients (SRTR). (2012). OPTN/SRTR 2010 Annual Data Report. Rockville, MD: Department of Health and Human Services, Health Resources and Services Administration, Healthcare Systems Bureau, Division of Transplantation.

Pickering, L. K. (Ed.). (2009). *Red book: 2009 report of the committee on infectious diseases* (26th ed., pp. 560–569). Elk Grove Village, IL: American Academy of Pediatrics.

Sun, A., Lam, C., & Wong, D. A. (2012). Expanded newborn screening for inborn errors of metabolism: Overview and outcomes. *Advances in Pediatrics*, *59*, 209–245.

Therrell, B. L., Buechner, C., Lloyd-Puryear, M.A., van Dyck, P.C., & Mann, M.Y. (2008). What's new in newborn screening? *Pediatric Health*, *2*(4), 411–429.

United Network for Organ Sharing. (2005). Critical pathway for pediatric organ donation. Retrieved from http://www.unos.org/resources/donorManagement.asp?index=2

Zargar, S. A., Yattoo, G. N., Javid, G., Khan, B. A., Shah, A. H., Shah, N. A., ... Shafi, H. M. (2004). Fifteen-year follow-up of endoscopic injection sclerotherapy in children with extrahepatic portal venous obstruction. *Journal of Gastroenterology and Hepatology*, *19*(2), 139–145.

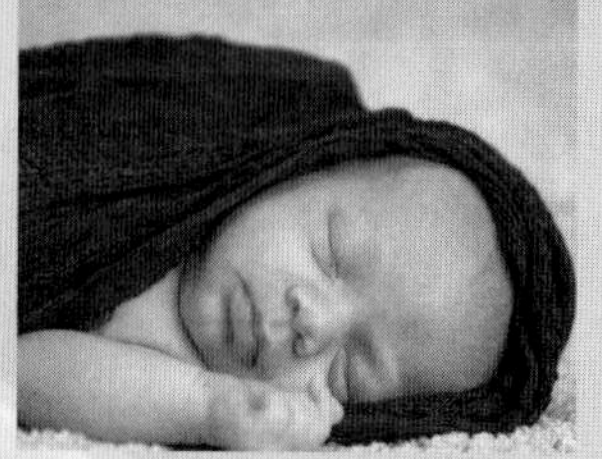

CHAPTER

28

Extremely-Low-Birth-Weight (ELBW) Infant

■ Shahirose S. Premji

The extremely-low-birth-weight (ELBW) infant, one who is born weighing less than 1,000 g, is a frequent resident of most neonatal intensive care units (NICUs) these days. The survival rate for ELBW infants has improved (Doyle, Roberts, Anderson, & Victorian Infant Collaborative Study Group, 2011; Kilbride, 2004) as a result of advances in technology, organization of perinatal care (Roze & Breart, 2004), and obstetrical interventions (e.g., antenatal corticosteroid use) (Kilbride, 2004). Survival rates to hospital discharge range from 26.5% to 87.8% (Guillen et al., 2011); the variations may be explained by strategies used to report rates (i.e., denominator bias) or differences in available resources particularly in developing countries (Ballot, Chirwa, & Cooper, 2010). Greater survival, however, has not always been associated with increased quality-adjusted survival (Kilbride, 2004). We must look to the future in anticipation, not of change in the limit of viability, but rather of evidence-based strategies to improve the quality of perinatal, neonatal, and postdischarge care with the goal to improve the long-term outcome of ELBW (Roze & Breart, 2004). This chapter reviews the challenges facing an ELBW infant and their family. It provides evidence to support neonatal interventions.

EVIDENCE-BASED NEONATAL NURSING CARE

Many years ago, all preterm infants were viewed as "low birth weight or small infants," and their care usually reflected a variation on general pediatric care. Over the past 45 years, it has become clear that preterm infants are a heterogeneous population who require very specialized treatment depending on their birth weight (Silverman, 1992). The definition of low birth weight now includes very low birth weight (VLBW), as an infant who is born weighing less than 1,500 g, and ELBW. Whatever the reasons for the ELBW status, these neonates require highly specialized care if they are to survive and thrive. In the 1950s and 1960s health care professionals realized that neonates, especially those who were sick and premature, required care based on an understanding of the disorders and disease and identification of rigorously evaluated treatment (Silverman, 1992). Examples such as retrolental fibroplasias secondary to the introduction of unrestricted oxygen therapy and kernicterus resulting from the use of sulfisoxazole underscore the importance of evidence-based practice (Silverman, 1992). Nurses' use of research in practice is not only slow but unpredictable; consequently, moving evidence to practice will be important to improving neonatal outcomes (Cumming, Hutchinson, Scott, Norton, & Estabrooks, 2010; Straus, Graham, Mazmanian, 2006).

IMPACT OF BIRTH OF ELBW INFANTS

Decision Making in the Delivery Room

Appropriate for gestational age infants less than 23 weeks gestation and less than 500 g birth weight are considered too immature to survive based on data collected over the past 10 to 15 years (Seri & Evans, 2008). For example, the EPICure study undertaken in the United Kingdom found that less than 1% of infants born at 22 to 23 weeks gestation survived and were discharged from hospital (Costeloe, Hennessy, Gibson, Marlow, & Wilkinson, 2000). In contrast, the majority of infants born greater than and equal to 25 weeks gestation and greater than and equal to 600 g survive and about half without severe long-term disabilities (Seri & Evans, 2008). At ELBW, particularly between 500 and 599 g defined as the "gray zone," there is uncertainty about survival and outcome (Seri & Evans, 2008). As a result, issues related to moral status (Smith, 2005), and judgments about survival and unacceptable quality of life pose a dilemma for health care professionals, parents, and society (Powell, Parker, Dedrick, Barrera, & Salvo, 2012; Seri & Evans, 2008).

An ELBW infant gains status as a patient and in a social sense as a member of a family once the infant is born. Health care professionals owe the ELBW infant a duty of ethical treatment and care because of this status (Smith, 2005). Whether to resuscitate and to initiate and continue intensive care raises questions related to the primacy of the newborn's best interest, respect for persons and legal rights, and the health care providers' consideration of ethical principles of beneficence, nonmaleficence, autonomy, justice, and futility. Ethical principles are difficult to implement in practice (Lorenz, 2003; Powell et al., 2012; Seri & Evans, 2008; Wilder, 2000). Treatment decisions for the ELBW infant reflect varied opinions on the proper approach to resuscitation and initiation of intensive care for these infants. The best interest of the child, which supports the universal right to life, is regulated by law in many countries (e.g., United States of America, United Kingdom, and Canada) (Albersheim, 2008; Kopelman, 2005; Schoonakker & Smith, 2007) and supported by the Hippocratic Oath and professional medical organizations (Haward, Kirshenbaum, & Campbell, 2011). Clinicians would therefore be inclined to initiate all necessary life support at least temporarily, to permit assessment of the harm-to-benefit ratio based on projected suffering and burden as determined by current data or "best guess" (Smith, 2005). This approach includes an opportunity for survival while minimizing risk of long-term disability if the child is incorrectly judged to be nonviable and survives (Wilder, 2000).

The best interest standard is, however, difficult to apply for decision making in the delivery room, given the subjective nature of appraising the mortality and morbidity of infants in the "gray zone" or threshold of viability. Additionally, care providers must consider parents' or guardians' expectations, values, and religious beliefs, as they are the primary caregivers and will have the ultimate responsibility of care (Haward et al., 2011; Kopelman, 2005; Schoonakker & Smith, 2007). A "negative" analysis of the best interest of the child has been proposed as it permits considerations of available options based on a range of moral, social, and legal issues. As well, it permits involvement of parents in decision making (Kopelman, 2005; Schoonakker & Smith, 2007). The American Academy of Pediatrics promotes involvement of parents early in the decision-making process regarding survival and disability; hence it incorporates parents' wishes to be involved in decision making (Schoonakker & Smith, 2007). A single approach or philosophy on care that is appropriate for all countries, cultures, or communities is an unreasonable expectation. Individual and societal values, long-term outcomes, associated physical, psychological, emotional, and financial costs, and finite resources will play a significant role in decision making regarding whether or not to resuscitate and continue care in ELBW infants. The marked variation in the frequency with which aggressive resuscitation is initiated in the zone of uncertainty is not surprising given the various ways in which competing values may be balanced by different individuals, cultures, and societies (Lorenz, 2003).

Ideally, a resuscitation plan should be in place prior to delivery. An individualized approach is recommended in management decisions regarding the aggressive resuscitation of ELBW infants (Powell et al., 2012). Statistical modeling is being employed to identify factors (e.g., higher birth weight, female sex, singleton gestation, antenatal corticoid steroids) that can assist clinicians in predicting morbidity and mortality and guide decision making (Powell et al., 2012; Tyson et al., 2008). In many instances though, there is often little time to make informed decisions about the reasonableness of resuscitation and initiation of intensive care (Powell et al., 2012). Contextual factors such as the woman's pain, labor, or deteriorating maternal or fetal condition, and inconsistent and conflicting information provided by multiple care providers pose a barrier to effective communication and decision making regarding resuscitation and delivery room care (Tomlinson, Kaempf, Ferguson, & Stewart, 2010). A standardized evidence-based approach to counseling that included recommendations for and against treatment was well received by patients who found the process useful and consistent and information understandable. More importantly, patients were comfortable with the decisions they made for self and their families (Tomlinson et al., 2010).

Ethical decisions regarding the extent of resuscitation efforts should be based on multiple factors including gestational age, birth weight, sex of the fetus, and the infant's condition at birth, survival and morbidity data, and the parents' wishes. Information should be provided in a consistent manner, and a multidisciplinary approach will ensure that a range of concerns and areas of clinical care are addressed (American College of Obstetricians and Gynecologists [ACOG], 2002). The plan should be based on consensus decision making by parents and all health care professionals involved in the provision of care to the mother and ELBW infant (Powell et al., 2012; Wilder, 2000).

Survival of ELBW Infants

Data based on gestational age are more appropriate than data based on birth weight for projecting survival and future disability in infants. However, unreliable gestational age estimates, and earlier reporting practices of rounding off gestational age to the nearest week of gestation, can have a significant impact on survival statistics (Ho & Saigal, 2005). Population-based studies examining survival by gestational age report marked variation in survival rates among different geographic areas. These variations are likely a reflection of management styles such as proactive versus less aggressive resuscitation and initiation of intensive care, and manner in which outcomes are reported (e.g., duration of survival) (Haward et al., 2011; Ho & Saigal, 2005; Lorenz, 2004). Table 28.1 illustrates the variation in survival rates of ELBW around the world by comparing countries such as the United States, Europe, Canada, and Japan. As is evident with each additional week of gestational age, there is a large improvement in survival rates (Haward et al., 2011). At comparable gestational age and birth weight, mortality rates are higher for males compared to females (ACOG, 2002).

TABLE 28.1

SURVIVAL RATES TO HOSPITAL DISCHARGE AMONG INFANTS BORN 22 TO 25 WEEKS GESTATION

Cohort	Year	Denominator	22 weeks	23 weeks	24 weeks	25 weeks
NICHD (United States) (Stoll et al., 2010)	2003–2007	Live births	6%	26%	55%	72%
VON (Multinational) (Hobar et al, n.d.)	2009	Live births	5%	33%	61%	–
Canadian Neonatal Network (Chan et al., 2001)	1996–1997	Population-based	1%	17%	44%	68%
EPIBel (Vanhaesebrouck et al., 2004)	1999–2000	Population-based	0%	6%	29%	56%
EPICure (United Kingdom, Ireland) (Wood, Marlow, Costeloe, Gibson, & Wilkinson, 2000)	1995	Population-based (LB + SB)	1%	11%	26%	44%
EXPRESS (Sweden) (Express Group, 2009)	2004–2007	Live births Population-based	12% 7%	54% 34%	71% 60%	82% 73%
Norwegian Infant Study (Markestad et al., 2005)	1999–2000	Admission to NICU Population-based	0 0	39% 16%	60% 44%	80% 66%
Switzerland (Fischer, Steurer, Adams, Berger, & Swiss Neonatal Network, 2009)	2000–2004	Population-based	0%	5%	30%	50%
Japan: Single Center (Iijima, Arai, Ozawa, Kawase, & Uga, 2009) Japan: Multicenter (Kusauda et al., 2006)	1991–2006 2003	Live births	25% 36%	47% 78%	50% 75%	–

EPIBel, extremely preterm infants in Belgium; EPICure, extremely preterm infant cohort in the United Kingdom and the Republic of Ireland; EXPRESS, extremely preterm infants in Sweden study; LB, live birth; NICHD, National Institutes of Health Center for Child Health and Human Development; NICU, neonatal intensive care unit; SB still birth; VON, Vermont Oxford Network.

Morbidity in ELBW Infants

Chronic lung disease, necrotizing enterocolitis (NEC), retinopathy of prematurity, and disabilities in mental and psychomotor development, neuromotor function, or sensory and communication function are major neonatal morbidities associated with ELBW (ACOG, 2002; Hakansson, Farooqi, Holmgren, Serenius, & Högberg, 2004; Ho & Saigal, 2005).

■ Chronic Lung Disease

Chronic lung disease, the most prevalent morbidity in ELBW infants, occurs in 57% to 70% of infants at 23 weeks gestational age. At 24 weeks gestational age, rates of chronic lung disease range from 33% to 89%, and at 25 weeks gestational age ranges from 16% to 71%. Chronic lung disease is a major morbidity influencing later development, given its association with poor nutrition and growth, poor feeding skills, prolonged hospitalization, and episodes of nosocomial infection. The "new BPD" (bronchopulmonary dysplasia, a form of chronic lung disease) that occurs primarily in ELBW infants is thought to have a qualitatively different pathogenesis marked by immaturity and alveolar hypoplasia rather than the hyperoxic barotrauma or volutrauma typically seen in surfactant deficient lungs (Narendran et al., 2003).

Early delivery room or prophylactic surfactant prior to stabilization with CPAP regardless of respiratory status has demonstrated beneficial outcomes such as reduced delivery room intubations, days on mechanical ventilation, fewer infants discharged home on oxygen, use of postnatal steroid, lowered oxygen saturation goals, and decreased incidence and severity of bronchopulmonary dysplasia (Geary, Caskey, Fonseca, & Malloy, 2008; Meyer, Mildenhall, & Wong, 2004; Narendran et al., 2003). However, a recent systematic review concluded that there are no clear benefits of using prophylactic surfactant when infants are routinely managed on CPAP. With routine application of CPAP as standard of practice, the risk of chronic lung disease or death was lower with selective treatment with surfactant when compared to prophylactic use of surfactant (Rojas-Reyes, Morley, & Soll, 2012). Dexamethasone treatment has been found to have no effect on chronic lung disease and is associated with gastrointestinal perforation and decreased growth in ELBW infants (Stark et al., 2001). More importantly, a systematic review reported a dramatic increase in neurodevelopmental impairment in preterm infants treated with glucocorticoids in the postnatal period (Barrington, 2001).

■ Necrotizing Enterocolitis

Necrotizing enterocolitis (NEC), an acquired gastrointestinal disease that complicates the neonatal course of survivors, affects 1 to 3 infants per 1,000 live births (Guthrie et al., 2003; Lee & Polin, 2003). ELBW infants are particularly susceptible and have a higher incidence of NEC; however, the clinical presentation is relatively similar to that for other affected neonates. The cause of NEC remains unclear but most likely represents a complex interaction of factors with a final common pathway of intestinal ischemia. In epidemiologic studies, prematurity is consistently identified as an independent determinant of NEC (Lee & Polin, 2003). Other factors include feeding practices, intestinal ischemia, and bacterial colonization (Kliegman, 1990). Hallmarks of NEC include pneumatosis intestinalis, hepatic portal venous gas, perforation, and pneumoperitoneum; these are evident on abdominal x-ray (Meerstadt & Gyll, 1994; Snapp, 1994). Manifestations of NEC include abdominal distention, residuals, vomiting, bloody stools, metabolic acidosis, cellular destruction, and gut necrosis. Treatment focuses on medical stabilization and interventions including bowel rest, gastric decompression, broad-spectrum systemic antibiotics, and parenteral nutrition. Infants with perforation either are operated on or have a peritoneal drainage (Lee & Polin, 2003). The catastrophic nature of NEC and the fragility of ELBW infants are evident in the overall mortality of the disease, which is approximately 50% (Blakely et al., 2005). Once NEC develops, the long-term consequences may include growth delay and severe neurodevelopmental delay (Salhab, Perlman, Silver, & Sue Broyles, 2004). Consequently, prevention of NEC has been the primary focus resulting in numerous approaches being proposed to prevent NEC (Neu & Walker, 2011).

Provision of small volumes of exclusive human milk (Meinzen-Derr et al., 2009) or human milk fortified with a human milk–derived fortifier (Sullivan et al., 2010) has been found to be safe (i.e., lower incidence of NEC). Standardized feeding regimens have been introduced in an attempt to reduce the incidence of NEC by minimizing variations in enteral feeding practices. A systematic review and meta-analysis of observational studies ("before" and "after") reported a reduced the incidence of NEC after the introduction of a standardized feeding regimen (Patole & de Klerk, 2005). A retrospective cohort study reported an association between prolonged duration of initial (i.e., in the first 3 postnatal days) antibiotic course and increased risk of NEC or death (Cotton et al., 2009). Although prophylactic enteral probiotic supplementation reduced the incidence of severe NEC (i.e., stage II or greater) (typical relative risk 0.35, 95% CI 0.24, 0.52) in preterm infants data for ELBW infants could not be extrapolated. Consequently, recommendations cannot be made regarding use of probiotics for prevention of NEC in ELBW infants (AlFaleh, Anabrees, Bassler, & Al-Kharfi, 2011). Use of oral immunoglobulin (Foster & Cole, 2011) as a preventative strategy for NEC is not supported in preterm or low-birth-weight infants; however, the strategy has not been studied exclusively in ELBW infants.

■ Retinopathy of Prematurity

Retinopathy of prematurity (ROP), a vascular proliferative disorder of the immature retina (i.e., abnormal growth of retinal capillaries during vascularization), causes acuity defects, refractive errors (particularly myopia), gaze abnormalities, and blindness (Andersen & Phelps, 2009). Vascularization of the retina is complete by 40 weeks gestational age (Brion, Bell, & Raghuveer, 2008). The developing retinal capillaries are susceptible to injury; hence preventative strategies (e.g., control of exogenous oxygen delivery) are aimed at reducing stress contributing to injury, while interdictive approaches (e.g., cryosurgery or laser ablation) are aimed at controlling or arresting progression of neovascularization (Phelps & Watts, 2009).

In developed countries, the population at risk for blinding retinopathy of prematurity has changed, with studies (Hardy et al., 2004) suggesting that ELBW are at greatest risk of advanced stages of retinopathy of prematurity requiring treatment (Gilbert et al., 2005). In contrast, in low- and moderate-income countries, it is the larger, more mature infants that are at risk of developing severe retinopathy of prematurity (Gilbert et al., 2005). To facilitate earlier identification and timely intervention for prethreshold retinopathy of prematurity in at-risk infants (i.e., ELBW), it is recommended that the timing of an eye exam be based on chronologic age of 4 to 6 weeks rather than 31- to 33-week postconceptional age being used (Subhani, Combs, Weber, Gerontis, & DeCristofaro, 2001). The American Academy of Pediatrics, Section on Ophthalmology, American Academy of Ophthalmology, and American Association for Pediatric Ophthalmology and Strabismus (2006) recommend the use of the international classification system (2005) to classify findings on retinal exams. Subsequent eye examinations, depending on the results, occur at least every 2 weeks until the retina is fully vascularized. Continued ophthalmologic follow-up of ELBW infants with severe retinopathy of prematurity is essential as retinopathy of prematurity may represent a lifelong disease, as evidenced by the number of eyes, both cryotherapy-treated and noncryotherapy-treated, that developed retinal detachment, blindness, and other related complications between ages 10 and 15 (Cryotherapy for Retinopathy of Prematurity Cooperative Group, 2005; Palmer et al., 2005).

In premature infants, factors such as change in oxygen exposure have been proposed to cause distribution in the vascularization. In a systematic review, supplementation with vitamin E, an antioxidant agent, was not supported given that there was an increased risk of sepsis and reduced risk of severe retinopathy and blindness among VLBW infants who were given vitamin E supplements (Brion et al., 2008). Darlow and Graham (2011) found that with vitamin A supplementation fewer infants required oxygen at 36 weeks postmenstrual age (numbers needed to treat 13, 95% CI 7, 100). Supplementation with vitamin A, the precursors of which have antioxidant properties, has been shown in a systematic review to be a potential protective therapy for retinopathy of prematurity in ELBW infants as there was a trend toward reduced incidence of retinopathy of prematurity in treated infants (Darlow & Graham, 2011). Askie, Henderson-Smart, and Ko (2009) performed a systematic review of studies of unrestricted oxygen use and outcomes in premature infants. They found that if oxygen levels were not monitored closely, morbidity in this population rose. Oxygen levels, therefore, must be watched and controlled carefully; however the optimal range of oxygen levels remains unknown (Askie et al., 2009).

Cryotherapy and laser therapy are standard care for threshold retinopathy of prematurity (Cryotherapy for Retinopathy of Prematurity Cooperative Group, 2005). Given the substantial proportion of eyes treated with cryotherapy that developed retinal detachment and unfavorable distance visual acuity, current research is focusing on early treatment for retinopathy of prematurity (Hardy et al., 2004; Subhani et al., 2001). A systematic review by Andersen and Phelps (2009) has reported early treatment with peripheral retinal ablation to be effective for treating eyes determined to be at high risk for a poor outcome or prethreshold retinopathy of prematurity. Treatment resulted in reduced risk of adverse structural outcome at 12 months and 5½ years with corresponding reduction in adverse acuity. Further research is required to assess whether the benefits of treatment will persist into adult life.

■ Neurodevelopment

Major neurologic impairments include cerebral palsy, motor impairment, visual and hearing impairments, and cognitive deficits (Ho & Saigal, 2005; Wood et al., 2000). Significant variation in neurodevelopmental outcomes is reported in single-center, multicenter, and national cohorts of extremely preterm children (Haward et al., 2011). Variability in morbidity reported by single-center, multicenter, and national cohorts of extremely preterm children (Haward et al., 2011) is striking (Lorenz, 2003) may be due to chronological age at evaluation, varying criteria for defining and reporting neurologic impairments (i.e., instruments to measure disability and functional capacity) (Haward et al., 2011; Ho & Saigal, 2005), differences in center demographics, antenatal interventions, and neonatal clinical practice or interventions (Vohr et al., 2004). Infants have been reported to have developmental lags without defined impairment (Ho & Saigal, 2005).

A study of 219 ELBW survivors admitted between 1992 and 1995 to Rainbow Babies and Children's Hospital in Cleveland, Ohio, and assessed at 8 years of age reported the following outcomes: (1) major neurosensory impairment, including cerebral palsy, deafness, and blindness (16%); (2) asthma requiring therapy (21%); (3) functional limitations including delay in growth or development, mental or emotional delay, need to reduce or inability to participate in physical activities, difficulty seeing, hearing, speaking, or communicating, and inability to play or socialize with others (64%); (4) one or more compensatory dependence needs, including prescribed medication, life-threatening allergic reactions, prescribed special diet, special equipment to see, hear, or communicate, and need for help or special equipment for walking, feeding, dressing, washing, and toileting (48%); and (5) services needed above routine, including visiting a physician regularly for a chronic condition, nursing care or medical procedures, occupational or physical therapy, special school arrangements, or an individualized education program (65%). The findings of this study may not be representative of all ELBW survivors, as this was not a population-based study. A recent population based study of ELBW found up to 50% prevalence of neurodevelopmental disability that remained throughout childhood (Johnson et al., 2009).

The ELBW infant follow-up group of the Vermont Oxford Network (VON) examined data from 33 North American VON centers for 1998, noting severe disability in 34% of infants (n = 3,567) assessed at 18 to 24 months' corrected age (Mercier et al., 2010). Despite improvements in perinatal interventions, extremely preterm infants are still at an increased level for adverse outcomes at 18 to 22 months corrected age (Hintz, Kendrick, et al., 2011). Neurodevelopmental outcomes for infants born at less than 25 weeks estimated gestation age remained unchanged between infants born between 1991 and 2001 versus those born between 2002 and 2004: moderate-to-severe cerebral palsy (adjusted odds ratio (aOR) 1.52, 95 Confidence Interval (CI) 0.86, 2.71); $p = 0.15$), mental developmental index less than 70 (aOR 1.3, 95% CI 0.91, 1.87; $p = 0.15$), and neurodevelopmental impairment diagnosed in 50% of surviving infants (aOR 1.4, 95% CI 0.98, 2.04; $p = 0.07$) (Hintz, Kendrick, et al., 2011). Neurodevelopmental and cognitive impairments have been found to remain stable between 6 and 11 years of age, with minimal shifts in severity of disability (Johnson et al., 2009). The proportion of ELBW survivors with adverse outcomes increases with decreasing gestational age (Haward et al., 2011), with poor chances of intact outcomes for infants 23 and 24 weeks gestation. At comparable gestational age and birth weight, disability rates (e.g., cerebral palsy) are higher for males than for females (ACOG, 2002; Johnson et al., 2009). Gestational age and sex have independent effects on neurodevelopmental outcomes (Haward et al., 2011).

Severe brain injury as evidenced by abnormal cerebral ultrasound findings predicts major morbidity such as quadriparesis and severe cerebral palsy in ELBW infants (Kuban et al., 2009). Interventions such as prophylactic indomethacin therapy have been used in clinical practice to reduce the occurrence of severe intraventricular hemorrhage or periventricular leukomalacia, which are significant short-term predictors of neurodevelopmental morbidity in ELBW infants. Although prophylactic administration of indomethacin reduces the incidence of severe intraventricular hemorrhage (Schmidt et al., 2007), it does not improve neurodevelopmental outcomes (Fowlie, Davis, & McGuire, 2010; Schmidt et al., 2001). Magnesium sulfate given to mothers at risk of preterm birth has been shown to have neuroprotective effects; improving long-term outcomes of infants born preterm (Doyle, 2012); however the most effective regimen remains to be determined (Bain, Middleton, & Crowther, 2012). The Caffeine for Apnea of Prematurity (CAP) trial, which enrolled infants less than 1,250 g, initially reported reduced rates of cerebral palsy and cognitive delay at 18 months of age; however, rates of disability were no different at 5 years corrected age (Schmidt et al., 2012).

Among other contributing factors, the neurodevelopmental morbidity has been partially attributed to the stressful nature of the intensive care unit (Gorski, 1991). Neurodevelopment can be promoted if the potential impact of the environment is recognized and interventions including one or more elements such as control of external stimuli (e.g., light, noise, minimal stimulation), clustering of care activities, and positioning or swaddling are implemented. There is evidence that this broad category of interventions, referred to as developmental care, offers the following benefits to preterm infants: improved short-term growth and feeding outcomes, decreased respiratory support, decreased length and cost of hospital stay, and improved neurodevelopmental outcomes to 24 months corrected age (Symington & Pinelli, 2009).

COMPLICATIONS OF BEING BORN AT ELBW

In the immediate neonatal period, ELBW infants are more susceptible to all the possible complications of premature birth because of their very vulnerable state of development. The balance of this chapter is an overview, a quick reference for typical problems experienced by ELBW infants and some of the outcomes for these infants. The chapter also addresses the key areas for care where nurses need to contribute to the scientific basis for practice.

Thermoregulation

Cold stress is associated with increased mortality and morbidity (e.g., hypoglycemia, respiratory distress, and metabolic acidosis) in premature infants (Hazan, Maag, & Chessex, 1991; McCall, Alderdice, Halliday, Jenkins, & Vohra, 2010). The incidence of hypothermia or temperature less than 36.4°C or 97.6°F varies between centers, and quality improvement data indicate rates greater than 56% for infants less than 750 g (Bhatt et al., 2007). In the first 12 hours of life, ELBW are not able to conserve heat, given poor vasomotor control (Knobel, Holditch-Davis, Schwartz, & Wimmer, 2009). A high body surface area-to-body weight ratio (Lyon, Pikaar, Badger, & McIntosh, 1997), and decreased ability to produce heat because of decreased brown fat stores and decreased glycogen supply, makes ELBW infants particularly vulnerable to hypothermia (defined as less than 36.5°C) (Knobel, Wimmer, & Holbert, 2005; McCall et al., 2010; Sauer, Dane, & Visser, 1984). Provision of warmth is the first step in the resuscitation of the newborn because the risk of cold stress is greatest at birth (Knobel et al., 2005). A systematic review (McCall et al., 2010) found that early intervention in the delivery room, particularly the application of plastic wraps (for infants less than 28 weeks gestational age) or transwarmer mattresses (infants less than 1,500 g) within 10 minutes after birth, prevents hypothermia, keeping infants warmer on admission to the NICU. These early interventions are in addition to "routine" care implemented immediately after birth such as drying the infant thoroughly, especially the head, removing any wet blankets, wrapping infant in a prewarmed blanket, and prewarming any contact surfaces. Further research is required to facilitate firm recommendations of these early interventions in clinical practice for ELBW.

The "gold standard" for nursing preterm infants in incubators or under radiant warmers is to maintain the body temperature at which the metabolic rate reaches the minimum or thermoneutral temperature (Rieger-Fackeldey, Schaller-Bals, & Schulze, 2003). In the first week of life, this thermoneutral temperature is dependent on gestational age and postnatal age, after which time it depends on body weight and postnatal age (Sauer et al., 1984). However, for ELBW infants, this optimal body temperature is not known (Rieger-Fackeldey et al., 2003). A study of ventilator-dependent ELBW infants in the early postnatal age (day 2–14) reported pronounced and consistent changes in spontaneous breathing secondary to minor changes in core body temperature within a range commonly accepted in routine clinical care in the NICU. The observed changes to body temperature are of uncertain clinical significance (Rieger-Fackeldey et al., 2003).

Respiratory Distress Syndrome

Respiratory distress syndrome (RDS), a common problem among ELBW infants, has a pathogenesis dominated by surfactant deficiency. Surfactant deficiency leads to decreased lung compliance, reduced alveolar ventilation, atelectasis, and alveolar hypoperfusion, which clinically manifests as grunting respirations, retractions, nasal flaring, cyanosis, and increased oxygen requirement shortly after birth. Clinical management includes supplemental oxygen, CPAP, and/or ventilatory support, and the clinical course may be complicated by air leaks, significant shunting through the patent ductus arteriosus (PDA), or bronchopulmonary dysplasia (Rodriguez, Martin, & Fanaroff, 2002; Rojas-Reyes et al., 2012).

Prophylactic (delivery room) and rescue (after established RDS) administration of surfactant reduces mortality associated with RDS in preterm infants (Rojas-Reyes et al., 2012). Prophylactic administration of surfactant has been reported to decrease the incidence of pneumothorax, the risk of pulmonary interstitial emphysema, and the risk of bronchopulmonary dysplasia (Rojas-Reyes et al., 2012). However, these differences were no longer evident when comparing infants routinely being managed on CPAPs who received prophylactic versus rescue surfactant treatment. In fact, the risk of chronic lung disease or death was lower in the latter (Rojas-Reyes et al., 2012). Prophylactic administration of synthetic surfactant when compared to animal-derived surfactant has been noted to show a trend toward decreased mortality in the neonatal period and at 36 weeks postmenstrual age. No significant differences in risk of bronchopulmonary dysplasia were found between groups (Pfister, Soll, & Wiswell, 2009).

Endotracheal suctioning for mechanically ventilated patients in the NICU is customary nursing practice aimed at reducing buildup of secretions and tube obstruction, which can cause discomfort, hypoxemia, hypercapnia, and lobar collapse. Closed suctioning, that is, suctioning without disconnecting intubated ventilated neonates, may have certain short-term benefits, for example, reduction in episodes of hypoxia (typical relative risk 0.48, 95% CI 0.31, 0.74), smaller percentage change in heart rate (weighted mean difference 6.77, 95% CI 4.01, 9.52), and fewer number of infants experiencing bradycardia (typical relative risk 0.38, 95% CI 0.15, 0.92) (Taylor, Hawley, Flenady, & Woodgate, 2012). There is currently a paucity of research on procedures such as preoxygenation, endotracheal suctioning without disconnection from the ventilator, increased mechanical ventilation, manual ventilation, and use of normal saline instillation for suctioning, which are part of the protocols for endotracheal suctioning. The potential serious side effects associated with these procedures warrant development of evidence-based protocols for endotracheal suctioning (Pritchard, Flenady, & Woodgate, 2010; Taylor et al., 2012).

Hyperbilirubinemia

Among ELBW infants, differences in neurodevelopmental outcomes have been attributed to differences in maximum levels of serum bilirubin levels and duration of phototherapy (Mazeiras et al., 2012). High levels of bilirubin are associated with kernicterus, a form of brain damage with sequelae such as deafness, mental retardation, and cerebral palsy. In ELBW infants kernicterus can occur at low levels of serum bilirubin (Moll, Goelz, Naegele, Wilke, & Poets, 2011), and many clinicians have been inclined to initiate phototherapy at low serum bilirubin levels (less than 7–10 mg/dL) (i.e., aggressive phototherapy) (Ambalavanan & Whyte, 2003). These studies, however, may be biased toward overestimating bilirubin toxicity because most problems that cause developmental delay are also associated with hyperbilirubinemia (Ambalavanan & Whyte, 2003). A randomized controlled trial examining the benefits or harms of aggressive phototherapy versus conservative phototherapy at 18 to 22 months found no significant difference in the rate of death or neurodevelopmental impairment. However, subgroup analysis showed reduced death or neurodevelopmental impairment, and a significant reduction in the rates of hearing loss and profound neurodevelopmental impairment without an increase in the rate of death or other adverse outcomes (e.g., cerebral palsy, mental development index score). Although aggressive phototherapy reduced neurodevelopmental impairment in infants weighing 501 to 750 g at birth, the rate of death was higher thereby counterpoising the benefits of aggressive phototherapy treatment (Morris et al., 2008). When comparing risk-adjusted outcomes between ELBW who received phototherapy with those who did not receive phototherapy, phototherapy was not independently associated with death or neurodevelopmental impairment (Hintz, Stevenson, et al., 2011). However, the rate of profound delay as measured by Bayley Scales Mental Developmental Index less than 50 was higher in infants 501 to 750 g birth weight who did not receive phototherapy (Hintz, Stevenson, et al., 2011).

In VLBW infants, phototherapy may increase insensible water loss (Bell, Neidich, Cashore, & Oh, 1979) secondary to heat generated by the phototherapy equipment (Kjartansson, Hammarlund, & Sedin, 1992), thereby complicating fluid management. Other known harmful effects of phototherapy include an increase in the incidence of PDA (Rosenfeld et al., 1986), as well as a potential increase in the incidence of retinopathy of prematurity (Yeo, Perlman, Hao, & Mullaney, 1998). The benefits and known and unknown adverse effects of phototherapy need to be weighed in decision making regarding initiation of phototherapy at low serum bilirubin levels (Ambalavanan & Whyte, 2003). Nurses' vigilance in monitoring input and output and signs and symptoms of PDA can guide medical decision making regarding risks and benefits of phototherapy, as well identify adverse consequences of phototherapy in the event treatment is initiated.

Apnea of Prematurity

Apnea is generally defined as periodic pauses in respirations lasting greater than 20 seconds duration, or shorter pauses associated with cyanosis, pallor, hypotonia, or bradycardia. However, varied definitions are also found with the proposed duration of pause being shorter (e.g., 15 seconds) (Spitzer, 2012). A proposed pathophysiologic mechanism thought to contribute to apnea of prematurity (AOP) involves immaturity of reflex pathways initiated by hypercapnia, hypoxia, and upper airway afferents (Martin, Abu Shaweesh, & Baird, 2004). Nevertheless, there are multiple etiologic factors such as intracranial hemorrhage, infection, gastroesophageal reflux (GER), anemia or hypoxemia, metabolic disorder, drug therapy, and temperature instability that may contribute to apnea. AOP is a diagnosis of exclusion in infants less than 37 weeks gestational age (Martin et al., 2004; Stokowski, 2005). There is uncertainty about the long-term consequence of recurrent AOP; however concern relates to the impact of multiple prolonged hypoxemia and reflex bradycardia on organ systems such as the brain leading to brain injury and poor neurodevelopmental outcome (Henderson-Smart & De Paoli, 2011; Janvier et al., 2004).

The incidence of AOP increases as gestational age decreases. In ELBW infants, apneic and bradycardic episodes persist beyond term gestation, most likely secondary to the higher incidence of chronic lung disease. These persistent apneic and bradycardic episodes complicate and contribute to variability in management decisions related to discharge planning and may prolong hospital stays (Eichenwald, Aina, & Stark, 1997). Clinical interventions for AOP include tactile stimulation, oscillating mattress (kinesthetic stimulation), provision of thermoneutral environment, methylxanthine therapy, CPAP or ventilatory support, nasal CPAP or NIPPV, and olfactory stimulation (Lemyre, Davis, & De Paoli, 2008; Marlier, Gaugler, & Messer,

2005; Martin et al., 2004; Osborn & Henderson-Smart, 2010; Stokowski, 2005). Although some of these interventions such as methylxanthines (Henderson-Smart & De Paoli, 2011), doxapram (Henderson-Smart & Steer, 2011), and NIPPV (Lemyre et al., 2008) have been shown in a systematic review to be effective in reducing the number of apneic and bradycardic episodes in preterm infants, more research is required before these interventions can be recommended as standard therapy in ELBW infants who are a subgroup of preterm infants.

Although current practice standards require nurses to document apnea/bradycardia episodes in order to facilitate management decisions, these records underestimate the frequency of events when compared to recordings (Razi, Humphreys, Pandit, & Stahl, 1999). Nurses spend a significant amount of time monitoring, assessing, and managing apneic and bradycardic episodes, given that nearly all ELBW infants experience AOP. There is a need to develop evidence-based criteria for a minimal safe observation period between the time of last apneic episode and hospital discharge (Eichenwald et al., 1997). Furthermore, a clear understanding of the impact of use of technology (e.g., home monitoring) on hospital discharge, subsequent rehospitalization, postdischarge morbidities (Eichenwald et al., 1997), and family functioning and coping is required.

PDA

Premature infants, particularly ELBW infants, have a significant incidence of persistent PDA, a vascular connection between the aorta and pulmonary artery (Dollberg, Lusky, & Reichman, 2005). Reliable diagnosis of PDA in the first 4 days of life depends on echocardiography because of poor specificity of clinical signs (e.g., murmur, wide pulse pressure, bounding pulses, and increased precordial activity) (Skelton, Evans, & Smythe, 1994). A cardiac murmur is more reliable after this time (Skelton et al., 1994). Metabolomics entails the measure of low-molecular-weight metabolites to determine the phenotype of a cell, tissue, or organism. Preliminary findings suggest that "the metabolomics analysis of the first urine passed by preterm infants can predict the persistent patency of the ductus arteriosus at 3 to 4 days of life, as demonstrated by echocardiography performed by an expert cardiologist" (Fanos, Antonucci, Barberini, Noto, & Atzori, 2012, p. 107). Consequently, metabolomics may facilitate diagnosis of PDA (Fanos et al., 2012).

In a small proportion of ELBW infants, the PDA may close spontaneously or persist without clinical consequences. Nevertheless, approximately 55% of ELBW infants require pharmacological treatment as they are symptomatic (e.g., evidence of left to right shunting, difficulty weaning mechanical ventilation, or increased mechanical support because of worsening pulmonary status) (Koch et al., 2006; Richards, Johnson, Fox, & Campbell, 2009). Treatment decisions for a diagnosed PDA are based on the clinical significance or clinical effect, the criteria for which vary among neonatologists (Wyllie, 2003). Infants with persistent PDA experience increases in mortality and morbidities such as more prolonged and severe RDS, chronic lung disease, and NEC (Dollberg et al., 2005) that may be attributed to their prematurity or PDA (Koch et al., 2006).

Prophylactic treatment circumvents the challenges of deciding whether or not a PDA is significant (Wyllie, 2003). Prophylactic administration of indomethacin, a nonselective cyclooxygenase reduces the incidence of symptomatic PDA and the need for surgical duct ligation. Adverse effects of indomethacin, including NEC, excessive bleeding, or sepsis, were no different between preterm infants receiving prophylactic indomethacin and controls. The incidence of oliguria was increased; however, this was not associated with major renal impairment. Although prophylactic administration of indomethacin reduces the incidence of severe intraventricular hemorrhage, it did not improve neurodevelopmental outcomes (Fowlie et al., 2010; Schmidt et al., 2001). Furthermore, approximately 64% of preterm infants will be medicated unnecessarily (Wyllie, 2003). Values attached by health care providers and parents to the benefits and risks of prophylactic treatment with indomethacin will guide the implementation of this intervention (Fowlie et al., 2010). According to Fanos, Pusceddu, Dessi, and Marciallis (2011), indomethacin prophylaxis should be abandoned as it "unethically exposes newborns who will never have a persistent patent ductus arteriosus to the side effects of drugs" and "cannot be recommended for the prevention of long-term morbidities and mortality, especially in centers where severe intraventricular hemorrhage is comparable to the national average and surgical complications are minimal" (p. 2146). Similarly, ibuprofen, also a cyclooxygenase inhibitor, unnecessarily compromises the infant's renal and gastrointestinal systems without conferring benefits in those ELBW infants with spontaneous closure of PDA. Consequently, prophylactic ibuprofen is not recommended (Fanos et al., 2011; Ohlsson & Shah, 2011). Advantages of prophylactic surgical closure of PDA include reduced incidence of stage II and III NEC; however, no reductions were noted in mortality or bronchopulmonary dysplasia. Again, given the rate of spontaneous closure of patent ductus arteriosus in ELBW infants and potential risks associated with surgery, prophylactic surgical closure is not recommended (Fanos et al., 2011; Ohlsson & Shah, 2011).

Both ibuprofen and indomethacin are effective in closing a PDA diagnosed either clinically or by echocardiogram at less than 28 days. No statistically significant difference was noted in failure of ductal closure, all causes of mortality, neonatal mortality, infant mortality and common neonatal morbidities (e.g., chronic lung disease, intraventricular hemorrhage, retinopathy of prematurity, and infection). Ibuprofen was deemed superior based on biochemical and physiological data suggesting that it has less adverse effects on organs (e.g., kidneys, gastrointestinal system, and brain) (Ohlsson, Walia, & Shah, 2010). Other interventions include fluid restriction and use of diuretics; however, there is little evidence to support their routine use in clinical practice (Wyllie, 2003). Furosemide, which increases prostaglandin production, is often given in conjunction with indomethacin to prevent indomethacin-related toxicity. Current evidence does not support this practice (Brion & Campbell, 2008). Surgical closure is undertaken when medical intervention fails or is contraindicated (Malviya, Ohlsson, & Shah, 2008; Wyllie, 2003).

Nursing care of the ELBW infants includes assessing, documenting, and reporting clinical signs of PDA such as bounding pulses, increased heart rate, and increasing pulse pressure (Koch et al., 2006). Nurses should monitor trends in oxygenation requirements and ventilation support in order to promote timely identification of infants with worsening pulmonary status. Reviewing weekly patterns will ensure that subtle increases in oxygen or ventilation needs over the course of a few days are not missed. Recording when radiographic examination(s) or echocardiograms have been ordered and completed will ensure findings are interpreted and treatment decisions are made promptly. Nurses should be familiar with contraindications of pharmacological treatments for patient ductus arteriosus in order to prevent or reduce risk of harm. ELBW infants receiving treatment should be monitored for oliguria, evidence of active bleeding, and NEC; as such, clinical or biochemical (e.g., creatinine) changes should be reported, as this will assist the medical team to modify treatment regimens in ELBW infants experiencing complications secondary to treatment.

Hypotension

Hypotension clinically manifests as low blood pressure, reduced cutaneous perfusion, and metabolic acidosis (Osborn & Evans, 2009a, b). It is unclear what drop in blood pressure constitutes hypotension in ELBW infants (Ambalavanan & Whyte, 2003); hence the threshold for treatment with crystalloids or cardiotropic medications varies among clinicians (Sehgal, 2011). A recent prospective study of infants born at less than 28 weeks gestational age showed that hypotension in the first 24 hours following birth was not associated with ultrasound findings suggesting cerebral white matter damaged and diagnosis of cerebral palsy at 24 months corrected age (Logan et al., 2011). ELBW infants with hypotension but prior to treatment were found to have similar cerebral blood flow velocity as infants in the control group matched for gestational age and birth weight that had normal blood pressure (Lightburn, Gauss, Williams, & Kaiser, 2009). Sehgal (2011) asserts that hypotension alone may not reduce perfusion of organs such as the brain, heart, kidneys, and gastrointestinal system in ELBW infants.

Strategies for management of hypotension include volume expansion, inotropes, or corticosteroids (Osborn & Evans, 2009a, b). Generally, corticosteroids are used as a last-chance therapy in managing hypotension (Ibrahim, Sinha, & Subhedar, 2011). Use of corticosteroids is supported based on our current understanding of pathophysiology (e.g., adrenocortical insufficiency, lower levels of cortisol concentration) (Ibrahim et al., 2011; Sasidharan, 1998). Of particular concern in ELBW is the extra sodium load administered with each bolus, which may impact fluid and electrolyte management thereby compromising outcomes (Barrington, 2011). In preterm infants without cardiovascular compromise, evidence does not support the routine use of early volume expansion (Osborn & Evans, 2009a). Dopamine has been shown to be more effective than albumin (Osborn & Evans, 2009b) and dobutamine (Subhedar & Shaw, 2009), but no firm recommendations can be made, as there is a paucity of evidence regarding effects on systemic oxygen delivery or cerebral perfusion and long-term benefit of dopamine (Barrington, 2011; Osborn & Evans, 2009b; Subhedar & Shaw, 2009). According to Barrington (2011), the extremely low-gestational-age newborn (ELGAN) study published by O'Shea et al. (2009) demonstrates that treatment for hypotension (i.e., fluid boluses or inotrope/vasopressors) was not guided by the degree of illness or degree of hypotension but rather by "fashion and taste" (p. F317). Barrington (2011), based on the review of recent publications on hypotension in ELBW including the Logan et al. (2011) study, concluded:

- Many infants with low blood pressure have normal systemic flow
- There is no clear evidence that infants with numerically low blood pressures but without evidence of shock have worsened outcomes
- There is no evidence that treating numerically low blood pressures improves outcomes
- There is no evidence base to determine the choice of one intervention over another (p. F317)

According to Sehgal (2011), in EBLW infants multiple factors may contribute to hemodynamic instability (e.g., PDA, pulmonary vascular resistance, and myocardial function) as such, a varied approach to care may be more appropriate than consensus based protocols. "A physiology-driven approach" framework is proposed using point-of-care echocardiography that will permit assessment of the ductus arteriosus, the muscles of the heart, and pulmonary and systemic hemodynamics Together with clinical context, this approach will help clinicians identify the etiology of cardiovascular compromise and permit individualized treatment decisions for ELBW infants (Sehgal, 2011, p. 1237). Since clinical context will continue to be an important marker, nurses must systematically assess the ELBW infants' cardiovascular health by monitoring heart rate, capillary refill time, blood pressure, difference in pulse pressure, quality of pulses (i.e., bounding), presence of murmur(s), and precordial activity.

Fluid and Electrolytes

In ELBW, the first days after delivery are characterized by fluid shifts resulting from both physiologic changes and pathophysiologic events. "Physiologic weight reduction," the contraction of the extracellular compartment of body water, can be exacerbated as a result of insensible water loss (water lost from skin surface and the respiratory tract) and sensible water loss (water lost through the urine and stool). Insensible water losses are extremely high and variable, making it challenging to predict total fluid intake. Given that the ELBW infant's kidneys have limited ability to compensate for varying water and solute intake (i.e., to adjust the concentration of urine), dehydration, fluid overload, and electrolyte imbalance are common events during the immediate postnatal period (Bell & Acarregui, 2010; Gaylord, Wright, Lorch, Lorch, & Walker, 2001; Lorenz, Kleinman, Ahmed, & Markarian, 1995).

A Cochrane systematic review concluded that restricted water intake in which physiological needs are met reduced risk of PDA and NEC but increased postnatal weight loss. Since there was a trend toward an increased risk of dehydration, although the difference was not significant, it would be important to monitor infants closely for dehydration. Certain complications such as bronchopulmonary dysplasia, intracranial hemorrhage and adverse events such as death were reduced with restricted fluid intake, though differences were not statistically significant when compared with liberal fluid intake (Bell & Acarregui, 2010). Since ELBW infants were not well represented in this systematic review, a restrictive fluid management strategy cannot be universally applied to ELBW infants (Bell & Acarregui, 2010).

Some NICUs use swamping (piping highly humidified air into the isolette) when the infant is under a radiant warmer in an effort to reduce insensible water losses and promote thermoregulation. Incubators with the ability to regulate and deliver precise levels of humidification have been introduced in the NICU with the aim of reducing transepidermal water loss. Retrospective studies revealed that using humidified incubators in ELBW infants led to improved fluid management (Gaylord et al., 2001; Kim, Lee, Chen, & Ringer, 2010). High humidity is often provided to reduce water loss; however, the optimal level and duration of humidity remains unknown (Sinclair & Sinn, 2009). High humidity may increase the risk of nosocomial infection in ELBW infants who are already compromised. New incubators have advanced systems of humidification (e.g., sterile humidity in gaseous vapor state) to minimize risk of infection. High humidity may decrease the amount of light energy or irradiance delivered by phototherapy devices and thus may reduce the efficacy of phototherapy treatment (de Carvalho, Torrao, & Moreira, 2011).

Fluid requirements of ELBW infants must be monitored closely by nurses, as fluid disturbances can affect overall risk of death (Bell & Acarregui, 2010) and exacerbate morbidities such as PDA, congestive heart failure (Bell, Warburton, Stonestreet, & Oh, 1980), NEC, and bronchopulmonary dysplasia (Bell & Acarregui, 2010). Daily weights, regular monitoring of electrolytes, strict documentation of fluid intake and output, cumulative fluid balance recordings, and graphic trends of growth should be maintained to facilitate decisions related to fluid management in ELBW infants. ELBW infants receiving high humidity, as well in those receiving phototherapy, should be observed closely for signs and symptoms of infection. The irradiance of light should be monitored on an ongoing basis to ensure effectiveness of phototherapy treatment.

Metabolic Considerations

In ELBW infants, maintaining normoglycemia is difficult because of insufficient glycogen stores, stress, high metabolic rates, and variability in fluid requirements. Parenteral nutrition further elevates the risk of hyper- and hypoglycemia in ELBW infants (Arsenault et al., 2012). Hyperglycemia has been associated with increased risk of death (Hays, Smith, & Sunehag, 2006; Kao et al., 2006), intraventricular hemorrhage (Hays et al., 2006), NEC, late-onset sepsis (Kao et al., 2006), and prolonged hospital stay (Hays et al., 2006). Routine use of insulin infusions to prevent hyperglycemia reduced the risk of hyperglycemia in VLBW infants, as well as ELBW infants. However, the systematic review concluded that given the increased risk of death before 28 days and hypoglycemia, routine use of insulin infusion to prevent hyperglycemia is not recommended (Sinclair, Bottino, & Cowett, 2011). At present there is no consensus regarding cutoff values for hypoglycemia, nor is there strong evidence to provide guidance about specific approaches to treatment (Arsenault et al., 2012). A blood glucose concentration persistently less than 36 mg/dL (2.0 mmol/L) or, in a symptomatic infant, a blood glucose concentration less than 45 mg/dL (2.5 mmol/L) is considered an indication for clinical intervention (Cornblath et al., 2000; Kalhan & Parimi, 2001). Rapid or high-concentration boluses are not advisable, because rebound hypoglycemia can occur. Clinical management of hypoglycemia and hyperglycemia with devices such as the continuous glucose-monitoring sensor may prove beneficial in ELBW infants (Beardsall et al., 2005).

Nutrition

In ELBW infants, endogenous nutritional stores are limited as their bodies are primarily water. These endogenous nutritional stores are quickly depleted under conditions of starvation as metabolic needs are high. As a result, early nutrition is imperative to ensure the infants' continued survival. Nourishing ELBW infants is an important clinical concern, particularly in the first weeks of life, as significant nutritional deficits (e.g., protein and energy) may accrue over the hospitalization, resulting in postnatal or extrauterine growth restriction (Ehrenkranz, 2010; Ehrenkranz et al., 2006; Embleton, Pang, & Cooke, 2001). Early patterns of growth have been shown to have an independent effect on growth and neurodevelopment, including cognition and behavior (Ehrenkranz et al., 2006; Stephens et al., 2009; Ziegler, Thureen, & Carlson, 2002). ELBW infants are at an increased risk of poor somatic growth, with the poorest growth being seen in those infants who have co-morbidities (e.g., feeding problems, respiratory illness, neurologic and developmental difficulties) (Wood et al., 2003). Malnutrition also impacts the structure (e.g., number of number) and function (e.g., neurotransmitter levels) of the brain and development of the retina (Uauy & Mena, 2001).

Although little is known about the optimal requirement and quality of nutrition, nutritional goals for ELBW infants include weight gain that is similar both in rate and composition to the normal fetus at the same postmenstrual age (Adamkin, 2006). Early aggressive nutrition, defined as providing nutrition at or beyond the established standards (Ziegler et al., 2002), has been the focus in hopes of promoting adequate nutrition and limiting the negative consequences associated with nutritional deficits. Given that ELBW infants may be slow to tolerate the introduction of enteral feeds because of delayed gastric emptying and immaturity of intestinal motor activity, aggressive parenteral nutrition should be established soon after birth (within a few hours) (Ziegler et al., 2002). Parenteral nutrition with 2.5 to 3.0 g/kg/d protein intake should be the target, with a stepwise increase commencing when energy intakes reach 70 kcal/kg/d. Protein requirements of about 4 g/kg/d is believed to be physiologic, and the increased blood urea nitrogen suggests effective utilization of amino acids and is in keeping with the high fetal urea productions noted in the human fetus (Adamkin, 2006; Ziegler et al., 2002). However, this higher amount of protein is necessary when enteral nutrition is not provided for long periods of time and should be used with care as efficacy and safety have not been examined in a systematic way (Ziegler et al., 2002). Provision of high-protein and energy intake to ELBW infants was shown to limit catabolism and improve both growth and neurodevelopmental outcomes in ELBW infants (Maggio et al., 2007; Stephens et al., 2009).

Intravenous lipids should be commenced within 24 hours of birth as this provides essential fatty acids and an exogenous source of long-chain polyunsaturated fatty acids. ELBW infants are prone to essential fatty acid deficiency as they have little adipose tissue at birth and are unable to produce adequate amounts of long-chain polyunsaturated fatty acids (Uauy & Mena, 2001; Ziegler et al., 2002). Twenty percent lipid emulsion provides lower phospholipid content and as a result long-chain polyunsaturated fatty acids; hence 10% lipid emulsion is preferred in the first few days until lipid intake is sufficiently advanced (i.e., 2.0 g/kg/d) (Ziegler et al., 2002). Although lipid emulsions can displace bilirubin from albumin binding sites, slow infusion rates (less than 150 mg/kg/hr), combined with slow increases in stepwise fashion to 3.0 g/kg/d should limit adverse effects (Ziegler et al., 2002). Aggressive intake of amino acids and intralipid administration of 3.5 g/kg/d of amino acids and 3 g/kg/d of intralipid are being advocated immediately after birth (within 1 hour) in VLBW infants and have been shown to be effective and safe (Ibrahim, Jeroudi, Baier, Dhanireddy, & Krouskop, 2004).

Use of trophic feeding or minimal enteral nutrition, defined as small-volume feeding of less than 24 mL/kg/d shortly after birth, is intended to achieve a biologic effect on the gastrointestinal system of VLBW infants in whom nutritional feeding is delayed (Bombell & McGuire, 2009). Although trophic feeding is well supported based on our understanding of the anatomic and physiologic disadvantages of delaying feeding (Premji, Paes, Jacobson, & Chessell, 2002), there is insufficient evidence regarding beneficial or harmful effects to make recommendations to inform clinical practice. Initiating trophic feedings within 48 hours of birth permits assessment of physiologic stability in ELBW infants (Premji et al., 2002). For ELBW infants, the continuous tube feeding method may be more energy efficient, as a subgroup analysis of infants included in a systematic review suggested that infants weighing less than 1,000 g gained weight significantly faster when fed by this method (Premji & Chessell, 2011). Further research is required to discern the benefits and risk of continuous tube feeding methods in ELBW infants.

ELBW infants are at increased risk of NEC, and earlier studies have demonstrated an association between timing of enteral feeding and rapid increases in feedings and NEC. Current evidence provides limited guidance regarding the effect of delayed (i.e., no advancement in first 5 days) versus earlier progression of feeding beyond trophic feeds on clinical outcomes in VLBW infants (Morgan, Young, & McGuire, 2011). Furthermore, slow advancement of feedings (i.e., 15–20 mL/kg) in VLBW infants results in delay in regaining birth weight and reaching full enteral feedings and does not reduce the risk of NEC. Numerous detrimental effects of total parenteral nutrition are cited in the literature, including metabolic complications, infection, and changes in the structural integrity and function of the gastrointestinal system. Consequently, more studies need to examine advancing feeding volumes in ELBW infants. Given that information regarding safety is unclear, a feeding advancement of not more than 30 mL/kg/d has been advocated (Premji et al., 2002). Refinement of feeding strategies that facilitate quick transition from parenteral to minimal enteral nutrition to progressive enteral nutrition and advancement of feedings that meet the specific needs of ELBW infants should be the focus of future research.

Human milk is considered the best feeding substrate for premature infants as it confers biologic (e.g., easier to digest and absorb), immunologic (e.g., lower rate of infection and incidence of NEC), and developmental (e.g., improved intelligence quotient) advantages (Lucas & Cole, 1990; Lucas, Morley, Cole, Lister, & Leeson-Payne, 1992; Schanler, 1995). A cohort study of 1,035 ELBW infants reported higher Mental Development Index scores at 18-months correct age in infants who received more breast milk versus formula during hospitalization in the NICU (Vohr et al., 2006). However, preterm human milk does not have sufficient quantities of protein, sodium, phosphate, and calcium to meet estimated needs for growth. Fortification of human milk is therefore essential to maintain adequate growth, nutrient retention, and biochemical homeostasis (Atkinson, 2000; Schanler, 1995). Commercially available fortifiers come in liquid or powder form. Potential complications of fortification include distended abdomen, increased osmolarity, and bacterial contamination. In a systematic review, protein supplementation of human milk in relatively healthy preterm infants resulted in short-term growth; however, the adverse effects of protein supplementation could not be discerned (Kuschel & Harding, 2009). Nurses should support mothers to express breast milk soon after birth, as well as assist mothers to maintain adequate milk supply by encouraging mothers to pump at least 8 to 12 times in a day. Strategies such as kangaroo care, which may facilitate milk production and growth of the infant, should be routine aspects of care.

Currently there is controversy with respect to concurrent feeding and indomethacin therapy. The reduced mesenteric diastolic blood flow associated with indomethacin therapy may be counteracted by minimal enteral nutrition, thereby exerting a protective influence on the gastrointestinal system. However, clinical practice varies between units, with some following the conventional wisdom of withholding enteral feeding during indomethacin therapy in order to prevent NEC (Premji et al., 2002). A study is currently underway assessing the efficacy and safety of feeding during indomethacin or ibuprofen therapy in infants 23 weeks to 33 weeks gestational age (NCT00728117).

Patole and de Klerk (2005) propose that clinical variation in practice determines risk of NEC. Neonatologists' lack of comfort with initiating and advancing protein and energy intake contributed to significant differences in practices, despite institution of guidelines of aggressive protein and energy intake (Stephens et al., 2009). Nursing management of feeding is also inconsistent, and variability in the practice of withdrawing feeding and management of feeding residuals (Hodges & Vincent, 1993) and selection of feeding route (e.g., nasogastric versus orogastric) (Birnbaum & Limperopoulos, 2009) has been shown. A better understanding is required of nursing practice related to tube feeding in order to facilitate a standardized systematic evidence-based approach founded on the current state of scientific knowledge (Premji, 2005).

Physiologic, behavioral, and neurologic immaturity contributes to feeding problems experienced by ELBW infants. A prerequisite to safe and successful oral feeding is effective sucking behaviors and intact gag and cough reflexes (Medoff-Cooper & Ray, 1995; Shaker, 1990). Transitioning ELBW infants from tube feeding to oral feeding is a major challenge for nurses, as no criteria exist to guide practice (Hawdon, Beauregard, Slattery, & Kennedy, 2000; Pickler & Reyna, 2003), and hence the practice is variable and based on custom (McCain, Gartside, Greenberg, & Lott, 2001). An evidence-based neonatal oral feeding protocol has been developed to create positive feeding experiences while assisting high-risk infants to achieve full oral feedings (Premji, McNeil, & Scotland, 2004). Infant characteristics (not postconceptional age) are the primary determinants used to plan physiologically appropriate feeding experiences for each stage—preoral stimulation, nonnutritive sucking, and nutritive sucking—of progression to oral feeding. The mainstay of this protocol is a professional resocialization in the way nurses view and engage in feeding interactions, with emphasis on the quality of the feeding interaction rather than the quantity of milk consumed by the infant. For continued improvement in nutritional management of ELBW infants, it is imperative that nurses engage in protocol appraisal and self-appraisal of practice, and that they review new evidence.

Gastroesophageal Reflux

Another complication related to digestion is gastroesophageal reflux (GER) disease, a maturational phenomenon caused by transient lower esophageal sphincter relaxation (Ambalavanan & Whyte, 2003; Omari et al., 2004). Placement of a feeding tube across the gastroesophageal junction has been shown to increase the incidence of GER (Peter, Wiechers, Bohnhorst, Silny, & Poets, 2002). Other factors that may influence the presence of GER include supine position and large volume of fluid intake. Clinical signs of GER include visible regurgitation, and infants may cry, be irritable, or have altered sleeping patterns (e.g., remain awakened) (Poet & Brockmann, 2011). GER is also considered a risk factor for aspiration and subsequent pneumonia (Ambalavanan & Whyte, 2003). The association between chronic lung disease and GER is thought to be due to greater diagnostic suspicion in infants with chronic lung disease (Fuloria, Hiatt, Dillard, & O'Shea, 2000; Poet & Brockmann, 2011). GER does not appear to increase the risk of delayed growth (less than 10th percentile) or development (Bayley Mental Developmental and Psychomotor Developmental Indices of less than 70) in VLBW infants (Fuloria et al., 2000). GER is considered pathologic based on the quality rather than quantity of the refluxate (Poet & Brockmann, 2011). GER is difficult to diagnose, as current techniques of esophageal pH monitoring cannot reliably detect GER in preterm infants. This is because frequent feeding causes esophageal acidification to pH less than 4 (Grant & Cochran, 2001; Omari et al., 2004). Consequently, the contribution of GER to neonatal morbidity and the efficacy of therapies for GER are difficult to evaluate.

The association between GER and AOP is biologically plausible as the refluxate can stimulate laryngeal chemoreceptors; hence it is not surprising that studies (e.g., Omari, 2009) have demonstrated a relationship between GER and apnea. There are studies (e.g., Peter, Sprodowski, Bohnhorst, Silny, & Poets, 2002) that also show no temporal relationship between apnea and GER in preterm infants (Peter, Sprodowski, et al., 2002). Poet and Brockmann (2011) concluded, given the lack of consistent evidence and the fact that anti-reflux medications have not been useful in managing AOP, that apneas are not related to GER. Pharmacologic measures (e.g., metoclopramide, domperidone) (Ambalavanan & Whyte, 2003) should be used sparingly, as the consequence of GER remains to be established in ELBW infants (Poet & Brockmann, 2011). Prone and left lateral positioning reduced the number and duration of reflux episodes (Corvaqlia et al., 2007; Ewer, James, & Tobin, 1999). At present, there is lack of consensus with regard to optimal management of GER in ELBW infants, as there are few randomized controlled trials to guide practice.

Anemia

The primary cause of anemia, particularly in the first 2 weeks of life, is phlebotomy losses resulting from intensive laboratory testing. Other causes include an inability to increase erythropoietin concentration and erythropoiesis, and severely limited blood volume based on body weight (Ohls, 2002). In the preterm infant, typically there is a physiologic fall in hemoglobin and hematocrit levels by approximately 6 weeks of age. The decline in hematocrit in ELBW infants is associated with clinical findings necessitating packed red blood cell transfusion, and hence is not considered "physiologic" (Aher & Ohlsson, 2010). It is uncertain what hematocrit levels precipitate clinical signs of anemia of prematurity and what is the minimal acceptable level for infants requiring ventilatory support (Ohls, 2002). Low hemoglobin and hematocrit levels often guide decisions regarding blood transfusion (Aher & Ohlsson, 2010). As a result of more stringent transfusion guidelines (i.e., lower threshold for transfusion), the numbers of blood transfusions have decreased over the past decade (Maier et al., 2000). No statistically significant differences were noted in death or neurodevelopmental impairment between those maintained at low hemoglobin levels (i.e., restrictive) versus those with high hemoglobin levels (i.e., liberal). Although infants in the restrictive group had lower hemoglobin levels in the first few weeks of life, at 18-months corrected age, these differences were no longer evident (Whyte et al., 2009). Post hoc analysis, however, revealed significantly higher rates of cognitive delay (i.e., Mental Development Index score less than 85) in the restrictive hemoglobin group (Whyte et al., 2009). In contrast, a retrospective study of ELBW infants revealed that the number of blood transfusions was significantly associated with severity of retinopathy of prematurity (Englert, Saunders, Purohit, Hulsey, & Ebeling, 2001). Other benefits of reducing the number of packed red blood cell transfusions include reduced risk of transmission of viral infections, reduced risk of incompatibility, and reduced cost (Aher & Ohlsson, 2010).

A meta-analysis reported that administration of recombinant erythropoietin in the first week of life resulted in a moderate reduction in the proportion of VLBW infants requiring blood transfusion. Subgroup analysis revealed that ELBW infants were less likely to avoid transfusion if treated with recombinant erythropoietin (Kotto-Kome, Garcia, Calhoun, & Christensen, 2004). Though a recent Cochrane systematic review concluded that early erythropoietin, that is, administration of erythropoietin before 8 days of age, is not recommended as there is no strong evidence for its neuroprotective role: no impact on mortality, limited clinical importance of reduction in blood cell transfusions, volume of red blood cells transfusions, and significant increase in the rate of retinopathy of prematurity (stage ≥ 3) (Ohlsson & Aher, 2010). Consequently, strategies or interventions (e.g., point-of-care devices) that reduce phlebotomy losses and blood transfusions throughout the infant's hospital stay warrant further investigation (Madan et al., 2005; Moya, Clark, Nicks, & Tanaka, 2001). Additionally, the nurse must act as an advocate to eliminate unnecessary laboratory monitoring.

Infection

Infections are frequent complications of ELBW, with approximately 50% to 65% of infants having at least one infection during hospitalization. There are multitudes of nonspecific signs and symptoms of sepsis, namely, temperature instability, apnea and bradycardia, feeding intolerance, abdominal distention, lethargy, septic shock, and increased need for oxygen or ventilatory support (Craft, Finer, & Barrington, 2009). Infection rates increase with decreasing birth weight and gestational age and are associated with increased mortality and poor neurodevelopmental and growth outcomes in childhood (Schlapbach et al., 2011; Stoll et al., 2004; Tolsma et al., 2011). The ELGAN study, which followed 1,059 infants born at less than 28 weeks gestational age, identified definite late neonatal bacteremia as an independent risk factor for retinopathy of prematurity (Tolsma et al., 2011).

Early-onset infection (before 72 hours) is due to maternal factors (congenital) and is uncommon, but can be life threatening (Ambalavanan & Whyte, 2003). Risk of early-onset sepsis (e.g., group B streptococcal) may be decreased with intrapartum antibiotic prophylaxis, but there is concern that it may mask infection, with onset of signs of sepsis taking longer. In almost all ELBW infants, antibiotics (ampicillin or penicillin and aminoglycoside) for suspected sepsis are initiated after birth, and if the infant is asymptomatic and culture is negative, antibiotic therapy is discontinued after 48 to 72 hours. It is unclear what impact the frequent and empiric use of antibiotics has on the incidence and resistance pattern of late-onset bacterial infection (Ambalavanan & Whyte, 2003). Prior use of broad-spectrum antibiotics has been associated with invasive candidiasis, which in ELBW infants may be fatal, ranking second among the leading causes of infection-related deaths in ELBW infants (Benjamin et al., 2010). Guidelines for early-onset sepsis recommending limited use of broad-spectrum antibiotics, as well as reduced duration of treatment, were found to be effective (i.e., did not "increase the risk of infectious relapse") when implemented for infants less than 35 weeks gestational age, and near term and term infants. Their efficacy and safety need to be established in ELBW infants (Labenne, Michaut, Gouyon, Ferdynus, & Gouyon, 2007, p. 593).

Late-onset sepsis (after 72 hours), referred to as nosocomial infection, is an acquired infection with coagulase-negative staphylococci being the most common cause of bacteremia (Craft et al., 2009). According to Craft et al. (2009), the risk of acquired infection is high because ELBW infants have an immature immune system; they often lack the protection of passive immunity, they have poor epidermal and gastrointestinal barrier function, and they may have central arterial or venous catheters (e.g., umbilical lines and percutaneous central venous catheters). Evidence-based practices that prevent or control the spread of bacterial and viral infections such as hand hygiene are not always adhered to in practice. These variations in practice may explain the different rates of infection reported in the literature by different NICUs (Higgins, Baker, & Raju, 2010). In ELBW infants, oral lactoferrin may reduce the incidence of late-onset sepsis (Pammi & Abrams, 2011), while pentoxifylline given as an adjunct to antibiotic treatment may reduce mortality without adverse effects (Haque & Pammi, 2011), but more research is required before these strategies can be routinely adopted in practice. Similarly, vancomycin for prophylaxis against sepsis has been found to be effective in reducing the incidence of sepsis, although further research is required as organisms may develop resistance to vancomycin (Craft et al., 2009).

Skin breakdown, another pathway for infection, occurs more frequently in ELBW infants, and it is proposed that topical ointment therapy may serve as a protective barrier leading to improved skin integrity and a decreased risk of nosocomial infection (Conner, Soll, & Edwards, 2009). Application of a preservative-free emollient ointment improves skin condition and reduces transepidermal water loss, but is associated with adverse outcomes. The risk of coagulase-negative staphylococcal infection and any nosocomial infection (e.g., bacterial and fungal organism) increased with the application of ointment (Conner et al., 2009). Other potential strategies to minimize skin breakdown, thereby reducing the risk of infection, include use of as little tape as possible, and changing the infant's position frequently to prevent abrasions and pressure areas. It is important to remember that other treatments, procedures, and conditions may aggravate the problem (e.g., steroid therapy; use of blood products, leading to thrombocytopenia or lymphocytopenia; invasive procedures; changes in the pH of the skin as a result of bathing practices). Renal function is compromised in ELBW infants. It is imperative that nurses give medications (particularly drugs that are nephrotoxic such as gentamicin) with careful consideration of renal function. If renal function is compromised, a toxic level of this drug can be reached quite quickly, leading to permanent renal and auditory damage. The nurse should consider where the drug is metabolized and cleared through the body. If the site is the renal system and if output is severely diminished, use of the medication may need to be suspended temporarily.

Given the spectrum of issues that may be encountered by an ELBW infant, an individualized approach to care is crucial. Consistent and sound clinical reasoning based on history and physical examination, comprehensive data (e.g., essential laboratory findings), and knowledge (e.g., research evidence) should guide nursing practice decisions. Moreover, parents' wishes should be considered in making judgments about best practices, as they hold the ultimate moral and legal authority to make decisions about the infant's treatment. The ethical imperative is shared decision making (Penticuff & Arheart, 2005).

FAMILIES OF ELBW INFANTS

The birth of an ELBW infant generates a cascade of parental emotions and fears beginning with decisions related to resuscitation and to uncertainty regarding survival of the infant (Sydnor-Greenberg & Dokken, 2000). An interpretive phenomenological analysis of mothers' lived experience of giving birth to an ELBW infants revealed that "being the mother" entailed being worried and scared about the uncertainty of the outcome and thinking the worst (Schenk & Kelley, 2010). Parental grief over the death of an ELBW infant, loss of a desired child, loss of pregnancy, or past losses may be adversely influenced by external factors. Nursing behaviors can influence this grief, which is a multidimensional complex process (Golish & Powell, 2003; Sydnor-Greenberg & Dokken, 2000).

Effective communication that incorporates support (physical or social) and teaching will assist parents to find their own unique paths to meaningful involvement (Sydnor-Greenberg & Dokken, 2000). It is important that nurses realize that there will be individual differences depending on the race, religion, nationality, and cultural background of the families. Although it may seem daunting at times, nurses should attempt to accurately interpret and respond to various behaviors by parents to facilitate meaningful involvement in caring for their infant (Sydnor-Greenberg & Dokken, 2000). Principles of family-centered care combined with principles of developmental care are an excellent framework to encourage families to participate as fully as possible in caring for and making decisions about their infant, and to form mutually beneficial and supportive partnerships in the NICU (Lester et al., 2011).

A crucial element in caring for ELBW infants is to engage families to participate collaboratively in deciding on appropriate care. The ability of the families to understand accurately their infant's medical condition, prognosis, and treatment options is dependent on the health care professional's ability to take a participatory approach to care (Penticuff & Arheart, 2005). Interventions that facilitate effective communication, collaborative care, and shared decision making warrant closer scrutiny by evaluating their efficacy.

SUMMARY

This chapter presented a brief overview of the mortality and morbidities associated with being born ELBW, care required for the problems encountered by ELBW infants, and potential areas for future research. There are many unknowns; however, there is hope; a trust in the future of life. Nurses, physicians, other health care providers, and parents can make a difference if they are aware of the potential problems and know how to detect or recognize them early.

CASE STUDY

Michael was born at 23 weeks by VD to a 23-year-old G2P1 mother HBsAg-negative, VDRL nonreactive, GBS-negative after failed tocolysis X 3 hours. Apgars 2/8. Intubated and given Surfactant in DR. Transported to NICU in incubator.

Admission Assessment

- GENERAL: 778g, TPR: 96, HR 168, RR 60 (ventilated), BP 24
- SKIN: mottled, cool, extensive bruising on both legs
- HEENT: normocephalic, fontanelle soft and flat, palate intact
- NECK: no masses, clavicles intact
- LUNGS: BBS equal, coarse rales
- CV: RRR, no murmur, CFT 4 seconds
- ABD: soft, flat, liver palpable at RCM, UAC in place, two arteries, one vein visible
- GENITALIA: normal preterm male genitalia, patent anus
- EXT: Moves all extremities, pulses X 4
- NEURO: poor tone, appropriate for gestational age (AGA) 23 weeks
- IMPRESSION: 23-week, preterm AGA, male newborn with respiratory distress

Questions to Consider

What is the first differential diagnosis for Baby Michael?
Respiratory distress secondary to surfactant insufficiency versus sepsis versus hypothermia

What will the initial management plan include?

1. Ventilatory support at lowest settings needed to maintain oxygenation; wean as possible using O2 saturations and ABG

2. Incubator with temperature and humidity control
3. IV fluids
4. Monitor blood pressure; consider bolus
5. Ampicillin and Gentamicin
6. Talking to parents

What diagnostic tests will likely be ordered?

1. CBC with differential
2. Blood culture
3. ABG
4. Bedside glucose
5. Blood chemistries, bilirubin levels
6. Chest x-ray

On day 2 of life, Michael's parents ask you, "Is he going to be okay?" What would you tell them?

There is no answer to this question, because we don't know all the answers. That is a good way to begin your answer. The editors hope that reading this book will better prepare you to answer these and other questions.

EVIDENCE-BASED PRACTICE BOX

Use of Human Milk in the Early Neonatal Period

Human milk is recognized as the ideal nutrition for preterm neonates because of the protection it confers to ELBW through its biologic and immunologic properties (Higgins et al., 2012). For ELBW infants, prevention of NEC is important, as it is a leading cause of mortality and morbidity. Neonates fed human milk have lower rates of NEC overall and those who develop NEC have lower mortality and late-onset sepsis, compared to neonates fed preterm formula (Schanler, Lau, Hurst, & Smith, 2005; Vohr et al., 2007). Human milk has a dose–response relationship in reducing the risk of NEC in the first 14 days to 28 days of life (Meinzen-Derr et al., 2009; Vohr et al., 2007). The amount of human milk received in early life is also related to health outcomes in later life (e.g., 30 months of age) in a dose–response fashion (Vohr et al., 2007). Slower weight gain in infants who were fed human milk did not preclude them from being discharged earlier (Schanler et al., 2005). Overall weight gain at 18 months was found to be no different in those receiving human milk when compared to those receiving formula in early life (Vohr et al., 2006). Human milk also reduces risk of atopy and rates of rehospitalization, and promotes developmental outcomes (Higgins et al., 2012; Vohr et al., 2007). Although donor human milk is associated with a lower risk of NEC when compared to formula feeding, no conclusions can be made given the quality of the evidence (Boyd, Quigley, & Brocklehurst, 2007).

References

Boyd, C. A., Quigley, M. A., & Brocklehurst, P. (2007). Donor breast milk versus infant formula for preterm infants: Systematic review and meta-analysis. *Archives of Disease in Childhood, Fetal and Neonatal Edition, 92*(3), F169–F175.

Higgins, R. D., Devaskar, S., Hay, W. W., Jr., Ehrenkranz, R. A., Greer, F. R., Kennedy, K., . . . Sherman, M. P. (2012). Executive summary of the workshop "Nutritional Challenges in the High Risk Infant." *Journal of Pediatrics, 160*(3), 511–516.

Meinzen-Derr, J., Poindexter, B., Wrage, L., Morrow, A. L., Stoll, B., & Donovan, E. F. (2009). Role of human milk in extremely low birth weight infants' risk of necrotizing enterocolitis or death. *Journal of Perinatology, 29*, 57–62. doi:10.1038/jp.2008.117

Schanler, R., Lau, C., Hurst, N. M., & Smith, E. O. (2005). Randomized trial of donor human milk feeding versus preterm formula as substitutes for mothers' own milk in the feeding of extremely premature infants. *Pediatrics, 116*(2), 400–406.

Vohr, B., Poindexter, B., Dusick, A., McKinley, L. T., Higgins, R. D., Langer, J. C., . . . National Institute of Child Health and Human Development National Research Network. (2007). Persistent beneficial effects of breast milk ingested in the neonatal intensive care unit on outcomes of extremely low birth weight infants at 30 months of age. *Pediatrics, 120*(4), e953–e959.

Vohr, B., Poindexter, B. B., Dusick, A. M., McKinley, L. T., Wright, L. L., Langer, J. C., . . . NICHD Neonatal Research Network. (2006). Beneficial effects of breast milk in the neonatal intensive care unit on the developmental outcome of extremely low birth weight infants at 18 months of age. *Pediatrics, 118*(1), e115–e123.

ONLINE RESOURCES

ELBW Follow-Up
http://www.vtoxford.org/research/elbw/elbw.aspx

John D. Lantos MD-Ethical Issues Around the Care of ELBW Infants
http://vimeo.com/20937433

Neil Finder MD-CPAP vs. Surfactant in the ELBW Infant
http://vimeo.com/21309386

Panel Discussion on Golden Hour Management of ELBW
http://vimeo.com/21319275

REFERENCES

Adamkin, D. H. (2006). Nutrition management of very low-birth weight infant: II. Optimizing enteral nutrition and postdischarge nutrition. *Neoreviews, 7*, e608–e614.

Aher, S. M., & Ohlsson, A. (2010). Late erythropoietin for preventing red blood cell transfusion in preterm and/or low birth weight infants (Cochrane Review). *The Cochrane library* (issue 4). John Wiley & Sons, Ltd.

Albersheim, S. (2008). Ethical consideration at the threshold of viability. *BC Medical Journal, 50*, 509–511.

AlFaleh, K., Anabrees, J., Bassler, D., & Al-Kharfi, T. (2011). Probiotics for prevention of necrotizing enterocolitis in preterm infants (Cochrane Review). In *The Cochrane library*, issue 3. John Wiley & Sons.

Ambalavanan, N., & Whyte, R. K. (2003). The mismatch between evidence and practice. Common therapies in search of evidence. *Clinics in Perinatology, 30*, 305–331.

American Academy of Pediatrics, Section on Ophthalmology, American Academy of Ophthalmology, & American Association for Pediatric Ophthalmology and Strabismus. (2006). Screening examination of premature infants for retinopathy of prematurity. *Pediatrics, 117*, 572–576.

American College of Obstetricians and Gynecologists. (2002). Perinatal care at the threshold of viability. ACOG Practice Bulletin No 38. *International Journal of Gynecology and Obstetrics, 79*, 181–188.

Andersen, C., & Phelps, D. L. (2009). Peripheral retinal ablation for threshold retinopathy of prematurity in preterm infants (Cochrane Review). In *The Cochrane library*, issue 1. John Wiley & Sons.

Arsenault, D., Brenn, M., Kim, S., Gura, K., Compher, C., Simpser, E., . . . Puder, M. (2012). A.S.P.E.N. clinical guidelines: Hyperglycemia and hypoglycemia in the neonate receiving parenteral nutrition. *Journal of Parenteral and Enteral Nutrition, 36*, 81–95.

Askie, L. M., Henderson-Smart, D. J., & Ko, H. (2009). Restricted versus liberal oxygen exposure for preventing morbidity and mortality in preterm or low birth weight infants (Cochrane Review). In *The Cochrane Library*, issue 3. John Wiley & Sons.

Atkinson, S. A. (2000). Human milk feeding of the micropremie. *Clinics in Perinatology, 27*, 235–247.

Bain, E., Middleton, P., & Crowther, C. A. (2012). Different magnesium sulphate regimens for neuroprotection of the fetus for women at risk of preterm birth (Cochrane Review). In *The Cochrane library*, issue 2. John Wiley & Sons.

Ballot, D. E., Chirwa, T. F., & Cooper, P. A. (2010). Determinants of survival in very low birth weight neonates in public sector hospital in Johannesburg. *BMC Pediatrics, 10*, 30.

Barrington, K. J. (2001). The adverse neuro-developmental effects of postnatal steroids in the preterm infant: A systematic review of RCTs. *BMC Pediatrics, 1*(1), e1.

Barrington, K. J. (2011). Low blood pressure in extremely preterm infants: Does treatment affect outcome? *Archives of Disease in Childhood: Fetal and Neonatal Edition, 96*, F316–F317.

Beardsall, K., Ogilvy-Stuart, A. L., Ahluwalia, J., Thompson, M., & Dunger, D. B. (2005). The continuous glucose monitoring sensor in neonatal intensive care. *Archives of Disease in Childhood: Fetal and Neonatal Edition, 90*, F307–F310.

Bell, E. F., & Acarregui, M. J. (2010). Restricted versus liberal water intake for preventing morbidity and mortality in preterm infants (Cochrane Review). In *The Cochrane library*, issue 6. John Wiley & Sons.

Bell, E. F., Warburton, D., Stonestreet, B. S., & Oh, W. (1980). Effect of fluid administration on the development of symptomatic patent ductus arteriosus and congestive heart failure in premature infants. *New England Journal of Medicine, 302*, 598–604.

Bell, F. B., Neidich, G. A., Cashore, W. J., & Oh, W. (1979). Combined effect of radiant warmer and phototherapy on insensible water loss in low-birth-weight infants. *Journal of Pediatrics, 94*, 810–813.

Benjamin, D. K., Jr., Stoll, B. J., Gantz, M. G., Walsh, M. C., Sánchez, P. J., Das, A., . . . Eunice Kennedy Shriver National Institute of Child Health and Human Development Neonatal Research Network. (2010). Neonatal candidiasis: Epidemiology, risk factors, and clinical judgment. *Pediatrics, 126*, e865–e873.

Bhatt, D. R., White, R., Martin, G., Van Marter, L. J., Finer, N., Goldsmith, J. P., . . . Ramanathan, R. (2007). Transitional hypothermia in preterm newborns. *Journal of Perinatology, 27*, S45–S47.

Birnbaum, R., & Limperopoulos, C. (2009). Nonoral feeding practices for infants in the neonatal intensive care unit. *Advances in Neonatal Care, 9*, 180–184.

Blakely, M. L., Lally, K. P., McDonald, S., Brown, R. L., Barnhart, D. C., Ricketts, R. R., . . . NEC Subcommittee of the NICHD Neonatal Research Network. (2005). Postoperative outcomes of extremely low birth-weight infants with necrotizing enterocolitis or isolated intestinal perforation: A prospective cohort study by the NICHD Neonatal Research Network. *Annals of Surgery, 241*, 984–999.

Bombell, S., & McGuire, W. (2009). Early trophic feeding for very low birth weight infants (Cochrane Review). In *The Cochrane library*, issue 3. John Wiley & Sons.

Brion, L. P., Bell, E. F., & Raghuveer, T. S. (2008). Vitamin E supplementation for prevention of morbidity and mortality in preterm infants (Cochrane Review). In *The Cochrane library*, issue 4. John Wiley & Sons.

Brion, L. P., & Campbell, D. (2008). Furosemide for prevention of morbidity in indomethacin-treated infants with patent ductus arteriosus. In *The Cochrane library*, issue 4. John Wiley & Sons.

Chan, K., Ohlsson, A., Synnes, A., Lee, D. S., Chien, L. Y., Lee, S. K., & the Canadian Neonatal Network. (2001). Survival, morbidity, and resource use of infants of 25 weeks gestational age or less. *American Journal of Obstetrics & Gynecology, 185*(1), 220–226.

Conner, M. J., Soll, R., & Edwards, W. H. (2009). Topical ointment for preventing infection in preterm infants (Cochrane Review). In *The Cochrane library*, issue 1. John Wiley & Sons.

Cornblath, M., Hawdon, J. M., Williams, A. F., Aynsley-Green, A., Ward-Platt, M. P., Schwartz, R., & Kalhan, S. C. (2000). Controversies regarding definition of neonatal hypoglycemia: Suggested operational thresholds. *Pediatrics, 105*, 1141–1145.

Costeloe, K., Hennessy, E., Gibson, A. T., Marlow, N., & Wilkinson, A. R. (2000). The EPICure study: Outcomes to discharge from hospital for infants born at the threshold of viability. *Pediatrics, 106*, 659–670.

Corvaqlia, L., Rotatori, R., Ferlini, M., Aceti, A., Ancora, G., & Faldella, G. (2007). The effect of body positioning on gastroesophageal reflux in premature infants: Evaluation by combined impedance and pH monitoring. *Journal of Pediatrics, 151*, 591–596.

Cotton, C. M., Taylor, S., Stoll, B., Goldberg, R. N., Hansen, N. I., Sánchez, P. J., . . . NICHD Neonatal Research Network. (2009). Prolonged duration of initial empirical antibiotic treatment is associated with increased rates of necrotizing enterocolitis and death for extremely low birth weight infants. *Pediatrics, 123*, 58–66.

Craft, A. P., Finer, N. N., & Barrington, K. J. (2009). Vancomycin for prophylaxis against sepsis in preterm neonates (Cochrane Review). In *The Cochrane library*, issue 1. John Wiley & Sons.

Cryotherapy for Retinopathy of Prematurity Cooperative Group. (2005). 15-year outcomes following threshold retinopathy of prematurity: Final results from the multicenter trial of cryotherapy for retinopathy of prematurity. *Archives of Ophthalmology, 123*, 311–318.

Cumming, G. G., Hutchinson, A. M., Scott, S. D., Norton, P. G., & Estabrooks, C. A. (2010). The relationship between characteristics of context and research utilization in a pediatric setting. *BMC Health Services Research, 10*, 168. Retrieved from http://www.biomedcentral.com/1472-6963/10/168

Darlow, B. A., & Graham, P. J. (2011). Vitamin A supplementation to prevent mortality and short- and long-term morbidity in very low birth weight infants (Cochrane Review). In *The Cochrane library*, issue 10. John Wiley & Sons.

de Carvalho, M., Torrao, C. T., & Moreira, M. E. (2011). Mist and water condensation inside incubators reduce the efficacy of phototherapy. *Archives of Disease in Childhood Fetal and Neonatal Edition, 96*, F138–F140.

Dollberg, S., Lusky, A., & Reichman, B. (2005). Patent ductus arteriosus, indomethacin and necrotizing enterocolitis in very low birth weight infants: A population-based study. *Journal of Pediatric Gastroenterology and Nutrition, 40*, 184–189.

Doyle, L. W. (2012). Antenatal magnesium sulfate and neuroprotection. *Current Opinion in Pediatrics, 24*(2), 154–159.

Doyle, L. W., Roberts, G., Anderson, P. J., & Victorian Infant Collaborative Study Group. (2011). Changing long-term outcomes for infants 500–999 g birth weight in Victoria, 1979–2005. *Archives of Disease in Childhood, Fetal and Neonatal Edition, 96*, F443–F447.

Ehrenkranz, R. A. (2010). Early nutritional support and outcomes in ELBW infants. *Early Human Development, 86*, S21–S25.

Ehrenkranz, R. A., Dusick, A. M., Vohr, B. R., Wright, L. L., Wrage, L. A., & Poole, W. K. (2006). Growth in the neonatal intensive care unit influences neurodevelopmental and growth outcomes of extremely low birth weight infants. *Pediatrics, 117*, 1253–1261.

Eichenwald, E. C., Aina, A., & Stark, A. R. (1997). Apnea frequently persists beyond term gestation in infants delivered at 24 to 28 weeks. *Pediatrics, 100*, 354–359.

Embleton, N. E., Pang, N., & Cooke, R. J. (2001). Postnatal malnutrition and growth retardation: An inevitable consequence of current recommendations in preterm infants? *Pediatrics, 107*, 270–273.

Englert, J. A., Saunders, R. A., Purohit, D., Hulsey, T. C., & Ebeling, M. (2001). The effect of anemia on retinopathy of prematurity in extremely low birth weight infants. *Journal of Perinatology, 21*, 21–26.

Ewer, A. K., James, M. E., & Tobin, J. M. (1999). Prone and left lateral positioning reduce gastro-oesophageal reflux in preterm infants. *Archives of Disease in Childhood, Fetal and Neonatal Edition, 81*, F201–F205.

Express Group. (2009). One year survival of extremely preterm infants after active perinatal care in Sweden. *JAMA, 301*, 2225–2233.

Fanos, V., Antonucci, R., Barberini, L., Noto, A., & Atzori, L. (2012). Clinical application of metabolomics in neonatology. *The Journal of Maternal-Fetal and Neonatal Medicine, 25*, 104–109.

Fanos, V., Pusceddu, M., Dessi, A., & Marciallis, M. A. (2011). Should we definitively abandon prophylaxis for patent ductus arteriosus in preterm newborns? *Clinics (Sao Paulo), 66*(12), 2141–2149.

Fischer, N., Steurer, M. A., Adams, M., Berger, T. M., & Swiss Neonatal Network. (2009). Survival rates of extremely preterm infants: (Gestational age < 26 weeks) in Switzerland: Impact of the Swiss guidelines for the care of infants born at the limit of viability. *Archives of Disease in Childhood, Fetal and Neonatal Edition, 94*, F407–F413.

Foster, J. P., & Cole, M. (2011). Oral immunoglobulin for preventing necrotizing enterocolitis in preterm and low birth weight neonates (Cochrane Review). In *The Cochrane library*, issue 7. John Wiley & Sons.

Fowlie, P. W., Davis, P. G., & McGuire, W. (2010). Prophylactic intravenous indomethacin for preventing mortality and morbidity in preterm infants (Cochrane Review). In *The Cochrane library*, issue 7. John Wiley & Sons.

Fuloria, M., Hiatt, D., Dillard, R. G., & O'Shea, T. M. (2000). Gastroesophageal reflux in very low birth weight infants: Association with chronic lung disease and outcomes through 1 year of age. *Journal of Perinatology, 20*(4), 235–239.

Gaylord, M. S., Wright, K., Lorch, K., Lorch, V., & Walker, E. (2001). Improved fluid management utilizing humidified incubators in extremely low birth weight infants. *Journal of Perinatology, 21*, 438–443.

Geary, C., Caskey, M., Fonseca, R., & Malloy, M. (2008). Decreased incidence of bronchopulmonary dysplasia after early management changes, including surfactant and nasal continuous positive airway pressure treatment at delivery, lowered oxygen saturation goals, and early amino acid administrational: A historical cohort study. *Pediatrics, 121*, 89. doi:10.1542/peds.2007–0225

Gilbert, C., Fielder, A., Gordillo, L., Quinn, G., Semiglia, R., Visintin, P., . . . International NO-ROP Group. (2005). Characteristics of infants with severe retinopathy of prematurity in countries with low, moderate, and high levels of development: Implications for screening programs. *Pediatrics, 115*, e518–e525.

Golish, T. D., & Powell, K. A. (2003). "Ambiguous loss": Managing the dialectics of grief associated with premature birth. *Journal of Social and Personal Relationships, 20*, 309–334.

Gorski, P. A. (1991). Promoting infant development during neonatal hospitalization: Critiquing the state of the science. *Children's Health Care, 20*, 250–257.

Grant, L., & Cochran, D. (2001). Can pH monitoring reliably detect gastro-esophageal reflux in preterm infants? *Archives of Disease in Childhood, Fetal and Neonatal Edition, 85*, F155–F157.

Guillen, U., DeMauro, S., Ma, L., Zupancic, J., Wang, E., Gafni, A., & Kirpalani, H. (2011). Survival rates in extremely low birth weight infants depend on the denominator: Avoiding potential for bias by specifying denominators. *American Journal of Obstetrics and Gynecology, 205*(4), 329.e1–329.e7.

Guthrie, S. O., Gordon, P. V., Thomas, V., Thorp, J. A., Peabody, J., & Clark, R. H. (2003). Necrotizing enterocolitis among neonates in the United States. *Journal of Perinatology, 23*, 278–285.

Hakansson, S., Farooqi, A., Holmgren, P. A., Serenius, F., & Högberg, U. (2004). Proactive management promotes outcomes in extremely preterm infants: A population-based comparison of two perinatal management strategies. *Pediatrics, 114*(1), 58–64.

Haque, K. N., & Pammi, M. (2011). Pentoxifylline for treatment of sepsis and necrotizing enterocolitis in neonates. In *The Cochrane library*, issue 10. John Wiley & Sons.

Hardy, R. J., Good, W. V., Dobson, V., Palmer, E. A., Phelps, D. L., Quintos, M., . . . Early Treatment for Retinopathy of Prematurity Cooperative Group. (2004). Multicenter trial of early treatment for retinopathy of prematurity: Study design. *Controlled Clinical Trials, 25*, 311–325.

Haward, M. F., Kirshenbaum, N. W., & Campbell, D. E. (2011). Care at the edge of viability: Medical and ethical issues. *Clinics in Perinatology, 38*, 471–492.

Hawdon, J., Beauregard, N., Slattery, J., & Kennedy, G. (2000). Identification of neonates at risk of developing feeding problems in infancy. *Developmental Medicine and Child Neurology, 42*, 235–239.

Hays, S. P., Smith, E. O., & Sunehag, A. L. (2006). Hyperglycemia is a risk factor for early death and morbidity in extremely low birth-weight infants. *Pediatrics, 118*, 1811–1818.

Hazan, J., Maag, U., & Chessex, P. (1991). Association between hypothermia and mortality rate of premature infant–revisited. *American Journal of Obstetrics and Gynecology, 164*, 111–112.

Henderson-Smart, D. J., & De Paoli, A. G. (2011). Methylxanthine treatment for apnoea in preterm infants (Cochrane Review). In *The Cochrane library*, issue 1. John Wiley & Sons.

Henderson-Smart, D. J., & Steer, P. (2011). Doxapram treatment for apnea in preterm infants (Cochrane Review). In *The Cochrane library*, issue 1. John Wiley & Sons.

Higgins, R. D., Baker, C. J., & Raju, T. N. (2010). Executive summary of the workshop on infection in the high-risk infant. *Journal of Perinataology, 30*, 379–383.

Hintz, S. R., Kendrick, D. E., Wilson-Costello, D. E., Das, A., Bell, E. F., Vohr, B. R., . . . NICHD Neonatal Research Network. (2011). Early-childhood neurodevelopmental outcomes are not improving for infants born at <25 weeks' gestational age. *Pediatrics, 127*, 62–70.

Hintz, S. R., Stevenson, D. K., Yao, Q., Wong, R. J., Das, A., Van Meurs, K. P., . . . Eunice Kennedy Shriver National Institute of Child Health and Human Development Neonatal Research Network. (2011). Is phototherapy exposure associated with better or worse outcomes in 501- to 1000-g-birth-weight infants? *Acta Pediatrica, 100*, 960–965.

Ho, S., & Saigal, S. (2005). Current survival and early outcomes of infants of borderline viability. *NeoReviews, 6*(3), e123–e132.

Hobar, J. D., et al. (n.d.). *Very low birth weight (VLBW) database summary of infants 501–1500 grams*. Retrieved from https://nightingale.vtoxford.org/summaries.aspx

Hodges, C., & Vincent, P. (1993). Why do NICU nurses not refeed gastric residuals prior to feeding by gavage? *Neonatal Network, 12*, 37–40.

Ibrahim, H. M., Jeroudi, M. A., Baier, R. J., Dhanireddy, R., & Krouskop, R. W. (2004). Aggressive early total parental nutrition in low-birth-weight infants. *Journal of Perinatology, 24*, 482–486.

Ibrahim, H. M., Sinha, I. P., & Subhedar, N. V. (2011). Corticosteroids for treating hypotension in preterm infants (Cochrane Review). In *The Cochrane library*, issue 12. John Wiley & Sons.

Iijima, S., Arai, H., Ozawa, Y., Kawase, Y., & Uga, N. (2009). Clinical patterns in extremely preterm (22 to 24 weeks of gestation) infants in relation to survival time and prognosis. *American Journal of Perinatology, 26*, 399–406.

Janvier, A., Khairy, M., Kokkotis, A., Cormier, C., Messmer, D., & Barrington, K. J. (2004). Apnea is associated with neurodevelopmental impairment in very low birth weight infants. *Journal of Perinatology, 24*, 763–768.

Johnson, S., Fawke, J., Hennessy, E., Rowell, V., Thomas, S., Wolke, D., & Marlow, N. (2009). Neurodevelopmental disability through 11 years of age in children born before 26 weeks of gestation: The EPICure Study. *Pediatrics, 124*, e249–e257.

Kalhan, S. C., & Parimi, P. S. (2001). Disorders of carbohydrate metabolism. In A. A. Fanaroff & R. J. Martin (Eds.), *Neonatal-perinatal medicine: Diseases of the fetus and infant* (7th ed., pp. 3–12). St Louis, MO: Mosby.

Kao, L. S., Morris, B. H., Lally, K. P., Stewart, C. D., Huseby, V., & Kennedy, K. A. (2006). Hyperglycemia and morbidity and mortality in extremely low birth weight infants. *Journal of Perinatology, 26*, 730–736.

Kilbride, H. W. (2004). Effectiveness of neonatal intensive care for extremely low birth weight infants. *Pediatrics, 114*, 1374.

Kim, S. M., Lee, E. Y., Chen, J., & Ringer, S. A. (2010). Improved care and growth outcomes by using hybrid incubators in very preterm infants. *Pediatrics, 125*, e137–e145.

Kjartansson, S., Hammarlund, K., & Sedin, G. (1992). Insensible water loss from the skin during phototherapy in term and preterm infants. *Acta Paediatrica, 81*, 764–768.

Kliegman, R. M. (1990). Models of the pathogenesis of necrotizing enterocolitis. *Journal of Pediatrics, 117*, S2–S5.

Knobel, R. B., Holditch-Davis, D., Schwartz, T. A., & Wimmer, J. E., Jr. (2009). Extremely low birth weight preterm infants lack vasomotor response in relationship to cold body temperatures at birth. *Journal of Perinatology, 29*, 814–821.

Knobel, R. B., Wimmer, J. E., Jr., & Holbert, D. (2005). Heat loss prevention for preterm infants in the delivery room. *Journal of Perinatology, 25*, 304–308.

Koch, J., Hensley, G., Roy, L., Brown, S., Ramaciotti, C., & Rosenfeld, C. R. (2006). Prevalence of spontaneous closure of the ductus arteriosus in neonates at a birth weight of 1000 grams or less. *Pediatrics, 117*, 1113–1121.

Kopelman, L. M. (2005). Rejecting the baby Doe rules and defending a "negative" analysis of the best interest standard. *Journal of Medicine and Philosophy, 30*, 331–352.

Kotto-Kome, A. C., Garcia, M. G., Calhoun, D. A., & Christensen, R. D. (2004). Effect of beginning recombinant erythropoietin treatment within the first week of life, among very-low-birth-weight neonates, on "early" and "late" erythrocyte transfusions: A meta-analysis. *Journal of Perinatology, 24*, 24–29.

Kuban, K. C. K., Allred, E. N., O'Shea, T. M., Paneth, N., Pagano, M., Dammann, O., . . . ELGAN study investigators. (2009). Cranial ultrasound lesions in the NICU predict cerebral palsy at age 2 years in children born at extremely low gestational age. *Journal of Child Neurology, 24*, 63–72.

Kusauda, S., Fujimura, M., Sakuma, I., Aotani, H., Kabe, K., Itani, Y., . . . Neonatal Research Network. (2006). Morbidity and mortality of infants with very low birth weight in Japan: Center variation. *Pediatrics, 118*, e1130–e1138.

Kuschel, C. A., & Harding, J. E. (2009). Protein supplementation of human milk for promoting growth in preterm infants (Cochrane Review). In *The Cochrane library*, issue 1. John Wiley & Sons.

Labenne, M., Michaut, F., Gouyon, B., Ferdynus, C., & Gouyon, J. B. (2007). A population-based observational study of restrictive guidelines for antibiotic therapy in early-onset neonatal infections. *The Pediatric Infectious Disease Journal, 26*, 593–599.

Lee, J. S., & Polin, R. A. (2003). Treatment and prevention of necrotizing enterocolitis. *Seminars in Neonatology, 8*, 449–459.

Lemyre, B., Davis, P. G., & De Paoli, A. G. (2008). Nasal intermittent positive pressure ventilation (NIPPV) versus nasal continuous positive airway pressure (NCPAP) for apnea of prematurity (Cochrane Review). In *The Cochrane library*, issue 3. John Wiley & Sons.

Lester, B. M., Miller, R. J., Hawes, K., Salisbury, A., Bigsby, R., Sullivan, M. C., & Padbury, J. F. (2011). Infant neurobehavioral development. *Seminars in Perinatology, 35*, 8–19.

Lightburn, M. H., Gauss, C. H., Williams, D. K., & Kaiser, J. R. (2009). Cerebral blood flow velocities in extremely low birth weight infants with hypotension and infants with normal blood pressure. *Journal of Pediatrics, 154*, 824–282.

Logan, J. W., O'Shea, T. M., Allred, E. N., Laughon, M. M., Bose, C. L., Dammann, O., . . . ELGAN Study Investigators. (2011). Early postnatal hypotension is not associated with indicators of white matter damage or cerebral palsy in extremely low gestational age newborns. *Journal of Perinatology, 31*, 524–534.

Lorenz, J. M. (2003). Management decisions in extremely premature infants. *Seminars in Neonatology, 8*, 475–482.

Lorenz, J. M. (2004). Proactive management of extremely premature infants. *Pediatrics, 114*, 264.

Lorenz, J. M., Kleinman, L. I., Ahmed, G., & Markarian, K. (1995). Phases of fluid and electrolyte homeostasis in the extremely low birth weight infant. *Pediatrics, 96*, 484–489.

Lucas, A., & Cole, T. J. (1990). Breast milk and neonatal necrotizing enterocolitis. *Lancet, 336*, 1519–1523.

Lucas, A., Morley, R., Cole, T. J., Lister, G., & Leeson-Payne, C. (1992). Breast milk and subsequent intelligence quotient in children born preterm. *Lancet, 339*, 261–264.

Lyon, A. J., Pikaar, M. E., Badger, P., & McIntosh, N. (1997). Temperature control in very low birth weight infants during first five days of life. *Archives of Disease in Childhood, 76*, F47–F50.

Madan, A., Kumar, R., Adams, M. M., Benitz, W. E., Geaghan, S. M., & Widness, J. A. (2005). Reduction in red blood cell transfusions using a bedside analyzer in extremely low birth weight infants. *Journal of Perinatology, 25*, 21–25.

Maggio, L., Cota, F., Gallini, F., Lauriola, V., Zecca, C., & Romagnoli, C. (2007). Effects of high versus standard protein intake on growth of extremely low birth weight infants. *Journal of Pediatric Gastroenterology and Nutrition, 44*, 124–129.

Maier, R. F., Sonntag, J., Walka, M. M., Liu, G., Metze, B. C., & Obladen, M. (2000). Changing practices of red blood cell transfusions in infants with birth weights less than 1000 g. *Journal of Pediatrics, 136*(2), 220–224.

Malviya, M. N., Ohlsson, A., & Shah, S. (2008). Surgical versus medical treatment with cyclooxygenase inhibitors for symptomatic patent ductus arteriosus in preterm infants (Cochrane Review). In *The Cochrane library*, issue 4. John Wiley & Sons.

Markestad, T., Kaaresen, P. I., Rønnestad, A., Reigstad, H., Lossius, K., Medbø, S., . . . Norwegian Extreme Prematurity Study Group. (2005). Early death, morbidity, and need of treatment among extremely preterm infants. *Pediatrics, 115*, 1289–1298.

Marlier, L., Gaugler, C., & Messer, J. (2005). Olfactory stimulation prevents apnea in premature newborns. *Pediatrics, 115*, 83–88.

Martin, R. J., Abu Shaweesh, J. M., & Baird, T. M. (2004). Apnoea of prematurity. *Pediatric Respiratory Reviews, 5*, S377–S382.

Mazeiras, G., Rozé, J. C., Ancel, P. Y., Caillaux, G., Frondas-Chauty, A., Denizot, S., & Flamant, C. (2012). Hyperbilirubinemia and neurodevelopmental outcome of very low birth weight infants: Results from the LIFT cohort. *PLos One, 7*, e30900. doi:10.1371/journal.pone.0030900

McCain, G. C., Gartside, P. S., Greenberg, J. M., & Lott, J. W. (2001). A feeding protocol for healthy preterm infants that shortens time to oral feeding. *Journal of Pediatrics, 139*, 374–379.

McCall, E. M., Alderdice, F. A., Halliday, H. L., Jenkins, J. G., & Vohra, S. (2010). Interventions to prevent hypothermia at birth in preterm and/or low birth weight babies (Cochrane Review). In *The Cochrane library*, issue 3. John Wiley & Sons.

Medoff-Cooper, R., & Ray, W. (1995). Neonatal sucking behaviors. *Image—Journal of Nursing Scholarship, 27*, 195–200.

Meerstadt, P. W. D., & Gyll, C. (1994). *Manual of neonatal emergency X-ray interpretation*. London, UK: Saunders.

Meinzen-Derr, J., Poindexter, B., Wrage, L., Morrow, A. L., Stoll, B., & Donovan, E. F. (2009). Role of human milk in extremely low birth weight infants' risk of necrotizing enterocolitis or death. *Journal of Perinatology, 29*, 57–62.

Mercier, C. E., Dunn, M. S., Ferrelli, K. R., Howard, D. B., Soll, R. F., & Vermont Oxford Network ELBW Infant Follow-Up Study Group. (2010). Neurodevelopmental outcome of extremely low birth weight infants from the Vermont Oxford network: 1998–2003. *Neonatology, 97*, 329–338.

Meyer, M., Mildenhall, L., & Wong, M. (2004). Outcomes for infants weighing less than 1000 grams cared for with a nasal continuous positive airway pressure-based strategy. *Journal of Paediatrics and Child Health, 40*, 38–41.

Moll, M., Goelz, R., Naegele, T., Wilke, M., & Poets, C. F. (2011). Are recommended phototherapy thresholds safe enough for extremely low birth weight (ELBW) infants? A report on 2 ELBW infants with kernicterus despite only moderate hyperbilirubinemia. *Neonatology, 99*, 90–94.

Morgan, J., Young, L., & McGuire, W. (2011). Delayed introduction of progressive enteral feeds to prevent necrotizing enterocolitis in very low birth weight infants (Cochrane Review). In *The Cochrane library*, issue 3. John Wiley & Sons.

Morris, B. H., Oh, W., Tyson, J. E., Stevenson, D. K., Phelps, D. L., O'Shea, T. M., . . . NICHD Neonatal Research Network. (2008). Aggressive vs. conservative phototherapy for infants with extremely low birth weight. *New England Journal of Medicine, 359*, 1885–1896.

Moya, M. P., Clark, R. H., Nicks, J., & Tanaka, D. T. (2001). The effect of bedside blood gas monitoring on blood loss and ventilator management. *Biology of the Neonate, 80*, 257–261.

Narendran, V., Donovan, E. F., Hoath, S. B., Akinbi, H. T., Steichen, J. J., & Jobe, A. H. (2003). Early bubble CPAP and outcomes in ELBW preterm infants. *Journal of Perinatology, 23*, 195–199.

Neu, J., & Walker, W. A. (2011). Necrotizing enterocolitis. *New England Journal of Medicine, 364*, 255–264.

Ohls, R. K. (2002). Erythropoietin treatment in extremely low birth weight infants: Blood in versus blood out. *Journal of Pediatrics, 141*, 3–6.

Ohlsson, A., Walia, R., & Shah, S. S. (2010). Ibuprofen for the treatment of patent ductus arteriosus in preterm and/or low-birth-weight infants. Cochrane Database of Systematic Reviews, Issue 4, CD003481. doi:10.102/14651858.CD003481.pub4

Ohlsson, A., & Shah, S. S. (2011). Ibuprofen for the prevention of patent ductus arteriosus in preterm and/or low birth weight infants (Cochrane Review). In *The Cochrane library*, issue 7. John Wiley & Sons.

Ohlsson, A., Walia, R., & Shah, S. S. (2010). Ibuprofen for the treatment of patent ductus arteriosus in preterm and/or low birth weight infants (Cochrane Review). In *The Cochrane library*, issue 4. John Wiley & Sons.

Omari, T. I. (2009). Apnea-associated reduction in lower esophageal sphincter tone in premature infants. *Journal of Perinatology, 154*, 374–378.

Omari, T. I., Rommel, N., Staunton, E., Lontis, R., Goodchild, L., Haslam, R. R., . . . Davidson, G. P. (2004). Paradoxical impact of body positioning on gastroesophageal reflux and gastric emptying in the premature neonate. *Journal of Pediatrics, 145*, 194–200.

Osborn, D. A., & Evans, N. (2009a). Early volume expansion for prevention of morbidity and mortality in very preterm infants (Cochrane Review). In *The Cochrane library*, issue 3. John Wiley & Sons.

Osborn, D. A., & Evans, N. (2009b). Early volume expansion versus inotrope for prevention of morbidity and mortality in very preterm infants (Cochrane Review). In *The Cochrane library*, issue 1. John Wiley & Sons.

Osborn, D. A., & Henderson-Smart, D. J. (2010). Kinesthetic stimulation for preventing apnea in preterm infants (Cochrane Review). In *The Cochrane library*, issue 1. John Wiley & Sons.

O'Shea, T. M., Allred, E. N., Dammann, O., Hirtz, D., Kuban, K. C., Paneth, N., . . . ELGAN study Investigators. (2009). The ELGAN study of the brain and related disorders in extremely low gestational age newborns. *Early Human Development, 85*, 719–725.

Palmer, E. A., Hardy, R. J., Dobson, V., Phelps, D. L., Quinn, G. E., Summers, C. G., . . . Cryotherapy for Retinopathy of Prematurity Cooperative Group. (2005). 15-year outcomes following threshold retinopathy of prematurity: Final results from the multicenter trial of cryotherapy for retinopathy of prematurity. *Archives of Ophthalmology, 123*, 311–318.

Pammi, M., & Abrams, S. A. (2011). Oral lactoferrin for the prevention of sepsis and necrotizing enterocolitis in preterm infants. In *The Cochrane library*, issue 12. John Wiley & Sons.

Patole, S., & de Klerk, N. (2005). Impact of standardised feeding regimens on incidence of neonatal necrotising enterocolitis: A systematic review and meta analysis of observational studies. *Archives of Disease in Childhood, Neonatal and Fetal Edition, 90*, F147–F151.

Penticuff, J. H., & Arheart, K. L. (2005). Effectiveness of an intervention to improve parent-professional collaboration in neonatal intensive care. *Journal of Perinatal and Neonatal Nursing, 19*, 187–202.

Peter, C. S., Sprodowski, N., Bohnhorst, B., Silny, J., & Poets, C. F. (2002). Gastroesophageal reflux and apnea of prematurity: No temporal relationship. *Pediatrics, 109*, 8–11.

Peter, C. S., Wiechers, C., Bohnhorst, B., Silny, J., & Poets, C. F. (2002). Influence of nasogastric tubes on gastroesophageal reflux in preterm infants: A multiple intraluminal impedance study. *Journal of Pediatrics, 141*, 277–279.

Pfister, R. H., Soll, R., & Wiswell, T. E. (2009). Protein containing synthetic surfactant versus animal derived surfactant extract for the prevention and treatment of respiratory distress syndrome (Cochrane Review). In *The Cochrane library*, issue 1. John Wiley & Sons.

Phelps, D., & Watts, J. (2009). Early light reduction for preventing retinopathy of prematurity in very low birth weight infants (Cochrane Review). In *The Cochrane library*, issue 1. John Wiley & Sons.

Pickler, R. H., & Reyna, B. A. (2003). A descriptive study of bottle-feeding opportunities in preterm infants. *Advances in Neonatal Care, 3*, 139–146.

Poet, C. F., & Brockmann, P. E. (2011). Myth: Gastroestophageal reflux is a pathological entity in the preterm infants. *Seminars in Fetal and Neonatal Medicine, 16*, 259–263.

Powell, T. L., Parker, L., Dedrick, C. F., Barrera, C. M., & Salvo, D. D. (2012). Decisions and dilemmas related to resuscitation of infants born on the verge of viability. *Newborn and Infant Nursing Reviews, 12*, 27–32.

Premji, S. S. (2005). Standardised feeding regimens: Hope for reducing the risk of necrotizing enterocolitis. *Archives of Disease in Childhood, 90*, 192–193.

Premji, S. S., & Chessell, L. (2011). Continuous nasogastric milk feeding versus intermittent bolus milk feeding for premature infants less than 1,500 grams (Cochrane Review). In *The Cochrane library*, issue 11. John Wiley & Sons.

Premji, S. S., McNeil, D. A., & Scotland, J. (2004). Regional neonatal oral feeding protocol: Changing the ethos of feeding preterm infants. *Journal of Perinatal and Neonatal Nursing, 18*(4), 371–384.

Premji, S. S., Paes, B., Jacobson, K., & Chessell, L. (2002). Evidence-based feeding guidelines for very low-birth-weight infants. *Advances in Neonatal Care, 2*(1), 5–18.

Pritchard, M., Flenady, V., & Woodgate, P. (2010). Preoxygenation for tracheal suctioning in intubated, ventilated newborn infants (Cochrane Review). In *The Cochrane library*, issue 1. John Wiley & Sons.

Razi, N. M., Humphreys, J., Pandit, P. B., & Stahl, G. E. (1999). Predischarge monitoring of preterm infants. *Pediatric Pulmonology, 27*, 113–116.

Richards, J., Johnson, A., Fox, G., & Campbell, M. (2009). A second course of ibuprofen is effective in the closure of a clinically significant PDA in ELBW infants. *Pediatrics, 124*, e287–e293.

Rieger-Fackeldey, E., Schaller-Bals, S., & Schulze, A. (2003). Effect of body temperature on the pattern of spontaneous breathing in extremely low birth weight infants supported by proportional assist ventilation. *Pediatric Research, 54*, 332–336.

Rodriguez, R. J., Martin, R. J., & Fanaroff, A. A. (2002). Part 3: Respiratory distress syndrome and its management. In A. A. Fanaroff & R. J. Martin (Eds.), *Neonatal-perinatal medicine* (pp. 1001–1011). St Louis, MO: Mosby.

Rojas-Reyes, X. M., Morley, C. J., & Soll, R. (2012). Prophylactic versus selective use of surfactant in preventing morbidity and mortality in preterm infants (Cochrane Review). In *The Cochrane library*, issue 3. John Wiley & Sons.

Rosenfeld, W., Sadhev, S., Brunot, V., Jhaveri, R., Zabaleta, I., & Evans, H. E. (1986). Phototherapy effect on the incidence of patent ductus arteriosus in premature infants: Prevention with chest shielding. *Pediatrics, 78*, 10–14.

Roze, J. C., & Breart, G. (2004). Care of very premature infants: Looking to the future. *European Journal of Obstetrics, Gynecology, and Reproductive Biology, 117*, S29–S32.

Salhab, W. A., Perlman, J. M., Silver, L., & Sue Broyles, R. (2004). Necrotizing enterocolitis and neurodevelopmental outcome in extremely low birth weight infants < 1000 g. *Journal of Perinatology, 24*, 534–540.

Sasidharan, P. (1998). Role of corticosteroids in neonatal blood pressure homeostasis. *Clinics in Perinatology, 25*, 723–740.

Sauer, P. J., Dane, H. J., & Visser, H. K. (1984). New standards for neutral thermal environment of healthy very low birth weight infants in week one of life. *Archives of Disease in Childhood, 59*, 18–22.

Schanler, R. J. (1995). Suitability of human milk for the low-birth weight infant. *Clinics in Perinatology, 22*, 207–222.

Schenk, L. K., & Kelley, J. H. (2010). Mothering an extremely low birth-weight infant: A phenomenological study. *Advances in Neonatal Care, 10*, 88–97.

Schlapbach, L. J., Aebischer, M., Adams, M., Natalucci, G., Bonhoeffer, J., Latzin, P., . . . Swiss Neonatal Network and Follow-Up Group. (2011). Impact of sepsis on neurodevelopmental outcome in a Swiss national cohort of extremely premature infants. *Pediatrics, 128*, e348–e357.

Schmidt, B., Anderson, P. J., Doyle, L. W., Dewey, D., Grunau, R. E., Asztalos, E. V., . . . Caffeine for Apnea of Prematurity (CAP) Trial Investigators. (2012). Survival without disability to age 5 years after neonatal caffeine therapy for apnea of prematurity. *JAMA, 307*, 275–282.

Schmidt, B., Davis, P., Moddemann, D., Ohlsson, A., Roberts, R. S., Saigal, S., . . . Trial of Indomethacin Prophylaxis in Preterms Investigators. (2001). Long-term effects of indomethacin prophylaxis in extremely-low-birth-weight infants. *New England Journal of Medicine, 344*, 1966–1972.

Schmidt, B., Roberts, R. S., Davis, P., Doyle, L. W., Barrington, K. J., Ohlsson, A., . . . Caffeine for Apnea of Prematurity Trial Group. (2007). Long-term effects of caffeine therapy for apnea of prematurity. *New England Journal of Medicine, 357*, 1893–1902.

Schoonakker, B., & Smith, C. (2007). How do neonatologists approach early treatment decisions at the extremes of prematurity? *Obstetrics, Gynaecology and Reproductive Medicine, 17*, 249–251.

Sehgal, A. (2011). Haemodynamically unstable preterm infant: An unresolved management conundrum. *European Journal of Pediatrics, 170*, 1237–1245.

Seri, I., & Evans, J. (2008). Limits of viability: Definition of the gray zone. *Journal of Perinatology, 28*, S4–S8.

Shaker, C. S. (1990). Nipple feeding preterm infants: A different perspective. *Neonatal Network, 8*, 9–17.

Silverman, W. (1992). Foreword. In J. C. Sinclair & M. B. Bracken (Eds.), *Effective care of the newborn*. New York, NY: Oxford University Press.

Sinclair, J. C., Bottino, M., & Cowett, R. M. (2011). Interventions for prevention of neonatal hyperglycemia in very low birth weight infants. In *The Cochrane library*, issue 10. John Wiley & Sons.

Sinclair, L., Sinn, J. K. H. (2009). Higher versus lower humidity for the prevention of morbidity and mortality in preterm infants in incubators (Protocol). In *The Cochrane library*, issue 1. John Wiley & Sons.

Skelton, R., Evans, N., & Smythe, J. (1994). A blinded comparison of clinical and echocardiographic evaluation of the preterm infant for patent ductus arteriosus. *Journal of Paediatrics & Child Health, 30*, 406–411.

Smith, L. (2005). The ethics of neonatal care for the extremely preterm infant. *Journal of Neonatal Nursing, 11*, 40–58.

Snapp, B. (1994). NEC and NIBD similar but distinct. *NANN Central Lines, 10*, 1, 13.

Spitzer, A. R. (2012). Evidence-based methylxanthine use in the NICU. *Clinics in Perinatology, 39*, 137–148.

Stark, A. R., Carlo, W. A., Tyson, J. E., Papile, L. A., Wright, L. L., Shankaran, S., . . . National Institute of Child Health and Human Development Neonatal Research Network. (2001). Adverse effects of early dexamethasone in extremely-low-birth-weight infants. *New England Journal of Medicine, 344*, 95–101.

Stephens, B. E., Walden, R. V., Gargus, R. A., Tucker, R., McKinley, L., Mance, M., . . . Vohr, B. R. (2009). First-week protein and energy intakes are associated with 18-month developmental outcomes in extremely low birth weight infants. *Pediatric, 123*, 1337–1343.

Stokowski, L. A. (2005). A primer on apnea of prematurity. *Advances in Neonatal Care, 5*, 155–170.

Stoll, B. J., Hansen, N. I., Adams-Chapman, I., Fanaroff, A. A., Hintz, S. R., Vohr, B., . . . National Institute of Child Health and Human Development Neonatal Research Network. (2004). Neurodevelopmental and growth impairment among extremely low-birth-weight infants with neonatal infection. *Journal of the American Medical Association, 292*(19), 2357–2365.

Stoll, B. J., Hansen, N. I., Bell, E. F., Shankaran, S., Laptook, A. R., Walsh, M. C., . . . Eunice Kennedy Shriver National Institute of Child Health and Human Development Neonatal Research Network. (2010). Neonatal outcomes of extremely preterm infants from the NICHD Neonatal Research Network. *Pediatrics, 126*, 443–456.

Straus, S. E., Graham, I. D., Mazmanian, P. E. (2006). Knowledge translation: Resolving the confusion. *The Journal of Continuing Education in the Health Professions, 26*, 3–4.

Subhani, M., Combs, A., Weber, P., Gerontis, C., & DeCristofaro, J. D. (2001). Screening guidelines for retinopathy of prematurity: The need for revision in extremely low birth weight infants. *Pediatrics, 107*, 656–659.

Subhedar, N. V., & Shaw, N. J. (2009). Dopamine versus dobutamine for hypotensive preterm infants. *The Cochrane library* (issue 1). John Wiley & Sons.

Sullivan, S., Schanler, R. J., Kim, J. H., Patel, A. L., Trawöger, R., Kiechl-Kohlendorfer, U., . . . Lucas, A. (2010). An exclusively human milk-based diet is associated with lower rate of necrotizing enterocolitis than a diet of human milk and bovine-milk-based products. *Journal of Pediatrics, 156*, 562–567.

Sydnor-Greenberg, N., & Dokken, D. (2000). Coping and caring in different ways: Understanding and meaningful involvement. *Pediatric Nursing, 26*, 185–190.

Symington, A. J., & Pinelli, J. (2009). Developmental care for promoting development and preventing morbidity in preterm infants (Cochrane Review). In *The Cochrane library*, issue 1. John Wiley & Sons.

Taylor, J. E., Hawley, G., Flenady, V., & Woodgate, P. G. (2012). Tracheal suctioning without disconnection in intubated ventilated neonates (Cochrane Review). In *The Cochrane library*, issue 3. John Wiley & Sons.

Tolsma, K. W., Allred, E. N., Chen, M. L., Duker, J., Leviton, A., & Dammann, O. (2011). Neonatal bacteremia and retinopathy of prematurity: The ELGAN study. *Archives of Ophthalmology, 129*, 1555–1563.

Tomlinson, M. W., Kaempf, J. W., Ferguson, L. A., & Stewart, V. T. (2010). Caring for the pregnant women presenting at periviable gestation: Acknowledging the ambiguity and uncertainty. *American Journal of Obstetrics and Gyencology, 202*, 529.e1–529.e6.

Tyson, J. E., Parikh, N. A., Langer, J., Green, C., Higgins, R. D., & National Institute of Child Health and Human Development Neonatal Research Network. (2008). Intensive care for extreme prematurity moving beyond gestational age. *New England Journal of Medicine, 358*, 1672–1681.

Uauy, R., & Mena, P. (2001). Lipids and neurodevelopment. *Nutrition Reviews, 59*, S34–S48.

Vanhaesebrouck, P., Allegaert, K., Bottu, J., Debauche, C., Devlieger, H., Docx, M., . . . Extremely Preterm Infants in Belgium Study Group. (2004). The EPIBEL study: Outcomes to discharge from hospital for extremely preterm infants in Belgium. *Pediatrics, 114*, 663–675.

Vohr, B. R., Poindexter, B. B., Dusick, A. M., McKinley, L. T., Wright, L. L., Langer, J. C., . . . NICHD Neonatal Research Network. (2006). Beneficial effects of breast milk in the neonatal intensive care unit on the developmental outcome of extremely low birth weight infants at 18 months of age. *Pediatrics, 118*, e115–e123.

Vohr, B. R., Wright, L. L., Dusick, A. M., Perritt, R., Poole, W. K., Tyson, J. E., . . . Neonatal Research Network. (2004). Center differences and outcomes of extremely low birth weight infants. *Pediatrics, 113*, 781–789.

Whyte, R. K., Kirpalani, H., Asztalos, E. V., Andersen, C., Blajchman, M., Heddle, N., . . . PINTOS Study Group. (2009). Neurodevelopmental outcome of extremely low birth weight infants randomly assigned to restrictive or liberal hemoglobin thresholds for blood transfusion. *Pediatrics, 123*, 207–213.

Wilder, M. A. (2000). Ethical issues in the delivery room: Resuscitation of extremely low birth weight infants. *Journal of Perinatal and Neonatal Nursing, 14*, 44–57.

Wood, N. S., Costeloe, K., Gibson, A. T., Hennessy, E. M., Marlow, N., Wilkinson, A. R., & EPICure Study Group. (2003). The EPICure study: Growth and associated problems in children born at 25 weeks of gestational age or less. *Archives of Disease in Childhood Neonatal and Fetal Edition, 88*, 492–500.

Wood, N. S., Marlow, N., Costeloe, K., Gibson, A. T., & Wilkinson, A. R. (2000). Neurologic and developmental disability after extremely preterm birth. *New England Journal of Medicine, 343*, 378–384.

Wyllie, J. (2003). Treatment of patent ductus arteriosus. *Seminars in Neonatology, 8*, 425–432.

Yeo, K. L., Perlman, M., Hao, Y., & Mullaney, P. (1998). Outcomes of extremely premature infants related to their peak serum bilirubin concentrations and exposure to phototherapy. *Pediatrics, 102*, 426–431.

Ziegler, E. E., Thureen, P. J., & Carlson, S. J. (2002). Aggressive nutrition of the very low birth weight infant. *Clinics in Perinatology, 29*, 225–244.

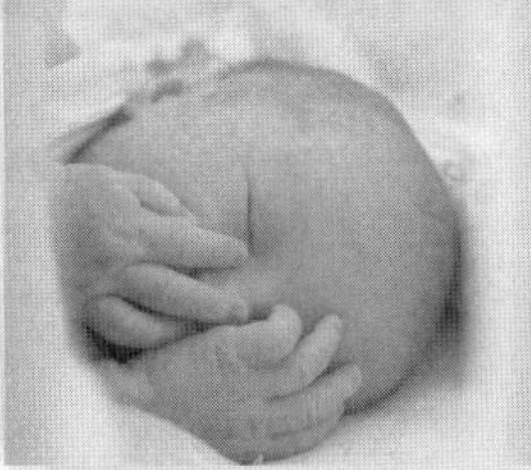

CHAPTER 29

The Late Preterm Infant

■ Maureen F. McCourt

Late preterm infants are infants born between 34 0/7 and 36 6/7 weeks and are increasing in number throughout the country and around the world. All preterm infant births are on the rise, with an increase of 33% in the last 25 years and almost all due to late preterm infant births (Martin et al., 2010; Martin, Osterman, & Sutton, 2010). Preterm births affect approximately 12.5% of all births, with 72% being late preterm infants (Martin et al., 2010).

There are two main etiological categories of late preterm births, spontaneous late preterm births and babies born after induction of labor or cesarean section. Spontaneous late preterm births result from complications of preterm labor and premature rupture of membranes. Inductions of labor or cesarean sections are indicated for many fetal and maternal factors, including maternal medical conditions, advanced maternal age, assisted reproductive techniques, multiple births, planned cesarean sections, and maternal request (Mohan & Jain, 2011).

Late preterm infants are of increasing interest to medical providers because they are larger in size than most premature infants but they are proving to have many challenges associated with immaturity and delayed transition. These infants' have higher rates of morbidity and mortality, as well as increased medical complications, neonatal intensive care unit (NICU) admissions, and prolonged hospitalization (Engle, 2011; Engle, Tomashek, Wallman, & the Committee on Fetus and Newborn, 2007; Ramachandrappa & Jain, 2009). Late preterm infants require closer monitoring and specialized medical and nursing care for this higher risk population with stricter discharge criteria and follow-up care. These infants have a higher rehospitalization rate and long-term sequelae. Additional research is needed to gain better understanding of late preterm infants. This knowledge will help to guide obstetrical and neonatal care to reduce the late preterm infant birth rate and provide specialized care to improve patient outcomes in the future. This chapter describes the late preterm infant and the challenges associated with their care.

DEFINITION

Since 1950 the definition for premature infants has been, "infants born before 37 completed weeks gestation (259th day) counting from the first day of the last menstrual period." This definition was established by the World Health Organization, and the American Academy of Pediatrics (AAP) and American Congress of Obstetricians and Gynecologists (ACOG) concur (Raju, Higgins, Stark, & Leveno, 2006). Within the premature infant category, there are subgroups with definitions including extremely preterm infants (infants less than 28 weeks) and very preterm infants (infants less than 32 weeks gestation). However, there is less clarity regarding infants born between 32 and 37 weeks gestation. In July 2005 the National Institute of Child Health and Human Development of the National Institutes of Health defined late preterm infants as infants born between 34 0/7 and 36 6/7 weeks (Raju et al., 2006). In developing this definition, many factors were taken into account, especially 34 weeks gestation being a maturational milestone in which surfactant is usually present. Labeling infants born between 34 0/7 and 36 6/7 weeks late preterm infants was critical in reminding caregivers that these infants are still premature and can develop physical and neurocognitive sequelae and will help discourage early elective deliveries and encourage specialized care optimizing outcomes (Martin, Fanaroff, & Walsh, 2011; Shapiro-Mendoza & Lackritz, 2012).

INCIDENCE AND EPIDEMIOLOGY

There has been an increase of 33% in the preterm birth rate between 1981 and 2006, which has almost entirely been due to late preterm infant births. In 2008, 12.5% of all births in the United States were infants less than 37 weeks. Of these infants, 72% were late preterm infants born between 34 and 36 weeks (Martin et al., 2010; Shapiro-Mendoza & Lackritz, 2012).

Of these late preterm births, multiple gestations have an elevated rate compared with singletons. Between 1990 and 2008, there was an increase in singleton births by 14.7%, and the rate increase for multiples was 27.4%. Studies from 1995 to 2000 showed congenital malformations are associated with late preterm births. Non-Hispanic Black mothers and maternal age less than 20 and greater than 35 years is also associated with increases in late preterm births (Shapiro-Mendoza & Lackritz, 2012).

ETIOLOGIC FACTORS CAUSING THE LATE PRETERM INFANT BIRTHS

The etiological factors contributing to late preterm births are complex and multifactorial. There are two main categories leading to late preterm births, including spontaneous late preterm births and induction of labor or cesarean section for maternal or fetal indications (Gyamfi-Bannerman, 2012; Mohan & Jain, 2011).

The first category, spontaneous late preterm births, relates to conditions where prevention of delivery is typically unavoidable. Maternal risk factors include preterm labor and premature rupture of membranes. This is especially prevalent when infection and inflammation are a concern. Research in the area of expeditious deliveries with preterm labor or PPROM versus expectant management to 37 weeks gestation is ongoing, in determining if these preterm deliveries are necessary or can be avoided (Gyamfi-Bannerman, 2012; Mohan & Jain, 2011).

The second category includes late preterm births related to inductions of labor and cesarean sections for maternal or fetal indications. The indications for delivery in this group include preeclampsia, eclampsia, IUGR, and planned cesarean sections. There has been a dramatic increase in cesarean sections due to increased fetal surveillance and interventions, increasing age of women giving birth, increase in multiple births due to fertility treatments, and heightened concerns of physicians and mothers regarding risks of vaginal births. Further research is needed to understand the impact of planned cesarean sections leading to preterm births and strategies for prevention (Mohan & Jain, 2011).

Other factors that impact late preterm births include maternal medical conditions, advanced maternal age, assisted reproductive technologies, and multiple births, which are all associated with preterm births. Gestational age assessments and obstetric practice guidelines can also impact late preterm births. Inaccurate gestational age assessment during elective deliveries can lead to late preterm deliveries, especially with maternal obesity and gestational diabetes. Presumption of fetal maturity at 34 weeks gestation and decreasing gestational age can also lead to increases in late preterm births (Engle & Kominiarek, 2008).

Decisions regarding obstetric intervention lie with the risks and benefits of continuing the pregnancy versus early delivery. Understanding the risks of a suboptimal uterine environment and the risks of late preterm infants is critical to help guide optimal clinical decision making. Further research in this area is necessary to guide clinical practice (Shapiro-Mendoza & Lackritz, 2012).

PATHOPHYSIOLOGIC IMMATURITY OF THE LATE PRETERM INFANT

Late preterm infants can be deceiving: They appear to be larger and mature, but are in fact physiologically and metabolically immature. Their immature systems can predispose them to medical complications, with increased morbidity and mortality rates. Below is a systematic review of their potential immature systems.

Respiratory

Late preterm infants are at higher risk for an immature respiratory system. These infants are at risk for an immature lung structure associated with the interruption of the transition from alveoli lined with cuboidal type II and flat type I epithelial cells (terminal sac period) to mature alveoli lined with thin type I epithelial cells (alveolar period). This can be associated with delayed intrapulmonary fluid absorption, surfactant deficiency and insufficiency, as well as inefficient gas exchange. Late preterm infants are often delivered by cesarean section, which occurs without the benefit of labor. Without labor, adrenergic and steroid hormones are not released that leads to a deficit in surfactant production and release. This leaves the late preterm infant at risk for respiratory disorders, including transient tachypnea of the newborn (TTN), respiratory distress syndrome (RDS), persistent pulmonary hypertension of the newborn (PPHN), and respiratory failure (Engle et al., 2007).

The late preterm infant can also have an increased risk of hypoxic respiratory depression, decreased central chemosensitivity to carbon dioxide, immature pulmonary irritant receptors, increased respiratory inhibition sensitivity to laryngeal stimulation, and decreased upper airway dilator muscle tone that can leave the infant at risk for apnea. Apnea in this group can also be due to central mediated apnea related to central nervous system immaturity (Engle et al., 2007).

Cardiac

There is less understanding of the cardiac pathophysiology in the late preterm infant. It appears these infants are at risk for cardiovascular structure and function immaturities leading to decreased cardiac reserve during times of stress. There can also be delayed ductal arteriosus closure and persistent pulmonary hypertension, which can complicate their recovery from respiratory disorders (Engle et al., 2007).

Metabolic

Immaturities can leave the late preterm infants with decreased stores of brown fat adipose and white adipose tissue, insufficient concentrations of hormones responsible for brown-fat metabolism and a decreased surface area to body weight. This results in an inability to generate heat combined with an increased loss of heat leading to thermoregulation issues with resultant hypothermia (Engle et al., 2007).

Late preterm infants have a decreased activity of hepatic uridine diphosphoglucuronate glycuronosyltransferase enzyme, which typically binds bilirubin to glucuronic acid, making it more soluble and more easily secreted in the stool and urine. These infants have a decreased stool frequency and are often dehydrated with a low urine output, making it difficult for bilirubin excretion. They also have an increased enterohepatic circulation related to immature gastrointestinal function and motility, with a decreased ability for hepatic uptake and conjugation of bilirubin. These factors leave late preterm infants at risk for elevated serum bilirubin levels, with resultant hyperbilirubinemia (Engle et al., 2007).

Late preterm infants also have an immature hepatic glycogenolysis and adipose tissue lipolysis, as well as hormone dysregulation and less hepatic gluconeogenesis and ketogenesis. This leaves them less able to respond to the abrupt loss of maternal glucose after birth with resultant hypoglycemia (Engle et al., 2007).

Gastrointestinal

Immature feeding patterns are a common occurrence when introducing enteral feeds in the late preterm infant. This is related to low oral motor tone with lower intraoral pressure during sucking and neuronal immaturity, with resultant poor coordination of sucking and swallowing patterns (Engle et al., 2007; Martin et al., 2011). These infants also have decreased peristalsis and sphincter control in the esophagus, stomach, and intestines. These immaturities lead to a compromised nutritional status (Raju et al., 2006).

Central Nervous System

Late premature infants are at risk for neurologic immaturity, with brain weights of only 65% and cerebral volume 53% compared with term infants. These infants have a cerebral cortex that is still smooth, gyri and sulci that are not fully formed, and incomplete myelination and interneural connections. If injury occurs during this neurological growth period the infant is at risk for white and gray matter injury, especially in the thalamic region and periventricular white matter. This leaves the late preterm infant at risk for neurologic disorders including poor development and long-term outcome (Martin et al., 2011).

MORBIDITY AND MORTALITY OF THE LATE PRETERM INFANT

Many studies have shown that late preterm infants are at increased risk for morbidity and mortality (Bird et al., 2010; Engle, 2011; Engle et al., 2007). Shapiro-Mendoza et al. (2008) found late preterm infants are seven times more likely to have neonatal morbidity during their birth hospitalization than their term infant counterparts. Cheng, Kaimal, Brucher, Halloran, and Caughey in 2011 researched singleton live births between 34 and 40 weeks of gestation. Infants at 34 weeks were found to be at greatest risk for hyaline membrane disease, mechanical ventilation use greater than 6 hours, and antibiotic use. At 35 weeks, infants had a greater use of surfactant, ventilation greater than 6 hours and NICU admission. Infants at 36 weeks had an overall higher risk of morbidities when compared to infants 37 to 40 weeks of gestation. The researchers concluded that, although the risk of neonatal complications decreases with increasing gestational age, neonatal complications are higher for late preterm infants than their term infant counterparts.

The morbidities the late preterm infants are at increased risk for include TTN, RDS, PPHN, respiratory failure, apnea, hyperbilirubinemia, hypoglycemia, hypothermia, feeding difficulties, and neonatal sepsis. These health issues place the infants at increased risk for admission to the NICU requiring treatments, including mechanical ventilation, intravenous fluids, and sepsis evaluation (Cheng, Kaimal, Bruckner, Halloran, & Caughey, 2011; Engle, 2011; Engle & Kominiarek, 2008; Raju et al., 2006).

Preterm infants also have higher mortality rates. Mathews and MacDorman (2011) found infant mortality rates were 3.6 times higher for late preterm infants than for infants born at 39 to 41 weeks. The three leading causes of infant mortality in all infants studied were congenital malformations, low birth weight and sudden infant death. Crump, Sundquist, Sundquist, and Winkleby (2011) found late preterm infants had a higher mortality rate when compared with term infants during early childhood and young adulthood. Causes of death in young adulthood were related to congenital anomalies, as well as respiratory, endocrine, and cardiovascular disorders. Tomashek, Shapiro-Mendoza, Davidoff, and Petrini (2007) found mortality rates to be three times higher in late preterm infants than term infants. Infant deaths for late preterm infants compared with term infants were six times higher between day 1 and 6, three times higher between day 7 and 27, and two times higher between day 28 and 365.

MEDICAL AND NURSING CARE OF THE LATE PRETERM INFANT

It is clear that late preterm infants are different from term infants and should be monitored more closely. Engle (2011) suggests infants born less than 35 weeks gestation or less than 2,300 g birth weight should be admitted to an area where they can be observed more closely than in a normal nursery. These infants are at increased risk for delayed transition and should have a physical exam and accurate gestational age assessment on admission. Vital signs and pulse oximeter checks should be done on admission and every 3 to 4 hours in the first 24 hours and every other shift thereafter. Strong feeding plans should be developed, with a formal breastfeeding evaluation done by a trained lactation consultant or neonatal nurse. Serum glucose monitoring should be done to assess for hypoglycemia. Transfer to a normal nursery or mother's room should be considered only when the late preterm infant shows signs of stability. If an oxygen hood is needed in excess of 40%, the infant should be transferred to a NICU or tertiary care facility for further management (Engle, 2011; Martin et al., 2011).

Late preterm infants are at increased risk for TTN, RDS, PPHN, respiratory failure, apnea, hyperbilirubinemia, hypothermia, hypoglycemia, feeding difficulties, neonatal sepsis, and NICU admission with a prolonged hospital stay as well as having mothers with increased emotional distress. These medical problems need careful assessment and treatment (Martin et al., 2011).

Respiratory Disorders

Late preterm infants are at increased risk for respiratory complications such as TTN, RDS, PPHN, respiratory failure, and apnea (Engle, 2011; Engle et al., 2007).

Researchers have found the incidence of RDS was 3.3% at 36 weeks gestation and 13.7% at 34 weeks gestation. The need for mechanical ventilation in this group was 2.3% and 6.3%, respectively (Cheng et al., 2011; Martin et al., 2011). Late preterm infants should be observed for respiratory symptoms, including tachypnea, retractions, nasal flaring, grunting, and cyanosis. Babies should be admitted to the NICU if respiratory disorders are suspected for monitoring, oxygen therapy, intubation, and surfactant as needed (Martin et al., 2011).

Late preterm infants are at higher risk for apnea. The incidence of apnea for late preterm infants is 4% to 7%, while term infant rates are less than 1% to 2% (Engle et al., 2007). Infants should be monitored for apnea and transferred to the NICU for an appropriate work-up and treatment as needed. It is important to rule out other causes of apnea such as sepsis. If central apnea is suspected, treatment options include monitoring of apnic events in mild cases and the use of caffeine for more persistent episodes of apnea.

Hyperbilirubinemia

Late preterm infants are at risk for hyperbilirubinemia and are two times more likely to develop significantly elevated bilirubin concentrations than term infants. Late preterm infants are also at increased risk of developing kernicterus since many infants are breastfeeding with inadequate maternal supports and insufficient follow-up. These infants should be observed for jaundice as well as have a risk assessment plan for jaundice. A predischarge bilirubin check should be done (serum or transcutaneous) with phototherapy as needed. Careful follow-up should be done to assess for jaundice since bilirubin levels are likely to peak at day 5 to 7 (Engle, 2011; Engle et al., 2007).

Hypoglycemia

Late preterm infants are at greater risk for hypoglycemia (Engle et al., 2007). It is important to prevent hypoglycemia because even moderate hypoglycemia can have serious neurodevelopment consequences in the late preterm infants (Laptook & Jackson, 2006). These infants should have their blood sugars monitored frequently, every hour for 4 hours or until greater than 50, twice. Late preterm infants should be monitored for symptoms of hypoglycemia, including poor feeding, hypothermia, crying, irritability, jitteriness, seizures, and apnea. Treatment will be necessary for a glucose level less than 40 to 50. These treatments include early enteral feeds, intravenous dextrose (2 mL/kg) bolus or maintenance IV fluids (GIR 4–6 mg/kg/min, Total Fluids 80 mL/kg/d), or a combination of these therapies (AAP, 2011; Engle, 2011).

Infants of diabetic mothers are often delivered early and will be at greater risk for hypoglycemia. Most institutions have glucose monitoring and protocols that should be followed as needed (AAP, 2011).

Hypothermia

Thermoregulation is a challenge for the late preterm infant. Laptook and Jackson (2006) found that infants weighing more than 2 kg and greater than 32 weeks had admission temperatures between 34.5°C and 36.5°C (94.1°F and 97.8°F). The late preterm infant's temperatures should be monitored closely after birth and every hour for 6 hours, then every 6 hours until discharge. The normal range is 36.5°C to 37.4°C (97.7°F–99.3°F) (Engle, 2011; Engle et al., 2007; Martin et al., 2011).

Infants' should be monitored for cold stress symptoms including tachypnea, poor color, cyanosis, pallor, mottling, altered pulmonary vasomotor tone, metabolic acidosis, and lethargy. Hypothermia can worsen respiratory transition and hypoglycemia. These symptoms combined with hypothermia can also suggest infection; therefore it is important to prevent these symptoms and an unnecessary costly work-up for sepsis (Martin et al., 2011).

It is important to keep the infant normothermic using strategies including skin-to-skin contact with the mother, keeping a dry hat on the infant, and using warm blankets in the delivery room. It is also important to keep the infant warm when weighing and to postpone a bath until stable (Engle, 2011; Engle et al., 2007; Mance, 2008; Martin et al., 2011).

Feeding Difficulties

The gastrointestinal tract of late preterm infants typically tolerates feedings, but these infants often have difficulty in coordinating sucking, swallowing, and breathing. Poor feedings can lead to weight loss, dehydration, hypoglycemia, and hyperbilirubinemia Feeding challenges place late preterm infants at risk for a prolonged hospital stay and rehospitalization (Cleaveland, 2010). It is important to evaluate feeding patterns and to provide appropriate interventions as needed, which may include occupational therapy consults and lactation support (Engle, 2011; Engle et al., 2007; Laptook & Jackson, 2006).

Early and Late Neonatal Sepsis

Late preterm infants are at increased risk for infection. Late preterm deliveries can often result from preterm labor and premature rupture of membranes with the etiology of infection. These infants undergo more sepsis work-ups than term infants as well as more antibiotic therapy. Providers should look at risk factors for sepsis and signs symptoms of infection, including temperature instability, lethargy, jitteriness, irritability, hypotonia, respiratory distress, hypotension, poor perfusion, poor feedings, vomiting, diarrhea, glucose instability, rashes, and jaundice. A complete blood count (CBC) with differential blood cultures and antibiotic therapy should be implemented with signs of infection. Appropriate length of treatment of antibiotics should be determined (Cohen-Wolkowiez et al., 2009; Martin et al., 2011).

Admission to NICU and Prolonged Hospital Stay

Late preterm infants are more likely to require admission to the NICU and prolonged hospitalization compared to term infants. The duration of the NICU hospital stay is inversely propositional to gestational age. Researchers have reported NICU admission rates of 6.7% to 96% at 34 weeks gestation, 42% to 80% at 35 weeks gestation, 22% to 43% at 36 weeks gestation and 6% to 12% for term infants. Median lengths of stay in the birth hospital at 34 weeks were 10 to 13 days, 35 weeks were 7 to 8 days, 36 weeks were 5 to 6 days, and 3 to 5 days for term infants. The percentage of infants who required hospitalization after their mothers' discharge were 75% for 34 weeks, 50% for 35 weeks, and 25% for 36-week infants (Engle, 2011). Common reasons for infant NICU stays include RDS, poor feeding, hypoglycemia, temperature instability, and hyperbilirubinemia (Engle, 2011; Martin et al., 2011; Ramachandrappa & Jain, 2009).

Increased Maternal Emotional Distress

Brandon et al. (2011) found mothers of late preterm infants have greater emotional distress than mothers of term infants. This emotional distress lasts at least 1 month after delivery. Mothers felt unprepared for the labor and delivery process and the poorer than expected infant health outcomes.

DISCHARGE AND FOLLOW-UP CARE AND REHOSPITALIZATION OF THE LATE PRETERM INFANT

Discharge

When planning discharge of the late preterm infant, criteria developed for both high-risk infants and healthy term infants should be considered. Discharge for term infants after a vaginal delivery is typically less than 48 hours. In 1995 the AAP recommended a minimum eligibility of 38 to 42 weeks gestation as discharge criteria for early discharge, less than 48 hours (AAP, Committee on Fetus and Newborn, 1995, 2004). Goyal, Fager, and Lorch (2011) found 40% of late preterm infants were discharged early, prior to 48 hours. The AAP continues to recommend discharge after 48 hours.

Engle et al. (2007) have recommended discharge criteria that reflect evidence of physiologic maturity feeding competencies, thermoregulation, maternal education, assessment and planned intervention for medical, family, environmental, and social risk factors, and follow-up arrangements. Important minimal discharge criteria should include: accurate gestational age determination, meeting of feeding-based competencies, thermoregulation and absence of medical illness, and social risk factors (usually after 48 hours); pediatric follow-up 24 to 48 hours after hospital discharge; vital signs within the normal range for 12 hours preceding discharge; passage of at least one stool spontaneously; 24 hours of successful feeding; a risk assessment for the development of severe hyperbilirubinemia and follow-up arranged as needed; physical exam with no abnormalities requiring hospitalization; no evidence of active bleeding at circumcision site for at least 2 hours, hepatitis B vaccine administration or an appointment for administration; metabolic screens according to state recommendations, passed car seat safety test; hearing assessment; and family environment and social risk factor assessment and parent training (AAP, Committee on Fetus and Newborn, 2008; Engle, 2011; Martin et al., 2011). Good discharge planning will allow a smooth transition for the infant from the hospital environment to home. It will also help reduce hospital readmissions.

Follow-Up Care

It is important to provide follow-up care for late preterm infants and resources for the family for healthy growth and rehospitalization prevention. Follow-up should begin in the hospital and be followed through once the late preterm infant is discharged.

Close follow-up should be provided by the primary care provider, making a visit 24 to 48 hours after hospital discharge. A risk assessment should be done for hyperbilirubinemia with strategies to avoid rehospitalization. Consultant follow-up including medical consultants, VNA, and early intervention should be used as needed.

It is important for the late preterm infants' mothers to obtain breastfeeding support from the pediatric nurse practitioner because often these infants are discharged early and lack sufficient time for breastfeeding support. These infants often have an immature suck swallow pattern that can lead to poor feeding, dehydration, hyperbilirubinemia, and rehospitalization (Ahmed, 2010; Radtke, 2011). Late preterm infants are at greater risk for breastfeeding associated rehospitalization compared to term infants (Radtke, 2011). Follow-up is critical for late preterm healthy growth and development.

Rehospitalization

There is an increased risk for rehospitalization of late preterm infants (Bird et al., 2010; Jain & Cheng, 2006). These infants have a 4.4% rehospitalization rate versus 2% for term infants and 2.7% to 3% for preterm infants less than 34 weeks (Escobar, Clark, & Greene, 2006). These hospital readmission rates were significantly higher for late preterm infants who were never admitted to the NICU or discharged early from the initial hospital stay (Escobar et al., 2006).

Medical reasons for rehospitalization of late preterm infants include hyperbilirubinemia (63%–71%), feeding difficulties (16%), and suspected sepsis (6%–20%) (Escobar et al., 2006) as well as RDS, apnea, vomiting, and crying (Jain & Cheng, 2006). Late preterm infants have an increased risk for rehospitalization due to respiratory illness. Rehospitalization rates to the Pediatric Intensive Care Unit for respiratory illnesses for late preterm infants in the first 2 years of life were 12% (Gunville et al., 2010).

Risk factors for readmissions include first born, breastfeeding infants, maternal complications during labor and complications during labor and delivery, public assistance, and East Asian heritage as well as never being admitted to the NICU. Strategies to reduce rehospitalization include identifying late preterm infants at risk, provision of breastfeeding support, appropriate hyperbilirubinemia screening, avoidance of early discharge, and promotion of accessible and frequent follow-up care (Jain & Cheng, 2006).

LONG-TERM OUTCOMES OF THE LATE PRETERM INFANT

Research has shown that late preterm infants have an increased risk of medical problems and poor health-related outcomes. They also have long-term adverse developmental outcomes, including cognitive delay with poor school performance as well as social and behavioral challenges (McGowan, Alderdice, Holmes, & Johnston, 2011; Talge et al., 2010; Woythaler, McCormick, & Smith, 2011). Although the absolute risk of poor long-term outcome in the late preterm infant population is low, it is significantly higher than their term counterparts (Engle, 2011).

Bird et al. (2010) found late preterm infants in the first year of life had an increased risk for poor health-related outcomes during the birth hospitalization. They found a statistically significant increase in health care utilization during the first year of life, including an increase in total hospital time and increased hospital and outpatient costs as well as overall total health care costs.

Kalia, Visintainer, Brumberg, Pici, and Kase (2009) reported finding that late preterm infants requiring NICU admission had increased needs for interventional therapies. Of the late preterm infants studied, 30% required early intervention services, 28% physical therapy, 16% occupational therapy, 10% speech therapy, and 6% special education. Woythaler et al. (2011) found late preterm infants have a poorer developmental outcome than term infants at 24 months of age, including more mild and severe mental and psychomotor developmental delays.

Late preterm infants were found to have an increased incidence of cerebral palsy (CP), developmental delay, and mental retardation (MR). These infants were three times more likely to be diagnosed with CP than their term counterparts and at a marginally higher risk for developmental delay and MR. Late preterm infants were not at increased risk for seizures noted in this study (Petrini et al., 2009).

Late preterm infants are at increased risk for poor school performance compared to their term counterparts. Morse, Zheng, Tang, and Rogh (2009) showed late preterm infants have a 3% greater risk for developmental delay during prekindergarten and kindergarten, with higher kindergarten suspension and retention rates. Baron et al. (2009) reported on late preterm infants admitted to the NICU having deficits in visuospatial, visuomotor, and executive function as well as action-verb relative deficits.

Talge et al. (2010) found late preterm infants exhibited poorer cognitive performance with IQ scores at age 6. They also found increased behavioral problems at age 6, including higher levels of internalizing and attention problems. Lipkind, Slopen, Pfieffer, and McVeigh (2012) found late preterm infants had an increased need for special education services and lower math and English scores in grade 3 when compared with term infants. Research by Chyi, Lee, Hitz, Gould, and Sutcliffe (2008) showed late preterm infants had poorer school performance, especially in reading skills, with an increased need for special education services when assessed between kindergarten and grade 5.

SUMMARY

In summary, late preterm infant births, infants born at 34 0/7 to 36 6/7 weeks, are on the rise. Late preterm deliveries are due to spontaneous preterm labor and inductions for fetal and maternal indications. These infants are at increased risk for physiologic immaturity, and higher morbidity and mortality rates. They also have more medical complications, NICU admissions, and prolonged hospitalizations. It is important to understand these risks and provide closer monitoring and expert medical and nursing care as well as stricter discharge criteria, follow-up care, and strategies to prevent rehospitalization. Late preterm infants are at increased risk of long-term sequelae. More research is needed in this population to understand how to prevent late preterm births and optimize care for successful outcomes.

CASE STUDY

Identification of the Problem. Baby boy M was born at 35 weeks gestation and developed respiratory distress at 4 hours of life in the normal newborn nursery.

Assessment: History and Physical Examination. Baby boy M was born at 35 weeks weighing 2,090 g to a 31-year-old G 1 P 0 now 1, blood type A positive, antibody screen negative, rapid plasma reagin nonreactive, Rubella immune, hepatitis B Surface Antigen negative, HIV negative, Group B streptococcus negative mother. This pregnancy was complicated by gestational diabetes, diet-controlled, and preterm labor. Maternal antibiotics were given. Labor persisted, and the infant was born by normal vaginal delivery. A nurse practitioner was at the delivery due to prematurity, and the infant emerged crying and was brought to the warmer. Routine drying and stimulation was provided and Apgars were 8 and 9. The infant transitioned nicely and was transferred to the normal nursery. At 4 hours of age the infant was tachypnea, grunting, retracting, and flaring and requiring face mask oxygen to keep saturations above 90%. The infant was transferred to the NICU. On admission to the NICU, the baby was noted to have a hood oxygen requirement of 25%, a dextrostix of 30, and a temperature of 36°C.

Physical Exam

- GENERAL APPEARANCE: Alert and active, mild distress
- HEAD: fontanelle soft and flat; no eye drainage, positive red reflex; ears normally set and rotated; nares patent; moist mucous membranes, palate intact
- SKIN: warm, well perfused, no lesions
- NECK: clavicles intact, no crepitus
- RESPIRATORY: lungs are clear to auscultation, breath sounds equal, expiratory grunting, nasal flaring, mild intercostal retractions, chest wall within normal limits, cry normal
- CARDIOVASCULAR: regular heart rate and rhythm without murmur, femoral pulses 2 plus bilaterally, well perfused, capillary refill less than 2 seconds
- ABDOMEN: soft, nontender, not distended, normal bowel sounds, no hepatosplenomegaly, three vessel umbilical cord
- GENITOURINARY: normal male genitalia, testes descended bilaterally, anus patent
- MUSCULOSKELETAL: no sacral dimple, no hip clunk, normal upper and lower extremities
- NEUROLOGIC: alert, moving all extremities times 4, normal tone and strength, Moro complete, normal grasp and suck, no focal deficits

Differential Diagnoses. Respiratory diagnoses: respiratory distress syndrome (RDS), transient tachypnea of the newborn (TTN), pneumonia, pulmonary hypertension

- Rule out sepsis
- Hypoglycemia
- Hypothermia

Diagnostic Tests

- Chest radiography
- Arterial blood gas
- Blood glucose and dextrostix monitoring
- CBC with differential
- Blood culture

Working Diagnosis. Baby M had a chest x-ray with prominent perihilar interstitial markings and fluid in the minor fissure, which is most consistent with TTN. He had a blood gas ph 7.40, pCO2 42, pO2 80 and a base excess of 1, which further supports the diagnosis. Baby M had a normal CBC with differential, a white blood count of 15.6, hematocrit of 17, and platelets of 211. The differential showed 46 neutrophils, 2 bands, 40 lymphocytes, 7 monocytes, and 5 eosinophils. The working diagnosis ruled out sepsis since the actual infection risk is low. The maternal group B streptococcus (GBS) status was negative, and the baby's physical exam was within normal limits except for the respiratory symptoms that point to TTN.

The dextrostix on admission to the NICU was 30. Baby M is a late preterm infant at risk for hypoglycemia due to metabolic immaturity. Additionally, baby M's mother had gestational diabetes, which puts the infant at risk for transient hypoglycemia.

Baby M had a temperature of 36°C, which is common in late preterm infants. Metabolic immaturities lead to transient hypothermia.

Development of Management Plan. The respiratory plan was to wean the oxygen as tolerated, keeping oxygen saturations greater than 90%. Baby M had an IV started due to his dextrostix of 30 and given a bolus of dextrose 10 in water (2 mL/kg) and started on maintenance IV fluids (GIR 5.6 mg/kg/min, total fluids of 80 mL/kg/d). Dextrostixs were to be performed every 1 to 3 hours until greater than 45. Baby M was placed on a warmer for his temperature of 36°C.

Implementation and Evaluation of Effectiveness
Baby M weaned to room air, and the respiratory symptoms resolved by 12 hours of life. Baby M's repeat dextrostix was 45 after the glucose bolus and IV fluids, with the resolution of the hypoglycemia. He started feeding at 24 hours of life and had difficulty with poor coordination of feeds and weight loss, which took 7 days to resolve. Baby M had difficulty maintaining his temperature and finally weaned to a crib after 4 days.

Outcome. Baby M experienced many of the typical medical complications related to late preterm infants' physiologic and metabolic immaturity, which resulted in a NICU admission and prolonged hospital stay. Baby M went home after a 7-day admission to the NICU. He will have close primary care provider follow-up to promote healthy growth and prevent rehospitalization.

EVIDENCE-BASED PRACTICE BOX

Late preterm infants are infants born between 34 0/7 and 36 6/7 weeks and are increasing in number throughout the country and around the world. These infants' have higher rates of morbidity and mortality, as well as increased medical complications, NICU admissions, and prolonged hospitalization (Engle, 2011; Engle et al., 2007; Ramachandrappa & Jain, 2009). Late preterm infants require closer monitoring and specialized medical and nursing care for this higher risk population with stricter discharge criteria and follow-up care. These infants have a higher rehospitalization rate and long-term sequelae.

It is clear that late preterm infants are different from term infants and should be monitored more closely. Late preterm infants are at increased risk for transient tachypnea of the newborn (TTN), respiratory distress syndrome (RDS), persistent pulmonary hypertension of the newborn PHN, respiratory failure, apnea, hyperbilirubinemia, hypothermia, hypoglycemia, feeding difficulties, neonatal sepsis, and NICU admission with a prolonged hospital stay as well as having mothers with increased emotional distress. These medical problems need careful assessment and treatment (Martin et al., 2011). Late preterm infants are more likely to require admission to the NICU and prolonged hospitalization compared to term infants.

When planning discharge of the late preterm infant, criteria developed for both high-risk infants and healthy term infants should be considered. Discharge for term infants after a vaginal delivery is typically less than 48 hours. In 1995 with a revision in 2004, the AAP recommended a minimum eligibility of 38 to 42 weeks gestation as discharge criteria for early discharge, less than 48 hours (AAP, Committee on Fetus and Newborn, 1995, 2004). Goyal et al. (2011) found 40% of late preterm infants were discharged early, prior to 48 hours. The AAP continues to recommend discharge after 48 hours.

Engle et al. (2007) have recommended discharge criteria that reflect evidence of physiologic maturity, feeding competences, thermoregulation, maternal education, assessment, and planned intervention for medical, family, environmental and social risk factors, and follow-up arrangements. Important minimal discharge criteria should include: accurate gestational age determination, meeting of feeding-based competencies, thermoregulation and absence of medical illness, and social risk factors (usually after 48 hours); pediatric follow-up 24 to 48 hours after hospital discharge; vital signs within the normal range for 12 hours preceding discharge; passage of at least one stool spontaneously; 24 hours of successful feeding; a risk assessment for the development of severe hyperbilirubinemia and follow-up arranged as needed; physical exam with no abnormalities requiring hospitalization; no evidence of active bleeding at circumcision site for at least 2 hours, hepatitis B vaccine administration or an appointment for administration; metabolic screens according to state recommendations, passed car seat safety test; hearing assessment; and family environment and social risk factor assessment and parent training (AAP Committee on Fetus and Newborn, 2008; Engle, 2011; Martin et al., 2011).

Good discharge planning will allow a smooth transition for the infant from the hospital environment to home. It will also help reduce hospital readmissions.

ONLINE RESOURCES

The Association of Women's Health, Obstetric and Neonatal Nurses (AWHONN) Late Preterm Infant Initiative
http://www.awhonn.org/awhonn/content.do?name=02_PracticeResources/2C3_Focus_NearTermInfant.htm

Caring for the Late Preterm Infant-Oklahoma Infant Alliance, endorsed by Council of International Neonatal Nurses
http://www.coinnurses.org/1_documents/resources/p_statement/LPI_Clinical_Guideline.ks.pdf

Council of International Neonatal Nurses (COINN) Position Statement on Care of the Late Preterm Infant.
http://www.coinnurses.org/1_documents/resources/p_statement/Position_Stat_Late_Preterm.pdf

Health Concerns of the Late Preterm Infant
http://preemies.about.com/od/preemiehealthproblems/a/LatePretermBirth.htm

REFERENCES

Ahmed, A. H. (2010). Role of the pediatric nurse practitioner in promoting breastfeeding for late preterm infants in primary care settings. *Journal of Pediatric Health Care, 24*(2), 116–122.

American Academy of Pediatrics Committee on Fetus and Newborn. (1995). Hospital stay for healthy term newborns. *Pediatrics, 96*(4 pt 1), 788–790.

American Academy of Pediatrics Committee on Fetus and Newborn. (2004). Hospital stay for healthy term newborns. *Pediatrics, 113*(5), 1434–1436.

American Academy of Pediatrics Committee on Fetus and Newborn. (2008). Hospital discharge of the high-risk neonate. *Pediatrics, 122*(5), 1119–1126.

American Academy of Pediatrics Committee on Fetus and Newborn. (2011). Postnatal glucose homeostasis in late-preterm and term infants. *Pediatrics, 127*(3), 575–579.

Baron, I. S., Erickson, K., Ahronovich, M. D., Coulehan, K., Baker, R., & Litman, F. R. (2009). Visuospatial and verbal fluency relative deficits in 'complicated' late-preterm preschool children. *Early Human Development, 85*(12), 751–754.

Bird, T. M., Bronstein, J. M., Hall, R. W., Lowery, C. L., Nugent, R., & Mays, G. P. (2010). Late preterm Infants: Birth outcomes and health care utilization in the first year. *Pediatrics, 126*, e311–e319.

Brandon, D. H., Tully, K. P., Silva, S. G., Malcom, W. F., Murtha, A. P., Turner, B. S., & Holditch-Davis, D. (2011). Emotional responses of mothers of late preterm and term infants. *Journal of Obstetric, Gynecologic & Neonatal Nursing, 40*(6), 719–731.

Cheng, Y. W., Kaimal, A. J., Bruckner, T. A., Halloran, D. R., & Caughey, A. B. (2011). Perinatal morbidity associated with late preterm deliveries compared with deliveries between 37 and 40 weeks of gestation. *BJOG: An International Journal of Obstetrics and Gynaecology, 118*(12), 1446–1454.

Chyi, G. J., Lee, G. H., Hintz, S. R., Gould, J. B., & Sutcliffe, T. L. (2008). School outcomes of late preterm infants: Special needs and challenges for infants born at 32–36 weeks' gestation. *Journal of Pediatrics, 153*(1), 25–31.

Cleaveland, K. (2010). Feeding challenges in the late preterm infant. *Neonatal Network, 29*(1), 37–41.

Cohen-Wolkowiez, M., Moran, C., Benjamin, D. K., Cotton, C. M., Clark, R. H., Benjamin, D. K., & Smith, P. B. (2009). Early and late onset sepsis in late preterm infants. *The Pediatric Infectious Disease Journal, 28*(12), 1052–1056.

Crump, C., Sundquist, K., Sundquist, J., & Winkleby, M. A. (2011). Gestational age at birth and mortality in young adulthood. *Journal of American Medical Association, 306*(11), 1233–1240.

Engle, W. A. (2011). Morbidity and mortality in late preterm and early term newborns: A continuum. *Clinics in Perinatology, 38*(3), 493–516.

Engle, W. A., & Kominiarek, M. A. (2008). Late preterm infants, early term infants, and timing of elective deliveries. *Clinics of Perinatology, 35*(2), 325–341.

Engle, W. A., Tomashek, K. M., Wallman, C., & the Committee on Fetus and Newborn. (2007). "Late-preterm" infants: A population at risk. *Pediatrics, 120*(6), 1390–1401.

Escobar, G. J., Clark, R. H., & Greene, J. D. (2006). Short-term outcomes of infants born at 35 and 36 weeks gestation: We need to ask more questions. *Seminar in Perinatology, 30*(1), 28–33.

Goyal, N. K., Fager, C., & Lorch, S. A. (2011). Adherence to discharge guidelines for late-preterm newborns. *Pediatrics, 128*(1), 62–71.

Gunville, C. F., Sontag, M. K., Stratton, K. A., Ranade, D. J., Abman, S. H., & Mourani, P. M. (2010). Scope and impact of early and late preterm infants admitted to the PICU with respiratory illness. *Journal of Pediatrics, 157*(2), 209–214.

Gyamfi-Bannerman, C. (2012). Late preterm birth: Management dilemmas. *Obstetric and Gynecology Clinics, 39*(2), 35–45.

Jain, S., & Cheng, J. (2006). Emergency department visits and rehospitalizations in late preterm infants. *Clinics in Perinatology, 33*(4), 935–945.

Kalia, J. L., Visintainer, P., Brumberg, H. L., Pici, M., & Kase, J. (2009). Comparison of enrollment in interventional therapies between late-preterm and very preterm infants at 12 months' corrected age. *Pediatrics, 123*(3), 804–809.

Laptook, A., & Jackson, G. L. (2006). Cold stress and hypoglycemia in the late preterm ("near term") infant: Impact on nursery of admission. *Seminars in Perinatology, 30*(1), 24–27.

Lipkind, H. S., Slopen, M. E., Pfeiffer, M. E., & McVeigh, K. H. (2012). School-age outcomes of late preterm infants in New York City. *American Journal of Obstetrics and Gynecology, 206*(3), e1–e6.

Mance, M. J. (2008). Keeping infants warm: Challenges of hypothermia. *Advances in Neonatal Care, 8*(1), 6–12.

Martin, J. A., Hamilton, B. E., Sutton, P. D., Ventura, S. J., Mathews, T. J., & Osterman, M. J. (2010). Births: Final data for 2008. *National Vital Statistics Report, 59*(1), 3–72.

Martin, J. A., Osterman, M. F., & Sutton, P. D. (2010). Are preterm births on the decline in the United States? Recent data from the National vital statistics system. *NCHS Data Brief, 39*, 1–8.

Martin, R. J., Fanaroff, A. A., & Walsh, M. C. (2011). *Neonatal-perinatal medicine diseases of the fetus and infant* (9th ed.). St. Louis, MO: Elsevier Mosby.

Mathews, T. J., & MacDorman, M. F. (2011). Infant mortality statistics from the 2007 period: Linked birth/infant death data set. *National Vital Statistics System, 59*(6), 1–30.

McGowan, J. E., Alderdice, F. A., Holmes, V. A., & Johnston, L. (2011). Early childhood development of late-preterm infants: A systematic review. *Pediatrics, 127*, 1111–1125.

Mohan, S. S., & Jain, L. (2011). Late preterm birth: Preventable prematurity? *Clinics in Perinatology, 38*(3), 1–7.

Morse, S. B., Zheng, H., Tang, Y., & Roth, J. (2009). Early school-age outcomes of late preterm infants. *Pediatrics, 123*(4), e622–e629.

Petrini, J. R., Dias, T., McCormick, M. C., Massolo, M. L., Green, N. S., & Escobar, G. J. (2009). Increased risk of adverse neurological development for late preterm infants. *Journal of Pediatrics, 154*(2), 159–160.

Radtke, J. V. (2011). The paradox of breastfeeding-associated morbidity among late preterm infants. *Journal of Obstetric, Gynecologic, & Neonatal Nursing, 40*(1), 9–24.

Raju, T. N., Higgins, R. D., Stark, A. R., & Leveno, K. J. (2006). Optimizing care and outcome for late-preterm (near-term) infants: A summary of the workshop sponsored by the National Institute of Child Health and Human Development. *Pediatrics, 118*(3), 1207–1214.

Ramachandrappa, A., & Jain, L. (2009). Health issues of the late preterm infant. *Pediatric Clinics of North America, 56*(3), 565–567.

Shapiro-Mendoza, C. K., & Lackritz, E. M. (2012). Epidemiology of late and moderate preterm birth. *Seminars in Fetal & Neonatal Medicine, 17*, 120–125.

Shapiro-Mendoza, C. K., Tomashek, K. M., Kotelchuck, M., Barfield, W., Nannini, A., Weiss, J., & Declercq, E. (2008). Effect of late-preterm birth and maternal medical conditions on newborn morbidity risk. *Pediatrics, 121*(2), e223–e232.

Talge, N. M., Holzman, C., Want, J., Lucia, V., Gardiner, J., & Brreslau, N. (2010). Later-Preterm birth and its association with cognitive and socioemotional outcomes at 6 years of age. *Pediatrics, 126*, 124–132.

Tomashek, K. M., Shapiro-Mendoza, C. K., Davidoff, M. J., & Petrini, J. N. (2007). Differences in mortality between late preterm and term singleton infants in the United States, 1995–2002. *Journal of Pediatrics, 151*(5), 450–456.

Woythaler, M. A., McCormick, M. C., & Smith, V. C. (2011). Late preterm infants have worse 24 month neurodevelopmental outcomes than term infants. *Pediatrics, 127*(3), e622–e629.

UNIT VI: ENVIRONMENTAL HEALTH AND FAMILY-CENTERED CARE IN THE NICU AND BEYOND

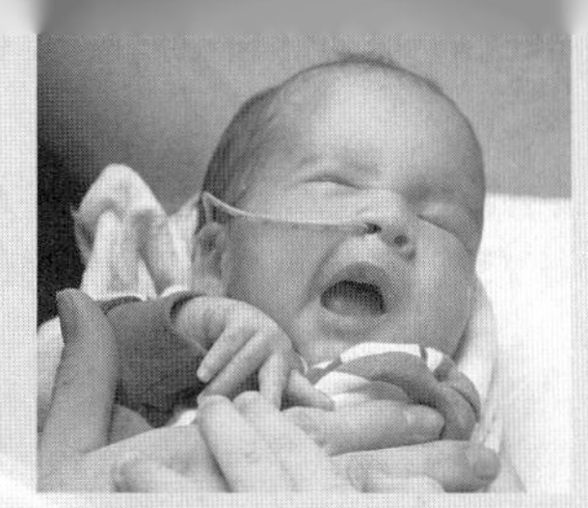

CHAPTER 30

Neurobehavioral Development

■ Diane Holditch-Davis and Susan Tucker Blackburn

The care of high-risk infants, both those born prematurely and those with medical, surgical, or developmental problems, has long been a major focus of nursing and health care. Advances in neonatal care have increasingly focused on the impact of the neonatal intensive care unit (NICU) environment on the infant's physiologic and neurobehavioral functioning, the provision of sensory input geared to meet the individual infant's needs and current level of developmental function, and mediating the effects of stress and overstimulation. Care in the NICU focuses on meeting the physiologic, neurobehavioral, and developmental needs of these infants, with attention to the social interactive consequences of the NICU environment. Improved understanding of these factors and of the pathophysiologic problems encountered by infants in the NICU, along with the development of new management strategies, technologies, and caregiving approaches, have markedly improved the outcome of high-risk infants.

Although tremendous progress has been made in reducing mortality and morbidity in high-risk infants, these infants, especially those born prematurely, are still vulnerable to a wide variety of neurodevelopmental problems. These problems include behavioral disorganization, attention deficit disorders, hyperexcitability, language problems, sensory/perceptual and higher-order cognitive problems, regulatory disorders, and school dysfunction (Adams-Chapman, 2009; de Jong, Verhoeven, & van Baar, 2012; Iacovidou, Varsami, & Syggellou, 2010; Larroque et al., 2008; Leppert & Allen, 2012; Stephens & Vohr, 2009). Adverse outcomes of high-risk infants may be related to a variety of factors, including immaturity, perinatal events, the early NICU environment, the home environment in which the child is raised, and parent–child interactions. The development of many of these infants is characterized by an unevenness that can lead to later difficulties.

Immature infants differ in two important ways from healthy full-term infants. First, these infants are born early and therefore must adapt to the extrauterine environment with bodily systems, including a central nervous system (CNS), that are not yet mature. Second, this interruption of intrauterine life significantly modifies the environment of the infant. Thus the preterm infant spends the last weeks or months of gestation in an environment—the NICU—that is very different from that of the uterus or the home of a healthy full-term infant. The NICU environment has similar implications for the more mature, although still vulnerable, ill full-term infant. For these infants, this environment is also abnormal and quite different from that experienced by healthy infants who go home with their parents soon after birth.

Neonatal nurses are very familiar with interpreting the physiologic status of infants and basing their interventions on physiologic changes. In recent years, nurses have placed increased emphasis on the importance of understanding the behaviors of infants under their care because behavior is the way infants communicate their needs and their responses to nursing interventions. However, two factors make this understanding difficult. First, newborn infants have limited behavioral repertoires. The same behavior may have different meanings in different situations, but busy neonatal nurses may not have the time necessary to correctly interpret infants' behaviors by comprehensively assessing both the infants' actions and the environmental stimulation. Second, the behaviors of critically ill infants are sometimes even more difficult to interpret because they lack the energy to display characteristic behavioral responses. Thus neonatal nurses can never rely totally on infants' behaviors to determine infants' needs, but in combination with physiologic parameters, understanding infant behavior enriches both nursing assessment and the evaluation of nursing interventions. In considering the vulnerabilities of ill and immature infants, it is useful to examine the implications of the state of CNS and sensory system development, neonatal neurobehavioral development, and sleeping and waking states—and their relevance for neonatal nursing.

FETAL AND NEONATAL CENTRAL NERVOUS SYSTEM DEVELOPMENT

As noted in Chapter 15, the development of the CNS can be divided into six overlapping stages (Table 15.1). These stages are important to consider in examining neurobehavioral development and the effects of the NICU environment because the stage of development influences the effect of any insult. In addition, several areas of the CNS, including predominately organizational processes, continue to undergo significant changes during the period when preterm infants are in the NICU, increasing their vulnerability to insult. Vulnerabilities include decreased inhibitory potential, slower nerve conduction and synaptic potential, inability to sustain high firing rates, incomplete cell differentiation, and decreased synaptogenesis and dendritic arborization. The stage of development is also reflected by the behaviors characteristic of immature infants such as altered state regulation, increased and decreased tone. alterations in primitive reflexes, increased irritability, immature inhibition, jerky movements, lower arousal, less able to sustain alert states, poorer coordination, altered autonomic regulation, and asymmetrical, uncoordinated posture and movement (Blackburn, 2012).

The first three stages of CNS development (dorsal induction, ventral induction, and neuronogenesis) are completed before the fourth month of gestation. The last three stages (neuron migration; organization, including synaptogenesis and arborization; and myelination) continue during the time many infants are in the NICU and have implications for the effects of the NICU environment and care. Areas of development during the last part of gestation that are particularly critical in considering neurobehavioral vulnerabilities of ill or immature infants include (1) autonomic homeostatic control, (2) alterations in the germinal matrix and migration of neurons and glial cells, (3) CNS organizational processes, (4) development of the neocortex, and (5) growth of the cortex and cerebellum (Blackburn, 2012; Volpe, 2008).

From about 28 to 32 weeks gestational age (GA), preterm infants begin to achieve some degree of physiologic homeostasis, with increasing control of the sympathetic system over their autonomic functioning. With increasing autonomic control, the infant develops greater autonomic stability. This autonomic stability can be seen, for example, in the decreasing incidence of apnea and bradycardia. As these infants move to greater cortical control over the next months, their development is characterized by periods of temporary organization followed by periods of disorganization as new levels of maturation and control are achieved. These periods of disorganization are reflected in the infant's sleep–wake patterns, proportion of transitional or indeterminate sleep, and fragmented behavioral responses, and reflexes.

The germinal matrix in the periventricular subependymal area is a site of origin for neuronal and glial cells. Neurons and glial cells migrate from the germinal matrix to their eventual loci within the CNS, where they further differentiate and take on unique and individual functions. Initially, the neurons migrate to areas deep within the cortex; later neurons migrate further toward the surface of the cortex. Thus neurons formed early come to lie in deeper layers of cortex and subcortex; those formed later are found in more superficial layers. The cortex generally has a complete component of neurons by 33 weeks gestation. Until 32 to 34 weeks GA, the fragile, poorly supported blood vessels in this area receive a significant proportion of cerebral blood flow (Volpe, 2008). Insults to this area before this period may lead to germinal matrix and intraventricular hemorrhage (Chapter 15).

Organization, or "the processes by which the nervous system takes on the capacity to operate as an integrated whole" (Blackburn, 2012), begins during the sixth month of gestation and extends many years after birth. Neuron growth and connections lead to development of brain sulci and gyri. A brain growth spurt occurs from 26 to 30 weeks, leading to more complex behaviors (Blackburn, 2012; Volpe, 2008). Organization of the CNS is critical for cortical and cognitive development. These processes may be particularly vulnerable to insults from the effects of the NICU environment (Bhutta & Anand, 2002; Sizun & Browne, 2006; Smith et al., 2011). Subplate neurons differentiate early and migrate to cortex from the germinal matrix to serve as guides for ascending and descending projections to target neurons. The subplate neurons provide critical connection sites for axons ascending from thalamus and other sites, until the neurons that these axons will eventually connect with have migrated from the germinal matrix. The subplate reaches its peak from 27 to 30 weeks (Blackburn, 2012; Volpe, 2008). Once cortical neurons have reached their eventual loci, they become arranged in layers and develop dendrites and axons that undergo extensive branching. The pattern of dendritic connections between neurons is a critical growth process that constitutes the "wiring" of the brain (also called arborization). These interconnections are critical for processing of impulses, cell-to-cell communication, and communication throughout the nervous system. Lack of connections can result in hypersensitivity, poorly modulated behaviors, and all-or-nothing responses, which can often be observed in preterm infants in the NICU. Similar behavior patterns can also be seen in some children in later infancy and childhood.

Organization also involves formation of connections or synapses between neurons and development of intracellular structures and enzymes for neurotransmitter production. Synaptogenesis is critical for integration across all areas of the nervous system. Synapses continue to restructure throughout development, and this process is thought to be the basis for memory and learning. Synaptogenesis is mediated by excitatory neurotransmitters such as glutamate. Glutamate acts on N-methyl-D-aspartate (NMDA) receptors to enhance neuronal proliferation, migration, and synaptic plasticity (Volpe, 2008). Another component of organization is reduction in the number of neurons and their connections through the death of many neurons and regression of dendrites and synapses. Neuronal death assists in elimination of errors within the nervous system, such as neurons that are improperly located, that fail to achieve adequate connections or that are underused (Koizumi, 2004; Volpe, 2008). For example, neuronal density in the visual cortex decreases from 620,000 neurons/mm^3 at 7 months gestation to 1,000,000 at term and 40,000 in the adult (Koizumi, 2004). Finally organization involves development of different types of glia cells, including astroglia, microglia, and oligodendrocytes (Volpe, 2008). Astroglia provide support for neurons, with axonal guidance, brain structural development and growth, blood–brain barrier function, and integration of information within the brain (Blackburn, 2012). Astroglia undergo rapid proliferation between 24 and 32 weeks gestation (Volpe, 2008). Oligodendrocytes are the cells that produce myelin within the CNS. These glia are particularly vulnerable to hypoxic and ischemic injury prior to 32 weeks gestation (premyelinating period) (Volpe, Kinney, Jensen, & Rosenberg, 2011). Damage to the premyelinating oligodendrocytes is a prominent feature in white matter injury in preterm infants (see Chapter 15).

Organizational processes and modification of neurons continue into adulthood but are particularly vulnerable during infancy. This ability of a neuron to change structure and function in response to external experiences and to store that information for memory and learning is referred to as neural (brain) plasticity (Blackburn, 2012; Limperopoulos, 2010). The neonate's brain is still under construction with enhanced plasticity. "Enhanced plasticity of the developing brain allows it to be influenced more strongly by the environment, than is the adult brain. However, this increased plasticity also creates selective brain vulnerability" (Limperopoulos, 2010, p. 94). The more immature the infant at birth, the greater the impact of neural plasticity. Sensory input influences later neuronal structure and function; for instance, an enriched environment during infancy improves developmental outcome by maximizing brain potential. This plasticity is both an advantage and a liability. Although sensory input may increase cellular processes and interconnections, the sensory environment may also produce undesired changes in structure and function (Blackburn, 2012). Thus the preterm infant in the NICU may be particularly vulnerable to these alterations.

Adverse neonatal experiences may alter brain development during this vulnerable time and thus later development. Neuronal differentiation and organization are controlled by the interaction of genes with the environment. Each neuron has many synaptic connections that allow the brain to integrate and organize information. There is initially an overproduction of neurons and nerve connections. Many of these neurons and connections are later eliminated. Whether a connection is retained or eliminated is influenced by the infant's early environment and experiences (Black, 1998). For example, the brain is more likely to strengthen and retain connections that are used repeatedly and to eliminate underused connections. Improper sensory input (too much or too little) or input that is inappropriate in terms of timing may alter brain development. Thus the environment of the immature infants in the NICU and in the early months following discharge is critical for brain development and later cognitive function with a risk of alterations in neuronal networks, wiring, function, and behavior with exposure to early inappropriate sensory input (Graven, 2011; Sizun & Browne 2006; Smith et al., 2011).

Preterm infants in the NICU experience a very different pattern and type of sensory input than they would encounter in utero, and different from what the brain is expecting at any given GA. This creates a mismatch between the sensory environment of the infant and the requirements of the CNS for growth and development (Lawhon & Als, 2010). Two types of neural plasticity have been proposed: experience-expectant and experience-dependent (Black, 1998). Experience-expectant plasticity is linked to the brain's developmental timetable. Thus specific sensory experiences and input are needed at specific times for neural development and maturation. Altered sequences or types of sensory input can modify or disrupt development. Experience-dependent plasticity involves interaction with the environment to develop specific skills for later use. This form of plasticity involves memory and learning and allows development of flexibility, adaptation, and individual differences in social and intellectual development (Black, 1998).

The cerebellum is also vulnerable to insults from the early environment. The cerebellum is important in cognition and interconnections between different areas of the brain, including the thalamus, parietal lobe, and prefrontal cortex. The cerebellum undergoes a critical growth spurt from 24 to 40 weeks gestation. This spurt includes an increase in dendritic arborization, which is complete earlier than many other areas of the brain (see Chapter 15). Insults may lead to altered cognitive function, language development, and behavioral development seen in some preterm infants (Limperopoulos et al., 2007; Volpe, 2008, 2009).

FETAL AND NEONATAL SENSORY DEVELOPMENT

The sensory systems develop in a specific sequence: somatosensory (tactile and proprioceptive), vestibular, chemoreceptive, auditory, and visual. During fetal life there is a lack of competing stimuli during rapid maturation of each system. For example, the infant develops chemoreception before the structures for hearing and vision are in place and after somatosensory and vestibular function has matured. Similarly, the hearing maturation in the fetus is most rapid during a time when vision is still immature and in an environment where vision is not being stimulated by light. Animal studies have demonstrated that out-of-sequence stimulation of one system interferes with development of not only that system but also other systems that are still immature (Blackburn, 2012; Lickliter, 2011). For example, in animal models inappropriate visual stimulation while hearing and vision are still developing may alter not only vision but also hearing development (Graven, 2011; Lickliter, 2011).

Somatosensory and vestibular sensations mature early. The fetus responds to touch around the mouth by 2 months of GA; hands become touch sensitive by 10 to 11 weeks. Nociceptors are found by 11 weeks, appearing first in the face, palms and soles, are seen in areas such as the trunk, arms and legs by 15 weeks, and are abundant by 20 to 22 weeks (Blackburn, 2012; Derbyshire, 2010). Vestibular stimulation is mediated by receptors in the ear that detect changes in directions and rate of head movement and rotation. Vestibular system maturation reaches structural maturation by 14 to 20 weeks gestation with responses to vestibular stimulation seen as early as 25 weeks gestation (Blackburn, 2012). Oral (taste) and nasal (smell) chemoreception develop during the second trimester. The taste buds appear by 7 to 8 weeks and receptors by 16 weeks. By term the infant has adult numbers of receptors. Nasal chemoreceptors develop from 7 to 20 weeks gestation and respond to the fragrant molecules in amniotic fluid. The composition of amniotic fluid varies with maternal diet and bathes both oral and nasal chemoreceptors. Exposure to substances from maternal diet may play a role in programming later dietary preferences (Beauchamp & Mennella, 2011; Lipchock, Reed, & Mennella, 2011). Fetal swallowing rates change with exposure to different taste in amniotic fluid (Beauchamp & Mennella, 2011; Lipchock et al., 2011). Preterm infants respond to different tastes and smells by at least 28 weeks gestation and possibly earlier (Cowart, Beauchamp, & Mennella, 2012; Lipchock et al., 2011). Nutrient odor may also influence nonnutritive. Term infants are able to detect, localize, and discriminate a variety of distinct odors and tastes. They respond preferentially to breast odors, their mothers' scents, and other odors associated with positive reinforcements (Cowart et al., 2012; Lipchock et al., 2011).

Auditory perception begins during fetal life and continues to develop until adolescence (Sanes & Bao, 2009). The structures of the auditory system, including the inner ear and cochlea, are mature enough to support hearing by approximately 20 weeks gestation. Fetal hearing is thought to begin at 24 to 25 weeks. In preterm infants, auditory evoked potentials can be recorded and responses to sound observed as early as 25 to 26 weeks (Blackburn, 2012; Werner, 2012). Auditory cortex development begins by the second trimester but is not mature until later in childhood (McMahon, Wintermark, & Lahav, 2012). Maturation of the cochlea and auditory nerve increase from 28 weeks on. Initially the hearing threshold is around 65 decibels (dB) with a range of 500 to 1,000 Hertz (Hz); increasing with increasing GA to a threshold of 20 to 25 dB and range of 500 to 2,000 Hz by term (Blackburn, 2012). Between 28 and 34 weeks, the preterm infant develops the ability to begin to orient to sound, turning the head in the direction of an auditory stimulus and showing evidence of arousal and attention (Glass, 2005; Gray & Philbin, 2004; McMahon et al., 2012). During the third trimester the cochlea continues to mature and develop its ability to hear sounds across frequencies. The hearing threshold decreases with GA. Infants have a preference for their own mothers' voices even before birth (Kisilevsky et al., 2009).

The eyes begin to develop early in the embryonic period (24–26 weeks) but continue anatomic and functional maturation into the third trimester and early infancy (Graven, 2011). Vision is the least mature sense at birth, and even full-term infants undergo significant continued maturation during infancy. The lens is initially cloudy; the second layer of the lens forms by 30 weeks followed by the third and fourth layers. Immature infants are very myoptic, and cone differentiation does not begin until after 30 to 32 weeks. By 22 weeks gestation, the layers of the retina have formed rod differentiation, and retinal vascularization begins by 25 weeks GA; myelination of the optic nerve begins at 24 weeks. By 26 weeks, visual cortex neurons are in place with rapid development of visual neuronal connections and processes between 28 and 34 weeks gestation (Blackburn, 2012; Glass, 2005). Prior to 28 weeks infants have little pupillary response. This response becomes more mature but is still sluggish between 30 and 34 weeks and is mature by 36 weeks (Glass, 2005; Graven, 2011). The visual cortex undergoes rapid dendritic and synaptic development between 24 and 34 weeks. By 34 to 36 weeks, the visual cortex is similar to that of the term infant, but still immature, with significant development in the first year after birth (Blackburn, 2012; Graven, 2011).

NEONATAL NEUROBEHAVIORAL DEVELOPMENT

To provide developmentally supportive, family-focused care for high-risk infants in the NICU, the nurse must understand behavioral and developmental issues as they affect the infant and the family. The term neurobehavioral "recognized bidirectionality—that biologic and behavioral systems dynamically influence each other and that the quality of behavior and physiologic processes is depending on neural feedback" (Lester & Tronick, 2004). In the past 25 years, our knowledge of early childhood development has been dramatically altered by an avalanche of new research in neurobiologic, behavioral, and social sciences that has led to major advances in understanding the conditions that influence the well-being and early development of infants and young children. A deeper understanding of the importance of early life experience and the highly interactive influences of genetics and the environment on the developing brain has deepened our understanding of the early years. Attention to the powerful influence of the role of early relationships and the capabilities of the development of emotions in young children has finally taken center stage. Add to this the changes in our social structures and changes in our families, culturally and economically, including the shifting of parenting roles, along with changes in the workplace and in child care services for the very youngest, and the continuing high levels of economic hardship in many families, and it becomes clear that a professional review and rethinking of policy and practice required dedicated attention and a thoughtful response (Shonkoff & Phillips, 2000).

One of the first requirements of early development is the process of acquiring the capacity to self-regulate.

This capacity refers to the mastery of tasks that were in the beginning carried out and accomplished by the mother's body while the infant was in the womb; after birth and the transition out of the womb, the task becomes the infant's job. This transition from external regulation to the ability to accomplish regulation on one's own is a lengthy process in infant development. The tasks involved initially include physiologic regulation such as maintaining normal body temperature, regulating day–night cycles, and learning to calm oneself and relax after basic needs are met. Later, self-regulation means controlling one's own emotions and managing to keep one's attention focused; this involves reacting and regulating one's range of developmental function (Shonkoff & Phillips, 2000). The process is deeply related to one's relationships with others. Parents become the "co-regulators" or extensions of the infant's internal regulatory systems working to regulate function in the young child just as he or she is working toward the same. This requires of caregivers the ability to read and understand the infant's needs and the sensitivity, knowledge, and energy to respond in helpful, satisfying ways. Parents must establish "regulatory connections" with young children and then shift the independent task of regulation gradually over to them, one domain and one day at a time, being forever watchful that the balance in the child is not seriously disrupted. The ways that infants and young children learn about self-management involves behavioral, emotional, and cognitive self-control, which must evolve for competent functioning.

During early child development (birth to 6 years) children become consistently independent and develop the ability to manage their own behavior. Two concerns related to these developmental processes are sleep behavior and crying behavior. Infants with serious medical conditions that require intensive care, including preterm or medically fragile infants, have more difficult transitions to regulatory competence. Immature sick newborns are much less able to organize and stabilize sleep, waking, and feeding. They tend to be unpredictable, to cry more, and to be fussier. They tend to make less eye contact, smile less, vocalize less, and show less positive affect, and they are generally more difficult and harder for parents to read. During the first 3 months after birth for a full-term newborn, the infant depends on the relationship with the primary caregiver. The infant takes on an extensive undertaking that requires that he or she learn to get to sleep without help, stop crying when consoled, respond to the caregiver, and establish day–night, wake–sleep rhythms. Once the rapid developmental changes of the first 3 months of life after full-term birth accomplish its developmental changes, the infant faces another level of regulation in controlling his or her emotions and behavior. Followed by the regulation of attention and the regulation of mental processes, a process known as executive function emerges and involves the ability to think, retrieve, and remember information, solve problems, and engage in complex activities, which involve oral language, reading and writing, math, and social behavior.

Early experiences clearly affect the development of the brain. Development begins during early fetal life and lays a foundation for all that is to follow. Als and colleagues (Als, 1986; Lawhon & Als, 2010) developed a model, the synactive theory of development, for understanding the organization of neurobehavioral capabilities in the development of the fetus and newborn infant. This model describes emerging behavioral organizational abilities of the neonate. This model is based on the assumption that infants actively communicate via their behavior, which becomes an important route for understanding thresholds of stress or stability. Behavior of the infant not only is the main route of communication but also provides the basis for the structure of developmental assessment and provision of developmentally appropriate care (Als, 1986).

This synactive theory of development provides a model through which one can specify the degree of differentiation of behavior and the ability of infants to organize and control their behavior. The focus is not on assessment of skills but on the unique way each individual infant deals with the world around her or him. The synactive theory of development specifies the range of neonatal behavior as the infant matures as well as the ability of the infant to regulate behavior. This model is based on the assumption that the infant's primary route of communicating both functional stability and the limits for stress is through behavior (Als, 1986; Lawhon & Als, 2010). For example, infants who extend their limbs after being turned to supine to have their diaper changed may be communicating that they cannot control their limbs and movement in that position. Containing the limbs of these infants helps them to develop control and reduces stress over the loss of control.

Infants are seen as being in continual interaction with their environment via five subsystems: autonomic/physiologic, motor, state/organizational, attentional/interactive, and self-regulatory. These subsystems mature simultaneously, and within each subsystem a developmental sequence can be observed. Thus at each stage of development, new tasks and organizations are learned against the backdrop of previous development. The subsystems are interdependent and interrelated. For example, physiologic stability provides the foundation for motor and state control; the infant cannot respond socially to caregivers until motor and state control is achieved. The loss of integrity in one subsystem can influence the organization of other subsystems in response to environmental demands. In the preterm, less organized infant, the systems interplay, continuously influencing each other. In the healthy full-term infant, these systems are synchronized and function smoothly. Thus full-term infants can regulate their autonomic, motor, state, and attentional systems with ease and without apparent stress. However, less mature infants tend to be able to tolerate only one or minimal activity at a time and may easily lose control if their individual thresholds are exceeded. Instability in the autonomic system can be seen in the pattern of respiration (pauses, tachypnea), color changes (red, pale, dusky, mottled), and various visceral signs (regurgitation, twitching, stooling). Organization of the motor system is assessed by observing the infant's tone and posture (flexed, extended, hyperflexed, flaccid); specific movement patterns of the extremities, head, trunk, and face; and level of activity.

The development of motor responses is closely linked to state organization (Als, 1999).

The state system is understood by noting the available range of states of consciousness (sleep to arousal, awake to alert, crying), how well each state is defined (in terms of behavioral and physiologic parameters), transitions between states, and the quality of organization of these states.

States may be poorly defined at first, especially in the immature infant. For example, jerky body twitches and fussing may accompany sleep and wake states. In addition, the immature infant may not be able to achieve clearly defined states as seen in the mature infant (see section on "Sleep–Wake States"). Initially, preterm infants tend to be unstable and fragile, with sudden changes in their autonomic, motor, and state systems. These infants often have minimal response to handling or other sensory input until a threshold is reached, then quickly develop a cascade of responses, ending in several color changes, flaccidity, bradycardia, and apnea. As the infant matures, the responses are more variable, and the infant is less likely to totally decompensate (Als, 1986, 1999). Changes within the autonomic, motor, and state systems at all stages of development not just are reactions to stress and overstimulation but can signal that the infant's tolerance threshold has been exceeded. By recognizing these signs early, the nurse can intervene to prevent mild to severe decompensation.

The attentional/interactive system involves the infant's ability to orient and focus on sensory stimuli, such as faces, sounds, or objects—that is, the external environment. This system also includes the range of abilities in states of consciousness: how well periods of alertness are defined and how transitions into and out of alertness are handled. At first, this alertness may be very brief, with a dull look or glassy-eyed stare. As this system matures, the infant is able to interact with greater ease and for longer periods. Social responsiveness requires that the infant have enough state control to sustain some awake and alert states (Als, 1986; 1999). The self-regulatory system includes behaviors the infant uses to maintain the integrity and balance of the other subsystems, to integrate the other systems, and to move smoothly between states. For example, some infants can tuck their limbs close to their body in an effort to gain control when stressed, whereas others seem to relax if they can brace a foot against the side of the crib.

In summary, the process of development appears to be that of stabilization and integration of some subsystems, which allows the differentiation and emergence of others that in turn provide feedback for the integrated system. In this process the whole system is reopened and transformed to a new level of more differentiated integration, from which the next newly emerging subsystem can further differentiate and press to actualization and realization (Als, 1986; 1999). By observing and assessing the newborn infant's responses to the caregiver and other aspects of the environment across these five subsystems of behavioral functioning, one can develop and implement a plan of care to support the infant's emerging neurodevelopmental organization and reduce stress. The NICU staff, especially nurses, play a significant role in shaping the environment and making caregiving more responsive to infants. This requires as careful observation and documentation of infant behavior as is given to physiologic status and development of an individualized plan of care. Infant responses to the environment will be influenced by factors such as state; basic needs (e.g., hunger); sensory threshold; parameters of the animate and inanimate environment, including readability, predictability, and responsivity; infant health status; and level of neurobehavioral maturity (Blackburn, 2012).

Infant behavioral responses include specific autonomic, motoric, and state cues, which indicate disorganization and stress and the need for immediate intervention, and stability and self-regulatory cues, which indicate that the infant is coping positively. Thus cues provide information about an infant's needs and status, handling of sensory input, stress and sensory overload, tolerance for stimuli, and need for rest and time-out. Table 30.1 provides examples of infant cues. A free online resource illustrating infant cues and infant sleep states was developed by the March of Dimes for parents of preterm infants. This resource, titled "Understanding Your Premature Infant" is available at http://www.marchofdimes.com/modpreemie/preemie.html. Although developed for parents, it is also useful for nurses and other health care providers.

Assessment of Neonatal Neurobehavioral Development

Developmental assessment of newborn functioning emerged with the awareness of the amazing capabilities of neonates. The newborn infant, who for years was thought to be nonreactive and incapable of social participation, is now seen as an active participant in social interaction and capable of self-regulation. Even with a greater understanding of newborn capabilities, researchers and clinicians have been unable to consistently predict the future course of an infant's development from early neurologic or behavioral assessments. Thus there is no one comprehensive assessment tool for all infants (El-Dib, Massaro, Glass, & Aly, 2011). Historically, two types of neonatal assessments have evolved—the neurologic examination and the behavioral examination. The neurologic examination assesses the function of the CNS and typically includes assessment of motor tone and reflex behaviors within the context of infant state. The behavioral examination complements and elaborates on the neurologic assessment. An assumption underlying the behavioral examination is that the observable behavior of an infant is a reflection of his or her underlying neurologic status. The behavioral examination seeks to describe the quality of behavioral performance. More recently, these two forms of assessment have been combined into the neurodevelopmental or neurobehavioral assessment.

The neurodevelopmental examination is important because it yields a large pool of early observable behavior, including information about the infant's neurologic status and abilities to cope and interact with the environment. In addition, data from this examination can assist the clinician in estimating maturity and in identifying and evaluating problems that could be precursors to later developmental problems. Because the neurodevelopmental examination

TABLE 30.1

EXAMPLES OF INFANT NEUROBEHAVIORAL CUES

Stability Cues/Engagement Cues	Stress Cues/Disengagement Cues
Alertness, attention, orienting to people and objects	Altered vital signs (heart rate, respiratory rate)
Arm and leg flexion	Arching
Eyes open, alert	Color changes or visceral signs such as spitting
Grasping	Diffuse states, rapid state changes
Hand to mouth activity	Finger splay
Modulated states and state transitions	Flaccid or hypertonic tone
Modulated tone and movement	Frantic activity
Self-consoling activities	Grimacing
Stable vital signs, color	Hand to face or ear
Stable visceral and motor signs	Staring, averting gaze
	Tremors or jitteriness

provides an immediate basis for determining the status of the infant's development, the results can be used for planning intervention strategies as well as for screening for infants in need of further diagnostic assessments.

Who Needs to Be Assessed?

All neonates and their caregivers can benefit from ongoing neurobehavioral assessment. These assessments provide information on the infant's behavioral capabilities, interactive qualities, and adaptations to the extrauterine environment. This information can be used in planning care, developing individualized intervention strategies, modifying care as the infant matures, and parent teaching and other activities to promote parent–infant interaction. However, for some infants, neurodevelopmental assessment is critical for documentation of neurodevelopmental status, screening, and early case finding.

Certain groups of infants are at increased risk for developmental disabilities and later cognitive impairment (Adams-Chapman, 2009; de Jong et al., 2012; Iacovidou et al., 2010; Larroque et al., 2008; Leppert & Allen, 2012; Stephens & Vohr, 2009). Infants that fall into the highest risk category include very-low-birth-weight (VLBW) infants and those with significant intracranial hemorrhages. Preterm infants with known sensory impairment and chronic illness are also at risk for later cognitive dysfunction. Infants with respiratory distress syndrome (RDS) are at greater risk if they also develop chronic lung disease. Severe bronchopulmonary dysplasia (BPD) is generally associated with a prolonged and complicated hospital course, increasing the risk for later neurodevelopmental problems. Preterm infants as a group are at greater risk than term infant of comparable postmenstrual ages. Preterm infants often exhibit manifestations of altered brain organization, including disrupted sleep, difficult temperament, both hyperresponsivity and hyporesponsivity to sensory input, prolonged attention to redundant information, inattention to novel stimuli, and poor quality of motor function. These precursors of learning problems in school are not fully explained by either the severity of illness among preterm infants or later conditions in the home environments (Glass, 2005).

Neurobehavioral Assessment in the NICU and Early Infancy

Neurobehavioral assessment can be performed at several different levels and is an essential part of comprehensive care of the high-risk infant in the NICU. Individuals such as Brazelton, Als, and their colleagues have sought to assess preterm and full-term newborn behavior and adaptations. Their work is based on an understanding of newborns as competent individuals with emerging developmental processes who are engaged in dynamic interactions and negotiations with their environment. As a result, several tools have been developed to describe and quantify neurobehavioral organization of both preterm and full-term newborns.

Tools for neurobehavioral and neuromotor assessment include: Amiel-Tison neurological assessment at term (ATNAT), assessment of preterm infants' behavior (APIB), Brazelton neonatal behavioral assessment scale (NBAS), neonatal intensive care unit network neurobehavioral scale (NNNS), Prechtl's assessment of general movements (GMs), neurobehavioral assessment of the preterm infant (NAPI), Dubowitz neurological assessment of the preterm and full-term infant (Dubowitz), neuromotor behavioral assessment (NMBA), and the test of infant motor performance (TIMP) (Als, Butler, Kosta, & McAnulty, 2005; Als, Lester, Tronick, & Brazelton, 1982; Amiel-Tison, 2002; Brazelton & Nugent, 2011; Campbell, 2005; Carmichael, Burn, Gray, & O'Callaghan, 1997; Dubowitz, Ricciw, & Mercuri, 2005; Einspieler & Prechtl, 2005; El-Dib et al., 2011; Korner & Constantinou, 2001; Lester & Tronick, 2004; Lester, Tronick, & Brazelton, 2004; Noble & Boyd, 2012; Snider et al., 2005). Several assessments for neurobehavioral assessment are described further. A recent analysis found that all of these measures "demonstrated adequate content and construct validity" (Noble & Boyd, 2012). The authors concluded that "in the absence of a criterion standard for neonatal neuromotor assessments, the NNNS and APIB have strong psychometric qualities with better utility for research. Similarly, the GMs, TIMP, and NAPI have strong psychometric qualities but better utility for clinical settings. The GM has best prediction of future outcome and the TIMP has best evaluative validity" (Noble & Boyd, 2012, p. 137).

The tools that are described here are the NBAS (Brazelton & Nugent, 2011); the APIB (Als et al., 1982; 2005), which is a component of the neonatal individualized development care and assessment program (NIDCAP, Boston: Children's Hospital) (Lawhon & Hedlund, 2008); the NICU Network Neurobehavioral Scale (NNNS) (Lester & Tronick, 2004; Lester et al., 2004; Salisbury, Fallone, & Lester, 2005); and the NAPI (Korner & Constantinou, 2001; Snider et al., 2005).

■ Brazelton Neonatal Behavioral Assessment Scale The NBAS is a comprehensive behavioral assessment of the healthy full-term neonate containing 6 clusters with 28 behavioral items and 18 reflex/motor items. The NBAS combines evaluation of basic reflex responses with the integration of motor capacity, state regulation, and interactive abilities (Brazelton & Nugent, 2011). Infants are followed through the various states of sleep, arousal, and wakefulness and assessed on their ability to self-regulate in the face of increasingly vigorous activity. A primary focus is observation of the infant's individual and unique ability to respond to outside stimulation while regulating responses to and coping with pleasurable or stressful situations. The infant's best performance is scored. The results are an assessment of the infant's ability to (1) organize states, (2) habituate to external stimulation, (3) regulate motoric activity in the face of increasing sensory input, (4) respond to reflex testing, (5) alert and orient to visual and auditory stimuli, (6) interact with a caregiver, and (7) self-console. Individuals planning to use the NBAS for clinical or research purposes must establish reliability with a recognized trainer. Training in the use of the NBAS is provided in various locations (http://www.brazelton-institute.com/intro.html).

The NBAS has been used in numerous studies of neonatal behavior, including investigations of cross-cultural differences, characteristics of drug-addicted infants, effects of obstetric medication, and aspects of maternal–infant interaction (Brazelton & Nugent, 2011). An especially valuable use of the NBAS for nurses and other clinicians is as an intervention. For example, when an NBAS is performed in front of the infant's parents, the parents become increasingly aware of and amazed at the remarkable abilities of their infant. An understanding of their newborn's capacity to interact visually, turn to their voices, regulate state and motor activity, and self-console expands the parents' perception of the infant as a unique, competent individual and enhances parent–infant interaction (Brazelton & Nugent, 2011). The newborn behavioral observations system (NBO) is another tool from this group that provides a series of 18 neurobehavioral observations for clinicians and parents to observe the infant together and determine the infant's capabilities and needs. Information on training is at http://www.brazelton-institute.com/clnbas.html.

In response to a need to identify the preterm infant's neurobehavioral repertoire, the NBAS was expanded and modified for use with low-birth-weight infants. Items were added to the original scale, including difficulty of elicitation of alerting, degree of facilitation necessary to support the infant, control over stimulation, robustness, endurance, degree of exhaustion, quality of alertness, and balance of tone (Brazelton & Nugent, 2011). These subscales are also useful in describing at-risk full-term infants, such as drug-exposed infants.

■ Assessment of Preterm Infant Behavior. The APIB was developed to respond to the need for a more discrete and comprehensive assessment of preterm infant functioning. The APIB is based on the synactive theory of development, which describes the early behavioral organization and development of the neonate. The APIB is particularly useful for the preterm and full-term high-risk infant from birth to 44 weeks postmenstrual age. The purpose of this assessment is to determine organization of the CNS and how infants cope with the intense environment of the NICU. The focus of the APIB is not only assessment of skill performance or specific responses to various stimuli but also the unique way each individual infant deals and interacts with the world around him or her. As described previously, infants are seen as being in continual interaction with their environment and as communicating their responsiveness via five subsystems (autonomic, motor, state, attentional, and self-regulatory) (Als, 1986; Als et al., 2005).

The APIB consists of six packages or sets of maneuvers adapted from the NBAS. The packages are organized to provide increasing input with which the infant must react, starting with stimulation while the infant is asleep to assess habituation. Subsequent packages move through maneuvers ranging from low and medium tactile manipulations to high tactile and vestibular handling. Throughout the assessment, the infant is continually observed for responses related to each of the five subsystems. Thus the infant is observed and scored on each of the five subsystems and for examiner facilitation (ability to use support) before, during, and after administration of the items in each package. These responses are called the system scores and range on a nine-point scale from organized (1) to disorganized (9).

The APIB has been used for research and clinical purposes. As a research tool, it has been used to describe and identify neonatal behavioral organization in preterm and other high-risk infants (Als, 1986; Als et al., 1982, 2005). Clinically, psychologists, neonatologists, neurologists, nurses, developmental specialists, and therapists have used the APIB in providing consultation in the NICU regarding developmental interventions for specific infants. The APIB is useful in determining an infant's degree of fragility and ability to tolerate different caregiving parameters. By measuring maturity of the five subsystems, one can determine maturity of each system and tolerance for handling as well as generate developmental care plans specific to each infant at that stage of development. The APIB is also useful in assessing infant readiness for changes in caregiving routines and in the physical and social environment. Assessing the degree of fragility and tolerance for activities can provide an invaluable piece of information about the infant's functional level and assist staff in making decisions about whether to protect the infant or to advance to the next level of care, as is illustrated in the following case.

A 28 weeks preterm infant had just been extubated and graduated to oxygen by nasal cannula and moved from the open bed to the incubator. An APIB revealed a responsive infant but one who was working extremely hard to regulate his system amid two major changes: extubation and change of physical environment. Although successful regulation was noted, it was also apparent that the infant was at maximal capacity in organizing himself. He showed efforts to tuck and maintain hand to mouth; however, he could not maintain these postures for long without help. It was apparent that the infant's threshold had been reached and that any more change or stress would have caused a loss of control in his system's integrity. Immediately after the assessment, the neonatologists ordered nipple feedings once a day. With this new demand, the examiner felt that this infant would exceed his threshold and be unable to regulate himself. The developmental specialist recommended waiting 1 week for the infant to stabilize and to integrate his new experiences before taking on any new demands. This recommendation was not followed, and feeding continued. Two days later, the developmental specialist returned and noted that the infant had a trial of nippling. He had desaturated, become bradycardic, required bag-and-mouth ventilation, and was considered to have "flunked" nippling. The order was terminated, with the plan to try again in a week. When feeding was reordered a week later, the infant tolerated it well.

Training in the APIB (http://www.nidcap.com) is extensive and requires knowledge of the NICU, including care practices and routines, staffing patterns, and typical infant experiences in that setting as well as physiologic limitations and medical problems. Interrater reliability, and concurrent and construct validity have been reported (Als et al., 2005).

■ Neonatal Individualized Development Care and Assessment Program. The NIDCAP incorporates several levels of developmental training in assessment techniques and intervention planning for high-risk preterm and full-term infants. Included in this program is an observation tool (level 1 NIDCAP naturalistic behavioral observation), which is extremely useful for the NICU nurse. This assessment involves an observation of the infant before, during, and after a routine caregiving episode. It provides the NICU nurse with information on the infant's individual cues for both stress and stable, organized function. The nurse can then structure the infant's experiences, including caregiving interventions and the physical and social environment, to support the infant at the current level of tolerance. This support includes an awareness of the timing of caregiving events, sequencing events and interventions to prevent or reduce stress as well as to enhance stable behavior. Support for parents in understanding their infant's unique behavior and needs is also provided (Lawhon & Hedlund, 2008, Lawhon & Als, 2010).

NIDCAP training (http://www.nidcap.com) involves didactic sessions and clinical demonstration of the observational tool, after which the trainee completes a specified number of observations on infants of different GA, postbirth age, and health status. This observation period is followed by an assessment of reliability for certification by the trainer. Individualized developmentally supportive care (see Chapters 31–34) as a total care concept, with care provided by NIDCAP certified or trained staff, has been demonstrated to result in a number of positive outcomes in various studies (Lawhon & Als, 2010; Lawhon & Hedlund, 2008).

■ NICU Network Neurobehavioral Scale (NNNS). The NNNS was developed for use with preterm and other at-risk infants such as those with perinatal drug exposure to measure the process of neurobehavioral organization, capturing both the normal range of behaviors and those present in high-risk infants (Lester & Tronick, 2004; Lester et al., 2004; Salisbury et al., 2005). The NNNS builds on several earlier assessments, including the neurological examination of the full-term newborn infant (Prechtl & Beintema, 1968), abstinence syndrome scoring, and several of the assessments described in this section (NBAS, APIB, and NAPI) (Lester & Tronick, 2004). The NNNS can be used with infants from about 30 weeks gestation to 46 to 48 weeks postmenstrual age and assesses both behavioral function and neurological integrity: (1) neurologic status (active and passive muscle tone, primitive reflexes, and CNS integrity); (2) behavioral state, sensory, and interactive responses; and (3) stress/abstinence scale. Items are administered only if the infant is in an appropriate state for that item. Administration of the assessment takes about 30 minutes (Lester & Tronick, 2004; Salisbury et al., 2005; Tronick & Lester, 2004). The scale can be used in clinical practice as well as research.

■ NAPI. The NAPI is an assessment developed at Stanford University to assess the differential maturity of infants between 32 weeks postconceptional age and term (Korner & Constantinou, 2001; Snider et al., 2005). Components include assessment of behavioral states, active tone, strength, reflexes, excitation and inhibition proneness, and orientation to visual and auditory stimuli. The NAPI has been used to monitor the developmental progress, to identify persistent lags in development, as an outcome measure in intervention studies and other studies, to describe individual differences in preterm infant development, and to identify infants with neurobehavioral alternations (Korner & Constantinou, 2001; Snider et al., 2005; Stephens & Vohr 2009). The reliability and validity of this test and normative data have been established. Training is available to learn to achieve reliability in administration and scoring of the examination (http://childdevelopmentmedia.com/infant-development-evaluation/70140psb.html).

Assessment Beyond Neonatal Development

As the infant matures, moves out of the neonatal period, and becomes a "long termer" in the NICU with chronic respiratory or other problems, neurodevelopmental assessments continue to provide important information (Spittle, Doyle, & Boyd, 2008). For the infant who requires prolonged hospitalization, a developmental assessment at the bedside can provide information on how the infant interacts with objects and people, organizes behavior, and copes with the environment as well as on the infant's neurologic status. No formal developmental assessments have been standardized for these NICU populations. Most developmental psychologists or specialists adapt items from other examinations such as the Bayley Scales of Infant Development II (Bayley, 1993) or the more recent Bayley Scales of Infant and Toddler Development (Bayley, 2005).

Because of the nature and severity of their illnesses, these infants may not be able to tolerate a complete examination at one session. To learn about the infant's behavioral capabilities and coping abilities adequately, the examiner must consider events that occurred for several hours before the assessment and be aware of the environment in which the infant normally lives and of his or her usual types of sensory experiences. Important areas of assessment include (1) availability of alerting, (2) ability to use interventions for consoling or developmental activities, (3) self-soothing capacity, (4) motor activities and strengths, (5) tolerance for handling (how long? with whom?), (6) degree of fragility, (7) degree of distractibility, (8) hand use, (9) parts of body available for use, and (10) respiratory capacity.

Sleep–Wake States

Another aspect of neurobehavioral development that is considered a part of any developmental program is sleep–wake states and how they affect responses to stimuli. Sleeping and waking states are clusters of behaviors that tend to occur together and represent the level of arousal of the individual, the individual's responsivity to external stimulation, and the underlying activation of the CNS. Three states have been identified in adults: wakefulness, non-REM (rapid eye movement) sleep, and REM sleep. In infants, it is also possible to identify states within waking and states that are transitional between waking and sleeping because infants are less able to make rapid changes between states than are adults. Infants also have more difficulty sustaining alertness when awake. Because the electrophysiologic patterns associated with sleeping and waking states in infants are somewhat different from those in adults (Heraghty, Hilliard, Henderson, Fleming, 2008), the sleep states are usually designated active and quiet sleep, rather than REM and non-REM sleep.

Neonatal nurses need to be aware of the infant's present sleep–wake state and typical sleep–wake patterns when making assessments because infant behavior and physiology are affected by state. The functioning of cardiovascular, respiratory, neurologic, endocrine, and gastrointestinal systems differ in different states. Moreover, sleeping and waking states affect the infant's ability to respond to stimulation. Thus infant responses to nursing interventions and to parental interactions depend to a great deal on the infant's state when the stimulation begins (Johnston, Stevens, Franck, Jack, Stremler, & Platt, 1999; Oehler, Eckerman, & Wilson, 1988). Timing routine interventions to occur when the infant is most responsive is an important aspect of some current systems of individualized nursing care (Als et al., 1986; Becker, Grunwald, Moorman, & Stuhr, 1991). Finally, studies have indicated that sleeping and waking patterns are closely related to neurologic status (Heraghty et al., 2008). Thus aberrant sleep–wake patterns could potentially be used to identify infants at risk for neurologic complications or poor developmental outcome.

■ **State Scoring Systems.** In adults, sleeping and waking are usually scored by electroencephalography (EEG). However, because of the neurologic immaturity of infants, EEG is less reliable and needs to be combined with observation. When EEG and behavioral scoring of states in preterm infants are compared, there is a high degree of agreement (Sahni, Schulze, Stefanski, Myers, & Fifer, 1995). Thus by directly observing infants, whether full term or preterm, and identifying global categories that are made up of a number of specific behaviors that tend to occur together and reflect a similar level of arousal and responsiveness to the environment, nurses can validly score sleeping and waking states in newborn infants. The behaviors that seem to be most important for scoring are respiration, eye movements, and motor activity (Brandon & Holditch-Davis, 2005; Tilmanne, Urbain, Kothare, Wouwer, & Kothare, 2009).

Nurse researchers currently use four standardized systems for scoring behavioral observations of sleep–wake states. The systems were developed by Brazelton (1984), Thoman (1990), Als et al. (1982), and Anderson (1999). These systems define states in very similar ways and are probably equally useful for clinical purposes. Table 30.2 presents a comparison of the state definitions used in these systems.

Clinicians and researchers differ in the ways they use these scoring systems. Neonatal nurses spend a lot of time observing infants and altering their care in response to infant behavioral changes. Experienced clinicians are undoubtedly already familiar with the characteristics of sleeping and waking states in these infants, even though they may be unable to name specific states. Thus all they need to do to include judgments of sleeping and waking states is to use the state definitions of any standardized scoring system to systematize their clinical impressions.

For research, however, it is essential that the investigator receive training in the use of a particular scale so that it is used reliably. Clinicians reading research need to understand the differences among the scoring systems so that they can better interpret the findings and understand reports using different names for the same sleep–wake state.

■ **Early State Scoring Systems.** Sleeping and waking scoring systems for infants originated in the work of neurologists, pediatricians, and behaviorists in the 1960s. The neurologists needed a way to systematize the observations they made along with EEG studies, and behaviorists and pediatricians were particularly interested in the waking states and the effect of state on responsiveness to stimulation. Wolff (1959, 1966), a pediatrician, conducted extensive observations of newborn infants in the hospital and at home. As the result of his observations, he proposed a seven-state system. Prechtl and Beintema (1968), pediatric neurologists, proposed a simple five-state system that could be used either to score observations made along with EEG or to ensure that motor reflexes were elicited under optimal conditions. Finally, a team of pediatricians and neurologists at the University of California at Los Angeles (UCLA) developed a manual to define the behavioral and EEG criteria for sleeping and waking (Anders, Emde, & Parmelee, 1971). Each of the state scoring systems currently in use is a refinement of these earlier systems.

■ Brazelton's State Scoring System. T. Berry Brazelton is a pediatrician from Harvard University in Cambridge, Massachusetts. He and his colleagues developed a state scoring system to be used as part of a behavioral evaluation of newborn infants, the NBAS (Brazelton, 1984; Brazelton & Nugent, 2011). The purpose of this tool was to assess the individuality of the infant within the interactional process. This state scale was derived both from Dr. Brazelton's clinical experiences and from the existing state systems of Prechtl and Beintema (1968) and Thoman (1975). Brazelton's state scoring system consists of six states: deep sleep, light sleep, drowsy, alert, considerable motor activity, and crying. During the administration of the NBAS, this scoring system is used to identify predominant states, state transitions, and the quality of the alertness. However, it can also be used for scoring sleep–wake states during other situations. By 1983, more than 100 papers had been published using the NBAS and Brazelton's state scale (Brazelton, 1984), and many more have been published since then.

Brazelton's state scoring system has a number of advantages that make it the scoring system of choice for clinicians and also useful for researchers. This state system is easy to learn because the differences between the states are fairly obvious and there are only six states. Because of the widespread use of Brazelton's state scoring system, individuals experienced with this scale are located in virtually every part of the United States. In addition, there are reliability-training centers located throughout the country for those who want to use the entire NBAS or plan to use the state scoring system in research. Thus obtaining training in this scoring system is relatively easy. Finally, most researchers and experienced clinicians are familiar with the state definitions from this scale so that findings of sleeping and waking observations made with this scoring system are readily understood.

On the other hand, this state scoring system does have some limitations for use in research. First, because of the small number of states, it is not always sensitive enough to identify differences between normal full-term infants and infants with perinatal complications. Moreover, the NBAS state scoring system is appropriate for use only with infants between 36 and 44 weeks GA. The sleeping and waking states of infants born before 36 weeks gestation and those born after 44 weeks gestation will not be completely captured with this system. For example, older infants frequently are motorically active and alert during play, but in Brazelton's system, alertness is scored only when the infant is motorically quiet. Young preterm infants are frequently unable to make much sound when crying; thus their cry periods would be scored as considerable motor activity.

■ Thoman's State Scoring System. Evelyn B. Thoman is a psychobiologist who worked at the University of Connecticut. Although trained as an experimental psychologist to work with animals, she became interested in the interactions between human infants and their mothers when she went to work with Dr. Anneliese Korner at Stanford University in 1969 and has been studying them ever since. She developed her first state scoring system in 1975 (Thoman, 1975) based on the work of Wolff (1966) and Korner (1972). Although some researchers continue to use this system today, it has undergone considerable revision (Thoman, 1990). The Thoman state scoring system consists of 10 sleeping and waking states: alert, nonalert waking activity, fuss, cry, daze, drowse, sleep–wake transition, active sleep, active–quiet transitional sleep, and quiet sleep. Dr. Thoman and others have shown that both acceptable interrater reliability and test–retest reliability can be obtained with her system (Holditch-Davis & Edwards, 1998a; Holditch-Davis, Scher, Schwartz, & Hudson-Barr, 2004; Holditch-Davis & Thoman, 1987; Thoman, Holditch Davis, & Denenberg, 1987). Predictive validity is demonstrated by evidence that early sleeping and waking behaviors scored on Thoman's scale are related to later developmental outcome (Holditch-Davis, Belyea, & Edwards, 2005; Thoman, Denenberg, Sieval, Zeider, & Becker, 1981).

Thoman's state scoring system has a number of advantages. The documented reliability and validity of this system is of value to researchers. The sleeping and waking states are differentiated enough that they can be used with infants with perinatal complications (Holditch-Davis et al., 2004; Holditch-Davis & Thoman, 1987; Thoman, Holditch-Davis, Graham, Scholz, & Rowe, 1988). This system has been used with preterm infants (Holditch-Davis et al., 2004) and with infants older than 1 month after term (Holditch-Davis, Miles, & Belyea, 2000). The states in this system can also be combined when an investigator does not need such fine discriminations.

This scoring system has two disadvantages. First, a 10-state system is somewhat more difficult to learn than a six-state system because it requires more subtle discriminations. However, individuals experienced in using a six-state system, such as Brazelton's, can readily learn this system. Also, because this state scoring system is not as widely used as Brazelton's, it is more difficult to obtain training in its use.

■ Als State Scoring System. Heidelise Als is a psychologist working at Harvard Medical School with Dr. Brazelton and his colleagues. For a number of years, she has worked

TABLE 30.2

APPROXIMATE EQUIVALENCE OF THE FOUR MAJOR SLEEP–WAKE STATE SCORING SYSTEMS

Brazelton	Thoman	Als	Anderson
6. Crying	Cry	6B. Lusty crying	12. Hard crying
		6A. Crying	11. Crying
5. Considerable motor activity	Fuss	5B. Considerable activity	10. Fussing
	Nonalert waking activity	5A. Active	9. Very restless awake
			8. Restless awake
4. Alert	Alert	4B. Bright alert	7. Alert inactivity
		4AH. Hyperalert	
		4AL. Awake and quiet	
3. Drowsy	Daze	3B. Drowsy	6. Quiet awake
	Drowse		5. Drowsy
	Sleep–wake transition	3A. Drowsy with more activity	4. Very restless sleep
2. Light sleep	Active sleep	2B. "Noisy" light sleep	3. Restless sleep
	Active–quiet transitional sleep	2A. Light sleep	2. Quiet sleep: irregular respiration
1.Deep sleep	Quiet sleep	1B. Deep sleep	1. Very quiet sleep
		1A. Very still deep sleep	

Note: Because the criteria used by these systems differ and because they are based on different conceptual frameworks, exact equivalence among them is not possible. Isolated instances of infant behavior may be scored quite differently than suggested by this table.

with these colleagues to modify the NBAS (Brazelton, 1984) to make it more appropriate for use with premature infants. The APIB is administered in much the same way as the NBAS, but the infant's behavior is scored in much greater detail so as to quantify not only the infant's skills but also the infant's reactivity and stress in response to environmental stimulation (Als et al., 1982; Pressler & Hepworth, 2002). Like the NBAS, the APIB is best administered to infants between 36 and 44 weeks GA, but the observational portion of the tool can be used with younger preterm infants (Als, 1986). The state scale from the NBAS has been expanded into a 13-state system by subdividing each of the 6 states so that the immature and unclear sleeping and waking states of premature infants can be more adequately described. These 13 states are very still deep sleep, deep sleep, light sleep, "noisy" light sleep, drowsy with more activity, drowsy, awake and quiet, hyper-alert, bright alert, active, considerable activity, crying, and lusty crying. The state subscale of the APIB has been shown to differentiate between premature and full-term infants after term (Als, Duffy, & McAnulty, 1988; Mouradian, Als, & Coster, 2000) and to correlate with electrophysiologic measures of brain activity (Duffy, Als, & McAnulty, 1990). In addition, the APIB and the state subscale are used to provide assessments that are the basis for planning individualized interventions as part of the NIDCAP (Als, 1986; Als et al., 1986; Pressler & Hepworth, 2002).

The Als state scoring system has a number of advantages and disadvantages for clinicians and researchers. First, a 13-state system is more difficult to learn than a 6-state system such as Brazelton's (Brazelton & Nugent, 1995). However, since the Als system was developed from the Brazelton states, individuals familiar with the Brazelton system should have no difficulty learning it, and when the complexity of the 13 states is not needed they can be collapsed to the 6 states from the NBAS. Second, inasmuch as the APIB, like the NBAS, was never intended for use with infants older than 1 month after term, the state scale may not adequately capture the states of older infants.

■ **Anderson's State Scoring System.** Gene Cranston Anderson is a doctorally prepared nurse researcher who worked at Case Western Reserve University in Cleveland, Ohio. She has long been interested in interventions that keep mother and infant together after birth, reduce infant crying, and promote feeding. She developed a 12-state scoring system, the Anderson behavioral state scale (ABSS), to be used with preterm infants based on her own observations of these infants (Anderson, 1999) and on the work of Parmelee and Stern (1972). Parmelee was one of the contributors to the UCLA state manual (Anders et al., 1971). The ABSS consists of very quiet sleep, quiet sleep with irregular respirations, restless sleep, very restless sleep, drowsy, quiet awake, alert inactivity, restless awake, very restless awake, fussing, crying, and hard crying. The states are arranged so that there is a linear relationship between the states and heart rate and energy consumption, with the states with the lowest numbers having the lowest mean heart rates. The ABSS has been used to show the effects of prefeeding nonnutritive sucking (Gill, Behnke, Conlon, McNeely, &

Anderson, 1988) and kangaroo care (Ludington, 1990) on preterm infant state patterns.

As with the other scoring systems, the ABSS has a number of advantages and disadvantages for clinicians and researchers. As the newest state scoring scale, it has had only limited use outside of nursing. Because the ABSS was designed for use with preterm infants, the utility of this scale for full-term infants and older infants is unknown, although its similarity to other state scoring systems suggests that it should be applicable for healthy full-term newborn infants. The ABSS may also be difficult to learn because of the complexity of 12 states. As Table 30.2 illustrates, the sleep states in this system differ markedly from the sleep states defined in other state scoring systems, so this is not a good scoring system to use if one is primarily interested in studying sleep states and wants to compare findings with other studies. Finally, the linear relationship between the states in this system and heart rate may make it the ideal choice for researchers who are primarily interested in studying the energy consumption of infants. However, this feature means the ABSS has a very different theoretical basis than the other state scales. The other state scoring systems differentiate among states based on qualitatively different aspects of the infant's behavior, but the ABSS emphasizes quantitative differences among the states, although more recently Anderson emphasized qualitative differences between states.

■ Description of Individual States. Because the definitions of sleep–wake states are so similar among these scoring systems (see Table 30.2), it is possible to describe in general the sleeping and waking states displayed by infants. For clarity's sake, generic state names will be used in all further descriptions. When they are not available, the state names from the Thoman system will be used. Each sleeping and waking state is made up of a different constellation of behaviors and serves a different function for the infant. Physiologic functioning is also different in each of these states.

Infants are most responsive to the environment when in the waking states, and, in particular, when alert. When the infant is alert, the eyes are open and scanning. Motor activity is typically low, particularly in full-term newborns, but premature infants and infants older than 1 month after term may be motorically active. Alertness is the state in which the infant exhibits focused attention on sources of stimulation (Brazelton & Nugent, 1995). Thus this is the best state in which to test reflexes (Prechtl & Beintema, 1968). Alertness has been suggested to be the optimal state for feeding (McCain, Gartside, Greenberg, & Lott, 2001; White-Traut, Berbaum, Lessen, McFarlin, & Cardenas, 2005). This state is also the one in which infants are most receptive to interactions with their parents and other adults. Yet alertness rarely occurs in the preterm period (Holditch-Davis, 1990; Holditch-Davis & Edwards, 1998a) and occurs relatively infrequently during the first month after term, only about 10% to 15% of the total day (Colombo & Horowitz, 1987).

Crying, another waking state, serves a communication function. However, the meaning of cries differs in different situations and may depend on their intensity (Fuller, 1991). Although crying that occurs when the infant is alone may elicit parental attention, crying that occurs during social exchanges may actually disrupt the parent–infant relationship. In full-term infants, crying during social interactions is related to the overall amount of maternal stimulation and to consistency in the patterning of maternal activities over weeks (Acebo & Thoman, 1995; Thoman, Acebo, & Becker, 1983). Studies have indicated that the intensity of crying is directly related to the heart rate of the infant (Ludington, 1990), and the higher the heart rate the greater the energy consumption of the infant (Woodson, Field, & Greenberg, 1983). In addition, this state is associated with decreased oxygenation in the bloodstream (Levesque, Pollack, Griffin, & Nielsen, 2000) and brain (Brazy, 1988).

The final waking state, nonalert waking activity, is characterized by periods when the infant is motorically active but not alert or crying. Usually the infant's eyes are open. One study of nonalert activity found that excess amounts of this state in full-term infants are associated with inconsistency in the patterning of states over weeks (Becker & Thoman, 1982), and, in turn, inconsistency in state patterning is related to poor developmental outcome (Thoman et al., 1981). Premature infants, after term, exhibit elevated levels of this state (Holditch-Davis & Thoman, 1987) and are known to be at increased risk of poor developmental outcome (Marlow, Wolke, Bracewell, Samara, & the EPICure Study Group, 2005; McGrath et al., 2005; Mwaniki, Atieno, Lawn, & Newton, 2012; Sullivan, Msall, & Miller, 2012). However, whether there is a relationship between these findings is unknown.

The states transitional between sleeping and waking have rarely been studied. In fact, the Prechtl scoring system omits them altogether on the grounds that they are not true states but just transitions between states (Prechtl & Beintema, 1968). However, newborn infants, both term and preterm, actually spend significant amounts of time in them, ranging from about 6% of the day at 29 weeks GA to 14% in the first month after term (Holditch-Davis, 1990; Holditch-Davis & Thoman, 1987). Thoman (1990) describes three states transitional between waking and sleeping: drowse, when the infant is quiet and appears sleepy with eyes opening and closing slowly; daze, when the infant is quiet with eyes that are open but dazed in appearance; and sleep–wake transition, when the infant exhibits mixed signals of waking and sleeping, is motorically active, and may appear to be waking up. Drowse and daze typically occur in the midst of periods of waking or as the infant is falling asleep. Sleep–wake transition typically occurs at the end of sleeping as the infant is awakening but may also occur in the middle of sleep, particularly in premature infants. Drowse, daze, and sleep–wake transition are often combined in research reports. However, studies have indicated that these states have different patterns of correlations with other states (Thoman et al., 1987). During the first month after term, premature infants have been found to spend significantly more time in sleep–wake transition and less time in drowse or daze than full-term infants (Holditch-Davis & Thoman, 1987). If these three states had been combined, these differences would have been missed. In addition, hospitalized preterm infants spend more time in sleep–wake transition when they are with nurses rather than parents but do not differ in the amount of drowsiness that occurs with these different caregivers (Miller & Holditch-Davis, 1992). They also exhibit more sleep–wake transition and less drowsiness during procedural care than during feeding and changing (Brandon, Holditch-Davis, & Belyea, 1999).

There are two major sleep states—active sleep and quiet sleep—although some state systems define a transitional state between them. In active sleep, the infant's respiration is uneven and primarily costal in nature. Sporadic motor movements occur, but muscle tone is low between these movements. Most behaviors, including hiccups, yawns, jitters, negative facial expressions (frowns and grimaces), and large movements, are less frequent in active sleep than waking but more frequent than in quiet sleep, but startles and jerks occur most frequently in active sleep (Holditch-Davis, Brandon, & Schwartz, 2003). The most distinct characteristic of this state is rapid eye movements that occur intermittently.

Active sleep is the most common state from birth throughout infancy, but it occurs during only about 20% of sleep in adults. Because of this dramatic developmental decrease and the frequent movements seen in infants during active sleep, many clinicians think of active sleep as a disorganized and primitive state. Surprisingly, this state has relatively recent phylogenetic origins, occurring only in birds and mammals. Thus it has been hypothesized to be necessary for brain development (Roffwarg, Muzio, & Dement, 1966). This hypothesis has received support in full-term infants (Denenberg & Thoman, 1981). In animal studies, prolonged deprivation of active sleep in infancy permanently altered brain functioning and resulted in hyperactivity, distractibility, and altered sexual performance (Mirmiran, 1986). Metabolic rates are higher in active than quiet sleep (Heraghty et al., 2008). Inasmuch as respiratory patterns are relatively unstable in active sleep (Elder, Larsen, Galletly, & Campbell, 2010; Holditch-Davis et al., 2004) and oxygenation is lower and more variable (Gabriel, Grote, & Jonas, 1980; Martin, Okken, & Rubin, 1979), the large amount of active sleep seen in young preterm infants (Holditch-Davis, Scher, Schwartz, & Hudson-Barr, 2004; Holditch-Davis & Edwards, 1998a) may contribute to their respiratory difficulties.

The other sleep state, quiet sleep, is characterized by a lack of body movements and the presence of regular respiration. A tonic level of motor tone is maintained in this state. Most behaviors, including hiccups, yawns, mouth movements, jitters, negative facial expressions, and large movements, are less frequent in quiet sleep than in waking or active sleep; the exception is sighs, which occur most frequently in quiet sleep (Holditch-Davis et al., 2003). The major purpose of quiet sleep seems to be rest and restoration. This state has been hypothesized to be necessary for healing (Adam & Oswald, 1984). Quiet sleep may also be needed for growth because it is in this state that growth hormone is secreted in adults. However, a study of full-term infants did not find any relationship between growth hormone secretion and quiet sleep (Shaywitz, Finkelstein, Hellman, & Weitzman, 1971). Oxygenation is higher during this sleep state (Gabriel et al., 1980; Martin et al., 1979) and respiration more regular (Elder et al., 2010). Thus quiet sleep may be beneficial for infants with respiratory problems.

The amount of quiet sleep is also very sensitive to the environment. Infant stimulation studies, for example, have found that quiet sleep is the state most likely to be increased by vestibular and kinesthetic interventions (Ingersoll & Thoman, 1994; Johnston, Stremler, Stevens, & Horton, 1997). The stimulation provided by routine nursing care, on the other hand, results in significantly less quiet sleep as compared with times when the preterm infant is undisturbed (Brandon et al., 1999), and the amount of this state is further reduced when the infant experiences painful or uncomfortable procedures (Holditch-Davis & Calhoun, 1989). Thus this is the state most likely to be affected by the NICU environment.

■ Effect of Physiologic Parameters on State. Physiologic functioning varies in different states. In turn, abnormalities in physiologic functioning can alter the sleeping and waking states of infants. This discussion focuses on the interrelationship of sleeping and waking and five areas of physiologic functioning of interest to neonatal nurses—perinatal illness, the CNS, circulatory system, respiration, and weight gain.

Perinatal Illness. The state patterns of infants who experienced perinatal complications may differ markedly from the state patterns of healthy full-term infants. Small-for-gestational-age full-term infants, for example, have more disorganized sleep as evidenced by more active sleep without rapid eye movements than healthy full-term infants (Watt & Strongman, 1985). They also exhibited poorer responsiveness during alertness as measured by the NBAS (Lester, Garcia-Coll, Valcarcel, Hoffman, & Brazelton, 1986).

The sleep of premature infants after term is known to differ from that of full-term infants of the same corrected ages, in that there is a decreased total amount of sleep, longer episodes of quiet sleep, more body movements, more frequent REM episodes, and somewhat lower correlation among the various behavioral criteria of the sleep states (Ellingson & Peters, 1980; Holditch-Davis & Thoman, 1987; Watt & Strongman, 1985). Premature infants show day–night differentiation in their sleeping and waking patterns at the same or an earlier postmenstrual age than full-term infants (Shimada, Segawa, Higurashi, & Akamatsu, 1993; Whitney & Thoman, 1994). In addition, their EEG patterns differ from those of full-term infants. Premature infants display longer bursts during trace alternans, earlier sleep spindle appearance, more immature EEG patterns, and poorer phase stability for EEG frequencies (Ellingson & Peters, 1980; Karch et al., 1982). Premature and full-term infants also differ on architectural, phasic, continuity, spectral, and autonomic measures (Scher,

Johnson, Ludington, & Loparo, 2011; Scher, Steppe, Dahl, Asthana, & Guthrie, 1992; Scher et al., 1994; Scher, Sun, Steppe, Guthrie, & Sclabassi, 1994). In particular, premature infants display shorter sleep state cycles, less quiet sleep, more arousals in quiet sleep, and less REM in active sleep (Scher et al., 2011). However, children born prematurely have similar rates of sleep problems from 5 months corrected age through 4 years of age (Wolke, Söhne, Riegel, Ohrt, & Osterlund, 1998).

The ways in which the waking states differ between full-term and premature infants of similar postmenstrual ages are less well established. Over prolonged observation periods, premature infants exhibited more alertness and nonalert waking activity and less drowsiness than full-term infants (Holditch-Davis & Thoman, 1987).

The severity of illness that the infant experiences during the perinatal period has relatively small additional effects on sleeping and waking. In general, critical illness has immediate effects on sleeping and waking patterns, but these effects disappear after the infant recovers as long as there are no neurologic complications and as long as infants are observed at the same ages corrected for GA at birth. Karch and colleagues (1982) studied healthy and ill preterm infants at comparable ages and found that ill infants exhibited more quiet sleep, more indeterminate sleep, and less wakefulness. The ill infants in this study were examined while on mechanical ventilation. Thus the state differences reflect the immediate influence of critical illness and mechanical ventilation. Preterm infants ill with RDS have been found to exhibit delayed state development but show state patterns comparable to those of healthy preterm infants once they recover (Holmes, Logan, Kirkpatrick, & Meyerl, 1979). Doussard-Roosevelt, Porges, and McClenny (1996) found that preterm infants with more medical complications showed more active sleep during brief sleep observations at 33 to 35 weeks than healthier preterm infants. Curzi-Dascalova et al. (1993) found that the longest sleep cycle of mechanically ventilated preterm infants was shorter than that of nonventilated infants. Holditch-Davis and Hudson (1995) used changes in sleep–wake states to identify a wide variety of acute medical complications in preterm infants, including hydrocephalus, sepsis, and cold stress. Infant medical complications also affected the scores of infants on standardized neurobehavioral assessments, but only on items requiring vigorous responses (e.g., vigor of crying, irritability, and motor development) and not on other state items, including alertness and percent sleeping (Korner et al., 1994). At term, preterm infants with medical complications showed lower sleep cyclicity scores than healthier preterm or term infants (Feldman, 2006).

Studies of infants who have recovered from their illnesses have found fewer differences. High and Gorski (1985) did not find any differences in the sleeping and waking patterns of convalescent premature infants differing in the severity of their previous illness. Likewise, Holditch-Davis (1990) found that the only difference in the development of sleeping and waking states in convalescent preterm infants was that more severely ill infants showed less fussing and somewhat poorer organization of quiet sleep. However, Holditch-Davis et al. (2004) found that longer mechanical ventilation was associated with more active sleep and less active sleep without REMs and that infants with lower birth weights had more regularity of respiration in quiet sleep. On the other hand, Brandon, Holditch-Davis, and Winchester (2005) found that longer mechanical ventilation was associated with less active sleep. Als et al. (1988) found no difference in the state organization of premature infants born at less than 33 weeks GA and premature infants born between 33 and 37 weeks GA when state organization was measured 2 weeks after term. In addition, scores on the NBAS state scale did not differ significantly between sick and healthy full-term infants at the time of hospital discharge (Holmes et al., 1982).

Infants with chronic lung disease are more likely than other premature infants to have oxygen desaturations when sleeping (Zinman, Blanchard, & Vachon, 1992). Yet how this illness affects sleeping and waking patterns is unclear. Holditch-Davis and Lee (1993) compared preterm infants with and without chronic lung disease from 32 to 36 weeks postmenstrual age on sleeping and waking during 4-hours observations in the intermediate care unit. The only difference between the infants with and without chronic lung disease was that infants with chronic lung disease had more irregular respiration in quiet sleep. Although many clinicians believe that infants with chronic lung disease are more sensitive to stimulation, there were also no differences in sleeping and waking when the infants with and without chronic lung disease were with caregivers (Holditch-Davis, 1995). However, at 36 weeks postmenstrual age, preterm infants with chronic lung disease had fewer periods of quiet sleep per hour and their EEG patterns differed as compared to preterm infants without this complication (Sommers, Tucker, & Laptook, 2011). At term age, premature infants with chronic lung disease were found to have less active sleep, more frequent arousals, and more frequent body movements in sleep than premature infants who never experienced any respiratory illnesses and performed more poorly on the interactive and motor clusters of the NBAS (Myers et al., 1992).

Treatments for perinatal illnesses also may affect the sleeping and waking states of preterm infants. For example, supplemental oxygen was associated with increased quiet sleep and total sleep time (Simakajornboon, Beckerman, Mack, Sharon, & Gozal, 2002). One study of preterm infants between 28 and 32 weeks postmenstrual age found that oxycodone was associated with a reduction in active sleep and an increase in sleep onset in quiet sleep as compared to a placebo, oral glucose, or swaddling by parents (Axelin, Kirjavainen, Salanterä, & Lehtonen, 2010). Prenatal magnesium sulfate affected the organization of sleep states leading to dysmaturity (a combination of accelerated and delayed state organization), whereas antenatal steroids had no effect (Black, Holditch-Davis, Schwartz, & Scher, 2006). Preterm infants whose mothers received antenatal phenobarbital did not differ in heart rate or sleep–wake states in the first 3 days of life from infants not receiving the medication, suggesting that the antenatal dosage was not sedating (McCain, Donovan, & Gartside, 1999).

Neurologic System. Because sleeping and waking states are assumed to reflect the underlying activation of the CNS, it is not surprising that a close relationship exists between sleep–wake states and CNS functioning. Four factors illustrate this interrelationship. First, sleeping and waking exhibit a large amount of development in the first year of life, the time of the most rapid CNS development. Sleeping and waking states affect neurologic responses. Infants with neurologic abnormalities exhibit abnormal sleeping and waking patterns. Finally, sleeping and waking states can be used to predict developmental outcome.

Development of Sleeping and Waking States. Infants exhibit definite developmental changes in their sleeping and waking state patterns throughout the first year of life. The age at which sleep–wake states first appear is unknown. The earliest study of sleeping and waking in preterm infants younger than 30 weeks GA found that these infants had only a single active sleep-like state (Dreyfus-Brisac, 1968), but these findings are questionable because all of the infants in this study were dying at the time of the state recordings. More recent studies of preterm infants have found that by 24 weeks GA, cycling between waking and sleeping can be identified by EEG in some preterm infants (Hellstrom-Westas, Rosen, & Svenningsen, 1991). By 25 to 27 weeks GA (the earliest age studied), infants exhibit distinct waking and sleeping states (Curzi-Dascalova et al., 1993; Holditch-Davis et al., 2004; Holditch-Davis & Edwards, 1998a; Scher, Johnson, & Holditch-Davis, 2005). However, before 30 weeks GA, the various behaviors associated with sleep and waking—eye movements, body movements, respiration, and muscle tone—are not well coordinated; not until at least 36 weeks GA do preterm infants exhibit the same degree of correlation between these parameters as do full-term infants (Curzi-Dascalova, Peirano, & Morel-Kahn, 1988; Parmelee & Stern, 1972). Studies of sleeping and waking states in fetuses conducted using observations made during ultrasound examinations have had similar findings (DiPietro, Hodgson, Costigan, Hilton, & Johnson, 1996).

Infants exhibit greater amounts of active sleep and indeterminate states during the preterm period and lower amounts of waking states than after term (High & Gorski, 1985; Holditch-Davis, 1990; Holditch-Davis & Edwards, 1998a; Holditch-Davis et al., 2004). Active sleep occupies as much as 60% to 70% of the day for young preterm infants (High & Gorski, 1985; Holditch-Davis & Edwards, 1998a; Holditch-Davis et al., 2004). The major developmental change during the preterm period is a decrease in the amount of sleep due to a decrease in active sleep (High & Gorski, 1985; Holditch-Davis & Edwards, 1998a; Holditch-Davis et al., 2004; Ingersoll & Thoman, 1999). In addition, quiet sleep and waking states, especially crying, increase (High & Gorski, 1985; Holditch-Davis & Edwards, 1998a; Holditch-Davis et al., 2004; Vles et al., 1992). The organization of the sleep states, as measured by the percentages of the state with typical state criteria, by the correlation between criteria, by the presence of definite sleep state cycles, also increases throughout the preterm period (Curzi-Dascalova et al., 1988; Feldman, 2006; Holditch-Davis & Edwards, 1998a; Holditch-Davis et al., 2004; Soubasi et al., 2009). The mean duration and frequency of episodes of each state also change over the preterm period: quiet waking, active waking, and sleep–wake transition episodes occurred more frequently than active waking and quiet sleep, but length of these periods increased over age (Holditch-Davis & Edwards, 1998b; Ingersoll & Thoman, 1999). These changes may be affected by gender as male preterm infants exhibited less active sleep, more drowsiness, and more waking than females (Foreman, Thomas, & Blackburn, 2008).

The sleeping and waking states of infants in the first month after term differ dramatically from those of preterm infants. Healthy full-term neonates sleep about 13 1/2 hours a day (Thomas & Foreman, 2005) and spend approximately 40% of the daytime in active sleep and 20% in quiet sleep (Holditch-Davis & Thoman, 1987). Slightly higher amounts of sleep states occur at night (Thoman & Whitney, 1989; Whitney & Thoman, 1994). Waking states make up the rest of the day, with alertness (14%) and drowsiness (13%) being the most common (Holditch-Davis & Thoman, 1987).

The major developmental trends exhibited by full-term infants in the first month are a decrease in active sleep and an increase in the amount of alertness (Denenberg & Thoman, 1981; Kohyama & Iwakawa, 1990). Moreover, the mean lengths of episodes of the sleep states change, with active sleep decreasing and quiet sleep increasing (Thoman & Whitney, 1989). Similar trends occur for premature infants during this period (Ariagno et al., 1997; Mirmaran, Baldwin, & Ariagno, 2003; Whitney & Thoman, 1994). In addition, both full-term and premature infants begin to show entrainment to a day–night schedule of sleeping and waking by about a month after term (Ariagno et al., 1997; Shimada et al., 1999).

Sleeping and waking states continue to develop throughout the first year. Waking periods become longer and more consolidated (Holditch-Davis, Tesh, Burchinal, & Miles, 1999; Louis, Cannard, Bastuji, & Challamel, 1997). The infant spends an increasing proportion of wakefulness in the alert state. The amount of time spent crying decreases (Michelsson, Rinne, & Paajanen, 1990; St. James-Roberts & Plewis, 1996). In addition, total sleep time decreases, with almost all of this decrease due to a decrease in active sleep time (Holditch-Davis et al., 1999; Kohyama & Iwakawa, 1990; Louis et al., 1997; St. James-Roberts & Plewis, 1996). The amount of quiet sleep remains the same or increases from term age on; thus by about 6 months of age, the amount of quiet sleep exceeds the amount of active sleep (Louis et al., 1997). In addition, the number of sleep episodes decreases and becomes consolidated primarily into nighttime, although most infants continue to exhibit some amount of night waking (Ottaviano, Giannotti, Cortesi, Bruni, & Ottaviano, 1996; Scher, 1991). By 1 year, the infant is taking about two daytime naps (Weissbluth, 1995) and sleeping about 10 to 12 hours through the night. Prematurely born infants may display shorter night sleep and more activity during the night than full-term infants (Asaka & Takada, 2010).

The nature of these changes depends somewhat on the caregiving environment. Thus breastfed infants exhibit less total sleep, longer sleep latency, more fragmented sleep, more non-REM sleep, and shorter duration of REM sleep than formula-fed infants do (Quillin & Glenn, 2004; Tikotzky et al., 2010; Schwichtenberg & Poehlmann, 2009). Also, 2-week-old and 6-month-old full-term infants with depressed mothers took longer to fall asleep and had more disrupted sleep than infants of nondepressed mothers (Armitage et al., 2009).

Other developmental changes during the first year affect the organization of sleep. The cycling between active and quiet becomes more consistent over the first few months, and by 4 months of age, the complete sleep cycle first exhibits a standard length of about 1 hour (Harper et al., 1981). Many preterm infants display hour-long sleep cycles by 36 weeks postmenstrual age (Borghese, Minard, & Thoman, 1995). The sleep states also develop the EEG patterns typical of adults. By 3 months of age, the EEG stages within quiet sleep can be identified, and this sleep state can now be called non-REM sleep (Ellingson & Peters, 1980).

Neurologic Responses. Infants exhibit different neurologic responses in different sleeping and waking states. The magnitude of neurologic reflexes is known to differ greatly in different states (Prechtl & Beintema, 1968). Therefore standardized infant assessments and neurologic examinations specify which states are optimal for testing each reflex (Brazelton & Nugent, 1995; Prechtl & Beintema, 1968). The amplitude, wave form, and latency of visual evoked potentials are different in different sleeping and waking states, with the greatest differences being between sleep and waking (Apkarian, Mirmiran, & Tijssen, 1991).

Neurologic Problems. The state patterns of infants with neurologic insults differ markedly from those of healthy infants. Infants with Down syndrome have been found to spend more time awake and to have abnormally long periods of quiet sleep (Prechtl, Theorell, & Blair, 1973). At term, using the NBAS, premature infants with intraventricular hemorrhage have been found to have lower arousal than healthy full-term infants (Anderson et al., 1989) and to be more likely to lack sleep–wake cycles than healthier preterm infants (Olischar, Klebermass, Waldhoer, Pollak, & Weninger, 2007). Full-term infants with hyperbilirubinemia show decreased amounts of wakefulness (Prechtl et al., 1973). As compared to full-term infants with only mild bilirubin elevations, infants with moderately elevated bilirubin values exhibit significantly lower scores in state regulation and range on the NBAS and exhibit minor neurologic abnormalities as shown by increased latency of brain-stem auditory evoked potentials (Vohr et al., 1990). Abnormal cry patterns have been found in infants who have neurologic injuries or hyperbilirubinemia or are at risk for sudden infant death syndrome (SIDS) (Corwin et al., 1995).

In addition, infants exposed prenatally to drugs or alcohol exhibit abnormalities in their state patterns, possibly as the result of neurologic insults caused by the drugs. For example, alcohol-exposed infants exhibit sleep disruptions and abnormal cries (Nugent, Lester, Greene, Wieczorek-Deering, & O'Mahony, 1996; Scher, Richardson, Coble, Day, & Stoffer, 1988). Newborn infants of mothers who smoked during pregnancy had higher cries than did infants whose mothers did not smoke (Nugent et al., 1996), and premature infants whose mothers smoked prenatally had altered sleep patterns–wake patterns (more active sleep, more waking after sleep onset), more motor activity in sleep, and altered peripheral chemoreceptors (decreased baseline activity in active sleep and increased response time in quiet sleep) (Stephan-Blancard et al., 2008, 2010). Infants exposed to marijuana have shorter, higher cries with more variation in frequency (Lester & Dreher, 1989) and exhibit a decrease in quiet sleep time (Scher et al., 1988). Methadone-exposed infants exhibit abnormal cries with short first expirations and are more irritable and less able to sustain a high-quality alert state (Huntington, Hans, & Zeskind, 1990; Jeremy & Hans, 1985). Infants experiencing opiate withdrawal exhibit more waking, more sleep fragmentation, and less quiet sleep (O'Brien & Jeffery, 2002). Infants who were exposed to cocaine or opiates during pregnancy showed more alertness and less quiet sleep than nonexposed infants (White-Traut et al., 2002). Infants who were prenatally exposed to cocaine showed less active sleep and more indeterminate sleep; they also showed less orientation and poorer state regulation, including more jitters, high-pitched cries, and hyperalertness, than drug-free infants (Bauer et al., 2005; Black, Schuler & Nair, 1993; Regalado, Schechtman, Del Angel, & Bean, 1995). On the other hand, Woods, Eyler, Behnke, and Conlon (1993) did not find any differences on the NBAS between cocaine-exposed and drug-free infants.

Prediction of Developmental Outcome. Finally, the organization of sleeping and waking, as indicated by individual state criteria or the overall patterning of states, can be used to predict the developmental outcome of infants. Greater amounts of quiet sleep in the preterm period relate to better alertness and orientation, less irritability, and better orientation to inanimate visual and auditory stimulation on the NAPI (Korner & Thom, 1990), an assessment similar to the APIB, at 32 and 36 weeks postmenstrual age (Brandon et al., 2005). In healthy preterm infants, lower spectral EEG energies predicted lower neurodevelopmental performance at 12 and 24 months (Scher, Steppe, & Banks, 1994). Low levels of trace alternans, an EEG pattern seen during quiet sleep in neonates, is predictive of lower intelligence quotients (IQs) in premature infants (Beckwith & Parmelee, 1986), and delayed maturity of EEG patterns of preterm infants was found to be associated with poor neurologic outcome (Ferrari et al., 1992; Hahn & Tharp, 1990). More sleep–wake transition, shorter sleep periods, and fewer arousals from quiet sleep during the first day of life in full-term infants are associated with lower developmental scores at 6 months (Freudigman & Thoman, 1993). Elevated amounts of intense bursts of rapid eye movements and long sleep-cycle lengths at 6 months are associated with developmental problems in full-term infants (Becker &

Thoman, 1982; Borghese et al., 1995) and low amounts of rapid eye movements were associated with lower Bayley mental development scores at 6 months corrected age in preterm infants (Arditi-Babchuk, Feldman, & Eidelman, 2009). Acoustic characteristics of infant cries have been used to predict developmental outcome in preterm infants and infants who were prenatally exposed to drugs (Huntington et al., 1990). Measures of sleep–wake states during the preterm period—including the total amount of sleep, the overall quality of state organization as compared with other infants, predominant pattern of state transitions, and sleep cycle length—have been found to predict Bayley scores at 6 months to 3 years corrected age (Borghese et al., 1995; DiPietro & Porges, 1991; Fajardo, Browning, Fisher, & Paton, 1992; Gertner et al., 2002; Holditch-Davis et al., 2005; Weisman, Aderka, Marom, Hermesh, & Gilboa-Schechtman, 2011; Whitney & Thoman, 1993). However, the amount of indeterminate sleep—any period not meeting the criteria for one of the five states defined by Prechtl and Beintema (1968)—in premature infants at term was not related to developmental status at 2 years (Maas et al., 2000). In apparently normal full-term infants, the stability of state patterns in the first month has been found to predict developmental outcome (Thoman et al., 1981). This finding has been replicated in premature infants after term (Whitney & Thoman, 1993) and in siblings of infants who died from SIDS (Thoman et al., 1988).

Circulatory System. Sleeping and waking states affect the infant's circulatory system. Overall, heart rate is higher in waking than sleeping states, and particularly during crying (Ludington, 1990; van Ravenswaaij-Arts, Hopman, & Kollee, 1989). Mean heart rates in the two sleep states are very similar, but heart rate is more variable in active sleep (Elder et al., 2010; Galland et al., 2000). This difference in variability is large enough that it is possible to differentiate between the two sleep states on the basis of heart rate variability (DeHaan, Patrick, Chess, & Jaco, 1977). Thus neonatal nurses need to be aware of the infant's state when determining heart rate, and routine vital signs probably should not be obtained while the infant is crying.

Sleeping and waking states also affect the infant's circulation. Cerebral blood flow is highest in waking (Greisen, Hellstrom-Vestas, Lou, Rosen, & Svenningsen, 1985). It is significantly higher in active sleep than in quiet sleep in full-term infants (Milligan, 1979), but not in infants less than term age (Greisen et al., 1985). Variability in cerebral blood flow velocity is lowest in quiet sleep, whereas marked fluctuations occur in active waking (fussing and nonalert waking activity; Ramaekers, Casaer, Daniels, Smet, & Marchal, 1989). Blood pressure is slightly higher when the infant is awake than when asleep (van Ravenswaaij-Arts et al., 1989) and lower in quiet sleep than active sleep (Witcombe, Yiallourou, Walker, & Horne, 2008).

Respiration. The effect of sleeping and waking states on the respiratory system is even greater than on the circulatory system. The nervous system controls of breathing differ in different states (Phillipson, 1978). During wakefulness, breathing is regulated by metabolic controls, general stimulation from the reticular activating system, and voluntary activities. In quiet sleep, metabolic controls predominate, and maintaining acid–base and oxygen homeostasis is the primary stimulus for breathing. Medullary respiratory center activity varies during active asleep depending on whether the infant is experiencing rapid eye movements and motor activity (phasic active sleep) or not (tonic active sleep), indicating that these two types of active sleep include different controls on breathing. During phasic active sleep, behavioral controls, similar to the voluntary controls in waking, predominate. In tonic active sleep, the major respiratory control results from direct stimulation of the state in a manner similar to the reticular stimulation of respiration during wakefulness. As a result of these different controls, infants exhibit higher respiratory rates and lower tidal volumes in phasic active sleep than in tonic active sleep (Haddad, Lai, & Mellins, 1982). In addition, the Hering-Breuer reflex is strong in active sleep in preterm infants (Hand et al., 2004).

Respiratory activity responds differently to chemical stimulation in different states. Baseline arterial oxygen and carbon dioxide levels are lower in active sleep than in either waking or quiet sleep (Gabriel et al., 1980; Martin et al., 1979; Mok et al., 1988), possibly because of hypoventilation or ventilation-perfusion inequalities in this state. Arousal in response to hypoxia differs in quiet sleep and active sleep, with some studies finding that it is slower in quiet sleep (Parslow, Harding, Adamson, & Horne, 2004) and others finding it slower in active sleep (Fewell & Baker, 1987). Response to hypercapnia is also different in different states. There is a shift to the right in the carbon dioxide response curve in quiet sleep as compared to waking (Cohen, Xu, & Henderson-Smart, 1991; Phillipson, 1978). This response is further reduced in tonic active sleep and is absent in phasic active sleep (Sullivan, 1980).

As a result of these differing neurologic controls on breathing, a number of respiratory variables in both full-term and preterm infants are influenced by sleep and waking states. Respiration rates are higher and more variable in active sleep (Elder, Campbell, Larsen, & Galletly, 2011; Holditch-Davis, Scher, & Schwartz, 2004). Active sleep has also been shown to result in hypoventilation in preterm infants because of central inhibition of spinal motoneurons (Schulte, Busse, & Eichhorn, 1977) and poor coordination between chest and abdominal muscles (Gaultier, 1990). Thus paradoxical movements of the chest wall and abdominal muscles during breathing are common during active sleep in preterm infants, and oxygen saturation is somewhat lower (Elder et al., 2011). However, it is not clear whether lung volume is decreased in active sleep in full-term infants. Expiratory volumes and flow rates are larger in waking than in sleeping infants (Lodrup, Mowinckel, & Carlsen, 1992).

The frequency of central apnea also differs between the two sleep states. Central apnea rarely occurs during waking. Most studies indicate that brief apneic pauses of less than 20 seconds in length occur more frequently in active sleep than quiet sleep in both full-term and preterm infants (Curzi-Dascalova, Bloch, Vecchierini, Bedu, & Vignolo, 2000; Holditch-Davis, Scher, & Schwartz, 2004; Vecchierini, Curzi-Dascolova, Ha, Bloch, & Gaultier, 2001). However, the frequency of periodic respiration (cyclic breathing alternating with brief apneic pauses) does not appear to differ between the sleep states (Holditch-Davis, Scher, & Schwartz, 2004). The mean length of apneic pauses is longer in quiet sleep (Holditch-Davis, Scher, & Schwartz, 2004). In addition, a variety of stresses, including an increase in body temperature and sleep deprivation, have been shown to increase apnea frequency, primarily in active sleep (Gaultier, 1994).

However, it cannot be concluded from these studies that pathologic apneas (apneic episodes longer than 20 seconds and usually associated with bradycardia and hypoxemia) are more common in active sleep because these studies rarely included episodes of pathologic apnea. Pathologic apnea is often too rare to permit statistical analyses comparing states (Holditch-Davis, Scher, & Schwartz, 2004). However, Tourneux et al. (2008) found that pathologic apnea with oxygen desaturation was more common in active sleep, whereas the frequency of pathologic apnea without desaturation did not differ between the sleep states. In addition, some association between active sleep and pathologic apnea is suggested by the fact that the methylxanthines, caffeine and theophylline, used to treat this condition are generally found to increase the amount of wakefulness and decrease the amount of sleep in addition to their direct effects on respiration (Brandon et al., 2005; Thoman et al., 1985). On the other hand, Hayes et al. (2007) found decreased waking, brief arousals, and movement bouts with caffeine or theophylline treatment. Infants have also been found to have greater respiration regularity in active sleep during treatment with theophylline and caffeine (Holditch-Davis, Scher, & Schwartz, 2004). Some studies have found that theophylline and caffeine had minimal effects on sleep–wake development (Curzi-Dascalova, Aujard, Gaultier, & Rajguru, 2002; Holditch-Davis & Edwards, 1998a), whereas others found theophylline is related to greater maturity of active sleep-quiet sleep cycles on EEG (Lee et al., 2010).

Weight Gain. Studies have found that obesity is related to shorter sleep duration in both adults and children, probably because of a bidirectional relationship in which inadequate sleep increases hunger and excess weight interferes with sleeping (Liu, Zhang & Li, 2012; Meyer, Wall, Larson, Laska, & Neumark-Sztainer, 2012). How early in life this relationship begins is unknown, but a recent study found that infants with shorter sleep durations were more likely to have higher weight-to-length ratios (Tikovtzky et al., 2009), suggesting that adequate sleep may protect against the development of obesity even in infancy.

■ Effect of Health Care Interventions on State. Sleeping and waking states are also affected by the types and timing of stimulation that the infant receives from the environment. Thus health care interventions have the potential to either promote state organization or to disrupt it. The effects of four common nursing interventions—routine NICU care, painful procedures, social interaction, and infant stimulation—on infant sleeping and waking are examined in this section.

■ Effect of Environmental Stimulation. The hospital provides stimulation that may be inappropriate for the development of premature infants and is likely to result in disorganized sleeping and waking patterns. The NICU provides infants with an extremely bright and noisy environment with little diurnal variation and frequent interventions for technical procedures, but little positive handling (Duxbury, Henly, Broz, Armstrong, & Wachdorf, 1984; Zahr & Balian, 1995). The sickest infants actually receive the most handling (High & Gorski, 1985; Zahr & Balian, 1995), even though they lack the physiologic reserves to cope with it. Premature infants may become hypoxic in response to virtually any form of stimulation. The severity of the negative physiologic responses to one procedure, endotracheal suctioning, has been related to the infant's state during the procedure (Bernert et al., 1997). Preterm infants who cried during suctioning had greater changes in oxygenation and heart rate than infants who slept through suctioning. Convalescent infants are handled less than ill infants but do experience social interactions as a greater percent of their care (High & Gorski, 1985).

Several of the aspects of routine NICU care are known to contribute to disruption of infant sleeping and waking patterns. Nursing and medical interventions frequently result in state changes. The frequency of these interventions in the NICU has been found to be as high as five times per hour (Duxbury et al., 1984). Preterm infants change their sleep–wake states about six times per hour, and 78% of these changes are associated with either nursing interventions or NICU noise (Zahr & Balian, 1995). Preterm infants are rarely able to sustain quiet sleep during nursing interventions (Brandon et al., 1999; Liaw et al., 2012) and usually awaken with each intervention. Thus, frequent nursing interventions are particularly likely to reduce the amount of quiet sleep (Liaw et al., 2012). Preterm infants normally spend only a small percentage of their time in waking states (High & Gorski, 1985; Holditch-Davis, 1990), but this percentage increases significantly when they are with nurses (Brandon et al., 1999; Liaw et al., 2012). Also, developmental changes in the amount of waking occur only over the time infants are with nurses, and the distribution of states differs depending on the nursing activity, with active waking more common and drowsiness less common during more intrusive care (Brandon et al., 1999). On the other hand, preterm infants showed more quiet sleep after nursing interventions than before them (Symanski, Hayes, & Akileshl, 2002), and bathing did not affect sleep–wake patterns (Lee, 2002).

Moreover, neonatal nurses and physicians often do not consider infant sleep–wake states and other infant cues when choosing the time for routine interventions. Although two studies found relationships between nursing care and sleeping and waking for groups of preterm infants (Barnard & Blackburn, 1985; Lawson, Turkewitz, Platt, & McCarton,

1985), these results probably represent infant reactions to nursing care or infants conditioned to anticipate regular nursing procedures rather than nurses responding to infant states. Infant activity has been found to decrease after nursing interventions (Blackburn & Barnard, 1985). Gottfried (1985) found that nurses responded to fewer than half the cries of convalescent premature infants. Yet a lack of responsiveness to infant cues may serve to slow the development of stable diurnal patterns of sleeping and waking that several investigators have suggested is the first task of infancy (Barnard & Blackburn, 1985). Full-term infants receiving responsive care develop day–night differentiation in their sleeping and waking in 5 to 7 days, whereas this differentiation is delayed when the care is not responsive (Sander, Stechler, Burns, & Lee, 1979).

In light of the recommendation by the American Academy of Pediatrics (AAP) (2011) that infants be placed on their backs to sleep, the effects of positioning on infant sleep–wake states also need to be considered. Full-term infants in the supine position show greater wakefulness, less quiet sleep, higher cerebral oxygenation levels, lower heart rates, higher rates of brief respiratory pauses, and better airway protection during sleep than when prone (Elder et al., 2010; Jeffery, Megevand, & Page, 1999; Skadberg & Markestad, 1997; Wong et al., 2011). Similar effects on sleeping and waking, heart rate, and oxygenation have been found in growing preterm infants and in preterm infants with chronic lung disease (Ariagno et al., 2003; Bhat et al., 2006; Chang, Anderson, & Lin, 2002; Horne, Bandopadhayay, Vitkovic, Cranage, & Adamson, 2002; Jarus et al., 2011; Saiki et al., 2009). In addition, respiration rates are more variable in a supine position in preterm infants, but not in full terms (Elder et al., 2011), and arousals are more common (Ariagno, van Liempt, & Mirmiran, 2006). On the other hand, lateral positioning was associated with an increase in quiet sleep (Liaw et al., 2012). Thus supine positioning is probably not appropriate for preterm infants with respiratory compromise.

However, in growing preterm infants, prone positioning was associated with a reduced ventilatory response to cardon dioxide as compared to supine position (Smith, Saiki, Hannam, Rafferty, & Greenough, 2010). Thus, in preterm infants who are no longer acutely ill, positioning decisions require balancing infant needs for rest and oxygenation with physiological changes with respiratory maturation and the need to provide an example for parents. Although prone sleeping has decreased after discharge for preterm infants, mothers of VLBW infants still tend to place their infants on their sides, rather than supine (Vernacchio et al., 2003).

Finally, the lighting of the NICU, as discussed earlier in this chapter, contributes to sleeping and waking problems in infants. Lighting in most NICUs is continuous, high-level, and fluorescent. The frequency of eye opening and waking states is related to the level of illumination in the NICU; less eye opening occurs when the lights are brightest (Moseley, Thompson, Levene, & Fielder, 1988; Robinson, Moseley, Thompson, & Fielder, 1989). Sudden decreases in lighting result in increased eye opening (Moseley et al., 1988). This finding supports the common nursing and parental intervention of shading infant eyes with one's hand to elicit alertness. In addition, infants exposed to NICUs that vary the intensity of lighting on a diurnal pattern open their eyes significantly more than those exposed to continuous illumination (Robinson et al., 1989).

In view of the problems with routine NICU care, several researchers have attempted to alter this environment to promote better sleeping and waking patterns in infants. When Gabriel, Grote, and Jonas (1981) consolidated nursing care so that convalescent premature infants were disturbed less often, the infants were awake less often and had longer sleep episodes. Fajardo, Browning, Fisher, and Paton (1990) cared for premature infants in a quiet, private room with a day-night cycle, demand feedings, and social interactions by the nurses. These babies showed an increase in the mean length of active sleep and an increase in the organization of sleep states as evidenced by a decreased number of state changes and increased number of enduring state episodes.

Als and colleagues (1986) developed a system of individualized interventions for preterm infants that included sensitivity to infant cues and careful avoidance of sleep disruptions. Their experimental infants did not exhibit different state patterns compared to the control infants, but the experimental infants did have fewer medical complications and improved performance on the APIB. A replication found improved state regulation and state stability as measured on the APIB (Buehler, Als, Duffy, McAnulty, & Liederman, 1995). Using a modification of Als intervention system, Becker, Chang, Kameshima, and Bloch (1991) also found improvements in infant morbidity but did not find differences in state behaviors on the NBAS at the time of hospital discharge; however, the experimental infants showed higher oxygen saturations, fewer disorganized movements, and more alertness during nursing care than did controls (Becker, Grunwald, Moorman, & Stuhr, 1993). Later studies found that infants receiving the intervention slept more than infants receiving traditional handling (Becker, Brazy, & Grunwald, 1997; Bertelle, Mabin, Adrien, & Sizun, 2005). However, other studies using Als intervention system did not find that it had any effect on sleep–wake states, either in the preterm period or after discharge (Ariagno et al., 1997; Westrup, Hellström-Westas, Stjernqvist, & Lagercrantz, 2002).

A number of researchers altered NICU lighting patterns. Mann, Haddow, Stokes, Goodley, and Rutter (1986) cared for preterm infants in a nursery in which light and noise intensities were reduced between 7:00 a.m. and 7:00 p.m. As compared with infants from a control nursery, the experimental infants were found to sleep more but not until after hospital discharge. Blackburn and Patteson (1991) compared preterm infants in a nursery with continuous lighting with infants in a nursery with lighting that was dimmed at night. Infants in cycled light exhibited less motor activity during the night and lower heart rates over the entire day than the control infants. When preterm infants in the intermediate care unit were given four half-hour nap periods a day during which their incubators were covered and they received no nursing or medical procedures, they exhibited less quiet waking and longer uninterrupted sleep bouts than preterm infants without naps (Holditch-Davis, Barham, O'Hale, & Tucker, 1995), and they experienced a more rapid decline in apnea and more rapid weight gain (Torres, Holditch-Davis, O'Hale, & D'Auria, 1997). Brandon, Holditch-Davis, and Belyea (2002) compared preterm infants who received care in near darkness with infants who received cycled light. Although there were no differences in state patterns (Brandon et al., 2005), the infants receiving cycled light showed more rapid weight gain (Brandon et al., 2002). In another study, preterm infants receiving cycled light showed earlier day–night patterning of activity than infants cared for in dim light (Rivkees, Mayes, Jacobs, & Gross, 2004). However, a third study found no differences in sleep or circadian patterns after discharge in infants exposed to dim lighting or cycled lighting (Mirmaran et al., 2003). All together, these findings suggest that neonatal nurses need to examine their routine practices to see if changes could be made to better promote stable sleeping and waking patterns in infants.

Painful Procedures. Infants in intensive care inevitably experience painful procedures. Neonatal nurses need to be alert to the effects of these procedures on infant sleeping and waking states. During painful procedures, infants are more likely to be awake and less likely to be in quiet sleep than during routine nursing care (Fearon, Kisilevsky, Hains, Muir, & Tranmer, 1997; Van Cleve, Johnson, Andrews, Hawkins, & Newbold, 1995). All but the youngest and sickest preterm infants are likely to cry (Johnston et al., 1999a; Van Cleve et al., 1995), although the length of time until the cry begins depends on the infant's sleeping and waking state at the beginning of the procedure (Grunau & Craig, 1987). Healthy full-term infants have the longest latency to cry when in quiet sleep, and young, preterm infants who are asleep at the beginning of the procedure and have recently undergone another painful procedure are the most likely to show only a minimal behavioral response to a painful procedure (Johnston et al., 1999a; Stevens, Johnston, & Horton, 1994). Immediately after the painful procedure, full-term infants are likely to remain awake (Anders & Chalemian, 1974). However, in preterm infants, this tendency is not any greater than the tendency to stay awake after routine handling (Holditch-Davis & Calhoun, 1989).

Nursing comfort measures also have the potential to minimize some of the state effects of pain without having negative effects on infant sleep. Yet how frequently practicing nurses actually use them is unclear. In one study, nurses were not found to use positive touches or talking any more frequently during painful procedures than during routine care (Holditch-Davis & Calhoun, 1989). Franck (1987) identified nine different comfort measures that nurses reported using to soothe infants who were receiving painful procedures (Chapter 23). To date, only a few of them have been studied. Tactile stimulation, music, and intrauterine sounds were found ineffective for both preterm and full-term infants when given during painful procedures (Beaver, 1987; Marchette, Main, & Redick, 1989). However, pacifiers were found to reduce crying and arousal in full-term and preterm infants when given during and after the procedure (Fearon et al., 1997). A sucrose-flavored pacifier was found to be even more effective than a plain pacifier in reducing the amount of crying by full-term and preterm infants during blood drawing and circumcision (Abad, Diaz, Domenech, Robayna, & Rico, 1996; Johnston et al., 1997; Johnston et al., 1999b). Swaddling has been shown to reduce arousals in sleep and increase REM sleep in full-term infants (Gerard, Harris, & Thach, 2002). Facilitated tucking—a modified form of swaddling in which the infant's arms and legs are contained in a flexed position next to the trunk—was effective in reducing responses to heelsticks (Corff, Seidemanm, Venkataraman, Lutes, & Yates, 1995). Preterm infants who received facilitated tucking during and after heelsticks exhibited less crying, less sleep disruption, and fewer state changes after the heelstick than without tucking (Corff et al., 1995; Obeidat, Kahalaf, Callister, & Froelicher, 2009). Rocking was not effective in reducing cry facial expressions in preterm infants in response to a heelstick, although the infants were in quiet sleep more (Johnston et al., 1997). Thus there is evidence that use of swaddling and pacifiers with sucrose can help reduce the sleeping and waking changes caused by painful procedures. However, additional research is needed to determine the effects of other comfort measures and how comfort measures affect more severe pain, such as postoperative pain.

Social Interaction. Sleeping and waking states are known to influence the interactions between full-term and premature infants and their mothers after term age, and in turn maternal interactions alter infant sleep–wake patterns. For example, infant crying may lead the mother to pick up the infant. At another time, a mother may awaken a sleeping infant for a feeding, thereby altering the infant's sleeping and waking patterns. Mothers have been found to exhibit different patterns of interactions when infants are in different states (Rosenthal, 1983). Aspects of the infant's state organization, including the degree to which he or she shows different patterns of crying and alertness in different situations, are related to the overall quality of the mother–infant interaction (Acebo & Thoman, 1995). A responsive style of mothering results in infants developing day–night differentiation in their sleeping and waking patterns sooner (Sander et al., 1979). In addition, maternal emotional stress has been found to relate to the amount of night sleeping that full-term infants exhibit at 4 and 12 months (Becker et al., 1991a).

Social interaction is known to affect sleep–wake patterns of premature infants after hospital discharge, and sleep–wake patterns in turn alter social interations. At 4 to 6 weeks corrected age, breastfed premature infants exhibited more crying, especially during daytime, than formula-fed infants did (Thomas, 2000). At 6 months corrected age, premature infants were more likely to be drowsy or asleep during feeding and alert during nonfeeding periods, and the behaviors of mothers differed during feeding and nonfeeding (Holditch-Davis et al., 2000). Mothers were more likely to engage in behaviors that involved close contact during feeding, such as holding, having body contact, and rocking their infants, whereas during nonfeeding periods, they were more likely to engage in more distal behaviors, such as gesturing and playing with the infant. Mothers who displayed more sensitive interactions or less negatiove affect had infants who took more naps and slept more in the daytime (Schwichtenberg & Poehlmann, 2009; Schwichtenberg, Anders, Vollbrecht, & Poehlmann, 2011). Conversely, preterm infants with higher sleep cyclicity scores at term were found to experience greater synchrony with their mothers at 3 months corrected age (Feldman, 2006).

Less is known about the effect of social interaction in the hospital on infant sleeping and waking states. Minde, Whitelaw, Brown, and Fitzhardinge (1983) found that ill preterm infants exhibited less eye opening—and thus probably less waking—when they were interacting with their mothers than did healthier preterm infants. Mothers report being aware of the sleeping and waking behaviors of their preterm infants—especially eye movements, orientation, and body movements—when they attempt to interact; they also report having used specific infant responses as guides to increase or decrease their interactive activity (Oehler, Hannan, & Catlett, 1993). Waking, eye opening, increased body movements, positive facial expressions, and calming encouraged increased interaction; body movements, negative facial expressions, and withdrawing discouraged maternal interaction. However, preterm infants exhibited the positive interactive behaviors rather small portions of the time with their mothers (Oehler, 1995).

Moreover, social stimulation affects the physiologic status of preterm infants. The variation in infant oxygen saturation during parent touching was related to behavioral state and GA, such that infants who were more aroused and awake at the beginning of touch and had younger GAs at birth showed greater variation in their oxygen saturations (Harrison, Leeper, & Yoon, 1991). Using a standardized protocol of social stimulation, Eckerman, Oehler, Medvin, and Hannan (1994) found that preterm infants of at least 33 weeks postmenstrual age responded to talking by eye opening and arousal, but when touching was added to the talking, the infants showed increased periods of closed eyes and negative facial expressions. Infants with more neurologic insults showed even greater negative responses to touching. This finding suggests that preterm infants are responsive to social stimulation of low intensity but that if the intensity of social stimulation is increased, they are no longer able to cope with it. Furthermore, medical complications further decrease infants' ability to cope with moderate-intensity social stimulation.

Preterm infants have also been found to respond differently to nurses and parents. In one study, preterm infants opened their eyes more when interacting with parents than when interacting with nurses (Minde, Ford, Celhoffer, & Boukydisl, 1975). In another study with sicker infants, preterm infants spent more time in active sleep and less time in sleep–wake transition when with their parents than when with nurses (Miller & Holditch-Davis, 1992). In both of these studies, parents and nurses behaved differently toward infants, with nurses more likely to engage in routine nursing and medical procedures and parents more likely to hold infants and provide positive social stimulation. These findings suggest that preterm infants respond to the less active, more social stimulation provided by parents at first by sleeping and then, as they mature, by awakening to engage in interaction. The early sleeping may serve to conserve energy consumption and promote growth.

Kangaroo care, a nursing intervention to promote mothers' holding their preterm infants in skin-to-skin contact, has been found, in many studies, to increase amount of sleeping—and especially quiet sleep—and decrease crying as compared with periods when the infant is alone in the incubator (Chwo et al., 2002; Ludington, 1990; Ludington-Hoe et al., 2006; Ludington-Hoe et al., 1999; Messmer et al., 1997; Scher et al., 2009). A few researchers, however, have not found any changes in state patterns during kangaroo care (de Leeuw, Colin, Dunnebier, & Mirmiran, 1991) or have found a decrease in active sleep and an increase in transitional sleep, but no change in quiet sleep (Bosque, Brady, Affonso, & Wahlberg, 1995). Studies using historical controls or allowing mothers to choose whether they wanted to provide kangaroo care found that infants receiving kangaroo care had more rapid maturation of sleep–wake states (longer bouts of quiet sleep and alertness and shorter bouts of active sleep) and higher orientation and state scores on the NBAS (Feldman & Eidelman, 2003; Ohgi et al., 2002).

Infant Stimulation. A number of the stimulation interventions used with infants are known to affect sleeping and waking states. In some cases, the goal of the intervention is to alter sleeping and waking states either to lower the infant's arousal so as to provide more energy for growth or to promote more mature state patterns. In other cases, the state effects are side effects of interventions that were designed to alter other aspects of the infant's functioning. This section examines the effects of several different types of infant stimulation interventions currently in use in NICUs.

Nonnutritive sucking is an intervention that has been variously used to soothe irritable infants and to promote feedings and growth. It is known to decrease restlessness and increase sleep time, particularly quiet sleep, in full-term and preterm infants (Liaw et al., 2012; Schwartz, Moody, Yarandi, & Anderson, 1987). The NBAS state scores were not altered in preterm infants offered regular nonnutritive sucking during tube feedings as compared to control infants (Field et al., 1982). Nonnutritive sucking is effective in reducing crying after painful procedures and promoting either alertness or sleeping (Fearon et al., 1997). When given to preterm infants just before feedings, nonnutritive sucking helps them to arouse into a quiet, waking state and then maintain this state, in which they are most likely to feed effectively (Gill et al., 1988; McCain, 1992, 1995; Pickler, Frankel, Walsh, & Thompson, 1996). Nonnutritive sucking is more effective in this arousal than stroking (McCain, 1992). When nonnutritive sucking was used as an intervention to bring preterms to a waking state before feeding, infants receiving the intervention took 5 fewer days to achieve full oral feedings than control infants (McCain et al., 2001). Other researchers did not find a change of state with nonnutritive sucking but did find that preterm infants who received nonnutritive sucking before feedings had higher feeding performance scores and more sleep after feedings (Pickler, Higgins, & Crummette, 1993).

Waterbeds are another infant stimulation intervention known to affect the sleeping and waking states of preterm infants. The purpose of this intervention is to provide compensatory vestibular-proprioceptive stimulation for preterm infants who are largely deprived of this form of stimulation in the NICU. Infants on waterbeds exhibit increased amounts of active and quiet sleep, less irritability, fewer state changes, and decreased crying (Deiriggi, 1990; Korner, Lane, Berry, Rho, & Brown, 1990). These effects are enhanced if the waterbed oscillates (Korner et al., 1990), but even infants on plain waterbeds exhibit more sleep than they do on regular incubator mattresses (Deiriggi, 1990). When infants have been on waterbeds for prolonged periods of time, state effects continue even during periods when the infant is off the waterbed, as evidenced by decreased irritability and increased alertness during a standardized APIB (Korner, Schneider, & Forrest, 1983). It has also been suggested that waterbeds reduce apnea (Korner, Guilleminault, Van den Hoed, & Baldwin, 1978). However, it is unlikely that this effect has clinical significance. When infants treated with theophylline for apnea of prematurity were placed on waterbeds, they showed the same state effects as found in infants without this complication, but they did not exhibit decreased apnea (Korner, Ruppel, & Rho, 1982).

Gentle touching is another form of infant stimulation. Harrison, Oliveet, Cunningham, Bodin, and Hicks (1996) provided 15 minutes of daily gentle human touch to preterm infants in the first 2 weeks of life. Infants had significantly less active sleep and motor activity during the periods of gentle touching. When the frequency of this intervention was increased to three times a day, preterm infants exhibited less active sleep, motor activity, and distress during gentle touching periods but did not differ from control infants on any outcome variable (Harrison, Williams, Berbaum, Stem, & Leeper, 2000). After gentle touching and after Yakson touch, a Korean process of gentle caresses, preterm infants exhibited greater sleep than infants in a control group (Im & Kim, 2009), and this effect was stronger for infants receiving Yakson touch (Im, Kim, & Cain, 2009).

Infant massage is another common infant stimulation technique. It provides both tactile and kinesthetic stimulation because it is necessary to move the infant to provide tactile stimulation to different parts of the body. The purpose of this type of stimulation is primarily to promote growth and augment development, but it also affects infant sleeping and waking states. White-Traut and Pate (1987) used the Rice Infant Sensomotor Stimulation, a 10-minute structured massage of the infant's entire body from head to toe, to provide extra stimulation for growing preterm infants. They found that during massage infants were more alert. In this study, however, infants were taken out of the incubator for the massage, so the state changes might have been the result of changes in the thermal environment. In another study, the intervention protocol was altered to be more contingent to infant cues (White-Traut, Nelson, Silvestri, Patel, & Kilgallon, 1993). Again, the experimental infants showed increased alertness during the intervention and continued to be alert for 30 minutes afterward. In another study, the massage intervention was compared with auditory stimulation alone; auditory stimulation along with massage; and auditory, massage, and rocking combined (White-Traut, Nelson, Silvestri, Cunningham, & Patel, 1997). Infants showed increasing alertness during the intervention in the massage and massage plus auditory groups, whereas the auditory group showed more quiet sleep. The massage, auditory, and rocking group showed minimal changes during the intervention but sustained alertness for 30 minutes afterward. The combined auditory, massage, and rocking intervention was then tested on preterm infants with periventricular leukomalacia (White-Traut et al., 1999). Infants who received this combined intervention showed an increase in alertness over the intervention period and were hospitalized for 9 fewer days. Increased alertness also resulted from this intervention when it was used with infants with prenatal substance exposure (White-Traut et al., 2002). A similar massage protocol that involved both tactile and kinesthetic stimulation resulted in preterm infants showing more mature electrical activity on the EEG (Guzzetta et al., 2011).

In other studies, stroking of the infant's body followed by passive flexion and extension of the extremities for 15 minutes three times a day for 5 to 10 days was shown to result in increased weight gain in preterm infants (Dieter, Field, Hernandez-Reif, Emory, & Redzepi, 2003; Scafidi et al., 1986, 1990), possibly because of increased vagal activity, gastric motility, and IGF-1 (Field, Diego, & Hernandez-Reif, 2011). During massage treatments, infants exhibited more active sleep (Scafidi et al., 1990), but whether these state effects persisted after the treatment period is less clear. In two studies, massage-treated infants exhibited better scores on the NBAS and spent less time asleep (Dieter et al., 2003; Scafidi et al., 1986), whereas in another, no differences in the state organization of treated and control infants were found (Scafidi et al., 1990). Infants receiving moderate pressure massage showed a greater decrease in active sleep, less agitated behavior, and less crying than infants receiving a light pressure massage (Field et al., 2004; Field, Diego, Hernandez-Reif, Deeds, & Figuereido, 2006).

Rocking is a form of infant stimulation usually performed in order to soothe the infant. It has been administered either directly while holding the infant or by placing the infant in special cribs or incubators modified to rock at specific speeds. The immediate effects of rocking are reduced crying (Byrne & Horowitz, 1981). However, the rhythm and direction of rocking are important in determining which of the other states the infant was most likely to exhibit (Byrne & Horowitz, 1981). Exposing preterm infants to rocking over a 2-week period had longer-lasting results (Cordero, Clark, & Schott, 1986). They exhibited increased quiet sleep and decreased active sleep.

In yet another study, preterm infants were placed in a nonrigid reclining chair twice a day for 3 hours from about 30 weeks postmenstrual age until hospital discharge (Provasi & Lequien, 1993). Sleeping and waking states were observed for a 2-hour period for control infants and two 2-hour periods for the experimental infants (once in their beds and once in the infant seat) shortly before discharge. Experimental infants spent more time in quiet sleep and active sleep and less time in quiet and agitated waking than the control infants, but no differences were found in the state patterns of the experimental infants when in their bed and in the infant seat.

Music has also been used as a form of infant stimulation in the NICU. Amon et al. (2006) found that preterm infants experiencing live music as compared to recorded music or no music showed a greater reduction in heart rate and more sleep 30 minutes after the intervention.

In a final type of infant stimulation, Thoman and Graham (1986) placed a "breathing" stuffed bear in the incubator with a preterm infant. The goal of this intervention was to provide a form of rhythmic stimulation that would help the infant organize his or her sleeping and waking patterns. In addition, this form of stimulation was voluntary. Because the bear took up only a small part of the incubator and babies were usually put to sleep in positions in which they were not in physical contact with the bear, infants could choose whether or not to remain in contact with the bear whenever their random movements brought them into contact with it. As compared with controls, experimental infants spent a much greater percentage of time in contact with the area of the incubator with the bear. By the end of the intervention period, experimental infants exhibited significantly increased quiet sleep time. This study has been replicated with two additional samples, and both have shown increased contact with the breathing bear as well as more quiet sleep and less active sleep than infants given a nonbreathing bear (Ingersoll & Thoman, 1994; Thoman, Ingersoll, & Acebo, 1991).

■ Usefulness of Neonatal Sleep–Wake States for Assessment. Sleeping and waking states are ubiquitous characteristics of neonates. The infant's behavioral and physiologic responses are filtered through neural controls mediated by the sleeping and waking states. Although it is certainly possible to give competent nursing care to high-risk infants without considering their sleep–wake states, recognizing specific states will enable the nurse to better interpret both physiologic and behavioral changes. By observing sleeping and waking, the nurse will be able to determine whether physiologic parameters are consistent with those expected in a particular state. Changes in sleeping and waking patterns can be used to help the nurse identify the need for interventions and to aid the evaluation of these interventions. Most importantly, by observing sleeping and waking behaviors, the nurse will come to know each infant better and thus be better able to provide individualized care. This knowledge of individual infants can then be shared with parents to help them develop positive interactions with their children.

SUMMARY

High-risk infants are both dependent on and vulnerable to their early environment—the NICU and intermediate nursery—to maintain their physiologic function, to promote growth and development, and to provide opportunities for the organization of state, behavioral, and social responsiveness. The immaturity and physiologic and neurobehavioral instability of these infants make them particularly vulnerable to environments that do not support their emerging organization and patterns or that do not attend to their cues and respond appropriately. Nurses can and do play a big role in controlling sleep in the NICU environment. It is important that parents are included in these efforts to promote positive sleep–wake patterns in the NICU and once the infant is home.

In summary, the goals in addressing the neurobehavioral needs of high-risk infants are the following:

1. Provide an environment that enhances and supports the infant's developing capabilities
2. Protect the infant from sensory overload and minimize stressors
3. Assist parents in understanding their infant's unique abilities
4. Help parents interact with their infant in ways appropriate to the infant's health status, state, and level of maturity

ONLINE RESOURCES

Brazelton Neonatal Behavioral Assessment Scale (NBAS) and Newborn Behavioral Observations system (NBO)
http://www.brazelton-institute.com/intro.html

The Center for Neurobehavioral Development (University of Minnesota)
http://www.cehd.umn.edu/icd/cnbd

Neonatal Individualized Development Care and Assessment Program (NIDCAP) including Assessment of Preterm Infant Behavior (APIB)
http://www.nidcap.com

Neurobehavioral Assessment of the Preterm Infant (NAPI)
http://childdevelopmentmedia.com/infant-development-evaluation/70140psb.html

Understanding Your Premature Infant (Resource illustrating infant cues and infant sleep states developed by the March of Dimes for parents of preterm infants)
http://www.marchofdimes.com/modpreemie/preemie.html

YouTube: Neurobehavioral Development of Young Children: Neuroscience and Early Trauma ~ Allan Schore, PhD
http://www.youtube.com/watch?v=6SK3vLc8wHo

REFERENCES

Abad, F., Diaz, N. M., Domenech, E., Robayna, M., & Rico, J. (1996). Oral sweet solution reduces pain-related behaviour in preterm infants. *Acta Paediatrica, 85*, 854–858.

Acebo, C., & Thoman, E.B. (1995). Role of infant crying in the early mother–infant dialogue. *Physiology and Behavior, 57*(3), 541–547.

Adam, K., & Oswald, I. (1984). Sleep helps healing [Editorial]. *British Medical Journal (clinical research edition), 289*(6456), 1400–1401.

Adams-Chapman, I. (2009). Insults to the developing brain and impact on neurodevelopmental outcome. *Journal of Communication Disorders, 42*, 256–262.

Als, H. (1986). A synactive model of neonatal behavioral organization: Framework for assessment of neurobehavioral development in the premature infant and for support of infants and parents in the neonatal intensive care environment. Part 1: Theoretical framework. *Physical and Occupational Therapy in Pediatrics, 6*(3–4), 3–53.

Als, H. (1999). Reading the premature infant. In E. Goldson (Ed.), *Nurturing the premature infant: Developmental interventions in the neonatal intensive care nursery* (pp. 18–85). New York, NY: Oxford University Press.

Als, H., Butler, S., Kosta, S., & McAnulty, G. (2005). The Assessment of Preterm Infants' Behavior (APIB): Furthering the understanding and measurement of neurodevelopmental competence in preterm and full-term infants. *Mental Retardation and Developmental Disabilities Research Review, 11*, 94–102.

Als, H., Duffy, F. H., & McAnulty, G. B. (1988). Behavioral differences between preterm and fullterm newborns as measured on the APIB System scores. *Infant Behavior and Development, 11*(3), 305–318.

Als, H., Lawhon, G., Brown, E., Gibes, R., Duffy, F. H., McAnulty, G., & Blickman, J. G. (1986). Individualized behavioral and environmental care for the very-low-birth-weight preterm infant at high risk for bronchopulmonary dysplasia: Neonatal intensive care unit and developmental outcome. *Pediatrics, 78*(6), 1123–1132.

Als, H., Lester, B. M., Tronick, E. C., & Brazelton, T. B. (1982). Manual for the assessment of preterm infant behavior (APIB). In H. E. Fitzgerald & M. Yogman (Eds.), *Theory and research in behavioral pediatrics* (Vol. 1, pp. 64–133). New York, NY: Plenum Press.

American Academy of Pediatrics Task Force on Sudden Infant Death Syndrome. (2011, November). *SIDS and other sleep-related infant deaths: Expansion of recommendations for a safe infant sleeping environment* (Technical Report). Retrieved from www.pediatrics.org/cgi/doi/10.1542/peds.2011-2285

Amiel-Tison, C. (2002). Update of the Amiel-Tison neurologic assessment for the term neonate or at 40 weeks corrected age. *Pediatric Neurology, 27*, 196–212.

Amon, S., Shapsa, A., Forman, L., Regev, R., Bauer, S., Litmanovitz, I., & Dolfin, T. (2006). Live music is beneficial to preterm infants in the neonatal intensive care unit environment. *Birth, 33*(2), 131–136.

Anders, T., Emde, R. & Parmelee, A. (Eds.). (1971). *A manual of standardized terminology, techniques and criteria for scoring of states of sleep and wakefulness in newborn infants.* Los Angeles, CA: UCLA Brain Information Service/BRI Publications Office.

Anders, T. F., & Chalemian, R. J. (1974). The effects of circumcision on sleep-wake states in human neonates. *Psychosomatic Medicine, 36*(2), 174–179.

Anderson, G. C. (1999). Kangaroo care of the premature infant. In E. Goldson (Ed.), *Nurturing the premature infant: Developmental interventions in the neonatal intensive care nursery* (pp. 131–160). New York, NY: Oxford University Press.

Anderson, L. T., Garcia-Coll, C., Vohr, B. R., Emmons, L., Brann, B., Philip, W. S., . . . Oh, W. (1989). Behavioral characteristics and early temperament of premature infants with intracranial hemorrhage. *Early Human Development, 18*(4), 273–283.

Apkarian, P., Mirmiran, M., & Tijssen, R. (1991). Effects of behavioural state on visual processing in neonates. *Neuropediatrics, 22*(2), 85–91.

Arditi-Babchuk, H., Feldman, R., & Eidelman, A. I. (2009). Rapid eye movement (REM) in premature neonates and developmental outcome at 6 months. *Infant Behavior and Development, 32*(1), 27–32.

Ariagno, R. L., Mirmiran, M., Adams, M. M., Saporito, A. G., Dubin, A. M., & Baldwin, R. B. (2003). Effect of position on sleep, heart rate variability, and QT interval in preterm infants at 1 and 3 months' corrected age. *Pediatrics, 111*(3), 622–625.

Ariagno, R. L., Thoman, E. B., Boeddiker, M. A., Kugener, B., Constantinou, J. C., Mirmiran, M., & Baldwin, R. B. (1997). Developmental care does not alter sleep and development of premature infants. *Pediatrics, 100*(6), e9. Retrieved from http://www.pediatrics.org/cgi/content/full/100/6/e9

Ariagno, R. L., van Liempt, S., & Mirmiran, M. (2006). Fewer spontaneous arousals during prone sleep in preterm infants at 1 and 3 months corrected age. *Journal of Perinatology, 26*(5), 306–312.

Armitage, R., Flynn, H., Hoffmann, R., Vazquez, D., Lopez, J., & Marcus, S. (2009). Early developmental changes in sleep in infants: The impact of maternal depression. *Sleep, 32*(5), 693–696.

Asaka, Y., & Takada, S. (2010). Activity-based assessment of the sleep behaviors of VLBW preterm infants and full-term infants at around 12 months of age. *Brain and Development, 32*(2), 150–155.

Axelin, A., Kirjavainen, J., Salanterä, S., & Lehtonen, L. (2010). Effects of pain management on sleep in preterm infants. *European Journal of Pain, 14*(7), 752–758.

Barnard, K. E., & Blackburn, S. (1985). Making a case for studying the ecological niche of the newborn. In B. S. Raff & N. W. Paul (Eds.), *NAACOG Invitational Research Conference. Birth defects: Original Article Series, 21*(3), 71–88.

Bauer, C. R., Langer, J. C., Shankaran, S., Bada, H. S., Lester, B., Wright, L. L., . . . Verter, J. (2005). Acute neonatal effects of cocaine exposure during pregnancy. *Archives of Pediatric and Adolescent Medicine, 159*(9), 824–834.

Bayley, N. (1993). *Bayley scales of infant development* (2nd ed.). San Antonio, TX: The Psychological Corporation.

Bayley, N. (2005). *Bayley scales of infant and toddler development* (3rd ed.). San Antonio, TX: Harcourt Assessment.

Beauchamp, G. K., & Mennella, J. A. (2011). Flavor perception in human infants: Development and functional significance. *Digestion, 83*(Suppl. 1), S1–S6.

Beaver, P. K. (1987). Premature infants' response to touch and pain: Can nurses make a difference? *Neonatal Network, 6*(3), 13–17.

Becker, P. T., Brazy, J. E., & Grunwald, P. C. (1997). Behavioral state organization of very low birth weight infants: Effects of developmental handling during caregiving. *Infant Behavior and Development, 20*, 503–514.

Becker, P. T., Chang, A., Kameshima, S., & Bloch, M. (1991). Correlates of diurnal sleep patterns in infants of adolescent and adult single mothers. *Research in Nursing and Health, 14*(2), 97–108.

Becker, P. T., Grunwald, P. C., Moorman, J., & Stuhr, S. (1991). Outcomes of developmentally supportive nursing care for very low birth weight infants. *Nursing Research, 40*(3), 150–155.

Becker, P. T., Grunwald, P. C., Moorman, J., & Stuhr, S. (1993). Effects of developmental care on behavioral organization in very-low-birth-weight infants. *Nursing Research, 42*(4), 214–220.

Becker, P. T., & Thoman, E. B. (1982). Waking activity: The neglected state of infancy. *Brain Research, 256*(4), 395–400.

Beckwith, L., & Parmelee, A. H., Jr. (1986). EEG patterns of preterm infants, home environment, and later IQ. *Child Development, 57*(3), 777–789.

Bernert, G., von Siebenthal, K., Seidl, R., Vanhole, C., Devlieger, H., & Casaer, P. (1997). The effect of behavioural states on cerebral oxygenation during endotracheal suctioning of preterm babies. *Neuropediatrics, 28*, 111–115.

Bertelle, V., Mabin, D., Adrien, J., & Sizun, J. (2005). Sleep of preterm neonates under developmental care or regular environmental conditions. *Early Human Development, 81*(7), 595–600.

Bhat, R. Y., Hannam, S., Pressler, R., Rafferty, G. F., Peacock, J. L., & Greenough, A. (2006). Effect of prone and supine position on sleep, apneas, and arousal in preterm infants. *Pediatrics, 118*(1), 101–107.

Bhutta, A. T., & Anand, K. J. (2002). Vulnerability of the developing brain. Neuronal mechanisms. *Clinics in Perinatology, 29*, 357–372.

Black, B., Holditch-Davis, D., Schwartz, T., & Scher, M. S. (2006). Effects of antenatal magnesium sulfate and corticosteroid therapy on sleep states of preterm infants. *Research in Nursing and Health, 29*(4), 269–280.

Black, J. E. (1998). How a child builds its brain: Some lessons from animal studies of neural plasticity. *Preventative Medicine, 27*, 168–171.

Black, M., Schuler, M., & Nair, P. (1993). Prenatal drug exposure: Neurodevelopmental outcome and parenting environment. *Journal of Pediatric Psychology, 18*(5), 605–620.

Blackburn, S. T. (2012). *Maternal, fetal and neonatal physiology: A clinical perspective* (4th ed.). Philadelphia, PA: Saunders.

Blackburn, S., & Barnard, K. E. (1985). Analysis of caregiving events in preterm infants in the special care unit. In A. Gottfried & J. Gaiter (Eds.), *Infants under stress: Environmental neonatology* (pp. 113–129). Baltimore, MD: University Park Press.

Blackburn, S., & Patteson, D. (1991). Effects of cycled lighting on activity state and cardiorespiratory function in preterm infants. *Journal of Perinatal and Neonatal Nursing, 4*(4), 47–54.

Borghese, I. F., Minard, K. L., & Thoman, E. B. (1995). Sleep rhythmicity in premature infants: Implications for developmental status. *Sleep, 18*, 523–530.

Bosque, E. M., Brady, J. P., Affonso, D. D., & Wahlberg, V. (1995). Physiologic measures of kangaroo versus incubator care in a tertiary-level nursery. *Journal of Obstetric, Gynecologic, and Neonatal Nursing, 24*(3), 219–226.

Brandon, D. H., & Holditch-Davis, D. (2005). Validation of an instrumented sleep-wake state assessment against biobehavioral assessment. *Newborn and Infant Nursing Reviews, 5*(3), 109–115.

Brandon, D. H., Holditch-Davis, D., & Belyea, M. (1999). Nursing care and the development of sleeping and waking behaviors in preterm infants. *Research in Nursing and Health, 22*, 217–229.

Brandon, D. H., Holditch-Davis, D., & Belyea, M. (2002). Preterm infants born at less than 31 weeks' gestation have improved growth in cycled light compared with continuous near darkness. *Journal of Pediatrics, 140*(2), 192–199.

Brandon, D. H., Holditch-Davis, D., & Winchester, D. M. (2005). Factors affecting early neurobehavioral and sleep outcomes in preterm infants. *Infant Behavior and Development, 28*(2), 206–219.

Brazelton, T. B. (1984). *Neonatal behavioral assessment scale* (2nd ed.). London: Spastics International Medical Publications, in association with William Heinemann Medical Books Ltd.; Philadelphia, PA: JB Lippincott Co.

Brazelton, T. B., & Nugent, J. (2011). *Neonatal behavioral assessment scale* (4th ed.). London, England: Mac Keith Press.

Brazy, J. E. (1988). Effect of crying on cerebral volume and cytochrome aa_3. *Journal of Pediatrics, 112*(3), 457–461.

Buehler, D. M., Als, H., Duffy, F. H., McAnulty, G. B., & Liederman, J. (1995). Effectiveness of individualized developmental care for low-risk preterm infants: Behavioral and electrophysiological evidence. *Pediatrics, 96*, 923–932.

Byrne, J. M., & Horowitz, F. D. (1981). Rocking as a soothing intervention: The influence of direction and type of movement. *Infant Behavior and Development, 4*(2), 207–218.

Campbell, S. K. (2005). *The test of infant motor performance. Test User's Manual* (Version 2.0). Chicago, IL: Infant Motor Performance Scales, LLC.

Carmichael, K., Burns, Y., Gray, P., & O'Callaghan, M. (1997). Neuromotor behavioural assessment of preterm infants at risk for impaired development. *Australian Journal of Physiotherapy, 43*, 101–107.

Chang, Y. J., Anderson, G. C., & Lin, C. H. (2002). Effects of prone and supine positions on sleep state and stress responses in mechanically ventilated preterm infants during the first postnatal week. *Journal of Advanced Nursing, 40*(2), 161–169.

Chwo, M. J., Anderson, G. C., Good, M., Dowling, D. A., Shia, S. H., & Chu, D. M. (2002). A randomized controlled trial of early kangaroo care for preterm infants: Effects on temperature, weight, behavior, and acuity. *Nursing Research, 10*(2), 129–142.

Cohen, G., Xu, C., & Henderson-Smart, D. (1991). Ventilatory response of sleeping newborn to CO_2 during normoxic rebreathing. *Journal of Applied Physiology, 71*(1), 168–174.

Colombo, J., & Horowitz, F. D. (1987). Behavioral state as a lead variable in neonatal research. *Merrill-Palmer Quarterly, 33*(4), 423–437.

Cordero, L., Clark, D. L., & Schott, L. (1986). Effects of vestibular stimulation on sleep states in premature infants. *American Journal of Perinatology, 3*(4), 319–324.

Corff, K. E., Seidemanm, R., Venkataraman, P. S., Lutes, L., & Yates, B. (1995). Facilitated tucking: A non-pharmacologic comfort measure for pain in preterm neonates. *Journal of Obstetric, Gynecologic and Neonatal Nursing, 24*, 143–147.

Corwin, M. J., Lester, B. M., Sepkoski, C., Peuker, M., Kayne, H., & Golub, H. L. (1995). Newborn acoustic cry characterisitics of infants subsequently dying of sudden infant death syndrome. *Pediatrics, 96*, 73–77.

Cowart, B. J., Beauchamp, G. K., & Mennella, J. A. (2012). Development of taste and smell in the neonate. In R. A. Polin, W. W. Fox, & S. H. Abman (Eds.), *Fetal and neonatal physiology* (4th ed., pp. 1899–1907). Philadelphia, PA: Saunders.

Curzi-Dascalova, L., Aujard, Y., Gaultier, C., & Rajguru, M. (2002). Sleep organization is unaffected by caffeine in premature infants. *Journal of Pediatrics, 140*, 766–771.

Curzi-Dascalova, L., Bloch, J., Vecchierini, M., Bedu, A., & Vignolo, P. (2000). Physiological parameters evaluation following apnea in healthy premature infants. *Biology of the Neonate, 77*, 203–211.

Curzi-Dascalova, L., Figueroa, J. M., Eiselt, M., Christova, E., Virassamy, A., d'Allest, A. M. . . . Dehan, M. (1993). Sleep state organization in premature infants of less than 35 weeks' gestational age. *Pediatric Research, 34*, 624–628.

Curzi-Dascalova, L., Peirano, P., & Morel-Kahn, F. (1988). Development of sleep states in normal premature and fullterm newborns. *Developmental Psychobiology, 21*(5), 431–444.

DeHaan, R., Patrick, J., Chess, G. F., & Jaco, N. T. (1977). Definition of sleep state in the newborn infant by heart rate analysis. *American Journal of Obstetrics and Gynecology, 127*(7), 753–758.

Deiriggi, P. M. (1990). Effects of waterbed flotation on indicators of energy expenditure in preterm infants. *Nursing Research, 39*(3), 140–146.

de Jong, M., Verhoeven, M., & van Baar, A. L. (2012). School outcome, cognitive functioning and behavioral problems in moderate and late preterm children and adults: A review. *Seminars in Fetal and Neonatal Medicine, 17*, 163–169.

de Leeuw, R., Colin, E. M., Dunnebier, E. A., & Mirmiran, M. (1991). Physiological effects of kangaroo care in very small preterm infants. *Biology of the Neonate, 59*(3), 149–155.

Denenberg, V. H., & Thoman, E. B. (1981). Evidence for a functional role for active (REM) sleep in infancy. *Sleep, 4*(2), 185–191.

Derbyshire, S. W. (2010). Foetal pain? *Best Practices and Research Clinical Obstetrics and Gynaecology, 24*, 647–655.

Dieter, J. N., Field, T., Hernandez-Reif, M., Emory, E. K., & Redzepi, M. (2003). Stable preterm infants gain more weight and sleep less after five days of massage therapy. *Journal of Pediatric Psychology, 28*(6), 403–411.

DiPietro, J. A., Hodgson, D. M., Costigan, K. A., Hilton, S. C., & Johnson, T. R. (1996). Fetal neurobehavioral development. *Child Development, 67*, 2553–2567.

DiPietro, J. A., & Porges, S. W. (1991). Relations between neonatal states and 8-month developmental outcome in preterm infants. *Infant Behavior and Development*, *14*(4), 441–450.

Doussard-Roosevelt, J., Porges, S. W., & McClenny, B. D. (1996). Behavioral sleep states in very low birth-weight preterm neonates: Relation to neonatal health and vagal maturation. *Journal of Pediatric Psychology, 21*, 785–802.

Dreyfus-Brisac, C. (1968). Sleep ontogenesis in early human prematurity from 24 to 27 weeks of conceptional age. *Developmental Psychobiology, 1*, 162–169.

Dubowitz, L., Ricciw, D., & Mercuri, E. (2005). The Dubowitz neurological examination of the full-term newborn. *Mental Retardation and Developmental Disabilities Research Review, 11*, 52–60.

Duffy, F. H., Als, H., & McAnulty, G. B. (1990). Behavioral and electrophysiological evidence for gestational age effects in healthy preterm and fullterm infants studied two weeks after expected due date. *Child Development, 61*(4), 271–286.

Duxbury, M. L., Henly, S. J., Broz, L. J., Armstrong, G. D., & Wachdorf, C. M. (1984). Caregiver disruptions and sleep of high-risk infants. *Heart and Lung, 13*(2), 141–147.

Eckerman, C. O., Oehler, J. M., Medvin, M. B., & Hannan, T. E. (1994). Premature newborns as social partners before term age. *Infant Behavior and Development, 17*(1), 55–70.

Einspieler, C., & Prechtl, H. F. R. (2005). Prechtl's assessment of general movements: A diagnostic tool for the functional assessment of the young nervous system. *Mental Retardation and Developmental Disabilities Research Review, 11*, 61–70.

Elder, D. E., Campbell, A. J., Larsen, P. D., & Galletly, D. (2011). Respiratory variability in preterm and term infants: Effect of sleep state, position and age. *Respiratory Physiology and Neurobiology, 175*(2), 234–238.

Elder, D. E., Larsen, P. D., Galletly, D., & Campbell, A. J. (2010). Cardioventilatory coupling in preterm and term infants: Effect of position and sleep state. *Respiratory Physiology and Neurobiology, 174*(1–2), 128–134.

El-Dib, M., Massaro, A. N., Glass, P., & Aly, H. (2011). Neurodevelopmental assessment of the newborn: An opportunity for prediction of outcomes. *Brain Development, 33*, 95–105.

Ellingson, R. J., & Peters, J. F. (1980). Development of EEG and daytime sleep patterns in low risk premature infants during the first year of life: Longitudinal observations. *Electroencephalography and Clinical Neurophysiology, 50*(1–2), 165–171.

Fajardo, B., Browning, M., Fisher, D., & Paton, J. (1990). Effect of nursery environment on state regulation in very-low-birth-weight premature infants. *Infant Behavior and Development, 13*(3), 287–303.

Fajardo, B., Browning, M., Fisher, D., & Paton, J. (1992). Early state organization and follow-up over one year. *Journal of Developmental and Behavioral Pediatrics, 13*(2), 83–88.

Fearon, I., Kisilevsky, B. S., Hains, S. M., Muir, D. W., & Tranmer, J. (1997). Swaddling after heel lance, age-specific effects on behavioral recovery in preterm infants. *Journal of Developmental And Behavioral Pediatrics, 18*, 222–232.

Feldman, R. (2006). From biological rhythms to social rhythms: Physiological precursors of mother-infant synchrony. *Developmental Psychology, 42*(1), 175–188.

Feldman, R., & Eidelman, A. I. (2003). Skin-to-skin contact (kangaroo care) accelerates autonomic and neurobehavioural maturation in preterm infants. *Developmental Medicine and Child Neurology, 45*(4), 274–281.

Ferrari, F., Torricelli, A., Giustardi, A., Benatti, A., Bolzani, R., Ori, L., & Frigieri, G. (1992). Bioelectric maturation in fullterm infants and in healthy and pathological preterm infants at term post-menstrual age. *Early Human Development, 28*(1), 37–63.

Fewell, J. E., & Baker, S. B. (1987). Arousal from sleep during rapidly developing hypoxemia in lambs. *Pediatric Research, 22*(4), 471–477.

Field, T., Diego, M., & Hernandez-Reif, M. (2011). Potential underlying mechanisms for greater weight gain in massaged preterm infants. *Infant Behavior and Development, 34*(3), 383–389.

Field, T., Diego, M. A., Hernandez-Reif, M., Deeds, O., & Figuereido, B. (2006). Moderate versus light pressure massage therapy leads to greater weight gain in preterm infants. *Infant Behavior and Development, 29*(4), 574–578.

Field, T., Hernandez-Reif, M., Diego, M., Feijo, L., Vera, Y., & Gil, K. (2004). Massage therapy by parents improves early growth and development. *Infant Behavior and Development, 27*, 435–442.

Field, T., Ignatoff, E., Stringer, S., Brennan, J., Greenberg, R., Widmayer, S., & Anderson, G. C. (1982). Nonnutritive sucking during tube feedings: Effects on preterm neonates in an intensive care unit. *Pediatrics, 70*(3), 381–384.

Foreman, S. W., Thomas, K. A., & Blackburn, S. T. (2008). Individual and gender differences matter in preterm infant state development. *Journal of Obstetric, Gynecologic, and Neonatal Nursing, 37*(6), 657–665.

Franck, L. S. (1987). A national survey of the assessment and treatment of pain and agitation in the neonatal intensive care unit. *Journal of Obstetric, Gynecologic, and Neonatal Nursing, 16*(6), 387–393.

Freudigman, K. A., & Thoman, E. B. (1993). Infant sleep during the first postnatal day: An opportunity for assessment of vulnerability. *Pediatrics, 92*, 373–379.

Fuller, B. F. (1991). Acoustic discrimination of three types of infant cries. *Nursing Research, 40*, 156–160.

Gabriel, M., Grote, B., & Jonas, M. (1980). Sleep induced pO_2 changes in preterm infants. *European Journal of Pediatrics, 134*(2), 153–154.

Gabriel, M., Grote, B., & Jonas, M. (1981). Sleep-wake pattern in preterm infants under two different care schedules during four-day polygraphic recording. *Neuropediatrics, 12*(4), 366–373.

Galland, B. C., Hayman, R. M., Taylor, B. J., Bolton, D. P. G., Sayers, R. M., & Williams, S. M. (2000). Factors affecting heart rate variability and heart rate responses to tilting in infants aged 1 and 3 months. *Pediatric Research, 48*, 360–368.

Gaultier, C. (1990). Respiratory adaptation during sleep in infants [Review]. *Lung, 168*(Suppl.), 905–911.

Gaultier, C. L. (1994). Apnea and sleep state in newborns and infants [Review]. *Biology of the Neonate, 65*(3–4), 231–234.

Gerard, C. M., Harris, K. A., & Thach, B. T. (2002). Spontaneous arousals in supine infants while swaddled and unswaddled during rapid eye movement and quiet sleep. *Pediatrics, 110*(6), e70. Retrieved from http://www.pediatrics.org/cgi/content/full/110/6/e70

Gertner, S., Greenbaum, C. W., Sadeh, A., Dolfin, Z., Sirota, L., & Ben-Nun, Y. (2002). Sleep-wake patterns in preterm infants and 6 month's home environment: Implications for early cognitive development. *Early Human Development, 68*, 93–102.

Gill, N. E., Behnke, M., Conlon, M., McNeely, J. B., & Anderson, G. C. (1988). Effect of nonnutritive sucking on behavioral state in preterm infants before feeding. *Nursing Research, 37*(6), 347–350.

Glass, P. (2005). The vulnerable neonate and the neonatal intensive care environment. In M. G. MacDonald, M. D. Mullett, & M. M. K. Shesia (Eds.), *Avery's neonatology: Pathophysiology and management of the newborn* (5th ed., pp. 111–128). Philadelphia, PA: Lippincott Williams & Wilkins.

Gottfried, A. W. (1985). Environment of newborn infants in special care units. In A. W. Gottfried & J. L. Gaiter (Eds.), *Infant stress under intensive care: Environmental neonatology* (pp. 23–54). Baltimore, MD: University Park Press.

Graven, S. N. (2000). Sound and the developing infant in the NICU: Conclusions and recommendations for care. *Journal of Perinatology, 20*, S88–S93.

Graven, S. N. (2011). Early visual development: Implications for the neonatal intensive care unit. *Clinics in Perinatology, 38*, 671–683.

Gray, L., & Philbin, M. K. (2004). Effects of the neonatal intensive care unit on auditory attention and distraction. *Clinics in Perinatology, 31*, 243–260.

Greisen, G., Hellstrom-Vestas, L., Lou, H., Rosen, I., & Svenningsen, N. (1985). Sleep-waking shifts and cerebral blood flow in stable preterm infants. *Pediatric Research, 19*(11), 1156–1159.

Grunau, R. V., & Craig, K. D. (1987). Pain expression in neonates: Facial action and cry. *Pain, 28*(3), 395–410.

Guzzetta, A., D'Acunto, M. G., Carotenuto, M., Berardi, N., Bancale, A., Biagioni, E., . . . Cioni, G. (2011). The effects of preterm infant massage on brain electrical activity. *Developmental Medicine and Child Neurology, 53*(Suppl 4), 46–51. doi:10.1111/j.1469-8749.2011.04065.x

Haddad, G. G., Lai, T. L., & Mellins, R. B. (1987). Determination of sleep state in infants using respiratory variability. *Pediatric Research, 21*(6), 556–562.

Hahn, J. S., & Tharp, B. R. (1990). The dysmature EEG pattern in infants with bronchopulmonary dysplasia and its prognostic implications. *Electroencephalography and Clinical Neurophysiology, 76*(2), 106–113.

Hand, I. L., Noble, L., Wilks, M., Towler, E., Kim, M., & Yoon, J. J. (2004). Hering-Breuer reflex and sleep state in the preterm infant. *Pediatric Pulmonology, 37*(1), 61–64.

Harper, R. M., Leake, B., Miyahara, L., Mason, J., Hoppenbrouwers, T., Sterman, M. B., & Hodgman, J. (1981). Temporal sequencing in sleep and waking states during the first 6 months of life. *Experimental Neurology, 72*(2), 294–307.

Harrison, L. L., Leeper, J., & Yoon, M. (1991). Preterm infants' physiologic responses to early parent touch. *Western Journal of Nursing Research, 13*(6), 698–713.

Harrison, L., Oliveet, L., Cunningham, K., Bodin, M. B., & Hicks, C. (1996). Effects of gentle human touch on preterm infants: Pilot study results. *Neonatal Network, 15*(2), 35–42.

Harrison, L. L., Williams, A. K., Berbaum, M. L., Stem, J. T., & Leeper, J. (2000). Physiologic and behavioral effects of gentle human touch on preterm infants. *Research in Nursing and Health, 23*, 435–446.

Hayes, M. J., Akilesh, M. R., Fukumizu, M., Gilles, A. A., Sallinen, B. A., Troese, M., & Paul, J. A. (2007). Apneic preterms and methylxanthines: Arousal deficits, sleep fragmentation and suppressed spontaneous movements. *Journal of Perinatology, 27*(12), 782–789.

Heraghty, J. L., Hilliard, T. N., Henderson, A. J., & Fleming, P. J. (2008). The physiology of sleep in infants. *Archives of Disease in Childhood, 93*(11), 982–985.

Hellstrom-Westas, L., Rosen, I., & Svenningsen, N. W. (1991). Cerebral function monitoring during the first week of life in extremely small low birthweight (ESLBW) infants. *Neuropediatrics, 22*(1), 27–32.

High, P. C., & Gorski, P. A. (1985). Recording environmental influences on infant development in the intensive care nursery: Womb for improvement. In A. W. Gottfried & J. L. Gaiter (Eds.), *Infant stress under intensive care: Environmental neonatology* (pp. 131–155). Baltimore, MD: University Park Press.

Holditch-Davis, D. (1990). The development of sleeping and waking states in high-risk preterm infants. *Infant Behavior and Development, 13*(4), 513–531.

Holditch-Davis, D. (1995). Behaviors of preterm infants with and without chronic lung disease when alone and when with nurses. *Neonatal Network, 14*(7), 51–57.

Holditch-Davis, D., Barham, L. N., O'Hale, A., & Tucker, B. (1995). The effect of standardized rest periods on convalescent preterm infants. *Journal of Obstetric, Gynecologic and Neonatal Nursing, 24*(5), 424–432.

Holditch-Davis, D., Belyea, M., & Edwards, L. (2005). Prediction of 3-year developmental outcomes from sleep development over the preterm period. *Infant Behavior and Development, 28*(2), 118–131.

Holditch-Davis, D., Brandon, D. H., & Schwartz, T. (2003). Development of behaviors in preterm infants: Relation to sleeping and waking. *Nursing Research, 52*(5), 307–317.

Holditch-Davis, D., & Calhoun, M. (1989). Do preterm infants show behavioral responses to painful procedures? In S. G. Funk, E. M. Tornquist, M. T. Champagne, L. A. Copp, & R. A. Wiese (Eds.), *Key aspects of comfort: Management of pain, fatigue, and nausea* (pp. 35–43). New York, NY: Springer.

Holditch-Davis, D., & Edwards, L. (1998a). Modeling development of sleep-wake behaviors: II. Results of 2 cohorts of preterms. *Physiology and Behavior, 63*(3), 319–328.

Holditch-Davis, D., & Edwards, L. (1998b). Temporal organization of sleep-wake states in preterm infants. *Developmental Psychobiology, 33*, 257–269.

Holditch-Davis, D., & Hudson, D. C. (1995). Using preterm infant behaviors to identify acute medical complications. In S. G. Funk, E. M. Tornquist, M. T. Champagne, & R. A. Wiese (Eds.), *Key aspects of caring for the acutely ill: Technological aspects, patient education, and quality of life* (pp. 95–120). New York, NY: Springer.

Holditch-Davis, D., & Lee, D. A. (1993). The behaviors and nursing care of preterm infants with chronic lung disease. In S. G. Funk, E. M. Tornquist, M. T. Champagne, & R. A. Wiese (Eds.), *Key aspects of caring for the chronically ill: Hospital and home* (pp. 250–270). New York, NY: Springer.

Holditch-Davis, D., Miles, M., & Belyea, M. (2000). Feeding and non-feeding interactions of mothers and prematures. *Western Journal of Nursing Research, 22*(3), 320–334.

Holditch-Davis, D., Scher, M., & Schwartz, T. (2004). Respiratory development in preterm infants. *Journal of Perinatology, 24*(10), 631–639.

Holditch-Davis, D., Scher, M., Schwartz, T., & Hudson-Barr, D. (2004). Sleeping and waking state development in preterm infants. *Early Human Development, 80*(1), 43–64.

Holditch-Davis, D., Tesh, E. M., Burchinal, M., & Miles, M. S. (1999). Early interactions between mothers and their medically fragile infants. *Applied Developmental Science, 3*, 155–167.

Holditch-Davis, D., & Thoman, E. B. (1987). Behavioral states of premature infants: Implications for neural and behavioral development. *Developmental Psychobiology, 20*(1), 25–38.

Holmes, D. L., Nagy, J. N., Slaymaker, F., Sosnowski, R. J., Prinz, S. M., & Pasternak, J. F. (1982). Early influences of prematurity, illness, and prolonged hospitalization on infant behavior. *Developmental Psychology, 18*(5), 744–750.

Holmes, G. L., Logan, W. J., Kirkpatrick, B. V., & Meyer, E. C. (1979). Central nervous system maturation in the stressed premature. *Annals of Neurology, 6*(6), 518–522.

Horne, R. S., Bandopadhayay, P., Vitkovic, J., Cranage, S. M., & Adamson, T. M. (2002). Effects of age and sleeping position on arousal from sleep in preterm infants. *Sleep, 25*(7), 746–750.

Huntington, L., Hans, S., & Zeskind, P. S. (1990). The relations among cry characteristics, demographic variables, and developmental test scores in infants prenatally exposed to methadone. *Infant Behavior and Development, 13*, 533–538.

Iacovidou, N., Varsami, M., & Syggellou, A. (2010). Neonatal outcomes of preterm delivery. *Annals of the New York Academy of Science, 1205*, 130–134.

Im, H., & Kim, E. (2009). Effect of Yakson and Gentle Human Touch versus usual care on urine stress hormones and behaviors in preterm infants: A quasi-experimental study. *International Journal of Nursing Studies, 46*(4), 450–458.

Im, H., Kim, E., & Cain, K. C. (2009). Acute effects of Yakson and Gentle Human Touch on the behavioral state of preterm infants. *Journal of Child Health Care, 13*(3), 212–226.

Ingersoll, E. W., & Thoman, E. B. (1994). The breathing bear: Effects on respiration in premature infants. *Physiology and Behavior, 56*(5), 855–859.

Ingersoll, E. W., & Thoman, E. B. (1999). Sleep/wake states of preterm infants: Stability, developmental change, diurnal variation, and relation with caregiving activity. *Child Development, 70*, 1–10.

Jarus, T., Bart, O., Rabinovich, G., Sadeh, A., Bloch, L., Dolfin, T., & Litmanovitz, I. (2011). Effects of prone and supine positions on sleep state and stress responses in preterm infants. *Infant Behavior and Development, 34*(2), 257–263.

Jeffery, H. E., Megevand, A., & Page, M. (1999). Why the prone position is a risk factor of sudden infant death syndrome. *Pediatrics, 104*, 263–269.

Jeremy, R. J., & Hans, S. L. (1985). Behavior of neonates exposed in utero to methadone as assessed on the Brazelton Scale. *Infant Behavior and Development, 8*(3), 323–336.

Johnston, C. C., Sherraud, A., Stevens, B., Franck, L., Stremler, R., & Jack, A. (1999a). Do cry features reflect pain intensity in preterm neonates? *Biology of the Neonate, 76*, 120–124.

Johnston, C. C., Stevens, B. J., Franck, L. S., Jack, A., Stremler, R., & Platt, R. (1999b). Factors explaining lack of response to heelstick in preterm newborns. *Journal of Obstetric, Gynecologic and Neonatal Nursing, 28*, 587–594.

Johnston, C. C., Stremler, R., Stevens, B., & Horton, L. (1997). Effectiveness of oral sucrose and simulated rocking on pain response in preterm neonates. *Pain, 72*, 193–199.

Karch, D., Rothe, R., Jurisch, R., Heldt-Hilderbrandt, R., Lübbesmeier, A., & Lemburg, P. (1982). Behavioural changes and bioelectric brain maturation of preterm and fullterm newborn infants: A polygraphic study. *Developmental Medicine and Child Neurology, 24*(1), 30–47.

Kisilevsky, B. S., Hains, S. M., Brown, C. A., Lee, C. T., Cowperthwaite, B., Stutzman, S. S., . . . Wang, Z. (2009). Fetal sensitivity to properties of maternal speech and sound. *Infant Behavior and Development, 32*, 59–71.

Kohyama, J., & Iwakawa, Y. (1990). Developmental changes in phasic sleep parameters as reflections of the brain-stem maturation: Polysomnographical examinations of infants, including premature neonates. *Electroencephalography and Clinical Neurophysiology, 76*(4), 325–330.

Koizumi, H. (2004). The concept of "developing the brain": A new natural science for learning and education. *Brain Development, 26*, 434–441.

Korner, A. F. (1972). State as variable, obstacle, and as mediator of stimulation in infant research. *Merrill-Palmer Quarterly, 18*(2), 77–94.

Korner, A. F., & Constantinou, J. C. (2001). *The neurobehavioral assessment of the preterm Infant: Reliability and developmental and clinical validity*. New York, NY: Guilford Press.

Korner, A. F., Guilleminault, C., Van den Hoed, J., & Baldwin, R. B. (1978). Reduction of sleep apnea and bradycardia in preterm infants on oscillating water beds: A controlled polygraphic study. *Pediatrics, 61*(4), 528–533.

Korner, A. F., Lane, N. M., Berry, K. L., Rho, J. M., & Brown, B. W., Jr. (1990). Sleep enhanced and irritability reduced in preterm infants: Differential efficacy of three types of waterbeds. *Journal of Behavioral and Developmental Pediatrics, 11*(5), 240–246.

Korner, A. F., Ruppel, E. M., & Rho, J. M. (1982). Effects of water beds on the sleep and motility of theophylline-treated preterm infants. *Pediatrics, 70*(6), 864–869.

Korner, A. F., Schneider, P., & Forrest, T. (1983). Effects of vestibular-proprioceptive stimulation on the neurobehavioral development of preterm infants: A pilot study. *Neuropediatrics, 14*(3), 170–175.

Korner, A. F., Stevenson, D. K., Forrest, T., Constaninou, J. C., Dimiceli, S., & Brown, B. W., Jr. (1994). Preterm medical complications differentially affect neurobehavioral functions: Results from a new neonatal medical index. *Infant Behavior and Development, 17*(1), 37–43.

Korner, A. F., & Thom, V. A. (1990). *Neurobehavioral assessment of the preterm infant*. Orlando, FL: The Psychological Corporation, Harcourt, Brace & Jovanovich.

Larroque, B., Ancel, P. Y., Marret, S., Marchand, L., André, M., Arnaud, C., . . . EPIPAGE Study Group. (2008). Neurodevelopmental disabilities and special care of 5-year-old children born before 33 weeks of gestation (the EPIPAGE study): A longitudinal cohort study. *Lancet, 37*, 813–820.

Lawhon, G., & Als, H. (2010). Theoretical perspective for developmentally supportive care. In C. Kenner & J. M. McGrath (Eds.), *Developmental care of newborns and infants* (2nd ed., pp. 19–42). Glenview, IL: National Association of Neonatal Nurses.

Lawhon, G., & Hedlund, R. E. (2008). Newborn individualized developmental care and assessment program training and education. *Journal of Perinatal and Neonatal Nursing, 22*, 133–144.

Lawson, K. R., Turkewitz, G., Platt, M., & McCarton, C. (1985). Infant state in relation to its environmental context. *Infant Behavior and Development, 8*(3), 269–281.

Lee, H. J., Kim, H. S., Kim, S. Y., Sim, G. H., Kim, E. S., Choi, C. W., . . . Choi, J. H. (2010). Effects of postnatal age and aminophylline on the maturation of amplitude-integrated electroencephalography activity in preterm infants. *Neonatology, 98*(3), 245–253.

Lee, H. K. (2002). Effects of sponge bathing on vagal tone and behavioural responses in premature infants. *Journal of Clinical Nursing, 11*, 510–519.

Leppert, M., & Allen, M. C. (2012). Risk assessment and neurodevelopmental outcomes. In C. A. Gleason & S. Devaskar (Eds.), *Avery's diseases of the newborn* (9th ed., pp. 920–936). Philadelphia, PA: Saunders.

Lester, B. M., & Dreher, M. (1989). Effects of marijuana use during pregnancy on newborn cry. *Child Development, 60*(4), 765–771.

Lester, B. M., Garcia-Coll, C., Valcarcel, M., Hoffman, J., & Brazelton, T. B. (1986). Effects of atypical patterns of fetal growth on newborn (NBAS) behavior. *Child Development, 57*(1), 11–19.

Lester, B. M., & Tronick, E. Z. (2004). History and description of the neonatal intensive care unit network neurobehavioral scale. *Pediatrics, 113*, 634–640.

Lester, B. M., Tronick, E. Z., & Brazelton, T. B. (2004). The neonatal intensive care unit network neurobehavioral scale procedures. *Pediatrics, 113*, 641–667.

Levesque, B. M., Pollack, P., Griffin, B. E., & Nielsen, H. C. (2000). Pulse oximetry: What's normal in the newborn nursery? *Pediatric Pulmonology, 30*, 406–412.

Liaw, J. J., Yang, L., Lo, C., Yuh, Y. S., Fan, H. C., Chang, Y. C., & Chao, S. C. (2012). Caregiving and positioning effects on preterm infant states over 24 hours in a neonatal unit in Taiwan. *Research in Nursing and Health, 35*(2), 132–145. doi:10.1002/nur.21458

Lickliter, R. (2011). The integrated development of sensory organization. *Clinics in Perinatology, 38*, 591–603.

Limperopoulos, C. (2010). Advanced neuroimaging techniques: Their role in the development of future fetal and neonatal neuroprotection. *Seminars in Perinatology, 34*, 93–101.

Limperopoulos, C., Bassan, H., Gauvreau, K., Robertson, R. L., Jr., Sullivan, N. R., Benson, C. B., . . . duPlessis, A. J. (2007). Does cerebellar injury in premature infants contribute to the high prevalence of long-term cognitive, learning and behavioral disability in survivors? *Pediatrics, 120*, 584–593.

Lipchock, S. V., Reed, D. R., & Mennella, J. A. (2011). The gustatory and olfactory systems during infancy: Implications for development of feeding behaviors in the high-risk infant. *Clinics in Perinatology, 38*, 627–641.

Liu, J., Zhang, A., & Li, L. (2012). Sleep duration and overweight/obesity in children: Review and implications for pediatric nursing. *Journal for Specialists in Pediatric Nursing, 17*(3), 193–204. doi:10.1111/j.1744-6155.2012.00332.x

Lodrup, K. C., Mowinckel, P., & Carlsen, K. H. (1992). Lung function measurements in awake compared to sleeping newborn infants. *Pediatric Pulmonology, 12*(2), 99–104.

Louis, J., Cannard, C., Bastuji, H., & Challamel, M. J. (1997). Sleep ontogenesis revisited: A longitudinal 24-hours home polygraphic study on 15 normal infants during the first two years of life. *Sleep, 20*(5), 323–333.

Ludington, S. M. (1990). Energy conservation during skin-to-skin contact between premature infants and their mothers. *Heart and Lung, 19*(5, Part 1), 445–451.

Ludington-Hoe, S. M., Anderson, G. C., Simpson, S., Hollingsead, A., Argote, L. A., & Rey, H. (1999). Birth-related fatigue in 34-36 weeks preterm neonates: Rapid recovery with very early kangaroo (skin-to-skin) care. *Journal of Obstetric, Gynecologic and Neonatal Nursing, 28*, 94–103.

Ludington-Hoe, S. M., Johnson, M. W., Morgan, K., Lewis, T., Gutman, J., Wilson, P. D., & Scher, M. S. (2006). Neurophysiologic assessment of neonatal sleep organization: Preliminary results of a randomized, controlled trial of skin contact with preterm infants. *Pediatrics, 117*(5), e909–e923.

Maas, Y. G. H., Mirmiran, M., Hart, A. A., Koppe, J. G., Ariagno, R. L., & Spekreijse, H. (2000). Predictive value of neonatal neurological tests for developmental outcome of preterm infants. *Journal of Pediatrics, 137*, 100–106.

Mann, N. P., Haddow, R., Stokes, L., Goodley, S., & Rutter, N. (1986). Effect of night and day on preterm infants in a newborn nursery: Randomised trial. *British Medical Journal: Clinical Research Edition, 293*(6557), 1265–1267.

Marchette, L., Main, R., & Redick, E. (1989). Pain reduction during neonatal circumcision. *Pediatric Nursing, 15*(2), 207–210.

Marlow, N., Wolke, D., Bracewell, M. A., Samara, M., & The EPICure Study Group. (2005). Neurologic and developmental disability at six years of age after extremely preterm birth. *New England Journal of Medicine, 352*(1), 9–19.

Martin, R., Okken, A., & Rubin, D. (1979). Changes in arterial oxygen tension during quiet and active sleep in the neonate. *Birth Defects: Original Article Series, 15*(4), 493–494.

McCain, G. C. (1992). Facilitating inactive awake states in preterm infants: A study of three interventions. *Nursing Research, 41*(3), 157–160.

McCain, G. C. (1995). Promotion of preterm infant nipple feeding with nonnutritive sucking. *Journal of Pediatric Nursing, 10*, 3–8.

McCain, G. C., Donovan, E. F., & Gartside, P. (1999). Preterm infant behavioral and heart rate responses to antenatal phenobarbital. *Research in Nursing and Health, 22*, 461–470.

McCain, G. C., Gartside, P. S., Greenberg, J. M., & Lott, J. W. (2001). A feeding protocol for healthy preterm infants that shortens time to oral feeding. *Journal of Pediatrics, 139*, 374–379.

McGrath, M. M., Sullivan, M., Devin, J., Fontes-Murphy, M., Barcelos, S., DePalma, J. L., & Faraone, S. (2005). Early precursors of low attention and hyperactivity in a preterm sample at age four. *Issues in Comprehensive Pediatric Nursing, 28*(1), 1–15.

McMahon, E., Wintermark, P., & Lahav, A. (2012). Auditory brain development in premature infants: The importance of early experience. *Annals of the New York Academy of Science, 1252*, 17–24.

Messmer, P. R., Rodriguez, S., Adams, J., Wells-Gentry, J., Washburn, K., Zabaleta, I., & Abreu, S. (1997). Effect of kangaroo care on sleep time for neonates. *Pediatric Nursing, 23*, 408–414.

Meyer, K. A., Wall, M. M., Larson, N. I., Laska, M. N., & Neumark-Sztainer, D. (2012). Sleep duration and BMI in a sample of young adults. *Obesity (Silver Spring), 20*(6), 1279–1287. doi:10.1038/oby.2011.381

Michelsson, K., Rinne, A., & Paajanen, S. (1990). Crying, feeding and sleeping patterns in 1 to 12-month-old infants. *Child: Care, Health and Development, 16*(2), 99–111.

Miller, D. B., & Holditch-Davis, D. (1992). Interactions of parents and nurses with high-risk preterm infants. *Research in Nursing and Health, 15*(3), 187–197.

Milligan, D. W. A. (1979). Cerebral blood flow and sleep state in the normal newborn infant. *Early Human Development, 3*(4), 321-328.

Minde, K., Ford, L., Celhoffer, L., & Boukydis, C. (1975). Interactions of mothers and nurses with premature infants. *Canadian Medical Association Journal, 113*(8), 741–745.

Minde, K., Whitelaw, A., Brown, J., & Fitzhardinge, P. (1983). Effect of neonatal complications in premature infants on early parent-infant interactions. *Developmental Medicine and Child Neurology, 25*(6), 763–777.

Mirmiran, M. (1986). The importance of fetal/neonatal REM sleep. *European Journal of Obstetrics, Gynecology, and Reproductive Biology, 21*(5–6), 283–291.

Mirmiran, M., Baldwin, R. B., & Ariagno, R. L. (2003). Circadian and sleep development in preterm infants occurs independently from the influences of environmental lighting. *Pediatric Research, 53*(6), 933–938.

Mok, J. Y., Hak, H., McLaughlin, F. J., Pintar, M., Canny, G. J., & Levison, H. (1988). Effect of age and state of wakefulness on transcutaneous oxygen values in preterm infants: A longitudinal study. *Journal of Pediatrics, 113*(4), 706–709.

Moseley, M. J., Thompson, J. R., Levene, M. I., & Fielder, A. R. (1988). Effects of nursery illumination on frequency of eyelid opening and state in preterm infants. *Early Human Development, 18*(1), 13–26.

Mouradian, L. E., Als, H., & Coster, W. J. (2000). Neurobehavioral functioning of healthy preterm infants of varying gestational ages. *Journal of Developmental and Behavioral Pediatrics, 21*, 408–416.

Mwaniki, M. K., Atieno, M., Lawn, J. E., & Newton, C. R. (2012). Long-term neurodevelopmental outcomes after intrauterine and neonatal insults: A systematic review. *Lancet, 379*(9814), 445–452.

Myers, B. J., Jarvis, P. A., Creasey, G. L., Kerkering, K. W., Markowitz, P. I., & Best, A. M., III. (1992). Prematurity and respiratory illness: Brazelton Scale (NBAS) performance of preterm infants with bronchopulmonary displasia (BPD), respiratory distress syndrome (RDS), or no respiratory illness. *Infant Behavior and Development, 15*(1), 27–42.

Noble, Y., & Boyd, R. (2012). Neonatal assessment for the preterm infant up to 4 months corrected age: A systematic review. *Developmental Medicine and Child Neurology, 54*, 129–139.

Nugent, J. K., Lester, B. M., Greene, S. M., Wieczorek-Deering, D., & O'Mahony, P. (1996). The effects of maternal alcohol consumption and cigarette smoking during pregnancy on acoustic cry analysis. *Child Development, 67*, 1806–1815.

Obeidat, H., Kahalaf, I., Callister, L. C., & Froelicher, E. S. (2009). Use of facilitated tucking for nonpharmacological pain management in preterm infants: A systematic review. *Journal of Perinatal and Nursing, 23*(4), 372–377.

O'Brien, C. M., & Jeffery, H. E. (2002). Sleep deprivation, disorganization and fragmentation during opiate withdrawal in newborns. *Journal of Paediatrics and Child Health, 38*(1), 66–71.

Oehler, J. M. (1995). Development of mother-child interaction in very low birth weight infants. In S. G. Funk, E. M. Tornquist, M. T. Champagne, & R. A. Wiese (Eds.), *Key aspects of caring for the acutely ill: Technological aspects, patient education, and quality of life* (pp. 120–133). New York, NY: Springer.

Oehler, J. M., Eckerman, C. O., & Wilson, W. H. (1988). Social stimulation and the regulation of premature infants' state prior to term age. *Infant Behavior and Development, 11*(3), 333–351.

Oehler, J. M., Hannan, T., & Catlett, A. (1993). Maternal views of preterm infants' responsiveness to social interaction. *Neonatal Network, 12*(6), 67–74.

Ohgi, S., Fukuda, M., Moriuchi, H., Kusumoto, T., Akiyama, T., Nugent, J. K., . . .Saitoh, H. (2002). Comparison of kangaroo care and standard care: Behavioral organization, development, and temperament in healthy, low-birth-weight infants through 1 year. *Journal of Perinatology, 22*(5), 374–379.

Olischar, M., Klebermass, K., Waldhoer, T., Pollak, A., & Weninger, M. (2007). Background patterns and sleep-wake cycles on amplitude-integrated electroencephalography in preterms younger than 30 weeks gestational age with peri-/intraventricular haemorrhage. *Acta Paediatrica, 96*(12), 1743–1750.

Ottaviano, S., Giannotti, F., Cortesi, F., Bruni, O., & Ottaviano, C. (1996). Sleep characteristics in healthy children from birth to 6 years of age in the urban area of Rome. *Sleep, 19*, 1–3.

Parmelee, A. H., Jr., & Stern, E. (1972). Development of states in infants. In C. D. Clemente, D. P. Pupura, & E. F. Mayer (Eds.), *Sleep and the maturing nervous system* (pp. 200–215). New York, NY: Academic Press.

Parslow, P. M., Harding, R., Adamson, T. M., & Horne, R. S. (2004). Effects of sleep state and postnatal age on arousal responses induced by mild hypoxia in infants. *Sleep, 27*(1), 105–109.

Phillipson, E. A. (1978). Control of breathing during sleep. *American Review of Respiratory Disease, 118*(5), 909–939.

Pickler, R. H., Higgins, K. E., & Crummette, B. D. (1993). The effect of nonnutritive sucking on bottle-feeding stress in preterm infants. *Journal of Obstetric, Gynecologic and Neonatal Nursing, 22*(3), 230–234.

Pickler, R. H., Frankel, H. B., Walsh, K. M., & Thompson, N. M. (1996). Effects of nonnutritive sucking on behavioral organization and feeding performance in preterm infants. *Nursing Research, 45*, 132–138.

Prechtl, H. F. R., & Beintema, J. (1968). *The neurological examination of the full-term newborn infant*. London: Spastics International Medical Publications, in association with William Heinemann Medical Books, Ltd.; Philadelphia, PA: JB Lippincott Co.

Prechtl, H. F., Theorell, K., & Blair, A. W. (1973). Behavioural state cycles in abnormal infants. *Developmental Medicine and Child Neurology, 15*(5), 06–615.

Pressler, J. P., & Hepworth, J. T. (2002). A quantitative use of the NIDCAP tool. *Clinical Nursing Research, 11*(1), 89–102.

Provasi, J., & Lequien, P. (1993). Effects of nonrigid reclining infant seat on preterm behavioral states and motor activity. *Early Human Development, 35*(2), 129–140.

Quillin, S. I. M., & Glenn, L. L. (2004). Interaction between feeding method and co-sleeping on maternal-newborn sleep. *Journal of Obstetric, Gynecologic and Neonatal Nursing, 33*(5), 580–588.

Ramaekers, V. T., Casaer, P., Daniels, H., Smet, M., & Marchal, G. (1989). The influence of behavioural states on cerebral blood flow velocity patterns in stable preterm infants. *Early Human Development, 20*(3–4), 229–246.

Regalado, M. G., Schechtman, V. L., Del Angel, A. P., & Bean, X. D. (1995). Sleep disorganization in cocaine-exposed neonates. *Infant Behavior and Development, 18*, 319–327.

Rivkees, S. A., Mayes, L., Jacobs, H., & Gross, I. (2004). Rest-activity patterns of premature infants are regulated by cycled lighting. *Pediatrics, 113*(4), 833–839.

Robinson, J., Moseley, M. J., Thompson, J. R., & Fielder, A. R. (1989). Eyelid opening in preterm neonates. *Archives of Disease in Childhood, 64*(7, Spec. No.), 943–948.

Roffwarg, H. P., Muzio, J. N., & Dement, W. C. (1966). Ontogenetic development of the human sleep-dream cycle. *Science, 152*, 604–619.

Rosenthal, M. K. (1983). State variations in the newborn and mother-infant interaction during breast feeding: Some sex differences. *Developmental Psychology, 19*(5), 740–745.

Sahni, R., Schulze, K. F., Stefanski, M., Myers, M. M., & Fifer, W. P. (1995). Methodological issues in coding sleep states in immature infants. *Developmental Psychobiology, 28*(2), 85–101.

Saiki, T., Rao, H., Landolfo, F., Smith, A. P., Hannam, S., Rafferty, G. F., & Greenough, A. (2009). Sleeping position, oxygenation and lung function in prematurely born infants studied post term. *Archives of Disease in Childhood: Fetal and Neonatal Edition, 94*(2), F133–F137.

St. James-Roberts, I., & Plewis, I. (1996). Individual differences, daily fluctuations, and developmental changes in amounts of infant waking, fussing, crying, and sleeping. *Child Development, 67*, 2527–2540.

Salisbury, A. L., Fallone, M. D., & Lester, B. (2005). Neurobehavioral assessment from fetus to infant: The NICU network neurobehavioral scale and the fetal neurobehavior coding scale. *Mental Retardation and Developmental Disabilities Research Review, 11*, 14–20.

Sander, L. W., Stechler, G., Burns, P., & Lee, A. (1979). Changes in infant and caregiver variables over the first two months of life: Regulation and adaptation in the organization of the infant-caregiver system. In E. B. Thoman (Ed.), *Origins of the infant's social responsiveness* (pp. 349–407). Hillsdale, NJ: Lawrence Erlbaum.

Sanes, D. H., & Bao, S. (2009). Tuning up the developing auditory CNS. *Current Opinion in Neurobiology, 19*, 188–199.

Scafidi, F. A., Field, T. M., Schanberg, S. M., Bauer, C. R., Tucci, K., Roberts, J., . . . Kuhn, C. M. (1990). Massage stimulates growth in preterm infants: A replication. *Infant Behavior and Development, 13*, 167–168.

Scafidi, F. A., Field, T. M., Schanberg, S. M., Bauer, C. R., Vega-Lahr, N., Garcia, R., . . .Kuhn, C. M. (1986). Effects of tactile/kinesthetic stimulation on the clinical course and sleep/wake behavior of preterm neonates. *Infant Behavior and Development, 9*(1), 91–105.

Scher, A. (1991). A longitudinal study of night waking in the first year. *Child: Care, Health and Development, 17*(5), 295–302.

Scher, M. S., Johnson, M. W., & Holditch-Davis, D. (2005). Cyclicity of neonatal sleep behaviors at 25 to 30 weeks' postconceptional age. *Pediatric Research, 57*(6), 879–882.

Scher, M. S., Johnson, M. W., Ludington, S. M., & Loparo, K. (2011). Physiologic brain dysmaturity in late preterm infants. *Pediatric Research, 70*(5), 524–528.

Scher, M. S., Ludington-Hoe, S., Kaffashi, F., Johnson, M. W., Holditch-Davis, D., & Loparo, K. A. (2009). Neurophysiologic assessment of brain maturation after an 8 weeks trial of skin-to-skin contact on preterm infants. *Clinical Neurophysiology, 120*(10), 1812–1818.

Scher, M. S., Richardson, G. A., Coble, P. A., Day, N. L., & Stoffer, D. S. (1988). The effects of prenatal alcohol and marijuana exposure: Disturbances in neonatal sleep cycling and arousal. *Pediatric Research, 24*(1), 101–105.

Scher, M. S., Steppe, D. A., & Banks, D. L. (1994). Lower neurodevelopmental performance at 2 years in healthy preterm neonates. *Pediatric Neurology, 11*, 121.

Scher, M. S., Steppe, D. A., Dahl, R. E., Asthana, S., & Guthrie, R. D. (1992). Comparisons of EEG sleep measures in healthy full-term and preterm infants of matched conceptional ages. *Sleep, 15*(5), 442–448.

Scher, M. S., Sun, M., Steppe, D. A., Banks, D. L., Guthrie, R. D., & Sclabassi, R. J. (1994). Comparison of EEG sleep state specific spectral values between healthy full-term and preterm infants at comparable postconceptional ages. *Sleep, 17*(1), 47–51.

Scher, M. S., Sun, M., Steppe, D. A., Guthrie, R. D., & Sclabassi, R. J. (1994). Comparisons of EEG spectral and correlation measures between healthy term and preterm infants. *Pediatric Neurology, 10*(2), 104–108.

Schulte, F. J., Busse, C., & Eichhorn, W. (1977). Rapid eye movement sleep, motoneurone inhibition, and apneic spells in preterm infants. *Pediatric Research, 11*(6), 709–713.

Schwartz, R., Moody, L., Yarandi, H., & Anderson, G. C. (1987). A meta-analysis of critical outcome variables in nonnutritive sucking in preterm infants. *Nursing Research, 36*(5), 292–295.

Schwichtenberg, A. J., Anders, T. F., Vollbrecht, M., & Poehlmann, J. (2011). Daytime sleep and parenting interactions in infants born preterm. *Journal of Developmental and Behavioral Pediatrics, 32*(1), 8–17.

Schwichtenberg, A. J. M., & Poehlmann, J. (2009). A transactional model of sleep-wake regulation in infants born preterm or low birthweight. *Journal of Pediatric Psychology, 34*(8), 837–849.

Shaywitz, B. A., Finkelstein, J., Hellman, L., & Weitzman, E. D. (1971). Growth hormone in newborn infants during sleep–wake periods. *Pediatrics, 48*(1), 103–109.

Shimada, M., Segawa, M., Higurashi, M., & Akamatsu, H. (1993). Development of the sleep and wakefulness rhythm in preterm infants discharged from a neonatal intensive care unit. *Pediatric Research, 33*(2), 159–163.

Shimada, M., Takahashi, K., Segawa, M., Higurashi, M., Samejim, M., & Horiuchi, K. (1999). Emerging and entraining patterns of sleep-wake rhythm in preterm and term infants. *Brain & Development, 21*, 468–473.

Shonkoff, J. P., & Phillips, D. A. (2000). *From neurons to neighborhoods: The science of early childhood development.* Washington, DC: National Academy Press.

Simakajornboon, N., Beckerman, R. C., Mack, C., Sharon, D., & Gozal, D. (2002). Effect of supplemental oxygen on sleep architecture and cardiorespiratory events in preterm infants. *Pediatrics, 110*(5), 884–888.

Sizun, J., & Browne, J. V. (2006). *Research on early developmental care in preterm neonates.* New Barnet, UK: John Libbey Publishing.

Skadberg, B. T., & Markestad, T. (1997). Behavior and physiological responses during prone and supine sleep in early infancy. *Archives of Disease in Childhood, 76*, 320–324.

Smith, A. P., Saiki, T., Hannam, S., Rafferty, G. F., & Greenough, A. (2010). The effects of sleeping position on ventilatory responses to carbon dioxide in premature infants. *Thorax, 65*(9), 824–828.

Smith, G. C., Gutovich, J., Smyser, C., Pineda, R., Newnham, C., Tjoeng, T. H., . . . Inder, T. (2011). Neonatal intensive care unit stress is associated with brain development in preterm infants. *Annals of Neurology, 70*, 541–549.

Snider, L., Tremblay, S., Limperopoulos, C., Majnemer, A., Filion, F., & Johnston, C. (2005). Construct validity of the Neurobehavioral Assessment of Preterm Infants. *Physical and Occupational Therapy in Pediatrics, 25*, 81–95.

Sommers, R., Tucker, R., & Laptook, A. (2011). Amplitude-integrated EEG differences in premature infants with and without bronchopulmonary dysplasia: A cross-sectional study. *Acta Paediatrica, 100*(11),1437–1441. doi:10.1111/j.1651-2227.2011.02393.x

Soubasi, V., Mitsakis, K., Nakas, C. T., Petridou, S., Sarafidis, K., Griva, M, . . . Drossou, V. (2009). The influence of extrauterine life on the aEEG maturation in normal preterm infants. *Early Human Development, 85*(12), 761–765.

Spittle, A. J., Doyle, L. W., & Boyd, R. N. (2008). A systematic review of clinimetric properties of neuromotor assessments for preterm infants during the first year of life. *Developmental Medicine and Child Neurology, 50*, 254–266.

Stéphan-Blanchard, E., Chardon, K., Léké, A., Delanaud, S., Djeddi, D., Libert, J. P., . . . Telliez, F. (2010). In utero exposure to smoking and peripheral chemoreceptor function in preterm neonates. *Pediatrics, 125*(3), e592–e599.

Stéphan-Blanchard, E., Telliez, F., Léké, A., Djeddi, D., Bach, V., Libert, J. P., & Chardon, K. (2008). In utero exposure to smoking and peripheral chemoreceptor function in preterm neonates. *Sleep, 31*(12), 1683–1689.

Stephens, B. E., & Vohr, B. R. (2009). Neurodevelopmental outcome of the premature infant. *Pediatric Clinics of North America, 56*, 631–646.

Stevens, B. J., Johnston, C. C., & Horton, L. (1994). Factors that influence the behavioral pain responses of premature infants. *Pain, 59*, 101–109.

Sullivan, C. E. (1980). Breathing in sleep. In J. Orem & C. D. Barnes (Eds.), *Physiology in sleep* (pp. 213–272). New York, NY: Academic Press.

Sullivan, M. C., Msall, M. E., & Miller, R. J. (2012). 17-year outome of preterm infants with diverse neonatal morbidities: Part 1-Impact on physical, neurological, and psychological health status. *Journal for Specialists in Pediatric Nursing, 17*(3), 226–241. doi:10.1111/j.1744-6155.2012.00337.x

Symanski, M. E., Hayes, M. J., & Akilesh, M. K. (2002). Patterns of premature newborns' sleep-wake states before and after nursing interventions on the night shift. *Journal of Obstetric, Gynecologic and Neonatal Nursing, 31*(3), 305–313.

Thoman, E. B. (1975). Early development of sleeping behaviors in infants. In N. R. Ellis (Ed.), *Aberrant development in infancy: Human and animal studies* (pp. 122–138). New York, NY: John Wiley & Sons.

Thoman, E. B. (1990). Sleeping and waking states in infancy: A functional perspective. *Neuroscience and Biobehavioral Reviews, 14*(1), 93–107.

Thoman, E. B., Acebo, C., & Becker, P. T. (1983). Infant crying and stability in the mother-infant relationship: A systems analysis. *Child Development, 54*(3), 653–659.

Thoman, E. B., Denenberg, V. H., Sieval, J., Zeider, L. P., & Becker, P. (1981). State organization in neonates: Developmental inconsistency indicates risk for developmental dysfunction. *Neuropediatrics, 12*(1), 45–54.

Thoman, E. B., & Graham, S. E. (1986). Self-regulation of stimulation by premature infants. *Pediatrics, 78*(5), 855–860.

Thoman, E. B., Holditch Davis, D., & Denenberg, V. H. (1987). The sleeping and waking states of infants: Correlations across time and person. *Physiology and Behavior, 41*(6), 531–537.

Thoman, E. B., Holditch-Davis, D., Graham, S. E., Scholz, J. P., & Rowe, J. C. (1988). Infants at risk for sudden infant death syndrome (SIDS): Differential prediction for three siblings of SIDS infants. *Journal of Behavioral Medicine, 11*(6), 565–583.

Thoman, E. B., Holditch-Davis, D., Raye, J. R., Philipps, A. F., Rowe, J. C., & Denenberg, V. H. (1985). Theophylline affects sleep-wake state development in premature infants. *Neuropediatrics, 16*(1), 13–18.

Thoman, E. B., Ingersoll, E. W., & Acebo, C. (1991). Premature infants seek rhythmic stimulation, and the experience facilitates neurobehavioral development. *Journal of Behavioral and Developmental Pediatrics, 12*(1), 11–18.

Thoman, E. B., & Whitney, M. P. (1989). Sleep states of infants monitored in the home: Individual differences, developmental trends, and origins of diurnal cyclicity. *Infant Behavior and Development, 12*(1), 59–75.

Thomas, K. A. (2000). Differential effects of breast- and formula-feeding on preterms' sleep-wake patterns. *Journal of Obstetric, Gynecologic and Neonatal Nursing, 29*, 145–152.

Thomas, K. A., & Foreman, S. W. (2005). Infant sleep and feeding pattern: Effects on maternal sleep. *Journal of Midwifery and Women's Health, 50*(5), 399–404.

Tikotzky, L., De Marcas, G., Har-Toov, J., Dollberg, S., Bar-Haim, Y., & Sadeh, A. (2010). Sleep and physical growth in infants during the first 6 months. *Journal of Sleep Research, 19*(1 Pt. 1), 103–110.

Tilmanne, J., Urbain, J., Kothare, M. V., Wouwer, A. V., & Kothare, S. V. (2009). Algorithms for sleep-wake identification using actigraphy: A comparative study and new results. *Journal of Sleep Research, 18*(1), 85–98.

Torres, C., Holditch-Davis, D., O'Hale, A., & D'Auria, J. (1997). Effect of standardized rest periods on apnea and weight gain of convalescent preterm infants. *Neonatal Network, 16*(8), 35–43.

Tourneux, P., Léké, A., Kongolo, G., Cardot, V., Dégrugilliers, L., Chardon, K., . . . Bach, V. (2008). Relationship between functional residual capacity and oxygen desaturation during short central apneic events during sleep in "late preterm" infants. *Pediatric Research, 64*(2), 171–176.

Tronick, E. Z., & Lester, B. M. (2004). *NICU network neurobehavioral scale manual.* Baltimore, MD: Brookes Publishing.

Van Cleve, L., Johnson, L., Andrews, S., Hawkins, S., & Newbold, J. (1995). Pain responses of hospitalized neonates to venipuncture. *Neonatal Network, 14*(6), 31–36.

Van Ravenswaaij-Arts, C. M., Hopman, J. C., & Kollee, L. A. (1989). Influence of behavioural state on blood pressure in preterm infants during the first 5 days of life. *Acta Paediatrica Scandinavica, 78*(3), 358–363.

Vecchierini, M. -F., Curzi-Dascolova, L., Ha, T. -P., Bloch, J., & Gaultier, C. (2001). Patterns of EEG frequency, movement, heart rate, and oxygenation after isolated short apneas in infants. *Pediatric Research, 49*, 220–226.

Vernacchio, L., Corwin, M. J., Lesko, S. M., Vezina, R. M., Hunt, C. E., Hoffman, H. J., . . . Mitchell, A. A. (2003). Sleep position of low birth weight infants. *Pediatrics*, 111(3), 633–640.

Vles, J. S., Van Oostenbrugge, R. J., Hasaart, T. H., Caberg, H., Kingma, H., Casaer, P. J., & Blanco, C. E. (1992). State profile in low-risk pre-term infants: A longitudinal study of 7 infants from 32-36 weeks of postmenstrual age. *Brain and Development, 14*(1), 12–17.

Vohr, B. R., Karp, D., O'Dea, C., Darrow, D., Coll, C. G., Lester, B. M., . . . Cashore, W. (1990). Behavioral changes correlated with brain-stem auditory evoked responses in term infants with moderate hyperbilirubinemia. *Journal of Pediatrics, 117*(2 Pt. 1), 288–291.

Volpe, J. J. (2008). *Neurology of the newborn* (5th ed.). Philadelphia, PA: Saunders.

Volpe, J. J. (2009). Cerebellum of the premature infant: Rapidly developing, vulnerable, clinically important. *Journal of Child Neurology, 24*, 1085–1104.

Volpe, J. J., Kinney, H. C., Jensen, F. E., & Rosenberg, P. A. (2011). The developing oligodendrocyte: Key cellular target in brain injury in premature infants. *International Journal of Developmental Neuroscience, 29*, 423–440.

Watt, J. E., & Strongman, K. T. (1985). The organization and stability of sleep states in fullterm, preterm, and small-for-gestational-age infants: A comparative study. *Developmental Psychobiology, 18*(2), 151–162.

Weisman, O., Aderka, I. M., Marom, S., Hermesh, H., & Gilboa-Schechtman, E. (2011). Sleep-wake transitions in premature neonates predict early development. *Pediatrics, 128*(4), 706–714.

Weissbluth, M. (1995). Naps in children: 6 months-7 years. *Sleep, 18*(2), 82–87.

Werner, L. (2012). Early development of the human auditory system. In R. A. Polin, W. W. Fox, & S. H. Abman (Eds.), *Fetal and neonatal physiology* (4th ed., pp. 1882–1898). Philadelphia, PA: Saunders.

Westrup, B., Hellström-Westas, L., Stjernqvist, K., & Lagercrantz, H. (2002). No indication of increased quiet sleep in infants receiving care based on the Newborn Individualized Developmental Care and Assessment Program (NIDCAP). *Acta Paediatrica, 91*, 318–322.

White-Traut, R. C., Berbaum, M. L., Lessen, B., McFarlin, B., & Cardenas, L. (2005). Feeding readiness in preterm infants: The relationship between preterm behavioral state and feeding readiness behaviors and efficiency during transition from gavage to oral feeding. *MCN, American Journal of Maternal Child Nursing, 30*(1), 52–59.

White-Traut, R. C., Nelson, M. N., Silvestri, J. M., Cunningham, N., & Patel, M. (1997). Response of preterm infants to unimodal and multimodal sensory intervention. *Pediatric Nursing, 23*, 169–175, 193.

White-Traut, R. C., Nelson, M. N., Silvestri, J. M., Patel, M. K., & Kilgallon, D. (1993). Patterns of physiologic and behavioral response of intermediate care preterm infants to intervention. *Pediatric Nursing, 1*(6), 625–629.

White-Traut, R. C., Nelson, M. N., Silvestri, J. M., Patel, M., Vasan, U., Han, B. K., . . . Bradford, L. (1999). Developmental intervention for preterm infants diagnosed with periventricular leukomalcia. *Research in Nursing and Health, 22*, 131–143.

White-Traut, R. C., & Pate, C. M. (1987). Modulating infant state in premature infants. *Journal of Pediatric Nursing, 2*(2), 96–101.

White-Traut, R., Studer, T., Meleedy-Rey, P., Murray, P., Labovsky, S., & Kahn, J. (2002). Pulse rate and behavioral state correlates after auditory, tactile, visual, and vestibular intervention in drug-exposed neonates. *Journal of Perinatology, 22*, 291–299.

Whitney, M. P., & Thoman, E. B. (1993). Early sleep patterns of premature infants are differentially related to later developmental disabilities. *Journal of Developmental and Behavioral Pediatrics, 14*(2), 71–80.

Whitney, M. P., & Thoman, E. B. (1994). Sleep in premature and full term infants from 24-hours home recordings. *Infant Behavior and Development, 17*, 223–234.

Witcombe, N. B., Yiallourou, S. R., Walker, A. M., & Horne, R. S. (2008). Blood pressure and heart rate patterns during sleep are altered in preterm-born infants: Implications for sudden infant death syndrome. *Pediatrics*, *122*(6), e1242–e1248.

Wolff, P. H. (1959). Observations on newborn infants. *Psychosomatic Medicine, 21*, 110–118.

Wolff, P. H. (1966). The causes, controls, and organization of behavior in the neonate. *Psychological Issues, 5*(1), 1–105.

Wolke, D., Söhne, B., Riegel, K., Ohrt, B., & Osterlund, K. (1998). An epidemiologic longitudinal study of sleeping problems and feeding experience of preterm and term children in southern Finland: Comparison with a southern German population sample. *Journal of Pediatrics*, 133(2), 224–231.

Wong, F. Y., Witcombe, N. B., Yiallourou, S. R., Yorkston, S., Dymowski, A. R., Krishnan, L., . . . Horne, R. S. (2011). Cerebral oxygenation is depressed during sleep in healthy term infants when they sleep prone. *Pediatrics, 127*(3), e558–e565.

Woods, N. S., Eyler, F. D., Behnke, M., & Conlon, M. (1993). Cocaine use during pregnancy: Maternal depressive symptoms and infant neurobehavior over the first month. *Infant Behavior and Development, 16*(1), 83–98.

Woodson, R., Field, T., & Greenberg, R. (1983). Estimating neonatal oxygen consumption from heart rate. *Psychophysiology, 20*(5), 558–561.

Zahr, L. K., & Balian, S. (1995). Responses of premature infants to routine nursing interventions and noise in the NICU. *Nursing Research, 44*(3), 179–185.

Zinman, R., Blanchard, P. W., & Vachon, F. (1992). Oxygen saturation during sleep in patients with bronchopulmonary dysplasia. *Biology of the Neonate, 61*(2), 69–75.

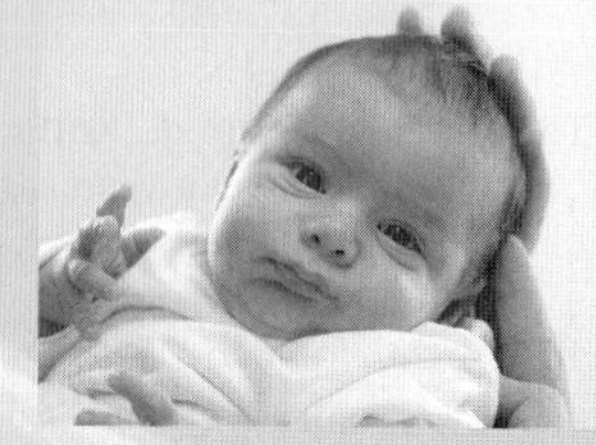

CHAPTER 31

The Neonatal Intensive Care Unit (NICU) Environment

■ Leslie Altimier and Robert D. White

THE NICU

The management of premature infants has advanced over the past three decades to the point that infants born as early as 22 weeks gestation now have a chance of survival in part due to technologic advances. This progress comes with great costs as these tiny patients are at a high risk for a variety of developmental problems, including cognitive deficits, poor academic achievement, and behavior disorders (Taylor, 2010). More focus is now directed to preterm and low-birth-weight infants who have mental health issues such as attention-deficit and attention-deficit-hyperactive disorders, anxiety disorders, and emotional disorders (Hack et al., 2009; Heinonen et al., 2010; Johnson et al., 2010; Vanderbilt & Gleason, 2010). A significant proportion of prematurely born children are now showing behaviors consistent with autism (Limperopoulos, 2009; 2010; Limperopoulos et al., 2008). Although the cause of these findings remains unclear, it is thought that early environmental influences on the brain during critically sensitive developmental periods account for these adverse outcomes (Browne, 2011).

Technology growth in the NICU environment has become increasingly stressful. From the first moments of life, the premature infant is subjected to noxious sounds, bright lights, and a multitude of painful procedures along with repetitive, nonnurturing handling. This altered sensory experience can have a negative impact on an infant's brain development. Infants that are exposed to repeated painful experiences can suffer negative short- and long-term consequences for brain organization during sensitive periods of development (Anand, 2000; Grunau et al., 2010). Seemingly typical handling and caregiving by the NICU staff such as bathing, weighing, and diaper changes indicate that these events were perceived as stress to the infant (Comaru & Miura, 2009; Liaw et al., 2009). As we strive to continue to improve our morbidity and mortality rates, we are challenged to enhance the neuroprotective strategies for these infants, thus demonstrating the need for a developmentally appropriate supportive environment that focuses on the interpersonal experiences of the preterm infant in the NICU.

Infants have demonstrated markedly improved outcomes when the stress of environmental overstimulation is reduced. This can be accomplished by incorporating neuroprotective strategies into the care of neonates as well as the design of a NICU. Neuroprotection has been defined as strategies capable of preventing cell death (McGrath, Cone, & Samra, 2011). Neuroplasticity refers to the ability of the brain to make short-term or long-term modifications to the strength and number of its synaptic neuronal connections in response to incoming stimuli associated with activity and experience. Neuroplasticity is a lifelong property of the human brain, although it is most prominent from birth until late childhood. It is thought that neuroplasticity peaks during early life because it is a period of rapid brain growth with the generation of excessive new synapses (synaptogenesis) and the activity-dependent and experience-dependent pruning of synapses. Neuroprotective strategies are interventions used to support the developing brain or to facilitate the brain after a neuron injury in a way that allows it to heal through developing new connections and pathways for functionality and by decreasing neuronal death (Pickler et al., 2010). Neuroprotective interventions (NPIs) that promote normal development and prevent disabilities include organizational, therapeutic, and environment-modifying measures such as family-centered developmental care (Bonnier, 2008; Altimier & Phillips, 2013). Along with the caregiving environment, the physical environment, including light, sound, temperature, activity, and space, has an impact on infant development (Altimier & Phillips, 2013).

NEONATAL BEHAVIORAL DEVELOPMENT

The neonate's neurologic system is in a highly active stage of development at birth. With volumes of research available demonstrating long-term disabilities in preterm-born children, understanding how we can better support the infant's fragile neurologic system to minimize these impairments can be the beginning of helping the infant to manage within the extrauterine environment (Butler & Als, 2008; Constable et al., 2008; Wolke, Samara, Bracewell, & Marlow, 2008).

Part of this support is the adoption of the conceptual framework and philosophy of developmental care and neuroprotection. The pioneering work by Sameroff, Brazelton, and Als found that assessing the individual infant's ability to cope with excessive stimulation provides the caregiver with information to modify each infant's environment and treatment strategies. When preterm infants were assessed and provided with developmentally supportive individualized care, Als (1986) saw significant outcome improvements, as shown by the following factors:

- Fewer days on the ventilator
- Earlier feeding success
- Shorter hospital stay
- A marked reduction in the number of complications
- Improved neurodevelopmental outcomes during the first 18 months of life

Improvements in medical outcomes as well as hospital costs were demonstrated by Liaw et al. (2009), Altimier, Eichel, Warner, Tedeschi, and Brown (2005) and Hendricks-Munoz et al. (2002) when developmental education and subsequent change of care practices were implemented. Altimier et al.'s (2005) results showed that a change in the physical NICU environment, as well as a comprehensive developmental care training program can be effective in improving the NICU environment and medical outcomes, decreasing length of stay (LOS), and decreasing hospital costs. The results by Hendricks-Munoz et al. (2002) showed that an alternative model of developmental care training can be effective in initiating immediate change in a NICU (Altimier et al., 2005; Hendricks-Munoz, 2002).

While early research focused on improved short-term physiological stability, evidence continues to mount demonstrating that a comprehensive program that addresses NICU design, unit policies, and staff training can positively impact preterm infant brain development and long-term outcome (NPA, 2010). Improved short-term medical outcomes, decreased length of hospitalization, and decreased hospital costs were all associated with developmental education and an improved NICU environment. A study by Louw and Maree (2005) demonstrated statistically significant improvement in the neonatal nurses' handling and positioning of preterm infants after formal exposure to developmental care principles and hands-on experience in the format of a workshop. Reports of young adult outcomes of very-low-birth-weight (VLBW; <1,500 g) children reveal that the neurodevelopmental sequelae and poor educational achievement evident during childhood persist into adulthood (Hack et al., 2004). The increase in psychopathology among VLBW survivors as young adults indicates a need for anticipatory guidance as well as early intervention that might help to prevent potential psychopathology (Hack et al., 2004, 2009).

The full-term healthy infant more often than not has a consistent nurturing caregiver as well as an appropriate variety of stimulation. The full-term infant with 40 weeks of intrauterine development is ready for a variety of sensory experiences, including visual, tactile, auditory, olfactory, and gustatory. Appropriate patterns of adaptation, cognitive learning, and motor control are formed when sensory information interacts with experience. On the other hand, a premature infant typically has numerous caregivers and is exposed to high levels of inappropriate sensory input that can alter adaptation patterns.

To better understand the correlation of early environmental factors to the developmental problems associated with prematurity and other high-risk events, it is essential to examine the environment in which these infants spend a critical period of their development. The neurologic and sensory systems do not exist as separate entities, but are interdependent and comprise the neurobehavioral and neurosensory development of the infant. Every sensory experience is recorded in the brain, leading to a behavioral response, thereby leading to yet another sensory experience. This cyclic interdependent action and reaction is the basis for neurobehavioral and neurosensory development. This chapter briefly reviews the neurologic development of the infant. It highlights the intrauterine environment (maternal womb) environment compared to the extrauterine (NICU) environment. The NICU environment is structured around the developmental core measures: healing environment (physical, sensory, and emotional), safeguarding sleep, minimizing stress and pain, positioning and handling, and partnering with families. Neuroprotective care related to each core measures is outlined by Altimier and Phillips (2013), first with the specific core measure. Each core measure has a related standard with defined infant characteristics, measurable goals, and corresponding neuroprotective interventions.

NEUROLOGIC DEVELOPMENT

The brain is the portion of the central nervous system (CNS) that receives messages; interprets, integrates, and organizes them; and sends out messages to produce motor, language, or emotional responses (Kranowitz, 1998). Neurologic development begins in the third week of gestation with the formation of the neural plate, neural folds, and neural tube. Once the tube is formed and becomes a closed system, different regions of the brain begin to develop. At 4 weeks gestation the brain differentiates into the forebrain, midbrain, and hindbrain. The forebrain translates input from the senses and is responsible for memory formation, thinking, reasoning, and problem solving. The midbrain functions as a relay station, coordinating messages to their final destination. Regulating the heart, breathing, and muscle movements is the function of the hindbrain. At 7 weeks gestation, the brain has the first detectable brain waves. By weeks 9 to 11, the basic brain structure is complete and brain mass increases rapidly (Kenner & King, 2010).

As these different regions of the brain begin to form, the development of the CNS is characterized by the following distinct overlapping processes: neuronal proliferation, neuronal and glial cell migration, organization, and myelination. These processes, especially organization and myelination, continue past birth (Blackburn, 2007).

There are three distinctive layers of the brain that develop as the brain matures: the brainstem, limbic system, and cerebral cortex (Lubbe & Kenner, 2008). The brainstem (medulla, cerebellum, and pons) is first fashioned around the 33rd day of gestation and is nearly complete around the seventh month of gestation (Ayres, 1987; Eliot, 1999; Rhawn, 1999). The brainstem receives sensory messages and relays the information to the cerebral cortex. It processes vestibular sensations necessary for hearing, balance, vision, and focusing attention (Lubbe & Kenner, 2008). It also regulates autonomic functions of internal organs, such as breathing, heartbeat, and digestion (Ayres, 1987; Kranowitz, 1998).

The limbic system (basal ganglia, hippocampus, amygdala, and hypothalamus) is located in the center of the brain. The cognitive brain (cerebrum) is known as the cerebral cortex and performs the most complex organizing of sensory input. The cerebral cortex is highly specialized and contains specific areas for dealing with voluntary functions in the body (Ayres, 1987; Eliot, 1999). Although the neurological system is one of the earliest systems to develop in the embryo, it is not fully matured until adulthood.

There are four areas of the nervous system function: autonomic, sensory, motor, and state regulation. These areas all develop before birth, yet maturation of these functions is not attained until after birth. Autonomic function includes self-regulation of respirations, heart rate (HR), temperature, and nutritional intake. The infant must adapt and respond to many changes simultaneously to survive in this new environment (Blackburn, 2007; Volpe, 2008). The sensory system (discussed later) begins before birth, but maturation of each system continues after birth. In utero, the sensory systems develop in precise order, and that order should be unaltered. Tactile (touch) develops first, then vestibular, followed by olfactory (smell), gustatory (taste), auditory (hearing), and visual (sight). Motor function (discussed under the Positioning and Handling section) also begins before birth and is the result of coordination between neurodevelopment and muscular development. State regulation patterns after birth are individual; however, attentional abilities are reflective of the infant's increasing ability to habituate to the environment (McGrath, 2008).

The development of the brain, both structure and function, is shaped by the influence and interaction of four major factors. These include genetic endowment, internal or endogenous stimulation and sleep, external experiences and stimulation of the sensory organs, and the environment. The brain architecture, cell differentiation, cell migration, primary or initial cell location, and response to initial stimulation are directed by the genes or genetic endowment. Outside stimulation of the environment can influence or alter the expression or effect of a given gene. Spontaneous brain activity that occurs in the absence of outside stimulation during fetal neurodevelopment (internal or endogenous stimulation and sleep) occurs primarily during the last 20 weeks of gestational life. External experiences and stimulation of the sensory organs occur with each sensory system. The initial stimulation is internal or endogenous; but at a critical or sensitive point in development, outside stimulation, and experience are needed for further development. Four components of the environment influence fetal, infant, and child development. These are the physical, chemical, sensory, and social/emotional environments. Events and stimuli from each of the four environments are capable of altering the course and outcome of developmental processes, which can be positive or negative (Graven & Browne, 2008a). (For more detailed information on neurobehavioral development and the neurologic system, see Chapter 30.)

INTRAUTERINE VERSUS EXTRAUTERINE ENVIRONMENT

Sensory Integration

Brain development in the fetus, neonate, and infant includes not just sensory systems but motor systems, social/emotional systems, and the cognitive system, which are connected and integrated during development. The maternal womb, or intrauterine environment, is conducive to positive sensory input, which is crucial for normal brain development in a developing fetus. The intrauterine environment protects the developing fetus against harsh outside stimulation while providing a variety of tactile, vestibular, chemical, visual, and auditory sensory stimuli in an integrated, multimodal fashion (Lickliter, 2011). The intrauterine environment of a developing fetus is characterized by generalized extremity flexion and containment, limited light and noise exposure, sleep cycle preservation, and unrestricted access to the mother via somatosensory auditory, and chemosensory pathways (NPA, 2010). The uterine wall provides secure boundaries for the developing fetus. Vestibular and tactile stimuli come from maternal and fetal movements and from contact with warm amniotic fluid as well as from contact with body parts and the wall of the uterus. Hormonal cycles of the mother provide rhythmic and cyclical stimulation. Nutritional needs of the fetus are met by the placenta. Auditory input includes maternal voice, bowel sounds, blood flow through the placenta and umbilical cord, and filtered sounds from the extrauterine environment, transmitted through liquid and solid media.

Prematurely born neonates are exposed to fluctuations in temperature, touch, light, sound, olfaction, oxygen, and nutrients that are very different from those they have experienced in utero. These negative sensory inputs replace the positive sensory inputs into the developing brain, which can permanently alter normal brain development. The developing brain is extremely sensitive to the appropriate levels of sensory stimuli and alterations can result in abnormal structural and functional development of the brain. This could account for the behavioral, cognitive, and functional deficits that many premature infants manifest (Rees, Harding, & Walker, 2011). Babies of low birth weight, or VLBW, many of whom are also small for gestational age, are at increased risk for auditory and visual impairment including sensorineural hearing loss and deficits in visual acuity, color vision, and contrast sensitivity. Additionally, long-term alterations in retinal function, subtle deficits in neural conduction in auditory pathways, and a reduction in the startle response, which is thought to indicate the ability of the CNS to filter out extraneous stimuli, have all been demonstrated (Bui et al., 2002; Rehn et al., 2002, 2004).

When an infant is born prematurely, the still-developing brain and sensory systems are affected by the continuous interplay of stimuli in the NICU. Events, stimuli, and environmental factors can support the processes of sensory development or create significant interference. Sensory interference may occur when immature sensory systems are stimulated out of turn or with inappropriate stimuli. It is essential that background neurosensory stimulation be kept at a level such that sensory systems can discriminate and accommodate meaningful signals or stimulation. This observation is especially true for sound, touch, smell, position, and comfort, which are part of early neurosensory development and in utero learning (or NICU learning) (Graven, 2006).

MODELS OF DEVELOPMENTAL CARE

Developmental care models are not new. They date back to Florence Nightingale in the 19th century with her theory on the importance of the nurturing, healing environment for the patient's restoration of health (Als, 1982, 1986; Altimier, 2011). Her focus was on the importance of a clean, well-lit, well-ventilated environment to provide the patient health and improve outcomes (Nightingale, 1860). Healing environments suggest that the hospital environment can make a difference in how quickly a patient recovers and that patients do experience a positive outcome in an environment that incorporates natural light, elements of nature, soothing colors, meaningful and varying stimuli, peaceful sounds, pleasant views, and a sense of beauty (Altimier, 2004).

The impact of the NICU environment on the infant's developing brain became evident to health care providers in the 1970s (Brazelton, 1974; Brazelton, Parker, & Zuckerman, 1976). Als synactive theory, building on the earlier work of Brazelton, interpreted the developmental process to be based on subsystem interaction between a neonate's internal functioning, the environment, and caregivers. The theory proposes that, at any given time in development, various subsystems interact with the environment. When there is imbalance within one subsystem, all other subsystems are affected (Als, 1982; Brazelton, 1974). The Universe of Developmental Care (UDC) model is a recent reformulation of neonatal developmental care theory. The UDC model was introduced in 2008 by Gibbins, Hoath, Coughlin, Gibbins, and Franck (2008) and portrays a patient- and family-centric environment within the health care universe. It extends the synactive theory with the concept of a shared surface interface, portrayed as the skin forming a link between the body/organism and environment in which care is rendered and received. The UDC approach recognizes the interactive link between all developing systems and the caregiver/family, while simultaneously providing a practical basis for formulating individualized patient care plans within the NICU's complex technological environment (Milford & Zapalo, 2010).

The Joint Commission identified opportunities to improve disease management and reduce mortality through the development of disease-specific core measure sets related to specific medical conditions. Coughlin, Gibbins, and Hoath (2009) proposed five core measures related to developmental cares that were nondisease specific medical conditions. These five core measures for developmental care are focused on care actions that are disease-independent, yet essential to promote healthy growth and development of the infant and family. The five core measures identified were protected sleep, pain and stress assessment and management, activities of daily living (positioning, feeding, and skin care), family-centered care (FCC), and the healing environment (Coughlin et al., 2009).

The Neonatal Integrative Developmental Care model simplified aspects from the UDC Model and incorporated concepts from the Core Measures of Neonatal Developmental Care. The core measures/neuroprotective principles are depicted as petals of a lotus with overlapping petals demonstrating the integrative nature of developmental care (Altimier, 2011). Further exploration of the literature by this author has resulted in the recategorization and expansion of the five neonatal CORE measures first introduced by Coughlin et al. (2009) to seven distinct developmental CORE Measures (Neuroprotective Practices) of Neonatal Care: Healing Environment, Safeguarding Sleep, Optimizing Nutrition, Minimizing Stress and Pain, Positioning and Handling, Protecting Skin, and most importantly, Partnering with Families (see Figure 31.1). These developmental CORE measures/neuroprotective practices of neonatal care will be highlighted throughout this chapter (Altimier & Phillips, 2013).

HEALING ENVIRONMENT

The NICU is where an extraordinary period of growth and development will take place for premature infants. Because the infant is no longer protected in the uterus, the physiologic and neuroprotective needs have dramatically changed. The healing environment encompasses the physical environment (space, privacy, and safety) as well as the sensory environment (noise, light, thermoregulation, and olfaction).

The physical environment involves not only space, but characteristics of space, which affect position, movement, motor development, and the ability to move. The chemical environment includes nutrition, nutritional factors, and

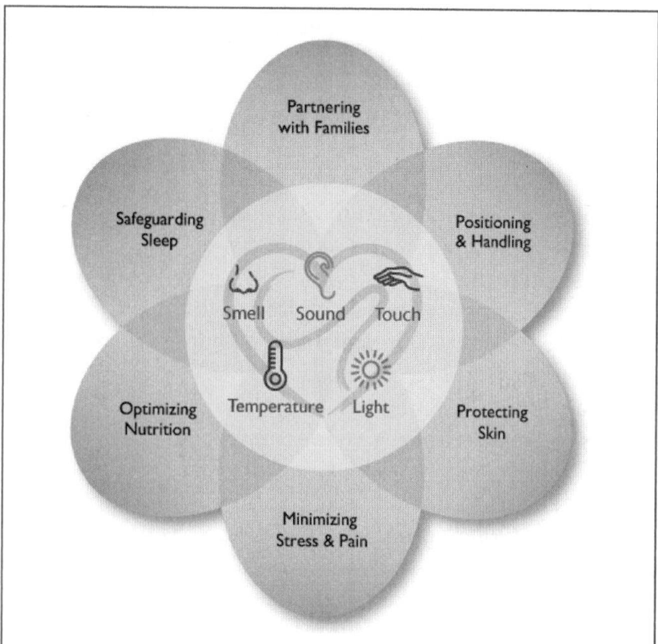

FIGURE 31.1 Neonatal integrative developmental care model. Courtesy of Philips Children's Medical Ventures.

toxin exposures. The factors from the chemical environment (nutrition and toxins) are most likely to create not only direct effects on the fetus or infant but also the epigenetic effects that alter gene expression. The sensory environment includes the exposures and experiencing of touch/temperature, movement, smell, noise/voice, and light/vision. The social/emotional environment attaches the social and emotional characteristics to sensory stimuli, which create memory circuits in the limbic (emotional development) and the social learning centers. These social/emotional stimuli associated with touch, smell, hearing, and vision, in addition to cortical changes, have direct effects in the areas of social and emotional learning and memory. All sensory stimuli carry social and emotional connections and characteristics. Adverse environmental factors can significantly interfere with health and appropriate neurodevelopment and neuroprocessing. Many environmental insults can result in lifelong alterations in brain development and function (Graven & Browne, 2008a).

Physical Environment (Space, Privacy, and Safety)

Toward Improving the Outcome of Pregnancy, published in 1976 by the March of Dimes, was a landmark publication written by a multidisciplinary committee to provide a rationale for planning and policy for regionalized perinatal care, as well as details of roles and facility design (Committee on Perinatal Health, 1976).

In 1992, a multidisciplinary NICU Committee, under the auspices of the Physical and Developmental Environment of the High-Risk Infant Project, first reached consensus on the first edition of recommended standards for NICU design. The purpose of this committee was to provide health care professionals, architects, interior designers, state health care facility regulators, and others involved in the planning of NICUs with a comprehensive set of minimum standards based on clinical experience and an evolving scientific database. The intent was to optimize design within the constraints of available resources, and to facilitate excellent health care for the infant in a setting that supports the central role of the family and the needs of the staff.

A way to promote the ideals of neurodevelopmental care and FCC is through appropriate environmental modifications or construction of new NICU facilities. The design should meet the neurodevelopmental needs of the infants, provide adequate space and facilities for FCC, and meet the needs of the NICU staff (Stevens, Helseth, & Kurtz, 2010).

One systematic review collectively linked a range of aspects of the physical environment of the NICU to the well-being of patients, family comfort, and the caregiving process. Single-family rooms were deemed superior compared to open-bay units for patient care and parent satisfaction (Domanico, Davis, Coleman, & Davis, 2010). Key factors associated with improved outcomes included increased privacy, increased parental involvement in patient care, assistance with infection control, noise control, improved sleep, decreased length of hospital stay, and reduced rehospitalization (Shahheidari, & Homer, 2012). Additionally, Shepley, Harris, and White (2008) demonstrated that the availability of individual patient rooms seemed to promote parental interaction with the baby and led to decreased rates of rehospitilization; positively influencing the outcomes for the infants.

The design of the NICU does impact outcomes for patients, families, and staff. When considering NICU design and unit configuration, it is important to remember that families and staff have different needs. Family needs include an emphasis on privacy and individualized care, whereas staff needs often emphasize efficiency and visibility. Single-family rooms are associated with shorter length of stay, increased privacy and opportunities for parental interaction, and fewer patient infections than those associated with open-bay wards. Parents also preferred the intimacy of a single-family room, and the noise levels were also decreased. Staff in single-family rooms expressed concerns about higher workloads due to decreased visibility of infants as well as diminished opportunities for staff interaction and communication (Shahheidari & Homer, 2012).Attention is given to the NICU configuration, the location within the hospital, minimum space, clearance, and privacy requirements for the infant space. Family, staff, administrative, and general support space is delineated. Attention is focused on illumination guidelines (ambient, day-lighting, and procedural) and acoustical guidelines (floor, wall, and ceiling surfaces). Electrical, gas, mechanical, isolation, ambient temperature, and ventilation recommendations likewise are outlined in the recommended standards. Specific guidelines around single-family rooms (SFRs) are outlined in Standard 6. Private (single-family) rooms allow improved ability to provide individualized and private environments for each baby and family when compared to multipatient rooms or pods. It has been suggested that caring for infants in individual private rooms in a NICU, in contrast to the open-bay environment, will lead to improved infant outcomes (McGrath, 2005). Decreased hospital-acquired infections, increased job satisfaction, and improved team support are some of the documented benefits from single-room NICUs (Walsh, McCullough, & White, 2006). The single-room NICU is a strategy that could address environmental concerns and minimize iatrogenic effects by reducing the risk of infection and stress on the preterm infant. The latest recommendations are now used worldwide and are available at http://www.nd.edu/~nicudes (White, Smith, & Shepley, 2013).

Sensory Environment (Tactile/Touch/Thermoregulation, Chemosensory [Gustatory and Olfactory]; Noise [Auditory], Light [Visual])

■ Tactile/Touch/Thermoregulation. The first principle of neonatal care is thermoregulation. The infant moves from a fluid-filled warm intrauterine environment to a dry cool environment. A major goal of neonatal care is to provide a neutral thermal environment in which an infant is neither gaining nor losing heat at the expense of energy expenditure. The physical environment (macroenvironment) should incorporate the following factors:

- Temperature: 72°F to 78°F (22°C–26°C)
- Relative humidity: 30% to 60%
- Air exchange six per hour (two with outside air exchange)
- All air filtered with at least the efficiency specified in the FGI (Facilities Guidelines Institute) guidelines (FGI, 2010).

To enhance the development of the preterm infant, frequent attention is often on the thermoregulatory (microenvironment) of the infant. The optimal environment for the infant is skin-to-skin caregiving by the mother, also known as kangaroo care (KC). Along with thermoregulatory properties, KC has demonstrated an improvement with breast milk feeding rates. There is also a clear relationship between KC and parental access to their infant in the NICU. Free access demonstrated a higher KC rate as well as breast milk feeding rate (de Vonderweid & Leonessa, 2009). When the parents are unavailable to skin-to-skin or skin-to-skin is not possible, thermoregulatory factors should focus on the infant's individual bed space (microenvironment), whether it is a radiant warmer, incubator, or open crib. To maintain a constant central temperature within narrow limits (36.5°C–37.5°C), VLBW infants or premature infants need to be cared for in either incubators or radiant warmers (Altimier, 2012). The trend in neonatal care has been toward the use of dual-function infant incubators. The dual functions available in these incubators are the radiant warmer mode (open-type incubator) and the incubator mode (closed-type incubator). This new technology allows for care of a critically ill premature infant in a highly humidified environment (incubator mode), which can then be switched to the radiant warmer mode during a treatment, procedure, or for family space. These high-tech incubators (available through Philip's Healthcare, Monroeville, PA, and GE Healthcare, Laurel, MD) are designed to provide the benefits of a humidified system while still permitting easy access to patients, an enclosed environment to decrease insensible water loss, and optimal protection from environmental change.

Attention should be given to equipment on the market that have dramatically decreased decibel levels, further enhancing the developing infant. Covers specifically made for incubators are available to minimize light reaching the infant's eyes. Positioning an infant in a midline, flexed, and contained position with the assistance of therapeutic positioning aids and swaddling decreases the surface area of the infant exposed to environmental air, thus reducing radiant and convective heat losses. Additionally, this flexed and contained position offers additional temperature stability for the infant by minimizing extraneous movement and energy expenditure (Altimier, 2012).

■ Chemosensory (Gustatory and Olfactory). Providing supports for mothers and infants to be together early in the NICU stay is essential in supporting the gustatory and olfactory sensory development. Providing odor and taste of the mother's milk has been shown to facilitate the infant's mouthing, sucking, arousal, and calming from irritability, especially in preparation for oral feeding (Rattaz, Goubet, & Bullinger, 2005; Sullivan & Toubas, 1998). Providing a pacifier with mother's milk has been shown to increase nonnutritive sucking, intake, and growth and to shorten the length of hospitalization (Als et al., 2003; Bingham, Abassi, & Sivieri, 2003; Chaze & Luddington-Hoe, 1984). Providing multisensory experiences such as combining odor and taste with proprioceptive and kinesthetic, visual and auditory input can potentiate sensory organization during feeding. Holding the baby close to the caregiver's body serves to provide this organized multisensory environment (Browne, 2008).

The olfactory system is functional by 28 weeks gestation (Liu et al., 2007). Olfaction (smell) is initiated by neural excitation in response to specific molecules in the immediate surroundings. Olfactory information (in the uterus and breast for the neonate) is transmitted directly from the nose to the cerebral cortex. Maternal odor influences neonatal behavior (Milford & Zapalo, 2010). A mother's scent has been found to facilitate state regulation and optimal feeding experiences for both term and preterm infants. Since olfaction is functional in the second trimester, sensory stimuli from the NICU environment rather than the mother may interfere with its development, as well as other sensory development and attachment (Schaal, Hummel, & Soussigan, 2004).

Neonates' sense of smell is stimulated primarily by unpleasant odors. A variety of odorous products, such as cleaners, skin preps, antibiotics, and alcohol (wipes and hand-gels), are often present in the typical NICU environment. Additionally, the neonate is exposed to fragrances or aftershave worn by staff members. Infants may respond to noxious olfactory stimuli with altered respirations, transient apnea, and/or an increased HR (Gardner & Goldson, 2002). Bartocci et al. (2000) found that the smell of NICU detergent, once detected by the neonate, elicited a response that decreases cerebral blood flow to the right hemisphere of the brain (Bartocci et al., 2000).

The emotional content of odors is highly plastic as it is modifiable by a few hours of mere exposure or by the pairings with reinforcers provided by caregivers (Liu et al., 2007). It has been shown that people can recall a scent with 65% accuracy after 1 year, because smells are processed by the same part of the brain that handles memories and emotions.

Enhancing the olfactory environment can be achieved through the utilization of olfactory NPIs. These positive NPIs may include maternal breast scent via a breast pad, soft cloth, or a Snoedel (Philips Children's Medical Ventures, Monroeville, PA). Pure sheep wool incorporated into the high-quality flannel doll absorbs the parents' scent and slowly releases it. Skin-to-skin contact helps to support the discrimination of maternal breast scent. Mouth care provided with breast milk helps the infant recognize the mother's smell and associates that smell with food and feeding when the infant is able to nipple feed.

Staff should not wear perfume, cologne, or aftershave in the NICU. Available unscented procedure preparation products should be used (Milford & Zapalo, 2010). Alcohol wipes should not be opened near an infant's head, and preferably, outside of the incubator environment. Cleaning products utilized in the NICU should be unscented. Laundry services should also use unscented products. The odor of tobacco on caregiver bodies and clothing as well as the odors of dry cleaning chemicals should be avoided (Lawhon & Als, 2010). Behaviorally, staff should be educated on this topic to prevent olfactory overstimulation.

■ Noise. At birth, ears are capable of discerning among more than 300,000 sounds. The brain processes sounds a thousand times faster than images and registers sounds even during sleep. The constant bath of noise affects everything from concentration to health. The word *noise* comes from *nausea*, the Latin word for sickness. Excessive noise levels in the NICU can damage the developing cochlea and delicate auditory structures, especially the hair cells of the cochlea, resulting in hearing loss and arousal (Moon, 2011). Arousal is important with premature infants who are unable to inhibit responses. High noise levels in NICUs affect infants as well as staff and families. Loud transient noise has been shown to cause immediate physiologic effects such as increased HR, blood pressure and respiratory rate (RR), apnea and bradycardia, hypoxia, and increased intracranial pressure (Wachman & Lahav, 2011). Additionally, noise contributes to sleep disturbance and hearing impairment, and decreases oxygen saturation, which have a negative impact on nervous system development (Chen, Chen, Wu, Huang, Wang, & Hsu, 2009; Domanico, Davis, Coleman, & Davis, 2010; Graven, 2006; Krueger, Shue, & Parker, 2007).

Both the facility itself and operations occurring in the NICU impact the acoustical environment. Heating and ventilation systems are a challenge in a unit that attempts to provide private, separate areas that require a full ceiling-to-floor separation. From a budgetary perspective, it may substantially increase the cost of the unit renovation or construction. Those units that have met the fiscal and physical challenges of providing adequate ventilation have done so in an attempt to provide a more homelike atmosphere.

Much of the therapy provided in the NICU is noisy, making it difficult to facilitate developmentally beneficial auditory stimuli. These high noise levels are often a result of equipment, alarms, nonacoustical finishes, communication devices, and talking, as well as the underlying heating, ventilation, and air conditioning system. NICU sound levels vary based on the hour of day and are often related to activities such as shift change and medical rounds (Krueger, Schue, & Parker, 2007). SFRs and larger clinical patient areas help reduce environmental noise because sound transmission declines geometrically as distances are increased (White, Smith, & Shepley, 2013).

The recommended guidelines for the acoustic environment state that:

> Infant rooms, staff work areas, and family areas shall be designed to produce minimal background noise and to contain and absorb as much transient noise as possible. The combination of continuous background sound and operational sound shall not exceed an hourly Leq of 45 dB [decibel] and an hourly L10 of 50 dB, both A-weighted slow response. Transient sounds or Lmax shall not exceed 65 dB, A-weighted, slow response in these rooms/areas. In staff work areas, family area, and staff lounge areas, the combination of continuous background sound and operational sound shall not exceed an hourly Leq of 50 dB and an hourly L10 of 55 dB levels, both A-weighted slow response. Transient sounds or Lmax shall not exceed 70 dB, A-weighted, slow response in these areas. (White, Smith, & Shepley, 2013)

Achieving these desired sound levels can help facilitate infant sleep and allow the baby to hear human voices at normal conversations (Philben, 2004). Both intensity and duration of sound exposure should be considered when evaluating the noise level in a NICU. Awareness of the impact of increased census and equipment on sound levels can influence health care personnel's ability to provide environmentally appropriate care to premature infants. Noise criterion ratings should be considered when selecting new equipment.

Infant bed areas should be situated to produce minimal background noise and to contain and absorb as much transient noise as possible. Many sound control features should be considered when designing a NICU. Evidence-based sound-reducing strategies have been shown to decrease decibel levels by 4 to 6 dB when planning environment management as part of a developmental, family-centered NICU (Byers, Waugh, & Lowman, 2006). The current air duct and ventilation system should be evaluated for noise as well as dust. Acoustic ceiling tiles in direct patient care areas should have a noise reduction coefficient rating of at least 0.90 for 80% of the entire surface area or an average NRC of 0.85 for the whole ceiling, including solid and acoustically absorptive surfaces (White, Smith, & Shepley, 2013). Porcelain sinks rather than stainless steel sinks can also minimize noise. Carpet decreases the noise level and promotes a homelike environment, yet rubber or vinyl flooring material directly at the bedside can ease the routine cleaning. Carpeting has been shown to be an acceptable floor covering in the hospital and the NICU and has obvious esthetic and noise-reduction appeal; however, it should be avoided in some areas, such as around sinks, isolation rooms, and soiled utility rooms. One important issue is the noise created by the equipment used to clean the carpet. When industrial-sized vacuum cleaners are used, the noise level frequently exceeds the recommended sound level in the immediate area of the infants. Utilization of a centralized vacuum system can limit noise levels and decrease dust levels. Other surfaces such as sound-absorbing wall surfaces and acoustical partitions may be used to additionally minimize noise.

Thoughtful design of traffic patterns and workspaces can help remove a great deal of unwanted noise. Beds that are built in a pod design rather than down a long hall can reduce staff travel time as well as decrease noise levels for the beds at the near end of the hallway (White, Smith, & Shepley, 2013). Additionally, patient care supplies, linen, and trash placed strategically on walls that access the hallway through sliding cupboards/doors help reduce traffic into the patient room/care area.

Background sound levels in the NICU may interfere with an infant's ability to discriminate speech of parents and other caregivers. Neonates are also exposed to vibration and noise when transported and when on high-frequency ventilation. Noise and vibration combined may have a synergistic effect. Telephones audible from the infant area should have adjustable announcing signals. Noise can be limited through use of communication devices such as personal wireless phones that are set to vibrate. This technology minimizes the need for hard wired phones placed close to the infant and can reduce the need for beepers, overhead paging systems, and intercoms.

Noise levels of equipment have been a challenge to minimize due to industrial design standards and alarm management parameters; however, more companies are focusing greater attention on the noise levels generated by such equipment. Including this parameter into purchasing decisions is worthwhile.

Dampening sounds from equipment, such as waste receptacles, sinks, paper-towel dispensers, and moveable equipment are suggestions for sound containment. Eliminating radios and all other unnecessary sounds; transferring infants from warmers to incubators with quiet motors as soon after admission as possible; and covering incubators with thick quilt/blankets with sound-absorbent material will also assist with sound abatement.

Fire alarms in the infant area should be restricted to flashing lights without an audible signal. The audible alarm level in other occupied areas must be adjustable.

Music therapy has been used in some units to calm and soothe the environment. There is not enough evidence to say what source, type, intensity, or duration of music may be beneficial to preterm infants. With such an emphasis to achieve the quietest environment possible for the developing neonate, there is much uncertainty as to what, if anything, should be introduced to provide developmental benefit when the parents are not present.

Some units are placing microphones in the ceiling above or on walls adjacent to infant care areas to determine the sound levels that are transmitted to the infant (decibel monitoring system). These microphones are wired to an alarm device that feeds a signal to a visual alarm if the sound level exceeds a predetermined level. This system helps alert staff and parents to sounds that exceed a reasonable level.

■ **Light.** Protecting the development of the visual system is important because visual problems continue to be common among NICU graduates who were born prematurely. Visual stimulation is not required at any point before term since the visual system is the last sensory system to develop functionally at term. The eyelids and iris control the amount of light entering the eye. Infants at or before 32 weeks gestation have thin eyelids and little or no pupillary constriction, which allows light to reach the retina much easier (Graven, 2011; LeVay, Wiesel, & Hubel, 1980). At 29 to 30 weeks gestation, sleep partitions into rapid eye movement (REM) and non-REM (NREM; slow-wave) sleep. Transition to regular sleep occurs around 30 to 34 weeks gestation (Graven, 2006). Protecting sleep cycles, and especially REM sleep periods, is critical for healthy visual development as any event or drug that disrupts REM sleep can impact visual development.

Endogenous brain activity stimulation (activity-independent) is created by spontaneous firing of neural cells in the retina, lateral geniculate nucleus (LGN), spinal cord, hippocampus, pons, cerebellum, cerebral cortex, and auditory systems which occurs at a particular time in their development. The endogenous stimulation of the visual system prepares the retina, LGN, and visual cortex for exogenous or outside stimulation. At 40 weeks gestation the human visual system has intact retinal development and pathways to the visual cortex. It is at this time that the visual system must have regular visual stimulation. Visual experiences for healthy visual development require ambient light (not direct light), focus, attention, novelty, movement, and after 2 to 3 months, color (Graven, 2006). The visual system develops in utero in the total absence of light and therefore, the visual system is not developmentally ready for external visual stimuli until birth at term. Three main areas of care in the NICU that can adversely affect visual development are interference with endogenous brain cell activity, sleep deprivation, and intense light exposure.

Lighting in the NICU should be adjusted to support each infant's best sleep and awake organization and to deliver care without impinging on the development, comfort, and care of other infants (Lawhon & Als, 2010). Lighting in the NICU needs to be adjustable to the infant's developmental stage. There needs to be a balance between dimmed ambient lighting, natural lighting, and brighter task lighting; yet, a baby should never be positioned facing directly into a light source. Only indirect ambient lighting should be utilized for preterm infants who cannot block out light through their thin eyelids, may not be able to turn away from light, and cannot communicate their needs (White, Smith, & Shepley, 2013). The focus of care for preterm infants 22 to 28 weeks gestation and/or VLBW infants should be on protecting the eyes from direct light and keeping ambient light exposure to low levels. Care of the 28 to 36 weeks gestation preterm infants should focus on protecting sleep cycles, especially REM sleep. During this time, intense stimulation from NICU noises, vibrations, and other disturbing stimuli of other sensory systems can greatly interfere with the processes of visual system development (Lickliter, 2011).

Ambient lighting levels in the infant care spaces shall be adjustable through a range of at least 1- to no more than 60-foot candles. Both natural and electric light sources need to have controls that allow immediate, sufficient darkening of any bed space for transillumination when necessary. No direct view of the electric light source or sun shall be permitted in the infant space. Use of multiple switches with individual dimmers to allow different levels of illumination is helpful. Procedural lighting should be available at each bedside to allow caregivers to evaluate a baby or to perform a procedure. This increased illumination should not increase light levels of adjacent babies. Illumination of support areas such as charting areas, medication preparation areas, and reception areas should be adequate to allow important or critical tasks to be performed. This light level should conform to Illuminating Engineering Society specifications (http://www.iesna.org). When possible, independent controls should be used to accommodate sleeping infants and working nurses (White, Smith, & Shepley, 2013).

Each infant room, care area, or adjacent staff work area should have at least one source of daylight visible. Windows provide a psychological benefit to NICU staff as well as families. Day-lighting is desirable for charting as well as the evaluation of infant skin tone. Exterior windows provide the recommended natural light and assist with diurnal cycling. However, serious problems with radiant heat loss or gain and glare can occur if infants are placed too close to external windows. External windows should be at least 2 feet away from the infant's bed and may be placed away from direct patient areas—for example, high up on the walls, as skylights, or in other locations that provide indirect light to the patient area. The latter might be a window in a hallway that secondarily allows light to pass into the NICU. All windows, including skylights, should have retractable covers for times when light is not desired. These windows should be insulated and have shading devices in a neutral color to minimize color distortion from transmitted light. Significant flexibility in lighting levels is required to accommodate the disparate needs of infants at various stages of development and at various times of the day, as well as the needs of caregivers.

Safeguarding Sleep

Sleep is an extremely important issue for the infant in the NICU. At approximately 28 weeks gestation, individual sleep patterns begin to emerge characterized by REM and NREM sleep periods. These periods become constant by 36 to 38 weeks gestational age. REM sleep dominates in the initial sleep cycles; REM and NREM are nearly equal as the infant approaches term, and by 8 months of age NREM sleep occupies nearly 80% of sleep time (Hobson, 1995). REM and NREM sleep cycling are essential for early neurosensory development, learning and memory, and preservation of brain plasticity for the life of the individual (Graven, 2006). Endogenous (arising from neurons within the neurosensory system) and exogenous (arising from outside the neurosensory system) stimuli are essential for neurosensory development. Patterns of endogenous stimulation occur only during REM sleep, thus making this period essential to the process of endogenous stimulation and the development of neurosensory systems. Once endogenous neurosensory systems are developed, they are readied for exogenous stimulation. Circadian rhythms are generated endogenously and are aligned with the environment by exogenous factors (Figueiro & White, 2013). For the visual system, the need for visual experiences does not occur until near term or 40 weeks gestational age. The environment of the fetus in utero and the preterm infant in the NICU requires appropriate levels of specific types of exogenous neurosensory stimuli for healthy early brain development (Graven, 2006; Graven & Browne, 2008b).

Preservation of "brain plasticity," the ability of the brain to constantly change its structure and function in response to environmental changes, is an essential process throughout childhood and adult life. Sleep deprivation (both REM and NREM) results in a loss of brain plasticity which is manifested by smaller brains, altered subsequent learning, and long-term effect on behavior and brain function. Facilitation and protection of sleep and sleep cycles are essential to long-term learning and continuing brain development through the preservation of brain plasticity (Maquet, Smith, & Stickgold, 2003).

Because REM sleep is essential for neurosensory as well as visual development, neuroprotective strategies for the NICU infant are to

- Protect the eyes from direct light exposure and maintain low levels of ambient light when not needed for care and procedures
- Provide some daily exposure to light, preferably including shorter wavelengths, for entrainment of the circadian rhythm (after 28 weeks gestation [Rivkees, 2004]).
- Protect sleep cycles, and especially REM sleep; avoid sleep interruptions, bright lights, loud noises, and unnecessary physical disturbing activities
- Avoid high doses of sedative and depressing drugs, which can depress the endogenous firing of cells, thus interfering with visual development, REM, and NREM sleep cycles
- Provide developmental care appropriate for the age and maturation of the infant (Graven, 2011)

Continuous bright lights in the NICU can disrupt sleep/wake states. Patients of any age who are trying to sleep find direct light unpleasant. Premature infants are photophobic; however, they will open their eyes with dim lights. If the light levels never change, infants never experience the diurnal rhythm necessary for development. Reducing light levels may facilitate rest and subsequent energy conservation, and promote organization and growth.

Special attention should be given to lighting as it relates to caregivers who work night shifts. Visual and circadian needs of staff are quite different from those of patients. Five characteristics of light important for both human visual and circadian systems are quantity, spectrum, timing, duration, and distribution. The visual system responds well to a light stimulus at any time of the day or night, and is not dependent on the timing of light. Timing of the light exposure, however, is critical for circadian development. The visual system responds to a light stimulus in milliseconds; yet, the duration of light exposure necessary to stimulate the circadian system can take minutes (Figueiro & White, 2013; Jewett, Rimmer, Duffy, et al., 1997; Khalsa, Jewett, Cajochen, & Czeisler, 2002; Rea, Figueiro, & Bullough, 2002).

Most babies should remain in a dimly lit environment at night, yet some staff may have difficulty staying alert, which could cause safety concerns. Shift-work disorder, a circadian sleep disorder characterized by sleepiness and/or insomnia, is associated with decreased productivity, impaired safety, diminished quality of life, and adverse effects on health, such as increased risk for metabolic syndrome, diabetes, cardiovascular disease, ischemic stroke, depression, obesity, gastrointestinal dysfunction, reproductive problems, and cancer (Antunes, Levandovski, Dantas, et al., 2010; Brown, Feskanich, Sanchez, et al., 2009; Drake, Roehrs, Richardson, et al., 2004; Figueiro & White, 2013; Knutsson & Boggild, 2010; Lawson, Rocheleau, Whelan, et al., 2012; Mahoney, 2010; Pan, Schernhammer, Sun, & Hu, 2011; Straif, Baan, Grosse, et al., 2007; Viitasalo, Lindstrom, Hemio, et al., 2012). Both the health of caregivers and the safety of infants need to be considered with all unit designs.

Minimizing Stress and Pain

The NICU is often a stressful environment for infants, parents, and staff. Sources of stress for infants include the physical environment, caregiver interventions, medical and surgical procedures, pain, distress, pathologic processes, temperature changes, handling, and multiple modes of stimulation, as well as separation from their parents. Consequences of neonatal stress include energy expenditure, altered healing and recovery, altered growth, and altered organization. Stress can also affect interactions and parenting. These stresses occur for the infant during a critical period of development. An infant's stress tolerance may be exceeded repeatedly, contributing to short- and long-term morbidity. Infants exposed to multiple invasive procedures in the NICU can have long-term changes in stress responsiveness and neurodevelopment (Anand, 2000).

Badr (2013) revealed from multiple studies, that preterm infants in the NICU could experience anywhere from 2 to 17 painful procedures per day. Painful interventions most studied included capillary blood sampling by heelstick or venipuncture, followed by endotracheal suctioning. A Cochrane review of six studies (n = 478) found that venipuncture was less painful than the heelstick procedure (Shah & Ohlsson, 2011). Because premature infants cannot manifest pain as well as mature infants, due to a lack of inhibitory control, they may be at an increased risk for negative brain alterations in both structure and function (Brummelte, Grunau, Chau, Poskitt, et al., 2012). Slater, Fabrizi, Worley, et al. (2010) found on EEG recordings that infants who were born prematurely and had experienced at least 40 days of intensive or special care, had increased neuronal response to noxious stimuli compared to healthy newborns at the same corrected age. It has also been suggested that intense or prolonged pain in premature infants may increase their risk for a brain injury by increasing intracranial pressure and oxygen desaturation leading to generation of free radicals that can damage fast-growing brain tissue (Bartocci, Bergqvist, Lagercrantz, & Anand, 2006; Bhutta & Anand, 2002; Ozawa, Kanda, Hirata Kusakawa, & Suzuki, 2011). NICU stressors and painful interventions may raise cortisol levels, limiting neuroplastic reorganization and therefore, learning and memory of motor skills. Pain and associated stress in the NICU setting may be inevitable; yet, differentiating the two is essential so that appropriate management of the infant can be achieved. Minimizing stress in preterm infants may have many neurologic benefits such as reducing the likelihood of programming abnormal stress responsiveness, which will help preserve existing neuroplastic capacity (Pitcher, Schneider, Drysdale, Ridding, & Owens, 2011).

Positioning and Handling

Developmentally appropriate or neuroprotective care includes both positioning and handling activities. In utero, the infant is contained in a circumferential enclosed space with 360° of well-defined boundaries. The brain of a third-trimester fetus is undergoing rapid development as cortical neurons layer, organize, specialize, and form vital connections and pathways. The formation of synaptic connections at this stage is vulnerable to circumstances and environment. The protection afforded by the consistency of the womb allows a much more controlled and predictable progression of this neuronal development than does the variable high-tech environment of the NICU. Conversely, the spontaneous resting posture of a third-trimester NICU infant often is flat, extended, asymmetrical with head to one side (usually the right), and with the extremities abducted and externally rotated (Hunter, 2010). Preterm and newly born sick infants abruptly lose the comfort and organizing boundaries of the womb while they simultaneously are exposed to invasive medical procedures. Over time, neuronal connections can be reinforced that favor this flattened, externally rotated, and asymmetrical resting posture as baseline for these infants.

Therapeutic positioning in the NICU can influence not only neuromotor development, but also physiologic function and stability, skin integrity, thermal regulation, bone density, and sleep facilitation/brain development (Hunter, 2010). Preterm infants left in unsupported extended positions frequently exhibit increased stress and agitation with decreased physiologic stability. Secure therapeutic positioning promotes improved rest and neurobehavioral organization. Body containment is an important factor because it increases the infant's feelings of security and self-control and decreases stress. Infants who are contained tend to be calmer, require less medication, and gain weight more rapidly. Placing the preterm infant in the prone position while in the NICU enables important achievements, such as longer periods of quality sleep and production of adaptive self-regulatory reactions (Jarus, Bart, Rabinovich, et al., 2011).

Although positioning is very important in the NICU, the astute bedside caregiver realizes that it is not just static position that affects neurodevelopmental outcomes, but caregiving and handling of the infant as well. Research has shown that developmental caregiving enhances the outcomes of high-risk infants who require neonatal intensive care. Handling of infants should be done with slow, modulated movements, with the infant's extremities flexed and contained. The idea of clustering care is now being modified because infants do not always tolerate all of the care that is being clustered into one caregiving period. Caregiving based on infant cues is an integral part of providing developmentally appropriate care. Infant-driven cues, rather than clustered care should be utilized for optimal caregiving practices. These cues provide communication about an infant's needs and status at any given time. Caregiving based on infant cues involves attention to messages from the infant that may indicate timing for interventions or opportunities for sensory input and interaction. These cues also indicate how the infant tolerates stimuli and stimulation. Frequent handling and touching can disturb sleep, leading to decreased weight gain, decreased state regulation, and more importantly detrimental effects on brain development. Attention to appropriate timing of caregiving according to the infant's sleep and arousal is important, as better sleep organization has been correlated with improved outcomes (Graven & Browne, 2008b). Gestational age, gravity, medical equipment, hard and flat surfaces, and inappropriate or too much handling are all factors that contribute to the altered development of the NICU infant. However, with appropriate handling, these factors may be minimized and outcomes enhanced. The majority of caregiving experienced by infants in NICUs involves medical or other caregiving interventions associated with high levels of sensory input. Infants should be handled gently without sudden changes in movement. Patterns of caregiving and handling in the NICU can profoundly affect the development of infant state organization and biologic rhythms. Children that were born prematurely have alterations in cortical development, functional connectivity, and patterns of neural activation in response to incoming stimuli. Because of this, their capacity for neuroplasticity is reduced and may contribute to common difficulties with learning and memory (Pitcher, Riley, & Ridding, 2011). A principle termed *activity-dependent development* refers to the influence of usage and repetition in formation of neural connections and pathways in the brain. It is hypothesized that if specific neurons are consistently fired together, they are strengthened and become dominant, causing a hard wiring for that response. In contrast, neurons that are not used or fired develop a weak neuronal connection, or may even disappear. Therefore, the consistency of the environment can strengthen or weaken a neuronal response. A preterm infant, when handled for reasons such as diaper change, hygiene, and feeding, or for diagnostic or therapeutic procedures, can react negatively for several minutes until he or she becomes exhausted. This results in an unnecessary expenditure of energy that can, at a later time, turn into physiological (bradycardia, tachycardia, drop in oxygen saturation, and apnea) or behavioral (flaccidity, fatigue, and difficulty sleeping) instability, and signs of distress and pain. Forming a "nest" provides postural, behavioral, and physiological stability to the newborn. Comaru and Miura (2009), researching postural support in preterm infants, demonstrated that although all babies displayed increased distress and pain scores during diaper changes, this was statistically less for babies nested compared to nonnested babies. Activity-dependent development is important to consider with the constant repetitive activities performed in the NICU by the bedside caregiver. This principle encourages the bedside caregiver to adapt all caregiving behaviors to alleviate as much aversive or negative sensory input from caregiving activities as possible. Nurses control caregiving routines by collaborating effectively with other disciplines to negotiate timing, intensity, and appropriateness of interventions, tests, and procedures. Continuous observation and response to infant cues require nurses to alter care routines according to developmentally supportive principles (Spruill, 2010). A paradigm shift from task-oriented and scheduled care to infant responsive care needs to occur to achieve optimal caregiving practices. The nurse must stay in the "present" or be "mindful" when interacting with the infant.

Skin-to-skin care or kangaroo care, the practice of holding a diaper-clad newborn or preterm infant on a parent's bare chest in an upright prone position, is an appropriate developmental plasticity intervention (Ludington-Hoe, 2010, 2013). This practice has been shown to foster autonomic and physiologic (HR functions, bradycardia, HR variability, RR and patterns, oxygenation, temperature, metabolism, and somatic growth), mental and motor developmental effects, and state development. Additionally, KC is an effective care practice as it relates to maternal–infant bonding, feeding, infection control, thermoregulation, and minimizing stress and pain (Ludington-Hoe, 2010). Maternal sounds and voice are calming auditory experiences for the infant (McMahon, Wintermark, & Lahave, 2012). Upon waking, looking at the mother's eyes and face are soothing, and are critical events for visual development prior to 40 weeks postmenstrual age (Graven, 2011). Physiological stabilization and behavioral calm ensue because the autonomic nervous system switches over from sympathetic (fight or flight status, stress activating mode) to parasympathetic control due to the release of oxytocin in the insular cortex following KC's pleasing touch stimulation of unmyelinated exquisitely sensitive c-afferent nerves that are in limited locales (chest, across the shoulders, and forearm) and only respond to pleasant touch (Bystrova, 2009; Morgan, Horn & Bergman, 2011).

Partnering With Families

The admission of an infant to the NICU is frequently a crisis for the family. The delivery is often unexpected, and the family unit is now separated. Their infant is attached to wires, cables, and equipment in a harsh NICU environment that is far different than the newly decorated home nursery they had planned. The environment can become comforting and inviting with attentive and compassionate caregivers who provide developmentally appropriate positioning and handling while partnering with parents. The concept of partnering with families in the NICU offers a philosophy of care that acknowledges that the family has the greatest influence over an infant's health and well-being. The family is integral to developmental care. All families, even those who are struggling with difficulties, bring important strengths to their infant's experiences in the NICU. Parents must be viewed as partners in the care of their infant, rather than visitors to the NICU. Creating an effective partnership between professionals and families has shown benefits such as decreased LOS, increased satisfaction for both staff and parents, and enhanced neurodevelopmental outcomes for infants (Cleveland, 2008). To measure the quality of developmental care delivered to premature infants in several Italian NICUs, Montirosso et al. (2012), created a scoring system, defined in terms of parental presence, infant interventions, and pain management, to assess how that care would affect their neurobehavioral outcomes at discharge. A higher score was found for infant-centered care, consisting of measures of parent involvement, including ability to room in, frequency and duration of KC, and nursing interventions aimed at decreasing infant energy expenditure and promoting autonomic stability (i.e., infant containment, reducing tactile stimulation), which led to better neurobehavioral outcomes at discharge in infants born 29 weeks gestation. Individualized family-centered developmental care is a framework for providing care that enhances the neurodevelopment of the infant through interventions that support both the infant and family unit. Effective partnerships must be based on mutual respect and value of family expertise, fully shared information, and joint decision making (Dallas, 2009).

Establishing family–professional partnerships in the NICU environment can be challenging. Because families are the constant in the infant's environment, helping families achieve a positive outcome from their NICU experience should be a priority while providing care (Boykova & Kenner, 2010). Equilateral respect among all members involved in the partnership will promote optimal patient care, enhance family satisfaction, and engage the health care team.

SUMMARY

As the preterm infant matures, the NICU environment the infant resides in plays a critical role in their future development. High-risk infants are both dependent on and vulnerable to their early environment, the NICU, to maintain their physiologic function, and to promote growth and development. Caregivers must be cautious when providing sensory input and must be sensitive to infant responses and abilities to tolerate stimuli.

Developmentally supportive care is sometimes perceived as "nice," yet optional. Consistent acceptance, practice, and accountability must be established to provide high-quality care for infants and families. Use of established guidelines, policies, and procedures to guide neonatal practice is essential. To provide developmentally supportive care and optimize the experience of neonates in intensive care, an understanding of their behavioral capabilities as well as their surrounding physical environment is essential. Health care professionals need to be cognizant of the growing body of research regarding the impact of the NICU environment on neurodevelopmental outcomes. Changes in developmental care can often begin with a few caregivers altering the way they care for premature infants. Role modeling, mentoring, and collaboration are keys in the promotion of optimal developmental care. An overarching goal is to achieve an efficient, peaceful, and satisfying environment for both administering and receiving care.

CASE STUDY

■ Identification of the Problem

- 25-week gestational age newly born premature infant boy weighing 950 g

■ Assessment: History and Physical Examination. Upon delivery, the infant was limp, cyanotic/pale, and apneic. The infant was successfully resuscitated following Neonatal Resuscitation Program© (NRP) guidelines; required 2 minutes positive pressure ventilation by T-piece resuscitator to initiate effective ventilation when spontaneous respirations were noted; infant received 10 minutes of continuous positive airway pressure via the T-piece resuscitator, prior to being transferred to the Neonatal Intensive care Unit (NICU).

■ Physical Examination on Admission to the NICU

- TEMPERATURE: 35.7°C, axillary HR: 180 beats/min
- RR: 56, shallow; saturations 88% to 92% in room air
- HEENT: WNL
- RESP: lung fields bilaterally clear and equal to bases; grunting
- CV: rate regular with no murmur noted; good peripheral perfusion, capillary blood refill less than 3 seconds, and strong peripheral pulses noted
- ABD: abdomen soft, flat, and nontender with no masses palpable; three-vessel cord; the anus appeared patent
- GENITOURINARY: normal male infant genitalia
- NEURO: appropriate responses, with eyes open and blinking; extremities well formed; decreased muscle tone

- SKIN: pale pink, thin, transparent, yet intact skin
- EXTREMITIES: well formed; 10 digits per extremity; low tone
- Umbilical arterial and venous catheters were placed for fluid management and laboratory specimen draws

■ **Differential Diagnoses.** The differential diagnosis includes:

1. Prematurity
2. Perinatal hypoxic-ischemic injury
3. Shock
4. Congestive heart failure
5. Sepsis screen

■ **Diagnostic Tests.** Head ultrasound at 24 hours of age

■ **Working Diagnosis.** Extreme prematurity

■ Development of Management Plan

- Place infant in radiant warmer/humidified incubator in midline, flexed, and contained position utilizing positioning aids (e.g., SnuggleUp, bendy, prone-plus, gel products) to maintain position
- Continuous monitoring of vital signs (VS), every 2 to 4 hours
- Maintenance fluid support; TPN (total parenteral nutrition) within 24 hours of life
- Respiratory support with CPAP (continuous positive airway pressure) as needed
- Antibiotics until cultures negative for 72 hours

■ Implementation and Evaluation of Effectiveness

Implementation of Management Plan (Immediately After Initial Assessment in the NICU)

- Infant was moved to a single private room where optimal dimmed lighting was utilized
- The infant was placed on the NeoPAP ventilator (CPAP of 5) within the first half hour of life
- The infant was converted to an 80% humidified incubator mode environment

■ Effectiveness of Management Plan

- Temperature was 36.7 at 1 hour of life
- Respiratory status stable by 2 hours of life
- Blood pressure was normal within 2 hours of life

■ **Outcome.** Extremely premature white male infant with stable VS. Anticipate lengthy NICU stay. Developmentally appropriate care will be individualized to meet the infant's needs at each developmental stage. Exogenous stimuli will be limited, with positive neuroprotective strategies introduced as tolerated and warranted.

EVIDENCE-BASED PRACTICE BOX

The design and operation of neonatal intensive care units (NICUs) have evolved from the 1960s to the 2000s to support and accommodate the changes in technology involved in meeting the physical and caregiving needs of preterm infants and their families. The equipment has changed, the space has enlarged, and caregiving practices have changed. Units historically were designed as large, open areas with visibility for the caregivers. Infants were in rows, close to each other with open space between bays. Technology has advanced with the ability to keep smaller and smaller infants alive. Small infants, less than 1,500 g occupy most patient days, with many stays being 3 months and longer. Although the survival rate has improved, the number of infants with evidence of neurological and learning problems continues to increase.

The focus on the environment of preterm infants and young neonates began in the 1970s but made little progress in changing the environment of the fetus or infant until the 1980s and 1990s. Even in 2012, it is estimated that less than half of the more than 1,000 NICUs in the United States and even fewer in Europe and Asia are able to maintain an environment and care practices that are supportive of early neurosensory and neuromotor brain development. These units support the physiology of care, but many fail to support the needs for healthy brain development, both neurosensory and neuromotor.

Although preterm birth accelerates the maturation of the lungs, kidneys, and gastrointestinal tract, it does not accelerate neuroprocesses, and under most conditions of care, it can seriously alter these processes. Processes under genetic control are thought to be important but not altered by the environment. With the studies of epigenetics, it is now clear that environmental factors can alter the expression of genes related to brain development without altering the DNA structure or code for the gene.

Alterations in the sensory environment including excess noise, bright lights, sleep deprivation, and poorly timed caregiving, all affect neurosensory development in the preterm infant. The physical environment, the nutritional environment, and the social/emotional environment also influence the processes involved in the early development of the neurosensory systems. Developmentally appropriate care provided in an environment that supports early brain development is essential for optimal outcome and the best possible long-term development. It is essential that all NICUs make changes necessary to have an environment and care practices that support the processes of early brain development (White, Smith, & Shepley, 2013).

ONLINE RESOURCES

Design Standardization in the Private Neonatal Intensive Care Unit Room
http://www.nainr.com/article/S1527-3369(10)00033-4/abstract
Environmental Impact on the Neonate
http://www.ncbi.nlm.nih.gov/pubmed/22013708
Evidence-Based Design—New Hanover Regional Medical Center NICU
http://www.youtube.com/watch?v=x8duUzagm5w
Neonatal Intensive Care Unit (NICU)
PRecommended Standards for Newborn ICU Design
https://www.nd.edu/~nicudes
Premature Baby Care
http://www.youtube.com/watch?v=_O0w8Lhekb0
http://www.uhhospitals.org/rainbow/services/neonatology/neonatal-intensive-care-unit-nicu

REFERENCES

Als, H. (1982). Toward a Synactive Theory of development: Promise for the assessment of infant individuality. *Journal of Infant Mental Health, 3*, 229–243.

Als, H. (1986). A synactive model of neonatal behavioral organization: Framework for the assessment and support of the neurobehavioral development of the premature infant and his parents in the environment of the neonatal intensive care unit. *Physical & Occupational Therapy in Pediatrics, 6*, 3–53.

Als, H., Gilkerson, L., Duffy, F., McAnulty, G., Buehler, D., Vandenberg, K., . . . Jones, K. J. (2003). A three-center, randomized, controlled trial of individualized developmental care for very low birth weight preterm infants: Medical, neurodevelopmental, parenting, and caregiving effects. *Journal of Developmental Behavioral Pediatrics, 24*, 399–408.

Altimier, L. (2004). Healing environments for patients and providers. *Newborn and Infant Nursing Reviews, 4*, 89–92.

Altimier, L. (2011). Mother and child integrative developmental care model: A simple approach to a complex population. *Newborn and Infant Nursing Reviews, 11*(3), 105–108. doi:10.1053/j.nainr.2011.06.004

Altimier, L. (2012). Thermoregulation: What's new? What's not? *Newborn and Infant Nursing Reviews, 12*(1), 51–63. doi:10.1053/j.nainr.2012.01.003

Altimier, L., Eichel, M., Warner, B., Tedeschi, L., & Brown, B. (2005). Developmental care: Changing the NICU physically and behaviorally to promote patient outcomes and contain costs. *Neonatal Intensive Care, 18*(4), 12–16.

Altimier, L., & Phillips, R. (2013). The Neonatal Integrative Developmental Care Model: Seven neuroprotective core measures for family-centered care. *Newborn and Infant Nursing Reviews, 13*(1), 9–22.

Anand, K. S. (2000). Pain, plasticity, and premature birth: A prescription for permanent suffering? *Nature Medicine, 6*, 971–973.

Antunes, L.C., Levandovski, R., Dantas, G., Caumo, W., & Hidalgo, M.P. (2010). Obesity and shift work: Chronobiological aspects. *Nutrition Research Reviews, 23*, 155–168.

Ayres, A. (1987). *Sensory integration and the child* (8th Print ed.). Prescott, AZ: Western Psychological Services.

Badr, L.K. (2013). Pain in premature infants: What is conclusive and what is not. *Newborn and Infant Nursing Reviews, 13*(2), 82–86.

Bartocci, M., Bergqvist, L.L., Lagercrantz, H., Anand, K.J.S. (2006). Pain activates cortical areas in the preterm newborn brain. *Pain, 122*, 109–117

Bartocci, M., Serra, G., Papiendieck, G., Winberg, J., Mustica, T., & Lagercrantz, H. (2000). Cerebral cortex response in newborn infants after exposure to the smell of detergent used in NICU: A near infrared spectroscopy study. *Pediatric Research, 47*, 388A.

Bhutta, A.T., & Anand, K.J. (2002). Vulnerability of the developing brain: Neonatel mechanisms. *Clinical Perinatology, 29*(3), 357–372.

Bingham, P., Abassi, S., & Sivieri, E. (2003). A pilot study of milk odor effect on nonnutritive sucking by premature newborns. *Archives Pediatric Adolescent Medicine, 157*, 72–75.

Blackburn, S. T. (2007). *Maternal, fetal & neonatal physiology: A clinical perspective* (3rd ed.). St. Louis, MO: Saunders.

Bonnier, C. (2008). Evaluation of early stimulation programs for enhancing brain development. *Acta Paediatrica (Oslo, Norway: 1992), 97*(7), 853–858.

Boykova, M., & Kenner, C. (2010). Partnerships in care: Mothers and fathers. In C. K. J. McGrath (Ed.), *Developmental care of newborns and infants: A guide for health professionals* (pp. 145–160). Glenview, IL: National Association of Neonatal Nurses.

Brazelton, T. (1974). Does the neonate shape his environment? *Birth Defects Original Article Series, 10*, 131–140.

Brazelton, T., Parker, W., & Zuckerman, B. (1976). Importance of behavioral assessment of the neonate. *Current Problems in Pediatrics, 7*, 1–32.

Brown, D.L., Feskanich, D., Sánchez, B.N., Rexrode, K.M., Schernhammer, E.S., & Lisabeth, L.D. (2009). Rotating night shift work and the risk of ischemic stroke. *American Journal of Epidemiology, 169*, 1370–1377.

Browne, J. V. (2008). Chemosensory development in the fetus and newborn. *Newborn and Infant Nursing Reviews, 8*(4), 180–186.

Browne, J. V. (2011). Developmental care for high-risk newborns: Emerging science, clinical application, and continuity from newborn intensive care unit to community. *Clinics in Perinatology, 38*(4), 719–729.

Brummelte, S., Grunau, R., Chau, V., Poskitt, K., Brant, R., Vinall, J., & . . . Miller, S. (2012). Procedural pain and brain development in premature newborns. *Annals of Neurology, 71*(3), 385–396. doi:10.1002/ana.22267

Bui, B., Rees, S., Loeliger, M., Caddy, J., Rehn, A., Armitage, J. A., & Vingrys, A. J. (2002). Altered retinal function and structure after chronic placental insufficiency. *Investigative Ophthalmology and Visual Science, 43*, 805–812.

Butler, S., & Als, H. (2008). Individualized developmental care improves the lives of infants born preterm. *Acta Paediatrica (Oslo, Norway: 1992), 97*(9), 1173–1175.

Byers, J. F., Waugh, W. R., & Lowman, L. B. (2006). Sound level exposure of high-risk infants in different environmental conditions. *Neonatal Network, 25*(1), 25–32.

Bystrova K. (2009). Novel mechanism of human fetal growth regulation: A potential role of lanugo, vernix caseosa and a second tactile system of unmyelinated low-threshold C-afferents. *Medical Hypotheses, 72*, 143–146.

Chaze, B., & Luddington-Hoe, S. (1984). Sensory stimulation in the NICU. *American Journal of Nursing, 84*, 68–71.

Chen, H-L., Chen, C-H., Wu, C-C., Huang, H-.J, Wang, T-M., & Hsu, C-C. (2009). The influence of neonatal intensive care unit design on sound level. *Pediatrics and Neonatology, 50*(6), 270–274.

Cleveland, L. (2008). Parenting in the neonatal intensive care unit. *Journal of Obstetrics, Gynecologic, and Neonatal Nursing, 37*(6), 666–691.

Comaru, T., & Miura, E. (2009). Postural support improves distress and pain during diaper change in preterm infants. *Journal of Perinatology, 29*, 504–507.

Committee on Perinatal Health. (1976). *Toward improving the outcome of pregnancy. Recommendations for the Regional Development of Maternal and Perinatal Services.* White Plains, NY: National Foundation-March of Dimes.

Constable, R. T., Ment, L., Vohr, B., Kesler, S. R., Fulbright, R. K., Lacadie, C., . . . Reiss, A. R. (2008). Prematurely born children demonstrate white matter miscrostructural differences at 12 years of age, relative to term control subjects: An investigation of group and gender effects. *Pediatrics, 121*, 306–316.

Coughlin, M., Gibbins, S., & Hoath, S. (2009). Core measures for developmentally supportive care in neonatal intensive care units: Theory, precedence and practice. *Journal of Advanced Nursing, 65*(10), 2239–2248. doi:10.1111/j.1365-2648.2009.05052.x

Dallas, C. (2009). Interactions between adolescent fathers and health care professionals during pregnancy, lqabor, and early postpartum. *Journal of Obstetrics, Gynecologic, and Neonatal Nursing, 38*(3), 290–299.

de Vonderweid, U., & Leonessa, M. (2009). Family centered neonatal care. *Early Human Development, 85*(Suppl. 10), S37–S38.

Domanico, R., Davis, D.K., Coleman, F., & Davis, B.O., Jr. (2010). Documenting the NICU design dilemma: Parent and staff perceptions of open ward versus single family room units. *Journal of Perinatology, 30*(5), 343–351.

Drake, C.L., Roehrs, T., Richardson, G., Walsh, J.K., & Roth, T. (2004). Shift work sleep disorder: Prevalence and consequences beyond that of symptomatic day workers. *Sleep, 27*, 1453–1462.

Eliot, L. (1999). *What's going on here? How the brain and mind develop in the first five years of life.* New York, NY: Bantam Books.

Figueiro, M.G., & White, R.D. (2013). Health consequences of shift work and implications for structural design. *Journal of Perinatology, 33*, S17-S23. doi:10.1038/jp.2013.7

Gardner, S., & Goldson, E. (2002). *The neonate and the environment* (5th ed.). St. Louis, MO: Mosby.

Gibbins, S., Hoath, S. B., Coughlin, M., Gibbins, A., & Franck, L. (2008). Foundations in newborn care. The universe of developmental care: A new conceptual model for application in the neonatal intensive care unit. *Advances in Neonatal Care (Elsevier Science), 8*(3), 141–147.

Graven, S., & Browne, J. V. (2008). Sensory development in the fetus, neonate, and infant: Introductions and overview. *Newborn and Infant Nursing Reviews, 8*(4), 169–172.

Graven, S. N. (2006). Sleep and brain development. *Clinics in Perinatology, 33*(3), 693–706.

Graven, S. N. (2011). Early visual development: Implications for the neonatal intensive care unit and care. *Clinics in Perinatology, 38*, 671–683. doi:10.1016/j.clp.2011.08.006

Graven, S. N., & Browne, J. V. (2008). Sleep and brain development: The critical role of sleep in fetal and early neonatal brain development. *Newborn and Infant Nursing Reviews, 8*(4), 173–179.

Grunau, R. E., Tu, M. T., Whitfield, M. F., Oberlander, T. F., Weinberg, J., Yu, W., . . . Scheifele, D. (2010). Cortisol, behavior, and heart rate reactivity to immunization pain at 4 months corrected age in infants born very preterm. *Clinical Journal of Pain, 26*(8), 698–704.

Guidelines for Design and Construction of Hospital and Health Care Facilities. (2010). Dallas, TX: Facilities Guidelines Institute.

Hack, M., Taylor, H., Schluchter, M., Andreias, L., Drotar, D., & Klein, N. (2009). Behavioral outcomes of extremely low birth weight children at age 8 years. *Journal of Developmental and Behavioral Pediatrics, 30*(2), 122–130.

Hack, M., Youngstrom, E. A., Cartar, L., Schluchter, M., Taylor, H. G., Flannery, D., . . . Borawski, E. (2004). Behavioral outcomes and evidence of psychopathology among very low birth weight infants at age 20 years. *Pediatrics, 114*(4 Part 1), 932–940.

Heinonen, K., Raikkonen, K., Pesonen, A. K., Andersson, S., Kajantie, E., Eriksson, J. G. . . . Lano, A. (2010). Behavioural symptoms of attention deficit/hyperactivity disorder in preterm and term children born small and appropriate for age: A longitudinal study. *BMC Pediatrics, 10*, 91.

Hendricks-Munoz, K. (2002). Developmental care: The impact of Wee Care developmental care training on short-term infant outcomes and hospital costs. *Newborn and Infant Nursing Reviews, 2*(1), 39–45.

Hobson, J. (1995). *The development of sleep.* New York, NY: Scientific American Library.

Hunter, J. (2010). Therapeutic positioning: Neuromotor, physiologic, and sleep implications. In C. K. J. McGrath (Ed.), *Developmental care of newborns and infants* (pp. 285–312). Glenview, IL: National Association of Neonatal Nurses.

Jarus, T., Bart, O., Rabinovich, G., Sadeh, A., Bloch, L., Dolfin, T., & Litmanovitz, I. (2011). Effects of prone and supine positions on sleep state and stress responses in preterm infants. *Infant Behavior & Development, 34*(2), 257–263. doi:10.1016/j.infbeh.2010.12.014

Jewett, M., Rimmer, D., Duffy, J., Klerman, E., Kronauer, R., & Czeisler, C. (1997). Human circadian pacemaker is sensitive to light throughout subjective day without evidence of transients. *American Journal of Physiology, 273*, R1800–R1809.

Johnson, S., Hollis, C., Kochlar, P., Hennessy, E., Wolke, D., & Marlow, N. (2010). Psychiatric disorders in extremely preterm children: Longitudinal finding at age 11 years in the EPICure study. *Journal of the American Academy of Child and Adolescent Psychiatry, 49*(5), 453–463, e451.

Kenner, C., & King, C. (Eds.). (2010). *Developmental care of newborns and infants* (2nd ed.). Glenview, IL: National Association of Neonatal Nurses.

Khalsa, S.B., Jewett, M.E., Cajochen, C., & Czeisler, C.A. (2003). A phase response curve to single bright light pulses in human subjects. *Journal of Physiology, 549*, 945–952.

Knutsson, A., & Bøggild, H. (2010). Gastrointestinal disorders among shift workers. *Scandinavian Journal of Work Environment Health, 36*, 85–95.

Kranowitz, C. A. (1998). *The out-of-sync child.* New York, NY: The Berkley Publishing Group.

Krueger, C., Schue, S., & Parker, L. (2007). Neonatal intensive care unit sound levels before & after structural reconstruction. *The American Journal of Maternal Child Nursing, 32*(6), 358–362.

Lawhon, G., & Als, H. (2010). *Theoretical perspective for developmentally supportive care* (2nd ed.). Glenview, IL: NANN.

Lawson, C.C., Rocheleau, C.M., Whelan, E.A., Lividoti Hibert, E.N., Grajewski, B., Spiegelman, D. et al. (2012). Occupational exposures among nurses and risk of spontaneous abortion. *American Journal of Obstetrics and Gynecology, 206*, 327 e1–e8.

LeVay, S., Wiesel, T., & Hubel, D. (1980). The development of ocular dominance columns in normal and visually deprived monkeys. *Journal of Comparative Neurology, 191*(1), 1–51.

Liaw, J., Yang, L., Chang, L., Chou, H. L., & Chao, S. C. (2009). Improving neonatal caregiving through a developmentally supportive care training program. *Applied Nursing Research, 22*(2), 86–93.

Lickliter, R. (2011). The integrated development of sensory organization. [Review Article]. *Clinics in Perinatology, 38*, 591–603. doi:10.1016/j.clp.2011.08.007

Limperopoulos, C. (2009). Autism spectrum disorders in survivors of extreme prematurity. *Clinics in Perinatology, 36*(4), 791–805.

Limperopoulos, C. (2010). Extreme prematurity, cerebellar injury, and autism. *Seminars in Pediatric Neurology, 17*(1), 25–29.

Limperopoulos, C., Bassan, H., Sullivan, N. R., Soul, J. S., Robertson, R. L., Moore, M., . . . du Plessis, A. J. (2008). Positive screening for autism in ex-preterm infants: Prevalence and risk factors. *Pediatrics, 121*(4), 758–765. doi:10.1542/peds.2007–2158

Liu, W., Laudert, S., Perkins, B., MacMillan-York, E., Martin, S., & Graven, S. (2007). The development of potentially better practices to support the neurodevelopment of infants in the NICU. *Journal of Perinatology, 27*, S48–S74.

Louw, R., & Maree, C. (2005). The effect of formal exposure to developmental care principles on the implementation of developmental care positioning and handling of preterm infants by neonatal nurses. *South Africa, 10*(2), 24–32.

Lubbe, W., & Kenner, C. (2008). Neonatal brain development. *Newborn and Infant Nursing Reviews, 8*(4), 166–167.

Ludington-Hoe, S. (2010). Kangaroo care is developmental care. In C. K. J. McGrath (Ed.), *Developmental care of newborns and infants: A guide for health professionals* (pp. 349–388). Glenview, IL: National Association of Neonatal Nurses.

Ludington-Hoe, S. (2013). Kangaroo care as a neonatal therapy. *Newborn and Infant Nursing Reviews, 13*(2), 73–75.

Mahoney, M.M. (2010). Shift work, jet lag, and female reproduction. *International Journal of Endocrinology, 2010*, 813764.

Maquet, P., Smith, C., & Stickgold, R. (2003). *Sleep and brain plasticity.* New York, NY: Oxford University Press.

McGrath, J. (2005). Single-room design in the NICU: Making it work for you. *Journal of Perinatal and Neonatal Nursing, 19*, 210–211.

McGrath, J. M. (2008). Supporting parents in understanding and enhancing preterm infant development. *Newborn and Infant Newborn Reviews, 8*(4), 164–165.

McGrath, J. M., Cone, S., & Samra, H. A. (2011). Neuroprotection in the preterm infant: Further understanding of the short- and long-term implications for brain development. *Newborn and Infant Nursing Reviews, 11*(3), 109–112. doi:10.1053/j.nainr.2011.07.002

McMahon, E., Wintermark, P., & Lahave, A. (2012). Auditory brain development in premature infants: The importance of early experience. *Annals of the New York Academy of Sciences, 1252*, 17–24.

Milford, C. & Zapalo, B. (Eds.). (2010). *The NICU experience and its relationship to sensory integration* (2nd ed., Vol. 3). Glenview, IL: National Association of Neonatal Nurses.

Montirosso,R., DelPrete, A., Bellù, R., Tronick, E. & Bergatti, R. (2012). Neonatal adequate care for quality of life (NEO-ACQUA) study group. Level of NICU quality of developmental care and neurobehavioral performance in very preterm infants. *Pediatrics, 129*(5). Available at: www.pediatrics.org/cgi/content/full/129/5/e1129

Moon, C. (2011). The role of early auditory development in attachment and communication. *Clinics in Perinatology, 38*, 657–669. doi:10.1016/j.clp.2011.08.009

Morgan, B.E., Horn, A.R., & Bergman, N.J.(2011). Should neonates sleep alone? *Biological Psychology, 70*, 817–825.

Nightingale, F. (1860). *Notes on nursing: What it is and what it is not.* New York, NY: Appleton & Company.

NPA (National Perinatal Association). (2010). *Position paper: NICU developmental care.* Salt Lake City, UT: Author.

Ozawa, M., Kanda, K., Hirata, M., Kusakawa, I., & Suzuki, C. (2011). Influence of repeated painful procedures on prefrontal cortical pain responses in newborns. *Acta Paediatrca, 100*(2), 198–203.

Pan, A., Schernhammer, E.S., Sun, Q., & Hu, F.B. (2011). Rotating night shift work and risk of type 2 diabetes: Two prospective cohort studies in women. *PLoS Medicine, 8*, e1001141.

Philben, M. (2004). Planning the acoustic environment of a neonatal intensive care unit. *Clinics in Perinatology, 31*, 331–352.

Pickler, R. H., McGrath, J. M., Reyna, B. A., McCain, N., Lewis, M., Cone, S., . . . Best, A. (2010). A model of neurodevelopmental risk and protection for preterm infants. *Journal of Perinatal & Neonatal Nursing, 24*(4), 356–365. doi:10.1097/JPN.0b013e3181fb1e70

Pitcher, J., Riley, A., & Ridding, M. (2011). Children born preterm have reduced long term depression (LTD)-like neuroplasticity. *Journal of Developmental Origins of Health and Disease, 2*(1), S145.

Pitcher, J., Schneider, L., Drysdale, J., Ridding, M., & Owens, J. (2011). Motor system development of the preterm and low birthweight infant. *Clinics in Perinatology, 38*, 605–625. doi:10.1016/j.clp.2011.08.010

Rattaz, C., Goubet, N., & Bullinger, A. (2005). The calming effect of a familiar odor on full-term newborns. *Journal of Developmental Behavioral Pediatrics, 26*, 86–92.

Rea, M., Figueiro, M., & Bullough, J. (2002). Circadian photobiology: An emerging framework for lighting practice and research. *Light Research Technology, 34*, 177–190.

Rees, S., Harding, R., & Walker, D. (2011). The biological basis of injury and neuroprotection in the fetal and neonatal brain. *International Journal of Developmental Neuroscience, 29*(6), 551–563. doi:10.1016/j.ijdevneu.2011.04.004

Rehn, A. E., Loeliger, M., Hardie, N. A., Rees, S. M., Dieni, S., & Shepherd, R. K. (2002). Chronic placental insufficiency has long-term effects on auditory function in the guinea pig. *Hearing Research, 166*, 159–165.

Rehn, A. E., Van Den Buuse, M., Copolov, D., Briscoe, T., Lambert, G., & Rees, S. (2004). An animal model of chronic placental insufficiency: Relevance to neurodevelopmental disorders including schizophrenia. *Neuroscience, 129*, 381–391.

Rhawn, J. (1999). Fetal brain and cognitive development. *Developmental Reviews, 20*, 81–98.

Rivkees, S.A. (2004). Emergence and influences of circadian rhythmicity in infants. *Clinics in Perinatology, 31*(2), 217–228.

Schaal, B., Hummel, T., & Soussigan, R. (2004). Olfaction in the fetal and premature infant: Functional status and clinical implications. *Clinics in Perinatology, 31*, 261–285.

Shah, V.S., & Ohlsson, A. (2011). Venepuncture versus heel lance for blood sampling in term neonates. *Cochrane Database of Systematic Reviews.* Oct. 5(10), CD001452

Shepley, M.M., Harris, D.D., & White, R. (2008). Open-bay and single-family room neonatal intensive care units—caregiver satisfaction and stress. *Environment and Behavior, 40*(2), 249–268.

Spruill, C. (2010). Caregiving and the caregiver. In C. K. J. McGrath (Ed.), *Developmental care of newborns and infants: A guide for health professionals* (pp. 75–92). Glenview, IL: National Association of Neonatal Nurses.

Stevens, D. C., Helseth, C. C., & Kurtz, J. C. (2010). *Achieving success in supporting parents and families in the neonatal intensive care unit* (2nd ed.). Glenview, IL: NANN.

Straif, K., Baan, R., Grosse, Y., Secretan, B., Ghissassi, F.E., Bouvard, V. et al. (2007). Carcinogenicity of shift-work, painting, and fire-fighting (on be half of the WHO International Agency for Research on Cancer Monograph Working Group). *Lancet Oncology, 8*, 1065–1066.

Sullivan, R., & Toubas, P. (1998). Clinical usefulness of maternal odor in newborns: Soothing and feeding preparatory responses. *Biology of the Neonate, 74*, 402–408.

Taylor, H. G. (Ed.). (2010). *Academic performance and learning disabilities.* Cambridge, UK: University Press.

Vanderbilt, D., & Gleason, M. (2010). Mental health concerns of the premature infant through the life span. *Child and Adolescent Psychiatric Clinics of North America, 19*(2), 211–228.

Viitasalo, K., Lindström, J., Hemiö, K., Puttonen, S., Koho, A., Härmä, M. et al. (2012). Occupational health care identifies risk for type 2 diabetes and cardiovascular disease. *Primary Care Diabetes, 6*, 95–102.

Volpe, J. J. (2008). *Neurology of the newborn* (5th ed.). Philadelphia, PA: Elsevier.

Wachman, E. M., & Lahav, A. (2011). The effects of noise on preterm infants in the NICU. *Archives of Disease in Childhood. Fetal and Neonatal Edition, 96*(4), F305–F309.

Walsh, W., McCullough, K., & White, R. (2006). Room for improvement: Nurses' perceptions of providing care in a single room newborn intensive care setting. *Advances in Neonatal Care, 6*, 261–270.

White, R. (2011). Designing environments for developmental care. *Clinics in Perinatology, 38*, 745–749. doi:10.1016/j.clp.2011.08.012

White, R. D, Smith, J. A., & Shepley, M. M. (2013). The physical environment of the newborn ICU: New recommended standards for newborn ICU design, eight edition. *Journal of Perinatology, 33*, S2–S16. doi:10.1038/jp.2013.10

Wolke, D., Samara, M., Bracewell, M., & Marlow, N. (2008). EPICure Study Group: Specific language difficulties and school achievement in children born at 25 weeks of gestation or less. *Journal of Pediatrics, 152*, 256–262.

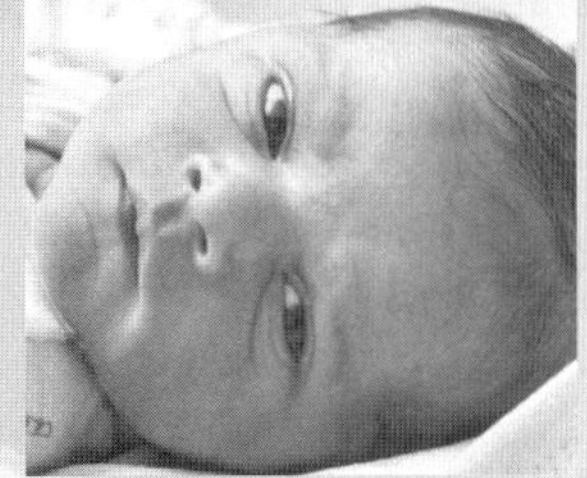

CHAPTER

32

Family: Essential Partner in Care

■ Jacqueline M. McGrath

Parents and families often enter the unfamiliar chaotic environment of the neonatal intensive care unit (NICU) for the first time exhausted, bewildered, and emotionally drained by the unexpected birth experience they have just encountered. In a recent qualitative study, Baum, Weidberg, Osher, and Kohelet (2012) reported how mothers who gave birth prematurely felt "somewhere between being pregnant and being a mother" and that this disconnect further added to their inability to reconnect and attach to their infant in the chaotic environment of the NICU. These ambivalent feelings decrease the mother's ability to be appropriately responsive and sensitive to her infant's needs and potentially lead to dyssynchrony within mother–infant interactions and overall poorer attachment (Baker & McGrath, 2011a; Flacking et al., 2012). Sometimes prenatal diagnosis provides the opportunity to enter and learn about the environment of the NICU prior to the birth of a high-risk infant. Although providing this information to families is helpful, if the birth is traumatic the context for what information the parents were provided prior to the birth may be lost (Beck, 2011). It does not matter which way a family enters the NICU; it is important to remember that at that initial moment a partnership must be formed between the family and professionals providing care for the infant (Baker & McGrath, 2009; Reis, Rempel, Scott, Brady-Fryer, & van Aerde, 2010). This relationship must continue as a true collaborative partnership for as long as it is in the best interest of the child (Ahmann, Abraham, & Johnson, 2004; Boykova & Kenner, 2010; McGrath, 2005a). Even with the added focus on the integration of family-centered care (FCC) that is prevalent in most NICUs today, families continue to report being extremely distressed by the NICU and their inability to parent their child in this environment (Baum et al., 2012; Liang & Freer, 2008).

Partnerships exist when there is a relationship between two or more parties that have a shared goal. Effective partnerships between professionals and families are based on mutual respect, valuing of family expertise, fully shared information, and joint decision making (Jones, Woodhouse, & Rowe, 2007). When parents are consistently well informed and involved as partners within the NICU team, ethical dilemmas can be potentially lessened and care decisions can be optimized in the best interest of the infant and their family (Boykova & Kenner, 2010; Coulter & Ellins, 2007; Ladd & Mercurio, 2003; Pillow, 2007). These partnerships between families and health professionals are essential and are the crux of caregiving interventions discussed within this chapter.

Change is the most certain event in life. A family experiencing the birth of an infant faces many changes. Some variations in lifestyle occur in the areas of employment, financial security, daily activities, relationships with others, and roles within the family. These changes have a major impact on each parent, family member, and on the family as a whole. When medical needs require admission of the infant to the NICU, the changes become even more significant because, for the most part, the needs of this "different" child or "different" birth have not been planned for or expected (Baum et al., 2012). For the family, these changes can be devastating and challenging to manage without full integration of the family into the NICU caregiving team. During this difficult time parents need more than support; they need to be true partners and an integral part of the process of caring for and parenting their child (Boykova & Kenner, 2010; Coulter & Ellins, 2007; McGrath, 2007b).

In the NICU, it is wholly impossible to provide excellent health care to the infant without partnering with the parents or family, or preferably both, in every aspect of care (Boykova, & Kenner, 2010; Stevens, Helseth, & Kurtz, 2010). Families provide the foundation for health concepts and are the child's portal to the health care system. Family beliefs and individual health values are highly correlated. Families are the constant for the child. The provision of individualized developmentally supportive care, of which FCC is a core principle, is pivotal to the long-term medical and developmental outcomes of the child (Aita & Snider, 2003; Montirosso et al., 2012). For these reasons, understanding the many influences of the context of family on the mental health status of each of its members is important for those caring for infants and children (Karatzias, Chouliara, Maxton, Freer, & Power, 2007; Poehlmann, Miller Schwichtenberg, Bolt, & Dilworth-Bart, 2009) (Box 32.1). Most professionals collaborating with children and families believe that a family-centered approach is the best option, because this type of care supports optimal outcomes for the child in concert with those derived from high-quality professional and technical care (Ahmann et al., 2004).

Clear definitions of family and the philosophy of FCC are critical to the foundation of the concepts presented in this chapter. Role theory is used to explain the issues families face during this challenging time. Factors that influence parenting behaviors include personal experiences, medical and nursing staff expectations, environmental conditions, and peer relationships. These factors can either promote or interfere with the development of an intact family unit (Morey & Gregory, 2012; Reis et al., 2010). A critically ill newborn complicates the attachment process (Brooks, Rowley, Broadbent, & Petrie, 2012), as well as the learning of parenting skills, and thus, an evidence-based framework is provided for understanding what families need in the neonatal setting. The chapter concludes with evidence-based FCC strategies that support optimal family functioning during the NICU experience and promote the discharge of intact families as the crisis of newborn intensive care begins to resolve. These strategies also include issues related to sibling adaptation and involvement of extended family members in the care and decision making related to the infant.

BOX 32.1

KEY ELEMENTS OF FAMILY-CENTERED CARE

The practice of family-centered care involves the following:

1. Recognizing the family as the constant in a child's life, whereas the service systems and those who work within each are always changing.
2. Facilitating family-professional partnerships and collaborations at all levels of health care provision.
3. Providing care for the individual child and their unique characteristics.
4. Families partnering and participating in program development, implementation, and evaluation.
5. Collaboration with families to contribute to policy formation.
6. Honoring the racial, ethnic, cultural, religious, and socioeconomic diversity of families.
7. Recognizing family strengths and individuality and celebrating those differences as valuable.
8. Respecting and supporting different methods of family coping with difficult situations and information.
9. Partnering and sharing with families, on a continuing basis and in a supportive manner, complete and unbiased information.
10. Encouraging and facilitating family-to-family support and networking.
11. Understanding and incorporating the developmental needs of infants, children, and their families into health care systems.
12. Implementing comprehensive policies and programs that provide emotional and financial support to meet the unique needs of families.
13. Designing accessible health care systems that are flexible, culturally competent, and responsive to family-identified needs.

Adapted from the Institute for Patient and Family-Centered Care (2011) and Johnson (2003, 2004).

FAMILY-CENTERED CARE

FCC is a philosophy of care in which the pivotal role of the family in the lives of children is recognized and respected (Johnson, 2003). According to this philosophy, families are supported in their natural caregiving and decision-making roles by building on their unique strengths as persons, and then as a family unit. FCC recognizes and promotes the normal patterns of a family's life at home and in the community. Rather than expecting the family to take on the medical culture of the institution, health care professionals recognize and reinforce the family's culture through a partnership formed in the best interests of the child. Parents and professionals are equals in a partnership committed to the child and to the development of optimum quality in the delivery of all levels of health care (Johnson, 2003, 2004; Malusky, 2005; Pillow, 2007). FCC strengthens the family unit through empowerment and advocacy by enabling the family to nurture and support their child's development (Cisneros-Moore, Coker, DuBuisson, Swett, & Edwards, 2003; Institute for Patient and Family-Centered Care, 2011) (Box 32.2).

From the child's perspective, FCC is safe and familiar; the infant/child is first and foremost a member of a family and care that is individualized to the family and is thus also individualized to the infant. When the framework of FCC is the foundation for caregiving, the family is visible, available, and supportive of their infant's needs because they are a collaborator and integral aspect of every decision that affects their child (Cartagena, Noorthoek, Wagner, & McGrath, 2012; Cooper et al., 2007; Malusky, 2005). Thus, their presence is noted in all aspects of care. The family members are an empowered partner in the caregiving of their child within the health care setting (Dunn, Reilly, Johnston, Hoopes, & Abraham, 2006; McGrath, 2006a, 2011). FCC begins wherever and whenever a family enters the health care system and continues through discharge. Families should encounter this philosophy of care before birth in antenatal care, continued it into the delivery room and beyond into the postpartum period (Hodnett, Gates, Hofmeyr, Sakala, & Weston, 2011; Lindner & McGrath, 2012; McGrath, 2006b). It is

BOX 32.2

FOUNDATIONAL PRINCIPLES OF FAMILY-CENTERED CARE

- Enabling: Building on family strengths to create opportunities and ways for families to use the abilities and competencies they already have to learn new ones to meet child and family needs
- Empowering: Acknowledging and respecting the fact that families have existing strengths and capabilities, and the professional builds on those strengths by supporting the family in meaningful decision making about issues that affect their welfare. Professionals who empower families interact and form partnerships with families in ways such that the family keeps or develops a sense of control over their own lives and are able to make positive changes to reinforce their own strengths, abilities, and actions

Adapted from the Institute for Patient and Family-Centered Care (2011) and Johnson (2003, 2004).

important to remember that families are not replaceable at any level in the overall development of the child. Within implementation of the philosophy of FCC, their impact always supersedes that of the health care system (Gooding et al., 2011).

DEFINITION OF FAMILY

The concept of whom and what comprises a family in North America is defined best by that family unit. Families expand, contract, and realign at a rapid pace to keep up with the rapidly changing demands of our world. Today, dual-career families, permanent single-parent households, unmarried couples, homosexual couples, remarried couples, and sole-parent adoptions are all accepted models of family, in addition to the "traditional" family units most common a century ago.

"Family" is a broad term that is best defined by the individual; however, in general, a family is made up of those people, both related and unrelated, who provide support, structure beliefs, and define values. Family has also been defined as a social system composed of two or more people who coexist in the context of expectations of reciprocal affection, mutual responsibility, and temporal duration (Kaakinen, Gedaly-Duff, Hanson, & Coehlo, 2009). Families provide the framework through which individuals enter and interact with society at large. For infants and children, families are the means to resources, education, and society. Again, it is important to remember that families bring their children to the health care system for care, and no matter how an infant comes to us, it comes with a family.

A family is defined by its members; "family" is an internal concept of how that particular group defines itself. It may be composed of family or friends; it may not depend on a blood bond but on the emotional tie or closeness felt among its members. It also may be an extended family that includes parents, grandparents, other relatives, and friends. Families today are not necessarily defined as they have been in the past and not according to gender-specific roles. Families also can be defined by considering the degree to which the following five attributes are present (these attributes also depend on the family's societal and cultural orientation) (Kaakinen et al., 2009).

1. A family is a social system or unit.
2. Family members may or may not be related by birth, adoption, or marriage.
3. A family may or may not include dependent children.
4. Families involve commitment and attachment.
5. Family members usually have roles and caregiving functions (e.g., protection, nourishment, and socialization).

ROLE THEORY

In the context of better understanding family dynamics, it is important to also review and examine role theory. Role theory, which first appeared in the literature in the 1930s, offers a framework for understanding families and identifying the roles that individuals play within the family. As a broad term, role theory represents a collection of concepts, subtheories, and research that address aspects of social behavior relevant to families. Over the years role theory has come to include two major theoretical perspectives: symbolic interaction and social structural role (Kaakinen et al., 2009). Within both perspectives, role is a basic concept in the attempt to explain social order and interpersonal relationships within the family and society.

The symbolic interaction theory relates to individuals who create and construct their personal environment as they interact with, shape, and adapt to their own social environment. These individual behaviors aid in constructing the meaning of roles. In contrast, social structural role theory has a broader base. It focuses on the ways in which society, social structure, and other social systems shape and determine an individual's behavior. Roles are social contexts with patterned behaviors that develop over time and are predetermined by social forces.

The term *role* has diverse uses. One definition of a role is overt and covert goal-directed patterns of behavior that result from individuals interacting with, shaping, and adapting to their social environment. Roles are dynamic, interactional, and reciprocal relationships among individuals; therefore values, attitudes, and behaviors influence these relationships. Each role has specific behaviors and expectations placed on it by society, and these expectations guide individuals as to when, where, and in what manner they are to perform within the role.

Each role also has specific demands. An individual learns these demands by maturing and advancing through the middle to later stages of the life cycle: (1) adolescence, (2) adulthood, (3) marriage and parenthood, and (4) middle and old age. Individuals respond to the demands of a role differently based on their maturity and current stage in the life cycle. For example, a single, adolescent girl would be expected to perform the maternal role differently from a married, adult woman.

Concepts within role theory identify seven areas of distress associated with roles: (1) role ambiguity, (2) role conflict, (3) role incongruity, (4) role overload, (5) role underload, (6) role overqualification, and (7) role underqualification. These terms are defined in Table 32.1. These defined areas of distress are responsible for producing role stress and strain. Role stress is defined as either internal or external pressure that generates role strain. As a consequence, feelings of frustration, tension, or anxiety are produced in either the individual or the reciprocal partners. When problems occur with a role, a person or group may need to modify or completely change roles. As an individual changes roles and learns a new role, the required behavioral changes can be stressful. However, not changing roles can result in intrapersonal and interpersonal role conflict, which can lead to further stress and anxiety. Parenting in the NICU can lead to role conflict since parents often feel they are not the ones parenting their child (McCann et al., 2008; Treyvaud et al., 2011).

The working mother is an example of role conflict and role overload problems. She struggles with her dual professional and maternal roles. A decision to quit work and devote all her time to mothering may contribute to a lack of self-worth or identity. A decision to continue both roles may generate feelings of guilt because the new mother feels she is neglecting her family's needs. Reducing her work hours is a behavioral change she may make to allow more time for her family. She thus receives the positive reinforcement of employment, yet has more time for family and her maternal role. If she does not modify her roles, she experiences further stress and anxiety. To be effective, role change requires several steps. Such change develops through gradual, continuous, and dynamic processes based on the individual's needs and those of relevant others. The steps to successful role change include identifying the role of the relevant other (or others), identifying the expectations of the new role, developing the abilities for it, taking on the new role, and modifying it.

TABLE 32.1

POTENTIAL ROLE PROBLEMS

Role	Potential Problems
Ambiguity	Expectations are vague or lack clarity
Conflict	Expectations are incompatible (conflicts exist between reality and expectations)
Incongruity	Self-identity and subjective values are grossly incompatible with role expectations
Overload	Too much is expected in the time available
Underload	Expectations are minimal and underuse the role occupant's abilities
Overqualification	Occupant's motivation, skills, and knowledge far exceed those required
Underqualification	Incompetence; the role occupant lacks one or more necessary resources (commitment, skill, knowledge)

Adapted from Lipson and Dibble (2005).

PARENTAL ROLE

Certain behaviors that are specific to both mothers and fathers define the role of the parent. Several factors influence these behaviors: cultural background, personality, previous parenting and life experiences, degree of attachment to the infant, and expectations that parents have of themselves and the infant or child. A child changes everything in the close-knit relationship of the couple. Both must take on a new role; they are not just partners sharing a relationship; they are now mothers and/or fathers as well. Feelings of inadequacy, conflict, and fatigue are often apparent during the transition and may adversely affect both existing relationships and those just developing between the parent and child (Brett, Staniszewska, Newburn, Jones, & Yaylor, 2011). Parenting remains the only major role for which there is little preparation in our society. Difficulties encountered in the early stages of parenting may adversely affect all relationships but most especially the marital relationship. These difficulties can arise even if the new child is not the first child in the family unit; each additional member of the family brings unique joys and challenges.

The situation in which a person must parent also influences behaviors. Parents faced with a crisis must modify their roles and adapt to the necessary changes encountered with the crisis. Role and behavior changes can cause considerable stress, especially if these changes occur abruptly (Treyvaud et al., 2011). Maternal depression is a well-known phenomenon encountered by many mothers both during pregnancy and in the postpartum period. Mothers who must encounter the NICU are at particularly high risk for developing depression (Barnard et al., 2011; Carvalho, Linhares, Padovani, & Martinez, 2009; Rogers, Kidokoro, Wallendorf, & Inder, 2012). Parents suffering from mental or physical illness or those who are chemically dependent can have limited coping abilities and social supports (Gray, Edwards, O'Callaghan, & Cuskelly, 2012). Screening at admission, and throughout the infant's stay in the NICU is important so that support and treatment can be provided for these at-risk mothers (Rogers et al., 2012). Other interventions might include getting the mothers more involved with their infants, helping them to connect with other mothers in similar situations, and finding resources for them in the community (Carvalho et al., 2009; Gray et al., 2012; Zelkowitz et al., 2011).

Single, adolescent, or first-time parents are also at a disadvantage. They may lack maturity and coping skills because of limited life experiences and unavailable or inappropriate social support systems. These disadvantaged situations may inhibit the development of the parent–infant relationship and thus impair parenting behaviors regardless of whether the infants are high-risk, preterm or full term (Gray et al., 2012). In addition, mothers and fathers parent differently and take on the role differently (Boykova & Kenner, 2010; Coulter & Ellins, 2007; Hynan, 2005). These differences are not wrong or right; they are just differences that need to be acknowledged and accepted. Parents who have experienced some type of loss through infertility may also have more difficulties parenting their infant in the NICU since their personal investment in having a child may be causing role strain accompanied by increased stress and anxiety (McGrath, (Abou) Samra, Zukowsky, & Baker, 2010). Sensitivity to these experiences and previous losses is important to understanding how best to support these parents in the NICU. Lastly, in the NICU mothers are often the focus and fathers can be easily overlooked and not well understood or supported (Boykova & Kenner, 2010; Cleveland, 2008; Davis, Mohay, & Edwards, 2003). Care of fathers in this high-risk situation is changing, but it still is an area where we need to improve and provide optimal care and support.

Infant-related factors can also interfere with parental attachment and subsequent parenting behaviors. An example is an infant born with a congenital anomaly. Many of these infants may be mentally or physically disabled for a lifetime, which interferes with the parents' expectations of their infant (Brooks et al., 2012; Flacking et al., 2012; Watson, 2010). A visible anomaly is particularly difficult for parents because society places such emphasis on appearance. An infant with an easily correctable anomaly is tentatively unacceptable to society, until the anomaly has been corrected. A visible, noncorrectable anomaly has a greater impact on the parents and other family members. This stigma may include preterm infants who have deficits related to their untimely birth, such as blindness, deafness, or severe respiratory compromise. These parents may suffer from "chronic sorrow," and the child may grow up hindered by "vulnerable child syndrome" (Allen et al., 2004; Bartlett, Nijhuis-van der Sanden, Fallang, Fanning, & Doralp, 2011; Major, 2003; (Abou) Samra & McGrath, 2009). It may be helpful to connect these families with support groups or other families with children with similar disabilities or diagnoses (Hurst, 2006; Liu, Chao, Haung, Wei, & Chien, 2010; Willis, 2008).

A life-threatening or terminal illness in a child is another situation that may interfere with parenting attachment and behaviors (Brooks et al., 2012). Parents may "hold back" their feelings for the child to try to protect themselves from loss and pain if the child dies (Ladd & Mercurio, 2003). This inability to attach to their infant interferes with the parenting experience and may affect the child's development if the child lives past the previously expected life span.

At any birth or interaction between a parent and their child, the nurse must identify adaptive and maladaptive parenting behaviors. Adaptive behaviors indicate that both the infant's and parent's needs are met, and thus the parent–child relationship can be established. Mothers and fathers have different ways of expressing their parental roles based on gender differences alone (Boykova & Kenner, 2010; Hynan, 2005; Mundy, 2010). Tables 32.2 and 32.3 identify mothering and fathering behaviors the nurse can use in assessing adaptive or maladaptive behavior. It is important to remember that these are guidelines and must be adapted individually to each parent based on his or her personality and the specific situation.

PARENTING DURING CRISIS

Taking on the parenting role is a major life task for a couple. The crisis of having a critically ill newborn in the NICU compounds the stress of that task. Whether the family unit attains growth from a positive resolution of this crisis or splinters because of a maladaptive adjustment largely depends on the partnership formed with caregiving and the quality of support provided (Aronson, Yau, Helfaer, & Morrison, 2009; Callahan & Hynan, 2002). The memory of what happens in the first days after a traumatic birth often stays with a family forever; just ask a mother to describe her birth experience, and she will talk for hours, explaining every detail (Baker & McGrath, 2009; Beck, 2011). Consequently, the relationships formed and interventions provided during the initial trauma can be critical to the adjustment and continued growth of the family unit (Barnard et al., 2011; Cleveland, 2008; Pinelli et al., 2008).

Parents' Reactions

Crisis can be defined as an upset of a steady state. It is a period of disequilibrium precipitated by an inescapable demand to which the person is temporarily unable to respond adequately. The birth of a critically ill infant represents two types of crises for parents. The birth of any infant is a developmental crisis, a natural transitional phase in the lives of a couple. When the infant is premature or ill, parents also experience an accidental and unexpected crisis. The meaning of the event for the family and the resources available to deal with the event are variables that determine the scope of the crisis (Amankwaa, 2005; Pinelli et al., 2008). With the technologic advances that have been made in medicine, some families are now able to better prepare for and make decisions about their child's prognosis and medical needs before birth. For example, many infants with gastroschisis or other anomalies are diagnosed during a prenatal ultrasound examination. In such cases, families have the opportunity to better plan for the birth and to make decisions with the health care team in a more conducive and supportive environment. The ability to anticipate the needs of the child reduces the sense of crisis for these families with the birth of the child.

Families of a premature or sick newborn react in different and individual ways. Some common reactions are

TABLE 32.2

GUIDELINES FOR ASSESSING ADAPTIVE AND MALADAPTIVE MOTHERING BEHAVIORS

Adaptive Behavior	Maladaptive Behavior
Delivery	
Attempts to position head to see infant as soon as delivered and while infant is on warming table	Does not position head to see baby
When shown infant:	When shown infant:
• Smiles	• Frowns
• Keeps eyes on infant, looking at all parts exposed	• Stares at ceiling
• Attempts a face-to-face position	• May not look at infant
• Uses fingertip touch on face and extremities	• Stares at baby without expression
• Asks to hold baby	• Does not assume en face position
• Partly opens blanket to see more of infant	• Does not touch baby
	• Does not ask to hold baby
	• Declines offer to hold baby
	• If infant is placed in her arms, lies still, and does not touch or stroke baby's face or extremities
• Talks to baby	• Does not talk to baby
• Asks questions about baby	• Asks few or no questions
Makes positive statements about baby: "She's so cute!" "He's so soft!"	Makes no comments or makes only negative statements: "She looks awful." "He's ugly."
May cry out of joy or relief that infant is normal or of desired sex.	May cry, appearing unhappy or depressed
May smile and cry at the same time. (To differentiate from crying out of disappointment, note facial expressions and verbal statements.)	When asked why she is crying, states she is disappointed in baby
Expresses satisfaction with or acceptance of infant's gender: "We really wanted a girl, but it's more important that he's healthy." "I can't believe it's a boy, at last!"	Expresses dissatisfaction with baby's gender: "Not another girl. I should have known better than to try again for a boy." "I don't even want to see him." May use profanity when told gender.
Predominant affect: appears pleased and happy	Predominant affect: appears sad, angry, or expressionless
Suddenly decides she wants to breastfeed	Suddenly decides against breastfeeding
First Week	
Initially uses fingertips on head and extremities. Progresses to using fingers and palm on infant's trunk. Eventually draws infant toward her, holding infant against her body	Uses fingertip touch without progressing to palm on trunk or drawing infant toward her body
Snuggles infant to neck and face	Does not hold infant to neck or face
Makes spontaneous movements, kissing, stroking, and rocking	Makes few or no spontaneous movements with infant
Attempts to establish eye contact by moving infant, assuming en face position, or shielding infant's eyes from light	Does not use en face position or attempt to establish eye-to-eye contact
Handles and holds baby at times other than when giving direct care	Handles baby only as necessary to feed or change diapers
Talks to infant	Does not talk to infant
Smiles at baby frequently; changes affect appropriately, such as when infant cries	Rarely smiles at baby or smiles all the time without change in affect
Makes many specific observations of infant: "Her eyes look like they might turn brown." "One foot turns in just a bit"	Makes no observations or makes few observations that are either general or negative
Discusses infant's characteristics, attempting to relate them to others in the family: "He has my ears but his daddy's chin"	Does not discuss infant's characteristics in relation to characteristics of family members
"She really doesn't look like either of us, she just looks like herself"	
With a positive manner, uses animal characteristics to describe baby: "She's just like a cuddly little kitten." "His hair feels like down"	In a negative or hostile manner, uses animal characteristics to describe: "She looks awful, just like a drowned rat." "He looks like an ape to me."
Asks questions about caring for infant discharge	Asks no questions about care

(continued)

TABLE 32.2

GUIDELINES FOR ASSESSING ADAPTIVE AND MALADAPTIVE MOTHERING BEHAVIORS

Adaptive Behavior	Maladaptive Behavior
First Few Weeks	
(if infant remains hospitalized after mother has been discharged)	
Calls every day or every other day	Calls less frequently than every other day or not at all
Visits a minimum of twice a week	Visits less frequently than twice a week or not at all
Visits for a minimum of 30 minutes	Visits for less than 30 minutes
Asks specific questions about infant's condition	Asks no specific questions
Asks appropriate questions frequently	Asks inappropriate questions
Spends most of visit looking at and handling infant	Spends most of visit observing unit activities and other infants (this may be normal behavior for the first one or two visits); has little or no interaction with infant during visits
Becomes involved with care when encouraged and supported by staff	When encouraged by staff to participate in care, refuses, terminates visit, or performs only minimal care
Although visits are frequent and last longer than 30 minutes, makes statements about missing infant (e.g., says that she misses infant at home or that she wishes she could visit more often and stay longer)	Makes no statements about missing infant, or states that she misses infant at home and wishes she could visit more often, but comments are not validated by frequent or lengthy visits
Expresses reluctance to terminate visit	Leaves nursery with little hesitation
Waits until infant is asleep before leaving; touches or talks to baby just before leaving; may stand outside window and look at baby before leaving unit	Frequently asks nurse to complete feeding or to change and settle infant
First Months	
Holds infant close to her body	Does not hold infant securely against her body
Supports infant's trunk and head in position of comfort	Head and body of infant are not well supported
Muscles in her arms and hands are relaxed and conform to curvature of infant's body	Shoulder, arm, and hand muscles appear tense; hands and fingers do not conform to infant's body
During feedings, holds infant in well-supported position against her body	Holds infant away from her body during feedings or props infant or bottle
Positions during feeding so eye-to-eye contact can occur	Position during feeding prevents eye-to-eye contact
Minimizes talking to infant while baby is sucking	Continues talking to infant during feeding even though infant is distracted and stops sucking
Refers to infant using given or affectionate name	Refers to infant in impersonal way (e.g., "the baby," "she," or "it")
Plays with infant at times unrelated to direct care	Handles infant mainly during caretaking activities
When infant is in infant seat, playpen, or crib, frequently interacts with baby	Leaves infant for long periods in infant seat, playpen, or crib, interacting only after infant becomes fussy
Places infant, when awake, in an area where baby can observe and interact with others	Leaves infant, when awake, alone for long periods in bedroom or isolated area
Occasionally leaves infant with someone else	Frequently leaves baby with someone else or refuses to leave baby with someone else
Uses discretion in selecting babysitter and provides instructions on baby's routines, likes and dislikes	Does not use good judgment in selecting babysitter; provides inadequate or no instructions for care
Provides infant with routine well-baby care. Carries out medical plan for management of specific problems or conditions (e.g., thrush, anemia, or ear infection). Makes additional phone calls or additional visits to physician.	Fails to provide infant with well-baby care, seeking medical assistance only after problems, or keeps all appointments and emergency room for imagined or insignificant problems
Remains close to infant during physical examinations and attempts to soothe baby if infant becomes distressed	Remains seated at a distance from the examination table; does not soothe infant during examination; frequently arranges for someone else to take infant for medical appointments
Makes positive statements about mothering role	Makes negative statements about mothering role

Modified from Hall-Johnson (1986).

TABLE 32.3

GUIDELINES FOR ASSESSING ADAPTIVE AND MALADAPTIVE FATHERING BEHAVIORS

Situation	Adaptive Behavior	Maladaptive Behavior
Touches child	Freely, uses whole hand	Infrequent, uses fingertips, rough
Holds child	Holds child close to his body, relaxed posture	Holds child distant from his body, unrelaxed
Talks to child	Shows positive manner and tone; uses appropriate language, speech, content	Uses curt, loud, inappropriate language or content
Facial expression	Makes eye contact, expresses spectrum of emotions	Makes limited eye contact, little change in expression
Listens to child	Active listener, gives feedback	Inattentive or ignores child
Demonstrates concern for child's needs	Active, involves others, seeks information	Indifferent, asks few questions
Aware of own needs	Expresses feelings about self in relation to child	Gives no expression about self
Responds to child's cues	Responds promptly to verbal, nonverbal cues	Has limited awareness and response
Relaxed with child	Shows relaxed posture, muscle tone	Shows rigid posture, tension, fidgeting
Disciplines child	Initiates reasonable, appropriate discipline	Does not initiate discipline or uses measures too severe or too lax
Spends time with, visits child	Routinely uses time so that child is involved	Has no routine, no emphasis on child during time spent
Plays with child	Uses appropriate level of play, active, both enjoy interaction	Uses inappropriate play, no obvious enjoyment
Gratification after interaction with child	Father states he is, appears gratified	Gives no statement or display of gratification
Initiates activity with child	Frequently	Infrequently
Seeks information and asks questions about child	Concerned, asks frequent, appropriate questions	Asks few questions, needs prompting
Responds to teaching	Positive, reinforces instructor, seeks more information	Has little interest
Knowledge of child's habits	Knowledgeable	Has little knowledge
Participates in physical care	Feeds, bathes, dresses child	Allows others to perform tasks
Protects child	Aware of environmental hazards, actively protects	Protective behaviors not exhibited
Reinforces child	Gives verbal-nonverbal responses to child's positive behaviors	Does not notice or acknowledge child's behavior
Teaches child	Initiates teaching	Shows no teaching behavior
Verbally communicates with mother about child	Uses positive, frequent verbal encounters	Gives negative, infrequent communication
Verbally and nonverbally supports mother	Demonstrates support; reassures, touches	Support not obvious
Mother supports father, father responds	Gives positive response	Responds negatively or gives no response
Speaks of other children	Responds when asked, initiates	Shows no interest, no initiation

Modified from Hall-Johnson (1986).

anxiety, guilt, fear, resentment, and anger. During the illness of a newborn, the parents must face many charged issues; two important ones are the loss of the perfect child they have anticipated and a fear that their infant may die (Beck, 2011; Cleveland, 2008). In general, excitement and a flurry of preparation surround the birth of a child. Family celebrations help parents share the anticipation of a new infant with friends and extended family members. Parents spend much time imagining what this child will look like and dreaming about the joys of parenting. The couple experience disappointment when the infant or pregnancy is not as anticipated. They may feel a sense of isolation from other couples who have a normal pregnancy or infant. They may even have feelings of isolation from each other or from close family members. The inability to produce a healthy infant or to protect the infant from the invasive and painful environment necessary to sustain the child's life may cause feelings of inadequacy. For many parents, the role the couple had thought they would assume seems impossible to attain in the environment of the NICU, where often it seems everyone else is making decisions about the fate of their infant (Cleveland, 2008; Ladd & Mercuiro, 2003; McGrath, 2007a). Parents seldom have had experience with the NICU before and the intensity of the situation is heightened even more by the fact that they and their infant are center stage.

To move forward with the attachment process, parents must reconcile their idealized image of the child with the actual infant. They mourn the loss of the perfect child that was expected and encounter anticipatory grief for the infant whose life may now be in jeopardy (Caeymaex et al., 2012; Dyer, 2005a; Shah, Clements, & Poehlmann, 2011). The birth of an ill or a premature infant often places parents in a state of disequilibrium; nothing is as it was before. For many parents hope is an important emotional concept during this time of crisis (Amendolia, 2010). Hope provides some equilibrium that things will get better for their infant and for themselves. However, hope can also lead parents to develop high expectations for their child that may be in conflict with the expectations of the health care team. These different expectations can lead to more conflict and role strain as families are trying to maneuver the difficult situation of the NICU and understand how to assume their parenting role and best support their child (Roscigno et al., 2012).

Mothers of premature infants have had the emotional work of pregnancy cut short and thus are often psychologically unprepared for the birth (Amankwaa, 2005; Beck, 2011; Dyer, 2005b). If the mother had felt ambivalent about the pregnancy, she may believe that the infant's illness is somehow punishment for those emotions. A mother may also feel guilty that she could not carry the infant to term, even if no reason can be found for the baby's premature birth.

Many parents of sick newborns go through identifiable stages of grief and loss with very emotional reactions (Dyer, 2005a). The initial response usually is one of overwhelming shock, characterized by irrational behavior, crying, and feelings of helplessness and despair. Families at this stage have difficulty with organization because their lives have been disrupted by the unexpected birth. They may feel as if everything is in chaos and the situation is out of their control. Substance abuse, adolescent pregnancy, clinical depression, and domestic violence can increase the chaos and vulnerability of these families (Cleveland, 2008). Parents also may feel guilt over the premature delivery or the infant's illness. Self-blame often characterizes these feelings ("If only I had stayed home that day I noticed the spotting"). Parents may try to escape the situation by using denial ("Everything will all be fine in just a few days"). At the bedside in these initial days, parents may focus on facts they can understand and avoid issues they do not. To health care providers, this may seem as if the parents aren't listening or that they are unwilling to hear the information provided, yet the parents are trying to cope with what to them is an overwhelming situation (Hardy & McGrath, 2008; McGrath, 2007a).

Intense feelings of resentment and anger follow denial. Parents may direct these feelings at themselves, the infant, members of the health care team, God, or even each other as parents. They may also experience feelings of ambiguity and may fear the infant's physical and mental outcome. For these reasons, they may avoid emotional involvement with the infant to protect themselves from the pain of possible loss. A lessening of the intense emotional reactions and an increased ability to begin caring for their infant's emotional and physical needs are characteristic of adaptation and of taking on the parenting role. Reorganization is the final stage; at this point, parents come to terms with their infant's problems. This can take a few days to several months. In some cases, these feelings of loss and grief may never be resolved (Caeymaex et al., 2012; Dyer, 2005b). Throughout these stages, often it is hope that helps parents to move forward and believe that a new day will bring better outcomes for their child (Amendolia, 2010).

Factors That Affect Parenting Skills

Certain factors affect a couple's ability to acquire parenting skills during the NICU experience (Box 32.3). Parents are unable to attach and detach at the same time; these two tasks are incongruent. Parents need time to detach or grieve for the lost perfect child before they can begin to attach to the ill infant. This adjustment may take days or even weeks, and for some parents attachment may never occur (Shah et al., 2011).

Parents in the NICU environment face physical and mechanical as well as psychological and emotional obstacles during this difficult time. In this chapter, we refer mostly to the psychosocial behaviors of parenting and becoming a family, but it is important to note that these behaviors also have implications for the parent's health and personal well-being (Howland, Pickler, McCain, Glaser, & Lewis, 2011). These physiologic issues cannot be ignored since parents who do not attend to their personal and physical needs are not as able to attend to the needs of their child. Miles and Brunssen (2003) have developed a parental stressor scale for the parent with an infant in the NICU. The scale measures parental perceptions of stressors

BOX 32.3

FACTORS THAT INFLUENCE FAMILY REACTIONS TO A CHILD'S HOSPITALIZATION OR ILLNESS

- Severity of the illness and the threat to the child
- Previous experience with illness or hospitalization (or both)
- Familiarity with the medical procedures involved in diagnosis and treatment
- Available support systems
- Available coping strategies of family members
- Number and degree of other family stresses
- Cultural or religious beliefs
- Communication patterns of family members

inherent to the NICU environment. Studies using this tool have found that an infant's appearance and experience of painful procedures, as well as the perceived severity of the child's illness, all contribute to the degree of stress experienced by parents (Franck, Cox, Allen, & Winter, 2005; Miles & Brunssen, 2003). A nurse who can properly identify the specific stressors with each parent or family has the opportunity to assist them in reducing those stressors and promoting adaptation for the family unit (Callahan & Hynan, 2002).

The nurse is potentially the principal barrier to parenting in the NICU, because the nurse can be seen as the gatekeeper of the infant (Latour, Hazelzet, Duivenvoorden, & van Goudoever, 2010). In reality, the baby belongs to the family and not to the medical team. For parents to attach to their infant, a welcoming, calming environment in which they feel comfortable is essential in the NICU (Box 32.4). This kind of environment encourages parents to grow in their primary caregiver role so they can develop skills needed to be advocates for their child. This advocacy is essential for the infant's continuing development, especially if the child has special needs (Franck et al., 2005). Meiers, Tomlinson, and Peden-McAlpine (2007) developed the Family Nurse Caring Belief Scale to examine nurses' beliefs about FCC activities. This instrument can be used to understand how nursing staff perceive their own delivery of FCC and as a means to examine changes in FCC in a particular NICU environment over time.

BOX 32.4

CREATING A WELCOMING ENVIRONMENT IN THE HOSPITAL FOR FAMILIES

1. When the opportunity presents before the birth, prepare the family for the infant's admission to the neonatal intensive care unit and hospital course.
2. Give a special orientation for families who have undergone an emergency admission.
3. Provide for the needs of families who have traveled long distances.
4. Make fathers as welcome as mothers.
5. Meet the needs of siblings and other family members.
6. Enable families to be together as much as possible; have open visiting hours 24 hours a day.
7. Encourage families to bring things from home that make their child feel more at home.
8. Provide privacy for visiting family.
9. Encourage family participation in the child's care.
10. Help the family stay in touch with extended family members and support givers in the community; isolation at the hospital is not helpful for the continued growth of the family.

Adapted from the Institute for Patient and Family-Centered Care (2011) and Johnson (2003, 2004).

Mothers and fathers react to stress and grief in different ways (Cleveland, 2008). A father may isolate himself and become engrossed in his work and may not share his feelings with the mother. A father often tries to be strong for the mother and may become protective, sometimes choosing to shield her from painful information (Hardy & McGrath, 2008; Hynan, 2005). The mother may view the husband's stoic behavior as cold and unfeeling. Both may have difficulty discussing the child because of their own grief or guilt feelings. Normal postpartum blues can increase the mother's sensitivity to this situation and lead to further depression (Callahan & Hynan, 2002). She may cry for no real reason and feel embarrassed about irrational behavior. Existing weaknesses in their relationship are often magnified. Parents are often separated in their feelings at this time, and fears may arise that their relationship is falling apart at a time when they each seem to need the other. Lack of communication can lead to isolation and feelings of resentment in each of the partners. Each may make assumptions about the other's feelings, resulting in misconceptions. The need to communicate and share in each other's experiences is especially true if the child has special needs or a developmental disability. These misconceptions, along with gender differences in coping, may continue for a lifetime if they are not recognized and shared during the neonatal period (Amankwaa, 2005; Poehlmann et al., 2009). Helping parents to understand that their feelings are not unusual is important to facilitate the sharing of these feelings with their partner. Some couples may require counseling during this time.

Other stressors in the family, such as the needs of other children, financial concerns, illness of family members, or marital stress, can complicate the situation (Pinelli et al., 2008). For example, factors that can influence the degree of stress perceived by the family include the availability of appropriate emotional and psychological support among family members and from friends and the availability and use of community resources (Pinelli et al., 2008). Maintaining a support system and using community resources and professional assistance are excellent coping strategies for dealing with the crisis. Coping abilities demonstrated during previous crises often can predict how parents will cope with the current crisis. In an acute crisis, the family may be unable to use the resources available adequately because of lowered self-esteem, reduced family cohesiveness, and impaired family communication. Interventions during this time should focus on helping the parents to recognize and use available coping strategies. Communication patterns could be impaired because of anger or emotion derived from the crisis situation (Pinelli et al., 2008). Therefore, at times the family may require outside assistance; they may be unable to use or maintain the community resources required without this support (Patterson, 1995).

A stressful situation has a specific meaning for each family and for each member of the family because of previous experiences and the family's perceptions of these demands and their personal capabilities. For example, a sepsis workup may not seem particularly stressful to the health care team but may be very stressful to parents and families (Newnam & McGrath, 2010). For some families, the least hint that their infant is sicker or more unstable can be devastating. Certain personality types thrive on stress and deal effectively with any crisis. Others are unable to deal with even the smallest crisis. For example, if a family acknowledges a stressor as a "challenge" or can bestow meaning on the situation, such as believing that "it is the Lord's will," adaptation will likely be more successful. Maladaptation results if the family interprets the stressor as threatening or undesirable. According to McCubbin and Patterson (1983), a stressful event has three levels of meaning within a family: the meaning of the stressful situation itself, the values inherent in the family identity, and the family's overall worldview (Patterson, 1995). The family's expectations for themselves and this new child affect parenting skills. Each partner within the couple draws on his or her own childhood experience for parenting role models. The meaning the stressor has to the family also depends on the family's identity, cultural beliefs, and worldview. The family's identity comprises the values of the family, which are seen in the routines and rituals that develop in individual families. Stressors may disrupt these routines and rituals, threatening the development, maturation, and stability of the family system (Patterson, 1995). The family's worldview is based on how the family interprets reality, its core belief system (religious and cultural beliefs), and its purpose in life. The way a family handles its problems or deals with change often is based on the family identity and worldview. The family worldview is the most stable of the three levels of meaning, but even it can be shattered by a severe crisis (Patterson, 1995).

The coping strategies are cognitive and behavioral components of the effort to handle the stressful event: that is, what the family "does" to handle the stress. These strategies can be emotion-focused (i.e., strategies for controlling the emotions the crisis has engendered, such as denial or anger) or problem-focused (i.e., action-oriented strategies to manage the crisis). Coping behaviors are learned, and families can use any or all of the major coping functions in a crisis situation. Emotion-focused strategies are used most often in the adjustment phase of a crisis, and problem-focused strategies are used more in the adaptation phase (Doucette & Pinelli, 2004).

CULTURAL PERSPECTIVES

Definitions

Some key definitions are important to an understanding of cultural perspectives.

- Ethnicity: a common ancestry through which individuals have evolved shared values and customs
- Culture: socially inherited characteristics, such as rituals, the thoughts, beliefs, behavior patterns, and traits inherent within a certain racial, religious, or social group
- Acculturation: changing one's cultural patterns and assimilating behaviors consistent with those of the society in which one lives. This task can be done by learning the language, intermingling socially, or developing friendships, or through marriage or relationships formed in school or workplaces.
- Religion: a belief in divine powers; a system of beliefs, practices, and rituals

The family has always been seen as the critical social unit for passing on beliefs and values in our society. Health care professionals must recognize and be sensitive to the influence of culture and ethnicity on a child's development and the family's response to illness or a chronic condition (Lipson & Dibble, 2005; Preyde, 2007). The family's cultural ties provide support and a sense of stability during times of upheaval and stress.

The meaning of family varies with the ethnic or cultural background of the family (Lipson & Dibble, 2005). The concept of immediate family in Anglo Americans means the nuclear family of mother, father, and children, although this is changing as other definitions of family are becoming increasingly acceptable in our society. For African American families, the definition of family usually means extended family within the community. For Italians, family means a very strongly knit group of family and friends extending over three or four generations. The Chinese family consists of all their ancestors and all their descendants. Mexican American families are often close-knit and have supportive communities that are multigenerational. Differences in family hierarchy can both positively and negatively influence young parents (Hurst, 2004). Understanding and appreciating the differences in the meaning of family across cultures and ethnic groups can assist the health care professional in promoting the family's health and supporting the family in times of illness or debilitating conditions (Ardal, Sulman, & Fuller-Thomson, 2011).

Ethnic or cultural groups differ in the meaning of illness and disability, and in when they seek health care (Lipson & Dibble, 2005). Although the nurse must recognize that each family and situation must be assessed individually, there are some general characteristics that may be helpful in understanding differences seen among ethnicities. In general, members of an Italian family rely on the family for help when ill and seek medical help only as a last resort. They use words and emotion to convey the meaning of an experience to others. The close-knit family is of vital importance, and the nurse must respect the family as a cohesive unit. In general, African Americans often have an underlying distrust of the health care system. To effectively work with African American families, the nurse must be supportive of the family or empower the family to solve their own problems. Racism and oppression have left their marks on these families, and health care providers must enable the family to be the advocate for the ill child, to cope constructively with problems, and to deal with an unknown future if disabilities persist (Hurst, 2006).

Members of some ethnic groups (e.g., Irish, African Americans, and Norwegians) consider illness to be the result of an individual's own sins, actions, or inadequacies. Native American Indians consider illness or disability the result of misconduct, for which the family is punished (Lipson & Dibble, 2005). The illness is part of the whole person. Native American Hawaiians view illness as an imbalance in the energy or harmony within the family. The illness is part of wellness, and this disharmony is a normal part of life. Anglo Americans view illness as stemming from a scientific cause that is outside the family. The illness is foreign and intrusive to the individual and the family. These traditional characteristics may be helpful in understanding the context of culture.

When a child is hospitalized, several important issues must be discussed with the family:

- What support the family wants
- Preferences regarding language, food, holidays, religion, and kinship
- Beliefs with regard to health, illness, and technologic advances
- Health practices (e.g., immunizations, annual physical examinations)
- Habits, customs, and rituals, which could affect their health

An understanding of family cultural differences can help the nurse provide care, determine the meaning of the illness or disability to the family, and assist the family in interventions appropriate to their culture (Brooks et al., 2012). This understanding also shapes parent and staff expectations of each other and of the ways in which care is provided. Taking the time to understand the regional cultural influences on families cared for in the NICU can facilitate communication between families and health care providers (Ichijima, Kirk, & Hornblow, 2011). Language can often be a barrier to providing care and understanding the needs of families. Providing appropriately supportive interpreters to families in the NICU is extremely important to supporting families and helping them to understand the needs of their infant (Matsuda & McGrath, 2011).

PROMOTING PARENTING IN THE NICU

A major nursing goal in the NICU for care of the family is to optimize parenting skills and discharge an intact family unit (Boykova & Kenner, 2012; McGrath, 2012). There are different ways to ease parental anxiety during the NICU experience. Open visiting policies, especially 24-hour visiting, provide the parents more opportunities to be with their infant while allowing them to deal with other responsibilities outside the NICU. Restricted visiting may imply that the staff is hiding details of the infant's condition. Unrestricted access to the infant allows the attachment and parenting processes to be fostered (Baker & McGrath, 2009; Franck & Spencer, 2003).

Facilitating the Attachment Process

The attachment process begins at birth. With a sick or premature infant, this process is often delayed until the parents can establish eye contact with and begin touching and caring for their infant. Bonding and attachment are enhanced by allowing the parents to touch and hold the infant as soon as the child's condition allows (Korja et al., 2008; Neu & Robinson, 2010). The preterm neonate's physical appearance, disorganized behavioral responses, and variable physiologic response to touch can cause much anxiety in the parents as they attempt to interact with their infant. However, it is important that the bedside nurse, who is well versed in what the sick or premature infant will tolerate, explain those maturational limitations to the parents. It is vital that parents understand an infant's immaturity and inability to respond or to tolerate eye contact or parental voice cues; otherwise parents may misinterpret cues or detach from their infant. Interventions that focus on helping parents to understand and respond sensitively to infant cues have been found to facilitate both the infant and the family (Melnyk et al., 2006; Zelkowitz et al., 2011). It also is important for the nurse to work with the parents to help them to recognize an infant's distress signals (e.g., hiccups, apnea, cyanosis, bradycardia, or mottling) so that parents can gauge their caregiving interactions by their infant's unique cues and behavior (Raines & Brustad, 2012; Zelkowitz et al., 2011).

Parent participation in the caregiving must begin at admission (Raines & Brustad, 2012). Soothing touch, providing containment, gentle infant massage, holding the infant, bathing, and skin-to-skin holding, or "kangaroo care," are just a few of the "high-touch" avenues for promoting parenting in the NICU (Korja et al., 2008; Neu & Robinson, 2010). Each of these supportive strategies should be provided to all infants in the NICU and reserved for families to implement with their infant. When parents are providing these interventions, there are physiologic and behavioral benefits for the infant as well as benefits to parents, including early bonding, increased confidence in parenting skills, and a sense of control. Parents who have the opportunity to participate in caregiving and getting to know their infant begin to have a sense of confidence that their infant is well cared for and may survive (Just, 2005; Pichler-Stachl et al., 2011; Prentice & Stainton, 2004; Reid, 2007). Nurses can use several key techniques to prepare parents for working with their infant and the technology in the NICU:

- Give constructive criticism
- Encourage parents to discuss their concerns and emotions
- Provide parents with information specific to their infant's care or condition
- Clarify information that parents have received through other channels
- Draw the parents' attention to positive points about their infant, including how the child responds to the parents
- Keep the channels of communication open by remaining nonjudgmental

Interventions with families must acknowledge the individuality of each member and of the family as a unit. Understanding that the needs of the whole are not equal to, greater than, or less than those of the parts is often a difficult concept for the neonatal nurse, who sometimes sees his or her role as involved more specifically with the care of the high-risk infant. Researchers repeatedly have found that hospital-based neonatal nurses view caring for families as not within their realm of practice (and certainly not the priority in their practice), but as something extra they do "when there is time" (Meiers et al., 2007; Mosqueda et al., 2012). These views are not congruent with developmentally supportive FCC practices. Optimal care requires that health care providers adopt a family-centered philosophy (Cisneros-Moore et al., 2003; Latour et al., 2010; Saunders, Abraham, Crosby, Thomas, & Edwards, 2003). Full implementation of a family-centered approach depends upon the support of the unit leadership and the institution. Staffing plans that allow health care providers, especially nurses, time in their schedules to work collaboratively with families must be a priority if developmentally supportive family-centered practices are truly fundamental to the philosophy of care in the NICU (Johnson, 2003, 2004; Sodomka, 2006).

Parents repeatedly have reported that they felt that health care professionals did not recognize them as the expert caregivers of their child and the constant in their child's life (Cescutti-Butler & Gavin, 2003; Jones et al., 2007; McKlindon & Schlucter, 2004). This perception may lead to mistrust in the developing partnership between the caregivers and the professionals and may intensify the stress for the parent and ultimately, the child during the hospitalization (McGrath, 2001). Acknowledging that parents are the experts and nurses are the consultants to whom parents come to for information or support is a shift that remains difficult for some professionals (Johnson, 2003, 2004). Parents are empowered by nurses when they are respected, involved in the plan of care, provided with complete, unbiased information, and given a sense of control in the health care setting (Baker & McGrath, 2011b; Johnson, 2003, 2004; McGrath, 2001; Pichler-Stachl et al., 2011). To support full integration and implementation, see Table 32.4 for evidence-based strategies and interventions that empower and support families during newborn intensive care.

TABLE 32.4

EVIDENCE-BASED FAMILY-CENTERED CARE STRATEGIES TO SUPPORT INFANTS AND FAMILIES IN THE NICU

Intervention	Level of Evidence	References
Encourage family to visit and spend as much time with their infant as possible	III	• Ahmann et al. (2004)
	IV	• Franck and Spencer (2003)
Facilitate and maintain a collaborative partnership with families	VI	• Figueroa-Altmann, Bedrossian, Steinmiller, and Wilmot (2005)
	IV	• McCormick, Escobar, Zgeng, and Richardson (2008)
	IV	• Meiers et al. (2007)
	VI	• Mundy (2010)
	V	• Reis et al. (2010)
Assisting the family to resolve guilt feelings	IV	• Caeymaex et al. (2012)
	IV	• Shah et al. (2011)
	VI	• Watson (2010)
Facilitate and provide opportunities for families to develop and sustain hope	VI	• Amendolia (2010)
	IV	• Roscigno et al. (2012)
Provide family with opportunities to learn about infant cues and behaviors to facilitate attachment and decrease sense of vulnerability	IV	• (Abou) Samra and McGrath (2009)
	IV	• Allen et al. (2004)
	IV	• Loo, Espinosa, Tyler, and Howard (2003)
	II	• Melnyk et al. (2006)
	II	• Tooten et al. (2012)
	II	• Zelkowitz et al. (2011)
Provide family with opportunities to hold and touch their child early in the NICU stay	IV	• Korja et al. (2008)
	II	• Neu and Robinson (2010)
Provide parents the choice to be present during procedures to support their child	IV	• Aronson et al. (2009)
	IV	• Axelin, Lehtonen, Pelander, and Salantera (2010)
	IV	• Mangureten et al. (2005)

(continued)

TABLE 32.4

EVIDENCE-BASED FAMILY-CENTERED CARE STRATEGIES TO SUPPORT INFANTS AND FAMILIES IN THE NICU (CONTINUED)

Intervention	Level of Evidence	References
Screen often and regularly for maternal depression and provide resources to support mothers as needed	IV	• Bartlett et al. (2011)
	II	• Barnard et al. (2011)
	VI	• Baum et al. (2012)
	VI	• Beck (2011)
	IV	• Callahan and Hynan (2002)
	II	• Carvalho et al. (2009)
	I	• Karatzias et al. (2007)
	V	• Poehlmann et al. (2009)
Facilitate parent presence and caregiving through communication that is welcoming and supportive	V	• Brett et al. (2011)
	III	• Brooks et al. (2012)
	VI	• Flacking et al. (2012)
	IV	• Pichler-Stachl et al. (2011)
	IV	• Raines and Brustad (2012)
Provide parents opportunities to participate in care through scheduling of caregiving to increase their presence	VI	• Baum et al. (2012)
	V	• Cleveland (2008)
	VI	• Davis et al. (2003)
Provide support to fathers and encourage them to participate in care	V	• Hynan (2005)
	VI	• Watson (2010)
Provide care that is culturally sensitive	VI	• Hurst (2004)
	IV	• Ichijima et al. (2011)
	II	• Preyde (2007)
Introduce the family to support systems in the form of families with children who are undergoing or have undergone similar experiences	VI	• Ardal et al. (2011)
	IV	• Domanico, Davis, Coleman, and Davis (2010)
	VII	• Gooding et al. (2011)
	VI	• Hurst (2006)
	III	• Liu et al. (2010)
	IV	• Treyvaud et al. (2011)
	III	• Willis (2008)
Provide the family with resources from the community (e.g., spiritual, economic, and social help, as well as information)	IV	• Doucette and Pinelli (2004)
	VI	• Hurst (2004)
	IV	• Pinelli et al. (2008)
Assist the family in recognizing and using their strengths and coping skills or facilitating development of new coping strategies to decrease stress in the NICU. Encourage the family to explore positive ways of coping with the situation	IV	• Gray et al. (2012)
	VI	• Howland et al. (2011)
	V	• Major (2003)
	IV	• Miles and Brunssen (2003)
	VI	• Watson (2010)
Facilitate positive perceptions of staff by families through staff communication styles	I	• Brett et al. (2011)
	IV	• Cescutti-Butler and Gavin (2003)
	III	• Cooper et al. (2007)
	VI	• Jones et al. (2007)
	IV	• Latour et al. (2010)
	III	• McCann et al. (2008)

(continued)

TABLE 32.4

EVIDENCE-BASED FAMILY-CENTERED CARE STRATEGIES TO SUPPORT INFANTS AND FAMILIES IN THE NICU (CONTINUED)

Intervention	Level of Evidence	References
Provide education for families that meets their needs and is provided in a supportive style	IV	• Coulter and Ellins (2007)
	IV	• Morey and Gregory (2012)
	II	• Shieh et al. (2010)

Rating System for the Hierarchy of Evidence
Level I: Evidence from a systematic review or meta-analysis of all relevant randomized controlled trials (RCTs), or evidence-based clinical practice guidelines based on systematic reviews of RCTs
Level II: Evidence obtained from at least one well-designed RCT
Level III: Evidence obtained from well-designed controlled trials without randomization
Level IV: Evidence from well-designed case-control and cohort studies
Level V: Evidence from systematic reviews of descriptive and qualitative studies
Level VI: Evidence from a single descriptive or qualitative study
Level VII: Evidence from the opinion of authorities and/or reports of expert committees

Adapted from Melnyk and Fineout-Overholt (2010).

Caretaking is a normal part of parenting. However, parents of sick or premature infants are often deprived of the time to prepare psychologically for caring for a high-risk infant and to develop the caretaking skills to feel confident (Just, 2005; Raines & Brustad, 2012). If nurses do not allow the family to become regularly involved in caretaking tasks, parents may feel inadequate or may resent the nurses. Positive reinforcement builds self-confidence in parenting abilities. Melnyk et al. (2006) have developed and tested the COPE (Creating Opportunities for Parent Empowerment) program to support and build confidence for parents in the NICU. This program empowers families through supportive education about preterm infant development.

Providing Information

Throughout the infant's illness, parents need accurate, timely information about their child's condition (Box 32.5). Loo et al. (2003) view parent learning as a process whereby parents focus on information that is provided when it is timely to the current needs of their infant. If the information provided is not timely and does not anticipate the needs of the parents as related to their relationship with their infant, it may not be helpful and may actually hamper the care (Baker & McGrath, 2011b). Information should be direct and honest and should not be contradictory; so limiting the number of professionals providing information is often helpful. Parents also appreciate the use of drawings and diagrams when their infant's condition is explained to them, and they appreciate being encouraged by staff members to ask questions. Presenting this information with some optimism allows the family some hope, and as discussed earlier hope is an important concept for coping with the NICU (Fox, Platt, White, & Hulac, 2005). Ideally, the information should be presented to both parents at the same time. It should be expressed

BOX 32.5

GUIDELINES FOR PROVIDING INFORMATION TO FAMILIES OF ILL INFANTS

Focus the teaching session so as to build confidence and foster independence in the family. Build from strengths of the parent; do not focus on weaknesses.

1. Begin by assessing what the family members already know.
2. Establish a working rapport with the family; work to ease their anxiety and fear and to convey confidence and assurance to family members.
3. Ask family members what they expect to learn from the session and provide information directed toward their concerns.
4. Initially, focus teaching on the diagnosis or current crisis.
5. Use language the family understands; avoid jargon.
6. Include the key characteristics of the plan of care and treatment.
7. Explain the ways in which the illness or medication regimen will affect daily life.
8. Use a variety of teaching materials and styles. All information should first be provided orally and reinforced with handouts to be taken home.
9. Keep the information simple and concrete; reinforce oral communication with handouts. Expect to repeat the information and do so readily.
10. Avoid fear tactics while providing information on both benefits and detrimental effects.
11. Use praise to instill confidence.
12. Include anticipatory guidance.

Adapted from Baker and McGrath (2011b); Menghini (2005); and Morey and Gregory (2012).

in simple terms with short explanations. The parents are under much stress, and this information may be unfamiliar (Brooks, Rowley, Broadbent, & Petrie, 2012, Loo et al., 2003; Menghini, 2005). Facts may need to be repeated several times before they are absorbed. Parents need a clear understanding of the information provided to make informed decisions about their infant's care. Family-friendly language in understandable terms should be used when delivering care and information (Baker & McGrath, 2011b; Menghini, 2005). Medical information from a primary caregiver, such as a neonatal nurse practitioner or primary physician, provides consistency, especially when the news is difficult or "bad" (Box 32.6). Families also need information about visiting hours, unit policies, equipment, procedures, and treatments their infant is receiving. Direct telephone access allows an update from their nurse or physician at all times. In support of oral communication, written information helps parents remember important facts. In addition, written communication also provides a place to refer to later when the information is more relevant to the care of the infant or when there are more questions (Baker & McGrath, 2011b; Menghini, 2005).

BOX 32.6

PROVIDING DIFFICULT INFORMATION

Although difficult information is most often provided by physicians, nurses often are part of the team, especially if the information will be painful to the family. Nurses must know how to support families in these difficult situations.

1. Whenever possible, bad news should be delivered with both parents present and/or supportive family members as deemed by the family.
2. Give unbiased information that is clear, direct, detailed, and understandable; during the discussion, get to the focus of the discussion quickly.
3. Provide the information with compassion and caring in a gentle but confident style; a private, quiet place free of distractions should be used for the discussion.
4. Personalize the information to this baby or child and this family. Use the child's name whenever possible.
5. Allow the family time to express feelings and ask questions. Provide support for those feelings and questions.
6. Provide information about resources and anticipatory guidance.
7. Arrange an opportunity for the family to meet another family who has experienced a similar situation or crisis.
8. Follow up with the family after an appropriate time to answer any latent questions or provide further support.

Adapted from Liang and Freer (2008).

Family Presence During Rounds

In many NICUs the practice of inviting family members to participate in medical rounds is becoming common (Aronson et al., 2009). Families are part of the decision-making process and as such are provided information so that they can, in collaboration with the medical/nursing team, decide when they would like to be present and make decisions for their child and when they feel they would rather not be involved (Mangureten et al., 2005; McGrath, 2006b; Pichler-Stachl et al., 2011). Through their presence in rounds, families are involved in the assessment of and planning for their child (Raines & Brustad, 2012; Reid, 2007; Reis et al., 2010). Caregiving issues related to scheduling of rounds, teaching of medical staff, and confidentiality for families during rounds are still unresolved and remain a concern for care providers (Ladd & Mercurio, 2003; Morey & Gregory, 2012). For the most part, units where these practices are now common have found that the partnership between the family and the medical team is worth the effort required to implement such decision-making relationships (Dunn et al., 2006). Providing for and facilitating the family's role as the constant in the child's life is the best approach for the child's long-term development. Critical pathways (see below) can also be used as an excellent means of providing education and anticipatory guidance to parents and families, especially when provision of information with skill building must be completed over a long hospitalization or by several staff members (Dunn et al., 2006).

Family Presence and Participation in Procedures

One of the fundamentals of FCC is the belief that the family is an active member of the caregiving team right from admission. Members of the caregiving team are not visitors. Parents are not asked to leave for rounds or procedures; they are invited to be as involved during procedures as they feel comfortable with; the degree of involvement would vary from parent to parent and family to family (Axelin et al., 2010). Parents need to have enough information to feel welcome and supportive of their child during procedures to be present. Presence during resuscitation is one of the areas where more and more NICUs are providing families the support to be present and supportive to their child; however, this means someone from the health care team needs to be supportive of parents during the event (Mangureten et al., 2005). Staff members may resist including families in these interventions because of the degree of risk to the infant. Nurses must also take into consideration that even though parent participation might lead to short-term physiologic losses for the infant, these losses might outweigh the long-term gains for the family and make a decision with the family that is in the best interest of the infant. Established protocols and education of both staff members and parents help with the transition to increased parental participation in the NICU (Just, 2005; Mundy, 2010).

Supporting Families With Caregiving Protocols

Critical pathways and caregiving protocols have been developed to aid in the organization and evaluation of nursing assessments and interventions with children and families. These pathways help promote continuity of care and aid the nurse in prioritizing the needs of the child and family. They are outcome-oriented and provide an excellent means of documenting nurses' actions. They can be used to enhance interaction between parents and their preterm infant. The pathway serves as a means to educate parents about the changing needs of their developing preterm infant. Implementation of the pathway increases parents' knowledge and responsiveness to their infant's behavior and helps parents develop independent, cue-based caregiving skills with their infant (Tooten et al., 2012; Zelkowitz et al., 2011). Other pathways have been developed with five areas of emphasis: environmental organization, the structure of caring and feeding (all of which relate more to the infant), and family involvement and education (which relate more to the needs of the family). Outcomes for infants include physiologic stability, behavioral organization, and establishing predictable behavioral patterns; outcomes for the family include enhancing social support, increasing knowledge, and increasing involvement in the infant's care while preparing for discharge (Boykova & Kenner, 2012; McGrath, 2012). Critical pathways also are an excellent means of providing education and anticipatory guidance to parents and families, especially when teaching must be done over a long hospitalization or by several staff members.

Family Conferences

Family conferences can be used to evaluate the intervention strategies and how well they were able to meet the family's goals. Collaboration during conferences allows all present the opportunity to examine individual perspectives and goals while negotiating and reevaluating strategies to increase satisfaction with the treatment plan (Brett et al., 2011; McCormick et al., 2008). The type of information communicated is also an important consideration. Health care professionals have often provided families with a lot of information about their infant in the here and now; what is sometimes missing is the "so what" of that information (Fox et al., 2005; McGrath, 2007b; Morey & Gregory, 2012; Reis et al., 2010). The result of this type of communication is that parents are not always provided with all the information they need to understand the whole situation for their child now and in the future so that appropriate participation in decision making can occur (McGrath, 2005a).

Facilitating Transfer to Another Facility

If the infant is transported from another facility or being transferred to another hospital, parents need time to be with their infant prior to the move and should go on the transport with the infant whenever possible (Fidler & McGrath, 2009; Rowe & Jones, 2008; van Manen, 2012). These brief interactions before a transport reduce inaccurate fantasies about the status of the neonate and promote bonding and attachment behaviors (Evans & Madsen, 2005; van Manen, 2012). Occasionally, the mother's condition is unstable, and she or a family member cannot visit the NICU. Instant pictures can be taken and given to the mother as soon as possible. Some NICUs are also using video conferencing to keep families better connected to their infant.

The number of nursing or medical personnel in nondescript surgical scrub outfits who interact with the parents can be overwhelming. Therefore introductions by name and position are important to families, and personnel should wear name tags to help further identify each staff member. Many institutions have adopted a primary nursing style of care where the number of caregivers is limited to a small group of professionals, to increase consistency of caregiving and information sharing. Families often feel more secure knowing that one nurse or team of nurses direct their baby's nursing care throughout the hospitalization, and this allows a trusting, collaborative relationship to be established (Box 32.7). A friendly approach facilitates open communication and demonstrates openness and approachability.

Using language that invites participation also is important (Box 32.8). The primary nurse can act as liaison between the family and the health care team. The liaison ensures that information about the infant's current

BOX 32.7

PRINCIPLES OF FAMILY–PROFESSIONAL COLLABORATION

Family–professional collaboration accomplishes the following:

- Promotes a relationship in which family members and professionals work together to ensure the best services for the child and family
- Recognizes and respects the knowledge, skills, and experience that families and professionals bring to the relationship
- Acknowledges that the development of trust is an integral part of a collaborative relationship
- Facilitates open communication so that families and professionals feel free to express themselves
- Creates an atmosphere in which the cultural traditions, values, and diversity of families are acknowledged and honored
- Recognizes that negotiation is essential in a collaborative relationship
- Brings to the relationship the mutual commitment of families, professionals, and communities to meet the requirements of children with special health needs and their families

Adapted from the Institute for Patient and Family-Centered Care (2011) and Liang and Freer (2008).

BOX 32.8

LANGUAGE THAT FACILITATES COLLABORATION

"Do you prefer us to call you by your first name or your last name?"

"Here's what I'm thinking, but I'm wondering how this will work for you."

"Tell me how can I help you."

"Our institution usually does ________ this way. Would that work for you?"

"These are the things I plan to provide for your child today. Would you like to provide some of these activities?"

"What goals do you have for your child's care?"

"How does your child look to you today?"

"Do you have any questions or suggestions about your child's care?"

"This sounds important; help me understand your concern."

"Who would you like to have included in discussions about your child's care?"

"Let's talk about how much you want to be consulted."

Adapted from Fox et al. (2005).

condition, any changes in condition, and long-term outcomes for the infant are communicated to the family. The liaison role becomes essential if the infant is transported back to a community hospital or to another unit in the same facility (Evans & Madsen, 2005; Fidler & McGrath, 2009; van Manen, 2012). Parents need to know what to expect in the new unit and to understand how this environment is now actually better suited to meet the changing needs of their infant. Otherwise, parental mistrust may develop (Evans & Madsen, 2005; McGrath, 2001).

■ **Preparing for Discharge.** As nurses prepare the infant for discharge from the NICU, it is important that the parents feel prepared to care for their infant (Boykova & Kenner, 2012). Building on the relationship already established, parents can be provided one last boost in confidence by allowing them to room in with sick newborns before discharge. Structured education has also been found to increase parent confidence and caring knowledge prior to discharge which could make the transition from hospital to home easier for families (Lopez, Anderson, & Feutchinger, 2012; Shieh et al., 2010). Parents feel secure knowing that nurses are close by if they are needed. This process also allows parents the assurance that they can care for their babies adequately.

Many times the neonatal intensive care hospitalization is the beginning of chronicity for the infant and the family. Parenting a chronically ill child is qualitatively different from parenting a normal child. Nurses must promote the parents' and family's role as the caregiver for the child by determining the family's mode of coping and supporting those strategies while promoting family adaptation to the chronic illness. A major goal of care for these families is to integrate the child back into the family unit rather than making the child with a chronic illness a "special nucleus" that becomes the only priority or focus of family needs.

FCC of an infant or child with any chronic illness is based on the premise that the family is the main source of support and caregiving for the child. The concept of FCC is in line with the Institute of Medicine's (IOM) core competency of providing patient-centered care, which in this instance of the neonate is the neonatal and family constellation (IOM, 2003). Thus FCC can be achieved through specific nursing strategies aimed at creating opportunities for families to use their own strengths and abilities to meet their child's and family's needs. Ultimately, family-centered interventions empower families to develop and maintain healthy lifestyles, leading to overall improvement of the family's quality of life.

Providing Support for Parents and Families

Parent networking can be a vital tool for promoting parenting. Knowing that other families have survived this crisis can be reassuring. Support groups generally are helpful; however, they are not appropriate for every situation (Hurst, 2006). Some couples need counseling so they can feel more comfortable with decision making and participation in care (McGreevey, 2006). The primary nurse plays a key role in assessing signs that the family is not coping and needs therapeutic counseling. Support groups or counseling helps families examine problems objectively and learn alternative behavior for adaptive coping (Ardal et al., 2011). The nurse also can assist parents in identifying additional means of support. Ideally, parents should be permitted to define their "family" as needed to provide support during this crisis, allowing family members to visit as unit policy dictates. Grandparents, extended family, neighbors, and friends may constitute this group (Greisen et al., 2009).

Grandparents are a source of support for many parents. However, grandparents may be forced into an uncomfortable role by seeing their own child in pain without a way to relieve that pain. Understanding the dynamics within the generations will be important to providing the best support to families. Grandparents are also trying to cope with this new crisis and may relive their own birthing experiences, which could result in associated anxieties and prevent them from being available to provide support for the parents (Frisman, Eriksson, Pernehed, & Morelius, 2012). Extended family members may be more helpful if discord exists between grandparents and the nuclear family (Greisen et al., 2009). Friends of the family can be an asset if they are effective listeners. They can offer to provide transportation for the mother and child care for siblings, or they can take over housekeeping chores to help alleviate family responsibilities. Just having someone to make telephone calls to other friends and family to update them on the infant's condition can be a great relief for the family.

Social workers involved early in the hospital stay provide parents with an objective person to discuss caregiving options and provide contact with community resources. Families are often reluctant to express dissatisfaction with their child's care to nurses. Social workers can help parents express concerns without fear of retaliation against their child. Clergy provide spiritual support for a family. Families often turn to religion for comfort and support at a time of crisis. It is important to offer these resources to parents and to provide the appropriate privacy to exercise their religious freedom.

PARENT AND STAFF EXPECTATIONS

When parents have a sick infant in the NICU, they have expectations. They expect excellent medical and nursing care for their child (Cescutti-Butler & Gavin, 2003; Cooper et al., 2007; Jones et al., 2007; Latour et al., 2010). They expect accurate and timely information throughout their child's illness, and they expect to be involved in decision making about the infant's care (Hardy & McGrath, 2008). They expect this relationship that is developing with the health care team will be a partnership and that the partnership will be honored in every interaction. The medical and nursing staff members, working as a team supportive of each other and the family, have the ability to instill confidence in parents through this partnership (Raines & Brustad, 2012). Parents develop advocacy skills through collaborative communications with the nursing and medial team (Hardy & McGrath, 2008; McGrath, 2011; McGrath & Hardy, 2008; McGreevey, 2006; Morey & Gregory, 2012). Conversely, members of the medical and nursing staffs have expectations of the infants and families within this partnership related to the care of the infant. Expectations for the family may include visiting regularly, respecting the routines of the NICU setting, and sharing information that may be helpful in the care of the infant (Meiers et al., 2007). Sometimes these expectations are unrealistic. For example, the staff may expect parents to visit more often, even though the parents live far from the hospital, have other children, must return to work, and have other responsibilities that may prevent more frequent visits (Franck & Spencer, 2003). Parents may also feel there is no role for them in the NICU if a collaborative partnership has not been established and the environment is not welcoming (Klegerg, Hellstrom-Westas, & Widstrom, 2007; Reis et al., 2010). Staff expectations for the infant may include wanting the infant to nipple-feed more often or be weaned from oxygen faster. It can be distressing to parents to think that the medical staff is not pleased with their infant's progress, even though this attitude may not be verbalized. For this reason, incongruities should be avoided both in actions and in communications (Hardy & McGrath, 2008; Reid, 2007). It seems reasonable to assume that parents who are partners, well informed, and participating in the care are less likely to experience these concerns (Baker & McGrath, 2009; McGrath, 2005a).

Staff members' attitudes are an important part of the development of positive parenting (Box 32.9). Staff behaviors and attitudes can inhibit or encourage parenting skills. Conflict about parenting roles can exist between parents and staff members, and this conflict may escalate into a struggle for control. Parents may view the staff members as acting as the infant's parents or the infant as belonging to the staff because staff members provide most of the care (Cescutti-Butler & Gavin, 2003; Jones et al., 2007). The staff members' pet names for the neonate further reinforce parents' fears. Nursing staff can help the family by encouraging them to personalize the infant's care and then following their lead with naming and dressing. Bringing in clothes, toys, and pictures of other family members and making recordings of family voices are ways parents contribute to caretaking.

Nurses who care for families need to provide support and promote the family as a unit; however, overinvolvement of nurses can be detrimental to the family unit. Establishing appropriate relationships with families in our care can sometimes be difficult. It is necessary to identify inappropriate nursing behaviors and correct them. Educating the nursing staff about the parenting process facilitates identification of inappropriate nursing behaviors (Box 32.10). The education can be initiated during orientation of new

BOX 32.9

KEY CONTENT OF FAMILY-CENTERED TRAINING PROGRAMS FOR HEALTH PROFESSIONALS

- Principles of family-centered care
- Cultural competence
- Child development
- Family systems
- Fostering communication with children and families
- Building of collaborative relationships with families
- Support for and strengthening of families in their caregiving roles
- Impact of hospitalization, illness, and injury on children and families, including the impact of health care costs on family resources
- Support for the developmental and psychosocial needs of children and families through hospital policies and programs
- Function and expertise of each discipline in the medical setting
- Multidisciplinary collaboration and team building
- Ethical issues and decision making
- Community resources for children and families

Adapted from Figueroa-Altmann et al. (2005) and McKlindon and Schlucter (2004).

BOX 32.10

BEDSIDE CAREGIVER BEHAVIORS THAT MAY BECOME BARRIERS TO POSITIVE PARENTING

- Infant "belongs" to the nurse and the NICU rather than to the family; nurse refers to assignments or primaries as "my babies."
- Family is not considered a member of the caregiving team; for example, they are asked to leave for rounds and shift report.
- Family is not asked about the characteristics of their infant or included in discussions related the infant. Families are not seen as the expert about their infant. They are talked about rather than talked with.
- Care is task oriented, and staffing is acuity based rather than based on meeting the needs of families. Families are not invited to participate in the child's care.
- Infant's schedule belongs to the nurse and the NICU rather than to the family, so that feeding and caregiving might occur when the family is unavailable to participate. Scheduling is inflexible.
- Family is seen as an adjunct to the infant and his or her care. They are not the client or patient. Spending time with families is not considered a priority but rather a luxury. Spending time with families is not seen as essential to providing care for the infant.

Compiled from Jones (2007); Latour et al. (2010); McCormick et al. (2008); and McGrath (2007b).

staff members and reinforced at intervals with continuing education workshops on the subject. Nurses must provide support while always acknowledging the boundaries of the family. Some families build walls and are so private about family matters that it is difficult to obtain enough information to meet family needs, whereas other families become overly dependent on the nursing staff, needing their support at every moment. Interventions that promote independent family decision making include the following (Johnson, 2003, 2004):

- Respecting the family as a unique unit
- Providing unbiased care to all families
- Providing as much continuity in the care provider as possible to promote family strengths
- Allowing the family to determine the implementation of the plan of care

With adequate staffing, nurses can better promote parenting in the NICU. Overworked nurses can become frustrated and stressed, overwhelmed by their own anxieties. These feelings may impede their ability to interact calmly and therapeutically with a fragile family unit. Nursing management considerations should include provision for adequate staffing to allow nurses the time and emotional energy to meet the needs of parents in crisis. Patient assignments should be evaluated not only for the technical care an infant requires but also for the psychosocial demands of the family. Institutional policies should be carefully evaluated as to how they meet the needs of families.

SIBLINGS

Siblings have needs, because they are an important part of the new infant's life. Sibling visits may help relieve anxieties and make the birth a reality. Siblings have a variety of responses to a newborn's arrival in the home, especially after a lengthy hospitalization. Family routines are disrupted by a "normal" birth and are further disturbed by an admission to the NICU and then again at the time of discharge. Siblings may feel displaced while parents are visiting the ill infant. Siblings often are left with babysitters when they have rarely had experience with caretakers outside the immediate family. Fathers who may be uncertain about their family role may embrace their familiar work role and spend more time on the job. In these ways routines are disrupted, and parents are less available for their other children. These feelings may result in a variety of acting-out experiences.

The birth of a new baby precipitates a family upheaval and the need for realignment of relationships and positions within the family constellation. Becoming a sibling is known to be a stressful or "crisis" experience for young children and can have an effect on their mental, emotional, and social development. The birth of a preterm or critically ill neonate who requires intensive care constitutes a further crisis for parents and consequently disrupts the equilibrium of the family system (Munch & Levick, 2001). Parents are reported to experience feelings of anxiety, grief, fear, anger, and guilt in response to the unanticipated events. Siblings are also affected and may experience helplessness, powerlessness, guilt, and anger in addition to the disruption of their daily routines and separation from their parents. The siblings may feel very alone because their worried parents are preoccupied with the newborn baby. Siblings feel like the forgotten family member at the very time they need attention most (Munch & Levick, 2001).

Addressing the needs of families of hospitalized patients has gained acceptance and support among nurses since the advent of the concept of FCC (Institute for Patient and Family-Centered Care, 2011; Johnson, 2003, 2004; Malusky, 2005; Pillow, 2007). All members of the family, parents and siblings, may exhaust their coping strategies and feel unsupported by those who are usually available emotionally and physically. The philosophy of FCC in the NICU is reported to encourage not only parent participation but also involvement of the well sibling or siblings in the family process. This involvement allows children to see their new sibling and to feel as if they are a part of the family process. Feelings of isolation may engender fantasies about what is taking place in the NICU. At any age, it is easier to cope with reality than with what can be imagined.

Increasing numbers of hospitals are allowing the participation of children at a sibling's birth, sibling contact with the infant at birth, sibling contact with the infant on the postpartum unit, and sibling visits in intensive care nurseries.

For nurses facing these challenges, the philosophy of FCC can provide a firm foundation in striving toward excellence in the practice of caring for children and families (Ahmann et al., 2004; Institute for Patient and Family-Centered Care, 2011; Sodomka, 2006). The development of a sibling–infant bond is vital to establishing and enhancing the relationship within the family unit. Holistic care surrounding childbirth may set up patterns or pathways that dramatically affect subsequent family interactions.

Some families feel they cannot be part of the care team. They either do not desire to provide care or cannot do so. Sometimes there is a tendency to label them as noncompliant with what the health care professional believes the family should do or how they should act. Before a label is used, find out from the parents why they do not want to participate. Is it because they fear they will hurt their child? Is it because they want to just be parents and not be responsible for the care? Is it a lack of understanding what is being asked of them? Based on their response, an individualized plan of care can be developed. For example, for the parent that is fearful about providing care, the health care team can provide education, psychological support, and be present to support caregiving activities. The key to success is to talk to the family, listen to their concerns/perspectives, and then tailor a plan to increase their participation as a care team member.

Sibling Visitation to the NICU

Sibling visitation in the hospital after the delivery of a newborn has become common practice. However, limited recent research exists that examines the consequences of permitting and prohibiting sibling visits in the NICU, despite the argument that sibling involvement is consistent with the concept of family-centered perinatal care. Early studies of NICU sibling visitation programs provided valuable descriptive data on siblings' responses to the sick neonate. NICU visits provided an opportunity for the older brother or sister to see, touch, and talk to the newborn. This exposure was reported to help the children integrate the reality of the experience, to prepare for the possible loss of the newborn, and in some cases to reverse regressive behavior that had begun during the newborn's hospitalization. However, the findings of these studies reflected the perceptions of providers and not necessarily those of the parents or siblings (Andrade, 1998; Gooding et al., 2011). More research is needed in this area. Some NICUs restrict sibling visitation during respiratory syncytial virus (RSV) season, whereas some do not have a strict policy for how visiting might still occur during this time of the year. The same is true for varicella exposures and how to safeguard the infants (Kellie, Makvandi, & Muller, 2011). Again, more research is needed in this area.

Implications for Practice

Nurses have a unique opportunity to support the development of positive sibling relationships in the NICU environment. Evolving models of comprehensive care no longer overlook or delegate the care and needs of the whole family. Research on the families of NICU neonates has demonstrated parents' desire for a family-centered approach to care (Cartagena et al., 2012). Siblings are an integral part of any family, and their adjustment or lack of adjustment to the birth of a newborn greatly affects the well-being of the whole family. Siblings' adjustment to the once-sick infant needs further exploration.

When the birth of a sibling is further complicated by the baby's being ill or at risk, professionals caring for the baby are in a position to reassure parents that siblings will respond to the neonate in various ways based on each child's personality, age, and interests. Professional reassurance can help parents realize that siblings cannot help feeling angry and displaced by the baby. The parents' ability to accept their older children's competitive feelings and yet continue to love them helps those children to integrate ambivalence. Support through this ambivalence facilitates acceptance of the baby and the baby's incorporation into the family. Increasing parents' knowledge about promoting positive sibling relationships through parent education programs may influence the parents' attitudes, thereby enhancing the future sibling relationship. In response to consumer demand, many hospitals have implemented sibling visitation and educational programs. This preparation can help siblings deal with the realities of the experience. Special attention from the NICU staff also can help siblings feel recognized, supported, and appreciated during this time of stress. Encouraging the sibling to gently touch and talk to the infant and allowing gifts of toys or even a drawing of themselves to be kept with the baby are activities that may foster attachment and growing connection with the newborn.

The death of a sibling usually has profound and lasting effects on surviving children. Surviving siblings, however young, may need some evidence that the baby existed—a visit to see the ill newborn in the incubator, a photograph, or a chance to participate in the funeral. Regardless of the child's age, it seems that the level of care offered to these siblings is crucial to determining the psychological and life adjustment of the bereaved child. Nurses need to be alert to the range and depth of childhood reactions. Many research findings discussed here can serve as invaluable guides to help NICU nurses promote and facilitate effective sibling interactions and positive involvement between the sick neonate and the siblings. An appropriate environment in which nurses can assist children in coping with the profound changes that affect the sibling bond should also be provided, because such efforts help siblings fully integrate this major event into their young lives.

Environmental Effects

A quiet, comforting atmosphere with low lighting helps calm both the infants and their families. External stimuli in the NICU must be controlled; unnecessary stimuli aggravate these infants' already overwhelmed immature nervous systems, and loud monitor alarms and excessive staff noise can be upsetting and unnerving to parents (McGrath, 2000). Jamsa and Jamsa (1998) found that parents in the NICU felt that the technologic environment was frightening and that it delayed their ability to parent their children. In general, the equipment made the families feel like outsiders. Their discomfort inhibited interaction with their child and delayed their participation in caregiving. These researchers suggested changes in the technology of the NICU, such as use of different kinds of alarm signals with diminished volume; wireless, handheld information terminals; and remote monitoring. Some of this technology already is appearing in the NICU. The technology used in the NICU must be continually reevaluated and designed with a parent- and consumer-based perspective (McGrath, 2000). Achieving a balance between the high-technology environment and the need of parents to touch their infant frequently helps foster parental self-confidence. This balance must be a priority for the neonatal nurse.

Recommendations for single rooms in the NICU and other acute care areas throughout the hospital setting are now included in the 2006 Guidelines for the Design and Construction of Hospital and Health care Facilities (http://www.aia.org/aah_gd_hospcons). These guidelines are based on several significant research studies where single rooms throughout the health care setting were found to offer higher occupancy rates, reduced transfer costs, and lower labor costs, even when the cost of new construction was calculated into the equation (McGrath, 2005b; McGrath, (Abou) Samra, & Kenner, 2011).

In addition, hospital-acquired infection and medication errors were reduced in these settings. Most patients and families also report better communication with health care professionals in single rooms because the provider often spends more time, answers questions more thoroughly, and is more compassionate and caring. Patient length of stay has been documented to be shorter in private single rooms, which again adds to the decrease in costs (please see the guidelines for more information about this research). This movement to single rooms in the hospital setting is also important for compliance with the patient and family privacy requirements under the Health Insurance Portability and Accountability Act of 2003, which includes speech privacy rulings.

So how do these guidelines affect the NICU? There is little research directly related to the effects of neonatal single-room design. Most units across the United States have always been equipped with a few isolation rooms that have been used for infants with highly infectious diseases and, more recently, to isolate extremely-low-birth-weight preterm infants who appear to be most overstimulated by the big open room environment of the NICU. With new construction, and a greater emphasis on individualized family-centered developmentally supportive care, more units have added more of these single rooms, and some units have chosen to move to an entirely single-room design (Baker & McGrath, 2010; McGrath, 2005b).

Research to support a less stressful NICU environment with lower lights and less noise and activity has demonstrated shorter lengths of stay, decreased iatrogenic effects, and increased deep sleep and alerting behaviors in the infant, which may provide greater opportunities for more normal cognitive development (Saunders et al., 2003). Moreover, in changing the environment to meet the needs of infants and families, the less stressful environment is often times more positive for caregivers and should have a positive impact on patient outcomes and a decrease in medication errors (Domanico et al., 2010; Pineda et al., 2012). The challenge in providing care in these designs is finding a balance between the needs of infants, families, and caregivers in the NICU. This may be best achieved in a single-room design, where areas in the unit can be designed to meet the needs of those who use them most and yet allow others to adjust their individualized areas or rooms to meet their needs (Baker & McGrath, 2010; Patterson, 1995). Evidence-based design standards for the NICU do exist and should be considered with any remodeling or new construction project (Cone & White, 2010; White, 2007). These guidelines should be used as a standard, especially when data are needed to support the need to invest upfront in more space, better traffic patterns, multiple kinds of lighting, and noise reduction materials. Paying attention to design is especially important for vulnerable infants who are at risk to develop disabilities. Research data also exist and should be used to support the need to choose colors and textures that increase health and well-being for all who interface in health care settings. For staff to transition to and work with ease in single-room designs, they must have access and become comfortable with central monitoring and communication systems that provide them knowledge about patient status even from remote locations. Work areas for nurses must also be near the private rooms and allow for interaction and teamwork among staff (Cone & White, 2010). More research is needed in this area and should be a focus for the future.

SUMMARY

The birth of any infant produces tremendous change in the lives of each member of the family. Normal adaptation can be complicated by the birth of a premature, critically ill infant or one with congenital anomalies requiring admission to the NICU. If the family does not have adequate coping strategies or resources, this crisis has the potential to produce much role stress and strain, which ultimately can weaken or destroy the family unit. The nurse plays an integral role in supporting and guiding the family to appropriate resources and services. By promoting adaptive rather than maladaptive roles, the nurse can ensure an intact family unit after the crisis of intensive care.

EVIDENCE-BASED PRACTICE BOX

John Jones was born at 33 weeks gestation. The nurses described him as a typical preemie with respiratory distress syndrome and intermittent apnea and bradycardia. He required continuous positive airway pressure (CPAP) for several days and then hood oxygen for a week. After being weaned to room air, he was moved to the transitional nursery, where he stayed for another week until he mastered sucking, swallowing, and breathing. John's mother visited often. Mrs. Jones kept John supplied with breast milk and the latest drawings from his two sisters, Suzie, age 6, and Becky, age 4. John's father visited once in a while on his way home from work but did not take an active role in caretaking. He said that he was afraid to hold John but that he would as soon as John got bigger and stronger. John was a cuddly little guy who had an uneventful recovery and was discharged after 3 weeks in the NICU.

Several days before discharge, John's mother confided in his primary nurse that she was about at the end of her rope because her husband was working longer hours and her daughters were acting up in ways they never had before. Becky had demonstrated regression behaviors of bed-wetting and thumb-sucking. She had also started carrying around her "blankie" again, something she had stopped doing long ago. Becky was particularly close to her mother, and after her mother's daily visit to the NICU, Becky would hit her mother, crying, "I hate you! I wish the baby would go away!" Mrs. Jones said that when she tried to console Becky, the child ran and hid under her bed, crying, "Leave me alone! You only love that baby!" If that weren't bad enough, Suzie had begun waking up with stomachaches and refusing to go to school. Suzie had always loved her teacher and classmates and now was frequently in trouble for misbehaving in class. When Mrs. Jones would make Suzie go to school, the little girl would cry and say, "I hate that baby! I'd like to run over him with Daddy's car!" Mr. Jones had withdrawn from family life and was spending long hours at work. Mrs. Jones was beside herself.

The nurse was able to reassure Mrs. Jones that the behaviors of her husband and daughters were typical. Although this reassurance didn't immediately alter the situation, at least Mrs. Jones knew that many families respond to NICU hospitalization in this way and that, given time, the family would reestablish equilibrium. Mrs. Jones was encouraged to take the weekend off from her NICU visiting routine. She was able to spend a couple of special days with her daughters and engage her husband in life outside the worries of the NICU.

However, this did not provide Mrs. Jones with emotional support or help with her feelings of being overwhelmed and depressed. The nurse was able to listen to her concerns and then put her in touch with a parent organization that had been formed to help support families through the transition home. The parent organization offered peer support from parents who had been through the experience. They were also able to help Mrs. Jones place the experience in its proper perspective.

The girls had enjoyed their weekend with their mother and were in a better frame of mind for the homecoming. Peer support helped Mrs. Jones so that she could in turn be available to her family. John was about ready for discharge and had progressed normally. Once John was home, Mrs. Jones included the girls in the baby's routine as much as possible by asking them to get his diapers and having them feed their dollies while she fed John. Suzie brought pictures of John to school for show and tell, and after Mrs. Jones called to speak to the teacher to explain the disruptions at home, Suzie gradually quit misbehaving. Becky continued to have problems with thumb-sucking and bed-wetting for several months while incorporating John into the family and establishing a new family routine.

ONLINE RESOURCES

Institute for Patient- and Family-Centered Care (IPFC): Institute supports the advancement and practice of patient- and family-centered care. Many resources are available to professionals and families on their website to support partnerships and collaborations at all levels of health care.
http://www.ipfcc.org

National Center for Cultural Competence: The primary focus of this center is increasing the capacity of health and mental health programs. Resources are available to support the design, implement, and evaluate culturally and linguistically competent service delivery systems. Other resources include self-assessment tools, publications, on-site training, and education.
http://www11.georgetown.edu/research/gucchd/nccc

NICU Family Support Program-March of Dimes
http://www.marchofdimes.com/baby/inthenicu_program.html

Preemie Voices
http://www.preemievoices.com

Preemieworld
http://www.preemieworld.com/blog

Voice4Patients: A consumer website devoted to empowering patients and families to be their own health care advocates. By raising the voices of patient and families, more immediate responses to concerns about patient safety and medical errors can be addressed. This website provides information on the "national epidemic of health care error" and offers links to useful resources and information on common medical conditions for patients and families.
http://www.voice4patients.com

REFERENCES

(Abou) Samra, H., & McGrath, J. M. (2009). Infant vulnerability and parent overprotection: Recommendations for health professionals. *Newborn and Infant Nursing Reviews, 9*(3), 136–138. doi:10.1053/j.nainr.2009.07.004

Ahmann, E., Abraham, M. R., & Johnson, B. H. (2004). *Changing the concept of families as visitors: Supporting family presence and participation*. Bethesda, MD: Institute for Patient and Family-Centered Care.

Aita, M., & Snider, L. (2003). The art of developmental care in the NICU: A concept analysis. *Journal of Advanced Nursing, 41*(3), 223–232.

Allen, E., Manuel, J., Legault, C., Naughton, M., Privor, C., & O'Shea, T. (2004). Perception of child vulnerability among mothers of former premature infants. *Pediatrics, 113*, 267–273.

Amankwaa, L. C. (2005). Maternal postpartum collapse as a theory of postpartum depression. *Qualitative Report, 10*(1), 21–38.

Amendolia, B. (2010). Hope and parents of the critically ill newborn: A concept analysis. *Advances in Neonatal Care, 10*(3), 140–144.

Andrade, T. M. (1998). Sibling visitation: Research implications for pediatric and neonatal patients. *Worldviews on Evidence-Based Nursing Presents the Archives of Online Journal of Knowledge Synthesis for Nursing, E5*, 58–64. doi:10.111/j.1524-475X.1997.00058.x

Ardal, F., Sulman, J., & Fuller-Thomson, E. (2011). Support like a walking stick: Parent-buddy matching for language and culture in the NICU. *Neonatal Network, 30*(2), 89–98.

Aronson, P. L., Yau, J., Helfaer, M. A., & Morrison, W. (2009). Impact of family presence during pediatric intensive care unit rounds on the family and medical team. *Pediatrics, 124*(4), 1119–1125.

Axelin, A., Lehtonen, L., Pelander, T., & Salantera, S. (2010). Mothers' different styles of involvement in preterm infant pain care. *Journal of Obstetric, Gynecologic, & Neonatal Nursing, 39*(4), 415–424.

Baker, B. J., & McGrath, J. M. (2009). Supporting the maternal experience in the neonatal ICU. *Newborn and Infant Nursing Reviews, 9*(2), 81–82. doi:10.1053/j.nainr.2009.03.002

Baker, B. J., & McGrath, J. M. (2010). Promoting parenting through single-room care in the NICU. *Newborn and Infant Nursing Reviews, 10*(2), 72–73.

Baker, B. J., & McGrath, J. M. (2011a). Maternal infant synchrony: An integrated review of the literature. *Neonatal, Paediatric and Child Health Nursing, 14*(3), 2–13.

Baker, B. J., & McGrath, J. M. (2011b). Parent education: The cornerstone of excellent neonatal nursing care. *Newborn and Infant Nursing Reviews, 11*(1), 6–7.

Barnard, R. S., Williams, S. E., Storfer-Isser, A., Rhine, W., Horwitz, S. M., Koopman, C., & Shaw, R. J. (2011). Brief cognitive-behavioral intervention for maternal depression and trauma in the neonatal intensive care unit: A pilot study. *Journal of Traumatic Stress, 24*(2), 230–234.

Bartlett, D. J., Nijhuis-van der Sanden, M. W. G., Fallang, B., Fanning, J. K., & Doralp, S. (2011). Perceptions of vulnerability and variations in childrearing practices of parents of infants born preterm. *Pediatric Physical Therapy, 23*, 280–288.

Baum, N., Weidberg, Z., Osher, Y., & Kohelet, D. (2012). No longer pregnant, not yet a mother: Giving birth prematurely to a very-low-birth-weight baby. *Qualitative Health Research, 22*(5), 595–606.

Beck, C. T. (2011). A metaethnography of traumatic childbirth and its aftermath: Amplifying causal looping. *Qualitative Health Research, 21*, 301–311. doi:10.1177/1049732310390698

Boykova, M., & Kenner, C. (2010). Partnerships in care: Mothers and fathers. In C. Kenner & J. M. McGrath (Eds.), *Developmental care of newborns and infants: A guide for health professionals* (2nd ed., pp. 145–160). Glenview, IL: National Association of Neonatal Nurses.

Boykova, M., & Kenner, C. (2012). Transition from hospital to home for parents of preterm infants. *Journal of Perinatal and Neonatal Nursing, 26*(1), 81–87.

Brett, J., Staniszewska, S., Newburn, M., Jones, N., & Yaylor, L. (2011). A systematic mapping review of effective interventions for communicating with, supporting and providing information to parents of preterm infants. *BMJ Open, 1*, e000023. doi:10.1136/bmjopen-2010-000023

Brooks, S., Rowley, S., Broadbent, E., & Petrie, K. J. (2012). Illness perception ratings of high-risk newborns by mothers and clinicians: Relationship to illness severity and maternal stress. *Health Psychology, 31*(5), 632–9. doi:10.1037/a0027591

Caeymaex, L., Jousselme, C., Vasilescu, C., Danan, C., Falissard, B., Bourrant, M.-M., . . . Speranza, M. (2012). Perceived role in end-of-life decision making in the NICU affects long-term parental grief response. *Archives of Diseases in Child and Fetal Neonatal Edition*, F1–F6. doi:10.1136/archdischild-F2 of F6 2011-301548

Callahan, J. L., & Hynan, M. T. (2002). Identifying mothers at risk for postnatal emotional distress: Further evidence for the validity of the perinatal posttraumatic stress disorder questionnaire. *Journal of Perinatology, 22*, 448–455.

Cartagena, D., Noorthoek, A., Wagner, S., & McGrath, J. M. (2012). Family centered care and nursing research. *Newborn and Infant Nursing Reviews, 12*(3), 118–119.

Carvalho, A. E. V., Linhares, M. B. M., Padovani, F. H. P., & Martinez, F. E. (2009). Anxiety and depression in mothers of preterm infants and psychological interventions during hospitalization in neonatal ICU. *The Spanish Journal of Psychology, 12*(1), 161–170.

Cescutti-Butler, L., & Gavin, K. (2003). Parents' perceptions of staff competency in a neonatal intensive care unit. *Journal of Clinical Nursing, 12*(5), 752–761.

Cisneros-Moore, K. A., Coker, K., DuBuisson, A. B., Swett, B., & Edwards, W. B. (2003). Implementing potentially better practices for improving family-centered care in neonatal intensive care units: Successes and challenges. *Pediatrics, 11*(4), e450–e460.

Cleveland, L. M. (2008). Parenting in the neonatal intensive care unit. *Journal of Obstetric, Gynecologic, & Neonatal Nursing, 37*(6), 666–691.

Cone, S., & White, R. D. (2010). Single-family room design in the newborn intensive care unit. In C. Kenner & J. M. McGrath (Eds.), *Developmental care of newborns and infants: A guide for health professionals* (2nd ed., pp. 93–103). Glenview, IL: National Association of Neonatal Nurses.

Cooper, L. G., Gooding, J. S., Gallagher, J., Sternesky, L., Ledsky, R., & Berns, S. D. (2007). Impact of family-centered care initiative on NICU care, staff and families. *Journal of Perinatology, 27*, S32–S37.

Coulter, A., & Ellins, J. (2007). Effectiveness of strategies for informing, educating, and involving patients. *British Medical Journal, 335*, 24–27.

Davis, L., Mohay, H., & Edwards, H. (2003). Mothers' involvement in caring for their premature infants: An historical overview. *Journal of Advanced Nursing, 42*(6), 578–586.

Domanico, R., Davis, D. K., Coleman, F., & Davis, B. O. (2010). Documenting the NICU design dilemma: Parent and staff perceptions of open ward versus single family room units. *Journal of Perinatology, 30*, 343–351.

Doucette, J., & Pinelli, J. (2004). The effects of family resources, coping, and strains on family adjustment 18 to 24 months after the NICU experience. *Advances in Neonatal Care, 4*(2), 92–104.

Dunn, M. S., Reilly, M. C., Johnston, A. M., Hoopes, R. D., & Abraham, M. R. (2006). Development and dissemination of potentially better practices for the provision of family-centered care in neonatology: The family-centered care map. *Pediatrics, 118*, S95–S107.

Dyer, K. (2005a). Identifying, understanding, and working with grieving parents in the NICU, Part I: Identifying and understanding loss and the grief response. *Neonatal Network, 24*(3), 35–46.

Dyer, K. (2005b). Identifying, understanding, and working with grieving parents in the NICU, Part II: Strategies. *Neonatal Network, 24*(4), 27–40.

Evans, R., & Madsen, B. (2005). Culture clash: Transitioning from the neonatal intensive care unit to the pediatric intensive care unit. *Newborn and Infant Nursing Reviews, 5*(4), 188–193.

Fidler, H., & McGrath, J. M. (2009). Neonatal transport: The family perspective. *Newborn and Infant Nursing Reviews, 9*(4), 187–190. doi:10.1053/j.nainr.2009.09.010

Figueroa-Altmann, A. R., Bedrossian, L., Steinmiller, E. A., & Wilmot, S. M. (2005). Improving partnerships with children and families: A model from the Children's Hospital of Philadelphia. *American Journal of Nursing, 105*(6), 72A–72C.

Flacking, R., Lehtonen, L., Thomson, G., Axelin, A., Ahlqvist, S., Moran, V. H., . . . The SCENE Group. (2012). Closeness and separation in the neonatal intensive care. *Acta Paediatrica, 101*(10), 1032–1037.

Fox, S., Platt, F. W., White, M. K., & Hulac, P. (2005). Talking about the unthinkable: Perinatal/neonatal communication issues and procedures. *Clinics in Perinatology, 32*, 157–170.

Franck, L. S., Cox, S., Allen, A., & Winter, I. (2005). Measuring neonatal intensive care unit-related parental stress. *Journal of Advanced Nursing, 49*(6), 608–615.

Franck, L. S., & Spencer, C. (2003). Parent visiting and participation in infant caregiving activities in a neonatal unit. *Birth, 30*(1), 31–35.

Frisman, G. H., Eriksson, C., Pernehed, S., & Morelius, E. (2012). The experience of becoming a grandmother to a premature infant—A balancing act, influenced by ambivalent feelings. *Journal of Clinical Nursing*. doi:10.1111/j.1365-2702.2012.04204.x

Gooding, J. S., Cooper, L. G., Blaine, A. I., Franck, L. S., Howse, J. L., & Berns, S. D. (2011). Family support and family-centered care in the neonatal intensive care unit: Origins, advances, impact. *Seminars in Perinatology, 35*, 20–28.

Gray, P. H., Edwards, D. M., O'Callaghan, M. J., & Cuskelly, M. (2012). Parenting stress in mother of preterm infants during early infancy. *Early Human Development, 88*(1), 45–49.

Greisen, G., Mirante, N., Haumount, D., Pierrat, V., Pallas-Alonso, C. R., Warren, I., . . . The European Science Foundation Network. (2009). Parents, siblings and grandparents in the neonatal intensive care unit: A survey of policies in eight European countries. *Acta Paediatrica, 98*, 1744–1750.

Hall-Johnson, S. (1986). *Nursing assessment and strategies for the family at risk* (2nd ed.). Philadelphia, PA: Lippincott.

Hardy, W., & McGrath, J. M. (2008). Supporting information-seeking behaviors of families in the 21century. *Newborn and Infant Nursing Reviews, 8*(3), 118–119. doi:10.1053/j.nainr.2008.06.013

Hodnett, E. D., Gates, S., Hofmeyr, G. J., Sakala, C., & Weston, J. (2011). Continuous support for women during childbirth. *Cochrane, CD003766*.

Howland, L. C., Pickler, R. H., McCain, N. L., Glaser, D., & Lewis, M. (2011). Exploring biobehavioral outcomes in mothers of preterm infants. *MCN: American Journal of Maternal Child Nursing, 36*(2), 91–97.

Hurst, I. (2004). Imposing burdens: A Mexican American mother's experience of family resources in a newborn intensive-care unit. *Journal of Obstetric, Gynecologic, & Neonatal Nursing, 33*(2), 156–163.

Hurst, I. (2006). One size does not fit all: Parents' evaluations of a support program in a newborn intensive care nursery. *Journal of Perinatal and Neonatal Nursing, 20*(3), 252–261.

Hynan, M. T. (2005). Supporting fathers during stressful times in the nursery: An evidence-based review. *Newborn and Infant Nursing Reviews, 5*(2), 87–92.

Ichijima, E., Kirk, R., & Hornblow, A. (2011). Parental support in neonatal intensive care units: A cross-cultural comparison between New Zealand and Japan. *Journal of Pediatric Nursing, 26*, 206–215.

Institute for Patient and Family-Centered Care. (2011). *Advancing the practice of patient- and family-centered care in hospitals: How to get started*. Bethesda, MD: Institute of Patient and Family-Centered Care.

Institute of Medicine. (2003). *Health professions education: A bridge to quality*. Washington, DC: National Academies Press.

Jamsa, K., & Jamsa, T. (1998). Technology in the neonatal intensive care: A study of parents' experiences. *Technology and Health Care, 6*(4), 225–230.

Johnson, B. H. (2003). Patient and family-centered care. *AHA News*. Bethesda, MD: Institute of Family-Centered Care.

Johnson, B. H. (2004). Families are allies for enhancing quality, patient safety. In: *AHA News*. Bethesda, MD: Institute of Family-Centered Care.

Jones, L., Woodhouse, D., & Rowe, J. (2007). Effective nurse parent communication: A study of parents' perceptions in the NICU environment. *Patient Education and Counseling, 69*, 206–212.

Just, A. (2005). Parent participation in care: Bridging the gap in the pediatric ICU. *Newborn and Infant Nursing Reviews, 5*(4), 179–187.

Kaakinen, J., Gedaly-Duff, V., Hanson, S., & Coehlo, D. (2009). *Family health care nursing: Theory, practice and research* (4th ed.). Philadelphia, PA: FA Davis.

Karatzias, T., Chouliara, Z., Maxton, F., Freer, Y., & Power, K. (2007). Post-traumatic symptomatology in parents with premature infants: A systematic review of the literature. *Journal of Prenatal and Perinatal Psychology and Health, 21*(3), 249–260.

Kellie, S. M., Makvandi, M., & Muller, M. L. (2011). Management and outcome of a varicella exposure in a neonatal intensive care unit: Lessons for the vaccine era. *American Journal of Infection Control, 39*(10), 844–848.

Klegerg, A., Hellstrom-Westas, L., & Widstrom, A.-M. (2007). Mother's perception of Newborn Individualized Developmental Care and Assessment Program (NIDCAP) as compared to conventional care. *Early Human Development, 83*, 403–411.

Korja, R., Maunu, J., Kirjavinen, J., Savonlahti, E., Hataja, L., Lapinleimu, H., . . . The PAPARI study group. (2008). Mother-infant interaction is influenced by the amount of holding in preterm infants. *Early Human Development, 84*, 257–267.

Ladd, R. E., & Mercurio, M. R. (2003). Deciding for neonates: Whose authority, whose interest? *Seminars in Perinatology, 27*(6), 488–494.

Latour, J. M., Hazelzet, J. A., Duivenvoorden, H. J., & van Goudoever, J. B. (2010). Perceptions of parents, nurses, and physicians on neonatal intensive care practices. *Journal of Pediatrics, 157*, 215–220.

Liang, I. A., & Freer, Y. (2008). Reorientation of care in the NICU. *Seminars in Fetal & Neonatal Medicine, 13*, 305–309.

Lindner, S. L., & McGrath, J. M. (2012). Family centered care in the delivery room environment. *Newborn and Infant Nursing Reviews, 12*(2), 70–72. doi:10.1053/j.nainr.2012.03.004

Lipson, J. G., & Dibble, S. L. (2005). *Culture and Clinical Care*. San Francisco, CA: USCF Nursing Press.

Liu, C.-H., Chao, Y.-H., Haung, C.-M., Wei, F.-C., & Chien, L.-Y. (2010). Effectiveness of applying empowerment strategies when establishing a support group for parent of preterm infants. *Journal of Clinical Nursing, 19*, 1729–1737.

Loo, K. K., Espinosa, M., Tyler, R., & Howard, J. (2003). Using knowledge to cope with stress in the NICU: How parents integrate learning to read the physiologic and behavioral cues of the infant. *Neonatal Network, 22*(1), 31–37.

Lopez, G. L., Anderson, K. H., & Feutchinger, J. (2012). Transition of premature infants from hospital to home life. *Neonatal Network, 31*(4), 207–214.

Major, D. A. (2003). Utilizing role theory to help employed parents cope with children's chronic illness. *Health Education Research, 18*(1), 45–57.

Malusky, S. K. (2005). A concept analysis of family-centered care in the NICU. *Neonatal Network, 24*, 25–32.

Mangureten, J., Scott, S. H., Guzetta, C. E., Clark, A. P., Vinso, L., Sperry, J., . . . Voelmeck, W. (2005). Effects of family presence during resuscitation and invasive procedures in a pediatric emergency department. *Journal of Emergency Nursing, 32*(3), 225–233.

Matsuda, Y., & McGrath, J. M. (2011). Working in a global village: Cultural competency and collaboration through interpreters. *Newborn and Infant Nursing Reviews, 11*(3), 102–104. doi:10.1053/j.nainr.2011.07.001

McCann, D., Young, J., Watson, K., Ware, R. S., Pitcher, A., Bundy, R., & Tutur, D. G. (2008). Effectiveness of a tool to improve role negotiation and communication between parents and nurses. *Paediatric Nursing, 20*(5), 15–19.

McCormick, M. C., Escobar, G. J., Zgeng, Z., & Richardson, D. K. (2008). Factors influencing parental satisfaction with neonatal intensive care among the families of moderately premature infants. *Pediatrics, 121*, 1111–1118.

McCubbin, H. I., & Patterson, J. (1983). The family stress process: The double ABCX model of adjustment and adaptation. In H. I. McCubbin, M. B. Sussman, & J. M. Patterson (Eds.), *Social stress and the family: Advances and developments in family stress theory and research* (pp. 7–37). New York, NY: Haworth.

McGrath, J. M. (2000). Developmentally supportive caregiving and technology: Isolation or merger of intervention strategies? *Journal of Perinatal and Neonatal Nursing, 14*(3), 78–91.

McGrath, J. M. (2001). Building relationships with families in the NICU: Exploring the guarded alliance. *Journal of Perinatal and Neonatal Nursing, 15*(4), 1–10.

McGrath, J. M. (2005a). Partnerships with families: A foundation to support them in difficult times. *Journal of Perinatal and Neonatal Nursing, 19*(2), 94–96.

McGrath, J. M. (2005b). Single room design in the NICU: Making it work for you. *Journal of Perinatal and Neonatal Nursing, 19*(3), 210–211.

McGrath, J. M. (2006a). Family presence during procedures: Breathing life into policy and everyday practices. *Newborn and Infant Nursing Reviews, 6*(4), 243–244. doi:10.1053/j.nainr.2006.09.008

McGrath, J. M. (2006b). Family-centered developmental care begins before birth: Little things can make a big difference. *Journal of Perinatal and Neonatal Nursing, 20*(3), 195–196.

McGrath, J. M. (2007a). "Will my baby be normal?" Helping families make informed decisions related to neonatal surgery. *Journal of Perinatal and Neonatal Nursing, 21*(1), 4–5.

McGrath, J. M. (2007b). Family caregiving: Synchrony with infant caregiving? *Newborn and Infant Nursing Reviews, 7*(1), 1–2. doi:10.1053/j.nainr.2006.12.003

McGrath, J. M. (2011). Strategies for increasing parent presence in the NICU. *Journal of Perinatal and Neonatal Nursing, 25*(4), 305–306. doi:10.1097/JPN.0b13e318235e584

McGrath, J. M. (2012). Strategies to support the transition to home. *Journal of Perinatal and Neonatal Nursing, 26*(1), 8–9. doi:10.1097/JPN.0b013e3182437255

McGrath, J. M., (Abou) Samra, H., & Kenner, C. (2011). Family centered developmental care practices and research: What will the next century bring? *Journal of Perinatal and Neonatal Nursing, 25*(2), 165–170. doi:10.1097/JPN.0b013e31821a6706

McGrath, J. M., (Abou) Samra, H., Zukowsky, K., & Baker, B. (2010). Parenting after infertility: Issues for families and infants. *MCN: The American Journal of Maternal Child Nursing, 35*(3), 157–164. doi:10.1097/NMC.0b013e3181d7657d

McGrath, J. M., & Hardy, W. (2008). Communication: An essential component of quality care. *Newborn and Infant Nursing Reviews, 8*(2), 64–66. doi:10.1053/j.nainr.2008.03.005

McGreevey, M. (Ed.). (2006). *Patients as partners: How to involve patients and families in their own care*. Oakbrook Terrace, IL: Joint Commission Resources, Inc.

McKlindon, D. D., & Schlucter, J. (2004). Parent and nursing partnership model for teaching therapeutic relationships. *Pediatric Nursing, 30*(5), 418–420.

Meiers, S., Tomlinson, P., & Peden-McAlpine, C. (2007). Development of the family nurse caring belief scale (FNCBS). *Journal of Family Nursing, 13*(4), 484–502.

Melnyk, B. M., Feinstein, N. F., Alpert-Gillis, L., Fairbanks, E., Crean, H. F., Sinkin, R. A., . . . Gross, S. J. (2006). Reducing premature infants' length of stay and improving parents' mental health outcomes with the Creating Opportunities for Parent Empowerment (COPE) neonatal intensive care unit program: A randomized, controlled trial. *Pediatrics, 118*, e1414–e1427.

Melnyk, B. M., & Fineout-Overholt, E. (2010). *Evidence-based practice in nursing and health care: A guide to best practice* (2nd ed.). Philadelphia, PA: Lippincott Williams & Wilkins.

Menghini, K. G. (2005). Designing and evaluating parent educational materials. *Advances in Neonatal Care, 5*(5), 273–283.

Miles, M., & Brunssen, S. H. (2003). Psychometric properties of the parental stressor scale: Infant hospitalization. *Advances in Neonatal Care, 3*(4), 186–196.

Montirosso, R., Del Prete, A., Bellu, R., Tronick, E., Borgatti, R., & The Neonatal Adequate Care for Quality of Life (NEO-ACQUA) Study Group. (2012). Level of NICU quality of developmental care and neurobehavioral performance in very preterm infants. *Pediatrics, 129*, e1129–e1137.

Morey, J. A., & Gregory, K. (2012). Nurse-led education mitigates maternal stress and enhances knowledge in the NICU. *MCN: American Journal of Maternal Child Health, 37*(3), 182–191.

Mosqueda, R., Castilla, Y., Perapoch, J., da la Cruz, J., Lopez-Maestro, M., & Pallas, C. (2013). Staff perceptions on newborn individualized developmental care and assessment program (NIDCAP) during its implementation in two Spanish neonatal units. *Early Human Development, 89*(1), 27–33. doi:10.1016/j.earlhumdev.2010.07.013

Munch, S., & Levick, J. (2001). I'm special too: Promoting sibling adjustment in the neonatal intensive care unit. *Health and Social Work, 26*(1), 45–49.

Mundy, C. A. (2010). Families in critical care; assessment of family needs in neonatal care units. *American Journal of Critical Care, 19*, 156–163.

Neu, M., & Robinson, J. A. (2010). Maternal holding of preterm infant during the early weeks after birth and dyad interaction at six months. *Journal of Obstetric, Gynecologic, & Neonatal Nursing, 39*(4), 401–414.

Newnam, K. M., & McGrath, J. M. (2010). Families and the sepsis work-up: Considering their fears. *Newborn and Infant Nursing Reviews, 10*(4), 160–162. doi:10.1053/j.nainr2010.09.004

Patterson, J. M. (1995). Promoting resilience in families experiencing stress. *Pediatric Clinics of North America, 42*(1), 47–63.

Pichler-Stachl, E., Pichler, G., Gramm, S., Zotter, H., Mueller, W., & Urlesberger, B. (2011). Prematurity: Influence on mother's locus of control. *Wien Klin Wochenschr: The Central European Journal of Medicine, 123*, 455–457. doi:10.1007/s00508-011-1601-8

Pillow, M. (Ed.). (2007). *Patients as partners: Toolkit for implementing national patient safety goal 13*. Oakbrook Terrace, IL: Joint Commission Resources, Inc.

Pineda, R. G., Stransky, K. E., Rogers, C., Duncan, M. H., Smith, G. C., Neil, J., & Inder, T. (2012). The single-patient room in the NICU: Maternal and family effects. *Journal of Perinatology, 32*, 545–551.

Pinelli, J., Saigal, S., Bill Wu, Y.-W., Cunningham, C., DiCenso, A., Steele, S., . . . Turner, S. (2008). Patterns of change in family functioning, resources, coping and parental depression in mothers and fathers of sick newborns over the first year of life. *Journal of Neonatal Nursing, 14*(5), 156–165.

Poehlmann, J., Miller Schwichtenberg, A. J. M., Bolt, D., & Dilworth-Bart, J. (2009). Predictors of depressive symptom trajectories in mothers of preterm or low birth weight infants. *Journal of Family Psychology, 23*(5), 690–704. doi:10.1037/a0016117

Prentice, M., & Stainton, M. C. (2004). The effects of developmental care of preterm infants on women's health and family life. *Neonatal, Pediatric and Child Health Nursing, 7*(3), 4–12.

Preyde, M. (2007). Mothers of very preterm infants: Perspectives on their situation and a culturally sensitive intervention. *Social Work in Health Care, 44*(4), 65–83.

Raines, D. A., & Brustad, J. (2012). Parent's confidence as a caregiver. *Advances in Neonatal Care, 12*(3), 183–188.

Reid, T. (2007). Perceptions of parent-staff communication in neonatal intensive care: The development of a rating scale. *Journal of Neonatal Nursing, 13*, 24–35.

Reis, M. D., Rempel, G. R., Scott, S. D., Brady-Fryer, B. A., & van Aerde, J. (2010). Developing nurse/patient relationships in the NICU through negotiated partnerships. *Journal of Obstetric, Gynecologic, & Neonatal Nursing, 39*(6), 675–683.

Rogers, C. E., Kidokoro, H., Wallendorf, M., & Inder, T. E. (2013). Identifying mothers of very preterm infants at-risk for postpartum depression and anxiety before discharge. *Journal of Perinatology, 33*(3), 171–176. doi:10.1038/jp.2012.75

Roscigno, C. I., Savage, T. A., Kavanaugh, K., Moro, T. T., Kirkatrick, S. J., Strassner, H. T., . . . Kimura, R. E. (2012). Divergent views of hope influencing communications between parents and hospital providers. *Qualitative Health Research, 22*(9), 1232–1246.

Rowe, J., & Jones, L. (2008). Facilitating transitions: Nursing support for parents during the transfer of preterm infants between neonatal nurseries. *Journal of Clinical Nursing, 17*, 782–798.

Saunders, R. P., Abraham, M. R., Crosby, M. J., Thomas, K., & Edwards, W. H. (2003). Evaluation and development of potentially better practices for improving family-centered care in the neonatal intensive care unit. *Pediatrics, 111*(4), e437–e449.

Shah, P. E., Clements, M., & Poehlmann, J. (2011). Maternal resolution of grief after preterm birth: Implications for infant attachment security. *Pediatrics, 127*(2), 284–292.

Shieh, S.-J., Chen, H.-L., Liu, F.-C., Liou, C.-C., Lin, Y.-in-H., Teng, H.-I., & Wang, R.-H. (2010). The effectiveness of structured discharge education on maternal confidence, caring knowledge and growth of premature newborns. *Journal of Clinical Nursing, 19*, 3307–3313.

Sodomka, P. (2006). Engaging patients and families: A high leverage tool for health care leaders. *Hospitals and Health Networks, 80*, 28–30.

Stevens, D. C., Helseth, C. C., & Kurtz, J. C. (2010). Achieving success in supporting parents and families in the neonatal intensive care unit. In C. Kenner & J. M. McGrath (Eds.), *Developmental care of newborns and infants: A guide for health professionals* (2nd ed., pp. 161–190). Glenview, IL: National Association of Neonatal Nurses.

Tooten, A., Hoffenkamp, H. N., Hall, R. A. H., Winkel, F. W., Eliens, M., Vingerhoets, A. J. J. M., & van Bakel, H. J. A. (2012). The effectiveness of video interaction guidance in parents of premature infants: A multicenter randomized controlled trial. *BMC Pediatrics, 12*, 76–97. doi:10.1186/1471-2431-12-76

Treyvaud, K., Doyle, L. W., Lee, K. J., Roberst, G., Cheong, J. L. Y., Inders, T., & Anderson, P. J. (2011). Family functioning, burden and parenting stress 2 years after a preterm birth. *Early Human Development, 87*, 427–431.

van Manen, M. (2012). Carrying: Parental experience of the hospital transfer of their baby. *Qualitative Health Research, 22*(2), 199–211.

Watson, G. (2010). Parental liminality: A way of understanding the early experiences of parents who have a very preterm infant. *Journal of Clinical Nursing, 20*, 1462–1471.

White, R. D. (2007). Recommended standards for the newborn ICU. *Journal of Perinatology, 27*(Suppl. 2), S4–S19.

Willis, V. (2008). Parenting preemies: A unique program for family support and education after NICU discharge. *Advances in Neonatal Care, 8*(4), 221–230.

Zelkowitz, P., Feeley, N., Shrier, I., Stremler, R., Westreich, R., Dunkley, D., . . . Papageogiou, A. (2011). The cues and care randomized controlled trial of a neonatal intensive care intervention: Effects on maternal psychological distress and mother-infant interaction. *Journal of Developmental and Behavioral Pediatrics, 32*(8), 591–599.

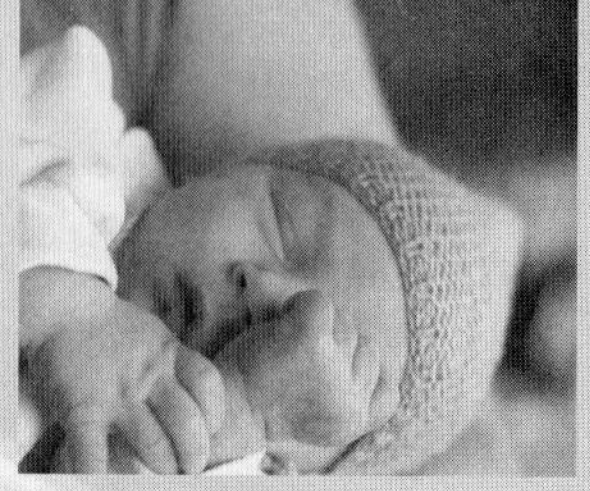

CHAPTER 33

Palliative and End-of-Life Care

■ Carole Kenner

In the neonatal intensive care unit (NICU), the assurance that "everything possible is being done" often is interpreted as meaning that the patient is receiving state-of-the-art technologic care. Yet the health care system fails both infants and their families when death occurs. The failure lies not in the infant's death itself, but rather in the neglect to emphasize state-of-the-art palliative care. Until it is evident that all dying infants receive highly skilled palliative care, as well as advanced technologic care, modern medicine cannot say that the best possible care has been provided to these infants and their families. This chapter focuses on the care of infants and their families who are facing life-threatening illnesses or are dying and the urgent need for exemplary neonatal and pediatric hospice and palliative care programs.

ETHICAL OBLIGATION TO PROVIDE OPTIMUM END-OF-LIFE CARE

It can be argued that all members of the health care team have an ethical obligation to plan and implement end-of-life (EOL) care; to provide highly skilled care at all times except at the EOL is to ignore the essence of comprehensive health care. The ethical dimensions of neonatal EOL care include an obligation to provide compassionate care; beneficent and nonmaleficent care, especially in regard to infant pain; and recognition of the moral authority of caring, informed parents as surrogate decision makers for their infants.

Compassionate Care at the EOL

More than a decade ago, Pellegrino and Thomasma (1993) argued that health care professionals have a special responsibility to provide compassionate care at the EOL. They identified compassion and temperance as among the essential virtues of medical practice and cautioned against overuse of high-technology equipment in place of human engagement with patients. They noted that particularly at the EOL, health care professionals can become so focused on technologic processes that they use them as "substitutes for human and compassionate care."

Palliative care is a global issue especially in the pediatric population. Variations in how children with life-threatening illnesses are treated are sometimes linked to cultural values and beliefs around the concept of death. Other barriers to access to such care are related to health policies (Fowler-Kerry, 2012). Fowler-Kerry outlines the new paradigm for pediatric palliative care emerging on a global stage. Even today, infants in the NICU frequently die while still intubated and connected to various pieces of equipment. A study of childhood deaths in Canadian hospitals found that the acuity of care was high before death and that most of the decisions about EOL issues were made very close to the actual time of death (McCallum, Byrne, & Bruera, 2000). In that study, most of the children were intubated at death (73%), and most died in the intensive care unit (83%). In the United States most pediatric deaths also occur in hospital intensive care units (Kerr, 2001), and there is evidence that children often suffer needlessly before death (Stephenson, 2000; Wolfe et al., 2000). Approximately 521,542 children die annually in the United States (Kochanek, Kirmeyer, Martin, Strobino, & Guyer, 2012). Most of these deaths take place in hospitals. In 2009 there were 26,531 deaths of children 1 year of age or less, with 55% linked to congenital malformations, genetic conditions, prematurity, low birth weight, maternal complications, accidental injuries, and sudden infant death (Kochanek et al., 2012). These figures have implications for neonatal care. A random survey of 30 NICUs across the United States indicated that, although most of these units had policies regarding postmortem and bereavement care services, none had procedural guidelines for EOL care. Since the late 1990s when this study was done, some progress has been made in the creation of policies and procedures (Carter et al., 2004). Books are available on the subject to guide the practitioner in working with children and their families during this very difficult period of their life (Carter, Levetown, & Friebert, 2011). Catlin and Carter (2002) developed a palliative care protocol that has assisted many perinatal and neonatal centers in the development of policies to assist with EOL and palliative care issues.

New approaches must be taken to establish compassionate EOL care for all infants in the NICU. This challenge is intensified in a system in which health care professionals are oriented toward active intervention with technologic devices rather than toward an acceptance of death (Jecker & Pagon, 1995; Kenner & Boykova, 2010). As Jecker and Pagon said, health care professionals are "applauded for acting, intervening, and forestalling death. Once set in motion, these active, goal-directed virtues can easily acquire a momentum of their own." These researchers urge an increased understanding and application of virtues such as patience, cautiousness, and humility in the perinatal setting. Some settings are developing a connection with perinatal hospices when a problem is detected prior to delivery that may result in a stillborn or "born dying" infant. One example of this is "Alexander's House" in Kansas City, Missouri (Pearce, 2006). Children's Hospital Medical Center, Cincinnati, Ohio, developed a perinatal hospice program called "Star Shine Hospice," another example of a hospice specifically focused on children (for more information go to http://www.cincinnatichildrens.org/service/s/starshine/default).

Wolfe (2000) advocates for compassionate EOL care for children. She identified the "principle of family" in pediatric EOL care: that is, an obligation to treat the whole family. Wolfe saw the health care staff as having an ethical obligation to "pursue comfort aggressively" and to fully engage the parents in the decision-making process for their child.

Obligation to Provide Beneficent Care

The widely accepted ethical principle of beneficence requires that health care professionals actively provide care that directly benefits their patients. As defined by Beauchamp and Childress (2001), the principle of beneficence encompasses both positive beneficence and actively providing benefit and utility, which requires a balancing of benefits and adverse effects. Professional codes of ethics require that nurses and physicians act in a manner that benefits those entrusted to their care. Health care professionals therefore are obligated to examine their actions with regard to intended beneficial outcomes while simultaneously considering the drawbacks or adverse consequences of their actions.

Obligation of Nonmaleficence

Health care professionals also have a legal and moral obligation to avoid inflicting harm on their patients (Beauchamp & Childress, 2001). Adherence to this ethical principle, known as nonmaleficence, may encompass the provision of life-sustaining treatment, as well as the cessation of such treatment. For example, when a treatment ceases to provide the intended benefit for a patient, it may be considered futile, and the health care professional therefore is no longer obligated to continue that treatment (Beauchamp & Childress, 2001). It also refers to the adequate management of pain and not inflicting undue harm from inadequate management.

Health care professionals who continue to provide futile and burdensome treatments may be viewed as doing more harm than good. The distinction is made by meticulously balancing the benefits and burdens to the patient. For critically ill infants in the NICU, procedures or treatments can be considered inhumane if they inflict pain or discomfort on the infant without actual benefit (Jecker & Pagon, 1995). Jecker and Pagon noted, "Medical interventions provided without benefit rob patients of their very humanity. Inhumanity implies that medical care aimlessly prolongs a patient's pain or suffering, making the use of medical technologies a torture or punishment. Inhumanity suggests a failure to empathize with the sufferings of patients."

Despite these arguments for humane care, burdensome, futile treatments sometimes still are given in the NICU. Weir (1984, 1995) has argued that death should not be considered the worst outcome for some infants, particularly when the chances for survival are remote or when physiologic survival is accompanied by unrelieved pain and suffering. In such cases, health care providers may be merely prolonging dying.

Recognition of Parents' Moral Authority

Parents have both the legal and moral authority to serve as surrogate decision makers for their infants. A growing body of literature supports parental decision-making authority, particularly for extremely premature or near-viable infants (Ho, 2003; Jecker & Pagon, 1995; Manning, 2005; Pinkerton et al., 1997; Raines, 1996); however, few studies have examined ways to empower parents to exercise this authority fully. Furthermore, a body of literature written by both parents and health care professionals suggests that parents may not be involved adequately in decisions about prolonged, aggressive treatments for their infants (Harrison, 1993; Pinch & Spielman, 1993, 1996; Raines, 1996; Stinson & Stinson, 1979). It can be argued that parents may not be as fully involved in decisions about their infant's care as they would like and have the authority to be, especially in cases in which aggressive therapies are of uncertain benefit to the infant. As Catlin and Carter (2002) point out, the real need in these instances is clear communication with parents and an understanding of how they wish to be involved in these decisions.

A consensus is growing among ethicists, clinicians, and families that when the benefits of life-sustaining therapies are questionable, parental involvement in treatment decision making is an ethical imperative (Harrison, 1993; Jakobi, Weissman, & Paldi 1993; Penticuff, 1987, 1988, 1995, 1998; President's Commission for the Study of Ethical Problems in Medicine and Biomedical and Behavioral Research, 1983). When life-sustaining therapies have proved futile, parents and professionals often are uncertain how to provide EOL care. The following quote is from Robert Stinson, father of Andrew, who was born in 1976 at 24 weeks gestation. At that time Andrew's survival was unprecedented. He underwent intensive care for

6 months, was critically ill throughout this time, and was resuscitated numerous times before his death.

"What they never understood was that one can care deeply enough about a child like Andrew to want his misery ended. Allowing Andrew to die naturally was what we wanted for him, not just to him. I thought often, when I did go in to see him, about his massive pain. He was sometimes crying then; a nearly soundless, aimless cry of pain, undirected and unlistened to except, I sometimes thought, by me. As often as I wanted to gather him into my arms, I wanted him to be allowed to die. What is the name for that?" (Stinson & Stinson, 1979).

Although the Stinsons' experience occurred many years ago, evidence suggests professionals do not always incorporate the parental perspective into care decisions (Harrison, 1993; King, 1992; Mehren, 1991; Pinch & Spielman, 1996; Raines, 1996), particularly with regard to burdensome, futile treatments (Yellin et al., 1998).

Burden of Treatment

The burden of treatment experienced by extremely premature infants in the NICU, especially those with minimal chance for survival, requires further ethical examination. In a national survey of physicians certified in neonatal-perinatal medicine, Yellin and colleagues (1998) found that many neonatologists believe that "there is an ethical or legal obligation to perform treatments that are not in the infant's best interests, regardless of parental preference." Yellin and coworkers concluded that because some neonatologists are unwilling to withdraw treatments, they may be overtreating some infants in the NICU. Unfortunately, this situation has not changed that much today (Kenner & Boykova, 2010).

The inordinate medical intervention that occurs for some infants stems from the lack of consensus surrounding the issue of futility (Avery, 1998; Penticuff, 1998). Penticuff (1998) identified harm that ensues for infants, families, the health care team, and society when there is no accepted definition of futility. Such harm includes "needless infant suffering through prolongation of the process of dying" and "psychologic entrapment of the medical team and the family," in which initial aggressive therapies lead inexorably to more aggressive therapies, with death as the only stopping point. An example is the controversy around treatment options for children with trisomy 13 and 18 where mixed opinions exist about how far treatment should go and how parents must be included in the decision making including decisions about palliative care (Carey, 2012).

Brody and colleagues (1997) call for compassionate clinical management during the withdrawal of intensive life-sustaining treatment for adult patients using a strategic approach with well-defined goals that dictate the plan of care. Once the goals have been identified, the team examines both the benefits and burdens of the proposed treatment plan with the family. With this approach, any treatment that is more burdensome than beneficial is limited or eliminated. Brody and coworkers identified pain and discomfort as components of treatment burden and said that there is "no sound rationale for withholding adequate analgesia or sedation" during EOL care. This is an area that requires further examination as it relates to critically ill neonates at the EOL.

The Institute of Medicine (IOM) identified five core competencies that guide patient care. These are: patient-centered care, interdisciplinary teams, evidence-based medicine, quality improvement, and information technology (Institute of Medicine [IOM], 2003). These all have relevance to palliative care, as it is patient and family focused and requires an integrated interprofessional team approach to provide quality care. Mullins and colleagues (2012) conducted a study funded by the National Institute for Nursing Research (NINR) (1 R21 NR010103-01A1) that examined the needs of parents of children newly diagnosed with cancer. Findings supported the needs parents had for clear messages from the health care team, for information to support positive coping and decrease stress (Mullins et al., 2012).

NEONATAL PAIN MANAGEMENT AT THE EOL

Only limited research is available on the provision of analgesia and sedation for infants at the EOL. One study focused on medications administered during life support (e.g., ventilator) withdrawal. Partridge and Wall (1997) conducted a retrospective chart review to examine the practice of opioid analgesia administration in one NICU at the time of life-support withdrawal. They found that of infants who had a known painful condition (e.g., acute abdominal or surgical pain) and were receiving analgesia before the decision was made to withhold further life-sustaining treatment, 84% received opioid analgesia during life-support withdrawal. An interesting finding of this study was that the infants who did not receive any analgesia at the time of life-support withdrawal had also not received any pain medication before the decision was made to discontinue life support. These findings suggest that analgesia is not being given to ease the possible suffering associated with withdrawal of life support, but rather to manage specific disease processes. (Additional aspects of neonatal pain management are discussed in Chapter 23.) It is recognized that even the smallest of patients have rights, and these include palliative care.

HOSPICE CARE

The use of hospice and palliative care has made a significant difference in EOL care for adults. However, the movement toward hospice care for neonates and young children has been slow to take hold. Hospice is both a philosophy and a system of compassionate, team-oriented care for individuals at the EOL. According to the National Hospice and Palliative Care Organization (2000), the guiding philosophy of hospice is that "each of us has the right to die pain free and with dignity, and that our families will receive the necessary support to allow us to do so." Hospice care can be provided in select hospitals, in individual hospice facilities, or in a person's home. Although there has been a national movement toward making hospice care available to most adults, there are few examples of hospice centers specifically designed for children and their families.

Pediatric Hospice Care

Although there are few pediatric hospices in the United States, those that exist provide exemplary care for children and their families. One example of a model program is the newly opened Kids Path Hospice and Palliative Care of Greensboro, North Carolina. At Kids Path, care is provided for children with acquired immune deficiency syndrome (AIDS), congenital anomalies, chromosomal disorders, and cancer (Kerr, 2001). It is the only children's hospice facility in North Carolina and among the fewer than 25 such facilities in the United States. Kids Path uses an interdisciplinary care team that includes a pediatric nurse practitioner (PNP), registered nurses (RNs), medical director, social worker, counselors, and a chaplain. This issue was addressed by the Oklahoma Attorney General's Task Force Report on the State of End-of-Life Health Care (Edmondson, 2005), where it was recognized that such specialized services are needed.

Barriers to Pediatric Hospice Service

Unfortunately, many barriers obstruct the availability and provision of hospice care to all children and families who could benefit from it. The National Hospice and Palliative Care Organization (2000) described psychologic, financial, educational, and regulatory barriers to pediatric palliative care (NHPCO, 2000). One of the psychologic barriers is the association of palliative care with the concept of giving up or going against hope (Kenner & Boykova, 2010). Families often avoid palliative care, rather than identifying with the life-enhancing benefits it offers. Financial barriers arise because the home-based, multidisciplinary care is often not reimbursed. The educational barriers for care providers are evident in the lack of palliative care training for most physicians and the avoidance of discussing hospice care with parents (Moody, Siegel, Scharbach, Cunningham, & Cantor, 2011). Some of these training issues can be addressed through simulated difficult conversations (Brown, Lloyd, Swearingen, & Boateng, 2012). Regulatory barriers also exist because the reimbursement system is based on the needs of adults. Ignoring the differences in care needs between children and adults creates barriers to hospice as an option for many families.

PEDIATRIC PALLIATIVE CARE

The American Academy of Pediatrics (AAP) issued guidelines in 2000 for the care of children with life-threatening and terminal conditions. The AAP recommended palliative care for infants when "no treatment has been shown to alter substantially the expected progression toward death." According to the AAP guidelines, palliative care incorporates control of pain, symptom management, and care of the psychologic, social, and spiritual needs of children and their families. The AAP also has established five principles of palliative care: (1) respect for the dignity of patients and families, (2) access to competent and compassionate palliative care, (3) support for the caregivers, (4) improved professional and social support for pediatric palliative care, and (5) continued improvement of pediatric palliative care through research and education. There is a section on Hospice and Palliative Medicine within the AAP that is updated on a regular basis. This section upholds the AAP (2000) guidelines and reinforces the need to enhance the quality of life for the child and family. It also stresses care coordination and a team approach while carrying out the five principles of care listed above (American Academy of Pediatrics [AAP], 2012).

Respect for the Dignity of Patients and Families

Respect for patients' and families' dignity means that information about palliative care should be provided, and the parents' ability to make their own choice of a program should be respected. Also, the plan of care must incorporate and respect the parents' expressed wishes for their child's care, specifically with regard to testing, monitoring, and treatment (AAP, 2000). This respect should consider religious beliefs and cultural values.

Access to Competent and Compassionate Palliative Care

Compassionate palliative care includes alleviation of pain and other symptoms and access to supportive therapies, such as grief counseling and spiritual support. This principle includes provision of adequate respite care for parents (AAP, 2000; Goldman, Hain, & Liben, 2012).

Support for the Caregivers

The AAP recognizes the importance of support for health care professionals involved in the child's care. This support may include paid funeral leave, peer counseling, or remembrance ceremonies (AAP, 2000).

Improved Professional and Social Support for Pediatric Palliative Care

The barriers discussed in this chapter can prevent families from obtaining pediatric palliative care. Health care professionals must help families overcome these obstacles (AAP, 2000).

Continued Improvement of Pediatric Palliative Care Through Research and Education

Health care professionals need continuing education on ways to provide comprehensive palliative care. Also, research is needed that focuses on the effectiveness of palliative care interventions and on models of pediatric palliative care delivery (AAP, 2000).

Incorporating Pediatric Palliative Care Into the NICU

The AAP recommends that palliative care begin at the time of diagnosis of a life-threatening or terminal condition (AAP, 2000). In the NICU, particularly for extremely premature neonates and for neonates with life-threatening anomalies, palliative care should begin at the time of admission. For many health care professionals, this requires a rather dramatic shift from providing intensive high-technology care to providing intensive palliative care. This is in direct contrast to another common tenet of neonatal care: that is that discharge planning should begin upon admission. At times, particularly during the early diagnostic phase, palliative care can be provided along with technologic care; this arrangement allows the staff to focus on symptom management and pain control while weighing the benefits and harm of treatment. It also provides for interdisciplinary team members who can provide the support the family needs.

Often, when a neonate is born at the edge of viability, the clinical course shows a downward trend. The neonate's physiologic parameters cause concern as evidence mounts that the organ systems are failing. This scenario represents the inevitable point at which intensive efforts to prolong life merely serve to prolong the infant's dying. In such cases, both infants and their families would benefit from a smooth transition to intensive palliative care. This requires a level of skilled care that is not always present in the NICU. The care providers must be able quickly to recognize the futility of sustained therapies and must be expert at providing palliative care to both infant and family. Unfortunately, as research has indicated, all too often infants and children die while still intubated (McCallum et al., 2000); suffer from pain that is inadequately controlled or untreated (Kenner & Boykova, 2010; Partridge & Wall, 1997); and have not received the benefits of palliative care measures (Byock, 1997; Goldman, 1998; Rushton, 2000; Stephenson, 2000). The National Association of Neonatal Nurses (NANN), the Association of Pediatric Oncology Nurses (APON), and the Society of Pediatric Nurses (SPN) have stated that this area of neonatal care is very important. Under the auspices of the National Leadership Academy on EOL Issues which is sponsored by Johns Hopkins University (http://www.son.jhmi.edu/newsandmedia/endoflife.html), these three organizations are adapting the Last Acts Precepts (http://www.lastacts.org) for neonatal and pediatric patients. The Last Acts organization provides support for health care professionals and families through publications and taking action on EOL issues. It believes that appropriate language must be included to reflect cases such as an infant who is literally born dying, as well as the family's unique needs in such cases. This collaboration is a milestone in efforts to recognize that neonatal and pediatric patients and their families deserve the same level of care that adults have received.

Worldwide recognition of the need for neonatal and pediatric palliative care is growing, thanks to funding from the Soros Foundation, the Robert Wood Johnson Foundation, City of Hope, Johns Hopkins University, the Association of American Colleges of Nursing, and other organizations that support educational efforts about EOL and palliative care. Nursing curricula are being revised to include content and competencies on EOL care. Training programs such as the End of Life Nursing Education Consortium (ELNEC) (http://www.aacn.nche.edu/elnec) are broadening nurses' knowledge in this specialty. A new training program was created by ELNEC that focuses on the pediatric population. This has been presented for the past several years in the United States and abroad. Modules that focus specifically on developmental issues regarding the concept of death and dying as well as how to assess for pain in the nonverbal child help health professionals to adapt materials to their settings. Organizations such as the International Association of Hospice and Palliative Care, the NHPCO, and the Hospice and Palliative Care Nurses Association, which traditionally have focused primarily on adult issues, have begun incorporating pediatric palliative care concerns into their initiatives. The inclusion of a chapter (Kenner & Boykova, 2010) on palliative care in the NICU in Dr. Betty Ferrell's palliative care textbook—the gold standard in palliative care—will increase the awareness of the need for EOL care in this population. All these actions bode well for the integration of EOL care into customary pediatric and neonatal care as a standard that is expected and demanded.

BEREAVEMENT

Grief is unique to each individual and varies in expression, duration, and meaning. Parents often move through the grief process differently. The infant's mother may express her grief by crying, whereas the father may express his grief by isolating himself.

For many parents, the grief process is lifelong. Significant life events can trigger grieving, as can such routine childhood milestones as seeing a neighbor's child get on the school bus for her first day of kindergarten or, many years later, receiving a high school graduation announcement for what would have been their child's class.

As parents progress through the first year after their loss, it is important to prepare them for the grief they are likely to experience in the future and to help them develop a plan for themselves. Every family is unique and determines their own milestone days, those days that bring special remembrance of their child. Milestone days may include the child's birthday, the anniversary of the child's death, or holidays. It sometimes is helpful for parents to schedule time off on these milestone days so that they can plan a special activity. Some parents may want to be alone and take a quiet walk together. Others may prefer to be surrounded by relatives or a few close friends. Still others may want to spend the day with another parent who has experienced similar grief.

The nurse should stress three important points to bereaved families: (1) grief is individualized; (2) grief is a process; and (3) family members should not hesitate to seek assistance with their grief, even years after the child's death.

SUMMARY

Even when death approaches quickly in the NICU, measures can be taken to ease the infant's transition and adequately assist the family. It is no longer enough to provide quality bereavement and postmortem care to infants and their families. Research into and evaluation of care guidelines are needed so that infants can receive the same quality of EOL care afforded other members of society. Neonatal nurses have been at the forefront of this movement and now have the opportunity to serve as leaders in the design and implementation of exemplary neonatal palliative care programs.

CASE STUDY

An infant was born at 24 weeks gestation to a family that had just moved to a new city and had no relatives in the area. This was a first baby for the family. Shortly after birth, it was recognized that the infant would probably not survive because, in addition to being premature, overwhelming sepsis was present. The care team (without the family) met. Some felt that the family needed to be given options immediately to call the palliative care team in for a discussion of treatment options, while other team members believed that a few more days should be given to the baby to see how the infant would respond to ventilation and antibiotic therapy. A consultation was done with the palliative care team who convinced the neonatal team to talk with the family, describe the infant's status, discuss the possible course, and ask them to be part of the team to make decisions about palliative care and in what form—in other words how aggressive they wanted the treatment to be, how in either case palliative care would be provided, how care would be coordinated, and how they as a family would be supported no matter what the outcome. Over the course of the next week, the infant continued to get progressively sicker, the family was supported by the palliative care team, and relatives were contacted via Internet means to ensure they could support the family and see the baby. The family planned the care and eventually made the decision to take the infant, whom they named Sarah Elizabeth, off the ventilator. They held and rocked the baby surrounded by staff they selected until the moment of death. The death was peaceful, and the palliative care team continued to follow up with the family for the next month. The team also debriefed the neonatal caregivers that worked closely with the family to ensure they were supported. The principles of dignity, respect, and need for caregiver support for both the family and professional staff were upheld.

EVIDENCE-BASED PRACTICE BOX

Much progress has been made since the early 2000s when protocols for perinatal and neonatal palliative care appeared. An instrument called the Perinatal Palliative Care Perceptions and Barriers Scale Instrument was developed by Drs. Charlotte Wool and Sally Northam. This instrument was developed and validated over time for use with nurses and physicians. The focus is to determine perceptions of the health professionals in order to develop staff/faculty training programs with the ultimate goal to provide better support of patients and families. This instrument can be used in a variety of ways and needs further testing to broaden its use.

Reference

Wool, C., & Northam, S. (2011). The Perinatal Palliative Care Perceptions and Barriers Scale Instrument©: Development and validation. *Advances in Neonatal Care, 11*(6), 397–403.

ONLINE RESOURCES

The Center to Advance Palliative Care (CAPC)
Palliative Care Tools, Training & Technical Assistance
http://www.capc.org/?gclid=COHm6OTcx7MCFUOK4Aodz38Atg

ELNEC-Pediatric Palliative Care
http://www.aacn.nche.edu/elnec/about/pediatric-palliative-care

Hospice and Palliative Care Nurses Association
http://www.hpna.org

IPAL_ICU The IPAL Project: Improving Palliative Care
Patient and Family Resources
http://www.capc.org/ipal/ipal-icu/patient-family-resources

Perinatal Hospice and Palliative Care: A Gift of Time
http://perinatalhospice.org/Perinatal_hospices.html

REFERENCES

American Academy of Pediatrics. (2000). Palliative care for children. *Pediatrics, 106*(2), 351–357.

American Academy of Pediatrics. (2012). *Section on hospice and palliative care.* Retrieved from http://www2.aap.org/sections/palliative/WhatIsPalliativeCare.html

Avery, G. B. (1998). Futility considerations in the neonatal intensive care unit. *Seminars in Perinatology, 22*(3), 216–222.

Beauchamp, T. L., & Childress, J. F. (2001). *Principles of biomedical ethics* (5th ed.). New York, NY: Oxford University Press.

Brody, H., Campbell, M. L., Faber-Langendoen, K., & Ogle, K. S. (1997). Withdrawing intensive life-sustaining treatment: Recommendations for compassionate clinical management. *New England Journal of Medicine, 336*(9), 652–657.

Brown, C. M., Lloyd, E., Swearingen, C. J., & Boateng, B. A. (2012). Improving resident self-efficacy in pediatric palliative care through clinical simulation. *Journal of Palliative Care, 28*(3), 157.

Byock, I. (1997). *Dying well: Peace and possibilities at the end of life.* New York, NY: Riverhead Books.

Carey, J. C. (2012). Current opinion: Perspectives on the care and management of infants with trisomy 18 and trisomy 13: Striving for balance. *Pediatrics, 24.* Retrieved from http://www.trisomy.org/striving-for-balance-carey-oct-2012-peds-opinions

Carter, B. S., Howenstein, M., Gilmer, M. J., Throop, P., France, D., & Whitlock, J. A. (2004). Circumstances surrounding the deaths of hospitalized children: Opportunities for pediatric palliative care. *Pediatrics, 114*(3), e361–e366.

Carter, B. S., Levetown, M., & Friebert, S. E. (2011). *Palliative care for infants, children, and adolescents: A practical handbook.* Johns Hopkins University Press.

Catlin, A., & Carter, B. (2002). Creation of a neonatal end-of-life palliative care protocol. *Journal of Perinatology, 22*(3), 184–195.

Edmondson, W. A. D. (2005). *The Oklahoma Attorney General's Task Force report on the state of end-of-life health care 2005.* Oklahoma City, OK: The Oklahoma Attorney General's Task Force.

Fowler-Kerry, S. (2012). Pediatric palliative care: A new and emerging paradigm. In C. Knapp, V. Madden, & S. Fowler-Kerry (Eds.), *Pediatric palliative care global perspectives* (pp. 449–451). The Netherlands: Springer.

Goldman, A. (1998). ABC of palliative care: Special problems of children. *British Medical Journal, 316*(7124), 49–52.

Goldman, A., Hain, R., & Liben, S. (2012). *Oxford textbook of palliative care for children.* Oxford: Oxford University Press.

Harrison, H. (1993). The principles for family-centered neonatal care. *Pediatrics, 92*(5), 643–650.

Ho, L. Y. (2003). Perinatal care at the threshold of viability—from principles to practice. *Annals of the Academy of Medicine of Singapore, 32*(3), 362–375.

Institute of Medicine. (2003). *Health professions education: A bridge to quality.* Washington, DC: National Academies Press.

Jakobi, P., Weissman, A., & Paldi, E. (1993). The extremely low birth weight infants: The twenty-first century dilemma. *American Journal of Perinatology, 10*(2), 155–159.

Jecker, N. S., & Pagon, R. A. (1995). Medical futility: Decision making in the context of probability and uncertainty. In A. Goldworth, W. Silverman, D. K. Stevenson, E. W. D. Young, & R. Rivers (Eds.), *Ethics and perinatology.* New York, NY: Oxford University Press.

Kenner, C., & Boykova, M. (2010). Palliative Care in the neonatal intensive care unit. In B. R. Ferrell & N. Coyle (Eds.), *Oxford textbook of palliative nursing* (3rd ed., pp. 1065–1097). New York, NY: Oxford Press.

Kerr, E. (2001). Kids Path cares for children coping with illness or loss. *MD News Piedmont Triad* (5), 24–26.

King, N. M. P. (1992). Transparency in neonatal intensive care. *Hastings Center Report, 22*(2), 18–25.

Kochanek, K. D., Kirmeyer, S. E., Martin, J. A., Strobino, D. M., & Guyer, B. (2012). Annual summary of vital statistics: 2009. *Pediatrics, 129*(2), 338–348. doi:10.1542/peds.2011–3435

Manning, D. (2005). Proxy consent in neonatal care—goal-directed or procedure-specific? *Health Care Analysis, 13*(1), 1–9.

McCallum, D. E., Byrne, P., & Bruera, E. (2000). How children die in hospital. *Journal of Pain and Symptom Management, 20*(6), 417–423.

Mehren, E. (1991). *Born too soon.* New York, NY: Doubleday.

Moody, K., Siegel, L., Scharbach, K., Cunningham, L., & Cantor, R. M. (2011). Pediatric palliative care. *Primary care, 38*(2), 327.

Mullins, L., Chaffin, M., Phipps, S., Hullmann, S., Fedele, D., & Kenner, C. (2012). A clinic-based interdisciplinary intervention for mothers of children newly diagnosed cancer: A pilot study. *Journal of Pediatric Psychology.* First published online September 3, 2012. doi:10.1093/jpepsy/jss093

National Hospice and Palliative Care Organization. (2000). *Compendium of pediatric palliative care.* New Orleans, LA: NHPCO.

Partridge, J. C., & Wall, S. N. (1997). Analgesia for dying infants whose life support is withdrawn or withheld. *Pediatrics, 99*(1), 76–79.

Pearce, E. W. J. (2006). *Perinatal hospice/supportive care for the dying unborn infant.* Supportive voice. Retrieved from http://www.careofdying.org/SV/PUBSART.ASP?ISSUE=SV99SU&ARTICLE=N

Pellegrino, E. D., & Thomasma, D. C. (1993). *The virtues in medical practice.* New York, NY: Oxford University Press.

Penticuff, J. H. (1987). Neonatal nursing ethics: Toward a consensus. *Neonatal Network, 5*(6), 7–16.

Penticuff, J. H. (1988). Neonatal intensive care: Parental prerogatives. *Journal of Perinatal and Neonatal Nursing, 1*(3), 77–86.

Penticuff, J. H. (1995). Nursing ethics in perinatal care. In A. Goldworth, W. Silverman, D. K. Stevenson, E. W. D. Young & R. Rivers (Eds.), *Ethics and perinatology.* New York, NY: Oxford University Press.

Penticuff, J. H. (1998). Defining futility in neonatal intensive care. *Nursing Clinics of North America, 33*(2), 339–352.

Pinch, W. J., & Spielman, M. L. (1993). Parental perceptions of ethical issues post-NICU discharge. *Western Journal of Nursing Research, 15*(4), 422–440.

Pinch, W. J., & Spielman, M. L. (1996). Ethics in the neonatal intensive care unit: Parental perceptions at 4 years postdischarge. *Advances in Nursing Science, 19*(1), 72–85.

Pinkerton, J. V., Finnerty, J. J., Lombardo, P. A., Rorty, M. V., Chapple, H., & Boyle, R. J. (1997). Parental rights at the birth of a near-viable infant: Conflicting perspectives. *American Journal of Obstetrics and Gynecology, 177*(2), 283–288.

President's Commission for the Study of Ethical Problems in Medicine and Biomedical and Behavioral Research. (1983). *Deciding to forego life-sustaining treatment.* Washington, DC: U.S. Government Printing Office.

Raines, D. A. (1996). Parents' values: A missing link in the neonatal intensive care equation. *Neonatal Network, 15*(3), 7–12.

Rushton, C. H. (2000). Pediatric palliative care: Coming of age. *Innovations in End-of-Life Care, 2*(2). (online journal).

Stephenson, J. (2000). Palliative and hospice care needed for children with life-threatening conditions. *Journal of the American Medical Association, 284*(19), 2437–2438.

Stinson, R., & Stinson, P. (1979). *The long dying of baby Andrew.* Boston, MA: Little, Brown.

Weir, R. F. (1984). *Selective nontreatment of handicapped newborns.* New York, NY: Oxford University Press.

Weir, R. F. (1995). Withholding and withdrawing therapy and actively hastening death II. In A. Goldworth, W. Silverman, D. K. Stevenson, E. W. D. Young & R. Rivers (Eds.), *Ethics and perinatology.* New York, NY: Oxford University Press.

Wolfe, J. (2000). Suffering in children at the end of life: Recognizing an ethical duty to palliate. *Journal of Clinical Ethics, 11*(2), 157–161.

Wolfe, J., Grier, H. E., Klar, N., Levin, S. B., Ellenbogen, J. M., Salem-Schatz, S., ... Weeks, J. C. (2000). Symptoms and suffering at the end of life in children with cancer. *New England Journal of Medicine, 342*(5), 326–333.

Yellin, P. B., Levin, B. W., Krantz, D. H., Shinn, M., Driscoll, J. M., & Fleischman, A. R. (1998). Neonatologists' decisions about withholding and withdrawing treatments from critically ill newborns. *Pediatrics, 102*(3), 757.

CHAPTER 34

Complementary and Integrative Therapies

■ Nadine A. Kassity-Krich and Jamieson E. Jones

The use of complementary and alternative medicine (CAM) is a growing trend in this country and abroad. This topic is included in a neonatal text because little research has been done in the area of CAM in the newborn; yet many of the families we serve use these therapies. In addition, some health care professionals are beginning to apply the concepts of holistic care and alternative modalities to this population. This emerging area of medicine has become so widespread that the National Institutes of Health (NIH) created the National Center for Complementary and Alternative Medicine (NCCAM). Monies are now set aside for in-depth research of CAM therapies. Health care professionals must recognize these therapies as well as the gaps in our scientific knowledge regarding CAM. In the neonatal unit, CAM therapies may soften the high-tech environment by adding the more nurturing elements one would expect around newborns. This chapter briefly describes some of the most popular and promising CAM therapies, explores how these options are used in the neonatal intensive care unit (NICU) and other infant populations, and identifies areas for further study.

CAM, the merging of complementary and alternative therapies with mainstream Western medicine, is often called integrative medicine. In integrative medicine, health professionals are expanding their view of Western medicine to a more holistic perspective. Two views are now being integrated—one that views disease as having specific causative agents and another that views the mind–body connection as a significant influence on health. In treating disease, practitioners of mind–body medicine look at many factors, including the nature of relationships—such as the relationship between parents and infants and the dynamic between healer and patient. This new integrative, holistic model has thus increasingly challenged our profession to broaden definitions of healing to include all aspects of relationships as part of health and wholeness.

In neonatal care, proponents of complementary therapies believe that the integration of CAM may minimize iatrogenic complications associated with prematurity or interventions to treat prematurity. The high-tech environment may overwhelm the infant with excessive stimulation. Alternatively, these infants may be touch-deprived from weeks in incubators. CAM therapies may provide balance to support the amazing technologic advances we have made.

Alternative medicine, like conventional medicine, has pros and cons, promotes good ideas and bad ones, and promises to hold both benefits and risks. To keep an open, skeptical mind will allow examination of our current medical model with its focus on the "cure" and allow us to broaden our perspective on healing and health. Nursing and nursing care is naturally compatible with CAM, since nursing care is based on a holistic approach. The operative word "care" connotes a friendlier, humanistic value than the word "cure" does. Caring (communication, sensitivity, holistic approach) is one of the hallmarks of our profession. Much of CAM is based on expanding these areas as well as broadening our awareness of many different subtleties in healing.

The complementary categories that were established by the NCCAM are used for discussion:

- Lifestyle Therapies (Developmental Care)
- Aromatherapy, Music, Light, Kangaroo Care (KC)
- Biomechanical Therapies
- Massage, Reflexology, Osteopathy/Cranial-Sacral (CS) Therapy
- Bioenergetic Therapies
- Acupuncture, Energy Healing, Healing Touch (HT), Reiki
- Biochemical Therapies
- Herbs and Supplements; Homeopathy and Galactagogues

Although some practices could fit in more than one category, the categories are useful for general description. For instance, some view homeopathy as a vibrational medicine because its effect is energetic rather than biochemical. Some also consider techniques that focus on environmental manipulation more alternative in nature. These fall into the realm of either family-focused care (Chapter 32) or the NICU environment (Chapter 31).

LIFESTYLE THERAPIES (DEVELOPMENTAL CARE)

General Developmental Care

Neurodevelopmental care includes any intervention undertaken to improve neurodevelopmental outcome. These include developmentally supportive NICU design (appropriate lighting and use of circadian light/dark cycles; low noise levels in the unit and incubator), nursing care plans (infant positioning and handling, feeding and bathing methods, speaking before handling), and pain management.

Research is needed to assess sensory overstimulation in preterm infants, as well as to demonstrate the efficacy of providing soothing sensory input to ameliorate the NICU experience for infants and their families. One benefit of all of these developmental therapies is they tend to encourage early participation by family members in caregiving, which has been shown to enhance bonding (Chapter 32).

Aromatherapy

The intent of aromatherapy is to alter a person's mood or behavior and to facilitate physical, mental, or emotional well-being through the use of aromatic and essential oils from herbs and flowers. People respond immediately and involuntarily to scents, which may release neurotransmitters in the brain and cause calming, sedating, pain-reducing, stimulating, or euphoric effects. For example, truck drivers are known to use peppermint aromatherapy to keep them awake during long night drives. A month-long Japanese study of aromatherapy found that when the air in an office for keypunch operators was scented with jasmine, error rates dropped 33%; the scent was also found to increase efficiency and relieve stress among employees. Could NICU staff use this anxiety-relief and stress reduction technique as well?

Aromatherapy is the fastest growing of all complementary therapies among the nursing field in the United States. It is only in the past few years that aromatherapy has become recognized by the U.S. State Boards of Nursing as a legitimate part of holistic nursing (Buckle, 2001). Lavender, of all the essential oils, has been the most studied by health care providers. Various studies mention the use of lavender on pillows in order to alleviate insomnia, as well as to help ICU patients cope with stress. Questions that arise include: if a newborn is having sleepless nights, might using olfaction mitigate this? Could we use lavender rather than sedatives for sleep? Could chamomile help regulate sleep–wake cycles? Could peppermint in incubators as "olfactory caffeine"—as a stimulant to minimize or eliminate apnea and bradycardia events in preemies? A French study recently published in *Pediatrics* demonstrates a 36% reduction in apnea with the introduction of the odor vanillin (used because of its weak trigeminal activation) when used in the treatment of apneas unresponsive to caffeine and doxapram (Marlier, Gaugler, & Messer, 2005).

Several recent articles address the role of olfaction as a tool in preterm infants. One article assessed the effects of familiar odors (maternal breast milk, amniotic fluid, etc.) used on healthy preterm infants during routine blood draws (heelsticks and venipuncture), noting a decrease in crying and grimacing compared to baseline in infants given various types of odorization (Goubet, Rattaz, Pierrat, Bullinger, & Lequien, 2003).

Researchers have reported that newborns have an acute sense of smell. Indeed, the natural odor that emanates from the mother forms part of the complex bonding process. Dr. Hisanobu Sugano, director of the Life Science Institute at Moa Health Science Foundation in Fukuoka, Japan, demonstrated through his numerous studies in subtle energies and aromatherapy that newborns could correctly identify their mothers' milk from nine other specimens. Several other experiments have shown that when used and unused breast pads are placed on either side of the newborn's head, the newborn will turn more often to the side of the used pad. Within a week after birth, the newborn can discern its mother's milk on a breast pad from the milk of other mothers. Surely babies are sensitive to the noxious odors of our environment from alcohol and Betadine swabs to the newest cousins of our skin cleansers. The calming or stimulating effects of CAM therapies could be a productive area for research. With the fragrance perception of newborns, is it possible to manipulate the scents to achieve effects from olfactory stimulants, anxiolytics, or enhanced attachment? In some cultures this process is already done. For instance, Filipino families often leave the mother's clothing in the newborn's crib to calm the child in her absence. Some suggestions might be to have the family bring in an article of the parent's clothing and place it in the bed in order to help calm and reassure the infant. Another would be to allow the infant to smell the breast milk container, reinforcing the mother's smell with feedings. Or place a small amount of milk on a pacifier for tube-fed babies. This fosters the formation of the nerve pathways and associations between smell/taste and feeding (McDowell, 2005).

A variety of aromatherapy oils are used for diaper rashes, such as lavender sitz baths, almond oils, and beeswax. Another oil is Brazilian guava, found to have analgesic effects, being investigated for use in babies. Some aromas are recommended for colic. They are believed to reduce infant anxiety as well as parental stress, which many feel plays a role in colic.

Music Therapy

For several years now, media attention has turned toward what is called the Mozart effect. This focuses on music as an auditory vehicle that can soothe and stimulate developing infants in utero as well as once they are born

(Campbell, 1997). Lullabies have been linked with infants throughout history; music therapy carries this tradition over into the NICU. For the past 10 years, music therapy has been used in the NICU to mediate stress and promote positive development. We know that by the 18th week of gestation, the auditory capabilities of the fetus are present. In utero, the uterine blood flow provides a soothing musical waterfall and the maternal heart beat a continuous tick-tock chant. Many studies have measured heart rate changes in the fetus when exposed to certain music in utero. The music and the tempo can assist with accelerating the heart rate in terms of bradycardia or decelerating the heart rate to help with stress-induced increases. Hospital noise differs markedly from in utero acoustics or the sound of soothing music (Ernst, 1996). Ambient noise in the NICU may cause distress, and attempts have been made to cover the noise in the NICU by using sound to negate other sounds. This is called sonic camouflage, or acoustic masking, aimed at sound reduction and minimization of vestibular stimulation.

Music has been shown to promote both neurologic development and language development if words accompany the music (Standley, 2001). Music with or without vocalization has been shown to soothe a crying infant or to decrease a heart rate and increase oxygen saturation levels. In the first meta-analysis of music therapy studies of premature infants, Standley reported that the observed state, heart and respiratory rates, oxygen saturation levels, weight gain, length of stay, feeding rate, and nonnutritive sucking rates were all positively influenced by music therapy (Standley, 2002). Recent literature on the pacifier-activated lullaby (PAL) allows the infant to coordinate music and sucking (Marwick, 2000). Music may even alleviate some of the distress infants sustain with suctioning (Chou et al., 2003) and heelsticks (Butt & Kisilevsky, 2000). It has been theorized that music therapy during performance of nursing interventions may enhance the infant's quality of life.

Based on experience rather than evidence from controlled studies, Standley (2001), a certified music therapist, suggests the following guidelines for music in the NICU:

- Music selection: sounds in the NICU should be soothing, constant, stable, and relatively unchanging to reduce alerting responses.
- Volume level: in the 65 to 70 decibel range is recommended.
- Maximum time per day for continuously playing music: 1.5 hours (alternating 45 minutes on and 45 minutes off). The different effects of live versus recorded music are still debated. The use of maternal vocalization is now a popular research focus. The long-term effects of missed exposure to maternal speech in late fetal life are not known.
- Approval for auditory stimuli: daily approval of the nurse providing care to the infant should be obtained for provision of music stimulation (adapted from Standley, 2001).

There are still many unanswered questions about the potential for sound therapy in our nurseries. Should we use it? Which types of music are best in particular situations? Is the therapeutic benefit of live music greater than recorded? Is Shostakovich better, Vivaldi, or the nurses' favorite radio station? Can music affect the caregivers' mood and behavior? Is there a "sonic caffeine"—a music or sound pattern that could ameliorate apnea and bradycardia in preterm infants?

Light Therapy

Research has demonstrated the scientific significance of phototherapy. Aside from the classically recognized effects of diminishing bilirubin and activation of vitamin D, numerous studies have shown this therapy's effect on thyroid stimulation alterations in renal and vascular parameters, increased gut transit times, and a host of other metabolic alterations. Hypothetically, other wavelengths of light may have physiologic effects. This hypothesis is the basis for the field of color and light therapy.

Regulation of ambient lighting in the NICU has been recognized as an important concern. Research in this area falls under the category of NICU design and environment and is discussed in Chapter 31. Constant exposure to light can result in disorganization of the infant's state (Jones, Kassity, & Duncan, 2001). For this reason, procedural lighting and blanket covers are used to shield infants in incubators from direct light. Research is needed to determine whether light therapy—exposing the infant to varying light cycles—alters circadian rhythms or physiologic stability through its effects on endocrine function. Assessing and broadening our current understanding could expand concepts of light, color, or other wavelengths for newborns as well as staff.

Kangaroo Care

KC was first described by Gene Cranston Anderson (1991) more than 20 years ago in the mountains of Bogotá, Colombia, yet the practice may be older than recorded history. In this practice, the newborn was placed skin-to-skin, usually on the chest between the mother's breasts to keep the baby warm. The effect of skin-to-skin care on physiologic stability and bonding has been investigated in many studies. Engler and Ludington (1999) conducted a survey of 1,133 NICUs in the United States to determine what percentage of those NICUs used KC. They found 82% of the units practiced some form of skin-to-skin care. To date, studies indicate that KC can positively affect both the mother (or caregiver) and the infant. When a parent holds the infant against his or her skin, the infant's breathing, oxygen saturation, and heart rate become more regular; the flexion and tone improve; and the sleep state becomes less disorganized (Ludington-Hoe, 2004). Various body positions also seem to affect gastric emptying and reflux. KC provides a sensory dialogue for the infant and caregiver as well as a method of central nervous system (CNS) regulation of the autonomic motor and state systems. Mounting evidence in favor of KC to promote physiologic stability has encouraged more studies with very immature, unstable infants (Eichel, 2001).

Infant Massage

Massage develops our first language, the expression of touch. There are many types of massage from gentle stroking, superficial friction, pressure, kneading, containment, vibration, and percussion to the more intense manipulations of Rolfing (Carroll, 2006). Fields (2000) has conducted infant massage research since the 1970s, much of which focused on the premature infant. Fields reported that massaged infants have a 47% greater weight gain and better organized sleep states; moreover, they are more responsive to social stimulation, have more organized motor development, and are commonly discharged 6 to 10 days earlier from the hospital. This allows the newborn to go home earlier, adding a significant cost savings.

Fields's study (2000) of cocaine-exposed newborns suggested that touch therapy increases vagal activity, which in turn releases the hormones gastrin and insulin, which may explain the weight gain in the premature infant. Massage stimulates the parasympathetic nervous system. If an infant is more attentive, it may follow that more stimulation from the parent is elicited, thus improving the dyad interactions and performance on the infant developmental assessment tools (Fields, 2000). "Touch promotes bonding and well being and is therefore an essential therapy for the benefit of parents, babies and health care professionals" (Feary, 2002). The efficacy of infant massage depends on respect and consideration for the infant's readiness. Massage should be state dependent; for example, the deep sleep state is not the best time for a massage. A time when the infant is fussy, however, may be the perfect time. Being aware of the baby and his or her receptivity and alertness is important in determining the best time for a massage rather than relying on a predetermined time. The type and amount of massage depends on the infant's gestational age, degree of illness or stability, and ability to engage. Fields (2000) has also suggested many benefits to the "massager"—such as lower stress hormone levels and decreased postnatal depression (Feary, 2002; Glover, Onozawa, & Hodgkinson, 2002). Some researchers have focused on massage as a way to reduce stress and to increase bonding and attachment when a parent performs massage. A significant emphasis has been placed on fathers performing massage as a bonding tool, as breastfeeding would be for the mother.

Research on the benefits of massage is increasing. Kirpatrick (personal communication, 2001) has found in her NICU experience that massage helps reduce postoperative edema through stimulation of cardiac and lymphatic activity and decreases the need for postoperative narcotics. Physical activity when combined with infant massage seems to stimulate bone growth and mineralization in premature infants. However, with osteopenia, which can be a major cause for morbidity in this population, further investigation is warranted (Aly et al., 2004).

Maternal administration of physical activity such as passive limb movements has been shown to enhance bone mineral acquisition in very-low-birth-weight (VLBW) infants. This could be a great way for a father to also feel included in the care of his baby. These care practices can also provide an opportunity for the infant to hear their parents' voices, as speech and language development is believed to be influenced by prenatal maternal speech.

A significant emphasis has been placed on fathers performing massage, as a bonding tool similar to what breastfeeding would be for the mother. It can also be a great way to get other family members, such as grandparents, involved. One day we may find that, just as important as the technologies of intensive care medicine, so will be the supportive touch of a parent in helping activate an optimal neurodevelopmental milieu. Data suggest benefits to the mother, as the masseuse, include lower stress hormone levels and decreased postnatal depression and anxiety.

Concerns have been raised as to whether infant massage can produce overstimulation and therefore adverse effects. Further research is needed, through controlled trials, to determine the benefits as well as the risks of this therapy.

Reflexology

Reflexology is an ancient form of healing, somewhat similar to traditional acupuncture. It is a healing method based on the principle that there are reflexes in the hands and feet specific to each organ, gland, function, and part of the human body. The goal of reflexology is to stop or reverse the negative chain reactions that occur within the mind–body and to restore the energy balance. According to the tenets of reflexologists, health problems occur when the flow of life energy (chi) is blocked or disturbed and that it is alleviated when the flow of chi is restored by manipulation of the reflex points. Applying pressure to these points can also bring about stress relief by improving circulation and minimizing pain. This modality can be considered the opposite of the heelstick blood draw; it involves the same area but a reverse technique. However, more research is needed in this area.

The presumed mechanisms in reflexology, from a Western medical perspective, are (1) that the treatment of reflex zones stimulates the body's blood flow; (2) that pressure to these points increases the body's production of endorphins; and (3) that it assists in the elimination of waste materials.

It is the opinion of this author that reflexology may be useful in a neonatal unit to help balance and soothe the patient's bioenergy, which might decrease periods of fussiness or disorganization. Reflexology may also benefit the infant by increasing blood flow to specific organ sites, increasing perfusion to the kidneys, and increasing cardiac output.

Osteopathy/CS Therapy

Osteopathy medicine is based on the premise that the body has within it an inherent therapeutic potency. The body is its own medicine chest. Most of the biomechanical manipulations in the pediatric osteopathic community fall under the healing category of CS therapy. A practitioner of CS therapy works with the subtle pressure fluctuations of the cerebral spinal fluid to optimize a patient's health. A practitioner of this discipline may gently realign cranial bones to bring them into the proper relationship.

A basic tenet of osteopathy is that many problems begin at birth. Birth (labor and delivery) is viewed as one of the most traumatic experiences and can produce skeletal strains that can cause problems throughout life. Recognition and treatment of these dysfunctions in the immediate postpartum period is considered an essential preventive measure. In the CS system, misalignment of structure that is not corrected can lead to potential alterations in function. The occipital area is believed to sustain most of the trauma during delivery. A study by Frymann (1998) explored the relationship between symptomatology in the newborn and the anatomic physiologic disturbances of the CNS. The study suggested that strains within the unfused fragments of the occipital bones produced problems in the nervous system, that is, vomiting, reflux, hyperactive peristalsis, colic, tremor, hypertonicity, and irritability.

Frymann (1998) reported that compression of the hypoglossal nerve could cause a newborn's failure to grasp the nipple and suck effectively. If left untreated, these newborns may exhibit tongue thrust and may have deviant swallowing patterns, speech problems, and even malocclusion. Problems such as sucking-swallowing difficulties and recurrent reflux after birth are so common that many mothers and doctors consider them to be normal. According to CS theory, these can be easily rectified. When the vagus nerve is compressed, for example, recurrent vomiting or reflux can occur. Decompress the condylar parts of the occiput, and the vomiting stops. In temporal bone development, misalignment may cause recurrent otitis media. If the sphenoids are involved, the child may have headaches. Until the structural cause of the problem is recognized and addressed, the underlying pathophysiology will not change. Osteopaths often feel that every child should be structurally evaluated after any type of trauma, especially birth.

This field presents some interesting opportunities for research. What portals of understanding could this field open in the search for intraventricular hemorrhage (IVH)? Could daily CS therapy assist in developing a more womb-like analogue for brain and spinal development? Could they palpate and help guide the developmental energies in the CS system by tuning in and tracking the system to retrace its normal developmental pattern, and bringing the memory of health to play? As osteopathy's founder, Dr. Andrew Still, once said, "To find health should be the objective of the doctor. Anyone can find a disease."

BIOENERGETIC THERAPIES

Acupuncture

Acupuncture is part of a complex system known as traditional Chinese medicine (TCM) that has been practiced in China for more than 2,000 years. This is an energy-based approach rather than a disease-oriented approach through the conventional diagnostic and treatment model. The main concept behind this philosophy is that of energy in the body. This energy is called chi (immeasurable by current instrumentation in Western science) (Freeman, 2001a), which underlies and supports all aspects of the physical body. This energy circulates throughout the body along specific pathways called meridians.

Obstructions in the flow of chi may cause disease. Acupuncturists rebalance the flow of energy by gently placing thin, solid, disposable, metallic needles into the skin along the meridians where chi is blocked. These needles either are briefly left in place or are stimulated with electricity, heat, laser, or moxibustion (burning of the moxa herb over the acupuncture point). Acupuncture has shown promising results in use for anesthesia, postoperative pain, and addiction recovery. In the West, acupuncture has been used since the early 1970s for various forms of addiction and withdrawal in expectant mothers, as well as for infants to help reduce the residual effects of drug exposure in cases of prenatal substance abuse (using the auricular location called the frustration point). This therapy is based on research done with acupuncture and withdrawal of drugs and alcohol (Janssen, Demorest, & Whynot, 2005).

Researchers are currently considering whether acupuncture can help treat colic, constipation, diminished postoperative urine output, apnea, and bradycardia as well as improve cardiac output and control of postoperative pain. Currently in China, acupuncture is used to treat infants with jaundice (augmenting hepatic chi), skin problems, teething, ear infections, constipation, conjunctivitis, and peripheral nerve injury.

Acupressure, which is similar to acupuncture, appears to be more popular in pediatric patients because it does not involve the use of needles. Acupressure involves applying pressure at acupuncture points along the 14 major energy meridians to promote the flow of chi. Numerous studies show that acupressure, like acupuncture, stimulates physical reactions in the body, such as changes in brain activity and blood chemistries, in addition to enhancing immune and endocrine functions (Jones & Kassity, 2001).

Healing Touch

Healing touch (HT) is an energy-based therapy developed by Mentgen and the American Holistic Nurses Association in the late 1980s. This therapy is considered experimental and requires parental consent and a certified practitioner. It is another therapy that reaches out to the human desire to be touched. It is a way to further humanize the health care relationship for the nurse as well as the patient. As noted previously, touch promotes healing and the formation of a bond.

During an HT session, infants are not to be disturbed. They usually are scheduled for at least two sessions per week that last from 15 to 40 minutes. HT consists first of a hand scan to assess the infant's condition. This assessment is done by gently and slowly moving a hand from head to toes, often 6 inches or more above the body, to detect changes in the infant's energy field. Once the assessment is completed, a variety of techniques can be used: energy field centering, comfort infusion, energy infusion or modulation, modified magnetic unruffling, spiral healing light, and halo. All of these methods use the hands-on technique or the movement of the hands over the body to balance the energy field of the infant.

Comfort infusion is a technique that parents can be taught. It is believed to relieve pain. Parents place the left palm over the infant, encouraging the pain to move through their palm, up through their body and drain out of their right hand. When parents no longer sense pain, the right hand is placed palm on or over the infant and the left one turned upward to infuse healing energy. This technique empowers parents to actively participate in care of their infants.

In any of these modes, the infant may be observed to calm down (if unsettled before HT), relax, and even fall into a sleep state. The spiral healing light uses a visualized light beam for those infants who are much compromised. A beam of healing light is visualized flowing through the crown chakra "energy center" down the arm and out the first two fingers and thumb as they are held together. Starting at the center of the infant's body, the beam is slowly directed in a clockwise spiral that expands to cover the whole body. The healing light touches every cell of the body and infuses healing energy. When the edges of the body are reached, the spiral is brought back to the center of the body while the practitioner visualizes the healing beam of light, thus giving the infant strength and energy to help the cells release excess fluid, carbon dioxide, bilirubin, or infection. When the center of the body is reached, a clear blue healing light is visualized as flowing through the practitioner's hand and is held over the infant's crown, thus washing away what has been released. Along with traditional medicine, HT promotes a calm, restful state and relieves discomfort, which helps support the body, mind, and spirit's natural healing process.

Energy-based healing is growing in popularity in hospitals and medical and nursing school curricula around the country. Results of HT studies support its use in depression, cancer, pain, and many other conditions. It also adds a spiritual dimension to our increasingly high-tech health care system.

Reiki

Reiki is another form of energy healing, in which energy is transferred from the hands of a practitioner to a patient using a sequence of hand positions above the body. Reiki relaxes and heals by clearing energy meridians and chakras (vortices of energy along the spine), thus restoring balance, relieving pain, and accelerating the healing process. Respiration slows; blood pressure decreases; emotional clearing and calming occur. Blockages are dissolved, and the vibrational frequency of the body is thought to increase.

Few studies of Reiki have been done in the United States. In one study from New Hampshire, more than 872 patients underwent a 15-minute Reiki treatment both before and after surgery (Alandydy & Alandydy, 1999). The patients reported an increased sense of relaxation, reduction in stress, and a possible enhancement of the natural healing ability of their bodies. Notably, no infants were included in the study; this is an area in need of further study.

Reiki treatments may be applicable for pregnancy and infancy in many situations. Simply increasing relaxation and improving the body's healing ability could be valuable in many circumstances surrounding pregnancy and birth. Further study is needed regarding the efficacy and safety of these techniques.

BIOCHEMICAL INTERVENTIONS

Homeopathy

The basic idea behind homeopathy is respect of the innate wisdom of the body. The premise is to honor the symptoms of illness that one's body experiences as it responds to defend, heal, or protect itself against stress or infection. The way a homeopath views this process is that the body's internal wisdom will defend and heal itself by choosing a beneficial response. Homeopathy is based on the "like cures like principle": A symptom in a patient is treated with a remedy that causes this same symptom, thus further stimulating the body's current responses (similar in philosophy to a vaccine). Homeopaths explain that when a truly effective therapy is underway, a temporary exacerbation of certain symptoms may appear. This idea contrasts with the suppression theory of conventional medicine, which homeopaths feel works on disease suppression rather than elimination. A homeopath's use of the principle of similars tries to minimize the wisdom of the body rather than suppress its symptoms (Ullman, 1999). Homeopathic remedies are an enigma to those unaware of the concepts of the energetic memory of water and the potentizing successions that enhance the memory of the water, but appear to physical science as a mere series of dilutions.

A review of 89 clinical studies showed that patients who were given a homeopathic medicine were 2.45 times more likely to improve than those who received placebos (Linde et al., 1997). These findings were based on the efficacy of homeopathic remedies in healing and treating a variety of conditions such as asthma, ear infections, postsurgical complications, sprains, rheumatoid arthritis, and those found around childbirth.

Homeopathy can be considered a catalyst to "jump start" the body and its healing process. Professional homeopaths prescribe medicine that is very patient specific and is based on that particular patient's past health history, past medical treatments, genetic inheritance, and the totality of the physical, emotional, and mental or spiritual symptoms. Unfortunately, titrating individualized medicine(s) for everyone, especially newborns, is not always easy. It sometimes takes more than a single visit to a homeopath to find the correct remedy to start the healing process (Linde et al., 1997). Chubby babies require different constitutional remedies than do small or low-birth-weight babies, as do babies who sleep through the night compared to those who do not. Some research on homeopathic remedies for pregnant women has been done. One must keep in mind that a mother who receives homeopathic remedies during pregnancy and childbirth will pass its benefits onto the fetus. Postnatal treatment of the mother will also benefit the child if he or she is breastfed (Linde et al., 1997). Infants who endure traumatic labors with bruising or other injury (i.e., postnatal IV infiltrates) are considered to benefit from a remedy called arnica, which aims to optimize the body's attempts to heal its wounds, both physical and psychological. In addition to arnica, *Hypericum perforatum* can be used for IV burns for the mother or newborn during hospitalization.

It is hypothesized that homeopathic remedies such as arnica, staphysagria, and calendula can help circumcised newborns heal from the physical and psychological trauma of circumcision. Chamomile is the most effective of many remedies suggested for colic and is also the most common remedy for teething pain in older infants. Other remedies for teething pain may include calcarea carbonica, calcarea phosphorica, and silicea. Magnesium phosphorica relieves the symptoms of gas, bloating, and burping. Nux vomica may be used when the woman has ingested alcohol or therapeutic or recreational drugs and the newborn exhibits colicky behavior. Aethusa is used for newborns who are intolerant of milk or who reflux shortly after milk has been ingested. Calendula given externally for diaper rash will soothe the newborn's bottom and help fight infection. In Europe, carbovege is a homeopathic remedy used for apnea and bradycardia in the infant. Homeopathy offers much to learn and information that can be assimilated into care to broaden the current medical understandings.

Herbal Medicine

The use of botanical medicine is ancient. Hippocrates (466–377 BC) integrated herbal medicine into his practice and teaching. The World Health Organization estimates that about 75% of the world population relies on botanical medicines; indeed, 30% of Americans also use botanical remedies, and the practice is growing in popularity (B. Barrett, Kiefer, & Rabago, 1999). It behooves health care professionals to be familiar with the expanding field of herbal medicine. Substances first isolated from plants account for approximately 25% of the Western pharmacopoeia, and another 25% is derived from modification of chemicals first found in natural products (B. Barrett et al., 1999; Freeman, 2001b). Digitalis, the ever-popular echinacea, and caffeine all are herbal and have effects and side effects (Boullata & Nace, 2000).

The bulk of phytomedicinal research has been conducted in Germany, where the medical and social culture is more accepting of herbal medicine. In Germany, millions of prescriptions are written for herbal medicines each year. In the United States herbal medicines are classified as food supplements and are often available without a prescription. They receive minimal regulatory governing from the Food and Drug Administration. Herbal remedies sold in the United States require no proof of efficacy, safety, potency, or standardization and may vary considerably from brand to brand (Gurley, Gardner, & Hubbard, 2000; Institution for Safe Medication Practices [ISMP], 1998; Klepser & Klepser, 1999). For instance, 24% of a sampling of more than 2,600 TCMs (herbs) at the Institute for Safe Medicine contained a therapeutic drug adulterant, and more than 50% contained two or more adulterants—including anti-inflammatory, analgesic, and diuretic agents (Huang, Wen, & Hsiao, 1997). Moreover, some Americans mistakenly believe that a natural herb is necessarily a safe herb. On the contrary, some are potent drugs (S. Barrett, 2004). In taking family history, nurses should ask whether any herbal substances are regularly used or were used during pregnancy. Knowing what, if any, herbal remedies nursing mothers use is essential, because the substances can be passed through breast milk to children.

Parents of neonates have been known to ask about aloe vera as a skin protectant or for its use with burns and skin irritations, as it has long been used as a folk remedy. Other creams made from comfrey, plantain, or marigold have been used for treatment of rashes and cradle cap. Calendula is used in Russia for conjunctivitis. Tree tea oil is an antifungal. Dandelion has diuretic properties, and chamomile is an antispasmodic, as are herbs such as valerian, fennel, aniseed, and cardamom. Peppermint stimulates bile flow and lowers lower-esophageal spinetic pressure. Milk thistle increases enterohepatic circulation. Tripola increases intestinal peristalsis. Kava can be used to induce oral numbness, which would be helpful with endotracheal tube discomfort. St. John's wort is used for nervous unrest and, more commonly, to treat depression. Immune stimulants such as echinacea and astragalus and all of the herbs in this discussion will surely be studied more extensively in adults before their use is standardized for children and infants. Caffeine is the leading herb therapy in the United States and is used for apnea and bradycardia in infants. Marked expansion can come out of phytomedicines if we remain open-minded to the worldwide wisdom accrued through its extensive use.

Galactagogues

Therapies in the management of inadequate breast milk supply are of special concern to neonatologists. Prescription galactagogues and increased fluid intake are traditional mainstays but many mothers prefer more natural therapies when breastfeeding. CAM therapies that have been used for centuries include: (a) herbal galactagogues such as Fenugreek, chaste tree, blessed thistle, fennel, trobangun leaves (most believed to work by antagonizing the dopamine receptor in increasing prolactin release) and (b) biomechanical galactagogues vary from massage, KC, and other relaxation therapies to auricular acupuncture which is used in China for the treatment of hypogalactia.

Research

Research on CAM is growing in neonatal care. Unfortunately, for a variety of reasons, little research has been done to support its use. As health care professionals, we can either help gain the evidence to support these practices or watch them be incorporated in possibly unsystematic, unhealthy ways. Currently, many in the medical community condemn these therapies without even making a genuine scientific inquiry into their efficacy. We need to encourage our researchers to conduct the studies necessary to move these modalities safely into the mainstream.

Other areas of research are evolving from multisensory interventions (White-Traut, 2004) to kinesthetic stimulation for preventing apnea (Henderson-Smart & Osborn, 2000). Multiple recent articles mention the use of probiotics in decreasing the incidence of necrotizing enterocolitis in VLBW infants. Examination of safety and efficacy through larger clinical trials will be needed (Kliegman & Willoughby, 2005).

Another area of CAM focus might be parents—for example, the development of "parent circles" that assist parents in gaining perspective on their situation is a complementary addition to the routines of an NICU (Pearson & Anderson, 2001).

Additionally, complementary ideas could be used to meet the often-overlooked needs of siblings. A program that includes this support might be very useful and is worthy of further study (Ballard, 2004). As research continues, CAM therapies may give us many new insights into the nature of the mind–body system and the overall complexities of health and healing. For instance, if no biochemical mechanisms exist in some CAM therapies, what are the mechanisms of action? If it is subtle energy, what can we do to measure it? Some scientists, for example, have begun to look at the heart rhythms and brain waves of energy healers to detect subtle changes in the overall patterning. In other cases, researchers are turning to double-blind studies to determine whether a CAM therapy is effective, even if the mechanism through which it works is not yet understood. CAM therapies have been traditionally viewed with suspicion by mainstream medicine. However, researchers and practitioners are looking increasingly at these therapies as new areas for scientific inquiry. Attaining reliable risk-benefit analysis and focusing on outcome research should be a long-term goal for practitioners interested in CAM therapies so that they may be used efficiently and without concern.

■ Cobedding. Cobedding of twins and higher order multiples (HOMs) is a growing practice. The rationale is that during their gestational development, multiple-gestation fetuses lived side by side. Once born, they are normally separated and put in a single bed, partly because of concerns over infection and because of the size of standard infant beds. Studies are underway that examine the effects of the practice of cobedding on physiologic stability, soothing, motoric organization, proprioceptive stimulation, and enhanced growth. One completed study (Altimier & Lutes, 2001) focused on premature twins and HOMs admitted to a large midwestern tertiary center. Twenty-three sets of twins, 4 sets of triplets, and 1 set of quadruplets were included. The control group consisted of 15 sets of twins, 7 sets of triplets, and 2 sets of quadruplets. A randomized control design was used on infants weighing less than 1,500 g. The following protocol was indicated:

- Twins and HOMs being cared for in the same NICU were put together when stability was achieved.
- Oxygen requirement was limited to nasal cannula only.
- IVs, gavage feeding, cardiopulmonary monitoring, pulse oximetry, and phototherapy were permitted.
- All equipment, clothing, and chart forms were color-coded to match each twin/multiple. The multiples wore hospital identification bands at all times.
- Positioning of multiples in the womb was replicated, if this was known. Otherwise, siblings were placed side by side, either facing each other, facing the other one's back, or in a head-to-toes position. Repositioning of one or more infants was considered if infant(s) appeared restless.
- One blanket was lightly swaddled around the multiples; hands were free to reach their own face or a sibling to facilitate each other's motor organization.
- Caregiving was clustered to address all infants' needs during the same interaction. (The infant in the most awake state received care first.)
- If one infant demonstrated temperature instability, the temperature probe was placed on that infant—otherwise on the smallest infant. All infants were dressed or undressed depending on their individualized thermoregulatory needs (used with permission from Altimier & Lutes, 2001).

The results demonstrated that the cobedded group had a more positive growth rate in weight and in head circumference than the control group. No differences in nosocomial rates or in thermal needs were noted between the two groups (Altimier & Lutes, 2001). Cobedding is considered a developmentally supportive care strategy (Nyqvist & Lutes, 1998). This therapy is being considered as part of some hospitals' quality improvement programs to support family-centered, developmental care for multiple gestation families (Polizzi, Byers, & Kiehl, 2003). Before this therapy is completely embraced, further research needs to determine the benefits and safety in this population of neonates. Recently, concerns have been raised again about the linkage between cobedding and sudden infant death syndrome (SIDS) (Burnett & Adler, 2006). The connection may be the tight swaddling of infants when cobedded. Until further research findings are released, this practice should be undertaken with caution, if at all.

SUMMARY

CAM may offer important potential for the NICU: Some evidence suggests that preterm neonates benefit from the soothing, calming properties of these therapies; these therapies may help the infants conserve energy and improve weight gain, and may augment bonding. CAM may also assist with consolation during painful procedures. It is exciting to observe the complexion of our profession changing so dramatically, from one so technically focused to the rebirth of a nurturant focus. The process can be inspiring as the search for a new sense of care is struggling to be born. The information given in this chapter is merely the tip of the iceberg. Further research to determine the benefits and risks of many of these therapies is needed. Complementary medicine may contribute to the increased effectiveness of clinical practice for enhanced patient and family care.

EVIDENCE-BASED PRACTICE BOX

Aromatherapy

Could aromatherapy be used as an adjunct to support respiratory and cardiac events in premature infants? Using fragrance as "olfactory caffeine," for example, could be a stimulant to minimize or eliminate apnea and bradycardia incidents in preemies.

A French study recently published in *Pediatrics* demonstrates a 36% reduction in apnea with the introduction of the odor vanillin (used because of its weak trigeminal activation) when used in the treatment of apneas unresponsive to caffeine and doxapram (Marlier et al., 2005). With the fragrance perception of newborns, it may be possible to manipulate the aromas to achieve effects from olfactory stimulants, anxiolytics, or even enhanced attachment.

The calming or stimulating effects of CAM modalities such as aromatherapy provide fertile ground for research. Although several other published articles address the role of olfaction as a technique in supporting preterm infants, this is an area that requires further exploration.

ONLINE RESOURCES

Complementary and Alternative Medical Therapies in Neonatology **http://www.accesspediatrics.com/abstract/6684772**

Complementary and Alternative Methods of Increasing Breast Milk Supply for Lactating Mothers of Infants in the NICU **http://www.ncbi.nlm.nih.gov/pubmed/20630837**

Varieties of Alternative Experience: Complementary Care in the Neonatal Intensive Care Unit **http://www.journals.lww.com/clinicalobgyn/Citation/2001/12000/Varieties_of_Alternative_Experience__Complementary.12.aspx**

REFERENCES

Alandydy, P., & Alandydy, K. (1999). Performance brief: Using Reiki to support surgical patients. *Journal of Nursing Care and Quality, 13*(4), 89–91.

Altimier, L., & Lutes, L. (2001). Co-bedding multiples. *Newborn and Infant Nursing Reviews, 1*(4), 205–206.

Aly, H., Moustafa, M. F., Hassanein, S. M., Massaro, A. N., Amer, H. A., & Patel, K. (2004). Physical activity combined with massage improves bone mineralization in premature infants: A randomized trial. *Journal of Perinatology, 24*(5), 305–309.

Anderson, G. C. (1991). Current knowledge about skin-to-skin (kangaroo) care for preterm infants. *Journal of Perinatology, 11*(3), 216–226.

Ballard, K. L. (2004). Meeting the needs of siblings of children with cancer. *Pediatric Nursing, 30*(5), 394–401.

Barrett, B., Kiefer, D., & Rabago, D. (1999). Assessing the risks and benefits of herbal medicine: An overview of scientific evidence. *Alternative Therapies, 5*(4), 40–49.

Barrett, S. (2004). *The herbal minefield.* Retrieved from http://www.quackwatch.org/01QuackeryRelatedTopics/herbs.html

Boullata, J. L., & Nace, A. M. (2000). Safety issues with herbal medicine. *Pharmacolotherapy, 20*, 257–269.

Buckle, J. (2001). The role of aromatherapy in nursing care. *Nursing Clinics of North America, 36*(1), 57–72.

Burnett, L. B., & Adler, J. (2006). *Pediatrics, Sudden infant death syndrome.* Emedicine. Retrieved from http://www.emedicine.com/EMERG/topic407.htm

Butt, M. L., & Kisilevsky, B. S. (2000). Music modulates behavior of premature infants following heel lance. *Canadian Journal of Nursing Research, 31*(4), 17–39.

Campbell, D. (1997). *The Mozart effect.* New York, NY: Avon Press.

Carroll, R. T. (2006). *Rolfing. The skeptic's dictionary.* Retrieved from http://skepdic.com/rolfing.html

Chou, L. L., Wang, R. H., Chen, S. J., & Pai, L. (2003). Effects of music therapy on oxygen saturation in premature infants receiving endotracheal suctioning. *Journal of Nursing Research, 11*(3), 209–216.

Eichel, P. (2001). Kangaroo care. *Newborn and Infant Nursing Reviews, 1*(4), 224–228.

Engler, A., & Ludington, S. M. (1999). Kangaroo care in the United States: A national survey. *Journal of Investigative Medicine, 47*(2), 168A.

Ernst, E. (1996). *Complementary medicine: An objective appraisal.* Oxford, UK: Butterworth-Heinemann.

Feary, A. M. (2002). Touching the fragile baby: Looking at touch in the special care nursery (SCN). *Australian Journal of Medical Herbalism, 9*(1), 44–48.

Fields, T. M. (2000). *Touch therapy.* St Louis, MO: Churchill Livingstone.

Freeman, L. W. (2001a). Acupuncture. In L. W. Freeman & G. F. Lawlis (Eds.), *Mosby's complementary and alternative medicine: A research-based approach.* St Louis, MO: Mosby.

Freeman, L. W. (2001b). Herbs as medical intervention. In L. W. Freeman & G. F. Lawlis (Eds.), *Mosby's complementary and alternative medicine: A research-based approach.* St Louis, MO: Mosby.

Frymann, V. M. (1998). *The collected papers of Viola M. Frymann, DO: Legacy of osteopathy to children.* Ann Arbor, MI: Edwards Brothers.

Glover, V., Onozawa, K., & Hodgkinson, A. (2002). Benefits of infant massage for mothers with postnatal depression. *Seminars in Neonatology, 7*(6), 495–500.

Goubet, N., Rattaz, C., Pierrat, V., Bullinger, A., & Lequien, P. (2003). The olfactory experience mediates response to pain in preterm newborns. *Developmental Psychobiology, 42*, 171–180.

Gurley, B. J., Gardner, S. F., & Hubbard, M. A. (2000). Content versus label claims in ephedra-containing dietary supplements. *American Journal of Health-Systems Pharmacy, 57*, 963–969.

Henderson-Smart, D. J., & Osborn, D. A. (2000). Kinesthetic stimulation for preventing apnea in preterm infants. *Cochrane Database of Systematic Reviews, 2*, CD000373.

Huang, W. F., Wen, K. C., & Hsiao, M. L. (1997). Adulteration by synthetic therapeutic substances of traditional Chinese medicines in Taiwan. *Journal of Clinical Pharmacology, 37*, 344–350.

Institution for Safe Medication Practices. (1998). *An overview of herbal medicines and adverse events. ISMP Medication Safety Alert! August 26, 1998.* Retrieved from http://www.ismp.org

Janssen, P. A., Demorest, L. C., & Whynot, E. M. (2005). Acupuncture for substance abuse treatment in the downtown eastside of Vancouver. *Journal of Urban Health, 82*(2), 285–295.

Jones, J., & Kassity, N. (2001). Varieties of alternative experience: Complementary care in the neonatal intensive care unit. *Clinical Obstetrics & Gynecology, 44*(4), 750–768.

Jones, J., Kassity, N., & Duncan, K. (2001). Complementary care alternatives for the NICU. *Newborn and Infant Nursing Reviews, 1*(4), 207–210.

Klepser, B. T., & Klepser, M. E. (1999). Unsafe and potentially safe herbal therapies. *American Journal of Health-Systems Pharmacy, 56*, 125–138.

Kliegman, R. M., & Willoughby, R. E. (2005). Prevention of necrotizing enterocolitis with probiotics. *Pediatrics, 115*(1), 171–172.

Linde, K., Clausius, N., Ramirez, G., Melchart, D., Eitel, F., Hedges, L. V., & Jonas, W. B. (1997). Are the clinical effects of homeopathy placebo effects? Meta-analysis of placebo-controlled trials. *Lancet, 350*(9081), 834–843.

Ludington-Hoe, S. M. (2004). Randomized controlled trial of kangaroo care: Cardiorespiratory and thermal effects on healthy preterm infants. *Neonatal Network, 23*(3), 39–48.

Marlier, L., Gaugler, C., & Messer, J. (2005). Olfactory stimulation prevents apnea in premature newborns. *Pediatrics, 115*(1), 83–88.

Marwick, C. (2000). Music hath charms for care of preemies. *Journal of the American Medical Association, 283*(4), 468–469.

McDowell, B. M. (2005). Nontraditional therapies for the PICU—part 1. *Journal for Specialists in Pediatric Nursing, 10*(1), 29–32.

Nyqvist, K. H., & Lutes, L. M. (1998). Co-bedding twins: A developmentally supportive care strategy. *Journal of Obstetric, Gynecologic, and Neonatal Nursing, 27*(4), 450–456.

Pearson, J., & Anderson, K. (2001). Evaluation of a program to promote positive parenting in the neonatal intensive care unit. *Neonatal Network, 20*(4), 43–48.

Polizzi, J., Byers, J. F., & Kiehl, E. (2003). Co-bedding versus traditional bedding of multiple-gestation infants in the NICU. *Journal of Healthcare Quality, 25*(1), 5–10.

Standley, J. M. (2001). Music therapy for the neonate. *Newborn and Infant Nursing Reviews, 1*(4), 211–216.

Standley, J. M. (2002). A meta-analysis of the efficacy of music therapy for premature infants. *Journal of Pediatric Nursing, 17*(2), 107–113.

Ullman, D. (1999). *Homeopathy A-Z*. Carlsbad, CA: Hay House.

White-Traut, R. (2004). Providing a nurturing environment for infants in adverse situations: Multisensory strategies for newborn care. *Pediatric Nursing, 30*(5), 394–401.

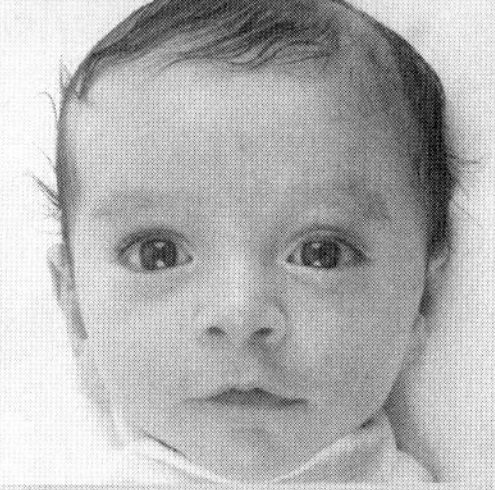

CHAPTER

35

Postdischarge Care of the Newborn, Infant, and Families

■ Marina Boykova, Carole Kenner, and Susan Ellerbee

The multiple problems that bring an infant to a neonatal intensive care unit (NICU) have been described, in depth, throughout the preceding chapters. Upon hospital discharge, high-risk infants require no less care as the health care needs of the initially sick infant often remain numerous and complex. Postdischarge and follow-up care focuses on the convalescing infant's growth, development, health promotion, disease prevention, chronic disease management, and care coordination. Importantly, parents also need care after hospital discharge. The transition from hospital to home for infants and their families is a very important time. This transition starts when the family begins to accept the role of the full-time caregiver outside the safety net of the hospital. The focus of this chapter is on the infant and parental care after hospital discharge.

POSTDISCHARGE CARE FOR HIGH-RISK INFANTS

The first challenge related to the appropriateness of postdischarge care is determining the infant and family's readiness for discharge. The American Academy of Pediatrics (AAP) classifies newborn patients into four groups before discharge: (1) preterm infant, (2) infant with special health care needs or dependence on technology, (3) infant at risk because of family issues, and (4) infant with anticipated early death (American Academy of Pediatrics & Committee on Fetus and Newborn, 2008). Consequently, discharge criteria as well as the postdischarge care depend on the different needs of these patient categories. In general, for high-risk infants to be discharged, they have to be physiologically stable; the decision is based on the clinical judgment of health professionals and determination of the infant's medical status.

The first category, preterm infants, can be discharged when oral feedings are sufficient to support appropriate growth; when they are able to maintain normal body temperature in a homelike environment without supplemental heat; and when sufficient mature respiratory control is present (AAP, 2008). However, apneic episodes are common in preterm infants before discharge; feedings and weight gain are also challenging issues (Radtke, 2011; Silberstein et al., 2009; Westerberg et al., 2010). Most preterm infants achieve physiological milestones by 34 to 36 weeks postconceptual age, but feeding and oxygen milestones are achieved last (Bakewell-Sachs, Medoff-Cooper, Escobar, Silber, & Lorch, 2009). Thus, observation up to 10 days without apnea before discharge is recommended (Lorch, Srinivasan & Escobar, 2011; Nivamat, 2012). For NICU infants, weight gain of 15 to 30 g/d must continue over a reasonable time (several days to 1 week), and it should occur in an open environment (crib); this gain should continue during the first 3 to 4 months of life and then decline to 5 to 15 g/d by the age of 12 to 18 months (Sherman, Aylward, & Shoemaker, 2011). To assure adequate and safe growth at home, 20 to 30 g (0.71–1.06 oz) of daily weight gain before discharge are desirable (LaHood & Bryant, 2007). Milk fortification, iron, vitamins, foliate, and vitamin D supplementation are often necessary. LaHood and Bryant (2007) recommended supplementation of milk feedings with fortifier, iron, and vitamins until the infant begins to gain 20 to 30 g daily (LaHood & Bryant, 2007).

For larger and healthier infants, 108 kcal/kg/d can be sufficient for adequate growth. For preterm infants, 120 to 130 kcal/kg/d can be required with increased protein (Casey, 2008; Sherman et al., 2011). Additional information on specific formulas and nutrition aspects is in Chapter 20 of this book.

There is a need to avoid excessive weight gain that may be associated with later health problems such as obesity, hypertension, and cardiovascular disease (Casey et al., 2011). Growth hormone has been recommended to improve growth patterns in preterm and small for gestational age infants; however, this therapy has been hypothesized to change insulin function, thus potentially leading to type 2 diabetes (Casey, 2008; Maiorana & Cianfarani, 2009). Nutritional aspects and standardized growth charts are presented in Chapter 20 of this book. Nutritional requirements vary according to the infant's past medical problems, status, and tolerance of feedings, thus individualized postdischarge instructions are necessary. Available growth charts are not always valid for preterm infants or infants with continuing health problems (Bertino et al., 2011; Casey, 2008; Tudehope, Gibbons, Cormack, & Bloomfield, 2012). Length, head circumference, and weight should always be considered together, and nutritional assessment of the infant is more than body measurements and may even require indirect calorimetry (Sherman et al., 2011). In general, frontal-to-occipital head circumference in preterm infants should be 0.7 to 1 cm/wk (in term infants 0.5 cm) in the immediate postnatal period; by 12 to 18 months it should decline to 0.1 to 0.4 cm/mo (Sherman et al., 2011). Increase in crown-to-heel length should be approximately 0.8 to 1.1 cm/wk in preterm infants (0.7–0.75 in term babies), and by the age of 12 to 18 months it should decline to 0.75 to 1.5 cm/mo (Sherman et al., 2011). Consult with a pediatric dietitian or infant nutrition specialist if there are concerns about growth failure and catch-up.

In the second category, the infant with special health care needs or dependence on technology will have differing needs than the average NICU graduate. This infant may not even be preterm but may be a late preterm or term infant who has had surgery, or developed chronic lung disease (CLD) or has congenital genetic condition or malformation, such as congenital heart disease (CHD). Depending on the exact condition, the infant may require more calories due to the "work of breathing" such as in case with CLD or CHD. With CLD, the infant may require 120 to 150 kcal/kg/d plus increased protein intake, fluid restriction, and electrolyte management, and control of vital functions (Sherman et al., 2011). An infant with cardiac disease again will often require fluid restriction and may need increased caloric intake as well. An infant with CLD will often require home oxygen therapy; appropriate parental teaching should be done before discharge. A pediatric pulmonologist should also be involved in postdischarge management of such patients; periodic evaluation of electrolyte status should also be performed due to use of diuretics in such infants.

The third category—an infant at risk because of family issues—focuses on the family and not just the infant. The infant may or may not be premature, but the family may have problems in adjusting to having a once sick infant now ready for discharge (discussed later in this chapter).

For infants in the fourth category—infants with anticipated early death—the aspects of the care are described in Chapter 33.

Follow-Up of High-Risk Infants

The follow-up appointments with primary care providers for high-risk infants should occur in accordance with the needs of the patient (American Academy of Pediatrics & The American College of Obstetricians and Gynecologists, 2012). For preterm infants and infants with early discharge from maternity unit (less than 48 hours after delivery), AAP (2012) as well as Canadian Pediatric Society (Whyte, 2010) recommend that the first appointment with the primary caregiver should occur in the first 2 to 4 days after discharge. In the immediate period after discharge, some of the high-risk infants should be examined weekly or semimonthly (American Academy of Pediatrics & the American College of Obstetricians and Gynecologists, 2012). Also, neurodevelopmental, behavioral, and sensory status should be assessed more than once during the first year "to ensure early identification of problems and referral for the appropriate interventions" (American Academy of Pediatrics & the American College of Obstetricians and Gynecologists, 2012). Infants born with birth weight less than 1,500 g, infants with hypoxic-ischemic encephalopathy (HIE), seizures, hypoxic cardiorespiratory failure, and multiple congenital anomalies should have standard neurodevelopmental tests at 1 and 2 years of corrected age. However, careful attention should be given to any NICU graduate. Infants who underwent major and minor surgeries (such as diaphragmatic hernia, major heart defects, pyloric stenosis, and even inguinal hernia) have been shown to have some degree of developmental delays (Walker, Holland, Halliday, & Badawi, 2012). Several risk factors can be identified for developmental delays in such surgical patients: genetic predisposition, prematurity, premorbid status, age at the time of surgery, duration of the procedure, and type of anesthetic/analgesic agents used (Walker et al., 2012). Purdy and Melwak (2012) have also suggested the following "red flags" for high-risk infant follow-up:

- Low Apgar score at 5 minutes (less than 4)
- Intraventricular hemorrhage more than Grade II, hydrocephalus
- HIE, abnormal neurologic exam (tremors, hypo/hypertonia), seizures
- Hyperbilirubinemia close to exchange transfusion levels
- Severe infections (sepsis, meningitis)
- Hypoglycemia requiring treatment
- Persistent pulmonary hypertension, extracorporeal membrane oxygenation, use of inhaled nitric oxide
- Discharge on apnea monitor and caffeine
- Infant of substance-abusing mother
- Congenital birth defects (such as Trisomy 21 or Down syndrome) (Purdy & Melwak, 2012)

Frequency of follow-up visits for the *well infant* varies with local and community practices as well as with the patient (American Academy of Pediatrics & the American College of Obstetricians and Gynecologists, 2012); however, it should be consistent with AAP's guidelines on preventive health care (AAP, 2008). The follow-up visit can take place at home or clinic; physical examination and measurements, developmental surveillance, psychosocial, and behavioral assessments are recommended at the infancy period at 1, 2, 4, 6, 9, and 12 months. In early childhood, these visits should take place at 15, 18, 24, and 30 months of age, and then at 3 and 4 years of age. Developmental screening is recommended at 9, 18, and 30 months of age

(AAP, 2008; see Figure 35.1). However, high-risk infants often require additional health check-ups.

Due to risks of visual impairments in NICU patients (i.e., retinopathy of prematurity, ROP), ophthalmic examinations should be performed. Infants ≤1,500 g or ≤32 weeks, infants with unstable clinical course, should have retinal screening (American Academy of Pediatrics Section on Ophthalmology, American Academy of Ophthalmology, & American Association for Pediatric Ophthalmology and Strabismus, 2006). By these recommendations, the first fundal examination in infants above 22 weeks of gestation should occur between 4 and 6 weeks of chronologic age or between 31 and 33 weeks postmenstrual age. Follow-up appointments should occur in 1- to 3-week intervals. Previously, it had also been recommended that preterm infants with or without ROP should be evaluated at 6 months of age and then yearly (American Academy of Pediatrics Section on Ophthalmology, 2001).

Hearing screening is also vitally important. Permanent hearing loss remains a serious complication of prematurity, certain neonatal diseases, or prolonged oxygen use (Robertson, Howarth, Bork, & Dinu, 2009). A recent study showed that only one third of infants were screened and followed up within the recommended timeframe (Holte et al., 2012). Munoz with colleagues also reported wide variations in tests used for infants as well as differences in waiting times (up to 5 months) (Munoz, Nelson, Goldgewicht, & Odell, 2011). In Massachusetts, 11% of infants were lost to follow-up and 25% of those with hearing loss did not receive early intervention (EI) services (Liu, Farrell, MacNeil, Stone, & Barfield, 2008). Hearing screening should be performed before discharge in any infant who was hospitalized for more than 5 days; auditory brainstem response (ABR, automated or not) is preferable so the auditory neuropathy is not missed (Delaney & Ruth, 2012). After discharge, an infant should be evaluated at 1 and 3 months of age; infants with identified hearing loss should be enrolled in EI programs by 6 months of age (American Academy of Pediatrics & Joint Committee on Infant Hearing, 2007). Very early enrollment, in the first 3 months, is beneficial for infants with hearing loss in terms of language development (Vohr et al., 2008); many states also recommend that at-risk children should be evaluated by an audiologist every 6 months for the first 3 years of life (Delaney & Ruth, 2012). In 2010, the American Academy of Pediatrics Task Force for Improving Newborn Hearing Screening, Diagnosis and Intervention developed guidelines for pediatric medical home providers; this guideline can be found at http://www.medicalhomeinfo.org/downloads/pdfs/Algorithm1_2010.pdf. The American Academy of Audiology (2011) has developed guidelines for hearing screening in the childhood (American Academy of Audiology, 2011) (available at http://www.cdc.gov). See Figure 35.2. Health professionals at follow-up clinics and primary care settings should pay careful attention to NICU patients. A study of Wang, Elliott, McGlynn, Brook, and Schuster (2008) revealed that infants less than 1,500 g on Medicaid health insurance did not receive recommended follow-up vision and hearing services. In this study, only 20% of children received hearing rehabilitation and only 23% received ophthalmologic exam between the ages of 1 and 2 years (Wang et al., 2008).

Immunizations

Appropriate immunizations should be given at discharge (American Academy of Pediatrics, 2012a; American Academy of Pediatrics & Committee on Fetus and Newborn, 2008). Vaccinations for preterm infants should be given according to the chronologic age; routine immunization schedules are not changed. The exception is hepatitis B immunizations in infants weighing less than 2,000 g: The first vaccine is given within 12 hours after birth, and then four vaccines are given at 1, 2, and 6 months of age (LaHood & Bryant, 2007). AAP (2012) recommends adding hepatitis B immunoglobulin to hepatitis B vaccine in infants of mothers with unknown HBsAg status. In infants who are heavier than 2,000 g and those mothers are HBsAg-positive, immunoglobulin should be added to hepatitis B vaccine, but no later than 1 week after birth (American Academy of Pediatrics, 2012a).

Vaccinations can be delayed if needed (i.e., due to the present medical conditions, transient illnesses, and rehospitalizations). However, careful attention should be given to the immunization schedule: A recent study reported that only 51% of NICU infants were given routine immunizations; 27% of infants had no vaccines at all (Navar-Boggan et al., 2011). The schedule for the recommended vaccinations and catch-up schedule for patients who start late, or more than 1 month behind, can be found at the Red Book online resource (American Academy of Pediatrics, 2012a). An accelerated 2- 3- 4-month schedule has also been suggested for preterm infants: presumably, protective concentrations can be achieved earlier, as well as sufficient cell memory can be induced with the additional dose given (Bonhoeffer, Siegrist, & Heath, 2006). Bonhoeffer et al. (2006) believe that the accelerated schedule with an additional dose and without correction for gestational age may help to protect preterm infants as early as possible within the safe postimmunization antibody titers. Please see recommended schedules for immunization in Figure 35.3.

To prevent respiratory infection, specifically respiratory syncytial virus (RSV) infection, a monoclonal antibody (palivizumab or Synagis® by Medimmune, Inc., Gaithersburg, MD) can be administered to infants. The proper use and dosage of the drug are of vital importance (Perrin & Bégué, 2012). RSV immunizations range from one dose to five doses. Palivizumab can be given at discharge, preferably 1 month before RSV season. During RSV season (November–March, sometimes April), fewer doses may be required (American Academy of Pediatrics, 2012b). Infants with CLD or CHD who are younger than 24 months of age and on the medical therapy, as well as preterm infants born before 32 completed weeks of gestation, are eligible for maximum five monthly doses. Maximum three doses can be given to preterm infants (32 weeks 0 days–34 weeks 6 days) with at least one risk factor and who were born 3 months before or during RSV season. Risk factors include siblings younger than 5 years of age and daycare

Each child and family is unique; therefore, these **Recommendations for Preventive Pediatric Health Care** are designed for the care of children who are receiving competent parenting, have no manifestations of any important health problems, and are growing and developing in satisfactory fashion. **Additional visits may become necessary** if circumstances suggest variations from normal.

Developmental, psychosocial, and chronic disease issues for children and adolescents may require frequent counseling and treatment visits separate from preventive care visits.

These guidelines represent a consensus by the American Academy of Pediatrics (AAP) and Bright Futures. The AAP continues to emphasize the great importance of **continuity of care** in comprehensive health supervision and the need to avoid **fragmentation of care.**

The recommendations in this statement do not indicate an exclusive course of treatment or standard of medical care. Variations, taking into account individual circumstances, may be appropriate.

	INFANCY								EARLY CHILDHOOD						
AGE[1]	PRENATAL[2]	NEWBORN[3]	3–5 d[4]	By 1 mo	2 mo	4 mo	6 mo	9 mo	12 m	15 mo	18 mo	24 mo	30 mo	3 y	4 y
HISTORY															
Initial/Interval	●	●	●	●	●	●	●	●	●	●	●	●	●	●	●
MEASUREMENTS															
Length/Height and Weight		●	●	●	●	●	●	●	●	●	●	●	●	●	●
Head Circumference		●	●	●	●	●	●	●	●	●	●	●			
Weight for Length		●	●	●	●	●	●	●	●	●	●				
Body Mass Index												●	●	●	●
Blood Pressure[5]		★	★	★	★	★	★	★	★	★	★	★	★	●	●
SENSORY SCREENING															
Vision		★	★	★	★	★	★	★	★	★	★	★	★	●[6]	●
Hearing		●[7]	★	★	★	★	★	★	★	★	★	★	★	★	●
DEVELOPMENTAL/BEHAVIORAL ASSESSMENT															
Developmental Screening[8]								●			●		●		
Autism Screening[9]											●	●			
Developmental Surveillance[8]		●	●	●	●	●	●		●	●		●		●	●
Psychosocial/Behavioral Assessment		●	●	●	●	●	●	●	●	●	●	●	●	●	●
Alcohol and Drug Use Assessment															
PHYSICAL EXAMINATION[10]		●	●	●	●	●	●	●	●	●	●	●	●	●	●
PROCEDURES[11]															
Newborn Metabolic/Hemoglobin Screening[12]		←	●	→											
Immunization[13]		●	●	●	●	●	●	●	●	●	●	●	●	●	●
Hematocrit or Hemoglobin[14]						★			●		★	★		★	★
Lead Screening[15]							★	★	●or★[16]		★	●or★[16]		★	★
Tuberculin Test[17]				★			★		★		★	★		★	★
Dyslipidemia Screening[18]												★			★
STI Screening[19]															
Cervical Dysplasia Screening[20]															
ORAL HEALTH[21]							★	★	●or★[21]		●or★[21]	●or★[21]	●or★[21]	●[22]	
ANTICIPATORY GUIDANCE[23]	●	●	●	●	●	●	●	●	●	●	●	●	●	●	●

	MIDDLE CHILDHOOD						ADOLESCENCE										
AGE[1]	5 y	6 y	7 y	8 y	9 y	10 y	11 y	12 y	13 y	14 y	15 y	16 y	17 y	18 y	19 y	20 y	21 y
HISTORY																	
Initial/Interval	●	●	●	●	●	●	●	●	●	●	●	●	●	●	●	●	●
MEASUREMENTS																	
Length/Height and Weight	●	●	●	●	●	●	●	●	●	●	●	●	●	●	●	●	●
Head Circumference																	
Weight for Length																	
Body Mass Index	●	●	●	●	●	●	●	●	●	●	●	●	●	●	●	●	●
Blood Pressure[5]	●	●	●	●	●	●	●	●	●	●	●	●	●	●	●	●	●
SENSORY SCREENING																	
Vision	●	●	★	●	★	●	★	●	★	★	●	★	★	●	★	★	★
Hearing	●	●	★	●	★	●	★	★	★	★	★	★	★	★	★	★	★
DEVELOPMENTAL/BEHAVIORAL ASSESSMENT																	
Developmental Screening[8]																	
Autism Screening[9]																	
Developmental Surveillance[8]	●	●	●	●	●	●	●	●	●	●	●	●	●	●	●	●	●
Psychosocial/Behavioral Assessment	●	●	●	●	●	●	●	●	●	●	●	●	●	●	●	●	●
Alcohol and Drug Use Assessment							★	★	★	★	★	★	★	★	★	★	★
PHYSICAL EXAMINATION[10]	●	●	●	●	●	●	●	●	●	●	●	●	●	●	●	●	●
PROCEDURES[11]																	
Newborn Metabolic/Hemoglobin Screening[12]																	
Immunization[13]	●	●	●	●	●	●	●	●	●	●	●	●	●	●	●	●	●
Hematocrit or Hemoglobin[14]	★	★	★	★	★	★	★	★	★	★	★	★	★	★	★	★	★
Lead Screening[15]	★	★															
Tuberculin Test[17]	★	★	★	★	★	★	★	★	★	★	★	★	★	★	★	★	★
Dyslipidemia Screening[18]		★		★		★	★	★	★	★	★	★	★	←		●	→
STI Screening[19]							★	★	★	★	★	★	★	★	★	★	★
Cervical Dysplasia Screening[20]							★	★	★	★	★	★	★	★	★	★	★
ORAL HEALTH[21]		●[22]															
ANTICIPATORY GUIDANCE[23]	●	●	●	●	●	●	●	●	●	●	●	●	●	●	●	●	●

1. If a child comes under care for the first time at any point on the schedule, or if any items are not accomplished at the suggested age, the schedule should be brought up to date at the earliest possible time.
2. A prenatal visit is recommended for parents who are at high risk, for first-time parents, and for those who request a conference. The prenatal visit should include anticipatory guidance, pertinent medical history, and a discussion of benefits of breastfeeding and planned method of feeding per AAP statement "The Prenatal Visit" (2001) [URL: http://aappolicy.aappublications.org/cgi/content/full/pediatrics;107/6/1456].
3. Every infant should have a newborn evaluation after birth, breastfeeding encouraged, and instruction and support offered.
4. Every infant should have an evaluation within 3 to 5 days of birth and within 48 to 72 hours after discharge from the hospital, to include evaluation for feeding and jaundice. Breastfeeding infants should receive formal breastfeeding evaluation, encouragement, and instruction as recommended in AAP statement "Breastfeeding and the Use of Human Milk" (2005) [URL: http://aappolicy.aappublications.org/cgi/content/full/pediatrics;115/2/496]. For newborns discharged in less than 48 hours after delivery, the infant must be examined within 48 hours of discharge per AAP statement "Hospital Stay for Healthy Term Newborns" (2004) [URL: http://aappolicy.aappublications.org/cgi/content/full/pediatrics;113/5/1434].
5. Blood pressure measurement in infants and children with specific risk conditions should be performed at visits before age 3 years.
6. If the patient is uncooperative, rescreen within 6 months per the AAP statement "Eye Examination in Infants, Children, and Young Adults by Pediatricians" (2007) [URL: http://aappolicy.aappublications.org/cgi/content/full/pediatrics;111/4/902].
7. All newborns should be screened per AAP statement "Year 2000 Position Statement: Principles and Guidelines for Early Hearing Detection and Intervention Programs " (2000) [URL: http://aappolicy.aappublications.org/cgi/content/full/pediatrics;106/4/798]. Joint Committee on Infant Hearing. Year 2007 position statement: principles and guidelines for early hearing detection and intervention programs. *Pediatrics.* 2007;120:898–921.
8. AAP Council on Children With Disabilities, AAP Section on Developmental Behavioral Pediatrics, AAP Bright Futures Steering Committee, AAP Medical Home Initiatives for Children With Special Needs Project Advisory Committee. Identifying infants and young children with developmental disorders in the medical home: an algorithm for developmental surveillance and screening. *Pediatrics.* 2006;118:405–420 [URL: http://aappolicy.aappublications.org/cgi/content/full/pediatrics;118/1/405].
9. Gupta VB, Hyman SL, Johnson CP, et al. Identifying children with autism early? *Pediatrics.* 2007;119:152–153 [URL: http://pediatrics.aappublications.org/cgi/content/full/119/1/152].
10. At each visit, age-appropriate physical examination is essential, with infant totally unclothed, older child undressed and suitably draped.
11. These may be modified, depending on entry point into schedule and individual need.
12. Newborn metabolic and hemoglobinopathy screening should be done according to state law. Results should be reviewed at visits and appropriate retesting or referral done as needed.
13. Schedules per the Committee on Infectious Diseases, published annually in the January issue of *Pediatrics.* Every visit should be an opportunity to update and complete a child's immunizations.
14. See AAP *Pediatric Nutrition Handbook,* 5th Edition (2003) for a discussion of universal and selective screening options. See also Recommendations to prevent and control iron deficiency in the United States. *MMWR.* 1998;47(RR-3):1–36.
15. For children at risk of lead exposure, consult the AAP statement "Lead Exposure in Children: Prevention, Detection, and Management" (2005) [URL: http://aappolicy.aappublications.org/cgi/content/full/pediatrics;116/4/1036]. Additionally, screening should be done in accordance with state law where applicable.
16. Perform risk assessments or screens as appropriate, based on universal screening requirements for patients with Medicaid or high prevalence areas.
17. Tuberculosis testing per recommendations of the Committee on Infectious Diseases, published in the current edition of *Red Book: Report of the Committee on Infectious Diseases.* Testing should be done on recognition of high-risk factors.
18. "Third Report of the National Cholesterol Education Program (NCEP) Expert Panel on Detection, Evaluation, and Treatment of High Blood Cholesterol in Adults (Adult Treatment Panel III) Final Report" (2002) [URL: http://circ.ahajournals.org/cgi/content/full/106/25/3143] and "The Expert Committee Recommendations on the Assessment, Prevention, and Treatment of Child and Adolescent Overweight and Obesity." Supplement to *Pediatrics.* In press.
19. All sexually active patients should be screened for sexually transmitted infections (STIs).
20. All sexually active girls should have screening for cervical dysplasia as part of a pelvic examination beginning within 3 years of onset of sexual activity or age 21 (whichever comes first).
21. Referral to dental home, if available. Otherwise, administer oral health risk assessment. If the primary water source is deficient in fluoride, consider oral fluoride supplementation.
22. At the visits for 3 years and 6 years of age, it should be determined whether the patient has a dental home. If the patient does not have a dental home, a referral should be made to one. If the primary water source is deficient in fluoride, consider oral fluoride supplementation.
23. Refer to the specific guidance by age as listed in Bright Futures Guidelines. (Hagan JF, Shaw JS, Duncan PM, eds. *Bright Futures: Guidelines for Health Supervision of Infants, Children, and Adolescents.* 3rd ed. Elk Grove Village, IL: American Academy of Pediatrics; 2008.)

KEY

● = to be performed ★ = risk assessment to be performed, with appropriate action to follow, if positive ←●→ = range during which a service may be provided, with the symbol indicating the preferred age

FIGURE 35.1 AAP recommendations for well-child follow-up care appointments.

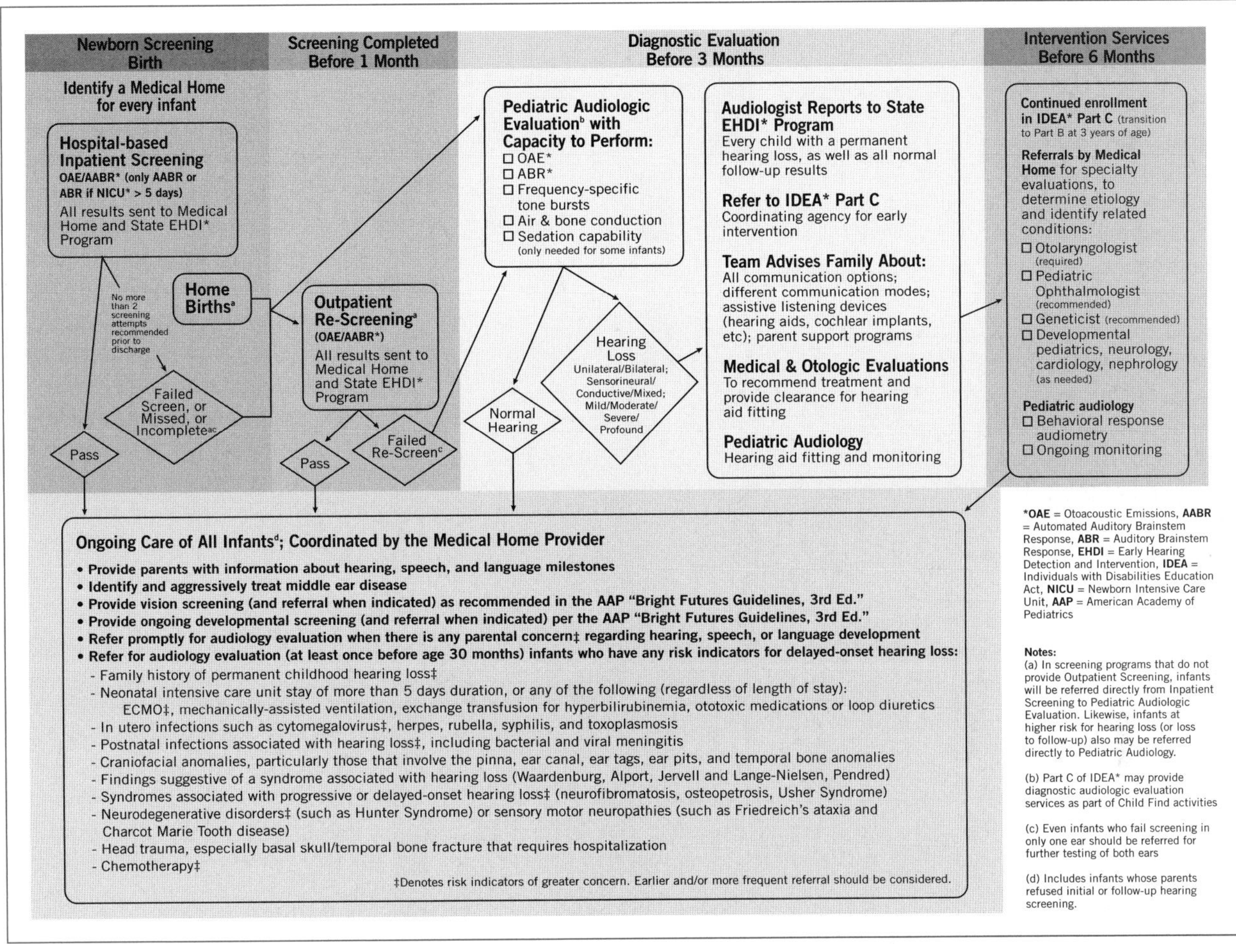

FIGURE 35.2 Early hearing detection and intervention (EHDI) guidelines for pediatric medical home providers. Adapted from AAP (2010).

attendance (American Academy of Pediatrics & Committee on Infectious Diseases, 2009). For preterm infants, infants with CLD or CHD, immunizations usually start November 1 for most geographic locations of the United States. For southern, north-central and southwest Florida, the recommended earliest day is July 1 and September 15, respectively. For preterm infants without CLD, the detailed dosage and timing can be found at the Red Book online resource (American Academy of Pediatrics, 2012b). Importantly, RSV seasons may vary from country to country and region to region; the reference to appropriate professional guidelines should be made.

EI Services

EI services have been available for many years. EI programs aim to prevent or improve biobehavioral and developmental problems of the infant. In the United States, EI service is covered under the Disabilities Education Act, part C, and infants through 35 months of age are eligible to participate (U.S. Department of Education, 2001). EI programs improve cognitive, behavioral, and physical outcomes in infants and preschoolers (Nordhov et al., 2010; Spencer-Smith et al., 2012); they have also been recognized as providing family support and decreasing parental stress, improving mother–infant interactions and feeding practices, and having positive effects on both maternal and infant outcomes (Brecht, Shaw, St. John, & Horwitz, 2012; Meijssen, Wolf, Koldewijn, van Baar, & Kok, 2011; Ravn et al., 2011; Walker et al., 2012; Wen, Baur, Simpson, Rissel, & Flood, 2011).

However, these programs are expensive and referral to them can be problematic. Nationally, EI services cost an estimated $611 million (Behrman & Butler, 2007); special education services associated with a higher prevalence of four disabling conditions (such as cerebral palsy, mental retardation, vision impairment, and hearing loss) add $1.1 billion or $2,200 per preterm infant (Behrman & Butler, 2007). In Massachusetts the program costs were estimated to be about 66 million in 2003 with a mean cost of $857 per infant involved in EI; however, for infants whose gestational age was 24 to 31 weeks, the costs were over $5,000, and for 32 to 36 weeks gestation they were $1,578 (Clements, Barfield, Ayadi, & Wilber, 2007). Additionally, criteria for these programs vary by state, and not all high-risk infants and their families are ever referred. Tang, Feldman, Huffman, Kagawa, and Gould (2012) found that 34% of infants that had high-risk conditions were not referred, even though they were eligible for EI programs (Tang et al., 2012).

Vaccine ▼ Age ▶	Birth	1 month	2 months	4 months	6 months	9 months	12 months	15 months	18 months	19–23 months	2–3 years	4–6 years
Hepatitis B[1]	**Hep B**	**HepB**					**HepB**					
Rotavirus[2]			**RV**	**RV**	**RV**[2]							
Diphtheria, tetanus, pertussis[3]			**DTaP**	**DTaP**	**DTaP**		*see footnote*[3]	**DTaP**				**DTaP**
Haemophilus influenzae type b[4]			**Hib**	**Hib**	**Hib**[4]		**Hib**					
Pneumococcal[5]			**PCV**	**PCV**	**PCV**		**PCV**				**PPSV**	
Inactivated poliovirus[6]			**IPV**	**IPV**			**IPV**					**IPV**
Influenza[7]									**Influenza (Yearly)**			
Measles, mumps, rubella[8]							**MMR**			*see footnote*[8]		**MMR**
Varicella[9]							**Varicella**			*see footnote*[9]		**Varicella**
Hepatitis A[10]									**Dose 1**[10]		**HepA Series**	
Meningococcal[11]								**MCV4 — see footnote**[11]				

Range of recommended ages for all children

Range of recommended ages for certain high-risk groups

Range of recommended ages for all children and certain high-risk groups

FIGURE 35.3 AAP immunization schedule, 2012.
From American Academy of Pediatrics (2012a).

Disparities in EI referral practices have also been documented: Referral was more likely in multiple-birth infants and less likely in infants more than 28 weeks of gestation, infants of Black non-Hispanic mothers and mothers without private insurance were also referred less than those White mothers or those with insurance (Barfield et al., 2008). Regional variation in EI participation/utilization has been also shown to be significant: Services are less likely to be delivered in the South of the United States (Grant & Isakson, 2012). McManus, McCormick, Acevedo-Garcia, Ganz, and Hauser-Cram (2009) found that both child characteristics (poverty) and state program (strict or liberal eligibility criteria) influenced EI participation: Nonpoor children, those who lived in states with strict eligibility criteria, were nearly as likely as poor children who lived in states with liberal eligibility criteria to receive EI services (McManus et al., 2009). In this study, the overall rate of EI participation was 45.7%, ranging from 23.1% to 83.3% across the states.

Another important issue is that some health professionals do not feel prepared to assess the high-risk infant and their families; thus referral may be inadequate because of insufficient knowledge and training of health professionals (Browne & Talmi, 2012). In Colorado, a statewide survey revealed that 77% of providers would like to have more education on infant evaluation, and 86% were interested in further education (Browne & Talmi, 2012). After implementing the collaborative educational programs where additional training and education were provided for health professionals involved in EI services (BABIES and PreSTEPS), the referral rate and service provision increased from 33% to 52% over a 1-year initiative (Browne & Talmi, 2012). The Zero to Three National Center for Infants, Toddlers, and Families is another nonprofit organization that provides training and education to professionals and families (http://www.zerotothree.org).

Moreover, long-term measurable outcomes of EI programs are often not precisely detectable, yet beneficial effects have been found in the most vulnerable children with complications (Orton, Spittle, Doyle, Anderson, & Boyd, 2009; Vanderveen, Bassler, Robertson, & Kirpalani, 2009; Verkerk et al., 2012). Another issue related to EI programs is that definition for a child with special health care needs (CSHCN) and the classification of an infant and family that need specialized care services are lacking an "at-risk" component (Newacheck, Rising, & Kim, 2006). In 1998, the Maternal and Child Health Bureau defined children with special health care needs as "children who have or are at risk for a chronic physical, developmental, behavioral, or emotional condition and who also require health and related services of a type or amount beyond that required by children generally" (McPherson et al., 1998). Obviously, NICU graduates and preterm infants do fit that definition: Many of them are discharged on home oxygen, specific medications, and feeding tubes, and may suffer long-term consequences of initial disease. Nationwide, in the United States the estimated number of CSHCN is 11,203,616 or 15.1% of the population; 14.8% of those have at least one unmet specific health need, and 23.4% have problems with getting referrals (National Survey of Children with Special Health Care Needs, 2009–2010, available at http://www.childhealthdata.org). Thus, health professionals should carefully consider all the problems with provision of adequate postdischarge care and undertake appropriate actions in benefits of NICU graduates, such as appropriate referral to specific treatments or EI services.

Resources for information in EI services include the National Early Childhood Technical Assistance Center (NECTAC), CB 8040, Chapel Hill, NC 27599–8040 (http://www.nectac.org) and the National Parent Technical Assistance Center Network (NPTAC) for building parental capacity in order to improve outcomes for children with disabilities (http://www.parentcenternetwork.org, PACER Center, 8161 Normandale Blvd, Minneapolis, MN 55437–1044).

Use of Services and Rehospitalizations as an Indicator of Adequacy of Postdischarge Care

The complexity of clinical health problems of NICU graduates including the late preterm infants (those born between 34 and 36 weeks gestation) is enormous (Mally, Bailey, & Hendricks-Muñoz, 2010). The associated costs of the hospital, posthospital care, and readmissions are enormous as well (Bird et al., 2010; Korvenranta et al., 2010; McLaurin, Hall, Jackson, Owens, & Mahadevia, 2009; Russell et al., 2007; Underwood, Danielsen, & Gilbert, 2007). Readmissions in this population can be twice as high as those in the term group even when there is good follow-up care (McLaurin et al., 2009). In today's health care market and with the move toward the creation of accountable care organizations (ACOs), the concerns are growing around increased expenditures related to readmissions. Even the healthiest premature infants have a readmission rate of almost 30% while the very immature infant may readmit at a rate of 50% (Escobar, Clark, & Greene, 2006; Ralser et al., 2012; Spicer et al., 2008). Readmission statistics are also related to mortality statistic. In infants less than 1,000 g and less than 27 weeks of gestation, De Jesus with coworkers found that post-NICU discharge mortality rate was 22.3 per 1,000 extremely-low-birth-weight infants, with African American race, unknown medical insurance, and prolonged hospital stay as risk factors (De Jesus et al., 2012). To understand the magnitude of this problem, it is important to notice that the overall infant mortality rate in the United States in 2010 was 6.15 per 1,000 live births (Hoyert & Xu, 2012). During the first year of life even late preterm infants are likely to require readmission more often than their term counterparts (McLaurin et al., 2009). Surgical patients also have high incidence of readmissions. South with colleagues reported 40% of NICU graduates with gastroschisis were readmitted, and 65% of readmissions occurred during the first year of life (South, Wessel, Sberna, Patel, & Morrow, 2011). Readmissions were not associated with gestational age, birth weight, or the length of hospital initial stay; one of the main reasons was abdominal distention/pain. In children with CHDs, readmissions occurred in one in five infants within 1 month postdischarge (Mackie, Ionescu-Ittu, Pilote, Rahme, & Marelli, 2008). The first weeks and months following discharge are the times of highest risk for readmissions especially if the mother is a teenager (Boykova & Kenner, 2012; Escobar et al., 2006; Ray, Escobar, & Lorch, 2010; Spicer et al., 2008; Wade et al., 2008). Emergency room visits are much more costly than primary care visits, yet families often feel they need the expertise of an acute care facility (Boykova & Kenner, 2012). The use of the hospital versus primary care services needs further research, as does the impact of parents' readiness for the transition to home on readmissions. To date, most of the research following discharge from a NICU has focused on the physiologic stability of the infant and the ongoing health issues in relationship to readmissions, and not parental transition/readiness. Providing care for parents after discharge is just as important as providing family-centered care in the NICU.

Family Care

The concept of the family as a unit is another point addressed in care-by-parents or transition units (Costello & Chapman, 1998). The father and siblings are often forgotten during discharge preparation. Most fathers want to participate in the care and decision making for a healthy or sick/premature newborn (Bolzan, Gale, & Dudley, 2004). The responses of fathers are sometimes different from those of mothers (Deave & Johnson, 2008; Rowe & Jones, 2010; Sloan, Rowe, & Jones, 2008). Siblings must also adjust to the infant, who may not seem real to them until they are able to visit the infant in the NICU (Gaal et al., 2010). Many units now encourage sibling visits to help ease the infant into the family well before the actual discharge. The change in NICU design to more single rooms and the inclusion of family areas or transition areas afford the family more opportunities to stay together as a family unit. This design provides the family with more of a home-like atmosphere while offering more privacy to them (White, 2010). This concept of care needs to continue following the discharge.

CARE FOR PARENTS AFTER HOSPITAL DISCHARGE

Parenting and caring of the vulnerable infant upon coming home can be very challenging for parents. AAP (2008) guidelines state that the "infant may be discharged before one of the infant's physiological competencies has been met, provided the health care team and the parents agree that it is appropriate, and suitable plans have been made to provide the additional support needed to ensure safe care at home" (American Academy of Pediatrics & Committee on Fetus and Newborn, 2008, p. 1121). AAP guidelines for hospital discharge (2008) also state that parents should be actively involved and prepared for caring for a baby at home. Preparedness of the parents for discharge and postdischarge as well as professional support are vital to ensure a successful transition home. However, it has repeatedly been shown that mothers rarely recall all the information given to them by health professionals within the hospital: Stress related to their infant's hospitalization and at the time of discharge makes advice and teaching overwhelming (Kenner & Lott, 1990; Loo, Espinosa, Tyler, & Howard, 2003; McKim et al., 1995). Smith with colleagues found that 12% of families feel unprepared for discharge; those families were more likely to report feeding problems, difficulties in obtaining supplies, and the inability of the pediatrician to access the discharge summary (Smith, Dukhovny, Zupancic, Gates, & Pursley, 2012; Smith, Young, Pursley, McCormick, & Zupancic, 2009). The hospitalization and discharge of high-risk and preterm infants always hold certain risks for the health of the infant. These times should be considered as serious challenges for parents.

NICU Experience

Giving birth to a sick or small infant interferes with the development of the role of the parent. Try to remember the first time you walked into the NICU. What were your thoughts and feelings? We know what ours were—an overwhelming urge to flee. Time seemed to be running. People were rushing and talking loudly; alarms were buzzing, intercoms were blaring, and doors were slamming. We suddenly felt tense, on edge, and fearful of our ability to survive in such an environment. Then we walked over to an incubator and peered in at a premature infant—born at 28 weeks gestation and weighing less than 1,000 g—who looked as though she had been through a war. Scratches and cuts were visible. Tape cut into the infant's face to hold an endotracheal tube in place. The right arm was pinned to the bed to hold an intravenous line in place, and her legs were restrained to prevent dislodgment of an umbilical arterial line that was being used for blood gas sampling. Our hearts sank. We could never be responsible for providing care to this type of infant. We tried to summon the courage to walk—if not run—out of there. We were almost immobilized—yet we recognized some of the ventilators, intravenous pumps, and monitors. Surely, with this passing acquaintance, we could learn to work in this environment and actually care for the critically ill infant. Now more than 30 years later, the units are quieter, and they look more like a home environment. Attention is paid to lighting and noise, and parents are an integral part of the environment. Yet the sense of overwhelming responsibility still resides in new health professionals.

If we feel that way, what do parents feel? Their feelings are much more intense. They have the additional fear of death of a family member, a vulnerable infant whose birth should be celebrated and yet a dense of doom clouds the birth experience. For the most part parents lack the knowledge about the medical diagnosis, equipment, treatments, and routines necessary to support neonates—their baby. In the last few decades, research has repeatedly shown that the NICU environment is extremely stressful for parents and can lead to alterations in their role both inside and outside the hospital that can last a lifetime if there is no attention/intervention (Holditch-Davis, Miles, Burchinal, & Goldman, 2011; Miles, 1989; Miles, Holditch-Davis, & Shepherd, 1998; Watson, 2011) The mothers must, in addition, make a physiological and psychological postpartum adjustment. They are also in need of care, yet most mothers when asked express the need to put aside their own time for healing to focus on their infants. For the fathers, the NICU experience is also stressful; the need to run between two units (the postpartum and the NICU) is an added stress even if these units are in the same institution. Constraints of work are also impressive (Hollywood & Hollywood, 2011; Mackley, Locke, Spear, & Joseph, 2010; Sloan et al., 2008). The parents' concern for their partners and their children often forces them between the two. For the family with other children at home, the stress becomes even greater. Who can take charge of the children? How long will it be necessary for another person to help with family responsibilities? Is someone who can or will step in to help even be available? These are very real family concerns that continue to exist after hospital discharge of the former NICU infant. New challenges also occur—questions about care to give to the infant, infant development, and the future. Along with these concerns comes the assumption of the new parental role. This role adjustment occurs for both first-time and experienced parents. It requires a change from a previous functional pattern to a new one. This change marks a developmental passage or transition.

Transition

Throughout life, events necessitate change. These life changes are often viewed as turning points. In the case of a NICU family, these turning points are the birth of a sick or preterm infant, hospitalization, and discharge from hospital and the transition to home. All these events require a new role acceptation (to accept the reality, facts about their infant's health), an adjustment or change in role, a setting of new priorities, and an examination of expectations. Taking on a new role requires energy, commitment, and most of all a change in the pattern of functioning—thus a transition. Transition involves change—leaving behind the familiar and trying something new. There are at least three transition processes for parents of NICU infants: transition to parenthood, transition to home, and transition to primary health care settings.

■ **Transition to Parenthood.** The role of parent is a good example of the transition process. For parents of a NICU infant, the transition to parenthood may have two time points—one associated with becoming parents at the time of birth and the other occurring at the time of discharge. Two important processes can be impeded in NICU parents, specifically mothers, while in the hospital: maternal role attainment (MRA) and attachment. These disturbances have consequences that may extend beyond the immediate posthospital discharge period, and both mothers and fathers can be struggling with certain problems (Hollywood & Hollywood, 2011; Jackson, Ternestedt, & Schollin, 2003; Mackley et al., 2010; Sloan et al., 2008).

Once a pregnancy is confirmed, the mother and father begin the task of examining their individual roles. For first-time parents, this means considering what it will be like to be a mother or father to a dependent infant. For parents with other children, the new infant will bring a unique personality and another dimension to the already formed family unit. This infant, too, will require role adjustment on the part of the parents. Acquisition of the maternal role and maternal identity, as described by Rubin (1984) and Mercer (1995), focused on mothers of healthy, term infants (Rubin, 1984). When the infant is premature or sick and does not fit the image of the desired child, women lose their normal frame of reference for the development of their own role expectations and the expectations of their infants as well. Later, MRA had been replaced with the new term, Becoming a Mother (BAM), as a more inclusive and comprehensive concept where maternal confidence and identity continue to grow or can be disrupted with a child's developmental challenges and life's realities (Mercer, 2004). Decreased MRA was observed with medically fragile infants due to high levels of worry in mothers and less responsiveness of infants (Miles, Holditch-Davis, Burchinal, & Brunssen, 2011); parenting quality has been shown to be influenced more by MRA than by child illness severity (Holditch-Davis et al., 2011).

The immediate process of attachment, a formation of a relationship between a parent and her or his newborn infant, occurs with wanting the pregnancy, positive maternal feelings, seeing the infant soon after birth, and immediate contact with the infant after birth (Bialoskurski, Cox, & Hayes, 1999). Delayed and problematic attachment occurs with a premature infant, uncertain outcomes, a handicapped child, poor maternal health, prolonged care that limits the family's ability to touch, hold, and protect their infant, a poor attitude in the partner, a lack of social support, drug dependency, and a taking-one-day-at-a-time attitude (Zabielski, 1994). Attachment, which is considered a dyadic process, becomes a triadic relationship in the NICU, in which NICU personnel—especially nurses—can alter the process. The mother of a premature infant is also a premature mother. Not only are the binding-in and claiming processes affected, but the mother herself is a "preemie" as well. Her pregnancy has ended before her own expectations were met and needs were fulfilled. Recent review of literature revealed that interactive and therapeutic relationships between a nurse and a mother foster the process of BAM; moreover, instructions without nurse input are not effective (Mercer & Walker, 2006). Nurses can hinder or facilitate a mother's attachment to her infant by encouraging mother–infant touch or by forbidding it. Provision of accurate information about the infant's care, health status, and ongoing communication can facilitate the formation of attachment (Cox & Bialoskurski, 2001). Nurses at the NICU were named as the best source of information that helped parents to understand infants' medical conditions (Kowalski, Leef, Mackley, Spear, & Paul, 2006). Research has also shown that a decrease of maternal stress as well as a decrease of early separation during hospitalization can prevent the development of distorted attachments in mothers of preterm infants (Korja, Latva, & Lehtonen, 2012). Also, those mothers can form balanced attachments with their infants, and maternal–infant interaction may be more positive and of higher quality than in mothers of full-term infants if maternal stress is managed and their interaction is fostered prior to and following discharge (Korja et al., 2009, 2012).

In addition to possibly affected attachment and development of parental role, the actual assumption of the new parental role can be quite overwhelming. Even when a healthy newborn is brought into a family, stress and even crisis can occur (Emmanuel & St John, 2010; Miller & Sollie, 1980). Some researchers and clinicians view transition to parenthood as a *crisis* rather than just a developmental passage to a new functional level. Since the 1970s, research has shown that families see birth hospitalization and bringing home a premature or ill infant who has been in the NICU as a crisis (Affleck & Tennen, 1991; Caplan, Mason, & Kaplan, 1965; Saigal, 1999). Even parents of low-risk premature infants suffer from distress (Jones, Rowe, & Becker, 2009). During hospitalization, parents often suffer from acute stress disorder (Jubinville, Newburn-Cook, Hegadoren, & Lacaze-Masmonteil, 2012) which can exist for a longer time after discharge as posttraumatic stress disorder (PTSD) (Shaw et al., 2009). Symptoms of PTSD include (1) reexperiencing the phenomenon (NICU traumatic experience), (2) avoiding thoughts, feelings, places, and people associated with the event, and (3) hyperarousal symptoms (such as irritability, startling easily, anger, difficulties with sleeping) (Mowery, 2011). A national survey showed that 9% of new mothers experience PTSD (Beck, Gable, Sakala, & Declercq, 2011). Higher levels of PSTD are often observed in parents of NICU and preterm infants (Ahlund, Clarke, Hill, & Thalange, 2009; Brandon et al., 2011; Elklit, Hartvig, & Christiansen, 2007; Kersting et al., 2004) that can last for months and years (Holditch-Davis, Bartlett, Blickman, & Miles, 2003; Kersting et al., 2004). Even if the infant requires no special equipment postdischarge or does not suffer from the initial neonatal disorder, the family may still experience PTSD related to the initial hospitalization and long-term consequences of initial psychological trauma for family. Recent research showed that parents of high-risk newborns often had higher levels of PTSD symptoms and depression; for an entire family, parenting of high-risk neonates led to fewer years of education of family members, higher unemployment, lower incomes, distortion of marital relationships, and family strain (Placencia & McCullough, 2012). Fortunately, the negative effects of neonatal hospitalization on family functioning, quality of life, and child behavior have been shown to decrease with time, and the family may adjust well, even with a neurosensory-impaired child. Rautava, Lehtonen, Helenius, and Sillanpaa (2003) followed 170 Finnish preterm infants and their families for 12 years. At 3 years of age, children in a high-risk group were reported as having more sleep and behavioral problems than children in a low-risk group; all of these differences disappeared by the time the children were 12 years old (Rautava et al., 2003). In the study of Saigal, Pinelli, Streiner, Boyle, and Stoskopf (2010) that examined the impact of illness in young adults born with extremely low birth weight at the age of 20 years, mothers reported that caring for their child with neurosensory impairment had even brought their family closer together (Saigal et al., 2010). What is important is helping families to cope with initial transitions after hospital discharge.

Two other major problems can occur when parenting high-risk and preterm infants who were hospitalized after birth. These problems are vulnerable child syndrome (VCS) and compensatory parenting. Parental responses to their infant are mediated by the infant's illness, the hospitalization, and "near miss" events. The VCS is one such response that has an impact on both the infant and parents. Green and Solnit (1964) hypothesized that, when children are expected to die prematurely or were seriously injured, the result is a disturbed psychosocial development of the family, based on the parent–child relationship (Green & Solnit, 1964). Because the child is seen as "vulnerable," parents overprotect the child, make more visits to health care providers for relatively minor illnesses, and may discipline the child in a gentler manner, which may result in behavior problems (Kokotos & Adam, 2009; Levy, 1980; Pearson & Boyce, 2004). It has been shown that even neonatal jaundice and inpatient phototherapy can contribute to the VCS development because the infant is labeled as sick and vulnerable by the parents (Usatin, Liljestrand, Kuzniewicz, Escobar, & Newman, 2010). What is important is the fact that VCS is a family disorder cyclically affecting both parents and children. Allen et al. (2004) found higher maternal perception of child vulnerability was associated with worse developmental outcomes and lower adaptive functioning in preterm infants less than 32 weeks of gestation with CLD at 1-year adjusted age. The mothers who perceived their children as more vulnerable were more anxious, more depressed, and perceived a greater impact of the illness on the family; longer hospitalization and maternal anxiety at discharge predicted higher perception of child vulnerability (Allen et al., 2004). Another study in depressed mothers of very-low-birth-weight infants suggested that VCS could be the reason for restricting preschool activities and negative maternal views of their infants' social abilities (Silverstein, Feinberg, Young, & Sauder, 2010). Research has shown that maternal adaptation during the neonatal period and maternal self-inefficacy beliefs about feeding the infant predicted mother's later perceptions of infant's vulnerability at the first 4 months of corrected age (Teti, Hess, & O'Connell, 2005). Thus, maternal attachment, development of parental role, and perception of the infant influence the entire postdischarge care and well-being of the family and infant.

Compensatory parenting is another disturbance when parenting an initially hospitalized child. This parenting style is compensation for feeling sorry for or guilty about having an infant in the NICU (Miles & Holditch-Davis, 1995). Parents try to provide special experiences for their infants born preterm and avoid other experiences; sometimes more stimulation to foster development with these children is provided. At the same time they have shielded their children from other life situations to protect them from further hurt, viewing them as "special" and "normal" at the same time (Miles & Holditch-Davis, 1997).

Disturbances in parenting occurring in parents are tightly related to parental psychological well-being. Anxiety and depression have been documented in parents of high-risk and preterm infants, both in the hospital and postdischarge (Doering, Moser, & Dracup, 2000; Gennaro, 1988; Obeidat, Bond, & Callister, 2009). At discharge, 43% of mothers of preterm infants had moderate to severe anxiety, and 20% had clinically significant levels of depression (Rogers, Kidokoro, Wallendorf, & Inder, 2012). Importantly, maternal anxiety at the NICU was shown to be predictive of adverse interactive behaviors, lower child cognitive development, and behavioral problems in infants less than 1,500 g at 24 months of age (Zelkowitz, Na, Wang, Bardin, & Papageorgiou, 2011; Zelkowitz, Papageorgiou, Bardin, & Wang, 2009).

Fortunately, it has also been reported that depression and anxiety decrease over time; however, correlates of depression can be different at discharge and a few months later (Carter, Mulder, Frampton, & Darlow, 2007; Mew, Holditch-Davis, Belyea, Miles, & Fishel, 2003; Padovani, Carvalho, Duarte, Martinez, & Linhares, 2009). In addition, on a positive note, a recent study showed that participation in EI programs was not limited by depressive symptoms in mothers (Feinberg, Donahue, Bliss, & Silverstein, 2012).

"Searching for normalcy" and grief are other aspects of parental challenges. May (1997) found that mothers are searching for normalcy in their lives through caring of the low-birth-weight infants when they are at home; the main theme of this study included learning caregiving, maintaining vigilance for infant's progress, normalizing with caregiver burden, and help seeking. Contradictory feelings of joy and grief are also present in parents of preterm infants who lost the "ideal child" and are often unable to communicate that feeling of loss (Golish & Powell, 2003). Unresolved grief may lead to insecure attachment and inadequate interactions between mother and baby (Shah, Clements, & Poehlmann, 2011). What is important here is that the normal grief response can become a chronic sorrow in parents who have a child with permanent, progressive, or cyclic health problems; this chronic sorrow can even become a pathological grief (Gordon, 2009).

■ **Transition to Home.** Although the NICU discharge is the overriding goal for the health care professional and the family, the actual transition to home can be a time of crisis for the family. Transition to home can be even more difficult for parents than the period of infant's hospitalization because parents are moving from a safe hospital environment to home and taking all the responsibilities for the care of their vulnerable infant. For many parents, the NICU reinforces learned helplessness. Parents express the need to understand their role and what is expected of them in relationship to their infants' care needs; yet they feel "in the way" and unable or incapable of caring for their infants. Thus, they learn to be helpless. The picture changes, however, at the time of discharge when parents move from the safety net of the hospital to independent caregiving at home and accepting total responsibility for their infants. The parents are told: "Now it is your turn." It is no wonder that this discharge can be cognitively appraised as being a stress and early parenting problems, possible risks in relationship development, can affect family and infant (Anderson, Riesch, Pridham, Lutz, & Becker, 2010; Lutz, Anderson, Riesch, Pridham, & Becker, 2009). Parents should be a part of the NICU health care team in order to fully understand what is wrong with their infant and to feel able to make decisions. When given the opportunity to discuss their concerns, parents are vocal about their feelings regarding their NICU care and preparation for discharge. One family stated, "The only time that the physicians really asked us our opinion or told us about the baby's condition was when they were obligated to get informed consent for an experimental treatment." Another family said, "We would ask the nurses about the baby's apnea, but they said they had to check with the physicians and they would have to talk to us." Other comments included, "I never understood why nurses just came over and turned off our baby's sounding alarms without seemingly looking at the baby."

Preparedness for discharge is vital. Information is critical to the successful transition home. A recent study showed that 12% of families were not prepared for discharge (Smith et al., 2012). Or, even when they report that they are prepared at discharge, parents were observed to be naively confident in caregiving and, in fact, were unable to provide proper care at home (Hess, Teti, & Hussey-Gardner, 2004). It can be assumed that inadequacy of caregiving and skills when caring for vulnerable infants may affect the health status of an infant and lead to readmissions or overuse of health care services. This assumption needs further research.

Transition to home can be especially challenging for parents if the infant requires technology at home or has specific health care needs. All the health and care needs of the infant often require advanced knowledge and skills from parents and primary health care providers. It has been shown that 19% of moderately preterm infants were discharged home with ongoing medical needs and the use of durable medical equipment such as apnea monitors, oxygen, or feeding tubes (Kirkby, Greenspan, Kornhauser, & Schneiderman, 2007). All these ongoing health care needs require additional support and education of parents postdischarge. Feeding issues (tube feedings, food intolerance, breastfeeding problems, formula selection) bring enormous stress on parents (Lutz, 2012). A decade of research showed that needs in informational support in parents of infants is very high, both in healthy and sick, both in the hospital and afterward (Brazy, Anderson, Becker, & Becker, 2001; De Rouck & Leys, 2009, 2011; Kenner, 1990; Kenner et al., 1993; Kenner & Lott, 1990; McKim, 1993; McKim et al., 1995; Perlman et al., 1991; Radecki, Olson, Frintner, Tanner, & Stein, 2009; Yee & Ross, 2006). Parents often feel unprepared (Sneath, 2009), and it is even worse with adolescent mothers (Boss, Donohue, & Arnold, 2010). Importantly, knowledge and skills needed by parents sometimes differ from those provided by health professionals (Brazy et al., 2001; Drake, 1995) and fulfilling individual information needs of parents is vital. Even assuming that some infants have to be rehospitalized due to medical conditions and parent education might have little effect in such cases (Klein, 2011), transition from hospital to home remains to be dependent on the levels of parental knowledge and skills, competency and confidence in caring for an infant, and availability of professional and social supports. Yet, there is limited research on transitional problems in parents of NICU patients, as well as solid theoretical frameworks and validated measurement tools. Some concepts of transition for parents of NICU infants are presented in Figure 35.4. One of the available models and instruments is described below.

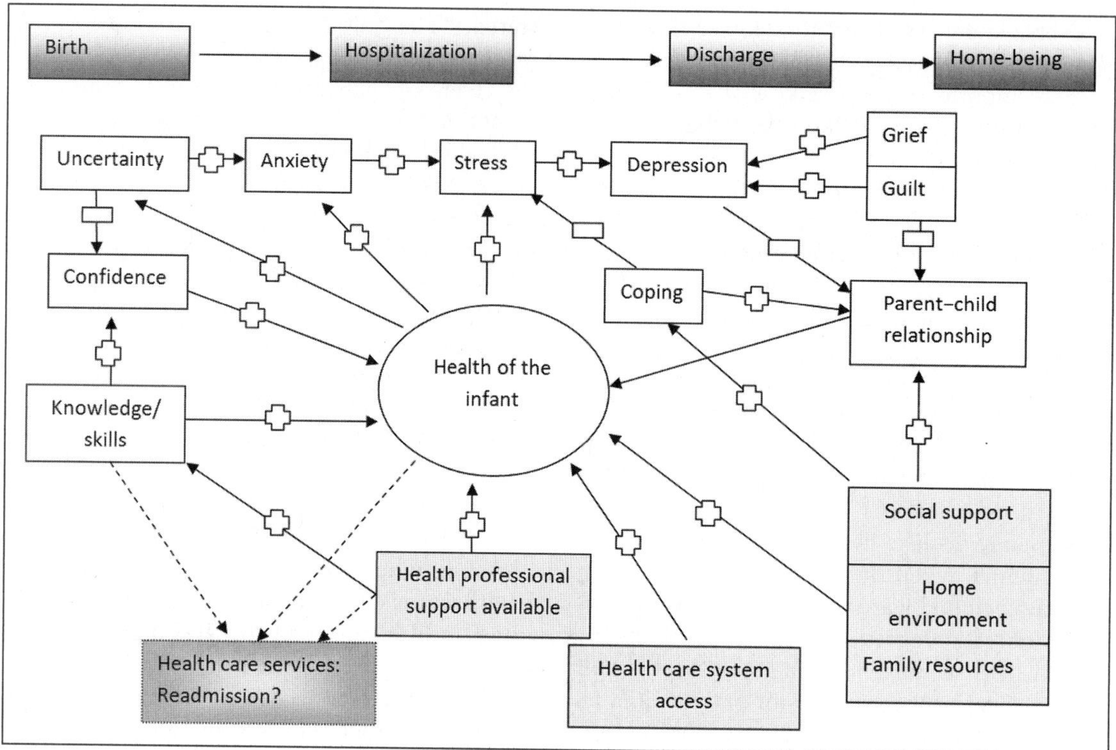

FIGURE 35.4 Concepts involved in transition derived from the literature and possible relationships among parental challenges, knowledge, infant health, professional support, and readmissions.

■ Example of Theoretical Framework on Parental Transition From NICU to Home. One theoretical model has been developed for parents of NICU patients who transitioned from hospital to home—the Transition Model developed by Kenner with colleagues (Flandermeyer, Kenner, Spaite, & Hostiuck, 1992a, 1992b; Kenner, 1988, 1990; Kenner & Lott, 1990). A series of studies were conducted on parents of both term and preterm infants after hospital discharge. Five main parental transitional challenges were identified in the immediate postdischarge period. These categories are Informational Needs, Parent–Child Role Development, Stress and Coping, Social Interaction, and Grief.

Informational Needs. The informational needs of parents include:

1. How to provide routine newborn care (feeding, bathing, for example)
2. How to recognize normal newborn characteristics, both physical and behavioral (amount of "normal" crying)
3. How to keep the infant healthy after discharge (i.e., immunizations)
4. How to recognize if their infant is not well; sleeping and awake periods
5. Infant development and prognosis for future
6. Equipment used on their infant at home if any. During home follow-up, parents, particularly mothers, want more information about feeding, formula, breastfeeding, elimination patterns, weight gain, and the infant's breathing pattern.

Parent–Child Role Development. This category refers to the parents and children's role expectations that are influenced by the development of relationships and interactions with an infant, which can be impaired by the infant's initial illness or special health care needs and interfere with development of parental role. For anyone making a transition or entering a new level of functioning or a new stage of life, certain expectations about what is to come exist. New parents of healthy infants make adjustments in how they carry out the tasks of daily living once their newborn is at home. When a problem with the infant that requires more attention or special care arises, parents may have to set aside their expectations of their roles and feel inadequate in parenting and making health care decisions for the infant. The parents may feel that they are not "real" parents and not capable of parenting and caring for their infant; that the physician's permission is necessary to make even the smallest change in the infants' routines that had been established in the hospital.

Stress and Coping. Stress and coping are related to alterations in parental role, uncertainty and anxiety caused by health problems of the infant, and parental perceptions of their abilities to care and cope with challenges at home. The expected feelings of joy and the months of anticipation of discharge to home are replaced by sharply contrasting feelings of fear, anxiety, caregiver's tiredness, and overwhelming stress. Coping abilities that have to be present to overcome the stress of discharge depend on resources available (informational, material, and social).

Social Interaction. Social Interaction category includes parents' ability to socialize after their infant is born sick or preterm. Often, parents isolate themselves due to health care risks for their infant (such as RSV infection) or limit their social activities because of misunderstanding about their infant's health issues or if their infant is technology-dependent. On the other hand, family and friends may be frightened to approach the parents for fear of doing or saying the wrong thing, thus isolating parents of a vulnerable infant. Social interaction depends on social support from the parental informal network, and the recipient (McKim et al., 1995) determines support from health care professionals, which can be viewed positively or negatively as perception of the support.

Grief. Grief found in parents of NICU infants is related to loss of the image of "ideal" infant and fear of the infant's ultimate death that influences relationships between parent and infant within the family as a whole and social interaction. Parents express the loss of their expected child once the reality of the neonatal problem shattered their hopes and fantasies. As time goes on, parents continue to grieve but in the form of anticipating that the infant would eventually die if he or she would be sick enough to require special care or have developmental problems. The process of grief and the period of mourning begin once the infant does not meet the parents' expectations of the fantasy or ideal child. If the parents have other children, they may speak of how different this child is from their other children or how different the infant is from their expectations. Another component of grief is the loss of the expected parenting role—that is, their normal role. Some or all of the social rituals that socialize mothers into their impending role and prepare them for their new responsibilities—such as baby showers, parenting classes, and birth announcements—may often have been absent with the birth of a premature or ill infant. Friends and family who would normally be happy to help celebrate the joyous occasion of birth with the exuberant parents may feel uncomfortable and helpless around them, thus withdrawing needed psychological support.

These categories form the basis for transition to home and have not changed in almost three decades (Boykova & Kenner, 2012). These five categories of parental concerns represent the taxonomy for transitional care follow-up. All concepts are interrelated, and relationships between them are reciprocal, with Informational Needs being the core category. The main feature of the model is that transition is viewed as a process, not the product or outcome of changes that were brought to parents with the birth of a vulnerable child. Hospitalization of an infant is the key factor that might influence postdischarge transition to home. This assumption was confirmed in other studies: Kenner (1988) and Bagwell (1990) found that parents from Level II and III units had similar concerns after hospital discharge; Boykova (2008) did not find any correlation between parental transitional concerns and birth weight or gestational age of former NICU infants (see the depiction of the model in Figure 35.5).

The Transition Model has a specific multidimensional tool for the measurement of transition challenges in parents of NICU infants—the Transition Questionnaire.

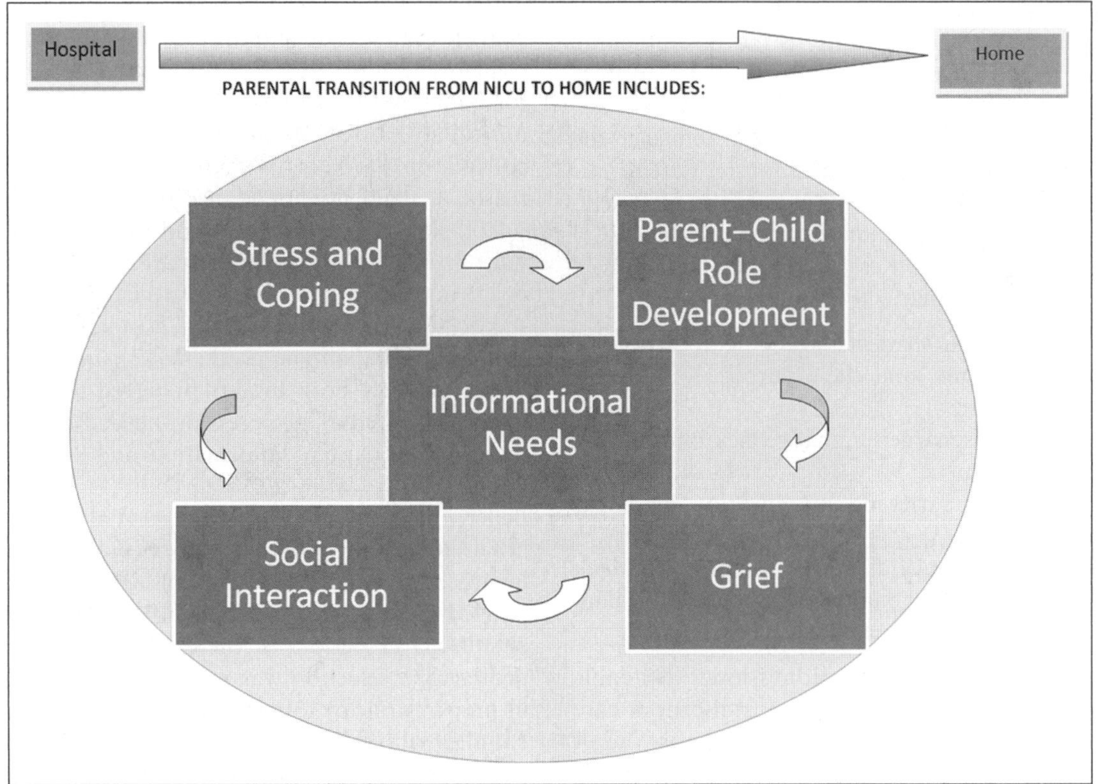

FIGURE 35.5 Hypothesized depiction of the concepts in the Transition Model.
From Kenner (1988, 1994).

Transition Questionnaire. The Kenner Transition Questionnaire (Boykova & Kenner, 2012) consists of four parts:

1. Thirty-seven statements in Likert-scale format that measure parental concerns and perceptions postdischarge
2. Three multiple-choice-format items considering certain informational needs in parents
3. Three open-ended questions related to parental concerns after discharge that they might have had
4. Demographic information part of the tool, consisting of 21 items about parent and infant

Several items are negatively worded in order to decrease response bias; 17 items have to be reversed when scoring. Scores on each item of the Likert scale–format are summed for the total score, as well as for subscales. The possible range of scores is 37 to 185, with the larger score reflecting fewer problems after discharge. The dimensions of the instrument are Informational Needs (6 items), Stress and Coping (15 items), Parent–Child Role Development (9 items), Grief (4 items), and Social Interaction (3 items). The item readability level is the fifth grade; time to complete the tool is approximately 15 to 25 minutes. Examples of the items are (1) "I feel competent in caring for my child," (2) "I have trouble sleeping at night because I worry about my child," (3) "I believe no one really understands how I feel," (4) "The people I live with have been supportive of me," (5) "I cannot control my child's health." The development of the instrument has been described elsewhere; both the Transition Model and instrument warrant further development and validation (Boykova & Kenner, 2012).

Transition to Primary Health Care. The third type of transition in parents and infants in the postdischarge period is the transition to the primary health care settings. Continuity of care, comprehensiveness, timeliness, and appropriateness of posthospital care can influence the health of an infant and family tremendously. Often, parents have difficulties in finding primary care providers who would be experienced and knowledgeable about NICU populations' needs and risks. Research in the population of adult patients has shown that:

1. Less than half of the patients are able to list their diagnoses, medications, and their purpose or adverse effects after discharge
2. Up to 20% of the discharge summaries lack information about hospital treatment
3. Up to 40% of summaries do not mention discharge medications
4. Ninety-two percent of discharge summaries lack information of patient or family counseling (Kripalani et al., 2007; Makaryus & Friedman, 2005)

The linkage between patient readmissions, avoidable complications, and appropriateness of postdischarge care has been well documented in the population of adult patients. The Transitional Care Model of Dr. Mary Naylor with colleagues from the University of Pennsylvania is an example of a practice model that has been proven to be effective and efficient in the population of elder/older patients with various medical conditions (Naylor, Aiken, Kurtzman, Olds, & Hirschman, 2011; Naylor et al., 2004, 2011). This model provides in-hospital planning and home follow-up for chronically ill high-risk patients, with a transitional care nurse as an assigned leader and coordinator for a multidisciplinary transitional care team of medical doctors, social workers, discharge planners, pharmacists, and other members of health care teams (Naylor et al., 2009).

Less is known about parents of NICU infants after discharge. A recent online survey on parents of preterm infants (*N* = 52, 99.9 were mothers) conducted with the help of the moderator of the blog from PreemieWorld, Deb Descenza, revealed that only 44.2% of parents participated in transitional care/follow-up programs (Boykova, 2012, data from pilot study, unpublished). Parents often had difficulties with getting appointments and finding specialists who would manage their infant's medical problems after discharge (such as pulmonologist, pediatrician, dietitian, developmental specialist, lactation specialist). Despite the expansion of developmental and family care principles all over the globe during recent decades, in this pilot study 77.1% of parents had been separated from their infants during hospital stay, and 41.7% could do only a small amount of caregiving while in the hospital. At least one rehospitalization after discharge occurred in 52.4% of cases. However, parents who were participating in transitional care programs were very satisfied with health care. And yet, attendance can be a problem. In Canada, where health care coverage is universal, Ballantyne, Stevens, Guttmann, Willan, and Rosenbaum (2012) found that attendance in follow-up programs decreased during the first 12 months from 84% to 74%, and the higher withdrawal from the programs occurred after NICU discharge, followed by withdrawal after the first appointment (Ballantyne et al., 2012). The reasons provided by mothers for nonattendance were not completely clear, as they were not fully reported. From the limited data this study could collect from mothers (two thirds did not voluntarily provide reasons), main nonattendance reasons were preference to be followed closer to home or by different health care provider (pediatrician). Hypothesized reasons were reluctance of having the child assessed (especially when a disability is suspected), elevated depression, socioeconomic differences, and PTSD (Ballantyne et al., 2012). In Australia, parents of prematurely born infants preferred to use services that were instrumental in accessing needed services, provided there was consistent information and supported parental self-efficacy in caring for their child (Pritchard, Colditz, & Beller, 2008). In this study, parents also highly evaluated NICU follow up programs and were less reluctant to follow recommendations; the use of help lines was not helpful and led to confusion and an increase in anxiety in the early postdischarge period. At the discharge point, helping with pediatrician selection was found to be assistive for parents in preparation for taking baby home (Smith et al., 2009). Families who felt unprepared to go home at the discharge point were more likely to report that their pediatrician could not access the infant's discharge summary and that they were not able to obtain needed feeding supplies for their infant (Smith et al., 2012). Unpreparedness for discharge, in addition to inadequate continuity of care and limited knowledge of primary health care providers, can be related to the overuse of services or avoidable readmissions. Three months postdischarge was reported as a period when parents use health care services most (Spicer et al., 2008). Wade et al. (2008) found that preterm infants during the first year after NICU discharge had frequent pediatric visits and prescription medications (mean 20 visits and 5.5 medications); surprisingly and unfortunately, half of the highest using infants were relatively healthy (who did not have CLD, necrotizing enterocolitis, or severe intraventricular hemorrhages). These findings dictate better continuity of care in the postdischarge period. Better care coordination of postdischarge services is needed in order to provide support to the family unit, ease the transition to the home, and promote positive growth and development of the infant.

Strategies to Help Families Postdischarge

Many interventions can alleviate a crisis for a family of a NICU or premature infant in a postdischarge period. Some approaches and strategies are described below.

■ Discharge Teaching and Information Giving. The NICU nurse—in the role of primary nurse, clinical nurse specialist, or neonatal nurse practitioner—can advocate for positive parental discharge. Recognizing parents' need for information about their infants and the required at-home care facilitates development of a collaborative, interdisciplinary plan of care, including discharge and follow-up. This type of collaborative plan should include the parents' demonstrating competence and comfort with routine newborn care. The nurse should ensure that the parents are completely comfortable with bathing, feeding, and diapering their infant and with administering any special care procedures, such as medication or oxygen therapy. Information given to parents about feeding patterns of preterm infants should include differences and similarities between term and preterm infants. Preterm infants often have shorter periods of sustained sucking, whether receiving feedings from the breast or bottle. Signs of adequate intake are similar for both groups: exhibiting feeding cues on a regular basis, seven to 10 feeds per 24 hours, and five to six wet diapers, and two to three stools per 24 hours. Pre- and postdischarge interventions have been shown to be effective for the duration of breastfeeding, promoting exclusive breastfeeding and improving maternal satisfaction (Ahmed & Sands, 2010); if available, a board-certified lactation consultant (BCLC) should assist the mother, as continued support of the breastfeeding mother is essential to decreasing the risk of early weaning. The parents also need to be taught how the NICU infant's temperament may differ from that of a healthy newborn. Parents need to be informed and reminded that even though their infant is 6 months old by chronologic age, she or he may be only 3 months old by conceptional age. Thus the infant may act more like a 3-month-old than like a 6-month-old.

Comprehensive discharge teaching has also been advocated in NICUs for a long time (American Academy of Pediatrics & Committee on Fetus and Newborn, 2008; Schlittenhart, Smart, Miller, & Severtson, 2011; Shieh et al., 2010). Quality of discharge teaching provided by nurses is vital. Good discharge teaching includes all this as well as developmental information and has positive outcomes on parental levels of anxiety and depression, as well as hospital expenditures. Melnyk and coworkers have developed a specific educational-behavioral program for parents of NICU infants, the Creating Opportunities for Parent Empowerment (COPE), which works in the hospital and postdischarge. The program consists of audio taped information and workbooks for parents; parents are taught about behavior and development and caring for their infant. Teaching parents occurs in four phases, the first of which starts at a NICU. This program has been proven to be effective and efficient; the cost savings for health care systems are estimated more than $2 billion per year if the program would be routinely implemented in NICUs across the country (Forsythe & Willis, 2008; Melnyk, Crean, Feinstein, & Fairbanks, 2008; Melnyk & Feinstein, 2009). Parenting Preemies is another program that helps parents to ease the transition to home, with educational materials, follow-up telephone calls, and home visits lasting 10 weeks (Willis, 2008). Such programs bring needed support and reassurance to parents, as well as contributing to continuity of care. Importantly, advice on financial issues, insurance coverage, and available programs is often needed, too (Discenza, 2009).

■ Communication and Continuity of Care. Parents often report that they feel supported and reassured if a professional in addition to family or friends advise them. However, many parents also express the frustration of trying to build rapport with medical and nursing staff in primary health care settings. Follow-up nurses, nurse practitioners, should recognize that it could be difficult to build trust and rapport with parents who have suffered and been traumatized by their infant's hospitalization and health problems. Communication is the key element to successful relationships. Nurses are expert communicators, as the art of nursing has revolved around the ability to convey care and personal attention to the patient. Unfortunately, because of today's health care crisis, nursing shortages have resulted in staff mixes and use of unskilled personnel, coupled with economic constraints resulting in shortened hospital stays; nurses are also falling into the trap of assembly-line health care delivery. However, nurses have the advantage of being able to identify and assess a family's needs and to convey these needs to other health care team members. Being an advocate for the family is an essential part of preparing a family for discharge. Follow-up, in essence, is allowing an open line of communication among health care professionals, the health care delivery system, and the family. It allows a partnership to develop between the health care team and the family. It gives the family back some control. Follow-up moves the family away from the learned helplessness acquired in the hospital to a more participative role. Families who want to vent feelings and concerns often seek out nurses—as long as the family feels that the nurses care enough to be concerned. Parents need to be able to openly express their concerns without fear of being judged as "bad" parents.

Nonverbal cues can get in the way of communication. The nurse's expertise, knowledge, and use of medical terminology without explanations all convey the nurse's need to be in control. Someone has to be in control, but relinquishing some control to the family does not lessen one's credibility as a professional. It conveys to the family that they have a role in their infant's care and that they are important, too. Importantly, nurses also need to convey information and coordinate the data between physicians, social workers, counselors, and other members of the health care team who work with the family. Application of the nursing process may sound trite, but it is important in terms of not only collecting data but also using the data to identify problems, make nursing diagnoses, and develop a plan of care before and after discharge. Communication among the health care team members including the parents has a positive impact on the parents before and after discharge (Discenza, 2012; Yee & Ross, 2006). Collaboration among pediatric medical follow-up, parent support or psychosocial assessments at home, and obstetrical follow-up for the mother is essential. Each health care professional has something to contribute to the family's overall well-being. It is essential not to compete but to work with other professionals for the good of the family. It also means that each profession must share information that it receives from the family.

■ **Social and Material Support.** After discharge, social support from family members, relatives, and friends (informal social networks) is vital. Social support is an important aspect of coping and managing stress; if support is not provided, family functioning and health may suffer. Once the social support needs of the NICU family have been identified, a plan of action must be implemented. Helpful resources might be parent support groups, parent hotlines, referral to financial resources, or home care agencies. Balancing infant care with other demands is difficult, at best, and maternal *fatigue* is often a major issue when the infant comes home (Corwin, Brownstead, Barton, Heckard, & Morin, 2005; Garel, Dardennes, & Blondel, 2007; Lee & Kimble, 2009). Acknowledgments of the mother's own physical discomfort convey a caring and supportive attitude. The caring attitude by health care professionals, the friendly hug, and the taking time to talk with the parents, even if it was about something other than their infant's problems, can have positive effects on parental well-being and ease their stress. Moreover, it has been shown in mothers of healthy infants that provision of psychosocial support in the postpartum period decreased the risks of readmissions (Barilla, Marshak, Anderson, & Hopp, 2010). The availability of a phone number and the potential for a home visit are always viewed as positive by parents. For many parents, the home visit provides a way to vent feelings that otherwise might be suppressed around family and friends; home visits also provide needed reassurance for parents in caring (McKim, 1993; McKim et al., 1995). Unfortunately, with the current health care insurance coverage in the United States, few visits are actually made, but are still available in some places and countries. In many cases, parents appreciate even a telephone call from NICU personnel.

■ **Screening.** Another important aspect of postdischarge care could be screening for depression, PTSD, and parenting disturbances. Screening for postpartum depression in NICU parents has been long recommended since depression is a known risk following a high-risk birth (Beck, 2003; Gray, Edwards, O'Callaghan, & Cuskelly, 2012; Horowitz, Murphy, Gregory, & Wojcik, 2009). Gray et al. (2012) found that parenting stress was heavily influenced by maternal depression. As described in this chapter, continued stress, feelings of failure, and grieving for the loss of the fantasy child all have the potential for leading to maternal and paternal depression. Parental anxiety and the depressive symptoms should be assessed in the postdischarge period and be part of routine follow-up care (American Academy of Pediatrics & Committee on Fetus and Newborn, 2008; Horowitz et al., 2009; Segre, O'Hara, Arndt, & Beck, 2010). Psychological counseling and other needed treatments should be available for parents. In addition, VCS needs to be considered by those providing post-hospital care.

■ **Home Care.** With the shift from acute-care hospitals to providing home care for infants, even technology-dependent infants, the postdischarge transitions can be even more challenging for parents than before. Some families are expected to set up a "mini" intensive care in the home, even providing lung ventilation or intravenous medications. There are several types of home care.

Types of Home Care. Home care, for most practical purposes, is classified as short-term, long-term, or hospice care. Other programs involve respite care, which is relief care for parents, day care, which is at a specialized place that provides care for high-risk infants during daylight hours; and foster care, which refers to a family or individual that takes in a child to live in their house that is not their own when the birth family cannot provide care.

Short-term Care. Short-term care is considered by many health care services to be less than 6 months in duration. Short-term care of an infant at home may include phototherapy for hyperbilirubinemia, administration of supplemental oxygen to treat respiratory distress, home monitoring for apnea of the premature infant, medication administration for various neonatal conditions, and alternative feeding methods such as gavage for nutritional support. The primary caregivers in the home usually attend to these treatment modalities. Parents and families are carefully instructed in the use of any equipment placed in the home to administer health care. Extensive teaching before hospital discharge must convey the precise reasons for the therapy, the necessity for close observation of the infant by the caregivers, and the importance of communication and supervision by the primary care physician. In situations of short-term home care, the condition is usually self-limiting, and the home therapy can be discontinued at a predetermined endpoint.

Long-term Care. The point at which care becomes long-term is determined by the nature of the health care needs of the individual. The providers of extended care and the insurers paying for the care also arbitrarily set the period for long-term care. In general, long-term care indicates that the duration of the condition and the need for care will exceed 6 months. Long-term home care addresses situations for children with disease processes such as bronchopulmonary dysplasia (BPD), short-bowel or short-gut syndrome, CHD, physical and cosmetic defects, neurologic and metabolic disorders, and numerous other prolonged pathologic conditions. On discharge, these children may require home care services performed by professional home care agencies or programs. Families gradually become integrated into the health care routine. The family's responsibility changes as the infant's condition changes. The primary care physician must be closely involved and should be able to rely comfortably on the caregiver's judgment for making assessments and alterations in the home care plan. Long-term home care requires open communication among the family, community physicians, tertiary resources, community health care providers, home medical equipment providers, and financial providers. Many hospital records are now incorporating discharge notes, especially nursing case management notes or orders for the actual discharge and home care follow-up plan. These notes are a good vehicle for communication among the community health care providers and the discharging hospital.

Hospice Care. Congenital anomalies are the leading cause of infant mortality in the United States and are also a major contributor to childhood morbidity, long-term disability, and loss of years of potential life. The proportion of infant deaths attributed to birth defects has remained significantly high. The human immunodeficiency virus (HIV) epidemic is improving but it still takes its toll on the neonatal population. Those infants require specialized home care and in some instances palliative care. In addition, with technologic advances the ability to prolong lives has increased. Infants who are born dying do go home, where they need end-of-life (EOL) or palliative care. When it becomes clear that an infant will no longer benefit from acute intervention, plans for health care should focus on physical and emotional comfort. The transition from acute care to palliative care involves the concept of hospice. Hospice care is a philosophy of caring when cure is no longer a reasonable expectation. This care is not strictly a kind of terminal care, but rather an effort to maximize current quality of life without giving up all interest in a cure. Hospice provides comfort measures and emphasizes alleviation of symptoms. Whether the infant is terminally or chronically ill, the ultimate goal is to provide an environment that comforts the child and supports the family.

Criteria for Home Care. Some hospitals throughout the country are developing specialized outreach and home care services as an extension of their inpatient services. Regardless of how services are to be provided, the decision to facilitate early discharge from hospital care to home care must be based on standards that are safe and that provide effective ongoing therapy. The infant, the family, the home equipment, and the follow-up health care system must meet criteria for discharge to home care.

Infant Criteria. The infant's home health care needs must be assessed as to technical feasibility and medical requirements. Nutritional support must be evaluated. How does the infant feed and how frequently? How often does the infant require gavage feedings, and which feeding techniques are required? Pharmacologic support assessment must be evaluated. What medication does the infant need and how often? What are the desired and adverse effects of these drugs? Does the infant require supplemental oxygen, respiratory therapy treatments, or chest physical therapy? The assessment of the level of care required must be matched to the ability and skills of the home care providers. It must be determined before discharge that care in the home will be safe and meet the needs of the infant and family.

The specific criteria for discharge of special groups of children—such as those with BPD, short-bowel or short-gut syndrome, neurologic disease, cardiac disease, and other pathologic conditions—are addressed in the preceding chapters.

Family Criteria. The assessment of the family's commitment to home care is perhaps the most critical factor determining the success or failure of home health care. After extensive discharge teaching, skills development, and repeated occasions of caregiving, the family must want the child at home and under their care. They must be willing and able to devote the time and energy required to meet the physical and emotional needs of the child. These factors are essential for the well-being of the family unit. To prepare families for the discharge of their sick or high-risk infant, NICU personnel must begin teaching them as soon as the neonate is admitted to the unit. Once the family is confident and capable of meeting the needs of the infant, a home assessment should be completed. Basic facilities such as heat, water, telephone, electricity, and transportation must be available. Appropriate support systems must be set up in the home, including the technology necessary for the delivery of care. The operation of phototherapy lights or blankets, oxygen delivery systems, portable suction equipment, respiratory and cardiac monitoring systems, ventilators, and numerous other devices must be thoroughly understood by the caregivers. Clear instructions need to be given to the family members by the providers of the home care technology. Ideally, the parents should bring the equipment to the hospital, or the equipment company can help transport it to the hospital before discharge. The rationale is that the parents can be taught on their own equipment. If a problem arises, it can usually be identified before the infant's discharge. The parents should spend at least 24 hours providing total care before discharge. This time under a health professional's supervision helps the family gain confidence in their caregiving abilities. They can also be reassured that they have the proper equipment.

Home Equipment Criteria. The most common equipment needs for neonates are cardiopulmonary monitoring, oxygen, suction, and feeding implements. The family's first decision is how to select a home care equipment company. Hospital discharge planners or the nurse responsible for the discharge can make recommendations. Once the supplier has been selected and the necessary equipment identified, parent education can begin, including neonatal cardiopulmonary resuscitation (CPR). The parents should be given written instructions to take home and a checklist for the CPR procedure that can be clearly posted. If parents cannot read, visual charts outlining the steps should be made available.

A cardiopulmonary monitor is the most common equipment needed in the home. Infants who should be placed on this type of monitoring are those whose sibling died of sudden infant death syndrome (SIDS) or who are at risk for SIDS, such as premature infants. These infants are usually monitored for several months. An infant on home oxygen or one who has neurologic impairment is at risk for apneic or bradycardic episodes or desaturation, thus requiring pulse-oximetry. Most of the cardiopulmonary monitors have built-in memory or pneumography capabilities that allow trends and strips to be viewed by home care nurses. Often, parents struggle with alarm limits and sounds, and appropriate teaching should be done before discharge. Parents need to understand alarm delays or oversensitivity, when to change probes, and how to respond.

If parents have an infant who requires home respiratory support, the family will need a ventilator, with oxygen and air tanks. An air compressor, and oxygen concentrator may also be needed. Portable or stationary oxygen devices vary in size and the amount of time that they will last. Humidification and suctioning equipment is needed for patients with ventilation support or tracheostomies. Parents should be taught how to perform suctioning, how often, and how to adjust suction when an illness occurs that may put the infant at risk for cross-contamination. Suctioning should be performed according to individual needs of a patient and to the physician or nurse practitioner's orders. Signs that indicate the need for suctioning are the same as those used by health professionals in the NICU: restlessness, decreased color, coughing, increased respiratory effort, or sounds of congestion. Humidification of the airway is necessary for infants with artificial airways, regardless of whether they are on oxygen. If the airway is not humidified, mucous membranes may dry and crack, creating areas that may become infected.

These examples of home care and monitoring are the most common. Specific instructions are needed regarding which equipment is necessary and how to use it in each situation; the equipment should be obtained from the home health care agency that is to provide care, the hospital equipment vendors, and the home health care equipment vendors. Information on home use of ventilators can be obtained from the Home Mechanical Ventilation Resource Center of the American College of Chest Physicians (http://www.chestnet.org). If parents are primary caregivers, they should keep a log of the timing of the suctioning and the type of secretions obtained. Time of medication administration and feeds also should be recorded. An emergency backup unit must be available—whether it is housed in the home or at immediate dispatch from the equipment company does not matter, as long as it is available for times when equipment failures occur with the portable device. Battery backup is also necessary. Ideally, the nurse should make a home visit before the discharge to assess the home environment for safety hazards. For example, is the house/apartment too hot or cold? Either condition can lead to apneic spells. Are there exposed wires in the house? Peeling paint? Open flames used for cooking when oxygen is going to be used in the house? Are there any strong or chemical odors that may be harmful to a child with respiratory compromise? Is there an emergency phone? Have utility companies been notified? Is there a backup plan in case of a power outage? Is there a plan for continued health promotion, such as immunizations? All aspects of the home and the community setting should be considered when discharging the infant and family.

SUMMARY

Postdischarge care is vital for an infant and family, and no less than intensive care provided in the hospital. Former NICU infants may suffer from numerous health problems and may have numerous health care needs. Parents are in need as well. The crisis of hospitalization and discharge has no time limit because it is so individual. Three major transitions can be identified in parents of former NICU and preterm infants: transition to parenthood, transition to home, and transition to primary health care settings; all transitions can bring challenges to infant and family. Parental role alteration, anxiety, depression, and an increased need for professional and social supports are tremendous. Medical follow-up of NICU infants as well as helping parents to deal with postdischarge challenges are vital in order to promote infant health, development and family well-being. The outcome of transition (i.e., readmissions, health status of the infant, parenting style disturbances) will depend on whether resources are available to support the individuals undergoing postdischarge challenges and may influence the whole life span of infant and family. Application of the interventions as close to the time of the discharge as possible is vital. The crisis of neonatal hospitalization, difficulties in caregiving and parenting of initially sick or small infant can be alleviated by appropriate interventions and strategies. These are: appropriate discharge teaching, parental participation in transitional care programs, adequacy and timeliness of follow-up, access and attendance to transitional programs and follow up, provision of timely and appropriate resources for family and infant, continuity and coordination of care, case management, and access to home care to name a few. Close collaboration and open communication between health care providers and family is required, as well as informational and technical assistance. The absence of these can lead to a less than optimal environment for the infant and child to grow.

CASE STUDY

This case study applies the Kenner Transition Model to the care of a technology-dependent infant.

In recent years the number of technology-dependent infants discharged home has increased, because of the many early discharge programs available and the survival of extremely-low-birth-weight infants with chronic conditions. Although a fair amount has been written about setting up early discharge programs and the positive financial rewards associated with early discharge, little research is available to look at the effects of having a technology-dependent infant at home.

Spangler-Torok (2001) studied mothers receiving and caring for their technology-dependent infants in the home and applied the concepts of transition to this unique population. The experiential descriptions were from eight mothers, aged 17 to 42, who were the primary caretakers of their technology-dependent infants. All of the mothers were interviewed within the first 4 weeks of receiving their infant into the home. Although this was a phenomenological study, it provides support for the concepts of the Kenner Transition Model.

■ **Information Needs.** Mothers in this study understood the need to learn about care and equipment so that the infant could be discharged. Mothers described moving from learning care to making judgments regarding the infant's health. Gathering information is a way of seeking control of the situation. The mothers in this study sought information to make an overwhelming experience more manageable. The mothers described initial fear of caring for the infant at home and their ability to move beyond the fear and do what is needed to be done. As more information was gathered, mothers described using their judgment in making infant health decisions. When receiving and caring for a technology-dependent infant in the home, more information seems to give mothers more control, confidence, and peace of mind.

■ **Grief.** The mothers in this study feared the infant becoming ill and requiring rehospitalization. Several of the mothers voiced concern that the infant might die. Mothers grieved over the loss of the "ideal" pregnancy and infant. Mothers would report that they were managing the home care experience, "but this is not what I planned for." Mothers grieved about the life their infants would have and vowed to give them "as normal a life as possible." Mothers worried about what others would think: "Will they think it was something I did while I was pregnant that caused this to happen to the baby?" Mothers felt the need to "warn" others that the baby was different before they approached the infant.

■ **Parent–Child Role Development.** Once they were at home, mothers in this study believed that they were getting to know their infants and that their infants were getting to know them as their mothers. Mothers reported learning things about their infants that they didn't know until they were home, such as when their fussy times were. Mothers believed that as they learned more about infant preferences and health-related behaviors, they were able to make appropriate adjustments to infant care. Regardless of whether they had other children, the mothers saw a need to adjust the parenting role and expectation to accommodate the premature infant. They realized that this infant was different and required special care—in some instances, more vigilant care. They discussed how the increased needs of this infant took time away from other children and spouses, but acknowledged that being home was easier than extended hospital visits. Most of the mothers in this study quit their jobs or school to care for the infant, which they would not have planned to do if the infant had been healthy. The mothers discussed lifestyle changes since the infant came home from the hospital such as decreased number of outings, staying indoors more, and limiting visitors to the home.

■ **Stress and Coping.** Mothers in this study acknowledged that receiving and caring for a technology-dependent infant in the home is a lot of work. One mother stated it is "a ton of work . . . 10 times more work than a normal infant." Mothers report that more time is needed with infant care as well as with supplemental tasks such as dealing with insurance companies, managing supplies, and checking equipment. A lot of time is required to prepare the infant for outings, and time is needed for the infant to readjust to home after outings. Mothers reported problems with infant digestion and temperament when away from home. "She may require 2 or 3 days to recover from an outing to the doctor's office." All of the mothers described the extra work and time the infant required, but most felt it was worth it to have the infant home with them. This initial anxiety decreases as the infant's respiratory status improves and the infant becomes less dependent on oxygen therapy (Zanardo & Freato, 2001).

Two mothers described being overwhelmed with infant care in the home and felt they faced too many demands. One mother felt torn between caring for the infant and spending time with her other children. She is "only one person" and can "only be in one place at a time." She appreciates the break the home nurses provide but feels guilty that her infant receives care from others. Another mother describes frustration in dealing with the equipment. She has a "hard time looking" at the feeding tube but is less bothered by the tracheotomy. She gets angry when her husband gravitates toward Holly, the "normal" twin, and leaves all the work for Grace to her. This mother is afraid that her infant will pick up on her frustration with the equipment and feel that she doesn't love her.

■ **Social Interaction.** Several mothers in this study attributed their ability to care for this infant at home to the support of family and friends. Mothers stated they could focus on infant care because others were handling household chores and running errands for them. One mother described how strangers who heard of their situation were delivering food to them. The same mother felt that their experience was probably easier than others because "so many people have pitched in to do things." In describing her experience, one mother stated, "We just needed a lot of family." Having people come and help seems to make the experience more manageable for some of the mothers. One mother described being supported by the home care nurses. "It's wonderful to have the nursing staff here, because when you want to break down and cry, they're there to tell you, rub your hand, or your shoulder and say, 'you're doing a good job, don't think that you're not; you are.'" She is thankful for them and uses the nurses for other things so that she can spend time with the infant.

Although some mothers spoke of the assistance they received, others described the lack of support from family and friends. A mother spoke of being "annoyed" with her husband. She discussed how supportive they were of each other during their infant's hospitalization and that she had assumed that would continue once they were home. She was disappointed by her husband's lack of support and assistance with infant care and home management. "Hey, we have special circumstances here, this isn't just your average baby and you need to help me," she said. Another mother describes a lack of support from husband, children, and friends. She says her husband helps with the cooking, but it takes her three times as long to clean up. Although her 12-year-old daughter is old enough to help, she doesn't. She also wonders why friends have not come to see her. She believes they are afraid to see the baby and therefore do not visit. She sometimes feels alone in her responsibility for the baby.

The experiences of the mothers caring for infants who require technology support lend credence to the Kenner Transition Model. The mothers reported a need for information, they grieved for the loss of the healthy child, and found they needed to adjust their parenting roles. They felt stressed and overwhelmed. These are all concepts in the Kenner Model. Other studies report similar findings (McLean et al., 2000; Zanardo & Freato, 2001).

EVIDENCE-BASED PRACTICE BOX

For more than 30 years issues around the transition home, discharge coordination, and follow-up care have been researched. The reality is that for parents of a premature or sick newborn, life changes with a NICU stay. The discharge while anticipated is not easy. The transition home even with follow-up appointments, programs in place, and written discharge instructions is not easy for most families. There is fear that the baby will become sick again; fear the baby might die; fear that the health professionals in primary care or the community will not know what to do like NICU professionals. Research studies published in 2011 to 2012 continue to support the need for more research in the area of transition from hospital to home and the need for a clearer understanding of the actual follow-up that is being done—the adherence to suggested follow-up visits and programs (Ballantyne et al., 2012; Hutchinson, Spillett, & Cronin, 2012; Lopez, Anderson, & Feutchinger, 2012; Murdoch & Franck, 2011; Smith et al., 2012). Murdoch and Franck (2011) identified six themes from mothers transitioning with their infants to home following a NICU stay: apprehension, confidence, responsibility, awareness, normalcy, and perspective. One or more of these themes have been reported in transition research studies for more than three decades. In light of health care reform and the emphasis on health promotion, the time is right to use this evidence to create better follow-up programs and adherence to these needed health visits.

ONLINE RESOURCES

American Academy of Audiology Childhood Hearing Screening Guidelines for Children Age 6 Months Through High School
http://www.cdc.gov/ncbddd/hearingloss/documents/AAA_Childhood%20Hearing%20Guidelines_2011.pdf

American Academy of Pediatrics 2012 Immunization Schedule Update
http://www.aapnews.aappublications.org/content/33/2/1.2.full

American Academy of Pediatrics Recommendations for Preventive Pediatric Health Care Bright Futures/American Academy of Pediatrics
http://www.brightfutures.aap.org/pdfs/AAP%20Bright%20Futures%20Periodicity%20Sched%20101107.pdf

Apnea of Prematurity
http://emedicine.medscape.com/article/974971-overview

Bright Futures
http://www.brightfutures.org

European Foundation for the Care of Newborn Infants
http://www.efcni.org

Institute for Patient- and Family-Centered Care
http://www.ipfcc.org

Late Preterm Infants Multidisciplinary Guidelines for the Care of the Late Preterm Infants
http://www.nationalperinatal.org/lptguidelines.php

March of Dimes Leaving the NICU: Preparing for Discharge
http://www.marchofdimes.com/prematurity/21284 _11221.asp

March of Dimes NICU Family Support Program
http://www.marchofdimes.com/baby/inthenicu_program.html

National Center for Medical Home Implementation
http://www.medicalhomeinfo.org/about

National Dissemination Center for Children with Disabilities
Overview of Early Intervention
http://nichcy.org/babies/overview
Neonatal Follow-up Programs, The Children's Hospital of wPhiladelphia
http://www.chop.edu/service/neonatology/our-programs/neonatal-follow-up
Newborn Hearing Screening
http://emedicine.medscape.com/article/836646-overview#sw2aab6b4
NICU Discharge Instructions
http://www.womenandinfants.org/newbornhealth/nicu/discharge-instructions.cfm
NICU Follow-Up
http://emedicine.medscape.com/article/1833812-overview
NICUniversity
http://www.nicuniversity.org
PreemieVoices
http://www.zerotothree.org
Preemieworld
http://www.preemieworld.com/blog
Program for Technology-Dependent Children-Golisano Children's Hospital, University of Rochester Medical Center
http://www.urmc.rochester.edu/childrens-hospital/pulmonology/technology-dependent.aspx
Transition to home from the Newborn Intensive Care Unit: Applying the Principles of Family-Centered Care to the Discharge Process
http://www.ncbi.nlm.nih.gov/pubmed/16915057
Zero to Three: National Center for Infants, Toddlers, and Families
http://www.zerotothree.org

REFERENCES

Affleck, G., & Tennen, H. (1991). The effect of newborn intensive care on parents' psychological well-being. *Child Health Care, 20*(1), 6–14.

Ahlund, S., Clarke, P., Hill, J., & Thalange, N. K. (2009). Post-traumatic stress symptoms in mothers of very low birth weight infants 2–3 years post-partum. *Archives of Women's Mental Health, 12*(4), 261–264. doi:10.1007/s00737-009-0067-4

Ahmed, A. H., & Sands, L. P. (2010). Effect of pre- and postdischarge interventions on breastfeeding outcomes and weight gain among premature infants. *Journal of Obstetric, Gynecologic, and Neonatal Nursing, 39*(1), 53–63. doi:10.1111/j.1552-6909.2009.01088.x

Allen, E. C., Manuel, J. C., Legault, C., Naughton, M. J., Pivor, C., & O'Shea, T. M. (2004). Perception of child vulnerability among mothers of former premature infants. *Pediatrics, 113*(2), 267–273.

American Academy of Audiology. (2011). *Childhood hearing screening guidelines*. Retrieved December, 2, 2012, from www.cdc.gov/ncbddd/hearingloss/documents/aaa_childhood-hearing-guidelines_2011.pdf

American Academy of Pediatrics. (2008). *Recommendations for preventive pediatric health care*. Retrieved from http://www.aap.org/en-us/professional-resources/practice-support/financing-and-payment/Documents/Recommendations_Preventive_Pediatric_Health_Care.pdf

American Academy of Pediatrics. (2012a). *Infectious disease presentation slides: Immunization schedules*. Retrieved from http://aapredbook.aappublications.org/site/misc/slides.xhtml

American Academy of Pediatrics. (2012b). *Infectious disease presentation slides: Respiratory syncytial virus*. Retrieved from http://aapredbook.aappublications.org/site/misc/slides.xhtml

American Academy of Pediatrics & the American College of Obstetricians and Gynecologists. (2012). *Guidelines for perinatal care* (7th ed.). Elk Grove Village, IL: American Academy of Pediatrics.

American Academy of Pediatrics & Committee on Fetus and Newborn. (2008). Hospital discharge of the high-risk neonate. *Pediatrics, 122*(5), 1196–1126. doi:10.1542/peds.2008-2174

American Academy of Pediatrics & Committee on Infectious Diseases. (2009). Policy statement—Modified recommendations for use of palivizumab for prevention of respiratory syncytial virus infections. *Pediatrics, 124*(6), 1694–1701. doi:10.1542/peds.2009-2345

American Academy of Pediatrics & Joint Committee on Infant Hearing. (2007). Principles and guidelines for early hearing detection and intervention programs. *Pediatrics, 120*(4), 898–921. doi:10.1542/peds.2007-2333

American Academy of Pediatrics Section on Ophthalmology. (2001). Screening examination of premature infants for retinopathy of prematurity. *Pediatrics, 108*(3), 809–811.

American Academy of Pediatrics Section on Ophthalmology, American Academy of Ophthalmology, & American Association for Pediatric Ophthalmology and Strabismus. (2006). Screening examination of premature infants for retinopathy of prematurity. *Pediatrics, 117*(2), 572–576. doi:10.1542/peds.2005-2749.

American Academy of Pediatrics Task Force for Improving Newborn Hearing Screening Diagnosis and Intervention. (2010). Early hearing detection and intervention (EHDI) guidelines for pediatric medical home providers. Retrieved December, 14, 2012, from www.medicalhomeinfo.org

Anderson, L. S., Riesch, S. K., Pridham, K. A., Lutz, K. F., & Becker, P. T. (2010). Furthering the understanding of parent–child relationships: A nursing scholarship review series. part 4: Parent–child relationships at risk. *Journal for Specialists in Pediatric Nursing, 15*(2), 111–134. doi:10.1111/j.1744-6155.2009.00223.x

Bagwell, G. A. (1990). Parent transition from a special care nursery to home: A replicative study. Unpublished master's thesis. University of Cincinnati College of Nursing, Cincinnati, Ohio.

Bakewell-Sachs, S., Medoff-Cooper, B., Escobar, G. J., Silber, J. H., & Lorch, S. A. (2009). Infant functional status: The timing of physiologic maturation of premature infants. *Pediatrics, 123*(5), e878–e886. doi:10.1542/peds.2008-2568

Ballantyne, M., Stevens, B., Guttmann, A., Willan, A. R., & Rosenbaum, P. (2012). Transition to neonatal follow-up programs: Is attendance a problem? *Journal of Perinatal and Neonatal Nursing, 26*(1), 90–98. doi:10.1097/JPN.0b013e31823f900b

Barfield, W. D., Clements, K. M., Lee, K. G., Kotelchuck, M., Wilber, N., & Wise, P. H. (2008). Using linked data to assess patterns of early intervention (EI) referral among very low birth weight infants. *Maternal and Child Health Journal, 12*(1), 24–33. doi:10.1007/s10995-007-0227-y

Barilla, D., Marshak, H. H., Anderson, S. E., & Hopp, J. W. (2010). Postpartum follow-up: Can psychosocial support reduce newborn readmissions? *Maternal Child Nursing Journal, 35*(1), 33–39.

Beck, C. T. (2003). Recognizing and screening for postpartum depression in mothers of NICU infants. *Advances in Neonatal Care, 3*(1), 37–46.

Beck, C. T., Gable, R. K., Sakala, C., & Declercq, E. R. (2011). Posttraumatic stress disorder in new mothers: Results from a two-stage U.S. national survey. *Birth, 38*(3), 216–227. doi:10.1111/j.1523-536X.2011.00475.x

Behrman, R. E., & Butler, A. S. (Eds.). (2007). *Preterm birth: Causes, consequences, and prevention*. Washington, DC: National Academies, Institute of Medicine Committee on Understanding Premature Birth and Assuring Healthy Outcomes.

Bertino, E., Di Nicola, P., Giuliani, F., Coscia, A., Varalda, A., Occhi, L., & Rossi, C. (2011). Evaluation of postnatal growth of preterm infants. *Journal of Maternal-Fetal and Neonatal Medicine*. doi:10.3109/14767058.2011.601921

Bialoskurski, M., Cox, C. L., & Hayes, J. A. (1999). The nature of attachment in a neonatal intensive care unit. *Journal of Perinatal and Neonatal Nursing, 13*(1), 66–77.

Bird, T. M., Bronstein, J. M., Hall, R. W., Lowery, C. L., Nugent, R., & Mays, G. P. (2010). Late preterm infants: Birth outcomes and health care utilization in the first year. *Pediatrics, 126*(2), e311–e319. doi:10.1542/peds.2009-2869

Bolzan, N., Gale, F., & Dudley, M. (2004). Time to father. *Social Work in Health Care, 39*(1–2), 67–88.

Bonhoeffer, J., Siegrist, C. A., & Heath, P. T. (2006). Immunisation of premature infants. [Review]. *Archives of Disease in Childhood, 91*(11), 929–935. doi:10.1136/adc.2005.086306

Boss, R. D., Donohue, P. K., & Arnold, R. M. (2010). Adolescent mothers in the NICU: How much do they understand? *Journal of Perinatology, 30*(4), 286–290. doi:10.1038/jp.2009.160 Boykova, M. (2008). Follow-up care of premature babies in Russia: Evaluating parental experiences and associated services. *Infant, 4 (4),* 101-105.

Boykova, M. (2008). Follow-up care of premature babies in Russia: Evaluating parental experiences and associated services. *Infant, 4*(4), 101–105.

Boykova, M., & Kenner, C. (2012). Transition from hospital to home for parents of preterm infants. *Journal of Perinatal and Neonatal Nursing, 26*(1), 81–87. doi:10.1097/JPN.0b013e318243e948

Brandon, D. H., Tully, K. P., Silva, S. G., Malcolm, W. F., Murtha, A. P., Turner, B. S., & Holditch-Davis, D. (2011). Emotional responses of mothers of late-preterm and term infants. *Journal of Obstetric, Gynecologic, and Neonatal Nursing.* doi:10.1111/j.1552-6909.2011.01290.x

Brazy, J. E., Anderson, B. M., Becker, P. T., & Becker, M. (2001). How parents of premature infants gather information and obtain support. *Neonatal Network, 20*(2), 41–48.

Brecht, C. J., Shaw, R. J., St. John, N. H., & Horwitz, S. M. (2012). Effectiveness of therapeutic and behavioral interventions for parents of low-birth-weight premature infants: A review. *Infant Mental Health Journal, 33*(6)651–665. doi:10.1002/imhj.21349

Browne, J. V., & Talmi, A. (2012). Developmental supports for newborns and young infants with special health and developmental needs and their families: The BABIES model. *Newborn and Infant Nursing Reviews, 12*(4), 239–247. doi:10.1053/j.nainr.2012.09.005

Caplan, G., Mason, E. A., & Kaplan, D. M. (1965). Four studies of crisis in parents of prematures. *Community Mental Health Journal, 1*(2), 149–161.

Carter, J. D., Mulder, R. T., Frampton, C. M., & Darlow, B. A. (2007). Infants admitted to a neonatal intensive care unit: Parental psychological status at 9 months. *Acta Paediatrica, 96*(9), 1286–1289. doi:10.1111/j.1651-2227.2007.00425.x

Casey, P. H. (2008). Growth of low birth weight preterm children. *Seminars in Perinatology, 32*(1), 20–27. doi:10.1053/j.semperi.2007.12.004

Casey, P. H., Bradley, R. H., Whiteside-Mansell, L., Barrett, K., Gossett, J. M., & Simpson, P. M. (2011). Evolution of obesity in a low birth weight cohort. *Journal of Perinatology, 32,* 91–96. doi:10.1038/jp.2011.75

Clements, K. M., Barfield, W. D., Ayadi, M. F., & Wilber, N. (2007). Preterm birth-associated cost of early intervention services: An analysis by gestational age. *Pediatrics, 119*(4), e866–e874. doi:10.1542/peds.2006-1729

Corwin, E. J., Brownstead, J., Barton, N., Heckard, S., & Morin, K. (2005). The impact of fatigue on the development of postpartum depression. *Journal of Obstetric, Gynecologic, and Neonatal Nursing, 34*(5), 577–586. doi:10.1177/0884217505279997

Costello, A., & Chapman, J. (1998). Mothers' perceptions of the care-by-parent program prior to hospital discharge of their preterm infants. *Neonatal Network, 17*(7), 37–42.

Cox, C., & Bialoskurski, M. (2001). Neonatal intensive care: Communication and attachment. *British Journal of Nursing, 10*(10), 668–676.

Deave, T., & Johnson, D. (2008). The transition to parenthood: What does it mean for fathers? *Journal of Advanced Nursing, 63*(6), 626–633. doi:10.1111/j.1365-2648.2008.04748.x

De Jesus, L. C., Pappas, A., Shankaran, S., Kendrick, D., Das, A., Higgins, R. D., . . . Walsh, M. C., for the Eunice Kennedy Shriver National Institute of Child Health and Human Development Neonatal Research Network. (2012). Risk factors for post-neonatal intensive care unit discharge mortality among extremely low birth weight infants. *Journal of Pediatrics, 161*(1), 70–74. doi: 10.1016/j.jpeds.2011.12.038

Delaney, A., & Ruth, R. (2012). *Newborn hearing screening.* Retrieved from http://emedicine.medscape.com/article/836646-overview

De Rouck, S., & Leys, M. (2009). Information needs of parents of children admitted to a neonatal intensive care unit: A review of the literature (1990–2008). *Patient Education and Counseling, 76*(2), 159–173. doi:10.1016/j.pec.2009.01.014

De Rouck, S., & Leys, M. (2011). Information behaviour of parents of children admitted to a neonatal intensive care unit: Constructing a conceptual framework. *Health, 15*(1), 54–77. doi:10.1177/1363459309360785

Discenza, D. (2009). NICU parents' top ten worries at discharge. *Neonatal Network, 28*(3), 202–203.

Discenza, D. (2012). Preemie parent frustration: Dealing with insensitive comments. *Neonatal Network, 31*(1), 52–53. doi:10.1891/0730-0832.31.1.52

Doering, L. V., Moser, D. K., & Dracup, K. (2000). Correlates of anxiety, hostility, depression, and psychosocial adjustment in parents of NICU infants. *Neonatal Network, 19*(5), 15–23.

Drake, E. (1995). Discharge teaching needs of parents in the NICU. *Neonatal Network, 14*(1), 49–53.

Elklit, A., Hartvig, T., & Christiansen, M. (2007). Psychological sequelae in parents of extreme low and very low birth weight infants. *Journal of Clinical Psychology in Medical Settings, 14*(3), 238–247. doi:10.1007/s10880-007-9077-4

Emmanuel, E., & St John, W. (2010). Maternal distress: A concept analysis. *Journal of Advanced Nursing, 66*(9), 2104–2115. doi:10.1111/j.1365-2648.2010.05371.x

Escobar, G. J., Clark, R. H., & Greene, J. D. (2006). Short-term outcomes of infants born at 35 and 36 weeks gestation: We need to ask more questions. *Seminars in Perinatology, 30*(1), 28–33. doi:10.1053/j.semperi.2006.01.005

Feinberg, E., Donahue, S., Bliss, R., & Silverstein, M. (2012). Maternal depressive symptoms and participation in early intervention services for young children. *Maternal and Child Health Journal, 16*(2), 336–345. doi: 10.1007/s10995-010-0715-3

Flandermeyer, A., Kenner, C., Spaite, M. E., & Hostiuck, J. (1992a). Transition from hospital to home. Part II. *Neonatal Network, 11*(5), 62–63.

Flandermeyer, A., Kenner, C., Spaite, M. E., & Hostiuck, J. (1992b). Transition from hospital to home: Part III. *Neonatal Network, 11*(6), 84–85.

Forsythe, P. L., & Willis, V. (2008). Parenting preemies: A unique program for family support and education after NICU discharge. *Advances in Neonatal Care, 8*(4), 221–230. doi:10.1097/01.ANC.0000333710.83517.19

Gaal, B. J., Pinelli, J., Crooks, D., Saigal, S., Streiner, D. L., & Boyle, M. (2010). Outside looking in: The lived experience of adults with prematurely born siblings. *Qualitative Health Research, 20*(11), 1532–1545. doi:10.1177/1049732310375248

Garel, M., Dardennes, M., & Blondel, B. (2007). Mothers' psychological distress 1 year after very preterm childbirth: Results of the EPIPAGE qualitative study. *Child: Care, Health and Development, 33*(2), 137–143.

Gennaro, S. (1988). Postpartal anxiety and depression in mothers of term and preterm infants. *Nursing Research, 37*(2), 82–85.

Golish, T. D., & Powell, K. A. (2003). "Ambiguous loss": Managing the dialectics of grief associated with premature birth. *Journal of Social and Personal Relationships, 20*, 309.

Gordon, J. (2009). An evidence-based approach for supporting parents experiencing chronic sorrow. *Pediatric Nursing, 35*(2), 115–119.

Grant, R., & Isakson, E. A. (2012). Regional variations in early intervention utilization for children with developmental delay. *Maternal and Child Health Journal*. doi:10.1007/s10995-012-1119-3

Gray, P. H., Edwards, D. M., O'Callaghan, M. J., & Cuskelly, M. (2012). Parenting stress in mothers of preterm infants during early infancy. *Early Human Development, 88*(1), 45–49. doi:10.1016/j.earlhumdev.2011.06.014

Green, M., & Solnit, A. J. (1964). Reactions to the threatened loss of a child: A vulnerable child syndrome. Pediatric management of the dying child, part III. *Pediatrics, 34*, 58–66.

Hess, C. R., Teti, D. M., & Hussey-Gardner, B. (2004). Self-efficacy and parenting of high-risk infants: The moderating role of parent knowledge of infant development. *Journal of Applied Developmental Psychology, 25*(4), 423–437. doi: 10.1016/j.appdev.2004.06.002

Holditch-Davis, D., Bartlett, T. R., Blickman, A. L., & Miles, M. S. (2003). Posttraumatic stress symptoms in mothers of premature infants. *Journal of Obstetric, Gynecologic, and Neonatal Nursing, 32*(2), 161–171.

Holditch-Davis, D., Miles, M. S., Burchinal, M. R., & Goldman, B. D. (2011). Maternal role attainment with medically fragile infants: Part 2: Relationship to the quality of parenting. *Research in Nursing and Health, 34*(1), 35–48. doi:10.1002/nur.20418

Hollywood, M., & Hollywood, E. (2011). The lived experiences of fathers of a premature baby on a neonatal intensive care unit. *Journal of Neonatal Nursing, 17*(1), 32–40. doi:10.1016/j.jnn.2010.07.015

Holte, L., Walker, E., Oleson, J., Spratford, M., Moeller, M., Roush, P., . . . Ou, H. (2012). Factors influencing follow-up to hewborn hearing screening for infants who are hard of-hearing. *American Journal of Audiology, 21*(2), 163–174. doi:10.1044/1059-0889(2012/12-0016)

Horowitz, J. A., Murphy, C. A., Gregory, K. E., & Wojcik, J. (2009). Community-based postpartum depression screening: Results from the CARE study. *Psychiatric Services, 60*(11), 1432–1434. doi:10.1176/appi.ps.60.11.1432

Hoyert, D. L., & Xu, J. (2012). Deaths: Preliminary data for 2011. *National Vital Statistics Reports, 61*(6), 1–65.

Hutchinson, S. W., Spillett, M. A., & Cronin, M. (2012). Parent's expereinces during their infant's transition from neonatal intensive care unit to home: A qualitative study. *Qualitative Report, 17*(Article 23), 1–20.

Jackson, K., Ternestedt, B. M., & Schollin, J. (2003). From alienation to familiarity: Experiences of mothers and fathers of preterm infants. *Journal of Advanced Nursing, 43*(2), 120–129.

Jones, L., Rowe, J., & Becker, T. (2009). Appraisal, coping, and social support as predictors of psychological distress and parenting efficacy in parents of premature infants. *Children's Health Care, 38*(4), 245–262. doi:10.1080/02739610903235976

Jubinville, J., Newburn-Cook, C., Hegadoren, K., & Lacaze-Masmonteil, T. (2012). Symptoms of acute stress disorder in mothers of premature infants. *Advances in Neonatal Care, 12*(4), 246–253. doi:10.1097/ANC.0b013e31826090ac

Kenner, C. (1988). *Parent transition from newborn intensive care unit to home* (Doctoral dissertation). Indiana University, Indianapolis, IN.

Kenner, C. (1990). Caring for the NICU parent. *Journal of Perinatal and Neonatal Nursing, 4*(3), 78–87.

Kenner, C., Flandermeyer, A., Spangler, L., Thornburg, P., Spiering, D., & Kotagal, U. (1993). Transition from hospital to home for mothers and babies. *Neonatal Network, 12*(3), 73–77.

Kenner, C., & Lott, J. W. (1990). Parent transition after discharge from the NICU. *Neonatal Network, 9*(2), 31–37.

Kersting, A., Dorsch, M., Wesselmann, U., Lüdorff, K., Witthaut, J., Ohrmann, P., . . . Arolt, V. (2004). Maternal posttraumatic stress response after the birth of a very low-birth-weight infant. *Journal of Psychosomatic Research, 57*(5), 473–476. doi:10.1016/j.jpsychores.2004.03.011

Kirkby, S., Greenspan, J., Kornhauser, M., & Schneiderman, R. (2007). Clinical outcomes and cost of the moderately preterm infant. *Advances in Neonatal Care, 7*(2), 80–87.

Klein, L. (2011). Effectiveness of parent education on late preterm infants' readmission rates. *Journal of Obstetric, Gynecologic, and Neonatal Nursing, 40*(s1), S110–S111. doi:10.1111/j.1552-6909.2011.01243_31.x

Kokotos, F., & Adam, H. M. (2009). The vulnerable child syndrome. *Pediatrics in Review, 30*(5), 193–194. doi:10.1542/pir.30-5-193

Korja, R., Latva, R., & Lehtonen, L. (2012). The effects of preterm birth on mother–infant interaction and attachment during the infant's first two years. *Acta Obstetricia et Gynecologica Scandinavica, 91*(2), 164–173. doi:10.1111/j.1600-0412.2011.01304.x

Korja, R., Savonlahti, E., Haataja, L., Lapinleimu, H., Manninen, H., Piha, J., & Lehtonen, L. (2009). Attachment representations in mothers of preterm infants. *Infant Behavior and Development, 32*(3), 305–311. doi:10.1016/j.infbeh.2009.04.003

Korvenranta, E., Lehtonen, L., Rautava, L., Hakkinen, U., Andersson, S., Gissler, M., . . . PERFECT Preterm Infant Study Group. (2010). Impact of very preterm birth on health care costs at five years of age. *Pediatrics, 125*(5), e1109–e1114. doi:10.1542/peds.2009-2882

Kowalski, W. J., Leef, K. H., Mackley, A., Spear, M. L., & Paul, D. A. (2006). Communicating with parents of premature infants: Who is the informant? *Journal of Perinatology, 26*(1), 44–48. doi:10.1038/sj.jp.7211409

Kripalani, S., LeFevre, F., Phillips, C. O., Williams, M. V., Basaviah, P., & Baker, D. W. (2007). Deficits in communication and information transfer between hospital-based and primary care physicians: Implications for patient safety and continuity of care. *The Journal of the American Medical Association, 297*(8), 831–841. doi:10.1001/jama.297.8.831

LaHood, A., & Bryant, C. A. (2007). Outpatient care of the premature infant. *American Family Physician, 76*(8), 1159–1164.

Lee, S.-Y., & Kimble, L. P. (2009). Impaired sleep and well-being in mothers with low-birth-weight infants. *Journal of Obstetric, Gynecologic, and Neonatal Nursing, 38*(6), 676–685. doi:10.1111/j.1552-6909.2009.01064.x

Levy, J. C. (1980). Vulnerable children: parents' perspectives and the use of medical care. *Pediatrics, 65*(5), 956–963.

Liu, C. L., Farrell, J., MacNeil, J. R., Stone, S., & Barfield, W. (2008). Evaluating loss to follow-up in newborn hearing screening in Massachusetts. *Pediatrics, 121*(2), e335–e343. doi:10.1542/peds.2006-3540

Loo, K. K., Espinosa, M., Tyler, R., & Howard, J. (2003). Using knowledge to cope with stress in the NICU: How parents integrate learning to read the physiologic and behavioral cues of the infant. *Neonatal Network, 22*(1), 31–37.

Lopez, G. L., Anderson, K. H., & Feutchinger, J. (2012). Transition of premature infants from hospital to home life. *Neonatal Network, 31*(4), 207–214.

Lorch, S. A., Srinivasan, L., & Escobar, G. J. (2011). Epidemiology of apnea and bradycardia resolution in premature infants. *Pediatrics, 128*(2), e366–e373. doi:10.1542/peds.2010-1567

Lutz, K. F. (2012). Feeding problems of neonatal intensive care unit and pediatric intensive care unit graduates: Perceptions of parents and providers. *Newborn and Infant Nursing Reviews, 12*(4), 207–213. doi:10.1053/j.nainr.2012.09.008

Lutz, K. F., Anderson, L. S., Riesch, S. K., Pridham, K. A., & Becker, P. T. (2009). Furthering the understanding of parent-child relationships: A nursing scholarship review series. Part 2: Grasping the early parenting experience—the insider view. *Journal for Specialists in Pediatric Nursing, 14*(4), 262–283.

Mackie, A. S., Ionescu-Ittu, R., Pilote, L., Rahme, E., & Marelli, A.J. (2008). Hospital readmissions in children with congenital heart disease: A population-based study. *American Heart Journal, 155*(3), 577–584. doi:10.1016/j.ahj.2007.11.003

Mackley, A. B., Locke, R. G., Spear, M. L., & Joseph, R. (2010). Forgotten parent: NICU paternal emotional response. *Advances in Neonatal Care 10*(4), 200–203. doi:10.1097/ANC.0b013e3181e946f0

Maiorana, A., & Cianfarani, S. (2009). Impact of growth hormone therapy on adult height of children born small for gestational age. *Pediatrics, 124*(3), e519–e531. doi:10.1542/peds.2009-0293

Makaryus, A. N., & Friedman, E. A. (2005). Patients' understanding of their treatment plans and diagnosis at discharge. *Mayo Clinic Proceedings, 80*(8), 991–994.

Mally, P. V., Bailey, S., & Hendricks-Muñoz, K. D. (2010). Clinical issues in the management of late preterm infants. *Current Problems in Pediatric and Adolescent Health Care, 40*(9), 218–233. doi:10.1016/j.cppeds.2010.07.005

May, K. M. (1997). Searching for normalcy: Mothers' caregiving for low birth weight infants. *Pediatric Nursing, 23*(1), 17–20.

McKim, E. (1993). The difficult first week at home with a premature infant. *Public Health Nursing, 10*(2), 89–96.

McKim, E., Kenner, C., Flandermeyer, A., Spangler, L., Darling-Thornburg, P., & Spiering, K. (1995). The transition to home for mothers of healthy and initially ill newborn babies. *Midwifery, 11*(4), 184–194.

McLaurin, K. K., Hall, C. B., Jackson, E. A., Owens, O. V., & Mahadevia, P. J. (2009). Persistence of morbidity and cost differences between late-preterm and term infants during the first year of life. *Pediatrics, 123*(2), 653–659. doi:10.1542/peds.2008–1439

McLean, A., Townsend, A., Clark, J., Sawyer, M. G., Baghurst, P., Haslam, R., & Whaites, L. (2000). Quality of life of mothers and families caring for preterm infants requiring home oxygen therapy: A brief report. *Journal of Pediatrics and Child Health, 36*(5), 440–444.

McManus, B., McCormick, M. C., Acevedo-Garcia, D., Ganz, M., & Hauser-Cram, P. (2009). The effect of state early intervention eligibility policy on participation among a cohort of young CSHCN. *Pediatrics, 124*(Suppl. 4), S368–S374. doi:10.1542/peds.2009-1255G

McPherson, M., Arango, P., Fox, H., Lauver, C., McManus, M., Newacheck, P. W., . . . Strickland, B. (1998). A new definition of children with special health care needs. *Pediatrics, 102*(1 Pt 1), 137–140.

Meijssen, D., Wolf, M. J., Koldewijn, K., van Baar, A., & Kok, J. (2011). Maternal psychological distress in the first two years after very preterm birth and early intervention. *Early Child Development and Care, 181*(1), 1–11.

Melnyk, B. M., Crean, H. F., Feinstein, N. F., & Fairbanks, E. (2008). Maternal anxiety and depression after a premature infant's discharge from the neonatal intensive care unit: Explanatory effects of the Creating Opportunities for Parent Empowerment program. *Nursing Research, 57*(6), 383–394. doi:10.1097/NNR.0b013e3181906f59

Melnyk, B. M., & Feinstein, N. F. (2009). Reducing hospital expenditures with the COPE (Creating Opportunities for Parent Empowerment) program for parents and premature infants: An analysis of direct healthcare neonatal intensive care unit costs and savings. *Nursing Administration Quarterly, 33*(1), 32–37. doi:10.1097/01.NAQ.0000343346.47795.13

Mercer, R. T. (2004). Becoming a mother versus maternal role attainment. *Journal of Nursing Scholarship, 36*(3), 226–232.

Mercer, R. T., & Walker, L. O. (2006). A review of nursing interventions to foster becoming a mother. *Journal of Obstetric, Gynecologic and Neonatal Nursing, 35*(5), 568–582. doi:10.1111/j.1552-6909.2006.00080.x

Mew, A. M., Holditch-Davis, D., Belyea, M., Miles, M. S., & Fishel, A. (2003). Correlates of depressive symptoms in mothers of preterm infants. *Neonatal Network, 22*(5), 51–60.

Miles, M. S. (1989). Parents of critically ill premature infants: Sources of stress. *Critical Care Nursing Quarterly, 12*(3), 69–74.

Miles, M. S., & Holditch-Davis, D. (1995). Compensatory parenting: How mothers describe parenting their 3-year-old, prematurely born children. *Journal of Pediatric Nursing, 10*(4), 243–253.

Miles, M. S., & Holditch-Davis, D. (1997). Parenting the prematurely born child: Pathways of influence. *Seminars in Perinatology, 21*(3), 254–266.

Miles, M. S., Holditch-Davis, D., Burchinal, M. R., & Brunssen, S. (2011). Maternal role attainment with medically fragile infants: Part 1. Measurement and correlates during the first year of life. *Research in Nursing and Health, 34*(1), 20–34. doi:10.1002/nur.20419

Miles, M. S., Holditch-Davis, D., & Shepherd, H. (1998). Maternal concerns about parenting prematurely born children. *American Journal of Maternal Child Nursing, 23*(2), 70–75.

Miller, B. C., & Sollie, D. L. (1980). Normal stresses during the transition to parenthood. *Family Relations, 29*(4), 459–465.

Mowery, B. D. (2011). Post-traumatic stress disorder (PTSD) in parents: Is this a significant problem? *Pediatric Nursing, 37*(2), 89–92.

Munoz, K., Nelson, L., Goldgewicht, N., & Odell, D. (2011). Early hearing detection and intervention: Diagnostic hearing assessment practices. *American Journal of Audiology, 20*(2), 123–131. doi:10.1044/1059-0889(2011/10-0046)

Murdoch, M. R., & Franck, L. S. (2011). Gaining confidence and perspective: A phenomenological study of mothers' lived experiences caring for infants at home after neonatal unit discharge. *Journal of Advanced Nursing.* doi:10.1111/j.1365-2648.2011.05891.x

Navar-Boggan, A. M., Halsey, N. A., Escobar, G. J., Golden, W. C., & Klein, N. P. (2011). Underimmunization at discharge from the neonatal intensive care unit. *Journal of Perinatology, 32*, 363–367. doi: 10.1038/jp.2011.111

Naylor, M. D., Aiken, L. H., Kurtzman, E. T., Olds, D. M., & Hirschman, K. B. (2011). The care span: The importance of transitional care in achieving health reform. *Health Affairs, 30*(4), 746–754. doi:10.1377/hlthaff.2011.0041

Naylor, M. D., Bowles, K. H., McCauley, K. M., Maccoy, M. C., Maislin, G., Pauly, M. V., & Krakauer, R. (2011). High-value transitional care: Translation of research into practice. *Journal of Evaluation in Clinical Practice.* doi:10.1111/j.1365-2753.2011.01659.x

Naylor, M. D., Brooten, D. A., Campbell, R. L., Maislin, G., McCauley, K. M., & Schwartz, J. S. (2004). Transitional care of older adults hospitalized with heart failure: A randomized, controlled trial. *Journal of the American Geriatrics Society, 52*(5), 675–684.

Naylor, M. D., Feldman, P. H., Keating, S., Koren, M. J., Kurtzman, E. T., Maccoy, M. C., & Krakauer, R. (2009). Translating research into practice: Transitional care for older adults. *Journal of Evaluation in Clinical Practice, 15*(6), 1164–1170. doi:10.1111/j.1365-2753.2009.01308.x

Newacheck, P. W., Rising, J. P., & Kim, S. E. (2006). Children at risk for special health care needs. *Pediatrics, 118*(1), 334–342. doi:10.1542/peds.2005-2238

Nivamat, D. J. (2012). *Apnea of prematurity*. Retrieved from http://emedicine.medscape.com/article/974971-overview

Nordhov, S. M., Rønning, J. A., Dahl, L. B., Ulvund, S. E., Tunby, J., & Kaaresen, P. I. (2010). Early intervention improves cognitive outcomes for preterm infants: Randomized controlled trial. *Pediatrics, 126*(5), e1088–e1094. doi:10.1542/peds.2010-0778

Obeidat, H. M., Bond, E. A., & Callister, L. C. (2009). The parental experience of having an infant in the newborn intensive care unit. *The Journal of Perinatal Education, 18*(3), 23–29. doi:10.1624/105812409X461199

Orton, J., Spittle, A., Doyle, L., Anderson, P., & Boyd, R. (2009). Do early intervention programmes improve cognitive and motor outcomes for preterm infants after discharge? A systematic review. *Developmental Medicine and Child Neurology, 51*(11), 851–859.

Padovani, F. H. P., Carvalho, A. E. V., Duarte, G., Martinez, F. E. M., & Linhares, M. B. M. (2009). Anxiety, dysphoria, and depression symptoms in mothers of preterm infants. *Psychological Reports, 104*(2), 667–679. doi:10.2466/pr0.104.2.667-679

Pearson, S. R., & Boyce, W. T. (2004). Consultation with the specialist: The vulnerable child syndrome. *Pediatrics in Review, 25*(10), 345–349. doi:10.1542/pir.25-10-345

Perlman, N. B., Freedman, J. L., Abramovitch, R., Whyte, H., Kirpalani, H., & Perlman, M. (1991). Informational needs of parents of sick neonates. *Pediatrics, 88*(3), 512–518.

Perrin, K. M., & Bégué, R. E. (2012). Use of palivizumab in primary practice. *Pediatrics, 129*(1), 55–61. doi:10.1542/peds.2010-2991

Placencia, F. X., & McCullough, L. B. (2012). Biopsychosocial risks of parental care for high-risk neonates: Implications for evidence-based parental counseling. *Journal of Perinatology, 32*(5), 381–386. doi:10.1038/jp.2011.109

Pritchard, M. A., Colditz, P. B., & Beller, E. M. (2008). Parental experiences and preferences which influence subsequent use of post-discharge health services for children born very preterm. *Journal of Paediatrics and Child Health, 44*(5), 281–284.

Purdy, I. B., & Melwak, M. A. (2012). Who is at risk? High-risk infant follow-up. *Newborn and Infant Nursing Reviews, 12*(4), 221–226. doi:10.1053/j.nainr.2012.09.011

Radecki, L., Olson, L. M., Frintner, M. P., Tanner, J. L., & Stein, M. T. (2009). What do families want from well-child care? Including parents in the rethinking siscussion. *Pediatrics, 124*(3), 858–865. doi:10.1542/peds.2008–2352

Radtke, J. V. (2011). The paradox of breastfeeding-associated morbidity among late preterm infants. *Journal of Obstetric, Gynecologic, and Neonatal Nursing, 40*(1), 9–24. doi:10.1111/j.1552-6909.2010.01211.x

Ralser, E., Mueller, W., Haberland, C., Fink, F.-M., Gutenberger, K.-H., Strobl, R., & Kiechl-Kohlendorfer, U. (2012). Rehospitalization in the first 2 years of life in children born preterm. *Acta Paediatrica, 101*(1), e1–e5. doi:10.1111/j.1651-2227.2011.02404.x

Rautava, P., Lehtonen, L., Helenius, H., & Sillanpaa, M. (2003). Effect of newborn hospitalization on family and child behavior: A 12-year follow-up study. *Pediatrics, 111*(2), 277–283.

Ravn, I. H., Smith, L., Lindemann, R., Smeby, N. A., Kyno, N. M., Bunch, E. H., & Sandvik, L. (2011). Effect of early intervention on social interaction between mothers and preterm infants at 12 months of age: A randomized controlled trial. *Infant Behavior and Development, 34*(2), 215–225. doi:10.1016/j.infbeh.2010.11.004

Ray, K. N., Escobar, G. J., & Lorch, S. A. (2010). Premature infants born to adolescent mothers: Health care utilization after initial discharge. *Academic Pediatrics, 10*(5), 302–308. doi:10.1016/j.acap.2010.07.005

Robertson, C. M., Howarth, T. M., Bork, D. L., & Dinu, I. A. (2009). Permanent bilateral sensory and neural hearing loss of children after neonatal intensive care because of extreme prematurity: A thirty-year study. *Pediatrics, 123*(5), e797–e807. doi:10.1542/peds.2008-2531

Rogers, C. E., Kidokoro, H., Wallendorf, M., & Inder, T. E. (2012). Identifying mothers of very preterm infants at-risk for postpartum depression and anxiety before discharge. *Journal of Perinatology, 33*(3),171–176.

Rowe, J., & Jones, L. (2010). Discharge and beyond: A longitudinal study comparing stress and coping in parents of preterm infants. *Journal of Neonatal Nursing, 16*(6), 258–266. doi:10.1016/j.jnn.2010.07.018

Rubin, R. (1984). *Maternal identity and the maternal experience*. New York, NY: Springer.

Russell, R. B., Green, N. S., Steiner, C. A., Meikle, S., Howse, J. L., Poschman, K., . . . Petrini, J. R. (2007). Cost of hospitalization for preterm and low birth weight infants in the United States. *Pediatrics, 120*(1), e1–e9. doi:10.1542/peds.2006-2386

Saigal, S. (1999). Maternal psychological distress and parenting stress after the birth of a very low-birth-weight infant. *Journal of Pediatrics, 135*(3), 397.

Saigal, S., Pinelli, J., Streiner, D. L., Boyle, M., & Stoskopf, B. (2010). Impact of extreme prematurity on family functioning and maternal health 20 years later. *Pediatrics, 126*(1), e81–e88. doi:10.1542/peds.2009-2527

Schlittenhart, J. M., Smart, D., Miller, K., & Severtson, B. (2011). Preparing parents for NICU discharge. *Nursing for Women's Health, 15*(6), 484–494. doi:10.1111/j.1751-486X.2011.01676.x

Segre, L. S., O'Hara, M. W., Arndt, S., & Beck, C. T. (2010). Nursing care for postpartum depression, part 1: Do nurses think they should offer both screening and counseling? *American Journal of Maternal Child Nursing, 35*(4), 220–225. doi:10.1097/NMC.0b013e3181dd9d81

Shah, P. E., Clements, M., & Poehlmann, J. (2011). Maternal resolution of grief after preterm birth: Implications for infant attachment security. *Pediatrics, 127*(2), 284–292. doi:10.1542/peds.2010-1080

Shaw, R. J., Bernard, R. S., Deblois, T., Ikuta, L. M., Ginzburg, K., & Koopman, C. (2009). The relationship between acute stress disorder and posttraumatic stress disorder in the neonatal intensive care unit. *Psychosomatics, 50*(2), 131–137. doi:10.1176/appi.psy.50.2.131

Sherman, M. P., Aylward, G. P., & Shoemaker, C. T. (2011). *Follow-up of the NICU patient*. Retrieved from http://emedicine.medscape.com/article/1833812-overview

Shieh, S. J., Chen, H. L., Liu, F. C., Liou, C. C., Lin, Y. i. H., Tseng, H. I., & Wang, R. H. (2010). The effectiveness of structured discharge education on maternal confidence, caring knowledge and growth of premature newborns. *Journal of Clinical Nursing, 19*(23–24), 3307–3313. doi:10.1111/j.1365-2702.2010.03382.x

Silberstein, D., Geva, R., Feldman, R., Gardner, J. M., Karmel, B. Z., Rozen, H., & Kuint, J. (2009). The transition to oral feeding in low-risk premature infants: Relation to infant neurobehavioral functioning and mother-infant feeding interaction. *Early Human Development, 85*(3), 157–162. doi:10.1016/j.earlhumdev.2008.07.006

Silverstein, M., Feinberg, E., Young, R., & Sauder, S. (2010). Maternal depression, perceptions of children's social aptitude and reported activity restriction among former very low birthweight infants. *Archives of Disease in Childhood, 95*(7), 521–525. doi:10.1136/adc.2009.181735

Sloan, K., Rowe, J., & Jones, L. (2008). Stress and coping in fathers following the birth of a preterm infant. *Journal of Neonatal Nursing, 14*(4), 108–115. doi:10.1016/j.jnn.2007.12.009

Smith, V. C., Dukhovny, D., Zupancic, J. A., Gates, H. B., & Pursley, D. M. (2012). Neonatal intensive care unit discharge preparedness: Primary care implications. *Clinical Pediatrics*, 1–8. doi:10.1177/0009922811433036

Smith, V. C., Young, S., Pursley, D. M., McCormick, M. C., & Zupancic, J. A. (2009). Are families prepared for discharge from the NICU? *Journal of Perinatology, 29*(9), 623–629. doi:10.1038/jp.2009.58

Sneath, N. (2009). Discharge teaching in the NICU: Are parents prepared? An integrative review of parents' perceptions. *Neonatal Network, 28*(4), 237–246.

South, A. P., Wessel, J. J., Sberna, A., Patel, M., & Morrow, A. L. (2011). Hospital readmission among infants with gastroschisis. *Jornal of Perinatology, 31*(8), 546–550. doi:10.1038/jp.2010.206

Spangler-Torok, L. (2001). *Maternal perceptions of the technology-dependent infant* (Doctoral dissertation), University of Cincinnati, OH.

Spencer-Smith, M. M., Spittle, A. J., Doyle, L. W., Lee, K. J., Lorefice, L., Suetin, A., . . . Anderson, P. J. (2012). Long-term benefits of home-based preventive care for preterm infants: A randomized trial. *Pediatrics, 130*(6), 1094–1101. doi:10.1542/peds.2012-0426

Spicer, A., Pinelli, J., Saigal, S., Wu, Y. W., Cunningham, C., & DiCenso, A. (2008). Health status and health service utilization of infants and mothers during the first year after neonatal intensive care. *Advances in Neonatal Care, 8*(1), 33–41. doi:10.1097/01.ANC.0000311015.56263.6f

Tang, B. G., Feldman, H. M., Huffman, L. C., Kagawa, K. J., & Gould, J. B. (2012). Missed opportunities in the referral of high-risk infants to early intervention. *Pediatrics, 129*(6), 1027–1034. doi:10.1542/peds.2011-2720

Teti, D. M., Hess, C. R., & O'Connell, M. (2005). Parental perceptions of infant vulnerability in a preterm sample: Prediction from maternal adaptation to parenthood during the neonatal period. *Journal of Developmental and Behavioral Pediatrics, 26*(4), 283–292.

Tudehope, D., Gibbons, K., Cormack, B., & Bloomfield, F. (2012). Growth monitoring of low birthweight infants: What references to use? *Journal of Paediatrics and Child Health, 48*(9), 759–767. doi:10.1111/j.1440-1754.2012.02534.x

Underwood, M. A., Danielsen, B., & Gilbert, W. M. (2007). Cost, causes and rates of rehospitalization of preterm infants. *Journal of Perinatology, 27*(10), 614–619. doi:10.1038/sj.jp.7211801

Usatin, D., Liljestrand, P., Kuzniewicz, M. W., Escobar, G. J., & Newman, T. B. (2010). Effect of neonatal jaundice and phototherapy on the frequency of first-year outpatient visits. *Pediatrics, 125*(4), 729–734. doi:10.1542/peds.2009–0172

U.S. Department of Education. (2001). *To assure the free appropriate public education of all children with disabilities: Twenty-third annual report to congress on the implementation of the individuals with disabilities act*. Washington, DC.

Vanderveen, J. A., Bassler, D., Robertson, C. M., & Kirpalani, H. (2009). Early interventions involving parents to improve neurodevelopmental outcomes of premature infants: A meta-analysis. *Journal of Perinatology, 29*(5), 343–351. doi:10.1038/jp.2008.229

Verkerk, G., Jeukens-Visser, M., Houtzager, B., Koldewijn, K., van Wassenaer, A., Nollet, F., & Kok, J. (2012). The infant behavioral assessment and intervention program in very low birth weight infants; outcome on executive functioning, behaviour and cognition at preschool age. *Early Human Development, 88*(8), 699–705. doi:10.1016/j.earlhumdev.2012.02.004

Vohr, B., Jodoin-Krauzyk, J., Tucker, R., Johnson, M. J., Topol,D., & Ahlgren, M. (2008). Early language outcomes of early-identified infants with permanent hearing loss at 12 to 16 months of age. *Pediatrics, 122*(3), 535–544. doi:10.1542/peds.2007-2028

Wade, K. C., Lorch, S. A., Bakewell-Sachs, S., Medoff-Cooper, B., Silber, J. H., & Escobar, G. J. (2008). Pediatric care for preterm infants after NICU discharge: High number of office visits and prescription medications. *Journal of Perinatology, 28*, 696–701.

Walker, K., Holland, A. J., Halliday, R., & Badawi, N. (2012). Which high-risk infants should we follow-up and how should we do it? *Journal of Paediatrics and Child Health, 48*(9), 789–793. doi:10.1111/j.1440-1754.2012.02540.x

Wang, C. J., Elliott, M. N., McGlynn, E. A., Brook, R. H., & Schuster, M. A. (2008). Population-based assessments of ophthalmologic and audiologic follow-up in children with very low birth weight enrolled in Medicaid: A quality-of-care study. *Pediatrics, 121*(2), e278–e285. doi:10.1542/peds.2007-0136

Watson, G. (2011). Parental liminality: A way of understanding the early experiences of parents who have a very preterm infant. *Journal of Clinical Nursing, 20*(9–10), 1462–1471. doi:10.1111/j.1365-2702.2010.03311.x

Wen, L. M., Baur, L. A., Simpson, J. M., Rissel, C., & Flood, V. M. (2011). Effectiveness of an early intervention on infant feeding practices and "tummy time": A randomized controlled trial. *Archives of Pediatrics and Adolescent Medicine, 165*(8), 701–707. doi:10.1001/archpediatrics.2011.115

Westerberg, A. C., Henriksen, C., Ellingvag, A., Veierod, M. B., Juliusson, P. B., Nakstad, B., . . . Drevon, C. A. (2010). First year growth among very low birth weight infants. *Acta Paediatrica, 99*(4), 556–562. doi:10.1111/j.1651-2227.2009.01667.x

White, R. D. (2010). Single-family room design in the neonatal intensive care unit-challenges and opportunities. *Newborn and Infant Nursing Reviews, 10*(2), 83–86.

Whyte, R. (2010). Safe discharge of the late preterm infant. *Paediatrics and Child Health, 15*(10), 655–666.

Willis, V. (2008). Parenting preemies: A unique program for family support and education after NICU discharge. *Advances in Neonatal Care, 8*(4), 221–230. doi:10.1097/01.ANC.0000333710.83517.19

Yee, W., & Ross, S. (2006). Communicating with parents of high-risk infants in neonatal intensive care. *Paediatrics and Child Health, 11*(5), 291–294.

Zabielski, M. T. (1994). Recognition of maternal identity in preterm and fullterm mothers. *Maternal Child Nursing Journal, 22*(1), 2–36.

Zanardo, V., & Freato, F. (2001). Home oxygen therapy in infants with bronchopulmonary dysplasia: Assessment of parental anxiety. *Early Human Development, 65*(1), 39–46.

Zelkowitz, P., Na, S., Wang, T., Bardin, C., & Papageorgiou, A. (2011). Early maternal anxiety predicts cognitive and behavioural outcomes of VLBW children at 24 months corrected age. *Acta Paediatrica*. doi:10.1111/j.1651-2227.2010.02128.x

Zelkowitz, P., Papageorgiou, A., Bardin, C., & Wang, T. (2009). Persistent maternal anxiety affects the interaction between mothers and their very low birthweight children at 24 months. *Early Human Development, 85*(1), 51–58.

UNIT VII: NEONATAL CARE IN THE NEW MILLENNIUM: CHALLENGES AND OPPORTUNITIES

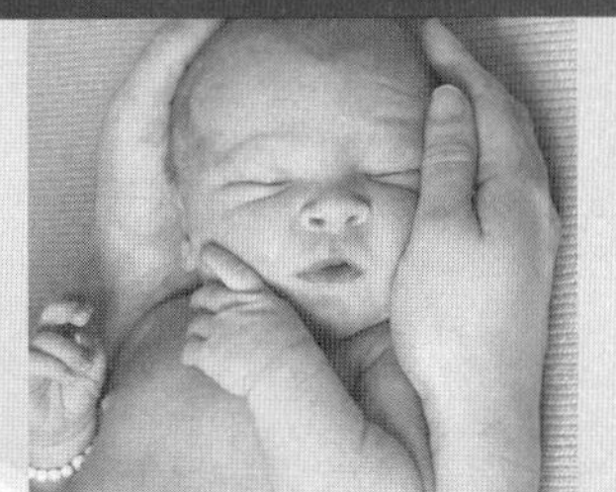

CHAPTER 36

Trends in Neonatal Care Delivery

■ Carole Kenner and Jana L. Pressler

This chapter briefly identifies some of the current trends in neonatal care. Today's neonatal care is shaped by the onslaught of Institute of Medicine (IOM) reports on patient safety, quality, technology, consumer involvement, and the need for an interdisciplinary approach to care. Fiscal constraints coupled with fierce competition have put serious dents in the perinatal regionalization model of care delivery with well-defined levels of care. The Affordable Care Act, which became law in March 2010, has the potential to impact coverage for women and children since it changes funding for Medicaid. While some states continue to argue about the legality of this law, changes are already occurring. In 2010 the IOM released *The Future of Nursing: Leading Change, Advancing Health Report*, which clearly identified nurses as the backbone of health care delivery and key players in health care reform. As McGrath (2011) noted, changes in health care will reconfigure neonatal health care. One growing area of change is in follow-up and family-centered care that is in line with the IOM's (2003) recommendation for patient-focused care. Scientific breakthroughs in genetics and technologic advances already have pushed the definition of viability and have brought with it the long-term consequences of comorbidities that can last a lifetime. The demand for evidence to support nursing practice is growing expeditiously.

LEVELS OF CARE

In the early 1990s, the report *Toward Improving the Outcome of Pregnancy: The 90s and Beyond (TIOPII)* (Committee on Perinatal Health, 1993) illustrated the need for levels of care and a regionalization plan for education and practice. The need to have high-risk perinatal care that also provided educational outreach to the community was embraced. The definitions for levels of care were incorporated in the work by the American Academy of Pediatrics (AAP) and the American College of Obstetrics and Gynecology (ACOG) in *Guidelines for Perinatal Care* (AAP/ACOG, 2007). *Toward Improving the Outcome of Pregnancy III* (TIOPIII; MOD, 2010), like TIOPII, emphasizes the need for preconception health through infancy to impact maternal infant outcomes. TIOPIII (MOD, 2010) builds on quality, safety, and performance initiatives for health professionals and health care delivery systems. Application of evidence-based care guidelines is a cornerstone of this work. Endorsed by the IOM, the theme of quality of care and safety will continue for many years. Similarly, addressing the other key themes is dependent on not only health care financing, but also differing health care needs and health care providers' understanding of what is needed and ongoing. The five key TIOPIII (MOD, 2010) themes are:

1. Assuring the uptake of robust perinatal quality improvement and safety initiatives
2. Creating equity and decreasing disparities in perinatal care and outcomes
3. Empowering women and families with information to enable the development of full partnerships between health care providers and patients and shared decision making in perinatal care
4. Standardizing the regionalization of perinatal services
5. Strengthening the national vital statistics system (MOD, 2010 p. ix)

The AAP Committee on Fetus and Newborn (COFN) (2004a, 2004b) acknowledges that, as the specialty of neonatal care has become more complex and as smaller and smaller infants have and are continuing to survive, the three levels of care (i.e., primary, secondary, tertiary) are inadequate for describing the care required. Further, some of the most highly specialized technologies are not needed in every community. Uniformity of care and integration of services are critical to the quality and outcome factors today.

Box 36.1 reflects the proposed definitions for levels of care. The COFN has contributed to each edition of the TIOPIII. The COFN (2011), in preparation for

BOX 36.1

PROPOSED UNIFORM DEFINITIONS FOR CAPABILITIES ASSOCIATED WITH THE HIGHEST LEVEL OF NEONATAL CARE WITHIN AN INSTITUTION

Level I Neonatal Care (Basic)

Well-newborn nursery has the capabilities to

- Provide neonatal resuscitation at every delivery
- Evaluate and provide postnatal care to healthy newborn infants
- Stabilize and provide care for infants born at 35 to 37 weeks gestation who remain physiologically stable
- Stabilize newborn infants who are ill and those born at less than 35 weeks gestation until transfer to a facility that can provide the appropriate level of neonatal care

Level II Neonatal Care (Specialty)

Special care nursery: Level II units are subdivided into two categories on the basis of their ability to provide assisted ventilation including continuous positive airway pressure

Level IIA has the capabilities to

- Resuscitate and stabilize preterm or ill infants before transfer to a facility at which newborn intensive care is provided
- Provide care for infants born at greater than 32 weeks gestation and weighing greater than or equal to 1,500 g (1) who have physiologic immaturity such as apnea of prematurity, inability to maintain body temperature, or inability to take oral feedings or (2) who are moderately ill with problems that are expected to resolve rapidly and are not expected to need subspecialty services on an urgent basis
- Provide care for infants who are convalescing after intensive care

Level IIB has the capabilities of

- A level IIA nursery and the additional capability to provide mechanical ventilation for brief durations (<24 hours) or continuous positive airway pressure

Level III (Subspecialty) NICU

Level III NICUs are subdivided into three categories.

Level IIIA NICU has capabilities to

- Provide comprehensive care for infants born at greater than 28 weeks gestation and weighing greater than 1,000 g
- Provide sustained life support limited to conventional mechanical ventilation
- Perform minor surgical procedures such as placement of central venous catheter or inguinal hernia repair

Level IIIB NICU has the capabilities to provide

- Comprehensive care for extremely low-birth-weight infants (≤1,000 g and ≤28 weeks gestation)
- Advanced respiratory support such as high-frequency ventilation and inhaled nitric oxide for as long as required
- Prompt and on-site access to a full range of pediatric medical subspecialists
- Advanced imaging, with interpretation on an urgent basis, including computed tomography, magnetic resonance imaging, and echocardiography
- Pediatric surgical specialists and pediatric anesthesiologists on-site or at a closely related institution to perform major surgery such as ligation of patent ductus arteriosus and repair of abdominal wall defects, necrotizing enterocolitis with bowel perforation, tracheoesophageal fistula or esophageal atresia, and myelomeningocele

Level IIIC NICU has the capabilities of

- A level IIIB NICU and also is located within an institution that has the capability to provide extracorporeal membrane oxygenation (ECMO) and surgical repair of complex congenital cardiac malformations that require cardiopulmonary bypass.

From the Committee on Fetus and Newborn (2004a).

publication of the seventh edition of the *Guidelines for Perinatal Care*, has recommended inclusion of content in this new edition on:

1. Continuous quality improvement
2. Patient safety
3. Interhospital transfer of pregnant women and neonates
4. Neonatal complications and management of the high-risk neonate
5. Compassionate and comfort care
6. Assessment of the late preterm
7. Glucose and pulse oximetry screening for critical congenital heart disease (CCHD)
8. Hypoxic-ischemic encephalopathy (HIE) and use of hypothermia as a treatment for HIE
9. Discharge to home—including discharge of infants dependent on technology
10. Recognition of the need for evidence to support vitamin D supplementation and iron supplements for preterm infants are new areas included in the updated guidelines.

Congenital heart diseases to be included in universal newborn screening have been discussed. The Centers for Disease Control and Prevention (CDC, 2012) identifies CCHD to be comprised of seven distinct defects; hypoplastic left heart syndrome, pulmonary atresia (with intact septum), tetralogy of Fallot, total anomalous pulmonary venous return, transposition of the great arteries, tricuspid atresia, and truncus arteriosus. These defects represent about 17% to 31% of all congenital heart diseases that are found in newborns (Kemper et al., 2011; Knapp, Metterville, Kemper, Prosser, & Perrin, 2010). The rationale for including this type of congenital heart disease screening in the universal newborn screening is that the symptoms of these conditions might not be apparent in the neonate prior to hospital discharge (CDC, 2012).

Another area of significant concern is high-risk follow-up. As more infants are surviving, the relative lack of consistency of how follow-up is conducted or who is eligible to receive follow-up care serves as a gap in care providers' knowledge. Toward this end, in June 2002 the National Institute of Child Health and Human Development (NICHD), National Institute of Neurologic Disorders and Stroke (NINDS), and CDC convened a workshop to begin to examine this gap. They also recognized that differences in data collection methods have led to difficulties with comparing outcomes both within and across centers (NICHD, NINDS, & CDC, 2004). To improve long-term developmental and physical neonatal outcomes, neonatal follow-up care must be clearly defined with levels corresponding to NICU levels of care. In the next decade this seminal work will shape the post-NICU experience for neonates and their families. Since 2002 many articles have been published on the lack of uniformity of guidelines for hospital discharge for newborns, the lack of qualified providers available for follow-up and early intervention programs in spite of referrals to high-risk clinics, a lack of parent preparedness for infant discharge, and the need for more research studies on the postdischarge outcomes of infants who were born extremely low birth weight, technology dependent, or who have had surgery (De Jesus et al., 2012; Dobson & Hunt, 2012; Fink, 2011; Pinto et al., 2012; Smith, Dukhovy, Zupancic, Gates, & Pursley, 2012; Trzaski, Hagadorn, Hussain, Schwenn, & Wittenzellner, 2012). In addition, it has been pointed out that often mothers never bring their infants back for the first neonatal follow appointment postdischarge (Ballantyne, Stevens, Guttmann, Willan, & Rosenbaum, 2012) yet the reasons for this lack of follow-up are unknown, creating another knowledge gap (Ballantyne et al., 2012). An additional area of concern is the missed opportunities for immunizing infants prior to discharge. Navar-Boggan, Halsey, Escobar, Golden, and Klein (2012) found that 27% of infants who were discharged from the NICU at or before 2 months of age had not received any vaccinations. The reasons for this problem of underimmunization are in urgent need of further study. Family-centered care and the need to include the family in care during the NICU stay, as well as the growing recognition for the need to teach families about developmental care both within and outside the hospital, continue to be at the forefront of neonatal care. Schlittenhart, Smart, Miller, and Severtson (2011) have developed an evidence-based comprehensive teaching tool for parents of infants discharged from the NICU. This tool exemplifies the trend for more evidence-based guidelines for discharge preparedness.

DEVELOPMENTAL CARE

Developmental outcomes have been at the forefront of care for many years, but today there is also a movement toward supporting and advocating *individualized family-centered care*. This care coincides with the IOM's (2001) emphasis on patient-focused care as a method to increase quality. Another aspect of this care supports IOM's initiative in interprofessional or interdisciplinary care and that is developmentally supportive care. Individualized family-centered care incorporates knowledge of growth and development; factors that interfere with positive growth such as prematurity, environmental noise, and lighting levels; the interface with physiologic responses to stress-inhibited growth factors and increases in cortisol levels; and positioning, to name only a few of the focal topics. Chapter 31 gives more in-depth information on individualized family-centered care.

The NICU environment and its impact on development from a long-term perspective have spawned growth in the use of Recommended Standards for Newborn ICU Design (White, 2007) throughout the world (for more information, see Chapter 31). These recommendations come from an interdisciplinary group of architects, institutional planners, developmental specialists, nurses, physicians, and parents. The use of such standards to renovate or build new NICUs will increase, as will the overall incorporation of individualized, family-centered, developmental care. One sign of this is the publishing of an interdisciplinary book on this subject, *Developmental Care of Newborns and Infants* by Kenner and McGrath (2010). This second edition contains levels of evidence to indicate how developmental interventions are supported by scientific studies. The recognition of neurobehavioral stability and the links to developmental care and long-term outcomes are increasing (Montirosso et al., 2012). Follow-up studies of formerly sick and premature infants are important, as they are used to examine developmental outcomes, the need for developmental care from the time of NICU admission, and the potential costs associated with physiologic complications and sequelae that might be reduced or avoided with developmental care. Developmental surveillance and screenings are needed if problems are to be detected early (Thomas, Cotton, Pan, & Ratliff-Schaub, 2012).

NEONATAL STATISTICS

Neonatal statistics are difficult to follow because of the lack of consistent terminology about the age of the fetus, neonate, and infant. To address that problem, the AAP COFN (2004a, 2004b) developed definitions of gestational, postmenstrual, chronologic, and corrected ages. These definitions are presented in Table 36.1.

According to the National Center on Health Statistics, the U.S. preterm birth rate fell in 2010 for the first time in many years to 11.99% (2011). In part, this was probably due to one or more of the following factors:

- The cesarean delivery rate decreased to 32.8% of all births
- A decrease occurred in low-birth-weight (<2,500 g) infants at 8.15%
- The rate of very-low-birth-weight (<1,500 g) infants stayed steady at 1.45% (National Vital Statistics Reports, 2011)

TABLE 36.1

AGE TERMINOLOGY DURING THE PERINATAL PERIOD

Term	Definition	Units of Time
Gestational age	Time between the first day of the last menstrual period and day of delivery	Completed weeks
Chronologic age	Time since birth	Days, weeks, months, years
Postmenstrual age	Gestational age plus chronologic age	Weeks
Corrected age	Chronologic age reduced by the number of weeks born before 40 weeks gestation	Weeks, months

From the Committee on Fetus and Newborn (2004b).

The U.S. neonatal mortality rate was reported at 4.19 deaths per 1,000 live births in 2009, down 1.9% from the previous year. Even more impressive, postneonatal deaths through the first year of life were reported at 2.24 deaths per 1,000 live births, a decrease of 3.4% from 2008 (U.S. Department of Health and Human Services, Health Resources and Services Administration, Maternal and Child Health Bureau, 2011). In 2007, over the course of 1 year, the infant mortality rate in the United States rose from 6.7 to 6.8 per 1,000 live births (MOD, 2012). According to the Central Intelligence Agency (CIA, 2012), the infant mortality rate in 2012 was still high, at 5.98 (6.6%) deaths per 1,000 live births. These data represent a less than optimal outcome than expected for a resource-rich country such as the United States. The factors that impact these data continue to reflect the health disparities and underinsured status of many women and children in the United States (MOD, 2012).

The March of Dimes (MOD), World Health Organization the Partnership for Maternal, Newborn and Child Health, Save the Children, and World Health Organization published a report, *Born Too Soon* (WHO, 2012), endorsed by more than 40 international organizations, including the Council of International Neonatal Nurses (COINN). This report represents landmark collaboration between governmental and nongovernmental agencies whose sole purpose of working together is to address Millennium Development Goals—especially #4—to improve outcomes of newborns and infants. The statistics are alarming: 15 million infants worldwide are born preterm; over 1 million children die each year due to prematurity, and prematurity is the leading cause of neonatal deaths and the second leading cause of death of all children under 5 years of age (WHO, 2012). The importance of these findings is that health care professionals must increase awareness of the serious morbidities associated with prematurity as the MOD and others have done and begin to put resources behind preconception health if one believes that maternal health is inextricably linked to prematurity and other complications. There is also growing recognition that late preterm birth (34–36 6/7 weeks) must be treated as a preterm birth, with special needs for late preterm infants to receive appropriate care. For example, mortality rates of late preterm infants are higher if there is a congenital heart defect found than if the same is found in a term infant (Swenson, Dechert, Schumacher, & Attar, 2012). There also is a need for more uniform guidelines for care for the late preterm infant. A national guideline for care of late preterm infants is being developed based on many organizations working together to bring consensus to this topic. Long-term school performance outcomes represent another area needing research since early findings indicate poor school performance at 5 years among both early and late preterm infants (Quigley et al., 2012).

Another area requiring additional research is readmissions following a NICU stay. Most of the research to date has focused on physiologic problems, yet the psychosocial needs and readiness of parents for discharge may also be impacting these figures. For example, re-hospitalizations during the first 2 years of life following a premature birth are often related to respiratory problems (Ralser et al., 2012). But how many other formerly premature infants are readmitted due to parental stress? This is an area of science that needs more emphasis and greater expansion.

MATERNAL/FETAL NEONATAL UNITS

Fetal surgery has been performed for more than three decades. The outcomes of these fetuses/infants have improved as best practices have evolved (Partridge & Flake, 2012; Shue, Harrison, & Hirose, 2012). Until recently, fetuses that remained in utero until a viable birth occurred were cared for in an "everyday" NICU. Now there is recognition of the need for more specialized care for infants who received surgery while in utero. Maternal/fetal/neonatal subunits or additions to NICUs have been developed for providing specialized care. Prototypes of this model are found at Children's Hospital of Philadelphia (CHOP) and Cincinnati Children's Hospital. These units include perinatal/neonatal/pediatric physician specialists who are familiar with fetal surgery, genetics, pediatric surgery, and the needs of the neonate and family after birth (http://www.fetalcarecenter.org). These units are growing throughout the United States and address the need for more collaboration between maternal/fetal specialists and neonatal/pediatric specialists.

GENETICS

Genetic breakthroughs as a result of the Human Genome Project (HGP) are influencing health and health care. Genomics, the term that refers to the interaction between genetic makeup and the environment, is gradually shaping how health is promoted. The U.S. Surgeon General, along with the work of the National Human Genome Research Institute (NHGRI) (http://www.genome.gov), advocates the use of the Family History Tool that incorporates health history in the traditional sense along with genetic history. Use of this tool coupled with knowledge of newborn screening tests will influence how health professionals plan and implement newborn care. One of the newer areas of emphasis by NHGRI is severe combined immunodeficiency syndrome (SCID), which appears to be related to several genetic mutations that may be preventable in the future (http://www.genome.gov/13014325). As another example, if an infant is born to a family with a history of diabetes, then the development of healthy eating habits to avoid obesity and other risk factors for diabetes should begin in the neonatal period. A genomics thrust then changes how care is planned and how it needs to be individualized. It also emphasizes the need for individualized family-centered care.

Another aspect of genetics is the controversy over the number of tests that a newborn should have, to prevent long-term complications of neonatal conditions and to improve quality of life. The MOD advocates up to 30 tests, whereas some state newborn screening programs suggest only 4. The question then becomes: Just because the test can be run and is minimally invasive, should it be done? Who decides? What are the ramifications—is there any danger of insurance discrimination? These ethical questions are at the heart of the debate about newborn screening and the intersection with genetic testing. There are websites and organizations dedicated to providing consumer-friendly information for parents on these topics to help them decide a course of action. Two good sources of information are KidsHealth for Parents (http://www.kidshealth.org/parent/system/medical/genetics.html) and the MOD (http://www.marchofdimes.com/pnhec/298_834.asp).

Another site that focuses on policy and newborn screening is the Genetics and Public Policy Center (http://www.dnapolicy.org/policy.gt.php). For general information on the HGP and resources for health professionals and families, see: (http://www.ornl.gov/sci/techresources/Human_Genome/home.shtml). Advances in genetic frontiers will continue to change neonatal care and improve outcomes. Areas of growing research include the use of stem cells for treatment of chronic lung disease, epigenetics, and linkages between maternal-fetal programming and behavioral outcomes (New York Academy of Sciences and Cincinnati Children's Hospital Medical Center, 2012), epigenetics and regulation of interuterine growth (Zinkhan et al., 2012), epigenetics and impact on later-life obesity (Rhee, Phelan, & McCaffery, 2012), biomarkers for neurologic problems including brain injury (Merhar, 2012), and stress markers in the development of necrotizing enterocolitis (Perrone et al., 2012). These are just a few of the new frontiers in neonatal care in the United States and abroad.

GLOBALIZATION

Recommendations for NICU standards and professional programs such as Neonatal Resuscitation, S.T.A.B.L.E. (Sugar & Safe Care, Temperature, Airway, Blood Pressure, Lab Work, and Emotional Support [http://www.stableprogram.org]), and Helping Babies Breathe supported by the AAP (http://www.helpingbabiesbreathe.org) are being used globally. Neonatal care issues are international. This era of globalization is changing the way care practices and outcomes are viewed. Protocols for care are developed so that they can be adapted for cultural sensitivity, technology availability, and geographic needs. The push toward evidence-based practice and the use of Cochrane reviews, the Joanna Briggs Institute Collaborative Systematic Reviews, and Vermont Oxford materials all are bringing neonatal care to a level that is supported by scientific findings rather than primarily by tradition. This movement is global and is being influenced by hospitals seeking Magnet status that espouses evidence-based practice guidelines to ensure quality care and more positive outcomes. As this influence continues, there will be shifts in how care is implemented. The COINN (http://www.coinnurses.org) is partnering with other organizations such as the European Foundation for the Care of Newborn Infants (http://www.efcni.org), the White Ribbon Alliance for Safe Motherhood (http://www.whiteribbonalliance.org), and many others worldwide to address policy, care, education, and research initiatives that touch the lives of mothers, fathers, newborns, and their siblings. These collaborations with the use of social media tools, listservs, and blogs will only increase in the next few years. Evidence-based guidelines for care are being adapted for use worldwide. One example of a growing global area of concern is palliative care for infants.

PALLIATIVE AND END-OF-LIFE CARE

There is an increasing awareness of the need for effective pain management. The Joint Commission on Accreditation of Healthcare Organizations (JCAHO) has declared pain as the fifth vital sign across the life span. For neonates, pain management is complicated by the patient's nonverbal status and the need to rely on physiologic parameters to measure pain and pain management responses. There is a need for more evidence to support pain management as seen in Chapter 23. One area that has increased the recognition of this gap in our neonatal care knowledge is palliative and end-of-life care.

Whether anyone likes to acknowledge it or not, some children are born dying. There are infants who cannot be saved despite the availability of sophisticated technology, and others who have life-threatening illnesses and who can survive. Those in the latter group, like all patients, deserve comfort or palliative care. (Chapter 33 reports on this new frontier of neonatal care.)

HEALTH INSURANCE PORTABILITY AND ACCOUNTABILITY ACT

Passage of the Health Insurance Portability and Accountability Act (HIPAA) of 1996 represented a major change in health information and how it could be disclosed to other agencies and persons. The privacy rule was enacted to protect an individual from having personal health information disclosed in such a way as to potentially bring harm or result in insurance discrimination (U.S. Department of Health and Human Services, 2012). The rule outlines how, when, and to whom information can be released and how it can be used (U.S. Department of Health and Human Services, 2012). As a result of this law, information regarding health and condition can only be disclosed with permission from the family (U.S. Department of Health and Human Services, 2012). Health care providers can provide information to other providers as needed and within the confines of the law. For example, electronic medical records are now common; information entered on mobile devices is also common, but the transmission should be encrypted and protected from accidental release. Transmission of information to insurance companies, governmental agencies, or for billing purposes must be in compliance with HIPAA (U.S. Department of Health and Human Services, 2012). It is beyond the scope of this chapter to discuss the law and the privacy rule in detail but health care providers must become familiar with the aspects that affect their practice. Health professionals have been fired and students dismissed from nursing programs for sharing information on social media boards or for looking at the medical records of patients whom they are not directly caring for at the present time. Discussing private health information is a violation of the privacy rule. Many health care agencies and some educational institutions are developing policies regarding the sharing of protected, identifiable information.

Technology advances and sharing of information will increase. Families use the Internet to share information with family members about their infant while in the NICU. They surf the net for information to understand their infant's condition. They are encouraged to use their infant's personal health information to be a partner in the care. Health providers share information from inpatient to outpatient and specialty services and in efforts to provide better care coordination and promote patient safety. All of these actions are good but must be considered within the context of HIPAA where it applies. Researchers must also abide by the HIPAA regulations and ensure that information and data are de-identified and protected from indiscriminate sharing.

Population Health

The National Institutes of Health (NIH) has expanded funding to support development of the Centers for Population Health and Health Disparities. These centers focus on developing strategies to address disparities to include the social determinants of health–social, behavioral, genetic, environmental, and biological. There are many practical applications for population health for neonatal/family care. Population health refers to actions or factors such as maternal factors that impact the health outcomes of the infant. Preconception health, factors that relate to prematurity and neonatal illness, are examples of areas that fit within population health. Brindle, Flageole, and Wales (2012) examined maternal factors that might affect the health outcomes of infants with gastroschisis. This study was conducted in Canada and found that younger women who used drugs during pregnancy in rural or very isolated regions of Canada, were giving birth to infants with gastroschisis (Brindle et al., 2012). This study is an example of population health and the linkages with social determinants and with specific neonatal conditions. This type of research will grow as health care includes more population management, including follow-up care for neonates and their families.

SUMMARY

This chapter has briefly highlighted some of the recent trends in neonatal care. With of all the new breakthroughs in care, it is hard to imagine what the next decade will bring.

ONLINE RESOURCES

Genetics & Public Policy Center
http://www.dnapolicy.org/policy.gt.php

Helping Babies Breathe supported by the American Academy of Pediatrics
http://www.helpingbabiesbreathe.org

KidsHealth for Parents
http://kidshealth.org/parent/system/medical/genetics.html

March of Dimes
http://www.marchofdimes.com/pnhec/298_834.asp

REFERENCES

American Academy of Pediatrics & American College of Obstetrics and Gynecology. (2007). *Guidelines for perinatal care* (6th ed.). Elk Grove Village, IL: Authors.

Ballantyne, M., Stevens, B., Guttmann, A., Willan, A. R., & Rosenbaum, P. (2012). Transition to neonatal follow-up programs: Is attendance a problem? [Research Support, Non-U.S. Gov't]. *Journal of Perinatal and Neonatal Nursing, 26*(1), 90–98. doi:10.1097/JPN.0b013e31823f900b

Brindle, M. E., Flageole, H., & Wales, P. W. (2012). Influence of maternal factors on health outcomes in gastroschisis: A Canadian population-based study. *Neonataology, 102*(1), 45–52.

Centers for Disease Control and Prevention. (2012). Screening for critical congenital heart defects. *Pediatric Genetics*. Retrieved from http://www.cdc.gov/ncbddd/pediatricgenetics/pulse.html

Central Intelligence Agency. (2012). The world factbook: Country comparison: Infant mortality rate. Retrieved from https://www.cia.gov/library/publications/the-world-factbook/rankorder/2091rank.html

Committee on Fetus and Newborn. (2004a). American Academy of Pediatrics (AAP) policy statement: Organizational principles to guide and define the child health care system and/or improve the health of all children. *Pediatrics*, *114*(5), 1341–1347.

Committee on Fetus and Newborn. (2004b). American Academy of Pediatrics (AAP) policy statement: Organizational principles to guide the child health care system and/or improve the health of all children. *Pediatrics*, *114*(5), 1362–1364.

Committee on Fetus and Newborn. (2011, October 16). *Report from the Committee on Fetus and Newborn. Presented at American Academy of Pediatrics (AAP) National Conference and Exhibition (NCE)*, Boston, MA.

Committee on Perinatal Health. (1993). *Toward improving the outcome of pregnancy: The 90s and beyond*. White Plains, NY: March of Dimes Birth Defects Foundation.

De Jesus, L. C., Pappas, A., Shankaran, S., Kendrick, D., Das, A., Higgins, R. D., & Human Development Neonatal Research Network. (2012). Risk factors for post-neonatal intensive care unit discharge mortality among extremely low birth weight infants. *Journal of Pediatrics*, doi:10.1016/j.jpeds.2011.12.038

Dobson, N. R., & Hunt, C. E. (2012). Interinstitutional variability in home care interventions after neonatal intensive care unit discharge. [Comment Editorial]. *The Journal of Pediatrics, 160*(2), 187–188. doi:10.1016/j.jpeds.2011.09.033

Fink, A. M. (2011). Early hospital discharge in maternal and newborn care. [Historical Article]. *Journal of Obstetric, Gynecologic, and Neonatal Nursing, 40*(2), 149–156. doi:10.1111/j.1552-6909.2011.01225.x

Institute of Medicine. (2001). *Crossing the quality chasm: The IOM health care quality initiative*. Washington, DC: National Academies Press.

Institute of Medicine. (2003). *Health professions education: A bridge to quality*. Washington, DC: National Academies Press.

Kemper, A. R., Mahle, W. T., Martin, G. R., Cooley, W. C., Kumar, P., Morrow, W. R., & Howell, R. R. (2011). Strategies for implementing screening for critical congenital heart disease. *Pediatrics, 128*(5), e1259–e1267. doi:10.1542/peds.2011-1317.

Kenner, C., & McGrath, J. M. (2010). *Developmental care of newborns & infants: A guide for health professionals* (2nd ed.). Glenview, IL: National Association of Neonatal Nurses (NANN).

Knapp, A. A., Metterville, D. R., Kemper, A. R., Prosser, L., & Perrin, J. M. (2010). *Evidence review: Critical congenital cyanotic heart disease*. Retrieved from http://www.hrsa.gov/advisorycommittees/mchbadvisory/heritabledisorders/nominatecondition/reviews/cyanoticheart.pdf

March of Dimes (MOD). (2010). *Toward improving the outcome of pregnancy III (TIOPIII): Enhancing perinatal health through quality, safety and performance initiatives*. White Plains, NY: MOD.

March of Dimes. (2012). *Peristats*. White Plains, NY: MOD.

McGrath, J. M. (2011). Expert opinion-neonatal healthcare: What does the future hold? *Journal of Perinatal and Neonatal Nursing, 25*(3), 219–221.

Merhar, S. (2012). Biomarkers in neonatal posthemorrhagic hydrocephalus. *Neonatology, 101*(1), 1–7. doi:10.1159/000323498.

Montirosso, R., Del Prete, A., Bellu, R., Tronick, E., Borgatti, R., & Neonatal Adequate Care for Quality of Life Study Group. (2012). Level of NICU quality of developmental care and neurobehavioral performance in very preterm infants. [Research Support, N.I.H., Extramural Research Support, Non-U.S. Gov't]. *Pediatrics, 129*(5), e1129–e1137. doi:10.1542/peds.2011-0813

National Institute of Child Health and Human Development (NICHD), National Institute for Neurologic Disorders and Stroke, and the Centers for Disease Control and Prevention. (2004). Follow-up care of high-risk infants. *Pediatrics*, *114*(5), 1377–1397.

National Vital Statistics Reports. (2011). Births: Preliminary data for 2010. *60*(2). Retrieved from http://www.cdc.gov/nchs/data/nvsr/nvsr60/nvsr60_02.pdf

Navar-Boggan, A. M., Halsey, N. A., Escobar, G. J., Golden, W. C., & Klein, N. P. (2012, May). Under-immunization at discharge from the neonatal intensive care unit. [Research Support, Non-U.S. Gov't]. *Journal of Perinatology, 32*(5), 363–367. doi:10.1038/jp.2011.111. Epub 2011 Aug 11.

New York Academy of Sciences and Cincinnati Children's Hospital Medical Center. (2012). Fetal programming and environmental exposures: Implications for prenatal care and pre-term birth. Retrieved from http://www.nyas.org/Events/Detail.aspx?cid=0080f200-94a0-412f-b4f9-d5a19971f489.

Partridge, E. A., & Flake, A. W. (2012). Maternal-fetal surgery for structural malformations. *Best Practice & Research Clinical Obstetrics & Gynaecology*. doi:10.1016/j.bpobgyn.2012.03.003

Perrone, S., Tataranno, M. L., Negro, S., Cornacchione, S., Longini, M., Proietti, F., & Buonocore, G. (2012). May oxidative stress biomarkers in cord blood predict the occurrence of necrotizing enterocolitis in preterm infants? [Research Support, Non-U.S. Gov't]. *Journal of Maternal-Fetal and Neonatal Medicine, 25*(Suppl. 1), 128–131. doi:10.3109/14767058.2012.663197

Pinto, N. M., Lasa, J., Dominguez, T. E., Wernovsky, G., Tabbutt, S., & Cohen, M. S. (2012). Regionalization in neonatal congenital heart surgery: The impact of distance on outcome after discharge. *Pediatric Cardiology, 33*(2), 229–238. doi:10.1007/s00246-011-0116-4

Quigley, M. A., Poulsen, G., Boyle, E., Wolke, D., Field, D., Alfirevic, Z., & Kurinczuk, J. J. (2012). Early term and late preterm birth are associated with poorer school performance at age 5 years: A cohort study. [Research Support, Non-U.S. Gov't]. *Archives of Disease in Childhood. Fetal and Neonatal Edition, 97*(3), F167–F173. doi:10.1136/archdischild-2011-300888

Ralser, E., Mueller, W., Haberland, C., Fink, F. M., Gutenberger, K. H., Strobl, R., & Kiechl-Kohlendorfer, U. (2012). Rehospitalization in the first 2 years of life in children born preterm. *Acta Paediatrica, 101*(1), e1–e5. doi:10.1111/j.1651–2227.2011.02404.x

Rhee, K. E., Phelan, S., & McCaffery, J. (2012). Early determinants of obesity: Genetic, epigenetic, and in utero influences. *International Journal of Pediatrics, 2012*, 463850. doi:10.1155/2012/463850

Schlittenhart, J. M., Smart, D., Miller, K., & Severtson, B. (2011). Preparing parents for NICU discharge: An evidence-based teaching tool. *Nursing for Women's Health, 15*(6), 485–494. doi:10.1111/j.1751-486X.2011.01676.x

Shue, E. H., Harrison, M., & Hirose, S. (2012). Maternal-fetal surgery: History and general considerations. *Clinics in Perinatology, 39*(2), 269–278. doi:10.1016/j.clp.2012.04.010

Smith, V. C., Dukhovny, D., Zupancic, J. A., Gates, H. B., & Pursley, D. M. (2012). Neonatal intensive care unit discharge preparedness: Primary care implications. *Clinical Pediatrics (Phila), 51*(5), 454–461. doi:10.1177/0009922811433036

Swenson, A. W., Dechert, R. E., Schumacher, R. E., & Attar, M. A. (2012). The effect of late preterm birth on mortality of infants with major congenital heart defects. *Journal of Perinatology, 32*(1), 51–54. doi:10.1038/jp.2011.50

Thomas, S. A., Cotton, W., Pan, X., & Ratliff-Schaub, K. (2012). Comparison of systematic developmental surveillance with standardized developmental screening in primary care. *Clinical Pediatrics (Phila), 51*(2), 154–159. doi:10.1177/0009922811420711

Trzaski, J. M., Hagadorn, J. I., Hussain, N., Schwenn, J., & Wittenzellner, C. (2012). Predictors of successful discontinuation of supplemental oxygen in very low-birth-weight infants with bronchopulmonary dysplasia approaching neonatal intensive care unit discharge. *American Journal of Perinatology, 29*(2), 79–86. doi:10.1055/s-0031-1295646

U.S. Department of Health and Human Services, Health Resources and Services Administration, & Maternal and

Child Health Bureau. (2011). *Child health USA 2011*. Rockville, MD: U.S. Department of Health and Human Services.

U.S. Department of Health and Human Services. (2012). Health information. summary of the HIPAA privacy rule. Retrieved from http://www.hhs.gov/ocr/privacy/hipaa/understanding/summary/index.html

White, R. (2007). *Recommended standards for newborn ICU design: Report of the seventh consensus conference on newborn ICU design*. Retrieved from http://www.nd.edu/~nicudes

World Health Organization (WHO). (2012). *Born Too Soon: The global action report on preterm birth*. Retrieved from http://www.who.int/pmnch/media/news/2012/201204_borntoosoon-report.pdf

Zinkhan, E. K., Fu, Q., Wang, Y., Yu, X., Callaway, C. W., Segar, J. L., & Lane, R. H. (2012). Maternal Hyperglycemia Disrupts Histone 3 Lysine 36 Trimethylation of the IGF-1 Gene. *Journal of Nutrition and Metabolism, 2012*, 930364. doi:10.1155/2012/930364

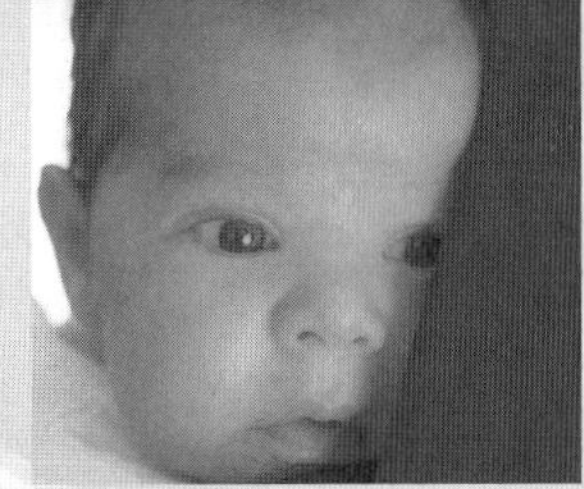

CHAPTER 37

Neonatal Care Using Informatics

■ Susan K. Newbold, Willa H. Drummond, and Tony C. Carnes

Hospitals have successfully used information technology (IT) in past decades to support administrative and financial functions. Recent governmental mandates to reform health care have awakened the interest of many hospitals and provider practices to the value of using IT to support patient care. Effective use of information technologies in neonatal intensive care units (NICUs) or any intensive care unit (ICU), may greatly improve patient care, and patient outcomes, reduce clinician workload, as well as decrease costs. Adoption of computerized technologies holds great promise as computer systems improve each year. Full functionality requires the integration of health care systems through adherence to emerging industry standards for computer-to-computer communication, health care data vocabularies, and quality management. This chapter focuses on the current status and near future advances of NICU IT and provides guidance for choosing and evaluating information systems (IS) for the NICU.

BACKGROUND INFORMATION

The evolution of informatics began in the late 1950s as health care and computer technology began to blend. According to Collen (1995), the term *medical informatics* first appeared in 1974 and became pervasive in the 1980s with the introduction of microcomputers and networked computers. One suggestion is that informatics was created as a new field with the first computerization of a cardiac catheterization laboratory by Dr. Homer Warner, Sr. Informatics expanded quickly as external technological innovations diffused throughout the heath care environment. Informatics pioneers were first classified as a subgroup of bioengineering. Many new names for the field appeared: medical computer science, medical information processing, and medical computer technology. Over time, health care professionals began substituting the term "health" for "medical" because informatics is a broad term that pertains to many health care disciplines, not just medicine. By the 1980s, the terms "clinical," "health," and "nursing" informatics surfaced. Saba and McCormick (2011) contend that the field of informatics emerged in nursing in the 1980s. The nursing profession was searching for a commonly accepted definition for each new and complex domain of knowledge. Various subgroups attempted to define their "domains" in order to clarify their differences and similarities (Collen, 1995). After several definitions were created for "generic" medical informatics, a consensus definition was written by the Long-Range Planning Committee of the National Library of Medicine (NLM) as:

> Medical informatics attempts to provide the theoretical and scientific basis for the application of computer and automated ISs to biomedicine and health affairs. . . . Medical informatics studies biomedical information, data, and knowledge—their storage, retrieval, and optimal use for problem solving and decision making. It touches on all basic and applied fields in biomedical science and is closely tied to modern IT, notably in the areas of computing and communication. (Linderg, 1987)

The consensus definition has not been seriously challenged since.

Nursing informatics (NI) has evolved rapidly from the predominately physician-populated field of medical informatics. In 1988, Judith Graves and Sheila Corcoran, authors of "The Study of Nursing Informatics," defined NI as "a combination of computer science, information science, and nursing science designed to assist with the management and processing of data, information, and knowledge to support the practice of nursing and the delivery of nursing care" (Graves & Corcoran, 1988).

Graves and Corcoran's classic definition considered functional components (i.e., "management and processing"), combined with conceptual components (i.e., "data, information and knowledge"), and then recognized the "process" whereby the functional components operate on the conceptual components. In short, Graves and Corcoran believe that NI should be more concerned with how the data are structured and organized than with the content of the data.

Lindberg's definition of informatics, along with that of Graves and Corcoran hint at the enormity of this relatively young field of health care. In this early stage of development, informatics continues to morph and to grow rapidly. The two strongest influences on the informatics field are evolving health care and advances in technology. Informatics attempts to merge these two dynamic influences to better the delivery of health care.

A workgroup sponsored by the American Nurses Association (ANA) (2008) utilized the Graves and Corcoran concept to create this well-accepted definition of NI:

> NI is a specialty that integrates nursing science, computer science, and information science to manage and communicate data, information, knowledge, and wisdom in nursing practice. NI supports consumers, patients, nurses, and other providers in their decision-making in all roles and settings. This support is accomplished through the use of information structures, information processes, and IT.

Landmark legislation in 2010 advanced electronic health records (EHRs) extensively in the United States. The Health Information Technology for Economic and Clinical Health Act (HITECH), passed in 2009, offered financial incentives for meeting the first of a series of tests of the "meaningful use" of health care IT. It is expected that there will be three stages to be achieved to realize maximum incentive payments to eligible providers and to avoid financial penalty. As of this writing, the requirements for Stage II are being adopted. In Stage II, the goal is to increase health information exchange between providers and promote patient engagement by giving patients secure online access to their health information.

The Healthcare Information Management Systems Society (HIMSS) Analytics offers an eight-stage U.S. EMR Adoption Model^{SM} that reveals how facilities have progressed with the implementation of EHRs. As of mid-2012, 42.4% of the 5,303 facilities reporting indicate they have ISs that support nursing/clinical documentation (flow sheets), clinical decision support systems (error checking), and picture archival communication systems outside of radiology. Only 13.3% of those facilities report having computerized provider order entry (CPOE), clinical decision support (clinical protocols), (HIMSS Analytics, 2012). Only 1.7% of facilities have a complete electronic medical recorder.

SPECIAL CONSIDERATIONS FOR THE EHR IN SUPPORTING PEDIATRIC AND NEONATAL PATIENT CARE

Lowry et al. (2012) published *A Human Factors Guide to Enhance EHR Usability of Critical User Interactions When Supporting Pediatric Patient Care*. They highlight clinically important special considerations for pediatric patients that are often not understood by those selecting ISs for the adult population.

- Weight-based dosing in the NICU is far more complex and difficult to standardize.
- Sophisticated rounding strategies and accurate weight measurements are used to avoid over- or underdosing, especially for infants who weigh less than 1,000 g.
- Patients can share the same birth date with multiple siblings, so identification can be an issue.
- Alerts can be challenging due to the need for both age and weight-based alerts. Age-based dosing considerations in neonates also must consider gestational age, elapsed days since birth, and "adjusted chronologic age" for growing very-low-birth-weight babies.

TYPES OF ISs

According to McGonigle and Mastrian (2012), the term "IS" refers to "the manual and/or automated components of a system of users or people, recorded data, and action used to process the data into information for a user, group of users, or an organization." Others argue that ISs also include those manual data management systems that still exist in parallel today. More specifically, clinical ISs are ISs that provide access to and methods for recording and managing clinical data. Some examples include paper and electronic flow sheets, daily notes, physician orders, pharmaceutical systems, as well as many others.

FLOW SHEET REPLACEMENT AND CLINICAL MONITORING

Critical care bedside clinicians are "hands-on" providers. The care environment is complex and filled with many simultaneous processes that inform medical decision making. ICUs are often crowded with both people and devices. Care providers are often summoned from one task to a more urgent one in seconds, making computer use/access/logoff difficult or impossible with existing systems. Clinical data acquisition and integration at most ICU bedsides still depend on pen-and-paper flow sheet methods and workarounds. This practice is very time consuming and creates an "information overload" of poorly organized, often illegible data, which can lead to oversights and potentially avoidable errors (Palma, Brown, Lehmann, & Longhurst, 2012; Salanova, Llorens, & Cifre, 2012).

Real-time integration of machine and ancillary data into a user-defined presentation format to support bedside patient care is an unmet dream of most intensive care doctors and practitioners. Past attempts to computerize aspects of ICU bedside physiologic data management have led to sophisticated, free-standing commercial bedside physiologic monitoring and treatment systems (monitors, ventilators, pumps, flowmeters). Each machine relates to a subset of the patient's overall problems (cardiac, respiratory, brain, etc.). Unfortunately, these existing bedside machines have no formal open communication standards with today's computers although we are moving toward adopting standards.

A second challenge for NICU computerization is acquiring and integrating important off-site ancillary data such as that from laboratory, pharmacy, and radiology departments. Computer tools to obtain, analyze, and present patient data trends and information important for clinical caregivers in complicated ICU situations are emerging and are becoming commercially available, usually as "templates" that require local programming.

As flow sheet replacement systems evolve, more complete solutions are being developed to reduce the drawbacks that have prevented the adoption of many of the early electronic flow sheet systems. The more complete solutions enable real-time temporal integration and storage of clinical patient information derived from many different clinical data sources. They have effective interfaces to analyze and display this data both for immediate patient care and for clinical research and quality assurance initiatives. Some of these new systems have touchscreen interfaces available that provide a single point of contact for viewing patient data that is stored in EHR systems, laboratory systems, and pharmacy systems along with data collected from the output of attached bedside machines. This type of automated integration greatly reduces the amount of bedside clinical patient data that must be reentered by the bedside nurse. Time-sensitive graphical displays provide a convenient mechanism for caregivers to review current and historical data about the patient so clinicians can quickly grasp a more complete picture of a critical care patient's status. With real-time integrated systems, many critical transients (e.g., apnea and bradycardia episodes) or trends (e.g., loss of heart rate variability) are harder to overlook in situations where multiple simultaneous events compete for a caregiver's time, such as crisis situations during transport or in the ICU. The most complete of these automated flow sheet systems improve upon current practices by:

1. Integrating important data from the EHR, laboratory, pharmacy, and bedside devices, then displaying the temporal information clearly and compactly at the patient bedside or point of care.
2. Capturing and integrating patient parameters (vital signs, labs, etc.) into a daily note system.
3. Enabling remote access to integrated patient data, just as if the clinician were at the point of care.
4. Interfacing patient data collected during transport with the patient electronic record.
5. Providing deidentified or scrubbed patient information securely to a data warehouse for supporting a broad range of quality assurance, medical, pharmaceutical, and bioinformatics research activities.
6. On the near-term horizon, the automatically captured, integrated data can be used for suggestive diagnostics, protocol adherence, and smart alert notifications.

Current paper-based flow sheet standards have been seemingly adequate throughout history. However, it is evident that a properly designed automated flow sheet system could decrease time collecting, communicating and analyzing patient data. This saved time can then allow clinicians to focus more on treatment and patient care; to date the dream remains elusive.

INTERDISCIPLINARY NOTES: DAILY DOCUMENTING CHALLENGES

Every day, in every ICU, many different notes must be generated that outline the care being provided for the patient by the nurse, the doctor, the respiratory therapist, and others on the care team (pharmacists, social workers, physical therapists, etc.). Generating these notes, from the initial history and physical (H&P), to the daily progress note, to the final discharge note, has often been problematic and is very time consuming.

The information contained in many of these notes is used both for communicating and documenting daily care and eventually for billing. Over the years, attempts to generate a "readable" note have taken on several forms. Traditionally, a clinician would record a few key words when moving from patient to patient or use a preprinted card with check boxes to record appropriate information. Later, in a more private, less chaotic space, the clinician may try to recall everything about the encounter and create a narrative note. The clinician might type the note, but this data entry method has slowed, and often disgruntled, clinicians. More often, the clinician would dictate the encounter narrative to a dictation service. Some number of hours or days later, a complete note would appear for the clinician to sign and place in the chart, as a prerequisite for reimbursement. The dictation is expensive for the hospital. The delay in returning the dictation to the care venue, plus the delay in signing, compounds ongoing operational problems of timely coordination of daily communication between different caregivers, especially in a cross-disciplinary teamwork-based NICU.

Several companies have developed "voice recognition" systems to overcome the delay-related issues. In some disciplines with "limited" vocabulary and quiet work environments, (e.g., radiology), voice recognition systems have achieved some popularity. If voice recognition systems can be made to work well, the daily note is theoretically available as soon as the clinician finishes speaking; edits can be made immediately. The usual drawback of such systems is that the "vocabulary" to be recognized must be greatly restricted in order for the system to work well. In addition, each clinician using the system must "train" the system to recognize their personal speech patterns. Extraneous noise can greatly influence the accuracy of the word recognition, so the dictation must be done in a relatively quiet environment, which is difficult to attain in the daily life of most NICUs. To achieve this, the clinician must, once again, be removed from the point of care to record the encounter. This can lead to errors and often requires first written, then verbal narration of facts in hopes to precisely record the encounter. Increasing point-of-care clinician absence can lead to team communication gaps, errors and redundant "documentation" potentially causing decreased accuracy, and wasting precious time duplicating facts. This dysfunctional workflow situation leads to increased caregiver frustration and therefore decreased product usage. However, when used in an optimal setting, voice recognition systems often excel.

Types of daily note systems based on templates are gaining popularity. A template is a document either in paper or electronic format that contains commonly used clinical data elements in a predefined format. The idea behind these templates is that the format of the template (e.g., daily note) is fairly static for a given patient type (neonate, cardiac, transplant, etc.). One of the more tedious tasks when using this writing system is gathering parameters (such as blood pressure, O_2Sat, and heart rate from the flow sheet) and retyping them. Another downfall is that the users could begin to rely on only those predefined elements within the template, thereby potentially missing unusual findings or situations. Templates that utilize a note system configured to accept bedside data from an automated data acquisition system can greatly reduce the time needed to generate daily notes, and often can increase completeness and comprehensibility of the daily note.

CPOE/MANAGEMENT

Meaningful use and the HITECH legislation are directed toward advancing CPOE. Some facilities are calling the practice computerized provider order management (CPOM). The promise of these systems includes reduction in errors through improved legibility, immediate cross-checking for prescription interactions, other error alerts, and more immediate fulfillment of orders. Currently only about 13.3% of hospitals are using CPOE or CPOM according to HIMSS Analytics, 2012. Poor training and system usability seem to be the root causes of problems with the early use of CPOE (Kuperman & Gibson, 2003). Although some hospitals have experienced failures implementing CPOE systems, there are also many hospitals with successful implementations. Among these success stories, studies have indicated benefits such as a reduction in medical errors, improved quality of patient care, and a positive effect on costs of health care are directly related to CPOE systems (Chapman, Lehmann, Donohue, & Aucott, 2012; Mekhjian et al., 2002; Saathoff, 2005). For neonates, the CPOE systems are rudimentary and often require extreme caregiver time and attention to dealing with difficult computer system navigation and workarounds, including defining pharmacy compounding, and so on, details that are usually unfamiliar to bedside clinicians. CPOE implementations themselves are often locally adapted from adult systems, leaving gaps and internal coding (e.g., rounding rules for 500 g infants) that may be inconsistent with optimizing clinical care in the NICU.

Chapman et al. (2012) studied the implementation of CPOE in a NICU. They conducted a one process-focused hospital study to determine if CPOE impaired or enhanced workflow in the NICU. By comparing the timing of administration of antibiotics before and after CPOE implementation, they concluded that CPOE in the NICU did not significantly improve antibiotic administration times, but the time to pharmacy verification was improved. This suggested further work was needed to investigate admission workflow which they deemed to be a complex process.

PHARMACY

Several pharmacy-related electronic ISs have been introduced in recent years that have reduced medication errors, thereby preventing harm to our tiniest patients. Many ICUs have adopted electronic dispensing systems to help ensure that the ordered medicine is given to the correct patient. Barcode medication administration is in the process of being widely adopted and the level of adoption stands at 11.5% (HIMSS Analytics, 2012). With such a system, barcode labels on the medication are scanned along with a barcode identification band on the patient, ensuring that the appropriate medication is given to the appropriate patient in the right dose at the right time and the correct route. If all is correct, the nurse or other health professional gives the medication and records the event in the electronic record. These systems require barcodes to be assigned to a patient and to each prescription filled by the pharmacy. In order for these systems to be most effective, a medication history must be made available to the pharmacy plus someone must be available to enter the historical data, both at admission and after every "transition of care" (e.g., a trip to the operating room and back).

OTHER SYSTEMS

In addition to the systems outlined, many other computerized systems exist within hospital settings that provide data regarding a patient's condition. Imaging systems to store and display x-ray, computed tomography (CT) scans, and magnetic resonance imaging (MRI) results are widely available. Laboratory systems that can send information to the EHR or store the results locally are being used by most modern hospitals.

An underlying layer of complexity with all of the mentioned systems is the hardware that is used to display the data. For example, most hospitals ISs are "hardwired," requiring a clinician to view and document patient data at a stationary computer. A rapidly emerging option is to make most interfaces "wireless," allowing mobile access to patient information. Wireless solutions include laptop personal computers, tablets, personal computers, and smart phones.

The problem with having so many different ISs is that ensuring accurate communication between systems is difficult. Such difficulties as code differences among systems, multiple logins, variable security protocols, and reducing data redundancy all point to a more complex integration problem. Lack of computer communication standards to express the broad spectrum of neonatal and perinatal diseases and transitional difficulties compounds the problem set.

INTEGRATING COMPUTER IS

Integration issues can be likened to language barriers. Suppose the organization's flow sheet system was in Spanish, the daily notes system in Russian, and the pharmacy system in Chinese. Obviously, communication would be difficult unless one spoke all three languages or had interpreters. In informatics, the "interpreter" that would make the above systems communicate is called an interface. Currently, interfaces are necessary because each independent system (flow sheet, daily notes, pharmacy, laboratory, etc.) within a hospital needs to communicate patient information with each other and the end users. Although interfaces are currently necessary as an interim solution, they are not perfect. In ICUs, optimal clinical care depends on clear integration of many different kinds of time-stamped clinical data. The data needed to support bedside clinical decision making is generated in many departments throughout the hospital. Caregivers, including nurses, respiratory therapists, doctors, social workers, and physical therapists, all contribute a specific set of important clinical observations to the overall clinical data matrix.

Current hospital ISs integrate critical clinical information and convey it to the caregiving team via myriad ways. Communication efforts are evolving, using both formal and informal methods, including charting on large paper flow sheets, printed laboratory reports, verbal reports, dictation, and handwritten/typed progress notes to name a few. Interestingly, some of these methods that are paper based exist within a partially computerized system due to poor integration and virtually no interface capability between departments. Current practices using paper are notorious for being time consuming, illegible, and laborious. They are also error prone, only allow limited access (only one user can view at any one time), create storage nightmares, and have data redundancy. The problem is complicated because any new computer systems installed often are not able to integrate with the original, or "legacy" systems, some of which were developed as far back as the 1970s. Thus, in many complex cases, the daily paper flowsheet creates a compact visual document that can be scanned in seconds for emerging and multisystem problems by experienced criticalists. Existing computer systems' screen displays require much clicking, rolling, and scrolling, which often obscures the temporal relationship of complex patient condition changes ("crashes"). Optimizing future systems with a higher level of integration and more cognitively appropriate and compact screen display would obviously work to correct many of these problems (Palma et al., 2012).

The ideal future method of communication would automate and integrate, in real time, all bedside information, laboratory results, medications, daily notes, and order entry directly into a centralized system. This centralized system would also have a decision support element that notices trends occurring in the patient, alerting the clinician and recommending possible interventions. Additionally, this type of system provides data to hospital administrators so that optimizing decisions can be made regarding staffing, billing, materials management, and quality assurance to name a few. This same system could also be used to push data to registries to assist hospitals with compliance mandates as well as assist in identifying best treatment patterns.

To make the leap from current to future systems, hospitals are faced with hundreds of different products from which to choose. Prior to 1996, many of the larger products boasted they were a "complete system," but they did not use standardized communication methods. The companies creating these products were unable to come to an agreement as to a unified common standard, and as a result the government created laws and national standards in an attempt to mandate that a common communication standard be developed.

INTERCOMMUNICATION STANDARDS AND HIPAA

Background of HIPAA

The Health Insurance Portability and Accountability Act of 1996 (HIPAA) (P.L. 104–191, Title II, Subtitle F) is one of the largest pieces of health care legislation in history. According to Friedrich (2001), HIPAA was passed with three main goals: (1) to improve access to health insurance, (2) to reduce fraud and abuse, and (3) to increase the efficiency and effectiveness of the health care system. The initial goal of increasing accessibility is two fold. One aspect is related to making health insurance portable and continuous for those changing employment locations. The second aspect deals with deterring insurance companies from rejecting individuals with preexisting health conditions. Friedrich also explained that the second goal of HIPAA related to fraud and abuse, and the third goal related to increasing the efficiency and effectiveness of health care, fall under the Administrative Simplifications section of HIPAA (2001). The Administrative Simplifications involve the development of standards and regulations for accessing, transmitting, and storing medical data. Friedrich (2001) states that there are two broad types of regulations: standards related to electronic transmission of data and those intended to ensure the security and privacy of patient information.

The HIPAA legislation mandated that specific code sets and computer communication strategies (both called "standards") be decided and implemented by specific dates, now all past. The start dates for use of HIPAA mandated coding and interconnection strategies were between 2003 and 2005. The foundational work for completing health care computer communication standards is in progress now. No one "standard" was, or is, completely finished. Standards-setting groups meet regularly. These groups are mostly voluntary. Overcoming the proprietary interests of vendors that have a large vested interest in proprietary (secret) software, communication strategies, and clinical expression codes did require the federal HIPAA legislation. New systems will be required to be "HIPAA-Compliant."

HIPAA Mandates: Codes Set Standards

Before HIPAA, there were no communication standards in place for health care providers and payers to transfer information electronically. More than 400 different formats for electronic transactions had been created for communications between providers and health plans (U.S. Department of Health and Human Services, 2000). HIPAA reduced the number to eight clinical code sets and two electronic transaction/computer communication standards for health care administrative and financial communications (U.S. DHHS, 2000). Congress made major operational modifications to the original plan in response to comments, problems, and evolving situations in May 2002 (U.S. Department of Health and Human Services, 2002).

Codes in HIPAA-defined health care rules are precisely formatted numbers and letters that match some clinical concept, such as a diagnosis, medication, or treatment. Communication standards provide a specific place assignment where programmers insert needed coded information, such as a patient identifier, whether they are writing a lab system, a clinical system, or an administrative system. The Health Level 7 (HL7) and ASC_X12N computer communication standards provide a uniform programming structure, so different vendors of clinical, lab, or hospital ISs can send medical and administrative information to each other, without data loss and with clearly defined meaning.

A "code set" is any organized system of codes for listing data elements, such as tables of terms, medical diagnosis codes, and medical procedure codes (U.S. DHHS, 2002). Code sets now defined under the HIPAA legislation are considered code set standards. Examples of these include International Classification of Diseases, 9th or 10th edition, Clinical Modification (ICD-9-CM), Health Care Financing Administration Common Procedural Coding Systems (HCPCS), Current Procedural Terminology (CPT), Current Dental Terminology (CDT), and National Drug Code (NDC). ICD-9-CM is used for diagnoses and hospital patient services codes. According to the American Recovery and Reinvestment Act (ARRA) of 2009, the Stage II Meaningful Use aspects of the HITECH legislation include converting from ICD-9 to the more complex ICD-10 by October 2014. To report supplies, durable medical equipment, and generic drugs under Medicare plans HCPCS is employed (U.S. DHHS, 2002). CPT is mandated for coding physician services. Dental services are coded under CDT, and NDC (National Drug Code) is used only for medications and drug systems for retail pharmacies (U.S. DHHS, 2002).

Computer communication standards defined under HIPAA include ASC_X12N and HL7. ASC_X12N, Version 4010 (Accredited Standards Committee, 2005) is used for health claims, attachments and encounters, payment and remittance advice, claim status, eligibility, referrals, health care enrollment, health plan premium payments, and first report of injury. This communication standard condenses more than 400 transaction formats, with one set of specific transaction standards that are formatted in one language (U.S. DHHS, 2000). HL7 is an accredited Standards Developing Organizations (SDOs) that produces standards (sometimes called specifications or protocols) for a particular health care domain such as pharmacy, medical devices, imaging, or insurance (claims processing) transactions. HL7's domain is clinical and administrative data (HL7, 2005).

As one can see, the elements defining the aforementioned code set standards are independent, not interdependent. Problems therefore quickly arose with initial attempts to apply HIPAA administrative code set standards to computerized clinical medical records. According to Chute (2002), most HIPAA approved code set standards such as ICD-9 and CPT could lose more than half the underlying, detailed clinical information because these code sets were originally established for billing purposes. Loss of pertinent clinical details needed for bedside care and communication can be detrimental for the patient, the providers, and the institution. Because of the obvious need for standard vocabularies in the clinical setting (medical, nursing, and laboratory), the Office of the National Coordinator for Health Information Technology (ONCHIT) was established in late 2004 to coordinate these efforts (Office of the National Coordinator, 2012). The hoped-for outcome of these efforts is rapid development of complete clinical code set standards for care-based computerized patient records.

Different from the above HIPAA-defined code set standards, clinical code set standards either in use, or nearly ready for release, are Systematized Nomenclature of Medicine Clinical Terms (SNOMED), Nursing Intervention Classification (NIC), Nursing Outcome Classification (NOC), North America Nursing Diagnosis Association (NANDA), and Logical Identifier Names and Codes (LOINC). "The SNOMED CT core terminology contains over 366,170 health care concepts with unique meanings and formal logic-based definitions organized into hierarchies" (SNOMED, 2005). NIC, NOC, and NANDA are independent code sets used for nursing diagnoses, treatments, and outcomes documentation. Each of the three has issues such as an inability to combine and link unique concepts as a single concept, poor coding, and an inability to reduce concepts to an anatomic level. Informatics nurses are currently working to harmonize several terminologies so that nurses can document the nursing processes in a standard manner. Lastly, LOINC, which facilitates "the exchange and pooling of results, such as blood hemoglobin, serum potassium, or vital signs, for clinical care, outcomes management, and research is utilized in structuring documentation" (Logical Observation Identifiers Names and Codes, 2012).

HIPAA Mandates: Identifiers

Identifiers are numbers assigned to health care providers (individuals, groups, or organizations) that deliver medical services, other health services, or medical supplies. The final rule for the National Provider Identifier (NPI) was published January 2004 (Centers for Medicare and Medicaid Services, 2005). However the proposed rules for assigning unique identifiers to employers and health plans are not yet fully operational. Employee identification numbers (EINs) are under scrutiny because the number to be used was determined by the Internal Revenue Service (IRS) to be the taxpayer identifying number, also known as the social security number (SSN). This was thought to be a good idea since most employees should already have a SSN assigned prior to being hired in an organization. However, the use of the SSN has caused controversy because health information and financial information will be directly linked to the same number. Additionally there are duplicate SSNs. National Health Plan Identifiers (NHPIs) are also undetermined at this time (CMS, 2005).

HIPAA Mandates: Privacy

Before HIPAA, legal protection of patients' privacy and confidentiality was fragmented across state, federal, and commercial insurance systems, which left many gaps in patient privacy (Hebda & Czar, 2004). Evolving, implementing and testing patient privacy rules under HIPAA law is an ongoing process. The effective compliance date was April 14, 2003.

The Privacy Rule was constructed in hopes of protecting verbal, written, or electronic personal health information (PHI) that can be traced to an individual. This PHI refers to any record containing any of the 18 elements defined as personal health data (e.g., name, birth date, SSN, address, etc.). The rule protects not only PHI within the walls of the hospital but also PHI while in transit to other locations (Friedrich, 2001). The rule applies to health plans, health care clearinghouses, and those health care providers who electronically conduct financial and administrative transactions (U.S. Department of Health and Human Services, 2001). Consent must be obtained from the patients prior to any release of their private information for treatment, payment, or other health care operations. Patients will have the right to restrict the use and disclosure of their information, and the option to file formal complaints if their privacy has been violated. All shared data must be stripped of PHI information unless sharing is authorized by the patient. In addition, patients must have full access to their medical records (U.S. DHHS, 2001). Since some of these elements are also vital statistics (e.g., date and time of birth), that are a matter of public record, *and* of extreme clinical importance for babies' health care management (e.g., developmental milestones), the problem for follow-up, other communication, and research is obvious to pediatricians. However, since adults have no such issues, the situation in standards' setting groups is stalled, because vendors of adult systems would have difficulty and expense "retrofitting" their software to support the date/time aspect for neonates. Currently, progress toward full utility for neonates is slow and/or stalled.

HIPAA Mandates: Security

Security regulations refer to technical protection of computerized PHI transmitted electronically within and among provider and payer organizations. Security standards have three categories: (1) administrative security (e.g., access controls and contingency plans); (2) technical security mechanisms (e.g., authorizations and audit controls); and (3) physical security (e.g., limit physical access to workstations) (Hirsch, 2003). Although these three categories are different, the security measures proposed in each category require similar forms of intervention.

For clinical users, HIPAA has created a very unstable and tenuous balance between security and usability (Dawes, 2001). For example, many paper-based units have removed all charts from the bedside, including flow sheets, to keep the patient's data more secure. This poses a workflow problem especially in an ICU because that information is needed at the bedside. In computerized systems, excess security has become a burden because hospitals are requiring excessive password usage to gain access to EHRs. In an emergency this process tends to delay patient care when it is needed most. Log-in times range from 30 to 75 seconds in usual times, across most NICUs. A nurse accessing the computer for charting, and so on may thus "waste" about an hour a day simply waiting for computer access.

HIPAA Mandates: Penalties

According to the U.S. Department of Health and Human Services, there are two types of penalties: civil and federal criminal (U.S. DHHS, 2001). For a civil penalty, the minimum fine for failure to comply with a standard is $100 per violation with a maximum of $25,000 for identical violations per year for each requirement violation. Criminal charges start at $50,000, with a maximum of 1 year in prison for wrongful disclosure (U.S. DHHS, 2001).

Clearly, there are numerous layers of complexity when considering clinical ISs. There are various types of ISs available for all aspects of the delivery of patient care. When reviewing any IS, it is critical to consider if and how these systems communicate or integrate with one another. Whether the NICU is in the process of replacing an entire EHR, or a smaller change such as an automated flow sheet, it is important to use a formal process to evaluate and select the system that is the best fit for the organization.

IS EVALUATION, SELECTION, AND IMPLEMENTATION

Bedside caregivers in the NICU need to have an understanding of general guidelines for evaluation, selection, and implementation of ISs into their hospital organization. Bedside caregivers, not just administrative staff, *must* play an integral role in the extensive and elaborate process of hospital IS selection and installation. Bedside caregivers who interact with the clinical IS on a daily basis are called "end users." End users help to define the requirements of the system in the early stages of evaluation and to give input during the selection process. End-user satisfaction is the key to the successful implementation of a system. Below we give a brief overview of these important processes to ensure that modern-era bedside caregivers have an understanding of their roles and expectations during a NICU IS selection and implementation.

RESEARCHING IS SOLUTIONS

Many hospital organizations are initiating the switch from paper-based charting systems to electronic charting systems. Some facilities currently have systems and are changing vendors, hardware, and software. This type of project is a massive undertaking for a hospital, financially, logistically, and culturally. Therefore, for future purchases, most hospitals are beginning to develop structured planning, purchasing, and implementation processes in an effort to avoid future project failures.

The first stage in the system evaluation/selection process is to logically identify and list the problems with the current system in a structured format (e.g., a spreadsheet). It is important to research alternative technological solutions or enhancements to the identified problem(s). Often a multidisciplinary (IT, clinical, and administrative representation) approach to these early, interdisciplinary "brainstorming" sessions yields enough ideas to structure a more substantial search. Initially, a Request for Information (RFI) can be directed to vendors that specialize in clinical ISs. The vendor will in turn reply with introductory product information. An RFI is a standard and affordable business process that is used to collect information about the capabilities of various products. The RFI is normally formatted so it can be used as an initial assessment tool for comparing vendors (Hunt, Sproat, & Kitzmiller, 2004).

Once the vendor list is at a manageable size, a more detailed comparison process begins, using a Request for Proposal (RFP). The main purpose of the RFP is to document the vendor's claims in terms of system functionality, support, training, cost, and implementation approach, including staff education and postinstallation support plans for the early months of the "go-live." The hospital's IT or ISs department will likely compose this document with input from all affected parties. At this step, input from the end users (practicing clinicians) is vital. An RFP should be created for each individual unit that includes its unique workflow issues. When you use an individualized approach, it is harder for the vendor to provide broad, generic answers that may be technically capable, but do not really address your unit's specialized requirements, and ultimately may be either unusable, unsafe, or both.

One of the most essential sections of the RFP describes the system's functional and technical requirements. Functional requirements are developed using input from bedside caregivers based on the daily workflow needs and data management goals for the specific unit. These detailed requirements are listed by the requesting hospital in a table/database format. Technical requirements pertain to issues such as network and hardware specifications that are required to make the system run (Hunt et al., 2004). Vendor response columns should be provided so the vendor can specifically address each requirement in terms of the technical details defining how their system meets each specification. Each requesting hospital should provide a predetermined response key for the vendor to use. The preestablished response key assists the purchasing team in cross-vendor comparisons.

In addition to the functional and technical requirements, the implementation and maintenance plan for the proposed system should be requested of the vendor. In the RFP response, the vendor should provide, in writing, their plan for implementation, training, and support of their system (Hunt et al., 2004). These components can make or break the success of the system. Finally, the RFP should request a detailed cost matrix of all aspects of the vendor's system and its implementation, including costs, plans and options for peri-go live testing and tuning and roll-out staging.

The completed RFP is sent out, and formal proposal replies are expected within weeks. If composed appropriately, the RFP will require the vendors to verify that they meet the details of the request. Their responses will contain information that will allow a thorough evaluation and selection process.

EVALUATION AND SYSTEM SELECTION

As the vendor proposals return, it is important for the IS or Informatics Department to begin the evaluation process. A metric scoring scale can be applied to the objective sections of the submitted proposals. The objective sections include the functional, technical, and financial requirements. The scoring scale allows the hospital to evaluate the vendor's systems objectively and consistently. A numerical weight value will be assigned to each response. For example, a response of "Not available" should receive a weighted score of zero, whereas a response of "Available and already successfully installed in a similar health care facility" should receive the highest weight on the response key scale. All objective sections of each vendor's proposal are scored based on their responses. Then a summary table can be created to display the final numeric results and ranking of each vendor.

Financial comparisons evaluate whether the requesting hospital can afford the high-scoring vendors. Typically, the financial department of the hospital assists in this phase. Several financial evaluation tools are commonly used. A cost-benefit analysis (CBA) is traditionally done by comparing the cost of each system to the proposed benefits. However, the CBA is purely an estimation approach and incorporates such concepts as "intangible" benefits that are difficult to quantify for parallel comparisons. A second approach is a cost-effectiveness analysis (CEA), including a Payback Analysis, a Return on Investment (ROI) estimation, and Net Present Value (NPV) assessment. The ROI and Payback Analysis are both methods that determine the time for each system to repay its costs. Once a system pays for itself, cost savings for the hospital will begin. The NPV calculates the value of each system at any given time, thus determining the profitability in current dollars. Typically, the financial department performs these analyses. End users who are active in the selection process should be familiar with commonly used comparison methods.

Once the objective scoring is complete and the cost analyses are done, vendors should be ranked according to their scored percentages. This ranking acts as a consistent comparison tool to determine which vendor best meets the hospital's desired criteria. This process is important because the purchasing organization must be able to quantify necessary functions for their desired system.

Finalist vendors' products can be further evaluated in many ways. Reference checks by telephone interviews of the specific vendor's clients to get an overall feel of client satisfaction with the vendor's installed system is one way to evaluate a finalist (Hunt et al., 2004). A standard questionnaire is another useful telephone tool that can again compare client feedback on an equal basis. There are several web-based agencies that conduct and publish results of satisfaction surveys that can be helpful to a buyer.

The next step is to conduct on-site vendor demonstrations. Demonstrations are necessary for end users to test whether their functional requirements can actually be met. A demonstration evaluation test tool should be created to assess how each system functions in the context of actual daily workflow for the particular unit. Part of the tool should use test case scenarios that are unique to the unit and also taxing to a system. An example of such a scenario may be to "demonstrate the admission of unnamed triplets where two were born before midnight and one was born after midnight." The demonstration tool should also assess usability and functionality of clinical documentation. For example, "What happens if a nurse is documenting an assessment but gets called away from the bedside before finishing? Is his or her work saved and time-stamped?"

The final step of product evaluation is to conduct site visits at other hospitals. Select similar hospital units that currently use the IS of interest. To obtain a true picture of how the system functions, it is best to conduct these site visits without the vendor present, which also allows the end users to express how they feel about the system and how it will fit into their workflow (Hunt et al., 2004). The site visit team should be multidisciplinary for gathering feedback from various perspectives, including different types of end users (i.e., nurses, respiratory therapists, doctors, informatics specialists). The site visit team should use the same evaluation tools that were used in the vendor demonstration to observe and evaluate the installed product function during real-life scenarios in real time. It is also important for the site visit team to note the physical layout of the unit and how the system fits into the staff's workflow. For example, is there a computer terminal in each patient room, or do the staff share one terminal per several patients? If the computers are mobile, do they easily fit into each patient room, or do the visitors have to leave before they can pass through the door? The site visit team can apply the onsite observations to their own NICU. In addition to environment and workflow observations, a site visit questionnaire can be created to gather more structured information from current end users.

As the evaluation process closes, a final decision-making team should review (1) subjective and objective information; (2) reference telephone interviews; (3) demonstration evaluation tool results; and (4) site visit feedback from questionnaires. Hospitals usually select a finalist and a runner up vendor. The two finalist vendors' supporting information is presented to the project steering committee (i.e., the final decision makers.) This committee will likely include representation from high-level executives (CEO), financial personnel (CFO), nursing (CNO), medical (CMO), IS/Informatics (CIO), chief medical information officer (CMIO), chief nursing informatics officer (CNIO), and so on. Once the selection is made and contract negotiations are finished, the implementation phase will begin.

IMPLEMENTATION

The key to a successful system conversion (i.e., switching the old system out and bringing the new system in without clinical disruption) is a well-thought-out implementation plan. A project implementation team should include end-user representation from every shift, IT personnel, and vendor representation. Administrative representatives who are people-oriented problem solvers are valuable team members. End users that are bedside caregivers are integral to the install because they provide functional knowledge for both the system design team and the training team. IT team members can provide technical services and schedule planning tools to ensure a smooth transition. Team members from the vendor facilitate local customization efforts and training based on their full understanding of their system's inner workings.

The implementation team is responsible for (1) installing hardware and software; (2) educating themselves with 100% of the system's functions; (3) customizing the system; (4) testing the system; (5) creating implementation and user documentation; (6) educating users hospital wide; (7) overseeing the actual system conversion; and (8) conducting the post-implementation evaluation. Typically the first five steps precede the live conversion. These steps make the system mesh with the subtle nuances of the hospital and/or the particular unit (i.e., the NICU). The last three steps rely heavily on end-user participation. The success of the system conversion is based on actual usability by the intended users in the clinical environment.

Before the installation of the hardware (monitors, keyboards, etc.) and software (instructions for the computer), the IT staff on the implementation team should verify the physical layout of the unit, check, and supplement power sources, lighting, noise, and privacy limitations. IT staff should walk through the unit with all end user representatives while they visualize and verbalize issues unique to the unit. This step ("cognitive walkthrough") helps prevent surprises and delays during the systemwide installation process.

Meanwhile, the vendor representatives of the implementation team should initiate system education and training of the end users within the team. The first end users trained will eventually become the trainers (Hunt et al., 2004). The end-user trainers need to know the operation of the system, its limitations, and backup plans in the event of an unexpected system shutdown. They must also understand how to log formal "issues and complaints" across all shifts to ensure continuous system quality improvement.

System customization, the third responsibility of the implementation team, ensures that the system is tailored to meet the unit's workflow needs. For example, the NICU may want to integrate the hospital laboratory list within the new system, so they can view the results of ordered laboratory tests, and specifically and concisely check only "abnormal values" across a 60-patient census list. It is important for the implementation team to determine that all customization/modification requests are sensible. Sometimes the customization process becomes unrealistic as individual end users' desires expand. For example, one user may want to view vital signs with heart rate as the initial value, while another user may prefer the temperature first. A few systems reaching market allow individual customization at this level, without changing the overall configuration for others. But currently an entire NICU usually must form a consensus of how the standard data is to be represented. Keep in mind that many small modifications to the system usually are needed within the first 6 months of the installation. Expect to give the vendor reasonable time to make those changes.

System testing is a very important responsibility of the implementation team and the vendor, working together. As customization occurs, it is important to verify the system is working properly with the new changes. The testing steps should be done by members of the team, not affiliated with the vendor. Each module of the system should be thoroughly tested for functionality using formal scenarios from actual clinical situations. Outlier management is important. Most NICU patients are "outliers" compared to the larger child and adult population. Thus, scenarios should include a sample of the most complex, as well as common cases managed on the unit. Technically, the flow of data between modules should be verified and validated. System response times should be tested at peak volume of staff using the system simultaneously and should be monitored and tuned at intervals. Performance tends to degrade as use and data intensity increase over time. All system tests must be fully documented for historical and legal purposes.

As the system is being customized, modified, and thoroughly tested in the NICU, the implementation team begins to create and revise the system's documents. User guides and educational material are created during this phase. Typically, materials already supplied by the vendor will need to be updated/modified due to local changes made to the product. The hospital education department should be included at this phase to aid with hospital-wide training and 24/7/365 educational dissemination.

The hospital-wide end-user education phase should start a few weeks before the go-live (conversion) date. The users need to know what to expect of the system, the rollout, and testing and tuning processes. They should feel prepared for the upcoming change. Choose several "super users" who are computer savvy end users, who are eager to help roll out the new system, and who are liked and respected by colleagues. In terms of system training, a diffusion approach tends to be the most successful. With the diffusion approach, super users, once trained, can train their coworkers with enthusiasm and during real-life scenarios/situations. It is best if the initial exposure to the system is in a quiet, comfortable, and well-lit area. Distractions should be kept at a minimum so that the training material can be fully absorbed. This session should not exceed 2 hours. If more time is needed, then subsequent sessions should be scheduled. After exposure to the system, move the users to the patient care setting. After go-live (see below), trainers should be available in the unit around the clock until the end users are comfortable navigating and using the system. Overtime pay for off-hours training builds positive attitudes.

When the implementation team has completed all planning, testing, documentation, and training steps, it is time for the final conversion or go-live step. There are several types of go-live options that have led to successful system conversions, including (1) parallel conversion; (2) pilot conversion; (3) phased conversion; and (4) crash conversion. The parallel method involves running both the old and new system at the same time until the users are comfortable with the new system. This approach is time consuming and expensive, but is safe in terms of bridging documentation gaps. The pilot conversion involves changing only one unit at a time. This approach is timely and effective for some organizations. The phased conversion involves installing application modules individually throughout the hospital. This phased conversion takes a considerable amount of time, but may ease the users into the system at a more comfortable rate. The crash approach involves shutting off the old system and turning on the new system overnight. This approach can be quite stressful for the end users and may lead to poor patient care. However, if the staff are adequately trained and are comfortable with the new system, this approach may be optimal, especially if the new system solves many preexisting problems. Each hospital should weigh the pros and cons of each approach heavily before choosing the best go-live scenario. Do not attempt massive inpatient conversions over holiday weekends, unless the hospital 24/7 critical care services can be closed down, or shifted to other hospitals for the duration.

There should be a postimplementation evaluation several months after the system conversion. Samples of the people directly involved in the conversion should provide feedback on the go-live process and on the system performance. This feedback may uncover gaps in the system use, or performance. Structured feedback may also aid in the redesign of subsequent system conversion approaches. The postimplementation evaluation results should also be analyzed to evaluate operating costs, benefits, and system stability.

The implementation process requires careful planning and much work. Without a solid multidisciplinary implementation team, the system conversion could fail, costing the hospital millions of dollars. The implementation team's stepwise responsibilities are critical to the ultimate success of the system. By following the eight implementation guidelines outlined above, a hospital should be able to avoid pitfalls and complete a successful implementation.

SUMMARY

The intensive care environment has always depended on the most advanced technologies to care for patients. Traditionally these technologies have been limited to bedside devices. It is inevitable that the device-based technology expand to include ISs. ISs, such as the electronic medical record, are necessary to capture the data that these devices report throughout the ICU. With the help of advanced computer systems we can view and analyze patient data in ways that traditional paper-based methods cannot permit. As we evolve into the information age in health care, it is important that bedside caregivers have an understanding of the pros and cons of various types of ISs, the importance of an integrated system, as well as the complexities that arise when implementing them into your hospital unit.

ONLINE RESOURCES

American Nursing Informatics Association
https://www.ania.org/ Health IT.gov
http://www.healthit.gov/policy-researchers-implementers/health-it-rules-regulations?utm_source=google&utm_medium=cpc&utm_campaign=privacy_and_legal

Health Information Management System Society
http://www.himss.org/ASP/index.asp

Online Journal of Nursing Informatics
http://www.ojni.org

U.S. Department of Health and Human Services
http://www.hhs.gov

RECOMMENDED READING

American Organization of Nurse Executives. (2012). *Position paper: Nursing informatics executive leader*. Retrieved from http://www.aone.org

Ball, M. J., Douglas, J. V., DuLong, D., Newbold, S. K., Sensmeier, J. E., Skiba, D. J., . . . Kiel, J. M. (Eds.). (2011). *Nursing informatics: Where technology and caring meet* (4th ed.). New York, NY: Springer-Verlag.

CIN: Computers, informatics, nursing. Hagerstown, MD: Lippincott Williams & Wilkins.

Hannah, K., Ball, M., & Edwards, M. (2010). *Introduction to nursing informatics* (3rd ed.). New York, NY: Springer.

Healthcare Information Management Systems Society. (2011). *Position Statement on transforming nursing practice through technology & informatics*. Retrieved from www.himss.org

Institute of Medicine & Committee of the Robert Wood Johnson Foundation Initiative on the Future of Nursing. (2011). *The future of nursing: Leading change, advance health*. Washington, DC: National Academy Press.

Logical Observation Identifiers Names and Codes. (2012). Retrieved from http://www.loinc.org

McCartney, P., & Barnes, J. (2012). *Perinatal nursing informatics guide for clinical health information technology*. Washington, DC: Association of Women's Health Obstetrics and Neonatal Nurses.

Moorman, J. R., Rusin, C. E., Lee, H., Guin, L. E., Clark, M. T., Delos, J. B., . . . Lake, D. E. (2011). Predictive monitoring for early detection of subacute potentially catastrophic illnesses in critical care. *Conference Proceedings: IEEE Engineering in Medicine and Biology Society, 55*, 15–18.

Online Journal of Nursing Informatics (OJNI). Kittanning, PA. Retrieved from http://www.ojni.org

Rikli, J., Huizinga, B., Schafer, D., Atwater, A., Coker, K., & Sikora, C. (2009). Implementation of an electronic documentation system using microsystem and quality improvement concepts. *Advances in Neonatal Care, 9*(2), 53–60.

Staundinger, B., Hob, V., & Ostermann, H. (2009). *Nursing and clinical informatics: Socio-technical approaches*. Hershey, PA: Information Science References.

The TIGER initiative. Retrieved from http://thetigerinitiative.org

REFERENCES

The Accredited Standards Committee X12. (2005). *About ASC X12*. Retrieved from http://www.x12.org/x12org/about/index.cfm

American Nurses Association. (2008). *Nursing informatics: Scope and standards of practice*. Silver Spring, MD: Author.

American Recovery and Reinvestment Act. *Recovery.gov*. Retrieved from www.recovery.gov

Centers for Medicare and Medicaid Services. (2005). *HIPAA administrative simplications–identifiers*. Retrieved from http://www.hhs.gov/ocr/privacy/hipaa/administrative/index.html

Chapman, A. K., Lehmann, C. U., Donohue, P. K., & Aucott, S. W. (2012). Implementation of computerized provider order entry in a neonatal intensive care unit: Impact on admission workflow. *International Journal of Medical Informatics, 81*(5), 291–295. doi: 10.1016/j.ijmedinf.2011.12.006

Chute, C. G. (2002, November). *Medical concept representation: From classification to understanding*. Presented at AMIA Symposium 2002, San Antonio, Texas.

Collen, M. F. (1995). *A history of medical informatics in the United States: 1950's to 1990*. Indianapolis, IN: Hartman Publishing.

Dawes, B. (2001). Patient confidentiality takes on a new meaning. *AORN Journal, 73*(3), 596, 598, 600.

Friedrich, M. J. (2001). Health care practitioners and organizations prepare for approaching HIPAA deadlines. *Journal of the American Medical Association, 286*(13), 1563–1565.

Graves, J. R., & Corcoran, S. (1988). Identification of data element categories for clinical nursing information systems via information analysis of nursing practice. Proceedings of the Annual Symposium on Computer Application in Medical Care. November 9, 358–363.

Health Information Technology for Economic and Clinical Health Act. (2009). Title XIII of the American Recovery and Reinvestment Act of 2009 (Pub.L. 111–5).

Health Insurance Reform: Modifications to Electronic Data Transaction Standards and Code Sets (45 CFR Part 162)

Health Level 7 International. *Learn about HL7*. Retrieved from http://www.hl7.org

Healthcare Information Management Systems Society Analytics. (2012). Retrieved from http://www.himssanalytics.org/emram/index.aspx

Hebda, T., & Czar, P. (2004). *Handbook of informatics for nurses and healthcare professionals* (4th ed.). Upper Saddle River, NJ: Pearson Education.

Hirsch, R. (2003). On HIPAA-the HIPAA security rule. *Healthcare Informatics, 20*(4), 56.

Hunt, E. C., Sproat, S. B., & Kitzmiller, R. R. (2004). *The nursing informatics implementation guide*. New York, NY: Springer.

Kuperman, G. J., & Gibson, R. F. (2003). Computer physician order entry: Benefits, costs, and issues. *Annals of Internal Medicine, 139*(1), 31–39.

Linderg, D. A. B. (1987). *NLM long range plan. Report of the Board of Regents*. Bethesda, MD: National Library of Medicine.

Lowry, S. Z., Quinn, M. T., Ramaiah, M., Brick, D., Patterson, E. S., Zhang, J., . . . Gibbons, M. C. (2012). *A human factors guide to enhance EHR usability of critical user interactions when supporting pediatric patient care*. National Institute of Standards and Technology. Retrieved from http://dx.doi.org/10.6028/NIST.IR.7865

McGonigle, D., & Mastrian, K. G. (2012). *Nursing Informatics and the foundation of knowledge* (2nd ed.). Burlington, MA: Jones & Bartlett Learning.

Mekhjian, H. S., Kumar, R. R., Kuehn, L., Bentley, T. D., Payne, B., & Ahmad, A. (2002). Immediate benefits realized following implementation of physician order entry at an academic medical center. *Journal of the American Medical Informatics Association, 9*(5), 529–539.

Office of the National Coordinator for Health Information Technology. (2012). Retrieved from http://www.healthit.gov

Palma, J. P., Brown, P. J., Lehmann, C. U., & Longhurst, C. A. (2012). Neonatal informatics: Optimizing clinical data entry and display *Neoreviews, 13*(2), 81–85.

Palma, J. P., Van Eaton, E. G., & Longhurst, C. A. (2011). Neonatal informatics: Information technology to support handoffs in neonatal care. *Neoreviews, 12*, 393–396.

Saathoff, A. (2005). Human factors considerations relevant to CPOE implementations. *Journal of Healthcare Information Management, 19*(4), 71–78.

Saba, V. K., & McCormick, K. A. (2011). *Essentials of nursing informatics* (5th ed.). New York, NY: McGraw-Hill.

Salanova, M., Llorens, S., & Cifre, E. (2012, June 25). The dark side of technologies: Technostress among users of information and communication technologies. *International Journal of Psychology*. [Epub ahead of print].

SNOMED International. (2005). SNOMED CT. Retrieved from http://www.ihtsdo.org/snomed-ct/

U.S. Department of Health and Human Services. (2000, last updated). *Frequently asked questions about electronic transaction standards adopted under HIPAA*. Retrieved from http://aspe.hhs.gov/admnsimp/faqtx.htm#whynational

U.S. Department of Health and Human Services. (2001, May 9). *Protecting the privacy of patients' health information*. Retrieved from http://aspe.os.dhhs.gov/admnsimp/final/pvcfact2.htm

U.S. Department of Health and Human Services. (2002, May 31). Health Insurance Reform: Modifications to Electronic Data Transaction Standards and Code Sets (45 CFR Part 162).

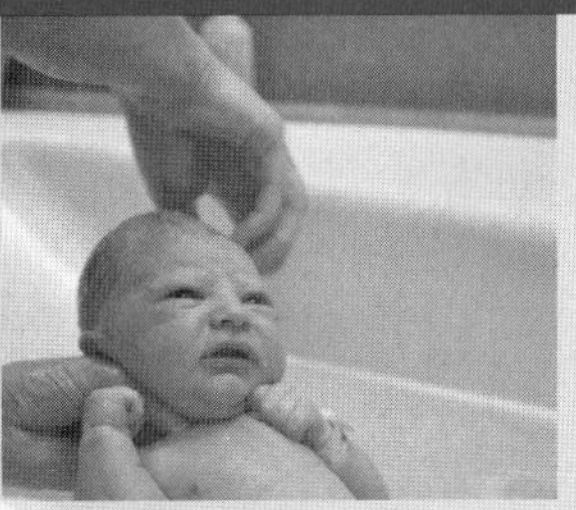

Human Genetics and Genomics: Impact on Neonatal Care

CHAPTER 38

■ Judith A. Lewis

Pick up a newspaper, listen to a radio, or watch the news and you will hear the word genetics. Today, with the human genome sequence completed, we know that genomics plays a significant role in every clinical facet of health care. Whereas genetics refers to the study of a single gene, genomics refers to the study of all genes in a particular organism, including their interaction with each other and the environment (http://www.genome/gov/glossary).

Genomics is a broader term and includes genetics, although the terms often are used interchangeably when talking about the science of heredity. This chapter discusses genetics and genomics and their impact on neonatal care.

INCIDENCE OF GENETIC CONDITIONS

Approximately 120,000 infants in the United States, or about 1 in 33, are born with a birth defect (CDC, 2008). These include structural and metabolic disorders, congenital infections, and other environmental causes such as perinatal substance abuse. Thus some newborns have birth defects that have a genetic basis, whereas other newborns suffer from a genetic disease. The distinction is that a genetic disease results from an aberration in the infant's deoxyribonucleic acid (DNA), such as occurs with cystic fibrosis and sickle cell anemia (Scheuerle, 2001).

For many neonatal nurses, genetic mechanisms and the role of genes in disease were not part of basic nursing education. Typically, little information about genomics was included in the curricula beyond the Mendelian laws of single-gene inheritance. With the exponential increase in genomic information, an expanded knowledge base is required. Families can easily obtain highly technical (and sometimes wrong) information about their infant's condition and the possible genomic basis for that condition. Health professionals must be knowledgeable about genomics and certain that families clearly understand their infant's condition. This chapter discusses genomics as it relates to neonatal and infant care.

HISTORICAL PERSPECTIVE

Long before DNA was discovered or any of the intracellular contents of cells were known, scientists noted that the basic traits of certain organisms were passed down to succeeding generations with varying degrees of constancy. This observation was noted not only among human beings and other "higher order" species of animals but also among plants and simple forms of animal life. In general, the physical characteristics of offspring usually resembled the physical characteristics of the parent organism. This fact was explained as a basic "mixing" of maternal and paternal characteristics in the formation of a new individual or new generation. More difficult to explain was how a child could resemble or have a specific characteristic found only in a more remote family member, such as a great grandmother or an uncle, rather than in one of the parents. In observing variations in inheritable characteristics over many generations among plants, Gregor Mendel, a 19th-century botanist, proposed a mechanism that essentially involved the "strength" of some characteristics to explain variations in patterns of inheritance. Even at this point, no one cell structure was identified as responsible for the transmission of these patterns of inheritance.

In the late 19th century, biologists discovered small "chromatic elements" in the nucleus of a cell that stained differently from other cell components. In addition, these elements, called chromosomes, were present only at specific times in the cell cycle. It was determined that chromosomes were composed of homologous pairs that split longitudinally during cell division. Chromosomes were thought to be responsible for Mendelian heredity. One half of each pair of chromosomes was derived from the maternal gamete and the other half from the paternal gamete.

In 1914 researchers discovered that chromosomes disappeared during the interphase of the cell cycle, only to reappear at mitosis in the same number and with the same morphologic features as at the previous mitosis. As a result of these observations, chromosome formation was speculated to be an organized process from one cell generation to another and not merely a result of random meshing of nuclear material. It was observed that when the chromosomes were abnormal in shape or number, subsequent development was abnormal. This led to the hypothesis that chromosomes were the carriers of heredity and that aberrations in chromosomes (both numeric aberrations and structural aberrations) would result in aberrant development. Normal functioning of cells and whole organisms depended on the equilibrium of this genetic material.

Even though these concepts were proposed more than 70 years ago, testing was limited by the dearth of technologic advances in cytogenetics (the analysis of chromosomes and their genes) and molecular genetics until relatively recently. Cytogenetic advancements occurred first and led to a means of diagnosing some specific genetic abnormalities. The early cytogenetic work increased the precision and clinical application of molecular genetic advancements.

HUMAN GENOME PROJECT

The human genome project (HGP) revealed that our human DNA contains approximately 3 billion DNA base pairs, which reside in the 23 pairs of chromosomes within the nucleus of all our cells. Each of our 23 pair of chromosomes contains hundreds to thousands of genes, which carry the instructions for making proteins. Each of the estimated 30,000 genes in the human genome makes an average of three proteins (The Human Genome Project Completion: Frequently Asked Questions, 2010). The genetic code directs the body's cells in how to perform, what to produce, and even when to die. It carries the "recipes" for the body's proteins, the building blocks of all tissues. When one of these recipes fails or is altered, so is the structure of the body. In some cases, this alteration is so subtle that only the cellular level or genotype is affected. In other cases, however, the mistake results in a disease or structural defect, such as occurs with neurofibromatosis or some forms of cancer.

A genomic map now shows which genes are located on what chromosome, and a region on the chromosome where defective genes are located (National Human Genome Research Institute [NHGRI], 2001). Although a condition may be known to be dependent on these defective genes for expression, the genes surrounding the defective ones may or may not be affected. However, the location gives the health professional a starting point to do some detective work about possible health risks.

Through the efforts of the HGP, science has gained knowledge of the specific locations of genes on specific chromosomes; this creates the opportunity to design therapies directly targeted to the defective gene. Pharmacogenomics, the science correlating individual genetic variation and drug response (Talking Glossary), has developed drugs to treat a person's unique genomic makeup. Gene therapy will also take into account the interaction of the environment with an individual's genome. For example, exposure to second-hand smoke is linked to asthma, but asthma also has a genomic basis. So the interaction of genes with exposure to cigarette smoke may result in disease—asthma. Such specific knowledge also gives health professionals the opportunity to predict the likelihood that specific family members will develop certain conditions. Prenatal teaching or preconception education becomes more important in light of this new information. True health promotion, and in some cases disease prevention, can be a reality. Dr. Barton Childs (1998) refers to this move away from the disease model to consideration of genetic foundations as using a genetic lens to view health.

With scientific advances in genomics, health professionals have raised many concerns about the ethical dilemmas and legal issues arising from the HGP. The Ethical, Legal, and Social Implications (ELSI) Branch of the HGP supports studies that analyze situations that present ethical and legal situations for health professionals and the children and families they serve.

Similar issues are being raised by advances in newborn screening and testing. Most screening is also genetic testing, as many of the conditions have a genetic underpinning. Tandem mass spectrometry (MS/MS) permits testing for more than 30 disorders. The ethical dilemma becomes: Should testing be done for conditions that have a poor prognosis or no effective treatment (Kenner & Moran, 2005)? Among the concerns to emerge were whether the tests should be mandatory or remain voluntary, and who would have access to the information. Discrimination in insurance coverage when a genetic problem is found is also a major ethical issue (Kenner & Moran, 2005). Another important dilemma in newborn screening is the variation among states in the newborn screening panel. Little and Lewis (2008) discuss the ethical issues related to potential disparities as well as the issue of informed consent in the area of routine newborn screening programs.

Nurses must continue to advocate for infants and families; to do this, they must have a solid grounding in genomic knowledge, including foundational genetics starting at the molecular level. Knowledge of the molecular level starts with the structure of the DNA molecule and includes the coding pattern for a protein.

DNA

DNA is composed of two very long chains (strands) of interlocking nucleotides (Figure 38.1). Each nucleotide is composed of a molecule of any one of the following four bases: adenine (A), guanine (G), thymine (T), and cytosine (C). Adenine and guanine are purine bases; thymine and cytosine are pyrimidine bases. These bases are attached to a five-carbon sugar (a pentose arrangement called a ribose), which is connected to a phosphate group.

The phosphate groups actually provide the linkage between the individual bases, forming the long strands. The phosphate connections therefore are the actual "backbone" of the DNA strand.

In human beings, DNA does not exist as a single strand; rather, the DNA is double stranded in an antiparallel arrangement. The two strands are not directly physically connected; instead, a number of relatively weak ionic forces hold the two strands in proximity. These ionic forces are different for the two groups of bases, and these differences are responsible for adenine always pairing with thymine and guanine always pairing with cytosine. Thus the two strands of DNA are lined up together and are composed of interacting bases that form base pairs. Because the bases are specific in their attractions, the two strands of DNA are complementary in terms of their nucleotide sequence. If the sequence of one DNA strand is known, the sequence of the complementary DNA strand can be accurately predicted.

In its native state during the reproductive resting state of the cell (G0), the double-stranded DNA has a loosely coiled helical (double strand) arrangement. At various times in the cell cycle, the DNA becomes more tightly packed together by further coiling at well-regulated intervals around protein substances called histones; this gives the DNA the appearance of beads on a string. The complex of DNA wound around each histone is called a nucleosome. In addition to the histone proteins that come into contact with the DNA at specific points in the strand and at certain times in the cell cycle, nonhistone proteins are associated with the DNA.

During cell division, the DNA must become even more tightly packed together to form dense structures called chromosomes. Each chromosome is composed of a relatively large section of DNA containing many genes. The basic structure of chromosomes is presented in Figure 38.2. Most of the nomenclature currently used to describe specific areas or features of chromosomes is derived from the 1971 Paris Conference of the International Human Genetics Congress.

Chromatids are the two long structures that make up the two longitudinal halves of the chromosome, present during metaphase of cell division. Chromatids on the same chromosome are called sister chromatids. The point at which the two sister chromatids are joined is called the centromere. Many chromosome features are described in relation to the centromere. The portions of the chromatids above the centromere are shorter than those below the centromere and are called the p arms (or "short" arms). The portions of the chromatids below the centromere are called the q arms (or "long" arms). The distal ends of the chromosome are called the telomeres or the terminals.

Normally, human beings have 46 chromosomes (23 different pairs) in all cells except mature red blood cells and the mature sex cells (sperm and ova). This number, called the diploid number of chromosomes for human beings, constitutes the genome, or the complete set of human genes. Of the 23 pairs, 22 pairs are autosomes,

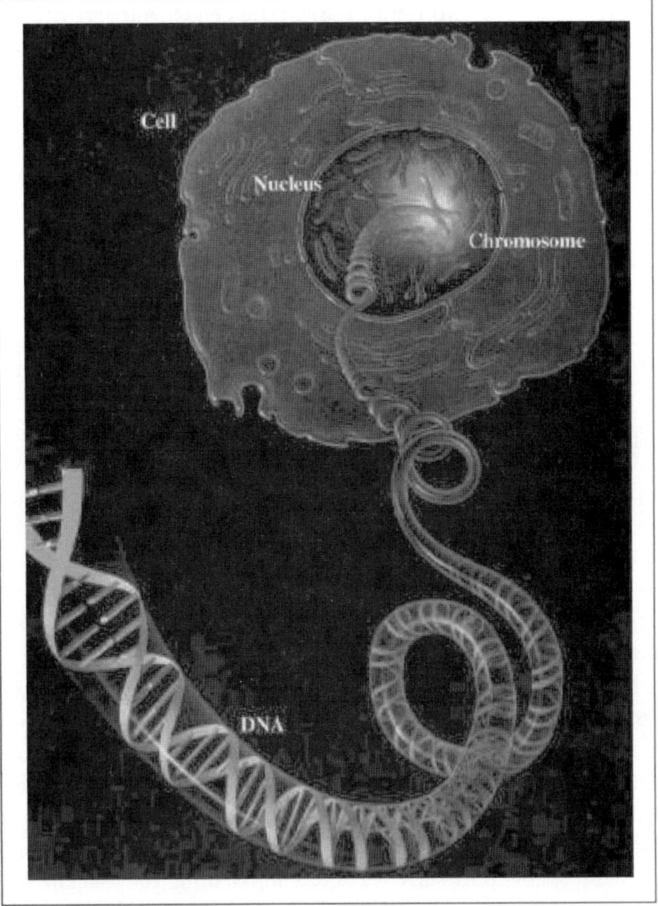

FIGURE 38.1 DNA is composed of two very long chains (strands) of interlocking nucleotides.
Courtesy National Human Genome Research Institute, Bethesda, MD.

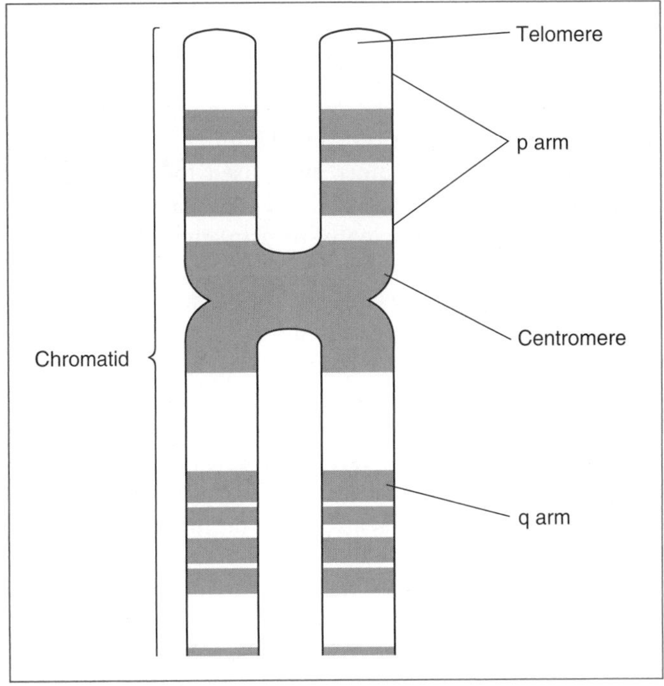

FIGURE 38.2 The basic structure of chromosomes.

which code for and regulate somatic cell development and function. The last pair are the sex chromosomes, which code for and regulate sexual development and function. Mature red blood cells have no nucleus and therefore have no chromosomes. Mature sex cells (gametes) have only 23 chromosomes (half of each pair). This number is known as the haploid number of chromosomes.

Genetic Testing

The chromosomes of an individual can be studied through a process called chromosome analysis (karyotyping). This process involves obtaining a sample of sterile, living tissue that is capable of relatively rapid cell division. Blood lymphocytes or skin fibroblasts are most often used for this purpose. The tissue is incubated with nutrient fluids at 37°C for several hours to several days to encourage more cells to enter the reproductive cycle and proceed to the mitotic phase. The dividing cells are artificially trapped in the metaphase stage of mitosis, fixed with preservative, placed on microscope slides, stained, and evaluated under the microscope. Microscopic photographs of metaphase chromosomes are made, and from these photographs the chromosomes are karyotyped, that is, grouped in sequences of pairs according to the size of the chromosome pairs and the positions of the centromeres. Each group begins with the largest pair of chromosomes that has the centromeres most centrally located. Subsequent chromosome pairs are ordered according to descending size and more distally located centromeres. Analysis of the photographed karyotype can determine numeric chromosome aberrations. However, this method of chromosome analysis is haphazard because specific individual chromosomes cannot be identified precisely. There are approximately 1,000 genes on each chromosome, but only about 100 genes in each band (i.e., the light and dark areas of the chromosome that appear using laboratory techniques) (Scheuerle, 2001).

A more sophisticated chromosome analysis is obtained when standard cytogenetic techniques are combined with the process of banding. Giemsa banding (G-banding) is the banding technique most often used for chromosome analysis. In G-banding, the fixed slides are exposed to a proteolytic enzyme (usually trypsin), which selectively digests areas of the chromosome, and the slide is then stained with Giemsa stain. The areas in which protein has been digested do not take up the stain, which leaves a white space (negative band) on the chromosome. The areas in which protein was not digested do take up the stain, leaving a dark area (positive band) on the chromosome. As a result of this process, each chromosome pair has a unique banded or striped appearance, which permits absolute identification of specific chromosomes (Figure 38.3).

Chromosome analysis that uses banding techniques can identify structural chromosomal abnormalities within individual chromosomes, as well as numeric chromosome abnormalities. However, even this technique has severe limitations, because the smallest chromosome area that can be observed under standard light microscopy has at least 10,000 base pairs. Many genetic disorders are known to involve deletions or rearrangements of genes much smaller than 10,000 base pairs.

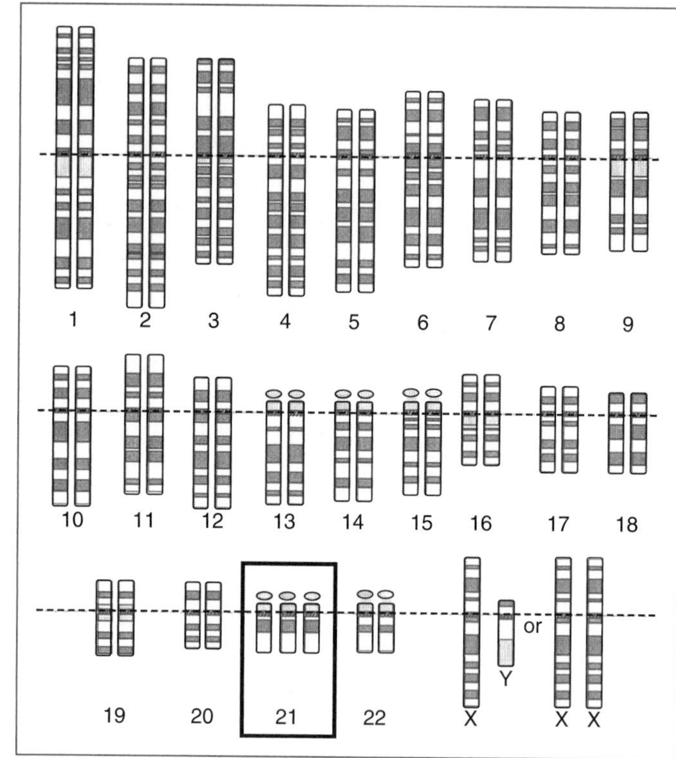

FIGURE 38.3 Each chromosome pair has a unique banded or striped appearance, which permits absolute identification of specific chromosomes.
Courtesy National Human Genome Research Institute, Bethesda, MD.

Molecular testing is also used to determine whether an aberration is present; this technique involves examining the DNA directly. Another form of testing involves examining the gene directly; this test requires knowledge of which gene alteration results in a specific disease process. A mutation that results in sickle cell anemia, for example, can be detected by this method of analysis, which uses allele-specific oligonucleotide (ASO) techniques (Scheuerle, 2001). The direct mutation technique depends on knowledge of the sequence of base pairs that is altered in a suspected disease. This technique can detect fragile X or a breakable area of a chromosome (Scheuerle, 2001). Linkage testing is used when one or more family members have a known genetic problem and the health professional wants to determine if the condition exists in the infant. The results of linkage testing are not considered diagnostic in the first person affected, but rather only after a second possibly affected family member has been identified. This testing is useful for diseases such as cystic fibrosis and Duchenne's muscular dystrophy.

Blood tests for DNA analysis are also used. These have been popularized for paternity issues and for use in criminal cases. The test is considered diagnostic. Protein tests performed on blood examine the structure of the protein.

The test helps when a suspected protein structural defect is believed to be involved in the defect or disease, such as Ehlers-Danlos syndrome, osteogenesis imperfecta, and Marfan syndrome. Each of these conditions is a connective tissue or protein abnormality (Scheuerle, 2001).

Biochemical screening is used when a defect in the metabolic enzymes is suspected. Measurement of amino or organic acids results in identification of an abnormality. The technique is considered a screening test and must be followed by direct measurement of the enzymes for diagnostic purposes.

Cellular Division

For human beings, development begins when one haploid egg is fertilized by a single haploid sperm. The result of this union is a single cell containing the entire human genome, 23 pairs of chromosomes, half of each pair from the maternal gamete (egg or ovum) and half from the paternal gamete (sperm). For the one-celled organism to develop successfully into a complete human being, cell division by duplication is necessary. Duplication divisions occur through the process of mitosis.

Mitosis

Mitosis permits duplication division of one cell to form two daughter cells, which are identical to each other and to the original cell. The complete process of cellular reproduction, including actual mitosis, involves four phases, which collectively are called the cell cycle (Figure 38.4). The primary purpose of the processes involved in mitosis is to ensure that each daughter cell precisely inherits the exact human genome. Although the process of mitosis usually results in an equal division of all cellular structures and contents for the two daughter cells, it is absolutely essential for function that the genetic material inherited by each daughter cell be identical to that of the original cell. The DNA synthesis phase, therefore, is a critical stage of cell division.

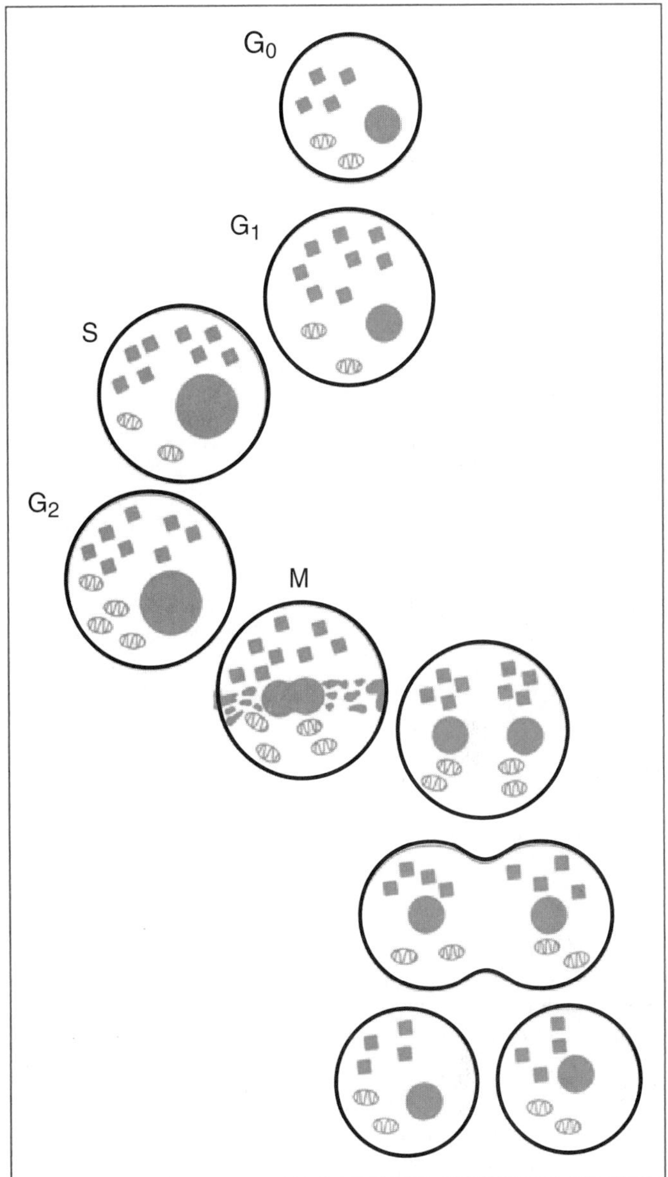

FIGURE 38.4 The cell cycle.

The cell cycle is actually a model depicting various activities that cells must accomplish for successful cell division that results in high-fidelity duplication. It is important to remember that the cell cycle refers only to the reproductive cycle of a cell; it does not take into consideration the cell's total life cycle. After development is complete, most cell types do not spend much time in the actual reproductive cycle. Rather, they exist as functional cell citizens that are performing all their specific and appropriate duties except reproduction. This nonreproductive state is called G0. Normal cells leave this state and enter the reproductive cycle only if (1) they are a specific cell type that is capable of cell division (some cells, such as neurons, skeletal muscle cells, and cardiac muscle cells, do not divide after development is complete); and (2) the particular cell type is needed for normal growth or replacement of dead or damaged cells.

■ **G1 Phase.** On entering the G1 phase of the cell cycle, the cell is committed to divide; this is an irreversible step for normal cells. At this time, the cell takes on added nutrients to form energy substances needed for the strenuous processes involved in actual cell division. In addition, the cell increases the fluid and membrane content to accommodate the needs of two cells.

■ **S Phase.** For each daughter cell to inherit the proper human genome, the DNA content of the original cell must first duplicate itself. The process of making more DNA to form a new cell is called DNA synthesis (S phase of the cell cycle), and it occurs entirely within the nucleus. The original strands of DNA temporarily loosen from the tight helical arrangement. The loosened strands separate into two single strands so that each single strand can be used as a template for the new DNA (Figure 38.5). A series of enzymes is required for this process.

To achieve duplication, the DNA strands relax; the strands unwind from the histones; and the helix

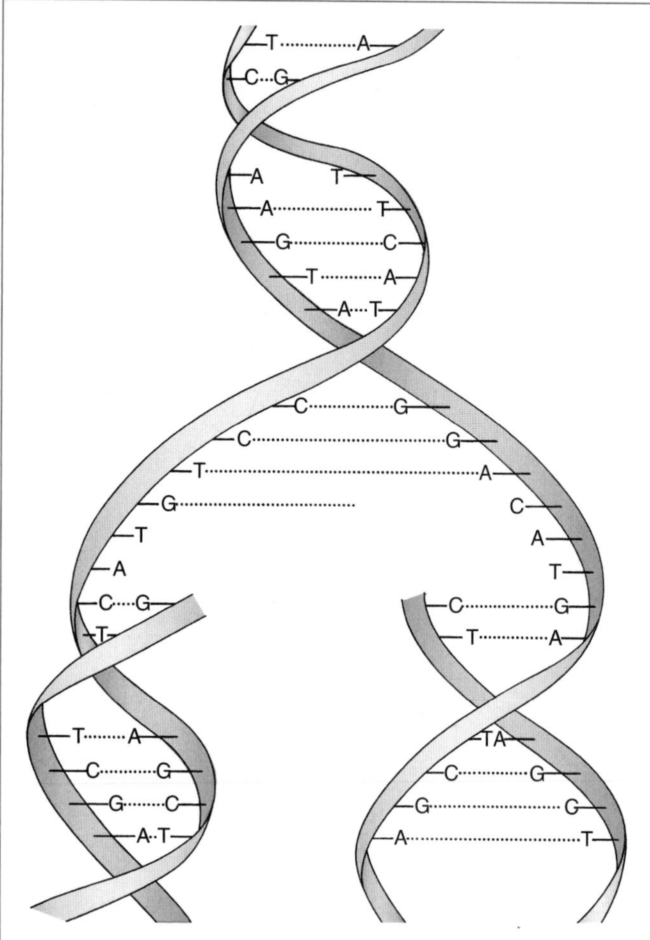

FIGURE 38.5 The loosened strands separate into two single strands so that each single strand can be used as a template for the new DNA.

straightens out slightly. An additional enzyme enters the straightened area and separates the two strands over a limited area. Another enzyme enters and prevents the two strands from rejoining. A different enzyme attaches itself to one strand, travels down it, "reads" the base sequence of this strand, and forms a new strand of DNA that is complementary to the one being read. This process is called the semiconservative mode of DNA synthesis because it results in two identical double helices, each containing one original strand of DNA and one newly created strand of DNA.

After the strands of DNA have been duplicated (replicated), they return to supercoiled chromosomes and line up so that they are ready to be pulled apart (split) during the M phase of the cell cycle. This splitting permits the two sets of DNA to become part of two new cells instead of just one cell.

■ G2 Phase. The G2 phase of the cell cycle is characterized by intense protein synthesis. The cell synthesizes all the enzymes and other complexes necessary to carry out the actual division of the cell, as well as the proteins needed for the regular "housekeeping" duties of the cell. Increased numbers of various organelles also are synthesized to meet the needs of two future cells.

■ M Phase. The actual part of the cell cycle in which two new cells are formed from the original cell is called mitosis, and it is the only time when the DNA is organized into chromosomes. This phase is further divided into subphases.

From the time the cell's DNA is duplicated in the S phase through the G2 phase, the cell's nucleus is said to be in interphase. During interphase, the DNA is loosely coiled into nucleosomes and is widely dispersed throughout the nucleus. Only the nucleolus and two centrioles are distinguishable under standard light microscopy. At this time the two centrioles each begin to form a daughter centriole. As the cell leaves the G2 phase and begins the M phase, the DNA begins to condense. In early prophase, long spaghetti-like strands of newly formed chromosomes are discernible. Throughout prophase, the DNA continues to condense until recognizable chromosomes are present. Later in prophase, the centrioles move to opposite poles of the cell and begin to synthesize spindle fibers. During prometaphase, these spindle fibers attach to the kinetochores of chromosomes on or near the centromeres, and the nuclear membrane begins to disintegrate. During metaphase of mitosis, the chromosomes are in the most compact and readily visible structural forms. The chromosomes line up in the middle of the cell along the equatorial plane. At this point the cell enters anaphase of mitosis, during which the two sister chromatids of each chromosome are pulled apart toward the pole to which each is attached. This process is called nucleokinesis, indicating that the nucleus has moved and separated into two nuclei within the one cell. Under normal conditions, the chromosomes separate in such a way that the two daughter cells receive genetic components that are identical to each other and identical to those of the originating cell. The spindle fibers continue their pulling motion, and the cell begins cytokinesis, or the separation of the single cell body into two separate cell bodies, each with one nucleus. Cytokinesis is completed during telophase of mitosis, and at this time the DNA begins to loosen from the compacted chromatids. When the nuclear material is completely dispersed throughout the nucleus with only the centrioles and nucleolus discernible, the two new daughter cells are in interphase.

During early embryonic development, the initial fertilized egg with 46 chromosomes undergoes many duplication divisions, resulting in a large, hollow ball of cells (blastocyte), each with the same amount and organization of genetic material in its nucleus and exactly the same appearance and function. Although individual genes can undergo mutations after conception that result in altered gene expression, the actual genetic fate of this future human being, determined at the time of conception, is irreversible and cannot be changed.

At this point, these early embryonic cells are called undifferentiated because none of these cells has yet taken on the specific appearance (morphologic characteristics) and function or functions of the mature cell type it eventually will become. Obviously, something has to change during the course of development, because normal human infants are not born as large balls of undifferentiated cells.

Between 8 and 10 days after conception, the human embryonic cells initiate the steps that lead to differentiation. In response to an unknown signal or signals, each cell commits itself to a specific maturational outcome. At the time of commitment, the cell has not taken on any differentiated features or functions, but it now positions itself within a group that eventually will take on specific morphologic characteristics and functional behavior. The process of commitment involves turning off specific genes that regulated and directed the early rapid growth and turning on other specific genes that control the expression of particular differentiated functions. The uncommitted, pluripotent cell is referred to as the stem cell. Stem cell transplants are used to treat leukemia and other forms of autoimmune suppression. Stem cell research has sparked considerable controversy over the use of fetal tissue in such experimental situations. Time, debate, negotiation, and perhaps legislation will surround these complex issues.

It is critical to remember that all differentiated somatic cells (body cells, not including sex cells) retain all the genes in the human genome. At one time the differences in appearance and function between cell types were explained by the theory that different cells actually "lost" the genes they did not need and retained only those required to reproduce and to perform special functions. We now know that this is not the way differentiation occurs and is maintained. Instead, all cells (excluding the sex cells) retain all genes. However, genes are selectively expressed or repressed in different cell types. For example, the gene for insulin is present in all cells; however, only in the beta cells of the pancreas is the insulin gene expressed, or "turned on," to meet the body's need for insulin production. There is nothing wrong with the insulin genes in other cell types (e.g., in skin cells or skeletal muscle cells); simply put, because the special functions of these other cells do not include the production of insulin, the insulin gene in these cells is maintained in a repressed, or "turned-off," state. This turning off of early embryonic genes appears to be accomplished through the activity of special repressor genes that function solely to repress the activity of the early embryonic genes so that they can no longer be freely expressed. This knowledge offers potential for future genetic treatment for many diseases.

Meiosis

The process by which early embryonic cells destined to become mature sex cells achieve maturation is somewhat different from that for somatic cells. Early in development, the committed sex cells continue to undergo mitotic cell division to increase their overall numbers. The cells resulting from these mitotic divisions continue to be diploid. Before the sex cells can completely mature, however, they must reduce their chromosome complement to the haploid rather than the diploid number through meiotic cell division. Meiosis is the form of cell division that reduces the genetic complement of the cells by half, an actual reduction division that is different from the duplication division of mitosis. The result of meiosis is the production of new daughter cells that are identical to each other (in terms of their autosomes) but different from the originating cell. This process is necessary for gametogenesis, the final formation of sex cells. To accomplish this, the entire process of meiosis involves two completely separate series of cell divisions, one stage of which closely resembles a mitotic cell division. As a result of meiosis, four haploid cells are formed from a single diploid precursor sex cell.

As the precursor gametes (sex cells) prepare to become haploid gametes, each diploid precursor undergoes one round of DNA replication (synthesis), just as mitotic cells do in the S phase of mitosis. At this point in the process, the diploid precursor cell is now tetraploid (4N), with twice the normal number of chromosomes (92).

The cell now enters prophase of the first meiotic division. Each chromosome has two sister chromatids joined only at the centromere. Early in prophase, or meiosis I, the chromosomes condense and coil up, and the homologous pairs of chromosomes form a synapse. During synapse the homologous pairs of chromosomes associate with each other, lying side by side to form a tetrad with four chromatids. Because they are so close and because they are not yet compacted completely, some "crossing over" of genetic material occurs, both from the chromatids on the same chromosome (sister chromatids) and from the chromatids on the homologous pair (nonsister chromatids). Many genes are located on each chromatid. This crossing over of genetic material from nonsister chromatids has the effect of randomly "reshuffling" the maternally and paternally derived genes within the chromatids of homologous pairs, producing a wide variety of new combinations.

All the autosomes undergo this reshuffling process during synapse. The sex chromosomes have only a few limited exchanges at the telomeres. This limitation of exchanges is necessary because the chromatids of the X and Y chromosomes are different, each with unique areas. By not exchanging unique areas, the integrity of the sex chromosomes is maintained. In this way, the species continues with only two genders.

After synapse the two centrioles in the cell move to opposite poles on the nucleus and begin to form spindles. The synaptic pairs of chromosomes further condense and move to the equatorial plane of the nucleus, where metaphase of meiosis I begins; this stage is similar to metaphase in mitosis. The newly created spindles attach to the centromeres of the chromosomes. Contraction of the spindles causes whole chromosomes to be separated from chromosome pairs, but the newly reorganized chromatids of each chromosome remain together (anaphase I). At this point, disjunction occurs as the chromosomes form dyads or pairs of sister chromosomes, and the cell completes cytokinesis so that two new cells with 46 chromosomes each are formed. However, because of the crossing over that occurred during synapse and because the new chromosomes randomly assort into pairs, the two newly created cells do not contain the identical gene complement of the precursor sex cell that began the process of meiosis. The new combination of chromosomes cannot be equally separated by maternal and paternal origin. Although the two new cells each contain 22 pairs of autosomes and one pair of sex chromosomes, some of the pairs may be composed wholly of maternally derived chromosomes; others may be composed wholly of paternal chromosomes; and still others may be composed of varying combinations of maternal and paternal genetic material.

These two cells, which contain 46 chromosomes each (two copies of each chromatid), now spend some time in interphase before completing meiosis. The amount of time spent in interphase varies, with secondary oocytes remaining considerably longer in interphase (years) than secondary spermatocytes. No further duplication or synthesis of DNA occurs in these cells.

Meiosis is completed after the second meiotic division. In meiosis II, the two new interphase diploid cells created in meiosis I enter prophase and begin condensing their DNA so that chromatids are formed. The centrioles in each of the two nuclei separate to opposite poles and form spindles that attach to the centromere of each chromosome. The cells now enter metaphase as the nuclear membrane begins to disintegrate.

The chromosomes in each of the two cells move to the equatorial plane and line up. The spindles separate the chromatids. Each pair of chromosomes has four chromatids. When these chromatids separate, one chromatid from each chromosome is segregated to each new daughter cell; each daughter cell therefore receives two chromatids from each pair of chromosomes. However, because the four chromatids segregate independently to the two daughter cells, there is no guarantee that each daughter cell will receive a chromatid from each chromosome of the chromosome pair. It is highly likely that for some chromosome pairs, the daughter cell will inherit two chromatids from one chromosome of a pair and none from the other chromosome.

The result of the entire process of meiosis is the formation of four haploid gamete cells from one diploid precursor sex cell. The crossing over of genetic material from homologous pairs of chromosomes during synapse with random assortment of chromatids in meiosis I, followed by independent segregation of chromatids in meiosis II, has some intriguing consequences. Even though all gametes are descended from the same clone of precursor sex cells and have identical genetic constitutions, the reshuffling of paternal and maternal whole genes and alleles (recessive as well as dominant) can result in hundreds or even thousands of possible minor variations in the genetic makeup of the gametes. Given this range of possibilities, the astounding fact is not that brothers and sisters sometimes do not resemble each other, but rather that they ever do.

PROTEIN SYNTHESIS

All cells that make protein have in their DNA the code for that protein, the actual gene for that protein. The unique DNA pattern (gene) for a specific protein is first converted into a piece of ribonucleic acid (RNA). RNA is similar to DNA, but instead of containing thymine (T), RNA contains uracil (U). Proteins are formed by the linkage of individual nitrogen units, called amino acids, into a linear strand. There are 22 different amino acids; each has a unique three-base code sequence, called a codon, that identifies the DNA and RNA recipe specific for that amino acid. Some amino acids have only one codon, whereas others have as many as four different but closely related codons:

Amino Acid	RNA Codon
Methionine	AUG
Alanine	GCU, GCC
Valine	GUU, GUC, GUA, GUG
Phenylalanine	UUU, UUC

The total number of amino acids in a specific protein and the exact order in which they are connected determine the nature and activity of the protein. The making of protein, or protein synthesis, is similar to some of the steps in DNA synthesis, although carried out on a smaller scale. The cell must loosen the area of DNA that contains the amino acid code (gene) for a specific protein such as insulin. The DNA in the region of the gene to be read loosens and unwinds slightly from the histones, using enzymes that are similar to those involved in DNA synthesis. Once the appropriate area of DNA has unwound and the two strands are separated and held open, a special RNA enzyme binds to the gene area of the DNA and reads it. When the enzyme recognizes a "start" signal, it moves along the strand and synthesizes a new strand of RNA complementary to the gene area of the DNA. When the enzyme reaches the end of the gene sequence, a "stop" signal tells the enzyme to stop making new RNA. The newly created RNA strand moves away from the gene. The DNA closes back together and recoils into the normal helical formation. The new piece of RNA is called messenger RNA (mRNA or sometimes just the "message") because it contains the special coded pattern sequence (the message) for building the specific protein (in this case, insulin).

After the mRNA has been transcribed from the gene, the mRNA interacts with two other types of RNA. Individual amino acids are present inside the cytoplasm, waiting to be properly aligned to form a protein, in a process called translation. Substances called ribosomes, which are made up of special bunches of ribosomal RNA, also are present, along with yet another type of RNA called transfer RNA (tRNA).

Transfer RNAs are adapter molecules that assist in bringing the correct amino acid into the lineup at the proper time. Each tRNA can carry or hold only one amino acid at a time, and the tRNA has an anticodon that is complementary to that specific amino acids codon. Therefore, because each tRNA can bind to only one of the 22 different amino acids, there must be at least 22 different types of tRNA. In the cytoplasm, the ribosome attaches to the mRNA strand and begins the reading process along the strand. When a three-base code is read and interpreted by the ribosome as a specific codon for a specific amino acid, the ribosome allows the tRNAs to come in and attempt to match their anticodons to the codon. When the correct tRNA matches up with the codon on the mRNA, that tRNA releases its amino acid and allows the amino acid to bind to the growing protein strand. This process is repeated all the way down the mRNA until all the correct amino acids are aligned in the right order to make the specific protein.

PATTERNS OF INHERITANCE

Mendel and others established general rules or concepts concerning the inheritance of specific traits governed by single genes. Much of the preliminary information was obtained through observation and manipulation of many generations of plant reproduction; however, these concepts proved to be generally accurate and applicable for the transmission of some human traits.

Mendelian Laws of Gene Expression

Mendel's work explained the concept of dominant and recessive traits. Through his observations of different types of garden peas, Mendel determined that specific varieties of peas had unique traits. For example, one variety of peas always produced wrinkled seeds when fertilized with pollen from the same pea type, whereas another variety of peas always produced smooth seeds when fertilized with pollen from its same pea type. Modeling out this information yielded the following table, in which P1 indicates the original parent generation; F1 indicates the first-generation offspring or progeny; F2 indicates the second-generation offspring or progeny; F3 indicates the third-generation offspring or progeny; and so forth for succeeding generations. Each generation of progeny was fertilized with pollen from the same generation.

Generation	Smooth Seeds	Wrinkled Seeds
P1	Smooth × smooth	Wrinkled × wrinkled
	↓	↓
F1	All smooth seeds	All wrinkled seeds
	↓Self-pollination	↓Self-pollination
F2	All smooth seeds	All wrinkled seeds
	↓Self-pollination	↓Self-pollination
F3	All smooth seeds	All wrinkled seeds
	↓Self-pollination	↓Self-pollination
F4	All smooth seeds	All wrinkled seeds

When Mendel experimented with cross-pollination (cross-breeding) of pea varieties, the inheritance of the traits came out differently than expected. The following model depicts Mendel's results when he fertilized a smooth pea variety with the pollen of a wrinkled pea variety.

P1	Smooth × wrinkled
F1	All smooth seeds Self-pollination
F2	Smooth and wrinkled seeds (3:1 ratio of smooth to wrinkled)

Mendel's explanation for this observation was that the trait for seed texture was determined by the inheritance of a pair of hereditary elements, now known as gene alleles (an allele is any possible alternative form of a gene) and that the relative "strength" of these two alleles varied. This variation in strength resulted in variable expression of the trait when the pair of hereditary elements was mixed (heterogeneous). When both parent seeds had the same hereditary element or genotypes (homogeneous), all the offspring in succeeding generations had the same appearance, or phenotype, of the expression of that element. For homogeneous pairs, the phenotypes and the genotypes were identical. When the parent seeds were heterogeneous for a particular hereditary element, the first-generation offspring expressed only the stronger or dominant element, even though both elements were present in all offspring. In this situation, the phenotype was different from the genotype; that is, the appearance of the peas in the F1 generation was smooth even though the hereditary elements for texture of these peas was heterozygous and consisted of one gene allele for smooth texture and one gene allele for wrinkled texture. The mixed appearance of the peas in the second self-fertilized generation led Mendel to determine that the hereditary element (gene allele) for smooth texture was dominant and the hereditary element for wrinkled texture was recessive.

Dominant traits could be expressed in the phenotype when the genotype for that trait was either homogeneous or heterogeneous, but recessive traits could be expressed in the phenotype only when the genotype for that trait was homogeneous.

Further experimentation with cross-pollination of plants led to the finding of codominance or incomplete dominance. In cross-pollinating red roses with white roses in the parental generation, Mendel predicted that only the dominant color trait would be expressed in the F1 generation, with both colors being expressed in the F2 generation (in a 3:1 ratio). Because red was a stronger, bolder color, Mendel expected that the first-generation flowers from this cross-pollination would all be red. Instead, the roses in the first-generation progeny were all pink, indicating that the gene for red and the gene for white were equally dominant. Roses in the second generation of this cross-pollination were red, pink, and white in a 1:2:1 ratio. Therefore in codominance, the phenotype accurately expresses the genotype. Red roses must have two red gene alleles (homogeneous), pink roses must have one red gene allele and one white gene allele (heterogeneous), and white roses must have two white gene alleles (homogeneous).

Traits or characteristics regulated by a single gene with multiple alleles are instances where the Mendelian rules for patterns of inheritance apply.

Patterns of Traits Inherited by Single-Gene Transmission

A single gene, whether dominant or recessive, may control a trait. The locations of many genes have been specifically identified, or mapped, on human chromosomes. Even without establishing a gene's chromosomal location, it is possible to determine genetic transmission through multiple generations of a family, as specific patterns that indicate whether the gene is dominant, recessive, located on an autosomal chromosome, or located on one of the sex chromosomes. This information can be elucidated without identifying the specific gene through the use of family pedigree analysis. Determination of inheritance patterns for a specific trait allows more accurate prediction of the risk of trait transmission.

A pedigree graphically represents a person's medical and biologic history (Olsen, Dudley-Brown, & McMullen, 2004). It is a schematic drawing of a family history (Figure 38.6), which allows a pictorial representation of patterns of inheritance over many generations.

Construction of a pedigree involves the use of symbols denoting standardized pedigree nomenclature (Bennett et al., 1995). The pedigree usually is started with the proband, the individual who draws medical (genetic) attention to the family. The proband usually is indicated with an arrow.

In analyzing a pedigree, the answers to the following specific questions are noted:

1. Is any pattern of inheritance present, or does the trait appear sporadic?
2. Is the trait transmitted equally or unequally to males and females?
3. Is the trait present in every generation, or does it skip a generation?

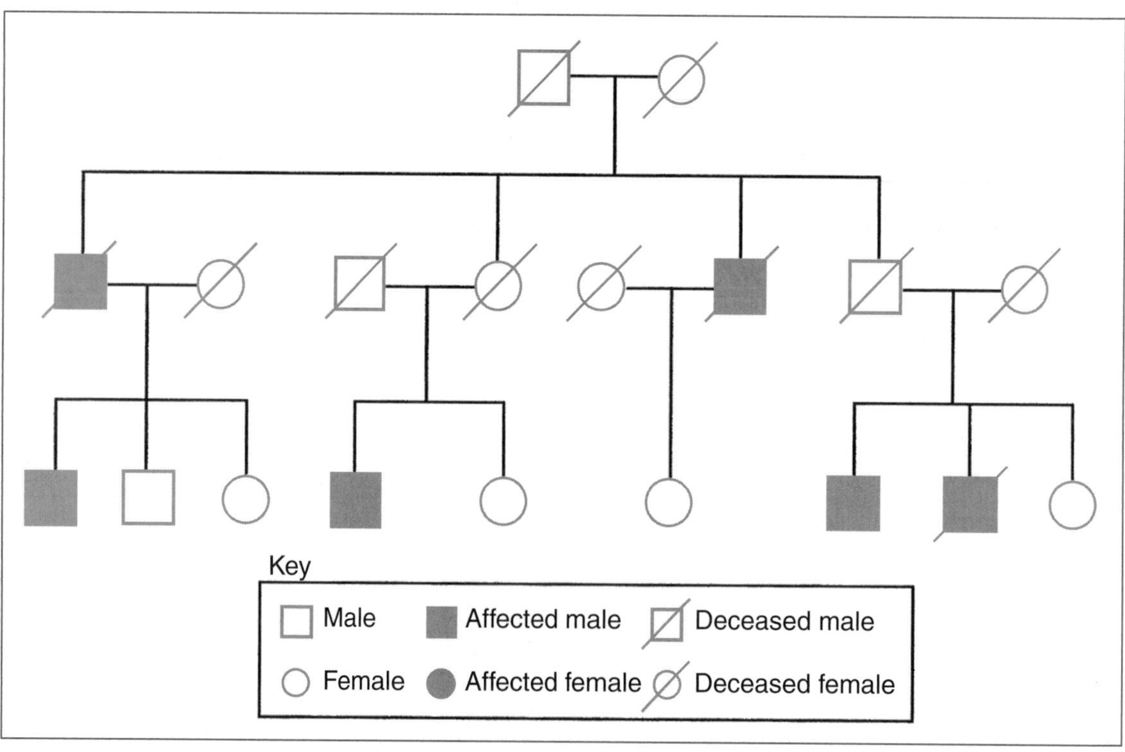

FIGURE 38.6 A pedigree.
Courtesy National Human Genome Research Institute, Bethesda, MD.

4. Do only affected individuals have children affected with the trait, or can unaffected individuals also have children who express the trait?

Construction of a pedigree as part of history taking:

- Facilitates note taking, increasing the accuracy of the history and serving as a means to organize collected information
- Serves as a means of communication, allowing information collected by one health team member to be shared with other professionals working with the individual or family so that information is not repeated
- Provides a means for professionals working with an individual or family to visualize and validate the relationships of affected individuals within a family scope. Creating a visual image of relationships may assist family members in clarifying who is or is not a blood relative of an affected individual.
- Facilitates the emergence of patterns of inheritance for a specific trait in a specific family
- Enhances analysis of gene expression and transmission of more than one trait through linkage studies
- Helps to identify individuals at risk within a kinship more accurately (these individuals then can undergo examination or receive counseling)

The four types of inheritance patterns associated with traits controlled by a single gene are autosomal dominant, autosomal recessive, sex-linked dominant, and sex-linked recessive. Figure 38.7 shows a variety of typical pedigrees for a number of inherited traits. Each of these inheritance patterns is defined by specific criteria.

Traits With an Autosomal Dominant Pattern of Inheritance

Autosomal dominant single-gene traits require that the gene controlling the trait be located on an autosomal (nonsex) chromosome, and the trait usually is expressed even when the gene is present on only one chromosome of a chromosome pair. A typical autosomal dominant

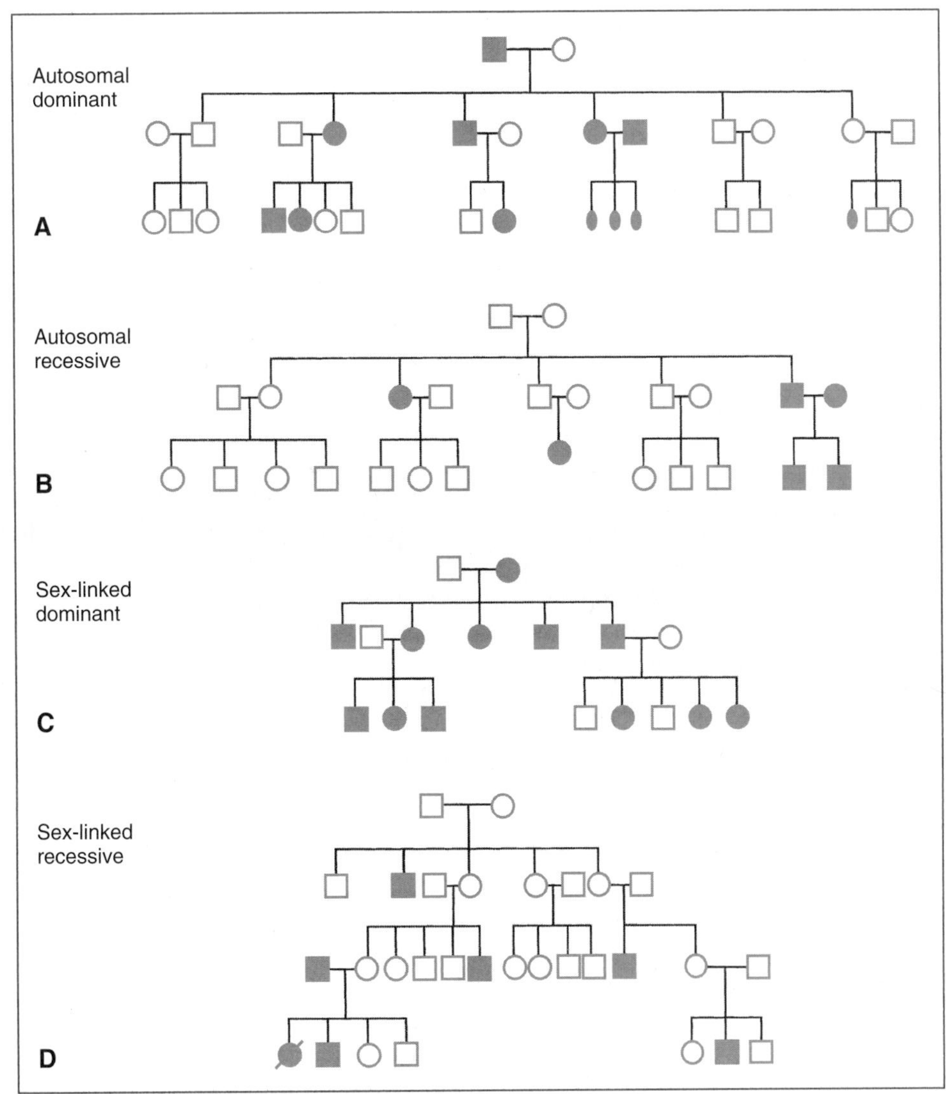

FIGURE 38.7 Variety of typical pedigrees for a number of inherited traits.

pattern of inheritance that meets all the defining criteria would be:

1. The trait appears in every generation with no skipping. When the trait is a result of a new mutation (de novo), this criterion is demonstrated only in the branch of the pedigree stemming from the person who first exhibited the new mutation.
2. The risk for affected individuals to have affected children is 50% with each pregnancy.
3. Unaffected individuals do not have affected children; therefore their risk is 0%.
4. The trait is found equally in males and females.

Autosomal dominant patterns of inheritance are associated with many normal variations in body structure, such as brown eye color, widow's peak hairline, and curly hair. In addition, this pattern of inheritance has been demonstrated in a variety of genetically transmitted problems, including achondroplasia, familial hypercholesterolemia, Huntington's disease, dentinogenesis imperfecta, brachydactyly, allergic hypersensitivity, Marfan syndrome, and familial hypercalcemia.

Traits With an Autosomal Recessive Pattern of Inheritance

Autosomal recessive single-gene traits require that the gene controlling the trait be located on an autosomal chromosome, and the trait can be expressed only when the gene is present on both chromosomes of a chromosome pair. A typical autosomal recessive pattern of inheritance that meets all the defining criteria would be:

1. The trait appears in alternate generations of any one branch of a kinship.
2. The trait or characteristic usually first appears only in siblings (progeny of unaffected parents) rather than in the parents themselves.
3. Approximately 25% of a kinship is affected and expresses the trait.
4. The children of an affected father and an affected mother are always affected (risk is 100% for each pregnancy). Two affected individuals cannot have an unaffected child.
5. Unaffected individuals who are carriers (have the gene on only one chromosome of a chromosome pair) and do not express the trait themselves can transmit the trait to their offspring if their mate either is a carrier or is affected. The risk of a carrier having a child who expresses the trait is 25% with each pregnancy when the carrier is married to another carrier, 50% with each pregnancy when the carrier is married to an affected individual, and 0% with each pregnancy when the carrier is married to a noncarrier. The risk of the unaffected carrier having a child who is a carrier for the trait is 50% with each pregnancy.
6. The trait is found equally in males and females.

Autosomal recessive patterns of inheritance are associated with many normal characteristics and variations in body structure and function, such as blue eye color, straight hair, and the Rh-negative blood type. In addition, this pattern of inheritance has been demonstrated in a variety of genetically transmitted conditions, including albinism, sickle cell anemia, cystic fibrosis, phenylketonuria, Tay-Sachs disease, Hurler's syndrome, Bloom syndrome, Fanconi's anemia, galactosemia, and hyperextensible thumb.

For some of these diseases, the carrier has no symptom of the trait, and in other conditions the carrier does not express the full-blown condition but may express a milder form when predisposing environmental or personal events are present. For example, carriers of sickle cell disease (SCD) may have some sickling of their red blood cells under conditions of extreme hypoxia, although the sickling is never as severe or widespread as it is in the person who is homozygous for SCD. For the most part SCD is not a single-gene mutation. Research has identified many versions of SCD that involve modifier genes such as those responsible for beta-globin genotype, fetal hemoglobin (HbF), beta S gene cluster haplotype, and alpha-thalassemia, as well as interaction with the environment in order to produce the disease (Kenner, Gallo, & Bryant, 2005).

Sex-Linked Patterns of Inheritance

Some genes are present only on the sex chromosomes. The Y chromosome appears to have few genes that are not also present on the X chromosome. However, the X chromosome has many single genes that do not appear to be present elsewhere in the human genome. For all intents and purposes, then, the discussion of sex-linked patterns of inheritance is really a discussion of X-linked patterns of inheritance.

Because X chromosomes are distributed unequally between males and females (1:2 ratio, respectively), the X-linked chromosome genes likewise are distributed unequally between the two genders. Males have only one X chromosome and are said to be hemizygous for any gene on the X chromosome. As a result, X-linked recessive genes have a dominant expressive pattern of inheritance in males and a recessive expressive pattern in females. This difference in expression occurs because males do not have a second X chromosome to balance the expression of any recessive gene on the first X chromosome.

■ **Dominant Patterns.** For a sex-linked (X-linked) dominant single-gene trait to be expressed, the gene controlling the trait must be located on only one of the X chromosomes. A typical sex-linked dominant pattern of inheritance meets certain criteria that are obvious in the pedigree. The defining criteria are:

1. There is no carrier status; all individuals with the gene are affected.
2. Female children of affected males are all affected (risk is 100%), whereas male children of affected males are unaffected (risk is 0%). Therefore the overall risk of an affected male having affected children is 50% for each

pregnancy, since the probability of having a female is also 50%. It is the inheritance of the trait by female offspring of affected males that defines the problem as X-linked dominant, because the inheritance pattern among the offspring of affected females is identical to an autosomal dominant pattern.
3. The trait appears in every generation.
4. For homozygous females, the risk of having an affected child is 100% with each pregnancy, and offspring of both genders are affected equally. For heterozygous females, the risk of having an affected child is 50% with each pregnancy, and children of both genders are equally at risk.
5. In the general population, X-linked dominant problems affect twice as many females as males, but heterozygous females usually express a milder form of the problem than do hemizygous males.

Common X-linked dominant problems include fragile X and hypophosphatemia.

■ Recessive Patterns. X-linked recessive single-gene traits are among the best-defined inherited health problems. This pattern of inheritance requires that the gene controlling the trait be present on both X chromosomes for the trait to be fully expressed in females (females must be homozygous for the trait) and on only one of the X chromosomes for the trait to be expressed in males (males must be hemizygous). A typical sex-linked recessive pattern of inheritance meets all the following defining criteria:

1. Expression, or incidence, of the trait is much higher among males in a kinship (and in the general population) than among females.
2. The trait cannot be transmitted from father to son because the father contributes only the Y chromosome to his son's sex chromosome pair.
3. Transmission of the trait occurs from father to all daughters (who are all carriers but either do not express any of the trait or express it in a very mild form).
4. Female carriers have a 50% risk (with each pregnancy) of transmitting the gene to their offspring. Female offspring who inherit the trait are carriers, and male offspring who inherit the trait are affected.

Sex-linked recessive inheritance patterns may be responsible for normal variation of some secondary female sex characteristics. This pattern of inheritance also has been associated with a variety of disorders, including hemophilia (A and B), Duchenne's muscular dystrophy, ichthyosis, Lesch-Nyhan syndrome, and color blindness. For some of these disorders, females who are heterozygous for the gene express no overt symptoms (such as color blindness). For other disorders, female heterozygotes express some mild aberrations (e.g., increased bleeding tendency in carriers of hemophilia). Few females who express homozygosity have been found; it may be that homozygosity related to sex-linked recessive diseases leads to such a severe disorder that it is lethal in embryonic or early fetal life.

Multifactorial Inheritance

The use of the term *multifactorial* refers to the new understanding of the interaction of the genome with the environment. As genetic knowledge increases, it is recognized that few conditions are really single-gene conditions, as described above with SCD.

Gene Variation and Nontraditional Inheritance

In addition to variation in the expression of single genes, a single gene may be responsible for the expression of many effects that appear unrelated. This concept, known as pleiotropy, probably involves changes or aberrations in regulatory genes rather than in structural genes. One example of pleiotropy is Marfan syndrome. This syndrome is transmitted as an autosomal dominant trait, but its expression involves a variety of aberrations in unrelated tissue types. These aberrations include excessive growth of long bones, the presence of or predisposition to development of an aortic aneurysm, and severe nearsightedness.

Some heritable problems are associated with more than one gene. For example, congenital deafness or Usher's syndrome is an outcome associated with a variety of abnormal genes, although not all of the genes have to be abnormal for deafness to result (Kenner et al., 2005). When more than one gene is responsible for a specific characteristic or trait, the trait is controlled through polygenic expression. Cleft palate and neural tube defects are other examples of developing tissues that require polygenic expression for normal development and that can develop abnormally if any of the required genes is not normal.

Mitochondrial Disorders

Mitochondria, intracellular organelles involved in energy production, have their own DNA (mtDNA) distinct from nuclear DNA (nDNA), discussed earlier in this chapter. A unique finding about mtDNA is that it is inherited exclusively through the maternal line. Each cell has numerous mtDNA molecules, so a single cell with an mtDNA mutation may also have other mtDNA without the mutation, a condition termed *heteroplasmy*. This heterogeneity in DNA composition contributes to variable expression in mitochondrial diseases. Conditions attributed to mtDNA mutations include Leber hereditary optic neuropathy (LHON), Kearns-Sayre disease, deafness, and Alzheimer's disease.

CHROMOSOMAL ABERRATIONS

As discussed previously, chromosomes are formed during the metaphase of mitosis from tightly packed, supercoiled DNA. Each chromosome contains hundreds of genes; detectable aberrations of any chromosome can result in aberration in the structure or expression of one or more genes.

Numeric Aberrations

The normal diploid number of human chromosomes at metaphase of mitosis is 46: that is, 23 pairs. Some individuals have missing or extra whole chromosomes. This type of aberration usually is the result of abnormal or delayed disjunction (nondisjunction) in gamete formation during meiosis I or meiosis II. Instead of all gametes having 23 chromosomes each, some gametes have 24, some have 22, and some have the normal 23. When a 24-chromosome gamete is united with a 23-chromosome gamete of the opposite sex during fertilization, the resulting individual has 47 chromosomes. One chromosome set contains three copies of a chromosome instead of the normal two copies; this situation is called a trisomy. When a 22-chromosome gamete from one parent is united with a 23-chromosome gamete of the other parent during fertilization, the resulting individual has 45 chromosomes. One chromosome set contains only one copy of a chromosome instead of the normal two copies; this is called a monosomy. Whenever the individual has more or fewer chromosomes than normal, some malformations and abnormal developmental processes are expressed. Nondisjunction is most commonly associated with advanced maternal age at the time of conception, presumably as a result of primary oocytes spending years in prophase of meiosis I. It is important to note, however, that nondisjunction can occur at any age.

In theory, nondisjunction can occur within any chromosome pair. However, nondisjunction of some chromosome pairs leads to embryolethal consequences. The most common chromosomal aberration found among all conceptuses is a missing X chromosome, or Turner syndrome (45,XO). Most conceptuses with a chromosome constitution of 45,XO do not survive beyond the embryonic period. The most common chromosomal aberration observed among newborns is trisomy 21 (Down syndrome) (47,XX or XY, 21). Other syndromes of trisomy that can be observed among newborns are trisomy 13, trisomy 15, trisomy 18, and sex chromosome trisomies (47,XXX; 47,XXY; 47,XYY). Trisomy 16 has been identified in embryonic and early fetal wastage, but this abnormality does not usually lead to a fully developed newborn. Autosomal monosomes may be conceived but rarely survive to the stage of birth, although monosomy 21 has been reported among newborns.

All individuals with autosomal trisomies experience some degree of mental retardation. In addition, each trisomy is associated with a specific set of abnormalities, malformations, and unique developmental patterns. This is why individuals with trisomy may share heritable characteristics with their normal family members (e.g., hair color and texture, skin tone, eye color), but many of their structural features tend to resemble those of unrelated individuals who have the same trisomy.

Individuals with missing or extra whole sex chromosomes tend to be intellectually normal and have fewer recognizable physical malformations compared with individuals with autosomal numeric aberrations. Somewhat controversial is the finding that these individuals have behavioral patterns that are not completely normal, such as attention deficit problems and other learning disorders.

Structural Aberrations

Structural aberrations can occur in one of two ways: (1) parts of chromosomes can break off and either become lost or attach themselves to other chromosomes, resulting in translocation of chromosomal material from one chromosome to another; or (2) one whole chromosome can become joined to another whole chromosome, a translocation of chromosomes called robertsonian translocation.

When chromosomes are broken and translocated to other chromosomes, the total amount of chromosomal material may be balanced (normal) or unbalanced (abnormal). If the total amount of chromosomal material present in the individual's cells is balanced, even though it is not located in the usual positions, the individual phenotypically is normal. Problems do not arise until this individual reproduces. Because some of this individual's gametes are not normal (i.e., not balanced) as a result of random assortment and independent segregation of chromatids during gametogenesis, the person is at risk for having chromosomally unbalanced and abnormal offspring. This individual should be referred for genetic counseling. The same situation is true for individuals with robertsonian translocations. As long as the normal amount of chromosomal material is present in all the individual's cells, the individual is phenotypically normal, even though the chromosomes' locations might be abnormal.

PRENATAL TESTING AND SCREENING

For an increasing number of heritable conditions, prenatal screening is available for determining if a fetus is affected. The issue of prenatal diagnosis is complex. Many of the tests are expensive, carry some degree of risk to the pregnancy, and cannot always provide conclusive results. Tests may be performed directly on fetal cells or indirectly on products synthesized by the fetus, or by imaging. Some tests are even done before implantation.

Preimplantation Genetic Diagnosis

Preimplantation genetic diagnosis (PGD) is used with in vitro fertilization (IVF), oftentimes to determine if the zygote has any readily detectable genetic abnormalities. The cells from the zygote are biopsied and analyzed using a polymerase chain reaction (which consists of a series of events or reactions that occur as a substance moves down the strands of DNA) or fluorescence in situ hybridization (FISH) (see explanation later in this chapter). The FISH test can detect conditions such as Duchenne's muscular dystrophy, cystic fibrosis, and severe combined immunodeficiency (SCID) (Harris & Verp, 2001). More commonly, tests are performed on fetal cells or enzymes.

Fetal Ultrasonography

Fetal ultrasonography involves the use of high-frequency sound waves that are reflected differently in various media and in tissues of different densities. With computer enhancement, ultrasonography can provide a relatively detailed image of the embryo and fetus. Interpretation of the images produced has been refined to such a degree that even minor structural aberrations can be detected.

Ultrasonography often is used to locate the placenta, cord, embryo or fetus, amniotic fluid pockets, and other associated structures before more invasive diagnostic procedures are performed. Fetal ultrasonography can provide information about fetal age, the amount of amniotic fluid present, and a variety of structural abnormalities (Hata et al., 1998), including the following:

- Neural tube defects (spina bifida, encephaloceles, microcephaly, anencephaly, hydrocephaly)
- Skeletal dysplasia (fractures, disproportions, bowing)
- Gastrointestinal anomalies (gastroschisis, atresias, tracheoesophageal fistulas)
- Congenital heart disease (coarctation of the aorta, transposition of the great vessels); echocardiograms can be performed in conjunction with ultrasonography to determine chamber and valvular abnormalities, hypoplastic ventricles, and septal defects
- Genitourinary problems (horseshoe kidneys, polycystic kidneys, exstrophy of the bladder, Potter's syndrome or sequence)
- Cystic hygromas

Tests on Fetally Derived Cells

A wide variety of tests can be performed directly on fetal cells. The most common methods of obtaining fetal cells are through amniocentesis and chorionic villus sampling (CVS).

■ Chromosome Analysis by Amniocentesis. Amniocentesis is an invasive procedure in which the amniotic cavity is accessed under sterile conditions through the abdominal wall of the mother. This procedure usually is performed in conjunction with fetal ultrasonography to minimize the risk of puncturing vital fetal structures with the relatively large-bore amniocentesis needle. The ideal gestational age for safe amniocentesis is 16 weeks after conception has occurred. At this time considerable amniotic fluid is present, and the fetus is capable of shedding many viable cells. Once the needle is in place, approximately 20 mL of amniotic fluid is withdrawn. Some viable fetal cells will be present in the fluid. This test sometimes is referred to as midtrimester testing, because it is used from 15 to 20 weeks gestation.

Early amniocentesis, which is performed before 14 weeks gestation, also is used. Usually, not enough fetal cells are obtained to ensure an adequate sample size for most tests, so cells are cultivated in tissue culture, then tested. The tests most often performed include chromosome analysis, enzyme analysis, tests for the presence or absence of a specific biochemical product, and examination of genes using molecular probes.

■ Chromosome Analysis by CVS. Chromosome analysis can also be performed on fetal tissue obtained through CVS. This technique involves removing a piece of tissue from the growing placenta after its location has been identified through ultrasonography. The needle can be inserted either through the cervical os (more common method) or by transabdominal puncture. This procedure can be performed during the first trimester, as early as 9 to 10 weeks gestation.

■ Enzyme Analysis. Some genetic metabolic diseases are caused by a deficiency of a specific enzyme in the fetus. Often these children are normal at birth because maternal enzymes crossed the placenta and performed the specific function in the fetus. However, after birth, maternal enzymes can no longer be used. The pathway affected by the missing or inactive enzyme malfunctions, and the body begins to demonstrate abnormal buildup of products or abnormal metabolism.

Fetal cells cultured for several weeks without the influence of maternal enzymes can express the same metabolic abnormalities that the child would show after birth. Enzyme analysis of the cells or culture fluid (or both) can determine whether a specific enzyme is present at all or whether it is present in normal concentrations. Some genetic metabolic problems that can be identified through enzyme analysis of fetal cells are Tay-Sachs disease, Hurler's syndrome, metachromatic leukodystrophy, galactosemia, and homocystinuria.

■ Alpha-Fetoprotein. Alpha-fetoprotein (AFP) is normally synthesized in measurable quantities only during embryonic and fetal life. In the early embryo, the yolk sac synthesizes AFP; later the fetal liver and gastrointestinal cells assume this function. AFP is present in fetal blood and in some extracellular fluids, and it serves the same function that albumin does in human blood after birth. Because the fetal and maternal circulations are integrated, substances made by the fetus that are small enough move down their concentration gradients into maternal serum. AFP also is present in fetal urine and therefore in amniotic fluid. The synthesis of AFP is well regulated, and the pattern of normal amniotic fluid levels specific to gestational age is known. Variation from this normal pattern is associated with developmental problems.

AFP can be measured in the amniotic fluid (requiring amniocentesis) or in maternal serum. The maternal serum alpha-fetoprotein (MSAFP) test is one of the more commonly used prenatal screening tests. The accuracy of both the amniotic fluid and MSAFP measurements requires exact identification of gestational age at the time the fluid or serum is obtained. An AFP value is considered elevated if it is at least twice the mean for that specific gestational age. The most common problem associated with elevated AFP is an open neural tube defect (the open tube provides a means for extra AFP to leak into the amniotic fluid). A lower than normal AFP value also has been associated with fetal developmental problems, although this phenomenon shows more variability. The most common condition consistently associated with low AFP is Down syndrome, although the phenomenon is not consistent enough to be used as the only screening test for Down syndrome. Other conditions associated with low AFP are gestational diabetes and spontaneous abortion.

■ Multiple Marker Screen. The multiple marker screen, or quad screen, is more sensitive for aneuploidy than is AFP by itself. This screen can detect changes in the maternal AFP, human chorionic gonadotropin (hCG), unconjugated estriol (uE3), and dimeric inhibin-A (DIA). These biologic markers are particularly useful in detecting conditions such as trisomies. The same factors that can affect AFP levels, of course, can cause inaccurate results in the multiple screen, including wrongly estimated dates of confinement and multiple gestations (twins).

The multiple marker screen is performed between 15 and 20 weeks gestation. If an abnormality is found, ultrasonography should be used to confirm the problem. The exact mechanism involved in the alteration marker levels when a chromosomal problem exists is unknown, although it probably relates to a problem with the fetal liver (Harris & Verp, 2001).

■ Percutaneous Umbilical Blood Sampling (PUBS) PUBS is another test that can be useful from 18 weeks gestation. It requires use of ultrasonography to visualize the positioning of the catheter into the umbilical cord. Blood is withdrawn and tested for genetic abnormalities. PUBS is an invasive procedure through which fetal blood can be obtained for karyotyping, but FISH is replacing PUBS in many perinatal centers.

■ FISH. FISH uses DNA probes that resemble chromosomal sequences or regions. These probes are fluorescent, and when they bind with areas in or on the chromosome, they are visible. FISH probes were first developed for several of the most common numerical chromosome abnormalities (i.e., 13, 18, 21, and X and Y) (Harris & Verp, 2001). The conditions for which they are used include Prader-Willi syndrome and aneuploidy (Harris & Verp, 2001).

■ Other Molecular or DNA Probes. In some cases the actual gene associated with a specific problem has been identified, and molecular probes complementary to the gene have been made. These probes can be used to determine whether the gene is present in fetal cells. Use of molecular probes does not require dividing fetal cells, although a sufficient volume of cells is necessary. In some cases, enough fetal cells can be obtained through amniocentesis or CVS so that the test can be performed directly on the DNA of the tissue. At other times, a greater volume of fetal cells is required, and the fetal cells must be grown in culture before the DNA can be extracted and probed.

Many molecular probes are commercially available, which makes testing more accessible and less costly. Genetic metabolic diseases for which molecular probes are commercially available include cystic fibrosis, hemophilia B, Huntington's disease, retinoblastoma, SCD, and thalassemia. Testing for genetic metabolic diseases for which probes are not commercially available can be performed in genetic research centers.

NEWBORN TESTING AND SCREENING

Advances in genetic technology have resulted in increased testing capability for numerous disorders, including infections, genetic disease, and metabolic disorders with a single blood spot (American College of Obstetricians and Gynecologists [ACOG], 2003; Banta-Wright & Steiner, 2004). Individual state statutes vary widely in the number of tests mandated, from as few as four to as many as 30 (U.S. National Newborn Screening and Genetics Resource Center, 2006).

Although many tests are currently available for newborn screening, for some of the identified diseases there are no effective treatments. Nationwide universal testing for 29 "core panel" conditions has been recommended (American College of Medical Genetics [ACMG], 2005), along with 25 "secondary targets," conditions that are part of the differential diagnosis of a core panel condition (table available at http://www.mchb.hrsa.gov/screening). Twenty-three of the 29 core conditions can be tested with a single blood spot using MS/MS (ACMG, 2005). However, debate continues about tests in the screening panel because most states are not prepared with a system of notification for follow-up and treatment when infants have positive test results. Unfortunately, molecular technology has eclipsed health care provider preparation in genomic knowledge. Nursing must respond to this gap in order to provide quality care in response to parental questions about testing, results, risk interpretation, and follow-up. In addition, nurses must be educated in order to contribute knowledgably to the many ethical and legal issues that have been raised about newborn testing, such as storing blood spots for future testing, cost effectiveness of universal testing, parental consent for testing, and privacy protection (Little & Lewis, 2008).

FAMILY HISTORY TOOL AND NURSING

Today there is recognition that a three-generation family history is essential for good health. To focus attention on the importance of family health history, U.S. Surgeon General Richard H. Carmona launched a national public health campaign in 2004 to encourage all American families to learn more about and record their family health history using Centers for Disease Control and Prevention's (CDC) Family History Tool (Yoon et al., 2002) or the U.S. Department of Health and Human Services "My Family Health Portrait" (U.S. DHHS, 2005). Recognition of the significance of accurate health history is a byproduct of the HGP. Nurses are often the professionals involved in taking a health history that could result in a pedigree. Typical information obtained for the three-generation family history and pedigree includes age and year of birth; age and cause of death for those deceased; ethnic background of each grandparent; relevant health information; illnesses and age at diagnosis; information regarding prior genetic testing; information regarding pregnancies including infertility, spontaneous abortions, stillbirths, and pregnancy complications; and consanguinity issues (Bennett, 1999). Together, history and pedigree have the capacity to demonstrate linkages between current health and future health risks. For example, SCD and its alterations at the cellular level may put the infant at risk as a teenager or adult for stroke. Understanding this risk, nurses can plan efforts for health promotion.

SUMMARY

Neonatal nurses must keep abreast of new genomic knowledge and prenatal/neonatal testing that can be done to impact long-term health (Williams, Tripp-Reimer, Schutte, & Barnette, 2004). Many health problems have genetic aspects for perinatal and neonatal nursing, such as prenatal screening and diagnosis, assistance with infertility testing and intervention, diagnosis of congenital syndromes and associations and metabolic disease, identification of reproductive hazards in the workplace and the surrounding environment both for health professionals and for the public, identification of congenital problems that occur secondary to substance abuse, and fetal therapy and surgery and the neonatal implications of such procedures (Feetham, Thomson, & Hinshaw, 2005; Jenkins, Grady, & Collins, 2005; Loescher & Merkle, 2005; Olsen et al., 2003). All health professionals at every level of education must have knowledge of genomics. In 2001 the National Coalition of Health Professional Education in Genetics (NCHPEG) published a list of core competencies, which are considered necessary for all health professionals in all disciplines (Jenkins, 2001). The nursing profession led this movement, recognizing the importance of genomics to all areas of nursing practice. A list of the genetics core competencies is available (http://www.nchpeg.org). A nurse with a subspecialty in genomics may act as a genetic counselor, informing families of their genetic risks, providing information, and giving support during the initial diagnosis and through follow-up. However, the holistic nature of nursing, which takes in biopsychosocial needs, extends beyond just counseling measures as they often are defined; it includes a broader perspective of care. The six roles of the professional nurse—advocate, practitioner, collaborator, investigator, educator, and leader—are all essential in working with patients and families with genetic and congenital disorders.

The nurse can also act as an advocate for the family and refer them to community resources such as genetics clinics, family support groups, or specialized home health care services. Access to care is an important aspect of advocacy for these families. The neonatal nurse involved in community-based follow-up care has a special need for updated genomic information. Prenatal and newborn screening and early identification of genetic, congenital, or familial problems often occur in this practice setting. This nurse is also involved in the treatment of the actual disease, such as phenylketonuria or cystic fibrosis, and must help educate the family about the need for complying with treatment and for continuing follow-up care. The nurse should also be aware of community resources, for both the public and the professional, that provide treatment, support, and education for such medical-genetic disorders. A list of available web-based resources is provided in Table 38.1. NCHPEG developed interprofessional core competencies (http://www.nchpeg.org). A nursing group led by Dr. Jean Jenkins and colleagues adapted these to reflect the nursing profession and care. It was published in 2012 and reflects the competencies in genetics and genomics for nurses with graduate degrees (Greco, Tinley, & Seibert, 2012).

TABLE 38.1

WEBSITES FOR GENOMIC RESOURCES AND PROFESSIONAL ORGANIZATIONS

Name	Website	Description
American College of Medical Genetics (ACMG)	http://www.acmg.net	Education and resources for professionals in medical genetics
American Medical Association (AMA)	http://www.ama-assn.org/ama/pub	Information about genetics and genetic resources; professional organization for medical doctors
American Nurses Association	http://www.nursingworld.org	Registered nurses' professional organization; continuing education; genetic articles; ethical issues; standards of practice
American Society of Human Genetics (ASHG)	http://www.ashg.org	Professional organization of human geneticists; genetics professional information and research
Association of Women's Health, Obstetric and Neonatal Nurses	http://www.awhonn.org	Clinical position statement
Centers for Disease Control (CDC) Office of Genomics and Disease Prevention (OGDP)	http://www.cdc.gov/genomics	Genetics information and research; tool for family history; public health priorities; common questions
Cincinnati Children's Hospital Genetics Education Program for Nurses (GEPN)	http://www.cincinnatichildrens.org/ed/clinical/gpnf	Modularized learning online for those practicing nurses or faculty who want to gain more genetic knowledge

(continued)

TABLE 38.1

WEBSITES FOR GENOMIC RESOURCES AND PROFESSIONAL ORGANIZATIONS (CONTINUED)

Name	Website	Description
Dolan DNA Learning Center	http://www.dnalc.org	Educational resources for children, parents, professionals
Ethical, Legal and Social Implications (ELSI) Research Institute	http://www.genome.gov/10001618	Federal program to fund research related to ELSI of genomic research
Gene Tests	http://www.ncbi.nlm.nih.gov/sites/GeneTests/?db=GeneTests	Free genetics information, disease reviews, international directory of laboratories and clinics
Genetic Alliance	http://www.geneticalliance.org	Coalition for genetic advocacy
Genetic and Rare Diseases (GARD) Information Center	http://rarediseases.info.nih.gov	Provides information specialists to answer consumer questions about rare diseases
Genetic Education Materials (GEM) Database	http://www.gemdatabase.org/GEMDatabase/index.asp	Searchable listing of public health genetics policy documents and clinical genetics educational materials
Genetic Resources on the Web (GROW)	http://www.nih.gov/sigs/bioethics/grow.html	Forum for organizations/professionals who desire high-quality information availability on the Internet
Genetics	http://www.ghr.nlm.nih.gov	National Library of Medicine website for consumer information about genetics
Genetics and Public Policy	http://www.dnapolicy.org	Genetic technology and public policy information Center
Genetics Education Center, University of Kansas	http://www.kumc.edu/gec	Genetics education; links to large number of Internet resources
Harvard Medical School, Department of Continuing Education	http://cme.med.Harvard.edu	Professional online continuing education
Health Resources and Services Administration (HRSA)	http://www.hrsa.gov	Federal resource for research funding, policy development
International Society of Nurses in Genetics (ISONG)	http://www.isong.org	Nursing organization devoted to genetics; genetics education, practice, and resources
March of Dimes	http://www.marchofdimes.com	Professional and consumer education about genetics, newborn screening, prevention of birth defects
National Coalition in Health Professional Education in Genetics (NCHPEG)	http://www.nchpeg.org	Multiprofessional organization supporting core education in genetics. Core competencies in higher education of professionals
National Guideline Clearinghouse	http://www.guideline.gov	Searchable site for guidelines relating to genetics
National Human Genome Research Institute (NHGRI)	http://www.genome.gov	Research and news about genomics
National Newborn Screening and Genetics Resource Center (NNSGRC)	http://genes-r-us.uthscsa.edu	Information on newborn screening by state; genetic resources
National Society of Genetics Counselors (NSGC)	http://www.nsgc.org	Professional organization of genetics counselors; genetic information; tools for collecting family history
Online Mendelian Inheritance	http://www.ncbi.nlm.nih.gov/entrez/query.fcgi?db=OMIM	Database of human genes and genetic disorders in man (OMIM)
Secretary's Advisory Committee on Genetics, Health and Society (SACGHS)	http://www4.od.nih.gov/oba/SACGHS.HTM	Committee of professionals and interested individuals representing public stakeholders in genetics issues
World Health Organization	http://www.who.int/genomics/en	Worldwide genomics progress (WHO) Genetics Resource Centre
U.S. Department of Energy Office of Science Genome Programs	http://www.doegenomes.org	Federal programs related to genomics

CASE STUDY

A White, male 39-week infant was born to a 23-year-old mother who had no complications during pregnancy. This was a first baby for the mother. Over the course of the first few days of life the infant became less and less responsive. On day 3 the infant was transferred to a tertiary center for evaluation. Upon arrival, the infant failed to respond to voice or touch. A genetics consult was requested. Through extensive testing the infant was determined to have an error of metabolism that regulated amino acid metabolism. With this information nutritionists, geneticists, neonatologists, and nurse practitioners worked to determine a formula that the infant could metabolize. The neonatologists and nurses worked with the mother to help explain what was happening to her baby. The geneticist went over the genetic risk for any future children she might have. Within 48 hours of the diagnosis, the infant awoke and was discharged within 1 week.

EVIDENCE-BASED PRACTICE BOX

An exploding area of genetics is referred to as epigenetics. This term refers to alterations in either the genotype or phenotype. The implications for neonates are tremendous. Areas of research include maternal use of antiepileptic drugs during pregnancy and the changes that occur in neonatal DNA (Smith et al., 2012); cardiorespiratory changes and epigenetics (Lagercrantz, 2012) and impact of epigenetics on a neonate experiencing maternal separation and environmental stress (Samra, McGrath, Wehbe, & Clapper, 2012). These are just a few areas that are examining epigenetic changes and the lifelong impact on the neonate's health.

References

Lagercrantz, H. (2012). Are cardiorespiratory complications a question of epigenetics? *PNAS*, *109*(7), 2192–2193.

Samra, H., McGrath, J., Wehbe, M., & Clapper, J. (2012). Epigenetics and family-centered developmental care for the preterm infant, *Advances in Neonatal Care*, *12*(5S), S2–S9.

Smith, A. K., Conneely, K. N., Newport, D. J., Kilaru, V., Schroeder, J. W., Pennell, P. B., . . . Brennan, P. A. (2012). Prenatal antiepileptic exposure associates with neonatal DNA methylation differences. *Landes Bioscience*, *7*(5), 458–463.

ONLINE RESOURCES

American Nurses Association Essential Genetic and Genomic Competencies for Nursing with Graduate Degrees
http://www.nursingworld.org/MainMenuCategories/EthicsStandards/Genetics-1/Essential-Genetic-and-Genomic-Competencies-for-Nurses-With-Graduate-Degrees.pdf

American Society of Human Genetics
http://www.ashg.org

Association of Women's Health, Obstetrics, and Neonatal Nursing
http://www.awhonn.org

Centers for Disease Control and Prevention
http://www.cdc.gov/genomics

Cincinnati Children's Hospital
http://www.cincinnatichildrens.org

Dolan DNA Learning Center
http://www.dnalc.org

Ethical, Legal and Social
http://www.genome.gov/10001618

(GEM) Database
http://www.gemdatabase.org/GEMDatabase/index.asp

Gene Tests
http://www.ncbi.nlm.nih.gov/sites/GeneTests/?db=GeneTests

Genetic Alliance
http://www.geneticalliance.org

Genetic Education Materials
http://www.gemdatabase.org

Genetic and Rare Diseases
http://www.rarediseases.info.nih.gov

Genetic Resources
http://www.nih.gov/sigs/bioethics

Genetics
http://www.ghr.nlm.nih.gov

Genetics Education
http://www.cincinnatichildrens.org/education/clinical/nursing/genetics/default

Genetics Education Center
http://www.kumc.edu/gec

Genetics and Public Policy
http://www.dnapolicy.org

Harvard Medical School
http://www.cme.med.Harvard.edu

Health Resources and Services Administration
http://www.hrsa.gov

International Society of Nurses
http://www.isong.org

March of Dimes
http://www.marchofdimes.com

National Coalition in Health
http://www.nchpeg.org

National Guideline
http://www.guideline.gov

National Human Genome
http://www.genome.gov

National Newborn Screening
http://www.genes-r-us.uthscsa.edu
National Society of Genetics
http://www.nsgc.org
Online Mendelian Inheritance
http://www.ncbi.nlm.nih.gov/entrez
Secretary's Advisory Committee
http://www4.od.nih.gov/oba
U.S. Department of Energy
http://www.doegenomes.org
World Health Organization
http://www.who.int/genomics/en

REFERENCES

American College of Medical Genetics. (2005). *Newborn screening: Toward a uniform screening panel and system*. Retrieved from http://www.mchb.hrsa.gov/screening/

American College of Obstetricians and Gynecologists. (2003). ACOG committee opinion number 287, October 2003: Newborn screening. *Obstetrics and Gynecology*, *102*(4), 887–889.

Banta-Wright, S. A., & Steiner, R. D. (2004). Tandem mass spectrometry in newborn screening: A primer for neonatal and perinatal nurses. *Journal of Perinatal and Neonatal Nursing*, *18*(1), 41–60.

Bennett, R. L. (1999). *The practical guide to the genetic family history*. New York, NY: Wiley-Liss.

Bennett, R. L., Steinhaus, K. A., Uhrich, S. B., O'Sullivan, C. K., Resta, R. G., Lochner-Doyle, D., . . . Hamanishi, J. (1995). Recommendations for standardized human pedigree nomenclature. Pedigree Standardization Task Force of the National Society of Genetic Counselors. *American Journal of Human Genetics*, *56*(3), 745–752.

Centers for Disease Control. (2008). Update on overall prevalence of major birth defects—Atlanta, Georgia, 1978–2005. *MMWR*, *57*(01), 1–5.

Childs, B. (1998). Medicine through a genetic lens. In M. Hager (Ed.), *The implications of genetics for health professional education*. New York, NY: Josiah Macy, Jr. Foundation.

Feetham, S., Thomson, E. J., & Hinshaw, A. S. (2005). Nursing leadership in genomics for health and society. *Journal of Nursing Scholarship*, *37*(2), 102.

Greco, K. E., Tinley, S., & Seibert, D. (2012) *Essential genetic and genomic competencies for nurses with graduate degrees*. Silver Spring, MD: American Nurses Association and International Society of Nurses in Genetics.

Harris, C. M., & Verp, M. S. (2001). Prenatal testing and interventions. In M. B. Mahowald, V. A. McKusick, A. S. Scheuerle, & T. J. Aspinwal (Eds.), *Genetics in the clinics: Clinical, ethical, and social implications for primary care*. St Louis, MO: Mosby.

Hata, T., Aoki, S., Hata, K., Miyazaki, K., Akahane, M., & Mochizuki, T. (1998). Three-dimensional ultrasonographic assessments of fetal development. *Obstetrics and Gynecology*, *91*(2), 218–223.

Jenkins, J. (2001). *Core competencies in genetics essential for all health care professionals*. Rockville, MD: National Coalition for Health Professional Education in Genetics (NCHPEG).

Jenkins, J., Grady, P. A., & Collins, F. S. (2005). Nurses and the genomic revolution. *Journal of Nursing Scholarship*, *37*(2), 98–101.

Kenner, C., Gallo, A. M., & Bryant, K. D. (2005). Promoting children's health through understanding of genetics and genomics. *Journal of Nursing Scholarship*, *37*(4), 308–314.

Kenner, C., & Moran, M. (2005). Newborn screening and genetic testing. *Journal of Midwifery and Women's Health*, *50*(3), 219–226.

Little, C. M., & Lewis, J. A. (2008). Newborn screening. *Newborn and Infant Nursing Reviews*, *8*(1), 3–9.

Loescher, L. J., & Merkle, C. J. (2005). The interface of genomic technologies and nursing. *Journal of Nursing Scholarship*, *37*, 111–119.

National Human Genome Research Institute. (2001). *About the human genome project. The Human Genome Research Project: From maps to medicine*. Retrieved from http://www.genome.gov/12011238

Olsen, S., Dudley-Brown, S., & McMullen, P. (2004). Case for blending pedigrees, genograms, and ecomaps: Nursing's contribution to the "big picture." *Nursing and Health Sciences*, *6*(4), 295.

Olsen, S. J., Feetham, S. L., Jenkins, J., Lewis, J. A., Nissly, T. L., Sigmon, H. D., & Thomson, E. J. (2003). Creating a nursing vision for leadership in genetics. *MEDSURG Nursing*, *12*(3), 177–183.

Scheuerle, A. E. (2001). Diagnosis of genetic disease. In M. B. Mahowald, V. A. McKusick, A. S. Scheuerle, & T. J. Aspinwal (Eds.), *Genetics in the clinics: Clinical, ethical, and social implications for primary care*. St Louis, MO: Mosby.

Talking glossary of genetic terms. (2012). Retrieved from http://www.genome.gov/Glossary/index.cfm

The Human Genome Project Completion: Frequently Asked Questions. (2010). Retrieved from http://www.genome.gov/11006943

U.S. Department of Health and Human Services. (2005). *U.S. Surgeon General's family history initiative*. Retrieved from http://www.hhs.gov/familyhistory

U.S. National Newborn Screening and Genetics Resource Center. (2006). *National Screening Status Report*. Washington, DC. Retrieved from http://genes-r-us.uthscsa.edu/nbsdisorders.pdf

Williams, J. K., Tripp-Reimer, T., Schutte, D., & Barnette, J. J. (2004). Advancing genetic nursing knowledge. *Nursing Outlook*, *52*, 73–79.

Yoon, P. W., Scheuner, M. T., Peterson-Oehlke, K. L., Gwinn, M., Faucett, A., & Khoury, M. J. (2002). Can family history be used as a tool for public health and preventive medicine? *Genetics in Medicine*, *4*(4), 304–310.

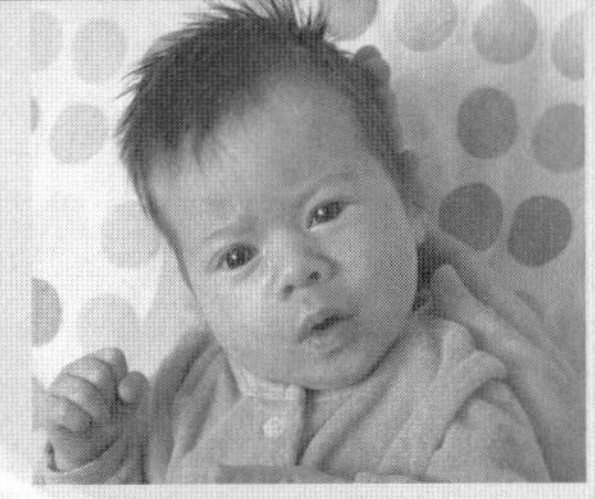

CHAPTER 39

Trends in Neonatal Research and Evidence-Based Practice

■ Lynda Law Wilson and Kathleen R. Stevens

There is a growing call for nurses to lead quality improvement and transformation of health care through research and evidence-based practice (EBP). Experts point to the critical role that nurses have in leading interprofessional groups in producing safe, quality health care (Institute of Medicine [IOM], 2001, 2011). Conducting research and integrating results into clinical decision making are vital to this task.

Some type of knowledge guides every clinical decision and action taken by a nurse. The underlying rationale for a nursing intervention may come from past experiences, trial and error, authority, a nursing procedure manual, a textbook, or, most reliably, science produced through systematic inquiry (research). Nurses, along with most health professionals, have embraced EBP as the knowledge foundation that assures the greatest likelihood that the chosen intervention will produce the intended outcome for the patient or the most accurate diagnosis of the condition. Progress, however, is sometimes held back by deeply rooted conventions in clinical decision making. In the past, nursing care policies often represented a source of knowledge known as authority, the policy makers' own clinical experience, tradition ("we have always done it this way"), internal or external benchmarks, and textbooks. Moving from tradition to EBP will increase the success of nursing care in assisting patients and families to better health.

The quality of care and resulting patient outcomes improve when the selection of interventions is based on research results. Quality of care is defined as "the degree to which health care to individuals and populations increase the likelihood of desired health outcomes and are consistent with current professional knowledge" (IOM, 2013). The definition implies the nurse's application of cause-and-effect interventions known to be effective in resolving the health issue. This definition also underscores key challenges in the research-to-evidence-to-practice quest: There must be an available body of research-produced knowledge; intervention research validates the likelihood that a given nursing intervention will produce the targeted health outcome; the care provided must align with what is known to be effective, as demonstrated through research.

The focus of this chapter is on linking neonatal nursing practice and research in such a way that the strongest knowledge—that derived from research—is put into practice—known as best practice. The chapter presents the basis of EBP, models of evidence-based quality improvement, various research roles for neonatal nurses, clinical problems amenable to research, and current trends in neonatal nursing research.

EVIDENCE-BASED NEONATAL NURSING PRACTICE

Not all sources of knowledge are highly reliable nor does care based on various sources consistently produce the desired patient outcome. Experience and trial and error are good teachers; however, the knowledge gained through these approaches contains bias. That is, it is unknown whether results are due to the intervention or to something other than the intervention that is outside of the nurse's awareness. Additionally, results from one situation may not be generalizable, that is, applicable to another situation or client. Clinical decisions drawn on experience and trial and error will not likely be the most effective in producing the patient outcome because these sources do not expose the full truth or validity of the broader reality. Also, knowledge resulting from trial and error (experience), not framed in explanatory models (theories), does little to advance the scientific foundation for practice.

The key premise of EBP is that research studies produce the most reliable source of knowledge upon which to base clinical decisions. Today, the measure of "best practice" is that interventions are based on "best evidence," that is, scientific findings. However, putting research into practice is fraught with several hurdles. The work within the EBP paradigm has overcome a number of hurdles in applying research results in practice. EBP has produced new ways of applying research evidence in clinical decision making to ensure the best outcome that science knows how to produce. Individual clinician decisions about care as well as agency policies about care standards should reflect the best evidence produced to date. The end result of applying state-of-the-science patient care is that health care status goals are effectively and efficiently met within the context of preferences of the patient and health care provider (Sackett, Straus, Richardson, Rosenberg, & Haynes, 2000). This rapidly advancing movement of EBP embodies new methods and represents a new paradigm of research application in clinical care. The care environment in neonatal nursing will exhibit many aspects of EBP in which the entire health care team is engaged.

WHAT IS EBP?

EBP is a process through which scientific evidence is identified, appraised, converted, and applied in health care interventions (Stevens, 2004). A still-widely-adopted definition of EBP is that it is the integration of best research evidence, clinical expertise, and patient preference. The objective of EBP is the application of the best available evidence in clinical care in order to increase the likelihood that the desired patient outcome is achieved.

Although evidence and knowledge can be drawn from a variety of sources, best evidence is specifically identified as evidence drawn from scientific investigation, or research (Guyatt, Rennie, Meade, & Cook, 2008). Using research evidence as the basis for care is best because it allows the nurse to gauge the certainty and predictability of the care in producing the intended outcome. Implementation of evidence into clinical decision making produces more accurate diagnosis, maximally effective and efficient intervention, and most favorable patient outcomes. These ends can be accomplished through EBP methods, processes, and models.

A MODEL OF EVIDENCE-BASED NURSING

Evidence-based nursing can be described as the process of establishing research-based practice (RBP) by transforming research knowledge through a number of forms, into practice and patient outcomes. Nurse scientists developed the ACE Star Model of Knowledge Transformation to explain the transformation necessary to enhance the clinical utility of research results by reducing the volume and complexity of research knowledge, converting one form of knowledge to the next, and incorporating a broad range of sources of knowledge throughout the EBP process (Stevens, 2004). The Star Model provides a framework in which to consider the transformation that takes place from a single research report from a form with low clinical utility (e.g., statistical test results in a primary research report) into a form that has high utility in clinical decision making and is firmly integrated into clinical practice. Knowledge transformation through five related forms is depicted as a five-point process (Figure 39.1). The forms of knowledge in this transformation are primary research, evidence summary, translation, integration, and evaluation (Stevens, 2004). Each form moves progressively forward in its usefulness for clinical decisions at the point of care, ending with measuring the impact of the evidence-based improvement.

Point One on the Star Model is represented by single, primary research studies. This is the knowledge form with which we are familiar—individual reports of research studies. Over the past four decades, nurse researchers have produced literally thousands of research studies on a wide variety of nursing clinical topics. Although primary research is requisite to EBP, such research does not hold a great deal of stable, accessible, clinical utility in clinical

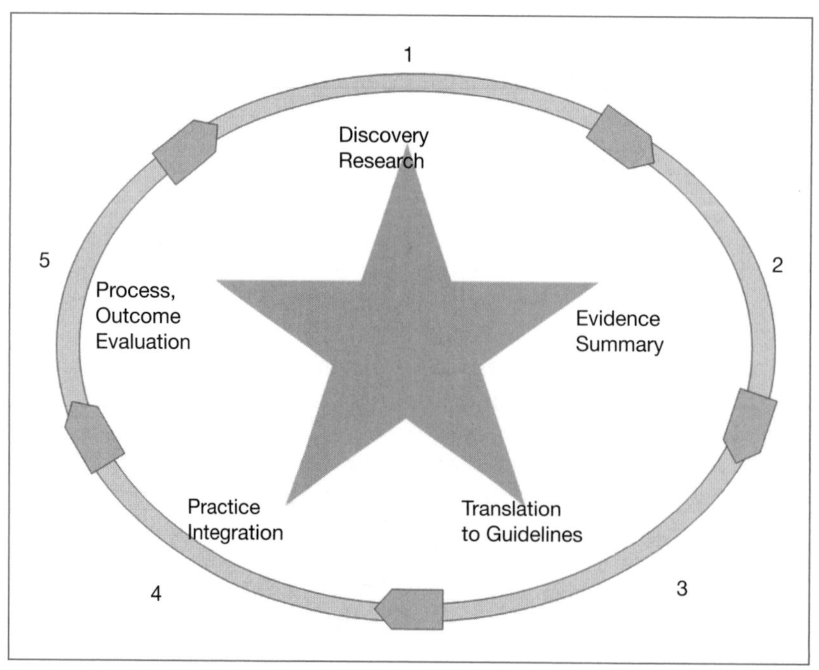

FIGURE 39.1 ACE Star Model of Knowledge Transformation.

decision making. The body of primary research on any given topic will likely include both strong and weak study designs, small and large samples, and conflicting or converging results, leaving the clinician uncertain about which study is the best reflection of cause and effect in selecting effective interventions. In addition, the body of research on a given clinical topic may number in the hundreds and, as such, are not useful for clinical decision making. In considering the form of knowledge on Point One for clinical decision making, two hurdles are evident: the volume and complexity of research literature.

The EBP solution is to transform these single research studies into clinically useful knowledge in Point Two of the Star Model using an evidence summary approach (Stevens, 2004). In this second stage of knowledge transformation, all primary research on a given clinical topic is systematically gathered, screened, and summarized into a single statement about the state of our knowledge on the topic. This summary step is considered the key step for moving research into practice (IOM, 2008). Systematic reviews (SRs) transform research knowledge in a number of notable ways and offer distinct advantages, as are summarized in Box 39.1. Evidence summaries communicate the latest scientific findings in an accessible form for the clinical nurse to readily apply the research in clinical decisions and create clinical unit policies. When developing an evidence summary, reviewers keep in mind that nonsignificant findings are as important to practice as positive results. However, nonsignificant findings tend not to be published and so are underrepresented in the literature.

Evidence summaries are performed by a number of groups and are called by several terms, such as evidence synthesis, SRs, and integrative reviews. The most widely used methods in rigorous evidence summary produce an SR that reflects the methods established in the mid-1990s (Higgins & Green, 2011). An SR is a type of evidence summary that uses a rigorous scientific approach to combine results from a body of primary research studies into a clinically meaningful whole. The SR is a research design that produces new knowledge through synthesis and typically uses the statistical procedure, meta-analysis, to combine findings across multiple studies. In this way, evidence summaries remove the obstacle of voluminous and rapidly expanding bodies of research literature. SRs are rated as the strongest evidence for best practice. At the same time, if summaries are not systematically developed, there is a risk of drawing erroneous conclusions about whether or not an intervention actually works. If this is the case, nurses may chose interventions that do not work or may be unaware of interventions that do work.

BOX 39.1

ADVANTAGES OF SRs

An SR accomplishes the following:

Reduces large quantities of information to a manageable form

Integrates existing information for decisions about clinical care, economic decisions, future research design, and policy formation

Increases efficiency in time between research and clinical implementation

Establishes generalizability across participants, across settings, and treatment variations and different study designs

Assesses consistency and explains inconsistencies of relationships across studies

Increases power in suggesting the cause-and-effect relationship

Reduces bias from random and systematic error, improving true reflection of reality

Provides better continuous updates of new evidence

Adapted from Mulrow (1994).

Developing sound evidence summaries requires specialized scientific skill and extensive resources—often over a year's worth of scientific teamwork. If done to rigorous standards, evidence summaries will review research across all relevant disciplines and across the globe, screen studies for relevance and quality of design, use multiple reviewers to abstract findings, and analyze the results to combine findings and examine the extent of bias in the set of research studies. For this reason, evidence summaries are often conducted by scientific and clinical teams that are specifically prepared in the methodology.

Once evidence summary is conducted, the knowledge can be transformed into Point Three of the Star Model through translation. In this stage, experts are called on to consider the evidence summary, fill in gaps with consensus expert opinion, and merge research knowledge with expertise to produce clinical practice guidelines (CPGs). This process translates the research evidence into clinical recommendations. New standards for developing CPGs specify processes that will produce high-quality, trustworthy guidelines, assuring that recommendations reflect current knowledge. A number of clinical specialty organizations produce guidelines. For example, the Association of Women's Health, Obstetric, and Neonatal Nurses (AWHONN) developed an excellent example of a CPG (Association of Women's Health Obstetric and Neonatal Nurses, 2010) The association combined research evidence and clinical expertise to produce evidence-based guidelines on assessment and care of the late preterm infant by locating and explicating the evidence, rating the strengths of evidence, including evidence-based recommendations, and publishing the guideline. Other, less rigorously developed guidelines are present throughout health care—in the form of clinical pathways, nursing care standards, and unit policies. Trustworthy CPGs reflect several characteristics: A specified process is followed during guideline development; the guideline identifies the evidence upon which each recommendation is made, whether it is research or expert opinion; and the evidence is rated using a strength-of-evidence rating scale (Graham, Mancher, Wolman, Greenfield, & Steinberg, 2011).

Once guidelines are produced, integration is accomplished through change at both the individual clinician and organizational level. Point Four of the Star Model encompasses integration of the CPG into practice at individual provider, microsystem, and system levels. Planned change approaches often are used to overcome resistance and move the individual and organization to a higher standard of practice based on evidence. Guidance for planned change is provided by several principles and theories: Because quality is a system property, systems must be changed with EBP; adoption of new practices can be amplified using principles from theories such as Rogers' theory of diffusion of innovation (Rogers, 1995). In neonatal nursing, as advances emerge, it is essential that all members of the health care team be actively involved in making quality improvement changes. Nurses will be leaders and followers in contributing to such improvement at their individual level of care as well as the system level of care.

Point Five, evaluation, is the fifth stage in knowledge transformation. Practice changes are followed by evaluation of the impact on a wide variety of outcomes, including effectiveness of the care in producing desired patient outcome; population outcomes; efficiency and cost factors in the care (short and long term), and satisfaction of providers and patients alike. Evaluation of specific outcomes has risen to a high level of public interest, given our new awareness that American health care is neither safe nor effective (IOM, 1999). As a result, quality indicators have been established for health care improvement and for public reporting (e.g., Agency for Healthcare Research and Quality (Agency for Healthcare Research and Quality [AHRQ], 2011).

WHAT ARE THE MAJOR FEATURES OF EBP?

It is especially important to consider individual provider and organizational factors that influence the adoption of practice evidence when the evidence was generated in very different health care environments or contexts. It may not be effective, for example, to apply practice guidelines that were developed in the United States to neonatal units in Latin America or Africa because psychosocial and health delivery systems vary in such a way that the knowledge is not generalizable.

Barriers to implementing RBP are removed by using evidence syntheses as the basis for clinical recommendations. SRs "efficiently integrate valid information and provide a basis for rational decision making" in clinical care (Mulrow, 1994). Only in rare instances will a single research study offer highly reliable answers to a clinical question (Eden, Levit, Berg, & Morton, 2011). It is most feasible for the nurse to use research evidence that has been summarized in the form of an SR. Because conducting evidence syntheses is a new, resource-intensive, and rigorous process, it is beyond the capacity of the typical clinician. For this reason, awareness of existing sources of synthesized evidence is critical for the clinician. Box 39.2 presents examples of evidence summaries from the *Cochrane Library of Systematic Reviews*. In addition, Table 39.1 describes other credible sources for evidence summaries. In some cases, conclusions from the evidence summary support current practice and increase confidence that the nursing care will produce the desired outcome. In other cases, the evidence points to a needed change in practice. In either case, examining current practice in light of state of the science is becoming an expectation for health care.

SOURCES OF EVIDENCE FOR PRACTICE

Recognizing that work needs to be done to translate research into practice, a number of entities are adding to the collection of forms of knowledge available to clinicians. This work is spurred by influential agencies such as the IOM and the AHRQ. Each of the Star Model points is now populated by several resources, pointing nurses to useful forms of knowledge for clinical decision making.

BOX 39.2

EXAMPLES OF EVIDENCE SUMMARIES OR PROTOCOLS ON NEONATAL NURSING CARE IN THE *COCHRANE DATABASE OF SYSTEMATIC REVIEWS*

Chang, A. S. M., Berry, A., & Sivasangari, S. (2008). Specialty teams for neonatal transport to neonatal intensive care units for prevention of morbidity and mortality (Protocol). *Cochrane Database of Systematic Reviews, (4), Art. No.: CD007485.* doi:10.1002/14651858.CD007485

Gray, P. H., & Flenady, V. (2011). Cot-nursing versus incubator care for preterm infants. *Cochrane Database of Systematic Reviews, (8), Art. No.: CD003062.* doi:10.1002/14651858.CD003062.pub2

Hodnett, E. D., Gates, S., Hofmeyr, G. J., Sakala, C., & Weston, J. (2011). Continuous support for women during childbirth. *Cochrane Database of Systematic Reviews, (2). Art. No.: CD003766.* doi:10.1002/14651858.CD003766.pub3

Jardine, L. A., Inglis, G. D. T., & Davies, M. W. (2011). Strategies for the withdrawal of nasal continuous positive airway pressure (NCPAP) in preterm infants. *Cochrane Database of Systematic Reviews, (2), Art. No.: CD006979.* doi:10.1002/14651858.CD006979.pub2

Lewin, S., Munabi-Babigumira, S., Glenton, C., Daniels, K., Bosch-Capblanch, X., van Wyk, B. E., . . . Scheel, I. B. (2010). Lay health workers in primary and community health care for maternal and child health and the management of infectious diseases. *Cochrane Database of Systematic Reviews, (3), Art. No.: CD004015.* doi:10.1002/14651858.CD004015.pub3

(*continued*)

Mills, J. F., & Tudehope, D. (2001). Fibreoptic phototherapy for neonatal jaundice. *Cochrane Database of Systematic Reviews, (1), Art. No.: CD002060.* doi: 10.1002/14651858.CD002060

Papatsonis, D., Flenady, V., & Liley H. (2009). Maintenance therapy with oxytocin antagonists for inhibiting preterm birth after threatened preterm labour. *Cochrane Database of Systematic Reviews, (1), Art. No.: CD005938.* doi:10.1002/14651858.CD005938.pub2

Pillai Riddell, R. R., Racine, N. M., Turcotte, K., Uman, L. S., Horton, R. E., Din Osmun, L., . . . Gerwitz-Stern, A. (2011). Non-pharmacological management of infant and young child procedural pain. *Cochrane Database of Systematic Reviews, (10), Art. No.: CD006275.* doi:10.1002/14651858.CD006275.pub2

Vickers, A., Ohlsson, A., Lacy, J., & Horsley, A. (2004). Massage for promoting growth and development of preterm and/or low birth-weight infants. *Cochrane Database of Systematic Reviews, (2), Art. No.: CD000390.* doi: 10.1002/14651858.CD000390.pub2

TABLE 39.1

ALPHABETICAL LIST OF SOURCES OF SYSTEMATIC REVIEWS ON THE INTERNET

Systematic Review Source	Address
Agency for Healthcare Research and Quality	http://www.ahrq.gov
Cochrane Collaboration	http://www.cochrane.org/cochrane/cc-broch.htm#CC (introductory information)
Joanna Briggs Institute	http://www.joannabriggs.edu.au/Home
Sigma Theta Tau International's Worldviews on Evidence-Based Nursing	http://onlinelibrary.wiley.com/journal/10.1111/(ISSN)1741-6787
U.S. Preventive Services Task Force	http://www.ahrq.gov/clinic/uspstfix.htm

Adapted from Stevens and Pugh (1999).

Synthesis work is conducted by several organized agencies. Because the conduct of a SR requires specialized scientific methods and significant resources, it is usually a sponsored activity conducted by groups of scientists. The leading agencies in this work are the Cochrane Collaboration (a global collaborative headquartered in the United Kingdom) and the AHRQ (a federally funded agency in the United States). Another source of evidence summaries is the Joanna Briggs Institute, headquartered in Adelaide, South Australia, that has centers for EBP and conducts SRs around the world. In turn, these agencies disseminate the evidence summaries for use by clinicians, health policy makers, and consumers of health care.

Point Three of the Star Model is populated by several agencies that develop or provide large collections of CPGs. The AHRQ supports the National Guidelines Clearinghouse, a searchable collection of almost 2,000 CPGs, most with strong evidential foundations. In the United Kingdom, the National Institute for Health and Clinical Excellence (NICE) develops evidence-based guidelines for health care providers, as well as for patients and caregivers. There is growing interest in promoting global collaboration in the development and evaluation of EBP guidelines. One organization that has formed to promote such collaboration is the Guidelines International Network, with members from 46 countries and an international guidelines library that contains more than 7,400 documents (Guidelines International Network, 2012). Another excellent resource for evidence-based neonatal care is the Vermont Oxford Network, which was established in 1988 and now includes 9,000 neonatal units worldwide. Member institutions participate in research and also have the option of participating in a quality improvement neonatology collaborative to identify and implement best practices in neonatal care (Vermont Oxford Network, 2012).

Point Four of the Star Model is now populated by the AHRQ Healthcare Innovations Exchange, with the goal of speeding integration of new and better ways of delivering and improving quality of health care. Almost 600 innovations are profiled, along with adopter's guidelines and tools for adopting and sustaining the innovation. Point Five, evaluation, is populated by a number of initiatives to measure and track the quality and safety of care. Quality indicator initiatives include the AHRQ National Healthcare Quality and Disparities Reports and National Database of Nursing Quality Indicators. System-level indicators include surveys of the agency's culture of patient safety and attainment of "never" events.

SKILLS ESSENTIAL IN EMPLOYING EBP

The skills required to accomplish EBP range from the frontline clinician's openness to credible changes in practice to the statistician's performing meta-analysis. At each clinician level and discipline, there are crucial competencies needed in terms of skills, attitudes, and actions. Although the principles and goals of EBP are obvious, the paradigm requires a shift in the way that nurses have traditionally perceived research and clinical decision making. Through an iterative process with an expert panel, national consensus about essential competencies for EBP in nursing has been established (Stevens, 2009). Table 39.2 provides examples of these competencies for the staff nurse level, organized by the five points of the Star Model. The competencies are organized across three levels of clinical practice: entry (staff nurse), intermediate (e.g., CNS or midlevel manager), and advanced (e.g., doctoral nurse participating in a SR team). In addition, the competencies span the five points of the Star Model.

HOW TO EMPLOY EBP

With the new insights into effective clinical decision making that EBP has provided, the question becomes, "How is EBP employed?" Although a number of methods are being developed, tested, and adopted, several guiding principles are apparent.

In today's trends, adoption of EBP is connected to clinical effectiveness and patient safety. EBP is connected to the agency's goal of improving care and outcomes. In clinical settings, often the administrative and managerial teams come to a conclusion that the agency will adopt an initiative: to employ EBP throughout their health care. The commitment requires time, leadership, engagement across all stakeholders, and resources, so several planning stages are helpful in making the initiative a success. These are as follows.

1. The plan for employing EBP may initially include announcements, persuasion for buy-in from all vested interests, and identification and mobilization of resources. Of the many resources needed, *time* in the clinician's workday is a key resource. Other resources can be drawn from existing departments such as the quality assurance department, the medical librarian, and academicians from collaborating universities.
2. To focus the EBP effort, clinical priority topics are identified and set out as the first targets for evidence-based quality improvement. To be successful, the organization and health care team are involved. Criteria useful for selecting priority topics are those established by the IOM to identify national priorities for health care improvement (IOM, 2003). These are: (1) *impact* in terms of burden on patient, family, health care system, and society; (2) evidence that already exists for *improvability* but is not yet used in standard care; and (3) *inclusiveness*, reflecting applicability to patients across the life span and settings.
3. Evidence is located. A comprehensive search is essential, and professional information management skills are valuable. Beginning with a search for evidence summaries is often productive in locating reviews that have already been completed. Locating other forms of knowledge, such as primary research and CPGs is also important in this step.
4. Critical appraisal of the evidence can be accomplished by an evidence team. Using existing checklists, the validity and strength of the evidence are rated.
5. An evidence-based CPG is adapted from an existing one or developed by the team. This CPG development process should be standardized to ensure that evidence is explicated and rated in all CPGs that are introduced into practice.
6. Quality indicators are selected, and baseline assessments are made.
7. A comprehensive plan for change, adoption of innovation, and integration into practice is developed and implemented.
8. The targeted quality indicators are measured once again and compared to baseline assessment. These outcome measures should include patient outcomes, health status (population) indicators, and cost impact. The impact on the care process is also measured to determine if clinical practice has been true to the prescribed CPG. Feedback from quality audits is effective in stabilizing the change to the new standard of care.

GLOBAL CONSIDERATIONS IN EBP

Implementing EBP may be challenging to nurses who live in low-resource countries that have limited access to the Internet and thus have limited opportunities to review the literature or identify evidence to guide practice. One resource that can help to improve access to information

Table 39.2

THE FIVE POINTS OF THE STAR MODEL AND SAMPLE COMPETENCIES FOR NURSES

Star Point	Competency
1. Original Research	Recognize ratings of strength of evidence when reading literature including web resources
2. Evidence Summary	List advantages of SRs as strong evidential foundation for clinical decision making
3. Translation	Use specified databases, access CPGs on various clinical topics
4. Integration	Assist in integrating practice change based on EB CPGs
5. Evaluation	Participate in EB quality improvement processes to evaluate outcomes of practice changes

Adapted from Stevens (2009). Reprinted with permission.

resources is the eGranary database of digital resources (Widernet, 2012). eGranary was founded in 2001 to provide access to Internet resources for the estimated seven out of eight people worldwide with limited Internet access. With support from numerous partner institutions and volunteers, digital and web-based resources are copied onto the eGranary server (after obtaining copyright permission), and these resources are then available to those who purchase the reasonably priced server. As an example of the capability of eGranary to disseminate knowledge, the University of Alabama at Birmingham Sparkman Center for Global Health has worked with numerous partners to develop a portal of more than 500 resources. This portal supports evidence-based nursing practice in Zambia and other English-speaking countries (eGranary Digital Library, 2012). Another resource to improve access to evidence for nurses in low-resource countries who have Internet access is the Health Internet Access to Research Initiative (HINARI) Access to Research in Health Program, set up by the World Health Organization (WHO) together with major publishers; this program enables developing countries to gain access to one of the world's largest collections of biomedical and health literature. It provides free or low-cost Internet access to more than 8,000 journals and online resources to not-for-profit institutions in low-resource countries (HINARI Access to Research in Health Program, 2012).

USING RESEARCH TO CHANGE NEONATAL NURSING PRACTICE

Identifying Problems for Neonatal Research

Neonatal nurses can use findings from research as well as other evidence to improve and change neonatal nursing practice. As noted above, the first step in developing an EBP protocol or procedure is the identification of a clinical problem to be addressed. Nurses might identify a problem of concern in their individual clinical setting.

Nurses in the clinical setting are often in the best position to identify and articulate highly relevant research questions and, through partnering with scientists, are able to carry out research studies that directly improve the delivery of nursing care. The types of questions posed by clinical nurses range from basic physiologic mechanisms in neonatal health to comparisons of efficacy between various interventions to identification of new phenomena as the topic for new programs of research. Ideas for research come from many different sources, including an individual nurse's experience, the nursing or health literature, discussions of social or health issues, or theory (Burns & Grove, 2009). With today's increased emphasis on quality and safety, research topics also emerge from quality assurance audits in the clinical unit, agency-wide interest in system support for quality and safety, and national recommendations for health care delivery changes.

Researchers and professional organizations sometimes conduct surveys or convene expert panels to identify research priorities. These priorities can also help researchers identify researchable problems. For example, the Strategic Plan for the National Institute of Nursing Research (NINR) identified five areas that will be the focus of research investment between 2011 and 2016: (a) enhancing health promotion and disease prevention; (b) improving the quality of life by managing the symptoms of acute and chronic illness; (c) improving palliative and end-of-life care; (d) enhancing innovation in science and practice; and (e) developing the next generation of nurse scientists. NINR promotes interdisciplinary research using a variety of methods including intervention studies, translational research programs, and research to evaluate costs, outcomes, and quality of care (National Institute of Nursing Research, 2011). In parallel, the Improvement Science Research Network (ISRN) established research priorities in improving health care delivery, which work in tandem with the NINR clinical research topics (ISRN, 2010). The ISRN Research Priorities underscore a new goal for nursing research, which is to discover which improvement interventions are effective in changing health care delivery. The broadly stated ISRN Research Priorities include (a) transitions and coordination in care across health care delivery segments; (b) high-performing clinical systems and microsystems; (c) evidence-based quality improvement and best practices; and (d) learning organizations and culture of quality and patient safety (ISRN, 2012).

Box 39.3 lists topics of current research interest questions for neonatal nurses. Many of these research questions are derived from the concern about the prevention of iatrogenic complications of treatments. Others emerge from systematic observation of clinical phenomena or from frustration with current practices.

The Role of Neonatal Nursing Organizations

Neonatal nursing organizations also assist with the identification of neonatal research priorities and development of EBP Guidelines. For example, in 1990 the AWHONN convened a panel of nurse experts to identify areas with sufficient research to develop research-based protocols that could be tested in multiple settings (Gennaro, 1994). Members of the AWHONN Research Committee recommended that the organization fund an EBP project to evaluate the best method for transition of preterm infants to open cribs and appointed a group of six neonatal nurse researchers to conduct the project (Meier, 1994). After reviewing the literature on the topic, the group held a series of meetings and ultimately developed a weaning protocol that was subsequently tested with 270 infants from 10 different hospitals (Medoff-Cooper, 1994). The evidence of this project suggested that preterm infants could be moved to an open crib at lower weights than had been suggested by results of previous studies. The AWHONN project is an excellent example of the contributions that clinical professional associations can make to the development of EBP guidelines. This project illustrates several points in the Star Model: evaluation of original research related to thermoregulation, developing a practice guideline based on a review and synthesis of the existing research, and evaluating the outcome of the EBP guideline.

BOX 39.3

SOME CURRENT NEONATAL NURSING RESEARCH QUESTIONS

Skin Care

How can epidermal damage from tape removal be reduced?

Can the permeable skin of preterm infants be used to deliver medication?

How can the barrier properties of the skin be improved to prevent infection and water loss?

Which cleansing agent and bathing techniques are best for preterm and full-term infants?

Do emollients prevent transepidermal water loss and dermatitis in premature infants?

What is the reliability and validity of the neonatal skin condition score?

Nutrition

How can breastfeeding practices be promoted among mothers of premature infants?

What are the most effective methods of feeding preterm infants?

What are the effects of kangaroo care on breast milk production?

Is weight gain improved with demand versus scheduled feeding?

How can intravenous access be improved and complications minimized?

Instruments and Procedures

What is the effect of routine care tasks, such as bathing, suctioning, on cerebral blood flow velocity?

Which pulse oximeters are most effective in reducing the effects of motion artifact?

Do temperature probe covers contribute to nosocomial infections by providing an environment for skin microbe colonization?

What is the effect of draw-up volume on the accuracy of electrolyte measurements from neonatal arterial lines?

Effect of the Environment and Supplemental Stimulation

What is the impact of light, noise, and handling on infants in the NICU?

What is the appropriate level of stimulation for preterm infants?

What is the effect of supplemental massage and gentle touch on preterm infants?

What are the effects of music therapy on preterm infants?

What is the effect of cycled lighting on preterm infants?

What is the most appropriate method of positioning preterm infants to promote neuromuscular development?

Extracorporeal Membrane Oxygenation (ECMO)

Is the initial training and ongoing education of ECMO specialists sufficient to maintain emergency management skills?

What are the long-term effects of ECMO's use?

What are the neurodevelopmental outcomes of infants who were treated with ECMO?

Endotracheal Tube Stabilization and Maintenance

How can slippage of the endotracheal tube within the trachea be measured?

How can movement of the endotracheal tube be minimized?

Is there a difference in the incidence of nosocomial infections, bronchopulmonary dysplasia, or frequency of suction when using closed versus open tracheal suctioning in neonates?

Management of Pain

How can neonatal pain be assessed?

When is pharmacologic treatment appropriate?

What factors influence preterm infants' responses to painful procedures?

Are there long-term consequences of unrelieved pain experienced in the neonatal period?

What is the most effective method for weaning the infant from analgesics?

Does the use of premedication prior to intubation result in fewer signs of physiologic distress during intubation compared to intubation without premedication?

What are effective nonpharmacologic pain-management techniques for use with neonates?

What are the analgesic effects of oral sucrose and pacifier use on preterm infants during painful procedures?

Thermoregulation

Which techniques are most effective in minimizing insensible water loss and maintaining thermoregulation in the extremely premature infant?

What are the optimal procedures for maintaining thermoregulation when transferring infants from incubators or warmers to open cribs?

What are the effects of skin-to-skin holding (kangaroo care) on thermoregulation of preterm infants?

Positioning and Holding

Which positions are most effective in promoting optimal oxygenation and in minimizing postural deformities?

What are the effects of skin-to-skin holding of high-risk infants?

What are the effects of containment and swaddling of preterm infants?

(*continued*)

How often should infants' positions be changed?

Under what conditions is the prone position linked to sudden infant death syndrome?

What factors influence parents' decisions about sleep positions of their infants?

Developmental Care

What are the outcomes of developmental care?

What are the effects of developmental care training programs on the care delivered by NICU staff?

What are valid and reliable measures of stress in preterm infants?

Is measurement of heart rate variability or vagal tone a reliable means for assessing stability or stress in preterm infants?

Effects of Cocaine

How is the behavior of a cocaine-exposed infant different from that of the nonexposed infant?

What is the appropriate level of environmental stimulation for these infants?

What types of intervention programs are effective for families of cocaine-exposed infants following hospital discharge?

Effective Parent Teaching Techniques

What are the most effective teaching methods for instructing parents in the care of their newborns?

Is computer-assisted instruction effective?

What type of posthospital follow-up is most helpful to parents of infants who are released from the NICU?

Are postdischarge telephone follow-up programs effective in promoting breastfeeding of preterm infants discharged from the NICU?

What are parents' perceptions of a parental care-by-parent program before NICU discharge of their infants?

Family Issues

What nursing interventions help to reduce stressors experienced by families who have infants in the NICU?

What is the incidence of depression among parents of preterm infants?

What interventions help grieving parents?

What interventions help to promote attachment and adaptive parenting between parents and preterm infants and between parents and infants with serious health problems?

What are the outcomes associated with participation in a parent support group for parents of preterm infants?

What are parents' perceptions of the NICU follow-up clinic?

Staff Education

What is the most effective method of orientation of new NICU nurses?

How should formal classroom teaching and clinical preceptorship be integrated?

Are self-paced learning modules an effective teaching methodology for neonatal nurses?

Can neonatal nurses use expert systems to support decision making?

Delivery of Nursing Care

What is the most effective model for delivery of nursing care in the NICU?

Can nonprofessional staff be used in the NICU to support the professional nurse?

Does the use of critical pathways facilitate "costing out" nursing services?

What is the effect of a structured neonatal resuscitation program on delivery room resuscitation practices?

What are the best strategies to promote use of evidence-based practice guidelines in the NICU setting?

Retention of Nurses in the Critical Care Setting

What are the factors that increase job satisfaction for nurses working in the NICU?

How do NICU nurses cope with stress?

What factors increase the likelihood that nursing jobs will be retained?

Do neonatal nurses perceive technology in the NICU as sources of stress?

AWHONN has implemented two other RBP initiatives to enhance evidence-based neonatal nursing care: (a) development of a protocol for neonatal skin care in association with the National Association of Neonatal Nurses (NANN); and (b) development of guidelines for care of late preterms (Medoff-Cooper, Bakewell-Sachs, Buus-Frank, & Santa-Donato, 2005). In the neonatal skin care project, a group of researchers reviewed extant literature to develop a CPG and data collection tools that were implemented by 51 sites involving 2,820 infants in all levels of care. Results of the study indicated that the use of the clinical guideline resulted in improved skin condition of neonates in intensive, secondary and well-baby nurseries. Nurses also were better able to identify risk factors for impaired skin integrity in neonates.

The Late Preterm Infant Initiative (LPTI) project was launched in April 2005 by AWHONN to develop a research-based guideline (RBG) for infants born between 34 and 37 weeks postmenstrual age. The initiative was based on a conceptual framework that focuses on neonatal physiologic functional status, nursing care practices, the neonatal care environment, and the role of the family (Medoff-Cooper et al., 2005). A sample of 15 geographically and demographically diverse sites participated in implementing and evaluating the RBG. The focus of this initiative is to enhance awareness of the special needs of the near-term infant among health care providers and consumers, and promote universal adoption of a practice guideline for care of these infants. For more information on this initiative, readers can go to the AWHONN website at http://www.awhonn.org/awhonn/content.do?name=03_JournalsPubsResearch/3G6_LatePreterm.htm.

The NANN has published position statements on various practice issues on its website, such as medication safety in the neonatal intensive care unit (NICU), palliative care for newborns and infants, the use of human milk and breastfeeding in the NICU, co-bedding of twins or higher-order multiples, and prevention of bilirubin encephalopathy and kernicterus (National Association of Neonatal Nurses, 2012).

Barriers and Facilitators to Implementing Neonatal Nursing EBP

Several studies have been conducted to evaluate the extent to which neonatal nurses are implementing EBP guidelines such as the AWHONN/NANN guidelines. For example, Johnson and Maikler evaluated the implementation of the skin care guidelines in a sample of 136 nurses from 26 hospitals, and identified several barriers to implementing the guidelines in practice: perception by some nurses that traditional practices were superior to the practices proposed by the evidence-based guidelines, difficulty in reading and understanding research evidence, lack of authority to implement the protocols, and lack of physician support (Johnson & Maikler, 2001). Wallin, Boström, Harvey, Wikblad, and Ewald (2000) conducted a similar study in Sweden to determine the extent to which national guidelines on evidence-based nursing care were being implemented in Swedish neonatal units. A total of 13 evidence-based guidelines were developed in cooperation with 42 of the 45 neonatal units in Sweden, and the guidelines were presented in a report that summarized the evidence supporting each guideline, as well as suggested measures for auditing the implementation of the guideline. Findings from this study indicated that 14.3% of the neonatal units were not using the guidelines at all, and there was variable implementation of the guidelines in the other units. Factors that were associated with guideline implementation included the extent to which the units were using a quality improvement method, the length of experience of the nurse manager, the level of research experience in the unit, and the availability of nursing staff resources.

Melnyk, Fineout-Overholt, Stone, and Ackerman (2000) surveyed 160 nurses and found that only 46% of these nurses identified their current practices as evidence-based. Factors associated with increased evidence-based care were nurses' beliefs about the importance of EBP, knowledge of EBP, length of practice as an advanced practice nurse, use of the *Cochrane Database of Scientific Reviews*, or the National Guideline Clearinghouse, and having a mentor to model EBP. Barriers to EBP included lack of time and heavy patient loads, lack of appreciation for the value of research, difficulty searching for and retrieving studies, difficulty reading, understanding, and evaluating research reports, institutional barriers, and limited autonomy or control over one's own practice. Institutional barriers include inadequate staffing and failure to reward nurses who initiate change based on findings from research.

To address the barriers to EBP effectively, neonatal nurses must receive education regarding the research process, have the opportunity to participate in research projects (in data collection or as research participants), and participate with colleagues in sessions to stimulate the formulation of questions from their clinical experience. One can begin by asking the question "why?" of every NICU nursing practice. Lack of resources—including time, money, and consultation—can be more difficult to address. In many institutions, the conduct of nursing research is still viewed as a frill and not central to the delivery of patient care. In such a setting, nurses who wish to conduct research may initially need to invest their own time and even money. However, once the research process has demonstrated clinical relevance, additional resources are often made available. Collaboration with colleagues within the institution, schools and universities, and industry can enhance resources. Writing grants with colleagues for the purposes of obtaining funds to support research is often the only way that clinical research can be conducted (Holtzclaw, Kenner, & Walden, 2009).

Mariano et al. (2009) evaluated the effects of mentoring on the EBP of a sample of 20 NICU nurses. Although the researchers were not able to demonstrate changes in EBP of the nurses, they did report changes in the NICU as a result of the project.

There is a need for ongoing research to monitor the extent to which neonatal nurses use evidence-based guidelines in practice, and to identify facilitators and barriers to such implementation that should be addressed to ensure continuous quality improvement in neonatal nursing care. In order to facilitate data collection for these studies, it is important to identify core measures that can be collected and recorded by neonatal units and that can be used to evaluate implementation of EBP guidelines. For example, Coughlin, Gibbins, and Hoath (2009) developed a set of such core measures that could be used to evaluate the implementation of evidence-based guidelines for developmentally supportive care in neonatal care. The core measures represent five categories of developmental care that were identified based on an extensive literature review of effective developmental care practices: protected sleep, pain and stress assessment/management, developmentally supportive activities of daily living, family-centered care, and the healing environment.

Conducting Research in Neonatal Nursing

Scientific substantiation of neonatal nursing and neonatal care requires collaboration with other nurses and health professionals. The clinical nurse is often the first to recognize and identify trends in newborn and infant care problems for which there is no apparent evidential base. With the guidance and assistance of other nurses, nurse specialists, and physicians, a collaborative investigation may be used to explore the problem. The combination of expertise from multiple disciplines can make a highly effective research team.

Research is a formal, systematic inquiry or examination of a given problem. The outcome or goal of research is to discover new information or relationships or to verify existing knowledge. Other less formal definitions of research focus on the understanding of an event by logically relating it to other events. Some types of research are designed to predict events by relating them empirically to antecedents in time.

Still other types of research attempt to control or manipulate an event or procedure to determine its impact on other phenomena (Burns & Grove, 2009). Quality assurance and quality improvement activities often lead to the design and conduct of research. Nurses are often introduced to issues related to objective data collection through quality assurance audits. Issues of clinical consequence that are identified through quality assurance screening can lead to the articulation of research questions. Research principles can also be used in the evaluation of new procedures, protocols, and products. Evaluation is often an integral part of NICU nursing, but it is performed subjectively. Using research methodology to perform evaluation promotes scientific objectivity.

Why Do Research?

Using the research process to discover new information or to confirm empirical knowledge allows the growth and evolution of nursing practice. Without research, nursing care would be based simply on tradition. The practice of nursing would change slowly and grow little because things would be done the way they have always been done. The failure to conduct research regarding neonatal care has taught us some sobering lessons. Judgments of efficacy based on observation of small numbers of infants or of treatments based on the principle "if a little is good, more is better" have resulted in significant morbidity and mortality for neonates. Increasing the risk of dehydration by withholding early feedings, misuses of oxygen therapy, and vitamin K are examples (Ramachandrappa & Jain, 2008). From these experiences, the use of clinical research trials to evaluate new therapies scientifically before widespread application has become more common in neonatal care. The research process also provides a vehicle for challenging accepted routines and theories. Nurses caring for neonates often identify issues for which inadequate scientific information on which to base clinical judgments does not exist.

Research Roles for Neonatal Nurses

The many different research roles for neonatal nurses include research consumer, participant, facilitator/coordinator, and investigator (Harrison, 2001). There is variability in the research roles that are considered appropriate for nurses across the globe. In some countries with limited opportunities for nurses to pursue doctoral degrees, nurses prepared at the master's level are expected to serve as research investigators, whereas in the United States, this role is generally reserved for nurses with doctoral-level education (Harrison, Hernandez, Cianelli, Rivera, & Urrutia, 2005a).

In the United States, the American Association of Colleges of Nursing (AACN) has published a series of "Essentials" guidelines that outline competencies for nurses in baccalaureate, master's, and Doctor of Nursing Practice (DNP) programs. The competencies related to research suggest that nurses prepared at the baccalaureate level use evidence to guide their practice (American Association of Colleges of Nursing, 2008). Nurses prepared at the master's level translate evidence to improve practice (American Association of Colleges of Nursing, 2011). Nurses prepared at the DNP level conduct application-oriented scholarly projects as opposed to the knowledge-generating research expected of nurses in PhD programs. DNP nurses are prepared to lead EBP initiatives (American Association of Colleges of Nursing, 2006). The American Nurses Association (ANA) asserts that all nurses are responsible for assuming various research activities and roles as appropriate to their education (American Nurses Association, 2010). The ANA has also created a research toolkit that is available online to help nurses provide evidence-based care (American Nurses Association, 2012).

All neonatal nurses should be knowledgeable consumers of research, should read reports of research, and ensure that their practice is research or evidence-based. To be a knowledgeable research consumer, the nurse must be a critical reader of research articles. A rigorous critique of research should also be carried out before one tries to use the findings in a practice situation. Strategies that might be implemented to assist nurses with developing critical appraisal skills include journal clubs or workshops (Horsley et al., 2011).

Another key research role for every neonatal nurse is to serve as an advocate for infants and families who are research participants to ensure that their rights are protected and that their safety is ensured. Thomas (2005) reviewed safety and ethical issues related to research with vulnerable infants and their families, and suggested that neonatal nurses may serve an important role by reporting any safety concerns to the Institutional Review Board (or ethics committee) that originally approved the study.

Nurses can also participate in research as data collectors or clinical research coordinators (CRCs). CRCs assume primary responsibility for implementing clinical studies and protocols that are critical for the successful implementation of any study (McKinney & Vermeulen, 2000). With the rapid expansion of global research, there is a growing demand for well-prepared CRCs, although there is considerable variability in the specific responsibilities, training, and titles of nurses who work in clinical research (Jones, Jester, & Harrison, 2006; Jones, Wilson, Carter, & Jester, 2009). The International Association of Clinical Research Nurses (CRNs) was formed to support the professional and educational needs of CRNs, and is working to identify specific competencies and standards to guide the educational preparation of CRNs (International Association of Clinical Research Nurses, 2012). The Association for Clinical Research Practitioners (ACRP) has a certification program for CRCs as well as for Clinical Research Associates. (For information see the ACRP website at http://www.acrpnet.org.) Several nursing schools have started master's level programs to prepare nurses for these roles (Harrison, Hernandez, Cianelli, Rivera, & Urrutia, 2005b) (see, for example, the website for the University of Alabama at Birmingham School of Nursing for a description of one such program; University of Alabama at Birmingham School of Nursing, 2012).

Another method of participating in the research process is to perform secondary analyses on data that were collected to answer another research question. Often answers to other research questions can be extracted from a single database without having to collect new data. Caution, however, must be used in the design of secondary analysis studies to minimize threats to validity and reliability inherent in the method.

Neonatal nurses may also promote research by coordinating research committees, promoting research utilization, coordinating research activities in the NICU, and providing educational programs to help nurses understand and use findings from research.

CURRENT TRENDS IN NEONATAL NURSING RESEARCH

Over the past 30 years, there has been a tremendous increase in the quantity and quality of descriptive as well as experimental and quasi-experimental studies focused on preterm or other high-risk infants and their families. Holditch-Davis and Black (2003) reviewed nursing research on the care of the preterm infant and identified 17 nurse researchers who had developed programs of neonatal research, meaning that the researcher had at least five publications since 1990 and was the first author on at least three of these publications. These programs of research had four themes: infant responses to the NICU environment, pain management, infant stimulation, and infant behavior and development. Holditch-Davis and Black suggested that these research programs had many strengths, including interdisciplinary focus and clinical relevance, but recommended that more studies should focus on the clinically ill infant and be based on a developmental science perspective.

Another trend in neonatal research is the publication of reports of EBP projects in the NICU. For example, Pollock and Franklin (2004) described an ongoing project to implement developmentally sensitive care in the NICU. Smith (2005) described the process of developing, implementing and evaluating a feeding guideline for very-low-birth-weight infants. Other examples of NICU EBP projects include: (a) evaluation of the use of heparinized saline versus normal saline for the maintenance of intravenous access in neonates (Cook, Bellini, & Cusson, 2011); (b) evaluation of the effect of toys in the NICU microenvironment on nosocomial infection rates (Hanrahan & Lofgren, 2004); and (c) proposing evidence-based guidelines for kangaroo care in the NICU (Ludington-Hoe, 2011).

An important source of funding for nursing research is the NINR, an institute within the U.S. Department of Health and Human Services (DHHS) National Institutes of Health (NIH). Abstracts of research funded by the NIH can be searched and retrieved in the Research Portfolio Online Reporting Tools (RePORT) database (National Institutes of Health, 2012a). A query using the keywords "neonatal nursing" resulted in a listing of 39 abstracts of research funded by the NIH (National Institutes of Health, 2012b). Table 39.3 lists examples of these funded studies.

There are many opportunities for neonatal nurses to implement EBP projects to improve the quality of care for patients and families. Sharing experiences by presentations at professional meetings or publication in the professional literature will contribute to the growing body of information about EBP and the implementation of evidence-based neonatal nursing practice.

SUMMARY

With more and more hospitals and health care organizations going for Magnet status and the inclusion of evidence-based clinical guidelines for care in these institutions research, research utilization, and EBP reviews and guidelines will continue to grow. This chapter has highlighted some of the ways neonatal nursing and care is being impacted by research and EBP.

Table 39.3

EXAMPLES OF STUDIES RELATED TO NEONATAL NURSING FUNDED BY THE NATIONAL INSTITUTES OF HEALTH IN 2011

Principal Investigator	Organization	Title of Study
Danilyn Mag-Akat Angeles	Loma Linda University	Pain and hypoxia in premature infants
Brenda J. Baker	Virginia Commonwealth University	Understanding late preterm mothers and infants
Beth Black	University of North Carolina Chapel Hill	End-of-life care after severe fetal diagnosis
Heather Elser	Duke University	Development of cerebral oxygenation in premature infants
Sheila Gephart	University of Arizona	Validating a necrotizing enterocolitis (NEC) risk index for neonates
Ruth E. Grunau	University of British Columbia	Pain in preterm infants: Development and effects
Barbara Medoff-Cooper	Children's Hospital of Pennsylvania	Transitional telehealth home care: REACH
Joseph Moorman	University of Virginia	Neonatal apnea: Online risk score from new analyses of bedside monitor waveforms
Rita Pickler	Virginia Commonwealth University	Patterned experience for preterm infants; feeding readiness in preterm infants
Jeannette A. Rogowski	University of Medicine/Dentistry of New Jersey	The effects of nursing on NICU patient outcomes
Suzanne Thoyre	University of North Carolina Chapel Hill	Guiding mothers to co-regulate oral feeding with very preterm infants

From the National Institutes of Health (2012b).

EVIDENCE-BASED PRACTICE BOX

For the past 20 years, neonatal researchers have conducted studies to assess the effects of music and music therapy provided to preterm infants in the NICU. Hodges and Wilson (2010) published an integrative review of 35 of these studies, which is an example of an evidence summary (the second category in the five-point Star Model noted in Table 39.2). The authors concluded that comparison of results from the studies was difficult because of the wide variations in type of music, volume, duration, and gestational ages of the infants. However, despite the limitations, findings from many of the studies suggested positive effects of music on increasing oxygen saturation levels, reducing heart rates and arousal, and improving parent–infant interaction in hospitalized preterm infants. The authors made specific recommendations about future research to address the limitations of existing studies and provide evidence for practice.

REFERENCES

Agency for Healthcare Research and Quality. (2011). *2011 National healthcare quality and disparities reports*. Rockville, MD: United States Department of Health and Human Services.

American Association of Colleges of Nursing. (2006). *The essentials of doctoral education for advanced nursing practice*. Washington, DC: Author.

American Association of Colleges of Nursing. (2008). *The essentials of baccalaureate education for professional nursing practice*. Washington, DC: Author.

American Association of Colleges of Nursing. (2011). *The essentials of master's education in nursing*. Washington, DC: Author.

American Nurses Association. (2010). *Nursing: Scope and standards of practice*. Silver Spring, MD: Author.

American Nurses Association. (2012). Research toolkit. Retrieved from http://www.nursingworld.org/MainMenuCategories/ThePracticeofProfessionalNursing/Improving-Your-Practice/Research-Toolkit

Association of Women's Health Obstetric and Neonatal Nurses. (2010). *Assessment and care of the late preterm infant. Evidence-based clinical practice guideline*. Retrieved from http://www.guideline.gov/content.aspx?id=24066&search=association+of+women%e2%80%99s+health%2c+obstetric%2c+and+neonatal+nurses

Burns, N., & Grove, S. K. (Eds.). (2009). *The practice of nursing research: Appraisal, synthesis, and generation of evidence* (6th ed.). Philadelphia, PA: Saunders.

Cook, L., Bellini, S., & Cusson, R. M. (2011). Heparinized saline vs normal saline for maintenance of intravenous access in neonates: An evidence-based practice change. *Advances in Neonatal Care (Elsevier Science), 11*(3), 208–215. doi:10.1097/ANC.0b013e31821bab61

Coughlin, M., Gibbins, S., & Hoath, S. (2009). Core measures for developmentally supportive care in neonatal intensive care units: Theory, precedence and practice. *Journal of Advanced Nursing, 65*(10), 2239–2248. doi:10.1111/j.1365-2648.2009.05052.x

Eden, J., Levit, L., Berg, A., & Morton, S. (2011). *Finding what works in health care: Standards for systematic reviews*. Washington, DC: National Academies Press.

eGranary Digital Library. (2012). Zambia nursing and midwifery. Retrieved from http://www.widernet.org/digitallibrary/portals/PortalViewer.asp?PortalPageID=492

Gennaro, S. (1994). Research utilization: An overview. *Journal of Obstetric, Gynecologic, & Neonatal Nursing, 23*(4), 313–319.

Graham, R., Mancher, M., Wolman, D. M., Greenfield, S., & Steinberg, E. (Eds.). (2011). *Clinical practice guidelines we can trust*. Washington, DC: National Academies Press.

Guidelines International Network. (2012). Introduction. Retrieved from http://www.g-i-n.net/about-g-i-n

Guyatt, G., Rennie, D., Meade, M., & Cook, D. (2008). *Users guide to the medical literature: A manual for evidence-based clinical practice*. New York, NY: McGraw-Hill Professional.

Hanrahan, K. S., & Lofgren, M. (2004). Evidence-based practice: Examining the risk of toys in the microenvironment of infants in the neonatal intensive care unit. *Advances in Neonatal Care (Elsevier Science), 4*(4), 184–205.

Harrison, L. L. (2001). Research roles for neonatal nurses. *Central Lines, 17*(1), 18–20.

Harrison, L. L., Hernandez, A. R., Cianelli, R., Rivera, S., & Urrutia, M. (2005a). Competencias en investigación para diferentes niveles de formación de enfermeras: Una perspectiva latinoamericana. *Ciencia y Enfermería, XI*(1), 59–71.

Harrison, L. L., Hernandez, A. R., Cianelli, R., Rivera, S., & Urrutia, M. (2005b). Perspectives of Latin American nursing professors and leaders about research competencies needed by nurses with different levels of academic preparation. *International Journal of Nursing Education Scholarship, 2*(1), 24.

Higgins, J. P. T., & Green, S. (2011). In T. C. Collaboration (Ed.), *Cochrane handbook for systematic reviews of interventions version 5.1.0*. Retrieved from www.cochrane-handbook.org

HINARI Access to Research in Health Program. (2012). About HINARI. Retrieved from http://www.who.int/hinari/about/en/

Hodges, A. L., & Wilson, L. L. (2010). Effects of music therapy on preterm infants in the neonatal intensive care unit. *Alternative Therapy Health Medicine, 16*(5), 72–73.

Holditch-Davis, D., & Black, B. P. (2003). Care of preterm infants: Programs of research and their relationship to developmental science. *Annual Review of Nursing Research, 21*, 23–60.

Holtzclaw, B. J., Kenner, C., & Walden, M. (2009). *Grant writing handbook for nurses* (2nd ed.). Sudbury, MA: Jones and Bartlett.

Horsley, T., Hyde, C., Santesso, N., Parkes, J., Milne, R., & Stewart, R. (2011). Teaching critical appraisal skills in healthcare settings. *Cochrane Database of Systematic Reviews (11)*.

Improvement Science Research Network. (2010). *Research priorities*. Retrieved from http://www.isrn.net/sites/isrn-drupal/files/documents/ISRNSummit_Research_Priorities_508_web.pdf

Improvement Science Research Network. (2012). Research priorities. Retrieved from http://www.improvementscienceresearch.net/research

Institute of Medicine. (1999). *To err is human: Building a safer health system*. Washington, DC: National Academies Press.

Institute of Medicine. (2001). *Crossing the quality chasm: Healthcare for the 21st century*. Washington, DC: National Academies of Science.

Institute of Medicine. (2003). *Priority areas for national action: Transforming health care quality*. Washington, DC: National Academies of Science.

Institute of Medicine. (2008). *Knowing what works in health care: A roadmap for the nation*. Washington, DC: National Academies Press.

Institute of Medicine (2011). *The future of nursing: Leading change, advancing health*. Washington, DC: The National Academies Press.

Institute of Medicine (2013). Crossing the quality chasm: The IOM health care quality initiative. http://www.iom.edu/Global/News%20Announcements/Crossing-the-Quality-Chasm-The-IOM-Health-Care-Quality-Initiative.aspx. Accessed May 20, 2013.

International Association of Clinical Research Nurses. (2012). About us. Retrieved from http://iacrn.memberlodge.org/Default.aspx?pageId=505167

Johnson, F. E., & Maikler, V. E. (2001). Nurses' adoption of the AWHONN/NANN neonatal skin care project. *Newborn & Infant Nursing Reviews, 1*(1), 59–67.

Jones, C. T., Jester, P. M., & Harrison, L. (2006). Clinical research in low resource countries. *Research Practitioner, 7*(6), 188–199.

Jones, C. T., Wilson, L. L., Carter, S., & Jester, P. M. (2009). Development and implementation of a distance-learning certificate program in clinical research coordination for coordinators at international sites. *Southern Online Journal of Nursing Research, 9*(3), 1–16.

Ludington-Hoe, S. M. (2011). Thirty years of kangaroo care science and practice. *Neonatal Network, 30*(5), 357–362.

Mariano, K. G., Caley, L. M., Eschberger, L., Woloszyn, A., Volker, P., Leonard, M. S., & Tung, Y. (2009). Building evidence-based practice with staff nurses through mentoring. *Journal of Neonatal Nursing, 15*(3), 81–87.

McKinney, J., & Vermeulen, W. (2000). Research nurses play a vital role in clinical trials. *Oncology Nursing Forum, 27*(1), 28.

Medoff-Cooper, B. (1994). Transition of the preterm infant to an open crib. *Journal of Obstetric, Gynecologic & Neonatal Nursing, 23*(4), 329–335.

Medoff-Cooper, B., Bakewell-Sachs, S., Buus-Frank, M. E., & Santa-Donato, A. (2005). The AWHONN Near-Term Infant Initiative: A conceptual framework for optimizing health for near-term infants. *Journal of Obstetric, Gynecologic & Neonatal Nursing, 34*(6), 666–671.

Meier, P. P. (1994). Transition of the preterm infant to an open crib: Process of the project group. *Journal of Obstetric, Gynecologic & Neonatal Nursing, 23*(4), 321–326.

Melnyk, B. M., Fineout-Overholt, E., Stone, P., & Ackerman, M. (2000). Evidence-based practice: The past, present, and recommendations for the millennium. *Pediatric Nursing, 26*(1), 77–81.

Mulrow, C. (1994). Rationale for systematic reviews. *British Medical Journal, 309*, 597–599.

National Association of Neonatal Nurses. (2012). Position statements. Retrieved from http://www.nann.org/education/content/poststmnts.html

National Institute for Health and Clinical Excellence. Retrieved from http://www.nice.org.uk. Retrieved May 20, 2013.

National Institute of Nursing Research. (2011). *Bringing science to life: NINR strategic plan*. Bethesda, MD: Author.

National Institutes of Health. (2012a). NIH RePORTER. Retrieved from http://projectreporter.nih.gov/reporter.cfm

National Institutes of Health. (2012b). Project search results for neonatal nursing. Retrieved from http://projectreporter.nih.gov/reporter_searchresults.cfm

Pollock, T. R., & Franklin, C. (2004). Use of evidence-based practice in the neonatal intensive care unit. *Critical Care Nursing Clinics of North America, 16*(2), 243–248.

Ramachandrappa, A., & Jain, L. (2008). Iatrogenic disorders in modern neonatology: A focus on safety and quality of care. *Clinics in Perinatology, 35*(1), 1–34.

Rogers, E. M. M. (1995). *Diffusion of innovations* (4th ed.). New York, NY: The Free Press.

Sackett, D. L., Straus, S. E., Richardson, W. S., Rosenberg, W., & Haynes, R. B. (2000). *Evidence-based medicine: How to practice and teach EBM* (2nd ed.). Edinburgh: Churchill Livingstone.

Smith, J. R. (2005). Early enteral feeding for the very low birth weight infant: The development and impact of a research-based guideline. *Neonatal Network, 24*(4), 9–19.

Stevens, K. R. (2004). ACE star model: Cycle of knowledge transformatio. Retrieved from http://www.acestar.uthscsa.edu/

Stevens, K. R. (2009). *Essential competencies for evidence-based practice in nursing*. San Antonio, TX: University of Texas Health Science Center.

Stevens, K. R., & Pugh, J. A. (1999). Evidence-based practice and perioperative nursing. *Seminars in Perioperative Nursing, 8*(3), 155–159.

Thomas, K. A. (2005). Safety: When infants and parents are research subjects. *Journal of Perinatal & Neonatal Nursing, 19*(1), 52–58.

University of Alabama at Birmingham School of Nursing. (2012). Clinical research management options. Retrieved from http://www.uab.edu/nursing/student-information/acad-prog/non-degree-options/crm-certificate

Vermont Oxford Network. (2012). What is the Vermont Oxford Network? Retrieved from http://www.vtoxford.org/about/about.aspx

Wallin, L., Boström, A. M., Harvey, G., Wikblad, K., & Ewald, U. (2000). National guidelines for Swedish neonatal nursing care: Evaluation of clinical application. *International Journal for Quality in Health Care, 12*(6), 465–474.

Widernet. (2012). Welcome to the Widernet project. Retrieved from http://www.widernet.org

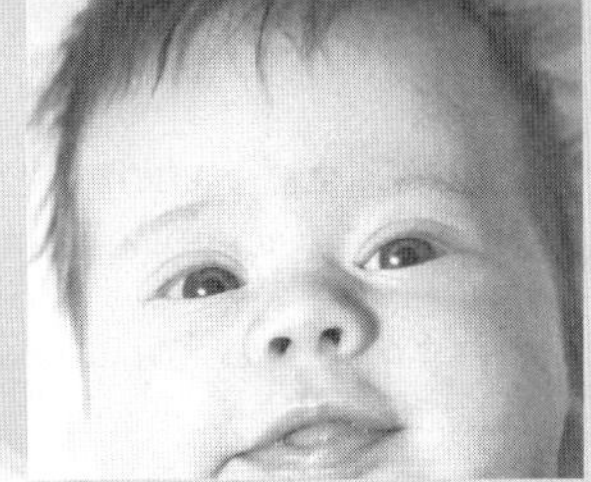

CHAPTER

40

Legal and Ethical Issues in Neonatal Care

■ Tanya Sudia-Robinson

In the high-technology and often high-tension milieu of the neonatal intensive care unit (NICU), nurses and other health care professionals inevitably encounter ethical issues. However, ethical issues involving neonates are not limited to the NICU. Neonatal nurses are providing comprehensive care in an increasingly complex environment for a very diverse population. These challenges will continue to bring ethical issues to the forefront of neonatal care and will require thoughtful reflection.

Ethical issues are often intertwined with legal considerations, further adding to their complexity. Neonatal nurses and advanced practice neonatal nurses are well positioned for leadership roles in managing ethical and legal issues in the neonatal care settings. This chapter provides an overview of ethical and legal issues that can arise across the spectrum of neonatal care, as well as approaches to recognizing and managing these issues.

RECOGNIZING ETHICAL ISSUES IN NEONATAL CARE AND THE NICU

The NICU and care of neonates can be laden with ethical issues (Cavaliere, Daly, Dowling, & Montgomery, 2011; Kuschel & Kent, 2011; Orzalesi, 2010). The blurred boundaries for viability, coupled with parental preferences and legal considerations, can lead to ethical issues across the spectrum of neonatal care. One of the challenges facing neonatal nurses is effectively recognizing ethical issues in the midst of providing complex care.

Some neonatal care issues with ethical implications may be more readily recognizable than others. For example, consider the case of a neonate experiencing deteriorating multisystem organ failure whose parents wish to continue aggressive care. The NICU team may be recommending increased palliative and supportive care measures with a deceleration in other measures. This type of heart-wrenching scenario unfortunately continues to occur and is recognized as a classical NICU ethical issue. It is important for neonatal nurses to examine other neonatal care ethical issues that are not as easily recognizable.

Parents may express care preferences that are deemed nonpermissible because they fall outside usual care practices and may be believed to be potentially harmful to the neonate. For example, parents may want to burn incense in the mother's hospital room in the presence of their newborn. While hospital policy will likely dictate no candles or other flaming substances for the security of all persons in the building and in consideration of the health of the neonate, it would not be in the family's best interest to end the interaction with a discussion of what is not permissible and why. Rather, it would be important for this neonate's nurse to talk further with the parents about their request. Engaging the parents in dialogue about the issue can provide insight into their beliefs and practice preferences. Through this process, the neonatal nurse and parents together can determine an acceptable alternative. The neonatal nurses' actions will demonstrate respect for their role as parents as well as their preferences. Perhaps most significant, though, is that the neonatal nurse will have established a supportive relationship with the parents as opposed to what could have quickly become an unintended adversarial relationship.

Situations such as the one just described may raise questions among neonatal nurses regarding how to best recognize and manage situations that extend beyond clinical care. To assist in understanding the development of ethical issues, an overview of key ethical principles follows.

ETHICAL PRINCIPLES

It is important for neonatal nurses to understand the ethical principles that can help guide their actions when they encounter an ethical situation. Beauchamp and Childress (2009) specify four key principles for biomedical ethics: autonomy, beneficence, nonmaleficence, and justice.

Each of these principles is presented along with examples demonstrating how neonatal nurses can apply them to everyday practice.

The principle of autonomy focuses on an individual's independence and the right to make decisions. In neonatal care, the decision makers are the parents rather than the actual patient. To respect the principle of autonomy, neonatal nurses and other team members should engage the parents in decision making about the neonate's plan of care to the fullest extent possible. For example, it may be medically indicated for a neonate to undergo surgical ligation of a patent ductus arteriosus. Prior to the surgical team obtaining informed consent for this surgery, the neonatal nurse and other team members can provide ample opportunity for the parents to consider the information provided to them to ensure that all of their questions are addressed.

Beneficence, or doing well, is a principle that along with nonmaleficence (avoiding causing harm) represents optimal nursing care. Neonatal nurses are consistently engaged in care that meets best practice standards for promoting the well-being of the neonate. Adequate positioning, promotion of rest, and other supportive care measures demonstrate care delivery in a beneficent manner. Similarly, the avoidance of causing intentional harm to a neonate illustrates nonmaleficent behavior. Consideration of these two ethical principles provides a supportive foundation for delivering the best possible care.

The ethical principle of justice can be viewed in a multitude of ways in health care incorporating varying components of equity, allocation, rationing, and access (Beauchamp & Childress, 2009). An examination of justice in neonatal care can focus on the actual process of care delivery. While neonatal nurses are not responsible for the broader issues of access to care, they are in a position to ensure that the neonates within their care receive similar attention and that the care is prioritized based on need. Providing care to all neonates without regard for extraneous factors such as socioeconomic status and ethnicity represents an important component of the principle of justice in neonatal care.

MANAGING ETHICAL ISSUES: RESOLUTION STRATEGIES

There are various approaches to managing the types of ethical issues that can arise in neonatal settings. While each neonatal care unit or hospital may have a standardized resolution pathway already in place, it can be helpful to explore alternate approaches. Among the ethical issue-resolution strategies available to neonatal nurses are engaging in nursing and/or health care team ethics rounds; debriefing discussions; and consultation and collaboration with hospital ethics committees.

Nursing Ethics Rounds

Among the strategies that neonatal nurses may find helpful when faced with ethical issues are engaging in nursing ethics rounds and team discussions. Nursing ethics rounds (Robichaux, 2012) can assist neonatal nurses to recognize and manage developing issues. Ethics rounds can provide an opportunity for addressing developing issues before they expand in complexity and become emotionally laden for all involved individuals. Additionally, through ethics rounds, neonatal nurses can engage in dialogue and elicit support from team members for any identified issues or care-based concerns.

Debriefing Discussions

Following a particularly complex or emotionally laden care situation, it can be beneficial for all members of the health care team to participate in debriefing discussions. These discussions can be requested by any team member, but should be scheduled when the key care providers can be in attendance. It is also helpful to ensure that any providers with dissenting opinions or conflicted views are included in open and nonjudgmental dialogue. The session should include a discussion of the salient ethical issues in the case, allowing all team members to identify their perceived areas of discomfort. For those team members who continue to have unresolved discomfort or distress, additional individualized support needs can be identified and enacted.

Collaborating With Hospital Ethics Committees

Hospital ethics committees generally operate in an advisory capacity and can provide guidance with the ethical issues of cases but not serve in a legal advisory capacity (Mercurio, 2011). In situations where different members of the health care team and/or the parents have conflicting perspectives on what will be the best course of action, it can be helpful to obtain the perspectives of individuals not directly involved with the case. Additionally, it is important to consider the perspective of the organization and explore the means to involve others from the organization in the clinical decision-making process as warranted (Bean, 2011).

Aside from providing perspectives on actual cases, ethics committees can assist in a consultative manner to garner perspective on potential issues before they arise. Ethics committees can also assist with reviews of past cases or tenuous situations by examining other pathways than the one taken and laying the foundation for future resolution strategies.

SUPPORT FOR THE FAMILY

While neonatal nurses often become engaged in close relationships with families of the neonates they care for, the family may begin to feel isolated when ethical issues arise. It is during these challenging times that neonatal nurses can exhibit leadership in ensuring that families remain engaged to the fullest extent possible. Supporting families in the NICU encompasses a multitude of actions on behalf of the neonate's parents as well as siblings and extended family members. The neonatal nurse may serve as an advocate for grandparent visitation or assist parents in explaining the complexities of the NICU to the neonate's siblings. Perhaps most importantly, neonatal nurses support parents through ensuring their role in various components of decision making (Kavanaugh, Moro, & Savage, 2010;

Sudia-Robinson, 2011b); respecting their role regardless of opposing treatment perspectives (Sudia-Robinson, 2011a); and speaking on their behalf (Spence, 2011) whenever necessary.

Decision Making

One means of demonstrating respect for parents is involving them in decision making (Rushton, 2007). In order for parents to truly participate in decision making, they must have the necessary information. Information for decision making should be presented to parents in a manner that is easily understandable, yet at an appropriate level for their education and background experiences. While all parents need baseline information, the kinds of questions that parents ask will provide a good indication of their desire and readiness for additional information. Additionally, by providing information in as objective a manner as possible, parents will be in a better position to share their values and perspectives rather than being overly influenced by those of the health care team (Kuschel & Kent, 2011).

Cultivating an invitational atmosphere will foster dialogue and provide an avenue for parents to be active participants in the decision-making process (see Box 40.1). By assuming that all parents have questions regarding some aspect of their neonate's care, neonatal nurses will keep the door to dialogue open. Invitational atmospheres for dialogue allow parents to ask as many or as few questions as they like. An open atmosphere for questions also provides opportunities for parents to ask questions at a time when they are ready to receive the information. For example, some parents can become overwhelmed when a large amount of information is presented during a single conversation. However, when they are given time to process the information, their questions will emerge and they can further engage in dialogue and decision making. For some parents, the role they play in determining outcomes may not even be as important as the opportunity to engage in the decision-making process (Gallagher, Marlow, Edgley, & Porock, 2011). Ethically sound decisions, collaboratively determined to be in the best interest of the infant, represent best practice (Orzalesi, 2010).

BOX 40.1

INVITATIONAL QUESTIONS AND STATEMENTS

Avoid yes/no response questions:

Is there anything you want to know about your baby's progress?

Replace with:

What else would you like to discuss regarding your baby's progress?

Other open-ended questions:

What else can I provide more information about?

What questions would you like to ask?

Invitational statements:

This is a lot of information. Let's pause so that you can ask questions.

We presented possible care options. Let's discuss your thoughts about each of them.

Tell me the questions you would like to ask the neonatal care team.

Determining Parental Preferences

While it is important to cultivate an open environment for parental engagement in various aspects of care for their neonate, it is equally important to determine their preferences for such involvement. Some parents will want to be very involved in decision making while others indicate a preference for varying degrees of delegation. Parental involvement should not be viewed as an all-or-none phenomenon, but rather on a continuum that may change over the course of the neonate's hospitalization (Gillam & Sullivan, 2011). Neonatal nurses can play a key role in assessing parental preferences of involvement in care decisions both at the onset and at key time intervals, such as when the neonate's condition significantly improves or becomes increasingly complex.

Opposing Points of View

In the increasingly complex care environment of NICUs, there will inevitably be varying perspectives on care decisions between parents and the health care team. Parents may hold different points of view regarding the overall treatment plan or specific components of care. Neonatal nurses can assist in bridging these differences by engaging parents in conversation about these issues and their preferences. Learning more about their perspective and desired outcomes can lead to improved communication and enhanced decision making (Gillam & Sullivan, 2011; Sudia-Robinson, 2011b).

In situations where parents and the health care team are in disagreement about major care issues, it is important for the neonatal nurse to foster continued parental engagement in decision making to the greatest extent possible. For example, a situation may arise where despite the parents' expressed preferences, continued aggressive care is deemed appropriate. The parents can still be encouraged to be involved in other decision making about the care of their neonate such as touch time scheduling. Neonatal nurses can ask parents about their preferences in the scheduling of limited touch times, ensuring that some of those times are when the parents indicate that they can be present at the bedside. Sometimes even relatively minor decision-making opportunities can help restore respect for their role as parents and enhance feelings of connection with their neonate.

SUPPORT FOR THE NEONATAL NURSE

While neonatal nurses are actively engaged in supporting neonates, their parents, and extended family members, they may neglect their personal needs for health and well-being. Attention to personal care needs is especially important for nurses working in settings that can be physically, mentally, and emotionally challenging. Neonatal nurses need to advocate for their own needs just as they do for the needs of the neonates and families they care for. Actively expressing their needs and taking steps to support themselves, colleagues, and other members of their team are key components of self-sustainability and effective care delivery. Without adequate support, untoward issues can arise for neonatal nurses and other team members. Additionally, during particularly challenging patient and family situations, neonatal nurses may find themselves feeling undue stress with related manifestations, such as compassion fatigue and moral distress.

Compassion Fatigue

Compassion fatigue and emotional exhaustion among nurses have been attributed to a variety of factors including stressful work environments, additional nursing care responsibilities and priority conflicts, extensive and intensive work hours, role responsibilities, and emotionally laden patient care situations (Boyle, 2011; Garcia & Calvo, 2011; McGibbon, Peter, & Gallop, 2010; Potter et al., 2010; Yoder, 2010). This is an evolving area of interest among both nurse administrators and researchers as they strive to develop interventions to support nurses who have experienced compassion fatigue and to develop preventive measures. For neonatal nurses, potential mitigating interventions include on-site professional counseling services; art therapy; rotating patient assignments; extra days off; spiritual support; grief resolution; and self-care goals with specified plans to achieve them (Boyle, 2011; Coetzee & Klopper, 2010; Yoder, 2010).

Moral Distress

Moral distress among nurses and other health care professionals can occur when they cannot enact what they perceive as the right or correct thing to do (Callister & Sudia-Robinson, 2011; Pauly, Varcoe, Storch, & Newton, 2009). Acknowledging feelings of moral distress in oneself as well as recognizing moral distress among team members is an important component in the process of ethical care delivery. Signs of moral distress can include feeling conflicted about care decisions and uncomfortable with a lack of involvement in care decisions. Attention to these feelings is important for both the neonatal team morale and overall care delivery (Janvier, Nadeau, Deschenes, Couture, & Barrington, 2007).

The American Association of Critical Care Nurses (AACN) presented a framework for nurses to manage moral distress, referred to as the 4 A's: ask, affirm, assess, and act (AACN, 2008). The first A, ask, focuses on the nurse asking oneself questions to determine if distress is present within oneself and/or the health care team. Next, through affirming, the nurse validates the feelings of distress by exploring with others. The third step involves assessing the source of the distress and determining that an action plan is needed. Through the fourth step, the nurse develops and implements an action plan. The 4 A's framework is circular rather than linear, indicating the need to revisit steps as the plan unfolds and to develop additional strategies as needed.

Strategies that neonatal nurses can utilize to manage moral distress within themselves and team members include verbalizing their concerns and feelings of distress through story telling (Austin, Kelecevic, Goble, & Mekechuk, 2009) and other means of sharing with team members. Further, journal clubs focused on the review of ethical issues and case studies can help neonatal nurses be better prepared when confronted with ethical issues (Garity, 2009).

SUMMARY

Neonatal nurses are uniquely positioned to serve as leaders and supporters of all aspects of ethical care delivery. Assisting parents to express their preferences for care delivery and providing support for those preferences to the greatest extent possible are components of practicing within an ethical context. Through the delivery of highly skilled bedside care to facilitating parental involvement in care-based dialogue and decision making, neonatal nurses enact key advocacy roles for neonates and their parents.

REFERENCES

American Association of Critical Care Nurses. (2008). *The 4A's to rise above moral distress*. Aliso Viejo, CA: Author.

Austin, W., Kelecevic, J., Goble, E., & Mekechuk, J. (2009). An overview of moral distress and the paediatric intensive care team. *Nursing Ethics, 16*(1), 57–68. doi:10.1177/096973308097990

Bean, S. (2011). Navigating the murky intersection between clinical and organizational ethics: A hybrid case taxonomy. *Bioethics, 25*(6), 320–325. doi:10.1111/j.1467-8519.2009.01783.x

Beauchamp, T., & Childress, J. (2009). *Principles of biomedical ethics*. New York, NY: Oxford University Press.

Boyle, D. A. (2011). Countering compassion fatigue: A requisite nursing agenda. *Online Journal of Issues in Nursing, 16*(1), 1–20. doi:10.3912/OJIN.Vol16No01Man02

Callister, L. C., & Sudia-Robinson, T. (2011). An overview of ethics in maternal-child nursing. *MCN, 36*(3), 154–159. doi:10.1097/NMC.0b013e3182102175

Cavaliere, T. A., Daly, B., Dowling, D., & Montgomery, K. (2011). Moral distress in neonatal intensive care unit RNs. *Advances in Neonatal Care, 46*(4), 256–268.

Coetzee, S. K., & Klopper, H. C. (2010). Compassion fatigue within nursing practice: A concept analysis. *Nursing and Health Sciences, 12*, 235–243. doi:10.1111/j.1442-2018.2010.00526.x

Gallagher, K., Marlow, N., Edgley, A., & Porock, D. (2011). The attitudes of neonatal nurses towards extremely preterm infants. *Journal of Advanced Nursing, 68*(8), 1768–1779. doi:10.1111/j.1365-2648.2011.05865.x

Garcia, G. M., & Calvo, J. C. A. (2011). Emotional exhaustion of nursing staff: Influence of emotional annoyance and resilience. *International Nursing Review, 59*, 101–107.

Garity, J. (2009). Fostering nursing students' use of ethical theory and decision-making models: Teaching strategies. *Learning in Health & Social Care, 8*(2), 114–122. doi:10.1111/j.1473-6861.2009.00223.x

Gillam, L., & Sullivan, J. (2011). Ethics at the end of life: Who should make decisions about treatment limitation for young children with life-threatening or life-limiting conditions? *Journal of Paediatrics and Child Health, 47*, 594–598. doi:10.1111/j.1440-1754.2011.02177.x

Janvier, A., Nadeau, S., Deschenes, M., Couture, E., & Barrington, K. J. (2007). Moral distress in the neonatal intensive care unit: Caregiver's experience. *Journal of Perinatology, 27*, 203–208.

Kavanaugh, K., Moro, T. T., & Savage, T. A. (2010). How nurses assist parents regarding life support decisions for extremely premature infants. *Journal of Obstetric and Neonatal Nursing, 39*, 147–158.

Kuschel, C. A., & Kent, A. (2011). Improved neonatal survival and outcomes at borderline viability brings increasing ethical dilemmas. *Journal of Paediatrics and Child Health, 47*, 585–589. doi:10.1111/j.1440-1754.2011.02157.x

McGibbon, E., Peter, E., & Gallop, R. (2010). An institutional ethnography of nurses' stress. *Qualitative Health Research, 20*(10), 1353–1378. doi:10.1177/1049732310375435

Mercurio, M. R. (2011). The role of a pediatric ethics committee in the newborn intensive care unit. *Journal of Perinatology, 31*, 1–9. doi:10.1038/jp.2010.39

Orzalesi, M. (2010). Ethical problems in the care of high risk neonates. *The Journal of Maternal-Fetal and Neonatal Medicine, 23*(S3), 7–10. doi:10.3109/14767058.2010.510647

Pauly, B., Varcoe, C., Storch, J., & Newton, L. (2009). Registered nurses' perceptions of moral distress and ethical climate. *Nursing Ethics, 16*(5), 561–573. doi:10.117/0969733009106649

Potter, P., Deshields, T., Divanbeigi, J., Berger, J., Cipriano, D., Norris, L., & Olsen, S. (2010). Compassion fatigue and burnout: Prevalence among oncology nurses. *Clinical Journal of Oncology Nursing, 14*(5), E56–E62. doi:10.1188/10.CJON.E56-E62

Robichaux, C. (2012). Developing ethical skills: From sensitivity to action. *Critical Care Nurse, 32*(2), 65–72.

Rushton, C. H. (2007). Respect in critical care: A foundational ethical principle. *AACN Advanced Care, 18*(2), 149–156.

Spence, K. (2011). Ethical advocacy based on caring: A model for neonatal and paediatric nurses. *Journal of Paediatrics and Child Health, 47*, 643–645. doi:10.1111/j.1440-1754.2011.02178.x

Sudia-Robinson, T. (2011a). Ethical implications of newborn screening, life-limiting conditions, and palliative care. *MCN, 36*(3), 188–196. doi:10.1097/NMC.0b013e318210214c

Sudia-Robinson, T. (2011b). Neonatal ethical issues: Viability, advance directives, family centered care. *MCN, 36*(3), 180–185. doi:10.1097/NMC.0b013e3182102162

Yoder, E. A. (2010). Compassion fatigue in nurses. *Applied Nursing Research, 23*, 191–197. doi:10.1016/j.apnr.2008.09.003

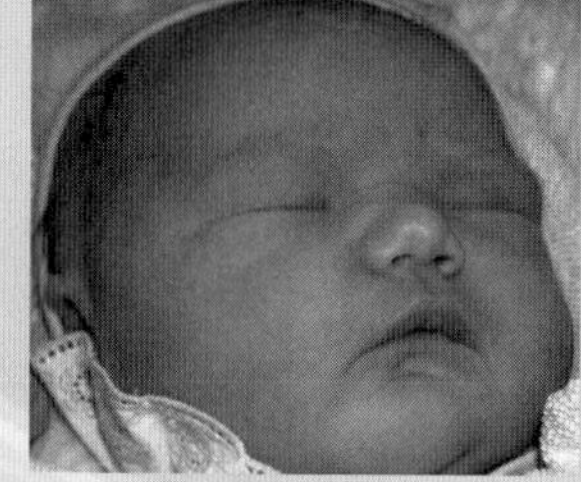

CHAPTER

41

Neonatal Care From a Global Perspective

■ Carole Kenner and Marina Boykova

In 2005, *The Lancet* published the "Neonatal Survival" issue (Lawn, Cousens, Zupan, & Lancet Neonatal Survival Steering Committee, 2005). This report called for action worldwide to address the United Nations Millennium Development Goals, especially #4 to reduce mortality of children less than 5 years of age. Why a call for action by perinatal and neonatal specialists who care for children in the first year of life? Why call this edition the Neonatal Survival and not child survival? The reason is that almost 50% of the deaths of children under 5 years of age is attributable to the neonatal period (Lawn et al., 2005). Most of the causes, including infection, intrapartal complications, and prematurity, are preventable (Lawn, Kerber, Enweronu-Laryea, & Cousens, 2010). In 2010, a progress report was released stating that the deaths in this population had been reduced from 4 million annually to 3.6 million (Lawn et al., 2010). The health burden for mortality under 5 years of age is primarily in India, Nigeria, Democratic Republic of the Congo, Pakistan, and China (United Nations, 2011). The global community responded by producing an action plan for implementation of strategies that would continue the progress. The World Health Organization (WHO, 2012), specifically the Partnership for Maternal Newborn & Child Health–WHO, led the Child Survival Call to Action. This initiative was in collaboration with UNICEF. Over 700 leaders participated in Washington, DC, in this historic meeting (http://www.who.int/pmnch/media/news/2012/20120614_childsurvival_call/en/index.html). Over the past decade, one key ingredient in improving health outcomes has been nursing. It is recognized that a strategy is to strengthen the education and training of neonatal and pediatric nurses. The March of Dimes, the Partnership for Maternal, Newborn, & Child Health, Save the Children, and the WHO issued a report in 2012, *Born Too Soon* (Group, Kinney, Howson, McDougall, & Lawn, 2012). In that report there is also a call to action citing that, to date, 15 million babies worldwide are born prematurely, with 60% of these births occurring in Africa and South Asia. The United States is in the top 10 countries that are the highest contributors to preterm births (Group et al., 2012). The call to action lists four shared actions. **Invest:** Ensure preterm interventions and research given proportional focus, so funding is aligned with health burden. **Implement:** Plan and implement preterm birth strategies at global and country levels and align on preterm mortality reduction goal. Introduce programs to ensure coverage of evidence-based interventions, particularly to reduce preterm mortality. **Innovate:** Perform research to support both prevention and treatment agendas. Pursue implementation research agenda to understand how best to scale-up interventions. **Inform:** Significantly improve preterm birth reporting by aligning on consistent definition and more consistently capturing data. Raise awareness of preterm birth at all levels as a central maternal, newborn, and child health issue. The overarching message is: Continued support for "Every Woman Every Child" and other reproductive, maternal, newborn, and child health efforts, which are inextricably linked with preterm birth. Ensure accountability of stakeholders across all actions (Group et al., 2012, p. 7). There is much work to be done globally to decrease morbidity and mortality of mothers, neonates, and children. Nurses are key to making a difference. Raising awareness of the factors that contribute to these rates, improved education and training of health professionals and community health workers, and a commitment to raise the standards of maternal–child care are the cornerstones to changing the global picture. To this end, this chapter is dedicated to the efforts that are at work to change neonatal nursing and neonatal and child outcomes. It also presents exemplars of neonatal nursing and its struggles as well as its opportunities.

A STRONG GLOBAL VOICE FOR NEONATAL NURSING

The Council of International Neonatal Nurses (COINN) was founded in 2005 by national neonatal nursing organizations that believed that a strong voice for neonates and their families was essential. These national members felt that already-strong organizations were needed to work together to help nurses in countries where there were no national organizations. Many times there were only a few nurses, and obviously they could not be trained or specialized in just neonatal care. These nurses, so few in number, needed to provide care across the life span. The founding groups were the National Association of Neonatal Nurses (NANN) in the United States, the National Neonatal Association (NNA) of the United Kingdom, the College of Australian Neonatal Nurses, formerly the Australian Association Neonatal Nurses Association, the New Zealand Association of Neonatal Nurses (NZANN) or Neonatal Nurses College of Aotearoa, and the Canadian Association of Neonatal Nurses (CANN). Over the next 7 years other national organizations joined, including the Danish Neonatal Nurses, Netherlands Innovation & Research-Dutch NICUs, Finnish Society of Neonatal Nurses-Finland, Sociedad Española de Enfermeria Neonatal (SEEN)-Spain. COINN helped launch organizations in Southern Africa–Neonatal Nursing Association of Southern Africa (NNASA), India-Indian Association of Neonatal Nurses (IANN), a network in Russia, and is beginning to discuss such work in Kenya and Brazil. Other areas of the world have offered regional representatives who can link nurses together in their region of the world. Through these efforts, over 60 countries are now represented by COINN. Why is this type of nongovernmental, nonprofit organization important?

COINN'S Role in Global Health

COINN has joined forces with many partners worldwide to address the issues of newborn health standards, neonatal nursing recognition as a specialty, and the need for lifelong learning for those caring for mothers and babies. COINNs partners are the 99nicu Forums, Caring Bridge, European Foundation for the Care of Newborn Infants, the Healthy Newborn Network, as an affiliate of the International Council of Nurses and the Partnership for Safe Motherhood and Newborn Health, the Partnership for Maternal Newborn & Child Health–WHO, and the White Ribbon Alliance for Safe Motherhood, to name a few. COINN has issued position statements on the Care of the Late Preterm Infant, Care of the Well Term Infant, Child Health, Poverty and Breastfeeding, Ethical Migration of Neonatal Nurses, Neonatal Nursing Education, and Routine Screening for Intimate Partner Violence. COINN has endorsed documents from other organizations that are helping to shape health policy and standards of care at both a national and global level. Some examples of the global perspective and why many issues are the same worldwide are presented in the next sections.

European Foundation for the Care of Newborns and Infants

The European Foundation for the Care of Newborn and Infants (EFCNI) was founded in 2008 to address the issues surrounding premature infant birth and their families. Since that time this organization has formed alliances with non-governmental and governmental organizations, including the March of Dimes, European Parliament, and many others to promote policy changes in the European Union. COINN has endorsed some of their more recent reports. They have issued several landmark reports and white papers. Their Benchmarking Report of 2010 (EFCNI, 2010) highlighted successful ingredients for changing the prematurity rates and outcomes.

Key factors that determine an effective and successful approach to tacking prematurity include:

> National neonatal health policy/program
> Formal dialogue between government, health care professionals, and parents
> Comprehensive data collection on prevalence/morbidity/mortality/cost burden based on standardized definitions and common measurement criteria (e.g., through registries)
> Comprehensive data collection on neonatal intervention outcomes/neonatal service management based on common measurement criteria (EFCNI, 2010, p. 7)

EFCNI issued a white paper in 2012 on caring for newborns and infants. This white paper is a call to action to address the provision of quality and safe maternal infant care (EFCNI, 2012). Thirteen key recommendations were made. While the focus was on Europe, the reality is that these recommendations fit with any country.

The 13 key recommendations made in this white paper identify that action is needed at both European and national level in order to:

1. Recognise the issues of maternal and newborn care and aftercare as a public health priority, particularly the health of preterm infants and infants with illnesses
2. Acknowledge the potential long-term health consequences of preterm birth and newborns with illnesses that need to be tackled
3. Address health inequalities in maternal and newborn care within all EU Member States
4. Conduct national audits on maternal, newborn care and aftercare services and establish multidisciplinary task forces for developing national best practice guidelines
5. Implement national policies and guidelines for high-quality preconceptional, maternal and newborn care and aftercare. These policies and guidelines should include the principles highlighted in this White Paper
6. Provide equal and early access for parents to complete and accurate information, education and counseling
7. Harmonise education and training of healthcare providers

8. Provide social and financial support for parents and families
9. Develop and implement strategies for public awareness and education
10. Harmonize cross-border maternal and newborn healthcare
11. Monitor outcomes and implement audit procedures in maternal, newborn and aftercare services
12. Implement European-wide standardized datasets for pregnancy and preterm birth outcomes
13. Invest in comprehensive research to tackle the challenge of preterm birth and its potential long-term consequences (EFCNI, 2012, pp. 5–6)

RUSSIAN EXAMPLE

Neonatal nurses in Russia have worked hard to raise the status of nursing in their country. They have a very strong Russian Nurses Association that has been a member of the International Council of Nurses for almost a decade. This group is working to raise the standards of nursing and supports exchanges with other countries. At the same time Russian neonatal nurses have formed a network to address the specific care and educational needs of neonates and their caregivers. For example, Children's Hospital #1 in Saint Petersburg developed collaboration in the early 1990s. Neonatal teams went back and forth between Russia and Oakland Children's Hospital, Oakland, California. Through this exchange infection rates as well as neonatal mortality rates dropped significantly (Kenner, Sugrue, Mubichi, Boykova, & Davidge, 2009). Medical leadership in Saint Petersburg supported neonatal nurses going to England to gain bachelor's and master's degrees. The administration supported a neonatal nurse educator at the unit level. Unfortunately, such efforts were not common in Russia, and some places have even eliminated unit educators. On the positive side, Russia has free follow-up care for mothers and babies, including home visits. This country has also supported changing the role of nurses to a more professional level. In the past it was not uncommon for nurses to sweep and scrub the floors and empty trash in addition to providing care.

INDIAN EXAMPLE

Indian neonatal nurses and neonatologists recognized that there was a growing problem of sicker, smaller babies requiring care. The Neonatology Forum of India, which represents the doctors, encouraged the neonatal nurses to work together with them and seek help from COINN to form a national organization. In 2007, this call to action resulted in the formation of the Indian Neonatal Nurses Association. The 2007 COINN International Conference of Neonatal Nurses hosted by the Indian Neonatal Nurses Association brought together over a 1,000 nurses and doctors from around the global. Why was this important? At one session during the conference, the president of COINN and a local neonatologist facilitated a discussion of the state of neonatal nursing in India. There it was revealed that even though it might be considered a Level II or intermediate care unit, the ratio was 75 babies to one nurse. The staffing was at critical levels as the nursing shortage was growing. Nurses were frustrated they could not provide the care they wanted so desperately to give. While, of course, this staffing was not the case everywhere in India, the neonatal outcomes were not good. For example in the *Born Too Soon* report (Group et al., 2012), India is reported to have had just over 27 million births in 2010, with 13 in 1,000 live births being preterm resulting in over 875,000 neonatal deaths. These figures are just for premature births and not other neonatal problems. With the sanction of the Ministry of Women's and Children's Health, the India Neonatal Nursing Association was launched in 2007. Since that time this organization with COINN has advanced neonatal nursing. *Saving Newborn Lives* in conjunction with COINN gave awards to three nurses to attend the International Conference hosted by the Neonatal Nursing Association of Southern Africa and COINN in Durban, South Africa in 2010. One of the awardees was from the Indian group. Participating in such conferences and having organizations work collaboratively are making a difference. The following sections provide exemplars of work going on globally to change neonatal care and education.

SOUTH AFRICAN EXAMPLE

For many years, the challenge of maternal–child health in sub-Saharan Africa has been highlighted. The highest neonatal death rates worldwide are still found in this region. The rate of premature births in South Africa in 2010 was 8/1,000 live births, with total births just over 1 million; neonatal deaths due just to prematurity was over 18,000 (Group et al., 2012). Neonatal nurses had enjoyed a time when their specialty was recognized by the nursing council; however, as the nursing shortage grew, the need for more generalized training grew. Thus neonatal specialized training was only supported at an institutional or unit level. The neonatal nurses brought the minister of health and *Saving Newborn Lives* to the international conference with COINN. From that meeting there were media releases to support the need for more education and training, as well as for nurses working with nongovernmental and governmental agencies to improve neonatal outcomes. Policy changes are slow but with this organized voice and now thanks to the media coverage, more recognition of the vital role nurses play in improving outcomes, progress is being made (Kenner, Boykova, & Eklund, 2011; Kenner et al., 2009). Educational outreach is growing, as are the requests for neonatal nurses to work at the policy table to change neonatal care. Southern Africa, South Africa in particular, must be viewed within the context of a change in health care delivery due to the increasing impact of HIV. As hospitals got overcrowded with patients with HIV/AIDS, South Africa developed community-based programs such as home visits and palliative care (Zelnick, 2011). Need for nurses grew at a time that wages and work conditions grew worse (Zelnick, 2011). Nurses, including neonatal nurses, began migrating to other countries, contributing to the brain drain (Zelnick, 2011). This migration, coupled with the growing needs for generalist nurses, has led to tensions for specialized education, especially in the area of maternal–child outcomes.

BRAZILIAN EXAMPLE

In June 2012, the Brazilian neonatal nursing community came together in the second annual meeting *Congresso Brasileiro de Enfermagem Neonatal* held in Fortaleza, Brazil. Almost 1,000 nurses and doctors were in attendance. Amazing work is going on there. A national repository exists to collect data on maternal–child outcomes. Interprofessional teams are beginning to emerge in the educational institutions as well as the practice arena. The nurses are working with policy makers to ensure that the standards of nursing and care are raised. Brazilian nurses are gaining opportunities for more autonomy in practice. They are viewed by many doctors as the key to changing the outcomes for the country. Prematurity rates have decreased over the past decade, and there is more emphasis being placed on breastfeeding, nutrition, and developmental care. Infectious disease is still a problem, as it is globally. They have formed a national research network that encompasses public health initiatives. Brazil is considered one of the BRIC countries—Brazil, Russia, India, and China. This refers to the growing economies in these countries and the important role they will have in changing global markets. For health this means that more countries will want to invest in BRIC and therefore will need a healthy workforce to draw workers from and to maintain. According to UNICEF, the younger than 5 years of age mortality rate in 1990 was 59 in 1,000 live births, but by 2010 the rate was 19 in 1,000 live births (UNICEF, 2012a). The neonatal mortality rate in 2010 was 17 per 1,000 live births (UNICEF, 2012a). Definite progress is being made in this country. This progress demonstrates the impact of improved nutrition, promotion of breastfeeding, increased support for reproductive health efforts, a strong public health model that includes examining differences between risk and poor populations and the factors that contribute to the differences, provision of public safe water, increased awareness of prematurity and rationale for decreasing elective cesarean sections, as well as monies to support vaccinations and treatment for infectious diseases including pneumonia and diarrhea (Holtz, 2013).

JAPANESE EXAMPLE

Japan is a global economic and technological force. Yet neonatal nurses in Japan have a limited role. Nurses in Japan oftentimes are not permitted to do any invasive procedures such as start intravenous therapy; they cannot easily question a doctor's authority, nor can they always contribute to the assessment (Kenner et al., 2011). Tides are changing as nurses and doctors are being invited to lecture and work in Japan to raise the awareness of Western techniques and care standards (Kenner et al., 2011). Gradually policies are changing through these exchanges. Collaborative efforts are under way to gather groups already working in Japan to address common issues such as neonatal care standards rather than working individually (Kenner et al., 2011).

RWANDAN EXAMPLE

Rwanda is a changing country. Neonatal mortality rates are 29 in 1,000 live births (UNICEF, 2012b). The amazing change is in the younger than 5 years of age mortality rate that moved from 163 in 1,000 live births in 1990 to 91 in 1,000 live births in 2010 (UNICEF, 2012b). How did this change come about? Over the past two decades, governmental and nongovernmental agencies have worked together to change the tides of health in this country. Recently, EOSVISIONS, COINN, and One Good Deed worked together with the Rwandan Ministry of Health and the Kigali Health Institute to provide neonatal education, specifically Helping Babies Breathe (http://www.helpingbabiesbreathe.org) from the American Academy of Pediatrics and S.T.A.B.L.E. Program developed by Dr. Kris Karlson Park City, Utah (http://www.stableprogram.com) (EOSVISIONS, 2012). This collaboration is new, but represents another step in raising the education of neonatal health providers.

These are just some examples of challenges as well as opportunities to impact neonatal nursing care and education. There are other broader issues that are also impacting neonatal nursing.

FUNDING FOR NURSING EDUCATION

A major factor in neonatal nursing care is neonatal nursing education. This education is linked to how a country finances medical and nursing education. Many countries fund medical education under the Department or Ministry of Education. But nursing education is often funded under the Ministry of Health. Obviously if a country has poor health outcomes and there is increasing political pressure to improve these outcomes, a country will put more financial resources into the care than into education that is competing for the same dollar (Kenner et al., 2009). Mexico, for example, changed this mode of funding several years ago. Nursing education is now funded under education and not health. This is one example of a policy initiative that needs to continue to be addressed on a country level. COINN and other organizations are raising the awareness of this issue.

SUMMARY

Global issues in neonatal nursing care and education are at the forefront of the Millennium Development Goals work. It is critical that nurses continue to see a role in changing standards of care for mothers and babies, raise the educational level of neonatal nurses, and work at policy tables to change public and health policies.

CASE STUDY

A 39-week infant was born in a remote village in Central America. The infant was transported by ambulance to a large metropolitan hospital that has an intensive care unit. The infant was diagnosed with a congenital heart defect that could be repaired with surgery. The only pediatric cardiac surgeon was unavailable as he had been in an accident and recovery was expected to take several weeks. The infant was maintained with oxygen in hopes he could survive until the surgeon was well. Transport of the infant out of the region for medical treatment was not possible. This case is replicated in many parts of the world with small variations on a regular basis.

EVIDENCE-BASED PRACTICE BOX

In 2005, Lawn and colleagues published *The Lancet "Neonatal Survival Series,"* which that stated over 4 million children younger than 5 years old died annually. By 2010 (Lawn et al., 2005), reported this number to have been reduced to 3.6 million. The health burden for this mortality is highest in India, Nigeria, Democratic Republic of the Congo, Pakistan, and China (United Nations, 2011).

Several strategies were used to reduce this mortality. For example, Lee and colleagues (2011) report that, of the 136 million babies born annually worldwide, about 8% require help to breathe, while 814,000 neonatal term infant deaths are due to intrapartum-related events resulting in asphyxia. Therefore, this research team conducted a systematic review of neonatal resuscitation and tactile stimulation and the link to neonatal mortality and morbidity whether in term, preterm, hospital, or home birth situations. GRADE criteria were used to determine mortality rate estimates for the Lives Saved Tool (LiST). A Delphi panel was used for effect size determination when there appears to be low-level evidence to support an intervention that was strongly recommended. The findings were that there were 24 neonatal resuscitation studies involving mortality reports, but none included use of immediate newborn assessment and stimulation as the only interventions. The conclusions following the Delphi panel was that in health care facilities neonatal resuscitation reduces term intrapartum-related death by as much as 30% but is less effective on preterm infant outcomes. In the community use of low or no technology resuscitation (basic), immediate newborn assessment, and stimulation also had less dramatic effects than in health care institutions with term infants. Further research is needed examining these practices.

Reference

Lee, A. C., Cousens, S., Wall, S. N., Niermeyer, S., Darmstadt, G. L., Carlo, . . . Lawn, J. E. (2011). Neonatal resuscitation and immediate newborn assessment and stimulation for the prevention of neonatal deaths: A systematic review, meta-analysis and Delphi estimation of mortality effect. *BMC Public Health, 11* (Suppl. 3): S12.

ONLINE RESOURCES

Council of International Neonatal Nurses
http://www.coinnurses.org
EOSVISIONS
http://www.eos-visions.com
Helping Babies Breathe
http://www.helpingbabiesbreathe.org
Save the Children's Videos
http://vimeo.com/41435895
Saving Newborn Lives
http://www.savethechildren.org/site/c.8rKLIXMGIpI4E/b.6234293/k.6211/Saving_Newborn_Lives.htm
The S.T.A.B.L.E. Program
http://www.stableprogram.com
UNICEF
http://www.unicef.org

REFERENCES

EFCNI. (2012). *Caring for tomorrow: EFCNO white paper on maternal and newborn health and aftercare services*. Karlsfeld, Germany.

EOSVISIONS. (2012). EOS Neonatal Health Programs. New York, NY.

European Foundation for the Care of Newborns and Infants. (2010). *EU Benchmarking Report 2009/2010: Too little too late? Why Europe should do more for preterm infants*. Karlsfeld, Germany: Author.

Group, B. T. S. E. S., Kinney, M. V., Howson, C. P., McDougall, L., & Lawn, J. E. (2012). *Executive summary for Born Too Soon: The global action report on preterm birth*. Geneva, Switzerland: World Health Organization.

Holtz, C. (2013). *Global health care: Issues and policies* (2nd ed.). Burlington, MA: Jones & Bartlett.

Kenner, C., Boykova, M., & Eklund, W. (2011). Impact on neonatal nursing globally: Exemplars of how US neonatal/perinatal nurses can get involved. *The Journal of Perinatal and Neonatal Nursing, 25*(2), 119–122. doi:10.1097/JPN.0b013e31821a6d8a

Kenner, C., Sugrue, N., Mubichi, F., Boykova, M., & Davidge, R. (2009). Global infant mortality/morbidity: A clinical issue, a global organizational approach [Review]. *Critical Care Nursing Clinics of North America, 21*(1), 1–9, doi:10.1016/j.ccell.2008.09.001

Lawn, J. E., Cousens, S., Zupan, J., & Lancet Neonatal Survival Steering Committee, T. (2005). 4 million neonatal deaths: When? Where? Why? [Research Support, Non-U.S. Gov't Research

Support, U.S. Gov't, Non-P.H.S.]. *Lancet, 365*(9462), 891–900. doi: 10.1016/S0140-6736(05)71048-5

Lawn, J. E., Kerber, K., Enweronu-Laryea, C., & Cousens, S. (2010). 3.6 million neonatal deaths--what is progressing and what is not? [Review]. *Seminars in Perinatology, 34*(6), 371–386. doi: 10.1053/j.semperi.2010.09.011

Lee, A. C., Cousens, S., Wall, S. N., Niermeyer, S., Darmstadt, G. L., Carlo, W. A., . . . Lawn, J. E. (2011). Neonatal resuscitation and immediate newborn assessment and stimulation for the prevention of neonatal deaths: A systematic review, meta-analysis and Delphi estimation of mortality effect. *BMC Public Health, 11* (Suppl. 3): S12.

United Nations. (UN). (2011). *Child mortality*. Report from the United Nations. New York, NY: Author.

UNICEF. (2012a). *Brazil statistics*. Retrieved from http://www.unicef.org/infobycountry/brazil_statistics.html

UNICEF. (2012b). *Rwanda statistics*. New York, NY: Author.

Zelnick, J. R. (2011). *Who is nursing them? It is us*. Amityville, NY: Baywood Publishing Company, Inc.

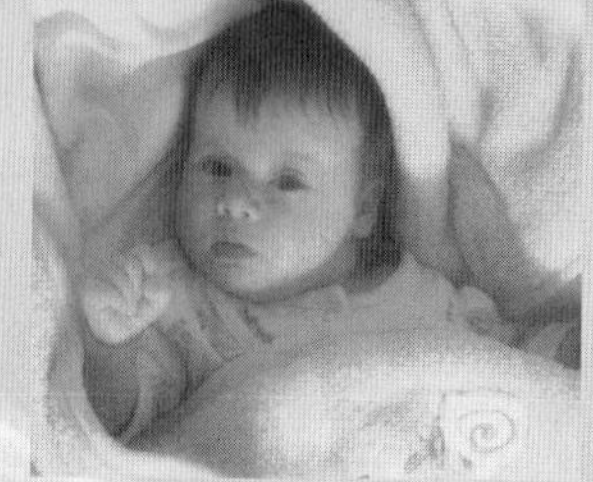

CHAPTER

42

Competency-Based Education and Continued Competency

■ Debra A. Sansoucie

There has never in the history of this nation been a greater public focus on health care. Along with this increased awareness has come a mounting expectation for safe and quality care. Among the initiatives that have taken on growing importance in improving the quality of health care is the competence of its providers. Competence and competency-based education (CBE) are not new concepts for the nursing profession. At the First Annual Nurse Educator Conference in November 1977, Dr. Dorothy Del Bueno described "competency-based education" and its applicability to nursing education related to its emphasis on adult learning principles, criterion-based performance measures, and educational outcomes (Del Bueno, 1978). In addition to the considerable confusion about what CBE actually entailed and the controversy about its value, Dr. Del Bueno understood that introducing CBE into existing nursing education programs could prove to be logistically difficult (Del Bueno, 1978). Almost 35 years later, educators are still debating the suitability of CBE for nursing education and the feasibility of its implementation. Nursing has historically demonstrated a commitment to assuring competency that relied on initial licensure, testing, continuing education, codes of ethics, and comprehensive certification programs designed to protect public safety (American Nurses Association [ANA], 2001). During the 1990s, however, the ability of all health care professionals to assure a safe and effective workforce came under increased public scrutiny. In 1999, the Institute of Medicine (IOM) recommended the implementation of periodic reexamination and re-licensure of physicians, nurses, and other health care providers based on competence and knowledge of safety practices (Institute of Medicine [IOM], 1999).

In response to the escalating concern, the Joint Commission on Accreditation of Healthcare Organizations (JCAHO) issued standards requiring documentation of the clinical competency of all nursing staff (JCAHO, 1999). Hospitals were tasked to develop systems for assessing initial and continuing competence for their nursing staff at a time when downsizing was resulting in the loss of both unit-based educators and clinical nurse specialists (CNS). Particularly affected were critical care units, such as the neonatal intensive care unit (NICU), which were already short staffed and had high nursing turnover rates.

As this movement toward documentation of minimal competencies for hospital nurses was developing, educational institutions were looking at terminal program objectives and the ways in which these might translate into minimal competency statements for graduates. By this time, CBE had gained acceptance in the nursing education community. Because it offered a potential bridge between education and practice, it was hoped that CBE would help to close the gap between a new nurse graduate's education for practice and actual practice requirements.

This chapter traces the evolution of the competency movement in health care, discusses the advantages and disadvantages of CBE, and describes the impact of the competency movement on neonatal nursing practice and education.

DEVELOPMENT OF THE COMPETENCY MOVEMENT

Hospital-based or diploma programs that used an apprentice model to integrate classroom learning and clinical performance dominated the American educational system for nurses until the late 1960s and early 1970s (Chapman, 1999). Subsequently, the growing importance of higher education shifted nursing education from the hospital-based training program to the academic school or university and transferred responsibility for the competence of the new graduate nurse from the hospital or employer to the university and its educators (Bechtel, Davidhizar, & Bradshaw, 1999). University-based nursing education gained in popularity, and the hospital-based programs began to disappear.

As the new paradigm for nursing education evolved, so did an enormous shift in the health care arena. Patients in hospitals were sicker, older, and more knowledgeable about the care they received. The gap between the knowledge and skills nursing students learn and use safely under supervision in the academic setting, and those needed to function safely and independently in the practice setting, became increasingly evident. According to Lenburg (1999a), "Employers are experiencing a widening gulf between the competencies required for practice and those new graduates learned in their education programs." Gaps in competency forced employers to spend more money on human resource time and expertise in orienting new nurses, thus adding to the cost of health care. As inpatient costs continued to escalate, hospitals began to place greater emphasis on strategies to reduce expenses. Hospital administrators realized that they could no longer afford expensive orientation programs that correlated with little improvement in objective performance outcomes (Hartshorn, 1992).

An early classic study published in the book, *On Competence: A Critical Analysis of Competence-Based Reforms in Higher Education*, paved the way for recommendations to reform the education of professionals in American universities and colleges (Grant, 1979). Grant's thoughts on competence are still relevant:

> Perhaps the most immediately plausible explanation for concern over competence is that levels of competence once thought at least tolerable for a society moving at a slower pace are quite inadequate for a society whose internal management is growing steadily more complicated. Consider, too, the amount of knowledge that individuals must master to conduct themselves competently and to have the self-confidence that comes from believing themselves competent. Today, in fact, belief in one's own competence is no longer enough, and a demand for demonstrated competence now motivates much of education. (pp. 19–20)

Also still applicable is Grant's definition of CBE: It is

> ... a form of education that derives a curriculum from an analysis of a prospective or actual role ... and attempts to certify student progress on the basis of demonstrated performance in some or all aspects of that role. (p. 6)

Eventually government became concerned about the issue of education and competency. In 1986 the National Governors Association took action to change the meaning and methods of documenting accountability and competence in higher education (Lenburg, 1999a). As a result of these changes, the purpose and methods of learning and practice in the United States refocused on outcomes and outcomes assessment.

Academia, responding to the increasing pressure to assure the competency of university graduates, dedicated the entire September/October 1990 issue of *Change*, the journal of the American Association of Higher Education, to addressing the problems of competence and higher education (Lenburg, 1999a, 1999b). As the competency movement continued to evolve, educators began to adopt concepts and strategies related to continuous quality improvement from the realms of business and industry (Lenburg, 1999a, 1999b). Teachers were challenged to alter the traditional lecture format to include more active, collaborative learning methods focused on expanding competencies that graduates would be expected to use in the workplace, such as assessment, critical thinking, communication, and leadership. Academic accreditation agencies such as the National League for Nursing (NLN) and the Commission for Collegiate Nursing Education (CCNE) also began to incorporate outcomes into their accreditation criteria (CCNE, 1998; NLNAC, 1997). In response to recommendations from the U.S. Department of Education, these criteria were changed to place even more emphasis on competence with the creation of the NLN Accreditation Commission (NLNAC) in 1996 (NLNAC, 1997).

Concern about the need for validation of initial and continuing competency among nursing and other health care providers began to reach beyond the walls of academia into other prominent organizations in the health care industry. In 1996, the Citizens Advocacy Center (CAC), an organization of public members of health care regulatory and governing boards, posed a compelling question: "Can the public be confident that health care professionals who demonstrated minimum level of competence when they earned their license continue to be competent years and decades after they have been in practice?" In an attempt to answer this question, the CAC held a 2-day meeting on the topic of continued competence of health care professionals. The proceedings of this conference, published in 1997, called for stronger measures to assure the public of the continued competence of health care workers and to remove those who may not be competent (Citizens Advocacy Center [CAC], 1997). The Pew Health Professions Commission report in 1995 recommended that states "require each board to develop, implement, and evaluate continuing competency requirements to assure continuing competence of regulated health professions" (Pew Health Professions Commission, 1995). A subsequent report called for states to require that health care professionals "demonstrate their competence in the knowledge, judgment, technical skills, and interpersonal skills relevant to their jobs throughout their careers" (Pew Health Professions Commission, 1998). These reports proposed periodic reviews of professional competence at intervals not to exceed 7 years. In addition to mandatory continuing education, the commission advocated repeat testing of professionals using the initial licensing examination or a new examination in the specialty or practice area, chart and/or peer review, and acceptance of professional credentialing such as certification and recertification.

In response to the findings of the Pew Taskforce on Health Care Workforce Regulation, the National Council of State Boards of Nursing (NCSBN) issued a position paper titled *Assuring Competence: A Regulatory Responsibility*. Competence was defined in this paper as "the application of knowledge and the interpersonal, decision-making, and psychomotor skills expected for the nurse's practice role within the context of public health, safety, and welfare." The NCSBN went on further to address the issue of ensuring competency validation at the state regulatory level (National Council of State Boards of Nursing [NCSBN], 1998).

Perhaps the strongest driving force of the competency movement came in the form of three successive reports from the IOM. In its seminal report, *To Err Is Human: Building a Safer Health Care System*, the IOM exposed a safety crisis in health care revealing the staggering estimate that as many as 98,000 people die in hospitals each year due to preventable medical errors. The IOM introduced the public to the concept of "professional competence" identifying competencies that should be included in the education of all health care professionals (IOM, 1999). In 2001, the IOM published *Crossing the Quality Chasm: A New Health System for the 21st Century*. This report condensed the principles of change into six guiding aims: health care should be safe, effective, patient-centered, timely, efficient, and equitable (IOM, 2001). In its third report, *Health Professions Education: A Bridge to Quality*, the IOM identified core competencies needed for health care professionals. The report suggested that "All health professionals should be educated to deliver patient-centered care as members of an interdisciplinary team, emphasizing evidence-based practice, quality improvement approaches and informatics" (Institute of Medicine [IOM], 2003).

Building on the momentum created by the IOM reports, the National Postsecondary Education Cooperative (NPEC) Working Group on Competency-Based Initiatives in Postsecondary Education (U.S. Department of Education, 2002) undertook to examine the use of competency-based initiatives in the United States. The resulting report, *Defining and Assessing Learning: Exploring Competency-Based Initiatives*, established a set of "strong principles" or key considerations for defining and measuring competencies. The overarching goal of this project was to create a hands-on resource for educators who sought to develop, implement or refine competency-based programs. Utilizing a case study approach, 12 "principles of strong practice" were identified (U.S. Department of Education, 2002):

- A senior administrator is the public advocate, leader, and facilitator for creating an institutional culture that is open to change, willing to take risks, and fosters innovations by providing real incentives for participants.
- The appropriate stakeholders fully participate in identifying, defining, and reaching a consensus about important competencies.
- Competencies are clearly defined, understood, and accepted by relevant stakeholders.
- Competencies are defined at a sufficient level of specificity that they can be assessed.
- Multiple assessments of competencies provide useful and meaningful information that is relevant to decision making or policy-development contexts.
- Faculty and staff fully participate in making decisions about the strongest assessment instruments that will measure their specific competencies.
- The precision, reliability, validity, credibility, and costs are all considered and examined in making selections about the best commercially developed assessments and/or locally developed approaches.
- The competency-based educational initiative is embedded within a larger institutional planning process.
- The assessments of competencies are directly linked with the goals of the learning experience.
- The assessment results are used in making critical decisions about strategies to improve student learning.
- The assessment results are clear and reported in a meaningful way so that all relevant stakeholders fully understand the findings.
- The institution experiments with new ways to document students' mastery of competencies that supplement the traditional transcript (pp. viii–xi).

Given the challenges currently facing the health care industry regarding patient safety and quality of care, preparing competent nursing graduates, while a crucial first step, is no longer enough. The need to address challenges posed by assuring and evaluating continuing competence has been acknowledged as an increasingly critical goal. Nursing leaders in education, administration, and practice have been confronted with the need for identifying and implementing strategies to evaluate competency throughout an individual's career trajectory. While quality and safety of health care remain in the forefront of the national agenda, the movement toward CBE and continuing competency validation will continue to gain strength and momentum in nursing.

COMPETENCE AND COMPETENCY

What is competence? What is competency? Is there a distinction between the two? Is competence measurable? Benner (1982) defined nursing competency as the ability to perform a task with desirable outcomes under the varied circumstances of the real world. In her work *From Novice to Expert* (1984), Benner positioned competence at the midpoint of a continuum ranging from novice to advanced beginner, to competent, to proficient, and finally to expert. According to Benner (1984), competent practitioners are consciously able to plan their actions but lack speed. It is interesting to note that the stage of being a "competent" practitioner is not the final one. Two stages (proficient and expert) come after the development of competence. The National Council for State Boards of Nursing (NCSBN, 2005) defined competency as "the application of knowledge and the interpersonal, decision-making, and psychomotor skills expected for the practice role, within the context of public health" (p. 81). In its *Position Statement on Professional Role Competence*, the American Nurses Association (ANA, 2008) maintains that "an individual who demonstrates 'competence' is performing successfully at an expected level" (p. 3). The ANA further states that "competency is an expected level of performance that integrates knowledge, skills, abilities, and judgment" (p. 3). The International Council of Nurses (ICN) describes competence as the "effective application of a combination of knowledge, skill and judgment demonstrated by an individual in daily practice or job performance" (International Council of Nurses [ICN], 2009, p. 6).

The terms are indeed interconnected and are often used interchangeably. McMullan et al. (2003) distinguished between competence and competency, noting that competence is focused on the *description* of the required action or behavior, while competency is focused on the *behavior* that underpins the competent performance.

Health care institutions are demanding more than ever that educators assure competent practitioners as outcomes of their educational institutions. However, the ANA (2008) maintains that assurance of competence is also the shared responsibility of the profession, nurses, professional organizations, credentialing and certification entities, regulatory agencies, employers, and other key stakeholders. The ANA asserts that competence is definable, measurable, and can be evaluated but that it is also situational and dynamic; that is, context determines what competencies are necessary. Competency is also seen as both an outcome and an ongoing process (ANA, 2008). The ANA *Standards of Practice* and *Standards of Professional Performance* "are authoritative statements by which the nursing profession describes the responsibilities for which its practitioners are accountable" (ANA, 2004, p. 1). The ANA includes measurement criteria that list key indicators of competent practice that must be met for each standard (ANA, 2004). Evaluation tools that capture data related to a nurse's knowledge base and actual performance should be applicable to the specific context and outcome of the competence evaluation. Evaluative tools and methods may include direct observation, patient records, portfolio, demonstrations, skills lab, certification, credentialing, simulation exercises, virtual reality testing, targeted continuing education with outcomes measurement, employer skills validation, and practice evaluation. The ANA warns, however, that no single tool or method can guarantee competence (ANA, 2008).

As noted by the ANA (2008), competence is situational and contextual. It is also both an outcome and an ongoing process. The new graduate nurse or the experienced nurse who is changing practice areas cannot reasonably be expected to be competent at the onset of employment in an acute care environment such as the NICU. It is reasonable to expect, however, that both will acquire both initial and ongoing competency if provided with appropriate orientation and opportunities for continuing education. As the professional organization for neonatal nurses and nurse practitioners (NPs), the National Association of Neonatal Nurses (NANN) and the National Association of Neonatal Nurse Practitioners (NANNP), a division of NANN, hold responsibility for setting the national standard for initial and continued competence for practitioners in the neonatal population focus. To this end, NANNP published a position statement in 2010, *Standard for Maintaining the Competence of Neonatal Nurse Practitioners*, which included recommendations for evaluation and documentation of continued competence for neonatal nurse practitioner (NNP) practice:

- Orientation of the novice NNP should provide several assessment points, utilizing multiple evaluative tools and methods, throughout the period of orientation.
- Evaluation of the experienced NNP should be based on the core competencies of NNP practice and should be conducted at least annually.
- A professional portfolio should be developed by both novice and experienced NNPs to provide evidence of individual learning and experience.
- State boards of nursing should request that ongoing competencies be part of the annual evaluation process (National Association of Neonatal Nurses [NANNP], 2010a).

NANNP concluded that "evidence-based care of the critically ill neonate is continually evolving and NNPs must maintain their competence throughout their career as they progress from novice to expert" (NANNP, 2010a, p. 283).

CBE

What is it? To understand CBE, one must first understand what the word *competency* actually means in an educational setting. Although the term is frequently used in education, there is no common understanding of its meaning. According to Tilley (2008), there is no clear and accepted definition of competency across nursing education and practice. Despite differences in definitions, however, the common goal is to ensure that nurses have the knowledge, skills, and abilities required to practice in a particular setting.

CBE may be broadly interpreted as a conceptual framework on which a total curriculum may be built, or more narrowly as a framework for an individual learning module. The term *performance-based learning* may also be used to denote a framework for learning systems that seek to document that a learner has attained a given competency or set of competencies (Voorhees, 2001). Regardless of terminology used, competency-based models rely on measurable assessment. The competency must be clear, transparent, and measurable, and all parties to the learning process should understand the outcomes of the learning experience (Voorhees, 2001).

The definition of competency used by the NPEC work group to build their conceptual learning model is "a combination of skills, abilities, and knowledge needed to perform a specific task" (U.S. Department of Education, 2002, p. 1). Traits and characteristics are the innate qualities of individuals upon which further experiences can be built. These are the foundation for learning. Skills, abilities, and knowledge that are developed through learning experiences build upon that foundation. Competencies result from integrative learning experiences in which skills, abilities, and knowledge interact to form learning. Lastly, demonstrations are the results of applying competencies. This is the level at which performance can be assessed. Figure 42.1 depicts the interrelationships of these terms with competencies (U.S. Department of Education, 2002, p. 1).

In order to assure that learners attain the skills, abilities, and knowledge that are critical to the role for which they are preparing, competencies must contain three key components: a description of the competency; a means of measuring or assessing the competency; and a standard by which the individual may be deemed to be competent (U.S. Department of Education, 2002). Nursing competencies may be divided into core and population-focused competencies. Core competencies are the skills and knowledge required for the minimum safe level of nursing performance. Population-focused competencies are the skills and knowledge required for the minimum safe level of nursing care for a specific patient population.

Although some competencies are mandated by accreditation agencies such as The Joint Commission (TJC), most nursing competencies are derived from standards of practice developed by professional nursing organizations. The National Clinical Nurse Specialist (CNS) Competency Task Force (2010) has developed and validated core competencies for CNS that are comprehensive, entry-level competencies expected for newly graduated CNS. CNS core competencies include Direct Care; Consultation; Systems Leadership; Collaboration; Coaching; Research; and Ethical Decision Making, Moral Agency, and Advocacy. These competencies reflect CNS practice across all specialties, populations, and settings (National CNS Competency Task Force, 2010). The National Organization of Nurse Practitioner Faculties (NONPF) has developed both core and population-focused nursing competencies for NPs. The most recent version of the *Nurse Practitioner Core Competencies* was published by NONPF in April 2011 and amended in 2012 (National Organization of Nurse Practitioner Faculties [NONPF], 2012). The competencies were revised from those previously published (NONPF, 2006) to reflect the emergence of the Doctor of Nursing Practice as the recommended educational entry level for NP practice (NONPF, 2008a, 2008b); to build upon previous work that identified knowledge and skills essential to DNP competencies (American Association of Colleges of Nursing [AACN], 1996, 2006; NONPF & National Panel, 2006); and to maintain consistency with the recommendations of the IOM report on *The Future of Nursing* (IOM, 2011). The core competencies include Scientific Foundation; Leadership; Quality; Practice Inquiry; Technology and Information Literacy; Policy, Health Delivery System; Ethics; and Independent Practice (NONPF, 2012). The nine core competencies are expected outcomes for an NP graduate, regardless of population focus, and are "acquired through mentored patient care experiences with emphasis on independent and interprofessional practice; analytic skills for evaluating and providing evidence-based, patient centered care across settings; and advanced knowledge of the health care delivery system" (NONPF, 2012, p. 1).

The core competencies can be adapted to fit specific population-foci within nursing. NONPF recently established the 2011–2012 Population-Focused Competencies Task Force to adapt the core competencies to each NP population focus that is recognized by the *APRN Consensus Model: Licensure, Accreditation, Certification and Education* (APRN Consensus Work Group & the National Council of State Boards of Nursing APRN Advisory Committee, 2008). These NP population foci include Family, Adult-Gerontology, Neonatal, Pediatrics, Women's Health, and Psychiatric Mental Health. The adult-gerontology and pediatric population foci have further

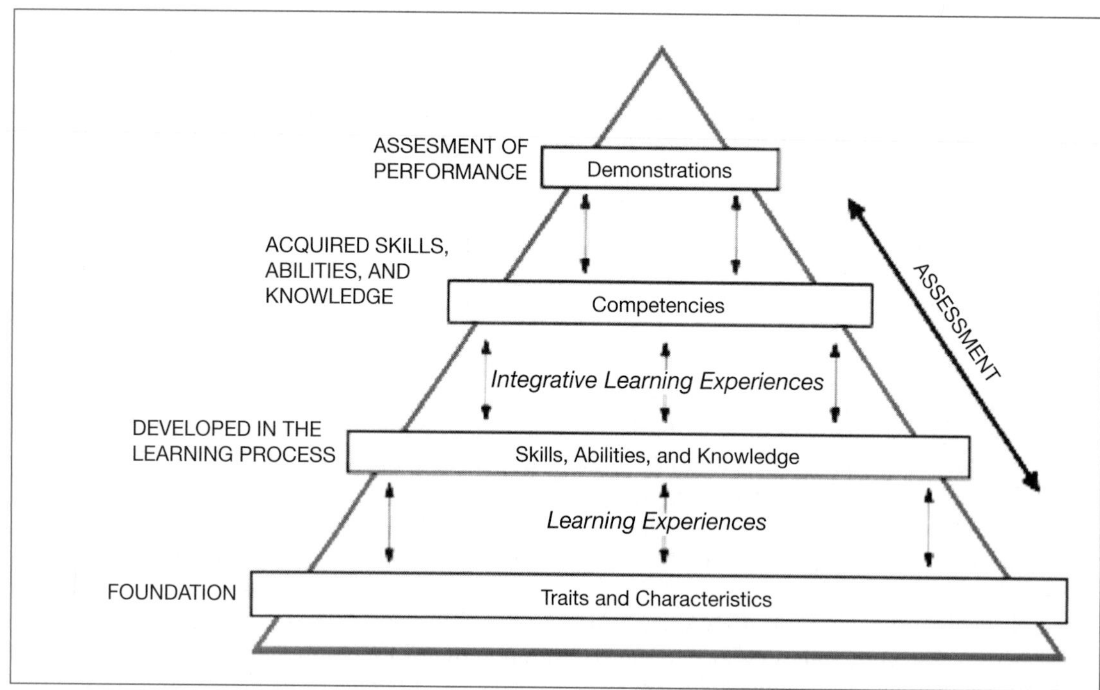

FIGURE 42.1 Conceptual framework for competency assessment.
From the U.S. Department of Education, National Center for Education Statistics (2002).

competency distinctions for acute versus primary care NP practice (NONPF, 2011). Organizations that are specific to each population focus, such as NANN and NANNP, have a multifaceted role in the development of their own specialized nursing competencies. Such organizations are responsible for developing specific educational standards and clinical guidelines on which professional nursing practice is based. Accordingly, NANN published *Education Standards and Curriculum Guidelines for Neonatal Nurse Practitioner Programs* in 2009 (National Association of Neonatal Nurses [NANN], 2009). These standards were revised from those previously published by NANN in 2002 to reflect evolving national guidelines and recommendations (NONPF, 2006; National Task Force for Quality Nurse Practitioner Education, 2008). *The Education Standards and Curriculum Guidelines* provide a framework on which new NNP programs may be developed and evaluated, as well as a self-study tool for existing NNP programs. Professional nursing organizations are also responsible for monitoring issues that affect the practice of nursing, such as the development of an appropriate health care policy, and for supporting research to link nursing interventions to patient outcomes. Finally, they support individual competence by providing educational opportunities for nurses to maintain their skills and knowledge, by influencing changes in state nurse practice acts, and by participating in the credentialing process as appropriate (Weinstein, 2000; Whittaker, Smolenski, & Carson, 2000).

One of the best-known approaches to CBE is the Competency Outcomes and Performance Assessment (COPA) model developed by Lenburg for the New York Regents College Nursing Program (Lenburg, 1999b). In the COPA model, traditional course objectives, lectures, and evaluation methods are replaced with outcomes that are more outcomes oriented and consistent with contemporary practice needs. This is achieved by developing and implementing competency outcomes, interactive learning strategies, and psychometrically sound performance assessment methods. Implementation of this model is governed by four key questions: What are the essential competencies and outcomes for contemporary practice? What are the indicators that define those competencies? What are the most effective ways to learn those competencies? What are the most effective ways to document that learners have achieved the required competencies?

According to Lenburg, there are eight core practice competencies, each having subset skills (Table 42.1). The traditional learning objectives focused on the learning process. Competency statements focus on the outcomes the institution desires in its graduates or employees. These statements are measurable performance outcomes that lend themselves to criterion-referenced performance evaluations. Objective evaluations based on psychometric concepts are developed to document learner competence for the core practice competencies. The psychometric concepts include critical elements, objectivity, sampling, acceptability, comparability, consistency, flexibility, and systematized conditions (Table 42.2).

Objective evaluations are developed for didactic and clinical learning. Didactic evaluations are called competency performance assessments (CPAs); clinical evaluations are called competency performance examinations (CPEs) (Luttrell, Lenburg, Scherubel, Jacob, & Koch, 1999). CPAs are used to evaluate didactic learning and classroom projects, such as poster presentations and written papers. CPEs are used in the clinical setting. They are often more exacting because the professional, legal, and ethical aspects of care all must be taken into account

An element critical to the success of the COPA model of education is periodic program evaluation to determine the effectiveness of the learning plan in achieving the desired learning outcomes. This periodic review also allows for routine updates as practice or unit procedures change.

TABLE 42.1

LENBURG'S CORE PRACTICE COMPETENCIES AND EXAMPLES OF SUBSET SKILLS

Core Competency	Subset Skill Examples
Assessment and intervention skills	Assessment
	Monitoring
	Therapeutic treatments
Communication skills	Oral
	Written
	Computer (information systems)
Critical thinking skills	Problem solving
	Evaluation
	Prioritizing
	Diagnostic reasoning
Human caring and relationship skills	Respect for cultural diversity
	Ethics
	Interpersonal relationships with patients, colleagues, and family
	Patient advocacy
Management skills	Delegation and supervision
	Materials resource management
	Accountability
	Quality improvement
Leadership skills	Professional accountability
	Role behaviors
	Risk taking
	Collaboration
Teaching skills	Health promotion
	Health restoration
	Group teaching
	Individual teaching
Knowledge integration skills	Nursing and related disciplines
	Liberal arts
	Natural and social sciences

Modified from Lenburg (1999b).

TABLE 42.2

PSYCHOMETRIC CONCEPTS USED WITH COMPETENCY PERFORMANCE ASSESSMENTS

Concept	Definition
Critical elements	Statements that collectively define competence for a particular skill; these are single, discrete, observable behaviors that are mandatory to demonstrate competence for the skill
Objectivity	A procedure that minimizes subjectivity on the part of the assessor (evaluator); two components are used: (1) a written statement of what is expected (e.g., the content of a particular skill or critical element) and (2) the consensual agreement of all directly involved in any aspects of the testing process
Sampling	The process of selecting the most frequently encountered or most essential skills for the test
Acceptability	The determination of what percentage of skills will be considered passing (i.e., 85% must be achieved for acceptable performance)
Comparability	The development of procedures to ensure that each test episode is essentially the same with regard to extent and difficulty
Consistency	The development of procedures to ensure that the testing process is the same regardless of who administers the examination
Flexibility	The ability to adapt when the performance examination is given in an actual clinical environment rather than as a simulation
Systematized conditions	The development of procedures for determining the actions to be taken in the event of unanticipated situations in the clinical environment so that evaluators (faculty) respond in a manner that is objective, comparable, and consistent

Modified from Lenburg (1999b).

A major concern regarding CBE is the measurability and standardization of clinical evaluation tools. According to the COPA model, the criterion-referenced outcomes used as performance indicators would give faculty and clinical instructors more confidence in their evaluations. Another advantage of the COPA model is that students could be moved through curricula as they demonstrate competencies, rather than on the basis of "seat time" amassed in a particular course. Passing a course would thus depend on mastery of the selected competencies, regardless of the length of the course of study (Kenner & Fernandes, 2001). Theoretically, this would allow teachers to spend more time with students having difficulty grasping course concepts while those with a firm understanding of those concepts could be allowed to progress. Despite the seeming advantages, there may also be drawbacks related to deployment of faculty resources and satisfying regulatory requirements for specified number of hours spent in class or clinical preceptorship. Most professional organizations and national certifying bodies for NPs require a minimum number of hours spent in either didactic education, clinical education, or both. Validation of competency versus completion of a defined minimum number of required hours for certification within a population focus continues to be a topic of conversation and controversy among nursing leaders.

Ensuring the competency of new nursing staff requires an organized approach to orientation of the unit and a system of verification and validation of knowledge and skills. Because nurses have a variety of educational and experiential backgrounds, the traditional orientation involving lectures and procedural manuals is no longer an efficient and effective strategy (Dunn et al., 2000). Competency-based orientation (CBO) is one form of CBE and is the preferred model for orientation in many institutions because it allows for the variation in nurses' backgrounds. CBO is "the simultaneous integration of the knowledge, skills, and attitudes that are required for performance in a designated role and setting" (Alspach, 1984). Ideally, this type of orientation would be an extension of a generic, competency-based curriculum followed by the academic institutions, adapted to fit the clinical or practice setting.

CBO has many advantages. One major advantage is the shortened orientation for experienced nurses (Marrone, 1999; O'Grady & O'Brien, 1992; Stewart & Vitello-Cicciu, 1989). In the current economic environment, this can result in significant savings for the unit and the institution. Other advantages include (1) measurable performance standards; (2) increased quality control (because performance standards are consistent); (3) elimination of repetitive classroom lectures and presentations; (4) adaptability of the length of orientation to the needs of the new graduate or the experienced nurse; (5) personal accountability on the part of orientees for their own learning (or lack of it); and (6) treatment of orientees as adult learners (Alspach, 1984; Chaisson, 1995; Marrone, 1999; Mikos-Schild, 1999; O'Grady & O'Brien, 1992; Staab, Granneman, & Page-Reahr, 1996). The educator becomes the facilitator of the process rather than the master teacher and gatekeeper of learning (Mikos-Schild, 1999). As unit resources, preceptors serve as expert role models and facilitate the learning of the orientee.

As the spotlight on competency in both nursing education and clinical practice continues to intensify, especially as it relates to patient safety and quality of care, best practices for implementation of CBE are certain to remain a focus of continuing dialogue.

IMPLICATIONS FOR NEONATAL NURSING

Because neonatal nursing is a population-focused area of practice, most graduate nurses complete their basic nursing education with little or no clinical experience in the NICU. This places the burden of developing practice competence on the unit and the hospital. As a result of the projected nursing shortage, many NICUs will be employing new graduate nurses at a time when the supply of seasoned neonatal nurses may be diminished. The traditional orientation approach of classroom learning followed by a period of joint clinical practice with an assigned preceptor may not be possible. As the competition for new graduate nurses intensifies, many hospitals are developing internship or externship programs.

Internships and externships for the new graduate nurse are a viable option for NICUs. Most newly graduated nurses recognize the paucity of their knowledge and skills for intensive care units and want some type of formalized educational program to become staff nurses in these areas. Depending on the availability of staff development instructors and experienced nurses willing to assume preceptor responsibilities, many internship and externship programs offer a mix of traditional classroom teaching and CBE. To maximize resources, hospitals often combine nurse interns and externs for the classroom work. For example, a large tertiary hospital may offer a maternal–child nursing option, whereas a children's hospital may offer a critical care option. In the former case, the interns and externs may take classes together on maternity and pediatric nursing. In the latter case, the interns may be in class for the critical care core content.

CBE is also well suited to orientation for new graduate nurses and for experienced nurses who are changing their focus area. For the seasoned staff nurse who switches from adult intensive care, the orientation can focus on the neonatal-specific aspects of critical care. The orientation program for this nurse can be individualized to allow credit for knowledge and skills previously learned. An experienced staff nurse who switches from the well-baby nursery to the NICU will need focused education on the critical care aspects of newborns, because she or he already has a knowledge base about concerns common to well and critically ill newborns such as thermoregulation and hypoglycemia.

Orientation of new graduates into the role of the NNP presents with its own set of challenges. As the baccalaureate to DNP educational pathway becomes more common, there will be an increasing number of newly graduated NNPs with very little NICU experience. Even experienced NNPs are responsible for maintaining validation of required competencies. In an effort to meet this critical need, the National Association of Neonatal Nurses [NANNP] (2010b) developed a *Competencies and Orientation Tool Kit for Neonatal Nurse Practitioners*. The goal of this tool kit is to establish consistent expectations concerning competencies for NNPs at varying levels, from novice to expert, and to provide a method of evaluating their competence. Ultimately, the intention is to assure the public that the NNP possesses the knowledge, skill, and clinical judgment required for providing safe, effective care (NANNP, 2010b).

COMPETENCY VALIDATION

Hospitals are required to document the initial and continued competency of their nursing staff. Competency validation is essential to ensure that the nurse continues to maintain the level of expertise necessary to provide safe care and that he or she has the knowledge needed to provide the best possible care for the particular problems of patients (Gunn, 1999).

The frequency of validation may vary according to the specific skill. The interval for validation of such skills as neonatal resuscitation is determined by the national standard, as set by the Neonatal Resuscitation Program (American Heart Association and American Academy of Pediatrics (AHA/AAP) Neonatal Resuscitation Steering Committee, 2011). Other skills are usually validated annually or as required by accreditation criteria set forth by TJC. Although there is little written regarding the number of procedures required for an NNP to obtain and maintain competence, the types and number of procedures done by an NNP depend on the practice site and patient population. While variations among practice sites may make achieving and maintaining skill competency a challenge, it is vitally important that NNPs maintain competence in certain procedures. NANNP (2010b) recommends the following guidelines for maintaining procedural competence: basic procedural and clinical reasoning skills for neonatal resuscitation, including endotracheal intubation, umbilical catheter placement, and needle thoracostomy, must be mandatory for all NNPs; maintenance of a procedural skills log documenting procedures performed, including success rates and complications, should be reviewed as part of an NNP's annual evaluation; and education and evaluation of competence for any procedure should be standardized to include use of universal precautions, use of the time-out, review and discussion of informed consent issues, procedural review, and assessment and management of the infant's comfort and pain. Minimal competence should be defined as performing a preset number of procedures as described in Tables 42.3 and 42.4, or by a procedural review (NANNP, 2010b).

Competency validation can be achieved through a variety of mechanisms, including chart or record review, simulation, 360-degree evaluation, portfolio, procedure or case logs, or patient survey (NANNP, 2010b). For many skills, a combination of methods is used; for example, validation of neonatal resuscitation skills includes objective examinations and performance evaluations. TJC stresses that use of a self-assessment, such as a skills checklist, does not constitute a competency assessment when used as the sole assessment method (The Joint Commission [TJC], 2009).

TABLE 42.3

BASIC SKILLS REQUIRED FOR ALL NNPs

Procedure	Minimum to Establish Competence Within Time Frame Designated by Institution (Usually 3–6 Months)	Minimum to Maintain Competency Annually
Intubation	Three supervised (successful) procedures	Three procedures
Umbilical line	Three supervised procedures	Three procedures or procedural review
Thoracostomy	Performance in skills lab and review of didactic content	Procedural review

Adapted from the National Association of Neonatal Nurse Practitioners (2010b).

TABLE 42.4

OTHER PROCEDURES THAT MAY BE REQUIRED

Procedure	Minimum to Establish Competence Within Time Frame Designated by Institution (Usually 3–6 Months)	Minimum to Maintain Competence Annually
Lumbar puncture	Three supervised procedures	Three procedures or procedural review
Bladder tap	Three supervised procedures	Three procedures or procedural review
Peripheral arterial stick and arterial line placement	Three supervised procedures	Three procedures or procedural review
PICC line placement	Three supervised procedures	Three procedures or procedural review
Exchange transfusion	One supervised procedure	Three procedures or procedural review
Chest-tube insertion	Three supervised procedures	Procedural review. If the NNP is unable to place a chest tube in 2 years, then a skills lab or simulation is required
Intra-osseous access	Three supervised procedures	Three procedures or procedural review
Circumcision	Three supervised procedures	Three procedures or procedural review

PICC, peripherally inserted central catheter.
Adapted from the National Association of Neonatal Nurse Practitioners (2010b).

CONTINUING COMPETENCE

According to the ANA (2008), assurance of continued competence is the shared responsibility of the profession, individual nurses, professional organizations, credentialing and certification entities, regulatory agencies, employers, and other key stakeholders. Maintaining individual competence is the professional obligation of every neonatal nurse. This obligation is spelled out clearly by the ANA in its position statement on *Professional Role Competence* (ANA, 2008): "The public has a right to expect registered nurses to demonstrate professional competence throughout their careers. ANA believes the registered nurse is individually responsible and accountable for maintaining professional competence" (p. 1).

Certification is a process that functions on a continuum through a nurse's career that is supported by *lifelong* learning and ongoing professional development. Voluntary certification is an excellent mechanism for staff nurses, CNS, and NPs to document their ongoing competence in neonatal nursing. In addition to measuring knowledge that is unique to a specific population, national certification examinations require documentation of ongoing education to maintain the certified nurse's expertise. Examinations for neonatal critical care nurses and neonatal critical care nurse specialists are available through the American Association of Critical Care Nurses (AACN) Certification Corporation (AACN, 2012). The National Certification Corporation (NCC) offers several examinations for neonatal nurses. These include examinations for both neonatal intensive care nursing and low-risk neonatal nursing care. Subspecialty areas, such as electronic fetal monitoring and neonatal pediatric transport, are also available to certified nurses (National Certification Corporation [NCC], 2012). In recognition of the expanding knowledge base needed to function in an increasingly complex health care environment, NCC replaced their Certification Maintenance Program with the Professional Development Certification Maintenance Program (National Certification Corporation [NCC], 2009). The focus of the new program is to determine that each certified nurse has maintained knowledge of the core competencies related to the certification specialty role. A specialty assessment evaluation is being utilized to identify targeted individual-specific continuing education needs to address knowledge gaps and provide a learning plan that the certified nurse can follow to meet certification maintenance requirements (NCC, 2009). The program is being implemented in two stages, with full implementation in 2014. NCC notes that this approach "brings greater accountability and transparency to the certification maintenance process while providing employers and the public a valid measure of assurance regarding the ongoing competency of nurses certified by NCC" (NCC, 2009, p. 2).

SUMMARY

Ensuring the competence of neonatal nurses and advanced practice nurses are major concerns of hospitals, regulators, insurance companies, and the public. Changes in the health care industry as a result of managed care, mergers of provider institutions such as hospitals, and significant reorganization within the delivery system have placed new demands on the nursing profession to ensure the ongoing competence of its members. Individually and collectively, nurses are challenged by the need to keep current in the midst of a knowledge and technology explosion, by the demand from payers for greater productivity and efficiency in health care, and by consumers' growing sophistication regarding the consequences brought about by incompetent providers. Standards of nursing practice and accreditation criteria from professional nursing organizations and agencies such as TJC are used to develop nursing competencies.

CBE provides a mechanism for contemporary nursing to provide a cost-effective, quality approach to nursing education. The competency-based approach is also well suited to individualizing orientation programs to meet the unique needs of nurses who have significantly different backgrounds and levels of experience. CBE shifts the focus of learning from the traditional model of objectives and classroom teaching to a new model based on achievement of specified competencies and outcomes.

Validation of competency is essential to ensure that the nurse continues to maintain the level of expertise necessary to provide safe, effective, quality care. A variety of methods and evaluative tools are currently used to validate nursing knowledge, and skills may include direct observation, patient records, portfolio, demonstrations, skills lab, certification, credentialing, simulation exercises, virtual reality testing, targeted continuing education with outcomes measurement, employer skills validation, and practice evaluation. While there are a variety of methods available, no single tool or method can guarantee competence.

Assurance of continued competence is the shared responsibility of the profession, professional organizations, credentialing and certification entities, regulatory agencies, employers, and other key stakeholders. Ultimately, however, maintaining competence is the professional obligation of each individual nurse. Continued competence is an ongoing process throughout a nurse's career that must be supported by lifelong learning and ongoing professional development. Each nurse is individually responsible and accountable for maintaining professional competence.

ONLINE RESOURCES

Competency-Based Education in the Health Professions: Implications for Improving Global Health
http://www.deepblue.lib.umich.edu/bitstream/2027.42/85362/1/CompBasedEd.pdf

Health Professionals for a New Century: Transforming Education to Strengthen Health Systems in an Interdependent World
http://www.healthprofessionals21.org

Interprofessional Education Collaborative. Core Competencies for Interprofessional Collaborative Practice
http://www.aacn.nche.edu/education-resources/ipecreport.pdf

National Organization of Nurse Practitioner Faculties. Competencies for Nurse Practitioners
http://www.nonpf.com/displaycommon.cfm?an=1&subarticlenbr=14

EVIDENCE-BASED PRACTICE BOX

Nursing is a complex combination of theory and practice that must be successfully integrated by nursing students in order for them to attain competence. Competence assessment methods must therefore be capable of measuring both knowledge and skills. The portfolio has been identified as a valuable means of assessment, enabling students to demonstrate achievement of competencies by presenting evidence from a variety of sources that display their experience, strengths, abilities, and skills. McCready (2007) published a review of the literature on the portfolio as a tool for the assessment of competence in nursing education. The author selected 14 articles for review based on predetermined inclusion and exclusion criteria. The evidence showed that portfolio assessment can enhance learning; however, it remained inconclusive as to whether the portfolio can measure competence. The author also noted that while the evidence on the portfolio as a means of assessment continues to expand, future research in this area should focus on qualitative rather than quantitative methodologies in keeping with the holistic nature of the portfolio itself.

Reference

McCready, T. (2007). Portfolios and the assessment of competence in nursing: A literature review. *International Journal of Nursing Studies, 44*, 143–151.

REFERENCES

Alspach, J. G. (1984). Designing a competency-based orientation for critical care nurses. *Heart Lung, 13*(6), 655–662.

American Association of Colleges of Nursing. (1996). *The essentials of master's education for advanced practice nursing.* Retrieved from http://www.aacn.nche.edu/Education/pdf/MasEssentials96.pdf

American Association of Colleges of Nursing. (2006). *The essentials of doctoral education for advanced nursing practice.* Retrieved from http://www.aacn.nche.edu/publications/position/DNPEssentials.pdf

American Association of Critical Care Nurses. (2012). *Certification.* Retrieved from http://www.aacn.org/DM/MainPages/CertificationHome.aspx?menu=Certification

American Heart Association and American Academy of Pediatrics (AHA/AAP) Neonatal Resuscitation Steering Committee. (2011). *Textbook of neonatal resuscitation* (6th ed.). Elk Grove Village, IL: AAP.

American Nurses Association. (2001). *Working paper on continuing professional nursing competence.* Washington, DC: Author.

American Nurses Association. (2004). *Nursing: Scope and standards of practice.* Washington, DC: Author.

American Nurses Association. (2008). *Professional role competence.* Washington, DC: Author.

American Nurses Association Expert Panel. (2000). *Continuing competence: Nursing's agenda for the twenty-first century.* Washington, DC: Author.

APRN Consensus Work Group & the National Council of State Boards of Nursing APRN Advisory Committee. (2008). *Consensus model for APRN regulation: Licensure, accreditation, certification and education.* Retrieved from https://www.ncsbn.org/7_23_08_Consensue_APRN_Final.pdf

Bechtel, G. A., Davidhizar, R., & Bradshaw, M. J. (1999). Problem-based learning in a competency-based world. *Nurse Education Today, 19*(3), 182–187.

Benner, P. (1982). From novice to expert. *American Journal of Nursing, 82*(3), 402–407.

Benner, P. (1984). *From novice to expert: Excellence and power in clinical nursing practice.* Menlo Park, CA: Addison-Wesley.

Chaisson, S. F. (1995). Role of the CNS in developing a competency-based orientation program. *Clinical Nurse Specialist, 9*(1), 32–37.

Chapman, H. (1999). Some important limitations of competency-based education with respect to nurse education: An Australian perspective. *Nurse Education Today, 19*(2), 129–135.

Citizens Advocacy Center. (1997). *Continuing professional competence: Can we assure it? Proceedings of a citizen's advocacy center conference, December 16–17, 1996.* Washington, DC: Author.

Commission for Collegiate Nursing Education (CCNE). (1998). *Standards for accreditation of baccalaureate and graduate nursing education programs.* Washington, DC: Author.

Del Bueno, D. J. (1978). Competency based education. *Nurse Educator, 3*(3), 10–14.

Dunn, S. V., Lawson, D., Robertson, S., Underwood, M., Clark, R., Valentine, T., ... Herewane, D. (2000). The development of competency standards for specialist critical care nurses. *Journal of Advanced Nursing, 31*(2), 339–346.

Grant, G. (1979). *On competence: A critical analysis of competence-based reforms in higher education.* San Francisco, CA: Jossey-Bass.

Gunn, I. P. (1999). Regulation of health care professionals. Part 2. Validation of continued competence. *CRNA: The Clinical Forum for Nurse Anesthetists, 10*(3), 135–141.

Hartshorn, J. C. (1992). Characteristics of critical care nursing internship programs. *Journal of Nursing Staff Development, 8*(5), 218–223.

Institute of Medicine. (1999). *To err is human: Building a safer health system.* Washington, DC: The National Academy of Sciences.

Institute of Medicine. (2001). *Crossing the quality chasm: A new health system for the 21st century.* Washington, DC: The National Academy of Sciences.

Institute of Medicine. (2003). *Health professions education: A bridge to quality.* Washington, DC: The National Academy of Sciences.

Institute of Medicine. (2011). *The future of nursing: Leading change, advancing health.* Washington, DC: The National Academy Press.

International Council of Nurses. (2009). *ICN framework of competencies for the nurse specialist.* Geneva, Switzerland: ICN.

Joint Commission on Accreditation of Healthcare Organizations. (1999). *Comprehensive accreditation manual for hospitals: The official handbook.* Oakbrook Terrace, IL: Author.

Kenner, C., & Fernandes, J. H. (2001). Knowledge management and advanced nursing education. *Newborn and Infant Nursing Reviews, 1*(3), 192–198.

Lenburg, C. B. (1999a). Redesigning expectations for initial and continuing competence for contemporary nursing practice. *Online Journal of Issues in Nursing, 4*(2), Manuscript 1. Retrieved from http://www.nursingworld.org/MainMenuCategories/ANAMarketplace/ANAPeriodicals/OJIN/TableofContents/Volume41999/No2Sep1999/RedesigningExpectationsforInitialandContinuingCompetence.aspx

Lenburg, C. B. (1999b). The framework, concepts, and methods of the competency outcomes and performance assessment (COPA) model. *Online Journal of Issues in Nursing, 4*(2), Manuscript 2. Retrieved from http://www.nursingworld.org/MainMenuCategories/ANAMarketplace/ANAPeriodicals/OJIN/TableofContents/Volume41999/No2Sep1999/COPAModel.aspx

Luttrell, M. F., Lenburg, C. B., Scherubel, J. C., Jacob, S. R., & Koch, R. W. (1999). Redesigning a BSN curriculum: Competency outcomes for learning and performance assessment. *Nursing and Health Care Perspectives, 20*(3), 134–141.

Marrone, S. R. (1999). Designing a competency-based nursing practice model in a multicultural setting. *Journal for Nurses in Staff Development, 15*(2), 535–562.

McMullan, M., Endacott, R., Gray, M. A., Jasper, M., Miller, C. M. L., Scholes, J., & Webb, C. (2003). Portfolios and assessment of competence: A review of the literature. *Journal of Advanced Nursing, 41*(3), 283–294.

Mikos-Schild, S. (1999). Competency-based orientation. *Today's Surgery Nurse, 21*(3), 3–17.

National Association of Neonatal Nurses. (2009). *Education standards and curriculum guidelines for neonatal nurse practitioner programs.* Glenview, IL: Author.

National Association of Neonatal Nurse Practitioners. (2010a). Standard for maintaining the competence of neonatal nurse practitioners. *Advances in Neonatal Care, 10*(6), 282–286.

National Association of Neonatal Nurse Practitioners. (2010b). *Competencies and orientation toolkit for neonatal nurse practitioners.* Glenview, IL: Author.

National Certification Corporation. (2009). *Continuing competency initiative.* Retrieved from http://www.nccwebsite.org/resources/docs/final_ncc_continuing_competency_web.pdf

National Certification Corporation. (2012). *Certification exams.* Retrieved from http://www.nccwebsite.org/Certification

National CNS Competency Task Force. (2010). *Clinical nurse specialist core competencies: Executive summary.* Retrieved from http://www.aacn.org/WD/Certifications/Docs/corecnscompetencies-execsumm.pdf

National Council of State Boards of Nursing. (1998). *Assuring competence: A regulatory responsibility.* Chicago, IL: Author.

National Council of State Boards of Nursing. (2005). *Business book: NCSBN 2005 annual meeting.* Chicago, IL: Author.

National League for Nursing Accreditation Commission. (1997). *Accreditation manual and interpretive guidelines*. New York, NY: Author.

National Organization of Nurse Practitioner Faculties. (2006). *Domains and core competencies of nurse practitioner practice*. Washington, DC: Author.

National Organization of Nurse Practitioner Faculties. (2008a). Eligibility for NP certification for nurse practitioner students in doctor of nursing practice programs. In *Clinical education issues in preparing nurse practitioner students for independent practice: An ongoing series of papers*. (2010). Retrieved from http://www.nonpf.org/associations/10789/files ClinicalEducationIssuesPPRFinalApril2010.pdf

National Organization of Nurse Practitioner Faculties. (2008b). Clinical hours for nurse practitioner preparation in doctor of nursing practice programs. In *Clinical education issues in preparing nurse practitioner students for independent practice: An ongoing series of papers*. (2010). Retrieved from http://www.nonpf.org/associations/10789/files/ClinicalEducationIssuesPPRFinalApril2010.pdf

National Organization of Nurse Practitioner Faculties. (2011). *Statement on acute care and primary care nurse practitioner practice*. Washington, DC: Author.

National Organization of Nurse Practitioner Faculties. (2012). *Nurse practitioner core competencies*. Washington, DC: Author.

National Organization of Nurse Practitioner Faculties and National Panel for NP Practice Doctorate Competencies. (2006). Retrieved from http://www.nonpf.org/associations/10789/files/DNP%20NP%20competenciesApril2006.pdf

National Task Force on Quality Nurse Practitioner Education. (2008). *Criteria for evaluation of nurse practitioner programs* (3rd ed.). Washington, DC: National Organization of Nurse Practitioner Faculties.

O'Grady, T. P., & O'Brien, A. (1992). A guide to competency-based orientation: Develop your own program. *Journal of Nursing Staff Development, 8*(3), 128–133.

Pew Health Professions Commission. (1995). *Reforming health care work force regulation: Policy considerations for the twenty-first century*. San Francisco, CA: Author.

Pew Health Professions Commission. (1998). *Strengthening consumer protection: Priorities for health care work force regulation: Report of the pew health professions commission*. San Francisco, CA: Author.

Staab, S., Granneman, S., & Page-Reahr, T. (1996). Examining competency-based orientation implementation. *Journal of Nursing Staff Development, 12*(3), 139–143.

Stewart, S. L., & Vitello-Cicciu, K. M. (1989). Designing a competency-based orientation program for the care of cardiac surgery patients. *Journal of Cardiovascular Nursing, 3*(3), 34–41.

The Joint Commission. (2009). *Competency assessment standards: FAQ details*. Retrieved from http://www.jointcommission.org/standards_information/jcfaqdetails.aspx?StandardsFaqId=31&ProgramId=1

Tilley, D. D. S. (2008). Competency in nursing: A concept analysis. *The Journal of Continuing Education in Nursing, 39*(2), 58–64.

U.S. Department of Education, National Center for Education Statistics. (2002). *Defining and assessing learning: Exploring competency-based initiatives, NCES 2002-159*. Washington, DC: NCES.

Voorhees, R. A. (2001). *Measuring what matters: Competency based learning education models in higher education*. San Francisco, CA: Jossey-Bass.

Weinstein, S. M. (2000). Certification and credentialing to define competency-based practice. *Journal of Intravenous Nursing, 23*(1), 21–28.

Whittaker, S., Smolenski, M., & Carson, W. (2000). Assuring continued competence—policy questions and approaches: How should the profession respond? *Online Journal of Issues in Nursing*. Retrieved from http://www.nursingworld.org/MainMenuCategories/ANAMarketplace/ANAPeriodicals/OJIN/TableofContents/Volume52000/No3Sept00/ArticlePreviousTopic/ContinuedCompetence.html

UNIT VIII NEONATAL DIAGNOSTIC AND CARE PROTOCOLS

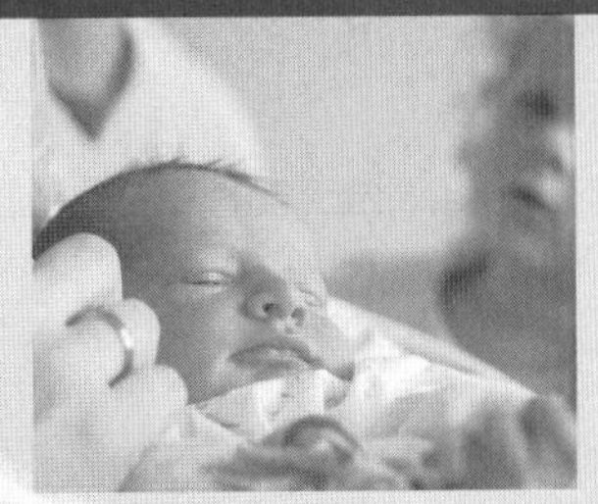

Diagnostic Processes

1

■ Samual Mooneyham

Care of the neonate typically involves numerous diagnostic procedures and tests to identify dysfunction related to birth, prematurity, illness, or congenital malformations. This chapter highlights the commonly used methods for developing a medical or surgical diagnosis in the newborn and infant. The nursing implications for appropriate assessment of preprocedural and postprocedural care also are discussed.

Diagnostic imaging has assumed an increasingly important role in neonatal diagnosis and the assessment, evaluation, and follow-up of neonatal care. Technologic advances since the 1970s have resulted in a variety of imaging modalities that demonstrate not only the internal structure but also the function of organ systems in the fetus and neonate. The spectrum of diagnostic imaging methods includes radionuclide imaging, ultrasonography, and magnetic resonance imaging (MRI), as well as conventional roentgenologic techniques. With such an array of imaging modalities available, complex, problem-oriented decision making is required to determine which techniques should be used and which omitted in a particular clinical situation. In addition, diagnostic imaging examinations are expensive, with ultrasonography being the least expensive and MRI the most expensive. As the public, the government, private insurers, and the health care system have become increasingly cost conscious, health care providers have faced growing pressure to make efficacious and cost-effective decisions about the use of imaging examinations.

The selection of a particular imaging examination should be based on the inherent patient risks, the likelihood that the examination will establish or refute a working diagnosis, the potential benefit to the patient, and the risk of liability if the examination is requested or if the examination is not requested (Juhl, Crummy, & Kuhlman, 1998; Swischuk, 1997a, 1997b). In selecting an imaging examination, the clinician must carefully consider how much the examination will affect the certainty of the differential diagnosis and whether the information derived from the examination will alter the diagnostic approach or choice of treatment. Diagnostic certainty never reaches 100%. Because of the cost, imaging examinations with a low diagnostic yield or those that only duplicate information that can be obtained from other, less expensive methods must be omitted. The acceptable level of compromise depends on the specific clinical problem, the type of imaging abnormality, and the experience of the radiologist (Swischuk, 1997b). To minimize the risks and maximize the diagnostic benefit from any imaging examination, the diagnostic procedure must be tailored to the specific clinical problem under consideration. For these reasons, diagnostic approaches vary among radiologists and institutions (Hilton & Edwards, 2006; Swischuk, 1997a, 1997b).

The roles of the nurse, neonatologist, nurse practitioner, and radiologist are critically interrelated in diagnostic imaging. It is essential that the history, clinical presentation, physical examination, and laboratory data be understood so that the imaging modalities selected are the ones properly indicated for the diagnostic evaluation and subsequent therapy of the individual newborn.

After the neonatologist or nurse practitioner orders a diagnostic imaging examination, the radiologist evaluates whether the examination is indicated, what views should be obtained, what sequence of examinations is necessary, and whether contrast or supplementary examinations are needed (Juhl et al., 1998; Swischuk, 1997a, 1997b).

Nurses should be aware of the rationale for the selection and sequencing of these diagnostic evaluations, the indications for various imaging modalities, the need for patient preparation, and the biophysical principles involved in producing the image. The nurse ensures that the correct newborn undergoes the procedure, monitors the newborn during and after the procedure, and minimizes changes in the thermal environment. The nurse may also be responsible for preparing information about the infant that is essential to the interpretation of imaging examinations. For example, the gestational, postnatal, and corrected gestational ages are important considerations when interpreting bone density, and the perinatal history is an important consideration when interpreting intracranial calcifications or hemorrhages (Swischuk, 1997a). In addition, the nurse must often act as a liaison between the medical staff and the parents. The relationship the nurse establishes with the family often provides an opportunity to inform the parents of the benefits and risks of the procedure and allows the parents to express their questions and concerns. Armed with a thorough understanding of these concepts, the nurse is able to coordinate the acquisition of diagnostic information with minimal disruption to patient care. A knowledge of patient preparation, proper positioning, and the potential risks of each procedure forms the basis of the care plans and parent teaching. These plans of care and acknowledgment of risks facilitate the development of unit policies and procedures.

DIAGNOSTIC IMAGING IN INFANTS

Diagnostic imaging in newborns and infants is unique, differing in several ways from the procedures used for older children and adults. Infants and newborns are not just small adults for whom smaller films and less exposure are all that is required. Significant differences exist, not just in size, but also in the origin and imaging appearance of disease entities, anatomic proportions, exposure factors, radiation protection, and methods of immobilization (Hilton & Edwards, 2006; Huda, Chamberlain, Rosenbaum, & Garrisi, 2001; Swischuk, 1997a, 1997b).

Conditions Requiring Diagnostic Imaging

Pathologic conditions commonly encountered in adults often are not found in infants, and many abnormal conditions are exclusive to the newborn period. Examples of these pathologic conditions are the congenital abnormalities of the newborn, such as atresias of the gastrointestinal (GI) tract, severe congenital heart defects, surgical causes of respiratory distress, spina bifida, and bilateral choanal atresia. These lesions, which are lethal if left untreated, often are symptomatic in the first days after birth. Medical problems related to premature and postmature birth, intrauterine growth disturbances, nonlethal developmental defects, genetic abnormalities, and perinatal asphyxia are of greatest concern in the newborn period. In addition, malignant tumors, such as neuroblastoma and Wilms' tumor, may appear in the newborn period and up to approximately 4 years of age. Certain infections, such as cytomegalovirus, toxoplasmosis, and syphilis, have a distinct radiographic and ultrasonographic presentation if exposure occurred in utero rather than in the neonatal period (Hilton & Edwards, 2006; Martin, Fanaroff, & Walsh, 2011; Swischuk, 1997a, 1997b).

Anatomic Proportions

The anatomic proportions of infants are very different from those of adults, and the younger the infant, the more marked the differences. A thorough knowledge of these proportions is essential for correct patient positioning to limit field exposure and for accurate interpretation of diagnostic imaging (Dowd & Tilson, 1999; Hilton & Edwards, 2006). It is important that not only the area in question, but the whole of the area in question, appear in the imaging field.

As shown in Figure I.1, the newborn's head is large in proportion to the body, and the cranial vault is large in proportion to the area of the face. The neck is short, and the diaphragm is high. The kidneys are low, about midway between the diaphragm and symphysis pubis. The abdomen is large because of the relative size of the liver and stomach. The pelvic cavity is very small, and the bladder extends above the symphysis pubis. The chest, pelvis, and limbs are small in proportion to the abdomen (Hilton & Edwards, 2006; Swischuk, 1997a, 1997b).

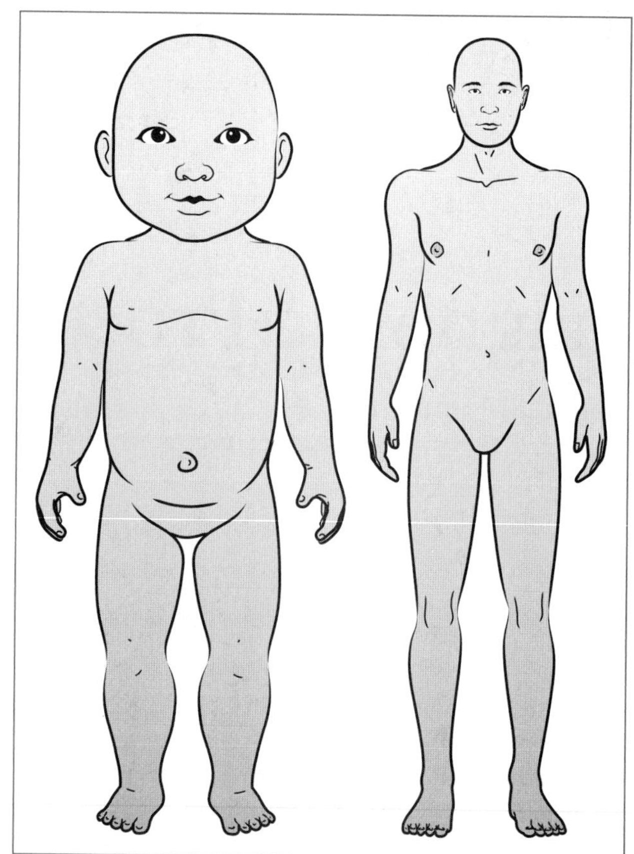

FIGURE I.1 Proportional anatomic differences between a neonate and an adult.

In an anteroposterior (AP) projection, the neonate's lungs appear wider than they are long and much higher up in the thoracic cavity than is normally expected (Hilton & Edwards, 2006; Swischuk, 1997a, 1997b). The diaphragm is located just below the level of the nipples. On a lateral projection, the posterior aspect of the lungs may extend to twice the depth of the anterior part (Swischuk, 1997a, 1997b).

The newborn's abdomen bulges laterally wider than the pelvis, and the bulge contains abdominal organs displaced by the large liver and stomach. Care must be taken to include this area of the abdomen in the imaging field (Hilton & Edwards, 2006; Swischuk, 1997a, 1997b). Irradiation should encompass the smallest possible body area consistent with production of the necessary information (Dowd & Tilson, 1999). Often the field is too large, particularly in premature infants and newborns. Arms and legs should not appear on the abdominal film, nor should half the skull and abdomen appear on a chest film (Figure I.2) (Hilton & Edwards, 2006; Martin et al., 2011; Swischuk, 1997a, 1997b).

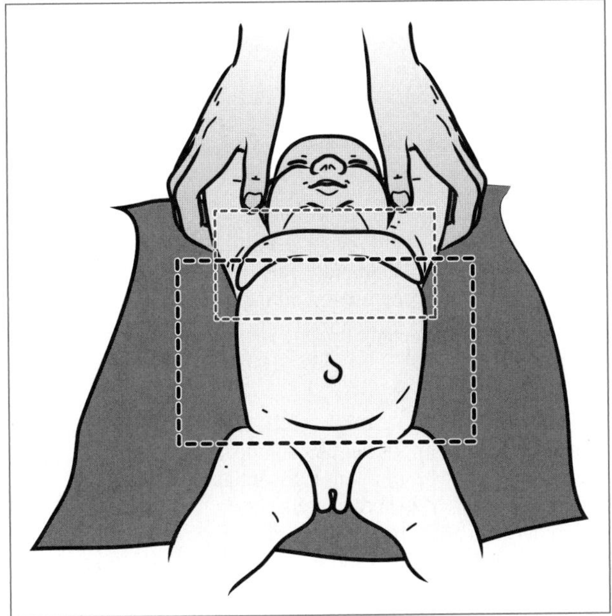

FIGURE I.2 Neonatal radiographs should be limited to only the area of interest. Total body radiographs should be avoided. The top box (*light dashed lines*) defines the area of interest for an anteroposterior chest radiograph. The bottom box (*heavy dashed lines*) defines the area of interest for an anteroposterior abdominal film. The gonad shield has been omitted for illustrative purposes.

TYPES OF DIAGNOSTIC IMAGING

Diagnostic imaging methods are limited to the demonstration of pathologic features no smaller than a few millimeters in diameter, whereas biochemical and histologic methods document disease at a molecular or cellular level. It is commonly thought that diagnostic imaging provides only anatomic information; however, a significant amount of physiologic data may be derived from studies such as barium examinations or urography, as well as from dynamic radionuclide, ultrasonographic, and molecular imaging (Abramoff, Van Gils, Jansen, & Mourits, 2000; Bushong, 2013; Weissleder & Mahmood, 2001; Weissmann & Seidel, 2000).

The four major diagnostic imaging methods are x-ray (roentgenologic) imaging, radionuclide imaging, ultrasonographic imaging, and MRI (Bushong, 1999, 2000, 2003, 2013; Juhl et al., 1998; Treves, 1995). This chapter discusses each of these imaging modalities in relation to the biophysical principles responsible for producing the image, the potential risks of the procedure, and the nursing care of the newborn or infant undergoing such an examination. Table I.1 summarizes the types of diagnostic imaging commonly used for neonates.

TABLE I.1

DIAGNOSTIC IMAGING METHODS COMMONLY USED FOR NEONATES

Technique	Indications and Advantages	Limitations	Potential Risks	Comments	Cost
Roentgenologic Techniques					
Radiographic imaging	Most frequently used initial diagnostic screening mode	Detects only four different levels of photon absorption (air, fat, water, and mineral); two-dimensional (2D) projection of three-dimensional (3D) structures	Ionizing radiation; thermal stress of cool film plate	Proper positioning of infant is essential; child must be monitored during procedure	$
Xeroradiographic imaging	Used to evaluate soft tissue structures	Tissue structures defined by relative amounts of air, fat, water, and minerals; seldom used since advent of newer diagnostic imaging methods	Higher level of ionizing radiation than with routine radiographs	Proper positioning of infant is essential; child must be monitored during procedure	$$
Fluoroscopic imaging	Used to evaluate motion or function of cardiovascular, gastrointestinal, and genito-urinary systems; may be used to guide therapeutic or diagnostic procedures	Images rely on greater radiation and/or movement of contrast material; improper diagnostic sequencing may delay informational yield; contrast material may have physiologic consequences	Much higher level of ionizing radiation than with routine radiographs; thermal stress of cool radiology environment	Proper positioning of infant is essential; child must be monitored during procedure	$$-$$$$

(continued)

TABLE I.1

DIAGNOSTIC IMAGING METHODS COMMONLY USED FOR NEONATES (CONTINUED)

Technique	Indications and Advantages	Limitations	Potential Risks	Comments	Cost
CT	Used to provide detailed, superior characterization of various soft tissue densities that cannot be detected by conventional radiographs	Motion artifact may cause blurring of scans; radiation dose depends on scan time; contrast material may have physiologic consequences	Ionizing radiation; thermal stress of cool environment	Proper positioning of infant is essential; child must be monitored during procedure	$$$
Ultrasound imaging	Does not use ionizing radiation, but rather uses sound waves to depict anatomic and functional motion of tissue; sound waves can be directed in a beam in a variety of planes; portable; different graphic displays are available	Ultrasound technique is operator dependent; does not provide as much information on organ function such as urography; reveals less anatomic detail than CT; scan is adversely affected by the presence of bone and air	Thermal stress may occur with application of cool scanning gel to infant's skin; there are no known deleterious effects from clinical use of ultrasound imaging	Proper positioning of infant is essential; child must be monitored during procedure	$
Radionucleotide imaging	Used to trace anatomic proportions and a wide range of physiologic functions in virtually every organ in the body; amount of ionizing radiation emitted by injected agent is significantly less than the amount required for corresponding radiograph	Diagnostic yield depends on uptake of radionucleotide by different organs; radionucleotides are rarely organ specific; limited anatomic resolution	Thermal stress during nucleotide scanning	Proper positioning of the infant is essential; maximum radiation exposure is not always the organ of interest; child must be monitored during procedure	$$
PET and SPECT	Both techniques have greater sensitivity and qualifications of the distribution and density of radioactivity to depict the "metabolic" function of tissue; 3D imaging is possible with computer reconstruction; dose of nucleotide is the same; artifactual lesions can be eliminated; amount of ionizing radiation emitted by injected agents (carbon 11, oxygen 15, nitrogen 13) is significantly less than the amount required for corresponding radiograph	PET scanning requires access to a cyclotron to produce the positrons used in scans	Thermal stress during nucleotide scanning	Proper positioning of infant is essential; child must be monitored during procedure	$$$$$$

(*continued*)

TABLE I.1

DIAGNOSTIC IMAGING METHODS COMMONLY USED FOR NEONATES (CONTINUED)

Technique	Indications and Advantages	Limitations	Potential Risks	Comments	Cost
MRI	Uses magnetic fields and radio waves to produce images; the region of the body scanned can be controlled electronically, and hardware does not limit scanning sites; scans are free of high-intensity artifacts; newer scanning techniques can quantify many pathologic conditions	Availability and cost; limited use in unstable infants on life support; monitoring equipment must be free from interference with magnetic field	Does not use ionizing radiation to produce images; limited access to infant during procedure	Proper positioning is essential; must be monitored during procedure	$$$$$$

X-Ray Imaging (Roentgenology)

The principles of conventional radiography have not changed since the discovery of x-rays in the late 1800s. However, the equipment and techniques have become far more sophisticated; current radiographic methods include tomography, fluoroscopy, computed tomography (CT), and digital radiography.

Roentgenologic Biophysical Principles

X-rays are a form of electromagnetic energy that travel at the speed of light (about 300,000 km [186,000 miles] per second). Other forms of electromagnetic energy include gamma rays, radio waves, microwaves, and visible light (Figure I.3). Only x-rays and gamma rays have enough energy to produce an ion pair by separating an orbital electron from its parent atom (Alpen, 1998; Bushong, 1999, 2000, 2003, 2013; Juhl et al., 1998). The amount of radiation present is measured by detection of such ionization. Radiation exposure is measured either in units of coulombs per kilogram (C/kg) or in roentgens (1 R/258/C/kg). Although the roentgen is no longer an official scientific unit, it is still widely used in radiology. The rad is the unit of measure for the amount of radiation absorbed by the body (Alpen, 1998; Bushong, 2013; Dowd & Tilson, 1999; Juhl et al., 1998).

When an x-ray beam is directed toward a part of the body, differential absorption of the x-ray photons by different types of body tissue occurs. A beam of x-ray photons is variously attenuated as it passes through the body tissues, producing a shadow image that is recorded on photographic film; the absorbed x-ray photons interact with the tissue, causing ionization in the body (Alpen, 1998; Bushong, 2013; Dowd & Tilson, 1999; Juhl et al., 1998). Bone and metal fragments absorb x-ray photons and therefore appear white on the radiographic film, whereas air-containing structures, such as lungs and gas-filled bowel, absorb few x-ray photons and appear black. Soft tissues and blood vessels appear as intermediate shades of gray.

A radiograph gives a two-dimensional projection of three-dimensional structures. An x-ray tube is positioned to direct the x-ray beam through the part of the neonate to be examined so as to record different views or projections on the film. This simple imaging technique can distinguish only among air, fat, and tissues with densities approximately equal to those of water or metals, but it continues to be enormously valuable and is still the diagnostic imaging method most often used in neonatal care.

X-ray photons are generated in the tungsten anode of the tube when it is bombarded by a stream of high-energy electrons emitted from the cathode (Figure I.4) (Alpen, 1998; Bushong, 2013; Dowd & Tilson, 1999; Juhl et al., 1998). The energy, or penetrating power, of the resulting x-ray photons is a function of the electron energy, which is controlled by the voltage gradient across the cathode-anode gap. In diagnostic radiology, this gradient usually is 60 to 120 kV (Bushong, 2013; Dowd & Tilson, 1999; Hilton & Edwards, 2006; Juhl et al., 1998). Low kilovoltage x-rays have poor penetrating ability, whereas higher kilovolt-age x-rays have deeper penetrating ability. The kilovoltage across the cathode-anode gap, therefore, controls the penetration of the x-ray beam.

The milliamperage (mA) indicates the amount of current applied to the cathode filament (Alpen, 1998; Bushong, 2013). The greater the current, the more electrons are produced for transmission across the cathode-anode gap, and the greater the number of x-ray photons generated by the anode in a finite time. The product of the exposure time and the milliamperage given to the cathode filament controls the amount, or dose, of x-rays and is expressed in milliampere-seconds (mAs) (Alpen, 1998; Bushong, 2013; Dowd & Tilson, 1999; Juhl et al., 1998).

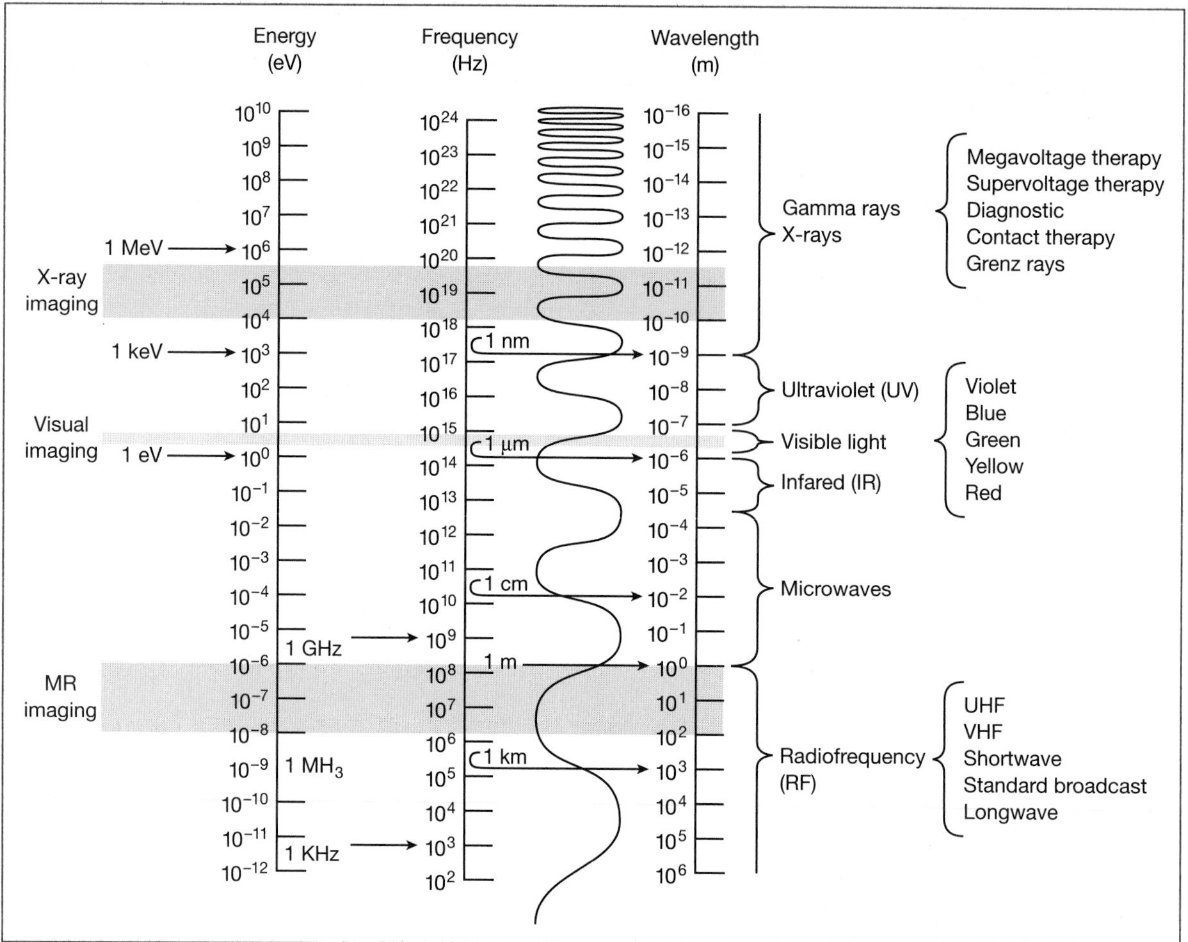

FIGURE I.3 The electromagnetic spectrum extends over 25 orders of magnitude. The chart illustrates the values of frequency, energy, and wavelength and identifies some common regions of the spectrum.
Adapted from Bushong (2013).

Early radiographs required an exposure time of as long as 30 minutes to produce a satisfactory image (Bushong, 2013; Juhl et al., 1998). It is not surprising, then, to find reports of radiation injury in the early days of radiology. Reports of superficial skin and tissue damage, hair loss, and anemia were common among patients and their physicians because of the prolonged exposure times and the low-energy radiation that was available. The development of an interrupterless transformer by H.C. Snook in 1907 and progressive improvements in the cathode ray tube resulted in a marked decline in reports of radiation injury. Since that time, improvements in film sensitivity and fluorescent screens have further reduced exposure times, to the point where the average exposure time for a chest radiograph is approximately one-twentieth of a second (Alpen, 1998; Bushong, 2013; Dowd & Tilson, 1999; Juhl et al., 1998). The short exposure time diminishes image blurring caused by involuntary and cardiovascular motion and reduces the neonate's exposure to radiation. However, it also is important to limit the cross-sectional area of the x-ray beam to the region of interest to reduce unnecessary irradiation of adjacent organs (Alpen, 1998; Bushong, 2013; Dowd & Tilson, 1999; Juhl et al., 1998).

Conventional radiographic images commonly have been recorded with large-size photographic film enclosed in an aluminum or plastic lightproof cassette. The film is compressed between fluorescent screens that emit visible light when exposed to x-rays. The fluorescence from the phosphor screens, rather than the direct effect of x-rays on the photographic emulsion, produces most of the image on the film (Alpen, 1998; Bushong, 2013; Juhl et al., 1998). Other diagnostic imaging methods also use ionizing radiation.

■ **Xeroradiography.** Xeroradiography is a radiographic imaging technique used to evaluate soft tissue. With this technique, the electrical charge of a photoconductive plate is altered in proportion to the intensity of the transmitted radiation image (Alpen, 1998; Bushong, 2013; Dowd & Tilson, 1999; Juhl et al., 1998). The image is recorded on the plate rather than on x-ray film. With soft tissue structures that differ only slightly in density, this method provides much better contrast than conventional radiography. It also provides an "edge effect" at the margins of discontinuous structures and therefore is indicated for the detection of nonmetallic foreign bodies and for evaluation of complex upper airway abnormalities in the neonate (Hilton & Edwards, 2006; Juhl et al., 1998; Swischuk, 1997a). Despite these benefits, the risks associated with this imaging technique must be considered. The radiation exposure involved is 6 to 12 times greater than that with conventional radiographs

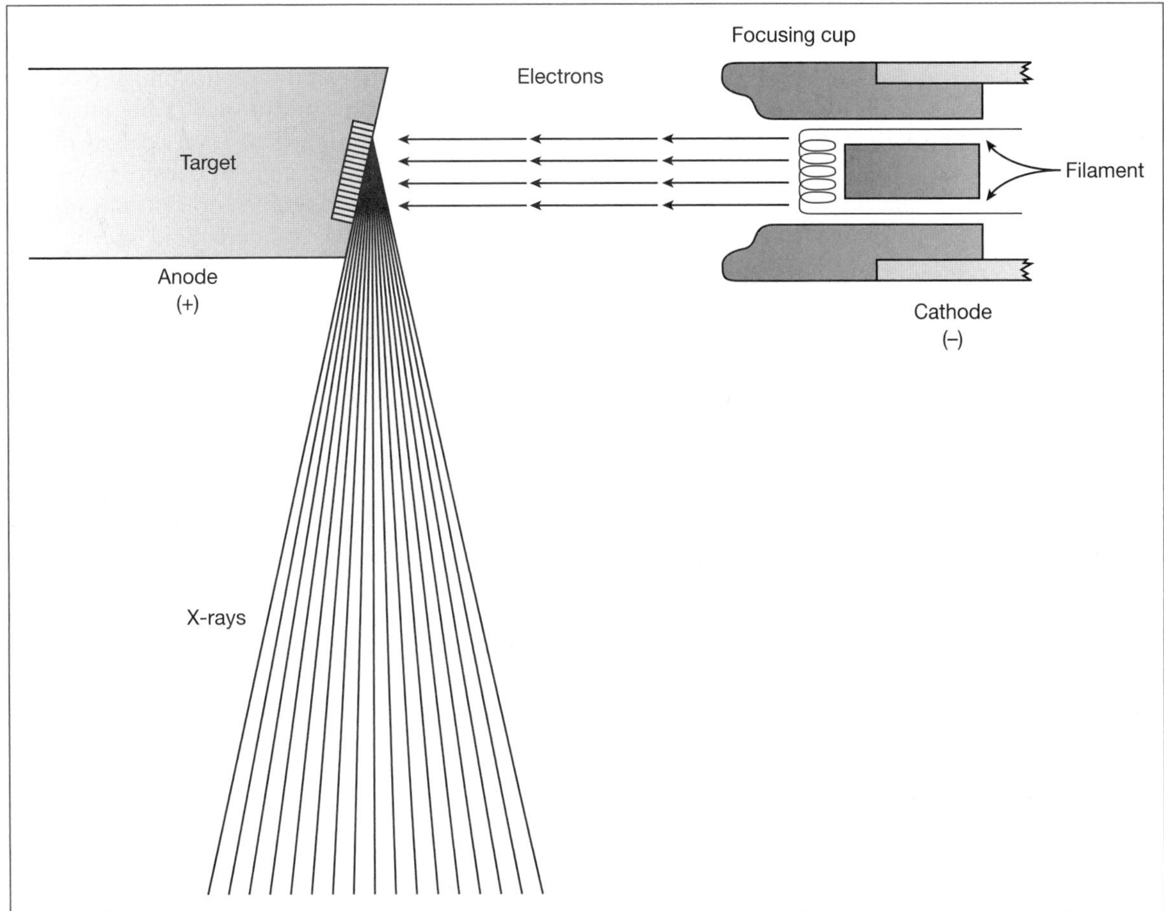

FIGURE I.4 Generation of x-ray photons in a tungsten anode-cathode tube.

(Alpen, 1998; Hilton & Edwards, 2006; Juhl et al., 1998; Swischuk, 1997a).

■ Fluoroscopic Imaging. Thomas Edison developed the fluoroscope in 1898 (Bushong, 2013). He focused on the use of fluorescent materials in this new imaging modality. During the period of his investigation, Edison analyzed the fluorescent properties of more than 1,800 materials, including zinc cadmium sulfide and calcium tungstate, both of which are still used. Edison halted his research in this area when his assistant and long-time friend, Clarence Dally, suffered severe x-ray burns that required bilateral upper extremity amputation. Dally's subsequent death in 1904 is considered the first x-ray fatality (Bushong, 2013; Dowd & Tilson, 1999; Juhl et al., 1998).

Fluoroscopic imaging is a radiologic technique used to evaluate the motion of an organ system. After passing through the patient, the fluoroscopic x-rays interact with the input phosphor of the image intensifier tube. The input phosphor converts the incident x-rays into visible light, which causes the photocathode to emit electrons (Alpen, 1998; Bushong, 2013; Dowd & Tilson, 1999; Juhl et al., 1998). These electrons are accelerated and focused by electrodes in the image intensifier onto the output phosphor to produce visible light that can be viewed directly through an optical system or by a television system (Alpen, 1998; Bushong, 2013; Dowd & Tilson, 1999). Fluoroscopic images can be recorded on film or videotape. Videotape recording of fluoroscopy has become essential. It is easier and safer to rerun videotape several times to evaluate dysfunction than to prolong the radiation exposure from fluoroscopy.

During a fluoroscopic examination, the anatomic structure may be evaluated by obtaining a spot film, which is produced by photographing the output phosphor on 100- or 105-mm film. This type of intensifier optical-coupled spot film camera reduces the radiation dose to the infant by at least 75% compared with a conventional spot film device (Bushong, 2013; Dowd & Tilson, 1999; Juhl et al., 1998; National Council on Radiation Protection and Measurements [NCRP], 1993a, 1993b, 1993c). Videotapes are used to record motions, and spot films are used to document anatomy. Although fluoroscopy has many advantages, the radiation dose delivered in 1 minute of fluoroscopy is equivalent to that of more than thirty 105-mm spot films or more than eight conventional radiographs (Alpen, 1998; Dowd & Tilson, 1999; NCRP, 1993a, 1993b, 1993c).

Electronic intensification of the faint fluoroscopic image allows fluoroscopy to be performed in subdued lighting. Improved intensifier systems have made invasive catheter studies, such as cardiac angiography, much easier to perform (Bushong, 2013; Dowd & Tilson, 1999).

Fluoroscopically guided cytologic biopsy of the lung, bone, pancreas, and lymph nodes has become possible with percutaneous needle insertion. With the aid of fluoroscopy, arteriovenous malformations can be embolized; arterial stenoses can be dilated with balloon catheters; and plastic stents can be inserted to provide drainage through biliary strictures (Hilton & Edwards, 2006; Swischuk, 1997a). These surgical-radiologic procedures are needed for only a relatively small proportion of neonates; however, all fluoroscopic procedures depend on high-quality image intensification, and all require cooperation among the neonatal, surgical, and radiologic teams to achieve the best results.

■ Conventional X-Ray Tomography. Tomography is a radiologic method of imaging a "slice" of tissue at a specific level. Coordinated movement of the x-ray tube and film cassette gives a defined image in the two-dimensional plane of interest, whereas the structures in front of or behind this plane are blurred out (Alpen, 1998; Bushong, 2000; Juhl et al., 1998). Tomography is useful in many circumstances, but its usefulness has been overshadowed by the development of CT.

■ Computed Tomography. CT was first developed in 1961 by William H. Oldendorf, and by 1973 it had become a recognized diagnostic imaging tool (Bushong, 2000). CT scanning obtains cross-sectional images rather than the shadow images of conventional radiography. Conventional radiography is based on variable attenuation of the x-ray beam as it passes through tissue. Because only the sum total of this attenuation is available for recording on the film, conventional radiography can detect only differences of 10% attenuation (Bushong, 2000, 2013; Juhl et al., 1998). Conventional radiographs, therefore, cannot produce a detailed characterization of various soft tissue densities. The densities that can be visualized on conventional radiographs are air, fat, soft tissue, and bone. CT passes multiple, highly collimated beams through the same cross-sectional slice of tissue at different angles during different intervals of time. In CT scanning, a fan x-ray beam from a source rotating about the infant passes through the body, and the exit transmission of x-ray beam intensity is monitored by a series of detectors (Alpen, 1998; Bushong, 2000). The x-ray beam "cuts a slice" from 3 to 13 mm thick through the infant. The exit transmission at any angle can be used to calculate the average attenuation coefficient along the length of the x-ray beam. By measuring the exit transmission at a large number of angles around the infant, a complex series of mathematic equations can be solved by computer to calculate and determine the mass attenuation coefficient of small (approximately 0.5 × 0.5 × 10 mm) volume elements, or voxels. The final cross-sectional image is made up of a display of the gray scale value of every voxel, which can be projected on a cathode ray tube and recorded photographically (Alpen, 1998; Bushong, 2000, 2013; Juhl et al., 1998). Bone is the densest, absorbs the largest amount of x-rays, and appears white; air is the least dense and appears black; soft tissues are displayed as intermediate shades of gray. CT scanning has the ability to separate spatial and contrast resolution and is much more sensitive to tissue densities than conventional radiographs. CT can distinguish differences in attenuation coefficients as small as 0.1%; it also detects changes in density in very small areas of tissue and allows identification of various components of soft tissue, such as subarachnoid space, white matter, gray matter, and ventricles (Alpen, 1998; Bushong, 2000, 2013; Juhl et al., 1998). CT of the body is technically more difficult than cranial examination because of cardiac and respiratory motion; however, a modern body scanner can complete a scan in 2 to 4 seconds, which reduces movement artifact. In the neonate, the rapid heart and respiratory rates limit the usefulness of this technique for thoracic examination.

With CT the density, or contrast resolution, depends on the radiation dose and scan time (Alpen, 1998; Bushong, 2000, 2013; Juhl et al., 1998). As the radiation dose (i.e., scan time) increases, the number of photons collected in each area increases and the statistical noise decreases, resulting in better contrast resolution. CT demonstrates tissue structure with precise clarity, showing superior anatomic detail compared with conventional radiographic imaging (Alpen, 1998; Bushong, 2013; Juhl et al., 1998). CT permits two-dimensional visualization of entire anatomic sections of tissue, which aids the determination of the extent of the disease or malformation. Anatomic and physiologic information can be visualized despite overlying gas and bone. Contrast enhancement can measure blood flow and help define pathologic abnormalities (Bushong, 2000; Swischuk, 1997a, 1997b). Bolus injection of contrast material allows excellent visualization of vascular structures.

As good as CT is as an imaging modality, it is still not a radiologic microscope; CT does have its drawbacks. It also uses ionizing radiation, and because the computers require a cool room for proper equipment performance, the neonate's environment is altered significantly, a circumstance that must be considered.

■ Digital Radiography and Digital Vascular Imaging. Digital radiography is the term used to describe techniques that use computers to produce projectional images similar to those of conventional radiography (Bushong, 2013). Although standard CT instruments have been designed to produce two-dimensional images of two-dimensional body slices, they can also be used to project three-dimensional structures into two-dimensional images that are similar to conventional radiographs. These projections do not have the fine detail of conventional radiographs, but because the pictorial data are stored in the computer, the image can be manipulated and subtle features can be enhanced (Bushong, 2013).

Another method of digital radiography converts the image intensifier picture to digital signals that can be stored and manipulated. The most important use of this method is to obtain digital subtraction images of the heart and major arteries from data recorded before and after the injection of angiographic contrast material (Bushong, 2013). This method is much less invasive than catheterization, although the technique is new and the equipment is expensive. It has been used on a very limited basis in the neonate.

Radiographic Contrast Agents

Plain radiography can differentiate only four kinds of body tissue: tissue containing gas (lung and bowel), fatty tissue and tissue containing calcium (bone or pathologic calcifications), and tissues of water density (solid organs, muscle, and blood). To demonstrate blood vessels that are in solid organs or surrounded by muscle or to demonstrate other hollow structures, artificial radiographic contrast agents must be introduced. The contrast medium may be negative or positive and may be injected, swallowed, or administered as an enema (Hilton & Edwards, 2006; Swischuk, 1997a, 1997b).

Negative contrast media absorb less radiation than adjacent soft tissues and therefore cast a darker radiographic image. Gases such as air, oxygen, and carbon dioxide can be used as negative contrast media. Because negative media provide a limited amount of contrast for conventional radiography, they are seldom used (Martin et al., 2011; Swischuk, 1997a, 1997b).

Positive contrast media use elements with a high atomic number, which absorb much more radiation than surrounding soft tissues and therefore cast a lighter image. Barium and iodine are the two elements currently used. Barium sulfate, a relatively stable, nontoxic compound, is the major contrast agent used for outlining the walls of the GI tract. Iodine-containing salts that are excreted by the kidneys are used for a wide variety of urographic and angiographic studies. The kidneys also excrete the newer nonionic, iodine-containing media. Because of their lower osmolality, these agents are less painful than iodine-containing salts when injected into arteries, and they are rapidly replacing the older contrast agents (Box I.1) (Hilton & Edwards, 2006; Martin et al., 2011; Swischuk, 1997a, 1997b).

BOX I.1

RADIOPHARMACEUTICALS USED IN NEONATAL DIAGNOSTIC IMAGING

- Technetium 99m
  Sulfur or tin colloid: used for imaging liver, spleen, bone marrow, ventilation, and gastrointestinal bleeding
  Albumin microspheres: used for imaging lung perfusion
  Pyrophosphate, diphosphate: used for imaging skeletal and myocardial infarcts
  Pertechnetate: used for imaging thyroid, brain, and gastrointestinal tract
  Diethylenetriaminepentaacetic acid (DTPA) glucoheptonate: used for imaging kidney and brain
  Hepatoiminodiacetic acid (HIDA): used for imaging biliary system
- Iodine 131: used for imaging thyroid and fibrinogen and for clot localization
- Xenon 131, krypton 81 m: used for imaging lung ventilation
- Thallium 201: used for imaging myocardial perfusion and for testicular localization

Ionizing Radiation Interactions With Tissue

When an infant undergoes a radiologic procedure, most of the radiation passes through the infant's body and strikes the fluorescent screens encompassing the film. The roentgen (or C/kg) is a measure of how many x-rays were present. For the infant, the more important quantity is the number of x-rays that stop in the body and how much energy they deposit. The radiation dose (rad) is a measure of the energy deposited. X-rays that pass through the infant are attenuated by photoelectric absorption and Compton scattering (Alpen, 1998; Bushong, 2013; Dowd & Tilson, 1999; Juhl et al., 1998).

Photoelectric absorption involves the complete interaction and absorption of the incoming x-ray photon by the atom. The photon energy is transferred to one of the orbital electrons, which is then ejected as a photoelectron (Alpen, 1998; Bushong, 2013). The ejected electron leaves a vacancy in one of the inner orbits, and an outer orbit electron immediately fills this vacancy. The difference in binding energies between the outer orbit and the inner orbit is released as a characteristic x-ray (Alpen, 1998; Bushong, 2013; Dowd & Tilson, 1999; Juhl et al., 1998). The attenuation of the photoelectric effect depends on the atomic number of the material and the amount of incoming energy. The photoelectric interaction declines rapidly with increasing energy and increases rapidly with increasing atomic number (Alpen, 1998; Bushong, 2013). This is why lead is such an effective shield and bone is so much more absorptive than soft tissue.

Compton scattering is the phenomenon in which only part of the energy of the incoming x-ray photon is transferred to the atom; this reduces the energy of the original photon and produces a scattered electron (Bushong, 2013). The scattered electron has a range of less than 1 mm in tissue. The reduced-energy x-ray photon can do exactly what the original x-ray photon could do; it can interact with another atom, causing a photoelectric effect and transferring all its energy to set an electron in motion, or it can itself undergo the Compton effect, scattering an electron and creating a new x-ray photon that has still further reduced energy (Alpen, 1998; Bushong, 2013; Juhl et al., 1998). Through these two processes, all the energy eventually is transferred to electrons to set them into high-velocity motion. At low photon energies (<60 kV), photoelectric interactions predominate. At approximately 140 kV, the photoelectric and Compton interactions transfer equal energy to tissue; at more than approximately 200 kV, most of the energy transfer to tissue is through the Compton interaction (Alpen, 1998; Bushong, 2013; Dowd & Tilson, 1999). Most neonatal diagnostic radiographs use photon energies between 60 and 100 kV (Hilton & Edwards, 2006; Martin et al., 2011; Swischuk, 1997a, 1997b).

X-ray photons with energies greater than 1.02 million electron volts (meV) cause both a photoelectric and a

Compton effect and have an additional capability as well. In the vicinity of the atom, the incoming x-ray photons disappear and, in the process, create new matter in the form of one electron and one positron (Alpen, 1998; Bushong, 2013; Dowd & Tilson, 1999). A positron is a particle of the same size and mass as an electron, but the positron has one unit of positive charge. To create this pair, exactly 1.02 meV of energy is consumed in the conversion of energy into matter. If the incoming x-ray photon has more energy than 1.02 meV, the residual energy is distributed equally to the electron and the positron in the form of kinetic energy (Alpen, 1998; Bushong, 2013; Dowd & Tilson, 1999).

The effects of the electron when placed in high-velocity orbit are the same as those previously described for the photoelectric and Compton effects. The positron effects are different. The positron expends some of its energy interacting with atoms of the material in which it has been set in motion. Eventually it meets an electron, and the two annihilate each other. When this occurs, both the electron and the positron disappear and two gamma rays appear each with 0.51 meV of energy (Alpen, 1998; Bushong, 2013; Dowd & Tilson, 1999; NCRP, 1993a, 1993b, 1993c).

With ionizing radiation, electrons are removed from their atoms and endowed with energies 14 to 20,000 times greater than those in ordinary biochemical reactions (Alpen, 1998; Bushong, 2013; Dowd & Tilson, 1999; Juhl et al., 1998). These electrons can maraud through tissue for some distance and can break any kind of chemical bond in the body (Bushong, 2013; Dowd & Tilson, 1999; NCRP, 1993a, 1993b, 1993c). In biochemical systems the reactions are carefully controlled, often by a special geometric juxtaposition of the reactants. A high-speed electron is akin to a bull in a china shop; it can break anything, anywhere. Once it has ripped an electron out of an atom in a molecule, the molecule itself is placed at such a high energy level that it can produce all kinds of chemical reactions that would never have been possible without ionizing radiation (Alpen, 1998; Bushong, 2013; Dowd & Tilson, 1999; NCRP, 1993a, 1993b, 1993c).

X-rays and gamma rays are identical in nature except that, in general, x-rays are made in high-voltage machines, whereas gamma rays originate from the nuclei of atoms. Radiations emitted from such naturally unstable atoms as uranium commonly are more energetic per unit than x-ray photons. For example, gamma rays commonly are measured in millions of electron volts (meV) per photon, whereas x-rays commonly are measured in 50 to 100 kiloelectron volts (keV) (50,000–100,000 electron volts). Gamma rays from unstable nuclei do all the things that x-rays do; that is, they can undergo photoelectric and Compton effects, and they can produce high-energy electrons and positrons (Bushong, 2013; Dowd & Tilson, 1999).

Other radiation decay products also create particulate radiation called alpha and beta rays. Beta rays are not truly rays but high-speed electrons emitted from the nuclei of decay products of uranium (Alpen, 1998; Bushong, 2013; Dowd & Tilson, 1999). Once emitted from the nuclei, beta particles act the same as any high-speed electron. Alpha rays are also not rays and are unlike beta particles. Alpha particles are emitted from the nuclei of uranium. Alpha particles are the "stripped" nuclei of helium and consist of any two protons. Ultimately, the two protons find two electrons in the environment and become helium gas. Most beta particles have energies of about 1 meV, although they are always accompanied by beta particles of lesser energies ranging down to nearly zero. Alpha particles, however, have energies of about 5 meV (Alpen, 1998; Bushong, 2013; Dowd & Tilson, 1999). X-rays and gamma rays, which pass through the body and do not produce effects on tissue, have no biologic effect. However, alpha and beta particles interact at every millimeter along their path through tissue, so that if they gain access to tissue, biologic harm is guaranteed (Bushong, 2013; Dowd & Tilson, 1999; NCRP, 1993a, 1993b, 1993c).

Biologic damage from ionizing radiation depends on the amount of energy deposited in a particular tissue. X-rays and gamma rays produce harmful effects only to the extent that they put high-speed electrons in motion. If the same number of electrons is put in motion by gamma rays from plutonium or from deposited radionuclide or by agents from external x-rays, the biologic effects are the same (Bushong, 2013; Dowd & Tilson, 1999; NCRP, 1993a, 1993b, 1993c).

Factors Affecting Radiographic Quality

Interpretation of a neonatal radiograph requires a rapid evaluation to determine whether the radiograph is technically satisfactory. Several factors determine the technical quality of a radiograph, including film exposure, phase of respiration, motion, tube angulation, and infant positioning. If one of these factors is unsatisfactory, the film may be misinterpreted. When nurses have an understanding of these factors, the technical quality of radiographs is improved.

■ **Film Exposure.** A reasonable criterion for judging film exposure is satisfactory visualization of the dorsal intervertebral disk spaces through the entire cardiothymic silhouette (Hilton & Edwards, 2006; Martin et al., 2011; Swischuk, 1997a, 1997b). If the film is underexposed, the dorsal disk spaces are lost, and the lungs and other structures have a homogeneous, "whitewashed" appearance. If the film is overexposed, the pulmonary vascular markings are progressively lost until the lungs have a black, "burned out" appearance (Hilton & Edwards, 2006; Swischuk, 1997a, 1997b).

■ **Phase of Respiration.** The phase of respiration at the time the film is obtained affects the appearance of the radiograph considerably (Figure I.5). On an expiratory film, the heart may appear grossly enlarged, the lung fields may appear opaque (which may simulate diffuse atelectasis), and the diaphragm is located above the seventh rib (Hilton & Edwards, 2006; Swischuk, 1997a, 1997b). On an inspiratory film, the diaphragm is at the eighth rib, the cardiothymic diameter is normal, and the pulmonary vascularity is prominent. The right hemidiaphragm is slightly higher than the left. If the right hemidiaphragm is at or above the level of the seventh rib, the film was obtained in the expiratory phase or the infant has hypoaerated (Hilton & Edwards, 2006; Swischuk, 1997a, 1997b).

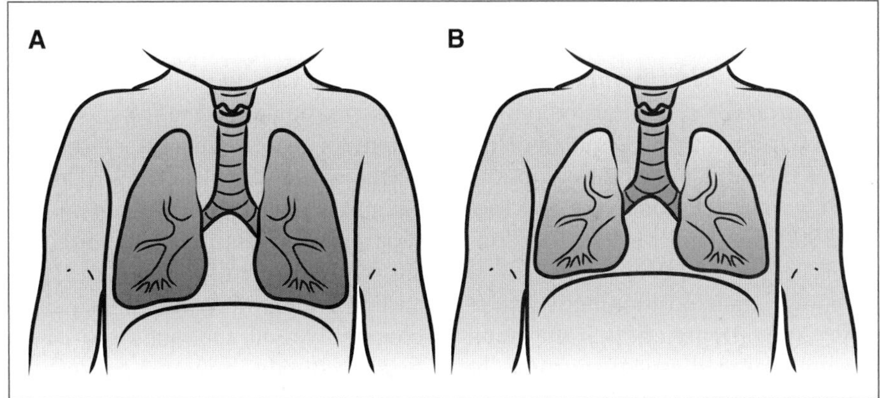

FIGURE I.5 Differences in appearance between inspiration (A) and expiration (B) in a neonatal chest radiograph. On full inspiration, the diaphragm is located at the eighth rib, and the lungs appear larger and darker. During expiration, the diaphragm is at or above the seventh rib, and the lung fields appear smaller and lighter. The heart size may also appear larger on expiratory films.

■ **Motion.** If the infant moves just as the radiograph is made, the resulting film is blurred. Motion causes blurring of the hemidiaphragms, the cardiovascular silhouette, and all fine pulmonary detail (Hilton & Edwards, 2006; Swischuk, 1997a, 1997b). Movement blur on diagnostic images can be prevented by fast imaging and adequate immobilization.

■ **Speed.** A short exposure time is essential for obtaining clear images. This can be achieved by limiting the duration of exposure to the energy source and by increasing the use of computed imaging.

■ **Immobilization.** The nursing staff is primarily responsible for ensuring adequate immobilization during diagnostic imaging. Inadequate immobilization is an important cause of poor quality on neonatal images. Proper immobilization techniques improve image quality, shorten the examination time, and eliminate the need for repeat studies (Hilton & Edwards, 2006; Swischuk, 1997a, 1997b). Proper immobilization may be less traumatic than manual restraint alone. An immobilization board may be required, or tape, foam rubber blocks and wedges, towels, diapers, or clear plastic acetate sheets may be used.

Physical risks to neonates are associated with immobilization. The type of restraint or an ill-designed immobilization device may cause trauma. Tape or plastic sheets may cause skin and soft tissue damage if not applied and removed carefully. Also, thermal stress may be a factor when a neonate is placed on a noninsulated board or film cassette. The nurse should position and immobilize the infant properly so that the technician can center the tube, position the beam, and make the exposure. If the nurse and the technician work together, superior results are achieved with greater speed and less disruption than if they worked separately.

Infants lie still only when they are very ill. Otherwise, they greatly resent being forcibly restrained, especially in an unusual position. A number of immobilization devices are available, but the best means is a pair of adequately protected adult hands (Hilton & Edwards, 2006; Swischuk, 1997a, 1997b).

■ **Tube Angulation.** Another factor that affects radiographic quality is angulation of the x-ray tube, along with improper field limitation. Often on neonatal films, the infant's chest appears mildly lordotic, with the medial clavicular ends projected on or above the dorsal vertebrae. This results in a rather peculiar chest configuration. The preossified anterior arcs of the upper ribs are positioned superior to the posterior arcs (Figure I.6). The lordotic projection tends to increase the apparent transverse cardiac diameter,

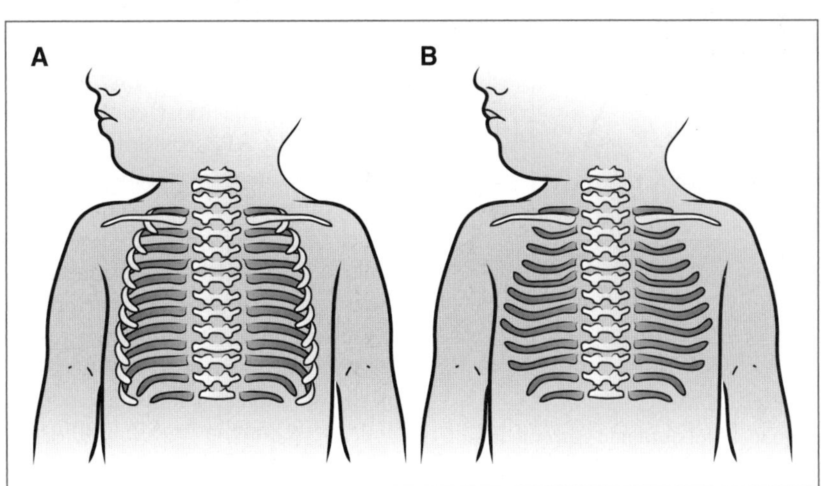

FIGURE I.6 Skeletal position in a normally positioned radiograph (A) and in a film obtained with cephalad positioning of the x-ray tube (B).

making it difficult to determine the size of the heart. Lordotic projections result when the x-ray tube is angled cephalad, when the x-ray beam is centered over the abdomen, or when an irritable infant has arched the back at the time of the film exposure. If the x-ray tube is angled caudad or the x-ray beam is centered over the head, the anterior rib arcs are angulated sharply downward in relation to the posterior arcs (Hilton & Edwards, 2006; Swischuk, 1997a, 1997b).

■ **Infant Positioning.** Proper infant positioning is important to radiographic quality and interpretation. If the infant is rotated, a false impression of a mediastinal shift may be created (Figure I.7). The direction and degree of rotation can be estimated by comparing the lengths of the posterior arcs of the ribs from the costovertebral junction to the lateral pleural line at a given level. The infant is rotated toward the side with the greatest posterior arc length (Hilton & Edwards, 2006; Swischuk, 1997a, 1997b).

Another measurement for determining the degree of rotation is the distance from the medial aspect of the clavicles to the center of the vertebral body at the same level. If the infant is properly positioned, the medial aspects of the clavicles should be equidistant from the center of the vertebral body (Hilton & Edwards, 2006; Swischuk, 1997a). The distance is greater on the side toward which the infant is rotated. On a lateral view, rotation can be readily determined by observing the amount of offset between the anterior tips of the right and left sets of ribs.

Before any chest film is interpreted, these factors must be systematically evaluated. Through experience this evaluation becomes automatic, and the film can be scanned rapidly.

Radiologic Projections

Radiologic projections are the geometric views of the radiograph, and they vary among institutions and radiologists. They can be customized to the specific infant or clinical condition. For example, the skull may require a simple AP film to make the diagnosis of a fracture, whereas a complete skull series may be necessary for evaluation of congenital malformations. In the neck and upper airway, a lateral film in inspiration with the infant's head extended may be sufficient for the evaluation of stridor, or a xeroradiograph of the soft tissue structures of the neck may be required. Because the radiation dose is much greater with a xeroradiograph than with a plain lateral neck film, the indications for this examination should be clear (Swischuk, 1997b).

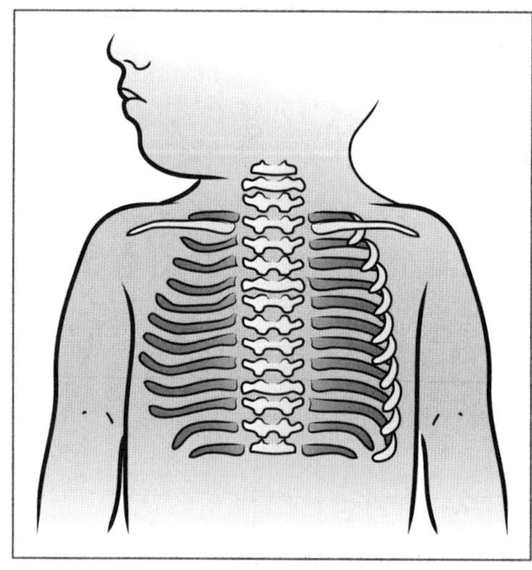

FIGURE I.7 Skeletal configuration in a film obtained with the infant rotated to the right.

For evaluation of the spine, the AP projection is most commonly used. Oblique views of the spine usually are difficult to obtain in infants because it is difficult to position and immobilize babies. Also, the diagnostic information gained does not outweigh the risk of the greater radiation exposure required to obtain such views. For evaluation of congenital hip dysplasia, an AP view of the entire pelvis and both hips is required. Gonadal exposure should be minimized with proper shielding during radiographic examination of the hips. Assessment of skeletal maturation in the infant requires an AP film of the left hemiskeleton, and a long bone series requires a film of the upper and lower extremities (Hilton & Edwards, 2006; Swischuk, 1997a, 1997b).

Chest radiographs are the most frequently performed diagnostic imaging procedure in the neonatal intensive care unit (NICU). In most cases an AP projection from a supine position is satisfactory for evaluating the infant's chest, heart, lung fields, endotracheal tube, line placement, and pneumothorax (air leak complications related to mechanical ventilation). The cross-table view allows verification of pleural chest tube being placed anteriorly or posteriorly. Lateral decubitus is used to evaluate small pneumothorax and small pleural fluid collection; these can be hard to see on an AP view. The upper right reveals abdominal perforation, which shows free air under the diaphragm (rarely used). Lateral projections of the chest often are poorly positioned, have diminished technical quality, and require greater radiation exposure of the infant. For the experienced radiographer, an AP film in the supine position is sufficient in most cases. In rare cases, a lateral chest film with esophageal barium contrast may be requested for evaluation of the left atrium of the heart (Gomella, Cunningham, & Eyal, 2009; Hilton & Edwards, 2006; Swischuk, 1997a, 1997b; Verklan & Walden, 2004).

Abdominal x-ray films also are frequently obtained in the NICU. The most commonly used radiographic projections are the AP, cross-table lateral, and left lateral decubitus views. Because the infant's abdomen is relatively cylindric, a lateral view provides more information than it does in an older child or adult. AP views define the gas pattern, intestinal displacement, some masses, ascites, and placement of lines such as umbilical catheters or intestinal tubes, whereas the cross-table lateral view is recommended in the diagnosis of abdominal perforation and the left lateral decubitus view is for diagnosis of intestinal perforation, free intra abdominal air (Gomella et al., 2009; Hilton & Edwards, 2006; Swischuk, 1997a).

Exposure Factors in Infancy

Numerous radiographic variables are involved in x-ray exposure. The x-ray machine, films, screens, types of cassette, and processing methods, as well as the radiologist's preference, may vary greatly from one department and institution to another. However, a few general principles can be stated:

1. Exposure time should be kept short to prevent movement blur and to limit the radiation dose.
2. Radiographic technicians should be knowledgeable about factors and variables that affect exposure so that repeat films occasioned by poor technique on the initial radiograph can be avoided.
3. A repeated infant x-ray is the major cause of the largest dose of unnecessary radiation (Hilton & Edwards, 2006; Swischuk, 1997a, 1997b); every possible precaution should be taken to ensure that the first attempt produces a film of diagnostic quality.
4. Before a repeat is done, the film should be shown to the radiologist or neonatologist who requested it; although the technical quality may not be ideal, the film may provide sufficient information.

Radiation exposure can also be reduced by using other diagnostic imaging modalities, when possible, that do not use ionizing radiation to create an image (e.g., ultrasonography, MRI) (Swischuk, 1997a, 1997b). If radiologic imaging is the best diagnostic approach for the infant's condition, it may be important to "customize" the examinations, to limit the area examined, and to reduce the number of follow-up films. The radiologist and technician should be knowledgeable about the rapid technologic advances in film-screen combinations, filtration, projections, and film processing, which can help produce a film of fine diagnostic quality while minimizing radiation exposure (Alpen, 1998; Swischuk, 1997a, 1997b).

Ideally, there would be no "routine" radiologic examinations, just problem-oriented procedures. However, there is a logical approach to radiographic examinations. Plain films should be obtained first. Then, if indicated, a dye contrast study (e.g., excretory urograph) should be performed, because the contrast material is rapidly eliminated from the body. Last, barium contrast studies should be obtained. Barium contrast studies are performed after the others because (1) barium interferes with any nuclear scintigraphic scans, body-computed tomograms, and ultrasonographic scans and (2) barium is slowly eliminated from the GI tract, which delays further diagnostic evaluation. Additional radiation exposure is possible if the barium must be completely eliminated before the next imaging procedure (Hilton & Edwards, 2006; Swischuk, 1997a, 1997b).

Adequate patient preparation is another means of reducing radiation exposure (Hilton & Edwards, 2006; Swischuk, 1997a, 1997b). If GI and genitourinary (GU) imaging are both to be performed, the GU examination should be scheduled first. Although each institution has its own policies, in preparation for a GU examination such as excretory urography, the infant should be kept on nothing by mouth (NPO) status for no longer than 3 hours; this can be accomplished by withholding the early morning feeding and scheduling the examination for 8 a.m. No preparation is necessary for excretory urography in infants with abdominal masses, trauma, or GU emergencies. If the infant has impaired renal function, the radiologist and the neonatologist should discuss the condition thoroughly so that the risks of this procedure are minimized. For an infant who has been feeding, the baby is prepared for a GI contrast study by keeping the child on NPO status for no longer than 3 hours before the examination. Generally, if a contrast study of the entire GI tract has been requested, the lower GI series is performed before the upper GI series (Hilton & Edwards, 2006; Swischuk, 1997a, 1997b). This allows time for elimination of the barium in the colon and prevents the barium from interfering with the diagnostic quality of the upper GI study. Colon preparation usually is unnecessary in the neonate and should be avoided in infants with an acute abdominal condition and in those suspected of having Hirschsprung disease (Swischuk, 1997a, 1997b).

Collaborative Care

■ **Radiation Protection.** Any radiation is considered harmful to the infant, and all efforts must be made to reduce radiation exposure without forgoing diagnostic information. Radiation exposure can have both genetic and somatic effects (Bushong, 2013; Dowd & Tilson, 1999; NCRP, 1993a, 1993b, 1993c). Reduction of radiation exposure should be the goal for sites that are sensitive genetically (gonads) and somatically (eyes, bone marrow). Although there is no evidence that somatic damage (e.g., carcinogenesis or cataracts) occurs as a result of low-dose diagnostic radiologic procedures, dose reduction should be accomplished for the site examined and for the rest of the body (Dowd & Tilson, 1999). Methods of reducing radiation exposure include performing examinations only when they are clinically indicated, selecting the appropriate imaging modality, using the lowest radiation dose that achieves an image of diagnostic quality, avoiding repeat examinations, reducing the number of films obtained, using appropriate projections with tight field limitation, ensuring proper positioning and immobilization, and shielding the gonads (Alpen, 1998; Dowd & Tilson, 1999; Hilton & Edwards, 2006; NCRP, 1993a, 1993b, 1993c).

If the gonads are not within the area of interest, gonadal exposure depends on the adequacy of field limitation. The maximum gonadal dose occurs when the gonads are unshielded and exposed to the primary x-ray beam. This dose declines rapidly as the distance from the gonads to the primary beam increases. Gonadal exposure in an AP film that includes the gonads can be reduced by 95% with proper contact shielding (Dowd & Tilson, 1999). The gonads should be shielded whenever they are within 5 cm of the primary x-ray beam.

Contact gonadal shields are easy to make from 0.5-mm thick lead rubber sheets, and they should be sized for gender and age (Figure I.8) (Swischuk, 1997a, 1997b). In males, proper positioning of the shield avoids obscuration of any

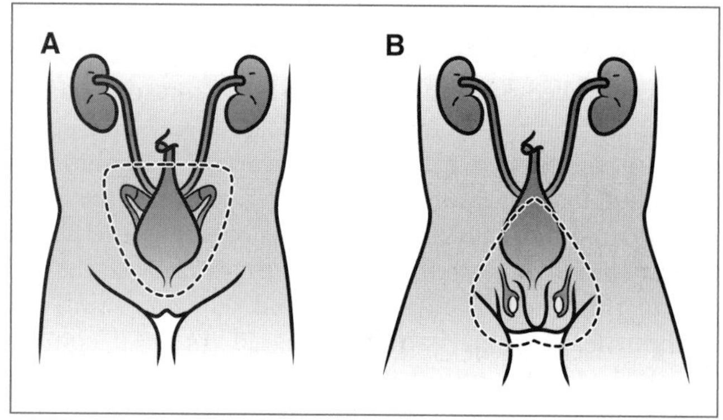

FIGURE I.8 Anatomic placement of gonad shield for female infants (A) and for male infants (B).

bony detail of the pelvis if the upper edge of the shield is placed just below the pubis and if the testicles have descended into the scrotum. In females, the position of the ovaries varies with bladder distention. Because of their anatomic location, the ovaries cannot be shielded without obscuring lower abdominal and pelvic structures. The lower margin of the gonad shield should be placed at the level of the pubis, and the upper margin should cover at least the lower margin of the sacroiliac joints (Hilton & Edwards, 2006; Swischuk, 1997a, 1997b).

■ **Radiation Safety.** The three ways to reduce radiation exposure of personnel are (1) shorten the duration of radiation exposure; (2) increase the distance from the radiation source; and (3) provide radiation shielding between the nurse and the radiation source (Alpen, 1998; Bushong, 2013; Dowd & Tilson, 1999; NCRP, 1993a, 1993b, 1993c). Portable radiologic examinations are the most common form of diagnostic imaging routinely performed in the NICU. During these procedures, there is a tendency for all the nurses to leave the room when an exposure is being produced; consequently, other infants may be left unattended for that short period. Because of this practice, parents have expressed fear about their infants facing environmental radiation hazards.

Using the example of an infant who receives two radiologic examinations per shift, the total dose outside a 30-cm (1 foot) radius of the primary beam is 70 microroentgens (μR). If the staff nurse worked a 250-day work year and held an infant who received two x-ray examinations per shift, the cumulative dose would be 18,000 μR (18 mrad) per year (1,000 μR = 1 mrad). This value is considerably lower than the background radiation in a building, which amounts to 100 to 150 mrad per year (Bushong, 2013; Dowd & Tilson, 1999).

Other radiologic studies done in the NICU have found that within 1.82 m (6 ft) of the target, an unshielded person receives 100 mrad *per hour of exposure.* Because the duration of exposure is approximately 0.1 second, the radiation dose is 0.003 mrad per exposure. This amount of radiation is far below the safety limit of 500 mrad per year. At this rate of radiation exposure, a full-time staff nurse would have to be exposed to more than 6,000 x-rays each day to reach the radiation safety limit per year (NCRP, 1993a, 1993b, 1993c).

It appears that if certain basic radiation precautions are observed, nurses and other NICU personnel need not leave the room during x-ray exposures. However, staff members should stay 30 cm (1 foot) or farther from the infant being radiographed. Care must be taken to ensure that if a horizontal beam film is obtained (e.g., in a cross-table lateral projection), no one is in the direct x-ray beam because the radiation dose in the primary beam is considerably higher than in the scattered portion. When a horizontal beam is used, it should not be directed at any other patient or person. Any employee within 30 cm (1 foot) of the incubator or one who is holding the infant for the exposure should wear a lead apron and gloves.

The x-ray beam must be confined to the area within the cassette's edges. An infant causes little scatter, but an adult's hands can easily come within the field of primary radiation and cause scatter. It is important to position and secure the infant properly while keeping the hands out of the x-ray beam. If correct radiographic technique is used, the dose to the nurse's lead-protected hands is approximately 0.01 mSv (millisieverts). The annual dose limit to the hands of nondesignated personnel is 500 mSv.

Table I.2 summarizes the process of systematic interpretation of radiographic images in the neonate.

Radionuclide Imaging

The use of radioisotopes has brought a new dimension to diagnostic imaging, because they can be used to trace a wide range of physiologic functions in virtually every organ in the body, thereby complementing conventional radiography and ultrasonographic imaging. The difference between conventional radiography and radionuclide imaging is that with the former, images are produced by the transmission of radiation, whereas with the latter, images are produced by the emission of radiation (gamma rays) previously introduced into the body and recorded on film or in a computer (Figure I.9) (Alpen, 1998; Bushong, 2013; Dowd & Tilson, 1999; Juhl et al., 1998; Treves, 1995).

Radionuclide studies yield both physiologic information and anatomic representations of the distribution of radioactivity, depending on the selective uptake of radionuclide by different organs of the body (Bushong, 2013; Dowd & Tilson, 1999; Treves, 1995). The primary disadvantage of radionuclide imaging is the limited anatomic resolution to diameters greater than 2 cm.

■ **Biophysical Principles.** Relatively small amounts of radioactivity are used in radionuclide imaging, and the radiation hazard is significantly smaller than for corresponding conventional radiographic investigations (Bushong, 2013; Dowd & Tilson, 1999; Treves, 1995). The radioactive substance injected usually is distributed throughout the body, and the site of maximum radiation is not always the organ under investigation (Bushong, 2013; Dowd & Tilson, 1999; Treves, 1995). For example, the thyroid gland selectively concentrates radioactive iodine, even if this compound is being used to study another organ. In this case, thyroid iodine uptake can be blocked pharmaceutically. The kidneys

TABLE I.2

RADIOGRAPHIC INTERPRETATION

Technical Evaluation	Characteristics
Film density and contrast	The intravertebral disk spaces should be visible through the cardiothymic silhouette. Underexposed films appear whitish with progressive loss of spaces; overexposed films have a "burned out" appearance with loss of pulmonary vascular markings.
Phase of respiration	The respiratory phase affects the appearance of the lung fields. During expiration, the cardiothymic silhouette appears larger, and the lung fields appear more opaque; the hemidiaphragms usually are at the level of the seventh rib. During inspiration, the cardiothymic silhouette is normal, pulmonary vascularity is seen, and the lung fields are clear. Adequate inspiration puts the right he midiaphragm at the level of the posterior eighth rib; the right hemidiaphragm usually is slightly higher than the left during basal breathing.
Motion	Radiology personnel must check for motion at the time the film is taken. Motion is detected by blurring of the hemidiaphragms and cardiothymic silhouette. Motion obscures all fine pulmonary vascular detail, which makes the films unsatisfactory for evaluation of the lung fields.
Tube angulation and patient positioning	Anteroposterior (AP) films of the newborn appear lordotic, with the medial ends of the clavicles projecting on or above the second dorsal vertebra. If the tube has been angled cephalad, the lordosis is exaggerated, with the anterior arcs of the ribs positioned superior to the posterior arcs. The cardiothymic silhouette appears larger because the view is through the transverse diameter of the heart. This occurs if the infant arches during the procedure or if the beam has been centered over the abdomen. Caudad angulation of the beam over the head results in distortion of the chest, with the anterior ribs arcs angled sharply downward in relation to the posterior arcs.
Rotation of the patient	Assessment of rotation is critical in determining whether mediastinal shift is present. Lateral rotation may lead to the false impression of a mediastinal shift. The trachea shifts toward the side of the rotation, and the contours of the heart are altered. The direction and degree of rotation are estimated by comparing the lengths of the posterior arcs of the ribs on both sides. The side with the longest posterior arc is the side to which the patient is rotated. Rotation also results in unequal lengths of the clavicles when they are measured from the medial aspects to the center of the vertebral body at the same level. The patient is rotated to the side with the longer clavicle.
Heart size and pulmonary vascularity	These features are difficult to determine in the newborn in the first 24 hours of life because of the dynamic cardiovascular alterations that occur during this period. Changes in the transitional circulation are associated with an increase in pulmonary blood flow and in blood return to the left atrium, a decrease in blood return and lower pressure in the right atrium, and changes in systemic and pulmonary arterial pressures. The newborn's heart size is relatively larger in the first 48–72 hours because of those rapid changes. Heart size can be accurately assessed only during basal breathing, because the size is significantly altered during phases of the cardiac cycle and during hyperexpansion of the lung. After the first 24 hours, a cardiothoracic ratio above 0.6 is the upper limit of normal. Fetal lung fluid is reabsorbed, and the air spaces are filled with air on inspiration. The resorption of lung fluid enhances the appearance of the pulmonary lymphatics, resulting in an apparent increase in vascularity at birth. Transient tachypnea of the newborn is characterized by perihilar streaky infiltrates with increased pulmonary vascularity and good lung inflation.
Cardiothymic silhouette	The cardiac configuration is difficult to determine in the newborn largely because of the variation in size and shape of the thymus. The aortic knob and main pulmonary artery are obscured by the thymus, which frequently has a wavy border. A tuck may be seen in the left lobe of the thymus at the lateral margin of the right ventricle, a feature called a sail sign. The apex of the heart has a more cephalad position and assumes a more caudal position over time. The elevation of the apex is due to the relative right ventricular hypertrophy of the fetus. After birth, as the left ventricle becomes more prominent, the cardiac apex descends. The thymus involutes rapidly under the stress of delivery and over the next 2 weeks of life may enlarge slightly.
Aeration of the lungs	Satisfactory inspiration positions the hemidiaphragms at the posterior arcs of the eighth rib. Expansion and radiolucency of the right and left sides are equal. If the sides are not comparable, a right and left lateral decubitus film should be obtained to evaluate for fluid levels or air. The lungs may bulge slightly through the ribs. On lateral projection, the hemidiaphragms should be smoothly domed. The AP and transverse diameters of the chest vary with age and disease. In a normal newborn, the AP and transverse diameters are equal. Over time, the transverse diameter increases, giving the chest cavity an oblong appearance. Air-trapping diseases produce a more rounded configuration, whereas hypoaeration results in a more flattened AP diameter. With hypoaeration, the right hemidiaphragm is located at the seventh rib, the posterior arcs have a more downward slope, and the transverse diameter of the chest is reduced. Laterally, hypoaeration results in increased doming of the diaphragm. With hyperaeration, the hemidiaphragm is located below the level of the ninth rib, the diaphragm is flattened, and the posterior rib arcs are horizontal. Hyperaeration also results in greater bulging of the lungs through the intercostal spaces and an increased diameter of the upper thorax.
Pulmonary infiltrates	Films should be evaluated for areas of increased pulmonary lucency or density. The characteristics and distribution of densities may lead to a diagnosis. Infiltrates should be described with regard to their distribution (unilateral, bilateral) and nature (alveolar, reticulated, diffuse, nondiffuse, patchy, streaky).

(*continued*)

TABLE I.2

RADIOGRAPHIC INTERPRETATION (CONTINUED)

Technical Evaluation	Characteristics
Mediastinal shift	The examiner evaluates for mediastinal shift by determining if the trachea, heart, and mediastinum are in normal position. In general, the shift occurs toward the side with the diminished lung volume or away from the hemithorax with the increased lung volume. Rotation of the patient must first be excluded.
Liver size	The edges of the liver should be clearly defined, and the size of the organ should correlate well with the size determined by palpation, especially when the intestines are filled with air. If insufficient gas is present in the abdomen, the size of the liver cannot be determined. Atelectasis obscures the upper margin of the liver. Radiographically, the size of the liver is not altered by the phase of respiration, as it is during palpation. Liver size may vary with progression of right-sided heart failure. The position of the liver may be altered by congenital malformations such as situs inversus.
Abdominal gas pattern	Swallowing air produces gas in the stomach. The gas pattern must be interpreted in light of the infant's history. In the newborn, stomach air is present, with progression of air through the small bowel at 3 hours of life and rectal air by 6 hours. With bowel obstruction, gaseous distention progresses until at some point the bowel is blocked; beyond that point there is a paucity of air or a gasless bowel. Lack of haustra in the colon makes it possible to distinguish the small and large bowels on the radiograph. A gasless abdomen may be seen with prolonged gastrointestinal decompression, severe dehydration, acidosis, oversedation, brain injury, diaphragmatic hernia, midgut volvulus, and esophageal atresia. Marked aerophagia may be due to mechanical ventilation, tracheoesophageal fistula, necrotizing enterocolitis, and mesenteric vascular occlusion. Free peritoneal air rises to the highest level and outlines superior structures; therefore it is best demonstrated on a left lateral decubitus film.
Catheter and tube positions	All catheter and tube positions should be evaluated and reported each time a radiograph is made. The position of these devices may provide clues to the underlying disease, and malpositioning of tubes and catheters may be life threatening. The trachea is positioned to the right in the midmediastinum, anterior and slightly to the right of the esophagus. The carina is located at T_4. In the right aortic arch, the trachea is found slightly to the left of the vertebral column. Endotracheal tubes optimally are placed in the midtrachea. If the tip is too low (below T_4) or too high (above the thoracic inlet), ventilation is suboptimal. Inadvertent esophageal intubation has occurred when the tip of the tube is below T_4 but is still in the midline or when the trachea can be visualized apart from the tube. Nasogastric (NG) tube placement should be reported. NG tubes may be too short (seen in the distal esophagus) or too long (seen in the duodenum or jejunum), or they may be coiled in the esophagus (tracheoesophageal atresia). The location of vascular catheters must be evaluated. Central catheters should be placed with the tip in the superior part of the inferior cava. Umbilical artery catheters ideally should be located in the high (T_6–T_9) or low (L3–L5) position, away from major arterial branches. Umbilical venous catheters should be positioned with the tip in the inferior vena cava and not in a hepatic branch.
Bony structures	The skeleton should be evaluated, especially the general configuration of the thoracic cage. Normally, over time, the cephalic portion of the thoracic cage becomes rounded and the transverse diameter increases. Hyperaeration exaggerates cephalic rounding, and the horizontal position of the rib arcs. Hypoaeration reduces the diameter of the upper thorax and increases the inferior slope of the rib arcs (bell-shaped thorax). The radiograph must be evaluated for fractures, dislocations, hypodensities, or other lucencies. Persistent elevation of the scapula and an ipsilateral elevated diaphragm (which occur secondary to phrenic nerve injury) may accompany Erb's palsy. Scans should be done for vertebral, rib, and other bony anomalies. Rib aplasia is associated with hemivertebrae, and complete or partial aplasia of the clavicles may be a manifestation of chromosomal abnormality. The proximal humeri can yield information related to congenital infections such as in rubella, syphilis, and cytomegalovirus infection. The bone density should be evaluated in relation to film penetration.

excrete the radioactive phosphonate agents used for skeletal scanning, and the maximum radiation dose is to the bladder mucosa (Dowd & Tilson, 1999; Treves, 1995). Promoting diuresis can reduce this dose effect. The radiation hazards in radionuclide imaging, therefore, are affected by the physiologic distribution of the agent and its physical half-life, the dose of radionuclide administered, and the pharmacologic half-life in the body (Dowd & Tilson, 1999; Treves, 1995).

■ **Choice of Nucleotide.** With nuclear diagnostic imaging, several factors help determine the amount of energy actually deposited in the tissue and may influence the choice of radionuclide. These factors include the following (Dowd & Tilson, 1999; Treves 1995):

- Route of entry
- Fraction of the administered dose that actually reaches the tissue
- Rate of biologic removal of the radionuclide
- Amount of radiation the tissue of interest receives from the portion of the radionuclide deposited in tissues other than the one of interest
- Number of microcuries of radionuclide taken in
- Careful calculation of the average energy of the beta particles emitted, of any ancillary gamma rays emitted, and of any loss of radiation out of the specific tissue
- Metabolic or other factors that might alter the distribution of the radionuclide in various tissues of the human population studied

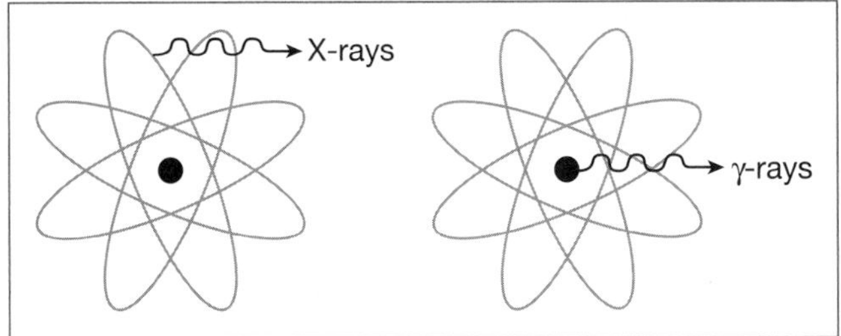

FIGURE I.9 X-rays are produced outside the nucleus of artificially excited atoms; gamma rays are produced inside the nucleus of radioactive atoms.

Estimation of the true dose of energy delivered to a specific tissue by radionuclide exposure, plutonium contamination, or external x-ray exposure, therefore, involves serious technical considerations and requires the efforts of physicists skilled in such measurements.

Nearly all radionuclides used in medicine are artificially produced in nuclear reactors. The most versatile of these compounds is technetium 99m (^{99m}Tc), which has many ideal physical properties, including the following (Dowd & Tilson, 1999; Treves, 1995):

1. It is nontoxic and nonallergenic
2. It is easily bound to other physiologic compounds
3. It is relatively inexpensive
4. It circulates in the blood, and small amounts accumulate in the gastric mucosa, salivary glands, and thyroid tissue
5. It is excreted primarily in the feces and urine but can also be found in sweat and tears
6. It does not accumulate in the brain (except in the choroid plexus) unless the blood–brain barrier has been disrupted
7. It has a short physical half-life (6 hours), long enough for tests to be completed while allowing high initial radio activities to be administered within an acceptable radiation hazard
8. It emits only gamma photons, which can be detected by the sodium iodide crystals of gamma cameras

Despite the wide use of technetium, it is not suitable for all investigations, and a number of alternative isotopes are available (Box I.1).

The ideal instrument for detecting the radiation emission of the radionuclide is the gamma camera. With this camera, images are rapidly acquired and dynamic studies are easily performed and quantified. Multiple views from various projections can be obtained. The camera consists of a large crystal of sodium iodide protected by a heavy lead collimator. The shielded crystal is placed over the target organ, and the gamma photons emitted from the body strike it and are converted into light scintillations. The pinhole and converging collimators allow the image to be magnified without loss of resolution. These light scintillations are manipulated electronically to define the distribution and intensity of the radioactivity. The final copy of the image is produced on film or stored on videotape or magnetic disk (Alpen, 1998; Bushong, 2013; Dowd & Tilson, 1999; Treves, 1995).

Because radiopharmaceuticals are rarely organ specific, interference from radioactivity outside the organ of interest is always a factor. Advances in computer processing similar to CT have been developed to eliminate this interfering background data, thereby increasing the accuracy of derived data. Two types of computer-enhanced radionuclide imaging are available: single photon emission computed tomography (SPECT) and positron emission tomography (PET). Both modalities have significant advantages over conventional planar radionuclide imaging in that (1) the sensitivity and qualification of the distribution and density of radioactivity are much greater; (2) three-dimensional imaging is possible with computer reconstruction; (3) the dose of radionuclide is the same; and (4) artifactual lesions can be eliminated (Bellenger et al., 2000; Bushong, 2001; Lewis et al., 2000; Swischuk, 1997a, 1997b; Tierney et al., 2001; Treves, 1995; Weisslleder, 2001).

■ Single Photon Emission Computed Tomography. With SPECT, a gamma camera is rotated 360° around the infant, and a series of equally spaced, cross-sectional images is obtained and stored in the computer. These images are used to reconstruct a series of cross-sectional slices at right angles to the axis of rotation of the camera. Each cross-sectional slice comprises a series of squares arranged in a matrix. Using a mathematic model, the computer can readily reconstruct these cross-sectional slices in other planes, such as the lateral or coronal plane. The image is then viewed directly from the computer screen or formatted on film. This type of computer-enhanced emission tomography scan uses the standard gamma-emitting radionuclides such as technetium, thallium, gallium, and iodine (Lewis et al., 2000; Treves, 1995).

■ Positron Emission Tomography. With PET, a different type of radiopharmaceutical, called a positron, is used. Positrons are the same size and shape as electrons but have a positive charge. Typical positrons used in this type of imaging are carbon 11, oxygen 15, and nitrogen 13. Using the metabolic nucleotide from oxygen, carbon, or nitrogen, PET scans create images that depict the "metabolic" function of tissue such as the brain (Bushong, 2013; Dowd & Tilson, 1999; Lin, Laine, & Bergmann, 2001; Treves, 1995; Weissleder & Mahmood, 2001). SPECT is widely available for general use, but PET scanning is available only at large university medical centers with access to a cyclotron, which can produce the short-lived positrons required for this imaging modality. Continued advances in particle physics enhance the development of the technique as a research tool in the study of cerebral blood flow and physiology. The recent substitution of fluorine in the glucose molecule has been very useful in the study of cerebral metabolism in neonates after intracranial hemorrhage (Peterson et al., 2000; Rushe et al., 2001; Swischuk, 1997a). Although this modality is not used frequently in clinical medicine, nurses should understand its potential as a research tool.

■ Collaborative Care. The care of a neonate undergoing a radionuclide scan requires knowledge about the patient's history and clinical manifestations, the type of nuclear scan requested, and the radiopharmaceutical used. In general, the doses of radiopharmaceuticals are based on the infant's body weight, and the total whole body irradiation is considerably less than that with a conventional radiograph. The infant poses no radioactivity hazard for the nursing staff or other neonates. Linen, diapers, and body excreta can be disposed of in the usual manner. Nurses should be aware that the radionuclide can concentrate in areas other than the organ of interest so that the proper agents for blocking thyroid iodine uptake can be administered or diuresis can be promoted.

Ultrasonographic Imaging

With neonates, ultrasonography frequently is used in the evaluation and treatment of internal anatomic structures. Unlike conventional radiography, ultrasonography does not involve the emission of ionizing radiation. Instead, sound waves are used to evaluate tissue densities, the movement of tissues, and blood flow (Bushong, 1999, 2013; Martin et al., 2011; Swischuk, 1997a, 1997b). The images can be recorded on videotape, photographic film, light-sensitive paper, or magnetic disk.

■ **Biophysical Principles.** By definition, ultrasound is any sound that has a frequency greater than 20,000 cycles per second (Hz), which exceeds the audible range of human hearing (20–20,000 Hz) (Bushong, 2013). Ultrasonography uses high-frequency sound waves (3.5–10 MHz). For echocardiography and Doppler studies, the ultrasound frequencies range in the millions of cycles per second (Bushong, 1999). Ultrasonography has the following advantages as a diagnostic tool (Bushong, 1999, 2013; Martin et al., 2011; Swischuk, 1997a, 1997b):

1. It emits no ionizing radiation and has no known deleterious somatic or genetic effects; therefore follow-up examinations may be repeated at will
2. Ultrasound waves can be directed as a beam
3. Sound waves obey laws of reflection and refraction
4. Ultrasound waves are reflected by objects of small size
5. Ultrasonography can be used in a variety of transverse, longitudinal, sagittal, or oblique planes
6. Ultrasonography is considerably less costly than either CT or MRI
7. Ultrasound equipment is easily portable
8. The examination is relatively painless and well tolerated
9. Sedation is rarely required
10. Ultrasonography relies on acoustic impedance of tissue to demonstrate anatomy
11. Ultrasonography is diagnostically accurate

The following are the principal disadvantages of ultrasonography (Bushong, 1999, 2013):

1. It is operator dependent
2. It does not provide as much information on organ function as urography
3. It has limited value as a screening procedure for "acute abdominal distress"; rather, the examination should focus on a particular area of interest
4. CT is superior in demonstrating the extent of disease, because ultrasonography demonstrates a smaller area of interest and less anatomic detail
5. Bone, excessive fat, and gas artifacts adversely affect ultrasonography

Because of these drawbacks, certain parts of the body, such as the brain, must be imaged through an ultrasound "window," such as the anterior fontanelle. In addition, because sound waves are poorly propagated through a gaseous medium, the transducer must have airless contact with the surface being examined, and parts of the body that contain large amounts of air are difficult to examine.

High-frequency sound passes through the body tissues at a fairly constant speed of approximately 1,500 m/sec, or 1.5 mm/μsec (Bushong, 1999, 2013). Using electronic mechanisms, it is possible to time the passage of an ultrasound impulse to within a fraction of a microsecond so that the distance between an ultrasound transducer and a reflecting interface of tissue can be determined to a fraction of a millimeter. The transducer converts electrical energy into ultrasonographic energy and acts as both the emitter of the initial impulse and the receiver of the reflected impulse.

The velocity of sound wave transmission is the product of the sound frequency and the wavelength. The speed at which sound is transmitted varies, depending on the density and compressibility of the medium (Bushong, 1999, 2013). The velocity of sound transmission is low in a gaseous medium because of the large compressibility and low density of the substance. Sound does not exist in the vacuum of outer space but is readily transmitted through objects of greater density, such as water or metal. This principle can be readily illustrated with the use of a tuning fork. When struck, the tuning fork vibrates and emits sound that can be easily heard. However, when the vibrating tuning fork is placed against the mastoid bone of the cranium, the sound is transmitted to the ear much more readily and is perceived as being louder.

Frequency and wavelength are inversely proportional in ultrasonography (Bushong, 1999, 2013). That is, as the ultrasound frequency increases, the wavelength decreases. The ability to distinguish objects of small size with ultrasonography is directly related to the sound wavelength. High-frequency ultrasonography uses short wavelengths and results in better image resolution than is seen with low-frequency, long-wavelength ultrasonography. This is the case because as the ultrasound frequency increases, the degree of interaction with the conducting medium increases, and absorption of the ultrasound beam is increased. Therefore at higher ultrasound frequencies, less tissue penetration occurs. For example, ultrasound examinations of the eye typically use frequencies of about 10 MHz, whereas an examination of deep structures of the abdomen uses frequencies of about 2.5 MHz (Bushong, 1999).

The frequency-dependent characteristic of ultrasonography results in its highly directional and collimated nature, which enhances its imaging ability (Bushong, 1999). As the frequency of sound increases, its dispersion from the source is reduced and its transmission becomes more like that of a collimated beam. This becomes apparent when experimenting with a household stereo. The woofers produce a low-frequency bass sound that fills the entire room with sound. A person's perception of these low-frequency sounds does not change, no matter where the person stands in the room. However, the higher frequency sound produced by the tweeters does not disperse as well in the room and can best be heard when the person is positioned directly in front of the speakers. In addition, low-frequency sounds seem at times to penetrate and reverberate in the body, which is not true with higher frequency sounds.

These same principles govern ultrasound transmission through tissue. At higher ultrasound frequencies, the beam becomes more collimated in a forward direction. As the ultrasound frequency is increased, the ability to distinguish small objects increases, but the penetrability of the beam decreases. For these reasons, the highest frequency transducer is chosen to provide the greatest depth for the tissue or organ imaged.

Ultrasonography also is useful as a diagnostic imaging method because it is reflected at tissue interfaces. A principle called sonic momentum describes the velocity of sound transmitted through tissue. Sound transmission through different tissues varies with sound velocity, the freedom of motion of the molecules (density), and the sound waves' compressibility. The way sound travels through a tissue often is referred to as the acoustic impedance of that tissue. As a sound wave travels through a homogeneous tissue, it continues in a straight line. When the sound wave reaches an interface between two tissues with different acoustic impedances, it undergoes reflection and refraction (Figure I.10) (Bushong, 1999, 2013). The amount of sound reflected depends on the degree of difference between the two tissues; the greater the disparity, the greater the reflection. Diagnostic ultrasound has little interest in the refracted wave but is primarily interested in the intensity of the reflected beam relative to the original sound wave (Bushong, 1999, 2013).

The major patterns of ultrasound reflection are anechoic, echoic, and mixed. An anechoic structure, which is described as sonar lucent, is a structure in which the acoustic medium is homogeneous and the sound waves are unimpeded. An anechoic structure may be fluid filled (bladder), cystic (hydronephrosis), or solid (lymphoma), as long as the tissue is homogeneous. Cystic structures usually have sharp echogenic margins anteriorly and posteriorly. Echoic structures are inhomogeneous and reflect sound waves. These tissues generally are solid and have a variety of densities (typical Wilms' tumor) or may be cystic (hemorrhagic Wilms' tumor). A mixed pattern of reflections has the combined qualities of anechoic and echoic tissues. In addition, ribs and calculi may cause imaging artifacts on an ultrasonographic image. These dense structures prevent further penetration of the ultrasound beam and cause a band-like region

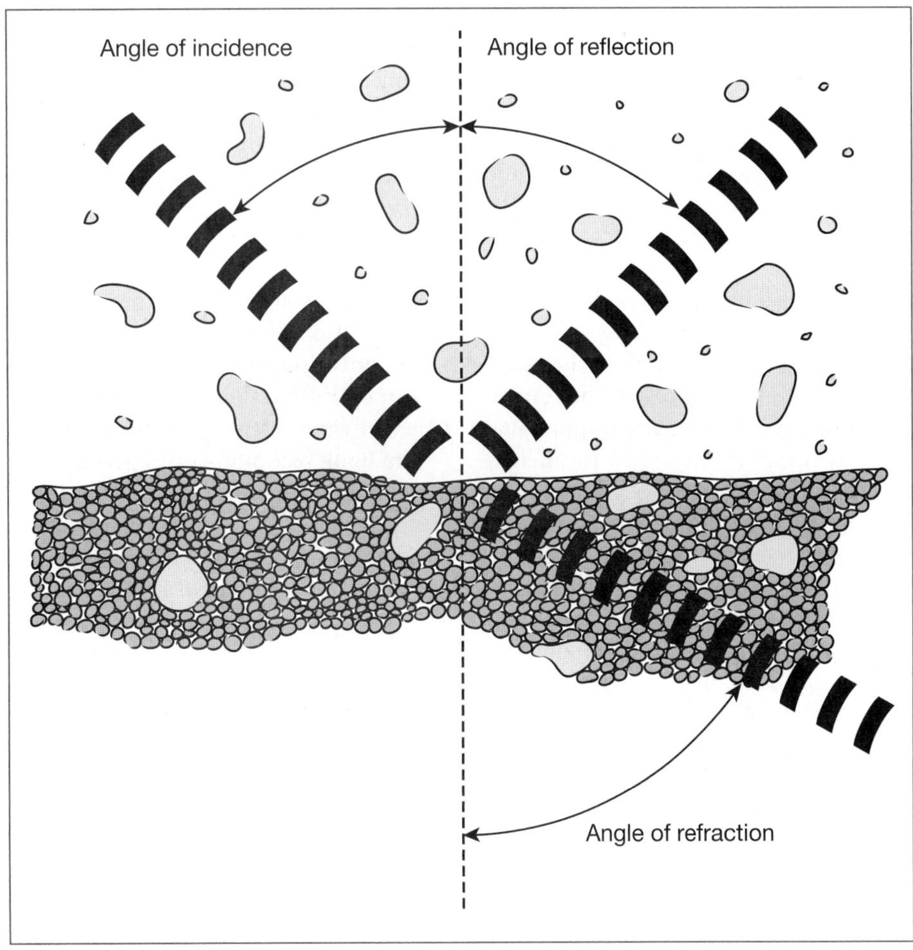

FIGURE I.10 The reflection and refraction of ultrasound.

of decreased sound transmission beyond that point, called acoustic shadowing (Bushong, 1999).

Applying these principles to clinical practice, it is known that ultrasound is propagated differently in various human tissues and is reflected from each acoustic interface (Bushong, 1999, 2013). A stationary interface results in a reflected ultrasound wave that has the same frequency as the transmitted wave. When the tissue interface is moving (e.g., the movement of red blood cells in a vessel), the reflected ultrasound wave has a shifted frequency directly proportional to the velocity of the reflecting blood cells, in accordance with a principle called the Doppler effect. If the movement of the blood cells is toward the transducer, the frequency of the reflected wave is higher than the transmitted frequency. Conversely, movement of blood away from the transducer results in a lower frequency of the reflected wave (Bushong, 1999, 2013). The difference between the transmitted frequency and the reflected frequency is called the Doppler shift. It is the principle of sound frequency shifts that allows the application of the mathematic relationship between the velocity of the target and the Doppler frequency to calculate flow. This is used most commonly in the echocardiographic evaluation of the heart and in cerebral blood flow determinations (Bushong, 1999, 2013).

■ **Modes of Ultrasonography.** Currently, there are five modes of ultrasonic imaging: two static modes (A-mode and B-mode), two dynamic modes (M-mode and real-time), and one Doppler mode. The two static and two dynamic modes use a pulse-echo transducer, which sends ultrasound waves for 0.0001 second and then waits for the reflected sound for 0.999 second. The first and most intense reflection of a sound wave occurs at the transducer-patient interface. At each succeeding tissue interface, reflection of the sound wave diminishes in intensity as the tissue is penetrated. The time required for the pulse to be reflected to the transducer and its returned intensity indicates the position of the interface; the reflection is indicated as a blip on the video display screen (Bushong, 1999, 2013).

In A-mode, ultrasonic images are displayed on the video screen as a series of vertical blips that represent the returning echoes. The distance between these blips is proportional to distances between the tissue interfaces, and the height of each blip is proportional to the intensity of the reflected beam. Thus distal reflections produce lower blips (Bushong, 1999). The main purpose of A-mode imaging is to measure depths of interfaces and to detect their separation accurately. A-mode ultrasonography is primarily used in echoencephalography to determine the cranial midline; it also is used for ultrasonically guided aspiration techniques such as amniocentesis. The advantages of A-mode are that it relies on axial resolution; it is relatively inexpensive; and it is easy to use. The primary disadvantage of this mode is that it requires frequent calibration (Bushong, 1999).

B-mode, or brightness mode, ultrasonic imaging displays information as dots, with the brightness of the dot corresponding to the distance of the reflecting interface from the transducer (Figure I.11 A and B). Advances in microcomputers and electromechanical coupling have resulted in a compound B-mode image (Bushong, 1999). This is achieved when the spatial position and direction of the ultrasound beam are coupled to the video display screen and the B-mode pulses are individually stored while the transducer is moved about the body. The image that appears on the video display screen, therefore, is the summation of many individual B-mode lines. The spatial resolution of this type of imaging varies considerably and depends on the transducer's characteristics and the electromechanical linkages available commercially. This mode of imaging has become widely used, especially for intracranial and abdominal examinations. The B-mode transducer can be moved linearly to provide a rectangular scan view, or it can be angled to provide a sector scan (Bushong, 1999).

M-mode, or motion mode, is an imaging process that incorporates pulse-echo ultrasonography to define tissue movement. If an ultrasound transducer is operated in A-mode over the heart, it detects a number of vertical blips from stationary objects, which indicate the motionless interfaces of the tissue. The amplitude of these blips is proportional to the intensity of the echo. The magnitude of the moving objects represents the degree of movement of tissue interface. If this A-mode scan is converted into a B-mode scan, the image is transformed into a number of dots, some of which are fixed and some of which are moving. If this image is driven on the x-axis according to time, as in a chart recording, a tracing of the dots results (Figure I.11C). The stationary dots trace a regular pattern according to the motion of the tissue interface. The y-axis is the depth of the tissue plane. This type of imaging is used primarily to monitor heart function and can be synchronized with the electrocardiograph (Bushong, 1999).

Real-time ultrasonic imaging is another dynamic form of examining tissues. Real-time is considered the ultrasonic fluoroscope and has several advantages over B-mode imaging, including the following:

1. Real-time ultrasonography units cost considerably less than B-mode units.
2. Acquisition of real-time images is much less dependent on operator skill.
3. Real-time examinations take less time because the imaging technique is relatively easy.
4. Portable versions of real-time units are readily available.

The transducer used for real-time ultrasonography is longer than the one used for B-mode imaging; therefore more gel is needed. The real-time transducer is moved over the surface until the anatomic region of interest is found. The dynamic image is recorded on videotape, and the examiner obtains stop-action frames by taking sequential photographs of the display. The disadvantages of real-time ultrasonography are that (1) the ultrasound beam interacts with tissue interfaces from only one direction, whereas B-mode transducers can move while storing the image from many directions, and (2) lateral resolution is superior in B-mode imaging compared with real-time imaging (Bushong, 1999).

The popularity of real-time ultrasonography as an imaging modality has generated three types of real-time transducer

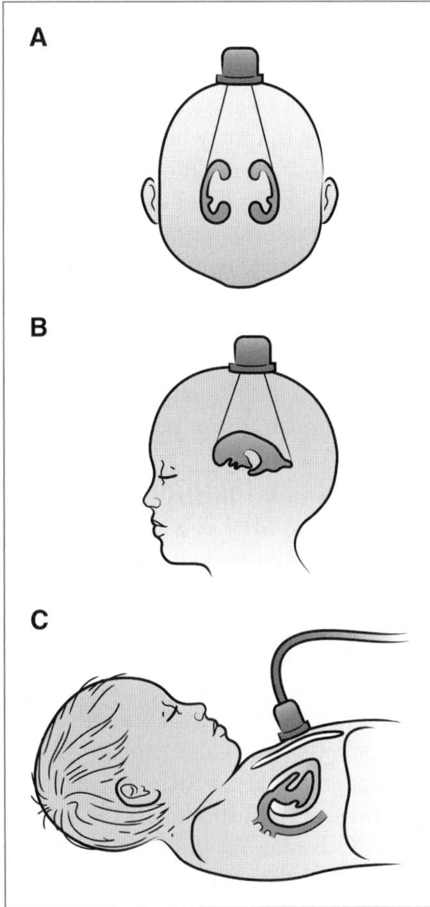

FIGURE I.11 (A) Ultrasound display pattern defining the sagittal sections of ventricular shape and size using brightness (B mode) imaging. (B) Ultrasound display pattern defining the shape and size of lateral ventricles in the neonate using B-mode imaging. (C) M-mode ultrasound display pattern produces a strip chart for tracing moving tissue interfaces such as appear in the heart.

devices—mechanical, linear array, and phased array—with displays that have distinct characteristics. The mechanical transducer was the first real-time device developed. This transducer is motorized so that the ultrasound beam is mechanically swept across the field in an oscillating fashion. Each sweep results in one image frame, and as many as 15 frames per second can be obtained. The transducer can be moved linearly for a rectangular view or in an angulated fashion for a sector view (Bushong, 1999). The mechanical transducer was not popular in the early days of real-time ultrasonography because of the limitation of frame rate per second, restricted field of view, and distortion. In recent years, manufacturers have improved this transducer by increasing the frame rate, expanding the viewing field, and reducing the distortion.

The linear array transducer device has a line of 32 transducers aligned in a single case. Because each transducer is only 2 mm wide, the overall length of the transducer case is 64 mm. In linear array, each transducer is energized in sequence from 1 to 32. This provides 32 image lines over the pulse of ultrasound, called sequential linear array. If four or five contiguous transducers are energized simultaneously, each pulse of the ultrasound results in four or five scan image lines, called segmental linear array. In a typical system, the transducers are fired in an overlapping pattern so that numbers 1 through 5, then 2 through 6, 3 through 7, and so on are segmentally, then sequentially energized (Bushong, 1999). This type of transducer device provides for greater image line density and improved image quality over sequential linear array devices. As with the mechanical devices, sequential and segmental linear array devices have poor lateral resolution.

Phased-array real-time ultrasonic imaging is similar to linear array in that it incorporates segmental excitation of the transducer elements. The transducers are segmentally sequenced and have programmable electronic circuitry to incorporate delay lines, so that the excitation and reception of the ultrasound waves by each element can be timed precisely. This delay allows a plane of sound waves from the transducer to be directed, or "phased." The result is a sector scan with a maximum sector angle of 90° (Bushong, 1999). The scan line rate, frame rate, and depth of scan can be selected. The electronic delay lines on the receiver circuitry allow some depth of focusing through synchronization of the returning reflected pulses. The transducer size is smaller than with linear array, and axial resolution is good. As with real-time imaging, lateral resolution is poor but can be improved with acoustic focusing.

■ Biologic Effects of Ultrasonography. Ultrasonic imaging was introduced into obstetric practice in 1966. Since that time, despite the widespread use of this imaging modality and the use of multiple scans during an individual pregnancy, there have been no reports of manifested injury or late effects in human beings (or fetuses) exposed to diagnostic levels of medical ultrasound (Bushong, 1999). In the laboratory, however, it has been shown that much higher levels of ultrasound can produce measurable tissue effects. The levels of ultrasound energy required to produce these effects are approximately 1,000 times greater than those used in diagnostic medical ultrasonography. In vitro, the mechanism of action of the ultrasonic effects on tissue is presumed to be increased tissue temperature, cavitation, and various viscous stresses on the tissue (Bushong, 1999, 2013).

The thermal effects of ultrasonography occur because of the molecular agitation and relaxation processes caused by the passing sound waves (Bushong, 1999, 2013). Extremely high levels of ultrasound are required to produce even a measurable increase in tissue temperature. The effects of the elevation in tissue temperature occur not only with ultrasonography but also with fever or hyperthermia. At the local tissue level, significant changes in tissue temperature, regardless of the cause, result in structural changes in macromolecules and membranes and alter the rates of biochemical reactions. The thermal effects of diagnostic medical ultrasonography do not result in any increase in tissue temperature.

High levels of experimental ultrasound can also result in alteration in the structure and function of macromolecules and cells without an increase in tissue temperature. These changes can result from cavitation, which occurs when tiny bubbles of gas are formed during the molecular relaxation after sound wave agitation (Bushong, 1999, 2013). As the cavitation increases, more energy is absorbed from the incident ultrasound beam. This is thought to cause disruption of molecular bonds and the production of free hydrogen and hydroxide radicals resulting from the dissociation of water vapor. Cavitation effects have not been observed with the levels of sound used in diagnostic medical ultrasonography (Bushong, 2013).

Every tissue has a specific density, and the density of tissues on either side of an interface may not be equal. As ultrasound waves interact along this tissue interface, the differences in density result in stress exerted on the tissue boundary. This tissue boundary stress results in small-scale fluid motions called microstreaming (Bushong, 1999). It is theoretically possible that microstreaming can disrupt membranes and cells in the region of the interface. Microstreaming has been observed in vitro only after exposure to extremely high levels of ultrasound.

Experimental evidence has shown that ultrasound in sufficiently high doses can degrade macromolecules and may produce chromosomal aberrations and cause cellular death. To induce these effects in living tissue, however, ultrasound intensities of 10 W/cm^2 exposure over considerable periods of time are necessary. The absolute minimum dose level that has been reported to have an observable effect in experimental specimens is 100 mW/cm^2, and then only after many hours of continuous ultrasonographic application (Bushong, 1999, 2013). The intensity range of diagnostic ultrasound is 1 to 10 mW/cm^2, and examinations using this modality frequently require only a few minutes of ultrasound exposure. There are no reports of human chromosomal effects or of changes in prenatal or neonatal death rates after exposure to ultrasound, nor is there evidence that ultrasound induces latent malignant disease. For these reasons, the use of ultrasonic imaging has grown in all areas of medicine, and its uses in neonatal care are increasing rapidly.

Indications for ultrasonography in neonatal intensive care commonly include evaluation of brain parenchyma and ventricular size, myocardial function and structure, cholelithiasis, choledochal cysts, intestinal duplication, renal neoplasms, urinary tract dilation and duplication, pelvic masses, and skeletal anomalies of the spine and hips (Martin et al., 2011).

■ **Collaborative Care.** The care of a neonate undergoing a diagnostic ultrasound examination ensures that any disruption of the infant's microenvironment is minimal. The infant's temperature can be maintained more easily if the ultrasound examination can be performed by using the transducer in the incubator. Although this method is technically more cumbersome for the ultrasonographer, cooperation between the ultrasonographer and the nurse facilitates the procedure. The transducer gel should be warmed to the same temperature as the infant's incubator to minimize heat loss. Heat loss caused by wet blankets or skin can be reduced by placing a diaper or other pad under the imaged area, as well as removing the gel quickly and drying the skin after the scan.

Having an understanding of the imaging examination to be performed allows the nurse to more accurately position the infant and move electrodes, tape, or other artifacts that limit the surface area to be scanned. The nurse's assistance in performing an ultrasound examination is important for monitoring the infant's tolerance of the procedure and for providing information that may be of diagnostic importance to the ultrasonographer. In addition, the nurse's presence at the bedside allows for immediate visual feedback and interpretation of the extent of the pathologic condition that may be present. This knowledge enables the nurse to better support the infant's parents as they make decisions on further diagnostic testing and treatment after their discussions with the medical staff. Interaction with the ultrasonographer at the bedside may also help the nurse to anticipate the infant's immediate and long-term future health care needs.

Magnetic Resonance Imaging

The theoretic basis for MRI is a development of research conducted since the 1940s for studying atomic nuclear structure, which resulted in the awarding of the Nobel Prize for physics in 1952 to Edward Purcell and Felix Block. In addition to the advances in atomic nuclear research, other developments were necessary, such as superconductivity and advances in computer programming, before this concept could be applied to diagnostic imaging.

As an imaging modality, MRI has several advantages over CT and ultrasound (Bushong, 2003, 2013; Huda et al., 2001; Lansberg, O'Brien, Tong, Moseley, & Albers, 2001; Peled & Yeashurun, 2001; Schierlitz et al., 2001):

1. Like ultrasonography, MRI does not use ionizing radiation to produce the image, but rather uses magnetic fields and radio waves.
2. The magnetic resonance image depends on three separate molecular parameters that are sensitive to changes in structure and bioactivity rather than on x-ray photon interaction with tissue electrons as in CT.
3. The region of the body imaged with MRI is not limited by the gantry geometry, as it is with CT, but can be controlled electronically, allowing imaging in transverse planes and in true sagittal, coronal, and oblique planes.
4. Magnetic resonance images are free of the high-intensity artifacts produced in CT scans by sharp, dense bone or metallic surgical clips.

The principal disadvantages of MRI are its high cost and limited availability. Its use for clinically unstable infants on life support also is restricted, because the strong magnetic field can interfere with monitoring devices, and access to the infant is limited during the procedure (Lansberg et al., 2001; Peled & Yeashurun, 2001; Schierlitz et al., 2001; Swischuk, 1997a, 1997b).

Despite the disadvantages of MRI, its clinical applications are rapidly expanding. The image quality is excellent, with the advances in the use of surface coils, and more sensitive head and body coils allow structures such as cranial nerves and small joints to be evaluated more precisely. The increased use of gating, fast scanning, and diffusion-weighted and magnetization transfer imaging have improved MRI evaluation of many tissues and structures and have identified many pathologic conditions that previously could not be quantified (Bushong, 1996, 2001; Fogel, Rychik, Chin, Hubbard, & Weinberg, 2001; Huppi et al., 2001; Nolte, Finsterbusch, & Frahm, 2000; Sinson et al., 2001; Swischuk, 1995).

■ Biophysical Principles. All particles in an atom have either a positive or a negative charge, or a "spin," like a tiny spinning top. The total spin of the protons and neutrons on the nucleus is the sum of the individual spins. Moving charges create magnetic fields; thus the nucleus of an atom develops north and south magnetic dipoles (Bushong, 2003, 2013; Dowd & Tilson, 1999; Juhl et al., 1998). In most materials such as soft tissue, these little spinning magnetic dipoles are randomly oriented (Figure I.12A). This random orientation causes all the spins and magnetic forces to cancel in the material so that the net magnetic force is zero. However, if the material is placed in a strong magnetic field, the magnetic dipoles align themselves, much like a compass needle aligns itself with the Earth's magnetic field. The alignment of these magnetic dipoles produces a net magnetic force or vector that is oriented parallel to the direction of the imposed magnetic field (Figure I.12B). Not all magnetic dipoles become aligned; some are in constant thermal motion so that nuclei are continually knocked out of alignment (Bushong, 2003, 2013; Juhl et al., 1998).

In MRI, the strong magnetic field is imposed to align the molecular magnetic dipoles, and radio frequency pulses then are applied. The known specific frequency of these radio waves displaces the net magnetic moment by an amount

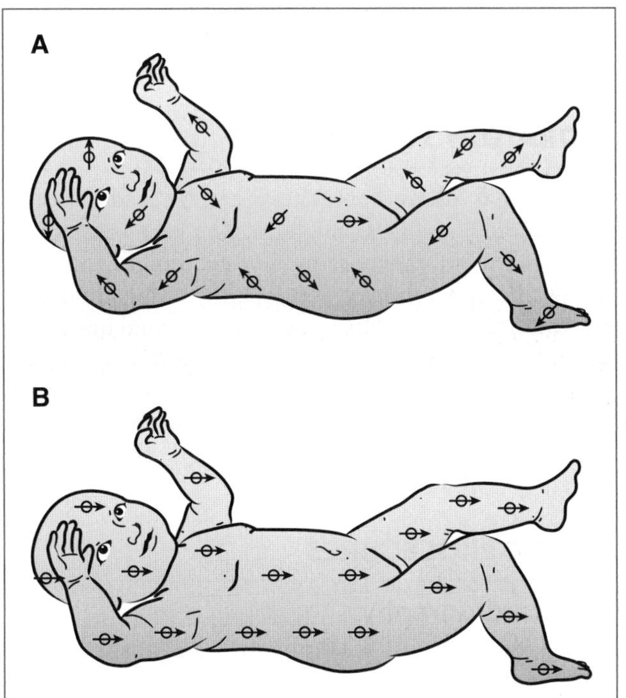

FIGURE I.12 (A) All the magnetic moments are randomly oriented in the body so that the net magnetic charge is zero. (B) Applied radio frequency pulses align the magnetic moments along a predetermined axis. The rate at which the atoms return to their "normal" magnetic moment after the radio frequency is stopped is characteristic for physiologic and pathologic tissues and is responsible for creating the magnetic resonance image.

determined by the strength and duration of the pulse. The frequency is directly proportional to the strength of the magnetic field and is known as the resonant frequency. After the pulse, the protons emit radio frequencies as they return to their original orientation. Therefore the frequency of signals emitted by the protons after the application with radio frequency waves reflects their position in the tissue. Although in theory any stable nuclei can be used, hydrogen is the most abundant and has the strongest resonance (Bushong, 2003, 2013; Juhl et al., 1998).

When protons are placed in a magnetic field, proton alignment does not occur instantaneously but rather increases exponentially with a time constant characterized by T_1, or spin-lattice relaxation time, which reflects the interaction of the hydrogen nucleus with its molecular environment (Bushong, 2003, 2013; Juhl et al., 1998). T_1 characterizes the return of the net magnetization from its displaced position to its normal vertical position resulting from spin-lattice interactions. To form an image, the radio frequency pulses must be applied repetitively. After each radio frequency pulse, the net magnetic force of the sample is reduced; therefore too rapid a radio frequency repetition depletes the magnetization of the tissue, and an image cannot be produced. Thus radio frequency pulses are sequenced with a certain time interval to allow the magnetic force to be reestablished. The longer the time interval, the greater the magnetic force and the longer the imaging time required (Bushong, 2003, 2013; Juhl et al., 1998).

After exposure to the radio frequency pulse has occurred, the signal emitted from the sample of protons decays exponentially with a time constant referred to as T_2, or spin-spin relaxation time. T_2 reflects the magnetic interactions between protons. It characterizes the exponential loss of signal caused by dephasing or desynchronization of magnetic force, which results from spin-spin interactions (Bushong, 2003, 2013; Dort et al., 2001; Juhl et al., 1998). The interval between the application of a radio frequency pulse and the emitted signal depends on the alignment and synchronization of magnetic dipoles. A strong magnetic force results in a long interval for the emitted signal after the pulse; this explains the contrast between tissues with different values of T_2 changes. T_1 is not equal to T_2, because each nucleus is not located within identical magnetic fields. Each hydrogen nucleus is subject to different local magnetic fields because of the presence or absence of other hydrogen nuclei (Bushong, 2003, 2013; Dort et al., 2001).

The third variable that affects image resolution with MRI is spin density. Spin density refers to the strength of the signal received from the nuclei before any of the decay processes have taken place (Bushong, 2003, 2013; Dort et al., 2001; Juhl et al., 1998). This strength is proportional to the number of nuclei within the detection volume of the scanner. Spin density is an indication of hydrogen concentration in the tissue.

A magnetic resonance image results from the mixture of these three properties (T_1, T_2, and spin density) unique to each tissue. The values of T_1 and T_2 for various tissues have been defined. A wide range of values exists among various types of tissue, and considerable differences have been documented between pathologic and normal tissue (Dort et al., 2001; Juhl et al., 1998). Each number defined for the relaxation times (T_1 and T_2) for various tissues depends on the primary external magnetic field and thus may vary from scanner to scanner. The visual projection of the magnetic resonance image is similar to that obtained in CT. By controlling the gradient field of radio frequency pulses, a series of projections at uniform angles through the tissue can be collected. The computer can then reconstruct the image and can emphasize the individual T_1, T_2, or spin density parameters to further define detail (Bushong, 2003, 2013; Dort et al., 2001; Juhl et al., 1998).

The spatial resolution of an MRI scan compares favorably to that with CT. If the object scanned is of high tissue contrast, a lesion as small as 1 mm can be defined. As more data are collected on this imaging modality, even greater spatial resolution and enhanced three-dimensional images are being obtained. As stronger magnetic fields are used, the emitted signals become stronger, and greater resolution may be possible using even higher radio frequency pulses (Bushong, 2003, 2013; Dort et al., 2001).

MRI is better able than CT to detect differences between low-contrast structures. The difference in T_1 and T_2 MRI between biologic tissues frequently is 10% or more. For example, on CT scans, the x-ray photon attenuation coefficient between gray and white matter is approximately 0.5%, whereas the differences in T_1, T_2, and spin density between gray and white matter are great, allowing for more accurate definition of these two tissues (Bushong, 2003, 2013; Dort et al., 2001). Thus MRI has become the diagnostic imaging mode of choice for certain neurologic conditions such as multiple sclerosis, cerebral infarctions, and periventricular leukomalacia. MRI may be useful in the early diagnosis of periventricular leukomalacia, before the characteristic cystic lesions have developed (Huppi et al., 2001; Krishnamoorthy, Soman, Takeoka, & Schaefer, 2000; Peterson et al., 2000; Sie, Barkhof, Lafeber, Valk, & van der Knaap, 2000; Tierney, Varga, Hosey, Grafman, & Braun, 2001).

■ Safety of Magnetic Resonance Imaging. MRI scanning uses three kinds of fields associated with the imaging process: (1) a static, moderately strong magnetic field; (2) a switched, weaker magnetic field gradient; and (3) radio frequency waves. The energies associated with the imaging process are approximately 10^{-8} eV/quantum, which are too weak to cause ionization or breakage of chemical bonds (Bushong, 2003, 2013; Dowd & Tilson, 1999). Energies associated with body temperature elevations are 100,000 to 1 million times greater; therefore these temperature effects are far more disruptive to chemical bonds than the energy associated with MRI (Bushong, 2003, 2013).

In the laboratory, biologic responses in animals, chromosomes, plant seeds, and molecular specimens have shown effects only after extremely high intensities of MRI energy. A dose–response relationship apparently exists, although the biologic threshold is exceedingly high. In human beings, tests for genetic damage have proved negative, and studies of workers in particle accelerators exposed to static magnetic fields six to seven times greater than those used with MRI have shown no detrimental effect (Bushong, 2003, 2013; Dowd & Tilson, 1999). Long-term studies of human beings exposed to radio frequency waves have not demonstrated any deleterious effect (Bushong, 2003, 2013; Dowd & Tilson, 1999).

The hazards of MRI relate primarily to any ferromagnetic objects (e.g., tools, oxygen cylinders, watches, bank cards, pens, and paper clips) that are accelerated toward the center of the magnetic field. The magnetic propulsion of these objects can result in projectile damage; therefore any patient with a pacemaker or an extensive metal prosthesis should be excluded from this imaging technique. In addition, MRI has not been fully tested with pregnant women.

■ Collaborative Care. The care of a neonate who requires an MRI scan includes careful preparation and elimination of any ferromagnetic objects brought near the magnetic field. The infant's condition must be clinically stable, because the strong magnetic field affects some monitoring devices, and visualization of the neonate is impossible during the scan. Surface respiratory monitors and possibly an esophageal stethoscope may be used. An MRI scan is degraded by motion; therefore the infant must be positioned comfortably and safely in the magnetic cylinders. Because the infant must remain motionless for several minutes, an MRI scan is best done after the infant has been fed and is sleeping. If the infant is unable to remain motionless for the duration of the scan, oral chloral hydrate sedation may be recommended.

LABORATORY VALUES

A wide variety of laboratory tests can be used in both the diagnosis and care of the newborn. The values given in this chapter represent the broader normal ranges, but values in a specific chapter may vary slightly, depending on the range the author considers to be within normal limits. Every attempt has been made to provide consistent diagnostic and laboratory values. However, many hospitals have compiled their own list of acceptable laboratory test values; therefore specific laboratories should be contacted when evaluating results (Tables I.3 through I.16).

CARDIAC PROCEDURES

Electrocardiography

Electrocardiography is a noninvasive diagnostic tool used with neonates. It is most useful in the diagnosis and management of cardiac arrhythmias or in conjunction with other diagnostic measures to evaluate cardiac function, specifically the circulatory demands placed on individual heart chambers. In the neonatal period, however, electrocardiography is less helpful in evaluating cardiac anomalies associated with significant ventricular enlargement (Flanagan, Yeager, & Weindling, 2005).

TABLE I.3

COMMON ELECTROLYTE AND CHEMISTRY VALUES

Parameter	Normal Value
Serum Electrolytes	
Sodium (Na)	135–145 mEq/L
Potassium (K)	4.5–6.8 mEq/L
Chloride (Cl)	95–110 mEq/L
Carbon dioxide (CO_2)	20–25 mmol/L
Serum Chemistries	
Blood urea nitrogen (BUN)	6–30 mg/dL
Calcium (Ca)	7–10 mg/dL
Creatinine (Cr)	0.2–0.9 mg/dL
Glucose (G)	40–97 mg/dL
Magnesium (Mg)	1.5–2.5 mg/dL
Phosphorus (P)	5.4–10.9 mg/dL

TABLE I.4

NORMAL HEMATOLOGIC VALUES

	Gestational Age (weeks)						
	28	34	Full-Term Cord Blood	Day 1	Day 3	Day 7	Day 14
Hemoglobin (g/dL)	14.5	15	16.8	18.4	17.8	17	16.8
Hematocrit (%)	45	47	53	58	55	54	52
Red cells (mm^3)	4	4.4	5.25	5.8	5.6	5.2	5.1
MCV (μm^3)	120	118	107	108	99	98	96
MCH (pg)	40	38	34	35	33	32.5	31.5
MCHC (%)	31	32	31.7	32.5	33	33	33
Reticulocytes (%)	5–10	3–10	3–7	3–7	1–3	0–1	0–1
Platelets ($\mu\ 10^3/mm^3$)			290	192	213	248	252

MCV, mean corpuscular volume; MCH, mean corpuscular hemoglobin; MCHC, mean corpuscular hemoglobin concentration.
Adapted from Klaus and Fanaroff (2001).

TABLE I.5

WHITE CELL AND DIFFERENTIAL COUNTS IN PREMATURE INFANTS

	Birth Weight					
	Under 1,500 g			1,500–2,500 g		
	1 week old	2 weeks old	4 weeks old	1 week old	2 weeks old	4 weeks old
Total count (×103/mm³)						
Mean	16.8	15.4	12.1	13	10	8.4
Range	6.1–32.8	10.4–21.3	8.7–17.2	6.7–14.7	7.0–14.1	5.8–12.4

(*continued*)

TABLE I.5

WHITE CELL AND DIFFERENTIAL COUNTS IN PREMATURE INFANTS (CONTINUED)

	Birth Weight					
	Under 1,500 g			1,500–2,500 g		
	1 week old	2 weeks old	4 weeks old	1 week old	2 weeks old	4 weeks old
Percentage of Total						
Polymorphs						
Segmented	54	45	40	55	43	41
Unsegmented	7	6	5	8	8	6
Eosinophils	2	3	3	2	3	3
Basophils	1	1	1	1	1	1
Monocytes	6	10	10	5	9	11
Lymphocytes	30	35	41	9	36	38

Adapted from Klaus and Fanaroff (2001).

TABLE I.6

SUMMARY OF NORMAL URINARY LABORATORY VALUES

	Age of Infant	Normal Value
Ammonia	2–12 months	4–20 μ Eq/min/m^2
Calcium	1 week	Under 2 mg/dL
Chloride	Infant	1.7–8.5 mEq/24 hours
Creatinine	Newborn	7–10 mg/kg/d
Glucose	Preterm Full-term	60–130 mg/dL 12–32 mg/dL
Glucose (renal threshold)	Preterm Full-term	2.21–2.84 mg/mL 2.20–3.68 mg/mL
Magnesium		180 ± 10 mg/1.73 m^2/dL
Osmolality	Infant	50–600 mOsm/kg
Potassium		26–123 mEq/L
Protein		Under 100 mg/m^2/dL
Sodium		0.3–3.5 mEq/dL (6–10 mEq/m^2)
Specific gravity	Newborn	1.006–1.008

Adapted from Ichikawa (1990).

TABLE I.7

ELECTROCARDIOGRAPHIC DATA PERTINENT TO THE NEONATE[a]

	Age			
Parameter	**Birth to 24 hours**	**1–7 days**	**8–30 days**	**1–3 months**
Heart rate (beats/min)	119 (94–145)	133 (100–175)	163 (115–190)	154 (124–190)
PR interval (sec)	0.1 (0.07–0.12)	0.09 (0.07–0.12)	0.09 (0.07–0.11)	0.1 (0.07–0.13)
P wave amplitude II	1.5 (0.8–2.3)	1.6 (0.8–2.5)	1.6 (0.08–2.4)	1.6 (0.8–2.4)

(continued)

TABLE I.7

ELECTROCARDIOGRAPHIC DATA PERTINENT TO THE NEONATE[a] (CONTINUED)

	Age			
Parameter	**Birth to 24 hours**	**1–7 days**	**8–30 days**	**1–3 months**
QRS duration (sec)	0.065 (0.05–0.08)	0.06 (0.04–0.08)	0.06 (0.04–0.07)	0.06 (0.05–0.08)
QRS axis (degrees)	135 (60–180)	125 (80–160)	110 (60–160)	80 (40–120)
R amplitude V_{4R} (mm)	8.6 (4–14.2)	—	6.3 (3.3–8.5)	5.1 (1.1–10.1)
R amplitude V_1 (mm)	11.9 (4.3–21)	—	11.1 (3.3–18.7)	11.2 (4.5–18)
R amplitude V_5 (mm)	10.2 (4–18)	10.7 (3.4–19)	11.9 (3.5–27)	13.6 (7.3–20.7)
R amplitude V_6 (mm)	3.3 (2.3–7)	5.1 (2.2–13.1)	6.7 (1.7–20.5)	8.4 (3.6–12.9)
S amplitude V_{4R} (mm)	3.8 (0.2–13)	—	1.8 (0.8–4.6)	3.4 (0–9.3)
S amplitude V_1 (mm)	9.7 (1.1–19.1)	—	6.1 (0–15)	7.5 (0.5–17.1)
S amplitude V_5 (mm)	11.9 (0.24)	6.8 (3.6–16.2)	4.8 (2.7–12.3)	4.7 (2–12.7)
S amplitude V_6 (mm)	4.5 (1.6–10.3)	3.3 (0.8–9.9)	2 (0.6–9)	2.4 (0.8–5.8)

[a] Mean (5th to 95th percentile).
Adapted from Fanaroff and Martin (1987) and Liebman and Plonsey (1977).

TABLE I.8

ACID–BASE STATUS

Determination	Sample Source	Birth	1 Hour	3 Hours	24 Hours	2 Days	3 Days
Vigorous Term Infants (Vaginal Delivery)							
pH	Umbilical artery	7.26					
	Umbilical vein	7.29					
PCO_2 (mmHg)	Arterial	54.4	38.8	38.3	33.6	34	35
	Venous	42.8					
O_2 saturation	Arterial	19.8	93.8	94.7	93		
	Venous	47.6					
pH	Left atrial		7.30	7.34	7.41	7.39	7.38
CO_2 content (mEq/L)	—	—	20.6	21.9	21.4	Temporal artery	Temporal artery
Premature Infants							
	Capillary (skin puncture)						
pH	<1,250 g				7.36	7.35	7.35
Pco_2 (mmHg)					38	44	37
pH	>1,250 g				7.39	7.39	7.38
Pco_2 (mmHg)					38	39	38

pH, hydrogen ion concentration; PCO_2, partial pressure of carbon dioxide; O_2, oxygen; CO_2, carbon dioxide.
Adapted from Schaffer (1971).

Echocardiography

Echocardiography, another noninvasive diagnostic procedure, commonly is used in the evaluation of the structure and function of the heart. This information can be important not only in the preoperative assessment of cardiac defects but also in the postoperative evaluation of procedures. High-frequency sound waves send vibrations to the structures in the heart, which reflect energy, which is transmitted into a visual image. Echocardiography may be used prenatally as early as 11 weeks gestation when used transvaginally or 18 weeks gestation when used transabdominally (Erenberg, 2011).

Single dimension echocardiography allows the evaluation of anatomic structures, including valves, chambers, and vessels. Two-dimensional echocardiography provides

TABLE I.9

SELECTED CHEMISTRY VALUES IN PRETERM AND FULL-TERM INFANTS

Constituent	Preterm Infant	Full-Term Infant
Alkaline phosphatase (U/L) (mean ± SD)[a]	207 ± 60 to 320 ± 142	164 ± 68
Ammonia (μg/dl)[b]		90–150
Base, excess (mmol/L)[b]		−10 to −2
Bicarbonate, standard (mmol/L)[c]	18–26	20–26
Bilirubin, total (mg/dl)		
Cord[c]	Under 2.8	Under 2.8
24 hours old	1–6	2–6
48 hours old	6–8	6–7
3–5 days old	10–12	4–6
1 Month or older	Under 1.5	Under 1.5
Bilirubin, direct (mg/dL)[c]	Under 0.5	Under 0.5
Calcium, total (mg/dL), week 1[d,e]	6–10	8.4–11.6
Ceruloplasmin (mg/dL)[b]		1–3 months: 5–18
Cholesterol (mg/dL)		
Cord[c]		45–98
3 days to 1 year old		65–175
Creatine phosphokinase (U/L)		
Day 1[f]		44–1150
Day 4		14–97
Creatine (mg/dL)	10 days: 1.3 ± 0.07 1 month: 0.6 ± 0.05	1–4 days: 0.3–1 Over 4 days: 0.2–0.4
Ferritin (μg/dL)		
Neonate[b]		25–200
1 month old		200–600
2–5 months old		50–200
Over 6 months old		7–142
Gamma-glutamyl transferase (GGT) (U/L)[g]		14–131
Glucose (mg/dL)		
Under 72 hours old[h,i]	20–125	30–125
Over 72 hours old	40–125	40–125
Lactate dehydrogenase (U/L)[g]		357–953
Magnesium (mg/dL)[e]		1.7–2.4
Osmolality (mOsm/L)[b]		275–295 (may be as low as 266)
Phosphorus (mg/dL)		
Birth[e]		4.5–8.7
Day 5		4.2–7.2
1 month old		4.5–6.5
Aspartate aminotransferase (SGOT/AST) (U/L)[h]		24–81
Alanine aminotransferase (SGPT/ALT) (U/L)[h]		10–33
Triglycerides (mg/dL)[c]		10–140
Urea nitrogen (mg/dL)[b]	3–25	4–12
Uric acid (mg/dL)[c]		3–7.5

(continued)

TABLE I.9

SELECTED CHEMISTRY VALUES IN PRETERM AND FULL-TERM INFANTS (CONTINUED)

Constituent	Preterm Infant	Full-Term Infant
Vitamin A (μg/dL) (mean ± SD) (under 10 μg/dL		
indicates very low hepatic vitamin A stores)[j]	16 ± 1	23.9 ± 1.8
Vitamin D		
25-hydroxycholecalciferol (ng/ml)[k,l,m]		20–60
1,25-dihydroxycholecalciferol (pg/ml)[k,l,m]		40–90

[a] Glass et al. (1982); [b] Tietz (1988); [c] Wallach (1983); [d] Meites (1975); [e] Nelson et al. (1987); [f] Drummond (1979); [g] Statlan et al. (1978); [h] Cornblath and Schwartz (1976); [i] Heck et al. (1987); [j] Shenai et al. (1981); [k] Cooke et al. (1990); [l] Lichtenstein et al. (1986); [m] Serum levels are affected by race, age, season, and diet.
Adapted from Fanaroff and Martin (2002).

more in-depth information about relationships between the heart and the great vessels (Flanagan et al., 2005).

Doppler echocardiography is used in various forms in the evaluation of characteristics of blood flow through the heart, valves, and great vessels. It can measure not only cardiac output but also flow velocity changes, as demonstrated in stenotic lesions. Regurgitation through insufficiently functioning valves can also be identified. Doppler studies can be used to show regurgitation through insufficiently functioning valves or to identify shunting, as through a patent ductus arteriosus (Zahka, 2011).

Cardiac Catheterization

Historically, cardiac catheterization in the neonate was used for the diagnosis of congenital heart disease. With the advent of more sophisticated echocardiography, especially Doppler echocardiography, cardiac catheterization is used increasingly as a therapeutic modality. The use of radiopaque dye allows for clarification of congenital heart disease and helps to provide data that cannot be obtained from echocardiography.

Immobilization and constant monitoring of the neonate are required during cardiac catheterization. The infant must be restrained to maintain supine positioning. Electrocardiographic electrodes must also be placed to provide constant monitoring of vital signs. Sedation may be considered to maintain proper positioning during the procedure.

A local anesthetic is administered at the insertion site. A radiopaque catheter is inserted into an arm or leg vessel by percutaneous puncture or cut-down. Under fluoroscopy, the catheter is visualized and passed into the heart. Contrast medium is injected through the catheter to allow visualization of the various cardiac structures. Selected chambers and vessels of the heart can be evaluated for size and function. Intracardiac pressures and oxygen saturations can also be measured during this procedure. The use of balloons during catheterization can facilitate procedures such as septostomy, angioplasty, and valvuloplasty (Erenberg, 2011; Flanagan et al., 2005).

After the necessary information has been obtained, the catheter is carefully removed. If a cut-down was performed, the vessel is ligated and the skin is sutured. Pressure should be applied over a percutaneous puncture site to enhance clot formation. For continued bleeding problems, pressure dressings may be applied to the insertion site; these must be checked frequently for active bleeding. After cardiac catheterization, the vital signs should be measured frequently and compared with precatheterization baseline values. Evaluation of localized bleeding or of signs of hypotension resulting in changes in heart rate and blood pressure is essential. Assessment of the insertion site and affected extremity for bleeding, color, peripheral pulses, temperature, and capillary refill should continue for at least 24 hours after the procedure. In addition, the nurse must monitor for complications of catheterization, including hypovolemia (as a result of bleeding or fluid loss during the procedure), infection, thrombosis, or tissue necrosis.

GENETIC TESTING

Chromosome Analysis

■ High-Resolution Karyotyping and Banding. Analysis of chromosome composition can assist in identification of various genetic disorders. A blood specimen is obtained from the infant and used to harvest an actual set of chromosomes. During active cell division, usually during metaphase, the chromosomes are photographed and then arranged in pairs by number. The chromosomes are also separated into regions, bands, and subbands. The end result, a karyotype with banding, is evaluated for the appropriate number of pairs, chromosome size, and structure. Specific genetic disorders can be associated with abnormal numbers of chromosomes (e.g., trisomy 21) or an abnormal chromosome structure, as in cri du chat syndrome, which reflects loss of part of the short arm of chromosome 5 (Kuller & Cefalo, 1996). Abnormal genes on the chromosomes can also cause genetic disorders, such as Duchenne muscular dystrophy, an X-linked recessive disorder.

High-resolution karyotype is widely used for infants with multiple congenital anomalies. This test consists of analysis of chromosomes from white blood cells. The cells are cultured, stimulated to divide, and cell division is halted with a mitotic inhibitor in the prometaphase stage. In this stage the chromosomes are at their longest length and the observed stained bands can reach 800 to 900. This test can take up to 2 weeks (Gomella et al., 2009).

Fluorescence In Situ Hybridization. Chromosomes can be further analyzed using fluorescence in situ hybridization

TABLE I.10

PLASMA ALBUMIN AND TOTAL PROTEIN IN PRETERM INFANTS FROM BIRTH TO 8 WEEKS

Gestation (weeks)	26	27	28	29	30	31	32	33	34	35	36	37	38	39	40	41	42
Albumin gm/dL																	
Reference range (95% confidence limits)	—	1.18–3.06	1.09–2.87	1.20–2.74	1.63–2.75	1.08–3.20	1.38–3.14	1.44–3.34	0.53–3.87	1.15–3.87	1.96–3.44	1.50–4.10	1.89–4.15	2.07–4.15	2.07–4.05	2.04–3.90	2.08–3.90
Corrected age																	
26–28 weeks gestation		2.13	2.10	2.58	2.29	2.39				2.73							
29–31 weeks gestation					2.02	2.14	2.44	2.44	2.54				2.82				
32–34 weeks gestation								2.35	2.42	2.46	2.38	2.44				3.35	
Total Protein gm/dL																	
Reference range (95% confidence limits)	—	1.28–7.94	3.03–5.03	2.18–5.84	2.64–5.80	3.26–5.66	3.63–5.81	3.57–5.87	3.57–6.59	1.52–8.62	3.85–6.91	4.69–6.95	3.32–9.16	4.17–8.25	4.26–8.08	3.73–8.47	3.24–8.76
Corrected age																	
26–28 weeks gestation		4.07	4.45	4.84	4.49	4.45				4.41							
29–31 weeks gestation					3.93	4.42	4.70	4.82	4.51				4.55				
32–34 weeks gestation								4.54	4.93	4.78	4.86	4.81				4.96	

Adapted from Fanaroff and Martin (2002) and Reading et al. (1990).

TABLE I.11

PLASMA-SERUM AMINO ACID LEVELS IN PREMATURE AND TERM NEWBORNS (μmol/L)

Amino Acid	Premature (First Day)	Newborn 16 (Before First Feeding)	16 days to 4 months
Taurine	105–255	101–181	
OH-proline	0–80	0	
Aspartic acid	0–20	4–12	17–21
Threonine	155–275	196–238	141–213
Serine	195–345	129–197	104–158
Asp + Glut	655–1155	623–895	
Proline	155–305	155–305	141–245
Glutamic acid	30–100	27–77	
Glycine	185–735	274–412	178–248
Alanine	325–425	274–384	239–345
Valine	80–180	97–175	123–199
Cystine	55–75	49–75	33–51
Methionine	30–40	21–37	31–47
Isoleucine	20–60	31–47	31–47
Leucine	45–95	55–89	56–98
Tyrosine	20–220	53–85	33–75
Phenylalanine	70–110	64–92	45–65
Ornithine	70–110	66–116	37–61
Lysine	130–250	154–246	117–163
Histidine	30–70	61–93	64–92
Arginine	30–70	37–71	53–71
Tryptophan	15–45	15–45	
Citrulline	8.5–23.7	10.8–21.1	
Ethanolamine	13.4–10.5	32.7–72	
Alpha-amino-*n*-butyric acid	0–29	8.7–20.4	
Methylhistidine			

Adapted from Klaus and Fanaroff (2001); Dickinson et al. (1965, 1970); and Behrman (1977).

TABLE I.12

URINE AMINO ACID LEVELS IN NORMAL NEWBORNS (μmol/L)

Amino Acid	μmol/day
Cysteic acid	Tr-3.32
Phosphoethanolamine	Tr-8.86
Taurine	7.59–7.72
OH-proline	0–9.81
Aspartic acid	Tr
Threonine	0.176–7.99
Serine	Tr-20.7
Glutamic acid	0–1.78
Proline	0–5.17
Glycine	0.176–65.3

(continued)

TABLE I.12

URINE AMINO ACID LEVELS IN NORMAL NEWBORNS (μmol/L) (CONTINUED)

Amino Acid	μmol/day
Alanine	Tr-8.03
Alpha-aminoadipic acid	
Alpha-amino-*n*-butyric acid	0–0.47
Valine	0–7.76
Cystine	0–7.96
Methionine	Tr-0.892
Isoleucine	0–6.11
Tyrosine	0–1.11
Phenylalanine	0–1.66
Beta-aminoisobutyric acid	0.264–7.34
Ethanolamine	Tr-79.9
Ornithine	Tr-0.554
Lysine	0.33–9.79
1-Methylhistidine	Tr-8.64
3-Methylhistidine	0.11–3.32
Carnosine	0.044–4.01
Beta-aminobutyric acid	
Cystathionine	
Homocitrulline	
Arginine	0.088–0.918
Histidine	Tr-7.04
Sarcosine	
Leucine	Tr-0.918

Adapted from Klaus and Fanaroff (2001); Meites (1997); and Fanaroff and Martin (1997).

TABLE I.13

CEREBROSPINAL FLUID VALUES OF HEALTHY TERM NEWBORNS

	Age			
Component	**Birth to 24 hours**	**1 day**	**7 days**	**Over 7 days**
Color	Clear or xanthochromic	Clear or xanthochromic	Clear or xanthochromic	
Red blood cells (cells/mm^3)	9 (0–1070)	23 (6–630)	3 (0–48)	
Polymorphonuclear leukocytes (cells/mm^3)	3 (0–70)	7 (0–26)	2 (0–5)	
Lymphocytes (cells/mm^3)	2 (0–20)	5 (0–16)	1 (0–4)	
Protein (mg/dL)	63 (32–240)	73 (40–148)	47 (27–65)	
Glucose (mg/dL)	51 (32–78)	48 (38–64)	55 (48–62)	
Lactate dehydrogenase (IU/L)	22–73	22–73	22–73	0–40

From Klaus and Fanaroff (2002); Naidoo (1968); and Neches et al. (1968).

TABLE I.14

CEREBROSPINAL FLUID VALUES IN VERY-LOW-BIRTH-WEIGHT INFANTS ON BASIS OF BIRTH WEIGHT

	≤1000 g		1001–1500 g	
	Mean ± SD	**Range**	**Mean ± SD**	**Range**
Birth weight (g)	763 ± 115	550–980	1278 ± 152	1,020–1,500
Gestational age (weeks)	26 ± 1.3	24–28	29 ± 1.4	27–33
Leukocytes/mm³	4 ± 3	0–14	6 ± 9	0–44
Erythrocytos/mm³	w	0–19,050	786 ± 1,879	0–9750
PMN leukocytes (%)	6 ± 15	0–66	9 ± 17	0–60
MN leukocytes (%)	86 ± 30	34–100	85 ± 28	13–100
Glucose (mg/dL)	61 ± 34	29–217	59 ± 21	31–109
Protein (mg/dL)	150 ± 56	95–370	132 ± 3	45–227

PMN, polymorphonuclear; MN mononuclear.
Modified from Rodriquez et al. (1990).

TABLE I.15

CEREBROSPINAL FLUID VALUES IN VERY-LOW-BIRTH-WEIGHT INFANTS (1,001–1,500 G) BY CHRONOLOGIC AGE

	Postnatal Age (days)					
	0–7		**8–28**		**29–84**	
Component	**Mean ± SD**	**Range**	**Mean ± SD**	**Range**	**Mean ± SD**	**Range**
Birth weight (g)	1,428 ± 107	1,180–1,500	1,245 ± 162	1,020–1,480	1,211 ± 86	1,080–1,300
Gestational age at birth (weeks)	31 ± 1.5	28–33	29 ± 1.2	27–31	29 ± 0.7	27–29
Leukocytes/mm³	4 ± 4	1–10	7 ± 11	0–44	8 ± 8	0–23
Erythrocytes/mm³	407 ± 853	0–2,450	1,101 ± 2,643	0–9,750	661 ± 1,198	0–3,800
PMN (%)	4 ± 10	0–28	10 ± 19	0–60	11 ± 19	0–48
Glucose (mg/dL)	74 ± 19	50–96	59 ± 23	39–109	47 ± 13	31–76
Protein (mg/dL)	136 ± 35	85–176	137 ± 46	54–227	122 ± 47	45–187

Modified from Rodriquez et al. (1990).

TABLE I.16

THYROID FUNCTION IN FULL-TERM AND PRETERM INFANTS

	Serum T_4 Concentration in Premature and Term Infants							Serum-Free T_4 Index in Premature and Term Infants		
	Estimated Gestational Age (weeks)									
	30–31	**32–33**	**34–35**	**36–37**	**Term**	**30–31**	**32–33**	**34–35**	**36–37**	**Term**
Cord										
Mean	6.5*	7.5‡	6.7‡	7.5	8.2			5.6	5.6	5.9
SD	1	2.1	1.2	2.8	1.8			1.3	2	1.1
N	3	8	18	17	17			12	10	14

(continued)

TABLE I.16

THYROID FUNCTION IN FULL-TERM AND PRETERM INFANTS (CONTINUED)

	Serum T_4 Concentration in Premature and Term Infants					Serum-Free T_4 Index in Premature and Term Infants				
	Estimated Gestational Age (weeks)									
	30–31	32–33	34–35	36–37	Term	30–31	32–33	34–35	36–37	Term
12–72 Hours Old										
Mean	11.5[‡]	12.3[‡]	12.4[‡]	15.5[†]	19	13.1[§]	12.9[§]	15.5[§]	17.1	19.7
SD	2.1	3.2	3.1	2.6	2.1	2.4	2.7	3	3.5	3.5
N	12	18	17	15	6	12	14	14	14	6
3–10 Days Old										
Mean	7.7[‡]	8.5[‡]	10[‡]	12.7[†]	15.9	8.3[§]	9[§]	12[¶]	15.1	16.2
SD	1.8	1.9	2.4	2.5	3	1.9	1.8	2.3	0.7	3.2
N	7	8	9	9	29	6	9	5	4	11
11–20 Days Old										
Mean	7.5[†]	8.3[‡]	10.5	11.2	12.2	8[#]	9.1[¶]	11.8	11.3	12.1
SD	1.8	1.6	1.8	2.9	2	1.6	1.9	2.7	1.9	2
N	5	11	9	9	8	5	8	8	5	8
21–45 Days Old										
Mean	7.8[‡]	8[‡]	9.3[‡]	11.4	12.1	8.4[#]	9[¶]	10.9		11.1
SD	1.5	1.7	1.3	4.2	1.5	1.4	1.6	2.8		1.4
N	11	17	13	5	5	11	17	5		5
46–90 Days Old			30–73				34–35			
Mean		9.6			10.2	9.4				9.7
SD		1.7			1.9	1.4				1.5
N		16			17	13				10

For comparison of premature and term infants (t test; * $p < 0.05$; ‡ $p < 0.001$; † $p < 0.005$; § $p = 0.001$; ¶ $p = 0.01$; # $p = 0.005$.
Adapted from Cuestas (1978).

(FISH) to detect syndromes that are not visible to the naked eye. The FISH process allows fluorescent-coated DNA probes to detect submicroscopic chromosomal deletions. It can be used with interphase and metaphase cells. This test is faster than high-resolution karyotyping (it still could take up to several weeks to complete). This test can provide a quick diagnosis to infants with trisomy 13, 18, 21, or Turner syndrome (Bajaj & Gross 2011; Gomella et al., 2009; Martin et al., 2011; McLean, 2005).

Bone marrow cells may be analyzed for chromosomes if a more rapid evaluation is required. Skin fibroblast analysis is required when an infant has been transfused, making lymphocyte analysis inaccurate. In cases such as stillbirth, tissue biopsy specimens can be used for chromosome testing because viable lymphocytes are absent (Hamilton & Wynshaw-Boris, 2009).

Sweat Chloride Test

The sweat chloride test is used to evaluate for and confirm the diagnosis of cystic fibrosis. During the procedure the skin is stimulated with pilocarpine and a small electrical current for 5 minutes. The sweat is collected on a 2 × 2-inch gauze pad or filter paper for 30 minutes. Over this 30-minute period, 75 mg of sweat must be produced to ensure an appropriate sweat rate (National Committee for Clinical Laboratory Standards, 1994). A sweat chloride level below 40 mEq/L is normal. Levels between 60 and 165 mEq/L are considered diagnostic for cystic fibrosis (Wilford & Taussig, 1998). Sweat tests can be inaccurate if an inadequate amount of sweat is produced; if the sweat evaporates; or if the patient has edema.

Comparative Genomic Hybridization or Chromosomal Microarray Analysis

The comparative genomic hybridization (CGH) and chromosomal microarray analysis (CMA) detects chromosomal deletions or duplication; this cytogenetic technique is relatively new. CGH/CMA compares reference standard DNA to the patient's DNA through a florescent technique. This test compares hundreds of regions across the entire genome to assess for the number of differences. It commonly assesses for microdeletion and microduplication, subtelomeric, and pericentromeric regions (Gomella et al., 2009).

Newborn Screening

Every infant born in a hospital in the United States under goes newborn screening. Newborn screening is done before leaving the hospital usually about day of 1 or 2. Some states require follow-up at about 2 weeks. All states are required to screen for 26 health conditions according to the March of Dimes (MOD) (2012). In addition, the MOD recommends that each state screens for 31. Some states are known to screen for 50 and more. For more information on newborn screens, see http://www.marchofdimesusa.org/baby/bringing-home_newbornscreening.html (*Newborn Screening*, 2012).

GASTROINTESTINAL PROCEDURES

Barium Enema

A barium enema is used in the evaluation of the structure and function of the large intestine. The diagnosis of disorders such as Hirschsprung disease and meconium plug syndrome can easily be supported by the use of this procedure.

For the enema procedure, either air or a contrast solution (e.g., barium sulfate) is instilled and a series of films are taken under fluoroscopy. The infant must be well restrained, starting in the supine position. As the contrast solution is instilled, its flow through the bowel is observed as the infant's position is changed. A series of abdominal x-ray films should be taken once the bowel has been filled with contrast solution. Follow-up films may also be necessary to document evacuation of the contrast solution from the bowel. Evaluation of the bowel is essential after this procedure to prevent constipation or obstruction. Assessment of bowel elimination is an important nursing concern after barium enema.

Upper Gastrointestinal Series With Small Bowel Follow-Through

As with the barium enema, barium sulfate or some other water-soluble contrast solution is used for the upper GI series with small bowel follow-through. However, the contrast solution is swallowed so that the upper GI tract can be examined. The three main areas examined are (1) the esophagus (for size, patency, reflux, and presence of a fistula or swallowing abnormality), (2) the stomach (for anatomic abnormalities, patency, and motility), and (3) the small intestine (for strictures, patency, and function).

Follow-up x-ray films may be desirable to evaluate both the emptying ability of the stomach and intestinal motility as the contrast material moves through the small bowel. Again, care of the infant includes assessment of temperature and cardiac and respiratory status throughout the procedure. The nurse should be alert for reflux or vomiting, which can be accompanied by aspiration. Evacuation of contrast material from the bowel remains a concern after upper GI series with small bowel follow-through and should be monitored by the nurse. It is also possible for fluid to be pulled out of the vascular compartment and into the bowel, resulting in hypotension. It is imperative that the health care team assess the infant for signs of these complications.

Rectal Suction Biopsy

Rectal biopsy is a procedure commonly used to help determine the presence or absence of ganglion cells in the bowel (the latter condition is seen in Hirschsprung disease). Before a rectal biopsy, it is essential to obtain bleeding times, prothrombin time, partial thromboplastin time, and platelet counts, as well as a spun hematocrit, to ensure that the infant is in no danger of excessive bleeding.

The infant is positioned supine with the legs held toward the abdomen. Small specimens of rectal tissue from the mucosal and submucosal levels are excised with a suction blade apparatus inserted through the anus into the bowel. The section of the pathology department that deals with the composition of ganglion cells evaluates the specimens.

Care of the infant after rectal suction biopsy should focus on assessments for bleeding or intestinal perforation. These assessments should include evaluation of vital signs for increased heart rate or decreased blood pressure, fever, persistent guaiac-positive stools, or frank rectal bleeding.

Liver Biopsy

Open or closed liver biopsy may be required for neonates. Open liver biopsy is a surgical procedure that requires general anesthesia, whereas a closed liver biopsy may be done using local anesthesia. As with the rectal biopsy, coagulation studies are essential, including bleeding time, platelet count, and spun hematocrit. Preoperative care may include sedation of the infant, requiring frequent monitoring of vital signs. Throughout the procedure, assessment of vital signs is essential for identifying changes in hemodynamics or respiratory status. After the procedure, assessment of vital signs for signs and symptoms of hemorrhage is essential. Indications of hemorrhage include decreases in the hemoglobin and hematocrit, which makes laboratory monitoring an important element of postbiopsy care. The biopsy site must be evaluated for signs of active bleeding, ecchymosis, swelling, or infection.

GENITOURINARY PROCEDURES

Cystoscopy

Cystoscopy permits direct visualization of the urinary structures, including the bladder, urethra, and urethral orifices, allowing diagnosis of abnormalities in the structure of the bladder and urinary tract.

Cystoscopy is performed using general anesthesia. Preparation of the urethral opening with an antiseptic solution is followed by sterile draping. The lubricated cystoscope is inserted through the urethra, and the urinary structures are examined.

As with any patient who has had anesthesia, postprocedural care includes vital sign assessment. However, particular attention should be paid to assessing for adequate urinary output, the presence of hematuria, and signs of infection (Pagana & Pagana, 2013).

Excretory Urography and Intravenous Pyelography

Excretory urography and intravenous pyelography complement cystoscopic evaluation because they allow the examiner not only to evaluate structures but also to focus on the function of those structures. Small amounts of contrast media are injected by the intravenous route, and as the contrast material is excreted through the urinary system, a sequence of x-ray films is taken. The configuration of organs and the rate of excretion of the contrast media are reflected in these films.

Excretory urography and intravenous pyelography are relatively safe for use in neonates and should cause no postprocedural complications.

Voiding Cystourethrogram

The purpose of a voiding cystourethrogram is to visualize the lower urinary tract after instillation of contrast media through urethral catheterization. The infant's bladder is emptied after catheterization and then filled with the contrast media. Serial films under fluoroscopy in a variety of positions are taken during voiding. After voiding, additional films are obtained. Pathologic results of a voiding cystourethrogram demonstrate residual urine in the bladder, such as with a neurogenic bladder, posterior valve obstructions, or vesicoureteral reflux.

As with cystoscopy, the infant should be evaluated for hematuria; the baby also should be checked for signs of infection (fever, cloudy or sedimented urine, foul-smelling urine) in the event of contaminated catheterization.

Electroencephalography

An electroencephalographic examination records the electrical activity of the brain. Numerous electrodes are placed at precise locations on the infant's head to record electrical impulses from various parts of the brain. This procedure can be important for diagnosing lesions or tumors, for identifying nonfunctional areas of the brain, or for pinpointing the focus of seizure activity.

The infant may require sedation during this procedure to prevent crying or movement. As much equipment as is safely possible should be removed to reduce electrical interference. Also, calming procedures, such as reducing light stimulation or warming the environment, may help quiet the infant during electroencephalography. The infant should be closely observed throughout the procedure for any signs of seizure activity.

RESPIRATORY PROCEDURES

Pulse Oximetry

Pulse oximetry is a widely used, noninvasive method of monitoring arterial blood oxygenation saturations (SaO_2). The SaO_2 is the ratio of oxygenated hemoglobin to total hemoglobin. A single probe, attached to an infant's extremity or digit, uses light emitted at different wavelengths, which is absorbed differently by saturated and unsaturated hemoglobin. The change in the light during arterial pulses is used to calculate the oxygen saturation. Pulse oximetry saturations reflect a more accurate measure of actual hemoglobin saturation. Saturations obtained by blood gas sample are calculated using a hemoglobin of 15 g% (Goetzman & Wennberg, 1999).

Proper placement of the probe should be assessed regularly, because movement, environmental light, edema, and diminished perfusion can reduce the accuracy of readings. The probe should be rotated every few hours to prevent skin breakdown at the site.

End-Tidal Carbon Dioxide Monitoring

End-tidal carbon dioxide (CO_2) monitoring is used routinely in pediatrics and in adult intensive care units. Its use in neonates, especially the smaller baby, is not yet practical as a continuing therapy because the adapters are heavy and create excess dead space in the ventilator system. End-tidal CO_2 monitoring is most useful during intubation procedures for determining if endotracheal intubation rather than esophageal intubation has occurred (Goetzman & Wennberg, 1999; Yorgin & Rhee, 1998).

Bronchoscopy

Bronchoscopy of the newborn is performed to visualize the upper and lower airways and to collect diagnostic specimens. The procedure can be done in the NICU using a flexible bronchoscope, or it can be performed under general anesthesia in the operating room using either a flexible or rigid bronchoscope. The flexible bronchoscope is preferable for examining the lower airways of an intubated patient or for examination of a patient with mandibular hypoplasia. A rigid bronchoscope is more advantageous in situations requiring removal of foreign bodies and for evaluation of patients with H-type tracheoesophageal fistula, laryngotracheoesophageal clefts, and bilateral abductor paralysis of the vocal cords (Wood, 1998). Examination of structures by direct visualization provides the opportunity to identify congenital anomalies, obstructions, masses, or mucous plugs and to evaluate stridor or respiratory dysfunction.

Bronchoscopy done at the bedside requires the nurse to assist with positioning, sedation, and monitoring of vital signs. Whether the infant undergoes flexible or rigid bronchoscopy, respiratory and cardiovascular monitoring should be continued in the immediate postprocedural period. Possible complications related to these procedures include bronchospasm, laryngeal spasms, laryngeal edema, or pneumothorax or bradycardia resulting in hypoxia.

SUMMARY

Marked technical advances over the past two decades have produced a variety of imaging methods for the diagnosis, treatment, and evaluation of neonates. Sizable expenditures have been directed toward improving image presentation and quality on the assumption that a trained clinical eye can make diagnostic use of the data provided. Investigations are useful only insofar as they reduce the diagnostic uncertainty. The final product of any radiologic imaging procedure is not a set of photographic pictures, but a diagnostic opinion that should be beneficial to the infant's management. Before initiating any imaging method, physicians should consider whether further information is really needed, and they should select the imaging technique that will give the required information with sufficient reliability and with minimal risk to the patient.

The value of any diagnostic imaging examination must be balanced against the potential hazards. In addition to care of the newborn during and after a procedure, nursing care of newborns and infants undergoing diagnostic procedures requires a knowledge of the expected outcomes and methods so that the best result possible is obtained. Nurses also must be knowledgeable about normal values for the laboratory tests commonly used in the care of newborns and infants.

REFERENCES

Abramoff, M. D., Van Gils, A. P., Jansen, G. H., & Mourits, M. P. (2000). MRI dynamic color mapping: A new quantitative technique for imaging soft tissue motion in the orbit. *Investigative Ophthalmology Visual Science, 41*(11), 3256–3260.

Alpen, E. L. (1998). *Radiation biophysics* (2nd ed.). San Diego, CA: Academic Press.

Bajaj, K., & Gross, S. (2011). Genetic aspects of perinatal disease and prenatal diagnosis. In R. Martin, A. Fanaroff, & M. Walsh (Eds.), *Neonatal-perinatal medicine* (9th ed.). St. Louis, MO: Elsevier Mosby.

Behrman, R. E. (1977). *Neonatal-perinatal diseases of the fetus and infant* (2nd ed.). St. Louis, MO: Mosby.

Bellenger, N. G., Burgess, M. I., Ray, S. G., Lahiri, A., Coats, A. J., Cleland, J. G., & Pennell, D. J. (2000). Comparison of left ventricular ejection fraction and volumes in heart failure by echocardiography, radionuclide ventriculography and cardiovascular magnetic resonance; are they interchangeable? *European Heart Journal, 21*(16), 1387–1396. doi:10.1053/euhj.2000.2011

Bushong, S. C. (1999). *Diagnostic ultrasound: Essentials of medical imaging series*. New York, NY: McGraw-Hill.

Bushong, S. C. (2000). *Computed tomography: Essentials of medical imaging series*. New York, NY: McGraw-Hill.

Bushong, S. C. (2003). *Magnetic resonance imaging: Physical and biological principles* (3rd ed.). St. Louis, MO: Mosby.

Bushong, S. C. (2013). *Radiologic science for technologists: Physics, biology, and protection* (10th ed.). St. Louis, MO: Elsevier Mosby.

Cooke, R., Hollis, B., Conner, C., Watson, D., Werkman, S., & Chesney, R. (1990). Vitamin D and mineral metabolism in the very low birth weight infant receiving 400 IU of vitamin D. *Journal of Pediatrics, 116*(3), 423–428.

Cornblath, M., & Schwartz, R. (Eds.). (1976). *Disorders of carbohydrate metabolism* (2nd ed.). Philadelphia, PA: WB Saunders.

Cuestas, R. A. (1978, June). Thyroid function in healthy premature infants. *Journal of Pediatrics, 92*(6), 963–967.

Dickinson, J. C., Rosenblum, H., & Hamilton, P. B. (1970). Ion exchange chromatography of the free amino acids in the plasma of infants under 2,500 gm at birth. *Pediatrics, 45*, 606.

Dort, J. C., Sadler, D., Hu, W., Wallace, C., La Forge, P., & Sevick, R. (2001). Screening for cerebellopontine angle tumours: Conventional MRI vs T2 fast spin echo MRI. *Canadian Journal Neurological Sciences, 28*(1), 47–50.

Dowd, S. B., & Tilson, E. R. (1999). *Practical radiation protection and applied radiobiology* (2nd ed.). Philadephia, PA: Saunders.

Drummond, L. M. (1979). Creatine phosphokinase levels in the newborn and their use in screening for Duchenne muscular dystrophy. *Archives of Disease in Childhood, 54*, 362–366.

Erenberg, F. (2011). Fetal cardiac physiology and fetal cardiovascular assessment. In R. Martin, A. Fanaroff, & M. Walsh (Eds.), *Neonatal-perinatal medicine* (9th ed.). St. Louis, MO: Elsevier Mosby.

Fanaroff, A., & Martin, R. (1987). *Neonatal-perinatal medicine: Diseases of the fetus and infant* (4th ed.). St. Louis, MO: Mosby.

Fanaroff, A., & Martin, R. (2002). *Neonatal-perinatal medicine: Diseases of the fetus and infant* (7th ed.). St. Louis, MO: Mosby.

Fanaroff, A. A., & Martin, R. J. (Eds.). (1997). *Neonatal-perinatal medicine: Diseases of the fetus and infant* (6th ed.). St. Louis, MO: Mosby.

Fanaroff, A. A., & Martin, R. J. (2002). *Neonatal-perinatal medicine* (7th ed.). Philadelphia, PA: WB Saunders.

Flanagan, M. F., Yeager, S. B., & Weindling, S. N. (2005). Cardiac disease. In M. G. MacDonald, M. D. Mullett, & M. K. Seshia (Eds.), *Avery's neonatology pathophysiology & management of the newborn* (6th ed.). Philadelphia, PA: Lippincott Williams & Wilkins.

Fogel, M. A., Rychik, J., Chin, A. J., Hubbard, A., & Weinberg, P. M. (2001). Evaluation and follow-up of patients with left ventricular apical to aortic conduits with 2D and 3D magnetic resonance imaging and Doppler echocardiography: A new look at an old operation. *American Heart Journal, 141*(4), 630–636.

Glass, E. J., Hume, R., Hendry, G. M., Strange, R. C., & Forfar, J. O. (1982). Plasma alkaline phosphatase activity in rickets of prematurity. *Archives of Disease in Childhood, 57*, 373–376.

Goetzman, B. W., & Wennberg, R. P. (1999). *Neonatal intensive care handbook* (3rd ed.). St. Louis, MO: Mosby.

Gomella, T. L., Cunningham, M. D., & Eyal, F. G. (2009). *Neonatology: Management, procedures, on-call problems, diseases, and drugs* (6th ed.). New York, NY: McGraw-Hill.

Hamilton, B. A., & Wynshaw-Boris, A. (2009). Basic genetics and patterns of inheritance. In R. K. Creasy, R. Resnik, J. D. Iam, C. J. Lockwood, & T. Moore (Eds.), *Creasy and Resnik's maternal-fetal medicine: Principles and practice* (6th ed.). Philadelphia, PA: Saunders Elsevier.

Heck, L. J., & Erenberg, A. (1987, January). Serum glucose levels in term neonates during the first 48 hours of life. *Pediatric Research, 110*(1), 119–122.

Hilton, S., & Edwards, D. K. III. (2006). *Practical pediatric radiology* (3rd ed.). Philadephia, PA: Saunders Elsevier.

Huda, W., Chamberlain, C. C., Rosenbaum, A. E., & Garrisi, W. (2001). Radiation doses to infants and adults undergoing head CT examinations. *Medical Physics, 28*(3), 393–399.

Huppi, P. S., Murphy, B., Maier, S. E., Zientara, G. P., Inder, T. E., Barnes, P. D., & Volpe, J. J. (2001). Microstructural brain development after perinatal cerebral white matter injury assessed by diffusion tensor magnetic resonance imaging. *Pediatrics, 107*(3), 455–460.

Ichikawa, I. (1990). *Pediatric textbook of fluids and electrolytes*. Baltimore, MD: Williams & Wilkins.

Juhl, J. H., Crummy, A. B., & Kuhlman, J. E. (1998). *Paul and Juhl's essentials of radiologic imaging* (7th ed.). Philadelphia, PA: Lippincott-Raven.

Klaus, M. H., & Fanaroff, A. A. (2001). *Care of the high-risk neonate* (5th ed.). Philadelphia, PA: WB Saunders.

Klaus, M. H., & Fanaroff, A. A. (2002). *Neonatal-perinatal medicine: Diseases of the fetus and infant* (6th ed.). St. Louis, MO: Mosby.

Krishnamoorthy, K. S., Soman, T. B., Takeoka, M., & Schaefer, P. W. (2000). Diffusion-weighted imaging in neonatal cerebral infarction: Clinical utility and follow-up. *Journal of Child Neurology, 15*(9), 592–602.

Kuller, J. A., & Cefalo, R. C. (1996). *Prenatal diagnosis and reproductive genetics*. St. Louis, MO: Mosby.

Lansberg, M. G., O'Brien, M. W., Tong, D. C., Moseley, M. E., & Albers, G. W. (2001). Evolution of cerebral infarct volume assessed by diffusion-weighted magnetic resonance imaging. *Archives of Neurology, 58*(4), 613–617.

Lewis, P. J., Siegel, A., Siegel, A. M., Studholme, C., Sojkova, J., Roberts, D. W., . . . Williamson, P. D. (2000). Does performing image registration and subtraction in ictal brain SPECT help localize neocortical seizures? *Journal of Nuclear Medicine, 41*(10), 1619–1626.

Lichtenstein, P., Specker, B. L., Tsang, R. C., Mimouni, F., & Gormley, C. (1986). Calcium-regulating hormones and minerals from birth to 18 months of age: A cross-sectional study. I. Effects of sex, race, age, season, and diet on vitamin D status. *Pediatrics, 77*, 883–890.

Liebman, J., & Plonsey, R. (1977). Electrocardiography. In A. J. Moss, F. H. Adams, & G. C. Emmanouilides. (Eds.), *Heart disease in infants, children and adolescents* (2nd ed.). Baltimore, MD: Williams & Wilkins.

Lin, J. W., Laine, A. F., & Bergmann, S. R. (2001). Improving pet-based physiological quantification through methods of wavelet denoising. *IEEE Transactions on Biomedical Engineering, 48*(2), 202–212.

March of Dimes. (2012). *Bringing baby home*. Retrieved from http://www.marchofdimesusa.org/baby/bringinghome_newbornscreening.html

Martin, R., Fanaroff, A., & Walsh, M. (2011). *Neonatal-perinatal medicine* (9th ed.). St. Louis, MO: Elsevier Mosby.

McLean, S. D. (2005). Congenital anomalies. In M. G. MacDonald, M. D. Mullett, & M. K. Seshia (Eds.), *Avery's neonatology pathophysiology & management of the newborn* (6th ed.). Philadephia, PA: Lippincott Williams & Wilkins.

Meites, S. (1975, January). Normal total plasma calcium in the newborn. *Critical Reviews of Clinical Laboratory Sciences,* 6(1), 1–18.

Meites, S. (Ed.). (1997). *Pediatric clinical chemistry: A survey of normals, methods, and instruments*. Washington, DC: American Association for Clinical Chemistry.

Naidoo, B. T. (1968, September 14). The cerebrospinal fluid in the healthy newborn infant. *South African Medical Journal, 42*(35), 933–935.

National Committee for Clinical Laboratory Standards. (1994). *Sweat testing: Sample collection and quantitative analysis: Approved guideline*. Wayne, PA: The Committee.

National Council on Radiation Protection and Measurements. (1993a). *Risk estimates for radiation protection* (NCRP Report No. 15). Bethesda, MD: National Council on Radiation Protection.

National Council on Radiation Protection and Measurements. (1993b). *Research needs for radiation protection* (NCRP Report No. 117). Bethesda, MD: National Council on Radiation Protection.

National Council on Radiation Protection and Measurements. (1993c). *A practical guide to the determination of human exposure to radiofrequency fields* (NCRP Report No. 119). Bethesda, MD: National Council on Radiation Protection.

Neches, W., & Platt, M. (1968). Cerebrospinal fluid LDH in 257 children. *Pediatrics, 41*, 1097–1103.

Nelson, N., Finnstrom, O., & Larsson, L. (1987). Neonatal reference values for ionized calcium, phosphate and magnesium. Selection of reference population by optimality criteria. *Scandinavian Journal of Clinical Laboratory Investigations, 47*(2), 111–117.

Newborn screening. (2012). Retrieved from http://www.marchofdimesusa.org/baby/bringinghome_newbornscreening.html

Nolte, U. G., Finsterbusch, J., & Frahm, J. (2000). Rapid isotropic diffusion mapping without susceptibility artifacts: Whole brain studies using diffusion-weighted single-shot steam MR imaging. *Magnetic Resonance in Medicine, 44*(5), 731–736.

Pagana, K. D., & Pagana, T. J. (2013). *Mosby's diagnostic and laboratory test reference* (11th ed.). St. Louis, MO: Elsevier Mosby.

Peled, S., & Yeshurun, Y. (2001). Superresolution in MRI: Application to human white matter fiber tract visualization by diffusion tensor imaging. *Magnetic Resonance in Medicine, 45*(1), 29–35.

Peterson, B. S., Vohr, B., Staib, L. H., Cannistraci, C. J., Dolberg, A., Schneider, K. C., . . . Ment, L. R. (2000). Regional brain volume abnormalities and long-term cognitive outcome in preterm infants. *Journal of the American Medical Association, 284*(15), 1939–1947.

Reading, R. F., Ellis, R., & Fleetwood, A. (1990). Plasma albumin and total protein in preterm babies from birth to eight weeks. *Early Human Development, 22*, 81.

Rodriquez, A. F., Kapian, S. L., & Mason, E. O. (1990). Cerebrospinal fluid values in the very low birth weight infant. *Journal of Pediatrics, 116*, 871.

Rushe, T. M., Rifkin, L., Stewart, A. L., Townsend, J. P., Roth, S. C., Wyatt, J. S., & Murray, R. M. (2001). Neuropsychological outcome at adolescence of very preterm birth and its relation to brain structure. *Developmental Medicine and Child Neurology, 43*(4), 226–233.

Schaffer, A. J. (1971). *Diseases of the newborn* (3rd ed.). Philadelphia, PA: WB Saunders.

Schierlitz, L., Dumanli, H., Robinson, J. N., Burrows, P. E., Schreyer, A. G., Kikinis, R., . . . Tempany, C. M. (2001). Three-dimensional magnetic resonance imaging of fetal brains. *Lancet, 357*(9263), 1177–1178.

Shenai, J. P., Chytil, F., Jhaveri, A., & Stahlman, M. T. (1981, August). Plasma vitamin A and retinol-binding protein in premature and term neonates. *Journal of Pediatrics, 99*(2), 302–305.

Sie, L. T., Barkhof, F., Lafeber, H. N., Valk, J., & van der Knaap, M. S. (2000). Value of fluid-attenuated inversion recovery sequences in early MRI of the brain in neonates with a perinatal hypoxic-ischemic encephalopathy. *European Radiology, 10*(10), 1594–1601.

Sinson, G., Bagley, L. J., Cecil, K. M., Torchia, M., McGowan, J. C., Lenkinski, R. E., . . . Grossman, R. I. (2001). Magnetization transfer imaging and proton MR spectroscopy in the evaluation of axonal injury: Correlation with clinical outcome after traumatic brain injury. *American Journal of Neuroradiology, 22*(1), 143–151.

Statlan, B.E., et al. (1978). *Clinical Chemistry, 24*, 1010.

Swischuk, L. E. (1997a). *Imaging of the newborn, infant, and young child* (4th ed.). Baltimore, MD: Williams & Wilkins.

Swischuk, L. E. (1997b). *Differential diagnosis in pediatric radiology* (3th ed.). Baltimore, MD: Williams & Wilkins.

Tierney, M. C., Varga, M., Hosey, L., Grafman, J., & Braun, A. (2001). PET evaluation of bilingual language compensation following early childhood brain damage. *Neuropsychologia, 39*(2), 114–121.

Tietz, N. W. (Ed.). (1988). *Textbook of clinical chemistry*. Philadelphia, PA: WB Saunders.

Treves, S. T. (1995). *Pediatric nuclear medicine* (2nd ed.). New York, NY: Springer.

Verklan, M., & Walden, M. (2004). *Core curriculum for neonatal intensive care nursing* (3rd ed.). St. Louis, MO: Elsevier Mosby.

Wallach, J. B. (1983). *Interpretation of pediatric tests*. Boston, MA: Little, Brown.

Weissleder, R., & Mahmood, U. (2001). Molecular imaging. *Radiology, 219*(2), 316–333.

Wiesmann, M., & Seidel, G. (2000). Ultrasound perfusion imaging of the human brain. *Stroke, 31*(10), 2421–2425.

Wilford, B. S., & Taussig, L. M. (1998). Cystic fibrosis: General overview. In L. M. Taussig & L. I. Landau (Eds.), *Pediatric respiratory medicine*. St. Louis, MO: Mosby.

Wood, R. E. (1998). Diagnostic and therapeutic procedures in pediatric pulmonary patients. In L. M. Taussig & L. I. Landau (Eds.), *Pediatric respiratory medicine*. St. Louis, MO: Mosby.

Yorgin, P. D., & Rhee, K. H. (1998). Gas exchange and acid-base physiology. In L. M. Taussig & L. I. Landau (Eds.), *Pediatric respiratory medicine*. St Louis, MO: Mosby.

Zahka, K. G. (2011). Approach to the neonate with cardiovascular disease. In R. Martin, A. Fanaroff, & M. Walsh (Eds.), *Neonatal-perinatal medicine* (9th ed.). St. Louis, MO: Elsevier Mosby.

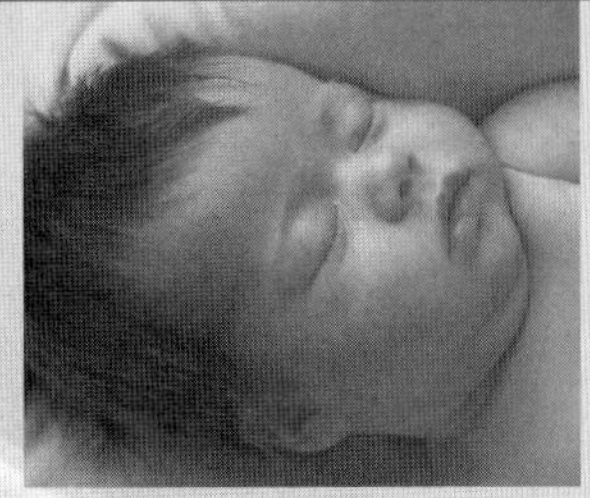

11

Developmental Care for the Sick and Preterm Infant

■ Caitlin Bradley and Rachel Ritter

While neonatal intensive care units and special care nurseries (NICU/SCN) have prolonged the lives of babies, they are no match for the intrauterine environment that perfectly meets the physiologic and developmental needs of the fetus through stimulation of senses, and the influence of maternal biorhythms (White, 2011). Disability and neurosensory impairment of NICU survivors is estimated at 5% to 15% for preterm infants and another 50% to 70% for infants born at less than 1.5 kg (Legendre, Burtner, Martinez, & Crowe, 2011; Spruill Turnage & Papile, 2012). To improve neurodevelopmental outcomes, and counter any discrepancies between the intrauterine environment and the NICU/SCN, the concept of developmental care was conceived.

Developmental care of infants was first introduced in the late 1970s. This eventually led to the more contemporary concept of individualized developmental care (IDC). IDC is a holistic approach to patient care delivery (Legendre et al., 2011), offering universally recognized benefits. It combines the delicate balance of providing the necessary medical and nursing care, while simultaneously maintaining sensitivity to the developmental needs of both the infant and the family. When IDC is delivered, the provider adapts to the dynamic needs of the infant–family team, and responds to the behavior and reactions of the neonate and the family.

Essential aspects of developmental care, such as providing boundaries and supporting the baby in flexion, are routinely provided by health care institutions delivering care to neonates. This is because developmental care is anecdotally felt to have both short- and long-term benefits. Short-term benefits include improved stability in patient condition and some report that the time to endotracheal extubation can be reduced (Pickler et al., 2010). Long-term benefits of developmental care include improved organization and better developmental outcomes (Pickler et al., 2010).

Many factors guide developmental care practice including (1) education and training of the health care providers and parents, (2) patient assessment, (3) equipment and resources, and (4) the infant's family (through a concept known as family-centered care [FCC]). Nurses are in a key position to serve as the primary force behind developmental care. However, the successful implementation of developmental care requires input and cooperation from all disciplines.

EDUCATION AND TRAINING OF HEALTH CARE PROVIDERS AND PARENTS

IDC is a philosophy of care guided by the infant's response to a stimulus as manifested by the infant's behavior and physiologic signs. Modifications in care are made by health care providers or parents in response to the dynamic changes of the infant. Sharp assessment skills are required to identify stress signs and respond to the infant in real time. To facilitate the delivery of IDC, common signs of stress in the neonate must be recognized by those caring for the infant. Health care providers and the family must receive adequate education to recognize the signs of stress and respond to it appropriately. Preparing those in contact with the infant will lead to earlier recognition of stress, which, in turn, will result in enhanced physiologic stability and improved outcomes.

Health Care Provider Education

Generally, basic nursing and medical education does not include developmental care of the sick neonate. Therefore the novice NICU/SCN provider must learn about developmental care as part of his or her workplace orientation through formal and informal instruction. Providers interested in expanding their knowledge base can do so through a number of different venues such as formal training programs, learning modules and conferences.

In 1986, the Newborn Individualized Developmental Care and Assessment Program (NIDCAP) (Als, Lawhon, & Brown, 1986) was unveiled, transforming NICU/SCN care. NIDCAP is certainly the most widely recognized formal training program, with national and international training centers and resources. NIDCAP provides rigorous training by experts in developmental care that leads to individual certification or unit-based certification. NIDCAP certification signifies that developmental care is a central focus or major goal of the individual or NICU/SCN. Individuals seeking NIDCAP certification must be prepared to spend a significant amount of time to gain and maintain the knowledge and expertise necessary to uphold the programs' standards. At minimum, health care institutions that wish to obtain NIDCAP certification must be (1) accredited, (2) have a NICU/SCN, and (3) employ at least one full-time employee with NIDCAP certification. To gain information on NIDCAP training centers and resources, one can visit http://www.nidcap.org/nidcap_training.aspx.

In addition to NIDCAP, a variety of training modules exist to facilitate training of developmental care skills. These training modules and conference information can be found in neonatal textbooks and online through nationally recognized groups such as the National Association of Neonatal Nurses (http://www.nann.org/education/content/education.html), Academy of Neonatal Nurses (http://www.academyonline.org/conference_schedule.html), Association of Women's Health Obstetrics and Neonatal Nurses (http://www.awhonn.org/awhonn/content.do;jsessionid=DDB2A13632825C1728226E93A49930C4?name=06_Events/06_Events_landing.htm), and internationally recognized groups such as the Council of International Neonatal Nurses (http://www.coinnurses.org/events.php). The learning modules are sometimes accompanied by posttests that can be used to confirm the acquisition of necessary information and developmental care skills.

Developmental care conferences, both national and international, are offered continuously throughout the year to health care providers. During these conferences health care providers are exposed to many types of programs and patient care devices to assist in providing developmental care. Moreover, conferences give health care providers the opportunity to network with other developmental care-minded individuals.

Parent Education

Parental involvement can alleviate the stress associated with their infant's hospitalization (Lanlehin, 2012) and helps to foster a partnership with parents to be active members of the health care team. Parent education is typically done at the bedside in real time using the infant's behavior as a guide. Educating parents in real time allows parents to receive immediate feedback from their infant about the effectiveness of their interventions.

Providers including nurses, nurse practitioners, physicians, and other multidisciplinary staff in the NICU/SCN should be equipped to provide parental education as it pertains to developmental care. Resources such as developmental care plans, books, and websites can help to supplement parental education. However, all reading materials should be prescreened by the health care provider to ensure that appropriate and accurate information is being given.

Multidisciplinary Approach

Health care providers caring for the neonate include, but are not limited to, nurses, nurse practitioners, physicians, speech therapy, occupational therapy, physical therapy, and dieticians. All providers, regardless of their discipline, are responsible for developmental care, and interventions among the providers should be consistent. Unit-based IDC education programs should address the whole interdisciplinary care team. Moreover, units dedicated to optimizing the infant's developmental care should provide educational offerings to the extended care team, including environmental services.

PATIENT ASSESSMENT

Goal of Developmental Care

In the NICU/SCN, infants use adaptive and maladaptive behaviors as they attempt to cope with the stimulation of this foreign environment. However, maladaptive behaviors can interfere with physiologic stability. IDC can help the premature or sick newborn cope with their surroundings and promote healthy adaption. The primary goal of IDC is the preservation of energy and the encouragement of self-regulation to achieve physiologic stability, weight gain, and optimal neurodevelopmental outcomes.

Recognition of Stress

The stress response of infants can be manifested very differently because infants are unique individuals. Also, because infants communicate nonverbally, the untrained observer may have difficulty recognizing the stress response. One infant may manifest stress through an autonomic mechanism such as irregular breathing, while another may exhibit an untoward motor response such as restlessness. Identifying stress requires time, training, and vigilance. By observing and "listening" to the infants' message, the health care provider and parent will be able to anticipate and intervene before the infant develops maladaptive (coping) behaviors.

Infants exhibit maladaptive behaviors through a disorganized fashion indicating that the infant is not coping well. If not corrected, these behaviors may become part of the infant's repertoire of routine stress responses (Legendre et al., 2011; Spruill Turnage & Papile, 2012). Moreover, maladaptive behaviors can be expressed by physiologic instability such as apnea which can be life threatening (Legendre et al., 2011; Spruill Turnage & Papile, 2012). A systems approach, divided into autonomic, motor and state systems, can be helpful to effectively assess the infant for signs of stress and the organization of behaviors (see Table II.1).

TABLE II.1

COPING BEHAVIORS: AUTONOMIC, MOTOR, AND STATE SYSTEMS

System Behaviors	Disorganized (Maladaptive)	Organization (Adaptive)
Autonomic System		
Respiratory	Tachypnea, irregular breathing pattern, apnea, bradypnea, sighing, gasping	Normal work of breathing, regular respiratory rate
Color	Pale, mottling, plethoric, cyanosis	Pink, no mottling
Visceral	Multiple coughs, sneezes, or yawns, hiccupping, gagging, grunting, straining, and vomiting	Absence of coughing, sneezing, yawning, hiccupping, gagging, grunting, straining, and vomiting
Related motor	Tremors, startles, twitching	Smooth movement, including flexion
Motor System		
Tone	Hypertonia, hypotonia, hyperflexion	Tone appropriate for postmenstrual age
Posture	Unable to maintain flexion, alignment	Flexion without supportive devices and smooth movement when stretching
Level of activity	Frequently moving, or no movement	Activity appropriate for postmenstrual age
State System		
Sleep	Restless, low cries, responsive to environment	Quiet, little response to environmental stimulus
Awake	Unfocused, gaze aversion, hyperalert with wide eyes, crying, eyes closed to avoid gaze, poor sleep times, difficult to console	Alert, focused on object or person, calms easily, consolable

From Brandon et al. (2007); Spruill Turnage and Papile (2012); and White (2011).

Responding to Stress

Pickler et al. (2010) report that when care is based on individual neurobehavioral responses, better regulation of motor and autonomic systems is observed (Pickler et al., 2010). Behavioral assessments should be done at regular intervals to observe the infant's response to the environment. This regular assessment of the infant serves as a baseline from which providers can identify individual stress responses.

Using the steps below, providers can gather detailed information about an infant's stress signs and response to interventions:

1. Observe behaviors
2. Intervene based on infant's behavioral cues (see Tables II.1 and II.2)
3. Observe responses to interventions
4. Adjust interventions as needed
5. Communicate and document the infant's stress response including adaptive and maladaptive behaviors, interventions used by the provider, and the responses to these interventions

Information gathered through these steps should be shared with the entire NICU/SCN team to ensure that IDC is seamless (Coughlin, Gibbins, & Hoath, 2009; Legendre et al., 2011; Nightlinger, 2011). The IDC plan should be displayed at each infant's bedside to optimize communication.

The Care Environment

NICU/SCN environments vary greatly from one institution to another, ranging from common rooms with multiple patients to newer units with private rooms. Private rooms afford greater control over the infant's environment and thus are becoming the new standard for providing ideal IDC. Regardless of the NICU/SCN design, however, each type of environment poses its own unique challenges (Brandon, Ryan, & Barnes, 2007). It is the responsibility of the care providers to examine their unit and implement changes to decrease light, sound, tactile, olfactory, and taste stimulation. For example, when seeking to reduce ambient noise, providers should take note of the location of the automatic paper towel dispensers. Automatic paper towel dispensers add high ambient noise and should not be placed near a patient's bed space. In addition, the location of the infant's bed space in relation to windows, doors and workstations, and exposure to light and sound will vary with placement of the bed space (see Table II.3).

EQUIPMENT AND RESOURCES

There are numerous devices available to aid in the developmental care of the sick newborn and/or preterm infant; some are used to maintain proper body alignment/position and others to promote self-regulation and appropriate sensory-motor experiences (Nightlinger, 2011). Whatever the

TABLE II.2

DECREASING STIMULATION IN THE NICU/SCN

Preventative measures during routine care:

- Avoid disruption of sleep through clustered care
- Speak to baby, quietly, prior to cares
- Use slow movements when moving baby during transitions
- Position hands close to mouth
- Hand containment
- Offer pacifier for nonnutritive sucking
- Nesting, boundaries, swaddling to maintain alignment, flexion and containment while still allowing for movement
- Reduce light, noise, and activity at the bedside (phones and pagers on vibrate)
- Kangaroo care and holding by family
- Offer and pace feedings based on baby's abilities

IDC in the ICU:

- Provide preventative measures as appropriate
- If unable to swaddle because of needed observation, positioning aids are helpful to provide boundaries and flexion and maintain alignment
- Covering of eyes when bright lights are needed during exams or interventions
- Encouraging quiet tones when speaking in the NICU/SCN environment
- Use of ear protection while exposed to NICU/SCN noise, such as mechanical ventilation or talking near the bedside
- Pharmacologic and nonpharmacologic treatment of pain
- During exams or intervention: swaddle or nest parts of the body not needed for exam or intervention

From Brandon et al. (2007); Nightlinger (2011); Spruill Turnage and Papile (2012); and White (2011).

TABLE II.3

ENVIRONMENTAL STIMULI

Sense	Recommendations
Light	For existing NICU/SCNs: Ambient lighting recommendations: 10–600 lux For new NICU/SCNs: Ambient lighting 10–20 lux Cover or shield eyes when not providing tactile stimulation Eyes should be covered when lights cannot be dimmed
Sound	Monitor random noise levels AAP recommends < 50 dBA to avoid physiologic stress and autonomic instability Avoid noise inside of closed isolette, such as music boxes. Encourage ability to hear mother's voice Limit the amount of talking, alarms, and other environmental noises around the infant's sleep space Provide ear protection when loud ambient noise is unavoidable
Touch	Kangaroo care: Recommended minimum of 1 hour Touch gently Avoid stroking the baby Offering containment with hands, nests/boundaries or by swaddling with a blanket

Taste/Oral	Nonnutritive sucking (NNS)
	  Offer pacifier
	  Use breast if mother has just pumped (unless gagging, retching, or grimacing is observed)
	Oral feeding is a complex task
	  Feeding maturation starts at 32 weeks, with nutritive suck at 32–36 weeks
	  Use readiness cues to guide oral feeding
	  Safe feeding requires coordination of suck, swallow, and breathing
	  Babies should be assessed for lip closure, cheek tone, sucking, posture, tone, reflexes, and movement
	Oral aversion develops over time due to negative stimulus in the mouth (endotracheal tube, suctioning)
	  Avoid offering pacifier *only* during times when infant is exposed to a painful stimuli
	  Consult speech therapy (early on) to provide interventions to avoid or minimize oral aversion
	Babies respond to breast milk and pleasant odors (smell of the mother or father)
	  Ask parents to bring a blanket or stuffed animal they've slept with
	Avoid noxious smells such as harsh detergents, cigarette smoke, and disinfectants
	  If parents smoke, encourage cessation
	  If they smoke, encourage them to shower and change after smoking

From Brandon et al. (2007); Spruill Turnage and Papile (2012); and White (2011).

purpose, proper positioning is important to both short-term and long-term development (Malusky & Donze, 2011; Nightlinger, 2011; Sweeney & Gutierrez, 2002).

Use of Positioning Devices

Many premature and sick infants lay flat and with their head to the side, are hypotonic, and exhibit low activity, predisposing them to a number of positional abnormalities such as limb extension, external rotation, and abduction of joints. This poor positioning predisposes infants to bone deformation, muscle shortening, and decreased joint mobility (Sweeney & Gutierrez, 2002). Some common positional deformities observed in the NICU/SCN include spinal curvature, hip abduction, scapular adduction, and positional head shape deformities (Sweeney & Gutierrez, 2002) (see Table II.4).

Ideally, a neonate's position should mimic the fetal position: flexed, contained, and midline (Nightlinger, 2011). Proper positioning promotes normal musculoskeletal development. Furthermore, neutral head alignment can decrease incidence of intraventricular hemorrhage (Malusky & Donze, 2011) by preventing changes to cerebral blood flow as well as promoting normal head shape development.

Positioning devices can be used to support and maintain proper body alignment with physiologic flexion in a neutral position. General rules to consider when positioning the NICU/SCN patient using supportive devices include (1) neutral head alignment or with chin slightly tucked, (2) scapular abduction with hands midline, (3) rounded lower back, and (4) symmetric hip flexion and neutral rotation (Sweeney & Gutierrez, 2002).

When using supportive devices, providers must be careful not to cause restriction of movement, as restrictive positioning can lead to joint compression, inadequate mechanical refinement, and the development of musculoskeletal abnormalities. Optimal positioning to promote musculoskeletal development in the NICU/SCN is described in Table II.4.

Always follow the manufacturer's instructions for the care and maintenance of any positioning devices used in the NICU/SCN. Clean the devices with the recommended cleaning agent to promote the integrity of the outer covering. Also, protective covers are recommended for some devices. These covers sometimes require special laundering. When special laundry services are not available, disposable covers should be used in their place to decrease the risk of infection transmission and to protect the

TABLE II.4

POSITIONING IN THE NICU/SCN

Body Part: Abnormal Alignment	Consequences and Limitations	Positioning for Prevention
Spinal: Exaggerated cervical lordosis and neck hyperextension	Difficulty with head centering, downward gaze and coordination of the hands to midline Impact: Head control development	Neutral midline neck position Avoid hyperextension
Extremity: Hip abduction	Shortened hip abductors Shortened iliotibial band Increased external tibial torsion Impact: Prevents movement in prone and sitting positions Impaired mobility, such as crawling, Development of out-toeing and wide gait	Maintain hips in neutral position with positional devices Rolls under legs while *supine* to encourage flexion and against thighs to prevent hip abduction While *prone,* place aid under hips to maintain pelvic tilt and hip flexion and support thighs with aid to prevent hip abduction
Extremity: Scapular adduction	Shoulder elevation and retraction Impact: Decreased movement of arms to midline Decreased arm and shoulder stability while prone Difficulty reaching Delayed rolling	Maintain rolled, rounded shoulders with rolls and positional devices Encourage hands to midline and mouth
Head: Dolichocephaly Scaphocephaly	Narrow head shape, anterior-posterior elongation Impact: Cosmetically unappealing Problems with vision, hearing Possible neurodevelopmental delay	Supine positioning and prone positioning
Head: Plagiocephaly	Occipital flattening Impact: Cosmetically unappealing Problems with vision, hearing Possible neurodevelopmental delay	Encourage head positioning on both sides while practicing back-to-sleep

From Kennedy and Long (2008) and Sweeney and Gutierrez (2002).

infant's skin as well as the device(s) shape and delicate construction.

Control of Stimulation

Development of the sensory and perceptual systems of infants occurs in a step-wise fashion: tactile and proprioceptive, vestibular, taste and smell, auditory, and finally visual (Nightlinger, 2011). NICU/SCN infants are frequently not prepared for the sensory input they are exposed to. Light, sound, touch, taste, and smell in the NICU/SCN are foreign to their developing systems. Care should be taken to minimize sensory and perceptual input before the baby is ready for the stimulation.

Environmental noise is a primary source of noxious stimuli in NICU/SCNs that is easily controlled. Isolettes are one of the main devices used to control sound as they provide a barrier to the outside world. Moreover, the padded portholes of isolettes allow access to the infant while concurrently ensuring a quiet environment when opening and closing. Thus, infants should be transferred to isolettes as soon as possible.

Also to reduce noise, ear covers can be employed when ambient sound levels are high, such as when an oscillator is being used for respiratory support and boundaries created with positioning devices can be used to decrease stimulation by blocking sound transmission.

Other sources of noise include phones and pagers. These items should be put on silent mode when near a patient's bedside.

Light is another frequently encountered source of noxious stimuli that can be easily reduced. To reduce light, isolettes can be covered, and light switches can be adapted, allowing lights to be dimmed. If dimming the lights is not a viable option, eye covers should be used when ambient lighting is greater than recommended, such as for phototherapy, examinations and procedures.

FAMILY-CENTERED CARE

FCC is the hallmark of high-quality neonatal and family care and an essential aspect of clinically sound care (McGrath, Samra, & Kenner, 2011). A primary function of the health care provider, regardless of discipline, is to partner with parents. Parents should be viewed as essential, active members of the baby's team and thus welcomed at the bedside 7 days per week, 24 hours a day. Parents should be encouraged to participate in rounds, attend regular family meetings, participate in caregiving that is individually appropriate for their infant, and be encouraged to advocate for their infant. They should be taught developmental care as soon as they are ready to participate in their infant's care. Encouraging parental participation fosters growth as a parent and as an advocate for their infant.

Furthermore, the development of a family advisory council or group has been shown to reveal important information of the parent experience (Landis, 2007). In these groups, family members share their NICU/SCN experience with staff members after hospital discharge. Information gained from this experience can be shared with staff to make positive changes in the NICU/SCN experience.

CONCLUSION

IDC is a holistic approach to patient care delivery (Legendre et al., 2011) with several goals, including achieving a balance between necessary medical and nursing care, promotion of the developmental needs of both the infant and family, preservation of energy, and the encouragement of self-regulation. Self-regulation, in turn, increases physiologic stability, weight gain, and optimal neurodevelopmental outcomes of NICU/SCN infants. To successfully integrate IDC into the NICU/SCN, education and training of the health care providers and parents are needed. This requires development of advanced infant assessment skills. Additionally, sufficient equipment, resources, and family involvement is essential to IDC's success. A major role of the bedside nurse is to facilitate developmental care; however, IDC requires a multidisciplinary approach, therefore all infant care providers, including the infant's parents, are responsible for its implementation.

While IDC is anecdotally felt to have both short- and long-term benefits, evidence to support its use is lacking. Nurses can fill this void by developing and participating in clinical studies whose aim it is to gain a better understanding of IDC.

REFERENCES

Academy of Neonatal Nurses: Conferences and Meetings. Retrieved from http://academyonline.org/conference_schedule.html

Als, H., Lawhon, G., & Brown, E. (1986). Individualized behavioral and environmental care for the very low birth weight preterm infant at risk for bronchopulmonary dysplasia: Neonatal intensive care unit and developmental outcome. *Pediatrics, 78*(6), 1123–1132.

Association of Women's Health Obstetrics and Neonatal Nurses. Retrieved from http://awhonn.org/awhonn/content.do;jsessionid=DDB2A13632825C1728226E93A49930C4?name=06_Events/06_Events_landing.htm

Brandon, D., Ryan, D., & Barnes, A. (2007). Effect of environmental changes on noise in the NICU/SCN. *Neonatal Network, 26*(4), 213–218.

Coughlin, M., Gibbons, S., & Hoath, S. (2009). Core measures for developmentally supportive care in neonatal intensive care units: Theory, precedence and practice. *Journal of Advanced Nursing, 65*(10), 2239–2248.

Council of International Neonatal Nurses. Retrieved from http://www.coinnurses.org/events.php.

Kennedy, E., & Long, T. (2008). The five essential elements for physical therapists providing services in the NICU/SCN. *Acute Care Perspectives, 17*(3), 2–6.

Landis, M. (2007). The many roles of families in "family centered care"-part IV. *Pediatric Nurse, 33*(3), 263–265.

Lanlehin, R. (2012). Factors associated with information satisfaction among parents of sick neonates in the neonatal unit. *Infant, 8*(2), 60–63.

Legendre, V., Burtner, P., Martinez, K., & Crowe, T. (2011). The evolving practice of developmental care in the neonatal unit: A systematic review. *Physical and Occupational Therapy in Pediatrics, 31*(3), 315–338.

Malusky, S., & Donze, A. (2011). Neutral head positioning in premature infants for intraventricular hemorrhage prevention: An evidence-based review. *Neonatal Network, 30*(6), 381–396.

McGrath, J., Samra, H., & Kenner, C. (2011). Family centered developmental care practices and research. *Journal of Perinatal and Neonatal Nursing, 25*(12), 165–170.

National Association of Neonatal Nurses. Retrieved from http://www.nann.org/education/content/education.html

Newborn Individualized Developmental Care and Assessment Program (NIDCAP). Retrieved from http://www.nidcap.org/nidcap_training.aspx

Nightlinger, K. (2011). Developmentally supportive care in the neonatal intensive care unit: An occupational therapist's role. *Neonatal Network, 30*(4), 243–248.

Pickler, R., McGrath, J., Reyna, B., McCain, N., Lewis, M., Cone, S., . . . Best, A. (2010). A model of neurodevelopment risk and protection for preterm infants. *Journal of Perinatal and Neonatal Nurses, 24*(4), 356–365.

Spruill Turnage, C., & Papile, L. (2012). Developmentally supportive care. In J. Cloherty, E. Eichenwald, A. Hansen, & A. Stark (Eds.), *Manual of neonatal care* (7th ed., pp. 166–177). Philadelphia, PA: Lippincott Williams & Wilkins.

Sweeney, J., & Gutierrez, T. (2002). Musculoskeletal implications of preterm positioning in the NICU/SCN. *Journal of Perinatal and Neonatal Nursing, 16*(1), 58–70.

White, R. (2011). The newborn intensive care unit environment of care: How we got here, where we're headed, and why. *Seminars in Perinatology, 35*, 2–7.

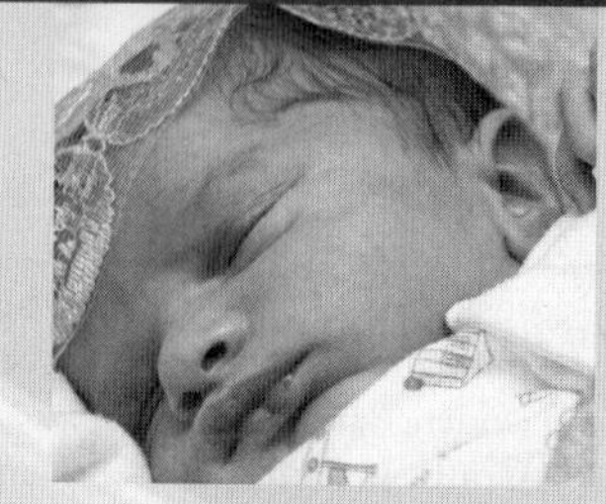

Neonatal Transport

III

■ Dorothy M. Mullaney

It has been estimated that there are over 65,000 transports of critically ill neonates in the United States each year (Karlsen, Trautman, Price-Douglas, & Smith, 2011). Neonatal transports have been described as a high-risk service due to the types of patients transported, the different environments the transport team must function in at each referring facility, the transport equipment itself, the mode of transportation, and the level of responsibility the transport team must assume as representatives of the receiving facility (American Academy of Pediatrics, Section of Transport Medicine, 2007; American Academy of Pediatrics & The American College of Obstetricians and Gynecologists, 2007; Bouchut, Van Lancker, Chritin, & Gueugniaud, 2011; Cornette, 2004a; Dulkerian, Douglas, & Taylor, 2011; Fenton, Leslie, & Skeoch, 2004; Leppälä, 2010). For the most part, neonatal transports represent a low-volume, high-acuity aspect of neonatal intensive care.

While in the process of providing expert care and stabilization to the neonate, members of the transport team are also expected to provide education to the team at the referring facility and communicate with the family in a manner that will form the basis of parent and family involvement in the care of their infant (Duritza, 2009; Hawthorne & Killen, 2006; Hogan & Logan, 2004; McNab, Richards, & Green, 1999; Steeper, 2002).

REGIONALIZATION OF NEONATAL CARE

The 1976 March of Dimes publication *Toward Improving the Outcome of Pregnancy, Recommendations for the Regional Development of Maternal and Neonatal Health Services* described the development of a regionalized perinatal health care system (Little, Horbar, Wachtel, Gluck, & Muri, 2010). The concept behind regionalization is to ensure effective and efficient patient flow with safe and quality care throughout the regional system (Rochefort & Lamothe, 2011; Staebler, 2011; Warner, Altimier, & Imhoff, 2002). These systems are generally defined geographically and within each geographic region there are facilities that provide varying levels of neonatal care, designated as Level I, Level II, Level III, or Level IV. The American Academy of Pediatrics ([AAP] 2004, 2012; AAP & ACOG, 2007) has defined these four levels of care as described in Table III.1. Any facility that cares for neonates, no matter their level designation, is expected to be capable of providing neonatal resuscitation and stabilizing an ill neonate until a transport team arrives to assume care (AAP, 2004). For the most part, the level III and level IV, or tertiary, facilities assume the responsibility of providing interfacility neonatal transports and outreach education for the regional program.

STABILIZATION BY THE REFERRING FACILITY

The first step in the transport process is recognizing the neonate who requires care at a higher level facility. The birth of an ill neonate requiring transport will be unexpected in most cases, and the local team must be able to quickly recognize this need and provide the appropriate initial care (Fenton et al., 2004). There are programs available, such as PCEP® (Kattwinkel et al., 2007), S.T.A.B.L.E.® (Karlsen, 2008), and ACoRN® (ACoRN Neonatal Society, 2009) that can be used as educational resources to train staff to care for unexpectedly ill neonates. Most regional programs will support one or two of these programs and the tertiary care unit should actively participate in training staff at the referring facilities to recognize and begin to stabilize the unexpectedly ill neonate.

Once a neonate had been identified as needing transport, the nurse practitioner or attending physician should contact the tertiary center to begin the transport process. While waiting for the transport team to arrive, the local team should continue with the stabilization process they have already begun, paying particular attention to thermoregulation, glucose homeostasis, maintaining oxygenation and ventilation, establishing vascular access if necessary and initiating antibiotic treatment if clinically indicated. In addition, the local team should continue to be in contact with the tertiary center while the transport team is en route if the neonate deteriorates or if any new issues are identified (Cornette, 2004b; Das & Leuthner, 2004; Wright, 2000).

TABLE III.1

LEVELS OF NEONATAL CARE
Level I—basic or primary care Well newborn nurseries
Level II—Special Care Nursery Provide care to neonates > 32 weeks gestational age and weigh > 1,500 g Provide continuous positive airway pressure (CPAP) Provide mechanical ventilation for up to 24 hours Provide convalescent care to neonates that have been in a tertiary neonatal unit
Level III—Neonatal Intensive Care Provide comprehensive care for neonates < 32 weeks gestation and weigh < 1,500 g Provide high-frequency ventilation and inhaled nitric oxide Onsite accessibility to pediatric subspecialists
Level IV—Regionalized Neonatal Intensive Care Provide Level III care Provide ECMO therapy Repair complex cardiac abnormalities requiring cardiopulmonary bypass

From AAP (2004, 2012) and AAP and ACOG (2007).

THE NEONATAL TRANSPORT PROGRAM

The American Academy of Pediatrics, Section of Transport Medicine (AAP, 2007) has stated that neonatal transports "should be performed expeditiously and safely by qualified personnel, with appropriate training and equipment" (p. 2). It is generally the responsibility of the tertiary center of the regional system to provide the neonatal transport service. The transport team should serve as an extension of the unit the neonate is going to and provide tertiary level care at the referring facility (Messner, 2011). The neonatal transport program should be tailored to meet the needs identified by the entire regional program. There are specific elements that should be part of every transport program, including an identified medical director and a neonatal or perinatal coordinator. In addition to providing neonatal transports, the regional program should have an educational mission and have a process for quality assurance for the transport team, the tertiary center, and the other facilities in the region (AAP, 2007; Cornette, 2004a; Lupton & Pendray, 2004; National Association of Neonatal Nurses [NANN], 2010; Woodward et al., 2002). An example of this type of regional outreach program is the New Hampshire Perinatal Program, which has been in existence for over 30 years and routinely provides educational opportunities and an on-site review of all shared patients at least yearly with all referring facilities (Frank et al., 1999).

TRANSPORT TEAM COMPOSITION

Many different transport team compositions have been described, and ultimately the team composition should be appropriate for the type of care the neonate requires (AAP, Section of Transport Medicine, 2007; Cornette, 2004a; Davies, Bickell, & Tibby, 2010; Fenton & Leslie, 2009; Fenton et al., 2004; Karlsen et al., 2011; Lee et al., 2002; Leppälä, 2010; Leslie & Stephenson, 2003; Lupton & Pendray, 2004; NANN, 2010). A recent national survey by Karlsen et al. (2011) identified 25 different types of neonatal transport team compositions. There were 335 respondents to this survey, and only one team did not include either an NNP or RN on the neonatal transport team.

The role of the NNP has been compared with the pediatric house-staff as a member of the transport team (Cornette, 2004a, 2004b; Fenton & Leslie, 2009; Fenton et al., 2004; Leslie & Stephenson, 2003). There is ample evidence that the care provided by NNPs is at least comparable and potentially improved due to the consistency and experience this role brings to the transport process. In addition, it is less and less frequent that pediatric house-staff are involved in neonatal transports, mainly due to restrictions on duty hours and limited clinical time spent in neonatal units. Because of these constraints, it is now generally recommended that pediatric house-staff not be part of the transport team unless they receive additional training (Fenton & Leslie, 2009; Woodward et al., 2002).

Lee et al. (2002) analyzed three different compositions of transport teams: an EMT team, an RN team, or a combined team of RN and RT. An MD would accompany any of these teams if the condition of the neonate warranted that level of care; however, the analysis did not show that the presence of a physician affected the outcome of the transport. The patient outcomes of the three types of teams were not significantly different. A cost analysis was performed and the RN team was found to be the most cost-effective model for most transports, followed by the combined team and then the EMT team.

The survey by Karlsen et al. (2011) classified the transport team as being either unit-based or dedicated. The two most common unit-based team compositions in this survey were RN-RT or RN-RT-NNP. The unit-based teams were staffed by neonatal intensive care personnel, who were responsible for patient care when not on transport, similar to the RN team and combined team in the cost analysis by Lee et al. (2002). Unit-based teams generally performed fewer than 200 transports per year.

Dedicated teams in this survey were most commonly composed of RN-RT or RN-RN. The dedicated teams usually had a volume of over 200 neonatal transports per year and covered a geographical distance of greater than 100 miles. Only about 37% of these teams transported neonates exclusively; 50% of the dedicated teams were combined neonatal/pediatric teams.

Fenton and Leslie (2009) have suggested that the professional background of the transport team members is less important than the training each member of the team receives in terms of providing excellent patient care, performing procedural skills, communicating with the family and referring facility providers, and being part of the quality assurance process of the regional transport system. The APP Section of Transport Medicine (2007) and the NANN (2010) have developed guidelines for the interprofessional training of the neonatal transport team. The composition of the transport team should always be appropriate for the level of care the neonate will require in order to ensure a safe, effective, and efficient transfer to the tertiary facility.

MODE OF TRANSPORTATION

Neonatal transports generally occur by ambulance, fixed wing aircraft, helicopter, or boat (AAP, Section of Transport Medicine, 2007; Karlsen et al., 2011; Leppälä, 2010; Lupton & Pendray, 2004; NANN, 2010). Other modes have been reported, including walking or riding in a rickshaw (Mori et al., 2007). If more than one mode of transportation is available, the decision should be based on the condition of the neonate and the distance to the tertiary facility. To ensure the safety of the transport team and neonate, weather conditions may also need to be taken into account.

In the survey by Karlsen et al. (2011), the majority of transports were by ground. Generally speaking, for shorter distances ground transport is the preferable mode. For distances that will require 2 hours or more of travel time one way, air transport may be more appropriate (Karagol, Zenciroglu, Ipek, Kundak, & Okumus, 2011; Lupton & Pendray, 2004). Transport by helicopter is the most costly and ambulance the least expensive (AAP, Section of Transport Medicine, 2007; Lupton & Pendray, 2004; Wright, 2000). Whatever mode of transportation is used, the team must be oriented to and comfortable with the configuration and equipment of the ground or air ambulance.

STABILIZATION BY THE TRANSPORT TEAM

Once the transport team has arrived at the referring facility, they should introduce themselves and receive a hand-off from the local team. This hand-off is critical, as it will inform the transport team about care already received, preventing unnecessary duplication of care and help guide the next steps (Wright, 2000). A successful hand-off will help expedite transporting the neonate to the tertiary facility safely. Table III.2 provides an example of information to be included in the hand-off to the transport team.

Once the hand-off is accomplished, the transport team should assess the neonate, continue with the stabilization, and provide any additional care to ensure a safe and efficient transfer to the tertiary center. It is essential that prior to transport, the neonate has a stable airway, receives any cardiovascular support needed, vascular access is ensured if necessary, and appropriate medications have been provided. Continued close attention should also be paid to thermoregulation and glucose homeostasis (Cornette, 2004b; Fenton et al., 2004; Leslie & Stephenson, 2003). Special consideration should be paid to ensuring that all tubes and catheters are in good position and secure; an accidental extubation or dislodgement of an umbilical line could result in destabilizing an already fragile neonate.

An important part of the role of the transport team is to anticipate any adverse clinical event that may occur while en route and try to minimize the possibility. This is best done by adequately stabilizing the neonate prior to departure from the referring facility.

TRANSPORT EQUIPMENT

The transport equipment allows the neonatal transport team to bring many aspects of the tertiary unit to the referring facility. The team members need to be comfortable using all the equipment, and as much as possible it should be standardized in terms of location, type, and so on. When choosing transport equipment, there are several important considerations. Safety should be an overriding concept and all equipment should meet all federal, state, and local regulations. The equipment should have the ability to run by both electricity and battery power. It will need to withstand changes in temperature and, if air transport is used, changes in altitude.

The transport isolette is the primary tool used by the neonatal transport team. It needs to be able to safely transport and keep warm a neonate weighing up to 5 kg. The neonate should be visible and easily accessible to the team throughout the transport. The transport isolette should have additional equipment mounted to it, including a cardiorespiratory monitor, IV pumps, air and oxygen tanks, oxygen blender for appropriate O_2 delivery, and a transport ventilator. There should also be space to add equipment if necessary, such as inhaled nitric oxide (AAP, Section of Transport Medicine, 2007; Cornette, 2004b; Fenton et al., 2004; Leppälä, 2010; Lupton & Pendray, 2004; Lutman & Petros, 2008; NANN, 2010).

In addition to the isolette and mounted equipment, the transport team will need to bring other smaller, but equally important, items that are usually kept ready to go in transport bags. This will allow the team to perform procedures and stabilize the neonate with equipment that is familiar to them. Each transport program should decide upon specific items brought, but Table III.3 lists some common equipment found in transport bags.

TABLE III.2

SAMPLE HAND-OFF FORM

Referring Hospital________________________ Referring Provider________________
Infant Data
Name_________________________________ Date of Birth__________________
Gestational Age__________________________ Birth Weight___________________
Reason for Transport____
____
Delivery Method____
Reason for Delivery____
Apgar Score 1 minute__________ 5 minutes____________ 10 minutes_______________
Resuscitation Included____
____

Maternal Data
Name_____________________________ Date of Birth __________________
Gravida _____ Para ______Term______ Ab ______ Preterm _____ Living_____
Prenatal Labs
Blood Group ______ Antibody______
Rubella _______ HBsAg ______ HIV_____ Syphilis ______ GBS ______
GC______ Chlamydia_______ CF screen ______
Other ____
Pregnancy Complications _______________________________________
____

Other Pertinent Information
Dad's Name ______________________ Date of Birth ____________________
____
____

Interventions by Referring Team
Procedures
____Intubation Size ETT_____ Insertion Marking_____
____UAC Size catheter____ Insertion Marking_____
____UVC Size catheter____ Insertion Marking_____
____PIV Size catheter____ Insertion Site_________
____Chest tube Size catheter____ Insertion Site_________
____CXR____
Ventilator Settings: PIP _____ PEEP _____ Rate _____ FiO_2_____
Vital Signs: HR_____ RR _____ BP _____ Temp _____ O_2 sat _____
Lab Work
Blood Gases__________________________________
____
____
CBC ____
Blood Culture _________________________________
Other Culture _________________________________
Type and Screen ______________________________
Medications
Name____________________ Dose___________ Time Given___________
Name____________________ Dose___________ Time Given___________
Name____________________ Dose___________ Time Given___________
Name____________________ Dose___________ Time Given___________

DOCUMENTATION

The regional transport service should have the ability to document all transport calls and advice given to the referring center. There should also be documentation regarding the time of phone calls and dispatch of the transport team. Leslie and Fenton (2012) have suggested that individual transports be defined as planned, unplanned, or time-critical. If a transport is designated as time-critical, the transport team should be able to be mobilized in 30 minutes or less.

The referring facility should provide the transport team with copies of the neonate's medical record that includes a delivery summary, initial presentation, and summary of the stabilization process, including laboratory values. A copy of the maternal history, including pertinent prenatal information, should also be included. Hard copies or CDs of x-rays or other imaging studies should also be available to the transport team (Cornette, 2004b; Das & Leuthner, 2004; Leppälä, 2010).

Prior to departure of the transport team it is imperative that consent forms authorizing the transport be obtained

TABLE III.3

TRANSPORT BAG EQUIPMENT

Medications
Antibiotics
Anticonvulsants
Code medications
Inotropic agents
Intravenous solutions
Dextrose 5% and 10%
Normal saline
Prostaglandins
Rapid sequence intubation medications
Surfactant
Respiratory Equipment
Endotracheal tubes
End-tidal carbon monoxide monitoring
Laryngoscope and blades
Resuscitation bag and masks
Laryngeal mask airways
CPAP prongs
Portable blood gas analyzer
Additional Equipment
Monitoring
ECG leads
O_2 saturation probes
Transducer
Temperature probes
Procedural
Umbilical catheter insertion
Chest tube insertion
Vascular Access
IV catheters
Intraosseous needles
Misc
Decompression tubes
Equipment for sterile procedures
Gown, mask, gloves, povidone-iodine, alcohol
Point of care glucose monitoring
Suction catheters
Tube and catheter stabilizing equipment
Reference manuals

and signed. There should be documentation of consent from the parents to transport their infant to the tertiary center. There may also be state, local, or third-party consent forms needing to be signed by the referring provider and a member of the transport team who is receiving care of the neonate (Cornette, 2004b; Lupton & Pendray, 2004).

Documentation by the neonatal transport team should include a flow sheet for vital signs, respiratory status, intake and output, and a brief description of interventions provided. A full note by the transport team leader describing the transport should be entered into the neonate's chart at the tertiary center. This note should include the time of arrival at the referring facility, time of arrival at the tertiary center, mode of transportation, and care given during the transport, both at the referring facility and en route. It is recommended that a copy of this note be sent to the referring provider as well as the neonate's primary care provider.

FAMILY-CENTERED CARE DURING TRANSPORT

The transport of a critically ill neonate is particularly stressful for parents who may or may not have anticipated the birth of an ill neonate and may not be able to immediately go to the receiving facility to fully participate in the care of their infant (Buchanan, 2009; Das & Leuthner, 2004; Dulkerian et al., 2011; Duritza, 2009; Franklin, 2006; Hawthorne & Killen, 2006; Hogan & Logan, 2004; Leppälä, 2010; McNab, Richards, & Green, 1999; Steeper, 2002; Wilman, 1997). It has been suggested that early parental participation in the care of their infant helps to foster the parent–infant relationship. Parental separation from their infant, which is inherent in the transport process, can adversely impact the successful development of this relationship (Franklin, 2006; Obeidat, Bond, & Callister, 2009). The neonatal transport team needs to be cognizant of this and try to facilitate parental involvement in the care of their infant during the transport process.

The first way parents participate in the care of their infant is by information sharing. Steeper (2002) has noted that there is a lack of information about how parents perceive the communication they receive about their infant during the transport process. Until more definitive information is available, the transport team should use the guidance of communication strategies already identified for parents whose infants are in a neonatal intensive care unit (Howland, 2007; Saunders, Abraham, Crosby, Thomas, & Edwards, 2003; Sharp, Strauss, & Lorch, 1992). This communication should begin when the local team identifies the need for transport. The parents should be informed of the reason the neonate needs to be transported for a higher level of care, the name of the facility he or she is going to, when it is expected the transport team will arrive, mode of transportation, and if it is possible for the mother to be transferred to the tertiary facility or if she can be discharged to travel to the receiving facility (Das & Leuthner, 2004; Leppälä, 2010; NANN, 2010; Wright, 2000).

For the parents and family of an ill neonate their first experience with the neonatal intensive care team will be the transport team. Most neonatal units pride themselves on providing family-centered care, realizing that the parents and family are not visitors to the neonatal unit, but a part of the team caring for the ill neonate. If this is truly believed, family participation in the care of their infant needs to begin during the transport process. Once the transport team arrives, they need to continue keeping parents informed as the local team has. The transport team needs to introduce themselves, and parents should be given the opportunity to stay with their infant during the stabilization by the transport team (NANN, 2010). Parents should be told what the assessments of the transport team are; any additional procedures to be done in the referring facility or that may be necessary during the transport process; and be given the opportunity to ask questions. If the parents have not been able to be present while readying the neonate for transport, the team should go to the mother's room so they can see and touch their infant prior to leaving the referring facility.

Many transport teams also provide the parents with some written information about the neonatal intensive care unit the neonate is going to that includes the phone number to the unit as well as a map for the parents to use. The team should ensure that the parents have a photograph of their infant; if not, the team should have the ability to provide one. Parents will also need information about the anticipated duration of the transport, and if they will not be accompanying the baby they should receive a phone call from the transport team once the infant has safely arrived in the neonatal intensive care unit.

CONCLUSION

The transport of an ill neonate from a Level I or Level II facility will always be a stressful and challenging experience. The transport process begins with the identification of the ill neonate, transitions through the transport team, and ends with admission to the neonatal intensive care unit. A well-developed regional neonatal or perinatal program helps to ensure the smooth transition of the neonate from the referring to the receiving facility. The goal of the neonatal transport team, a part of the regional program, is to provide high-quality, safe, efficient, and family-centered care to the ill neonate prior to arrival in the Level III unit.

REFERENCES

ACoRN Neonatal Society. (2009). ACoRN acute care of at-risk newborns. Retrieved from http://www.acornprogram.net

American Academy of Pediatrics, Committee on Fetus and Newborn. (2004). Policy statement: Levels of neonatal care. *Pediatrics, 114*, 1341–1347.

American Academy of Pediatrics, Committee on Fetus and Newborn. (2012). Policy statement: Levels of neonatal care. *Pediatrics, 130*, 587–597.

American Academy of Pediatrics, Section of Transport Medicine. (2007). *Guidelines for air and ground transport of neonatal and pediatric patients* (3rd ed.). Elk Grove Village, IL: American Academy of Pediatrics.

American Academy of Pediatrics & The American College of Obstetricians and Gynecologists. (2007). *Guidelines for perinatal care* (6th ed.). Elk Grove Village, IL: American Academy of Pediatrics.

Bouchut, J.-C., Van Lancker, E., Chritin, V., & Gueugniaud, P. Y. (2011). Physical stressors during neonatal transport: Helicopter compared with ground ambulance. *Air Medical Journal, 30*(3), 134–139. doi:10.1016/j.amj.2010.11

Buchanan, K. (2009). Failed neonatal transport. *Advances in Neonatal Care, 9*(2), 82–84.

Cornette, L. (2004a). Contemporary neonatal transport: Problems and solutions. *Archives of Diseases of Children Fetal Neonatal Edition, 89*, F212–F214. doi:10.1136/adc.2003.046201

Cornette, L. (2004b). Transporting the sick neonate. *Current Paediatrics, 14*, 20–25. doi:10.1016/j.cupe.2003.09.001

Das, U. G., & Leuthner, S. R. (2004). Preparing the neonate for transport. *Pediatric Clinics of North America, 51*, 581–598.

Davies, J., Bickell, F., & Tibby, S. M. (2010). Attitudes of paediatric intensive care nurses to development of a nurse practitioner role for critical care transport. *Journal of Advanced Nursing, 67*(2), 317–326. doi:10.1111/j.1365-2648.2010.05454.x

Dulkerian, S. J., Douglas, W. P., & Taylor, R. M. (2011). Redirecting treatment during neonatal transport. *Journal of Perinatal and Neonatal Nursing, 25*(2), 111–114. doi:10.1097/JPN.0b013e31821a20ab.

Duritza, K. (2009). Neonatal transport—A family support module. *Newborn and Infant Nursing Reviews, 9*(4), 212–218. doi:10.1053/j.nainr.2009.09.006

Fenton, A. C., & Leslie, A. (2009). Who should staff neonatal transport teams? *Early Human Development, 85*, 487–490.

Fenton, A. C., Leslie, A., & Skeoch, C. H. (2004). Optimizing neonatal transfer. *Archives of Diseases of Children Fetal Neonatal Edition, 89*, F215–F219. doi:10.1136/adc.2003.019711

Frank, J. E., Rhodes, T. T., Edwards, W. E., Darnall, R. A., Smith, B. D., Little, G. A., . . . Flanagan, V. A. (1999). The New Hampshire perinatal program: Twenty years of perinatal outreach education. *Journal of Perinatology, 19*(1), 3–8.

Franklin, C. (2006). The neonatal nurse's role in parental attachment in the NICU. *Critical Care Nursing Quarterly, 29*(1), 81–85.

Hawthorne, J., & Killen, M. (2006). Transferring babies between units: Issues for parents. *Infant, 2*(2), 44–46.

Hogan, D. L., & Logan, J. (2004). The Ottawa model of research use: A guide to clinical innovation in the NICU. *Clinical Nurse Specialist, 18*(5), 255–261.

Howland, L. C. (2007). Preterm birth: Implications for family stress and coping. *Newborn and Infant Nursing Reviews, 7*(1), 14–19.

Karagol, B. S., Zenciroglu, A., Ipek, M. S., Kundak, A. A., & Okumus, N. (2011). Impact of land-based neonatal transport on outcomes in transient tachypnea of the newborn. *American Journal of Perinatology, 28*(4), 331–336.

Karlsen, K. A. (2008). The S.T.A.B.L.E. program. Retrieved from http://www.stableprogram.org

Karlsen, K. A., Trautman, M., Price-Douglas, W., & Smith, S. (2011). National survey of neonatal transport teams in the united states. *Pediatrics, 128*. doi:10.1542/peds.2010–3796

Kattwinkel, J., Cook, L. J., Hurt, H., Nwacek, G. A., Short, J. G., & Crosby, W. M. (2007). Perinatal continuing education program (PCEP): Improving care for pregnant women and newborns. Retrieved from http://www.healthsystem.virginia.edu/internet/pcep

Lee, S. K., Zupancic, J. A. F., Sale, J., Pendray, M., Whyte, R., Brabyn, D., . . . Whyte, H. (2002). Cost-effectiveness and choice of infant transport systems. *Medical Care, 40*(8), 705–716. doi:10.1097/01.MLR.0000020930.04786.F9

Leppälä, K. (2010). Whether near or far . . . transporting the neonate. *Journal of Perinatal and Neonatal Nursing, 24*(2), 167–171.

Leslie, A., & Fenton, A. (2012). Categorizing neonatal transports. *Archives of Diseases of Children Fetal Neonatal Edition, 97*(1), F77.

Leslie, A., & Stephenson, T. (2003). Neonatal transfers by advanced neonatal nurse practitioners and paediatric registrars. *Archives of Diseases of Children Fetal Neonatal Edition, 88*, F509–F512.

Little, G. A., Horbar, J. D., Wachtel, J. S., Gluck, P. A., & Muri, J. H. (2010). Evolution of quality improvement in perinatal care. In Committee on Perinatal Health (Ed.), *Toward improving the outcome of pregnancy III* (pp. 9–18). White Plains, NY: March of Dimes.

Lupton, B. A., & Pendray, M. R. (2004). Regionalized neonatal emergency transport. *Seminars in Neonatology, 9*, 125–133. doi:10.1016/j.siny.2003.08.007

Lutman, D., & Petros, A. (2008). Inhaled nitric oxide in neonatal and paediatric transport. *Early Human Development, 84*, 725–729.

McNab, A. J., Richards, J., & Green, G. (1999). Family-oriented care during pediatric inter-hospital transport. *Patient Education and Counseling, 36*, 247–257.

Messner, H. (2011). Neonatal transport: A review of the current evidence. *Early Human Development, 87S*, S77.

Mori, R., Fujimaura, M., Shiraishi, J., Evans, B., Corkett, M., Negishi, H., & Doyle, P. (2007). Duration of inter-facility neonatal transport and neonatal mortality: Systematic review and cohort study. *Pediatrics International, 49*, 452–458.

National Association of Neonatal Nurses. (2010). *Neonatal nursing transport standards: Guidelines for practice* (3rd ed.). Glenview, IL: National Association of Neonatal Nurses.

Neonatology on the Web. (2005). A resource and learning tool of health care professionals. Retrieved from webmaster@neonatology.org

Obeidat, H. M., Bond, E. A., & Callister, L. C. (2009). The parental experience of having an infant in the newborn intensive care unit. *The Journal of Perinatal Education, 18*(3), 23–29. doi:10.1624/105812409X461199

Rochefort, C. M., & Lamothe, L. (2011). Forcing the system: A configuration analysis of a regional neonatal-perinatal health network. *Health Care Management Review, 36*(3), 241–251.

Saunders, R. P., Abraham, M. R., Crosby, M., Thomas, K., & Edwards, W. E. (2003). Evaluation and development of potentially better practices for improving family-centered care in neonatal intensive care units. *Pediatrics, 111*(4), e437–e444.

Sharp, M. C., Strauss, R. P., & Lorch, S. C. (1992). Communicating medical bad news: Parents' experiences and preferences. *Journal of Pediatrics, 121*, 539–546.

Staebler, S. (2011). Regionalized systems of perinatal care: Health policy considerations. *Advances in Neonatal Care, 11*(1), 37–42.

Steeper, S. (2002). Neonatal transportation: Exploring parental views. *Journal of Neonatal Nursing, 8*(6), 173–176.

Warner, B., Altimier, L., & Imhoff, S. (2002). Clinical excellence for high risk neonates: Improved perinatal regionalization. *Neonatal Intensive Care, 15*(6), 33–38.

Wilman, D. (1997). Neonatal transport: The effect on parents. *Journal of Neonatal Nursing, 3*(5), 16–22.

Woodward, G. A., Insoft, R. M., Pearson-Shaver, A. L., Jaimovich, D., Orr, R. A., Chambliss, R., & Westergaard, F. (2002). The state of pediatric interfacility transport: Consensus of the second national pediatric and neonatal interfacility transport medicine leadership conference. *Pediatric Emergency Care, 18*(1), 38–43.

Wright, J. D. (2000). Before the transport team arrives: Neonatal stabilization. *The Journal of Perinatal and Neonatal Nursing, 13*(4), 87–107.

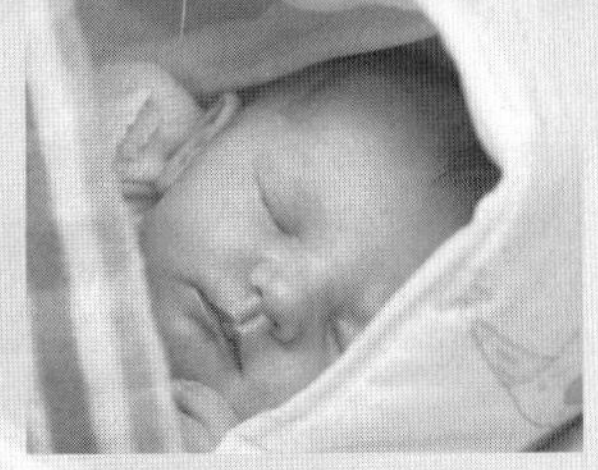

Introduction to Vascular Access

IV

■ Elizabeth L. Sharpe

As the threshold of viability is lowered, the challenge of nourishing the premature survivors has increased. Premature infants require optimal amounts of protein, carbohydrates, and fats to achieve growth, and the method of delivering these nutrients is crucial to their safe delivery. Current vascular access devices used with neonates include: umbilical catheters, peripherally inserted central catheters (PICCs), central venous catheters, midline catheters, and peripheral intravenous devices(see Table IV.1). The *selection of device* should consider the individual patient's needs weighed with risks versus benefits. These considerations include the chemical properties of the therapy such as osmolarity, pH and irritant or vesicant properties, and the intended duration of therapy. The Centers for Disease Control recommends using "a midline catheter or peripherally inserted central catheter (PICC), instead of a short peripheral catheter, when the duration of IV therapy will likely exceed six days" (O'Grady et al., 2011). Medications with a pH of less than 5 or greater than 9 and osmolarity greater than 600 mOsm/L or known irritants should be administered via central venous access (Alexander, Corrigan, Gorski, Hankins, & Perucca, 2010; INS, 2011).

PICCs are now commonly used to administer total parenteral nutrition and certain medications in neonatal intensive care. When properly maintained, PICCs provide reliable long-term access for delivery of parenteral nutrition and hyperosmolar or irritant medications, fewer interruptions in therapy, decreased incidence of painful procedures and stress to infants, and fewer opportunities for needlestick exposure to health care providers. The risks and disadvantages include: the need for radiographic confirmation of catheter tip location with insertion and following repositioning, specialized training required, risk for extravasation, phlebitis, pericardial and pleural effusion, occlusion, thrombosis, infection, and migration or dislodgement (see Table IV.2).

Indications for a PICC include the need for long-term parenteral nutrition or hyperosmolar medications. Typical patient profiles are extreme prematurity, diagnoses with delayed feedings, patients with congenital anomalies limiting vascular options, and those requiring long-term vascular access for nutrition or treatment. The most commonly used veins for PICC placement are the basilic, cephalic, greater and lesser saphenous, posterior auricular, and temporal. Other veins that may be cannulated include the external jugular, axillary, femoral, and popliteal. As venous anatomy progresses from distal toward the heat, the size of these vessels increases in diameter, creating the desired superior blood flow for optimal hemodilution to minimize vessel damage. In the upper extremity, the basilic and cephalic veins flow directly into the axillary vein, then the subclavian vein, then the brachiocephalic vein into the superior vena cava (SVC). In the head, the posterior auricular and temporal veins flow directly into the jugular vein, then into the subclavian vein, the brachiocephalic and the superior vena cava. For catheters inserted into the veins of the upper extremity or scalp, the optimal catheter tip location is in the SVC (FDA, 1989; INS, 2011; Pettit & Wyckoff, 2007). In the lower extremities, the greater and lesser saphenous veins flow directly into the femoral vein, then the iliac, then the inferior vena cava (IVC). For catheters inserted into the veins in the lower extremities, the optimal catheter tip location is in the IVC between the right atrium and diaphragm (Pettit & Wyckoff, 2007). Radiographic confirmation should be obtained following catheter insertion, any adjustments to reposition the catheter, and if a complication is suspected.

Insertion Procedure

- Evaluate needs and duration of intended therapy
- Discuss with family and obtain informed consent
- Perform physical assessment for vein selection
- Measure distance from intended insertion site to SVC for upper extremity or scalp vessels or IVC for lower extremity vessels
- Gather central line kit, catheter, introducer, sterile gloves, maximum sterile barriers and other needed supplies
- Prepare patient for procedure, including pharmacologic and developmental comfort measures
- Don hair covering and mask
- Perform hand hygiene
- Prepare sterile field and equipment
- Prepare catheter by flushing and trimming to premeasured length
- Position patient as developmentally appropriate

TABLE IV.1

TYPES OF INTRAVENOUS DEVICES

Type of Device	Intended Duration	Average Dwell Time	Type of Infusion	Optimal Tip Location
Peripheral intravenous (PIV)	Short term	15–54 hours (Pettit, 2003)	Nonirritant, isotonic solutions D12.5% or less	Peripheral
Midline (ML)	5–7 days	8.7 days to as much as 80 days (Leick-Rude & Haney, 2006; Wyckoff, 1999)	Nonirritant, isotonic solutions D12.5% or less	Upper portion of extremity, below axilla, above clavicle, away from areas of flexion
PICC	More than 6 days to long term	22 days to indefinitely (Liu et al., 2011)	Parenteral nutrition, vesicant therapy, infusates pH < 5 or > 9, > 600 mOsm/L > D12.5%	Lower 1/3 of SVC or IVC above level of diaphragm
Percutaneous central venous catheter	5–7 days	5–7 days	Parenteral nutrition, vesicant therapy, infusates pH < 5 or > 9, > 600 mOsm/L	Lower 1/3 of SVC or IVC above level of diaphragm

- Prepare insertion site by disinfecting skin with antimicrobial agent. Chlorhexidine gluconate or povidone iodine may be used. Chlorhexidine may be used with caution in premature infants or infants less than 2 months of age. These products may cause irritation or chemical burns.
- Utilize maximum sterile barrier precautions to isolate the extremity or insertion site
- Apply sterile tourniquet
- Insert introducer bevel up at 15°- to 30°-degree angle and observe for blood return. Remove the needle from over the sheath introducers.
- Remove tourniquet
- Place catheter in introducer lumen using nontoothed forceps and thread catheter in small increments
- Remove introducer per manufacturer's directions
- Apply gentle pressure to site until bleeding stops
- Verify inserted catheter length and any externally lying
- If a catheter with stylet is used, remove stylet at this time
- Aspirate to confirm blood return and flush to confirm patency
- Attach luer-lock extension tubing if not in catheter apparatus
- Secure catheter temporarily with skin closure tapes while awaiting radiographic confirmation
- Confirm catheter tip location in SVC or IVC
- Reposition catheter if not in SVC or IVC
- Obtain radiographic reconfirmation of catheter tip location
- Remove povidone iodine from skin and allow to dry
- Secure catheter to skin and apply sterile transparent occlusive dressing
- Document procedure, any repositioning, radiographic confirmation, premedication, catheter specifics, including brand and lot number, trimmed length, inserted length, and patient tolerance.

Points for Practice in PICC Maintenance

- Be sure that catheter tip location correlates with type of infusion
- No greater than D12.5 if catheter tip location is not central in SVC or IVC
- Change dressing if becomes loose, nonocclusive, moist, or soiled
- Maintain adequate minimum infusion rates to prevent occlusion
- Flush with no smaller than a 5 or 10 mL syringe per manufacturer's directions (INS, 2011)
- If heparin locking, flush with 1 mL normal saline and 1 mL 10 units/mL heparin every 6 hours (INS, 2008)

Central line–associated bloodstream infection (CLABSI) is defined as a primary bloodstream infection in a patient that had a central line within the 48-hour period before the development of the bloodstream infection and is not bloodstream related to an infection at another site (O'Grady et al., 2011). Numerous campaigns successfully directed at CLABSI prevention have included a bundled approach of simultaneously practiced strategies (Cooley & Grady, 2009; Curry, Honeycutt, Goins, & Gilliam, 2009; Kime, Mohsini, Nwankwo, & Turner, 2011). Some of these bundle components included: hand hygiene, maximum sterile barrier precautions for insertion, dedicated team, chlorhexidine for skin antisepsis, chlorhexidine-impregnated dressings, sterile tubing changes, needleless connector scrub hygiene, closed medication systems, and daily evaluation of line necessity for timely removal of the line when no longer needed. A care bundle is a group of practices that individually impact outcomes but when applied together, dramatically improve outcomes (IHI, 2012; Marschall et al., 2008). The implementation of evidence-based central line care across statewide collaboratives has significantly reduced CLABSIs (Schulman et al., 2011; Wirtschafter et al., 2011).

TABLE IV.2

PREVENTION AND MANAGEMENT OF PICC COMPLICATIONS

Complication	Risk Factors	Prevention	Management
CLABSI	Prematurity Inexperienced or untrained caregivers Multiple manipulations of catheter Prolonged dwell time Contamination of catheter hub or needleless connector	Central line bundle elements including: Specially trained personnel Maximum sterile barrier precautions Maintaining an occlusive dressing Meticulous catheter care Hub hygiene Chlorhexidine or povidone iodine for skin antisepsis Limiting breaks in line Daily review of line necessity	Intravenous antibiotic therapy Removal of catheter if unable to clear infection or if gram-negative bacilli, *staphylococcus aureus* or Candida (Benjamin et al., 2001)
Occlusion	Low flow rates less than 0.5 mL/hours Inadequate flushing	Flushing before and after incompatible medications Maintaining adequate minimum infusion rates (0.5 mL/hours–2 mL/hours)	Clearing agents specific to etiology may be used. Thrombolytics can be instilled according to manufacturer's directions.
Phlebitis	Catheter tip outside the SVC or IVC Rapid or traumatic insertion Cephalic or saphenous vein insertion Catheter mobility due to inadequate securement	Use smallest size catheter that will accommodate therapy Screen infusates for irritant or vesicant properties, hyperosmolarity or extreme pH (<5 or >9). Maintain secure occlusive dressing Position catheter tip in SVC or IVC Slow gentle insertion technique	Warm compresses over the vein every 4 hours and elevation of the extremity. Often resolves spontaneously. If it does not resolve or worsens after 24 hours, may need to discontinue the catheter.
Thrombosis	Catheter tip outside SVC or IVC Catheter mobility Left-sided insertion in upper extremity Protein C, protein S or antithrombin deficiencies	Use smallest size catheter that will accommodate therapy Position catheter tip in SVC or IVC	Options include: Venogram Antithrombolytics Removal of catheter
Extravasation	Catheter tip outside SVC or IVC Irritant or hyperosmolar infusions	Evaluate infusion needs in device selection Position catheter tip in SVC or IVC for optimal hemodilution Frequent, at least hourly site assessment	Radiographic confirmation of catheter tip location Treat specific to area of extravasation Remove catheter
Pericardial/pleural effusion	Catheter tip outside SVC or IVC Inadequate securement	Position catheter tip in SVC or IVC for optimal hemodilution Frequent, at least hourly site assessment Maintain secure dressing	Stop infusion Chest x-ray and echocardiogram for pericardial effusion Attempt to aspirate blood from catheter while awaiting imaging Withdraw catheter to proper position in SVC or IVC Repeat radiographic confirmation
Migration/dislodgement	Loose or inadequate dressings Tension on tubing and catheter	Frequent, at least hourly site assessment Maintain secure dressing	Reevaluate catheter tip location Determine if catheter tip location is appropriate for therapy required Consider catheter exchange or alternate site if new tip location is not satisfactory

Specially trained personnel play a key role in preventing and detecting complications. Personnel who care for patients with central lines should receive specialized training in catheter insertion, care, and maintenance. While not every complication is preventable, the effects can be minimized by early detection. Frequent monitoring of vascular access sites at least hourly can play a critical role in managing complications and producing positive outcomes.

EVIDENCE-BASED PRACTICE FOR PICCs

Health care providers caring for infants with vascular access should be aware of the risks of complications, especially infection, and incorporate the latest evidence-based practice directed at minimizing complications. In a report of 18 of every 100 babies experiencing an iatrogenic event with 87% of these preventable, 20% were due to catheters, and 15% due to nosocomial infection (Kugelman et al., 2008). Practices regarding insertion, catheter tip location, care, and maintenance have traditionally reflected primarily knowledge gained from the adult and pediatric population. Fortunately, new evidence specific to neonates continues to come forward to drive evidence-based care for vascular devices in infants. The benefit of decreased risk of complications associated with optimal catheter tip location has been demonstrated (Colacchio, Deng, Northrup, & Bizzarro, 2012). Some of these reflect the benefits of bundles and teams in decreasing infections (Cooley & Grady, 2009; Curry et al., 2009; Golombek, Rohan, Parvez, Salice, & LaGamma, 2002; Kime et al., 2011). The implementation of a team approach using specially trained personnel has been associated with desirable outcomes. Practices regarding catheter tip location, maintenance, and CLABSI prevention reflect emerging evidence of successful strategies that should be incorporated to continue to improve care outcomes.

TECHNOLOGICAL ADVANCES FOR PICCs

As technologic advances permit the miniaturization of equipment, greater options for PICC care are becoming available for safer insertion and maintenance of these tiny lifelines. The use of ultrasound, infrared technology, and modified Seldinger technique can facilitate PICC insertion and provide new solutions for locating and accessing challenging infant vasculature.

REFERENCES

Alexander, M., Corrigan, A., Gorski, L., Hankins, J., & Perucca, R. (2010). *Infusion nursing: An evidence-based approach* (3rd ed.). St. Louis, MO: Saunders Elsevier.

Benjamin, D. K., Jr., Miller, W., Garges, H., Benjamin, D. K., McKinney, R. E., Jr., Cotton, M., . . . Alexander, K. A. (2001). Bacteremia, central catheters, and neonates: When to pull the line. *Pediatrics, 107*(6), 1272–1276.

Colacchio, K., Deng, Y., Northrup, V., & Bizzarro, M. J. (2012). Complications associated with central and non-central venous catheters in a neonatal intensive care unit. *Journal of Perinatology: Official Journal of the California Perinatal Association, 32*(12), 941–946.

Cooley, K., & Grady, S. (2009). Minimizing catheter-related bloodstream infections: One unit's approach. *Advances in Neonatal Care: Official Journal of the National Association of Neonatal Nurses, 9*(5), 209–226; quiz 227–208.

Curry, S., Honeycutt, M., Goins, G., & Gilliam, C. (2009). Catheter-associated bloodstream infections in the NICU: Getting to zero. *Neonatal Network, 28*(3), 151–155.

FDA Drug Bulletin: Precautions Necessary with Central Venous Catheters. (1989).

Golombek, S. G., Rohan, A. J., Parvez, B., Salice, A. L., & LaGamma, E. F. (2002). "Proactive" management of percutaneously inserted central catheters results in decreased incidence of infection in the ELBW population. *Journal of Perinatology: Official Journal of the California Perinatal Association, 22*(3), 209–213.

IHI. (2012). How-to Guide: Prevent Central Line-Associated Bloodstream Infections. Retrieved from http://www.ihi.org

INS, I. N. S. (2008). Flushing Protocols.

INS, I. N. S. (2011). *Infusion nursing standards of practice.* Norwood, MA: Wolters Kluwer Lippincott Williams & Wilkins.

Kime, T., Mohsini, K., Nwankwo, M. U., & Turner, B. (2011). Central line "attention" is their best prevention. *Advances in Neonatal Care: Official Journal of the National Association of Neonatal Nurses, 11*(4), 242–248; quiz 249–250.

Kugelman, A., Inbar-Sanado, E., Shinwell, E. S., Makhoul, I. R., Leshem, M., Zangen, S., . . . Bader, D. (2008). Iatrogenesis in neonatal intensive care units: Observational and interventional, prospective, multicenter study. *Pediatrics, 122*(3), 550–555.

Leick-Rude, M., & Haney, B. (2006). Midline catheter use in the intensive care nursery. *Neonatal Network, 25*(3), 189–199.

Liu, H., Han, T., Zheng, Y., Tong, X., Piao, M., & Zhang, H. (2011). Analysis of complication rates and reasons for nonelective removal of PICCs in neonatal intensive care unit preterm infants. *Journal of Infusion Nursing, 32*(6), 336–340.

Marschall, J., Mermel, L. A., Anderson, D. J., Arias, K. M., Burstin, H., Calfee, D. P., . . . Yokoe, D. S. (2008). A compendium of strategies to prevent healthcare-associated infections in acute care hospitals. [Practice Guideline Research Support, Non-U.S. Gov't]. *Infection Control and Hospital Epidemiology: The Official Journal of the Society of Hospital Epidemiologists of America, 29*(Suppl. 1), S12–S21.

O'Grady, N. P., Alexander, M., Burns, L. A., Dellinger, E. P., Garland, J., Heard, S. O., . . . Saint, S. (2011). Guidelines for the prevention of intravascular catheter-related infections. *American Journal of Infection Control, 39*(4 Suppl. 1), S1–S34.

Pettit, J. (2003). Assessment of infants with peripherally inserted central catheters: Part 2. Detecting less frequently occurring complications [Case Reports Review]. *Advances in Neonatal Care: Official Journal of the National Association of Neonatal Nurses, 3*(1), 14–26.

Pettit, J., & Wyckoff, M. (2007). Peripherally inserted central catheters guideline for practice.

Schulman, J., Stricof, R., Stevens, T. P., Horgan, M., Gase, K., Holzman, I. R., . . . Saiman, L. (2011). Statewide NICU central-line-associated bloodstream infection rates decline after bundles and checklists. [Comparative Study Multicenter Study Research Support, Non-U.S. Gov't]. *Pediatrics, 127*(3), 436–444. doi:10.1542/peds.2010-2873

Wirtschafter, D. D., Powers, R. J., Pettit, J. S., Lee, H. C., Boscardin, W. J., Ahmad Subeh, M., & Gould, J. B. (2011). Nosocomial infection reduction in VLBW infants with a statewide quality-improvement model. *Pediatrics, 127*(3), 419–426. doi:10.1542/peds.2010-1449.

Wyckoff, M. (1999, Fall). Midline catheter use in the premature and full-term infant. *Journal of Vascular Access Devices, 4*(3), 26–29.

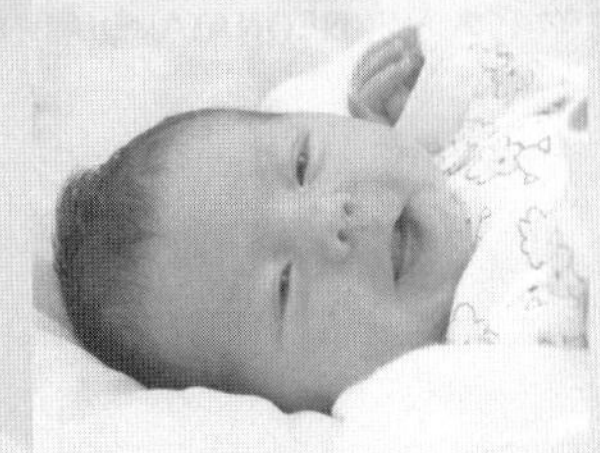

V

Age-Appropriate Care of the Premature and Hospitalized Infant

■ Mary E. Coughlin

The Joint Commission requires direct care providers to participate in education and training *specific to the needs of the patient population they serve*. These needs are not defined or derived from the patient's diagnosis but instead are based on the unique developmental human needs of the patient as a consequence of their diagnosis and hospitalization.

Age-appropriate care focuses on the developmental, holistic human needs of the patient. Referencing Maslow's hierarchy of needs[1] (Figure V.1), age-appropriate care integrates physiologic needs with the need for safety, love and belonging, esteem, and self-actualization framed by the psychosocial, developmental stage of the individual receiving care.

WHAT IS AGE-APPROPRIATE FOR THE PREMATURE AND HOSPITALIZED INFANT?

Erikson's Stages of Development

Eric Erikson,[2] a developmental psychologist, whose life work focused on the crisis of identity, put forth eight stages of psychosocial development.[3] His first stage, the period from birth to 2 years, looks at trust versus mistrust and asks the existential question of the infant: Can I trust the world? The outcome of this stage is framed by the maternal–infant relationship. For the premature and hospitalized neonate the mother parent figure and the neonatal clinician—primarily the nurse—share the "maternal" identity.

It is during this stage of development that establishing a secure attachment has lifelong implications for an individual's psychological and emotional integrity. Creating experiences that convey consistency through compassionate, communicative, and caring interactions is critical for a healthy psychoemotional and developmental future.

Developmentally Supportive Care

Heidelise Als and colleagues (1982) and Als, Duffy, and McAnulty (1988a, 1998b) described the complex relationship between the developing brain of preterm infants and the increasingly technological NICU environment and articulated an individualized approach to care based on the infant's capacity to interact with the surrounding environment. Specifically Als proposed that infant behaviors are a means of communication and that developmentally responsive health care professional examine the infant's responses to the environment and adjust their caregiving activities accordingly.

THE UNIVERSE OF AGE–APPROPRIATE CARE

A conceptual model is a descriptive model of a system based on qualitative assumptions about its elements, their interrelationships, and system boundaries. The universe of age-appropriate care (formerly the universe of developmental care—Gibbins, Hoath, Coughlin, Gibbins, & Franck, 2008) graphically represents a patient–centered model of care (Figure V.2). The orbital plane encircling the infant represents the physiologic systems of the body. It is a disturbance in one or more of these physiologic systems that prompts the patient to seek hospital level care. Surrounding this orbital reference point are the care planets. These care planets represent the shared care interface across which various care interactions occur that are deemed necessary to promote recovery and wellness. Overshadowing this matrix of celestial bodies is the family, however defined. The family is intimately and infinitely linked to the patient. Beyond the patient–family dyad is the health care community, the physical and systems environments.

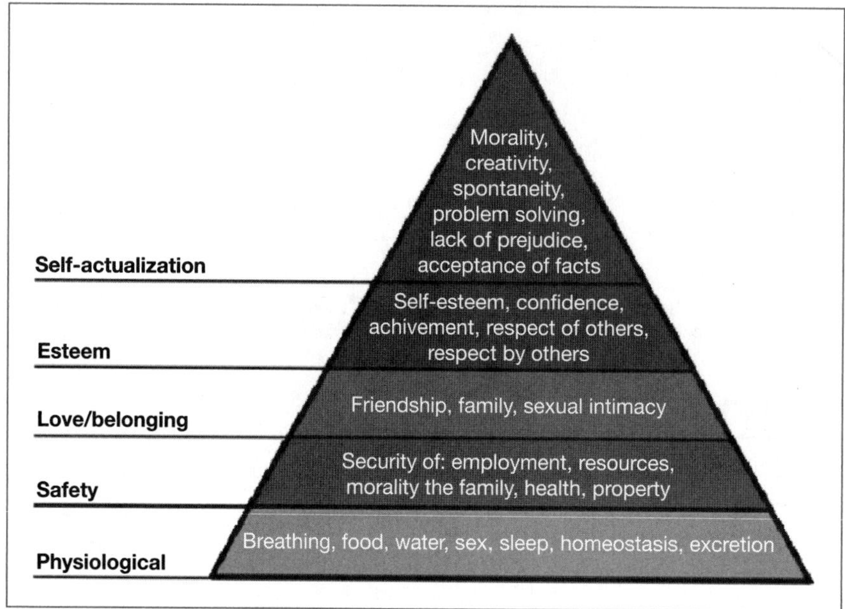

FIGURE V.1 Maslow's hierarchy of needs.

Extending across the entire universe is education—education for health care professionals, the family, and the patient.

This conceptual model aligns with the focus of global health care reform and the focus on quality, safety, and the patient experience of care.

CORE MEASURES FOR AGE-APPROPRIATE CARE

The core measures for age-appropriate care (formerly core measures for developmental care) represent disease-independent, evidence-based care strategies extrapolated from the literature related to developmental care and quality caring practices. These evidence-based care strategies have been organized into five core measure sets: (1) protected sleep, (2) pain and stress assessment and management, (3) activities of daily living, (4) family-centered care, and (5) the healing environment. The core measures for age-appropriate care align with the Institute of Medicine's Core Competencies to include patient centricity, interprofessional teamwork, evidence-based practice standards, and commitment to continuous quality improvement.

Protected Sleep

Sleep plays a critical role in synaptic development, learning, and memory, and as such, it is imperative that sleep is accurately assessed, supported, and protected during the hospital experience. The developmentally supportive clinician demonstrates age-appropriate competence with regard to sleep by individualizing care interactions based on the infant's sleep–wake cycle. This same clinician incorporates care interactions that support sleep (for example skin-to-skin interactions) and ensures that parents are educated on infant sleep needs both in hospital and postdischarge.

Pain and Stress Assessment and Management

Research suggests that premature and hospitalized infants have an increased vulnerability to pain and stress, with long-term psychological, behavioral, and physiological sequelae. The developmentally supportive clinician demonstrates age-appropriate competence with regard to pain and stress assessment and management ensures that pain and stress is assessed routinely with all care interactions. In addition, pain and stress is managed before, during, and after all procedural encounters and assessed until the infant returns to baseline. Family members are educated, informed, and involved in their infant's pain and stress management plan.

Age-Appropriate Activities of Daily Living

Postural stability, handling, feeding, and routine caregiving affect physiological integrity, sleep, functional mobility, neurodevelopment, and sensory processing. Activities of daily living include: (1) postural support and mobility, (2) alimentation, and (3) the preservation of mucosal and skin integrity. Looking at these activities through an age-appropriate lens, the competent clinician ensures postural integrity to promote comfort, safety, physiologic stability, and optimal neuromotor development; alimentation (whether via the oral route or enteral route) that is infant-driven, individualized, nurturing, and safe; and finally the preservation of mucosal and skin integrity—achieved through frequent assessment, evidence-based hygiene strategies and preventative measure that mitigate the risk for hospital-acquired injury.

Family-Centered Care

The infant–family relationship is vital for authentic survival that extends beyond hospitalization. The competent clinician providing age-appropriate care for the premature and hospitalized infant and their family respects and values patient–family preferences, listens to and clearly

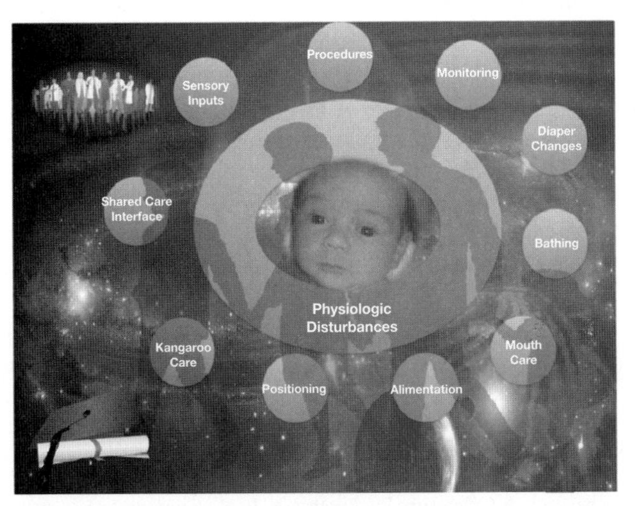

FIGURE V.2 The universe of age-appropriate care.

communicates and educates the family, facilitates shared decision making, and continuously promotes healthy parenting during the NICU stay that builds competence and confidence for postdischarge success. Assessing the emotional well-being of the parents and providing resources and support services that assist in short-term and long-term parenting, decision making, and parental well-being are key caring actions for the competent neonatal clinician.

The Healing Environment

The healing environment consists of the physical, human, and the organizational system. The physical environment includes the sensory milieu, the care space, and the aesthetics of the patient surroundings. The human environment is comprised of a collaborative interprofessional health care team that is patient focused with a commitment to excellence, safety and quality caring actions, attitudes, and behaviors that create a healthy work environment. Effective organizational systems focus on establishing a culture of safety through reliability, accountability, and sustainability of established age-appropriate, best-practice standards for the population served.

IMPLICATIONS OF THE PROVISION OF AGE-APPROPRIATE CARE FOR NEONATAL OUTCOMES

Implications of the provision of age-appropriate care for neonatal outcomes rely on the extent to which these evidence-based care strategies are incorporated into the culture of care in the newborn intensive care unit setting. Montirosso et al. (2012) concluded that infants exposed to high-quality infant-centered care demonstrated a higher capacity for attention and regulation and less excitability and hypotonicity with lower stress/abstinence NICU Network Neurobehavioral Scale (NNNS) scores than infants from low-care units. As the core measure sets are specifically infant and family centered, a positive association with these findings can be deduced.

Refer to Table V.1 for an outline of each core measure, corresponding clinical/systems impacts, and associated references.

SUMMARY

Early adverse life experiences have been shown to have a deleterious effect on physical and psychoemotional health on the infant–family dyad (Vanderbilt & Gleason, 2010). Mitigating risks and reducing complications associated with the NICU experience require the consistent reliable provision of evidence-based age-appropriate care for the premature and hospitalized infant.

Table V.1

OUTLINE OF CORE MEASURE, SYSTEM IMPACT, AND REFERENCES

Core Measure	Impacts	Reference
Protected sleep	• Neurosensory development • Preservation of brain plasticity—learning and memory • Immune function	Graven and Browne (2008), Imeri and Opp (2009), Colombo and De Bon (2011)
Pain and stress assessment and management	• Brain development • Oxidative stress • Brain structure and function	Smith et al. (2011), Brummelte et al. (2012), Slater et al. (2012)
Age-appropriate activities of daily living (postural integrity, alimentation, skin care)	• Movement and cognition • Self-regulation and autonomy • Barrier function	Koziol et al. (2011), Ross and Philbin (2011), Fluhr et al. (2010)
Family-centered care	• Length of stay • Parent role attainment • Parental confidence/competence	Ortenstrand et al. (2010), Franck et al. (2011), Gooding et al. (2011)
Healing environment (physical, human, systems)	• Brain development and neurosensory integrity • Patient safety and interprofessional collaboration • Systems/human factors	Ponte, Gross, Milliman-Richard, and Lacey (2010), White (2011), Reason (1995)

Neurodevelopmental outcomes for the premature individual are not only associated with gestational age at birth but also caregiving, family, and community experiences. Establishing consistency and reliability in the caregiving milieu of the newborn intensive care unit through the application of age-appropriate care strategies creates the substrate for favorable outcomes beyond the neonatal period.

NOTES

1. en.wikipedia.org/wiki/Maslow%27s_hierarchy_of_needs
2. en.wikipedia.org/wiki/Erik_Erikson
3. en.wikipedia.org/wiki/Erikson%27s_stages_of_psychosocial_development

REFERENCES

Als, H. (1982). Towards a synactive theory of development: Promise for the assessment of infant individuality. *Infant Mental Health Journal, 3*, 229–243.

Als, H., Duffy, F. H., & McAnulty, G. (1988a). Behavioral differences between preterm and fullterm newborns as measured with the APIB system scores: I. *Infant Behavior Development, 11*, 305–318.

Als, H., Duffy, F. H., & McAnulty, G. (1988b). The APIB, an assessment of functional competence in preterm and fullterm newborns regardless of gestational age at birth: II. *Infant Behavior Development, 11*, 319–331.

Brummelte, S., Grunau, R. E., Chau, V., Poskitt, K. J., Brant, R., Vinall, J., . . . Miller, S. P. (2012). Procedural pain and brain development in premature newborns. *Annals of Neurology, 71*(3), 385–396.

Colombo, G., & DeBon, G. (2011). Strategies to protect sleep. *Journal of Maternal-Fetal & Neonatal Medicine, 24*(Supp. 1), 30–31.

Fluhr, J. W., Darlenski, R., Taieb, A., Hachem, J. P., Baudouin, C., Msika, P., . . . Berardesca, E. (2010). Functional skin adaptation in infancy—almost complete but not fully competent. *Experimental Dermatology, 19*(6), 483–492.

Franck, L. S., Oulton, K., Nderitu, S., Lim, M., Fang, S., & Kaiser, A. (2011). Parent involvement in pain management for NICU infants: A randomized controlled trial. *Pediatrics, 128*(3), 510–518.

Gibbins, S., Hoath, S. B., Coughlin, M., Gibbins, A., & Franck, L. (2008). The universe of developmental care: A new conceptual model for application in the neonatal intensive care unit. *Advances in Neonatal Care, 8*(3), 141–147.

Gooding, J. S., Cooper, L. G., Blaine, A. I., Franck, L. S., Howse, J. L., & Berns, S. D. (2011). Family support and family centered care in the neonatal intensive care unit: Origins, advances, impact. *Seminars in Perinatology, 35*(1), 20–28.

Graven, S. N., & Browne, J. V. (2008). Sleep and brain development: The critical role of sleep in fetal and early neonatal brain development. *Newborn and Infant Nursing Reviews, 8*(4), 173–179.

Imeri, L., & Opp, M. R. (2009). How and why the immune system makes us sleep. *Nature Reviews Neuroscience, 10*, 199–210.

Koziol, L. F., Budding, D. E., & Chidekel, D. (2011). From movement to thought: Executive function, embodied cognition, and the cerebellum. *Cerebellum, 11*(2), 505–525.

Montirosso, R., Del Prete, A., Bellu, R., Tronick, E., Borgatti, R., & Neonatal Adequate Care for Quality of Life (NEO-ACQUA) Study Group. (2012). Level of NICU quality of developmental care and neurobehavioral performance in very preterm infants. *Pediatrics, 129*, e1129–e1137.

Ortenstrand, A., Westrup, B., Brostrom, E. B., Sarman, I., Akerström, S., Brune, T., . . . Waldenström, U. (2010). The Stockholm neonatal family centered care study: Effects on length of stay and infant morbidity. *Pediatrics, 125*(2), e278–e285.

Ponte, P. R., Gross, A. H., Milliman-Richard, Y. J., & Lacey, K. (2010). Interdisciplinary teamwork and collaboration: An essential element of a positive practice environment. *Annual Review of Nursing Research, 28*, 159–189.

Reason, J. (1995). Understanding adverse events: Human factors. *Quality in Healthcare, 4*(2), 80–89.

Ross, E. S., & Philbin, M. K. (2011). Supporting oral feeding in fragile infants: An evidence-based method for quality bottle-feedings of preterm, ill, and fragile infants. *Journal of Perinatal and Neonatal Nursing, 25*(4), 349–357.

Slater, L., Asmerom, Y., Boskovic, D. S., Bahjri, K., Plank, M. S., Angeles, K. R., . . . Angeles, D. M. (2012, April 30). Procedural pain and oxidative stress in premature neonates. *Journal of Pain*. doi: 10.1111/j.1475–4762.2011.01067.x

Smith, G. C., Gutovich, J., Smyser, C., Pineda, R., Newnham, C., Tjoeng, T. H., . . . Inder, T. (2011). Neonatal intensive care unit stress is associated with brain development in preterm infants. *Annals of Neurology, 70*(4), 541–549.

Vanderbilt, D., & Gleason, M. M. (2010). Mental health concerns of the premature infant through the lifespan. *Child and Adolescent Psychiatric Clinics of North America, 19*(2), 211–228, vii–viii.

White, R. D. (2011). The newborn intensive care unit environment of care: How we got here and where we're heading, and why. *Seminars in Perinatology, 35*(1), 2–7.

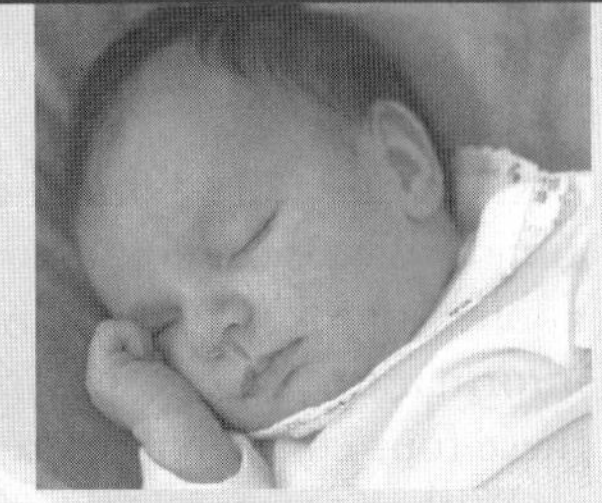

VI

Competency Education in the NICU

■ Wakako Eklund

The concept of competency has taken hold in health care for decades and continues to challenge health care organizations to consider the most cost-effective and yet, efficient method of developing an educational program to ensure the competency of the nursing staff and maintaining the competency of those who contribute to the quality of the care delivered for years to come. One of the historic phenomena that influenced the trend toward competency in education was the shift in nursing education from a hospital-based one to that of a university-based nursing education from the 1970s to the 1980s, which created the issue of how to prepare the graduates so that it would not add an excess burden to the health care delivery system (Lenburg, 1999). The statement by Lenburg in 1999 clearly describes a call for a partnership between the education and health care organizations.

> Competent practice, therefore, is more essential and mandatory than ever, as employers, consumers, insurance companies, and health care conglomerates expect more and different skills than in the past, which often goes far beyond those the faculty in schools of nursing currently emphasize, expect, or reward. The gap in expectations precipitates the urgent need for increased mutual respect, shared accountability and collaborative partnerships between those in nursing education and service more than ever before. Instead of each sector independently focusing just on its own responsibilities, which falls short of the collective need, educators and service leaders are urged to work collaboratively to establish core practice competencies and assessment methods and then hold those engaged in health care delivery accountable for them. (Lenburg, 1999)

In the unique setting of the NICU where highly technically dependent, extremely fragile infants are surviving at an increasingly early gestational age, where technological advancement is continuing with greater emphasis on evidence-based practice in the second decade of the 21st century, it would not be an overstatement to say that the burden placed on health care facilities is far greater than it once was during the earlier years of neonatal nursing in the United States.

In the standards published by the Joint Commission on Accreditation of Health Care Organizations (JCAHO) in 1999, JCAHO, for the first time, required that health care organizations document the clinical competency of the nursing staff (JCAHO, 1999). This led to the need for a clearly designed plan for education at the beginning, when hiring and maintenance of competence by continuing education throughout the course of an individual's employment.

It would surprise most readers to hear that the issue surrounding nurses competencce was controversial. In 1999, Lenburg stated, "Competence, assessment of competence, documentation of competent performance, and mandatory continuing competence are controversial topics receiving increasing emphasis in current manuscripts and conferences of all types and at all levels."

Society's awareness of safety and quality issues in the health care industry and the reports from the Institute of Medicine (IOM) with regard to quality and safety, such as *To Error Is Human: Building a Safer Health System* (IOM, 1999) further increased the heavy demand on health care organizations to drastically enhance the effort to achieve the goal for safer health care with higher quality. The report, *Crossing the Quality Chasm* emphasized that safety and quality did not suffer due to a single clinician's error, but rather due to the system's inability to translate the knowledge into practice by utilizing financial and human resources effectively (2001). IOM (2003a) also addressed nursing as the defense against preventable issues that are threatening patient safety. Competent nurses play an important role in maintaining a safe health care delivery system. IOM's (2003b) recommendation on the health professions' education addressed the core competencies required for all health care professionals no matter the specialty. The core competencies needed for health care professionals of the

21st century are patient-centered care, work in interdisciplinary teams, employment of evidence-based practice, application of quality improvements, and utilization of informatics. The following discussion demonstrates how these four competencies relate to the NICU environment.

With regard to the first core competency, patient-centered care, nurses have always been in the position to eagerly support the families, the neonatal units in general have not always advocated for the presence of the family and incorporation of their role into the plan of care. Increasing evidence indicates that family involvement is critical in optimizing both the quality of care and outcomes for both the infants and the parents (Bracht, O'Leary, Lee, & O'Brien, 2013, McGrath, Samra, & Kenner, 2011, O'Brien et al., 2013). Efforts must be made to maximize the presence of the family-centered-care philosophy by welcoming the family as the primary caregivers of their infants and part of the decision-making team. The second competency is to work in interdisciplinary teams. Neonatal intensive care is not possible without the collaboration of nursing, medicine, pharmacy, respiratory, and other professionals trained in specialty areas, such as physical, speech, or occupational therapy. Understanding various roles within the care team is necessary to create the team to care for the patients in the NICU. The fragile and vulnerable population who has no voice to speak out and advocate for themselves deserves highly motivated nursing professionals who are in tune with the evidence-based practice, in order to provide safe care and to strive toward quality improvements. The competency of utilization of informatics is evident in current neonatal settings. The skill in informatics contributes to the evidence-based practice by enhancing nurses' ability to research a topic, connect with the neonatal community on the Internet or in discussion groups, and access relevant journals. Informatics have also enhanced the data collection needed for nursing research and quality-impovement projects. Informatics is also fully incorporated into many NICUs today in nursing documentation systems and order entries.

After release of the historic IOM report (1999), the Agency for Healthcare Research and Quality (AHRQ), which is the health services research arm of the U.S. Department of Health and Human Services (HHS), responded with various efforts for funding and conducting research, designing and evaluating useful tools to enhance safety, and numerous other initiatives (AHRQ 2009).

One example focuses on the nurses and their potential in contributing to patient safety. In 2008, the AHRQ and the Robert Wood Johnson Foundation partnered and completed "Patient Safety and Quality: An Evidence Based Handbook for Nurses"; 22,000 copies of this book were distributed to nursing schools and clinicians who are working in the clinical field (AHRQ, 2008).

Nurses form the largest workforce in the health care organization; they are central to patient care and are also the force that drives quality improvements to achieve better outcomes. Nurses' abilities to utilize the knowledge, skills, and past experience in caring for the patients whose needs may be changing on the continuum depend largely on the individual organization's ability to train and educate them and to maintain the skill and knowledge level of the staff (AHRQ, 2008). The fact that nurses form the largest part of our workforce is very true in the care of the neonatal population. Without well-trained, competent nurses, who understand the changing needs of our vulnerable neonatal patients, no NICU can remain functional. The institutions and health care organizations are challenged to nurture and maintain this valuable workforce.

In 2010, the IOM partnered with the Robert Wood Johnson Foundation and published "The Future of Nursing: Leading Changed, Advancing Health" (IOM, 2010). One of the four key messages calls for nurses to "practice to the full extent of their education and training" (IOM, 2010).

Health care organizations are expected to provide general hospital education for the entire hospital staff, keeping the IOM core competencies in mind, and each unit-based educational program must be tailored to meet the specificities of the patient population cared for in the area.

In accordance with JCAHO requirements (1999), the competency of the nursing staff must be clearly documented at the beginning of the hiring process as well as annually. By successfully completing the designed program, an individual nurse is considered competent to assume the role of a neonatal nurse. Since little neonatal specialty education is offered in most undergraduate programs, there is an added challenge for neonatal intensive care units (NICUs) as they design educational programs to prepare new graduate nurses, as well as for experienced RNs who are new to the specific NICU environment and the unique patient population. Many units serve large populations of surgical patients and extremely-low-birth-weight (ELBW) infants. Yet, other NICUs may focus more on the slightly late preterm infants and not on ELBWs. A large number of Level III NICUs serve a wide range of patient populations, which necessitate extensive educational offerings.

Under cost containment efforts, funding dedicated to the education of nurses may be limited in many institutions, challenging those who design the educational plan (Bullock, Paris, & Terhaar, 2011). Various creative measures are used by educators to provide the foundational NICU-specific education. Often, advance practice neonatal nurses, such as clinical nurse specialists or neonatal nurse practitioners, partner with the unit educator to design and update the educational program.

The education needed to prepare a competent neonatal nurse is often provided through multiple modalities, such as didactic education, online tutorial, self-study module, digital material, as well as on-site preceptorship in order to help nurses apply the knowledge to practice. The following sections describe one example of how NICU nurses are trained using a combination of on-site training and other modalities of educational offerings. The primary focus of the discussion is placed on the new graduates' orientation design and the content required to prepare the nurses to become competent in Level III NICU setting.

COMPETENCY-BASED ORIENTATION PROGRAM AT THE LEVEL III NICU

The orientation educational program designed for competency in Level III NICU may begin with a set of courses essential to every RN who steps foot in the NICU. It would be helpful that new graduates gain neonatal-specific, hands-on simulation prior to taking on any patient assignments in the NICU. With the essential courses under their belts, the orientees enter the NICU better prepared to assume the care of the actual infant, starting with noncomplex, convalescent infants in a step-down unit. There are various approaches to providing the systematic didactic content and on-site training including simulation. The following provides a sample plan implemented at one Level III NICU.

REQUIREMENTS

The Neonatal Resuscitation Program (NRP), co-sponsored by the American Academy of Pediatrics and the American Heart Association, is an evidence-based educational approach to train health care providers with newborn-resuscitation skills (AAP, 2012). Although completion of this course does not automatically lead to individual competence in resuscitation skill, essential basic skills and knowledge needed as the foundation of neonatal resuscitation are provided in this program. Every nurse is required to receive the NRP training and receive the provider certificate before taking care of infants in the NICU. Highly simulation-oriented NRP will provide the new orientees opportunities to familiarize themselves with resuscitation equipment and other essential neonatal equipment and supplies as well as likely scenarios seen in delivery rooms prior to assuming the care of high-risk neonates. (See Chapter 22 for more information on simulation.)

A national program such as S.T.A.B.L.E.® (Karlsen, 2013) may fortify the foundational knowledge. S.T.A.B.L.E. is an educational program focusing on postresuscitation/pretransport stabilization care for sick neonates. The orientees are provided with a full day of the learner course, and the certificate must be maintained throughout the entire course of employment. Maintenance is due every 2 years. The name of this excellent educational program stands for **s**ugar/safety, **t**emperature, **a**irway, **bl**ood pressure, **l**ab work, and **e**motional support. The program is an effective introduction to basic neonatal pathophysiology. The course presents the learners with various situations and clinical presentations they will later face in an actual setting.

With the completion of NRP and the S.T.A.B.L.E. program, an orientee may benefit from a day in the NICU to become oriented to the physical setting and to observe what occurs in a day of life for infants and their families in the NICU. A set of DVDs covering a wide range of basic topics designed to provide helpful supplemental information was created by the unit educator of one NICU to provide supplemental material that anyone can view at his or her own pace. Each topic is short and not intended to replace the lecture material given in the low-risk and high-risk courses described later. This self-guided DVD or a similar program made available as short webinars or web-based tutorials, offer flexibility to learners. For those orientees who have taken NRP and S.T.A.B.L.E, but have not sat through the low-risk course described here have not been given information on pathologies frequently observed in the step-down units. These tutorials may provide a jump start or a review for the new nurses. The sample titles include:

- Infection Control
- What to Do in a Code
- Use of Developmental Aids
- How to Give a Good Report
- Feeding the Preterm Infant
- How to Care for Infants With Reflux

Low-Risk Course

■ Skill Lab. The early part of the orientation can also be dedicated to the necessary hands-on skill lab experience for the orientee. For example, set up can be created with a mannequin with a central line to actually handle intravenous tubing and to learn how to change the lines using sterile techniques. Unit-specific hands-on simulation experience can be created.

The low-risk course is offered over a 2-day period. This course outline is created and taught by a team of neonatal nurse practitioners (NNPs). The program was to is designed to meet the state neonatal nurse educational objectives (TN Perinatal Care System, 2011). The low-risk course is intended to provide the knowledge base essential to the nursing staff caring for infants in the step-down setting competently. Therefore, the courses are preferably offered at the beginning portion of the clinical preceptorship in the step-down NICU. Some orientees may take the course prior to the first day on unit orientation or after a few weeks spent in the step-down setting. The advantages to those who have already spent time in the unit is that the actual experience of having seen a few infants with specific issues could help digest the course material, and it may help with retention. It is not meant to guarantee that everything that a new graduate RN potentially encounters in the step-down NICU is taught in this course. However, the broad topics covered intend to provide a solid foundation in addition to the NRP and S.T.A.B.L.E. program upon which an orientee can further build his or her experience.

Day 1

- Maternal Risk Factors
- Fetal Circulation/Transition to Extrauterine Life
- Physical/Gestational Assessment
- Thermoregulation
- Neonatal Fluid Balance
- Neonatal Enteral Nutrition
- Newborn Screening
- Patterns of Newborn Jaundice
- Late Preterm Infants

Day 2

- Glucose Metabolism
- Sepsis

Gastrointestinal Conditions
Arterial Blood Gas
Respiratory Diseases and Modalities
Hematological Conditions
Cardiac Assessment of the Newborn
Commonly Used Medications in Neonatal Care
Consultation/Referral in Neonatal Care

■ Step-Down Unit Orientation. Discussion regarding the bedside orientation that is usually provided with one preceptor directly working with one orientee may be helpful. The new graduates are given approximately 5 weeks of clinical preceptorship in the step-down unit, depending on the pace of advancement per the clinical competency checklist that is formulated. The checklist describes the necessary concepts and skill set that must be demonstrated to competently care for the infants.

The orientee may begin by taking assignments from least complex to more complex in a stepwise fashion as mastery of skill and knowledge needed is observed by the preceptor. In this example of the orientation program, when the step-down unit orientation is completed, the orientee will temporarily come off the status of "orientee" to assume the role of step-down nurse with a mentor or a buddy available.

The preceptor and the orientee must mutually agree that she or he is ready, and if any extra time is needed, the orientation will need an extension. After approximately 2 months working in a full staff role in the step-down unit, the new graduate advances and takes the high-risk course and assumes the role of an orientee again, now in the high-risk side of NICU.

The time spent in the role of a staff nurse in the step-down unit for a few months after the step-down portion of the orientation may allow time for an individual to develop his or her new identity as a staff RN. Transition stress experienced by the new graduate as she or he transitions from a student role to an orientee role and then to a full staff role cannot be neglected. The National Council of State Boards of Nursing (NCSBN) now has a template for transition into practice for new graduates (2013). This model is being tested in many areas of the United States in order to ease the transition from school to career.

High-Risk Course

The high-risk course can be offered over a 2-day period. This course was also designed by a team of NNPs and is in accordance with the state neonatal nursing objectives (TN Perinatal Care System, 2011). The high-risk course attempts to expose nurses to an array of issues faced by the high-risk infants who are admitted to the high-risk NICU after either an in-house delivery or a transfer. Although it is not possible to cover every problem encountered in a NICU, this high-risk course serves as an excellent base for the new graduates to build their further knowledge and experience. The content of the high-risk course is:

Day 1
Grief/Attachment
Developmental Issues Regarding Neonatal Care
Retinopathy of Prematurity/Laser Therapy
Neurological Conditions of the Neonate
Electrolyte Disturbances
Neonatal Meningitis
Neonatal Parenteral Nutrition
Gastrointestinal Disorders

Day 2
Maternal Substance Abuse and Neonatal Abstinence Syndrome
Genitourinary Disorders
Immunizations for the NICU Baby
Advanced ABG Interpretation
Infrequent Hematologic Disorders in the NICU
Cardiac Disorders
More Respiratory Diseases and Their Treatments
Respiratory Syncytial Virus

High-Risk NICU Orientation

Each day of orientation it is preferable that one preceptor is paired with one orientee to take on the assignments. The competency checklist includes a wide range of specific skills, knowledge, and concepts, such as family-centered care and developmental care. An orientee advances from a stable infant on high-flow nasal cannula or CPAP and gradually progresses to a stable ventilated infant. Initial patient assignment and ways to advance through the orientation can be tailored individually based on the orientee's progress.

Additional supplemental material provided in short tutorials, either as DVDs or as webinars to enhance uniformity of information is alway helpful for new nurses. These materials can serve as reviews or simply to reinforce the content covered in the high-risk didactic course. Some of the topics include:

- Respiratory Therapy (various modalities)
- Central Line Care
- Chest Tube Care

During the high-risk NICU orientation, as the opportunities arise, information on delivery attendance, assisting with new admissions, and observing others with unusual situations can be offered to the orientee either as an observational experience or an actual participation.

High-risk infants enter the NICU in a wide range of sizes with a variety of problems, requiring broad categories of life-saving equipment. Perhaps there is no other specialty in nursing where patient size ranges as much as with the neonates. For example, a 450-g infant is one tenth the size of a larger infant weighing 4,500 g. This increases the challenge for learning as well as teaching. There is a need to become highly cognizant of the different sizes of tubing, catheters, medication dosages, and intravenous fluid infusion rates, not to mention the various developmental stages represented in the NICU patients that require attention and how to translate it into day-to-day care.

Translating the knowledge the orientees receive into the actual care of the infants and families requires time. There would be a need for opportunities for the orientee to reflect, with the preceptor's encouragement, on how theory and knowledge were applied to the management of a specific case to which one was assigned on any given day. Nurturing the new graduates to become competent in caring for the high-risk infants requires patience.

Becoming familiar with every situation is simply not achievable in a matter of a few months; however, experiencing as many situations as possible during orientation allows the orientee to widen the experience base that she or he can relate to and to reinforce the didactic knowledge received up to that point.

ANNUAL COMPETENCY

Completing the orientation checklist meets the competency requirements set forth by the facility; however, annual competency must be maintained. NRP and S.T.A.B.L.E. certification renewal is essential, although these are completed every 2 years. The annual competency for NICU contains requirements for staff to review knowledge of essential topics specific to the population, such as delivery room set up and care or maintenance of centrally inserted catheters. Infrequently performed procedures and skills must be included to allow periodic review and to maintain the competency. Other topics include professional practice issues, such as safety standards and privacy policies in the NICU. Additionally, annual competency often covers procedural skills or knowledge in the use of various equipment essential to the care of the ill infants.

If we do not use the skill or knowledge, it is not possible to polish it or maintain it. Efforts must be made to help the new nurses become increasingly comfortable with the environment and the scope of practice. For example, in order for the new nurses to grow in confidence and to improve the skill in the delivery room setting, experienced nurses are encouraged to invite the new staff to join when the NICU team attends deliveries. Advancing from an observer to a participant does not occur over night. Highly skilled nursing care is required in the NICU. Annual competency is a way to remind the staff where they may lack experience and what information must be reinforced to maintain the safety and quality standards.

CONCLUSION

Role transition from a newly graduated nurse to a competent nurse challenges the health care delivery system across the globe. Successful educational programs not only produce competent nurses essential for high-quality care and safe environments, but also a quality and stable workforce that leads to the next generation. Setting well-defined goals with accurate feedback, such as in the case of competency-based orientation, has positive effects on retention (Bullock et al., 2011; Beeman, Jernigan, & Hensley, 1999). Incorporating the mentorship or buddy system beyond the scope/time frame of the orientation period encourages the new nurses to continue to assimilate into the role of full-fledged staff nurse. Preceptorship is a time-limited relationship; however, mentoring has the potential to assist the novice nurse who is on her or his path to becoming an expert (Funderburk, 2008). Preceptor and mentor with the theoretical understanding of Benner's "Novice to Expert" model is an asset in competency building (Benner, 2001). Investing in quality orientation programs to educate new nurses has potential long-term gain, such as decreased turnover of new graduates, in addition to the immediate gain of producing nurses who contribute to creating a safe environment for infants and their families (Bullock et al., 2011).

The competency-based orientation program described in this chapter is by no means a prescription for success. Many organizations are highly challenged by the task and struggle to meet the educational needs of their new staff. Availability of support programs such as the "Foundation of Neonatal Care: A Comprehensive Competency-Based Orientation Program" (NANN, 2006) may be a valuable option.

Experienced neonatal nurses must keep in mind that if not for the effort of the educators and the preceptors, they may not have become neonatal nurses. We need a competent workforce, and in order to achieve that goal, more emphasis needs to be placed on easing the transition into a new role, whether that be a staff role or an advanced practice nurse. Future advanced practice neonatal nurses are found among staff nurses today. Investing in the future neonatal workforce begins with our investment in these new graduates.

ACKNOWLEDGMENT

Special gratitude to a colleague and the leader of the advanced practice team, Patti Scott, DNP, NNP-BC who invested a great amount of work for staff nursing education in her life during the past two decades not only in one facility, but over a large area of the state, as well as outside of the state.

REFERENCES

Agency for Healthcare Research and Quality. (2008). *Patient safety and quality. An evidence-based handbook for nurses*. Retrieved from http://www.ahrq.gov/qual/nurseshdbk/

Agency Health to Healthcare Research and Quality (2009). Advancing patient safety. A decade of evidence, design and implementation. AHRQ Publication, 9(10), 0084. Retrieved from http://www.ahrq.gov/professionals/quality-patient-safety/patient-safety-resources/resources/advancing-patient-safety/advancing-patient-safety.pdf

American Academy of Pediatrics (2012). Neonatal Resuscitation Program. NRP Course Description. Retrieved from http://www2.aap.org/nrp/instructors/about/about_coursedescrp.html

Beeman, K., Jernigan, C., & Hensley, P. (1999). Employing new grads: A plan for success. *Nursing Economics, 17*(2), 91–95.

Benner, P. E. (2001). *From novice to expert: Excellence in power and practice* (Commemorative ed.). Upper Saddle River, NJ: Prentice Hall.

Bracht, M., O'Leary, L., Lee, S. K., & O'Brien, K. (2013). Implementing family-integrated care in the NICU: a parent education and support program. [Research Support, Non-U.S. Gov't]. Adv Neonatal Care, *13*(2), 115–126. doi:10.1097/ANC.0b013e318285fb5b

Bullock, L. M., Paris, L. G., & Terhaar, M. (2011). Designing and outcome-focused model for orienting new graduate nurses. *Journal for Nurses in Staff Development, 27*(6), 252–258.

Funderburk, A. E. (2008). Mentoring: The retention factor in the acute care setting. *Journal of Nurses in Staff Development, 24*(3), E1–E5.

Institute of Medicine (IOM). (1999). *To error is human: Building a safer health system*. Washington, DC: Institute of Medicine and National Academies Press. Retrieved from http://www.nap.edu/openbook.php?isbn=0309068371

Institute of Medicine (IOM). (2001). *Crossing the quality chasm*. Washington, DC: National Academies Press. Retrieved from http://www.nap.edu/catalog.php?record_id=10027

Institute of Medicine (IOM). (2003a). *Patient safety: Achieving a new standard of care*. Washington, DC: National Academies Press.

Institute of Medicine (IOM). (2003b). *Health professions education: A bridge to quality*. Washington, DC: National Academies Press. Retrieved from http://www.nap.edu/catalog.php?record_id=10681

Institute of Medicine (IOM). (2010). *The future of nursing: Leading change, advancing health*. Retrieved from http://www.iom.edu/Reports/2010/The-Future-of-Nursing-Leading-Change-Advancing-Health.aspx

Joint Commission on Accreditation of Healthcare Organizations (JCAHO). (1999). *Comprehensive accreditation manual of hospitals: The official handbook*. Oakbrook Terrace, IL: JCAHO.

Karlsen, K. A. (2013). The S.T.A.B.L.E. program. Retrieved from http://www.stableprogram.org

Lenburg, C. B. (1999). Redesigning expectations for initial and continuing competency for contemporary nursing practice. *Online Journal of Issues in Nursing*.

McGrath, J. M., Samra, H. A., & Kenner, C. (2011). Family-centered developmental care practices and research: what will the next century bring? *Journal of Perinatal Neonatal Nursing, 25*(2), 165–170. doi:10.1097/JPN.0b013e31821a6706

National Council of State Boards of Nursing. (2013). Transition to practice engaging, experiencing, empowering. Retrieved from https://www.ncsbn.org/363.htm#why

NANN. (2006). Foundations of neonatal care: A comprehensive competency-based orientation program. CD-ROM. Retrieved from http://www.nann.org/pubs/content/foundations.html

O'Brien, K., Bracht, M., Macdonell, K., McBride, T., Robson, K., O'Leary, L., . . . Lee, S. K. (2013). A pilot cohort analytic study of Family Integrated Care in a Canadian neonatal intensive care unit. [Research Support, Non-U.S. Gov't]. BMC Pregnancy Childbirth, 13 Suppl 1, S12. doi:10.1186/1471-2393-13-S1-S12

Tennessee Perinatal Care System. (2011). Educational objectives for nurses levels I, II, III and neonatal transport nurses (4th ed.). Retrieved from http://health.state.tn.us/Downloads/Perinatal_2011.pdf

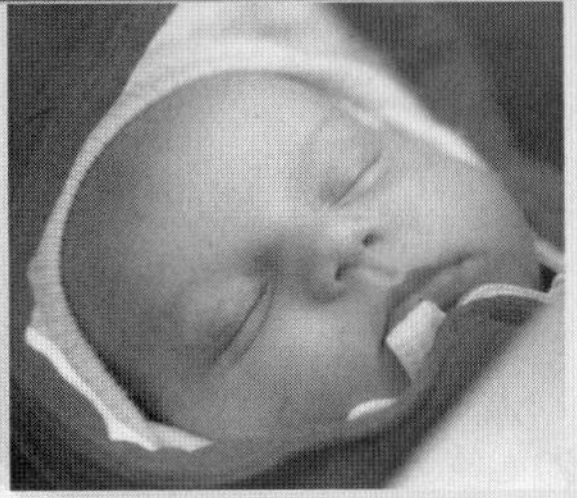

Transfusion Guidelines

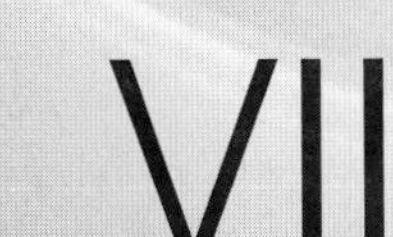

■ Gail A. Bagwell

- A central hematocrit should be obtained on admission, and no further hematocrits obtained unless specifically ordered.
- Transfusions generally should be considered only if acute blood loss of greater than 10% associated with symptoms of decreased oxygen delivery occurs or if significant hemorrhage of greater than 20% total blood volume occurs.
- In term and preterm infants, a transfusion should be considered if an immediate need for increased oxygen delivery to tissues is suspected clinically.
- Transfuse 20 mL/kg packed red cells unless the hematocrit is greater than 29% (0.29). A volume of 20 mL/kg also could be used if significant phlebotomy losses are anticipated in smaller infants whose hematocrits are greater than 29% (0.29). The volume may be administered in two 10-mL/kg aliquots.
- For infants receiving erythropoietin, considerations of the above guidelines should be made regarding the rate of decrease in hemoglobin or hematocrit, the infant's reticulocyte count, the postnatal day of age, the need for supplemental oxygen, and the overall stability of the infant.
- Central measurements of hemoglobin or hematocrit are preferred; alternatively, heelstick measurements may be obtained after warming the heel adequately. An infant meeting the following criteria should not be transfused automatically, but a transfusion should or can be considered for the following:

    1. A transfusion should be considered if acute blood loss of greater than 10% associated with symptoms of decreased oxygen delivery occurs or if significant hemorrhage of greater than 20% total blood volume occurs.
    2. For infants requiring moderate or significant mechanical ventilation, defined as mean arterial pressure (MAP) > 8 cm H_2O and FiO_2 > 0.40 on a conventional ventilator or MAP > 14 and FiO_2 > 0.40 on high-frequency ventilator, transfusions can be considered if the hematocrit is less than 30% (0.30) (hemoglobin <10 g/dL [100 g/L]).
    3. For infants requiring minimal mechanical ventilation, defined as MAP < 8 cm H_2O and/or FiO_2 < 0.40 on a conventional ventilator or MAP < 14 and/or FiO_2 < 0.40 on high-frequency ventilator, transfusions can be considered if the hematocrit is <25% (0.25) (hemoglobin <8 g/dL [80 g/L]).
    4. For infants receiving supplemental oxygen who do not require mechanical ventilation, transfusions can be considered if the hematocrit is less than 20% (0.20) (hemoglobin <7 g/dL [70 g/L]), and one or more of the following is present:

        - Greater than 24 hours of tachycardia (heart rate >180 beats/min) or tachypnea (respiratory rate > 60 breaths/min)
        - A doubling of the oxygen requirement from the previous 48 hours
        - Lactate > 2.5 mEq/L (2.5 mmol/L) or an acute metabolic acidosis (pH < 7.20)
        - Weight gain less than 10 g/kg/d over the previous 4 days while receiving greater than 120 kcal/kg/d
        - If the infant will undergo major surgery within 72 hours

    5. For infants who have no symptoms, transfusions can be considered if the hematocrit is less than 18% (0.18) (hemoglobin < 6 g/dL [60 g/L]) associated with an absolute reticulocyte count of less than 100_103/mcL (100_109/L) (<2%)

REFERENCE

Ohls, R. K. (2007). Transfusions in the preterm infant. *Neoreviews*, *8*, e377. doi:10.1542/neo8-9-e377

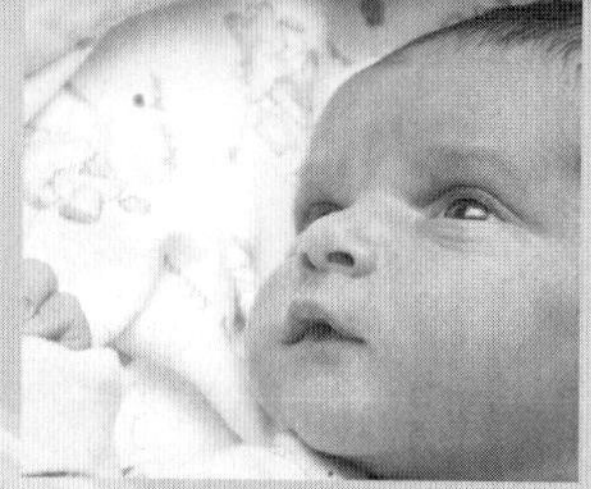

VIII

Management of Jaundice in the Newborn Nursery

■ Gail A. Bagwell

Nearly two thirds of the 4 million newborns born in the United States will develop clinical jaundice, but the majority will not develop any severe sequelae as a result of the hyperbilirubinemia. Knowing which neonate will or will not develop sequelae as a result of the hyperbilirubinemia is the challenge that health care professionals must face when caring for the newborn.

A major factor that makes a newborn more prone to developing more severe jaundice is prematurity. The more premature a baby is, the greater the risk. Several reasons for this is the premature infant liver has a delay in reaching maximum concentrations of uridine diphosphoglucouronate glucuronosyltransferase (UGT) the substance that helps with the breakdown of bilirubin. The premature baby may feed less than a term baby which leads to fewer bowel movements, another essential component in eliminating bilirubin from the body.

As stated earlier in this text, the sequelae related to hyperbilirubinemia are acute bilirubin encephalopathy (transient mild encephalopathy) and chronic bilirubin encephalopathy (Kernicterus). Kernicterus is a preventable disease, if a newborn's jaundice is recognized and managed properly. The American Academy of Pediatrics in 1994 developed guidelines for health care professionals to manage hyperbilirubinemia in the newborn and revised them in 2004. The 2004 guidelines can be found in Figure VIII.1. A study by Burke et al. (2009) showed that since the implementation of the AAP 1994 guidelines the incidence of hospitalizations with a diagnosis of kernicterus in the United States has decreased, showing that proper adherence to the AAP guidelines helps to prevent long-term sequelae of hyperbilirubinemia.

1 Newborn infant

2 Assess for jaundice every 8–12 hours

3 Is jaundice present ?

No

Yes

4 Has TcB or TSB been measured?

No

Yes

5 Is newborn ready for discharge?

No

Yes

Go to Box 2

6 Any risk factors or infant < 72 hours old?

No

Yes

7 Discharge and follow-up at physician discretion*

8 Follow up by 48–120 hours of age, exact timing depends upon age in hours (see recommendation 6.1.2) and presence of risk factors (see Table 2)

9 Is follow-up assured?

No

Yes

10 Measure TSB or TcB if not already done, assure plan for follow-up and/or management* according tobilirubin level

11 Discharge with planned follow-up*

12 Is age < 24 hours or does jaundice by visual assessment or TcB appear severe enough to require TSB or TcB?

No

Yes

13 Measure TSB or TcB and interpret by age in hours

14 Is TSB > 95th percentile (see Figure 2)

No

Yes

15 Evaluate TSB level, gestational age and hours of life. Treat if criteria for treatment met (see Figures 3,4)

16 Any repeat TSB drawn?

No

Yes

Go to Box 5

17 Is TSB level increasing across percentile line? (see Figure 2)

No

Yes

Go to Box 15

Go to Box 18

18 1. Evaluate cause.
2. Treat if criteria for treatment met (see Figures 3,4).
3. Repeat TSB in 4–24 hours

Go to Box 17

* Provide information and written guidelines about jaundice to parents of all newborns at discharge.

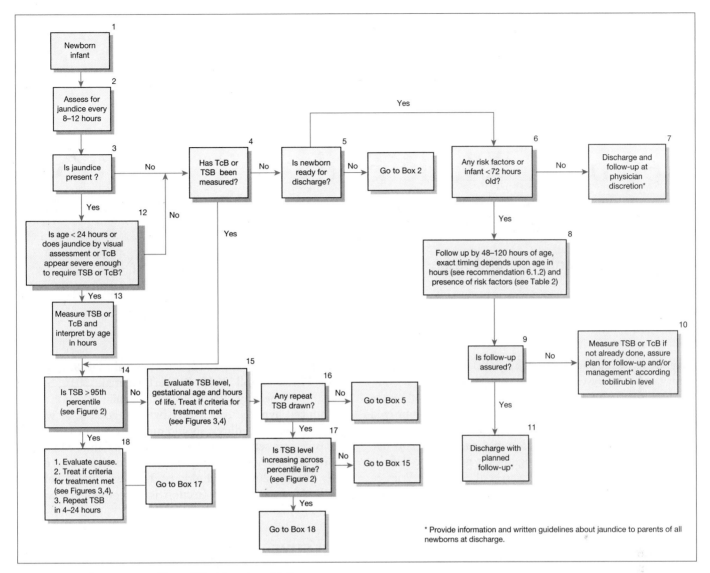

FIGURE VIII.1 Management of hyperbilirubinemia guidelines.
Adapted from *Pediatrics* (2004).

REFERENCES

American Academy of Pediatrics. (2004). Management of hyperbilirubinemia in the newborn infant 35 or more weeks of gestetion. *Pediatrics*, 114, 297–316.

Burke, B. L., Robbins, J. M., Biral, T. M., Hobbs, C. A., Nesmith, C., & Tifford, J. M. (2009). Trends in hospitalizations for neonatal jaundice and kernicterus in the United States, 1988–2005. *Pediatrics*, *123*(2), 524.

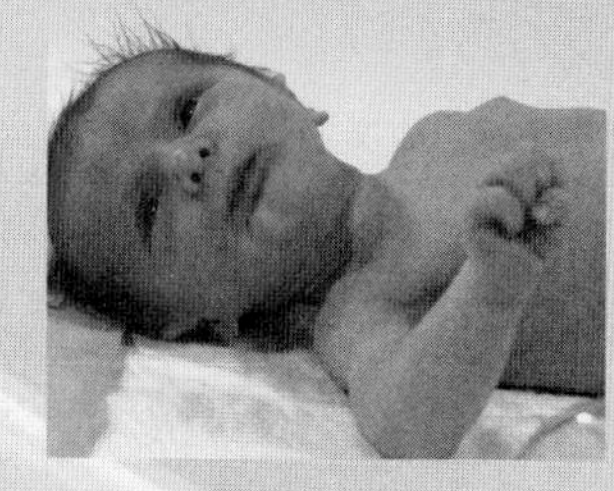

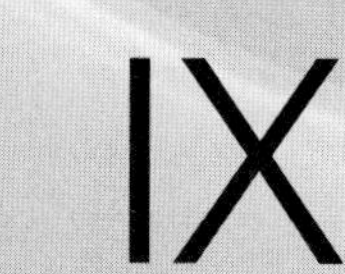

Newborn Whole-Body Cooling Protocol

IX

■ Georgia R. Ditzenberger and Susan Tucker Blackburn

Hypoxic ischemic encephalopathy (HIE) is an injury to the brain caused by systemic hypoxemia, ischemia, or a combination of the two conditions. The incidence of severe forms of HIE has declined markedly as a result of improved perinatal care; however, the insult is significant enough to cause transient organ dysfunction in 4 to 6 per 1,000 live births and result in death or significant neurologic deficits in 1 per 1,000 live births (Bonifacio et al., 2012; de Vries & Jongmans, 2010; Dickey et al., 2011; Roland & Hill, 2007; Wachtel & Hendrics-Munoz, 2011).

Most term infants with HIE manifest characteristic patterns of neurologic clinical signs over the first 72 hours post birth. The neurologic clinical signs have been used to characterized the severity of HIE into three stages, summarized in Chapter 15, Table 15.6.

Infants with HIE have multiorgan and multisystem problems arising from the original hypoxic and/or ischemic insult, and therefore require a coordinated team approach to management. Prompt identification and treatment of alterations in neurological, cardiovascular, pulmonary, gastrointestinal, and renal systems is exceedingly important to prevent or minimize further damage (Gunn, et al., 2008; Jacobs, et al., 2011; Kelen & Robertson, 2010; Stola & Perlman, 2008; Volpe, 2008; Wachtel & Hendricks-Munoz, 2011).

Management of term infants with HIE in terms of neurologic sequelae focuses on elimination of the cause of the original hypoxia, promotion of adequate cerebral perfusion, maintenance of adequate continuous glucose supply and improve brain oxygenation (Kelen & Robertson, 2010; Stola & Perlman, 2008; Volpe, 2008; Wachtel & Hendricks-Munoz, 2011). Induced mild hypothermia has been shown to provide neuroprotection and reduce the extent of tissue injury. Hypothermia, induced either by head-cooling protocol or by whole-body cooling protocol, is increasingly the treatment of choice for infants greater than or equal to 36 weeks gestation with moderate to severe HIE (Bonifacio et al., 2012; Hoehn et al., 2008; Laptook 2012; Pfister & Soll, 2010; Rutherford et al., 2010; Sarkar et al., 2009; Selway, 2010; Stola & Perlman, 2008).

Induced hypothermia, either by head-cooling or whole-body cooling procedures, should only be done in a neonatal intensive care setting (NICU), due to the heightened vulnerability of the newborn to rapid changes in all systems of the body (Barks, 2008; Reynolds & Talmage, 2011; Selway, 2010). Discussed in this section is a protocol for whole-body cooling.

OBJECTIVE

To provide whole-body cooling to eligible newborns with HIE.

POLICY

1. Eligibility for this therapy is assessed by the medical team through the inclusionary/exclusionary criteria determined by the neonatologists and/or neurologists; current eligibility criteria is summarized in Table IX.1)
2. The neonate will undergo whole-body cooling therapy to achieve and maintain esophageal temperature of 33.5°Celsius for 72 hours
3. After 72 hours is completed, the newborn will be rewarmed over a 6-hour period
4. A physician/NNP must enter an order to initiate the whole-body cooling therapy and again to initiate rewarming (Barks, 2008; Hoehn et al., 2008; Laptook, 2012; Long & Brandon, 2007; Selway, 2010; Simbruner, et al., 2010)

RISKS TO NEWBORN

1. Changes in blood pressure, either hypo- or hypertension
2. Abnormal clot formation

3. Skin impairment/breakdown
4. Metabolic acidosis (Sarkar et al., 2009)

EQUIPMENT AND SUPPLIES

1. Radiant warmer
2. Cooling unit of choice, with probe adaptor, connecting hoses
3. Newborn size (25" × 33") cooling blanket
4. Distilled/sterile water
5. Tape or transparent dressing to secure the esophageal probe in place

Setup of cooling unit of choice, per manufacturer's instructions

Precool the blanket on the radiant warmer and before placing the newborn on the blanket, per manufacturer's instructions

ESOPHAGEAL PROBE INSERTION AND SKIN TEMPERATURE PROBE

1. Soften the esophageal probe prior to insertion by placing it in a warm water bath for a few moments; do NOT use lubricants.
2. Nasal placement of the probe is preferred. Position the probe in the lower third of the esophagus; measure the distance from the nares to the ear to the sternum, subtract 2 cm and mark with indelible pen before inserting for ease in assessing probe position during cooling period.
3. Secure the probe by taping to the newborn's nose. Probe position should be confirmed with chest x-ray.
4. Secure the skin probe to the abdomen, not extremities, chest or back; do not use the radiant warmer skin temperature (the radiant warmer is OFF).
5. Connect the esophageal and skin probes to the appropriate probe cable attachments per manufacturer's instructions on cooling unit and/or monitoring device; the esophageal temperature probe must be connected to the cooling device, as this is the temperature used to control the water temperature to maintain a temperature steadystate. Attach the skin probe to an external temperature-monitoring device.

COOLING THE NEWBORN

1. An open radiant warmer with a precooled newborn size cooling blanket should be used for whole-body cooling. Place the newborn on the cooling blanket with the entire head and naked body exposed to the surface of the cooling blanket.
2. Turn the radiant warmer to OFF; all other exogenous heat sources should be OFF.
3. Do not place cloth blanket, diaper, wrap, flannel, and so on, between the newborn and the surface of the cooling blanket.
4. Once the newborn's esophageal temperature has reached the set point of 33.5°C, a single layer such as a *thin* receiving blanket may be placed between the newborn and the cooling blanket to prevent soiling of the cooling blanket. A small diaper covering as little of the perianal area as possible may be used—promote maximum exposure to the cooling blanket.

ASSESS/MONITOR NEWBORN STATUS

1. Assessment of the newborn's skin integrity, perfusion, and potential complications should be performed and documented with each hands-on assessment; contact the medical team immediately if integrity impairment is noted.
2. Monitor newborn's respiratory status; if not already intubated, the newborn may require intubation due to hypoventilation, hypoxemia, metabolic acidosis, and so on.
3. Monitor newborn for seizure activity; often newborns are placed on continuous electroencephalogram with/without video during the cooling therapy period.
4. Monitor blood pressure either with continuous arterial access (preferred) or by appropriate cuff on upper extremity every 15 minutes during the initial cooling process and then every ½ hour thereafter; notify medical team immediately if blood pressure changes.
5. Monitor changes in heart rate; often newborns become consistently bradycardic (<100 beats per minute) during cooling therapy (Barks, 2008; Long & Brandon, 2007; Reynold & Talmage, 2011; Simbruner, et al., 2010).

TEMPERATURE MONITORING

1. During body cooling, monitor the esophageal, skin, axillary, and blanket water temperatures every 15 minutes for the first 2 hours.
2. After all temperatures are stable, record all temperatures every hour for the remainder of the 72-hour period.

REWARMING THE NEWBORN

1. At the end of the 72-hour cooling period and after an order has been written, begin the gradual rewarming period; rewarm over a 6-hour period at the rate of 0.5°C per hour.
2. Use the esophageal probe temperature control to gradually warm the cooling blanket and thereby gradually warm the newborn.
3. At the end of the 6-hour rewarming period with the blanket, the newborn's thermoregulatory support will be returned to the radiant warmer servo-control with the skin probe already in place on the newborn's abdomen, to continue the rewarming process.
4. Turn off the blanket and remove it from under the newborn; keep the newborn on the radiant warmer.
5. Turn on the radiant warmer, set the skin-servo temperature 0.5°C higher than the newborn's surface skin temperature and gradually rewarm by 0.5°C to a skin temperature of 36.5°C.
6. Continue to care and monitor for the newborn on the radiant warmer per NICU protocol (Barks, 2008; Hoehn, et al., 2008; Long & Brandon; 2007; Pfister & Soll, 2010; Selway, 2010).

TABLE IX.1

CRITERIA TO DETERMINE ELIGIBILITY OF NEWBORNS WITH HIE FOR WHOLE-BODY COOLING

1.	Term >/= 36 weeks gestation
2.	No major congenital anomalies or known congenital anomalies
3.	Birth weight > 1800 g (not intra-uterine growth restricted)
4.	Is less than 6 hours of life when admitted to a neonatal intensive care unit
5.	Meets Sarnat Stage 2, moderate HIE, or Stage 3, severe HIE, assessment by neonatologist and/or pediatric neurologist

From Gancia and Pomero (2011) and Hoehn et al. (2008).

SELECTED READING

Barks, J. (2008). Technical aspects of starting a neonatal cooling program. *Clinics in Perinatology, 35*(4), 765–776.

Bonifacio, S. L., Gonzalez, E., & Ferriero, D. M (2012). Central nervous system injury and neuroprotection. In C. A. Gleason & S. Devaskar (eds), *Avery's diseases of the newborn* (pp. 869–891). Philadelphia, PA: Elsevier/Saunders.

de Vries, L. S., & Jongmans, M. J. (2010). Long-term outcome after neonatal hypoxic-ischaemic encephalopathy. *Archives of Disease in Childhood—Fetal and Neonatal Edition, 95*(3), F220–F224.

Dickey, E. J., Long, S.N., & Hunt, R. W (2011). Hypoxic ischemic encephalopathy—what can we learn from humans? *Journal of Veterinary Internal Medicine*, 25, 1231–1240.

Gancia, P., & Pomero, G. (2011). Brain cooling and eligible newborns: should we extend the indications? *Journal of Maternal-Fetal and Neonatal Medicine*, 24, 53–55.

Gunn, A. J., Wyatt, J. S., Whitelaw, A., Barks, J., Azzopardi, D., Ballard, R., . . . CoolCap Study Group. (2008). Therapeutic hypothermia changes the prognostic value of clinical evaluation of neonatal encephalopathy. *The Journal of Pediatrics, 152*(1), 55–58, 58.e1.

Hoehn, T., Hansmann, G., Bührer, C., Simbruner, G., Gunn, A. J., Yager, J., . . . Thoresen, M. (2008). Therapeutic hypothermia in neonates. Review of current clinical data, ILCOR recommendations and suggestions for implementation in neonatal intensive care units. *Resuscitation, 78*(1), 7–12.

Jacobs, S. E., Morley, C. J., Inder, T. E., Stewart, M. J., Smith, K. R., McNamara, P. J., . . . , Infant Cooling Evaluation Collaboration. (2011). Whole-body hypothermia for term and near-term newborns with hypoxic-ischemic encephalopathy: A randomized controlled trial. *Archives of Pediatrics & Adolescent Medicine, 165*(8), 692–700.

Kelen, D., & Roberson, N. J. (2010). Experimental treatments for hypoxic ischaemic encephalopathy. *Early Human Development*, 86, 369–377.

Laptook, A. R. (2012). The use of hypothermia to provide neuroprotection for neonatal hypoxic-ischemic brain injury. In J. Perlman (Ed.), *Neurology* (2nd ed., pp. 63–76). Philadelphia, PA: Saunders/Elsevier.

Long, M., & Brandon, D. H. (2007). Induced hypothermia for neonates with hypoxic-ischemic encephalopathy. *Journal of Obstetric, Gynecologic, & Neonatal Nursing, 36*(3), 293–298.

Pfister, R., & Soll, R. (2010). Hypothermia for the treatment of infants with hypoxic–ischemic encephalopathy. *Journal of Perinatology, 30*, S82–S87.

Reynolds, R., & Talmage, S. (2011). "Caution! Contents should be cold": Developing a whole-body hypothermia program. *Neonatal Network: The Journal of Neonatal Nursing, 30*(4), 225–230. Epub July 5, 2011.

Roland, E. H., & Hile, A. (2007). Neonatal hypoxic-ischemic and hemorrhagic cerebral injury. In G. M. Fenichel (ed), *Neonatal Neurology* (pp. 69–90). Philadelphia, PA: Churchill Livingstone/Eslevier.

Rutherford, M., Ramenghi, L. A., Edwards, A. D., Brocklehurst, P., Halliday, H., Levene, M . . . . Azzopardi, D. (2010). Assessment of brain tissue injury after moderate hypothermia in neonates with hypoxic-ischaemic encephalopathy: A nested substudy of a randomised controlled trial. *The Lancet Neurology, 9*, 39–45.

Sarkar, S., Barks, J., Bhagat, I., & Donn, S. (2009). Effects of therapeutic hypothermia on multiorgan dysfunction in asphyxiated newborns: Whole-body cooling versus selective head cooling. *Journal of Perinatology, 29*, 558–563.

Selway, L. D. (2010). State of the science: Hypoxic ischemic encephalopathy and hypothermic intervention for neonates. *Advances in Neonatal Care, 10*(2), 60–66.

Simbruner, G., Mittal, R. A., Rohlmann, F., Muche, R., & Participants nnnT. (2010). Systemic hypothermia after neonatal encephalopathy: Outcomes of neo.nEURO.network RCT. *Pediatrics, 126*(4), e771–e778.

Stola, A., & Perlman, J. (2008). Post-resuscitation strategies to avoid ongoing injury following intrapartum hypoxia-ischemia. *Seminars in Fetal and Neonatal Medicine*, 13, 424–431.

Tagin, M. A., Woolcott, C. G., Vincer, M. J., Whyte, R. K., & Stinson, D. A. (2012). Hypothermia for neonatal hypoxic ischemic encephalopathy: An updated systematic review and meta-analysis. *Archives of Pediatrics & Adolescent Medicine*. doi:10.1001/archpediatrics.2011.1772.

Wachtel, E. V., & Hendricks-Munoz, K. D. (2011). Current management of the infant who presents with neonatal encephalopathy. *Current Problems in Pediatric and Adolescent Health Care*, 41, 132–153.

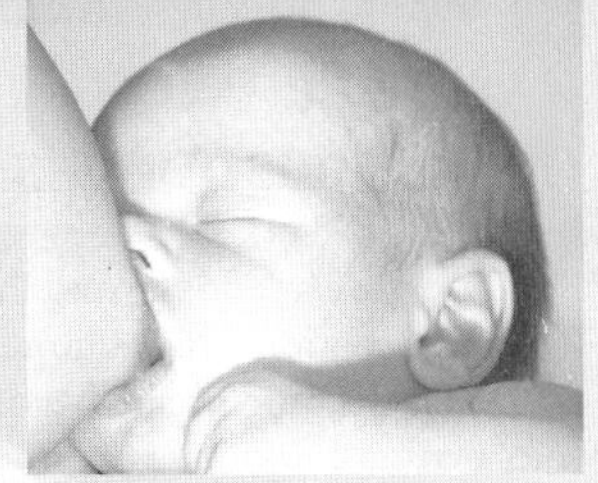

APPENDIX

A

Neonatal Nurses and Interconception Care

■ Merry K. Moos

Health care providers and policy makers are increasingly aware that efforts to prevent reproductive casualties that begin in prenatal care are starting too late to affect primary prevention (Centers for Disease Control and Prevention [CDC], 2006). As a result, preconception and interconception care have become a focus for health care interactions with women of childbearing age. Preconception and interconception health are defined as "Any intervention provided to women of childbearing age, regardless of pregnancy desire, to improve the health outcomes of women, newborns and children" (Dean et al., 2012). Knowledge of interconception care is important for NICU nurses because of their ongoing interactions with individual women when they visit their infants. This ongoing relationship allows the NICU nurse to observe the new mother's health status, her self-care practices, and her use of health and medical resources. Thus, the nurse may observe a woman becoming withdrawn, depressed, or anxious; she may observe that she is missing meals or stress eating; the nurse may note lack of sleep and lack of support.

Identification of a new mother's health care needs gives the NICU staff the opportunity to provide education, guidance, and support to the mother as they perform their usual care. NICU nurses can help identify maternal medical needs and health risks and assist new mothers in addressing their own health even as they focus on the well-being of their neonate.

Examples for each include:

- Strategies for taking care of self include encouraging:
  - Time away from unit to eat meals
  - Healthy snacks
  - Taking breaks to walk in and around the hospital
  - Talking about her feelings about the baby's situation and encourage discussing fears, concerns, self-blame with the unit social worker and with her usual provider
- Strategies for minimizing risks to women's own health and future reproductive outcomes include encouraging:
  - Women to maintain or become smoke free
  - Healthy approaches to stress reduction
  - Waiting the optimal time (18–60 months) before becoming pregnant again (Conde-Agudelo, Rosas-Bermudez, & Kafury-Goeta, 2006)
  - Postpartum visit with health care provider
  - Use of an over-the-counter (OTC) daily multivitamin with folic acid after prenatal vitamins are depleted
  - Follow up with their usual provider for any medical needs identified during pregnancy (e.g., premature infant born due to severe preeclampsia, respiratory distress syndrome related to mother's diabetes)
  - Early identification and referral for signs and symptoms of anxiety and depressive disorder
- Strategies for encouraging care with a woman's usual provider:
  - Ask mother how she is doing when she visits her newborn
  - Encourage making appointment with usual health care provider
  - Offer assistance from social worker or other help as needed

ONLINE RESOURCES

Before, Between and Beyond Pregnancy: The National Preconception Curriculum and Resources Guide for Clinicians **http://www.beforeandbeyond.org**

Information for women, families, and clinicians interested in preconception health can be accessed at
http://www.cdc.gov/preconception
http://www.marchofdimes.com/professionals/medicalresources.html

Preconception Health Promotion: The Foundation for a Healthier Tomorrow. A slide module for nurses on the content and evidence around preconception care. Content is available without cost and CNE credit is available for a fee.
http://www.marchofdimes.com/nursing

REFERENCES

Centers for Disease Control and Prevention (CDC). (2006). Recommendations for improving preconception health and health care: United States: A report of the CC/ATSDR Preconception Workgroup and the Select Panel on preconception Care. *Morbidity and Mortality Weekly Report (MMWR)*, *55*, 1–23.

Conde-Agudelo, A., Rosas-Bermudez, A., & Kafury-Goeta, A. C. (2006). Birth spacing and risk of adverse perinatal outcomes: A meta-analysis. *Journal of the American Medical Association*, *295*(15):1809–1823.

Dean, S., Bhutta, Z., Mason, M. E., Howson, C., Chandra-Mouli, V., Lassi, Z., & Imam, A. (2012). Care before and between pregnancy. In C. P. Howson, M. V. Kinney, & J. E. Lawn (Eds.), *Born too soon: The global action report on preterm birth*. Geneva Switzerland: World Health Organization.

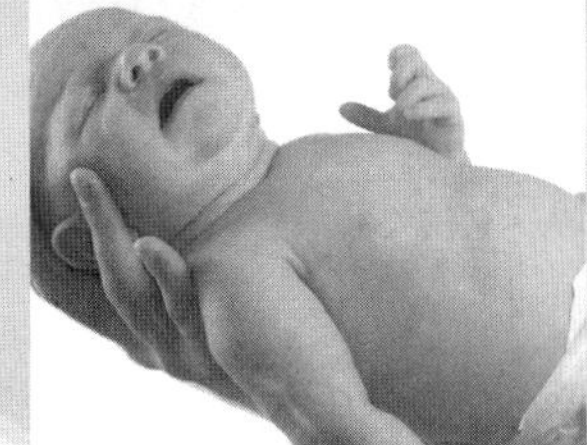

APPENDIX B

Conversion Table to Standard International (SI) Units

Component	Present Unit	×	Conversion Factor	=	SI Unit
Clinical Hematology					
Erythrocytes	per mm^3		1		$10^6/L$
Hematocrit	%		0.01		(1)vol RBC/vol whole blood
Hemoglobin	g/dL		10		g/L
Leukocytes	per mm^3		1		$10^6/L$
Mean corpuscular hemoglobin concentration (MCHC)	g/dL		10		g/L
Mean corpuscular volume (MCV)	μm^3		1		fL
Platelet count	$10^3/mm^3$		1		$10^9/L$
Reticulocyte count	%		10		10^{-3}
Clinical Chemistry					
Acetone	mg/dL		0.1722		mmol/L
Albumin	g/dL		10		g/L
Aldosterone	ng/dL		27.74		pmol/L
Ammonia (as nitrogen)	μg/dL		0.7139		μmol/L
Bicarbonate	mEq/L		1		mmol/L
Bilirubin	mg/dL		17.1		μmol/L
Calcium	mg/dL		0.2495		mmol/L
Calcium ion	mEq/L		0.50		mmol/L
Carotenes	μg/dL		0.01836		μmol/L
Ceruloplasmin	mg/dL		10.0		mg/L
Chloride	mEq/L		1		mmol/L
Cholesterol	mg/dL		0.02586		mmol/L
Complement, C_3 or C_4	mg/dL		0.01		g/L

(*continued*)

Component	Present Unit	×	Conversion Factor	=	SI Unit
Copper	μg/dL		0.1574		μmol/L
Cortisol	μg/dL		27.59		nmol/L
Creatine	mg/dL		76.25		μmol/L
Creatinine	mg/dL		88.40		μmol/L
Digoxin	ng/mL		1.281		nmol/L
Epinephrine	pg/mL		5.458		pmol/L
Fatty acids	mg/dL		10.0		mg/L
Ferritin	ng/mL		1		μg/L
α-Fetoprotein	ng/mL		1		μg/L
Fibrinogen	mg/dL		0.01		g/L
Folate	ng/mL		2.266		nmol/L
Fructose	mg/dL		0.05551		mmol/L
Galactose	mg/dL		0.05551		mmol/L
Gases					
PO_2	mm Hg (= torr)		0.1333		kPa
PCO_2	mm Hg (= torr)		0.1333		kPa
Glucagon	pg/mL		1		ng/L
Glucose	mg/dL		0.05551		mmol/L
Glycerol	mg/dL		0.1086		mmol/L
Growth hormone	ng/mL		1		μg/L
Haptoglobin	mg/dL		0.01		g/L
Hemoglobin	g/dL		10		g/L
Insulin	μg/L		172.2		pmol/L
	mU/L		7.175		pmol/L
Iron	μg/dL		0.1791		μmol/L
Iron-binding capacity	μg/dL		0.1791		μmol/L
Lactate	mEq/L		1		mmol/L
Lead	μg/dL		0.04826		μmol/L
Lipoproteins	mg/dL		0.02586		mmol/L
Magnesium	mg/dL		0.4114		mmol/L
	mEq/L		0.50		mmol/L
Osmolality	mOsm/kg H_2O		1		mmol/kg H_2O
Phenobarbital	mg/dL		43.06		μmol/L
Phenytoin	mg/L		3.964		μmol/L
Phosphate	mg/dL		0.3229		mmol/L
Potassium	mEq/L		1		mmol/L
	mg/dL		0.2558		mmol/L
Protein	g/dL		10.0		g/L
Pyruvate	mg/dL		113.6		μmol/L
Sodium ion	mEq/L		1		mmol/L
Steroids					
17-hydroxycorticosteroids	mg/24 h		2.759		μmol/d
17-ketosteroids	mg/24 h		3.467		μmol/d
Testosterone	ng/mL		3.467		nmol/L
Theophylline	mg/L		5.550		μmol/L
Thyroid tests					

(*continued*)

Component	**Present Unit**	×	**Conversion Factor**	=	**SI Unit**
Thyroid-stimulating hormone	μU/mL		1		mU/L
Thyroxine (T_4)	μg/dL		12.87		nmol/L
Thyroxine free	ng/dL		12.87		pmol/L
Triiodothyronine (T_3)	ng/dL		0.01536		nmol/L
Transferrin	mg/dL		0.01		g/L
Triglycerides	mg/dL		0.01129		mmol/L
Urea nitrogen	mg/dL		0.3570		mmol/L
Uric acid (urate)	mg/dL		59.48		μmol/L
Vitamin A (retinol)	μg/dL		0.03491		μmol/L
Vitamin B_{12}	pg/mL		0.7378		pmol/L
Vitamin C (ascorbic acid)	mg/dL		56.78		μmol/L
Vitamin D					
Cholecalciferol	μg/mL		2.599		nmol/L
25 OH-cholecalciferol	ng/mL		2.496		nmol/L
Vitamin E (alpha-tocopherol)	mg/dL		23.22		μmol/L
D-xylose	mg/dL		0.06661		mmol/L
Zinc	μg/dL		0.1530		μmol/L
Energy	kcal		4.1868		kj (kilojoule)
Blood pressure	mm Hg (= torr)		1.333		mbar

Modified from Young D. S. (1987). Implementation of SI units for clinical laboratory data. Style specifications and conversion tables. *Annuls of Internal Medicine, 106, 114.*

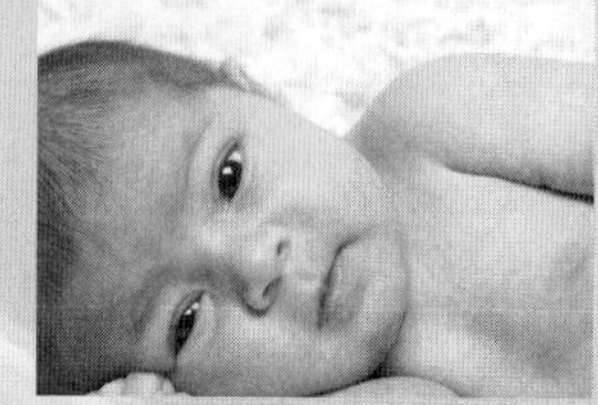

APPENDIX C

Frequently Used Reference Values and Conversions

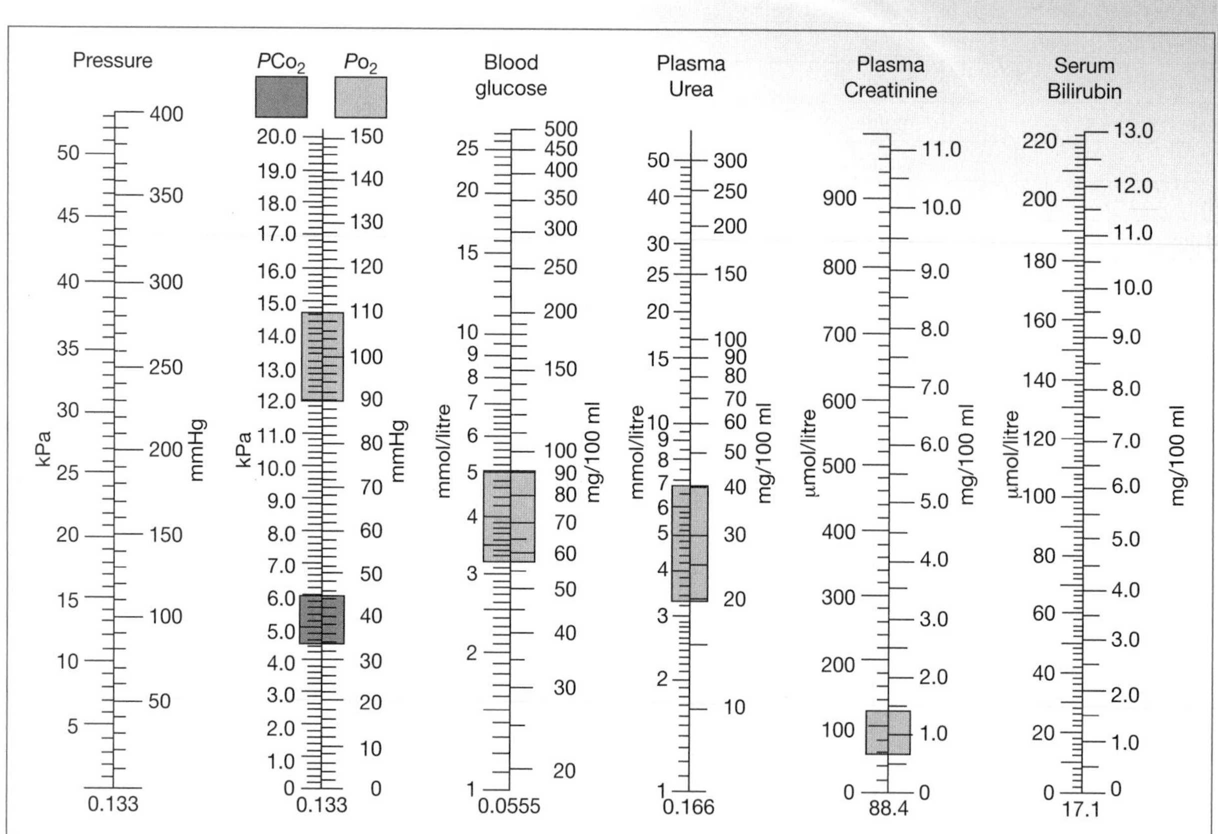

Note: Shading indicates the normal range where appropriate. To convert "old" to "new" units, multiply by the conversion factor at the foot of each column. Modified from Halliday, H. L., McClure, G., & Reid, M. (1985). *Handbook of neonatal intensive care* (2 ed.). Philadelphia, PA: WB Saunders.

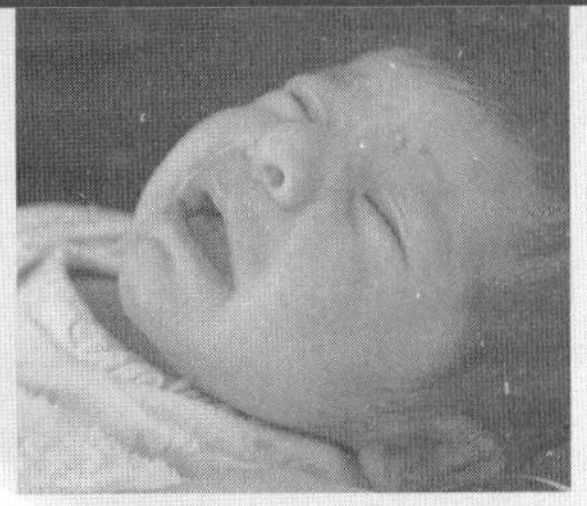

Index